NURSING DIAGNOSIS AND INTERVENTION IN NURSING PRACTICE

NURSING DIAGNOSIS AND INTERVENTION IN NURSING PRACTICE

Second Edition

CLAIRE CAMPBELL, R.N., M.S., F.N.P.

Practicing Family Nurse Practitioner
Adjunct Assistant Professor
University of Texas at Arlington School of Nursing
Arlington, Texas

Former Staff and Head Nurse, Medical-Surgical Nursing
Parkland Memorial Hospital
Dallas, Texas

Former Instructor
Texas Woman's University
Dallas, Texas

A Wiley Medical Publication
JOHN WILEY & SONS
New York • Chichester • Brisbane • Toronto • Singapore

Library of Congress Cataloging in Publication Data:
Campbell, Claire.
 Nursing diagnosis and intervention in nursing
practice.

 (A Wiley medical publication)
 Includes index.
 1. Nursing. 2. Diagnosis. I. Title. II. Series.

[DNLM: 1. Nursing process—Handbooks. WY 100 C187n]
RT41.C28 1984 610'.73 83–21836
ISBN 0–471–08427–1

Printed in the United States of America

10 9 8 7 6 5 4 3

To the Source of all our blessings
To Hugh, Clara, and loved ones
To my devoted colleagues
To all those entrusted to our care

Preface

This book is devoted to the nursing process, particularly to the development and identification of nursing diagnoses and interventions. Its focus is, with special emphasis, on patterns of nursing diagnosis. It is based on the concept that nursing diagnoses are determined from existing or potential health problems treated by professional nurses. These patient problems are identified in strictly nursing, rather than in medical, terms. For years, nurses have been using medical diseases as the basis of nursing treatment. But today, we are developing our own list of patient problems in an effort to establish a more precise nursing profession.

Nursing Diagnosis and Intervention in Nursing Practice is designed for professional registered nurses involved in clinical practice or education and for students learning nursing care. It describes a step-by-step system of analyzing and solving patient problems while providing nursing care. The book is intended to be a quick, practical source from which patient care plans can be made and to provide a common vocabulary of nursing practice until a standard nomenclature of nursing diagnosis can be developed.

Part One contains information about the changes that have occurred in nursing diagnosis development. It discusses some of the factors that affect change, charts the development of nursing diagnosis patterns, and analyzes results of a research study that supports the use of such patterns. It also includes a step-by-step description of how to formulate a nursing diagnosis using the pattern system.

Parts Two and Three list over 850 nursing diagnoses. Part Two contains those diagnoses that are predominantly nursing: problems solved by nurses more often than by other health professionals. Part Three contains dual diagnoses: problems solved by both nurses and practitioners of other health disciplines. Each diagnosis is presented in a manner consistent with the nursing process and includes appropriate assessment criteria and interventions.

Part Four is an alphabetical guide to the nursing interventions found in Parts Two and Three. Each intervention is followed by a definition, a rationale, the human needs fulfilled by the intervention, and any contraindications for its use. The interventions are divided into four categories: nursing treatments, nursing observations, health teaching, and medical treatments performed by nurses. Those that are usually performed by nurses only in emergencies are coded *ET*, meaning emergency treatment.

In an effort to save space, a few similarly stated nursing interventions appear in a combined form in Parts Two and Three. For example, *Measure the intake* and *Measure the output* appear as *Measure the intake and output*; *Observe for edema, Observe for impaired circulation*, and *Observe for inflammation* appear as *Observe for edema, impaired circulation, and inflammation*. When looking up combined interventions in Part Four, the reader must convert them to their original form. For example, if in Part Two or Three the statement reads *Observe for complaints of fatigue and weakness*, the reader will look in Part Four for *Observe for complaints of fatigue* and *Observe for complaints of weakness*. Although the nursing interventions have been worded consistently in an effort to clarify nursing functions, they are not intended for use in a recipe-type care plan. They are presented as alternatives from which the nurse can choose specific interventions appropriate to the individual patient in his or her unique health-related situation.

At the back of the book are several valuable reference tools. Appendix 1 contains a list of common etiology, and Appendix 2, a system of coding nursing diagnoses and interventions for computerized retrieval. A glossary, a bibliography, and a single index, incorporating both nursing diagnoses and interventions, complete the volume. Throughout the text when a general personal pronoun is required, *she* is used for the nurse and *he* for the patient; this scheme is used for the sake of brevity and is not intended to be sexist.

The system set forth in this book involves the use of basic diagnostic patterns to formulate nursing diagnosis statements. The system is designed to promote consistent use of terminology and ease in formulating nursing diagnoses. This book was written with the hope that nurses will find the use of nursing diagnoses a challenging and rewarding aspect of nursing practice.

Claire Campbell

Acknowledgments

This book originally evolved from the association of the following registered nurses and the author, all of whom were together in the pursuit of graduate studies:

Suzanne J. Beach, R.N., M.S., CNNA. Director, Department of Nursing, Children's Medical Center of Dallas, Dallas, Texas

Dolores Chumchal Berkovsky, R.N., M.S. Administrator, Residential Treatment Center, St. Theresa's Home, Forth Worth, Texas. Former Associate Professor of Nursing, Texas Christian University, Fort Worth, Texas

Cecilia M. Holland, R.N.C., M.S.N. Geriatric Nurse Practitioner, Supervisor, Nursing Home Care Unit, Veterans Administration Medical Center, Knoxville, Iowa. Former Staff Nurse, Sam Rayburn Memorial Veterans Center, Bonham, Texas, and Instructor of Nursing, Paris Junior College, Paris, Texas

Hazel M. Jay, R.N., M.Ed., M.S. Former Associate Dean, University of Texas at Arlington School of Nursing, Arlington, Texas; Director of Continuing Education, University of Texas, School of Nursing at Forth Worth, Fort Worth, Texas; and Assistant Professor, Texas Woman's University, College of Nursing, Dallas, Texas

Claire Jenkins Johnson, R.N., M.S., CCRN. Staff Nurse, ICU/CCU, Mississippi Baptist Medical Center, Jackson, Mississippi. Former Critical Care Nurse Consultant, Dallas, Texas, and Director, Critical Care Nursing Course, School of Allied Health Sciences, University of Texas Health Science Center at Dallas, Dallas, Texas

Anne Kuempel, R.N., B.S.N., M.S. Assistant Executive Director for Patient Services, St. David's Community Hospital, Austin, Texas. Former Assistant Executive Secretary, Board of Nurse Examiners for the State of Texas, Austin, Texas

Shirley J. Pinterich, R.N., M.S. Vice President, Nursing, Huguley Memorial Medical Center, Fort Worth, Texas. Former Associate Professor of Nursing and Chairman, Southwestern Adventist College, Keene, Texas, and Instructor of Nursing, Union College, Denver, Colorado

Mary K. Olson Robitaille, R.N., M.S. Chief, Enlisted Education Branch, U.S. Army Medical Department, U.S. Army Medical Department Personnel Support Agency, Washington, D.C. Former Chief Nurse, 32nd Combat Support Hospital, Federal Republic of Germany, and Nephrology Nurse Clinician, Brooke Army Medical Center, Fort Sam Houston, Texas

Wanda J. Thompson, R.N., F.N.P., Ed.D. Associate Professor, University of Texas at Arlington School of Nursing, Arlington, Texas. Former Assistant Professor of Nursing, Dallas Baptist College, Dallas, Texas

Linda S. White, R.N., M.S. Former Director, Accelerated Program in Nursing, University of Tennessee, College of Nursing, Memphis, Tennessee

Kathleen S. Winger, R.N., M.S. Former Associate Director of Nursing, St. Paul's Hospital, Dallas, Texas

As the study of nursing diagnoses and interventions progressed, other health professionals became involved. Without the consultant expertise and outstanding generosity of these nursing colleagues, this work could never have achieved completion:

Jane M. Baggett, R.N., B.S. Supervisor, Adolescent Service, Baylor University Medical Center, Dallas, Texas. Former Staff Nurse, Children's Medical Center and Timberlawn Psychiatric Hospital, Dallas, Texas

Jessie F. Bewley, R.N., M.S. Former Assistant Professor, Texas Woman's University, College of Nursing, Dallas, Texas, and Instructor of Nursing, Parkland Memorial Hospital School of Nursing, Dallas, Texas

Pauline Baker Boswell, R.N., B.S. Assistant Head Nurse, General Surgery, Presbyterian Hospital of Dallas. Former Head Nurse, General Surgery, Parkland Memorial Hospital, Dallas, Texas

Kathlene Brown, R.N., B.S.N., M.S. Associate Instructor, Baptist Memorial College of Nursing, San Antonio, Texas. Former Instructor, Baptist System School of Nursing, Little Rock, Arkansas; Director of In-Service Education, Baylor University Medical Center, Dallas, Texas; and Director of CCU, Good Samaritan Hospital, Phoenix, Arizona

Mary Reardon Castles, R.N., M.S.N., Ph.D. Professor and Director of Research, University of Missouri at St. Louis, St. Louis, Missouri

Bernadette Claus, R.N. Office Nursing, Southwest Clinic, Medical City Complex, Dallas, Texas. Former Staff Nurse, St. Paul's Hospital, Dallas, Texas

Cheryl Conatser, R.N., M.S. Clinical Nurse, Specialist in Pediatric Oncology, Children's Medical Center of Dallas. Former Instructor, Pediatric Nursing, El Centro College, Dallas, Texas, and Texarkana College, Texarkana, Texas

Linda J. Hawley, R.N., M.S. Assistant Professor, Community Health and Family Nursing, University of Texas at Arlington School of Nursing, Arlington, Texas

Judith Evelyn MacKenzie Henley, R.N., M.S. Assistant Professor, Texas Woman's University, School of Nursing, Dallas, Texas. Former Staff Nurse, Head Nurse, In-Service Instructor for Obstetric Units and Education Coordinator for Nursing Service, Parkland Memorial Hospital, Dallas, Texas

Nancy Vollmer Henley, R.N., M.S., M.A. Former Assistant Director of Nursing, Parkland Memorial Hospital, and Assistant Professor, Texas Woman's University, College of Nursing, Dallas, Texas

Patricia Lane, R.N., M.S. Independent Researcher in Surgical Specialties. Clinical Faculty at Texas Woman's University, Dallas, Texas. Former Staff Nurse, Emergency Room and Burn Intensive Care Unit, Parkland Memorial Hospital, Dallas, Texas

Teddy Langford, M.S.N., Ph.D. Dean, School of Nursing, Texas Tech University, Lubbock, Texas. Former Associate Dean of Education, University of Colorado School of Nursing, Denver, Colorado, and Vice President for Academic Affairs, University of Texas System School of Nursing, Austin, Texas

Louise Lorraine Lastelick, R.N., M.S. Mental Health Consultant and Counselor, Private Practice, Metro Mental Health Services, Richardson, Texas. Former Assistant Professor of Nursing, University of Southwestern Louisiana, Lafayette, Louisiana, and Assistant Supervisor, Neurosurgery Division, Baylor University Medical Center, Dallas, Texas

Margaret McClusky McElroy, R.N., M.S., Ph.D. Assistant Professor, Texas Woman's University, College of Nursing, Dallas, Texas. Former Instructor, St. Paul's Hospital School of Nursing, Dallas, Texas

Brenda J. McFadin, R.N., B.A. Administrative Supervisor, Baylor University Medical Center, Dallas, Texas

Jackie McFarlin, R.N., M.Ph., M.S., Ph.D. Assistant Professor, University of Texas at Arlington School of Nursing, Arlington, Texas. Former Assistant Professor at Baptist College School of Nursing, Dallas, Texas, and Arkansas Tech University, Russellville, Arkansas

Barbara Clark Mims, B.S.N., M.S.N., CCRN. Director, Nurse Internships and Critical Care Education, Parkland Memorial Hospital, Dallas, Texas. Former Staff Nurse, Cardiovascular Surgical ICU, Methodist Hospital, Houston, Texas, and Head Nurse of Respiratory ICU, Parkland Memorial Hospital, Dallas, Texas

Myrna R. Pickard, R.N., Ed.D. Dean, University of Texas at Arlington School of Nursing, Arlington, Texas. Former Nurse Administrator, John Peter Smith Hospital School of Nursing, Forth Worth, Texas

Ann Ruth Roberson, R.N., COHN, CFNP. Manager, Health Services Unit, Otis Engineering Corporation, Dallas, Texas. Former Staff and Head Nurse of Surgical Specialties, Parkland Memorial Hospital, Dallas, Texas

Patricia C. Scott, R.N., M.N. Staff Nurse, Veterans Administration Medical Center, Gainesville, Florida

Deanna L. Snow, R.N. Supervisor of Adult Psychiatry, Baylor University Medical Center, Dallas, Texas

Judy L. Spinella, R.N., M.S., C.E.N. Clinical Coordinator, Emergency Department, San Francisco General Hospital, San Francisco, California. Former Assistant Professor, University of Texas at Arlington School of Nursing, Arlington, Texas, and Staff Nurse, John Peter Smith Hospital, Forth Worth, Texas

Mary Lovatt Smith Tragus, R.N., M.S.N. Former Rehabilitation Specialist, International Rehabilitation Associates, Inc., and Instructor of Nursing, Texas Woman's University, College of Nursing, Dallas, Texas

Betty H. Wade, R.N., M.S.N. Associate Professor, Texas Woman's University, College of Nursing, Dallas, Texas. Former Staff Nurse, Head Nurse, Supervisor, Medical Nursing and Clinical Research Center, University of Alabama Hospitals and Clinics at Birmingham, Birmingham, Alabama

Carol Ware, R.N., B.S.N., M.B.A. Systems Analyst and Project Leader, Presbyterian Hospital of Dallas, Texas. Former Head Nurse, Medical-Surgical Unit, Parkland Memorial Hospital, Dallas, Texas

Nancy B. Watt, R.N., M.S., CNAA. Vice-President for Nursing, St. John's Regional Health Center, Springfield, Missouri. Former Assistant Administrator, Patient Care, Irving Community Hospital, Irving, Texas; and Assistant Director, Parkland Memorial Hospital, Dallas, Texas

Opal White, R.N., M.P.H., D.N.S. Former Professor, Texas Woman's University, College of Nursing, Dallas, Texas, and Professor and Coordinator, University of Colorado School of Nursing, Denver, Colorado

Frances Whited, R.N., B.S., M.S. Assistant Professor, Texas Woman's University, College of Nursing, Dallas, Texas. Former Staff Nurse, Dallas City Health Department, Dallas, Texas

Evelyn B. Wormser, R.N., M.S.N. Mental Health and Health Promotion Specialist, University of Texas at Arlington School of Nursing, Arlington, Texas. Private Practice in Counseling

To **Hazel M. Jay, R.N., M.Ed., M.S.,** and **Myrna R. Pickard, R.N., Ed.D.,** who directed and coordinated the study *Nursing Diagnosis Patterns: An Analysis of Registered Nurses' Responses*, we extend the deepest gratitude and appreciation for this outstanding effort. Through their expertise, significant information has been added to the concept of nursing diagnosis.

We would also like to extend sincere appreciation to each of the 1,064 nurses who participated in this study and to the nurse administrators who made arrangements for the project. The participating agencies, principal nurse administrators, and their research assistants were as follows:

All Saints Episcopal Hospital, Fort Worth, Texas, **Judy Jones, R.N., M.S.N.**

Arlington Community Hospital, Arlington, Texas, **Helen Mena, R.N., M.H.A., Margaret Denheyer, R.N., B.N.**

Arlington Memorial Hospital, Arlington, Texas, **Paula Thompson, R.N., B.S.N.**

Florida Hospital, Orlando, Florida, **Jack Northcutt, R.N., M.S.**

Fort Worth Osteopathic Medical Center, Fort Worth, Texas, **Marsha Cox, R.N., M.S.N., M.B.A.**

Glenview Hospital, Fort Worth, Texas, **Shelia Long, R.N., B.S.**

Hackettstown Hospital, Hackettstown, New Jersey, **Joyce Pifer, R.N., M.S.**

Harris Hospital, Fort Worth, Texas, **Cleta Brown, R.N., M.S.N.**

Huguley Memorial Medical Center, Fort Worth, Texas, **Shirley J. Pinterich, R.N., M.S., Reulita Vigilia, R.N., M.S.**

John Peter Smith Hospital, Fort Worth, Texas, **Jeanneane Cline, R.N., M.S.**

Loma Linda University Medical Center, Loma Linda, California, **Gertrude Haussler, R.N., M.S.**

Maine Medical Center, Portland, Maine, **Judy T. Stone, R.N., M.S., Linda Pearson, R.N., M.Ed.**

Medical Plaza Hospital, Fort Worth, Texas, **Gladys Haryol, R.N., B.S.N., Sean Meredith, R.N.**

Parkland Memorial Hospital, Dallas, Texas, **Elizabeth Good, R.N., M.S., Barbara A. Mims, B.S.N., M.S.N., CCRN**

Porter Memorial Hospital, Denver, Colorado, **Marlene Van Puymbrouck, R.N., M.S.**

St. David's Community Hospital, Austin, Texas, **Anne Kuempel, R.N., B.S.N., M.S., Jacqueline Clements, R.N., M.S.N.**

St. Joseph's Hospital, Fort Worth, Texas, **Jim Murphy, R.N., M.A., Kay Willis, R.N., M.S.**

Seton Medical Center, Austin, Texas, **Betty J. Thomas, R.N., M.S.N.**

Special appreciation is also extended to **Joan S. Reisch, Ph.D.,** Associate Professor of Internal Medicine and Health Care Sciences, and her staff at the University of Texas Health Science Center, Medical Computing Resources Center, Dallas, Texas.

With sincerest gratitude, we wish to thank **Mary Reardon Castles, R.N., M.S.N., Ph.D.,** for her guidance and direction during the early days when *Nursing Diagnosis and Intervention in Nursing Practice* was only an idea.

Sincere appreciation is also extended to **Saundra G. Haun** for her secretarial services; to **Richard R. Haun**, who, for several years, shuttled the manuscript between Dallas, Texas, and London, England; to **Elizabeth Ann Campbell** and **Michele Conway** for their assistance; and to the entire staff of John Wiley & Sons, Inc., especially nursing editor **Andrea Stingelin**.

Claire Campbell

Contents

**PART THREE
DUAL NURSING DIAGNOSES 707**

**PART FOUR
NURSING INTERVENTIONS 1415**

NURSING DIAGNOSIS AND INTERVENTION IN NURSING PRACTICE

PART ONE
NURSING DIAGNOSIS IN TRANSITION

1 NURSING DIAGNOSIS

THE CHALLENGE OF NURSING DIAGNOSIS

In today's complex world of health care, registered nurses are skilled, competent professionals who continue the work nurses have done for generations, providing a broad scope of services to both ill and well persons. In addition to the many contributions that the modern nurse has made, another challenge is being met. Nurses are adding to the scope of nursing knowledge by contributing to and becoming proficient at the identification of nursing diagnoses. Although professional nurses have for many years been making judgments about patient responses in health care situations, the challenge of formulating nursing diagnosis statements is relatively new.

Many factors have contributed to the development of nursing diagnosis:

Health needs of the consumer
Legislation that affects nursing diagnosis in all areas of professional nursing, including practice at advanced and specialized levels
Realities of current nursing practice
Curricula in schools of nursing
Differentiation of nursing and medical interventions
Patient problems, as exemplified in nursing literature
Standards of nursing practice
The North American Nursing Diagnosis Association

Health Needs of the Consumer

Health needs, as perceived by the consumer, have been more clearly defined because of the accessibility and availability of knowledge in scientific and technical fields. Consumers today enjoy a higher level of education and have access to more comprehensive information than previous generations enjoyed. Complete health care and health maintenance are considered essential. Consumers are knowledgeable about current health problems and how they are prevented and treated. They know how environment, lifestyle, and society in general influence health, and they seek to adapt in a manner compatible with a productive life and sound economics.

The emergence of an informed public and recent advances in technology have helped expand the number of health professions and the scope of each of their activities designed to integrate health services for the increased benefit of the patient. This, in turn, has increased the need for the nursing profession to state explicitly its contribution to health care—a need that can best be met through nursing diagnoses that state those problems that nurses solve. Nursing diagnoses make it easier for nursing to integrate its services with those of other health professionals and, at the same time, remain accountable for activities specific to nursing.

Legislation

The quest for health has prompted new legislation to protect consumers. Several states have rewritten their nursing practice acts to meet consumer and practitioner demands, and others are in the process of doing so.

The question of whether nursing diagnosis should be defined by law has provoked considerable debate. Professional nurses have endeavored to avoid implying medical diagnosis in the terminology used in nursing diagnoses. To imply medical diagnosis would not be permissible under the medical and nursing acts of most states, and it would serve no purpose to duplicate already existing health services.

If medical diagnoses are to be kept separate from nursing diagnoses, the differences between the two must be clearly defined. The Division of Library and Archival Services of the American Medical Association has suggested that a generally accepted definition of medical diagnosis is to be found in the *Attorney's Dictionary of Medicine and Word Finder.* The definition states that a medical diagnosis is "the determination of what kind of a disease a patient is suffering from, especially the art of distinguishing between several possibilities."[437:27]

Murchison and Nichols stated that "almost all courts would agree that [medical] diagnosis is the determination of a disease from its symptoms."[360:95] Such statements clearly indicate that the diagnosis of disease is considered a medical responsibility and has always been a part of medical practice. Since medical diagnosis is clearly the identification of disease, what then is nursing diagnosis?

The American Nurses' Association definition of nursing practice reads that "the practice of professional nursing means the performance for compensation of any acts in the observation, care and counsel of the ill, injured, or infirm or in the maintenance of health or prevention of illness of others or in the supervision and teaching of other personnel or in the administration of medications and treatments prescribed by licensed physicians or dentists, requiring for all these functions substantial, specialized judgment and skill based on knowledge and application of the principles of biological, physical and social sciences. The foregoing shall not be deemed to include acts of diagnosis [implying medical diagnosis] or prescription of therapeutic or corrective measures."[763:2]

These general components of nursing care provide areas for independent nursing diagnosis and nursing intervention. In addition to basic nursing care, the increased demands of the consumer for improved health services have placed new responsibilities on the nurse. Many diverse factors, such as isolated geographic areas, substandard communities, critical care units, and care specific to certain age groups, have contributed to the development of new nursing activities that are either more comprehensive or more specialized than nursing activities in the past.

The nurse in an expanded role performs physical examinations, identifies normal and abnormal findings, orders drugs, and initiates therapy not previously associated with nursing.[507:15-16] She treats uncomplicated and chronic illnesses, common childhood conditions, and minor injuries; manages normal pregnancy, labor, and delivery; and provides acute and emergency care.[257:507-510] The 1970 U.S. Department of Health, Education and Welfare "Report on Extending the Scope of Nursing Practice,"[763] stated that "the functions of nurses are changing primarily because nurses have demonstrated their competence to perform a greater variety of functions."[763:12] These changes in function tend to complicate the question of what the nurse can diagnose without infringing on the physician's medical diagnosis.

Nursing practice acts generally restrict the professional nurse by incorporating such statements as "the foregoing shall not be deemed to include acts of [medical] diagnosis or prescription of therapeutic or corrective measures."[765:3] A "Position on Nursing Practice" published by the Michigan Nurses' Association stated that nurses assist the patient with health problems that include "existing or potential deficits in the ability to breathe, eat, drink, eliminate, maintain hygiene and comfort, exercise and rest, insure safety from environmental hazards, communicate, express emotional and spiritual needs and learn."[257:159] The California Nurses' Association indicated that the professional nurse identifies "each person's physical, psychologic and social needs, and assists the individual and his family to achieve an optimal health regime and dignified death."[257:160] According to Mundinger and Jauron, the New York Nurse Practice Act describes nursing diagnosis as "human responses to actual or potential health problems."[643:94]

These definitions, which reflect the general professional and legislative approaches to nursing diagnoses, support the broad concept that a range of health care problems can be treated independently by nurses. Because of this broad concept, the question has arisen as to whether nursing diagnosis, which does not include the identification of diseases, involves the identification of signs and symptoms of disease.

Lesnik and Anderson indicated that professional nurses have several areas of independent function. One of these areas is "the observation of symptoms and reactions including symptomatology of physical and mental conditions and needs, requiring evaluation or application of principles based upon the biologic, the physical, and social sciences."[292:259] Murchison and Nichols stated that "the nurse is properly allowed the responsibility of judging the gravity of symptoms without engaging in [medical] diagnosis."[360:95] They were of the opinion that in such areas as diagnosis of dysrhythmias, "when the nurse judges that the patient exhibits ventricular fibrillation, she is merely observing a symptom, not diagnosing the disease suggested. In determining that the patient is suffering a true cardiac arrest, the nurse is exercising judgment as to the seriousness of the symptom, but is not ascertaining the nature of the disease."[360:94]

The foregoing statements support the concept that nurses do identify and evaluate signs and symptoms but do not diagnose the diseases that such data represent. The physician "infers from signs and symptoms the abnormalities in function and structure."[355:20] The nurse infers from signs and symptoms their effects on the patient's capacity to function as well as the person's ability to cope with the signs and symptoms themselves.[294:119]

It is essential that the scope and limits of nursing diagnosis be developed, not in terms of the minimum legal requirements of nursing performance, but in terms of the maximum legal extent of nursing practice. Even though this level is not currently encouraged in some states, the consumer's demand for maximum health care will support nursing practice designed to provide such care.

Realities of Current Nursing Practice

In the process of developing terminology for nursing diagnoses, the realities of current nursing practice must be considered. The nursing judgments that are being made and recorded in everyday contact with patients must be examined. In hospitals, community health agencies, or wherever the professional nurse may be, nursing judgments are being made and identified in nursing terms, even though such terms have not been compiled into a nomenclature of diagnoses. The realities of practice are a major source of nursing diagnosis terminology.

Curricula in Schools of Nursing

Prior and Silverstein suggested that "a nurse who meets the requirements for professional nursing practice . . . possesses a body of selective knowledge, relevant to the health sciences, drawn from the biologic, the physical, and psychosocial basic sciences and selected medical science knowledge."[218:95] The basic knowledge of the professional nurse determines the kind and number of nursing diagnosis that can be made. The extent of this basic knowledge is determined primarily by the curriculum to which the nurse has been exposed. That curriculum, in addition to its effects on the nurse's level of knowledge, is also reflected in nursing practice.

Differentiation of Nursing and Medical Interventions

In defining nursing diagnosis terminology, one must recognize that "nursing diagnoses are limited to areas of independent nursing action."[643:96] When a health problem is recognized by the nurse and treatment is initiated on the basis of standing medical orders, resolution of the problem is within the scope of medicine, not the scope of nursing, even though the nurse assists in resolving the problem.

Murchison and Nichols stated that "the differentiation of the doctor's diagnosis and a nursing diagnosis is based on the courses of action open to each professional after the decision from the observation is made."[360:97] The American Nurses' Association Committee on Legislation[778:2] and Lesnik and Anderson[292:260] agree that one of the six independent areas of nursing is "the application and the execution of nursing procedures and techniques."[292:260]

If the nurse is to be able to determine which health problems nursing can resolve, diminish, or prevent, a clear distinction must be made between those interventions that are nursing treatments applicable to nursing diagnoses and those that are medical treatments carried out by the nurse. It must be recognized that today, as in the past, physicians direct many nursing procedures and techniques. Traditionally, "the medical components of nursing care have included those aspects of medical treatment delegated by the physician to the nurse."[112:103] This medical component has long been prevalent in nursing activities. The physician's direction of some nursing treatments and the frequency with which nurses carry out medical treatments have led to the misconception by patients, nurses, and physicians that all nursing interventions are medical treatments, while in fact they are nursing treatments. A statement of a health problem is not a nursing diagnosis unless the nurse can independently treat the health problem. Therefore, nurses must clearly define what the nursing treatments are before they can determine which health problems fall within the nursing domain.

Patient Problems in Nursing Literature

In any attempt to compile a list of nursing diagnoses, one of the most significant resources is nursing literature. Nursing literature has been a consistent guide for nurses in their efforts to solve health problems. Even though the health problems recognized by nurses have not been stated in the form of nursing diagnoses, they have been expressed in such a way that they provide the basic terminology for nursing diagnoses.

Standards of Nursing Practice

In 1973, the Congress for Nursing Practice of the American Nurses' Association set forth *Standards of Nursing Practice*. These standards were designed for the purpose of guaranteeing quality of nursing services.[754:5] On the subject of nursing diagnosis, Standard II reads:

Nursing diagnoses are derived from health status data.

RATIONALE

The health status of the client/patient is the basis for determining the nursing care needs. The data are analyzed and compared to norms when possible.

ASSESSMENT FACTORS

1. The client's/patient's health status is compared to the norm in order to determine if there is a deviation from the norm and the degree and direction of deviation.
2. The client's/patient's capabilities and limitations are identified.
3. The nursing diagnoses are related to and congruent with the diagnoses of all other professionals caring for the client/patient.[754:5]

Standards of Nursing Practice recognizes nursing diagnosis as essential to the systematic method of nursing practice. It provides broad guidelines for the identification of problems that nurses solve.

The North American Nursing Diagnosis Association

As early as 1859, Florence Nightingale described nursing in the publication *Notes on Nursing*.[370:19] Throughout the years, nursing leaders have expressed many philosophies of nursing. The general approach has been to describe nursing in terms of nursing's functions rather than to identify problems that nurses solve.

In 1956, Gertrude Hornug suggested the use of the term *nursing diagnosis.*[89:24] Other leaders, such as Faye Abdellah, Dorothy Johnson, and Wilda Chambers, supported this view.[89:24] During the 1960s, there was increased awareness of and research in nursing diagnosis.

During the early 1970s, Gebbie and Lavin recognized the need for a classification system of nursing diagnosis.[89:25] They were instrumental in forming the National Conference on Classification of Nursing Diagnosis for the purpose of developing a taxonomy of nursing diagnoses. This group met first at St. Louis University School of Nursing in 1973[89:26] and again in 1975. Since their third meeting in 1978,[89:27] they have met every two years. In 1982, the group expanded to become the North American Nursing Diagnosis Association. Through their efforts, recognition of the need for nursing diagnosis has become worldwide.

NURSING DIAGNOSIS DEFINED

Nursing literature contains statements of what professional nurses believe nursing diagnosis to be. Gebbie and Lavin defined a nursing diagnosis as "the identification of those patient problems or concerns most frequently identified by nurses, problems which are usually identified by nurses before they are recognized by other health care workers, and problems which are amenable to some intervention which is available in the present or potential scope of nursing practice."[584:250] Komarita considered nursing diagnosis a "determination of the nature and extent of nursing problems presented by the individual patients or families receiving care,"[610:91] and Marriner indicated that a "nursing diagnosis is a statement of a conclusion based on scientific principles and indicating the patient's need for nursing care."[326:32] Mundinger and Jauron stated that a diagnosis "is essentially an inference about a state that is undesirable. . . . As nurses, we are responsible for diagnosing and treating human responses to health problems."[643:96]

At the 1976 American Nurses' Association biennial convention, the House of Delegates in its Resolution on the Classification System of Nursing Diagnosis stated that "nursing diagnosis describes actual or potential health problems which nurses are capable [of treating] and licensed to treat."[756:9] Gordon stated that "nursing diagnoses, or clinical diagnoses made by professional nurses, describe actual or potential health problems which nurses, by virtue of their education and experience, are capable of and licensed to treat."[196:2]

Criteria for Nursing Diagnosis

Specific standards are used to determine whether a patient problem is considered a nursing diagnosis. The criteria described here are those identified in the 1978 edition of *Nursing Diagnosis and Intervention in Nursing Practice*:[86:12]

> The diagnosis is a human response.
> The professional registered nurse can legally prescribe and carry out treatment for the problem independent of medical direction.
> The diagnosis occurs repeatedly in a significant number of patients.
> One or more human needs, as identified by Abraham Maslow, exist.
> The supporting data are such that they can be obtained and analyzed by the professional registered nurse in the light of nursing knowledge.
> The supporting data present two or more related facts.
> The diagnostic problem is not a specific disease identified as such in the standard medical classification systems.

The Purpose of Nursing Diagnosis

Nursing diagnoses are essential to the professional practice of nursing for many reasons:[86,196]

To increase the quality of patient care through patient care plans that reflect individual problems and needs

To use the nursing process in a logical, organized manner

To support a common core of communications among professional nurse colleagues

To identify clearly the existing body of scientific knowledge that is the framework of professional nursing

To provide more meaningful nursing records and to facilitate retrieval of those records

To use nursing diagnosis for certification of nurses in specialty areas

To secure compensation for nurses, based not on the present system of payment for performance of interventions, but on payment for problems nurses solve

To make nursing more visible and to more clearly differentiate the nursing role from the medical role

To plan staffing needs from the nursing diagnosis problems that need to be solved

The Difference Between Nursing Diagnoses and Nursing Goals

The nursing diagnosis is a statement of the person's response or behavior. This response is the problem that is causing the person difficulty and that brings him to seek nursing assistance. The nursing goal is a statement of the expected change in the person's response or behavior. This change should occur after nursing intervention. It is the expected outcome, stated in measurable terms. When this change occurs, the nurse will have assisted the person to a higher level of functioning.

Differences Between Nursing Diagnosis and Medical Diagnosis

Nurses and physicians have long recognized that their professional domains have common areas of overlapping problem identification and intervention methods. The nurse focuses on diagnostic problems concerning adaptation and limitations in illness and maintenance of wellness. The physician, in making a medical diagnosis, recognizes pathologic processes and focuses primarily on pathophysiologic etiology and organic unwellness.[125:8] Basic data are evaluated in order to identify the patient's problem and label it in terms of a specific disease.

Both disciplines use essentially the same reasoning process to arrive at diagnostic decisions. When looking at the problems that nurses and physicians solve, as described in the literature, it is evident that there are two kinds of diagnoses: *predominant diagnoses*, which are patient problems more often solved or treated by a single profession than any other profession; and *dual diagnoses*, which are patient problems commonly solved or treated by more than one health discipline. The diagnostic domains of nursing and medicine include both types of diagnoses:

Predominantly Nursing Diagnoses
Problems of:
   Comfort deficits
   Communication-of-needs deficits
   Hygiene deficits
   Self-mobility deficits
   Self-nutrition deficits
   Self-protection deficits
   Self-restorative deficits
   Self-therapy deficits
   Psychosocial adaptation

Predominantly Medical Diagnoses
Problems of:
   Disease or pathologic entities
   Trauma

Dual Diagnoses

Emergency conditions
Minor illnesses
Pain problems
Health maintenance problems
Suspected disease problems
Drug problems
Nutrition problems
Psychosocial nonadaptation
Rehabilitation problems
Spiritual problems
Wellness
Health resource problems

It has been established that nursing diagnoses are limited to those problems that nurses treat independently. In actual practice, nurses in expanded roles are making medical diagnoses as well. Working under physician protocol, the nurse identifies the medical problem and initiates treatment according to medical direction.

With this additional responsibility, nurses are making both nursing diagnoses and medical diagnoses. Nurses actually diagnose four types of patient problems:

Problems that only professional nurses have the authority to treat

Problems that nurses and members of another health profession, such as doctors, and paramedics, both have the authority to treat; such problems involve dual diagnoses   } Nursing diagnoses

Problems of case finding that are recognized by the professional nurse as medical problems and are referred to medicine for comprehensive evaluation and treatment

Problems that are medical problems that nurses can treat only under the direction of medical protocol   } Medical diagnoses

The fact that a nurse, using protocol, is treating a person with a medical diagnosis does not change that health problem to a nursing diagnosis. If, in the future, nurses are given legal license to treat certain medical problems independently, such diagnostic problems will become dual diagnoses and will then fall within the domain of nursing. An awareness of the different and common diagnostic domains of nursing and medicine supports unity between the two disciplines.

The Relevancy of Nursing Theory and Nursing Diagnosis Patterns

For years, nursing has been developing a body of knowledge that serves as a guide for the definition and practice of nursing.[187:2] A body of knowledge best serves society's expectations for professionalism when it represents more than an accumulation of ideas and speculations about the application of certain skills. The credibility and respectability of a discipline within the social arena of professionalism depend on the consistency of the discipline's knowledge, scientific orderliness, and translation into a uniquely valued form of practice fulfilling a distinct social need.

Beginning with an identified social dilemma, facts and information regarding the nature of the phenomenon embodying the unmet need and the phenomenon proposed by a discipline for meeting the need are gathered, described, and explained in order to es-

---

This section was written by Jackie McFarlin, R.N., Ph.D.

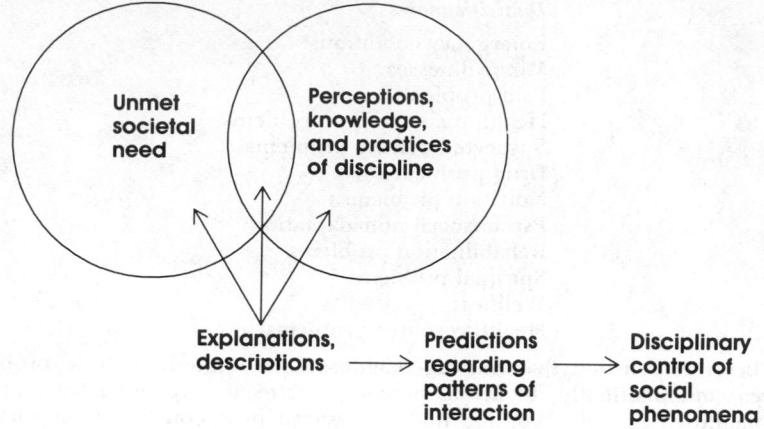

tablish valid patterns for predicting and controlling outcomes from the intersection of the two phenomena. The diagram illustrates this process.

Common sense knowledge, which is the sharing among practitioners of information descriptive of the realities held as factual by the discipline, prepares the way for a synthesis between society and the profession regarding meaningfulness of the nature of the profession.[440] Fact finding that is allowed to occur randomly creates a gap between society and the profession, ultimately weakening the profession's autonomy, power, and credibility.[344]

Efforts to improve consensus concerning description of the social and nursing phenomena encourage scientifically structured advances in knowledge that reveals and separates necessary events from accidental or nonessential events.[467:1] Necessary events in the interaction between social and nursing phenomena serve as content for typifying major attributes of the phenomena. Concepts used by nursing include persons, environment, health, and nursing actions.[187:2]

Specific concepts for each of these four categories have been described by various nursing theorists. The concepts within each theoretical framework represent building blocks for statements of interrelationship, hypotheses, and empirical generalizations that form the essence of the theory. For example, some theorists, such as Roy, conceptualize persons as adaptive beings, environment as a field of stimuli, and health as a continuum representing adaptive responses.[424] Orem prescribed nursing actions based on concepts such as self-care, agency, environmental resources, self-care demands, and self-care needs.[380]

For both these theorists and others, prescribed patterns for nursing action emerge from the theorists' interpretations of an interaction among conceptualized events symbolic of persons, their environment, health factors, and the nurse. Hypotheses are representative of the statements of the interrelationship and generate direction for empirical research that either confirms or refutes the reliability and credibility of the theory. Once the research data accentuate the theoretical perspective, intersubjectivity among practitioners regarding the predictive strength of the theory completes the translation of empirical generalizations into practice.

Translation of nursing theory into practice is strengthened not only through empirical research but also through the use of certain tools unique to nursing, such as patterns of nursing diagnosis. Nursing diagnosis patterns serve theory development primarily in two ways. First, diagnostic patterns are useful for structuring theoretically relevant hypotheses to be tested by empirical research. For example, nursing theorists Roy, Orem, and Rogers express conceptual interrelationships in terms of the person exchanging information with an environment in an effort to progress toward high levels of wellness. Nursing diagnosis patterns including *Potential for . . .* , *Instability of . . .* , *Incapacity to . . .* , and *Discomfort of . . .* provide specific criteria for relating the assessment data proposed by the theory to a clinical problem. Thus, the researcher can test hypotheses dealing with the validity of the nurse's perceptual information concerning person, environment, and health in formulating clinical judgments representing a less biased reality.

A second way diagnostic patterns strenghten nursing theory concerns the translation of theorized images into meaningful clinical events. Theorists Peplau, King, and Levine focus on the interpersonal interactions between the nurse as an environmental resource and persons who seek or need guidance in maintaining and achieving optimal levels of functioning. Nursing diagnosis patterns such as *Low self-esteem . . .* , *Role conflict . . .* , *Loneliness . . .* , *Grief reaction . . .* , and *Bonding interruption . . .* serve as tools that aid the practitioner in separating the essential, necessary events of a clinical situation from accidental temporary events. The registered nurse practicing in a clinical setting recognizes many aspects of a patient's behavior. Interpretation is based on the theoretical perspective and overall meaning of the behavior. Thus, nursing actions prescribed by the theory are consistent with the specific patient's problems, needs, goals, and potentials.

Because nursing diagnosis patterns are instrumental in expressing and translating the science and art of nursing, the consistency between particular patterns and selected nursing theories depends on the presenting issues in a given clinical event. A nurse basing practice on a specific theoretical nursing framework may use any of the patterns at various times, depending on the factors affecting specific clinical situations. Validity of the nursing diagnosis patterns as appropriate tools for use with selected nursing theories is measurable. Formulation of theoretically sound clinical judgments and specific diagnostic patterns are suited to the particular event.

The use of theory as a framework for explaining, describing, predicting, and controlling the clinical situation, together with the nursing diagnosis patterns, holds the potential for strengthening social acceptability, professional integrity, and scientific validity. Therefore, the body of knowledge identified by and for nursing will enhance the meaning of nursing and broaden the scope of practice.

Priorities in Nursing Diagnosis

Priorities in solving nursing diagnosis problems can be determined by modifying Maslow's hierarchy of needs as follows:[328:37-47]

> Physiologic needs
> Safety needs
> Belongingness needs
> Self-esteem needs
> Esteem-from-others needs
> Self-actualization needs

Physiologic needs, which are essential to life, always have first priority. Such needs must be met if a person is to sustain life and satisfy other needs. Safety needs may be of a physical or psychologic nature. Unless a person feels safe in the essential aspects of life, the potential for personal growth is greatly diminished. The need for positive relatedness to others falls under belongingness needs. Persons need to feel loved and unified with others and to communicate at the highest level possible. Self-esteem, esteem-from-others, and self-actualization needs all affect personal growth as an individual strives toward maturity. These needs, when achieved, lead to high levels of fulfillment.

Clarity of Diagnostic Statements

There are many current views on how to label or state a nursing diagnosis. If nurses are to use nursing diagnosis statements to communicate with one another, it is essential that the terminology reflect clarity of meaning and thought. According to John Dewey, there are three levels of thought:[132]

Abstract, which is theoretical and not practical
Intermediate, which is transitional between abstract and concrete and is used to proceed from one idea to the other
Concrete, which is applied to dealing with difficulties on a practical level

When examining levels of thought, we see that certain words convey more precise imagery:

Abstract	Flower
Intermediate	Rose
Concrete	Yellow rosebud

So it is with nursing diagnosis labels. The more precisely descriptive the diagnostic statement, the greater the potential for clear communications of the intended meaning:

Examples

Abstract	Fluid status
Intermediate	Fluid imbalance
Concrete	Fluid volume depletion related to burn wound
OR	
Abstract	Comfort deficit
Intermediate	Pain
Concrete	Headache related to laceration wound

Since concrete descriptions communicate more precise information, it is suggested that diagnostic labels be stated as concretely as possible.

Various Meanings of the Term *Problem*

In the nursing profession, the term *problem* is used in a variety of ways. There are several kinds of problems with which nurses become involved:

The *complaint problem* is the conclusion the person has arrived at as to what is troubling him and is the problem he presents to the professional.[125:16–17]
The *patient problem* is the conclusion the professional determines to be the patient's difficulty. "Nurses assess and formulate statements of patient problems which are known as 'nursing diagnosis.' "[333:7]
The *nursing problem* is any difficulty the nurse has in solving the defined patient problem.[5]
The *problem list* is a composite of all identified problems, both nursing and medical.[507]

Understanding the various meanings of *problem* clarifies the use of the term in its relationship to nursing.

Responsibility for Making Nursing Diagnoses

Nursing diagnoses are made by professional registered nurses. By virtue of their education, professional nurses have the capability to make judgments and use critical thinking. They are skilled in the use of the nursing process by which they identify nursing diagnoses. Gordon states that "standards and laws clearly dictate that this [nursing diagnosis] is a professional activity."[196:271] Other nursing personnel may provide information about the patient to the professional nurse and may assist in interventions related to the diagnosis. However, the process of diagnosing problems that nurses treat is clearly a professional activity.

Clinical Settings in Which Nursing Diagnoses Are Made

Nursing diagnoses are made anywhere the professional nurse practices:

Hospitals
Community health agencies
Clinics
Schools
Physicians' offices
Health maintenance organizations
Nursing homes
Hospices

Advantages of Using Nursing Diagnoses in Clinical Settings

Certain benefits are derived from using diagnoses when working with patients:

Nursing diagnoses set priorities for care.
Identification of a diagnostic problem provides a base from which a plan of care is determined.
The process of data gathering that leads to diagnosis conveys concern for the patient, which increases the patient's sense of security.
Identifying the problem in terms of a nursing diagnosis clarifies the specific problem for the person.
By identifying the problems that nurses are solving, the profession is clarifying for patients the service that nurses have to offer.

The challenge of nursing diagnosis has in some ways been met but still holds a future of growth for nurses. There is much to be done, and today's professional nurses are meeting that challenge.

2 NURSING DIAGNOSIS PATTERNS: AN ANALYSIS OF REGISTERED NURSES' RESPONSES

Myrna R. Pichard, R.N., Ed.D.
Hazel M. Jay, R.N., M.Ed., M.S.

THE DEVELOPMENT OF NURSING DIAGNOSIS PATTERNS

At a nursing diagnosis workshop held in San Antonio, Texas, in May 1980, Gordon indicated that there were patterns of nursing diagnosis yet to be described and essential criteria yet to be developed for each pattern. Those comments gave Campbell the incentive to research patterns of nursing diagnosis and the essential characteristics of each. First, the body of work done for the first edition of *Nursing Diagnosis and Intervention in Nursing Practice* was reviewed from a new perspective. The nursing diagnoses listed in the text were studied and then separated into groups. Gradually, certain consistencies became evident among the identifiable diagnostic patterns. Nursing literature was thoroughly reviewed for information suggesting diagnostic labels that would best characterize these patterns. In addition, practicing nurses were consulted about the more commonly used diagnostic labels and were asked to consider various nursing approaches that might suggest patterns.

It was from the recommendations of practicing nurses, combined with information from nursing literature, that the diagnostic patterns slowly evolved. For example, in 1979, Watt[777] developed a patient classification system at Irving Community Hospital, Irving, Texas, using the Delphi Technique. The findings of Watt's study resulted in a weighted acuity indicator for five categories of care: type I (minimal/self-care), type II (partial care), type III (complete care), type IV (intensive care level 1), and type V (intensive care level 2). The descriptions of each level of care indicated increasing complexity and became the basis of a flexible staffing system used to forecast and provide staff coverage on both a short-term and long-term basis. The patient characteristics identified by Watt were adapted for the essential criteria of the diagnostic patterns *Incapacity to . . . , Partial incapacity to . . .* , and *Instability of . . . .* Watt's patient classification system served as a guide for pattern identification based on actual clinical practice.

The nursing literature provided information about the kinds of problems nurses solve, such as those of insufficient health knowledge, physiologic conditions that require monitoring, and emotional responses resulting from the illness experience.

As data were gathered for pattern development, Campbell concentrated on those patterns believed to be predominantly nursing, that is, those patterns of patient problems solved more often by nurses than any other profession.

A review of the nursing process as outlined in the nursing literature suggested that each nursing diagnosis pattern consisted of essential criteria, a definition of the response, and a diagnostic label.[89:5 & 13, 196:235]

The *essential criteria* are the subjective and objective data that distinguish one diagnostic pattern from another and that are required to establish the diagnosis of that pattern. If the pattern is to be consistently used, its essential criteria must be appropriate for many patient situations. For example, if there is a pattern of *Incapacity to . . .*, the essential criteria must be suitable to *Incapacity to perform personal hygiene, Incapacity to dress self,* or *Incapacity to feed self.*

The *definition of the response* is a statement describing and explaining the meaning of the essential criteria. The definition was compiled from various views in nursing literature.

The *diagnostic label* is the title of the diagnostic pattern. The choice of labels was a different task. For some patterns, specific terminology was found to be in common use. For other patterns, the general concept was consistent, but the terminology was either inconsistent or unidentified. Labels were chosen from commonly used terminology or from diagnostic labels suggested by practicing nurses.

Many problems cited throughout nursing literature are listed in *International Classification of Diseases,* the *Standard Nomenclature of Disease and Operations,* and the *Diagnostic and Statistical Manual of Mental Disorders (DSM-III).* No attempt was made to alter these patterns specifically for use in nursing. Diagnostic statements such as *throbbing pain, hemorrhage, cardiogenic shock,* and *depressive reaction* are clearly understood by nurses, physicians, and other health care professionals. Such diagnostic statements were placed in the category of dual diagnoses.[86]

The implications of a classification system are extensive. Gordan has identified a number of areas in which the scope of practice might be more clearly defined. To define the problems that nurses identify, diagnose, and treat is the most concrete way of using nursing diagnoses. Communication could be improved by the use of a standardized language in nursing. Continuity of care could also be improved, with discharge summaries written in terms of the status of the problems nurses have treated. The nursing diagnoses could be communicated to follow-up agencies. Nursing diagnoses are relevant to nursing education, and many baccalaureate programs are using nursing diagnoses as the basis for organizing knowledge in the curriculum. Another major implication of adopting a standard classification system is that it would necessitate experimental research to determine the interventions necessary to attain specified outcomes.[618] The advantages for clinicians would be the use of more analytical approaches to clinical decision making, assistance in the selection of intervention strategies, and the identification of criteria for evaluation.[630] A number of issues are still to be considered, including whether nursing's efforts should be directed toward identifying nursing interventions or describing nursing phenomena, whether etiology should be included as a part of the nursing process, and whether nursing should develop its own classification system with a theoretical framework or should employ a classification system currently in use by health care institutions.[266]

THE DEVELOPMENT OF THE NURSING DIAGNOSIS QUESTIONNAIRE

The initial purpose of this study was to develop a questionnaire using the nursing diagnosis patterns and the associated assessment characteristics identified by Campbell to determine the extent to which nurses with different educational backgrounds agreed with the diagnostic labels, definitions, and criteria. In an effort to reach a population of nurses with different basic educational backgrounds, the questionnaire was administered to registered nurses in general hospital settings at selected geographic locations.

The specific purpose of the study was to determine the level of agreement of a group of registered nurses with the identified essential assessment criteria, definition, and diagnostic label. The registered nurses were graduates from baccalaureate program (BSN), associate degree programs (ADN), and diploma programs (Di).

Research Design

To meet the study's purpose, the investigators:

1. Selected general hospitals, the largest employer of the identified population, as the setting for data collection.
2. Used frequency distributions in describing the results.
3. Compared educational groups using chi-square contingency table analysis. If $p < 0.05$, this indicated disagreement among groups; and if $0.05 < p < 0.10$, this was accepted as a tendency toward disagreement among groups.[421]

Definition of Terms

The following terms were used in the study:

1. *Nursing diagnosis*, or clinical diagnosis made by a professional nurse, describes "actual or potential health problems which nurses, by virtue of their education and experience, are capable and licensed to treat."[196:2]
2. *Nursing diagnosis pattern*, Campbell stated, consists of a set of essential criteria, a definition of the response, a diagnostic label that describes the basic character-istics of a particular human response, and a label that can be applied to more than one nursing diagnosis statement.
3. *Essential criteria* are the subjective and objective data that distinguish one diag-nostic pattern from another and that are required to be present for the diagno-sis of that pattern.[86]
4. *Diagnostic label* is a descriptive word or phrase that represents the pattern of hu-man response and is the first part of the nursing diagnosis statement.
5. *Registered nurse* is a person licensed to practice nursing in the state of resi-dence.[630]
6. *Baccalaureate education (BSN)* for nurses refers to a college education with a ma-jor in nursing, which combines education in the theory and practice of nursing with general education in the humanities and the sciences.[365]
7. *Associate degree program in nursing (ADN)* is a 2-year program of study that pre-pares students to be eligible to take state licensure examinations to become registered nurses.[364]
8. *Diploma program in nursing (Di)* is usually under the control of a hospital and prepares a person to be eligible for licensure as a registered nurse.[366]
9. *Level I* denotes the higher administrative positions held by registered nurses. The titles used here are vice president, director of nursing service, and associ-ate and assistant administrators. The position requires responsibility for func-tions of planning, coordinating decision making, and directing the nursing service or educational activities.[325]
10. *Level II* denotes the middle-management positions held by registered nurses. The titles used were unit supervisor, head nurse, patient care coordinator, unit manager, staff development educator, and patient educator. The primary re-sponsibility for functions included supervision, delegation, and evaluation of personnel.[325]
11. *Level III* denotes the staff-level position. The registered nurse directs patient care responsibilities and performs professional nursing care in accordance with standard nursing procedures.[325]

Method and Procedure of Study

The study was conducted during a 3-month period in 18 general hospitals located in two areas of Texas and one area in each of the following states: California, Colorado, Florida, New Jersey, and Maine. Contact was made with the nurse administrator in each hospital, who helped decide on the time, place, and person to administer the questionnaire. Persons administering the questionnaires were usually assistant or associate nursing administrators or nursing staff development personnel, who selected the prospects that took part in the study. Those administering the questionnaire are referred to as research assistants in this discussion.

A nonprobability sampling approach was used. Subjects were not identified by name in order to maintain confidentiality and anonymity. All questionnaires were prenumbered, and the numbers were recorded for administrative purposes only. A cover letter was attached to each questionnaire, asking the subject to participate in the study. A total of 1,064 registered nurses who graduated from 4-, 3-, or 2-year nursing programs participated in the study.

Limitations

Several limitations were identified by the investigators:

1. The use of a Likert-type scale is more vulnerable to response sets.
2. The nonrespondents might bias the data, thereby influencing generalizations about the whole population.
3. The subjects in the study might not be representative of the registered nurse population.
4. The person administering the questionnaire might be known to the subjects, possibly influencing participation or the lack of participation in the study.
5. The nature of the study required that persons selected would volunteer and for this reason might respond differently than would nonvolunteers.
6. The study was designed to collect information describing a phenomenon with little control over extraneous variables.

Instrumentation

The questionnaire was developed using Campbell's unpublished essential assessment criteria, definitions, and diagnostic labels. Part I of the questionnaire addressed demographic data. Part II contained the directions and the nursing diagnosis patterns with essential criteria, definitions, and labels. The questionnaire used a Likert-type scale with five possible responses: *strongly agree* (SA), *agree* (A), *undecided* (U), *disagree* (D), and *strongly disagree* (SD).

Content validity was established by setting up a panel of registered nurse experts. The pretest was administered and written comments obtained. One of the concerns of the investigators was the length of the questionnaire, but during the pretest, the average time was 20 minutes, with the longest time recorded being 35 minutes. After the test, each of the patterns—including the essential criteria, definitions, and diagnostic labels—was discussed, as was the questionnaire format. The suggestions were taken into consideration to modify the tool.

DATA COLLECTION

Three methods were used in administering and collecting the questionnaire:

1. Participants were asked to complete parts I and II at a designated time and place of convenience. The protocol for the study included maintaining a record of the prenumbered questionnaires. The research assistants were responsible for returning the completed questionnaires on a designated date for pickup by the investigators.
   OR
2. The subjects were asked to go to a central area and complete the questionnaire. The primary investigator or investigators were usually present at these meetings.
   OR

3. Questionnaires were mailed. A time schedule was arranged to allow for delivery, administration, and return. Arrangements for the administration of the questionnaire to the out-of-state subjects were made with the top-level nurse administrator. Communication was by letter or telephone.

DATA ANALYSIS

The descriptive survey consisted of demographic variables and 46 nursing diagnosis patterns. To analyze the 46 responses by basic nursing education level, a chi-square analysis for contingency tables was used. The groups consisted of a relatively large number of nurses: BSN, 503; ADN, 250; and Di, 311.

Two responses were combined to allow for valid statistical analysis. Responses of *disagree* and *strongly disagree* were combined. This was done because the number of times the *strongly disagree* response was given was low.

Patterns That Were Not Accepted As Stated

Of all the nursing diagnosis patterns tested, the following were subject to disagreement among the three educational groups—BSN, ADN, Di—and were not accepted at the $p = 0.05$ level: no. 3, *Incapacity to . . .* ; no. 6, *Competence in . . .* ; no. 13, *Spiritual awareness . . .* ; no. 29, *Helplessness/powerlessness . . .* ; no. 30, *Hopelessness . . .* ; no. 37, *Misconception of self . . .* ; and no. 45, *Threatened body image . . .* (Table I).

TABLE I
Chi-square Analysis of the Frequency of Responses

Nursing Diagnosis		Chi-square	Degrees of Frequency	Significance Level
No.	Pattern			
3	Incapacity to (level 1, 2, or 3)	13.838	6	0.04
6	Competence in	15.429	6	0.02
13	Spiritual awareness	19.744	6	0.005
29	Helplessness/powerlessness	15.242	6	0.02
30	Hopelessness	14.954	6	0.03
37	Misconception of self	19.367	6	0.005
45	Threatened body image	21.543	6	0.005

NO. 3. NURSING DIAGNOSIS: INCAPACITY TO . . . (LEVEL 1, 2, OR 3)

DEFINITION

Incapable of self-care and requiring total assistance

ASSESSMENT DATA

Levels of Incapacity
1a. Attempts self-care but is unable to perform self-care
 b. Activity is slightly controlled
 c. Ambulatory but with assistance
2a. Makes no attempt at self-care
 b. Activity is greatly controlled
 c. Nonambulatory
3a. Makes no attempt at self-care
 b. Activity is rigidly controlled
 c. Nonambulatory

NURSING DIAGNOSIS PATTERN: Incapacity to . . . (no. 3)
SUMMARY OF NURSES' COMMENTS: The nurses were primarily concerned with the confusion

caused by the three levels in the pattern. Level 1 was less acceptable than levels 2 and 3. The overwhelming comment was that ambulatory status has no relation to a person's level of incapacity.

DISPOSITION: Changes were made in both the definition and assessment data to comply more fully with the nurses' suggestions. This nursing diagnosis pattern was retained because of the frequency with which it is mentioned in the literature. However, it should be resurveyed to determine if the changes show significant agreement among groups.

NO. 6. NURSING DIAGNOSIS: COMPETENCE IN . . .

DEFINITION

Person (or family) gives evidence of adequate ability, knowledge, or proficiency in the task of (specify the task)

ASSESSMENT DATA

1. Person (or family) relates being capable of handling his problem
2. Person (or family) demonstrates the ability to handle the problem or complete the task

---

NURSING DIAGNOSIS PATTERN: Competence in . . . (no. 6)

SUMMARY OF NURSES' COMMENTS: The nurses' primary concern was with assessment datum 1, *person (or family) relates being capable of handling his problem.* The group stated that verbalizing competence in a task was unacceptable and that competence in a task had to be determined by performance.

DISPOSITION: Semantic changes were made in both the definition and assessment data. Since nurses in community health are using this concept in actual practice, this pattern was kept. Registered nurses (BSN, ADN, and Di) should be resurveyed to determine if the changes will show significant agreement among groups.

NO. 13. NURSING DIAGNOSIS: SPIRITUAL AWARENESS . . .

DEFINITION

An evolving consciousness of the need for a relationship with a supreme being

ASSESSMENT DATA

1. Person recognizes that he is not sufficient to self
2. Relates having had little or no meaningful relationship with a supreme being
3. Recognizes and contemplates the existence of a supreme being higher than self, on whom one is essentially dependent

---

NURSING DIAGNOSIS PATTERN: Spiritual awareness . . . (no. 13)

SUMMARY OF NURSES' COMMENTS: The nurses expressed strong dislike for the use of the term *supreme being.* They preferred such terms as *belief system, faith,* and *divinity.* Assessment datum 2, *relates having had little or no meaningful relationship with a supreme being,* was the primary factor of nonacceptance in this pattern. The responses indicated that a person who did not have a meaningful relationship with a supreme being could still experience spiritual awareness. The respondents who disliked becoming involved in spiritual matters expressed negative opinions and objected to having to place a value judgment on a person's belief system.

DISPOSITION: Both the definition and assessment data were altered to reflect the respondents' comments. An attempt was made to broaden the scope of this pattern so that it would be suitable for any spiritual perspective. It should be included in a later survey to determine if the changes have significant agreement among the identified groups.

NO. 29. NURSING DIAGNOSIS: **HELPLESSNESS/POWERLESSNESS . . .**

DEFINITION

Feeling that one has no power or resources to control a situation and is vulnerable to whatever happens

ASSESSMENT DATA

1. Person verbalizes that he has little control over a situation
2. Feels there is nothing he can do to alter things
3. Feels subject to the mercy and power of others
4. Feels forced to accept whatever occurs
5. Manifests direct help-seeking behavior (seeking answers, talking to others, reading books)
   OR
6. Manifests indirect help-seeking behavior (acting out, withdrawal, somatic complaints)

NURSING DIAGNOSIS PATTERN: Helplessness/powerlessness . . . (no. 29)

SUMMARY OF NURSES' COMMENTS: The nurses expressed concern that the term *feels* used in assessment data 2, 3, and 4 was not measureable. A number of nurses stated that persons who feel helpless do not use help-seeking behavior.

DISPOSITION: The definition and assessment data were changed in accordance with the nurses' suggestions. Because of the likeness of this pattern to the pattern *Hopelessness . . .* , new references from the literature were used to clarify this pattern further. Since *Helplessness . . .* is a common nursing diagnosis, it was retained. The recommendation is to reexamine the pattern and determine the degree of agreement with registered nurse subjects.

NO. 30. NURSING DIAGNOSIS: **HOPELESSNESS . . .**

DEFINITION

The feeling that efforts are useless and ineffective

ASSESSMENT DATA

1. Believes that efforts toward a goal are futile
2. Feels extremely discouraged and fatigued
3. Relates having given up trying
4. Exhibits passive behavior (ceases all positive action)

NURSING DIAGNOSIS PATTERN: Hopelessness . . . (no. 30)

SUMMARY OF NURSES' COMMENTS: The nurses stated that this diagnostic pattern was not measureable and that it was too closely allied to *Helplessness. . . .* The respondents suggested additional objective data.

DISPOSITION: The literature was again reviewed and changes were made in the assessment data to more clearly differentiate *Hopelessness* . . . from *Helplessness* . . . . Additional objective data were added. This diagnostic pattern should be resurveyed to determine whether the changes show agreement among the groups.

NO. 37. NURSING DIAGNOSIS: MISCONCEPTION OF SELF . . .

DEFINITION

An inaccurate interpretation about oneself

ASSESSMENT DATA

1. Verbalizes perceived characteristics of self
2. Relates conclusions about self that are in error
3. Exhibits overt behavior appropriate to self-perception but inappropriate to the perception of others

---

NURSING DIAGNOSIS PATTERN: Misconception of self . . . (no. 37)

SUMMARY OF NURSES' COMMENTS: The nurses considered this pattern to be difficult to diagnose because the assessment data were based on the person's own perception and lacked measurable characteristics.

DISPOSITION: It was agreed that the abstract nature of this pattern was inadequately supported in nursing literature to justify its retention.

NO. 45. NURSING DIAGNOSIS: THREATENED BODY IMAGE . . . (DISTURBED BODY IMAGE, NEGATIVE BODY IMAGE)

DEFINITION

Feeling endangered by changes in one's physical body

ASSESSMENT DATA

1. Person has experienced a physical change in body sensation, size, function, or appearance
2. Relates the perception that the body is different than previously
3. Perceives the change as negative and unacceptable
4. Feels intensely threatened by the change
5. Exhibits withdrawal behavior (avoids looking at or touching the body part) or aggressive behavior (demands that others care for him; angry outbursts)
6. Has visible or verifiable body changes

NURSING DIAGNOSIS PATTERN: Threatened body image . . . (no. 45)

SUMMARY OF NURSES' COMMENTS: The nurses' primary objection was about the assessment data indicating that a physical change had occurred and was perceived as threatening. The nurses preferred that the assessment data reflect the thought that the person perceived a threat to the body, whether or not the threat actually existed.

DISPOSITION: The alternative patterns *Disturbed body image* . . . and *Negative Body Image* . . . were deleted as suggested in the nurses' comments. Also, changes in the assessment data were made to bring the pattern into greater accord with the nurses' suggestions. Since problems of body image are commonly found in nursing practice, the pattern was retained.

Patterns That Tended Not to Be Accepted As Stated

Nursing diagnoses no. 14, *Spiritual distress* . . . ; no. 25, *Fear of* . . . ; no. 34, *Withdrawal from* . . . ; and no. 46, *Body-image modification* . . . had a significance level between 0.05 and 0.10, indicating that there was a tendency toward disagreement among groups about accepting the pattern as stated (Table II).

TABLE II
Chi-square Analysis of the Frequency of Responses

Nursing Diagnosis		Chi-square	Degrees of Frequency	Significance Level
No.	Pattern			
14	Spiritual distress	11.887	6	.07
25	Fear of	11.707	6	.07
34	Withdrawal from	11.168	6	.08
46	Body-image modification	11.584	6	.07

NO. 14. NURSING DIAGNOSIS: SPIRITUAL DISTRESS . . .

DEFINITION

Troubled concern about threats to one's harmonious relationship with a supreme being

ASSESSMENT DATA

1. Person is experiencing a life change
2. Person relates having had positive spiritual/religious values
3. Expresses concern that the spiritual/religious values are being threatened

---

NURSING DIAGNOSIS PATTERN: Spiritual distress . . . (no. 14)

SUMMARY OF NURSES' COMMENTS: There was disagreement with assessment datum 1, that a life change had to be experienced for a person to be in spiritual distress. The nurses suggested that in assessment datum 2, the word *positive* be deleted. Some nurses strongly objected to nurses diagnosing spiritual problems.

DISPOSITION: Changes in definition and assessment data were made as suggested by the nurses' comments.

NO. 25. NURSING DIAGNOSIS: FEAR OF . . .

DEFINITION

A feeling of alarm and fright

ASSESSMENT DATA

1. Person experienced feelings of danger and threat
2. Describes or identifies the danger or threat
3. Manifests increased respirations; restlessness (pacing, sleeplessness, putting things in order); agressive behavior (damanding, controlling, attacking behavior), or withdrawal behavior (avoiding persons or situations)

NURSING DIAGNOSIS PATTERN: Fear of . . . (no. 25)

SUMMARY OF NURSES' COMMENTS: The respondents questioned assessment datum 2, *describes or identifies the danger or threat*, as being incorrect information. It was suggested that additional objective data was needed.

DISPOSITION: Assessment datum 2, which the respondents interpreted to be incorrect information, was further documented[471:74,105:406] and was not changed.

NO. 34. NURSING DIAGNOSIS: WITHDRAWAL FROM . . .

DEFINITION

Moving away from interactions with persons or situations that one cannot overcome

ASSESSMENT DATA

1. Perceives a threat
2. Desires to move away from and avoid the threat
3. Removes self from threatening persons or situations

NURSING DIAGNOSIS PATTERN: Withdrawal from . . . (no. 34)

SUMMARY OF NURSES' COMMENTS: The nurses expressed concern about assessment datum 1, *perceives a threat.* They described the statement as not measureable and too vague. The respondents suggested additional objective data.

DISPOSITION: Changes were made in the assessment data as suggested by the participating nurses.

NO. 46. NURSING DIAGNOSIS: BODY-IMAGE MODIFICATION . . .

DEFINITION

Adjusting to the perception of changes in one's physical body

ASSESSMENT DATA

1. Person has experienced a physical change in body sensation, size, function, or appearance
2. Relates the perception of the body as different than previously
3. Expresses a need to integrate the former body with the new
4. Perceives a sense of loss from the previous body image
5. Has visible or verifiable body changes

NURSING DIAGNOSIS PATTERN: Body-image modification . . . (no. 46)

SUMMARY OF NURSES' COMMENTS: The respondents requested that assessment datum 4, *perceives a sense of loss from the previous body image,* to include the words *a sense of loss or gain.*

DISPOSITION: Changes were made in the assessment data as suggested by the comments.

During the review of the nursing diagnoses patterns, three patterns needed to be relabeled or deleted besides the previously mentioned pattern *Misconception of self. . . .* The patterns were no. 1, *Full capacity to . . . ;* no. 15, *Spiritual modification . . . ;* and no. 38, *Delayed bonding. . . .* (Table III is a summary of all the revisions.)

NURSING DIAGNOSIS PATTERN: Full capacity to . . . (no. 1)

REASON FOR RELABELING: Despite the fact that this pattern showed significant agreement among groups, there were a number of comments that indicated concern regarding the title and problem. *Full capacity to . . .* is a positive statement of a person's ability. The diagnostic pattern *Competence in . . .* is also a positive statement but is open to broader usage. Therefore, to avoid repetition, *Full capacity to . . .* was eliminated, and *Competence in . . .* was considered an appropriate substitute.

TABLE III
Summary of Revisions Based on Comments and Critical Value of the Nursing Diagnosis Patterns

	Nursing Diagnosis	Significance			
No.	Pattern	Levels	Title	Definition	Assessment
1	Full capacity to	.2416	Deleted	—	—
2	Partial capacity to	.3088	X	X	X
3	Incapacity to	.0316	NC	X	X
4	Unknowledgeable about	.4754	NC	X	X
5	Unskilled at	.4055	NC	SC	X
6	Competence in	.0172	NC	SC	SC
7	Instability of	.3755	X	SC	X
8	Discomfort of	.3053	NC	X	X
9	Potential for	.1051	NC	NC	NC
10	Inability to	.1019	NC	NC	X
11	Difficulty	.8348	NC	SC	X
12	Positive screening cues for	.5035	NC	NC	NC
13	Spiritual awareness	.0031	NC	X	X
14	Spiritual distress	.0645	NC	X	X
15	Spiritual modification	.5837	Deleted	—	—
16	Abandoned feeling	.9255	NC	NC	X
17	Loneliness/isolated feeling	.3837	NC	NC	X
18	Ambivalence	.1023	NC	SC	X
19	Anger	.1494	NC	SC	X
20	Anxiety	.1106	NC	SC	X
21	Conflict	.3685	NC	SC	X
22	Depression	.1795	NC	NC	X
23	Dependency feelings	.7690	NC	NC	X
24	Embarrassment	.1265	NC	NC	X
25	Fear of	.0688	NC	NC	X
26	Frustration	.3394	NC	SC	X
27	Grief reaction	.1826	NC	NC	X
28	Guilt	.2150	NC	SC	X
29	Helplessness/powerlessness	.0185	NC	X	X
30	Hopelessness	.0206	NC	NC	X
31	Feeling rejected	.6561	NC	SC	X
32	Rejection of	.1825	NC	NC	X
33	Denial of	.8195	NC	SC	X
34	Withdrawal from	.0833	NC	SC	X
35	Disengagement/detachment	.3438	X	X	X
36	Low self-esteem	.3071	NC	SC	X
37	Misconception of self	.0036	Deleted	—	—
38	Delayed bonding	.1877	Deleted	—	—
39	Bonding interruption	.4038	X	X	X
40	Nonbonding	.1492	Determined to be maladaptive rather than adaptive		
41	Role conflict	.3583	NC	SC	X
42	Role modification	.1324	NC	NC	X
43	Regression	.1106	NC	X	X
44	Self-identity modification	.2828	NC	SC	X
45	Threatened body image	.0015	X	NC	X
46	Body-image modification	.0719	NC	SC	X

Abbreviations: NC = no change; SC = semantic change; X = change.

NURSING DIAGNOSIS PATTERN: Spiritual modification . . . (no. 15)

REASON FOR DELETION: Although this diagnosis showed sufficient agreement among groups, the participants' comments indicated considerable difficulty with the concept. Comments also indicated that the assessment data were redundant and belonged under *Spiritual awareness* . . . or *Spiritual distress.* . . . During the review process, the redundancy became apparent. The assessment data were incorporated in the *Spiritual awareness* . . . and *Spiritual distress* . . . patterns, and the *Spiritual modification* . . . was deleted.

NURSING DIAGNOSIS PATTERN: Delayed bonding . . . (no. 38)

REASON FOR DELETION: Even though this nursing diagnosis pattern has significant agreement among groups, the respondents considered the label too vague. Campbell had attempted to apply it to adult situations as well as to mother–child relationships ineffectively. It was decided that this pattern should be completely reworked and evaluated at a later date.

In addition to those patterns that were deleted or relabeled, the pattern *Nonbonding* . . . (no. 40), with a critical value of $p=0.2998$, was determined to be more characteristic of maladaptive than of adaptive behavior. It was moved to Part Three, "Dual Nursing Diagnoses," Chapter 28, "Psychosocial Nonadaption."

The nursing diagnosis patterns were found to be generally acceptable to the registered nurse participants. After the patterns were adjusted to reflect the suggestions and significance levels, each pattern was reviewed again for its suitability to multiple diagnostic situations. The accepted nursing diagnosis patterns are listed and discussed in Chapter 3.

Characteristics of the Sample

The number of registered nurses who participated in the study was 1,064. They received their various types of education in almost every state in the Union, including Alaska and Hawaii; only Rhode Island, Vermont, and Wyoming were not represented. The highest number of participants, totalling 581, were graduates from Texas nursing programs. Table IV summarizes the geographic regions in which the participants received either a BSN, ADN, or Di. The western region included Alaska, California, Hawaii, Oregon, and Washington; the mountain region, Colorado, Idaho, Nevada, and Utah; the southwestern region, Arizona, New Mexico, Oklahoma, and Texas; the central area, Illinois, Indiana, Iowa, Kansas, Missouri, Nebraska, Ohio, and Wisconsin; the northern region, Michigan, Minnesota, Montana, North Dakota, and South Dakota; the southern region, Alabama, Arkansas, Florida, Georgia, Kentucky, Mississippi, Louisiana, and Tennessee; and the eastern sector, Connecticut, Delaware, Maine, Maryland, Massachusetts, New Hampshire, New Jersey, New York, North Carolina, South Carolina, Pennsylvania, Virginia, and the District of Columbia. Registered nurses from other countries were included in the study as well. Table IV summarizes the geographic regions in which participants received either a BSN, an ADN, or a Di. There were 1,008 subjects from the United States and 56 subjects from other countries.

TABLE IV
Numbers of Subjects by Geographic Region or Country in Which Nursing Education Was Obtained (N=1064)

United States	No.	Other	No.
West	55	Scotland	5
Mountain	23	Philippines	10
Southwest	599	New Zealand	1
Central	91	Ireland	6
North	17	Hungary	1
South	89	Canada	6
East	134	England	26
Total	1,008	Thailand	1
		Total	56

There were 61 males and 1,003 females. The education level distribution was BSN, 503; ADN, 250; and Di, 311, and is shown in Table V.

TABLE V
Distribution of Registered Nurses According to Sex and Education

	BSN		ADN		Di	
Sex	No.	%	No.	%	No.	%
Female	474	94	226	90	303	97
Male	29	6	24	10	8	3
Total	503	100	250	100	311	100

Thirteen subjects indicated that they held bachelor degrees in other fields. The average age of the BSN was 31; ADN, 37; and Di, 45. The average length of practice for BSN was 7 years; for ADN, 14 years; and for Di, 24 years. A total of 33 persons failed to respond to this request for information. The summary is presented in Table VI.

TABLE VI
Distribution of Age and Years of Practice According to Education for Entire Group

Education	No.	Did Not Respond	Age (Mean)	Years of Practice
BSN	486	17	31	7
ADN	242	8	37	14
Di	303	8	45	24
Total	1,031	33		

The request for the number of years the subject lived in the state as a practicing nurse and the actual years of practice was confusing to more than 50% of the participants. Therefore, the frequency tabulations were confined to the years of nursing practice.

The present study did not attempt to determine if there was a difference in the responses of those with advanced degrees. There were 49 respondents with a master of science in nursing, 18 had a master's degree in another field, and three had earned doctorates. All respondents had responsibility for the functions as defined in levels I or II. The distribution of advanced degree and functional responsibility are noted in Table VII.

TABLE VII
Distribution of Registered Nurses with Advanced Degrees and Functional Responsibility

	All Groups		Level I		Level II	
Degree	No.	%	No.	%	No.	%
Master of science in nursing	49	70	39	67	10	83
Masters degree in another field	18	26	18	33	0	0
Doctorate	3	4	1	0	2	17
Totals	70	100	58	100	12	100

The functional responsibility of each basic education level indicated a higher number of the third level in all groups. No responses were recorded for the ADN at the first level. Table VIII includes registered nurses with advanced degrees.

Nurses who participated in the survey practiced in such areas as ambulatory care, coronary care, emergency room, medical–surgical nursing, infection control, medical nursing, nursing administration, obstetrics, operating room, orthopedics, outpatient clinic, pediatrics, quality assurance, recovery room, rehabilitation, surgical units, intensive care, hospice, in-service education, and psychiatric nursing.

TABLE VIII
Summary Data of Functional Responsibility

Level	All Groups		BSN		ADN		Di	
	No.	%	No.	%	No.	%	No.	%
I	44	4	23	4	0	0	21	7
II	223	21	109	22	33	13	81	26
III	797	75	373	74	216	87	208	67
Total	1,064	100	505	100	249	100	310	100

Implications

The use of nursing diagnosis patterns was of interest to a number of nurses. Of the 1,064 nurses who returned the questionnaire, 620 (58.3%) responded with individual comments. The researchers noted that a conceptual framework for nursing practice is often determined by the area of practice, and the consistent testing of diagnostic hypotheses is not easily identifiable in actual practice. Top-level nursing administrators are encouraging staff to use nursing diagnosis patterns. Nurses in two participating agencies had already begun the process by identifying the theoretical framework and the nursing patterns for selected practice areas. Although interest in nursing diagnosis was evident, there still appears to be a gap in the consistent application of nursing diagnoses.

While the study has provided insight into various diagnostic patterns, further research is indicated. Investigation of the following questions may elicit new data:

Does the conceptual framework of nursing curricula provide the theoretical orientation for nursing practice?

What are the barriers in putting the nursing diagnosis patterns into practice?

Is nursing more accepting of the phenomenon surrounding nursing practice or does nursing practice inhibit the phenomenona?

Research is also needed to identify and determine areas that are clearly nursing. Collaborative efforts by nurse educators and nurse practitioners are still needed in order to achieve greater relevancy and support for the nursing diagnosis.

3 STRUCTURE AND FUNCTION OF NURSING DIAGNOSIS PATTERNS

DIAGNOSTIC PATTERNS IN HEALTH PROFESSIONS

When a person seeks nursing care, he does so with the hope that the nurse will solve a problem that he cannot resolve alone. The function of the professional nurse is to recognize those problems that she is competent to solve. The identification of such problems depends on the nurse's expertise in sorting out and fitting together essential data. Expertise is enhanced when patterns of problems are quickly recognized and treated.

A *nursing diagnosis pattern* consists of a set of essential criteria, a definition, and a label that describes the basic characteristics of a particular human response and that can be applied to more than one nursing diagnosis statement. Nurses commonly deal with two kinds of patterns: patterns of nursing diagnosis and patterns of medical diagnosis. Historically, nurses have been taught the patterns of medical diagnosis. Every professional nurse is expected to recognize that the essential criteria of inflammation are swelling, redness, pain, heat, and loss of function and that the essential criteria of shock are hypotension, pallor, rapid, thready pulse, and rapid respirations. There are hundreds of patterns of medical diagnosis that both nurses and physicians are expected to recognize and treat. Within the whole of medical diagnosis, only a small portion of the total can legally be treated independently by nurses. Nevertheless, nurses have been taught medical diagnoses, the treatment of which makes up a large segment of nursing functions. Such diagnoses fall within the category of dual diagnoses, discussed in Part Three.

Patterns of nursing diagnosis have existed since the beginning of nursing. However, not until recently did professional nurses seek to clearly define the problems they solve. Most nurses recognize the characteristics of a person who is incapable of self-care or one who is without knowledge. In the past, such judgments were based on experience and intuition, but now nurses have the opportunity to more clearly articulate those problems that nurses solve and to determine the essential criteria for each pattern of nursing diagnosis.

In looking at these patterns, consideration was given to other health care professionals. Each pattern was evaluated to determine whether it was unique to nursing or shared with other professions. Through research of nursing literature, it became evident that absolute uniqueness is difficult to claim. A thorough study of any aspect of nursing will eventually demonstrate that other health professionals share at least some aspect of what is claimed to be nursing. Problems of incapacity in which the nurse gives assistance are also dealt with by occupational and physical therapists. Psychosocial problems in which nurses provide psychologic guidance and comfort also fall within the realm of social workers and psychologists. Nevertheless, certain aspects of health care are *predominantly nursing;* that is, in particular areas of health and illness care, the nurse is the primary care provider. The decision to classify a given area as predominantly nursing was made on the basis of confirmation in nursing literature and verification by the evident realities of nursing practice.

There are also patterns that apply to several health disciplines but that have not been labeled or have a label that is not compatible with nursing. For instance, both nurses and physicians screen for illnesses. Physicians have not identified the "finding of illness cues" as a pattern of diagnosis. If a physician finds cues that indicate diabetes mellitus, further studies are done to confirm or rule out the diagnosis. The nurse, however, cannot legally diagnose and treat diabetes mellitus. In screening, the nurse finds the illness cues and refers the person to the physician. This leaves the nurse without a diagnostic pattern which describes the case finding expertise of nurses.

In the area of patterns of psychologic responses, nurses use such terms as anxiety, fear, and grief as commonly as do physicians, psychologists, sociologists, and chaplins. However, nurses focus on very specific aspects of these emotions as they relate to the person's experience of illness and health care. No other profession but nursing has recorded in its literature adaptive emotional responses that nurses consistently treat. It is therefore appropriate to define and claim these patterns as predominantly nursing, since they are primarily the focus of nursing care.

COMPONENTS OF THE NURSING DIAGNOSIS PATTERN

Each nursing diagnosis pattern consists of the following elements:[89:5 & 13; 196:235]

Diagnostic label
Definition
Essential criteria or data

The *diagnostic label* is the descriptive word or phrase that represents the pattern. It is a statement of the person's basic response and the first part of the complete nursing diagnosis statement. The label is the core response used to describe the nursing diagnosis statement. It must not conflict with or have the same meaning as any other diagnostic label. Examples of labels are *Discomfort of . . .*, *Instability of . . .*, *Potential for . . .*, *Fear of. . . .*

The *definition* explains the meaning of the diagnostic label. It is clear and concise and expresses the essential nature of the human response.

The *essential criteria* consist of subjective and/or objective data that must be present for the pattern to exist. The essential criteria occur consistently in all problems that fall within the pattern. These criteria are used to differentiate one diagnostic pattern from another. Essential criteria are emphasized by a dot (•) in front of the statement. Nonessential criteria are not emphasized. All three components—the diagnostic label, definition, and essential criteria—equal the nursing diagnosis pattern.

LIST OF NURSING DIAGNOSIS PATTERNS

The following patterns were identified as a result of the study discussed in Chapter 2.

General Nursing Diagnosis Patterns
Discomfort of . . .
Difficulty . . .
Inability to . . .
Incapacity to . . .*
Partial incapacity to . . .
Instability of . . .
Potential for . . .
Positive screening cues for . . .
Spiritual awareness . . .*
Spiritual distress . . .
Unknowledgeable about . . .

---

*Diagnostic label requires retesting for an acceptable critical value.

Unskilled at . . .
Competence in . . .*

Psychosocial Nursing Diagnosis Patterns

Abandoned feeling . . .
Loneliness/isolated feeling . . .
Ambivalence . . .
Anger . . .
Anxiety . . .
Conflict . . .
Depression . . .
Dependency feelings . . .
Embarrassment . . .
Fear of . . .
Frustration . . .
Grief reaction . . .
Guilt . . .
Helplessness/powerlessness . . .*
Hopelessness . . .*
Feeling rejected . . .
Rejection of . . .
Withdrawal from . . .
Denial of . . .
Disengagement/detachment . . .
Low self-esteem . . .
Bonding interruption . . .
Role conflict . . .
Role modification . . .
Regression . . .
Self-identity modification . . .
Threatened body image . . .*
Body-image modification . . .

These diagnostic patterns reflect a broad spectrum and suggest that nursing is concerned with aspects of a person's life both in illness and in wellness. Although in numbers there are more psychosocial patterns than general patterns, this does not mean that nursing is primarily directed toward solving psychosocial problems. There were simply more possible human responses of a psychosocial nature that were identifiable. The human responses of *Discomfort of . . .*, *Incapacity to . . .*, *Instability of . . .*, *Spiritual distress . . .*, etc., are of equal significance, as nurses concern themselves with the whole person.

DESCRIPTION OF NURSING DIAGNOSIS PATTERNS

Each nursing diagnosis pattern has a label, definition, and specific essential criteria. The following is a list of the patterns that resulted from the study described in Chapter 2, and that are used throughout this text.

General Nursing Diagnosis Patterns

More than any other profession, nursing focuses on human discomfort. The pattern *Discomfort of . . .* refers to responses of the human senses. It includes hearing, seeing, smelling, touching, and tasting; the perception of heat and cold, and the physiologic

---

*Diagnostic label requires retesting for an acceptable critical value.

NURSING DIAGNOSIS PATTERN: DISCOMFORT OF . . .[159,423]

DEFINITION

Experiencing as distressful such physical sensations as cold, heat, dryness, wetness, pressure, loudness

ASSESSMENT DATA

Subjective Data
• Person relates experiencing the unpleasant sensation of (name the sensation)

Objective Data
• May exhibit behavior such as pulling at or removing a tight bandage, looking for a blanket when cold, crying when the diaper is wet, struggling with restraints

---

sensation of weakness. This pattern does not include diagnoses of pain. Pain is most definitely a discomfort, but discomfort is not necessarily a form of pain. The diagnostic criteria for specific types of pain are clearly outlied within the framework of medical diagnosis. Nurses independently treat pain under the dual diagnoses system. For this reason, the pattern *Discomfort of . . .*, focuses on distressful human sensation other than pain.

The ability to differentiate between the nursing diagnosis of discomfort and pain takes professional skill. The importance of such differential diagnosis is that the correct diagnosis leads to maximum patient comfort. The postsurgical patient may wince and cry out each time he moves the incised body part. This diagnosis could be *throbbing pain.* This same person may constantly wet his lips, complain of a sensation of cotton in his mouth, etc. This diagnosis would be *Discomfort of mouth dryness.* Through the recognition and treatment of both pain and discomfort, human misery is reduced.

NURSING DIAGNOSIS PATTERN: DIFFICULTY . . .[524]

DEFINITION

Person (or family) is only partially effective in achieving

ASSESSMENT DATA

Subjective Data
• Person (or family) relates that it is hard to attain a solution/goal
• Verbalizes unsuccessful methods attempted

Objective Data
• Person (or family) has demonstrated repeated efforts to attain the goal or solution
• Person (or family) may exhibit behavior or signs indicating that methods attempted are partially but not completely effective, e.g., called to make a clinic appointment but was told he would have to wait 6 weeks to see the doctor

---

Difficulty . . . is a nursing diagnosis pattern used in situations in which a person is working toward achieving a goal but is finding it very hard to do so. In such instances, nursing assistance can accelerate or make easier the achievement of the goal. For example, a person calls for a clinic appointment with the hope of being seen in a few days. When told he can have an appointment in 6 weeks, he has achieved his goal of making an appointment, but the time element has presented a difficulty and is unsatisfactory. Through assistive intervention, the nurse helps the patient obtain an early appointment. A diagnosis of *Difficulty utilizing community resources* would be appropriate here. *Difficulty . . .*

is used in hard-to-achieve situations and differs from the pattern *Partial incapacity to . . . ,* which is used for states of limited physical performance.

NURSING DIAGNOSIS PATTERN: INABILITY TO . . . [524]

DEFINITION
Person (or family) is ineffective in achieving

ASSESSMENT DATA
Subjective Data
- Person (or family) relates being unable to attain a solution/goal
- May or may not know of or have attempted solution methods

Objective Data
- Person (or family) may exhibit behavior or signs indicating that the solution/goal is not achieved, e.g., person does not keep a doctor's appointment because he cannot find transportation

---

Inability to . . . is a pattern of response observed when a person is completely ineffective in achieving a goal in a specific situation. This pattern differs from *Incapacity to . . .* in that the problem does not involve limitations in physical performance. The person may be capable of achieving the goal, but either the methods being used or uncontrollable stressors have prevented goal achievement. For example, take the case of a mother of three schoolchildren who becomes ill. She requires dressing changes and medications four times daily. No relatives are available to assist in the situation. The children attend school, and although they are capable of caring for their mother, the fact that they are not at home means they are not available to provide care to her during the day. A diagnosis of *Family inability to provide therapeutic care* would be appropriate here. The pattern *Inability to . . .* is used to describe situational goals that cannot be achieved.

NURSING DIAGNOSIS PATTERN: INCAPACITY TO . . . [380,777]

DEFINITION
Being incapable of activities of daily living and requiring total assistance with such activities

ASSESSMENT DATA
Subjective Data
- Person may or may not relate being unable to carry out self-care

Objective Data
- Person exhibits behavior such as minimal, ineffective, or no body movements, makes no attempt at self-care

---

Incapacity to . . . is a human response in which a person cannot perform those activities of daily living that he usually performs for himself. The essential criteria indicate that the person cannot physically do anything for himself, that he is completely dependent on others to perform those activities for him. If the person cannot bathe, feed, dress, or toilet himself, then the responses are *Incapacity to perform personal hygiene, Incapacity to feed self, Incapacity to dress self,* etc. *Incapacity to . . .* refers to the physical performance of self-care. It differs from the pattern *Inability to . . . ,* which is used in goal-achieving situations involving no physical limitations.

NURSING DIAGNOSIS PATTERN: **PARTIAL INCAPACITY TO . . .** [380,777]

DEFINITION

Being capable of but needing assistance with activities of daily living

ASSESSMENT DATA

Subjective Data
• Person relates attempts at self-care
• Requests assistance to complete self-care

Objective Data
• Person exhibits behavior such as struggling to retrieve objects for self-care, having difficulty reaching body parts or manipulating self-care objects, attempting self-care for only short periods before resting, dropping or spilling things

---

Partial incapacity to . . . is the response of a person who can physically perform some activities of daily living but cannot complete the task without some assistance. Help may be required in gathering the tools for the task or in performing the particular activity of daily living, such as bathing, feeding, and ambulating. *Partial incapacity to perform personal hygiene* and *Partial incapacity to ambulate* are nursing diagnoses that refer to limited physical performance. *Partial incapacity to . . .* differs from the pattern *Difficulty . . .* , which is used in hard-to-achieve situations in which physical capacity is sufficient.

NURSING DIAGNOSIS PATTERN: **INSTABILITY OF . . .** [249,777]

DEFINITION

Person presents unstable physiologic signs indicating a physiologic imbalance that threatens the integrity of the specific body system

ASSESSMENT DATA

Subjective Data
• Person may or may not relate symptoms

Objective Data
Level 1
• Person exhibits signs that are intermittently unstable and stable
• Signs may or may not indicate a life-threatening imbalance
• Signs of instability are (name the signs)

Level 2
• Person exhibits signs that are consistently unstable
• Signs indicate a life-threatening imbalance
• Signs of instability are (name the signs)

Instability of . . . is a human response in which a person exhibits physiologic or psychologic cues of disequilibrium. This response implies a state of frequent physiologic or psychologic change that threatens human balance. Instability is an actual state. It has two levels: non-life-threatening and life-threatening. Any disease or illness is considered a state of imbalance. Instability differs in that the person's condition is one of fluctuation and threat. The diagnosis of instability is not based on the medical diagnosis, but on the element of continuing change from that which is considered normal. For example, one person who has had a myocardial infarction may exhibit consistent vital signs that fall within normal limits. Although there is a potential for physiologic change, actual instability does not exist. Another person who has had a myocardial infarction may exhibit hypotension and dysrrythmias, characterizing a state of instability. In this case, the diagnoses would be *Instability of arterial pressure* and *Instability of cardiac rhythm*.

Nursing has been charged with the responsibility of observing and protecting patients during states of instability. Nurses assume this responsibility in all areas of nursing from intensive care to community health.

NURSING DIAGNOSIS PATTERN: POTENTIAL FOR . . .[196,295]

DEFINITION

The presence of stressors that increase the possibility of the occurrence of a problem

ASSESSMENT DATA

Subjective Data
• No actual symptoms of (name the potential problem)

Objective Data
• No actual signs of (name the potential problem)
• One or more stressors are present that increase the possibility of the problems occurring

---

Potential for . . . is a nursing diagnosis pattern in which no actual signs or symptoms are observed. The person is not currently exhibiting a response, but the possibility of an unfavorable response exists. For a potential problem to exist, there must be stressors that could cause the problem. Since a potential problem does not exhibit any signs or symptoms of an actual problem, the stressors cannot be listed under signs and symptoms. In order to make a diagnosis, the stressors must be listed somewhere in the assessment data. Logically, they fit under *Related Data*.

In an "actual" problem, the signs and symptoms suggest the diagnosis. The etiology (stressors) is not absolutely essential for a diagnostic conclusion but is most frequently used for intervention planning. In a potential problem, the stressors must be known in order to arrive at a diagnostic conclusion.

Two types of potential nursing diagnosis can be defined. First, there are potential problems associated with a person who is ill or who is undergoing diagnostic or treatment measures which involve possible complications or unfavorable reactions. Such responses have not yet occurred but could occur. The person who has just come from abdominal surgery has the *Potential for shock* and the *Potential for bleeding*. Although his condition is currently stable, the possibility exists that a complication could occur. With this pattern, as with that of *Instability of . . .* , it is the nurse who stays at the patient's bedside and monitors the person's condition until the potential threat is minimal or alleviated.

There are also potential problems that result from such factors as heredity, lifestyle, and environment. Generally speaking, these potential problems are associated with clusters of stressors that are known to lead to disease, as shown by population studies. Science has demonstrated that certain known patterns of high-risk factors usually cause disease or trauma. If the high-risk factors are altered or reduced, the potential for the problem's occurrence is diminished. In most situations, the person has some control over the risks and is amenable to learning about and altering them. For example, it is well known that if drinking alcohol, driving, and accelleration at an excessive speed occur, there is a *Potential for motor vehicle injury*. This type of potential problem is the concern of many health care professionals and some health agencies and is primarily an element of health maintenance.

Thus, the pattern *Potential for . . .* is one of possible, not actual, unfavorable responses. Nurses are intellectually astute in knowing what can occur and in recognizing the impending or actual onset of potential illness or injury problems.

NURSING DIAGNOSIS PATTERN: POSITIVE SCREENING CUES FOR . . .[295]

DEFINITION

Person exhibits significant abnormal clinical findings during brief testing

ASSESSMENT DATA

Subjective Data
• Person may or may not verbalize significant symptoms

Objective Data
• Exhibits, during screening, clinical findings that are not within the standard normal range

---

A primary aspect of nursing is to screen patients for disease and illness. The term *positive screening cues* means that a patient presents evidence indicating that it is highly likely that he has a certain disease or illness. The word *positive* is used to affirm that certain cues of disease are present. The use of the word *screening* indicates that a judgment is being made on the basis of some of the standard medical procedures used to verify a specific condition. The term *screening* is important to nursing from a legal aspect. By law, nurses cannot diagnose disease. To state that a person has diabetes mellitus is not within the domain of nursing, since nurses cannot independently treat disease. The word *screening* clarifies that the nurse has used diagnostic procedures to uncover that which most likely represents a disease entity. Finally, *cues* refers to signs and symptoms. In this diagnostic pattern, symptoms may or may not be presented by the patient. The nurse relies heavily on clinical findings rather than on symptoms.

Through the use of the nursing diagnosis *Positive screening cues for diabetes mellitus*, the nurse expresses that the patient exhibits signs and symptoms commonly associated with diabetes mellitus. In addition, the nurse communicates that the judgment made is based on screening and that it does not constitute a conclusive medical diagnosis.

One criterion for acceptance of a nursing diagnosis pattern is that there be appropriate, independent nursing intervention. The primary intervention in this pattern is *referral to a physician*. There has been some question as to whether referral can be considered a nursing intervention. While referral is not a procedural treatment, it is a nursing activity that promotes health and well-being. It is therapeutic in that it is supportive, communicates caring, and provides guidance toward health. Without the intervention of referral, the person's condition would be unconfirmed and untreated. Referral is an important aspect of patient care and is considered in this text to be a nursing intervention.

Health care professionals other than nurses use screening techniques. Physicians use screening to arrive at a medical diagnosis of a specific disease. Nonprofessional private or government agencies also screen for disease, but their screening is limited to procedural skills and is not based on in-depth knowledge.

Professional nurses use screening techniques based on their scientific knowledge of and judgments about health and illness. Nurses have always used screening techniques and referred patients for further diagnostic evaluation. Recognition of this nursing activity has gone relatively unnoticed. Through the use of the diagnostic pattern *Positive screening cues for . . .*, professional nurses will call attention to their diagnostic capabilities and their valuable contribution toward health care.

NURSING DIAGNOSIS PATTERN: SPIRITUAL AWARENESS . . .[157,771]

DEFINITION

An ongoing consciousness of a need for a more positive, spiritual force in one's life

ASSESSMENT DATA

Subjective Data
• Person verbalizes that he alone is not sufficient
• Relates a need for a more meaningful spiritual relationship
• May request spiritual assistance

Objective Data
• May exhibit behavior such as reading spiritual books, viewing or listening to spiritual programs, attending religious services, quiet contemplation

The pattern *Spiritual awareness . . .* reflects the vulnerability that many but not all people feel when ill or in a threatening situation. The person's response demonstrates a need for a more positive force in his life. He becomes profoundly aware of his desire for a greater source of inner strength. Perceiving the caring nature of the nurse, many patients comfortably confide such spiritual needs. Nurses recognize the existence of spiritual problems such as *Spiritual awareness related to a life situation* and intervene appropriately as they seek to treat the whole person.

NURSING DIAGNOSIS PATTERN: **SPIRITUAL DISTRESS** . . .[157,771]

DEFINITION

Troubled concern about threats to one's belief system

ASSESSMENT DATA

Subjective Data
• Person verbalizes definite spiritual/religious values
• Expresses concern that the values are being threatened
• May request assistance with spiritual matters

Objective Data
• May exhibit behavior such as sleeplessness, restlessness, demanding and controlling behavior, unusual quietness, crying

Spiritual distress . . . is a pattern that refers to a person's belief system. Illness often stimulates intense responses in which people cling to their spiritual beliefs. When the person feels his beliefs are threatened, he may convey this to a nurse. For example, certain foods are required to fulfill the obligations of certain belief systems. But illness can prevent a person from carrying out the spiritual rituals associated with required foods. A diagnosis of *Spiritual distress related to disrupted spiritual practices* is appropriate in this instance.

Nurses are instrumental in helping persons fulfill those beliefs essential to their total life. Some nurses prefer to delegate such problems to ministers, chaplains, and priest. Many nurses, however, find the spiritual realm of nursing challenging.

NURSING DIAGNOSIS PATTERN: **UNKNOWLEDGEABLE ABOUT** . . .[86,524]

DEFINITION

Lacking sufficient information

ASSESSMENT DATA

Subjective Data
• Person's discussion or questions indicate a need for additional information, clarification, or validation of information
OR

- Person's lack of questions or comments indicates not wanting information or not knowing enough to seek information
- When questioned directly, the person's response or lack of response indicates that he does not know

Objective Data
- May exhibit behavior such as acting inappropriately based on insufficient knowledge, not taking precautions

Being *Unknowledgeable about . . .* something is the response of a person who lacks information. He may ask questions about what he wants to know, or he may not know enough to ask a question. *Unknowledgeable about . . .* is the pattern that refers to knowledge that is not task oriented. There is simply a need for new or additional information. For example, when a person does not know how babies are born, he is *Unknowledgeable about childbirth.* If he does not know about the formation of kidney stones, he is *Unknowledgeable about renal calculi.* The *Unknowledgeable about . . .* pattern is used when only information and not a task is of importance.

NURSING DIAGNOSIS PATTERN: UNSKILLED AT . . .[86,524]

DEFINITION

Being nonproficient, with or without knowledge, in performing the specific task

ASSESSMENT DATA

Subjective Data
- Person's discussion or questions indicate a need for additional information, clarification, or validation of information about performing the task
    OR
- Person's lack of questions or comments indicates not wanting information or not knowing enough to seek information about performing the task

Objective Data
- Person cannot correctly demonstrate how to (name the task)

The nursing diagnosis pattern *Unskilled at . . .* is used when a person lacks information and is not proficient in a task. It is the added element of the task that differentiates this pattern from the *Unknowledgeable about . . .* response. When a person does not know how to care for a colostomy, he lacks information about the colostomy and lacks skill in the task of colostomy care. *Unskilled at colostomy care* communicates this double need for information and task competence. *Unskilled at managing drugs* indicates a response in which a person lacks information about drugs and lacks skill in drug administration. The nursing diagnosis pattern *Unskilled at . . .* is the basis for integrating information and tasks in health teaching.

NURSING DIAGNOSIS PATTERN: COMPETENCE IN . . .[524,775]

DEFINITION

Person (or family) gives evidence of adequate ability, knowledge, or proficiency in the handling of a problem or task

ASSESSMENT DATA

Subjective Data
- Person (or family) verbalizes ability and knowledge of how to handle his problem

> *Objective Data*
> • Person (or family) correctly demonstrates the ability to handle the problem or complete the task

Many nurses, especially those practicing in community health, diagnose a person's strengths. The pattern *Competence in . . . .* is used to state a person's adequacy and proficiency. For example, the patient who has adjusted satisfactorily from wellness to illness and eventually from illness to wellness demonstrates the response *Competence in psychologic adaptation.* The new mother who is learning about and satisfactorily caring for her infant exhibits the response *Competence in parenting.*

To be competent in health matters indicates wellness. The need for nursing care focuses on the maintenance of the strength through follow-up care. This response does not present a problem in the sense that something is wrong that must be corrected. The problem is that the competency must be maintained as an ongoing process. *Competence in . . .* speaks to a state of ability rather than one of inability. The professional approach of identifying strenghts is a distinct element in nursing practice. It assists the person seeking improved health to recognize his levels of adequacy. It supports the continuation of health practices on the basis of positive health attitudes.

Psychosocial Nursing Diagnosis Patterns

> ### NURSING DIAGNOSIS PATTERN: **ABANDONED FEELING . . .** [107,524]
>
> DEFINITION
> A feeling of having been deserted by another person whether the desertion is real or imagined
>
> ASSESSMENT DATA
> *Subjective Data*
> • Verbalizes that he has been forsaken
> • Expresses concern that the significant other will not return or will return too late
> *Objective Data*
> • *Children* may exhibit regressive behavior such as crying, bed wetting, thumb sucking, or returning to bottle-feeding. *Adults* appear alone, quiet, withdrawn, deep in thought, may exhibit anger or demanding behavior, may refuse to do anything until the person returns

When a person feels deserted, he is experiencing an *Abandoned feeling . . . .* He feels that significant others have left him, that they are not interested in a meaningful relationship with him, that a relationship has been broken with little probability of resumption. It is common for hospitalized children and elderly persons to feel abandoned by their loved ones. The death of a significant other often leaves the survivors with a sense of having been abandoned. This response is one of *Abandoned feeling related to absent significant other.*

An *Abandoned feeling . . . ,* in which the person feels forsaken, differs from *Loneliness . . . .* The lonely person feels separate from others. One can be lonely yet not abandoned. Nurses recognize such feelings and help the person work through the emotion. A caring nurse can greatly reduce the pain of real or imagined abandonment.

NURSING DIAGNOSIS PATTERN: LONELINESS/ISOLATED FEELING . . .[105,471]

DEFINITION

Feeling separate and remote from others

ASSESSMENT DATA

Subjective Data
• Relates a sense of distance from others
• May express a longing for human contact
• Relates that there is no one with whom he can currently share

Objective Data
• May exhibit behavior such as repeated requests or demands, prolonging conversations, frequent telephoning, reaching for another's hand, avoiding contacts, overemphasizing a lack of need for others, overactivity

---

Illness elicits the response *Loneliness . . .* because no one can experience the illness but the individual. In a sense he is isolated and separate from all others in his experience. He can look at others and know that he alone bears the pain and suffering. A diagnosis of *Loneliness related to physical loss* is appropriate in such instances.

When feeling lonely, the person may doubt his capacity to endure. He may question whether his strength is sufficient to meet the situation. Loneliness is often not expressed verbally and requires nursing skill to recognize behavioral cues. This pattern of diagnosis is common to everyone; those experiencing illness are especially vulnerable to loneliness.

NURSING DIAGNOSIS PATTERN: AMBIVALENCE . . .[432,471,524]

DEFINITION

The existence of two or more opposing emotions directed at an object

ASSESSMENT DATA

Subjective Data
• Relates being troubled by opposing emotions
• Verbalizes both positive and negative feelings or is unable to state feelings clearly

Objective Data
• May exhibit contradictory behavior such as anger and loving behavior, dependent and independent behavior

---

The pattern *Ambivalence . . .* refers to the response of experiencing two opposing emotions at the same time. The person experiences both positive and negative feelings toward an object or situation. *Ambivalence . . . ,* which focuses on emotions, differs from *Conflict . . . ,* which is primarily decision oriented. Health–illness situations arouse many opposing emotions, such as fear mingled with a desire to get well and anger at and dependency on loved ones or health care providers. Human responses commonly diagnosed by nurses are *Ambivalence related to recovery from illness* and *Ambivalence related to significant others.* Frequently, the patient is unaware of what he is experiencing. Nurses recognize, identify, and explore with the person this normal response of opposing emotions.

NURSING DIAGNOSIS PATTERN: ANGER . . .^{105,432,471,525}

DEFINITION

A feeling of resentment or hostility

ASSESSMENT DATA

Subjective Data
• Person may or may not verbalize or openly express anger
• When expressing anger, verbalizations reveal hostility or resentment

Objective Data
• Manifests physical findings such as facial flushing or pallor, rapid or deep respirations, rapid or pounding pulse, increased blood pressure, perspiration, trembling
• May exhibit behavior such as demanding and controlling behavior, clenching the jaw or fist, shouting, throwing or slamming objects, unusual quietness, avoiding persons or situations, somatic complaints

---

The pattern *Anger . . .* refers to a response of hostile or resentful feelings. In illness or loss, anger is often a normal response. It is a method of coping with a life interruption and a means of working through to acceptance of an unfavorable reality. Patients may respond with *Anger related to inflicted physical pain, Anger related to role loss, Anger related to loss of personal freedom,* etc. Nurses help the person recognize and cope with anger in a constructive rather than destructive manner. Such guidance leads the angry person toward self-enlightenment, hence personal growth.

NURSING DIAGNOSIS PATTERN: ANXIETY . . .^{105,471,432,525}

DEFINITION

A vague, ill-defined feeling of apprehension and uneasiness

ASSESSMENT DATA

Subjective Data
• Person relates experiencing feelings of threat or danger to self or others
• Unable to identify or describe what causes the feeling
• Usually verbalizes "I don't know why I'm upset," "I don't understand what's bothering me"

Objective Data
• Manifests physical findings such as facial flushing or pallor, rapid or deep respirations, rapid or pounding pulse, increased blood pressure, perspiration, trembling
• May exhibit behavior such as restlessness, sleep disturbances, anorexia, irritability, difficulty concentraing, making poor judgments, forgetfulness, rapid speech, demanding and controlling behavior, avoiding persons or situations

---

Anxiety . . . is a response to threat. It is a vague feeling of apprehension and uneasiness. When anxious, a person feels a sense of danger that cannot be clearly identified. Since the effect is vague, the person feels unsure of how to cope with it. Anxiety is a common emotional response to illness and disease. It can be an emotional response in which the self feels threatened, such as *Anxiety related to undefined threat.* It can be a physiologic response in which the body sends signals that all is not well within the systems, such as *Anxiety related to physiologic imbalance.*

The vagueness of *Anxiety* . . . differs from *Fear* . . . , which is a clearly defined threat. Patients often express their anxieties to the nurse. It is nursing's responsibility to assist the person to explore the anxiety and identify it in terms of a precise fear. Once the fear is identified, the person can cope with the threat. Nurses can reduce the degree of anxiety associated with illness by caring, showing concern, and sharing information with patients and families.

NURSING DIAGNOSIS PATTERN: CONFLICT . . .[105,432,471,525]

DEFINITION
A conscious or unconscious struggle between opposing choices or persons

ASSESSMENT DATA
Subjective Data
- Person relates thinking about the choice of options
- Discusses the pros and cons and states that the choices are both acceptable and unacceptable
- Prolongs making a decision

Objective Data
- May exhibit behavior such as restlessness, pacing, sleeplessness or fretful sleep, heavy smoking, anger, seeking others' opinions, unusual quietness, inability to take decisive action, tearfulness when asked for a decision

---

Both health and illness bring about situations that require important decision making. *Conflict* . . . is a frequent response of persons who must make decisions regarding their own health or illness or that of a significant other. *Conflict* . . . , which is decision oriented, differs from *Ambivalence* . . . , which focuses on opposing emotions. The person in conflict is confronted with both acceptable and unacceptable choices. Common responses, such as *Conflict related to health decisions for self* and *Conflict related to health decisions for a significant other*, are often observed.

NURSING DIAGNOSIS PATTERN: DEPRESSION . . .[105,471]

DEFINITION
A mental state of gloom and sadness

ASSESSMENT DATA
Subjective Data
- Person states feeling moody and sad
- Is preoccupied with a loss
- Expresses the wish that the loss be restored
- Complains of lack of energy, nervousness, early-morning insomnia, fretful or excessive sleep, changes in appetite

Objective Data
- May exhibit behavior such as slowed body movements, overactivity, unkempt appearance, decreased involvement in usual interests, irritability, restlessness, indifferent attitude, tearfulness, difficulty concentrating, poor posture

---

The pattern *Depression* . . . refers to an adaptive mood of sadness. This depression response is less intense than the nonadaptive depressive reaction seen in maladaptive behavior. The person experiences a slowing down or overactivity but is still able to function, whereas in depressive reaction, the capacity to function is severely jeopardized.

There are many theories concerning the causes and processes of depression. This pattern is based on the theory that depression, like grief, follows loss and separation. In *Depression* . . . the loss is not fully acknowledged and there is melancholia and a hope that the loss will be fully restored, while in a *Grief reaction* . . . the loss is acknowledged and followed by mourning and bereavement.

Persons attempting to adjust to physical losses and losses resulting from illness often experience depression, such as *Depression related to role loss*. Physiologic changes can also cause depression. Such responses are expressed as *Depression related to physiologic imbalance*. Nurses share their nursing expertise to help the person cope with the causes of depression and with the depression itself.

NURSING DIAGNOSIS PATTERN: DEPENDENCY FEELINGS . . . [105,471,525]

DEFINITION

Feeling the need to rely on others for support

ASSESSMENT DATA

Subjective Data
• Person verbalizes a need for protection
• Requests help from others
• Relates concern with matters of self

Objective Data
• May exhibit behavior such as being helpless, seeking reassurance, difficulty with decision making, demanding help, doing more than he is really able to or appearing uninterested in order to counteract the dependency feeling

---

Dependency feelings . . . normally occur when a person is unable to act on behalf of himself. In this pattern, the person's response includes a recognition of the need to rely on others. In societies in which independence is applauded, feelings of dependency are troublesome. Nurses recognize that dependency in illness, infancy, and old age is a normal response. One such response is *Dependency feelings related to physical loss*. Nurses convey acceptance of the person's dependency feelings and gradually support the person's return to independence. Recognition of this problem is essential to recovery from illness.

NURSING DIAGNOSIS PATTERN: EMBARRASSMENT . . . [471,524]

DEFINITION

A state of self-conscious uneasiness or noncomposure

ASSESSMENT DATA

Subjective Data
• Person may or may not relate experiencing self-consciousness
• Acknowledges feeling threatened with humiliation or loss of dignity

Objective Data
• May manifest physical findings such as facial flushing
• May exhibit behavior such as drooped shoulders, head held downward, inappropriate laughter, flustered speech, hiding the face, crying, angry outbursts, avoidance of embarrassing discussions or situations

---

This pattern of diagnosis refers to a response of self-conscious uneasiness. Embarrassment may be a fleeting response that quickly resolves itself during health or illness care. In such instances, it is not used as a nursing diagnosis. However, for some persons, *Em-*

barrassment . . . is a major problem during health or illness care. These persons are constantly guarding themselves against the threat of humiliation or indignity. They are troubled by responses such as *Embarrassment related to body exposure* and *Embarrassment related to natural body function.* This pattern is commonly seen in adolescence. When embarrassment is a significant problem to the patient, it warrants recognition by the nurse. Much can be done to minimize this distressing response when staff members work together to safeguard the person's dignity.

NURSING DIAGNOSIS PATTERN: FEAR OF . . .[105,471,525]

DEFINITION

A feeling of alarm and fright

ASSESSMENT DATA

Subjective Data
- Person experiences feelings of threat or danger
- Can describe or identify the threat or danger

Objective Data
- Manifests physical findings such as facial flushing or pallor, rapid or deep respirations, rapid or pounding pulse, increased blood pressure, perspiration, trembling
- May exhibit behavior such as restlessness, sleep disturbances, changes in eating habits, irritability, short attention span, making poor judgments, forgetfulness, rapid speech, demanding and controlling behavior, avoidance of persons or situations

---

Fear of . . . is a response to a specific danger. The person knows what he is afraid of. This factor makes fear easier to cope with than anxiety, which is vague. Illness arouses a multitude of specifically perceived dangers which affect every aspect of the person's life such as *Fear of burdening others, Fear of death, Fear of disfigurement, Fear of loss of lifestyle,* and *Fear of loss of sexuality.* Although fear is a normal response to the threat of illness, coping with it requires adaptive energy. All health care professionals are aware of the impact of this emotion on the ill person. Nursing, however, specializes in assisting persons to move through the illness experience with a minimum of fear.

NURSING DIAGNOSIS PATTERN: FRUSTRATION . . .[105,432,471,525]

DEFINITION

Feelings of irritation and tension when a desired goal is blocked

ASSESSMENT DATA

Subjective Data
- Person relates that a desired goal is delayed or unattainable
- Verbalizes irritability

Objective Data
- May exhibit behavior such as heavy sighing, frowning, shaking the head, clenching the hands

---

In illness situations, *Frustration* . . . is a common emotional response. The limitations imposed by illness create tensions when goal achievement is delayed or not possible. It is common for an ill person to experience *Frustration related to physical limitations.* The person's family may respond with *Frustration related to a dependent significant other.* This pattern of response is important for nurses to recognize. Nursing assistance and the reduction of externally imposed stressors can keep frustration to a minimum. Since severe frustrations may lead to hostile behavior, control of frustrating situations is essential to the recovery of ill persons.

NURSING DIAGNOSIS PATTERN: GRIEF REACTION . . . [105,471,525]

DEFINITION

Feelings of deep sorrow and distress

ASSESSMENT DATA

Subjective Data
• Person relates an initial feeling of shock and disbelief
• Later expresses anger
• Then acknowledges the loss and that the loss will not be restored
• Relates feeling unsettled, vaguely confused, and intensely sad

Objective Data
• May exhibit grieving behavior, such as weeping, saddened facial expression, decreased participation in external interests, withdrawal from persons or situations, seeking a substitute for the lost object

---

A *Grief reaction . . .* is a normal response to loss. It is an adaptive means of overcoming the stress of loss. *Grief reaction . . .*, which resolves the loss through acknowledgment, mourning, and bereavement, differs from *Depression . . .* . In depression, loss is not fully acknowledged, and there is melancholia with the hope that the loss will be restored. The grief response has three normal phases: the disequilibrium phase, in which the person experiences disbelief, mourning, and anger; the disorganization phase, in which the loss is recognized as permanent and the person feels poorly organized, has a sense of unreality, is restless, and experiences somatic complaints; and the reorganization phase, in which the person detaches himself from the lost person and moves on to new interrelationships. Illness brings about many responses to loss, such as *Grief reaction related to physical loss*, *Grief reaction related to role loss*, and *Grief reaction related to loss of a significant other*. Nurses recognize the grief reaction as a normal response to loss. They assist and support the person through the adaptive grief process.

NURSING DIAGNOSIS PATTERN: GUILT . . . [105,471,525]

DEFINITION

Blaming oneself for a particular action or omission

ASSESSMENT DATA

Subjective Data
• May or may not verbalize regret and remorse
• Blames self for causing a recent or past situation

Objective Data
• May exhibit behavior such as attempting to correct an error, doing nothing about the situation, being overly attentive, overactive, using self-punishing behavior, projecting blame, making excuses

---

The pattern *Guilt . . .* involves a response in which a person blames himself for a specific action or omission. In this pattern, guilt is a normal response and can lead to growth if the person learns from the situation. It differs from nonadaptive guilt, in which there is strong self-condemnation and self-devaluation. In health care situations, responses of guilt are often diagnosed such as *Guilt related to being a survivor, Guilt related to the birth of an imperfect child,* and *Guilt related to unsanctioned health therapy.* Nurses help persons to express their guilt feelings and to carry out measures that will resolve the guilt and reestablish peace of mind.

NURSING DIAGNOSIS PATTERN: HELPLESSNESS/POWERLESS-NESS . . .[213,471,525]

DEFINITION

Feeling that one has no power or resources to control a situation and is unable to manage alone

ASSESSMENT DATA

Subjective Data
- Person verbalizes that he has little control over a situation
- Relates being unable to handle the situation alone
- Expects others to help him cope effectively

Objective Data
- May exhibit behavior such as seeking answers by talking to others or reading, acting out, crying, somatic complaints

---

The helpless person feels he has no control over or cannot master a situation alone. In order to be secure, a person needs to feel he has effective coping mechanisms for maintaining physical and psychologic safety. In illness situations, there is an element of loss of control over what happens to the self or significant others. The person often finds that coping mechanisms that were effective in the past are not successful in the current situation. The person feels overwhelmed and uncertain. Nurses recognize such problems as *Helplessness related to physical loss* and *Helplessness related to health therapy.*

It is important to differentiate between *Helplessness . . . , Hopelessness . . . ,* and *Dependency feelings . . . . In Helplessness . . . ,* the person recognizes that he does not have the coping strengths or resources to successfully overcome a situation alone. He looks to others for aid or relief so that he can cope with his problem. *Hopelessness . . .* results when the helpless person is not assisted. The hopeless person believes that resolution of the problem is not possible. *Dependency feelings . . .* stem from having to rely solely on others to meet one's needs. It differs from helplessness in that the dependent person looks to others for protection and care rather than for new methods of coping.

Nurses can help the person experiencing helplessness to explore this problem, gain insight into new coping mechanisms, and support action to regain control of the situation.

NURSING DIAGNOSIS PATTERN: HOPELESSNESS . . .[213,471]

DEFINITION

The feeling that efforts are useless and ineffective

ASSESSMENT DATA

Subjective Data
- Verbalizes that efforts toward resolving a situation are futile
- Expresses feelings of extreme discouragement and negative expectations
- Relates having given up trying

Objective Data
- May exhibit behavior such as crying, saddened facial expression, indifferent attitude, unusual quietness, ceasing any further effort

---

The response *Hopelessness* . . . is one in which a person feels that efforts toward resolving a situation are futile. He sees no solution to the problem, has negative expectations, and gives up trying. Such responses include *Hopelessness related to physical loss* and *Hopelessness related to approaching death.*

Hopelessness . . . , *Helplessness* . . . , and *Depression* . . . are closely allied but different. In *Hopelessness* . . . , the person is convinced that there is no solution to the problem. In *Helplessness* . . . , the person feels he does not have the strengths or resources to cope effectively with the problem. He looks to others for aid or guidance so that he can cope successfully. The response of *Depression* . . . occurs when a person experiences a sense of gloom or sadness associated with a loss that he wants restored.

In *Hopelessness* . . . , the belief that efforts are futile may or may not be based on reality. When no solution to the problem actually exists, the nurse supports the person through his feeling of hopelessness, encouraging acceptance of the reality. When there are solutions to the problem that are unrecognized by the patient, the nurse assists in problem solving and in restoring a sense of hope.

NURSING DIAGNOSIS PATTERN: FEELING REJECTED . . .[105]

DEFINITION

Feeling that one is not acceptable to another/others

ASSESSMENT DATA

Subjective Data
- Person expresses feelings that others do not care about or approve of him
- Verbalizes thoughts that others do not see him as a person of worth

Objective Data
- May exhibit behavior such as acting out, somatic complaints, avoiding the person, unusual quietness, crying

---

When *Feeling rejected* . . . , a person perceives that he is unacceptable to and unworthy of the love of others. He arrives at this conclusion on the basis of how others react to him. An ill person is very sensitive to the reactions of others toward him. He is quick to perceive any cues of rejection and therefore easily feels rejected. A common problem is that of *Feeling rejected related to physical loss.* Many patients feel rejected as a result of intended, negative cues from significant others. Nurses assist the patient to express feelings about the rejection and to cope in such a way as to maintain self-esteem.

NURSING DIAGNOSIS PATTERN: REJECTION OF . . .[105]

DEFINITION

Feeling that a significant other or situation is not acceptable to oneself

ASSESSMENT DATA

Subjective Data
- Person relates that a significant other or situation is not acceptable to himself
- Expresses feelings of anger, disapproval, lack of interest

Objective Data
- Exhibits behavior such as spending less time with the person or in the situation, refraining from caressing, failing to fulfill his expected role, and intimidating, ridiculing, or abusing the other person

---

The pattern *Rejection of* . . . is a response in which one person exhibits nonacceptance of another and withholds love. In health care situations, it is most often family members or some significant other who rejects the ill or dependent person. The problem is often *Rejection of a significant other related to physical loss.* Nurses can be instrumental in supporting family unity by assisting members to explore and cope with their rejection of a loved one. By resolving this problem, the nurse also reduces the suffering of the person being rejected.

NURSING DIAGNOSIS PATTERN: **WITHDRAWAL FROM** . . .[105,432,471,525]

DEFINITION

Moving away from interactions with persons or situations

ASSESSMENT DATA

Subjective Data
• Person relates the perception of a threatening person or situation
• Expresses a need to move away from or avoid the threat

Objective Data
• May physically or emotionally remove himself by exhibiting behavior such as excessive sleeping, extended silence, turning away, pretending not to hear, avoiding eye contact, refusing to talk, avoiding associations with the person or situation

---

The pattern *Withdrawal from* . . . is a response in which a person moves away from or avoids a threat. Most threatening instances involve a choice of either an attack or withdrawal response. Withdrawal is often a most effective response. It is a means of avoiding what one prefers not to deal with. It can also be a way of reestablishing physical or psychologic equilibrium. In illness situations, withdrawal is often used as a method of conserving energy for healing. Such is reflected in the problem *Withdrawal from socialization.* Withdrawal that is a movement away from threat differs from *Disengagement/ detachment* . . . , which is a loss of interest in a terminating personal or situational relationship. Nurses recognize and support withdrawal as long as it is an adaptive response.

NURSING DIAGNOSIS PATTERN: **DENIAL OF** . . .[471,525]

DEFINITION

Being unable to admit the existence of certain facts

ASSESSMENT DATA

Subjective Data
• Person verbally rejects the occurring reality
    OR
• Ignores references made regarding the reality
• If confronted, does not want to openly discuss the issue

Objective Data
• May exhibit unrealistic behavior in response to the facts, such as refusing to seek medical help, using rationalization to support the denial, laughing and joking about the situation, yet functions well

---

Denial of . . . is a defense mechanism in which the person does not admit that which is factual. Denial offers psychologic protection against severe threat or danger. Denial is a normal, adaptive response when used as a temporary adjusting method. The pattern *Denial of* . . . focuses on the normal adaptive response and differs from pathologic, long-term maladaptive denial. In illness, trauma, and death, denial can be used as an effective adaptation mechanism. Nurses frequently identify such problems as *Denial of physical loss, Denial of approaching death,* and *Denial of loss of a significant other.* Nurses accept a person's use of denial. In time, the practitioner observes for cues that the denial is no longer needed and that the person is ready to face reality. Nurses diagnose this pattern and support the person through complete adaptation.

NURSING DIAGNOSIS PATTERN: DISENGAGEMENT/DETACH-MENT . . .[525]

DEFINITION

An attempt to release oneself or others from personal attachments or responsibilities

ASSESSMENT DATA

Subjective Data
- Person acknowledges that a relationship with another person, situation, or life itself is ending or has lost permanent or temporary significance
- Expresses feelings of decreased interest

Objective Data
- May exhibit behavior such as spending less time with significant persons or activities, decreasing approval-seeking or loving behavior, being cooperative without wholehearted involvement, exhibiting anger in an attempt to break the relationship

---

The response *Disengagement/detachment . . .* is one in which a person acknowledges that a relationship with another person or situation is ending. He then attempts to release himself from the attachment. The response *Disengagement/detachment related to approaching death* is a common one. Once there is acceptance that death is inevitable, both the dying person and family members gradually release themselves from their attachment to one another. This is a normal response recognized by nurses and supported whenever appropriate.

NURSING DIAGNOSIS PATTERN: LOW SELF-ESTEEM . . .[105]

DEFINITION

Having feelings of negative self-worth

ASSESSMENT DATA

Subjective Data
- Person relates certain unfulfilled expectations of self
- Makes self-depreciating remarks or is highly critical of others

Objective Data
- May exhibit behavior such as unkept appearance, poor posture, avoiding interaction with others, attempting overachievement, sustaining underachievement, crying, apologizing unnecessarily, refusal to participate in activities, angry outbursts, demanding and controlling behavior

---

The *Low self-esteem . . .* pattern refers to a response in which a person perceives himself as having little worth. The person has set up certain standards or expectations for himself that he has not been able to fulfill. Illness and injury frequently interfere with the achievement of self-expectations. The stress of health care increases tensions, which also interrupt the fulfillment of expectations. Problems such as *Low self-esteem related to physical loss* and *Low self-esteem related to loss of emotional control* are frequently observed by nurses. Temporary low self-esteem is a normal response to illness. Nurses recognize this and encourage the person to express such feelings about himself. With adequate, positive support, the patient can reestablish a sense of personal worth.

NURSING DIAGNOSIS PATTERN: **BONDING INTERRUPTION** . . .[207,313,414]

DEFINITION

Feeling cut off from relating to a significant other, expressions of emotional closeness and caring

ASSESSMENT DATA

Subjective Data
• Person verbalizes a strong attachment for another
• Relates wanting to enter into the feelings of and share intimately the experiences of the loved one
• Expresses a desire to make resources of strength, time, thought, etc., available to the loved one
• Relates feeling cut off from expressing care, concern, and responsibility for the loved one

Objective Data
• May exhibit behavior such as making frequent phone calls, visiting at unauthorized times, prolonging allowed visiting, sitting long hours in the waiting room, crying, attempting to assist with and/or supervise physical needs

---

Bonding Interruption . . . is a response experienced by both the ill person and family members. During times of crisis, significantly attached persons look to one another for support and strength. When separation is forced on them, the continuity of their normal attachment and caring behaviors is broken. The involved persons cannot give and receive the love and strength they normally share with each other. Each experiences a temporary loss of union with loved ones.

The current health care system forces the separation of significant others during illness crisis. Both the patient and significant others experience a *Bonding interruption.* . . . Nurses in all areas, but especially in intensive care and isolation units, recognize the response of *Bonding interruption related to health care.* Nurses make every effort to give the bonded persons the time and opportunity to share with one another their strengths and expressions of caring.

NURSING DIAGNOSIS PATTERN: **ROLE CONFLICT** . . .[105,424,471]

DEFINITION

A person's struggle with conflicting expectations of self or others about behavior in a particular role

ASSESSMENT DATA

Subjective Data
• Person relates certain different role expectations set by self or others
• Relates that the demands of the role are incompatible with his needs or are difficult to achieve

Objective Data
• May exhibit behavior such as avoiding or refusing to fulfill the expected role or trying to fit into the expected role despite conflict

The pattern *Role conflict . . .* is associated with several situations. There can be conflict between two or more people about their different role expectations for the same role, conflict over two mutually desirable roles when only one can be fulfilled, and conflict about a role that is incompatible with the person's abilities or needs. Illness often forces changes in a person's roles, bringing about role conflict.

Nurses identify such problems as *Role conflict related to an incompatible role* and *Role conflict related to forced role change.* The person in conflict often needs assistance in defining and exploring the problem as it relates to his health status or that of a significant other. The nurse encourages decision making about role choices and changes in role relationships. She also assists the person through role changes in different developmental phases.

NURSING DIAGNOSIS PATTERN: ROLE MODIFICATION . . .[471,524]

DEFINITION

Adjusting to changes in the expected role behaviors specific to one's responsibilities, position, or situation in life

ASSESSMENT DATA

Subjective Data
- Person recognizes changes in self or significant other that indicate a need for a role change
- Identifies the expected behaviors of the new or changed role
- May express awkwardness, uncertainty, or relief with the new role

Objective Data
- May exhibit behavior such as learning new skills and abilities, performing new role behaviors, assuming new responsibilities as in adolescence and young adulthood, releasing responsibilities as in illness or old age

---

Once a person decides to alter his role, he moves into the behavior pattern *Role modification. . . .* In role modification, there is an adjustment to changes in role expectations and relationships. The person may be coping with *Role modification related to loss/gain of a significant other* or *Role modification related to physical loss/gain.* During this modification of or change in role behavior, the nurse assists with or teaches the person the most effective, and sometimes new, role behaviors or skills. As the person reaches completion of role modification, nursing assistance is no longer needed.

NURSING DIAGNOSIS PATTERN: REGRESSION . . .[105,432,471,525]

DEFINITION

An attempt to protect oneself by using coping behavior appropriate at an earlier developmental level

ASSESSMENT DATA

Subjective Data
- Person relates feeling that the past was safe, that the present and future are unsafe
- Verbalizes primarily about self

Objective Data
- *Adults* exhibit behavior such as compliance with suggestions from others, accepting assistance, relinquishing responsibility to others, seeking reassurance, approval, and physical closeness. *Children* often return to earlier behavior patterns of bed wetting, thumb sucking, return to bottle-feeding, temper tantrums, baby talk

---

The pattern *Regression* . . . is a response in which a person uses behavior appropriate to an earlier developmental level. He perceives his current situation as one from which he wants to retreat to a less demanding level of function. Illness or injury sometimes causes a response such as *Regression related to physical loss*. Nurses recognize that such behavior is a mechanism for self-protection. Its temporary nature makes it adaptive. Reassurance from the nurse strengthens the person's feeling of safety. It restores his belief in his capacity to cope until the use of regression is no longer needed.

NURSING DIAGNOSIS PATTERN: SELF-IDENTITY MODIFICATION . . .[105,432]

DEFINITION

Adjusting to change in one's beliefs, attitudes, ideas, and feelings

ASSESSMENT DATA

Subjective Data
- Person has experienced a significant life change
- Relates perceiving self as different than previously
- Expresses a need to integrate the former self with the new by asking, Who am I? (my worth as a person), What am I? (my status as an individual in social groups), Why am I? (my philosophy of life)

Objective Data
- May exhibit behavior such as changing physical appearance, changing jobs, becoming involved in helping organizations, associating with different social groups, advancing educational level

---

Each individual moves through different developmental stages and through various life crises. As he does so, his ideas and feelings about himself change through the response *Self-identity modification*. . . . He is different today than he was yesterday because of life experiences. Throughout life, a person from time to time evaluates who he is, what he is, and why he is. As the answers to these questions change, he perceives a new self-identity. Major life changes or events alter self-identity. As nurses follow persons through the life cycle and illness, they recognize problems such as *Self-identity modification related to physical loss* and *Self-identity modification related to loss or gain of a significant other*. As the person attempts to adjust his self-identity to his changing self, the nurse encourages the expression of feelings and the acceptance of changes in beliefs and attitudes about himself.

NURSING DIAGNOSIS PATTERN: THREATENED BODY IMAGE . . .[105,471,525]

DEFINITION

Feeling endangered by changes in one's body that alter one's concept of the body

ASSESSMENT DATA

Subjective Data
- Person relates a change in body sensation, size, function, or appearance
- Verbalizes that the body is different than previously
- Expresses feeling threatened by the change

Objective Data
- Person has visible or verifiable body changes

> • May exhibit behavior such as avoiding looking at or touching the body part, facial expressions of displeasure when viewing the body, demanding that others care for him, covering up body parts

The pattern *Threatened body image* . . . refers to a response in which a person's perception of his physical self is threatened. He perceives changes in his body that are unacceptable and considered a danger to his self-concept. In illness or developmental cycles, body changes in structure or function are often dramatic. The person finds his changed body unfamiliar. He is aware that others respond to his body in a different way than previously. He may not want to look at or touch the changed body as long as he feels threatened. Nurses identify problems such as *Threatened body image related to natural body changes* and *Threatened body image related to physical loss*. Nurses help the person express feelings about the changed body and offer guidance that reduces the perception of changes as threatening.

NURSING DIAGNOSIS PATTERN: BODY-IMAGE MODIFICATION . . .[105,471]

DEFINITION

Adjusting one's concept of the body as a result of body changes

ASSESSMENT DATA

Subjective Data
• Person relates a change in body sensation, size, function, or appearance
• Verbalizes that the body is different than previously
• Relates a sense of loss or gain
• Expresses a need to integrate the former body with the new

Objective Data
• Person has visible or verifiable body changes
• May exhibit behavior such as looking at and touching the body part, caring for the body, using devices needed for improved body function, cautiously attempting increased activity, changing clothing to accommodate body changes, showing off body changes, appropriately decreasing acitivity

---

Once the person has overcome the threat of change in body structure and function, he attempts *Body-image modification.* . . . He begins to test the body for what it can and cannot do. He learns new ways to maximize body function and to improve body appearance. He gradually becomes familiar and comfortable with his changed body. The nurse identifies such problems as *Body-image modification related to physical loss* and *Body-image modification related to improved health status*. The practitioner assists the person as needed and teaches new methods of adaptation to changes in body structure and function. When the change in body image is consistent with the new body, nursing assistance is no longer needed.

The nursing diagnosis patterns described in this chapter reflect the problem areas in which nurses intervene. The patterns also reflect much of the subject matter found within nursing's body of knowledge. Chapters 4 and 5 describe how to use the diagnostic patterns within the nursing process to formulate nursing diagnoses.

4 NURSING DIAGNOSIS THROUGH THE NURSING PROCESS

THE NURSING PROCESS

Before the nursing process actually begins, the nurse and the patient discuss the patient's situation. If nursing assistance seems appropriate, the nursing process is activated. The initial nurse–patient contact is important because it sets the tone for the quality of the relationship throughout the episode of care.

The nursing process is a step-by-step system of problem solving that includes:[89,196,333]

ASSESSMENT
Data Collection
    Subjective Data (symptoms)
    Objective Data (signs)
    Related Data (significant data other than signs and symptoms)
Data Analysis
    Nursing Diagnosis
Common Etiology (stressors)

PLANNING
Unmet Needs
Expected Outcome (goals)

NURSING INTERVENTIONS
Nursing Treatments
Nursing Observations
Health Teaching
Medical Treatments Performed by Nurses

EVALUATION

ASSESSMENT

Comprehensive nursing assessment, carried out in a highly skilled manner, is essential in determining the relevant factors in the patient's situation. Assessment includes data collection, data analysis, and etiology.

Data Collection

Data collection is the process of gathering relevant information about the patient and his situation. Data are collected by means of the nursing history, physical examination, laboratory findings, and other significant information. The data base includes information concerning physiologic, behavioral, sociologic, spiritual, and environmental impairments and strengths.

55

Subjective data are obtained by talking with and listening to the patient and/or family to obtain a nursing history. The patient communicates his chief complaint, his past and current health status, and some information about how he perceives himself. He reveals the symptoms that he alone can feel and experience. Symptoms include sensations that cannot be observed by the examiner, abnormalities that cannot be confirmed by physical examination, and events that can be verified only by the patient.[125]

Objective data include those overt signs that the nurse can perceive through her own senses of seeing, hearing, feeling, and smelling. During a physical examination, the nurse gathers data through observation, percussion, palpation, and auscultation. Laboratory and other studies may be used to develop a complete data base. The patient's stated symptoms are verified by physical examination, and the examiner looks for physical findings not mentioned in the history.[125]

Related data include any information, other than signs and symptoms, that is significant to the person. Such information might include sociocultural factors, geographic location, age, sex, race, and the like.

Data Analysis

Data analysis is the process of putting collected data in order, selecting essential information, discarding nonessential data, and interpreting the meaning of the data. Each diagnosis has a set of essential criteria. That is, there must be at least two or more facts that present a pattern or set of manifestations specific to any one diagnosis. It is only by comparing the data that the patient presents with her own clinical findings that the nurse can exclude some data and accept other data in order to make a diagnosis. The nurse does not rely solely on the statements of the patient or simply accept the patient's conclusion; the nurse makes a professional judgment—a diagnosis—based on data analysis.

Diagnosing is a process of reviewing and assessing a series of findings. According to Gordon, *nursing diagnoses,* "or clinical diagnoses made by professional nurses, describe actual or potential health problems which nurses, by virtue of their education and experience, are capable of and licensed to treat."[196:2] Each nursing diagnosis is a human response that is the result of a stressor. It is a behavioral change and describes what has occurred within the individual, family, or community. Nursing diagnoses fall within two groups: predominantly nursing diagnoses and dual diagnoses.

Predominantly nursing diagnoses are patient problems more often solved or treated by nursing than any other profession. They are the problems that other health disciplines seldom, if ever, treat. The predominantly nursing diagnoses presented in Part Two have been structured from nursing diagnosis patterns. These patterns represent the kinds of problems that individuals look to nursing to solve. They form the basis for a nursing diagnosis statement.

Dual diagnoses are those patient problems that are commonly solved or treated by nursing, medicine, and other health disciplines. Gebbie and Lavin stated that "there is no prohibition against using a label from another field if we [nurses] use it with the characteristics and accuracy usually expected and it says what we want it to say."[584:253] The 1970 "American Medical Association Position Paper on Nursing" and the "U.S. Department of Health, Education and Welfare Report on Extending the Scope of Nursing Practice," stated that an "identical act or procedure may be the practice of medicine when carried out by a physician and the practice of nursing when carried out by a nurse."[257:295]

The diagnosis of disease is considered the exclusive prerogative of the physician, while the diagnosis of human responses is the prerogative of the nurse. Nevertheless, an area of dual responsibility and dual activity may be found in the mutual diagnosis and treatment of the signs, symptoms, and ill-defined conditions identified in the medical classifications. This duality does not constitute an infringement of one profession on the other; rather, it represents a cooperative effort between two professions seeking to provide health care.

An example of dual diagnosis is seen in *cardiac arrest;* the diagnosis can be arrived at by either the doctor or the nurse. Each practitioner can institute independent treatment procedures. Malnutrition, indigestion, and muscle spasms are other examples of conditions that may be identified and treated by either the doctor or the nurse.

The nursing diagnosis cannot be made on the nurse's assumption that a particular response is a problem for the patient. A response that is a problem for one person may have little or no effect on another individual. However, when a patient is unable to identify his problem or when his attention is focused on other problems that are less significant, the professional nurse guides the person in problem identification. Additional information on nursing diagnosis is presented throughout this text.

Common Etiology (Stressors)

Etiology is synonomous with the cause of a problem. If nursing diagnosis is to be accurate, the cause of the problem is to be considered. Stressors and their effect have been studied extensively. Muir[358:26] stated that stressors produce reactions or responses and that they result in a change arising from within the person or from the external environment. Selye[441] explained that from stressors, change is produced and that the stressor or causative agent is a stimulus or antagonist. Stressors may be the presence of a stress agent or the absence of an equilibrium factor.[441:51 & 305] Webster's dictionary states that a stressor is "something that brings about a result or effect":[524:124]

$$\text{STRESSOR} \xrightarrow{\text{yields}} \text{RESPONSE}$$

In identifying nursing diagnos is, there has been some confusion as to the difference between diagnostic responses and etiologic stressors. Stressors and responses have sometimes been used interchangeably:

Example

DENIAL   related to   ANXIETY
(response)   (response)

This diagnostic statement indicates that a response is causing a response. It would be more precise to write the diagnosis as *Denial of . . . related to threat of . . .* It is the threat that is the stressor. Anxiety is a response, and it is preferable not to use it as a stressor. If, by definition, a stressor is the cause of a response, it cannot be the response as well.

It is recommended that nursing diagnosis patterns of responses not be used as stressors for the following reasons:

If nursing diagnoses are to be structured correctly, causes and effects should not be interchangeable.
Interchanging responses and stressors brings about confusion in writing diagnostic statements.
To maintain a high level of professional diagnositc skill, precision is essential.

Since it is a function of nursing to reduce stressors, it is necessary to be able to clearly differentiate the stressor and the response.

However, there is one exception to the rule of avoiding the interchange of responses and stressors. Nurses do treat some medically oriented conditions that fall within the category of dual diagnosis. These dual diagnoses can be used as stressors for the nursing diagnosis pattern responses:

Example

INCAPACITY TO FEED SELF   related to   PAIN
(nursing diagnosis: a response)   (dual diagnosis: a stressor)
PAIN   related to   MYOCARDIAL INFARCTION
(dual diagnosis: a response)   (a disease: a stressor)

In this edition, an effort has been made to identify stressors as separate from diagnostic responses. It was possible to group the stressors into 13 categories:

Birth defects
Inherited factors
Diseases
Injuries
Signs and symptoms
Psychosocial factors
The human body itself
Health care (iatrogenic) factors
Developmental phases
Lifestyle
Situational factors
Environmental factors
Human error

A complete list of stressors under these categories is found in Appendix 1. Stressors are essential to the diagnostic statement because that which caused the patient's problem may affect the plan of intervention. Through knowledge of the etiology, the nurse can identify a precise nursing diagnosis.

PLANNING

Once the nursing diagnosis has been identified, the nurse begins to plan for intervention. The planning phase of the nursing process includes the identification of unmet needs and expected outcome (goals).

Unmet Needs

The term *human needs* refers to the absence of an essential component that is vital to an integrated body system.[328:35-38] In 1939, the physiologist Cannon[87:24] described homeostasis as an attempt by the body to maintain a state of constancy in its internal environment. Since that time, other physiologists have agreed with this theory. Guyton stated that "the term homeostasis is used by physiologists to mean maintenance of static, or constant, conditions in the internal environment. Essentially all the organs and tissues of the body perform functions that help to maintain these constant conditions."[203:3] Ganong concurred that "a large part of physiology is concerned with regulatory mechanisms which act to maintain the constancy of the internal environment."[182:18]

In 1954, Maslow[328:35-36] stated that each person has basic human needs that are vital to the integration of the homeostatic system. These needs are essential components, and they must be gratified if there is to be a healthy existence. He categorized them according to their priority, with the highest priority being assigned to those needs most important to maintaining life: the physiologic and safety needs. Maslow[328:37-47] believed that once these most basic needs were met, human beings could move forward to meet their needs for belonging, esteem, esteem from others, and self-actualization. Maslow's categories[328:37-47] followed this sequence of priority, in descending order:

Physiologic needs
Safety needs
Belongingness needs
Self-esteem needs
Esteem-from-others needs
Self-actualization needs

According to Maslow, basic need deprivation results in an unhealthy state in the individual.[328:57] Since the person in an unhealthy state becomes the concern of the professional nurse, nurses recognize human needs. Beland stated that "in illness the capacity of the individual to cope with disturbances in his environment, in such a manner that his needs are satisfied, is reduced."[35:46] She further described the functions of the nurse in helping the person maintain homeostasis. Such functions include "modifying the external environment, supporting the efforts of the patient to adapt or respond, and providing him with the materials required to maintain the constancy of his internal environment."[35:46] If homeostasis and need gratification are essential for health, then nurses who help patients fulfill unmet needs are simultaneously helping them resolve their health problems. Nurses also recognize that a person's awareness of his unmet needs is what forces him to acknowledge his health problems and compels him to attempt to solve them.

Professional nurses have long recognized that certain human needs take priority over others. Some needs must be met immediately, while others can be postponed, especially during an illness in which life itself is threatened. In the first edition of *Nursing Diagnosis and Intervention in Nursing Practice*, the concept of need deprivation was the focus of the development of nursing diagnoses. These diagnoses implied human-need deprivation. The nursing interventions applicable to each diagnosis were selected to fulfill the unmet human needs. Although the focus of this edition is on patterns of nursing diagnoses and not the human need concept, Maslow's need theory has been maintained throughout this work. The same priority ranking of needs is used in this text as in the earlier edition.

Priority Ranking of Subcategories of Maslow's Human Needs

Physiologic Needs

Oxygen, circulation (tissue oxygenation or perfusion)
Water–salt balance (fluid and/or electrolyte balance)
Food balance (nutritional balance)
Acid–base balance
Waste elimination (of food residue, urine, intestinal gases, nitrogenous and other toxic substances, carbon dioxide, and bronchopulmonary secretions)
Normal temperature
Sleep, rest, relaxation
Activity, exercise
Energy
Comfort
Stimulation
Cleanliness
Sexuality

Safety Needs

Protection from physical harm
Protection from psychologic threat
Freedom from pain
Physiologic or psychologic stability
Dependence
Predictable, orderly world

Belongingness Needs

Love and affection
Acceptance
Caring, or direct, communicating relationships
Approval from others

Unity with loved ones
Group unity or companionship

Self-Esteem Needs

Sense of usefulness
High evaluation of self
Sense of adequacy
Self-reliance
Goal achievement
Mastery and competence in skills, or continued competence in skills
Independence
Endurance

Esteem-from-Others Needs

Recognition/appreciation from others
Dignity
Importance, influence
Reputation of good character
Attention
Status
Control over others, self or situation

Self-Actualization Needs

Personal growth and maturity
Awareness of potential
Increased or continued learning
Full or continued development of potential
Identification of values or priorities
Spiritual, religious, or philosophic satisfaction
Increased creativity
Increased reality perception and/or problem-solving ability
Less rigid conventionality
Less of the familiar, more of the novel
Greater satisfaction in beauty
Increased pleasantness or pleasure
Less of the simple, more of the complex

Every person who is in a healthy state has unmet needs that can be fulfilled. Even when some needs are unsatisfied, a state of homeostasis may exist. But in the unhealthy state, deficiencies or failure to fulfill human needs can result in disequilibrium. It is essential that nurses recognize unfulfilled needs when making plans to help the patient restore health.

By identifying the human needs that present difficulties for the patient, the nurse perceives the significant factors involved in the problem. For instance, when a diagnosis of elevated body temperature is made, the patient's problem, as stated, is simply an overproduction of body heat. When the unmet needs of water–salt balance, normal temperature, sleep, rest, and comfort are recognized, the nurse has detailed information about the overall effects of the problem. One of the most important reasons why nurses recognize unmet needs relates to planning interventions. It is the nursing intervention that fulfills needs. Unless the nurse is aware of the unmet needs, it is unlikely that the interventions will be totally appropriate to the resolution of the problem. The diagram clarifies the relationship of unmet needs to nursing interventions.

Knowledge of unmet needs is essential in assisting the nurse in determining those nursing interventions that will be most beneficial to the patient.

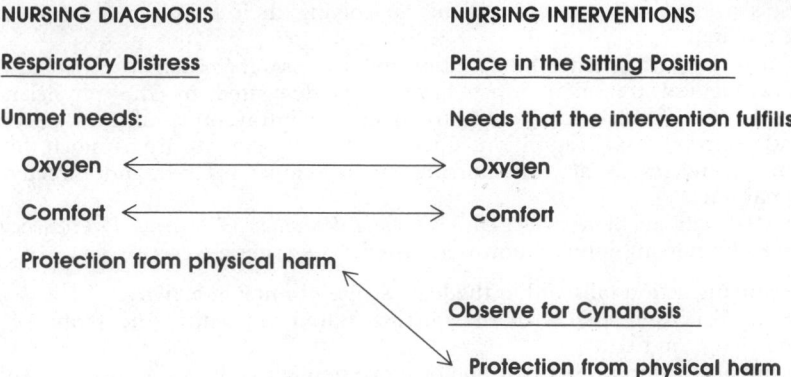

NURSING DIAGNOSIS	NURSING INTERVENTIONS
Respiratory Distress	Place in the Sitting Position
Unmet needs:	Needs that the intervention fulfills:
Oxygen	Oxygen
Comfort	Comfort
Protection from physical harm	
	Observe for Cynanosis
	Protection from physical harm

Expected Outcome (Goals)

In the planning process, the nurse identifies those aims of nursing care that nursing intervention should bring about. Goals, or expected outcomes, are determined early in nursing care, although they may not be accomplished for some time. Expected outcomes are mutually determined by the nurse and the patient. This cooperative factor increases the likelihood that the goals will be reached.

Marlene Mayers stated that an *expected outcome* is "synonymous with short-term behavioral objectives. One or more desired patient outcomes are written for each problem statement."[334:131] Mayers stated that the expected outcome must be stated in objective terms so it can be evaluated. She added that expected outcome need not always represent anticipated cure, since at times, cure is impossible. It is best to write the expected outcome in a realistic perspective of what can be achieved.[333:64] For potential problems, the expected outcome must be stated in terms of prevention or maintenance.[333:66] The expected outcome are the criteria for evaluation.[333:16]

NURSING INTERVENTIONS

Nursing interventions include activities that reflect nursing responsibility in the performance of health treatment: nursing treatments, nursing observations, health teaching, and medical treatments performed by nurses. A *nursing intervention* is a single-action nursing measure designed to fulfill the unmet human needs that are inferred from the patient's problem. If the nursing diagnosis indicates water–salt imbalance, then the nursing intervention must be such that the unmet need for water–salt balance is met. In order to determine and initiate nursing interventions, one must have a scientific background and extensive education in nursing. Such interventions may be carried out only by the professional nurse or by someone under direct supervision of the professional nurse. There are three categories of independently initiated nursing interventions: nursing treatments, nursing observations, and health teaching.

Nursing treatments consist of those single-action nursing measures that provide assistance, regulation of the internal or external environment, support in functioning, and comfort, as well as those that facilitate hygiene, improved or independent activity, and prevention of illness or injury through protective and precautionary measures. Nursing interventions that are considered to be emergency measures are identified in this text by the symbol (ET). *Nursing observations* consist of the single-action nursing measures of examining, checking, inspecting, and monitoring. *Health teaching* consists of those nursing measures that provide health information and explanation and teach skills performance. The professional nurse has sole responsibility for ordering and initiating the nursing treatments, nursing observations, and health teaching described previously. They are the nurse's avenue for assisting patients in solving their health problems within the realm of nursing.

The fourth kind of nursing intervention involves *medical treatments performed by nurses.* These are medical treatments that have been delegated by the physician to the nurse.[112:103] They include such medical treatments as intravenous infusion, peritoneal dialysis, and gastrointestinal aspiration. These medical treatments are as much the responsibility of the nurses as are the nursing interventions ordered and directed by the professional nurse.

In the 1978 edition of *Nursing Diagnosis and Intervention in Nursing Practice,* criteria for acceptance of a nursing intervention were listed. The criteria were:

> The nursing action falls within the legal scope of nursing activity.
> The rationale and effects of the nursing action are within the scope of nursing knowledge and skills.
> The nursing action must fulfill one or more unmet needs.

Each nursing intervention statement was structured as a single nursing action. The rationale for implementation and the contraindications were also identified. These are all listed in Part 4 of this text. This listing provides the nurse with a detailed explanation of each intervention.

While the full range of health interventions available to the patient were being reviewed, the question of which health interventions are nursing interventions and which are medical interventions arose. The literature was reviewed extensively to differentiate between the two. Nursing interventions are single-action treatments that are ordered by a professional nurse and carried out by a professional nurse or by a nursing assistant under professional nursing supervision. They are listed as follows:

Basic Nursing Treatments
Airway patency maintenance[73:50]
Alignment, body[72:133]
Ambulation, patient[306:1742]
Ambulation with mechanical aids[73:29]
Aseptic technique, maintenance of[73:818]
Baths, emollient: starch, bran, oatmeal[306:1756]
Bath, sitz[306:1755]
Bathing[423:184]
Bathing, sponge[73:726]
Bed-making[306:1743]
Binder applications[423:175]
Bladder irrigations, management of[73:469]
Bladder training[73:36]
Blakemore tube inflation and deflation[73:441]
Blood transfusion, management of[73:199]
Bowel elimination[72:473]
Bowel training[73:38]
Breast pump, use of[527:636–637]
Catheterization, urinary[306:1748]
Catheter, management of urinary[73:467]
Chest drainage, management of[72:260]
CircOlectric frames, placing on[73:757]
Cold applications[306:1754]
Cold packs[306:1754]
Cold sponges[306:1755]
Cough exercises[72:234]
Deep-breathing exercises[73:50]
Denture care[423:177]
Douche, vaginal[73:535]

Dressing and undressing, assistance with[523:163]
Dressings, nonmedicated wet[73:569]
Dressings, occlusive[73:571]
Dressings, wound[73:64]
Ear hygiene[72:745]
Eating assistance[306:1745]
Electrolytes, food and oral fluid replacement of[541:63]
Enemas[306:1747]
Environment, modification of[306:1742]
Expression of breast milk, manual[527:637]
Fluid replacement, oral[541:36]
Food appropriateness for eating, determining[272:104]
Food preference, assistance with[272:103]
Footboard, application of[72:168]
Gastric tube, management of[73:385]
Hair care[306:1744]
Heat applications, dry[306:1752]
Heat applications, moist[306:1752]
Hot packs[306:1754]
Hyperalimentation, management of[73:1086]
Intravenous infusion, management of[72:85]
Irrigations, nonmedicated low-pressure: eye, ear, nose[306:1749] ; wound[73:908]
Isolation technique[306:1757]
Isometric exercises[73:7]
Massage, back[73:799]
Massage, uterine fundus[73:1001]
Nail care[306:1744]
Nursing-care-related referrals[73:38]
Nutrition, maintaining balanced[272:103]
Nutritional supplements, nonprescription[72:671]
Oral hygiene[306:1746]
Oxygen therapy, management of[73:131]
Perineal care[73:537]
Positioning of the body[73:5]
Postmortem care[423:293]
Postural drainage[306:1752]
Predeath care[72:40]
Range-of-motion exercises[72:161]
Restraints[306:1746]
Skin care[306:1744]
Steam inhalation, nonmedicated[306:1751]
Stryker frame, placing on[73:763]
Teaching, patient[73:25]
Tracheostomy, management of[73:99]
Traction, management of[72:852]
Trochanter roll, application of[73:19]
Tube feedings, management of[73:19]
Urine elimination[72:473]

Emergency Nursing Treatments
Bivalve cast[73:778]
Cardiac compression, external[73:901]
Defibrillation[72:418]
Gastric lavage[423:440]
Intravenous infusion, initiation of[73:905]
Nasogastric intubation[73:911]

Oxygen therapy, initiation of[73:909]
Positive-pressure therapy, initiation of[73:902]
Pulmonary resuscitation[72:950]
Rotating tourniquets[73:282]
Splinting, fracture[73:916]
Tetanus prophylaxis[73:909]
Tracheostomy[73:933]

Additional Nursing Measures Performed by Nurses in the Expanded Role

Anesthetics, application of local[692:16]
Drugs, nonprescription[692:16]
Immunization[257:288]
Incision and extension of wounds not involved with major blood vessels, nerves, or tendons[692:16]
Management of common childhood conditions[257:508]
Management of the healthy newborn[257:509]
Management of uncomplicated labor and delivery[257:509]
Management of uncomplicated postpartum period[257:508]
Management of uncomplicated pregnancy[257:508]
Suture removal[73:64]
Suturing[692:16]

Medical Interventions

Aerosol inhalation, medicated[306:1724]
Anesthesia, administration of[478:607-610]
Back exercises, prescribing[73:800]
Bed rest, prescribing[452:781]
Blakemore tube insertion[72:524]
Blood transfusion, prescribing[72:94]
Braces, prescribing[72:175]
Burger exercises, prescribing[73:320]
Burger-Allen postural exercises, prescribing[72:329]
Cardiac compression[478:1043]
Cast application[452:318]
Cauterization[452:902]
Chemotherapy perfusion, prescribing[72:185]
Chest drainage, water-sealed[452:249]
Colostomy irrigation[272:272]
Contact lens, prescribing[72:721]
Contrast baths, prescribing[72:329]
Crutches, prescribing[72:174]
Crutch gait, prescribing[72:174]
Cutdown, arterial[306:1731]
Defibrillation[72:418]
Diets specific to diseases[306:1770]
Dressings, medicated wet[272:232]
Drugs, prescribing nasal spray and sublingual,[306:1724] intradermal,[306:1725] subcutaneous,[306:1727] intramuscular,[306:1728] intracardiac and intraarterial,[306:1731] intrathecal,[306:1732] rectal,[306:1733] aerosol inhalation,[306:1733] and vaginal[306:1734]
Ear irrigations, medicated[73:685]
Eye irrigations, medicated[73:685]
Endotracheal intubation[73:105]
Eyeglasses, prescribing[72:721]
Fluid and electrolyte replacement[72:83]
Gastric cooling[72:462]
Gastric gavage[423:450]

Hearing aids, prescribing[72:756]
Hemodialysis[452:1102]
Hyperalimentation, prescribing[73:1086]
Hypodermocylsis, prescribing[306:1728]
Hypothermia[452:1086]
Incision and drainage[423:715]
Intraarterial infusion[72:186]
Intravenous infusion, prescribing[306:1729]
Nasogastric and intestinal intubation and aspiration[306:1738]
Nebulization, medicated[306:1724]
Nutritional supplements, prescribing[72:669]
Operative procedures[478:517-606]
Orthotist, prescribing[72:175]
Oxygen therapy, prescribing[306:1725]
Pacemaker insertion[452:1048]
Paracentesis[306:1735]
Pericardicentesis[306:1736]
Peritoneal dialysis[452:1106]
Phlebotomy[452:579]
Phototherapy treatment[73:1130]
Postmastectomy exercises, prescribing[452:935]
Prosthesis, prescribing[72:175]
Pulmonary resuscitation[272:346]
Radiation therapy[72:201]
Radioisotope therapy[72:202]
Reduction of fractures and dislocations[423:816]
Splinting, fracture[73:916]
Suture removal[73:64]
Suturing[452:220]
Thoracentesis[306:1736]
Tidal drainage[272:319]
Tube feedings, prescribing[73:395]
Rotating tourniquets[452:611]
Tracheal aspiration[306:1741]
Traction, prescribing[452:327]
Tracheostomy[72:222]
Urinary bladder installations, medicated[272:319]

Since one of the six independent functions of nursing is "the application and execution of nursing procedures and techniques,"[292:260] professional nurses can initiate nursing interventions for the consumer's benefit without physician direction when those nursing treatments apply to health problems that fall within the nursing domain. Of the total number of nursing interventions that have been listed, 99.98% can be performed independent of physician direction. Only 0.02% of these nursing interventions are medical treatments performed by nurses.

The 1978 study also led to the conclusion that nursing interventions could be grouped into a few broad categories. The work of Matheney[329:99-100] and that of Maloney[318:63-66] were combined to produce seven nursing intervention categories, described as follows:

Nursing Intervention Categories
Assistive nursing intervention: one in which the nurse helps carry out those normal daily activities that cannot be carried out by the patient
Hygienic nursing intervention: one that is necessary for the maintenance of cleanliness
Rehabilitative nursing intervention: one that supports improved or independent activity and function in mobility; management of specific devices, supplies, and body al-

terations; retraining for bowel and bladder function; measures to ease work and conserve physical energy; clothing adjustments specific to health problems; budgeting; planning with the family and agencies; referral to resource persons; and involvement of the patient in community and social affairs

Supportive nursing intervention: one in which the nurse provides needed objects (oxygen, nutrition, fluids), facilitates processes or activities (elimination, body alignment, exercise, rest, sleep, entertainment), provides physical or psychologic comfort or healing measures, or simply maintains a healthy environment

Preventive nursing intervention: one in which the nurse provides protective or precautionary measures to avert physical or behavioral illness, injury, disease, or threat or to prevent complications or recurrences of physical or behavioral disorders, malfunctioning of therapeutic devices, or noneffective treatments

Observational nursing intervention: one in which the nurse examines, checks, inspects, and monitors physical and behavioral responses to illness, injury, and disease and their associated therapies

Educative nursing intervention: one in which the nurse provides satisfactory and accurate health information and explanation of treatment

Nursing interventions provide an opportunity for individualized care. Nurses consider all the options available for intervention as it relates to the specific diagnosis. When all alternatives have been considered, only those interventions deemed appropriate to the individual patient are initiated. Nursing provides unique plans of care for unique human beings. It is the quality of individualizing these interventions that is the mark of the professional nurse.

EVALUATION

After nursing intervention, the next step in the nursing process is evaluation. Nursing *evaluation* is an appraisal of the effectiveness of nursing actions. Once the nurse has selected and init iated appropriate nursing interventions, the unmet needs of the patient should be fulfilled. However, it must be determined whether the expected outcome, or goals, of the nursing interventions have actually been accomplished.

According to Mager,[316:44-53] standards for evaluating the accomplishment of nursing goals consist of:

Describing the goal
Selecting measurable criteria for goal evaluation
Appraising the degree to which the criteria were met

Goal description involves the statement of expected outcome. Only by knowing the specific changes that are expected to occur can it be determined whether those changes actually did occur. Selecting criteria for goal evaluation includes determining those specific criteria that will be the standards for evaluating each goal. After criteria are selected, the degree to which the criteria are met is appraised by both the nurse and the patient. Evaluation provides the professional nurse with information about whether the desired changes in the patient's condition were realized. The following shows the steps used in determining whether the expected outcome has been accomplished.

Steps in Evaluation

Determining nursing goals (expected outcome) before initiating nursing interventions
Selecting criteria for goal evaluation
Appraisal by the nurse and the patient as to the goal attainment

The nursing process consists of assessment, planning, intervention, and evaluation. It is the logical, well-organized, step-by-step process that guides nursing practice.

5 FORMULATING NURSING DIAGNOSES FROM DIAGNOSTIC PATTERNS

STEPS IN FORMULATING A NURSING DIAGNOSIS

With an understanding of the nursing process, the diagnostic patterns can be used to formulate a nursing diagnosis statement. Formulating a nursing diagnosis involves collecting subjective and objective data, determining which data are essential, interpreting essential data in terms of a diagnostic pattern, using the pattern title to begin the diagnostic statement, and completing the diagnostic statement with formula I or II, as described below. Once the diagnosis has been formulated, the nurse verifies the diagnosis and completes the nursing process through planning, intervention, and evaluation. This entire process can be broken down into nine steps.

Step 1. Collect the Data Base

Nursing history
Physical examination or objective data
Related data (such as age, sex, race, sociocultural factors, geographic location)

Step 2. Analyze the Data

Put the data in order
Determine which data are essential, significant, or abnormal
Disregard nonessential data

Step 3. Separate the Essential Data into Specific Problem Groups

Examples
Self-care problems
Information problems

Step 4. Review the Essential Criteria of the Nursing Diagnosis Patterns

Step 5. Interpret the Collected Essential Data in Terms of the Essential Criteria of the Diagnostic Patterns

Do the findings represent the pattern *Incapacity to . . .* , *Unskilled at . . .* , *Fear of . . .* , or one of the other patterns listed? If there is no appropriate pattern, perhaps there is a need for more data; or perhaps your diagnosis is a dual diagnosis.

Step 6. Use the Pattern Title as the First Part of the Behavioral Response the Person Is Exhibiting

Incapacity to . . .
Unskilled at . . .
Fear of . . .

Step 7. Complete the Diagnostic Statement with Nursing Diagnosis Formula I or II

    I.   RESPONSE + OBJECT OF RESPONSE + ETIOLOGY (STRESSOR)
        OR
    II.   RESPONSE + ETIOLOGY (STRESSOR)

Examples

I.

RESPONSE	+	OBJECT OF RESPONSE	+	ETIOLOGY (STRESSOR)
INCAPACITY TO (response)		PERFORM PERSONAL HYGIENE (object)	R/T*	PAIN (stressor)
FEAR OF (response)		PAIN (object)	R/T	DIAGNOSTIC PROCEDURE (stressor)
UNSKILLED AT (response)		DIABETIC INSULIN THERAPY (object)	R/T	LACK OF KNOWLEDGE (stressor)

II.

RESPONSE	+	ETIOLOGY (STRESSOR)
PHANTOM PAIN (response)	R/T	SURGICAL AMPUTATION (stressor)
EPISTAXIS (response)	R/T	CONTUSSION (stressor)
ANGER (response)	R/T	PHYSICAL LOSS (stressor)

OBJECT OF RESPONSE IN FORMULA I: Formula I requires an object and is used with diagnostic patterns that end with a preposition, with the exception of the pattern *Difficulty* . . . The object is a statement that further describes the pattern response. It is required to explain the full meaning of the response.

    The object may include terminology that seems to be the same as the stressor:

Example

FEAR OF   BURN INJURY   R/T   RADIATION THERAPY
(response)   (object)   (stressor)

If it were stated as

FEAR   R/T   RADIATION THERAPY
(response)   (stressor)

the statement would not communicate what the person is fearful of.

    In addition, a person could have several fears related to radiation therapy:

Fear of burn injury
Fear of impotence
Fear or hair loss } Related to radiation therapy
Fear of fetal injury

    The following patterns *do* require objects:

Discomfort of . . .
Difficulty . . .
Inability to . . .
Incapacity to . . .
Partial incapacity to . . .
Instability of . . .

---

*R/T is an abbreviation for *related to*.

Potential for . . .
Positive screening cues for . . .
Unknowledgeable about . . .
Unskilled at . . .
Competence in . . .
Fear of . . .
Rejection of . . .
Denial of . . .
Withdrawal from . . .

Formula II does not require the use of an object. These patterns are self-explanatory and require only a stressor to complete the statement. *Dual diagnosis* statements are also amenable to formula II. Hemorrhage, cardiac arrest, and the like are responses that are universally understood.

The following patterns *do not* require objects:

Abandoned feeling . . .
Loneliness/Isolated feeling . . .
Ambivalence . . .
Anger . . .
Anxiety . . .
Conflict . . .
Depression . . .
Dependency feelings . . .
Embarrassment . . .
Frustration . . .
Grief reaction . . .
Guilt . . .
Helplessness/Powerlessness . . .
Hopelessness . . .
Feeling rejected . . .
Regression . . .
Bonding interruption . . .
Disengagement/Detachment . . .
Role conflict . . .
Role modification . . .
Low self-esteem . . .
Threatened body image . . .
Body-image modification . . .
Self-identity modification . . .
Spiritual awareness . . .
Spiritual distress . . .

ETIOLOGY IN FORMULA I AND II: Guidelines for including the stressor in the diagnostic statement are as follows:

1. Avoid using the title of any nursing diagnosis pattern as a stressor.
2. A dual diagnosis statement may be used as a stressor for a nursing diagnosis pattern.
3. Stressors to be used with either a nursing diagnostic pattern or a dual diagnosis are listed in Appendix 1.

If, when making a nursing diagnosis, you find that there are *human responses* in the stressor column, evaluate if those responses could be either part of the problem's data base or associated with a different problem. Sometimes multiple stressors cause a single response, and in such instances there is both a primary and secondary stressor.

Parts Two and Three contain hundreds of nursing diagnosis statements. Some diagnostic labels are complete, with the etiology, and others are not. Limited space makes it impossible to list each diagnostic pattern separately with every possible stressor. In some instances, the nursing diagnosis statement is stated in such a way that the nurse must add the stressor:

Example

Incapacity to perform personal hygiene requires that a stressor be added, such as:

Incapacity to perform personal hygiene R/T *weakness*

In other instances, a stressor is listed, but in general terms. This was done to differentiate problems falling within a common pattern:

Example

Anger R/T *physical loss*

These diagnostic statements require more specific stressors when actually used in clinical practice, such as:

Anger R/T leg amputation
Anger R/T diabetes mellitus

Perhaps with further refinement of the list of stressors, greater consistency can be provided in the future.

Step 8. Verify That the Nursing Diagnosis Is a Problem for the Patient

If the patient is responsive and able, ask whether he perceives the response to be a problem.

Step 9. Complete the Nursing Process by

Identifying the unmet needs
Stating the expected outcome
Determining and initiating nursing interventions
Evaluating the plan of care

The following case study illustrates the application of diagnostic patterns to a specific situation. Many forms are available for data gathering. The one used here is based on Gordon's form for data gathering in *Nursing Diagnosis: Process and Application.*[196:333]

CASE STUDY

NURSING HISTORY

General Description of Client: Second admission of a 62-year-old, white woman within 1 year. She is alert and cooperative. Her medical diagnosis is diabetes mellitus and leukemia.

Health Perception–Health Management Data: States she "doesn't feel well at all." Feels she is "getting old very fast." States that during her last admission, she was taught how to give her own insulin injections and to calculate her diabetic diet. However, when she got home, "it all seemed so confusing." She takes her insulin and hopes the dosage is right.

Nutritional–Metabolic Data: Eats three times a day. Never eats sweets. Doesn't measure her diabetic food. Guesses pretty well what she's supposed to eat. Is able to stay up long enough to fix a meal.

Elimination Data: No elimination or urination problems. Does not take laxatives.

Activity–Exercise Data: Complains of weakness and pain in her back and hips. Has "hardly been able to walk for the past month." Finds it difficult to take care of herself and needs help.

Sleep–Rest Data: Sleeps 8 hours every night. Occasionally naps during the day. Stays in bed and reads or watches television quite often because she doesn't feel strong enough to stay up for long periods.

Cognitive–Perceptual Data: States that she has no hearing problems. Vision "is not what it used to be." She wears glasses, and sees well enough to read. Likes to learn about new things any time she has the opportunity.

Self-Perception–Self-Concept Data: States that she feels very weak. Finds it difficult to do the things she wants to do. Feels she is "not very clean" because she can bathe only twice a week when a neighbor comes to help her.

Role–Relationships Data: She lives alone. The neighbors take turns doing her grocery shopping. Her children live out of town, and she doesn't want to have to rely on them. The neighbors do what they can to help. Her husband left her several months ago because "he couldn't stand her sickness." She's unable to work any more because she's so weak. The rest of the family is well. She visited her sister 2 years ago and she was well.

Sexuality–Reproductive Data: Has two boys and a girl. Had no complications during pregnancy or childbirth.

Coping–Stress-Tolerance Data: States she has had many trials in her life, but "none have been too big to manage." She feels very sad many times and frequently cries since her husband left.

Value–Belief Data: Went to church every Sunday until she got sick. Believes that people are basically good; at least they are good to her.

PHYSICAL EXAMINATION

General Appearance: Appears unkempt. Hair is oily. Clothing is soiled. Poor oral hygiene.

Teeth: Has three lower teeth missing on the left side.

Hearing: Within normal limits, by Weber test and whisper test.

Vision: Corrected vision 20/30, both eyes, by Snellen chart.

Temperature: 98° F.

Pulse: rate, 80; rhythm, regular.

Respirations: Rate, 16; rhythm, regular; breath sounds, normal.

Blood Pressure: 130/70.

Weight: 170 lb. *Height:* 5'6".

Motor Function: Range of motion limited by pain and weakness.

Skin: Moist, warm skin. No lesions.

Gait: Unsteady.

Health Management Data, Objective: Unable to demonstrate correctly how to give her insulin. Cannot correctly calculate her diabetic diet.

GROUPING OF ESSENTIAL DATA

Subjective Data
Weakness and pain
Does not feel well
Bathes only twice a week } Self-care problem
Finds it difficult to care for self

Giving insulin and preparing diet are } Information problem
  confusing

Recent loss of husband, job, and health
Feels sad } Emotional problem
Cries frequently

Objective Data
Normal vital signs
Weight, 170 lb } Nutritional problem
Height, 5'6"

Moves slowly and cautiously
Poor oral hygiene
Hair oily } Self-care problem
General unkempt appearance
Clothing soiled

Unable to demonstrate insulin injections $\Big\}$ Information problem
Cannot calculate diabetic diet

Related Data

Age, 62 years
Sex, female
Race, white
Medical diagnosis diabetes mellitus and leukemia
Family, has two sons and one daughter

Nonessential Data

Visited her sister 2 years ago

Review the essential criteria for the nursing diagnostic patterns and the collected subjective and objective data. The collected data should match the essential criteria of certain patterns. Even if the patient's words were not exactly the same as the essential criteria of the pattern, the collected data should reflect the same content. Interpret the essential data in terms of nursing diagnostic patterns:

Problems	Patterns
The *self-care problem* is a response of	Partial incapacity to . . .
The *information problem* is a response of	Unskilled at . . .
The *emotional problem* is a response of	Grief reaction . . .
The *nutritional problem* does not match a nursing diagnostic pattern. It does match the *dual diagnosis pattern* of	Obesity . . .

Then use the nursing diagnostic pattern as the first part of the diagnosis, and complete the diagnostic statements:

Partial incapacity to perform personal hygiene R/T weakness and pain
Unskilled at managing diabetic diet R/T lack of knowledge
Unskilled at managing diabetic insulin therapy R/T lack of knowledge
Grief reaction R/T loss of health, husband, job
Obesity R/T diabetes mellitus

Having identified the nursing diagnosis, complete the nursing process by identifying unmet needs, stating expected outcome, initiating nursing interventions, and evaluating the plan of care.

CONVERTING THE NURSING PROCESS TO PROBLEM-ORIENTED CHARTING

Problem-oriented charting is a method devised by Weed[507] to organize health care records. Organized by this system, information about a patient is easily accessible and clearly understood. When using the nursing process, it is easy to convert it to problem-oriented charting, as shown by the diagram.

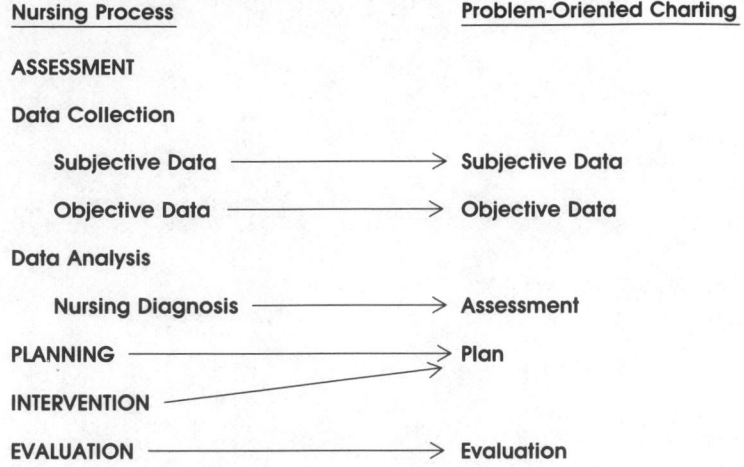

Nursing Process	Problem-Oriented Charting
ASSESSMENT	
Data Collection	
Subjective Data ——————→	Subjective Data
Objective Data ——————→	Objective Data
Data Analysis	
Nursing Diagnosis ——————→	Assessment
PLANNING ——————→	Plan
INTERVENTION	
EVALUATION ——————→	Evaluation

CODING NURSING DIAGNOSES AND INTERVENTIONS FOR INFORMATION SYSTEMS

In today's computerized world, many nurses find it necessary to code nursing diagnosis statements. Appendix 2 provides a suggested code for each problem. The dual diagnoses are coded according to the accepted numerical codes found in the *International Classification of Diseases* and the *Diagnostic and Statistical Manual of Mental Disorders*. Those nursing diagnoses formulated from the diagnostic patterns are coded according to the code of each pattern. This system can be used for organizing nursing diagnostic statements. Only when a taxonomy of nursing diagnoses is developed will there be a universally accepted coding system. Appendix 2 also includes a suggested system of coding nursing intervention categories.

INDIVIDUALIZING NURSING DIAGNOSES

Through the use of diagnostic patterns, nurses can maintain consistency in the basic context of nursing knowledge. *Incapacity to . . .* will consistently reflect a person's ineffective performance of self-care activities. *Instability of . . .* will consistently refer to a state of disequilibrium. But since human beings have unique characteristics and problems, it is imperative that nursing diagnoses reflect that individuality as well.

Diagnostic patterns are tailored to the individual by the addition of the object of the response and the stressor:

Incapacity to perform personal hygiene related to old age
Incapacity to ambulate related to Parkinson's disease

These diagnostic statements exemplify the consistent use of nursing diagnosis patterns individualized by the use of an object and a stressor appropriate to the individual patient and his unique problem.

PART TWO

PREDOMINANTLY NURSING DIAGNOSES

Part Two covers that sphere of knowledge and skill that nursing independently provides within the health care system and that nurses, more than practitioners of any other discipline, are educated to provide.

6 Nursing Diagnoses of COMFORT DEFICITS

Domain of Nursing Expertise: Comfort Deficits

This chapter covers that sphere of nursing knowledge and skill related to discomforts resulting from levels of incapacity, illness therapy, and the environment. Such discomforts cause physical distress, annoyance, irritation, and suffering. This domain includes discomfort due to self-care deficits.

Views of Nursing Leaders That Support This Domain of Nursing Expertise

Nurses should aim at preventing unnecessary suffering.

Florence Nightingale [370:6]

Nurses must be aware of and attend to or regulate the discomforting or deleterious effects of medical care measures performed or prescribed by the physician.

Dorothea Orem [380:50–51]

In nursing situations where the goal of life and health cannot be achieved, as in terminal illness, nurses give care and help individuals die with dignity.

Imogene King [267:84]

Nursing is service dedicated to encouraging and supporting people in an effort to restore their integrity with comfort, dignity and relative independence.

Ernestine Wiedenbach [516:25]

Our challenge is to consider man the physical being and his needs for physical comfort and safety within the framework of his total integrated being without any attempt at separation from the whole.

Valentia Fischer and Arlene Connally [156:11]

Discomforts Associated with Hearing Sensation

DISCOMFORT OF NOISE[108]

ASSESSMENT

Data Collection

Subjective Data
- Person relates experiencing the unpleasant sensation of:
  Loud, resounding sound
  A feeling of confusion

Objective Data
- May exhibit behavior such as irritability, demanding that the noise stop, restlessness, putting a pillow over the head, rapid blinking of the eyes, putting hands over the ears

Data Analysis

Nursing Diagnosis
DISCOMFORT OF NOISE: Experiencing as distressful the physical sensation of loud sounds or hypersensitivity to sound

Common Etiology (Stressors)
DISEASES: Any chronic or severe disease but especially brain abscess, brain tumor, encephalitis, meningitis, neuritis, tetanus
INJURIES: Any injury but especially cerebral concussion
SIGNS AND SYMPTOMS: Confusion, fatigue, fever, headache, irritability, pain, sleeplessness, unconsciousness (during which sound is perceived as greatly magnified)
PSYCHOSOCIAL FACTORS: Threat of chronic or severe stress
HEALTH CARE FACTORS: *Adverse effects of drug therapy:* Irritability from epinephrine or thyroid preparations, heavy drug sedation from sedatives (during which sound is perceived as greatly magnified)
DEVELOPMENTAL PHASES: Infancy (newborn), old age
ENVIRONMENTAL FACTORS: Loud noise, prolonged exposure to noise

PLANNING

Unmet Needs
Comfort, protection from physical harm

Expected Outcome
Person verbalizes feeling comfortable with the level of noise

NURSING INTERVENTIONS

Nursing Treatments
Place in a private room (located away from major activity)
Place in a heavily draped, carpeted room to reduce noise
Provide quiet (close the doors and windows, turn off the television and radio, speak softly when around the unconscious or heavily sedated person, place a "quiet" sign on the door)
Limit visitors (to one at a time and to short periods of time, be sure only one person in the room speaks at a time)
Turn off audible monitor signals
Provide a pleasant buffer sound to mask uncontrollable noise (soothing music, soft humming of electrical equipment such as a fan or air conditioner)

Nursing Observations

Observe for evidence of a favorable response to therapy (reduced irritability etc.)

Health Teaching

Recommend methods for noise reduction (closing doors and windows, carpeting floors and draping windows, wearing ear plugs or ear muffs)

EVALUATION

Record actual outcome

Discomforts Associated with Olfactory Sensation

DISCOMFORT OF BODY ODOR[362,451]

ASSESSMENT

Data Collection

Subjective Data

• Person relates experiencing the unpleasant sensation of:
  Odor from a body area
  Relates feeling dirty
  Wants to get away from the odor
  Complains of nausea, anorexia

Objective Data

• May exhibit behavior such as a disturbed facial expression, covering the nose

Data Analysis

Nursing Diagnosis

DISCOMFORT OF BODY ODOR: Experiencing as distressful the physical sensation of smelling an undesirable body odor

Common Etiology (Stressors)

DISEASES: Carcinoma, draining fistula, infection (pus-producing)

INJURIES: Burn wound

SIGNS AND SYMPTOMS: Diarrhea, excessive flatulence, incontinence, sweating, (diaphoresis), vomiting

HEALTH CARE FACTORS: *Medical procedures:* Odor from gastrointestinal tube, genitourinary tube, T-tube, wound drainage, draining-wound dressings. *Surgical procedures:* Colostomy, ileostomy, nephrostomy (drainage tube), ureterocolostomy, ureteroileostomy, ureterosigmoidostomy. *Therapeutic devices:* Soiled cast

HUMAN ERROR: Incomplete cleansing after elimination

PLANNING

Unmet Needs

Comfort, cleanliness

Expected Outcome

Person verbalizes feeling comfortable with the absence of or reduction of the offensive odor

NURSING INTERVENTIONS

Nursing Treatments

Bathe daily

AND
Bathe locally (whenever needed)
Provide clean clothing
Maintain clean, dry linen
Maintain adequate room ventilation
Change the dressing frequently
Control ileostomy and colostomy odor by deodorization (and cleanliness)
Control offensive odors by removing the source (soiled dressings, etc.)
Provide airtight drainage containers
Apply soda bicarbonate (baking soda) to an odiferous cast (sprinkle the baking soda generously onto the cast, leave it on 1 or 2 hours and then dust it off)
Use pleasant odors to mask unpleasant odors (use scented candles, wick or spray deodorizers, place bars of scented soap around the room)

Nursing Observations
Observe for evidence of a favorable response to therapy

Health Teaching
Explain the reason for and intended effect of the methods used
Recommend putting 1 or 2 drops of wintergreen oil in the vacuum cleaner bag (to freshen the air when the carpet is vacuumed)

EVALUATION
Record actual outcome

Discomforts Associated with Tactile Sensation

DISCOMFORT OF DRY MOUTH/LIPS/NARES[35]

ASSESSMENT
Data Collection
Subjective Data
• Person relates experiencing the unpleasant sensation of:
    Parched lips and mouth
    Stinging lips or nares
    Lips may feel hot and swollen

Objective Data
• May exhibit behavior such as frequent moistening of the lips with the tongue, rubbing the lips

Data Analysis
Nursing Diagnosis
DISCOMFORT OF DRY MOUTH/LIPS/NARES: Experiencing as distressful the physical sensation of dryness of the lips, mouth, and nasal mucosa

Common Etiology (Stressors)
SIGNS AND SYMPTOMS: Fever, mouth breathing
HEALTH CARE FACTORS: *Medical procedures*: Endotracheal intubation, unhumidified oxygen or compressed air, nasal packing, nasogastric suction or feeding. *Surgical procedures*: Tracheostomy

ENVIRONMENTAL FACTORS: *Environmental cold*: Low external temperature. *Environmental heat*: High external temperature. *Humidity*: Dry climate

PLANNING

Unmet Needs

Comfort, protection from physical harm

Expected Outcome

Person relates having moist, comfortable lips, mouth, nares

NURSING INTERVENTIONS

Nursing Treatments

Lubricate the lips (and external nares)
Refresh with a mouthwash
    OR
Swab the mouth with diluted glycerine
Administer vaporized air (or put a nebulizer in the room)
Clear nasal secretions
Moisten the mouth with cracked ice
Provide oral hygiene (at least three times a day)
Provide fresh drinking water
Give small, frequent drinks (unless contraindicated)
Give hard candy (to suck on)

Nursing Observations

Observe for evidence of a favorable response to therapy (moist, comfortable mouth, lips, and nares)

Health Teaching

Explain the reason for and intended effect of the therapy

EVALUATION

Record actual outcome

DISCOMFORT OF DRY SKIN[306,499]

ASSESSMENT

Data Collection

Subjective Data
• Person relates experiencing the unpleasant sensation of:
    Skin tightness
    Itching and burning
    Rough skin texture

Objective Data
• May exhibit behavior such as scratching or peeling the skin, restlessness
  Skin may be reddened and chapped or cracked

Data Analysis

Nursing Diagnosis
DISCOMFORT OF DRY SKIN: Experiencing as distressful the physical sensation of poorly moistened and lubricated skin

Common Etiology (Stressors)
DISEASES: Diabetes mellitus, myxedema, peripheral vascular insufficiency, varicose veins (advanced)

SIGNS AND SYMPTOMS: Edema
HEALTH CARE FACTORS: *Medical therapy*: Radiation therapy
DEVELOPMENTAL PHASES: Old age
ENVIRONMENTAL FACTORS: *Environmental cold*: Low external temperature. *Environmental heat*: Indoor heating. *Humidity*: Low environmental humidity. *Water*: Prolonged exposure to water. *Wind*: Prolonged exposure to high wind
HUMAN ERROR: Prolonged sun tanning

PLANNING
Unmet Needs
Comfort, protection from physical harm, increased learning
Expected Outcome
Person relates that skin feels comfortably moist and lubricated

NURSING INTERVENTIONS
Nursing Treatments
Bathe in warm water (avoid hot water, which dries the skin, and bathe less frequently, only as needed)
Clean the skin with a nondrying soap (such as Dove, Neutrogena, Alpha-Keri, Shepard's Soap)
OR
Add an emollient to the bath water (½ to 1 ounce of Alpha-Keri, Lubath, Nivea oil, mineral oil, or olive oil)
Lubricate the skin with baby oil, bath oil, or body lotion (while the skin is still slightly wet after bathing)
OR
Lubricate the skin with cocoa butter, diluted glycerine, lanolin, mineral oil, or olive oil
Maintain a cool room temperature (and use vaporized air)
Nursing Observations
Observe for evidence of a favorable response to therapy
Health Teaching
Advise against prolonged skin exposure to the sun, to water
Inform that the skin should be protected from wind burn
Advise against scratching (dry skin when it itches)
Explain the reason for and intended effect of the therapy

EVALUATION
Record actual outcome

DISCOMFORT OF THIRST[35,522]

ASSESSMENT
Data Collection
Subjective Data
• Person relates experiencing the unpleasant sensation of:
    Cotton in the mouth
    Tongue thickness
    Craving for fluid
  Frequently asks for fluids
  Intermittently asks how long it will be before he can have a drink

Objective Data
- May exhibit behavior such as moving the tongue about the mouth, irritability, restlessness

Data Analysis

Nursing Diagnosis

DISCOMFORT OF THIRST: Experiencing as distressful the sensation of having an intense desire for fluid intake

Common Etiology (Stressors)

DISEASES: Diabetes mellitus, diabetes insipidus, hyperparathyroidism, primary aldosteronism

INJURIES: Burn injury

SIGNS AND SYMPTOMS: Fever, dehydration, diarrhea, hemorrhage, hypernatremia, hyperhidrosis, mouth breathing, polyuria, uremia, paralysis, pain, weakness, etc., which prevent a person from obtaining fluids

HEALTH CARE FACTORS: *Medical therapy*: Nothing by mouth (NPO), radiation therapy, restricted fluid intake (limited amounts). *Adverse effects of drugs*: Anticholinergics, atropinelike drugs, diuretics, scopolamine. *Surgical procedure*: Wiring of a mandible fracture

SITUATIONAL FACTORS: Impending death

ENVIRONMENTAL FACTORS: *Environmental heat*: High external temperature

PLANNING

Unmet Needs

Comfort, fluid and electrolyte balance

Expected Outcome

Person relates having a moist, comfortable mouth
Person relates satisfaction with the relief of thirst

NURSING INTERVENTIONS

Nursing Treatments

Balance fluid intake to equal output (especially in diabetes mellitus, and increase the fluid intake by 500–1,500 cc during fever)
Moisten the mouth with cracked ice
Apply a cold, moist compress (to the lips)
Lubricate the skin (lips) with petrolatum
Swab the mouth with diluted glycerine
Distribute the fluid intake over 24 hours
Give small, frequent drinks
Provide fluid selection
Provide cold water for mouth rinsing but not swallowing (rinsing between drinks when fluid is restricted)
Refresh with a mouthwash (between drinks)
Give hard candy (to suck on)
Encourage decreased sodium-food intake (if thirst is chronic)
Provide oral hygiene (at least three times a day)

Nursing Observations

Observe for evidence of a favorable response to therapy
Measure the intake and output
Monitor blood studies for abnormal hematology (elevated hematocrit)
Monitor blood studies for abnormal chemistry

Health Teaching

Explain the reason for and intended effect of the therapy

EVALUATION

Record actual outcome

DISCOMFORT OF WETNESS[527]

ASSESSMENT

Data Collection

Subjective Data
• Person relates experiencing the unpleasant sensation of:
  A moist body area
  Cold, wet clothing or linens
  Chilling

Objective Data
• May exhibit behavior such as crying, standing with legs spread apart, removing clothing, rolling over and remaining on one side of the bed
  Skin may have a reddened, chapped appearance or a red rash

Data Analysis

Nursing Diagnosis
DISCOMFORT OF WETNESS: Experiencing as distressful the physical sensation of excessive skin moisture

Common Etiology (Stressors)
DISEASES: Cellulitis (purulent drainage), epistaxis, ruptured esophageal varices (bloody drainage), fistula (anal, rectal, or vaginal, causing fecal drainage), Parkinson's disease (drooling), obesity (sweat between overlapping skin surfaces)
INJURIES: Burn wound (serous drainage), cranial fracture (spinal fluid drainage), incision, laceration, puncture wound (serous or purulent drainage)
SIGNS AND SYMPTOMS: Seizures (excessive salivation), diaphoresis, incontinence
HUMAN BODY: *Body states:* Teething (drooling)
HEALTH CARE FACTORS: *Medical therapy:* Genitourinary drainage, T-tube drainage, wound drainage. *Surgical procedures:* Colostomy, ileostomy, nephrostomy (drainage tube), rhinoplasty, ureterocolostomy, ureteroileostomy, ureterosigmoidostomy
ENVIRONMENTAL FACTORS: *Environmental heat:* High external temperature. *Humidity:* High environmental humidity

PLANNING

Unmet Needs
Comfort, cleanliness, protection from physical harm, dependence

Expected Outcome
Person relates feeling comfortable and dry

NURSING INTERVENTIONS

Nursing Treatments
Bathe daily
  AND
Bathe locally (whenever needed)
Provide clean clothing (as needed)
Maintain dry, clean linen
Maintain dry skin
Lubricate the skin with petrolatum (to protect against enzymatic damage from saliva, diarrhea, fistula drainage)

Specific to Incontinence
Apply an external urinary catheter
  OR
Place a urinal at the perineum
Protect with absorbent padding
Clothe in disposable incontinent briefs

Protect with plastic pants

Apply cornstarch to the skin (as a skin-protective substance on areas of urinary contamination)

Toilet frequently

Change the wet diaper immediately

Specific to Local Drainage Tubes

Bandage with a draining-wound dressing

Change the dressing frequently

Specific to Diaphoresis

Clothe in flannel pajamas at night (for night sweats)

Protect with absorbent padding

Maintain a cool room temperature (to minimize sweating)

Apply cornstarch to the skin (as a skin-protective substance)

Dust the skin with an antiperspirant powder (in areas such as the feet)

Specific to Drooling

Protect with a plastic bib

Provide disposable tissue

Place in the side-lying position (when in bed)

Encourage decreased acid-food intake (for excessive salivation)

Nursing Observations

Inspect the skin for breakdown

Inspect for signs of irritation

Check the tube(s) for patency

Observe for evidence of a favorable response to therapy

Health Teaching

Instruct to maintain skin dryness, skin cleanliness (give specific instructions appropriate to the cause)

Instruct to immediately change wet diapers

Explain the reasons for and intended effect of the therapy

EVALUATION

Record actual outcome

Discomforts Associated with Pressure Sensation

DISCOMFORT OF INTRAABDOMINAL PRESSURE[73,306,451]

ASSESSMENT

Data Collection

Subjective Data

• Person relates experiencing the unpleasant sensation of:

   Abdominal tightness

   Intense fullness

May complain of nausea, anorexia, shortness of breath

Objective Data
- May exhibit behavior such as restlessness, holding the abdomen, moving with difficulty
  May have clinical findings such as dyspnea, vomiting, tight and shiny abdominal skin, increased abdominal circumference

Data Analysis

Nursing Diagnosis
DISCOMFORT OF INTRAABDOMINAL PRESSURE: Experiencing as distressful the physical sensation of tension within the abdominal cavity

Common Etiology (Stressors)
DISEASES: Abdominal tumor, Laennec's cirrhosis, paralytic ileus, uterine tumor
SIGNS AND SYMPTOMS: Ascites
HUMAN BODY: *Body states:* Pregnancy
HEALTH CARE FACTORS: *Medical therapy:* Peritoneal dialysis

PLANNING

Unmet Needs
Comfort, protection from physical harm, increased learning

Expected Outcome
Person relates increased abdominal comfort

NURSING INTERVENTIONS

Nursing Treatments
Change the patient's position frequently (side-lying positions, knee-flexed positions)
Give small, frequent feedings (instead of full meals)
Handle gently
Place in the sitting position (for respiratory distress)
Do not place in the flat position
Remove constrictive clothing
Arrange pillows comfortably (under or around the abdomen to reduce the pressure sensation)
Massage gently (give a relaxing back massage)
Lubricate the skin with lanolin, mineral oil, etc. (to relieve the tight abdominal skin)

Nursing Observations
Observe for evidence of a favorable response to therapy

Health Teaching
Explain the causes of the health problem
Explain the reason for and intended effect of the methods used

EVALUATION

Record actual outcome

DISCOMFORT OF INTRANASAL PRESSURE[73,278]

ASSESSMENT

Data Collection

Subjective Data
- Person relates experiencing the unpleasant sensation of:
  Nasal distention
  Air hunger
  Headache

Objective Data
• May exhibit behaviors such as pulling at the nasal pack, restlessness, sleeplessness, irritability

Data Analysis

Nursing Diagnosis
DISCOMFORT OF INTRANASAL PRESSURE: Experiencing as distressful the physical sensation of pressure within the nasal cavity

Common Etiology (Stressors)
HEALTH CARE FACTORS: *Medical therapy:* Nasal packing

PLANNING

Unmet Needs
Comfort, protection from physical harm, increased learning

Expected Outcome
Person verbalizes increased nasal comfort

NURSING INTERVENTIONS

Nursing Treatments
Elevate the head
  OR
Place in the sitting position
Do not place in the flat position
Feed unhurriedly (swallowing increases intranasal pressure when nasal packing is in place)
Give full-liquid foods (since chewing is difficult)
Provide oral hygiene (frequently)
Apply a cool, moist compress (to the forehead or across the nose and eyes)

Nursing Observations
Observe for dyspnea, choking
Observe for evidence of a favorable response to therapy

Health Teaching
Explain the reason for and intended effect of the therapy

EVALUATION

Record actual outcome

DISCOMFORT OF INTRAPULMONARY PRESSURE[73,219]

ASSESSMENT

Data Collection

Subjective Data
• Person relates experiencing the unpleasant sensation of:
    Severe tension within the thoracic cavity

Objective Data
• May exhibit behavior such as pulling off the ventilator nose clip or mask

Data Analysis

Nursing Diagnosis
DISCOMFORT OF INTRAPULMONARY PRESSURE: Experiencing as distressful the physical sensation of tension within the chest cavity

Common Etiology (Stressors)
HEALTH CARE FACTORS: *Therapeutic equipment:* Use of an intermittent positive-pressure breathing (IPPB) machine

PLANNING

Unmet Needs
Comfort, protection from physical harm, increased learning

Expected Outcome
Person verbalizes increased comfort and tolerance for ventilator pressure

NURSING INTERVENTIONS

Nursing Treatments
Attend the patient constantly (during treatment)
Reassure verbally
Limit IPPB treatments to short periods
Gradually increase the amount of ventilator pressure
Place in the sitting position
Do not place in the flat position
Refrain from strapping the ventilator mask in place
    AND
Refrain from using a ventilator nose clip

Nursing Observations
Observe for evidence of a favorable response to therapy

Health Teaching
Teach how to take positive-pressure breathing (if the person relaxes totally during inhalation, the pressure seems to be less)
Explain the reason for and intended effect of the therapy

EVALUATION
Record actual outcome

DISCOMFORT OF SKIN PRESSURE[73,306,451]

ASSESSMENT

Data Collection

Subjective Data
• Person relates experiencing the unpleasant sensation of:
    Numbness or tingling of the skin
    Skin heaviness
    Skin irritation

Objective Data
• May exhibit behavior such as restlessness, rubbing a skin area, distressful facial expression, lying very still
  Skin redness in the area of the discomfort

Data Analysis

Nursing Diagnosis
DISCOMFORT OF SKIN PRESSURE: Experiencing as distressful the physical sensation of tension against the skin

Common Etiology (Stressors)
HEALTH CARE FACTORS: *Medical and nursing therapy:* Bed rest, positioning. *Therapeutic devices:* Artificial limb, bandage, bedpan, brace, cast, cervical collar, crutches, prolonged sitting in a wheelchair, rotating tourniquets, safety restraints, tight bed covers, traction

PLANNING

Unmet Needs

Comfort, protection from physical harm, increased learning

Expected Outcome

Person verbalizes increased comfort in the skin area

NURSING INTERVENTIONS

Nursing Treatments

Specific for Bed Rest and Positioning
Position comfortably
Position with pillows (to reduce pressure)
Change the person's position frequently
Massage gently (the area of pressure)
Pad the bony prominences
Maintain body alignment

Specific for Bed Covers
Apply a bed cradle (to keep covers off the skin)

Specific for a Bedpan
Pad the bedpan
Provide a fracture bedpan
Remove the bedpan immediately following its use

Specific for a Cast
Pad the rough cast edges
Bivalve and spread the cast to relieve pressure (if necessary)

Specific for Restraints
Restrain the patient (loosely or with padding around the body area, using a nonslip knot)
Use a chest restraint (instead of a limb restraint)
Release restraints and walk the person periodically

Specific for Tourniquets
Apply rotating tourniquets (with padding between the skin and tourniquet)

Specific for Traction
Position comfortably (with the extremity in the center of the supporting frame)
Pad the rough traction connections (that touch the skin)
Massage gently (over the bony prominences)

Nursing Observations

Observe for evidence of a favorable response to therapy

Health Teaching

Specific for a Brace
Inform that clothing should be worn between the brace and the skin (to prevent pressure)
Explain how to recognize the outgrowth of a brace

Specific for a Cast
Explain how to pad rough cast edges

Specific for Crutches
Explain how to determine proper crutch length (to prevent pressure against the axilla)

Specific for Positioning
Instruct to change position frequently
Explain how to maintain body alignment

Specific for a Prosthesis
Instruct to gradually increase the wearing time of the prosthesis
Teach how to apply a stump sock

Specific for a Wheelchair
Instruct to do wheelchair push-ups (to reduce pressure on the buttocks)

EVALUATION

Record actual outcome

Discomforts Associated with Taste Sensation

DISCOMFORT OF DIMINISHED TASTE[125]

ASSESSMENT

Data Collection

Subjective Data
• Person relates experiencing the unpleasant sensation of:
   Dull or flat taste
   Most foods tasting the same

Objective Data
• May exhibit behavior such as decreasing food and fluid intake, irritability, excessive
   seasoning of food

Data Analysis

Nursing Diagnosis
DISCOMFORT OF DIMINISHED TASTE: Experiencing as distressful the physical sensation of decreased perception of the normal flavor of food and drinks

Common Etiology (Stressors)
DISEASES: Bell's palsy, chronic rhinitis
INJURIES: Basal skull fracture
HEALTH CARE FACTORS: *Surgical therapy:* Laryngectomy
DEVELOPMENTAL PHASES: Old age
LIFESTYLE: Cigarette/tobacco smoking

PLANNING

Unmet Needs

Comfort, protection from physical harm, increased learning

Expected Outcome

Person verbalizes increased taste sensation
Person maintains adequate food and fluid intake

NURSING INTERVENTIONS

Nursing Treatments

Provide an attractive meal tray (the pleasure of the visual senses can increase the plea-
   sure of the taste sense)
Give flavor-intensified food (food treated with monosodium glutamate, if not con-
   traindicated)
Give strongly seasoned foods (with lots of lemon and onion)
Provide food selection
Provide foods at their most appetizing temperature
Withhold food until the patient requests it
Discourage smoking

Nursing Observations
Observe for evidence of a favorable response to therapy

Health Teaching
Explain the causes of the problem (such as facial, glossopharyngeal, vagus, or cranial nerve impairment, temporal lobe lesion, nasal infection, frequent use of tobacco which deadens the tastebud receptors, injury to or disease of olfactory end organs or nerves leading to the cerebral cortex)

Explain the reason for and intended effect of the therapy

EVALUATION

Record actual outcome

DISCOMFORT OF UNPLEASANT TASTE[125]

ASSESSMENT

Data Collection

Subjective Data
• Person relates experiencing the unpleasant sensation of:
   A bitter, sour, salty, sweet, brackish, or metallic taste

Objective Data
• May exhibit behavior such as displeased facial expression, decreased food or fluid intake, refusal to take drugs

Data Analysis

Nursing Diagnosis
DISCOMFORT OF UNPLEASANT TASTE: Experiencing as distressful the physical sensation of an undesirable taste

Common Etiology (Stressors)
DISEASES: Brain tumor, bronchiectasis, cerebrovascular accident, pyorrhea, sinusitis
SIGNS AND SYMPTOMS: Frequent belching (eructation)
HEALTH CARE FACTORS: *Medical therapy:* Radiation therapy. *Drug therapy:* Aminophylline, antibiotics, brewer's yeast, potassium, etc.
HUMAN ERROR: Infrequent or inadequate oral hygiene

PLANNING

Unmet Needs
Comfort, increased learning

Expected Outcome
Person verbalizes improvement in taste
Person maintains adequate food and fluid intake

NURSING INTERVENTIONS

Nursing Treatments

General Measures
Provide oral hygiene (especially before meals and after productive coughing)
Season the food for individual taste (use less salt, more sweetener, stronger flavor, etc.)
Give hard candy (such as lemon drops, to disguise an unflavorable taste)

Specific to Drugs
Dilute the medication
Disguise drugs with fruit-flavored syrup
Do not disguise drugs in food
Follow distasteful drugs with fruit juice

Refrain from forcing distasteful drugs

Place drug tablets in a gelatin capsule

Moisten the mouth with cracked ice (before giving the medication, to deaden the sense of taste)

Give iced liquids (chilled liquid medicine is more easily tolerated)

Nursing Observations

Observe for evidence of a favorable response to therapy

Health Teaching

Recommend the use of mouthwash (the person's favorite flavor)

Recommend that the tongue be brushed

EVALUATION

Record actual outcome

Discomforts Associated with Thermal Sensation

DISCOMFORT OF COLD BODY SENSATION[306]

ASSESSMENT

Data Collection

Subjective Data

• Person relates experiencing the unpleasant sensation of:
  Chilliness
  Coolness

Objective Data

• May exhibit behavior such as hugging self, frequently raising the thermostat

Data Analysis

Nursing Diagnosis

DISCOMFORT OF COLD BODY SENSATION: Experiencing as distressful the physical sensation of insufficient body warmth

Common Etiology (Stressors)

DISEASES: Anemia, hypothyroidism (myxedema), Raynaud's phenomenon, Simmond's disease

SIGNS AND SYMPTOMS: Low body weight

HEALTH CARE FACTORS: *Diagnostic procedure:* Body exposure for diagnostic procedure

DEVELOPMENTAL PHASES: Old age

ENVIRONMENTAL FACTORS: *Environmental cold:* Low external temperature

PLANNING

Unmet Needs

Normal temperature, comfort, protection from physical harm, increased learning

Expected Outcome

Person verbalizes increased comfort and warmth

NURSING INTERVENTIONS

Nursing Treatments

Cover with warm blankets

Place a blanket directly against the skin (to avoid the chill of cold sheets)

Drape for warmth

Dress in warm clothing (preferably wool or flannel clothing, heavy sweaters, layered clothing that fits snugly around the neck, wrists, and ankles)

Decrease drafts

Keep the patient's windows closed

Maintain a warm room temperature (draped and carpeted rooms are warmest)

Place only warm hands and objects on the patient

Give warm liquids (coffee, tea, warm milk, chocolate, juices, boullion)

Refrain from giving iced liquids

Refrain from giving local cold applications

Discourage smoking (and alcoholic drinks, both of which constrict blood vessels and increase chilling)

Encourage moderate physical exercise (to promote circulation)

Nursing Observations

Observe for evidence of a favorable response to therapy

Health Teaching

Explain the reason for and intended effects of the methods used

EVALUATION

Record actual outcome

DISCOMFORT OF WARM BODY SENSATION[306]

ASSESSMENT

Data Collection

Subjective Data

• Person relates experiencing the unpleasant sensation of:
    Being hot

Objective Data

• May exhibit behavior such as restlessness, removing bed linens and clothing, fanning self

  May manifest physical findings of facial and neck flushing, sweating, increased pulse rate

Data Analysis

Nursing Diagnosis

DISCOMFORT OF WARM BODY SENSATION: Experiencing as distressful the physical sensation of excessive body warmth

Common Etiology (Stressors)

DISEASES: Thyrotoxicosis

SIGNS AND SYMPTOMS: Fever, weakness

HUMAN BODY: *Body states:* Menopause

SITUATIONAL FACTORS: Impending death

ENVIRONMENTAL FACTORS: *Environmental heat:* High external temperature. *Humidity:* High environmental humidity

PLANNING

Unmet Needs

Normal temperature, comfort, protection from physical harm, increased learning

Expected Outcome

Person verbalizes increased comfort and coolness

NURSING INTERVENTIONS

Nursing Treatments

Cover with lightweight blankets (when cover is necessary)
Dress in lightweight clothing
Give iced liquids
Refrain from giving hot liquids
Refrain from giving oral stimulants
Discourage the intake of oral stimulants
Refrain from giving local heat applications
Apply a cool, damp cloth to the face (especially during fever)
Place absorbent pads under the person (and over a plastic-covered or foam mattress, which holds heat)
Change the person's position frequently (to a cooler area of the bed, to air the skin surfaces)
Increase drafts
Maintain adequate room ventilation
Maintain a cool room temperature
Place by a window
Place in an uncrowded area
Discourage strenuous activities
Encourage active diversional activities (during menopausal hot flashes)

Nursing Observations

Observe for evidence of a favorable response to therapy

Health Teaching

Explain the reason for and intended effect of the methods used
Advise against exposure to intense heat
Explain the need to avoid overexertion
Recommend the use of lightweight clothing

EVALUATION

Record actual outcome

Discomforts Associated with Visual Sensation

DISCOMFORT OF LIGHT SENSITIVITY[371,522]

ASSESSMENT

Data Collection

Subjective Data
• Person relates experiencing the unpleasant sensation of:
    Eye irritation
    Excessive perception of brightness

Objective Data
• May exhibit behavior such as squinting
  May manifest physical findings of excessive tearing

Data Analysis

Nursing Diagnosis
DISCOMFORT OF LIGHT SENSITIVITY: Experiencing as distressful the physical sensation of glaring light

Common Etiology (Stressors)
DISEASES: Albinism, Colorado tick fever, conjunctivitis, corneal ulcer, hypoparathyroid-
ism, iritis, keratitis, measles, meningitis, retinitis, rickettsialpox, vitamin A deficiency,
Weil's disease, yellow fever
SIGNS AND SYMPTOMS: Photophobia
HEALTH CARE FACTORS: *Drug therapy:* Belladonna or atropine optic solution

PLANNING

Unmet Needs
Comfort, protection from physical harm, increased learning

Expected Outcome
Person verbalizes increased eye comfort

NURSING INTERVENTIONS

Nursing Treatments
Subdue the room lighting (lower the lamp light, draw the drapes, tilt the examination
lights away from the patient's face)
Provide sunglasses (when appropriate)

Nursing Observations
Inspect the eyes for pupil size, equality, and response to light (if appropriate, but when
doing so, shine the examination light across the pupil, not into it)
Observe for evidence of a favorable response to therapy

Health Teaching
Advise against letting light shine directly into the eyes
Explain the causes of the health problem (eye tissue irritation, drug side effects, etc.)

EVALUATION

Record actual outcome

DISCOMFORT OF RESTRICTED VISION[73,371,440]

ASSESSMENT

Data Collection

Subjective Data
• Person relates experiencing the unpleasant sensation of:
Not being able to visualize all or parts of the environment
Being able to only see the ceiling, the floor, or straight ahead

Objective Data
• May exhibit behavior such as holding the neck or head still, knocking things over
when reaching for what he cannot see

Data Analysis

Nursing Diagnosis
DISCOMFORT OF RESTRICTED VISION: Experiencing as distressful the physical sensation of being unable to have full vision of the environment despite adequate visual acuity

Common Etiology (Stressors)
INJURIES: Cervical sprain
SIGNS AND SYMPTOMS: Limited range of motion, pain
MEDICAL THERAPY: Body casting, traction
THERAPEUTIC EQUIPMENT: Brace, cervical collar, use of a respirator, safety restraints, Stryker
frame

PLANNING
Unmet Needs
Comfort, protection from physical harm, increased pleasure
Expected Outcome
Person verbalizes satisfaction with what he is able to see

NURSING INTERVENTIONS
Nursing Treatments
Reassure verbally (that the furniture, television, etc., will be rearranged to permit maximum visual field)
Provide prism eye glasses (to facilitate reading if the person can only look upward when lying flat)
Provide a wide mirror to reflect the room (tilt the mirror for maximum vision)
Illuminate the room adequately
Place objects within reach (and within sight)
Nursing Observations
Observe for evidence of a favorable response to therapy
Health Teaching
Explain the reason for and intended effect of the methods used

EVALUATION
Record actual outcome

Discomforts Associated with Energy Sensations

DISCOMFORT OF WEAKNESS[371,396,451]

ASSESSMENT
Data Collection
Subjective Data
• Person relates experiencing the unpleasant sensation of:
 Feeling hot
 Trembling legs
 Lightheadedness

Objective Data
• May exhibit behavior of moving slowly or with poor balance
 May manifest physical findings of sweating, rapid pulse, deep breathing
Data Analysis
Nursing Diagnosis
DISCOMFORT OF WEAKNESS: Experiencing as distressful the physical sensation of lack of strength

Common Etiology (Stressors)
DISEASES: Any disease
INJURIES: Any injury
SIGNS AND SYMPTOMS: Severe or prolonged pain

HUMAN BODY: *Natural body function:* Childbirth

HEALTH CARE FACTORS: *Diagnostic procedures:* Extensive or painful. *Medical therapy:* Bed rest, enemas, hemodialysis, peritoneal dialysis, radiation therapy, rehabilitation therapy, alcohol or drug withdrawal. *Drug therapy:* Chemotherapy. *Surgical therapy:* Surgery of any kind. *Convalescence:* Resumption of physical activity during convalescence

DEVELOPMENTAL PHASES: Old age

LIFESTYLE: Insufficient or unbalanced diet, insufficient rest and sleep

SITUATIONAL FACTORS: Situational crisis

PLANNING

Unmet Needs

Comfort, protection from physical harm, increased learning

Expected Outcome

Person verbalizes increased comfort despite weakness

NURSING INTERVENTIONS

Nursing Treatments

Encourage adequate rest (the person should rest for a while, get up for a short period, then rest again)

Encourage increased carbohydrate intake and increased fatty-food intake (for quick, short-term energy)

Encourage increased protein-food intake (for longer-lasting energy)

Give small, frequent feedings
  OR
Give snacks (between meals)

Give iced or cool liquids (to offset the warm feeling associated with weakness)

Dress in lightweight clothing (to keep the body cool and avoid expending energy to carry about heavy clothing)

Maintain a cool room temperature (for less energy consumption)

Nursing Observations

Observe for evidence of a favorable response to therapy

Health Teaching

Explain the reason for and intended effects of the methods used

EVALUATION

Record actual outcome

Self-Care Deficits in Managing Comfort

INCAPACITY TO MANAGE PAIN [310,625,626,627,628]

ASSESSMENT

Data Collection

Subjective Data

• Person may or may not relate being unable to carry out pain relief measure for self
  Relates that pain is currently being experienced

Objective Data

• Person exhibits behavior such as minimal, ineffective, or no body movement and makes no attempt to relieve his own pain

May exhibit restlessness, excessive perspiration, increased respirations, drawn facial expression, clenched teeth or hands, wrinkled forehead, still or flexed position, crying or moaning sounds

Data Analysis

Nursing Diagnosis

INCAPACITY TO MANAGE PAIN: Being incapable of providing pain relief for self and requiring total assistance with pain relief

Common Etiology (Stressors)

BIRTH DEFECTS: Blindness, Down's syndrome, hydrocephalus, developmental deficit

DISEASES: Autism, blindness, brain tumor, carcinoma, cataracts, cerebral palsy, cerebrovascular accident, congestive heart failure, Duchenne's muscular dystrophy, encephalitis, Friedreich's ataxia, Guillain-Barre syndrome, Laennec's cirrhosis, leukemia, manic-depressive psychosis, meningitis, mental retardation, multiple sclerosis, myasthenia gravis, organic brain syndrome, osteoarthritis, Parkinson's disease, posterolateral sclerosis, psychosis, pulmonary edema, renal failure, retinal detachment, rheumatoid arthritis, senility, Sydenham's chorea, typhoid

INJURIES: Burn wound, cerebral concussion, bone fracture, fracture and compression of the spinal cord, traumatic amputation

SIGNS AND SYMPTOMS: Blurred vision, confusion, diplopia, dizziness, dyspnea, fatigue, hallucinations, memory loss, pain, paralysis, rigidity, joint swelling, touch sensation loss, vertigo, weakness

HEALTH CARE FACTORS: *Drug therapy:* Narcotics, sedatives, tranquilizers. *Medical therapy:* Casting, traction. *Surgical procedures:* Amputation, replantation of digits, skin graft of hand, tenoplasty of hand. *Surgical incision:* Painful surgical incision. *Therapeutic devices:* Enforced immobility with safety restraints

DEVELOPMENTAL PHASES: Toddler, preschooler, old age

MAJOR PATHOPHYSIOLOGIC FACTORS CAUSING THE PROBLEM: Pain stimuli signal the body to protect itself; depending on its severity, pain causes the person to attempt to protect the body by such devices as immobility or unusual positioning; the expenditure of energy to cope with pain or the disease, condition, or therapy causing pain often results in weakness or impaired function, reducing the person's ability to manage the pain

PLANNING

Unmet Needs

Comfort, protection from physical harm, protection from psychologic threat, freedom from pain, dependence, increased learning

Expected Outcome

Verbal expressions of increased comfort

Quiet rest, peaceful facial expression, respiration rate 16–20 beats/minute (adult), relaxed positioning

NURSING INTERVENTIONS

Nursing Treatments

Acknowledge dependency

Anticipate needs (for pain relief before the person has to request it)

Approach unhurriedly

Handle gently

Communicate nurse sensitivity to the person's pain

Ask the person what makes him comfortable

Discuss possible pain-reducing measures (medication, heat, positioning, pressure relief)

Provide a pain-relief measure of the patient's choice

Reassure that the pain will subside or be relieved

Offer assurance of other measures if the pain-relief method fails

Provide an atmosphere of acceptance (if the person cannot tolerate much pain)

Give nonprescription drugs (if such is effective for pain relief)

Give the drug (narcotic) having the fewest side effects for the person, when drug choices are available

Give pain relief drugs on a regular, preventive schedule, not PRN

Give half the narcotic dose PO and half IM before converting to a full PO dosage

Ask the person to relate the onset of returning pain before the pain becomes severe

Refrain from equating sleep with the absence of pain (fatigue may have exhausted a person who is still feeling pain)

Nursing Observations

Before Giving Medications

Determine the physiologic factors that will increase or decrease drug absorption (absorption is decreased with impaired circulation, tissue damage, and obesity and is increased with rapid metabolism, in impaired renal function, in adolescents and young adults, in underweight persons, and in smokers)

Observe the level of arousal and the respiratory rate before giving an analgesic

Evaluate the pain for intensity and quality

Determine the urgency for pain relief (and administer accordingly)

After Giving Medication

Observe for complaints of pain duration (duration varies individually)

Observe for oversedation (difficulty in arousal, respiratory depression)

Observe for inadequate analgesic pain relief (pain that still exists 1 hour after the drug dose or that becomes severe before the next scheduled dose)

Evaluate the effectiveness of the pain-relief measure (the person verbalizes pain relief, exhibits freedom of movement, has a relaxed facial expression)

Health Teaching

Explain that it is acceptable to admit the existence of pain (if the person denies or minimizes the pain)

Explain how to use nondrug methods for pain relief (heat and cold applications, therapeutic soaks, positioning, relaxation, supportive bandages and garments)

Explain the reason for the delay in giving a pain-relief drug (if based on the prescribed hours of drug administration)

Explain how to describe pain (aching, burning, constrictive, cramping, stabbing, throbbing)

Explain the causes of pain (infection, inflammation, pressure)

Medical Treatments Performed by Nurses

Give the prescribed drugs (ask the physician to order aspirin or acetaminophen with analgesics (narcotics); combined, they affect both the peripheral nervous system and central nervous system for greater pain relief)

EVALUATION

Record actual outcome

PARTIAL INCAPACITY TO MANAGE PAIN[310,625,626,627,628]

ASSESSMENT

Data Collection

Subjective Data

• Person relates attempts at providing pain relief for self
• Requests assistance in managing pain
• Relates that pain is presently being experienced or that the pain is partially but not adequately relieved

Objective Data
- Person exhibits behavior such as struggling to reach the medication bottle, squinting in an effort to read the medication instructions

  May exhibit restlessness, excessive perspiration, increased respiration rate, drawn facial expression, wrinkled forehead, crying or moaning

Data Analysis

Nursing Diagnosis
PARTIAL INCAPACITY TO MANAGE PAIN: Being capable of but needing assistance with the management of pain

Common Etiology (Stressors)
BIRTH DEFECTS: Blindness, clubhand, Down's syndrome, developmental deficit

DISEASES: Aortic insufficiency, aortic stenosis, aplastic anemia, blindness, brain tumor, bursitis, carcinoma, cataracts, cerebral palsy, cerebrovascular accident, congestive heart failure, Duchenne's muscular dystrophy, encephalitis, Friedreich's ataxia, Guillain-Barré syndrome, herpes zoster, Hodgkin's disease, Laennec's cirrhosis, leukemia, manic–depressive psychosis, Meniere's disease, meningitis, mental retardation, migraine headache, mitral stenosis, multiple sclerosis, myasthenia gravis, organic brain syndrome, osteoarthritis, Parkinson's disease, pneumothorax, posterolateral sclerosis, psychosis, pulmonary edema, pulmonary stenosis, renal failure, retinal detachment, rheumatoid arthritis, senility, Sydenham's chorea, tricuspid stenosis, typhoid

INJURIES: Burn wound, cerebral concussion, dislocation, bone fracture, fracture and compression of the spinal cord, herniated intervertebral disc, traumatic amputation

SIGNS AND SYMPTOMS: Blurred vision, difficulty with concentration, confusion, diplopia, dizziness, dyspnea, fatigue, hallucinations, hyperactivity, malaise, memory loss, pain, paralysis, joint swelling, touch sensation loss, tremor, vertigo, weakness

HEALTH CARE FACTORS: *Drug Therapy*: Narcotics, sedatives, tranquilizers. *Medical Therapy*: Cast, intravenous infusion, traction, blood transfusion. *Surgical procedures*: Amputation, replantation of digits, tenoplasty of hand. *Surgical incision*: Painful surgical incision

DEVELOPMENTAL PHASES: Adolescence, old age

MAJOR PATHOPHYSIOLOGIC FACTORS CAUSING THE PROBLEM: Pain stimuli signal the body to protect itself; depending on its severity, pain causes the person to attempt to protect the body by such devices as immobility or unusual positioning; the expenditure of energy to cope with pain or the disease, condition, or therapy causing pain often results in weakness or impaired function, reducing the person's ability to manage the pain

PLANNING

Unmet Needs
Comfort, protection from physical harm, protection from psychologic threat, freedom from pain, dependence, increased learning

Expected Outcome
Verbal expressions of increased comfort

Quiet rest, peaceful facial expression, respiration rate 16–20 beats/minute (adult), relaxed positioning

NURSING INTERVENTIONS

Nursing Treatments
Acknowledge dependency

Anticipate needs (for pain relief before the person has to request it)

Approach unhurriedly

Handle gently

Communicate nurse sensitivity to the person's pain

Ask the person what makes him comfortable

Discuss possible pain-reducing measures (medication, heat, positioning, pressure relief)

Provide a pain-relief measure of the patient's choice

Reassure that the pain will subside or be relieved

Offer assurance of other measures if the pain-relief method fails

Provide an atmosphere of acceptance (if the person cannot tolerate much pain)

Give nonprescription drugs (if such is effective for pain relief)

Give the drug (narcotic) having the fewest side effects for the person, when drug choices are available

Give pain-relief drugs on a regular, preventive schedule, not PRN

Give half the narcotic dose PO and half IM before converting to a full PO dosage

Ask the person to relate the onset of returning pain before the pain becomes severe

Refrain from equating sleep with the absence of pain (fatigue may have exhausted a person who is still feeling pain)

Encourage self-performance (whenever possible)

Nursing Observations

Before Giving Medication

Determine the physiologic factors that increase or decrease drug absorption (absorption is decreased with impaired circulation, tissue damage, and obesity and is increased with rapid metabolism, in impaired renal function, in adolescents and young adults, in underweight persons, and in smokers)

Observe the level of arousal and the respiratory rate before giving an analgesic

Evaluate the pain for intensity and quality

Determine the urgency for pain relief (and administer accordingly)

After Giving Medication

Observe for complaints of pain duration (duration varies individually)

Observe for oversedation (difficulty in arousal, respiratory depression)

Observe for inadequate analgesic pain relief (pain that still exists 1 hour after the drug dose or that becomes severe before the next scheduled dose)

Evaluate the effectiveness of the pain-relief measures (the person verbalizes pain relief, exhibits freedom of movement, has a relaxed facial expression)

Observe for readiness to assume self-care

Health Teaching

Explain that it is acceptable to admit the existence of pain (if the person denies or minimizes the pain)

Explain how to use nondrug methods for pain relief (heat and cold applications, therapeutic soaks, positioning, relaxation, supportive bandages and garments)

Explain the reason for the delay in giving a pain-relief drug (if based on the prescribed hours of drug administration)

Explain how to describe pain (aching, burning, constrictive, cramping, stabbing, throbbing)

Explain the causes of pain (infection, inflammation, pressure)

Medical Treatments Performed by Nurses

Give the prescribed drugs (ask the physician to order aspirin or acetaminophen with analgesics (narcotics); combined, they affect both the peripheral nervous system and central nervous system for greater pain relief)

EVALUATION

Record actual outcome

7 Nursing Diagnoses of COMMUNICATION DEFICITS

Domain of Nursing Expertise: Communication Deficits

This chapter covers that sphere of nursing knowledge and skill related to problems of disrupted exchange and expression of information between persons. This domain involves recognition of a person's incapacity to relate basic needs to others during illness, therapy, and certain developmental changes. It includes nursing expertise in identifying individuals' needs despite their inability to communicate such needs.

Views of Nursing Leaders That Support This Domain of Nursing Expertise

As a comprehensive service, nursing includes . . . the maintenance of effective verbal and nonverbal communication.

Faye Abdellah[187:107 & 111]

Components of basic nursing include assisting the patient to . . . communicate with others in expressing emotions, needs, fears, etc.

Virginia Henderson[220:12]

Self-Care Deficits in Managing Communications

INCAPACITY TO COMMUNICATE NEEDS[69,216,448,512,679]

ASSESSMENT

Data Collection

Subjective Data
• Person cannot relate being unable to communicate
  May feel isolated

Objective Data
• Person exhibits behavior such as making no visible attempt to communicate, making
    ineffective gestures, writing illegibly

Data Analysis

Nursing Diagnosis
INCAPACITY TO COMMUNICATE NEEDS: Being incapable of expressing one's needs through the
    exchange of thoughts and ideas with others

Common Etiology (Stressors)
DISEASES: Brain tumor, cerebrovascular accident, Guillain-Barré syndrome, myasthenia
    gravis, subarachnoid hemorrhage, subdural hematoma
INJURIES: Cerebral concussion, drug overdose
SIGNS AND SYMPTOMS: Coma (diabetic, eclamptic, epileptic, hepatic, or uremic), syncope
HEALTH CARE FACTORS: *Drug Therapy:* Sedative (heavy sedation). *Medical therapy:* Electrocon-
    vulsive therapy. *Surgical therapy:* Anesthesia

PLANNING

Unmet Needs

Comfort, protection from physical harm, protection from psychologic threat, depen-
    dence, caring and communicating relationships

Expected Outcome

The person who cannot communicate will receive adequate communication from other
    persons

NURSING INTERVENTIONS

Nursing Treatments

Anticipate needs (all physical, psychosocial, spiritual needs must be foreseen by the
    nurse, since the person cannot communicate)
Talk with the patient (as though you expect him to hear what you say)
Refrain from saying anything you would not want the patient to hear
Touch the patient frequently (to communicate caring)

Nursing Observations

Observe the level of consciousness (to determine when his communication ability
    reaches partial incapacity)

Health Teaching

Explain the reasons for and intended effect of the therapy (to communicate caring and
    reduce emotional trauma)

EVALUATION
Record actual outcome

PARTIAL INCAPACITY TO COMMUNICATE NEEDS[69,216,448,512,679]

ASSESSMENT

Data Collection

Subjective Data
- Person relates attempts at communicating needs, requests assistance with communications

  May express feelings of frustration or anger

Objective Data
- Person exhibits behavior such as any of the following:

  Difficulty forming words or bringing forth voice sounds

  May be able only to blink the eyelids or shake the head for yes and no answers

  Difficulty organizing words into phrases and sentences

  Difficulty selecting the correct words to describe what he wants to say

  Spoken words jumbled and unrecognizable

  Simply repeats what has just been said

  Weak voice sounds

  Tremulous, jerky speech

  Lisping

  Slow, one-syllable-at-a-time speech

  Sing-song, writhing, up-and-down speech

  Thick-slurred speech

  Choppy, stuttering speech

  Uncoordinated speech with involuntary disorganized mouth and tongue movements

  Spastic, hesitant speech

  Cannot hear at all

  Can hear only with difficulty

  Can hear the spoken words of others clearly, but they are received as jumbled messages having no meaning

  Cannot hear messages sent from a close distance but hears distant messages well

  Cannot understand the language of the sender of the message

  Difficulty differentiating similarly shaped letters in a word

  Can visualize an object on paper but is unable to determine what it is

  Holds books and papers upside down or sideways

  May refuse to attempt to read

  Difficulty writing sentences that express a meaningful idea

  Difficulty writing legibly

Data Analysis

Nursing Diagnosis

PARTIAL INCAPACITY TO COMMUNICATE NEEDS: Being capable of but needing assistance with the expression of one's needs through the exchange of thoughts and ideas with others

Common Etiology (Stressors)

BIRTH DEFECTS: Cerebral palsy, cleft lip, cleft palate, deafness, developmental deficit, dyslexia

DISEASES: Aphasia, apraxia, autism, carcinoma, (laryngeal, tracheal and oral), cerebrovascular disease, deafness, Guillain-Barré syndrome, myasthenia gravis, organic brain syndrome, otosclerosis, Parkinson's disease, senility

INJURIES: Cerebral concussion, drug overdose, mandibular fracture, oral burn wound

SIGNS AND SYMPTOMS: Confusion, delusions, dysphagia, dyspnea (severe), hoarseness, laryngeal edema, laryngeal spasm, pain (especially severe)

HEALTH CARE FACTORS: *Diagnostic procedure:* Nasal intubation for diagnostic procedure, bronchoscopy, gastric analysis, gastroscopy. *Drug Therapy:* Sedative, tranquilizer drugs.

Medical therapy: Electroconvulsive therapy, gastric lavage, heated mist inhalation therapy, intermittent positive-pressure breathing, nasal packing, nasogastric suction, oxygen therapy. *Surgical therapy:* Anesthesia. *Surgical procedures:* Esophagectomy. parotidectomy, pharyngotomy, reconstruction procedure for mouth disorders (cleft, lip/palate, harelip), tongue excision, tonsilectomy, tracheostomy, tympanoplasty, vocal cordectomy, wiring of a mandibular fracture

DEVELOPMENTAL PHASES: Toddler, old age

LIFESTYLE: Foreign language

MAJOR PATHOPHYSIOLOGIC FACTORS CAUSING THE PROBLEM: Loss of communication abilities occurs when there is damage to the speech center of the brain, the temporal and frontal lobes; when there is paralysis or poor coordination of the muscles of articulation involving the lips or tongue; when auditory loss prevents a person from hearing his own voice; when air passing through a tracheostomy prevents stimulation of the vocal cords by normal passage of air over that organ; when weakness reduces respiratory volume, decreasing air flow over the vocal cords; when malformation of the tongue, mouth or palate prevents normal formation of speech through sound; when there is disease of the larynx; when there is disease or damage of the muscle-coordinating areas of the brain (extrapyramidal)

PLANNING

Unmet Needs

Comfort, protection from physical harm, protection from psychologic threat, dependence, acceptance, caring and communicating relationships, independence, increased learning

Expected Outcome

Adequate expression of messages with or without substitute speech methods, such as writing and gesturing

Good attention and appropriate action responses to messages sent

Correct feedback of messages received

NURSING INTERVENTIONS

Nursing Treatments

Anticipate needs (such as the need for food, fluids, elimination, wanted items, and clean linens, to reduce the person's frustration level)

Approach unhurriedly

Demonstrate calmness

Reassure verbally

Listen attentively

Provide an atmosphere of acceptance

Provide frequent contact with the person

Arrange geographic placement (so the patient can see the nurses)

Provide quiet

Ask simple, direct questions

Encourage simple signal-language during impaired communication

Limit communication to one person at a time

Give one direction at a time

Repeat the message until it is understood

Limit the conversation to short discussions

Use simple words and short sentences

Use single-word communications

Provide objects related to the message

Give important messages only when the patient is receptive

Wait for a response to one message before delivering another

Refrain from asking the patient to repeat the message too often

Refrain from shouting at persons with communication disorders

Allow time for thought comprehension

Limit patient use of the telephone (if comprehension or hearing is impaired)
Provide an alternative method of communication appropriate to the person's specific
  needs and abilities (such as picture cards of objects, words-and-phrases cards, writing
  pad and pencil, alphabet letters for word composition)
  OR
Communicate by gesture
  OR
Provide a language interpreter (if the person speaks a foreign language)
Avoid verbal communications (if the person is deaf and cannot lip-read)
Avoid written communication (if writing or word comprehension is impaired)
Offer reading material with familiar content (if reading reception is impaired)
Read to the patient
Correct misinterpreted messages immediately
Obtain feedback of the communicated message
Touch the patient judiciously (for he may misinterpret the intended message)
Solicit the family's assistance in understanding the patient's speech
Make a referral (to a speech therapist)

Nursing Observations
Observe performance level and problems involved in completing the task (of communi-
  cating)
Observe for an excessive stress level (resulting from the impaired communications)

Health Teaching
Advise that communications be delayed during fatigue
Describe those behaviors that usually occur in communication impairment (frustration,
  embarrassment, irritation)
Explain that communication should be encouraged despite impairment
Explain that ill persons are often hypersensitive
Expalin that one's face should be kept visible when speaking to a deaf person
Instruct to use simple words when speaking with persons having impaired communica-
  tion reception
Recommend the use of slow, distinct speech with persons having impaired communica-
  tion reception
Explain that questions need to be phrased for yes and no answers when there is im-
  paired speech delivery
Explain that the tracheostomy must be covered in order to speak
Recommend the use of a typewriter for a person unable to write
Explain the importance of correct message interpretation
Explain the causes of the health problem
Explain the reason for and intended effect of the therapy
Explain the importance of wearing a Medic Alert tag

EVALUATION
Record actual outcome

8 Nursing Diagnoses of HYGIENE DEFICITS

Domain of Nursing Expertise: Hygiene Deficits

This chapter covers that sphere of nursing knowledge and skill related to problems of limitations that render a person incapable of or ineffective in performing the cleanliness activities a person usually performs for himself or for dependent persons. Such limitations result from illness, injury, disability, infirmity, developmental changes, or knowledge deficits.

Views of Nursing Leaders That Support This Domain of Nursing Expertise

The unique function of the nurse is to "assist the individual, sick or well, in the performance of those activities contributing to health or recovery (or to a peaceful death) that he would perform unaided if he had the necessary strength, will or knowledge." The nurse is to assist the client to carry out the plan of care prescribed for him by the physician.

Virginia Henderson [220:34]

King defines nursing as a process of action, reaction, interaction, and transaction whereby nurses assist people of any age group, to meet their basic needs in performing activities of daily living and to cope with health and illness at some particular point in the life cycle.

Imogene King [267:20]

Nursing is conceptualized as an art and as a body of knowledge. Knowledge required for general or health nursing is described as sanitary knowledge or hygiene.

Florence Nightingale [379:66]

Nurses manage and maintain required self-care continuously for persons who are totally incapacitated. In other instances, nurses help persons to maintain required self-care by performing some, but not all, measures . . . guiding individuals as they gradually move toward self care.

Nursing is perhaps best described as the giving of direct assistance to a person, as required, because of the person's specific inabilities in self-care resulting from a situation of personal health. . . . It is the personal care which adults give to themselves, including attention to ordinary health requirements, and the following of the medical directives of their physicians.

Dorothea Orem [380:1-2, 379:69]

Self-Care Deficits in General Hygiene

INCAPACITY TO PERFORM PERSONAL HYGIENE[159,362,366]

ASSESSMENT

Data Collection

Subjective Data
• Person may or may not relate being able to carry out general hygiene

Objective Data
• Person exhibits behavior such as minimal, ineffective, or no body movement, makes no attempt at carrying out self-bathing or hair, nail, mouth, and skin care

Data Analysis

Nursing Diagnosis
INCAPACITY TO PERFORM PERSONAL HYGIENE: Being incapable of daily cleansing and care of the body and requiring total assistance with such activities

Common Etiology (Stressors)
BIRTH DEFECTS: Cerebral palsy, developmental deficit, Down's syndrome, duchenne's muscular dystrophy, hydrocephalus
DISEASES: Autism, blindness, brain tumor, cachexia, carcinoma, cerebrovascular accident, congestive heart failure, diabetic ketoacidosis, encephalitis, Friedreich's ataxia, Guillain-Barré syndrome, Hodgkin's disease, Laennec's cirrhosis, leukemia, major depression, meningitis, multiple sclerosis, myasthenia gravis, myocardial infarction, organic brain syndrome, osteoarthritis, Parkinson's disease, posterolateral sclerosis, psychosis, renal failure, retinal detachment, rheumatoid arthritis, senility, subarachnoid hemorrhage, subdural hematoma, Sydenham's chorea
INJURIES: Burn wound, cerebral concussion, bone fracture, fracture and compression of the spinal cord, poisoning, traumatic amputation
SIGNS AND SYMPTOMS: Confusion, convulsions, dizziness, dyspnea, hallucinations, memory loss, pain, paralysis, joint swelling, vertigo, weakness
HEALTH CARE FACTORS: *Drug therapy:* Narcotics, sedatives, tranquilizers. *Medical therapy:* Casting, traction. *Surgical therapy:* Surgery of any kind. *Surgical procedures:* Amputation, replantation of digits, tenoplasty of hand. *Surgical incision:* Painful surgical incision
DEVELOPMENTAL PHASES: Old age
MAJOR PATHOPHYSIOLOGIC FACTORS CAUSING THE PROBLEM: Incapacity to perform activities of daily living can result from any of the following: decreased cardiac output, impaired oxygenation of tissue cells, organ degeneration or damage, impaired transmission of impulses from nerves to muscles, accumulation of toxic metabolic by-products, disrupted cerebral chemical/neuronal balance, tissue function impaired by the inflammatory process, brain cell damage or deficient development

PLANNING

Unmet Needs
Comfort, cleanliness, dependence, increased learning

Expected Outcome
Clean hair, eyes, ears, nose, skin, nails, mouth, teeth
No unpleasant body or breath odor, no unpleasant taste

NURSING INTERVENTIONS

Nursing Treatments
Acknowledge dependency
Anticipate needs

Provide privacy
Drape for warmth
Bathe daily (unless the person is aged or has a skin disorder)
Brush and comb the hair
Brush and floss the teeth
Clean the dentures, the nails, the eyes
Clear nasal secretions
Apply after-bath powder (if not lubricating the skin)
Apply an antiperspirant to the axillary region
Lubricate the skin with baby oil, bath oil, or body lotion

Nursing Observations
Inspect the skin for breakdown
Inspect for signs of (skin) irritation
Test the skin for impaired feeling perception
Inspect the skin for infectious lesions and for color
Palpate the skin for temperature
Inspect for impaired circulation
Test motor function
Inspect the joints for abnormalities
Observe for readiness to assume self-care

Health Teaching
Explain the reason for and intended effect of the hygiene (personal comfort, prevention
of disease)

EVALUATION

Record actual outcome

PARTIAL INCAPACITY TO PERFORM PERSONAL HYGIENE[159,362,366]

ASSESSMENT

Data Collection

Subjective Data
• Person relates attempts at self-bathing and caring for hair, nails, mouth, and skin
• Requests assistance to complete self-care
  May complain of fatigue before completing hygiene

Objective Data
• Person exhibits behavior such as struggling to retrieve hygiene supplies, reaching body
  parts, or manipulating hygiene tools

Data Analysis

Nursing Diagnosis
PARTIAL INCAPACITY TO PERFORM PERSONAL HYGIENE: Being capable of but needing assistance
  with cleanliness and care of one's body

Common Etiology (Stressors)
BIRTH DEFECTS: Blindness, cerebral palsy, developmental deficit, Down's syndrome, Duchenne's muscular dystrophy
DISEASES: Aortic insufficiency, aortic stenosis, aplastic anemia, blindness, bursitis, cachexia,
  carcinoma, cataracts, cerebrovascular accident, congestive heart failure, diplopia, encephalitis, Friedreich's ataxia, Guillain-Barré syndrome, Hodgkin's disease, Laennec's
  cirrhosis, leukemia, major depression, manic–depressive psychosis, multiple sclerosis,
  myasthenia gravis, myocardial infarction, organic brain syndrome, osteoarthritis, Par-

kinson's disease, posterolateral sclerosis, psychosis, retinal detachment, rheumatoid arthritis, senility, Sydenham's chorea

INJURIES: Back strain, burn wound, cerebral concussion, dislocation, bone fracture, fracture and compression of the spinal cord, herniated intervertebral disc, traumatic amputation

SIGNS AND SYMPTOMS: Blurred vision, difficulty concentrating, confusion, diplopia, dizziness, dyspnea, memory loss, pain, joint swelling, vertigo, weakness

HEALTH CARE FACTORS: *Drug therapy:* Narcotics, sedatives, tranquilizers. *Medical therapy:* Casting, intravenous infusion, traction, blood transfusion. *Surgical therapy:* Surgery of any kind. *Surgical procedures:* Amputation, replantation of digits, tenoplasty of hand. *Surgical incision:* Painful surgical incision

DEVELOPMENTAL PHASES: Old age

MAJOR PATHOPHYSIOLOGIC FACTORS CAUSING THE PROBLEM: Partial incapacity to perform activities of daily living can result from any of the following: decreased cardiac output, impaired oxygenation of tissue cells, organ degeneration or damage, impaired transmission of impulses from nerves to muscles, accumulation of toxic metabolic by-products, disrupted cerebral chemical/neuronal balance, tissue function impaired by the inflammation process, brain cell damage or deficient development

PLANNING

Unmet Needs
Comfort, cleanliness, dependence, independence, increased learning

Expected Outcome
Clean hair, eyes, ears, nose, skin, nails, mouth, teeth
No unpleasant body or breath odor, no unpleasant taste
Person performs at expected level of independent self-care

NURSING INTERVENTIONS

Nursing Treatments
Provide assistance until the person is fully able to assume self-care
Provide privacy
Drape for warmth
Approach unhurriedly
Provide needed supplies
Assist with hygiene
Encourage self-performance (partial self-hygiene)

Nursing Observations
Observe performance level and problems involved in completing tasks

Health Teaching
Teach how to use assistive grooming devices
Explain the reason for and intended effect of the hygiene

EVALUATION
Record actual outcome

UNSKILLED AT PERSONAL HYGIENE[159,362,366]

ASSESSMENT

Data Collection

Subjective Data
• Person's discussion or questions indicate a need for additional information, clarification, or validation of information about performing the task of maintaining general hygiene

OR
* Person's lack of questions or comments indicates not wanting information or not knowing enough to seek information about performing the task of maintaining general hygiene
Person may not know:
Why hygiene is important
The methods used to achieve hygiene

Objective Data
* Person cannot correctly demonstrate how to:
Bathe
Apply antiperspirant
Clean the mouth, nails, ears, eyes, nares, hair
Lubricate the skin

Data Analysis

Nursing Diagnosis
UNSKILLED AT PERSONAL HYGIENE: Being nonproficient, with or without knowledge, in the performance of the specific task of practicing health habits of body and individual cleanliness

Common Etiology (Stressors)
HEALTH CARE FACTORS: Lack of or incorrect health instruction, lack of health-skill experience
DEVELOPMENTAL PHASES: Infancy, toddler, preschooler

PLANNING

Unmet Needs
Comfort, cleanliness, protection from physical harm, dependence, mastery and competence in skills, independence, increased learning

Expected Outcome
Clean hair, eyes, ears, nose, skin, nails, mouth, teeth
No unpleasant body or breath odor, no unpleasant taste
Correct verbal feedback of the information taught
Correct return demonstration of how to bathe, to apply antiperspirant, to clean the mouth, nails, ears, eyes, nares and hair, to lubricate the skin

NURSING INTERVENTIONS

Nursing Treatments
Provide temporary assistance until the skill is learned
Bathe daily
Apply an antiperspirant to axillary region
Brush and comb the hair
Shampoo the hair
Brush and floss the teeth
Clean the nails, dentures, ears, eyes
Clear nasal secretions
Lubricate the skin with baby oil, bath oil, or body lotion (after dampening the skin)
Encourage self-performance

Nursing Observations
Observe for readiness to assume self-care
Determine teaching effectiveness by testing, verbal feedback, and return demonstration

Health Teaching
Advise daily bathing
Recommend a daily change of clean clothing
Inform that clean linens are essential
Advise frequent hair brushing
Instruct to maintain skin cleanliness

Explain the need for nail cleanliness, the need for frequent hair shampooing
Teach how to brush and floss the teeth correctly
Inform that cleanliness is basic to health
Explain the reason for and intended effect of the hygiene

EVALUATION

Record actual outcome

UNSKILLED AT HYGIENE METHODS FOR DEPENDENT PERSON[159,366,444]

ASSESSMENT

Data Collection

Subjective Data

• Person's discussion or questions indicate a need for additional information, clarification, or validation of information about performing the task of keeping another person clean
  OR
• Person's lack of questions or comments indicates not wanting information or not knowing enough to seek information about performing the task of keeping another person clean

Objective Data

• Person cannot correctly demonstrate how to:
   Give a bed or tub bath, shampoo hair when the person is in bed or has limited mobility
   Give skin and nail care
   Provide oral hygiene
   Change the person's clothing
   Change bed linens when the bed is occupied

Data Analysis

Nursing Diagnosis

UNSKILLED AT HYGIENE METHODS FOR DEPENDENT PERSON: Being nonproficient, with or without knowledge, in the performance of the specific task of maintaining body cleanliness of a dependent person

Common Etiology (Stressors)

HEALTH CARE FACTORS: Lack of health instruction, lack of health-skill experience

PLANNING

Unmet Needs

Comfort, cleanliness, protection from physical harm, dependence, mastery and competence in skills, independence, increased learning

Expected Outcome

Clean hair, eyes, ears, nose, skin, nails, mouth, teeth
No unpleasant body or breath odor, no unpleasant taste
Correct verbal feedback of the information taught
Correct return demonstration of how to give a bed or tub bath, shampoo hair in or out of bed, give skin and nail care, change a person's clothes, change an occupied bed

NURSING INTERVENTIONS

Nursing Treatments

Provide temporary assistance until the skill is learned
Encourage the person or family to ask questions

Nursing Observations

Observe for readiness to assume self-care (of the dependent person)

Determine teaching effectiveness by testing, verbal feedback, and return demonstration

Health Teaching

Inform that cleanliness is basic to health

Advise daily bathing (unless the person is aged or has a skin disorder)

Teach how to give a bed bath

Inform that clean linens are essential

Recommend a daily change of clean clothing

Teach how to brush and floss the teeth correctly

Explain the need for nail cleanliness

Instruct to maintain skin cleanliness, to lubricate the skin, to inspect the skin

Advise frequent hair brushing

Explain the need for frequent hair shampooing

Explain how to shampoo the hair

Teach how to make an occupied bed

Recommend methods for preparing a sick room at home

Explain the reason for and intended effect of the hygiene

EVALUATION

Record actual outcome

Self-Care Deficits in Hygiene for Specific Body Parts

INCAPACITY TO PERFORM HAIR CARE[363,366]

ASSESSMENT

Data Collection

Subjective Data

• Person may or may not relate being unable to carry out hair care

Objective Data

• Person exhibits behaviors such as minimal, ineffective, or no body movement and makes no visible attempt at washing, combing, brushing hair, or applying conditioners

Data Analysis

Nursing Diagnosis

INCAPACITY TO PERFORM HAIR CARE: Being incapable of the care and cleanliness of one's hair and requiring total assistance with such activities

Common Etiology (Stressors)

BIRTH DEFECTS: Blindness, cerebral palsy, clubhand, developmental deficits, Down's syndrome, Duchenne's muscular dystrophy

DISEASES: Autism, blindness, cachexia, carcinoma, cataracts, cerebrovascular accident, congestive heart failure, diplopia, encephalitis, Friedreich's ataxia, Guillain-Barré syndrome, Hodgkin's disease, Laennec's cirrhosis, leukemia, major depression, manic–depressive psychosis, meningitis, multiple sclerosis, myasthenia gravis, myocardial infarction, organic brain syndrome, osteoarthritis, Parkinson's disease, posterolateral sclerosis, psychosis, retinal detachment, rheumatoid arthritis, senility, subarachnoid hemorrhage, subdural hematoma, Sydenham's chorea

INJURIES: Back strain, burn wound, cerebral concussion, dislocation, bone fracture, fracture and compression of the spinal cord, herniated intervertebral disc, poisoning, traumatic amputation

SIGNS AND SYMPTOMS: Difficulty concentrating, confusion, convulsions, diplopia, dizziness, dyspnea, hallucinations, memory loss, pain, paralysis, joint swelling, vertigo, weakness

HEALTH CARE FACTORS: *Medical therapy:* Casting, traction. *Surgical therapy:* Surgery of any kind. *Surgical procedures:* Amputation, replantation of digits, tenoplasty of hand. *Surgical incision:* Painful surgical incision

DEVELOPMENTAL PHASES: Old age

MAJOR PATHOPHYSIOLOGIC FACTORS CAUSING THE PROBLEM: Incapacity to perform activities of daily living can result from any of the following: decreased cardiac output, impaired oxygenation of tissue cells, organ degeneration or damage, impaired transmission of impulses from nerves to muscles, accumulation of toxic metabolic by-products, disrupted cerebral chemical/neuronal balance, tissue function impaired by the inflammatory process, brain cell damage or deficient development

PLANNING

Unmet Needs

Comfort, cleanliness, dependence, increased learning

Expected Outcome

Clean, brushed, combed, and manageable hair

NURSING INTERVENTIONS

Nursing Treatments

Acknowledge dependency
Anticipate needs
Handle gently
Brush and comb the hair (in a comfortable style)
Shampoo the hair
Moisten the hair with conditioning formula
Soften the hair with a cream rinse (or other patient-requested hair preparation)

Nursing Observations

Inspect the hair for abnormalities (dryness, thinning, matting, pediculi, and nits)
Palpate for tenderness (of the scalp)
Observe for readiness to assume self-care

Health Teaching

Teach how to use assistive grooming devices
Explain the reason for and intended effect of the care

EVALUATION

Record actual outcome

PARTIAL INCAPACITY TO PERFORM HAIR CARE[362,366]

ASSESSMENT

Data Collection

Subjective Data

• Person relates attempts at hair care
• Requests assistance to complete hair care
  May complain of fatigue before completing hair care

Objective Data
- Person exhibits behavior such as having difficulty retrieving supplies for hair care, reaching toward the head, and manipulating the comb, brush, hair spray, etc., and may spill shampoo, misdirect water when washing the hair

Data Analysis

Nursing Diagnosis

PARTIAL INCAPACITY TO PERFORM HAIR CARE: Being capable of but needing assistance with cleansing and grooming one's hair

Common Etiology (Stressors)

BIRTH DEFECTS: Cerebral palsy, clubhand, developmental deficit, Down's syndrome, Duchenne's muscular dystrophy

DISEASES: Blindness, bursitis, cachexia, carcinoma, cataracts, cerebrovascular accident, congestive heart failure, diplopia, encephalitis, Friedreich's ataxia, Guillain-Barré syndrome, Hodgkin's disease, Laennec's cirrhosis, leukemia, major depression, meningitis, multiple sclerosis, myasthenia gravis, myocardial infarction, organic brain syndrome, osteoarthritis, Parkinson's disease, posterolateral sclerosis, psychosis, retinal detachment, rheumatoid arthritis, senility, Sydenham's chorea

INJURIES: Burn wound, cerebral concussion, dislocation, bone fracture, fracture and compression of the spinal cord, traumatic amputation

SIGNS AND SYMPTOMS: Blurred vision, confusion, diplopia, dizziness, dyspnea, fatigue, hallucinations, memory loss, pain, joint swelling, vertigo, weakness

HEALTH CARE FACTORS: *Medical therapy:* Casting, intravenous infusion, traction, blood transfusion. *Surgical therapy:* Surgery of any kind. *Surgical procedures:* Amputation, replantation of digits, tenoplasty of hand. *Surgical incision:* Painful surgical incision

DEVELOPMENTAL PHASES: Old age

MAJOR PATHOPHYSIOLOGIC FACTORS CAUSING THE PROBLEM: Partial incapacity to perform activities of daily living can result from any of the following: decreased cardiac output, impaired oxygenation of tissue cells, organ degeneration or damage, impaired transmission of impulses from nerves to muscles, accumulation of toxic metabolic byproducts, disrupted cerebral chemical/neuronal balance, tissue function impaired by the inflammatory process, brain cell damage or deficient development

PLANNING

Unmet Needs
Comfort, cleanliness, dependence, independence, increased learning

Expected Outcome
Clean, brushed, combed, manageable hair
Person performs at an expected level of independent self-care

NURSING INTERVENTIONS

Nursing Treatments
Provide assistance until the person is fully able to assume self-care
Anticipate needs (for assistance)
Assist with hair hygiene (as needed)
Encourage self-performance

Nursing Observations
Inspect the hair for abnormalities (dryness, thinning, matting, pediculi, and nits)
Observe performance level and problems involved in completing tasks

Health Teaching
Teach how to use assistive grooming devices

EVALUATION
Record actual outcome

UNSKILLED AT HAIR CARE[362,366]

ASSESSMENT
Data Collection
Subjective Data
- Person's discussion or questions indicate a need for additional information, clarification, or validation of information about performing the task of cleaning and grooming the hair
  OR
- Person's lack of questions or comments indicates not wanting information or not knowing enough to seek information about performing the task of cleaning and grooming hair
  Person may not know:
    Why hair care is important
    The methods used to achieve hair care

Objective Data
- Person cannot correctly demonstrate how to:
    Comb and brush the hair
    Shampoo hair
    Apply softening and conditioning formulas

Data Analysis
Nursing Diagnosis
UNSKILLED AT HAIR CARE: Being nonproficient, with or without knowledge, in the performance of the specific task of cleansing and caring for the hair

Common Etiology (Stressors)
HEALTH CARE FACTORS: Lack of instruction, lack of health-skill experience
DEVELOPMENTAL PHASES: Infancy, toddler, preschooler

PLANNING
Unmet Needs
Comfort, cleanliness, protection from physical harm, dependence, mastery and competence in skills, independence, increased learning

Expected Outcome
Clean, brushed, combed, and manageable hair
Correct verbal feedback of the information taught
Correct return demonstration of how to brush, comb, shampoo, and condition hair

NURSING INTERVENTIONS
Nursing Treatments
Provide temporary assistance until the skill is learned
Brush and comb the hair (in a comfortable style)
Shampoo the hair
Soften the hair with a cream rinse
Moisten the hair with conditioning formula
Encourage self-performance

Nursing Observations
Inspect the hair for abnormalities (dryness, thinning, matting, pediculi, and nits)
Observe for readiness to assume self-care
Determine teaching effectiveness by testing, verbal feedback, and return demonstration

Health Teaching
Inform that cleanliness is basic to health
Advise frequent hair brushing
Advise limited use of hair spray
Explain the need for frequent hair shampooing

Explain how to shampoo hair
Recommend the use of dry shampoo (when unable to wash the hair)
Instruct to wash combs and brushes with each shampoo
Explain the reason for and intended effect of the hygiene

EVALUATION

Record actual outcome

INCAPACITY TO PERFORM NAIL CARE[362,366]

ASSESSMENT

Data Collection

Subjective Data
• Person may or may not relate being unable to carry out nail care

Objective Data
• Person exhibits behavior such as minimal, ineffective, or no body movement and makes no visible attempt at cleaning, shaping, and trimming nails

Data Analysis

Nursing Diagnosis
INCAPACITY TO PERFORM NAIL CARE: Being incapable of cleansing and caring for one's nails and requiring total assistance with such activities

Common Etiology (Stressors)
BIRTH DEFECTS: Blindness, cerebral palsy, clubhand, developmental deficit, Duchenne's muscular dystrophy
DISEASES: Autism, blindness, cachexia, carcinoma, cataracts, cerebrovascular accident, congestive heart failure, diplopia, Friedreich's ataxia, Guillain-Barré syndrome, Hodgkin's disease, Laennec's cirrhosis, leukemia, major depression, manic–depressive psychosis, multiple sclerosis, myasthenia gravis, myocardial infarction, organic brain syndrome, osteoarthritis, Parkinson's disease, posterolateral sclerosis, psychosis, retinal detachment, rheumatoid arthritis, senility, subarachnoid hemorrhage, subdural hematoma, Sydenham's chorea
INJURIES: Burn wound, cerebral concussion, bone fracture, fracture and compression of the spinal cord, traumatic amputation
SIGNS AND SYMPTOMS: Blurred vision, difficulty concentrating, confusion, diplopia, dizziness, dyspnea, hallucinations, memory loss, pain, joint swelling, vertigo, weakness
HEALTH CARE FACTORS: *Medical therapy:* Casting, traction. *Surgical therapy:* Surgery of any kind. *Surgical procedures:* Amputation. *Surgical incision:* Painful surgical incision
DEVELOPMENTAL PHASES: Old age
MAJOR PATHOPHYSIOLOGIC FACTORS CAUSING THE PROBLEM: Incapacity to perform activities of daily living can result from any of the following: decreased cardiac output, impaired oxygenation of tissue cells, organ degeneration or damage, impaired transmission of impulses from nerves to muscles, accumulation of toxic metabolic by-products, disrupted cerebral chemical/neuronal balance, tissue function impaired by the inflammatory process, brain cell damage or deficient development

PLANNING

Unmet Needs
Comfort, cleanliness, dependence, increased learning

Expected Outcome
Clean, shaped, trimmed nails
Unbroken, smooth cuticles

NURSING INTERVENTIONS

Nursing Treatments
Acknowledge dependency
Anticipate needs
Clean the nails
File the nails in one direction and only on the underside
Soak the nails in warm oil
Lubricate the skin (around the nails) with body lotion

Nursing Observations
Inspect the nails for abnormalities (deformities, thickness, splitting, discoloration), for signs of infection
Observe for cyanosis
Observe for readiness to assume self-care

Health Teaching
Explain the reason for and intended effect of the care
Teach how to use assistive grooming devices

EVALUATION

Record actual outcome

PARTIAL INCAPACITY TO PERFORM NAIL CARE[362,366]

ASSESSMENT

Data Collection

Subjective Data
• Person relates attempts at cleaning, shaping, and trimming nails
• Requests assistance to complete nail care

Objective Data
• Person exhibits behavior such as struggling to retrieve supplies for nail care or to manipulate scissors, emory board, etc.

Data Analysis

Nursing Diagnosis
PARTIAL INCAPACITY TO PERFORM NAIL CARE: Being capable of but needing assistance with cleansing and caring for one's nails

Common Etiology (Stressors)
BIRTH DEFECTS: Blindness, cerebral palsy, clubhand, developmental deficit, Down's syndrome, Duchenne's muscular dystrophy
DISEASES: Autism, blindness, cachexia, carcinoma, cataracts, cerebrovascular accident, congestive heart failure, dipoplia, Friedreich's ataxia, Guillain-Barré syndrome, Hodgkin's disease, Laennec's cirrhosis, leukemia, major depression, manic-depressive psychosis, multiple sclerosis, myasthenia gravis, myocardial infarction, organic brain syndrome, osteoarthritis, Parkinson's disease, posterolateral sclerosis, psychosis, retinal detachment, rheumatoid arthritis, senility, Sydenham's chorea
INJURIES: Burn wound, cerebral concussion, dislocation, bone fracture, fracture and compression of the spinal cord, traumatic amputation
SIGNS AND SYMPTOMS: Blurred vision, difficulty concentrating, confusion, diplopia, dizziness, dyspnea, hallucinations, memory loss, pain, joint swelling, vertigo, weakness
HEALTH CARE FACTORS: *Medical therapy*: Casting, intravenous infusion, traction, blood transfusion. *Surgical therapy*: Surgery of any kind. *Surgical procedures*: Amputation. *Surgical incision*: Painful surgical incision

DEVELOPMENTAL PHASES: Old age

MAJOR PATHOPHYSIOLOGIC FACTORS CAUSING THE PROBLEM: Partial incapacity to perform activities of daily living can result from any of the following: decreased cardiac output, impaired oxygenation of tissue cells, organ degeneration or damage, impaired transmission of impulses from nerves to muscles, accumulation of toxic metabolic by-products, disrupted cerebral chemical/neuronal balance, tissue function impaired by the inflammatory process, brain cell damage or deficient development

PLANNING

Unmet Needs

Comfort, cleanliness, dependence, independence, increased learning

Expected Outcome

Clean, shaped, trimmed nails
Unbroken, smooth cuticles
Person performs at an expected level of independent self-care

NURSING INTERVENTIONS

Nursing Treatments

Provide assistance until the person is fully able to assume self-care
Anticipate needs (for assistance)
Assist with nail hygiene (as needed)
Encourage self-performance

Nursing Observations

Inspect the nails for abnormalities (deformities, thickness, splitting, discoloration), for signs of infection
Observe for cyanosis
Observe for performance level and problems involved in completing tasks

Health Teaching

Teach how to use assistive grooming devices

EVALUATION

Record actual outcome

UNSKILLED AT NAIL CARE[362,366]

ASSESSMENT

Data Collection

Subjective Data

• Person's discussion or questions indicate a need for additional information, clarification, or validation of information about performing the task of nail care
  OR
• Person's lack of questions or comments indicates not wanting information or not knowing enough to seek information about performing the task of nail care

Objective Data

• Person cannot correctly demonstrate how to:
  Clean the nails
  Shape the nails
  Properly lubricate the nails
  Care for the cuticles

Data Analysis

Nursing Diagnosis

UNSKILLED AT NAIL CARE: Being nonproficient, with or without knowledge, in the performance of the specific task of cleansing and caring for one's nails

Common Etiology (Stressors)

HEALTH CARE FACTORS: Lack of health instruction, lack of health-skill experience

DEVELOPMENTAL PHASES: Infancy, toddler, preschooler, adolescent

PLANNING

Unmet Needs

Comfort, cleanliness, protection from physical harm, dependence, mastery and competence in skills, independence, increased learning

Expected Outcome

Clean, shaped, trimmed nails

Unbroken, smooth cuticle

Correct verbal feedback of the information taught

Correct return demonstration of how to clean, shape, and trim nails

NURSING INTERVENTIONS

Nursing Treatments

Provide temporary assistance until the skill is learned

Clean the nails

Soak the nails in warm oil

File the nails in one direction and only on the underside

Encourage self-performance

Nursing Observations

Inspect the nails for abnormalities (clubbing, splitting, discoloration)

Observe for readiness to assume self-care

Determine teaching effectiveness by testing, verbal feedback, and return demonstration

Health Teaching

Advise that lanolin be applied to brittle nails

Explain how to file the nails correctly, that nails should be soaked before trimming

Explain the need for nail cleanliness

Instruct to cut the toenails straight across

Explain the reason for and intended effect of the care (clean, healthy nails)

EVALUATION

Record actual outcome

INCAPACITY TO PERFORM ORAL HYGIENE[362,366,444]

ASSESSMENT

Data Collection

Subjective Data

• Person may or may not relate being unable to carry out oral hygiene

Objective Data

• Person exhibits behavior such as minimal, ineffective or no body movement and makes no attempt at brushing and flossing teeth, washing whole or partial dentures, moisturizing lips and oral cavity

Data Analysis

Nursing Diagnosis

INCAPACITY TO PERFORM ORAL HYGIENE: Being incapable of carrying out procedures to cleanse the mouth and requiring total assistance with such activities

Common Etiology (Stressors)

BIRTH DEFECTS: Blindness, cerebral palsy, developmental deficit, Down's syndrome, Duchenne's muscular dystrophy, hydrocephalus

DISEASES: Aplastic anemia, autism, blindness, brain tumor, cachexia, carcinoma, cataracts, cerebrovascular accident, congestive heart failure, diabetic ketoacidosis, diplopia, eclampsia, encephalitis, Friedreich's ataxia, Guillain-Barré syndrome, Hodgkin's disease, Laennec's cirrhosis, leukemia, major depression, manic–depressive psychosis, meningitis, multiple sclerosis, myasthenia gravis, myocardial infarction, organic brain syndrome, osteoarthritis, Parkinson's disease, posterolateral sclerosis, psychosis, pulmonary edema, renal failure, retinal detachment, rheumatoid arthritis, senility, subarachnoid hemorrhage, subdural hematoma, Sydenham's chorea

INJURIES: Burn wound, cerebral concussion, dislocation, bone fracture, fracture and compression of the spinal cord, herniated intervertebral disc, poisoning, traumatic amputation

SIGNS AND SYMPTOMS: Blurred vision, difficulty concentrating, confusion, diplopia, dizziness, dyspnea, hallucinations, pain, paralysis, joint swelling, vertigo, weakness

HEALTH CARE FACTORS: *Medical therapy*: Casting, intravenous infusion, traction, blood transfusion. *Surgical therapy*: Surgery of any kind. *Surgical procedures*: Amputation. *Surgical incision*: Painful surgical incision

DEVELOPMENTAL PHASES: Old age

MAJOR PATHOPHYSIOLOGIC FACTORS CAUSING THE PROBLEM: Incapacity to perform activities of daily living can result from any of the following: decreased cardiac output, impaired oxygenation of tissue cells, organ degeneration or damage, impaired transmission of impulses from nerves to muscles, accumulation of toxic metabolic by-products, disrupted cerebral chemical/neuronal balance, tissue function impaired by the inflammatory process, brain cell damage or deficient development

PLANNING

Unmet Needs

Comfort, cleanliness, protection from physical harm, dependence, increased learning

Expected Outcome

Clean mouth and teeth
No unpleasant mouth odor or taste
Moist oral mucous membranes
Firm gums

NURSING INTERVENTIONS

Nursing Treatments

Acknowledge dependency
Anticipate needs
Brush and floss the teeth
Brush the tongue (if coated)
Massage the gums (with the rubber tip on a toothbrush or soft plastic pick)
Clean the dentures
Insert and remove the dentures (as needed)
Safeguard the patient's dentures
Lubricate the lips
Refresh with a mouth freshner or a mouthwash
Swab the mouth with diluted glycerine

Nursing Observations

Inspect the teeth for abnormalities (caries, cracking, discoloration, poor alignment), the gums for abnormalities (bleeding, inflammation, receding, swelling, discoloration)

Observe for readiness to assume self-care

Health Teaching

Explain the reason for and intended effect of the hygiene (that brushing and flossing prevent cavities and gum problems)

Teach how to brush and floss the teeth correctly, how to clean dentures

Teach how to massage the gums (with the rubber tip on a toothbrush or soft plastic pick)

EVALUATION

Record actual outcome

PARTIAL INCAPACITY TO PERFORM ORAL HYGIENE[362,366,444]

ASSESSMENT

Data Collection

Subjective Data

• Person relates attempts at brushing and flossing the teeth, washing whole or partial dentures, moisturizing the lips and oral cavity
• Requests assistance to complete self-care
  May complain of fatigue before completing oral hygiene

Objective Data

• Person exhibits behavior such as having difficulty retrieving supplies for oral hygiene and manipulating toothbrush, toothpaste, etc.

Data Analysis

Nursing Diagnosis

PARTIAL INCAPACITY TO PERFORM ORAL HYGIENE: Being capable of but needing assistance with procedures to cleanse the mouth

Common Etiology (Stressors)

BIRTH DEFECTS: Blindness, cerebral palsy, clubhand, developmental deficit, Down's syndrome, Duchenne's muscular dystrophy

DISEASES: Autism, blindness, brain tumor, cachexia, carcinoma, cataracts, cerebrovascular accident, congestive heart failure, diplopia, Friedreich's ataxia, Guillain-Barré syndrome, Hodgkin's disease, Laennec's cirrhosis, leukemia, major depression, manic–depressive psychosis, meningitis, multiple sclerosis, myasthenia gravis, myocardial infarction, organic brain syndrome, osteoarthritis, Parkinson's disease, posterolateral sclerosis, psychosis, renal failure, retinal detachment, rheumatoid arthritis, senility, Sydenham's chorea

INJURIES: Burn wound, cerebral concussion, dislocation, bone fracture, fracture and compression of the spinal cord, traumatic amputation

SIGNS AND SYMPTOMS: Blurred vision, difficulty concentrating, confusion, diplopia, dizziness, dyspnea, fatigue, hallucinations, memory loss, pain, joint swelling, vertigo, weakness

HEALTH AND CARE FACTORS: *Drug therapy:* Narcotics, sedatives, tranquilizers. *Medical therapy:* Casting, intravenous infusion, traction, blood transfusion. *Surgical therapy:* Surgery of any kind. *Surgical procedures:* Amputation. *Surgical incision:* Painful surgical incision

DEVELOPMENTAL PHASES: Old age

MAJOR PATHOPHYSIOLOGIC FACTORS CAUSING THE PROBLEM: Partial incapacity to perform activities of daily living can result from any of the following: decreased cardiac output, impaired oxygenation of tissue cells, organ degeneration or damage, impaired transmission of impulses from nerves to muscles, accumulation of toxic metabolic by-products, disrupted cerebral chemical/neuronal balance, tissue function impaired by the inflammatory process, brain cell damage or deficient development

PLANNING

Unmet Needs
Comfort, cleanliness, dependence, independence, increased learning

Expected Outcome
Clean mouth and teeth
No unpleasant mouth odor or taste
Moist oral mucous membranes
Firm gums
Person performs at an expected level of independent self-care

NURSING INTERVENTIONS

Nursing Treatments
Provide assistance until the person is fully able to assume self-care
Anticipate needs (for assistance)
Assist with oral hygiene (as needed)
Encourage self-performance

Nursing Observations
Inspect the teeth for abnormalities (caries, cracking, discoloration, poor alignment), the gums for abnormalities (bleeding, inflammation, receding, swelling, discoloration)
Observe performance level and problems involved in completing tasks

Health Teaching
Explain the reason for and intended effect of the hygiene (that brushing and flossing prevent cavities and gum problems)
Teach how to brush and floss the teeth correctly, how to clean dentures
Teach how to massage the gums (with the rubber tip on a toothbrush or soft plastic pick)
Teach how to use assistive grooming devices

EVALUATION

Record actual outcome

UNSKILLED AT ORAL HYGIENE[362,366,444]

ASSESSMENT

Data Collection

Subjective Data
• Person's discussion or questions indicate a need for additional information, clarification, or validation of information about performing the task of oral hygiene
    OR
• Person's lack of questions or comments indicates not wanting information or not knowing enough to seek information about performing the task of oral hygiene
    Person may not know:
        Why oral hygiene is important
        The methods used to prevent tooth decay and gum disease

Objective Data
• Person cannot correctly demonstrate how to:
  Brush the teeth
  Floss the teeth
  Use mouthwash
  Use a water jet
  Clean dentures
  Care for braces or a wired jaw
  May have unclean teeth, breath odor, bleeding gums, or gum hyperplasia

Data Analysis

Nursing Diagnosis

UNSKILLED AT ORAL HYGIENE: Being nonproficient, with or without knowledge, in the performance of the specific task of cleansing the mouth and teeth and stimulating the gums

Common Etiology (Stressors)

HEALTH CARE FACTORS: Lack of health instruction, lack of health-skill experience
DEVELOPMENTAL PHASES: Toddler, preschooler

PLANNING

Unmet Needs

Comfort, cleanliness, protection from physical harm, dependence, mastery and competence in skills, independence, increased learning

Expected Outcome

Clean mouth and teeth
No unpleasant mouth odor or taste
Moist oral mucous membranes
Firm gums
Correct verbal feedback of the information taught
Correct return demonstration of how to brush and floss the teeth, use mouthwash and a water jet, and/or clean dentures

NURSING INTERVENTIONS

Nursing Treatments

Provide temporary assistance until the skill is learned
Brush and floss the teeth
Clean the dentures
Refresh with mouth freshener, a mouthwash
Swab the mouth with diluted glycerine
Lubricate the lips
Provide a drinking straw (to suck in mouthwash when jaws are wired)
Make a referral (to a dentist for stained or decaying teeth or for bleeding gums)
Discourage smoking
Encourage self-performance

Nursing Observations

Inspect the teeth for abnormalities (caries, cracking, discoloration, poor alignment), the gums for abnormalites (bleeding, inflammation, receding, swelling, discoloration)
Observe for readiness to assume self-care
Determine teaching effectiveness by testing, verbal feedback, and return demonstration

Health Teaching

Inform that cleanliness is basic to health
Advise early and consistent use of the toothbrush
Advise mouth rinsing when brushing is inconvenient
Recommend the use of dental floss
Recommend that the tongue be brushed (if coated)
Teach how to brush and floss the teeth correctly

Teach how to massage the gums (with the rubber tip on the toothbrush or a soft plastic pick)

Teach how to clean dental braces (use a soft toothbrush and water jet)

Teach how to clean dentures

Explain the reason for and intended effect of the hygiene

EVALUATION

Record actual outcome

INCAPACITY TO PERFORM SKIN CARE[362,366]

ASSESSMENT

Data Collection

Subjective Data
• Person may or may not relate being unable to carry out skin care

Objective Data
• Person exhibits behavior such as minimal, ineffective, or no body movement, makes no attempt at washing, drying, moisturizing, or massaging the skin

Data Analysis

Nursing Diagnosis

INCAPACITY TO PERFORM SKIN CARE: Being incapable of carrying out procedures involving cleanliness and care of the skin and requiring total assistance with such activities

Common Etiology (Stressors)

BIRTH DEFECTS: Blindness, cerebral palsy, developmental deficit, Down's syndrome, Duchenne's muscular dystrophy, hydrocephalus

DISEASES: Autism, blindness, cachexia, carcinoma, cataracts, cerebrovascular accident, congestive heart failure, encephalitis, Friedreich's ataxia, Guillain-Barré syndrome, Hodgkin's disease, Laennec's cirrhosis, leukemia, major depression, manic–depressive psychosis, meningitis, multiple sclerosis, myasthenia gravis, myocardial infarction, organic brain syndrome, osteoarthritis, Parkinson's disease, posterolateral sclerosis, psychosis, renal failure, retinal detachment, rheumatoid arthritis, senility, subarachnoid hemorrhage, subdural hematoma, Sydenham's chorea

INJURIES: Burn wound, cerebral concussion, dislocation, bone fracture, fracture and compression of the spinal cord, herniated intervertebral disc, poisoning, traumatic amputation

SIGNS AND SYMPTOMS: Blurred vision, difficulty concentrating, confusion, convulsions, diplopia, dizziness, dyspnea, hallucinations, memory loss, pain, paralysis, joint swelling, vertigo, weakness

HEALTH CARE FACTORS: *Medical therapy:* Casting, intravenous infusion, traction, blood transfusion. *Surgical therapy:* Surgery of any kind. *Surgical procedures:* Amputation. *Surgical incision:* Painful surgical incision

DEVELOPMENTAL PHASES: Old age

MAJOR PATHOPHYSIOLOGIC FACTORS CAUSING THE PROBLEM: Incapacity to perform activities of daily living can result from any of the following: decreased cardiac output, impaired oxygenation of tissue cells, organ degeneration or damage, impaired transmission of impulses from nerves to muscles, accumulation of toxic metabolic by-products, disrupted cerebral chemical/neuronal balance, tissue function impaired by the inflammatory process, brain cell damage or deficient development

PLANNING

Unmet Needs

Comfort, cleanliness, protection from physical harm, dependence, increased learning

Expected Outcome
Clean, moisturized, comfortable skin

NURSING INTERVENTIONS

Nursing Treatments
Acknowledge dependency
Anticipate needs
Bathe daily (unless the person is aged or has a skin disorder)
Maintain dry, clean skin
Do not allow overlapping skin surfaces to touch
Massage gently or vigorously
Lubricate the skin with baby oil, bath oil, or body lotion (after dampening the skin)
Lubricate the skin with cocoa butter, glycerine, lanolin, mineral oil, or olive oil (if the skin is very dry and after dampening the skin)
Change the patient's position frequently
Maintain dry, clean linen, wrinkle-free sheets
Place on a flotation mattress, a silicone pad, an alternating pressure mattress, a sheepskin

Nursing Observations
Inspect the skin for breakdown, for infectious lesions, for color
Inspect for signs of irritation
Observe for evidence of pressure on the skin
Test the skin for impaired feeling perception
Palpate the skin for temperature
Observe for readiness to assume self-care

Health Teaching
Instruct to maintain skin cleanliness, to lubricate the skin, to inspect the skin
Explain the reason for and intended effect of the care

EVALUATION

Record actual outcome

PARTIAL INCAPACITY TO PERFORM SKIN CARE[362,366]

ASSESSMENT

Data Collection

Subjective Data
• Person relates attempts at cleansing and lubricating the skin

Objective Data
• Person exhibits behavior such as having difficulty retrieving supplies for skin care and manipulating soap, lotion, etc.

Data Analysis

Nursing Diagnosis
PARTIAL INCAPACITY TO PERFORM SKIN CARE: Being capable of but needing assistance with cleansing and care of the skin

Common Etiology (Stressors)
BIRTH DEFECTS: Blindness, cerebral palsy, clubhand, developmental deficit, Down's syndrome, Duchenne's muscular dystrophy
DISEASES: Autism, blindness, brain tumor, cachexia, carcinoma, cataracts, cerebrovascular accident, congestive heart failure, diplopia, encephalitis, Friedreich's ataxia, Guillain-Barré syndrome, Hodgkin's disease, Laennec's cirrhosis, leukemia, major depression, manic–depressive psychosis, multiple sclerosis, myasthenia gravis, myocardial infarction, organic brain syndrome, osteoarthritis, Parkinson's disease, posterolateral sclero-

sis, psychosis, retinal detachment, rheumatoid arthritis, senility, Sydenham's chorea

INJURIES: Burn wound, cerebral concussion, dislocation, bone fracture, fracture and compression of the spinal cord, poisoning, traumatic amputation

SIGNS AND SYMPTOMS: Blurred vision, difficulty concentrating, confusion, diplopia, dizziness, dyspnea, fatigue, memory loss, pain, joint swelling, vertigo, weakness

HEALTH CARE FACTORS: *Drug therapy:* Narcotics, sedatives, tranquilizers. *Medical therapy:* Casting, intravenous infusion, traction, blood transfusion. *Surgical therapy:* Surgery of any kind. *Surgical procedures:* Amputation. *Surgical incision:* Painful surgical incision

DEVELOPMENTAL PHASES Old age

MAJOR PATHOPHYSIOLOGIC FACTORS CAUSING THE PROBLEM: Partial incapacity to perform activities of daily living can result from any of the following: decreased cardiac output, impaired oxygenation of tissue cells, organ degeneration or damage, impaired transmission of impulses from nerves to muscles, accumulation of toxic metabolic byproducts, disrupted cerebral chemical/neuronal balance, tissue function impaired by the inflammatory process, brain cell damage or deficient development

PLANNING

Unmet Needs
Comfort, cleanliness, dependence, independence, increased learning

Expected Outcome
Clean, moisturized, comfortable skin
Person performs at an expected level of independent self-care

NURSING INTERVENTIONS

Nursing Treatments
Provide assistance until the person is fully able to assume self-care
Anticipate needs (for assistance)
Assist with skin hygiene (as needed)
Encourage self-performance

Nursing Observations
Inspect the skin for breakdown, for infectious lesions, for color
Inspect for skin irritation
Observe for evidence of pressure on the skin
Test the skin for impaired feeling perception
Palpate the skin for temperature
Observe performance level and problems involved in completing tasks

Health Teaching
Instruct to maintain skin cleanliness, lubricate the skin (after dampening the skin), inspect the skin
Explain the reason for and intended effect of the care
Teach how to use assistive grooming devices

EVALUATION
Record actual outcome

UNSKILLED AT SKIN CARE[362,366]

ASSESSMENT

Data Collection

Subjective Data
• Person's discussion or questions indicate a need for additional information, clarification, or validation of information about performing the task of skin care
  OR

• Person's lack of questions or comments indicates not wanting information or not knowing enough to seek information about performing the task of skin care

Person may not know of those products that are best for skin care, of the importance of preventing skin trauma

Objective Data
• Person cannot correctly demonstrate how to:
    Cleanse the skin
    Lubricate the skin

Data Analysis

Nursing Diagnosis
UNSKILLED AT SKIN CARE: Being nonproficient, with or without knowledge, in the performance of the specific task of cleansing and caring for the skin

Common Etiology (Stressors)
HEALTH CARE FACTORS: Lack of health instruction, lack of health-skill experience
DEVELOPMENTAL PHASES: Infancy, toddler, preschooler, adolescent

PLANNING

Unmet Needs
Comfort, cleanliness, protection from physical harm, dependence, mastery and competence in skills, independence, increased learning

Expected Outcome
Clean, moisturized, comfortable skin
Correct verbal feedback of the information taught
Correct return demonstration of how to clean and lubricate the skin

NURSING INTERVENTIONS

Nursing Treatments
Provide temporary assistance until the skill is learned
Bathe daily (unless the person is aged or has a skin disorder)
Maintain dry, clean skin
Massage gently or vigorously
Lubricate the skin with baby oil, bath oil, or body lotion (after dampening the skin)
Lubricate the skin with cocoa butter, glycerine, lanolin, mineral oil, or olive oil (if the skin is very dry and after dampening the skin)
Encourage self-performance

Nursing Observations
Inspect the skin for breakdown, for infectious lesions, for color
Inspect for skin irritation
Observe for evidence of pressure on the skin
Test the skin for impaired feeling perception
Palpate the skin for temperature
Observe for readiness to assume self-care
Determine teaching effectiveness by testing, verbal feedback, and return demonstration

Health Teaching
Instruct to maintain skin cleanliness, to maintain skin dryness, to lubricate the skin (after dampening the skin), to inspect the skin (periodically)
Advise against piercing or squeezing the skin/lesions, against prolonged skin exposure to the sun, against prolonged skin exposure to water, against pulling off dead skin or scabs, against walking barefoot
Emphasize the danger of cutting calloused skin
Explain the importance of testing cosmetics for skin irritation
Explain the need to avoid mechanical trauma
Inform that skin should be protected from windburn

EVALUATION

Record actual outcome

INCAPACITY TO PERFORM FEMININE HYGIENE[143,362,366,451]

ASSESSMENT

Data Collection

Subjective Data
• Person may or may not relate being unable to carry out feminine hygiene

Objective Data
• Person exhibits behavior such as minimal, ineffective, or no body movement and makes no attempt at cleansing the perineum, at therapeutic vaginal douching, or at changing sanitary napkins or tampons

Data Analysis

Nursing Diagnosis
INCAPACITY TO PERFORM FEMININE HYGIENE: Being incapable of carrying out procedures associated with hygienic care of the female genitalia

Common Etiology (Stressors)
Diseases: Blindness, cachexia, carcinoma, cerebrovascular accident, congestive heart failure, Friedreich's ataxia, Guillain-Barré syndrome, Hodgkin's disease, Laennec's cirrhosis, leukemia, major depression, manic–depressive psychosis, multiple sclerosis, myasthenia gravis, myocardial infarction, organic brain syndrome, osteoarthritis, Parkinson's disease, posterolateral sclerosis, psychosis, rheumatoid arthritis, rickets, senility, Sydenham's chorea
INJURIES: Burn wound, bone fracture, fracture and compression of the spinal cord, traumatic amputation
SIGNS AND SYMPTOMS: Confusion, dizziness, dyspnea, hallucinations, memory loss, pain, paralysis, joint swelling, vertigo, weakness
HEALTH CARE FACTORS: *Medical therapy:* Casting, traction. *Surgical therapy:* Surgery of any kind. *Surgical procedures:* Amputation. *Surgical incision:* Painful surgical incision
DEVELOPMENTAL PHASES: Old age
MAJOR PATHOPHYSIOLOGIC FACTORS CAUSING THE PROBLEM: Incapacity to perform activities of daily living can result from any of the following: decreased cardiac output, impaired oxygentaion of tissue cells, organ degeneration or damage, impaired transmission of impulses from nerves to muscles, accumulation of toxic metabolic by-products, disrupted cerebral chemical/neuronal balance, tissue function impaired by the inflammatory process, brain cell damage or deficient development

PLANNING

Unmet Needs

Comfort, cleanliness, dependence, increased learning

Expected Outcome

A clean perineal area
No unpleasant perineal odor
No abnormal vaginal discharge

NURSING INTERVENTIONS

Nursing Treatments

Acknowledge dependency
Anticipate needs

Bathe (perineum) daily (or more frequently if needed)
Change the sanitary pads frequently
Administer a vaginal douche (when indicated for infection)
Provide clean clothing (especially undergarments)

Nursing Observations
Inspect the vagina for discharge
Inspect the skin for breakdown (excoriation), for infectious lesions
Inspect for bleeding
Observe for incontinence
Observe for readiness to assume self-care

Health Teaching
Explain the reason for and intended effect of the hygiene (comfort, prevention of infection and unpleasant odor)

EVALUATION
Record actual outcome

PARTIAL INCAPACITY TO PERFORM FEMININE HYGIENE [143,362,366,451]

ASSESSMENT

Data Collection

Subjective Data
• Person relates attempts at feminine hygiene
• Requests assistance to complete self-care
  May complain of fatigue before completing hygiene

Objective Data
• Person exhibits behavior such as having difficulty retrieving hygiene supplies, cleansing the perineum, changing sanitary napkins or tampons, or douching

Data Analysis

Nursing Diagnosis
PARTIAL INCAPACITY TO PERFORM FEMININE HYGIENE: Being capable of but needing assistance with procedures associated with hygienic care of the female genitalia

Common Etiology (Stressors)
DISEASES: Blindness, cachexia, carcinoma, cerebrovascular accident, congestive heart failure, Friedreich's ataxia, Guillain-Barré syndrome, Hodgkin's disease, Laennec's cirrhosis, leukemia, major depression, manic–depressive psychosis, multiple sclerosis, myasthenia gravis, myocardial infarction, organic brain syndrome, osteoarthritis, Parkinson's disease, posterolateral sclerosis, psychosis, rheumatoid arthritis, senility, Sydenham's chorea
INJURIES: Burn wound, bone fracture, fracture and compression of the spinal cord, traumatic amputation
SIGNS AND SYMPTOMS: Difficulty concentrating, confusion, dizziness, dyspnea, fatigue, hallucinations, memory loss, pain, joint swelling, vertigo, weakness
HEALTH CARE FACTORS: *Drug therapy:* Narcotics, sedatives, tranquilizers. *Medical therapy:* Casting, intravenous infusion, traction, blood transfusion. *Surgical therapy:* Surgery of any kind. *Surgical procedures:* Amputation. *Surgical incision:* Painful surgical incision
DEVELOPMENTAL PHASES: Old age
MAJOR PATHOPHYSIOLOGIC FACTORS CAUSING THE PROBLEM: Partial incapacity to perform activities of daily living can result from any of the following: decreased cardiac output, im-

paired oxygenation of tissue cells, organ degeneration or damage, impaired transmission of impulses from nerves to muscles, accumulation of toxic metabolic by-products, disrupted cerebral chemical/neuronal balance, tissue function impaired by the inflammatory process, brain cell damage or deficient development

PLANNING

Unmet Needs

Comfort, cleanliness, dependence, independence, increased learning

Expected Outcome

A clean perineal area
No unpleasant perineal odor
No abnormal vaginal discharge
Person performs at an expec:ed level of independent self-care

NURSING INTERVENTIONS

Nursing Treatments

Provide assistance until the person is fully able to assume self-care
Anticipate needs (for assistance)
Bathe (the perineum) daily (or more frequently if needed)
Change the sanitary pads/tampons frequently (preferably every 4 hours)
Administer a vaginal douche (when indicated for infection)
Provide clean clothing (especially undergarments)
Encourage self-performance

Nursing Observations

Inspect the vagina for discharge
Inspect the skin for breakdown (excoriation), for infectious lesions
Inspect for bleeding
Observe performance level and problems involved in completing tasks

Health Teaching

Explain the reason for and intended effect of the hygiene (comfort, prevention of infection and unpleasant odor)

EVALUATION

Record actual outcome

UNSKILLED AT FEMININE HYGIENE [143,362,366,451]

ASSESSMENT

Data Collection

Subjective Data
• Person's discussion or questions indicate a need for additional information, clarification, or validation of information about performing the task of feminine hygiene
  OR
• Person's lack of questions or comments indicates not wanting information or not knowing enough to seek information about performing the task of feminine hygiene
  Person may not know:
    Which products are recommended for use
    Precautions to take in order to avoid irritation and infection
    Signs of infection from tampons

Objective Data
- Person cannot correctly demonstrate how to:
  - Cleanse the perineum
  - Apply or change sanitary napkins or tampons
  - Administer a therapeutic vaginal douche
  May have unpleasant perineal odor

Data Analysis

Nursing Diagnosis
UNSKILLED AT FEMININE HYGIENE: Being nonproficient, with or without knowledge, in the performance of the specific task of hygienic care of the female genitalia

Common Etiology (Stressors)
HEALTH CARE FACTORS: Lack of health instruction, lack of health-skill experience
DEVELOPMENTAL PHASES: Adolescent

PLANNING

Unmet Needs
Comfort, cleanliness, protection from physical harm, dependence, mastery and competence in skills, independence, increased learning

Expected Outcome
A clean perineal area
No unpleasant perineal odor
No abnormal vaginal discharge
Correct verbal feedback of the information taught
Correct return demonstration of perineal cleansing, application and change of sanitary napkins or tampons, vaginal douching

NURSING INTERVENTIONS

Nursing Treatments
Provide temporary assistance until the skill is learned
Bathe (the perineum) daily (or more frequently if needed)
Change the sanitary pads/tampons frequently (preferably every 4–6 hours)
Administer a vaginal douche (when indicated for infection)
Provide clean clothing (especially undergarments)
Encourage self-performance

Nursing Observations
Observe the vagina for abnormal odor (indicating infection)
Observe for readiness to assume self-care
Determine teaching effectiveness by testing, verbal feedback, and return demonstration

Health Teaching
Advise daily bathing
Recommend a daily change of clean clothing (especially undergarments)
Recommend the wearing of cotton underpants (instead of synthetics)
Recommend that perfumed vaginal products be avoided (such as feminine hygiene sprays, prepackaged douches, deodorants and powders of any kind, perfumed tampons or sanitary pads)
Advise frequent sanitary pad/tampon change (at least every 4–6 hours)
Explain how to use toilet tissue correctly by cleansing from front to back
Advise moderation in douching (needed only for infection, not necessary after menstruation or intercourse)
Teach how to give a douche (when needed)
Teach how to apply sanitary pads
Teach how to insert tampons
Inform that a yellow, purulent vaginal discharge indicates inflammation (and requires medical attention)

Explain the reason for and intended effect of the hygiene (comfort, prevention of infection and unpleasant odor)

EVALUATION
Record actual outcome

Self-Care Deficits in Urinary/Bowel Elimination

INCAPACITY TO PERFORM TOILETING [362,366]

ASSESSMENT
Data Collection
Subjective Data
• Person may or may not relate being unable to carry out toileting activities

Objective Data
• Person exhibits behavior such as minimal, ineffective, or no body movement and makes no attempt at using toilet facilities, removing clothing for elimination, cleansing self with correct wiping, replacing clothing, flushing the toilet, or washing hands

Data Analysis
Nursing Diagnosis
INCAPACITY TO PERFORM TOILETING: Being incapable of carrying out the activities of and the hygiene associated with elimination of urinary and fecal wastes and requiring total assistance with such activities

Common Etiology (Stressors)
BIRTH DEFECTS: Cerebral palsy, developmental deficit, Down's syndrome, Duchenne's muscular dystrophy, hydrocephalus, meningomyelocele
DISEASES: Autism, carcinoma, cerebrovascular accident, congestive heart failure, diabetic ketoacidosis, encephalitis, Friedreich's ataxia, Guillain-Barré syndrome, Hodgkin's disease, Laennec's cirrhosis, leukemia, major depression, meningitis, multiple sclerosis, myasthenia gravis, organic brain syndrome, osteoarthritis, Parkinson's disease, posterolateral sclerosis, psychosis, renal failure, retinal detachment, rheumatoid arthritis, senility, subarachnoid hemorrhage, subdural hematoma, Sydenham's chorea
INJURIES: Burn wound, drug overdose, bone fracture, fracture and compression of the spinal cord, herniated intervertebral disc
SIGNS AND SYMPTOMS: Difficulty concentrating, confusion, hallucinations, memory loss, pain, paralysis, joint swelling, vertigo, weakness
HEALTH CARE FACTORS: *Drug therapy:* Narcotics, sedatives, tranquilizers. *Medical therapy:* Casting, traction. *Surgical therapy:* Major surgery of any kind. *Surgical incision:* Painful surgical incision
DEVELOPMENTAL PHASES: Old age
MAJOR PATHOPHYSIOLOGIC FACTORS CAUSING THE PROBLEM: Incapacity to perform activities of daily living can result from any of the following: decreased cardiac output, impaired oxygenation of tissue cells, organ degeneration or damage, impaired carbohydrate metabolism, impaired transmission of impulses from nerves to muscles, accumulation of toxic metabolic by-products, disrupted cerebral chemical/neuronal balance, tissue function impaired by the inflammatory process, brain cell damage or deficient development

PLANNING

Unmet Needs

Comfort, cleanliness, dependence, increased learning

Expected Outcome

Uses standard or substitute toilet facilities
Hands, perineal area, and anal area are clean
Body is clothed with clean, appropriate clothing

NURSING INTERVENTIONS

Nursing Treatments

Respond immediately to the patient's call
Toilet frequently
Provide a bedpan or a bedside commode
  OR
Place a urinal at the perineum
Remove the bedpan immediately after use
Provide toilet hygiene, clean clothing (as needed)
Provide privacy
Wash the patient's hands (after toileting)
Place air freshner in the room
Encourage self-performance

Nursing Observations

Observe for complaints of constipation; dysuria
Observe for incontinence
Inspect for stool abnormalities (blood, clay-colored, etc.)
Observe the urine for abnormal color, content, and odor
Observe for readiness to assume self-care

Health Teaching

Explain the reason for and intended effect of the care
Teach how to use assistive toileting devices

EVALUATION

Record actual outcome

PARTIAL INCAPACITY TO PERFORM TOILETING [362,366]

ASSESSMENT

Data Collection

Subjective Data
• Person relates attempts at placing self on the toilet facility and managing toilet hygiene
• Requests assistance to complete self-care
  May verbalize embarrassment

Objective Data
• Person exhibits behavior such as having difficulty getting to and positioning self to use the commode, bedpan, or urinal, having elimination accidents, and struggling to clean self after elimination; may have urine or feces on clothing, hands, perineum, legs, feet, bed

Data Analysis

Nursing Diagnosis

PARTIAL INCAPACITY TO PERFORM TOILETING: Being capable of but needing assistance with carrying out the hygiene associated with toileting

Common Etiology (Stressors)

BIRTH DEFECTS: Blindness, cerebral palsy, developmental deficit, Down's syndrome, Duchenne's muscular dystrophy

DISEASES: Aplastic anemia, autism, blindness, brain tumor, carcinoma, cerebrovascular accident, congestive heart failure, encephalitis, Friedreich's ataxia, Guillain-Barré syndrome, Hodgkin's disease, Laennec's cirrhosis, leukemia, major depression, manic-depressive psychosis, meningitis, mitral stenosis, multiple sclerosis, myasthenia gravis, organic brain syndrome, osteoarthritis, Parkinson's disease, posterolateral sclerosis, psychosis, pulmonary stenosis, retinal detachment, rheumatoid arthritis, senility, Sydenham's chorea

INJURIES: Burn wound, bone fracture, herniated intervertebral disc, traumatic amputation

SIGNS AND SYMPTOMS: Difficulty concentrating, confusion, diplopia, dizziness, dyspnea, edema, hallucinations, malaise, memory loss, pain, joint swelling, vertigo, weakness

HEALTH CARE FACTORS: *Drug therapy:* Narcotics, sedatives, tranquilizers. *Medical therapy:* Casting, intravenous infusion, traction, blood transfusion. *Surgical therapy:* Surgery of any kind. *Surgical procedure:* Amputation. *Surgical incision:* Painful surgical incision

DEVELOPMENTAL PHASE: Old age

MAJOR PATHOPHYSIOLOGIC FACTORS CAUSING THE PROBLEM: Partial incapacity to perform activities of daily living can result from any of the following: decreased cardiac output, impaired oxygenation of tissue cells, organ degeneration or damage, impaired transmission of impulses from nerves to muscles, accumulation of toxic metabolic by-products, disrupted cerebral chemical/neuronal balance, tissue function impaired by the inflammatory process, brain cell damage or deficient development

PLANNING

Unmet Needs

Comfort, cleanliness, dependence, independence, increased learning

Expected Outcome

Uses standard or substitute toilet facilities
Hands, perineal area, and anal area are clean
Body is clothed with clean, appropriate clothing
Person performs at an expected level of independent self-care

NURSING INTERVENTIONS

Nursing Treatments

Provide assistance until the person is fully able to assume self-care
Respond immediately to the patient's call
Arrange geographic placement (near a bathroom)
Dress in easily removable clothing
Toilet frequently
Provide a bedpan, a bedside commode, a urinal
Remove the bedpan immediately after use
Provide toilet hygiene, clean clothing (as needed)
Arrange easy access to the bed-positioning switch (if the patient uses the bedpan in bed)
Provide privacy
Wash the patient's hands (after toileting)
Place air freshener in the room
Encourage self-performance

Nursing Observations

Observe for complaints of constipation, dysuria
Observe for incontinence

Inspect for stool abnormalities (blood, clay-colored, etc.)
Observe the urine for abnormal color, content, and odor
Observe performance level and problem involved in completing task

Health Teaching

Explain the reason for and intended effect of the care
Teach how to use assistive toileting devices (higher commode seat)
Recommend safety devices (supporting bars on each side of the commode)

EVALUATION
Record actual outcome

Self-Care Deficits in Environmental Hygiene

UNSKILLED AT ENVIRONMENTAL CLEANLINESS[72,362,734]

ASSESSMENT

Data Collection

Subjective Data
- Person's discussion or questions indicate a need for additional information, clarification, or validation of information about performing the task of keeping the environment clean
  OR
- Person's lack of questions or comments indicates not wanting information or not knowing enough to seek information about performing the task of keeping the environment clean
  Person may not know that:
  Frequent dusting of furniture, walls, windows, and floors is necessary
  Dishes and utensils should be washed daily
  Bed linens should be washed/changed weekly
  Bathrooms require scrupulous cleaning
  Rodent and insect control is essential
  Animals must be clean and controlled

Objective Data
- Person cannot correctly demonstrate how to:
  Perform the methods used to maintain environmental cleanliness

Data Analysis

Nursing Diagnosis
UNSKILLED AT ENVIRONMENTAL CLEANLINESS: Being nonproficient, with or without knowledge, in the performance of the specific task of keeping the external surroundings free from soil or dust

Common Etiology (Stressors)
HEALTH CARE FACTORS: Lack of health instruction, lack of health-skill experience

PLANNING

Unmet Needs

Cleanliness, protection from physical harm, increased learning

Expected Outcome
Correct verbal feedback of the information taught
Correct return demonstration of the methods used to maintain environmental cleanliness

NURSING INTERVENTIONS

Nursing Treatments
Provide temporary assistance until the skill is learned
Encourage the person to ask questions

Nursing Observations
Determine teaching effectiveness by testing, verbal feedback, and return demonstration

Health Teaching
Inform that cleanliness is basic to health
Explain how to maintain environmental cleanliness (include damp-dusting furniture, garbage disposal, vacuuming, linen changes, scrubbing bathrooms daily, cleaning bathtubs after each use, insect and animal control, etc.)
Explain the reason for and intended effect of the methods used

EVALUATION
Record actual outcome

Self-Care Deficits in Clothing the Body

INCAPACITY TO DRESS SELF[362,366,444]

ASSESSMENT

Data Collection

Subjective Data
• Person may or may not relate being unable to dress self

Objective Data
• Person exhibits behavior such as minimal, ineffective, or no body movement and makes no attempt at dressing and undressing self

Data Analysis

Nursing Diagnosis
INCAPACITY TO DRESS SELF: Being incapable of clothing the body and of removing clothing and requiring total assistance with such activities

Common Etiology (Stressors)
BIRTH DEFECTS: Cerebral palsy, developmental deficit, Down's syndrome, Duchenne's muscular dystrophy, hydrocephalus
DISEASES: Autism, blindness, cachexia, carcinoma, cerebrovascular accident, congestive heart failure, depression, eclampsia, encephalitis, Friedreich's ataxia, Guillain-Barré syndrome, Hodgkin's disease, Laennec's cirrhosis, leukemia, major depression, manic–depressive psychosis, meningitis, multiple sclerosis, myasthenia gravis, myocardial infarction, organic brain syndrome, osteoarthritis, Parkinson's disease, posterolateral sclerosis, psychosis, renal failure, rheumatoid arthritis, senility, subarachnoid hemorrhage, subdural hematoma, Sydenham's chorea
INJURIES: Burn wound, cerebral concussion, bone fracture, fracture and compression of the spinal cord, poisoning, traumatic amputation

SIGNS AND SYMPTOMS: Confusion, dyspnea, hallucinations, memory loss, pain, joint swelling, weakness

HEALTH CARE FACTORS: *Medical therapy:* Casting, traction. *Surgical therapy:* Surgery of any kind. *Surgical procedures:* amputation. *Surgical incision:* Painful surgical incision

DEVELOPMENTAL PHASES: Old age

MAJOR PATHOPHYSIOLOGIC FACTORS CAUSING THE PROBLEM: Incapacity to perform activities of daily living can result from any of the following: decreased cardiac output, impaired oxygenation of tissue cells, organ degeneration or damage, impaired transmission of impulses from nerves to muscles, accumulation of toxic metabolic by-products, disrupted cerebral chemical/neuronal balance, tissue function impaired by the inflammatory process, brain cell damage or deficient development

PLANNING

Unmet Needs

Comfort, cleanliness, dependence, increased learning

Expected Outcome

Body is clothed with clean, comfortable, appropriate clothing

NURSING INTERVENTIONS

Nursing Treatments

Acknowledge dependency
Anticipate needs
Handle gently
Ask the patient what (clothing) makes him comfortable
Dress and undress the patient
Dress in personal clothing (whenever possible)
Provide clean clothing
Dress in nonrestrictive clothing
Make a referral (to National Self-Help Clearinghouse* for additional information)

Nursing Observations

Observe for clothing that restricts circulation or movement (and avoid the use of such)
Observe for readiness to assume self-care

Health Teaching

Advise against wearing restrictive clothing
Explain how to adjust clothing to meet health needs (oversized clothes facilitate ease in dressing, full skirts conceal colostomies, etc.)
Recommend the use of knots to distinguish clothing color for the visually impaired
Teach how to use assistive dressing devices

EVALUATION

Record actual outcome

PARTIAL INCAPACITY TO DRESS SELF[362,366,444]

ASSESSMENT

Data Collection

Subjective Data
- Person relates attempts at dressing self
- Requests assistance to complete self-care
  May complain of fatigue before completing self-dressing

---

*City University of New York, 33 W. 42nd Street, New York, NY 10036

Objective Data
• Person exhibits behavior such as struggling to button, zip, hook, tie, buckle, place arms in armholes, place feet and legs into pant legs, coordinate colors

Data Analysis

Nursing Diagnosis
PARTIAL INCAPACITY TO DRESS SELF: Being capable of but needing assistance with clothing the body and removing clothing

Common Etiology (Stressors)
BIRTH DEFECTS: Cerebral palsy, developmental deficit, Down's syndrome, Duchenne's muscular dystrophy

DISEASES: Autism, blindness, cachexia, carcinoma, cerebrovascular accident, congestive heart failure, Friedreich's ataxia, Guillain-Barré syndrome, Hodgkin's disease, Laennec's cirrhosis, leukemia, major depression, manic–depressive psychosis, multiple sclerosis, myasthenia gravis, myocardial infarction, organic brain syndrome, osteoarthritis, Parkinson's disease, poliomyelitis, posterolateral sclerosis, psychosis, rheumatoid arthritis, senility, Sydenham's chorea

INJURIES: Burn wound, bone fracture, fracture and compression of the spinal cord, poisoning, traumatic amputation

SIGNS AND SYMPTOMS: Confusion, dizziness, dyspnea, fatigue, hallucinations, memory loss, pain, joint swelling, vertigo, weakness

HEALTH CARE FACTORS: *Drug therapy:* Narcotics, sedatives, tranquilizers. *Medical therapy:* Casting, intravenous infusion, traction, blood transfusion. *Surgical therapy:* Surgery of any kind. *Surgical procedures:* Amputation. *Surgical incision:* Painful surgical incision

DEVELOPMENTAL PHASES: Old age

MAJOR PATHOPHYSIOLOGIC FACTORS CAUSING THE PROBLEM: Partial incapacity to perform activities of daily living can result from any of the following: decreased cardiac output, impaired oxygenation of tissue cells, organ degeneration or damage, impaired transmission of impulses from nerves to muscles, accumulation of toxic metabolic by-products, disrupted cerebral chemical/neuronal balance, tissue function impaired by the inflammatory process, brain cell damage or deficient development

PLANNING

Unmet Needs
Comfort, cleanliness, dependence, independence, increased learning

Expected Outcome
Body is clothed with clean, comfortable, appropriate clothing
Person performs at an expected level of independent self-care

NURSING INTERVENTIONS

Nursing Treatments
Provide assistance until the person is fully able to assume self-care
Anticipate needs (for assistance with zippers, buttons, shoestrings, etc.)
Ask the patient what (clothing) makes him comfortable
Assist with dressing and undressing
Provide clean clothing
Dress in easily removable clothing (buttons down the front, no tight snaps)
Dress in nonrestrictive clothing
Make a referral (to National Self-Help Clearinghouse for additional information)
Encourage self-performance

Nursing Observations
Observe for clothing that restricts circulation or movement (and avoid use of such)
Observe performance level and problems involved in completing tasks

Health Teaching
Advise against wearing restrictive clothing
Explain how to adjust clothing to meet health needs (oversized clothes facilitate ease in dressing, full skirts conceal colostomies)

Inform that when there is limited movement, the affected body side should be dressed first

Teach how to use assistive dressing devices

Explain that clothes should be laid out in the order of dressing for persons with impaired cerebral function

Recommend the use of knots to distinguish clothing color for the visually impaired

EVALUATION

Record actual outcome

UNSKILLED AT DRESSING SELF[238]

ASSESSMENT

Data Collection

Subjective Data

• Person's discussion or questions indicate a need for additional information, clarification, or validation of information about performing the task of clothing oneself

    OR

• Person's lack of questions or comments indicates not wanting information or not knowing enough to seek information about performing the task of clothing oneself

  Person may not know:

    Sequence of putting on and removing clothes

    Weight of clothing to be used during different seasons

  Note: No subjective data from infants/toddlers

Objective Data

• Person cannot correctly demonstrate how to:

    Put on and remove clothing

    Manage clothing that needs to be buttoned, zipped, hooked, tied, buckled, laced

    Coordinate the color of clothing

Data Analysis

Nursing Diagnosis

UNSKILLED AT DRESSING SELF: Being nonproficient, with or without knowledge, in the performance of the specific task of clothing the body and removing clothing

Common Etiology (Stressors)

HEALTH CARE FACTORS: Lack of health instruction, lack of health-skill experience

DEVELOPMENTAL PHASES: Infancy, toddler, preschooler

PLANNING

Unmet Needs

Comfort, cleanliness, dependence, mastery and competence in skills, independence, increased learning

Expected Outcome

Body is clothed with clean, comfortable, appropriate clothing

Correct verbal feedback of the information taught

Correct return demonstration of clothing self and removing clothing

NURSING INTERVENTIONS

Nursing Treatments

Approach unhurriedly (allowing at least 30 minutes for a child to dress himself)

Provide temporary assistance until the skill is learned

Anticipate needs (for assistance with zippers, buttons, shoelaces, etc.)

Provide clean clothing (lay clothes out in the order of dressing)

Provide the child with a play-practice doll or cloth that has a zipper, laces, buttons, and snaps

Provide frequent contact with the person (during efforts at dressing)

Encourage self-performance

Set limits on unacceptable behavior (such as tearing clothes, deliberate incorrect dressing)

Refrain from using punitive measures (when mistakes are made)

Offer praise (for successful self-dressing)

Nursing Observations

Observe performance level and problems involved in completing tasks

Health Teaching

Recommend a daily change of clean clothing

Explain that clothes should be laid out in order of dressing for small children

Recommend that independence be encouraged (as soon as the child resists being dressed by the mother)

Advise the child about the front and back of clothes, right and left shoe, armholes versus pants legs

EVALUATION

Record actual outcome

Self-Care Deficits in Hygiene Specific to Child Care

UNSKILLED AT BATHING/DRESSING INFANT[313,527]

ASSESSMENT

Data Collection

Subjective Data

• Person's discussion or questions indicate a need for additional information, clarification, or validation of information about performing the task of bathing and dressing an infant

  OR

• Person's lack of questions or comments indicates not wanting information or not knowing enough to seek information about performing the task of bathing and dressing an infant

Objective Data

• Person cannot correctly demostrate how to:

  Handle the infant during hygiene activities

  Give the infant a bath

  Dress the infant with the least discomfort to the child

  Apply a diaper properly for protection and comfort

Data Analysis

Nursing Diagnosis

UNSKILLED AT BATHING/DRESSING INFANT: Being nonproficient, with or without knowledge, in the performance of the specific task of bathing and dressing a newborn or small infant

Common Etiology (Stressors)
HEALTH CARE FACTORS: Lack of health instruction
SITUATIONAL FACTORS: Motherhood, fatherhood, grandparenthood, foster parenthood

PLANNING

Unmet Needs
Comfort, cleanliness, protection from physical harm, dependence, mastery and competence in skills, independence, increased learning

Expected Outcome
Clean infant hair, eyes, ears, nose, mouth, skin, nails, teeth, clothes, and linen, no unpleasant body odor
Correct verbal feedback of the information taught
Correct return demonstration of how to bathe, dress, and handle an infant

NURSING INTERVENTIONS

Nursing Treatments
Provide temporary assistance until the skill is learned
Encourage the parent or family to ask questions

Nursing Observations
Observe for readiness to assume self-care (of the infant)
Determine teaching effectiveness by testing, verbal feedback, and return demonstration

Health Teaching
Teach how to bathe an infant (bathe at the same time daily, use clean equipment and hands, never leave the child alone, avoid splashing water, keep the infant warm, start with the face and hair, then go to the body, limbs, and genital area, then apply lotion, avoid the use of powder)
Teach how to clean an infant's ears (clean with a washcloth, use mineral oil to soften hardened earwax)
Teach how to clean an infant's nose (use a washcloth, flexible cotton-tipped stick, or bulb syringe)
Teach how to dress an infant (gather clothing so it slips easily over the head, then dress the arms, avoid restrictive and excessive clothing)
Explain the reason for the intended effect of the hygiene

EVALUATION
Record actual outcome

UNSKILLED AT TOILET TRAINING A CHILD[238,313,460]

ASSESSMENT

Data Collection

Subjective Data
• Person's discussion or questions indicate a need for additional information, clarification, or validation of information about performing the task of training a child to control elimination
  OR
• Person's lack of questions or comments indicates not wanting information or not knowing enough to seek information about performing the task of training a child to control elimination

Person may not know:
   Correct age for toilet training a child
   Proper toilet training technique
   How to dress the child properly for training
   How much control the child is capable of maintaining

Objective Data
• Person cannot correctly demonstrate how to:
   Dress the child for toilet training
   Gain the child's cooperation during commode sittings

Data Analysis

Nursing Diagnosis
UNSKILLED AT TOILET TRAINING A CHILD: Being nonproficient, with or without knowledge, in the performance of the specific task of teaching a child bladder and bowel control

Common Etiology (Stressors)
HEALTH CARE FACTORS: Lack of health instruction
SITUATIONAL FACTORS: Motherhood, fatherhood, grandparenthood, foster parenthood

PLANNING

Unmet Needs
Comfort, dependence, mastery and competence in skills, independence, increased learning

Expected Outcome
Correct verbal feedback of the information taught
Correct return demonstration of how to dress the child for toilet training and to gain child cooperation during commode sittings

NURSING INTERVENTIONS

Nursing Treatments
Provide temporary assistance (with toilet training) until the skill is learned
Encourage the parent to ask questions

Nursing Observations
Determine teaching effectiveness by testing, verbal feedback, and return demonstration

Health Teaching
Advise that toilet training failures be ignored
Explain that a child should become accustomed to dry diapers during toilet training
Explain that commode sittings should be scheduled during toilet training
Explain that controlled elimination should be praised during toilet training
Inform as to the correct terminology for elimination (voiding, urinating, stool, bowel movement)
Inform that a child should be diapered only at night during toilet training
Inform that a child should be dressed in easily removable clothes for toileting
Inform that a child should be fully awakened during nighttime toileting
Inform that children are receptive to stages of toilet training at different ages (age 15–16 months can stay dry for 2 hours, age 18–24 months can notify when he wants to go to the bathroom, age 2–2½ years goes alone to the bathroom, age 3 years stays dry at night)
Inform that toilet training should be delayed until the child can sit up
Inform that toilet training should be limited to short periods daily

EVALUATION
Record actual outcome

UNSKILLED AT UMBILICAL CORD CARE[114,527]

ASSESSMENT

Data Collection

Subjective Data
- Person's (usually the mother) discussion or questions indicate a need for additional information, clarification, or validation of information about performing the task of caring for the infant's umbilical cord
  OR
- Person's lack of questions or comments indicates not wanting information or not knowing enough to seek information about performing the task of caring for the infant's umbilical cord

  Person may not know:
  The importance of umbilical cord care
  When the cord will come loose
  That the navel must be kept dry until the scab comes off
  Signs that should be reported

Objective Data
- Person cannot correctly demonstrate how to:
  Clean the infant's umbilicus
  Change the umbilical dressing (if one is needed)

Data Analysis

Nursing Diagnosis
UNSKILLED AT UMBILICAL CORD CARE: Being nonproficient, with or without knowledge, in the performance of the specific task of cleansing and caring for the healing umbilicus following birth

Common Etiology (Stressors)
HEALTH CARE FACTORS: Lack of health care
SITUATIONAL FACTORS: Motherhood, fatherhood, grandparenthood, foster parenthood

PLANNING

Unmet Needs
Comfort, cleanliness, protection from physical harm, dependence, mastery and competence in skills, independence, increased learning

Expected Outcome
A clean infant umbilicus
Correct verbal feedback of the information taught
Correct return demonstration of how to clean the infant's umbilical cord

NURSING INTERVENTIONS

Nursing Treatments
Provide temporary assistance until the skill is learned
Bathe (the umbilicus) daily
Change the dressing frequently (if present)
Moisten the dressing before removal
Clean with alcohol or with surgical soap
Maintain dry, clean skin
Expose the umbilical cord to air
Encourage self-performance (by the infant's mother)
Encourage the parent to ask questions

Nursing Observations
Inspect for bleeding, for edema, for drainage, for inflammation
Obtain a bacterial culture (if oozing occurs)

Observe for readiness to assume infant's care
Determine teaching effectiveness by testing, verbal feedback, and return demonstration

Health Teaching

Instruct to change wet diapers immediately (and to keep the diaper away from the umbilical cord so the cord is not exposed to urine)
Explain (to the mother) the reason for and intended effect of the hygiene
Teach (the mother) how to do umbilical care (gently wiping with alcohol)

EVALUATION

Record actual outcome

Family Self-Care Deficits in Providing Physical Care

FAMILY INABILITY TO PROVIDE PHYSICAL CARE[362,366,775]

ASSESSMENT

Data Collection

Subjective Data
• Family relates being unable to provide physical care for one or more members
• May or may not know of or have attempted solution methods
  May express feelings of frustration, anger, helplessness
  Verbalizes that family members do not participate in the care of the sick member(s)
  Reveals that no family member feels responsible for the physical care of its members
  May confirm that they are waiting for the nurse to do it

Objective Data
• Family or ill person exhibits behavior or signs indicating that physical care is not achieved, they make little or no attempt to care for the sick member, environmental disarray is evident, and the sick person appears unkempt, wears soiled clothing, and lies on dirty linen

Data Analysis

Nursing Diagnosis
FAMILY INABILITY TO PROVIDE PHYSICAL CARE: Being ineffective in providing for the usual activities of daily living for a family member who is no longer able to do so for himself

Common Etiology (Stressors)
PSYCHOSOCIAL FACTORS: Lack of interest of significant others, lack of knowledge about role expectations, lack of responsibility
HEALTH CARE FACTORS: Lack of health instruction, lack of health-skill experience
SITUATIONAL FACTORS: Chronic illness of a significant other; prolonged illness, injury, or hospitalization of a care provider; youth, old age, or death of a care provider; poverty

PLANNING

Unmet Needs

Protection from physical harm, dependence, group (family) unity, mastery and competence in skills, independence, increased learning

Expected Outcome

All family members are receiving adequate physical care as evidenced by well-kept appearance, clean clothing, clean environment, etc.

At least one family member is actively responsible for the physical care of the others

NURSING INTERVENTIONS

Nursing Treatments

Acknowledge dependency

Provide assistance until the family is fully able to assume self-care (of ill member(s))

Encourage self-performance (as a family unit)

Encourage the acceptance of interdependency (among family members)

Explore with the family their strengths and resources

Encourage family-shared responsibility

Nursing Observations

Observe for (family) readiness to assume self-care

Make a follow-up evaluation (if and when the family assumes self-care)

Health Teaching

Explain the reason for and intended effect of the care

Explain the importance of persons offering emotional support to one another

EVALUATION

Record actual outcome

FAMILY DIFFICULTY PROVIDING PHYSICAL CARE[362,366,775]

ASSESSMENT

Data Collection

Subjective Data

• Family relates it is hard to provide physical care for one or more members

• Verbalizes unsuccessful methods attempted

  May express feelings of frustration and anger

  Reveals that one or more family members are burdened with the strain of caring for the sick, while other members do nothing

  Verbalizes that some members receive care while others do not

Objective Data

• Family has demonstrated repeated efforts to provide care

• Family or ill person exhibits behavior or signs indicating that methods attempted are partially but not completely effective, for example:

  Family combs the dependent person's hair, but his clothing is soiled

  Meals may be served but are cold and of poor quality

Data Analysis

Nursing Diagnosis

FAMILY DIFFICULTY PROVIDING PHYSICAL CARE: A family is only partially effective in providing for the usual activities of daily living for a family member who is no longer able to do so for himself

Common Etiology (Stressors)

PSYCHOSOCIAL FACTORS: Lack of knowledge about role expectations

HEALTH CARE FACTORS: Lack of health instruction, lack of health-skill experience

SITUATIONAL FACTORS: Chronic illness of a significant other; prolonged illness, injury, or hospitalization of a care provider; youth, old age, or death of a care provider; poverty

PLANNING

Unmet Needs

Protection from physical harm, dependence, group (family) unity, mastery and competence in skills, independence, increased learning

Expected Outcome

All family members are receiving adequate physical care as evidenced by well-kept appearance, clean clothing, clean environment, etc.

At least one, and preferably all, family members are actively responsible for the physical care of the others

NURSING INTERVENTIONS

Nursing Treatments

Acknowledge dependency

Provide assistance until the family is fully able to assume self-care (as a unit)

Encourage self-performance (as a family unit)

Encourage the acceptance of interdependency (among family members)

Explore with the family their strengths and resources

Encourage family-shared responsibility

Discuss priority setting (with family members who do not share in physical care)

Nursing Observations

Make a follow-up evaluation (to determine whether the situation has improved)

Health Teaching

Explain the reason for and intended effect of the care

Explain the importance of persons offering emotional support to one another

EVALUATION

Record actual outcome

9 Nursing Diagnoses of MOBILITY DEFICITS

Domain of Nursing Expertise: Mobility Deficits

This chapter covers that sphere of nursing knowledge and skill related to problems of a person's limitations in moving from place to place and methods most readily available in achieving locomotion. Such restrictions of mobility result from illness, therapy, or developmental changes.

Views of Nursing Leaders That Support This Domain of Nursing Expertise

Components of basic nursing include assisting the patient to move and maintain desirable posture, walking, sitting, lying and changing from one position to another.

Virginia Henderson[220:12]

As a comprehensive service, nursing includes . . . the promotion of optimal activity.

Faye Abdellah[187:107 & 111]

Nursing is involved in "Universal Self-Care Requisites: The maintenance of a balance between activity and rest."

Dorothea Orem[380:42]

Self-Care Deficits in Mobility

PARTIAL INCAPACITY TO AMBULATE[108,477]

ASSESSMENT

Data Collection

Subjective Data
- Person relates attempts at walking
- Requests assistance with walking
  Complains of fatigue after limited ambulation

Objective Data
- Person exhibits behavior such as walking slowly, leaning toward one side while walking, holding onto chairs and railings, taking short, wide-based steps and swaying from side to side (waddling gait), raising the thigh excessively high, slapping the heel down before the foot (steppage gait), walking with choppy, stiff movements, dragging the toes, holding the legs together, while flexing the hips, knees, and joints (spastic gait), walking by crossing the legs (scissor gait), propelling the body forward with short, shuffling steps that become faster and faster (parkinsonian gait), walking by drooping one side of the body (limping gait), taking one or two normal steps and then one or two long, hopping steps (chorea gait), lifting the feet too high and placing them down with excessive force in a staggering, wavering, lurching walk (atactic gait), colliding with furniture, etc.

Data Analysis

Nursing Diagnosis
PARTIAL INCAPACITY TO AMBULATE: Being capable of but needing assistance with walking

Common Etiology (Stressors)
BIRTH DEFECTS: Cerebral palsy, clubfoot, congenital hip dislocation, Duchenne's muscular dystrophy, kyphosis, lordosis
DISEASES: Alcoholism, ankylosing spondylitis, blindness, bursitis, cachexia, carcinoma, cataracts, cerebrovascular accident, congestive heart failure, diplopia, Friedreich's ataxia, Guillain-Barré syndrome, Huntington's chorea, labyrinthitis, Meniere's disease, multiple sclerosis, myasthenia gravis, peripheral neuritis, osteoarthritis, Parkinson's disease, poliomyelitis, posterolateral sclerosis, retinal detachment, rheumatoid arthritis, rickets, Sydenham's chorea, central nervous system syphilis, tabes dorsalis
INJURIES: Back strain, burn wound, cerebral concussion, dislocation, bone fracture, herniated intervertebral disc, poisoning, traumatic amputation
SIGNS AND SYMPTOMS: Ataxia, backache, blurred vision, confusion, diplopia, dizziness, dyspnea, pain, joint swelling, touch-sensation loss, vertigo, weakness
HUMAN BODY: *Body state:* Body distortion during pregnancy (especially with multiple fetus)
HEALTH CARE FACTORS: *Drug therapy:* Narcotics, sedatives, tranquilizers. *Medical therapy:* Prolonged bed rest, casting. *Surgical therapy:* Surgery of any kind. *Surgical procedures:* Amputation, arthoplasty (hip or knee), bunionectomy, bursectomy, decompression of spinal cord, fasciotomy, fusion of bone or joint, graft of bone, laminectomy, reduction of dislocation or fracture, transplantation (bone, muscle, or tendon). *Surgical incision:* Painful surgical incision
DEVELOPMENTAL PHASES: Old age
MAJOR PATHOPHYSIOLOGIC FACTORS CAUSING THE PROBLEM: Partial incapacity to ambulate can result from any of the following: decreased cardiac output, impaired oxygenation of tissue cells, organ degeneration or damage, impaired transmission of impulses from nerves to muscles, accumulation of toxic metabolic by-products, disrupted cerebral chemical/neuronal balance, tissue function impaired by the inflammatory process, brain cell damage or deficient development

PLANNING

Unmet Needs

Activity and exercise, protection from physical harm, dependence, mastery and competence in skills, independence, increased learning

Expected Outcome

No evidence of physical injury during ambulation

Person performs at an expected level of independent self-care

NURSING INTERVENTIONS

Nursing Treatments

Provide assistance until the person is fully able to assume self-care

Approach unhurriedly

Assist with mobility (by physically supporting the person)

Attend the patient constantly (while ambulating)

Mobilize with a walker, a wheelchair, or a cane

Place in an uncrowded area

Minimize environmental barriers (such as clutter on the floor, obstructing furniture)

Limit the patient's mobility distance (to a short distance)

Encourage normal use of the involved limb

Apply a safety helmet to the head

Use a waist strap during mobility

Nursing Observations

Observe for mobility capabilities

Observe for complaints of weakness

Observe for abnormal gait

Test for impaired coordination

Observe performance level and problems involved in completing the task

Health Teaching

Explain the reasons for and intended effects of the methods used

Instruct to use a wide supportive stance for good body balance

Instruct to wear well-fitting shoes

Recommend the use of low-heeled shoes

Teach good body mechanics

Teach that weight-bearing should be done on the unaffected side

EVALUATION

Record actual outcome

INCAPACITY TO SIT UP[108,477]

ASSESSMENT

Data Collection

Subjective Data

• Person may or may not relate being unable to sit up

Objective Data

• Person exhibits behavior such as minimal, ineffective, or no body movement and makes no attempt at sitting up

Data Analysis

Nursing Diagnosis

INCAPACITY TO SIT UP: Being incapable of assuming or maintaining the sitting position and requiring total assistance with such activities

Common Etiology (Stressors)

BIRTH DEFECTS: Cerebral palsy, developmental deficit, Duchenne's muscular dystrophy; hydrocephalus

DISEASES: Cachexia, carcinoma, cerebrovascular accident, congestive heart failure, Friedreich's ataxia, Guillain-Barre syndrome, multiple sclerosis, myasthenia gravis, myocardial infarction, poliomyelitis, posterolateral sclerosis, subarachnoid hemorrhage, subdural hematoma, Sydenham's chorea

INJURIES: Burn wound, cerebral concussion, bone fracture, fracture and compression of the spinal cord, herniated intervertebral disc

SIGNS AND SYMPTOMS: Dizziness, pain, joint swelling, vertigo, weakness

HEALTH CARE FACTORS: *Medical therapy:* Casting, traction. *Surgical therapy:* Surgery of any kind. *Surgical incision:* Painful surgical incision

DEVELOPMENTAL PHASES: Old age

MAJOR PATHOPHYSIOLOGIC FACTORS CAUSING THE PROBLEM: Incapacity to sit up can result from any of the following: decreased cardiac output, impaired oxygenation of tissue cells, organ degeneration or damage, impaired transmission of impulses from nerves to muscles, accumulation of toxic metabolic by-products, disrupted cerebral chemical/neuronal balance, tissue function impaired by the inflammatory process, brain cell damage or deficient development

PLANNING

Unmet Needs

Comfort, protection from physical harm, dependence, independence, increased learning

Expected Outcome

Person is placed in the sitting position when he desires such and as needed for therapeutic reasons

NURSING INTERVENTIONS

Nursing Treatments

Place in the sitting position
Position with pillows
   OR
Prop with a back rest
Maintain body alignment (when in the sitting position)
Arrange easy access to the bed positioning switch
Sit the patient in an armchair (for support while sitting)
Dress in nonconstrictive clothing
Safeguard with siderails
Restrain the patient (around the waist, only if needed to prevent injury)

Nursing Observations

Observe for complaints of fatigue

Health Teaching

Explain the reason for and intended effect of the methods used

EVALUATION

Record actual outcome

PARTIAL INCAPACITY TO SIT UP[108,477]

ASSESSMENT

Data Collection

Subjective Data

• Person relates attempts at sitting up

- Requests assistance with sitting up
  Relates feeling unsteady when sitting up

Objective Data
- Person exhibits behavior such as falling forward or to one side when sitting and cannot sit up without some back support

Data Analysis

Nursing Diagnosis
PARTIAL INCAPACITY TO SIT UP: Being capable of but needing assistance with assuming and maintaining the sitting position

Common Etiology (Stressors)
BIRTH DEFECTS: Cerebral palsy, developmental deficits, Duchenne's muscular dystrophy
DISEASES: Aplastic anemia, carcinoma, cerebrovascular accident, congestive heart failure, encephalitis, Friedreich's ataxia, Guillain-Barré syndrome, Hodgkin's disease, Laennec's cirrhosis, leukemia, Meniere's disease, meningitis, multiple sclerosis, myasthenia gravis, myocardial infarction, osteoarthritis, Parkinson's disease, poliomyelitis, posterolateral sclerosis, rheumatoid arthritis, rickets, senility, subarachnoid hemorrhage, subdural hematoma, Sydenham's chorea
INJURIES: Back strain, burn wound, cerebral concussion, dislocation, bone fracture, fracture and compression of the spinal cord, herniated intervertebral disc
SIGNS AND SYMPTOMS: Backache, dizziness, dyspnea, pain, joint swelling, vertigo, weakness
HUMAN BODY: *Body state:* Body distortion during pregnancy
HEALTH CARE FACTORS: *Drug therapy:* Narcotics, sedatives, tranquilizers. *Medical therapy:* Prolonged bed rest, casting, traction. *Surgical therapy:* Surgery of any kind. *Surgical procedures:* Amputation, decompression of spinal cord, laminectomy. *Surgical incision:* Painful surgical incision
DEVELOPMENTAL PHASES: Old age
MAJOR PATHOPHYSIOLOGIC FACTORS CAUSING THE PROBLEM: Partial incapacity to sit up can result from any of the following: decreased cardiac output, impaired oxygenation of tissue cells, organ degeneration or damage, impaired transmission of impulses from nerves to muscles, accumulation of toxic metabolic by-products, disrupted cerebral chemical/neuronal balance, tissue function impaired by the inflammatory process, brain cell damage or deficient development

PLANNING

Unmet Needs
Comfort, protection from physical harm, dependence, independence, increased learning

Expected Outcome
Person demonstrates the ability to get into and maintain the sitting position with aid
Person performs at an expected level of independent self-care

NURSING INTERVENTIONS

Nursing Treatments
Provide assistance until the person is fully able to assume self-care
Position with pillows
   OR
Prop with a back rest
Maintain body alignment (when in the sitting position)
Arrange easy access to the bed positioning switch
Sit the patient in an armchair (for support while sitting)
Provide a trapeze bar and/or bed rope (to aid positioning)
Dress in nonconstrictive clothing
Safeguard with siderails
Restrain the patient (around the waist, only if needed to prevent injury)

Nursing Observations
Observe for complaints of fatigue
Observe performance level and problems involved in completing the task

Health Teaching

Explain the reason for and intended effect of the methods used

Teach good body mechanics

Explain how to maintain a correct sitting position

Explain how to use a bed rope (for pulling to a sitting position)

Teach how to use the forearm to push up from a lying position when hemiplegic

Explain methods for position change when in pain (for abdominal incision, raise bed, turn to lateral position and slowly sit up)

EVALUATION

Record actual outcome

PARTIAL INCAPACITY TO STAND UP[108,477]

ASSESSMENT

Data Collection

Subjective Data

- Person relates attempts at standing
- Requests assistance with standing

  May complain of leg weakness or unsteadiness

Objective Data

- Person exhibits behavior such as struggling to a standing position, swaying, using a bent posture, and leaning on a supportive object while standing

Data Analysis

Nursing Diagnosis

PARTIAL INCAPACITY TO STAND UP: Being capable of but needing assistance with moving from a sitting to a standing position

Common Etiology (Stressors)

BIRTH DEFECTS: Cerebral palsy, clubfoot, congenital hip dislocation, Duchenne's muscular dystrophy

DISEASES: Cachexia, carcinoma, cerebrovascular accident, congestive heart failure, encephalitis, Friedreich's ataxia, Guillain-Barré syndrome, Hodgkin's disease, Laennec's cirrhosis, leukemia, Meniere's disease, meningitis, multiple sclerosis, myasthenia gravis, myocardial infarction, osteoarthritis, Parkinson's disease, poliomyelitis, posterolateral sclerosis, rheumatoid arthritis, rickets, Sydenham's chorea

INJURIES: Back strain, burn wound, cerebral concussion, dislocation, bone fracture, herniated intervertebral disc, traumatic amputation

SIGNS AND SYMPTOMS: Diplopia, dizziness, dyspnea, pain, joint swelling, touch sensation loss, vertigo, weakness

HEALTH CARE FACTORS: *Medical therapy:* Casting. *Surgical therapy:* Surgery of any kind. *Surgical procedures:* Amputation, arthoplasty (hip or knee), bunionectomy, decompression of spinal cord, fusion of bone or joint, graft of bone, laminectomy, reduction of dislocation or fracture. *Surgical incision:* Painful surgical incision

DEVELOPMENTAL PHASES: Old age

MAJOR PATHOPHYSIOLOGIC FACTORS CAUSING THE PROBLEM: Partial incapacity to stand up can result from any of the following: decreased cardiac output, impaired oxygenation of tissue cells, organ degeneration or damage, impaired transmission of impulses from nerves to muscles, accumulation of toxic metabolic by-products, disrupted cerebral chemical/neuronal balance, tissue function impaired by the inflammatory process, brain cell damage or deficient development

PLANNING

Unmet Needs

Protection from physical harm, dependence, mastery and competence in skills, independence, increased learning

Expected Outcome

Person is able to stand with assistance
There is frequent position change and body movement
Person performs at an expected level of independent self-care
No evidence of physical injury

NURSING INTERVENTIONS

Nursing Treatments

Provide assistance until the person is fully able to assume self-care
Approach unhurriedly
Attend the patient constantly (while he attempts to or does stand)
Change the patient's position gradually (to a standing position)
Provide a low-height bed
Mobilize with either a cane or a walker
Dress in nonconstrictive clothing
Remove harmful objects from the environment
Secure all tubing, so there is no interference with mobility

Nursing Observations

Inspect for abnormal body movements
Observe for complaints of fatigue, of weakness
Observe performance level and problems involved in completing the task

Health Teaching

Explain the reason for and intended effect of the methods used
Instruct to use a wide supportive stance for good body balance and to wear well-fitting shoes
Recommend the use of low-heeled shoes
Teach good body mechanics
Teach that weight-bearing should be done on the unaffected side
Teach how to use a cane or walker for balancing and weight-bearing
Teach how to move from a sitting to a standing position if hemiplegic
Advise not to stand for prolonged periods
Recommend the use of a shower chair (when unable to stand in the shower)

EVALUATION

Record actual outcome

PARTIAL INCAPACITY TO TRANSFER BODY[108,477]

ASSESSMENT

Data Collection

Subjective Data
• Person relates attempts at transferring his body
• Requests assistance with the transfer

Objective Data
• Person exhibits behavior such as having difficulty raising the body off a bed or chair or propelling the body to a new surface

Data Analysis

Nursing Diagnosis

PARTIAL INCAPACITY TO TRANSFER BODY: Being capable of but needing assistance with moving self from the bed to the wheelchair, car, regular chair, bathtub, etc., or back to bed

Common Etiology (Stressors)

BIRTH DEFECTS: Cerebral palsy, Duchenne's muscular dystrophy

DISEASES: Cerebrovascular accident, Friedreich's ataxia, Guillain-Barré syndrome, multiple sclerosis, osteoarthritis, poliomyelitis, posterolateral sclerosis, rheumatoid arthritis, Sydenham's chorea

INJURIES: Bone fracture, fracture and compression of the spinal cord, herniated intervertebral disc, traumatic amputation

SIGNS AND SYMPTOMS: Pain, joint swelling, weakness

HEALTH CARE FACTORS: *Medical therapy:* Casting. *Surgical procedures:* Amputation, hip or knee arthoplasty, reduction of fracture. *Surgical incision:* Painful surgical incision

DEVELOPMENTAL PHASES: Old age

MAJOR PATHOPHYSIOLOGIC FACTORS CAUSING THE PROBLEM: Partial incapacity to transfer the body can result from impaired transmission of impulses from nerves to muscles.

PLANNING

Unmet Needs

Dependence, mastery and competence in skills, independence, increased learning

Expected Outcome

Person is able to transfer body weight with assistance
There is frequent position change and body movement
Person performs at an expected level of independent self-care
No evidence of physical injury

NURSING INTERVENTIONS

Nursing Treatments

Provide assistance until the person is fully able to assume self-care
Place on an orthopedic bed
   AND
Provide a trapeze bar, a low-height bed
Arrange easy access to the bed positioning switch
Provide a transfer board
Lift with a hydraulic hoist
Refrain from pulling the patient across the sheets
Suggest home adaptations appropriate to the health problem (hoist, transfer board, etc.)

Nursing Observations

Observe for fatigue
Observe performance level and problems involved in completing the task

Health Teaching

Explain the reasons for and intended effect of the methods used
Instruct to lock the wheelchair before transferring
Teach good body mechanics
Teach that weight-bearing should be done on the unaffected side
Teach muscle-strengthening exercises (do pushups off chair or firm surface to strengthen biceps and shoulder muscles)
Instruct that the nonhemiplegic leg be placed down first when getting out of bed
Teach how to move from a bed to a chair and how to get into a bathtub if hemiplegic
Teach how to transfer from a bathtub to a wheelchair, from a bed to a wheelchair, from a chair to a wheelchair, from a wheelchair to an automobile, from a wheelchair to a bathtub, from a wheelchair to a bed, from a wheelchair to a chair, and from an automobile to a wheelchair

Teach how to use the forearm to push up from a lying position if hemiplegic, how to use the unaffected leg to move the hemiplegic leg, and how to use a hydraulic hoist

EVALUATION

Record actual outcome

Self-Care Deficits in Exercise

INCAPACITY TO EXERCISE[138,362]

ASSESSMENT

Data Collection

Subjective Data
• Person may or may not relate being unable to perform exercise

Objective Data
• Person exhibits behavior such as minimal, ineffective, or no body movement and makes no attempt at carrying out range of motion of joints and limbs

Data Analysis

Nursing Diagnosis
INCAPACITY TO EXERCISE: Being incapable of carrying out repeated body movement in order to maintain body strength and function and requiring total assistance with such activities

Common Etiology (Stressors)
BIRTH DEFECTS: Cerebral palsy, developmental deficit, Duchenne's muscular dystrophy
DISEASES: Carcinoma, cerebrovascular accident, congestive heart failure, diabetic ketoacidosis, encephalitis, Friedreich's ataxia, Guillain-Barré syndrome, Hodgkin's disease, Laennec's cirrhosis, leukemia, major depression, meningitis, multiple sclerosis, myasthenia gravis, myocardial infarction, osteoarthritis, Parkinson's disease, poliomyelitis, posterolateral sclerosis, renal failure, rheumatoid arthritis, senility, subarachnoid hemorrhage, subdural hematoma, Sydenham's chorea
INJURIES: Burn wound, bone fracture, fracture and compression of the spinal cord, herniated intervertebral disc, poisoning
SIGNS AND SYMPTOMS: Pain, paralysis, joint swelling, weakness
HEALTH CARE FACTORS: *Medical therapy:* Therapeutic bed rest, casting, traction. *Surgical therapy:* Surgery of any kind. *Surgical incision:* Painful surgical incision
DEVELOPMENTAL PHASES: Old age
MAJOR PATHOPHYSIOLOGIC FACTORS CAUSING THE PROBLEM: Incapacity to perform exercise can result from any of the following: decreased cardiac output, impaired oxygenation of tissue cells, organ degeneration or damage, impaired transmission of impulses from nerves to muscles, accumulation of toxic metabolic by-products, disrupted cerebral chemical/neuronal balance, tissue function impaired by the inflammatory process, brain cell damage or deficient development

PLANNING

Unmet Needs

Exercise, protection from physical harm, dependence, increased learning

Expected Outcome

Performance of range-of-motion exercise and isometric exercises

NURSING INTERVENTIONS
Nursing Treatments
Exercise (limbs) in range of motion
Nursing Observations
Observe for complaints of fatigue, of pain
Test for the degree of muscle strength
Observe for readiness to assume self-care
Health Teaching
Explain the reason for and intended effect of the therapy
Teach how to do isometric exercises, range-of-motion exercises

EVALUATION
Record actual outcome

PARTIAL INCAPACITY TO EXERCISE[138,362]

ASSESSMENT
Data Collection
Subjective Data
• Person relates attempts at exercise
• Requests assistance to complete exercise

Objective Data
• Person exhibits behavior such as struggling to carry out range of motion of joints and
  limbs

Data Analysis
Nursing Diagnosis
PARTIAL INCAPACITY TO EXERCISE: Being capable of but needing assistance with carrying out
  repeated body movement in order to maintain body strength and function

Common Etiology (Stressors)
BIRTH DEFECTS: Cerebral palsy, developmental deficits, Duchenne's muscular dystrophy
DISEASES: Aplastic anemia, bursitis, carcinoma, cerebrovascular accident, congestive heart
  failure, encephalitis, Friedreich's ataxia, Guillain-Barré syndrome, Hodgkin's disease,
  Laennec's cirrhosis, leukemia, major depression, meningitis, myasthenia gravis, myo-
  cardial infarction, multiple sclerosis, osteoarthritis, Parkinson's disease, poliomyelitis,
  posterolateral sclerosis, renal failure, rheumatoid arthritis, rickets, senility, subarach-
  noid hemorrhage, subdural hematoma, sydenham's chorea
INJURIES: Burn wound, bone fracture, fracture and compression of the spinal cord, herniated intervertebral disc, poisoning
SIGNS AND SYMPTOMS: Pain, joint swelling, weakness
HEALTH CARE FACTORS: *Medical therapy:* Casting, traction. *Surgical therapy:* Surgery of any
  kind. *Surgical incision:* Painful surgical incision
DEVELOPMENTAL PHASES: Old age
MAJOR PATHOPHYSIOLOGIC FACTORS CAUSING THE PROBLEM: Partial incapacity to exercise can result from any of the following: decreased cardiac output, impaired oxygenation of tissue cells, organ degeneration or damage, impaired transmission of impulses from
  nerves to muscles, accumulation of toxic metabolic by-products, disrupted cerebral
  chemical/neuronal balance, tissue function impaired by the inflammatory process,
  brain cell damage or deficient development

PLANNING

Unmet Needs

Exercise, protection from physical harm, dependence, independence, increased learning

Expected Outcome

Person engages in range-of-motion and/or isometric exercises

NURSING INTERVENTIONS

Nursing Treatments

Provide assistance until the person is fully able to assume self-care

Exercise (limbs) in range of motion

Place a footboard at the feet (for leg exercises)

Provide a trapeze bar (to move the body and for arm exercises)

Remove constrictive clothing (for easy body movement)

Encourage self-performance

Nursing Observations

Observe for complaints of fatigue, of pain

Inspect the skin for color

Palpate the skin for temperature

Test for the degree of muscle strength

Observe performance level and problems involved in completing the task

Health Teaching

Explain the reason for and intended effect of the therapy

Teach how to do isometric exercises, range-of-motion exercises

EVALUATION

Record actual outcome

10 Nursing Diagnoses of SELF-NUTRITION DEFICITS

Domain of Nursing Expertise: Self-Nutrition Deficits

This chapter covers that sphere of nursing knowledge and skill related to problems that center on the individual's limitations in feeding self and dependent others, especially during illness, therapy, and developmental phases.

Views of Nursing Leaders That Support This Domain of Nursing Expertise

The role of the nurse . . . in institutional settings . . . is ensuring that the patient eats the food delivered to him.

Alice Rines and Mildred Montag [411:298–299]

By basic nursing care I mean helping the patient to eat and drink adequately.

Virginia Henderson [221:16]

Nursing is involved in "Universal Self-Care Requisites: The maintenance of a sufficient intake of water and food."

Dorothea Orem [380:42]

Self-Care Deficits in Food/Fluid Intake

INCAPACITY TO FEED/HYDRATE SELF [362,366]

ASSESSMENT

Data Collection

Subjective Data
• Person may or may not relate being unable to feed/hydrate self

Objective Data
• Person exhibits behavior such as minimal, ineffective, or no body movement, makes no attempt at feeding/hydrating self, is unable to manipulate a cup, glass, or utensils, is unable to bring food and fluid to the mouth, and is unable to open packaged foods and fluids

Data Analysis

Nursing Diagnosis
INCAPACITY TO FEED/HYDRATE SELF: Being incapable of supplying food or fluid to the mouth and requiring total assistance with such activities

Common Etiology (Stressors)
BIRTH DEFECTS: Blindness, cerebral palsy, developmental deficit, Down's syndrome, hydrocephalus, Duchenne's muscular dystrophy
DISEASES: Autism, blindness, brain tumor, carcinoma, cataracts, cerebrovascular accident, congestive heart failure, diplopia, encephalitis, Friedreich's ataxia, Guillain-Barré syndrome, Laennec's cirrhosis, leukemia, major depression, manic-depressive psychosis, meningitis, multiple sclerosis, myasthenia gravis, organic brain syndrome, osteoarthritis, Parkinson's disease, poliomyelitis, posterolateral sclerosis, psychosis, pulmonary edema, renal failure, retinal detachment, rheumatoid arthritis, senility, Sydenham's chorea, typhoid
INJURIES: Burn wound, cerebral concussion, bone fracture, fracture and compression of the spinal cord, poisoning, traumatic amputation
SIGNS AND SYMPTOMS: Blurred vision, confusion, diplopia, dizziness, dyspnea, fatigue, hallucinations, memory loss, pain, paralysis, rigidity, joint swelling, touch-sensation loss, vertigo, weakness
HEALTH THERAPY: *Drug therapy:* Narcotics, sedatives, tranquilizers. *Medical therapy:* Casting, traction. *Surgical procedures:* Amputation, replantation of digits, skin graft of hand, tenoplasty of hand. *Surgical incision:* Painful surgical incision. *Therapeutic devices:* Enforced immobility with safety restraints
DEVELOPMENTAL PHASES: Old age
MAJOR PATHOPHYSIOLOGIC FACTORS CAUSING THE PROBLEM: Incapacity to feed or hydrate self can result from any of the following: decreased cardiac output, impaired oxygenation of tissue cells, organ degeneration or damage, impaired transmission of impulses from nerves to muscles, accumulation of toxic metabolic by-products, disrupted cerebral chemical/neuronal balance, tissue function impaired by the inflammatory process, brain cell damage or deficient development

PLANNING

Unmet Needs
Fluid and electrolyte balance, nutritional balance, comfort, dependence, increased learning

Expected Outcome
Daily intake of essential food groups
Daily fluid intake of at least 2,000 cc if there are no fluid restrictions

NURSING INTERVENTIONS

Nursing Treatments

Acknowledge dependency

Anticipate needs

Approach unhurriedly

Arrange pleasant surroundings (at meals)

Provide an attractive meal tray

Provide food selection, fluid selection, fresh drinking water, foods at their most appetizing temperature

Grant special requests (when possible)

Position comfortably

Wash the patient's hands (before feeding)

Feed the patient

Feed unhurriedly (with normal-size bites)

Encourage self-performance (by having the patient hold crackers, bread, etc., when possible)

Nursing Observations

Observe for readiness to assume self-care

Health Teaching

Teach how to use assistive eating/drinking devices

EVALUATION

Record actual outcome

PARTIAL INCAPACITY TO FEED/HYDRATE SELF[362,366]

ASSESSMENT

Data Collection

Subjective Data

• Person relates attempts at bringing food or fluid to the mouth

• Requests assistance to complete self-care

  May complain of fatigue before completing self-feeding or hydration

Objective Data

• Person exhibits behavior such as having difficulty reaching food or fluid, struggling to
  open packaged foods or cut food, exhibiting unsteady manipulation of cups, glasses,
  plates, and eating utensils and possibly spilling food or fluid, having difficulty taking
  more than one or two drinks of fluid or bites of food at one sitting

Data Analysis

Nursing Diagnosis

PARTIAL INCAPACITY TO FEED/HYDRATE SELF: Being capable of but needing assistance with bringing food and/or fluid to the mouth

Common Etiology (Stressors)

BIRTH DEFECTS: Blindness, cerebral palsy, clubhand, developmental deficit, Down's syndrome, Duchenne's muscular dystrophy

DISEASES: Aortic insufficiency, aortic stenosis, aplastic anemia, blindness, brain tumor,
bursitis, carcinoma, cataracts, cerebrovascular accident, congestive heart failure, diplopia, encephalitis, Friedreich's ataxia, Guillain-Barré syndrome, herpes zoster, Hodgkin's disease, Laennec's cirrhosis, leukemia, major depression, manic–depressive
psychosis, Meniere's disease, meningitis, migraine headache, mitral stenosis, multiple
sclerosis, myasthenia gravis, organic brain syndrome, osteoarthritis, Parkinson's dis-

ease, pneumothorax, poliomyelitis, posterolateral sclerosis, psychosis, pulmonary edema, pulmonary stenosis, renal failure, retinal detachment, rheumatoid arthritis, rickets, senility, Sydenham's chorea, tricuspid stenosis, typhoid

INJURIES: Burn wound, cerebral concussion, dislocation, drug overdose, bone fracture, fracture and compression of the spinal cord, herniated intervertebral disc, poisoning, traumatic amputation

SIGNS AND SYMPTOMS: Blurred vision, difficulty concentrating, confusion, diplopia, dizziness, dyspnea, fatigue, hallucinations, hyperactivity, malaise, memory loss, pain, paralysis, joint swelling, touch sensation loss, tremor, vertigo, weakness

HEALTH THERAPY: *Drug therapy:* Narcotics, sedatives, tranquilizers. *Medical therapy:* Casting, intravenous infusion, traction, blood transfusion. *Surgical procedures:* Amputation, replantation of digits, tenoplasty of hand. *Surgical incision:* Painful surgical incision

DEVELOPMENTAL PHASES: Old age

MAJOR PATHOPHYSIOLOGIC FACTORS CAUSING THE PROBLEM: Partial incapacity to feed/hydrate self can result from any of the following: decreased cardiac output, impaired oxygenation of tissue cells, organ degeneration or damage, impaired transmission of impulses from nerves to muscles, accumulation of toxic metabolic by-products, disrupted cerebral chemical/neuronal balance, tissue function impaired by the inflammatory process, brain cell damage or deficient development

PLANNING

Unmet Needs

Fluid and electrolyte balance, nutritional balance, comfort, dependence, independence, increased learning

Expected Outcome

A daily intake of essential food groups
A daily fluid intake of at least 2,000 cc if there are no fluid restrictions
Person performs at an expected level of independent self-care

NURSING INTERVENTIONS

Nursing Treatments

Provide assistance until the person is fully able to assume self-care
Anticipate needs (for assistance)
Approach unhurriedly
Provide a convenient meal tray
Cut the food into bite size pieces
Open packaged foods
Protect with a plastic bib
Provide firm eating utensils, lightweight utensils, unbreakable objects (dishes)
Assist with feeding (as needed)
Fill the drinking cup or glass only half full (to avoid spilling)
Provide fresh drinking water, fluid selection
Provide frequent contact with the person (during the meal in case needs arise)
Provide privacy (during meals when spillage is caused by tremor)
Encourage self-performance

Specific to Hyperactivity
Provide finger foods
Feed by bottle or by cup (which can be carried about)
Provide food selection
Give small, frequent feedings and drinks

Nursing Observations

Observe for complaints of fatigue (while feeding self)
Observe and record the food intake
Measure the (fluid) intake
Observe performance level and problems involved in completing the tasks

Health Teaching

Teach how to use assistive eating/drinking devices
Recommend eating methods suggested for the visually impaired (use of forefinger to determine fluid level in glass, clock-placement of food on plate)

EVALUATION

Record actual outcome

UNSKILLED AT FEEDING/HYDRATING SELF[94,185,286]

ASSESSMENT

Data Collection

Subjective Data
• Person's (child's) discussion or questions indicate a need for additional information, clarification, or validation of information about performing the task of feeding self and drinking from a cup
  OR
• Person's (child's) lack of questions or comments indicates not wanting information or not knowing enough to seek information about performing the task of feeding self and drinking from a cup
Note: Usually no subjective data from infants/toddlers

Objective Data
• Person (child) cannot correctly demonstrate how to:
  Drink from a cup
  Eat with a knife, fork, spoon

Data Analysis

Nursing Diagnosis
UNSKILLED AT FEEDING/HYDRATING SELF: Being nonproficient, with or without knowledge, in the performance of the specific task of bringing food and/or fluid to the mouth

Common Etiology (Stressors)
PSYCHOSOCIAL FACTORS: Lack of guidance from parents
DEVELOPMENTAL PHASES: Infancy, toddler

PLANNING

Unmet Needs

Fluid and electrolyte balance, nutritional balance, comfort, dependence, mastery and competence in skills, independence, increased learning

Expected Outcome

A daily intake of essential food groups
A daily fluid intake appropriate to child's age
Person performs at an expected level of independent self-care
Correct return demonstration of feeding and hydrating self

NURSING INTERVENTIONS

Nursing Treatments

Provide temporary assistance until the skill is learned
Anticipate needs (for assistance)
Approach unhurriedly
Postpone feeding when the child is fatigued
Cut food into bite-size pieces
Open packaged foods
Protect with a plastic bib

Provide unbreakable objects (plastic dishes, utensils)
Assist with feeding (as needed)
Provide finger foods
Fill the drinking cup or glass only half full (to avoid spilling)
Provide frequent contact with the person (during the meal)
Encourage self-performance
Set limits on unacceptable behavior (such as throwing food)
Refrain from using punitive measures (when there is accidental spilling or messiness)
Offer praise (for successful self-feeding)

Nursing Observations
Observe performance level and problems involved in completing the tasks

Health Teaching
Recommend that independence be encouraged (as soon as the baby resists being fed by the mother)

EVALUATION
Record actual outcome

UNSKILLED AT FEEDING/HYDRATING DEPENDENT PERSON[362,366]

ASSESSMENT
Data Collection
Subjective Data
• Person's discussion or questions indicate a need for additional information, clarification, or validation of information about performing the task of feeding another person
    OR
• Person's lack of questions or comments indicates not wanting information or not knowing enough to seek information about performing the task of feeding another person
  Person may not know:
    Methods used to feed someone else
    Precautions to be taken when feeding a dependent person

Objective Data
• Person cannot correctly demonstrate how to:
    Put food in the mouth of a dependent person
    Offer fluids in comfortable amounts
    Position someone else for feedings

Data Analysis
Nursing Diagnosis
UNSKILLED AT FEEDING/HYDRATING DEPENDENT PERSON: Being nonproficient, with or without knowledge, in the performance of the specific task of feeding and providing fluid for a person unable to do so for himself

Common Etiology (Stressors)
HEALTH CARE FACTORS: Lack of health instruction, lack of health-skill experience

PLANNING

Unmet Needs

Fluid and electrolyte balance, nutritional balance, comfort, protection from physical harm, dependence, mastery and competence in skills, independence, increased learning

Expected Outcome

Correct verbal feedback of the information taught

Correct return demonstration of how to put food in dependent person's mouth and to offer fluids

NURSING INTERVENTIONS

Nursing Treatments

Provide temporary assistance until the skill is learned

Feed unhurriedly

Place in the sitting position (½ hour before, during, and ½ hour after meals)

Provide a drinking straw (if the dependent person can suck)

Encourage the person to ask questions

Nursing Observations

Observe for diet intolerance

Observe for readiness to assume self-care (of the dependent person)

Determine teaching effectiveness by testing, verbal feedback, and return demonstration

Health Teaching

Demonstrate how to feed a dependent person (position, feeding technique, etc.)

Instruct to elevate the head (½ hour before, during, and ½ hour after meals)

Instruct to feed unhurriedly

Recommend that food be cut into bite-size pieces

Recommend that food servings be in proportion to the appetite

Recommend rough-textured food that stimulates swallowing (toast instead of soft bread and baked instead of creamed potatoes)

Instruct to place food into the unaffected side of the mouth of hemiplegics

Instruct the person to use his tongue to move food from the buccal pockets

Explain that fluids should not be given to persons unable to swallow

Recommend a regular meal schedule

Explain the need for pleasant mealtimes

Explain the reason for and intended effect of the methods used

EVALUATION

Record actual outcome

PARTIAL INCAPACITY TO CHEW/SWALLOW FOOD OR FLUIDS[362,366]

ASSESSMENT

Data Collection

Subjective Data

• Person relates attempts to chew or swallow food or drink
• Requests assistance

  May complain of a lump-in-the-throat sensation, throat tightness, painful chewing/ swallowing at times, may verbalize a preference not to eat

Objective Data
- Person exhibits behavior such as slow chewing/swallowing, poor control of food in the mouth and esophagus, may cough when swallowing, may put only small amounts of food or fluid into the mouth at a time

  May have physical finding of decreased jaw movement or swallowing reflex

Data Analysis

Nursing Diagnosis

PARTIAL INCAPACITY TO CHEW/SWALLOW FOOD OR FLUIDS: Being capable of but needing assistance with effectively reducing food or small particles and controlling food or fluids as they pass through the mouth and esophagus into the stomach

Common Etiology (Stressors)

BIRTH DEFECTS: Cerebral palsy, cleft lip, cleft palate, developmental deficit, Down's syndrome, Duchenne's muscular dystrophy, esophageal atresia, tracheoesophageal fistula

DISEASES: Oral and throat carcinoma, cerebrovascular accident, diphtheria, encephalitis, esophageal hernia, esophageal stricture, Guillain-Barré syndrome, herpes simplex, major depression, multiple sclerosis, myasthenia gravis, Parkinson's disease, posterolateral sclerosis, pyorrhea, streptococcal pharyngitis, Sydenham's chorea, tetanus, tic douloureux, tonsillitis, trench mouth, trigeminal neuritis

INJURIES: Oral burn wound, mandibular fracture

SIGNS AND SYMPTOMS: Dysphagia, tonsillar edema, pain

HEALTH CARE FACTORS: *Medical Therapy:* Nasal packing. *Surgical procedures:* Laryngectomy, tongue excision, tracheostomy, wiring of a mandible fracture. *Therapeutic devices:* Dentures

MAJOR PATHOPHYSIOLOGIC FACTORS CAUSING THE PROBLEM: Partial incapacity to chew or swallow food can result from impaired transmission of impulses from nerves to muscles, tissue function impaired by the inflammatory process, or narrowing of the esophagus

PLANNING

Unmet Needs

Fluid and electrolyte balance, nutritional balance, comfort, protection from physical harm, dependence, independence, increased learning

Expected Outcome

A daily intake of essential food groups
A daily fluid intake of at least 2,000 cc if there are no fluid restrictions
Food intake with minimal discomfort and difficulty masticating
Swallowing without aspiration

NURSING INTERVENTIONS

Nursing Treatments

Approach unhurriedly
Place in the sitting position, or in the slight sitting position (with neck slightly flexed)
Cut the food into bite-size pieces
Feed unhurriedly
Give small, frequent feedings
Discourage talking while eating and drinking
Suction the airway (as needed)

Specific to Partial Incapacity to Chew

Give clear-liquid foods, full-liquid foods, soft foods, mechanically soft foods, puréed foods (as in appropriate)

Specific to Partial Incapacity to Swallow

Attend the patient constantly (while eating and drinking)
Give full liquid foods, puréed foods, soft foods
Refrain from giving hot liquids, from giving iced liquids
Moisten the mouth with cracked ice (until the swallowing reflex improves)
Refrain from distracting the patient while he swallows

Nursing Observations
Observe for airway obstruction
Observe and record the food/fluid intake

Health Teaching
Advise against gulping food and drink
Recommend thorough food chewing
Recommend rough-textured foods that stimulate swallowing (toast instead of soft bread, baked instead of creamed potatoes)
Instruct to place food into the unaffected side of the mouth of the hemiplegic
Instruct the person to use his tongue to move food from the buccal pockets
Advise not to partake of very hot or cold foods or drinks
Explain that fluids should not be given to persons unable to swallow
Explain the causes of the health problem
Explain the reason for and intended effect of the methods used
Inform that airway noise indicates obstruction
Describe those symptoms that should be reported (coughing, choking, wheezing)

EVALUATION

Record actual outcome

PARTIAL INCAPACITY TO SUCK FLUIDS[55,527]

ASSESSMENT

Data Collection

Subjective Data
• Care giver relates infant's difficult attempts to suck
• Requests assistance

Objective Data
• Infant exhibits behavior such as poor control of liquids sucked into the mouth, swallowing large amounts of air, sucking only one to six times and then ceasing to suck, or shows signs of sucked liquids spreading into the nose

Data Analysis

Nursing Diagnosis
PARTIAL INCAPACITY TO SUCK FLUIDS: Being capable of but needing assistance with drawing liquid into the mouth by suction movements of the tongue and lips

Common Etiology (Stressors)
BIRTH DEFECTS: Cleft lip, cleft palate
SIGNS AND SYMPTOMS: Choking, weakness

PLANNING

Unmet Needs
Fluid and electrolyte balance, nutritional balance, comfort, protection from physical harm, dependence

Expected Outcome
A daily fluid and formula intake appropriate to the child's age

NURSING INTERVENTIONS

Nursing Treatments
Hold the infant while feeding
Feed by rubber-tipped medicine dropper, by syringe, by bottle (as is appropriate; use a special long nipple)

Feed unhurriedly
Give small, frequent feedings
Stimulate the sucking reflex through jaw and lip pressure
Give a pacifier to the infant (to stimulate sucking between feedings)
Use a large-holed nipple for feeding (if the infant is able to control liquids)
Use a small-holed nipple for feeding (if the infant is unable to control liquids)
Suction the airway (as needed)

Nursing Observations
Observe for airway obstruction
Observe performance level and problems involved in completing the task
Measure the intake

Health Teaching
Teach how to bottle-feed an infant
Explain the causes of the health problem (child cannot create negative pressure for sucking with cleft lip and chokes easily)
Describe those symptoms that should be reported (coughing, choking, wheezing)

EVALUATION
Record actual outcome

Self-Care Deficits in Nutrition Specific to Child Care

UNSKILLED AT BOTTLE-FEEDING INFANT[313,527]

ASSESSMENT
Data Collection
Subjective Data
• Person's discussion or questions indicate a need for additional information, clarification, or validation of information about performing the task of feeding an infant with a bottle
  OR
• Person's lack of questions or comments indicates not wanting information or not knowing enough to seek information about performing the task of feeding an infant with a bottle
  Person may not know:
  Types of bottles and nipples to use
  Correct amounts to feed the infant
  How to encourage fluid intake
  Age at which to terminate bottle-feeding

Objective Data
• Person cannot correctly demonstrate how to:
  Hold the infant during feeding
  Hold the formula bottle
  Dispel gastric air which the infant has swallowed

Data Analysis

Nursing Diagnosis

UNSKILLED AT BOTTLE FEEDING INFANT: Being nonproficient, with or without knowledge, in the performance of the specific task of nourishing an infant with milk from a bottle

Common Etiology (Stressors)

HEALTH CARE FACTORS: Lack of health instruction

SITUATIONAL FACTORS: Motherhood, fatherhood, grandparenthood, foster parenthood

PLANNING

Unmet Needs

Nutritional balance, comfort, protection from physical harm, dependence, mastery and competence in skills, independence, increased learning

Expected Outcome

Correct verbal feedback of the information taught

Correct return demonstration of how to hold, feed, and bubble (burp) the infant

NURSING INTERVENTIONS

Nursing Treatments

Provide temporary assistance until the skill is learned

Hold the infant while feeding

Feed by bottle

Feed unhurriedly

Position the infant with the head elevated for burping (midway and after bottle-feeding)

Encourage the person to ask questions

Nursing Observations

Estimate the amount of feeding the baby will need

Observe infant for adequate sucking reflex

Observe for (parent) readiness to assume self-care (of the infant)

Determine teaching effectiveness by testing, verbal feedback, and return demonstration

Make a follow-up evaluation (for appropriate weight gain)

Health Teaching

Teach how to bottle-feed an infant (hold the infant with his head supported and turned slightly to one side, keep the neck of the bottle full at all times, keep the milk at room temperature)

Explain how to stimulate an infant to remain awake during feeding (change the infant's position, move the bottle, thump the infant's foot)

Recommend that infants be fed on a self-demand schedule

Explain how to distinguish crying from hunger and other causes (finger- and fist-sucking indicate hunger)

Describe the signs of infant readiness to be weened (restlessness, shorter feeding periods)

Explain the need for pleasant mealtimes

Explain the hazards of flat positioning and bottle propping during infant feeding (choking, ear infection)

Instruct that only water, not milk or juice, be given in the infant's bottle at bedtime (the sugar in milk and juices promotes tooth decay when remaining in the infant's mouth overnight)

Explain the reason for and intended effect of the methods used

EVALUATION

Record actual outcome

UNSKILLED AT BREAST-FEEDING INFANT[55,527]

ASSESSMENT

Data Collection

Subjective Data
* Person's (woman's) discussion or questions indicate a need for additional information, clarification, or validation of information about performing the task of breast-feeding
  OR
* Person's (woman's) lack of questions or comments indicates not wanting information or not knowing enough to seek information about performing the task of breast-feeding

  Woman may not know:
  When to start breast-feeding
  How often to breast-feed
  Preferable length of nursing periods
  Types of clothing appropriate for breast-feeding
  Dangers of taking drugs during breast-feeding
  Need for balanced nutrition

Objective Data
* Person (woman) cannot correctly demonstrate how to:
  Clean breast nipples
  Position self and infant for breast-feeding
  Stimulate infant during feeding
  Use nipple shields or padding

Data Analysis

Nursing Diagnosis
UNSKILLED AT BREAST-FEEDING INFANT: Being nonproficient, with or without knowledge, in the performance of the specific task of nourishing an infant with milk from the mother's breast

Common Etiology (Stressors)
HEALTH CARE FACTORS: Lack of health instruction
SITUATIONAL FACTORS: Motherhood

PLANNING

Unmet Needs
Nutritional balance, comfort, cleanliness, protection from physical harm, dependence, mastery and competence in skills, independence, increased learning

Expected Outcome
Correct verbal feedback of the information taught
Correct return demonstration of how to cleanse the nipples, to position self and infant for breast-feeding, to stimulate the infant during feeding, and to use nipple shields or padding

NURSING INTERVENTIONS

Nursing Treatments
Provide temporary assistance (with breast-feeding) until the skill is learned
Encourage the person to ask questions
Make a follow-up evaluation (for appropriate weight gain)

Nursing Observations
Inspect the breasts for abnormalities (engorgement, cracked or bleeding nipples)

Health Teaching
Explain the advantages and disadvantages of breast-feeding (breast milk is more nutritious than cow's milk, is free from bacteria, and seldom causes allergy; the procedure

requires a rigid home schedule for infant feeding, and lactation causes breast discomfort)

Correct misinformation regarding breast-feeding (breast size does not affect lactation and breasts will not lose shape if properly supported)

Explain how to prepare the breasts during pregnancy for postdelivery breast-feeding (breast massage, lanolin application, pulling on nipples)

Teach prenursing nipple hygiene (wash with warm water)

Teach how to breast feed an infant (in the sitting and semisitting position; bubble infant every 5 minutes; avoid hurrying)

Inform of the recommended length of infant nursing periods (10 minutes at first with gradual increase to 20 minutes)

Explain the hazards of flat positioning during infant feeding (infant choking, ear infection, dental caries)

Recommend that infants be fed on a self-demand schedule

Explain how to distinguish crying from hunger and other causes (finger- and fist-sucking indicates hunger)

Explain that mothers have a choice of single or double breast-feeding

Explain that nursing the infant on alternate breasts reduces breast tenderness

Inform that extended breast-sucking indicates hunger

Explain how to stimulate an infant to remain awake during feeding (change position, thump the infant's feet)

Teach how to express breast milk manually, how to express breast milk mechanically

Describe the signs of infant readiness to be weaned (restlessness, shortened feeding periods)

Recommend the use of a brassiere for breast support, the use of a nipple shield, the use of nipple padding

Explain how to adjust clothing to meet health needs (brassieres, blouses, dresses that open in front)

Explain the need for pleasant mealtimes (during breast-feeding)

Explain the reason for and intended effects of methods used

EVALUATION

Record actual outcome

UNSKILLED AT FEEDING INFANT SOLID FOOD[172,313]

ASSESSMENT

Data Collection

Subjective Data

• Person's discussion or questions indicate a need for additional information, clarification, or validation of information about performing the task of feeding solid food to an infant

OR

• Person's lack of questions or comments indicates not wanting information or not knowing enough to seek information about performing the task of feeding solid food to an infant

Person may not know:

Specific solid foods a child can eat at different ages

Appropriate amounts of food to offer

How to prepare foods for the child

Food preferences of the child

Correct sequence for introducing new foods

Necessity of positive attitudes toward new food

Objective Data
- Person cannot correctly demonstrate how to:
    Put food in the mouth of the infant
    Offer food and fluids in comfortable amounts
    Position the infant for feedings

Data Analysis

Nursing Diagnosis
UNSKILLED AT FEEDING INFANT SOLID FOOD: Being nonproficient, with or without knowledge, in the performance of the specific task of introducing solid foods to infants

Common Etiology (Stressors)
HEALTH CARE FACTORS: Lack of health instruction
SITUATIONAL FACTORS: Motherhood, fatherhood, grandparenthood, foster parenthood

PLANNING

Unmet Needs
Nutritional balance, comfort, dependence, mastery and competence in skills, independence, increased learning

Expected Outcome
Correct verbal feedback of the information taught
Correct return demonstration of how to put food into the infant's mouth and to offer fluids

NURSING INTERVENTIONS

Nursing Treatments
Provide temporary assistance until the skill is learned
Hold the infant while feeding
Feed unhurriedly
Place in the sitting position (while eating)
Encourage the parents to ask questions

Nursing Observations
Estimate the amount of feeding the baby will need
Observe for diet intolerance
Observe for (parent) readiness to assume self-care (of the infant)
Determine teaching effectiveness by testing, verbal feedback, and return demonstration
Make a follow-up evaluation (to determine proficiency in feeding the infant)

Health Teaching
Demonstrate how to feed an infant (positioning, putting the spoon well into the mouth, avoiding large portions)
Recommend a regular meal schedule
Explain the need for pleasant mealtimes
Advise that infants be started on solid foods no later than 6 months
Explain that premature infants require prescribed foods
Recommend the preferable age for introducing specific foods to children (cereals, age 1–4 months; fruits, age 2–4 months; vegetables, age 3–5 months; etc.)
Inform that new foods should be introduced to children at the beginning of the meal (acceptance is greatest while the child is hungry)
Inform that vegetables should be fed to children before fruits at the meal (naturally sweet foods deaden the appetite for additional food)
Recommend that children be introduced to a wide variety of food
Recommend that food servings be in proportion to the appetite
Teach the principles of good nutrition
Explain the reason for and intended effect of the methods used.

EVALUATION
Record actual outcome

UNSKILLED AT PREPARING INFANT FORMULA[55,313]

ASSESSMENT

Data Collection

Subjective Data
- Person's discussion or questions indicate a need for additional information, clarification, or validation of information about performing the task of fixing formula for an infant
  OR
- Person's lack of questions or comments indicates not wanting information or not knowing enough to seek information about performing the task of preparing formula for an infant
  Person may not know:
  Type formula to use
  Where to obtain formula and equipment

Objective Data
- Person cannot correctly demonstrate how to:
  Mix the formula preparation
  Prepare the bottles with formula

Data Analysis

Nursing Diagnosis
UNSKILLED AT FORMULA PREPARATION: Being nonproficient, with or without knowledge, in the performance of the specific task of making ready feedings for an infant

Common Etiology (Stressors)
HEALTH CARE FACTORS: Lack of health instruction
SITUATIONAL FACTORS: Motherhood, fatherhood, grandparenthood, foster parenthood

PLANNING

Unmet Needs
Fluid and electrolyte balance, nutritional balance, comfort, cleanliness, protection from physical harm, dependence, mastery and competence in skills, independence, increased learning

Expected Outcome
Correct verbal feedback of the information taught
Correct return demonstration of how to mix the formula and prepare bottles

NURSING INTERVENTIONS

Nursing Treatments
Provide temporary assistance (with formula preparation) until the skill is learned
Encourage patient questions

Nursing Observations
Determine teaching effectiveness by testing, verbal feedback, and return demonstration

Health Teaching
Teach how to prepare a formula (presterilized method, thermal method, or the use of prepackaged formulas)
Explain how to obtain supplies
Explain the reason for and intended effect of the methods used

EVALUATION

Record actual outcome

11 Nursing Diagnoses of SELF-PROTECTION DEFICITS

Domain of Nursing Expertise: Self-Protection Deficits

This chapter covers that sphere of nursing knowledge and skill related to the vulnerability of the unwell person to ineffective, inappropriate, or excessive physical or psychosocial responses that threaten the body's state of balance during illness and illness therapy, including the inability of the individual to protect himself in that vulnerable state.

Views of Nursing Leaders That Support This Domain of Nursing Expertise

While trying to help the body maintain its homeostatic state, the nurse must be aware of those signs and symptoms that may be indicative of a failure to respond to the threat of imbalance or a failure of the regulating mechanisms to return the body to a balanced state. The nurse must be aware of those signs and symptoms that indicate failure in the adaptive mechanisms.

Valentia Fischer and Arlene Connally [156:54]

A careful nurse will keep constant watch over her sick.

Observation is for the sake of saving life and increasing health and comfort.

Florence Nightingale [370:17 & 125]

Some medical care measures introduce hazards into the person's life. The use of these measures necessitates the use of protective care measures.

Dorothea Orem [380:50]

For certain human responses, we have norms to guide our judgments of what promotes integrity.

Behaviors which are currently adaptive but which may become maladaptive unless reinforced may be stated as potential problems.

Sister Callista Roy [424:28–29 & 33]

The most effective nursing involves continuous observation and interpretation of patient behavior.

Ida Jean Orlando [221:15]

Actual Threats of Acid–Base Nonhomeostasis

INSTABILITY OF ACID–BASE STATUS[1,78,230,249]

ASSESSMENT

Data Collection

Subjective Data
• Person may or may not relate the following symptoms:
  Weakness
  Anorexia
  Vomiting
  Paresthesia
  Abdominal pain

Objective Data

Level 1
• Person exhibits signs that are intermittently unstable and stable
• Signs may or may not indicate a life-threatening imbalance
• Signs of instability are:
  Arterial pH below 7.35 (acidosis)
    OR
  Arterial pH above 7.45 (alkalosis)
  Weak pulse or bounding pulse, wide pulse pressure
  Shallow respirations or deep, rapid respirations (Kussmaul)
  Hypotension
  Tetany
  Flushed, warm skin

Level 2
• Person exhibits signs that are consistently unstable
• Signs indicate a life-threatening imbalance
• Signs of instability are:
  Same as Level 1

Data Analysis

Nursing Diagnosis
INSTABILITY OF ACID–BASE STATUS (ACID–BASE INSTABILITY): Person presents unstable acid–base signs indicating a physiologic imbalance in the normal rate of hydrogen ion to bicarbonate ion in the blood

Common Etiology (Stressors)
DISEASES: Congestive heart failure, Cushing's syndrome, diabetes mellitus, eclampsia (toxemia of pregnancy), emphysema, Guillain-Barre syndrome, hepatitis, hyperventilation, myasthenia gravis, pneumonia, pneumothorax, pulmonary edema, renal failure, thyrotoxicosis

INJURIES: Starvation, poisoning

SIGNS AND SYMPTOMS: Dehydration, diarrhea, fever, pain (abdominal), shock, vomiting

HEALTH CARE FACTORS: *Drug therapy*: Adverse effects of drugs such as aspirin, antacids, corticosteroids, diuretics, sedatives, narcotics. *Medical therapy*: Intravenous infusion of sodium chloride or lactated Ringer's solution, nasogastric suction, administration of high concentrations of oxygen to persons with chronic obstructive pulmonary disease, prolonged continuous positive-pressure breathing. *Surgical therapy*: Anesthesia. *Surgical procedure*: Colostomy, ileostomy

HUMAN ERROR: Improper dosage of insulin, accidental or intentional overdose of drugs, improper settings on a mechanical ventilator

MAJOR PATHOPHYSIOLOGIC FACTORS CAUSING THE PROBLEM: Unstable acid–base states result from disturbances or inadequacies of pH regulatory mechanisms, such as inadequacies in chemical buffers, respiratory function, and kidney function; these mechanisms maintain a constant ratio of carbonic acid to bicarbonate (base), with the kidneys providing most of the control through excretion or retention of acids and bases. *Acidosis*: Develops from an alkali deficit and an acid excess (ketones result from excessive fatty acid metabolism; lactic acid excess is caused by anaerobic metabolism), and from retention of carbonic acid (hypoventilation). *Alkalosis*: Develops from a hydrogen deficit (gastric suction), from an alkali excess (ingestion of absorbable antacids), and from excessive excretion of carbonic acid (hyperventilation). *Metabolic acidosis*: Stimulates the respiratory center, and very deep breathing (Kussmaul) ensues as a compensatory mechanism (excretion of carbonic acid). *Metabolic alkalosis*: May result in hypoventilation as a compensatory mechanism. Electrolyte disturbances accompany both acidosis and alkalosis

PLANNING

Unmet Needs
Acid–base balance, protection from physical harm, physiologic stability

Expected Outcome
Critical changes in the acid–base values will be promptly identified

The acid–base status will improve to an acceptable level and ultimately become stabilized at the optimum level possible

Level 1

Person will receive frequent, intermittent nursing observation and monitoring, frequent reevaluation of status, and immediate adjustment of therapy

Level 2

Person will receive constant nursing observation and monitoring, constant reevaluation of status, and immediate ajdustment of therapy

NURSING INTERVENTIONS

Nursing Treatments
Connect the person to an ECG monitor (keep the ECG monitor alarms set and turned on)

Obtain a complete present and past history

Obtain a blood sample and send for analysis (electrolytes, arterial blood gases as requested by the physician)

Obtain a urine sample and send for analysis (glucose, pH, acetone)

Provide standby equipment (oxygen, mechanical ventilator, bag–valve–mask resuscitator, intravenous fluids) and drugs (sodium bicarbonate, potassium, calcium, diuretics)

Reassure verbally (that the nurse is nearby and will protect the person)

Consult with the physician (as needed, and discuss methods of intervention)

Provide the family with information about the patient's progress (frequently, or if a change in condition occurs)

Nursing Observations
Monitor blood studies for abnormal acid–base, for abnormal electrolytes

Test the urine for pH

Test the urine for sugar and acetone (if the person is in ketoacidosis)

Interpret laboratory results and notify the physician of abnormalities

Observe the ECG monitor (check the rhythm strip and determine the type, duration, and frequency of arrhythmia)

Observe for confusion (in ketoacidosis)

Observe for complaints of dizziness, pain, respiratory muscle weakness

Observe for tetany (in respiratory alkalosis)

Monitor the blood pressure
Inspect the chest for respiratory rate and rhythm
Palpate the pulse for rate, rhythm, and volume
Measure the intake and output
Measure the flow rate of the intravenous fluids
Observe for signs of physiologic stability (serum pH of 7.35–7.45, alert consciousness)

Health Teaching

Instruct to report any serious symptoms immediately (drowsiness, thirst, dizziness, numbness, nausea, abdominal pain, tetany)
Explain the reason for intended effect of the observation and monitoring

Medical Treatments Performed by Nurses

Administer intravenous fluids
Give the prescribed drugs

EVALUATION

Record actual outcome

Actual Threats of Body-Temperature Nonhomeostasis

INSTABILITY OF THERMOREGULATION [1,78,230,249]

ASSESSMENT

Data Collection

Subjective Data
• Person may or may not relate symptoms
  Complains of feeling hot or cold

Objective Data

Level 1
• Person exhibits signs that are intermittently unstable and stable
• Signs may or may not indicate a life-threatening imbalance
• Signs of instability are:
    Decreased or increased body temperature
    Flushed, warm skin or pale, cold skin
    Rapid pulse and respirations
     OR
    Slow pulse and respirations
    Diaphoresis or shivering
    Excessive drowsiness

Level 2
• Person exhibits signs that are consistently unstable
• Signs indicate a life-threatening imbalance
• Signs of instability are:
    Same as Level 1

Data Analysis

Nursing Diagnosis
INSTABILITY OF THERMOREGULATION (THERMOREGULATION INSTABILITY): Person presents an unstable body temperature level, indicating a physiologic imbalance between heat production and heat loss

Common Etiology (Stressors)

BIRTH STATUS: Premature infant, low-birth-weight infant

DISEASES: Brain tumor with pressure on the hypothalamus, severe moist gangrene, infection (resistant to treatment), meningitis, staphylococcal pneumonia, septicemia, thyrotoxicosis or thyroid storm, typhoid fever, yellow fever

INJURIES: Burn wound, cerebral injury (concussion, contusion, or hematoma) causing damage to or pressure on the hypothalamus, heat stroke

HEALTH CARE FACTORS: *Drug therapy:* Adverse effects of chemotherapy

DEVELOPMENTAL STAGES: Newborn, old age

ENVIRONMENTAL FACTORS: Prolonged exposure to environmental cold or heat, especially with high humidity

HUMAN ERROR: Excessive cooling of an infant by baths or exposure

MAJOR PATHOPHYSIOLOGIC FACTORS CAUSING THE PROBLEM: Instability of thermoregulation can result from abnormalities of the brain or toxic substances that affect the temperature-regulating center in the hypothalamus, or from exposure to excessive heat or cold; toxins called pyrogens (from bacteria or degenerating tissues) cause the hypothalamic thermostat to increase its setting, resulting in fever; when the thermostat setting is changed suddenly (as from certain bacterial pyrogens), the person experiences chills until the body's temperature reaches the new setting; when the temperature is above 106° F, the tissue cells (especially in the brain) are damaged and destroyed; when the body temperature is allowed to drop to 94° F, the hypothalamus begins to lose its effectiveness in regulating temperature, partly because the rate of cellular heat production is depressed; a low body temperature induces sleepiness or coma and depression of the central nervous system's heat-control mechanisms, thereby preventing shivering

PLANNING

Unmet Needs

Normal temperature, protection from physical harm, physiologic stability

Expected Outcome

Critical temperature changes will be promptly identified

The thermal status will improve to an acceptable level and ultimately become stabilized at the optimum level possible

Level 1

Person will receive frequent, intermittent nursing observation and monitoring, frequent reevaluation of status, and immediate adjustment of therapy

Level 2

Person will receive constant nursing observation and monitoring, constant reevaluation of status, and immediate adjustment of therapy

NURSING INTERVENTIONS

Nursing Treatments

Obtain a complete present and past history

Provide standby equipment (hypo- or hyperthermia blanket, intravenous fluids, defibrillator, immersion tub, bath thermometer) and drugs (antipyretics)

Provide quiet

Encourage adequate rest

Reassure verbally (that the nurse is nearby and will protect the person)

Consult with the physician (as needed, and discuss methods of intervention, such as drug therapy, intravenous fluids)

Provide the family with information about the patient's progress (frequently, or if a change in condition occurs)

Nursing Observations

Monitor the body temperature (rectal thermometer or readings from a core temperature probe)

Monitor the blood pressure

Inspect the chest for respiratory rate and rhythm

Palpate the pulse for rate, rhythm, and volume

Auscultate the chest for abnormal heart sounds (dysrhythmias)

Monitor the flow rate of the intravenous fluids

Observe for confusion, convulsions

Observe for complaints of chills, headache

Inspect the skin for color (redness, pallor), for abnormal perspiration (diaphoresis, no perspiration)

Observe for signs of physiologic stability (body temperature of approximately 98.6°F; warm, dry skin)

Health Teaching

Instruct to report any serious symptoms immediately (feeling very hot or cold)

Explain the reason for and intended effect of the observation and monitoring

Medical Treatments Performed by Nurses

Administer intravenous fluids

Give the prescribed drugs

Place on a hypo- or hyperthermia blanket

Administer humidified oxygen

EVALUATION

Record actual outcome

Actual Threats of Cardiovascular Nonhomeostasis

INSTABILITY OF ARTERIAL PRESSURE[26,73,78,230,249]

ASSESSMENT

Data Collection

Subjective Data

• Person may or may not relate the following symptoms:

Weakness

Headache

Lightheadedness

Faintness in the upright position

Objective Data

Level 1

• Person exhibits signs that are intermittently unstable and stable

• Signs may or may not indicate a life-threatening imbalance

• Signs of instability are:

Increased, decreased, or fluctuating blood pressure

Level 2

• Person exhibits signs that are consistently unstable

• Signs indicate a life-threatening imbalance

• Signs of instability are:

Same as Level 1

Data Analysis

Nursing Diagnosis

INSTABILITY OF ARTERIAL PRESSURE (ARTERIAL PRESSURE INSTABILITY): Person presents unstable blood pressure readings indicating a physiologic imbalance in the relationship between cardiac output and total peripheral resistance

Common Etiology (Stressors)

DISEASES: Anaphylactic shock, cardiac insufficiency or failure, eclampsia (toxemia of pregnancy), hemorrhage, essential hypertension, pheochromocytoma, renal insufficiency or failure

SIGNS AND SYMPTOMS: Increased intracranial pressure, quadriplegia (hyperreflexia), shock

HEALTH CARE FACTORS: *Drug therapy:* Adverse effects of drugs. *Surgical therapy:* Anesthesia (general or spinal)

MAJOR PATHOPHYSIOLOGIC FACTORS CAUSING THE PROBLEM: Instability of arterial pressure results from an imbalance between cardiac output and total peripheral resistance; cardiac output may be impaired by a deficient volume of blood returned to the right heart or by various pathologic conditions of the heart or its structures; total peripheral resistance depends primarily on the caliber of the arterioles; conditions that cause vasoconstriction or vasodilatation or that impair the arteriolar nerve supply, elasticity, or lumenal size will disrupt the regulatory mechanisms for arterial pressure; severely decreased cardiac output results in hypoxia of tissues and organs, with acidosis occurring from anaerobic metabolism; a marked increased peripheral resistance can cause hypertension, which in turn increases the workload of the heart and damages the arteries by the excessive pressure; cardiac, cerebral, and renal tissues are usually the first to show evidence of the arterial damage

PLANNING

Unmet Needs

Protection from physical harm, physiologic stability

Expected Outcome

Critical changes in the arterial pressure will be promptly identified

The arterial pressure will improve to an acceptable level and ultimately be stabilized at the optimum level possible

Level 1

Person will receive frequent, intermittent nursing observation and monitoring, frequent reevaluation of status, and immediate adjustment of therapy

Level 2

Person will receive constant nursing observation and monitoring, constant reevaluation of status, and immediate adjustment of therapy

NURSING INTERVENTIONS

Nursing Treatments

Obtain a complete present and past history

Provide standby equipment (oxygen, intravenous fluids, emergency drugs)

Encourage adequate rest

Reassure verbally (that the nurse is nearby and will meet the person's needs)

Elevate the head (in hypertension), or place in the foot-elevated head-lowered (Trendelenburg) position (in hypotension)

Maintain a normal room temperature (to decrease metabolism and oxygen consumption)

Consult with the physician (as needed, and discuss methods of intervention, such as fluids and drugs)

Provide the family with information about the person's progress (frequently, or if a change in condition occurs)

Nursing Observations

Monitor the blood pressure

Palpate the pulse for rate, rhythm, and volume

Monitor the pulse pressure

Monitor the mean arterial pressure

Monitor the flow rate of the intravenous fluids

Observe for signs of physiologic stability (systolic blood pressure 100–140 mm Hg, diastolic blood pressure 60–90 mm Hg, consistently stable blood pressure after 5–6 intermittent readings, normal pulse pressure, with a systolic pressure about 40 points higher than the diastolic pressure)

Health Teaching

Instruct to report any serious symptoms immediately (severe headache, pounding pulsations, dizziness, faintness)

Explain the reason for and intended effect of the observation and monitoring

Medical Treatments Performed by Nurses

Administer intravenous fluids

Give the prescribed drugs

EVALUATION

Record actual outcome

INSTABILITY OF CARDIAC RATE/RHYTHM [26,73,78,249]

ASSESSMENT

Data Collection

Subjective Data

• Person may or may not relate the following symptoms:

  Cardiac rate: Complaints of rapid pulse, report of sudden blackout or seizures

  Cardiac rhythm: Complaints of palpitations, dyspnea, fatigue

Objective Data

Level 1

• Person exhibits signs that are intermittently unstable and stable

• Signs may or may not indicate a life-threatening imbalance

• Signs of instability are:

  Cardiac rate: Increased, decreased, or fluctuating heart/pulse rate

  Cardiac rhythm: Apical–radial pulse deficit, venous distention, irregular heart rhythm audible on auscultation, arrhythmias documented by cardiac monitor or ECG

Level 2

• Person exhibits signs that are consistently unstable

• Signs indicate a life-threatening imbalance

• Signs of instability are:

  Same as Level 1

Data Analysis

Nursing Diagnosis

INSTABILITY OF CARDIAC RATE/RHYTHM (CARDIAC RATE/RHYTHM INSTABILITY): Person presents signs of an unstable cardiac rate/rhythm indicating a physiologic imbalance in the generation or conduction of the electrical impulses of the heart

Common Etiology (Stressors)

BIRTH DEFECTS: Congenital heart disease

BIRTH STATUS: Premature infant, low-birth-weight infant

DISEASES: Anemia (severe), congestive heart failure, diabetes mellitus, endocarditis, hepatic insufficiency, hypoglycemia, hypothyroidism, infection (severe), mitral value prolapse, myocarditis, myocardial infarction, pericarditis, renal insufficiency or failure, thyrotoxicosis

INJURIES: Any severe trauma

SIGNS AND SYMPTOMS: Bleeding (severe), dehydration (moderate, severe), fever (high), hypercapnia, hypoxia, pain (severe)

PSYCHOSOCIAL FACTORS: Threat of real or imagined danger

HEALTH CARE FACTORS: *Diagnostic procedures*: Angiography, cardiac catheterization. *Medical procedures*: Hemodialysis, plasmaphoresis. *Drug therapy*: Epinephrine, atropine, digitalis, diuretics. *Therapeutic equipment*: Malfunctioning cardiac pacemaker. *Surgical therapy*: Anesthesia. *Surgical procedures*: Any

DEVELOPMENTAL PHASES: Old age

LIFESTYLE: High caffeine or alcohol intake, smoking

MAJOR PATHOPHYSIOLOGIC FACTORS CAUSING THE PROBLEM: Instability of cardiac rate can be caused by a demand for increased tissue perfusion (infection, shock, pyrexia), resulting in sympathetic stimulation and increased rate; parasympathetic (vagal) stimulation (sleep, rectal distention, gastric dilatation) will decrease the heart rate; instability of cardiac rhythm may be the result of disturbed generation or conduction of the electrical impulses; factors that disturb the electrical activity include cardiac cell damage (ischemia, infarction), electrolyte imbalance (potassium, calcium), and temperature extremes (hypo- and hyperthermia); cardiac disease can result in combined rate and rhythm instability; extremely rapid and slow cardiac rates result in decreased cardiac output, possibly with the development of hypoxemia; serious arrythmias (complete heart block, ventricular tachycardia, ventricular fibrillation) cause a serious decrease in cardiac output; the effect of the other arrhythmias varies with the length and frequency of the episodes

PLANNING

Unmet Needs
Tissue oxygenation, protection from physical harm, physiologic stability

Expected Outcome
Critical changes in the cardiac rate and rhythm will be promptly identified
The cardiac rate and rhythm will improve to an acceptable level and ultimately become stabilized at the optimum level possible

Level 1
Person will receive frequent, intermittent nursing observation and monitoring, frequent reevaluation of status, and immediate adjustment of therapy

Level 2
Person will receive constant nursing observation and monitoring, constant reevaluation of status, and immediate adjustment of therapy

NURSING INTERVENTIONS

Nursing Treatments
Connect the person to an ECG monitor (keep the ECG monitor alarms set and turned on)
Obtain a complete present and past history
Obtain a blood sample and send for analysis (CBC, electrolytes, cardiac enzymes, arterial blood gases, as requested by the physician)
Provide standby equipment (oxygen, pacemaker, defibrillator, airway intubating equipment, AMBU-bag, emergency drugs)
Reassure verbally (that the nurse is nearby and will meet the person's needs)
Consult with the physician (as needed, and discuss methods of intervention such as drugs, cardioversion, vagal stimulation, pacemaker)
Provide the family with information about the person's progress (frequently, or if a change of condition occurs)

Nursing Observations
Auscultate the apical heartbeat for rate and rhythm
Auscultate the apical and palpate the radial pulses for a pulse deficit
Auscultate the chest for abnormal heart sounds

Observe the ECG monitor (check the rhythm strip and determine the type, duration, and frequency of arrhythmia)
Check the monitor electrodes for placement periodically
Auscultate the chest for adventitious sounds
Inspect the neck veins for distention
Monitor the blood pressure
Inspect the chest for respiratory rate and rhythm
Palpate the pulse for rate, rhythm, and volume
Monitor the pulse pressure (for narrowing)
Palpate for peripheral pulses
Inspect for impaired circulation (edema, cyanosis, pallor)
Monitor the flow rate of the intravenous fluids
Measure the intake and output
Measure the body weight (daily)
Monitor the body temperature
Observe for complaints of dizziness, fatigue, nervousness
Observe for heart failure (dyspnea, nonproductive cough, neck vein distention, nausea, chest pain, edema, gallop heart rhythm, rales at the base of the lungs)
Interpret laboratory results and notify the physician of abnormalities
Observe for signs of physiologic stability (*Cardiac rate*: 70–80 beats/minute, normal volume. *Cardiac rhythm*: Regular rhythm of heartbeat, equal apical–radial pulse, no venous distention, normal ECG rhythm strip. *Skin*: Pink, warm, dry skin)

Health Teaching
Instruct to report any serious symptoms immediately (pain, palpitations, dyspnea, etc.)
Explain the reason for and intended effect of the observation and monitoring

Medical Treatments Performed by Nurses
Administer intravenous fluids
Give the prescribed drugs
Defibrillate the heart muscle
Administer humidified oxygen

EVALUATION
Record actual outcome

INSTABILITY OF TISSUE PERFUSION [1,26,73,78,230,362]

ASSESSMENT

Data Collection

Subjective Data
• Person may or may not relate the following symptoms:
Cerebral perfusion
Complaints of:
  Dizziness
  Confusion

Myocardial perfusion
Complaints of:
  Chest pain
  Apprehension
Peripheral perfusion
Complaints of:
  Cool or cold extremities
  Sweating
  Pain

Objective Data

Level 1
- Person exhibits signs that are intermittently unstable and stable
- Signs may or may not indicate a life-threatening imbalance
- Signs of instability are:
    Pallor or cyanosis
    Blanching of lips, ear lobes, nail beds
    Edema
    Increased pulse rate
    Apical–radial pulse deficit
    Decreased blood pressure
    Pale, cold skin
    Diminished to absent pulses
    Abnormal pulse pressure (above or below 30–50 mm Hg)
    Pulsus paradoxicus (pulse volume is weaker with inspiration and stronger with expiration)
    Abnormal central venous pressure (above or below 6–10 cm H_2O)
    Abnormal pulmonary capillary wedge pressure (above or below 4–12 mm Hg)
    Increased or decreased cardiac output (above or below 4–6 liters/minute)

Level 2
- Person exhibits signs that are consistently unstable
- Signs indicate a life-threatening imbalance
- Signs of instability are:
    Same as Level 1

Data Analysis

Nursing Diagnosis
INSTABILITY OF TISSUE PERFUSION (TISSUE PERFUSION INSTABILITY): Person presents unstable circulatory signs indicating physiologic imbalance in the oxygenation of and nutrient supply to body tissue

Common Etiology (Stressors)
BIRTH DEFECTS: Congenital heart disease
BIRTH STATUS: Premature infant, low-birth-weight infant
DISEASES: Any major disease that affects the cardiovascular system (abdominal, aortic, cerebral, or thoracic aneurysm), anaphylactic shock, anemia (severe), arteriosclerosis, Buerger's disease, cardiac tamponade, cardiomyopathy, cardiovascular disease, cerebrovascular accident, diabetes mellitus, disseminated intravascular coagulopathy (DIC), endocarditis, esophageal varices, hemorrhage, hypertension, severe infection, myocardial infarction, myocarditis, phlebothrombosis, Raynaud's disease, septicemia, sickle cell anemia, thrombophlebitis, thyrotoxicosis
INJURIES: Blunt and penetrating wounds to the chest, burn wound, electric shock, flail chest, heat exhaustion, heat stroke, near drowning, traumatic amputation, venomous snakebite
HUMAN BODY: *Body states:* Pregnancy

HEALTH CARE FACTORS: *Diagnostic procedures*: Angiography, biopsy (kidney, liver, or lung), cardiac catheterization *Medical procedures*: Blood transfusion, hemodialysis, plasmophoresis. *Surgical therapy*: Anesthesia. *Surgical procedures*: Any. *Therapeutic equipment*: Malfunctioning pacemaker (mechanical)

DEVELOPMENTAL PHASE: Old age

MAJOR PATHOPHYSIOLOGIC FACTORS CAUSING THE PROBLEM: Instability of tissue perfusion results when there is a disturbance in cardiac pump effectiveness, blood vessel patency, volume of blood, or quality of the oxygen-carrying components of the blood; inadequate localized tissue perfusion is more commonly caused by diseased or injured blood vessels or by the local tissue themselves; tissue ischemia of moderate-to-rapid onset causes pain as well as pallor or cyanosis; the slower the onset of ischemia, the better the ability of the cells to adjust to the decreased availability of oxygen; prolonged ischemia leads to necrosis (infarction, gangrene) of the tissues; inadequate generalized tissue perfusion is more commonly the result of cardiac insufficiency or a deficit of blood volume or hemoglobin; the tissue and organ ischemia cause signs consistent with impaired function of the specific tissues and organs involved; tissue ischemia impairs the cellular metabolic processes, leading to anaerobic metabolism, which produces an excess of lactic acid; when a large area of tissue is ischemic, metabolic acidosis develops

PLANNING

Unmet Needs

Tissue oxygenation, protection from physical harm, physiologic stability

Expected Outcome

Critical changes in tissue perfusion will be promptly identified

Tissue perfusion will improve to an acceptable level and ultimately become stabilized at the optimum level possible

Level 1

Person will receive frequent, intermittent nursing observation and monitoring, frequent reevaluation of status, and immediate adjustment of therapy

Level 2

Person will receive constant nursing observation and monitoring, constant reevaluation of status, and immediate adjustment of therapy

NURSING INTERVENTIONS

Nursing Treatments

Connect the person to an ECG monitor (keep the ECG monitor alarms set and turned on)

Obtain a complete present and past history

Obtain a blood sample and send for analysis (CBC, electrolytes, cardiac enzymes, arterial blood gases, as requested by the physician)

Provide standby equipment (oxygen, defibrillator, intubation equipment, bag–valve–mask resuscitator) and drugs (morphine, lidocaine, etc.)

Reassure verbally (that the nurse is nearby and will meet the person's needs)

Consult with the physician (as needed, and discuss methods of intervention, such as fluids, drugs, cardioversion)

Provide the family with information about the person's progress (frequently, or if a change of condition occurs)

Nursing Observations

Monitor the central venous pressure (which measures the circulating blood volume, vessel tone, and efficiency of ventricular function)

Monitor the pulmonary artery (PA) pressure by Swan-Ganz catheter (which reflects the function of the left heart by measuring the back pressure in the pulmonary artery)

Monitor the pulmonary capillary wedge pressure (PCWP) by Swan-Ganz catheter (which provides the most accurate estimate of left ventricular pressure at the end of diastole and the average left atrial pressure)

Monitor the cardiac output (a reflection of heart rate × stroke volume)

Monitor the body temperature (for fever from infection caused by catheterization for monitoring)

Check the general functioning of the hemodynamic monitoring system (catheter patency and placement, balancing and calibration of the system, airtightness of the system)

Auscultate the apical heartbeat for rate and rhythm

Auscultate the chest for abnormal heart sounds (indicating arrhythmia)

Observe the ECG monitor (check the rhythm strip and determine the type and duration of cardiac abnormalities)

Check the monitor electrodes for placement periodically

Inspect the neck veins for distention

Palpate the pulse for rate, rhythm, and volume (all the peripheral pulses)

Observe for pulsus paradoxicus (a weak pulse volume on inspiration and a strong pulse on expiration)

Monitor the blood pressure

Monitor the pulse pressure (for narrowing)

Auscultate the chest for adventitious sounds

Inspect the chest for respiratory rate and rhythm

Check the oxygen flow rate (for correct concentrations of oxygen and check equipment for proper delivery of oxygen)

Monitor the flow rate of the intravenous fluids

Measure the intake and output

Measure the body weight (daily)

Monitor blood studies for abnormal hematology, electrolytes, cardiac enzymes

Monitor blood studies for arterial blood gases

Interpret laboratory results and notify the physician of abnormalities

Inspect for impaired circulation (cyanosis, edema, pallor)

Observe for complaints of (cardiac or muscle) pain

Inspect for bleeding (petechiae, ecchymosis, hematuria, bleeding from wound or orifices, etc.)

Monitor the internal counterpulsation intraaortic balloon apparatus

Monitor the external counterpulsation pressure-suit apparatus

Determine the cerebral perfusion pressure (PP) (which is equal to the mean arterial pressure, MAP, minus the intracranial pressure, ICP: $PP = MAP - CAP$)

Observe for heart failure (dyspnea, nonproductive cough, neck vein distention, nausea, chest pain, edema, gallop heart rhythm, rales at the base of the lung)

Observe for signs of physiologic stability (*Pulse*: Regular rate 70–80 beats/minute. *Blood pressure readings*: Systolic pressure 100–140 mm Hg; diastolic pressure 60–90 mm Hg. *Normal pulse pressure*: Systolic pressure about 40 points higher than the diastolic pressure. *Normal cardiac output*: Stroke volume × heart rate = cardiac output of 4–6 liters/minute; normal serum electrolytes, cardiac enzymes, arterial blood gases; urine output of at least 20–30 ml/hour. *Skin*: Pink, warm, dry skin)

Health Teaching

Instruct to report any serious symptoms immediately (pain, palpitations, sweating, coldness, numbness, tingling)

Explain the reason for and intended effect of the observation and monitoring

Medical Treatments Performed by Nurses

Administer intravenous fluids

Give the prescribed drugs

Administer humidified oxygen

EVALUATION

Record actual outcome

Actual Threats of Fluid and Electrolyte Nonhomeostasis

INSTABILITY OF FLUID AND ELECTROLYTE STATUS[73,230,249,362]

ASSESSMENT

Data Collection

Subjective Data

• Person may or may not relate the following symptoms:

Fluid volume deficit (thirst)

Fluid volume excess (weakness, apathy)

Electrolyte imbalance (*Sodium deficit*: Dull headache, abdominal cramps, anxiety, weakness, fatigue. *Sodium excess*: Thirst. *Potassium deficit*: Anorexia, weakness, flatulence, depression. *Potassium excess*: Weakness, nausea, intestinal colic, diarrhea, paresthesias. *Calcium deficit*: Abdominal, muscle, hand, or foot cramps; tingling at the fingertips. *Calcium excess*: Deep bone or flank pain, severe muscle aches. *Magnesium deficit*: Sometimes muscle cramps, paresthesias of feet and legs, painfully cold hands and feet in vasoconstriction)

Objective Data

Level 1

• Person exhibits signs that are intermittently unstable and stable

• Signs may or may not indicate a life-threatening imbalance

• Signs of instability are:

Fluid volume deficit (weight loss, elevated temperature, hypotension, narrow pulse pressure, rapid thready pulse, dry, coated, or fissured tongue, dry skin and mucous membranes, skin folds slow to assume normal position when pinched, highly concentrated urine, scanty urine output)

In infants (absence of tears, sunken fontanel)

Fluid volume excess (weight gain of more than 1 lb/day indicates fluid retention with 1 lb equal to approximately 450 ml, edema or ascites, normal or high blood pressure, rapid pulse and respirations, moist lung rales, excessive frothy saliva, diluted urine, excessive urine output, marked personality changes, i.e., strange behavior)

Electrolyte imbalance in levels of sodium, potassium, calcium, and magnesium (*Sodium deficit*: Oliguria or anuria, decreased skin elasticity, soft, shrunken tongue, sunken, soft eyeballs, glassy stare. *Sodium excess*: Flushed skin, tough and dry tongue, oliguria, anuria. *Potassium deficit*: Abdominal distention, intestinal ileus, soft, flabby muscles, ECG abnormality. *Potassium excess*: Irritability in which muscles contract when tapped or squeezed, flaccid paralysis later, ECG abnormality. *Calcium deficit*: Muscular twitching or contractions including corpopedal spasms and tentany, Chvostek's and Trousseau's signs. *Calcium excess*: Loss of muscle tone, muscle incoordination, constipation, vomiting. *Magnesium deficit*: Positive Chvostek's sign or Babinski sign, disorientation, hyperactive deep reflexes, tremor, convulsions)

Level 2

• Person exhibits signs that are consistently unstable

• Signs indicate a life-threatening imbalance

• Signs of instability are:

Same as Level 1

Data Analysis

Nursing Diagnosis
INSTABILITY OF FLUID AND ELECTROLYTE STATUS (FLUID AND ELECTROLYTE INSTABILITY): Person shows unstable fluid and electrolyte levels, indicating a physiologic imbalance of the ratio of concentration of electrolytes and the volume of water in the body's cellular and extracellular compartments

Common Etiology (Stressors)
BIRTH STATUS: Premature infant, low-birth-weight infant

DISEASES: Metabolic acidosis, alcholism, chorea, congestive heart failure, dysentery, eclampsia, fistula, malabsorption syndrome, malnutrition, pulmonary edema, renal insufficiency or failure

INJURIES: Burn wound, cerebral concussion or contusion, crushing injury, near drowning, heat exhaustion, heat stroke

SIGNS AND SYMPTOMS: Bleeding, dehydration, diarrhea, edema, vomiting

HEALTH CARE FACTORS: *Medical therapy:* Nasogastric suction, T-tube drainage, wound drainage, gastrostomy, jejunostomy or nasogastric feeding, intravenous infusions, peritoneal dialysis. *Surgical procedures:* Any

MAJOR PATHOPHYSIOLOGIC FACTORS CAUSING THE PROBLEM: Excess water in the extracellular fluid (ECF) compartment results in a shift of water (by osmosis) into the intracellular fluid (ICF) compartment; the dilutional effect of excess water in the cells, especially brain cells and muscle cells, results in pathologic signs and symptoms; conversely, the loss of water from the ECF stimulates a shift of water from the ICF into the ECF and results in manifestations of dehydration; electrolytes (electrically charged particles dissolved in the body water) are essential to many cellular control mechanisms and to cellular reactions; an excess or deficit of one or more electrolytes in either the ECF or ICF results in pathologic signs and symptoms; for example, a potassium–calcium imbalance prevents normal transmission of electro-chemical impulses in nerve and muscle fibers, a sodium imbalance causes disturbed inorganic metabolism and fluid imbalance, and a chloride–bicarbonate imbalance disrupts acid–base balance

PLANNING

Unmet Needs
Fluid and electrolyte balance, protection from physical harm, physiologic stability

Expected Outcome
Critical levels of fluid and electrolyte imbalance will be promptly identified

The fluid and electrolyte levels will improve to an acceptable level and ultimately become stabilized at the optimum level possible

Level 1

Person will receive frequent, intermittent nursing observation and monitoring, frequent reevaluation of status, and immediate adjustment of therapy

Level 2

Person will receive constant nursing observation and monitoring, constant reevaluation of status, and immediate adjustment of therapy

NURSING INTERVENTIONS

Nursing Treatments
Obtain a complete present and past history

Obtain a blood and urine sample and send for analysis (hematocrit, serum electrolytes, urine specific gravity, and osmolality as required by the physician)

Provide standby equipment (intravenous fluids, defibrillator) and drugs (potassium, calcium, sodium chloride, magnesium, sodium bicarbonate, glucose, insulin)

Connect the person to an ECG monitor (in potassium or calcium excess or deficit)

Reassure verbally (that the nurse is nearby and will protect the person)

Consult with the physician (as needed, and discuss intervention methods, such as fluids and drugs)

Provide the family with information about the patient's progress (frequently, or if a change in condition occurs)

Nursing Observations

Monitor blood studies for abnormal electrolytes, hematology; urine studies (for specific gravity, etc.)

Interpret laboratory results and notify the physician of abnormalities

Observe the ECG monitor (check the rhythm strip and determine the type, duration, and frequency of arrhythmias if such occurs)

Measure the body weight (daily for gain or loss)

Measure the intake and output (compute the 24-hour intake and output and check for significant differences)

Test for fluid deficit (*Skin turgor*: Pinched skin takes 30 seconds or more to flatten. *Mucous membrane moisture*: Finger will not glide smoothly across the buccal mucosa)

Monitor the central venous pressure (an increase indicates increased circulating blood volume, a decrease indicates blood or fluid loss)

Monitor the pulmonary artery (PA) pressure by Swan-Ganz catheter

Monitor the pulmonary capillary wedge pressure (PCWP) by Swan-Ganz catheter

Estimate the blood volume loss (if bleeding occurs)

Monitor the body temperature

Palpate the pulse for rate, rhythm, and volume

Inspect the chest for respiratory rate and rhythm

Monitor the blood pressure

Test for Chvostek's sign

Test for a positive Trousseau's sign

Observe for signs of physiologic stability (*Fluid balance:* Normal hematocrit, consistent weight level. *Electrolyte balance:* Normal serum electrolytes)

Health Teaching

Instruct to report any serious symptoms immediately (severe weakness, irritability, fatigue, tingling, muscle spasms, pain, vomiting, convulsions)

Explain the reason for and intended effect of the observation and monitoring

Medical Treatments Performed by Nurses

Administer intravenous fluids

Give the prescribed drugs

Give the prescribed diet and fluids

EVALUATION

Record actual outcome

Actual Threats of Neurologic Nonhomeostasis[1,78,249,691]

INSTABILITY OF INTRACRANIAL PRESSURE

ASSESSMENT

Data Collection

Subjective Data

• Person may or may not relate the following symptoms:

Headache

Nausea
Visual disturbances such as double or blurred vision
Hallucinations

Objective Data

Level 1
- Person exhibits signs that are intermittently unstable and stable
- Signs may or may not indicate a life-threatening imbalance
- Signs of instability are:
    Vomiting
    Papilledema
    Nystagmus
    Pupillary changes
    Ataxia
    Behavioral changes reflecting the level of consciousness, such as progressive lethargy, inattentiveness, irritability, agitation, confusion, impaired memory, disorientation
    Muscle weakness
    Difficulty communicating
    Seizures (sometimes)
    Slow, bounding pulse
    Widening pulse pressure (with increasing systolic pressure)
    Presence of Babinski sign (sometimes)
    Bulging fontanels (of young infants)

Level 2
- Person exhibits signs that are consistently unstable
- Signs indicate a life-threatening imbalance
- Signs of instability are:
    Same as Level 1

Data Analysis

Nursing Diagnosis
INSTABILITY OF INTRACRANIAL PRESSURE (INTRACRANIAL PRESSURE INSTABILITY): Person presents an unstable level of intracranial pressure, indicating a physiologic imbalance in the proportional volume of cerebrospinal fluid, blood, and brain mass

Common Etiology (Stressors)
DISEASES: Brain abscess or tumor, encephalitis, hydrocephalus, meningitis
INJURIES: Head trauma (such as intracranial hemorrhage, subdural or epidural hematoma, concussion, contusion, skull fracture), poisoning with drugs or lead
HEALTH CARE FACTORS: *Surgical procedures:* Carotid endarterectomy, craniofacial surgery, cranioplasty, craniotomy, transsphenoidal hypophysectomy
MAJOR PATHOPHYSIOLOGIC FACTORS CAUSING THE PROBLEM: The cranial contents consist of three components: the cerebrospinal fluid, the blood supply, and the brain tissues; because these components are contained in a rigid, bony vault, an increase in the volume of any one component requires an equalizing decreased volume of the others; in pathologic states, the increased pressure from severe brain edema, large hematoma, etc., can become too great for the compensatory mechanisms, forcing the brain downward; herniation of a portion of the temporal lobe through the tentorial opening causes pressure on the third cranial nerve, causing dilatation and fixation of the pupil on the same side of the lesion; herniation of the cerebellar tissue through the foramen ovale causes pressure on the brain stem, resulting in a slowing pulse rate, rising systolic pressure, respiratory irregularities, and loss of temperature regulation; pressure on the motor pathways in the cortex causes progressive muscle weakness on the opposite side of the lesion; the slower the onset of the increased pressure, the better the compensatory mechanisms function; the more rapid the onset of pressure, the more severe or permanent the brain damage

PLANNING

Unmet Needs
Protection from physical harm, physiologic stability

Expected Outcome
Critical levels of intracranial pressure will be promptly identified

The unstable intracranial pressure will improve to an acceptable level and ultimately become stabilized at the optimum level possible

Level 1

Person will receive frequent, intermittent nursing observation and monitoring, frequent reevaluation of status, and immediate adjustment of therapy

Level 2

Person will receive constant nursing observation and monitoring, constant reevaluation of status, and immediate adjustment of therapy

NURSING INTERVENTIONS

Nursing Treatments
Obtain a complete present and past history

Provide standby equipment and drugs (such as a ventricular tap and drill set(s) and osmotic diuretics)

Maintain a steady intravenous infusion flow rate (in order to prevent increased intracranial pressure from increased vascular volume; fluid flow rate is usually maintained at 50–60 ml/hour or less for adults with increased intracranial pressure)

Avoid activities that increase intracranial pressure (prone positioning; legs hyperflexed at the hips, head, at or below the heart level; arousing the person suddenly; flexing the neck so the veins are compressed, etc.)

Space necessary activities that increase intracranial pressure (turning, suctioning, painful procedures such as injections, checking for fecal impaction, etc.)

Elevate the head (20–30 degrees, provided there are no contraindications)

Eliminate undesirable light and noise

Reassure verbally (that the nurse is nearby and will protect the person)

Consult with the physician (as needed, and discuss interventions such as drugs and fluids)

Provide the family with information about the patient's progress (frequently, or if a change in condition occurs)

Nursing Observations
Observe the level of consciousness (degree of alertness, coherence, orientation)

Inspect the eyes for pupil size, equality, and response to light

Inspect the eyes for papilledema (its current level and signs of increased or decreased papilledema)

Test for the degree of muscle/motor strength (using the palmar-drift test for upper extremities and the extended-leg test for lower extremities or have the person lift the leg off the bed and push the foot against the nurse's hand)

Test the strength and equality of the hand grasps

Observe spontaneous body movements (for bilaterally equal movement or for apparent weakness on one side)

Observe for cyanosis (if the person is not well oxygenated cerebral vasodilatation will occur, further increasing the increased intracranial pressure)

Monitor the intracranial pressure (ICP) recordings (for levels above 200 mm H_2O or 15 mm Hg)

Determine the cerebral perfusion pressure (PP) (when the intracranial pressure increases, the cerebral perfusion pressure decreases)

Observe for development of Cushing's phenomenon (increased systolic blood pressure with a widened pulse pressure, decreased pulse rate, and respiratory changes, which indicates decreased cerebral perfusion pressure resulting from increased intracranial pressure)

Palpate the pulse for rate, rhythm, and volume
Monitor the blood pressure
Inspect the chest for respiratory rate and rhythm
Monitor the rectal temperature
Inspect the ears and nose for cerebrospinal fluid leakage
Observe for a halo sign (a circle of serosanguineous fluid near the head indicates spinal fluid leakage)
Inspect the head for Battle's sign (a bruised area on the temple and behind the ear indicates a possible skull fracture)
Observe for speech loss (impaired communication abilities)
Observe for complaints of visual disturbance (double vision, blurred vision)
Observe for complaints of headache, nausea
Observe for restlessness, memory impairment, irritability, vomiting
Observe for seizures (localized or generalized)
Observe for abnormal gait (if ambulatory)
Test and observe for nystagmus (spontaneous nystagmus often occurs when the intracranial pressure is great enough to involve the brain stem)
Monitor blood studies for abnormal electrolytes, for arterial blood gases
Interpret laboratory results and notify the physician of abnormalities
Measure the intake and output (include leaking cerebrospinal fluid in output)
Observe for signs of physiologic stability (*Intracranial pressure (ICP)*: 110–140 mm H_2O or 0–10 mm Hg. *Normal cerebral perfusion pressure*: No vomiting, headache, or papilledema)

Specific to Infants
Measure the circumference of the head (for increase in size)
Palpate the cranial suture line for separation
Palpate the fontanelles for bulging or tightness (do this when the child is not crying)
Observe the characteristics of the child's cry (high-pitched cry)

Health Teaching
Instruct to report serious symptoms immediately (such as severe headache, visual disturbances, vomiting, increasing drowsiness)
Instruct to avoid activities that increase intracranial pressure (overfeeding resulting in vomiting, straining to defecate or cough, bending over or straining to reach an object, etc.)
Explain the reason for and intended effect of the observation and monitoring

Medical Treatments Performed by Nurses
Administer intravenous fluids
Give the prescribed drugs
Administer humidified oxygen

EVALUATION
Record actual outcome

INSTABILITY OF NEUROMUSCULAR FUNCTION [1,78,249,691]

ASSESSMENT
Data Collection

Subjective Data
• Person may or may not relate the following symptoms:
  Weakness
  Fatigue

Difficulty chewing, swallowing, breathing, articulating words
Numbness or tingling
Pain
Decreased or loss of control of bowel and bladder sphincters

Objective Data

Level 1
- Person exhibits signs that are intermittently unstable and stable
- Signs may or may not indicate a life-threatening imbalance
- Signs of instability are:
  Abnormal motor function (impaired body movement, muscle weakness, decreased strength of hand grasp)
  Decreased, absent, or hyperactive deep reflexes
  Loss of touch sensation
  Abnormal posturing (decorticate or decerebrate posturing)

Level 2
- Person exhibits signs that are consistently unstable
- Signs indicate a life-threatening imbalance
- Signs of instability are:
  Same as Level 1

Data Analysis

Nursing Diagnosis

INSTABILITY OF NEUROMUSCULAR FUNCTION (NEUROMUSCULAR INSTABILITY): Person presents unstable neuromuscular signs indicating a physiologic imbalance in the electrical function of nerves and muscles

Common Etiology (Stressors)

BIRTH DEFECTS: Arteriovenous malformation

BIRTH STATUS: Premature infant, low-birth-weight infant

DISEASES: Cerebral aneurysm, cerebrovascular accident, encephalitis, Guillain-Barré syndrome, meningitis, multiple sclerosis, myasthenia gravis, Reye's syndrome

INJURIES: Cerebral concussion, contusion, hematoma; fracture and compression of the spinal cord; poisoning by drugs or other chemicals

SIGNS AND SYMPTOMS: Electrolyte imbalance (potassium, calcium, sodium, magnesium)

HEALTH CARE FACTORS: *Drug therapy*: Adverse drug effects, postoperative patients who have received neuromuscular blocking drugs (curare, Syncurine, Pavulon, Anectine, etc.) may show exacerbation of paralysis if certain antibiotics are given too soon (kanamycin, neomycin, tetracycline, lincomycin, streptomycin, colistin). *Surgical procedures*: Laminectomy; laminotomy, thymectomy

ENVIRONMENTAL FACTORS: *Chemical substances*: Inhalation of substance

MAJOR PATHOPHYSIOLOGIC FACTORS CAUSING THE PROBLEM: Disturbances of neuromuscular function can vary from mild weakness or incoordination to complete paralysis; causative lesions may involve the motor neurons of the cerebral cortex, internal capsule, brain stem, spinal cord, or peripheral nerves, or they may be located at the myoneural junction or in the muscle tissues; instability of neuromuscular function results from temporary damage or from a disturbance such as brain or nerve hypoxia attributable to limited pressure, inflammatory lesions, or electrolyte imbalance; prolongation or intensification of the damages or disturbance may result in permanent loss of function

PLANNING

Unmet Needs
Protection from physical harm, physiologic stability

Expected Outcome
Critical changes in neuromuscular function will be promptly identified
The unstable neuromuscular function will improve to an acceptable level and ultimately become stabilized at the optimum level possible

Level 1

Person will receive frequent, intermittent nursing observation and monitoring, frequent reevaluation of status, and immediate adjustment of therapy

Level 2

Person will receive constant nursing observation and monitoring, constant reevaluation of status, and immediate adjustment of therapy

NURSING INTERVENTIONS

Nursing Treatments

Obtain a complete present and past history

Provide standby equipment and drugs (airway intubation equipment, drugs such as prostigmine)

Encourage alternate rest and activity (by limiting unnecessary activity and spacing necessary activity with rest periods in between to prevent muscle tiring; rest periods are especially important if the person has myasthenia gravis or multiple sclerosis)

Give full-liquid foods

OR

Give soft foods (to persons with weak chewing and swallowing muscles)

Reassure verbally (that the nurse is nearby and will protect the person)

Consult with the physician (as needed, and discuss various aspects of therapy)

Provide the family with information about the patient's progress (frequently, or if a change in condition occurs)

Nursing Observations

Observe the level of consciousness (degree of alertness, coherence, orientation)

Test for the degree of muscle/motor strength (using the palmar-drift test for the upper extremities, the extended-leg test for lower extremities)

Test the strength and equality of the hand grasps

Test for range of motion (full or limited range of motion of joints)

Test for impaired coordination (ask the person to perform lap-patting)

Test for impaired balance (with closed eyes, the person should be able to stand with feet together with little or no swaying)

Test for sensory abilities of location and position (have the person identify the part of the body touched by cotton as well as the up or down position of the big toe)

Test for decreased vibratory sensation, for heat and cold perception

Test for abnormal deep-reflex responses (caused by spinal cord injury)

Test the cranial nerves (either all or specific nerve function)

Observe for dyspnea, incontinence, irritability, lethargy, muscle twitching, tremors, abnormal gait, speech loss (including difficulty articulating words)

Observe for complaints of dizziness, fatigue, malaise, numbness and tingling, weakness

Inspect the skin for color, the joints for abnormalities, the eyelids for drooping

Inspect the eyes for pupil size, equality, and response to light

Inspect for deformity

Test and observe for nystagmus (which often indicates a neurologic disorder)

Monitor the blood pressure

Palpate the pulse for rate, rhythm, and volume

Inspect the chest for respiratory rate and rhythm

Observe performance level and problems involved in completing activities of daily living

Specific for Infants

Test the infant for the Moro reflex (infant normally responds to stimuli with a wide, flinging motion of the arms; if the Moro reflex lasts beyond 4 months, it may indicate an inability to walk)

Test the infant for the neck-righting reflex (when an infant's head is turned, he will normally turn his whole body to maintain alignment with his head; this reflex disappears at 6–8 months of age, beyond which it may indicate an inability to walk)

Test the infant for the rooting reflex (when touched on the cheek, the infant normally turns his head in that direction seeking food; failure to do so indicates central nervous system or intracranial injury)

Observe infant for adequate sucking reflex (note whether sucking is strong and consistent)

Observe for signs of physiologic stability (alert responsiveness, pupil equality and equal responses to light, firm hand grasps, full range of motion of all muscles and joints)

Health Teaching

Instruct to report any serious symptoms immediately (irritability, numbness and tingling, muscle weakness)

Instruct to avoid activities that increase intracranial pressure (especially if the person has an aneurysm, cerebrovascular accident, or concussion; activities to avoid include coughing, straining at stool or while reaching for objects)

Advise against exposure to intense heat (such as hot baths/showers, electric blankets, hot environmental temperatures, if the person has multiple sclerosis)

Explain the reason for and intended effect of the observation and monitoring

Medical Treatments Performed by Nurses

Administer intravenous fluids

Give the prescribed drugs

EVALUATION

Record actual outcome

Actual Threats of Pulmonary Nonhomeostasis

INSTABILITY OF PULMONARY FUNCTION[78,249]

ASSESSMENT

Data Collection
Subjective Data
• Person may or may not relate the following symptoms:
    Shortness of breath
    Fatigue
    Complaints of apprehension

Objective Data

Level 1
• Person exhibits signs that are intermittently unstable and stable
• Signs may or may not indicate a life-threatening imbalance
• Signs of instability are:
    Abnormal respiratory rate (deviating from the following normal rates: *Newborn:* 30–50 breaths/minute. *2–12 years:* 20–30 breaths/minute. *12–20 years:* 12–20 breaths/minute. *Adults:* 15–17 breaths/minute)
    Abnormal respiratory rhythm

Increased muscular effort during breathing with use of accessory muscles of respiration, retraction, or stridor

Vigorous abdominal and diaphragmatic movement with little chest wall movement

Periodic or cyclic pattern of breathing (rapid, shallow breathing followed by short apneic period, etc.)

Depressed respirations (very shallow or slow breathing)

Tachycardia

Cyanosis

Diaphoresis

Patient aggressively changes position from recumbent to upright

Speaks between labored breaths

Nasal flaring

Restlessness

Irritability

Coughing

Heavy pulmonary secretions

Abnormal arterial blood gases (increased or decreased pH–acid–base level, HCO_3–bicarbonate level, PaO_2–arterial oxygen level, $PaCO_2$–arterial carbon dioxide level)

Abnormal pulmonary function studies (spirometry, vital capacity, expiratory reserve capacity, inspiratory capacity, functional residual capacity)

Level 2
• Person exhibits signs that are consistently unstable
• Signs indicate a life-threatening imbalance
• Signs of instability are:
    Same as Level 1

Data Analysis

Nursing Diagnosis

INSTABILITY OF PULMONARY FUNCTION (PULMONARY FUNCTION INSTABILITY): Person presents unstable respiratory signs indicating a physiologic imbalance of pulmonary ventilation, perfusion, and gas exchange

Common Etiology (Stressors)

BIRTH DEFECTS: Chylothorax, cystic fibrosis, hyaline membrane disease

BIRTH STATUS: Premature infant, low-birth-weight infant

DISEASES: Adult respiratory distress syndrome, asbestosis, asthma, atelectasis, bronchitis, bronchopneumonia, brucellosis, cancer of the lung, cardiac tamponade, cerebrovascular accident, congestive heart failure, croup, emphysema, Guillain-Barre syndrome, myasthenia gravis, pleural effusion, pneumoconiosis, pneumonia, pneumonitis, pneumothorax, pulmonary edema, pulmonary embolus, pulmonary stenosis, tetanus, tuberculosis

INJURIES: Cerebral concussion or contusion, near drowning, electric shock, flail chest, foreign body in larynx or pharynx, heat exhaustion, heat stroke, lung or myocardial contusion, poisoning, rib or sternal fracture, venomous snakebite

SIGNS AND SYMPTOMS: Abdominal distention, tenacious secretions, bronchospasms

HEALTH CARE FACTORS: *Diagnostic procedures:* Biopsy of the lung, bronchoscopy. *Medical therapy:* Disrupted closed-chest drainage. *Drug therapy:* Barbiturates, narcotics, sedatives. *Surgical therapy:* Anesthesia. *Surgical procedure:* Bullectomy, pneumonectomy, segmental resection, thoracotomy

ENVIRONMENTAL FACTORS: *Chemical substances:* Inhalation of substance

MAJOR PATHOPHYSIOLOGIC FACTORS CAUSING THE PROBLEM: Impaired pulmonary function results from pathologic factors that interfere with ventilation, perfusion, or diffusion, or a combination of these; insufficient ventilation and imbalance between ventilation and perfusion, from increased physiologic dead space, result in hypoxemia with hypercapnia; inadequate diffusion of oxygen across the alveolar–capillary membrane (or inadequate transfer to cells) results in hypoxemia not accompanied by hypercapnia; insufficient ventilation is primarily the result of inadequate neuromuscular mechanisms, such as drugs, anesthesia, head injury, and myasthenia gravis, or of inadequate lung or chest structures, such as lung disease, obstructing secretions, and flail chest; insufficient perfusion is primarily the result of damaged capillary beds (emphysema), obstruction (emboli), or hypotension (shock); insufficient gas exchange results from an imbalance of ventilation and perfusion and from an inadequate alveolar–capillary membrane, as in fibrosis

PLANNING

Unmet Needs

Oxygen, waste elimination (carbon dioxide), protection from physical harm, physiologic stability

Expected Outcome

Critical changes in respiratory status will be promptly identified

The unstable pulmonary status will improve to an acceptable level and ultimately become stabilized at the optimum level possible

Level 1

Person will receive frequent, intermittent nursing observation and monitoring, frequent reevaluation of status, and immediate adjustment of therapy

Level 2

Person will receive constant nursing observation and monitoring, constant reevaluation of status, and immediate adjustment of therapy

NURSING INTERVENTIONS

Nursing Treatments

Connect the person to an ECG monitor (keep the ECG monitor alarms set and turned on)

Connect the person to a respiratory monitor

Obtain a complete present and past history

Obtain a blood sample and send for analysis (CBC and arterial blood gases, as requested by the physician)

Provide standby equipment (oxygen, suction machine; pharyngeal, endotracheal, and tracheostomy tubes, trays; bag–valve–mask resuscitator, mechanical ventilator, defibrillator, chest tube drainage equipment) and drugs (respiratory stimulants, diuretics, and analgesics to control pain)

Encourage alternate rest and activity (by limiting unnecessary activity and spacing necessary activity with rest periods in between in order to decrease oxygen consumption)

Give small frequent feedings
  AND
Give full-liquid foods
  OR
Give soft foods (to persons with severe dyspnea)

Avoid overheating or chilling the person (to minimize oxygen consumption. Maintain a normal room temperature. Avoid heavy blankets and clothing, body exposure to chilling, etc.)

Reassure verbally (that the nurse is nearby and will protect the person)

Place in the (well-supported) sitting position (when dyspneic, unless contraindicated by hypotension)

Suction the airway (as needed)

Anticipate and provide for needs (to decrease the need for speaking and exertion, which increases oxygen consumption)

Consult with the physician (as needed, and discuss intervention methods such as oxygen, drugs)

Provide the family with information about the patient's progress (frequently, or if a change in condition occurs)

Nursing Observations

Inspect the chest for respiratory rate and rhythm

Inspect the chest for symmetrical expansion

Observe for cyanosis, dyspnea

Auscultate the chest for lung aeration, for adventitious sounds

Auscultate the chest for abnormal breath sounds (absent or diminished breath sounds, rales, rhonchi, wheezes)

Auscultate the chest for abnormal voice sounds (pectoriloquy, bronchophony, or egophony)

Percuss the chest for abnormal resonance

Percuss the posterior chest for decreased diaphragmatic descent

Monitor the oxygen saturation status by ear oximeter or transcutaneous monitor (which gives continuous readings of the status of the oxygen (O_2) and partial arteriolar pressure of oxygen (PO_2) and helps determine when adjustments of the fraction of inspired oxygen (FIO_2) is needed)

Interpret laboratory results and notify the physician of abnormalities (evaluate the arterial blood gases in terms of oxygenation, CO_2 elimination, and acid–base balance; in very long-term, chronic situations, the hemoglobin and hematocrit may increase as the body compensates its oxygen-carrying capacity)

Observe the ECG monitor (check the rhythm strip and determine the type, duration, and frequency of any arrhythmias that occur)

Monitor the cardiac output

Monitor the blood pressure

Palpate the pulse for rate, rhythm, and volume

Monitor the flow rate of the intravenous fluids

Observe for adequate hydration (warm, moist skin, consistent weight, rapid capillary refill, pinched skin that rapidly returns to normal position)

Monitor the body temperature

Check the mechanical ventilator for proper functioning (check the settings every hour)

Check the oxygen flow rate (for correct delivery of oxygen concentrations, and check equipment for proper delivery of oxygen)

Check the chest-bottle drainage for quantity and character

Measure the intake and output

Observe the level of consciousness (degree of alertness, coherence, orientation)

Observe for heart failure (dyspnea, nonproductive cough, neck vein distention, nausea, chest pain, edema, gallop heart rhythm, rales at the base of the lungs)

Observe for pulmonary edema (restlessness, cough with frothy sputum, dyspnea, cyanosis, distended neck veins, tachycardia, wheezing, bubbling rales, severe anxiety)

Observe for complaints of apprehension

Inspect the sputum for characteristics

Observe for signs of physiologic stability (normal arterial blood gases, pink, moist skin, patent airway with airflow through the mouth or nose, chest wall or abdominal movement with each respiration)

Health Teaching

Instruct to report any serious symptoms immediately (air hunger, hemoptysis, pain)

Explain the reason for and intended effect of the observation and monitoring

Medical Treatments Performed by Nurses

Administer intravenous fluids

Give the prescribed drugs

Administer manual or mechanical ventilation

Administer oxygen by nasal cannula (or as appropriate)

EVALUATION

Record actual outcome

Actual Threats of Renal Nonhomeostasis

INSTABILITY OF RENAL CLEARANCE [78,230,249]

ASSESSMENT

Data Collection

Subjective Data

• Person may or may not relate the following symptoms:
  Anorexia
  Nausea
  Vomiting

Objective Data

Level 1
• Person exhibits signs that are intermittently unstable and stable
• Signs may or may not include a life-threatening imbalance
• Signs of instability are:
  Increased serum creatinine (above 1.4 mg/100 ml) and blood urea nitrogen (above 20 mg/100 ml)
  Decreased urine creatinine clearance (less than 100 ml/minute)
  Protein in the urine
  Urine specific gravity below 1.010 or above 1.030
  Elevated serum potassium (in acute renal failure or during the oliguric phase of chronic renal failure)
  Polyuria, oliguria, or anuria
  Confusion, sometimes

Level 2
• Person exhibits signs that are consistently unstable
• Signs indicate a life-threatening imbalance
• Signs of instability are:
  Same as Level 1

Data Analysis

Nursing Diagnosis
INSTABILITY OF RENAL CLEARANCE (RENAL CLEARANCE INSTABILITY): Person presents an unstable renal profile indicating a physiologic imbalance in the excretion and concentrating functions of the kidenys

Common Etiology (Stressors)
BIRTH DEFECTS: Congenital kidney disease (polycystic disease, familial amyloidosis)
BIRTH STATUS: Premature infant, low-birth-weight infant
DISEASES: Congestive heart failure, diabetes mellitus, glomerulonephritis, hypernephroma, interstitial nephritis, lupus erythematosus, nephroblastoma, nephrosclerosis, nephrotic syndrome, polyarteritis nodosa, pyelonephritis, renal calculi, renal insufficiency or failure, rhabdomyolosis, tubular necrosis (from cardiac failure, etc.)
INJURIES: Burn wound, crushing injury, heat stroke, poisoning
SIGNS AND SYMPTOMS: Shock (hemorrhagic)
HEALTH CARE FACTORS: *Diagnostic procedures:* Kidney biopsy. *Medical therapy:* Blood transfusion reaction. *Drug therapy:* Nephrotoxic drugs. *Surgical therapy:* Anesthesia. *Surgical procedures:* Any major surgery
DEVELOPMENTAL PHASES: Old age
ENVIRONMENTAL FACTORS: *Chemical substances:* Inhalation of substance
MAJOR PATHOPHYSIOLOGIC FACTORS CAUSING THE PROBLEM: Renal function can be impaired by a wide range of pathophysiologic factors classified according to anatomic location. *Prere-*

nal factors: Impair function by decreasing renal perfusion and include decreased cardiac output (cardiac failure, arrhythmias, septic shock), decreased vascular volume (dehydration, hemorrhage), renal vascular obstruction (thrombosis, stenosis). *Intrarenal factors:* Primary renal pathology that damages or destroys one or more components of the nephrons or the adjacent tissues and includes glomerular disease or damage (immune reaction, diabetes, toxemia of pregnancy, nephrotic syndrome), tubular damage (ischemia, hemolysis, toxins), interstitial damage (infection, toxic chemicals), vascular damage (hypertensive disease), tumors or cysts. *Postrenal factors:* Impair function by obstruction and include renal calculi, neoplasm, stricture or stenosis

PLANNING

Unmet Needs

Waste elimination (nitrogenous and other toxic substances), protection from physical harm, physiologic stability

Expected Outcome

Critical changes in renal function will be promptly identified
The unstable renal function will improve to an acceptable level and ultimately become stabilized at the optimum level possible

Level 1
Person will receive frequent, intermittent nursing observation and monitoring, frequent reevaluation of status, and immediate adjustment of therapy

Level 2
Person will receive constant nursing observation and monitoring, constant reevaluation of status, and immediate adjustment of therapy

NURSING INTERVENTIONS

Nursing Treatments

Obtain a complete present and past history
Obtain a blood sample and send for analysis (renal profile including BUN, creatinine, protein, uric acid, CBC, and electrolytes as requested by the physician)
Obtain a urine sample and send for analysis (both routine and 24-hour analysis)
Catheterize with an indwelling urinary catheter (if requested by the physician to facilitate urine measurement)
Provide standby equipment (intravenous fluids, peritoneal dialysis tray, catheterization tray) and drugs (diuretics)
Reassure verbally (that the nurse is nearby and will protect the person)
Consult with the physician (as needed, and discuss interventions such as fluids and drugs)
Provide the family with information about the patient's progress (frequently, or if a change in condition occurs)

Nursing Observations

Monitor blood studies for abnormal renal function (elevated BUN, creatinine, decreased serum protein)
Monitor urine studies for abnormal renal function (creatinine clearance, protein, urea and urea clearance, uric acid, specific gravity)
Interpret laboratory results and notify the physician of abnormalities
Measure the body weight (daily for gain or loss)
Measure the intake and output (compute the 24-hour intake and output, check for a significant difference)
Monitor the blood pressure
Palpate the pulse for rate, rhythm, and volume
Inspect the chest for respiratory rate and rhythm
Monitor the body temperature
Observe for confusion (or other behavioral changes), muscle twitching, restless leg phenomenon, convulsions

Observe for complaints of pain (in the costovertebral angle, flank pain)

Observe the urine for abnormal color (very dark or pale), content (blood, pus, fatty droplets), and odor

Observe the urine by implementing the three-bottle procedure (put the person's first voiding in urine bottle no. 1, second voiding in bottle no. 2, and third voiding in bottle no. 3, then discard and clean bottle no. 1 for the fourth voiding and continue the rotating procedure, and check the characteristics of the urine by comparing the three specimens)

Observe the ECG monitor (for signs of hyperkalemia)

Observe for signs of physiologic stability (BUN, creatinine, protein, creatinine clearance within normal limits, adequate urinary output, normal urine studies)

Health Teaching

Instruct to report any serious symptoms immediately (confusion, twitching, polyuria, oliguria, or anuria)

Teach how to adjust the diet (both food and fluids according to dietary needs and restrictions)

Explain the reason for and intended effect of the observation and monitoring

Medical Treatments Performed by Nurses

Administer intravenous fluids

Give the prescribed drugs

Give the prescribed diet, the prescribed fluids

EVALUATION

Record actual outcome

Actual Threats of Reproductive Nonhomeostasis

INSTABILITY OF FETUS STATUS[50,388,527]

ASSESSMENT

Data Collection

Subjective Data

• Mother may or may not relate symptoms:
   Absence of fetal movement

Objective Data

Level 1

• Fetus exhibits signs that are intermittently unstable and stable
• Signs may or may not indicate a life-threatening imbalance
• Signs of instability are:
   Tachycardia of fetal heart rate, over 160 beats/minute
   Bradycardia of fetal heart rate, under 110 beats/minute
   Loss of variability, in which the internal monitor records a smooth instead of a dipping baseline
   Meconium (fetal stool) in the amniotic fluid when the membranes rupture

Level 2

• Fetus exhibits signs that are consistently unstable
• Signs indicate a life-threatening imbalance

• Signs of instability are:
  Same as Level 1

Data Analysis

Nursing Diagnosis

INSTABILITY OF FETUS STATUS (FETUS INSTABILITY): The unborn fetus presents unstable signs indicating a physiologic imbalance that threatens normal development and/or birth

Common Etiology (Stressors)

BIRTH STATUS: Potential premature infant, multiple gestation

DISEASES (MATERNAL): Anemia (severe), cardiovascular disease, diabetes mellitus, eclampsia, infection, hemorrhage, placental insufficiency, preeclampsia

INJURIES (MATERNAL): Any severe trauma

SIGNS AND SYMPTOMS: Edema, fever

HEALTH CARE FACTORS: *Drug therapy*: Adverse effects of any drug. *Medical therapy*: Fetal injury from amniocentesis. *Surgical therapy*: Anesthesia

MAJOR PATHOPHYSIOLOGIIC FACTORS CAUSING THE PROBLEM: Instability of fetal status is primarily caused by fetal hypoxia; this may result from mechanical causes such as compression of the umbilical cord by the fetal head or from functional causes such as placental insufficiency, maternal shock or severe anemia, or eclampsia; fetal hypoxia leads to serious acidosis; mild, chronic hypoxia results in fetal tachycardia; severe hypoxia causes fetal bradycardia and a relaxed anal sphincter, with meconium staining of the amniotic fluid

PLANNING

Unmet Needs

Protection from physical harm, physiologic stability

Expected Outcome

Critical changes in fetal status will be promptly identified

The unstable fetal status will improve to an acceptable level and ultimately become stabilized at the optimum level possible

Level 1

Person will receive frequent, intermittent nursing observation and monitoring, frequent reevaluation of status, and immediate adjustment of therapy

Level 2

Person will receive constant nursing observation and monitoring, constant reevaluation of status, and immediate adjustment of therapy

NURSING INTERVENTIONS

Nursing Treatments

Connect the mother to the fetal/maternal ultrasound monitor (placing and attaching the transducers against the abdomen)

Obtain a complete present and past history

Obtain a maternal blood sample and send for analysis (arterial blood gases will reveal the maternal acid–base status, which effects the fetus; send fetal blood sample if such has been obtained by the physician)

Place (the mother) in the side-lying position (to reduce the compression of the uterus on the vena cava)

Provide standby equipment and drugs (for both a vaginal delivery and a cesarean section, including suction machine, incubator, warm receiving blanket)

Maintain a warm room temperature (in the delivery room)

Withhold all drugs (which might depress the fetus)

Encourage (maternal) deep breathing (for relaxation and anxiety-reducing purposes)

Reassure (the mother and father) verbally (that the nurse is nearby and will protect both the mother and fetus)

Consult with the physician (as needed, and discuss intervention methods)

Provide the family with information about maternal/fetal progress (frequently, or if a change in condition occurs)

Nursing Observations

Observe the fetal/maternal ultrasound monitor (observe for tetanic uterine contractions and for a type II deceleration in fetal heart tones, which indicates fetal distress)

Time the uterine contractions

Palpate the uterus for contraction quality

Monitor the fetal heart sounds (with a fetoscope, and notify the physician if the fetal heart rate is below 110 or above 160 beats/minute)

Monitor the (maternal) blood pressure

Palpate the (maternal) pulse for rate, rhythm, and volume

Inspect the (maternal) chest for respiratory rate and rhythm

Monitor the (maternal) body temperature (for fever, indicating infection)

Monitor the flow rate of the intravenous fluids

Interpret laboratory results and notify the physician of abnormalities (a fetal blood pH of 7.25 or less should be reported immediately to the physician)

Inspect the amniotic fluid for meconium (which, when present, indicates fetal hypoxia)

Observe for signs of physiologic stability (normal fetal heart rate of 120–160 beats/minute, fetal movement, no meconium stools, normal fetal scalp blood pH above 7.25)

Health Teaching

Instruct (the mother) to report any serious symptoms immediately (absence of fetal movement, unexpected pain)

Explain the reason for and intended effect of the observation and monitoring

Medical Treatments Performed by Nurses

Administer intravenous fluids

Give the prescribed drugs

Administer humidified oxygen (to the mother at 7–8 liters)

EVALUATION

Record actual outcome

Actual Threats of Psychologic Nonhomeostasis

INSTABILITY OF PSYCHOLOGICAL BEHAVIOR[105,371,471]

ASSESSMENT

Data Collection

Subjective Data
• Person may or may not relate the following symptoms:
  Feels a severe decrease in capacity to function or to control behavior

Objective Data

Level 1
• Person exhibits signs that are intermittently unstable and stable
• Signs may or may not indicate a life-threatening imbalance
• Signs of instability are:
  Unpredictable, exaggerated, or uncontrolled behavior
  Noticeable changes in behavior or thinking

Level 2
- Person exhibits signs that are consistently unstable
- Signs indicate a life-threatening imbalance
- Signs of instability are:
   Same as Level 1

Data Analysis

Nursing Diagnosis
INSTABILITY OF PSYCHOSOCIAL BEHAVIOR (BEHAVIORAL INSTABILITY): Person presents unstable emotional or behavioral signs indicating a poorly integrated psychologic status

Common Etiology (Stressors)
DISEASES: Alcoholism, brain abscess or tumor, major depression, manic–depressive psychosis, obsessive–compulsive neurosis, organic brain syndrome, psychosis
SITUATIONAL FACTORS: Situational crisis/stress

PLANNING

Unmet Needs
Protection from physical harm and psychologic threat, psychologic stability

Expected Outcome
Critical changes in behavior will be promptly identified
The psychologic instability will improve to an acceptable level and ultimately become stabilized at the optimum level possible
Person will gain control and be able to maintain effective psychologic responses

Level 1
Person will receive frequent, intermittent nursing observation and monitoring, frequent reevaluation of status, and immediate adjustment of therapy

Level 2
Person will receive constant nursing observation and monitoring, constant reevaluation of status, and immediate adjustment of therapy

NURSING INTERVENTIONS

Nursing Treatments
Obtain a complete present and past history
Provide standby drugs (sedatives, tranquilizers)
Arrange pleasant surroundings, orderly surroundings
Provide quiet
Provide privacy
Provide seclusion (if needed, to prevent the person from harming himself or others)
Minimize environmental dangers (remove objects that might be used to harm the person or others)
Attend the person constantly
   OR
Provide frequent patient contact
Reassure verbally (that the nurse is nearby and will protect the person)
Consult with the physician or psychiatric nurse specialist (as needed)
Provide the family with information about the patient's progress (frequently, or if a change in condition occurs)

Nursing Observations
Determine the precipitating factors and the relieving factors (of the instability)
Identify abnormal perceptions (hallucinations, illusions)
Identify abnormal thought content (obsessive thoughts, autistic thinking, delusions about self or others)
Identify attention span abnormalities (short attention span)
Identify disturbing conversation topics
Identify the appropriate use of defense mechanisms, the inappropriate use of defense mechanisms

Identify the current dominant emotion (anger, grief, hopelessness)

Observe for evidence that the person is reaching out for emotional support

Observe for impaired conceptual thinking (confused, irrational thought), for impaired judgment (difficulty identifying and solving problems), and for memory impairment (difficulty with recall)

Evaluate the significance of emotional distress mannerisms

Evaluate the significance of nonverbal communication

Evaluate the safety of the environment (while the person is unstable)

Observe for signs of psychologic stability (independent functioning, control of behavior, satisfaction within self)

Health Teaching

Instruct to report any serious symptoms immediately (oncoming loss of control, intense anxiety, etc.)

Explain the reason for and intended effect of the observation and monitoring

Medical Treatments Performed by Nurses

Give the prescribed drugs

EVALUATION

Record actual outcome

Potential Threats to Acid–Base Homeostasis

POTENTIAL FOR METABOLIC ACIDOSIS[42,371,399]

ASSESSMENT

Data Collection

Subjective Data
• There are no actual symptoms of metabolic acidosis

Objective Data
• There are no actual signs of metabolic acidosis

Related Data
• There are one or more stressors present that increase the possibility that metabolic acidosis will occur

DISEASES: Addison's disease, alcoholism, anemia, congestive heart failure, Crohn's disease, diabetes mellitus, fistula (small bowel or pancreatic), hepatitis, malnutrition, myocardial infarction, renal insufficiency, thyrotoxicosis

INJURIES: Drug overdose (especially salicylates), poisoning

SIGNS AND SYMPTOMS: Dehydration, diarrhea, fever, hypoxia, shock

HEALTH CARE FACTORS: *Medical therapy*: Intestinal drainage by nasogastric suction, intravenous infusions of sodium chloride solutions or with potassium. *Drug therapy*: Carbonic anhydrase inhibitor therapy

LIFESTYLE: High-fat diet, liquid protein diet, low-carbohydrate diet, overvigorous exercise

Data Analysis

Nursing Diagnosis

POTENTIAL FOR METABOLIC ACIDOSIS: The presence of stressors that increase the possibility of the actual occurrence of an excessive accumulation of acids or loss of bicarbonate

PLANNING

Unmet Needs

Protection from physical harm, increased learning

Expected Outcome

No signs or symptoms of metabolic acidosis will occur
OR
If signs and symptoms occur, they will be promptly recognized as an *actual* problem and appropriately treated
Person will, when able, take appropriate precautions to prevent accumulation of acids and excessive loss of base

NURSING INTERVENTIONS

Nursing Treatments

Provide a balanced nutritional diet (if intake is poor)
Give high-sodium fluids orally (avoid high-chloride fluids)
AND
Encourage increased sodium-food intake (during prolonged, profuse sweating or impaired renal function where there is sodium loss)
Encourage increased carbohydrate intake (during fever)

Nursing Observations

Monitor blood studies for abnormal acid–base (decreased bicarbonate HCO_3, pH increased lactic acid in chronic cardiac problems)
Monitor blood studies for abnormal glucose (if the patient has diabetes)
Test the urine for pH (below 5.5)
Test the urine for sugar and acetone (if the patient has diabetes)
Monitor the pulse pressure (for widening)
Palpate the pulse for volume (bounding pulse)
Palpate the skin for temperature (increased warmth)
Inspect the skin for color (flushed appearance)
Inspect for dehydration
Observe for complaints of dizziness, malaise, pain (abdominal), thirst, weakness
Observe for restlessness, vomiting
Observe the breath for abnormal odors
Observe the level of consciousness

Health Teaching

Describe those symptoms that should be reported (weakness, malaise, nausea, vomiting, headache, drowsiness)
Teach the principles of good nutrition (in maintainng acid–base balance, such as increased carbohydrate intake during fever and increased sodium intake during diaphoresis, and in balancing nutritional intake and exercise with the diabetic's insulin dosage, etc.)
Explain why the potential problem could become actual (when carbohydrate reserves are depleted or there is poor nutritional intake, the body obtains its energy through protein and fat metabolism, which leads to acidosis; in fever, carbohydrate demands are increased while carbohydrate intake is usually decreased; impaired carbohydrate metabolism, as in diabetes, fails to control the blood sugar, which results in increased fat metabolism and the accumulation of blood ketones; adequate sodium is needed to combine with carbonic acid and maintain a normal pH level; in profuse sweating and impaired kidney function, the loss of sodium reduces the amount available to combine with carbonic acid)
Explain the reason for and intended effect of the preventive therapy

EVALUATION

Record actual outcome

POTENTIAL FOR METABOLIC ALKALOSIS[42,371,399]

ASSESSMENT

Data Collection

Subjective Data
• There are no actual symptoms of metabolic alkalosis

Objective Data
• There are no actual signs of metabolic alkalosis

Related Data
• There are one or more stressors present that increase the possibility that metabolic alkalosis will occur

DISEASES: Bartter's syndrome, Cushing's syndrome, milk alkali syndrome, primary aldosteronism, chronic respiratory acidosis

SIGNS AND SYMPTOMS: Vomiting (hydrochloric acid loss), diarrhea (potassium loss)

HEALTH CARE FACTORS: *Medical therapy*: Intravenous infusions with large doses of bicarbonate or lactated infusions, nasogastric suction (loss of hydrochloric acid). *Drugs*: Adverse effects of drugs such as corticosteroids, diuretics (increased renal excretion of potassium and chloride)

HUMAN ERROR: Excess intake of antacids (alkalis) or bicarbonates, especially with high milk intake, excessive ingestion of licorice (20–40 gm daily).

Data Analysis

Nursing Diagnosis
POTENTIAL FOR METABOLIC ALKALOSIS: The presence of stressors that increase the possibility of the actual occurrence of an excessive bicarbonate accumulation or loss of acid

PLANNING

Unmet Needs
Protection from physical harm, increased learning

Expected Outcome
No signs or symptoms of metabolic alkalosis will occur
  OR
If signs and symptoms occur, they will be promptly recognized as an actual problem and will be treated appropriately
The person will, when able, take appropriate precautions to prevent accumulation of bicarbonate and excessive loss of acid

NURSING INTERVENTIONS

Nursing Treatments
Give fruit juices (which are acidifying, such as cranberry, plum, prune)
Give high potassium fluids orally
  OR
Encourage increased potassium-food intake (when on diuretics or adrenocorticosteroids and during vomiting and diarrhea)
Refrain from giving bicarbonates, milk, carbonated beverages
Irrigate the gastric tube with saline (instead of plain water)

Nursing Observations
Monitor blood studies for abnormal acid–base (such as increased bicarbonate (HCO_3) level, increased pH, and decreased chloride level)
Test the urine for pH (above 7.42)
Observe for tremors (of the hands)
Inspect the chest for respiratory rate and rhythm
Observe for compaints of weakness, anorexia, headache
Observe for convulsions, irritability, restlessness, tetany, vomiting
Auscultate the abdomen for abnormal (decreased) bowel sounds

Health Teaching

Describe those symptoms that should be reported (lethargy, tetany, tremor, convulsions, vomiting, irritability, confusion, twitching)

Teach how to adjust the diet (for maintaining acid–base balance, such as use of acidifying juices, high potassium fluids, etc.)

Explain why the potential problem could become actual (alkalosis can result when there is excessive bicarbonate intake, incompatible nutritional intake and insulin dosage, or the administration of corticosteroids)

Explain the reason for and intended effect of the preventive therapy

Recommend that alkalis be used conservatively (such as absorbable antacids and milk)

EVALUATION

Record actual outcome

POTENTIAL FOR RESPIRATORY ACIDOSIS[42,371,399]

ASSESSMENT

Data Collection

Subjective Data
• There are no actual symptoms of respiratory acidosis

Objective Data
• There are no actual signs of respiratory acidosis

Related Data
• There are one or more stressors present that increase the possibility that respiratory acidosis will occur

DISEASES: Adult respiratory distress syndrome, asthma, atelectasis from airway obstruction, chronic bronchitis, chronic obstructive pulmonary disease (COPD), emphysema, Guillain-Barre syndrome, myasthenia gravis, severe pneumonia, large pneumothorax, poliomyelitis, pulmonary edema

INJURIES: Injuries to the central nervous system (specifically the medulla)

HEALTH CARE FACTORS: *Medical therapy*: Mechanical ventilation (with hypoventilation). *Drug therapy*: Adverse effects of drugs, depressants (hypnotics, narcotics, sedatives, etc.) *Surgical therapy*: Anesthesia

Data Analysis

Nursing Diagnosis
POTENTIAL FOR RESPIRATORY ACIDOSIS: The presence of stressors that increase the possibility of the actual occurrence of an abnormally high level of carbon dioxide accumulating in the blood

PLANNING

Unmet Needs

Protection from physical harm, increased learning

Expected Outcome

No signs or symptoms of respiratory acidosis will occur
  OR
If signs and symptoms occur, they will be promptly recognized as an actual problem and will be treated appropriately

The person will, when able, take appropriate actions to maintain adequate pulmonary ventilation

NURSING INTERVENTIONS

Nursing Treatments

Encourage deep breathing (frequently)

Encourage moderate physical exercise (not strenuous exercise)

Refrain from giving carbonated beverages
Withhold the oxygen therapy (if the blood O_2 level is elevated)
Suction the airway (to keep the airway clear of obstructing secretions)

Nursing Observations

Inspect the chest for respiratory rate, depth, and rhythm (depression)
Auscultate the chest for lung aeration
Monitor blood studies for abnormal gas exchange (increased CO_2)
Observe for complaints of headache, visual disturbance
Palpate the pulse for rate (tachycardia), rhythm, and volume
Observe the level of consciousness

Health Teaching

Instruct to increase fluid intake
Teach how to do abdominal breathing
Teach how to do resistive breathing exercises
Describe those symptoms that should be reported (headache, visual disturbances, tachycardia)
Teach how to do bronchopulmonary hygiene measures
Explain why the potential problem could become actual (excessive amounts of carbon dioxide, in the form of carbonic acid, accumulate when a pulmonary or neuromuscular disorder prevents adequate ventilation of the lungs or when a person breathes air containng above normal amounts of carbon dioxide)
Explain the reason for and intended effect of the preventive therapy

EVALUATION

Record actual therapy

POTENTIAL FOR RESPIRATORY ALKALOSIS[42,371,399]

ASSESSMENT

Data Collection

Subjective Data
• There are no actual symptoms of respiratory alkalosis

Objective Data
• There are no actual signs of respiratory alkalosis

Related Data
• There are one or more stressors present that increase the possibility of respiratory alkalosis occurring
DISEASES: Acidosis (metabolic), asthma, bacteremia (gram-negative), brain tumor, encephalitis, hepatic failure, hyperventilation (from anxiety), pneumonia
INJURIES: Drug overdose (aspirin), cerebral injury (medulla)
SIGNS AND SYMPTOMS: Fever
HEALTH CARE FACTORS: *Medical therapy:* Mechanical ventilation (with hyperventilation). *Drug therapy*: Adverse effects of drugs (stimulants)
ENVIRONMENTAL FACTORS: *Environmental heat*: High external temperature

Data Analysis

Nursing Diagnosis
POTENTIAL FOR RESPIRATORY ALKALOSIS: The presence of stressors that increase the possibility of the actual occurrence of excess carbon dioxide excretion

PLANNING

Unmet Needs

Protection from physical harm, increased learning

Expected Outcome

No signs or symptoms of respiratory alkalosis will occur
  OR
If signs and symptoms occur, they will be recognized as an actual problem and will be
  treated appropriately
The person will, when able, take appropriate actions to prevent hyperventilation

NURSING INTERVENTIONS

Nursing Treatments

Attend the patient constantly (if breathing rapidly or deeply)
Elevate the head ⎫
  OR   ⎬ To ease breathing
Place in the sitting position ⎭
Refrain from giving continuous positive pressure breathing (at a rapid rate or with ex-
  cessive pressure)
Provide a paper bag for breathing (and assist the person to breathe into the paper bag
  at regular intervals when unable to control breathing pattern)

Nursing Observations

Inspect the chest for respiratory rate, depth, and rhythm
Monitor blood studies for arterial blood gases (decreased Pco_2, increased pH)
Observe for complaints of dizziness, lightheadedness, numbness, and tingling, tinnitus
Observe for tetany, muscle twitching, tremors

Health Teaching

Explain why the potential problem could become actual (rapid or very deep respirations
  cause excessive loss of carbon dioxide, resulting in alkalosis)
Describe those symptoms that should be reported (numbness and tingling, muscle
  twitching, lightheadedness)
Advise that highly emotional situations be avoided (if the person is susceptible to hyper-
  ventilation)
Teach how to do breath-holding (and slow, relaxed breathing)
Explain how to use a paper bag to reduce hyperventilation (if it occurs)
Recommend that high altitudes be avoided (after cardiac damage)
Recommend methods for achieving total relaxation (to reduce anxiety-related hyperven-
  tilation; such as breathing-control techniques and listening to soft music)
Explain the reason for and intended effect of the preventive therapy

EVALUATION

Record actual outcome

Potential Threats to Body Temperature Homeostasis

POTENTIAL FOR HYPOTHERMIA[35,72,527]

ASSESSMENT

Data Collection

Subjective Data

• There are no actual symptoms of decreased body temperature

Objective Data

• There are no actual signs of decreased body temperature

Related Data

• There are one or more stressors present that increase the possibility that decreased body temperature will occur

BIRTH STATUS: Premature infant

DISEASES: Alcoholism, anemia, arteriosclerosis, diabetes mellitus, hypoglycemia, myxedema

INJURIES: Burn wound, fracture and compression of the spinal cord, starvation

HEALTH CARE FACTORS: *Health therapy*: Body exposure for therapy. *Medical therapy*: Therapeutic apheresis. *Surgical therapy*: Body exposure during surgery

DEVELOPMENTAL PHASES: Infancy (newborn), old age

LIFESTYLE: Insufficient or unbalanced diet

ENVIRONMENTAL FACTORS: *Environmental cold*: Low external temperature

Data Analysis

Nursing Diagnosis

POTENTIAL FOR HYPOTHERMIA (POTENTIAL FOR SUBNORMAL TEMPERATURE): The presence of stressors that increase the possibility of the actual occurrence of a body temperature below 96° F orally or 97° F rectally

PLANNING

Unmet Needs

Protection from physical harm, increased learning

Expected Outcome

No signs or symptoms of decreased body temperature will occur
 OR
If signs and symptoms occur, they will be promptly recognized as an actual problem and will be treated appropriately
Person (or care giver) verbalizes an understanding of and practices preventive methods

NURSING INTERVENTIONS

Nursing Treatments

Decrease drafts
Drape for warmth
Dress in warm clothing
Maintain a warm room temperature
Refrain from giving iced liquids
Refrain from giving local cold applications
Encourage increased protein-food intake (if the problem is chronic)
Encourage moderate physical exercise

Specific to the Newborn Infant

Maintain a warm body temperature for the newborn (wrap the infant in a dry, warm towel or blanket; warm hands before touching infant; place the infant on a dry, warm surface, in an open bed with radiant overhead heat, or next to the mother's warm skin)
 OR
Place the newborn in an incubator
Maintain a normal room temperature
 AND
Decrease drafts (in the delivery room)
Delay bathing (the infant until normal temperature is established)

Nursing Observations

Monitor the oral temperature
 OR
Monitor the rectal temperature
Check the environmental controls on the incubator periodically

Health Teaching
Describe those symptoms that should be reported (chills, low temperature)
Advise against exposure to inclement weather
Recommend the use of warm clothing
Explain why the potential problem could become actual (a decreased metabolic rate, inadequate nutrition, impaired peripheral nerve function, or poor tissue oxygenation can result in decreased body temperature)
Explain the reason for and intended effect of the preventive therapy

EVALUATION
Record actual outcome

POTENTIAL FOR FEVER[35,72]

ASSESSMENT

Data Collection

Subjective Data
• There are no actual symptoms of elevated body temperature

Objective Data
• There are no actual signs of elevated body temperature

Related Data
• There are one or more stressors present that increase the possibility of an elevated body temperature
DISEASES: Brain tumor, cerebrovascular accident, infection of any kind, herpes zoster, Hodgkin's disease, leukemia, thyrotoxicosis
INJURIES: Trauma of any kind, especially brain injury to the hypothalamus
SIGNS AND SYMPTOMS: Dehydration
HUMAN BODY: *Natural body function*: Childbirth
HEALTH CARE FACTORS: *Diagnostic procedures*: Invasive diagnostic procedures. *Medical therapy*: Invasive medical therapy such as chest tube drainage, urinary catheter drainage, hemodialysis, intravenous infusion, bladder irrigation, paracentesis, peritoneal dialysis, thoracentesis, blood transfusion; alcohol or drug withdrawal. *Drug therapy*: Adverse effects of drugs such as epinephrine, atropine (especially in children), Pro-Banthine (propantheline), immunization vaccines, allergy to drugs, especially antibiotics, antineoplastics, sulfonamides, barbiturates, thiouracils, iodides, and laxatives containing phenolphthalein, which can cause drug fever. *Surgical therapy*: Any surgery
ENVIRONMENTAL FACTORS: *Environmental heat*: High external temperature
HUMAN ERROR: Overdressing an infant in excessively warm clothing

Data Analysis

Nursing Diagnosis
POTENTIAL FOR FEVER (POTENTIAL FOR PYREXIA) (POTENTIAL FOR ELEVATED BODY TEMPERATURE): The presence of stressors that increase the possibility of the actual occurrence of a body temperature above 99.5° F orally or 100.5° F rectally

PLANNING

Unmet Needs
Protection from physical harm, increased learning

Expected Outcome
No signs or symptoms of elevated body temperature will occur
  OR
If signs and symptoms occur, they will be promptly recognized as an actual problem and will be treated appropriately

The person (or care giver) verbalizes an understanding of and practices preventive methods

NURSING INTERVENTIONS

Nursing Treatments

Balance fluid intake to equal output
Discourage the intake of oral stimulants
Cover with lightweight blankets (in cold or drafty environments)
Dress in lightweight clothing
Maintain a cool room temperature
Refrain from giving hot liquids
Refrain from giving local heat applications
Encourage moderate activity, moderate physical exercise (and recommend avoiding excessive activity or exercise)

Nursing Observations

Monitor the body temperature

Health Teaching

Describe the signs and symptoms that indicate the need for taking the temperature (hot dry skin, flushed face, malaise, convulsion in infant, chill in adult)
Describe those symptoms that should be reported (fever)
Explain why the potential problem could become actual (normally, the body responds with an elevated temperature when there is infection, increased metabolic rate, impaired circulation, central nervous system depression or damage, or dehydration)
Explain the reason for and intended effect of the preventive therapy

EVALUATION

Record actual outcome

Potential Threats to Cardiovascular Homeostasis

POTENTIAL FOR BLEEDING/HEMORRHAGE[278,371]

ASSESSMENT

Data Collection

Subjective Data

• There are no actual symptoms of bleeding or hemorrhage

Objective Data

• There are no actual signs of bleeding or hemorrhage

Related Data

• There are one or more stressors present that increase the possibility that bleeding or hemorrhage will occur

DISEASES: Abortion (natural), aneurysm (abdominal, aortic, cerebral, or thoracic), aplastic anemia, carcinoma, cerebrovascular accident, endometriosis, esophageal varices, gastric ulcer, hemophilia, hypertension, Laennec's cirrhosis, leukemia, scurvy, subarachnoid hemorrhage

INJURIES: Trauma of any kind

NATURAL BODY FUNCTION: Childbirth

BODY STATES: Menstruation, pregnancy

HEALTH CARE FACTORS: *Diagnostic procedures*: Angiography, blood analysis sampling (by venipuncture or arterial puncture), biopsy (kidney, liver, lung, muscle, skin), bronchoscopy, cardiac catheterization, colonoscopy, gastroscopy, proctosigmoidoscopy. *Medical or nursing therapy or procedures*: Hemodialysis, thoracentesis, exchange blood transfusion, therapeutic apheresis, withdrawal of intravenous infusion or blood transfusion needle. *Drug therapy*: Adverse effects of anticoagulant therapy, large doses of aspirin. *Surgical procedure*: Any. *Therapeutic equipment*: Placement on a bypass machine, chest tube and drainage apparatus

Data Analysis

Nursing Diagnosis

POTENTIAL FOR BLEEDING OR HEMORRHAGE: The presence of stressors that increase the possibility of the actual occurrence of blood loss through bleeding or hemorrhage

PLANNING

Unmet Needs

Protection from physical harm, increased learning

Expected Outcome

No signs or symptoms of bleeding/hemorrhage will occur
   OR
If signs and symptoms occur, they will be promptly recognized as an actual problem and will be treated appropriately
Person verbalizes an understanding of and practices preventive methods

NURSING INTERVENTIONS

Nursing Treatments

Apply a cold pack
   OR
Apply manual pressure over the potential bleeding area (if there is injury but bleeding has not started yet or when venipuncture or arterial puncture has been done)
Handle gently
Refrain from dislodging blood clots
Refrain from giving hot liquids or oral stimulants (which dilate blood vessels and increase circulation)
Give bland foods (to prevent erosion of esophageal varicies or gastric ulcer)
Withhold drugs (such as salicylates, which cause bleeding)

Specific to Potential Internal Bleeding
Place on complete bed rest
Refrain from jarring the bed
Change the person's position gradually

Specific to Potential Gum or Oral Bleeding
Brush the teeth with a soft toothbrush

Specific to Potential Bleeding from Blood Dyscrasis or Anticoagulant Therapy
Use small-gauge injection needles

Specific to Potential Uterine Bleeding
Massage the uterine fundus (at regular intervals after delivery)

Specific to Potential Bleeding from a Liver or Kidney Biopsy
Position with pillows (for maximum pressure against the puncture site; have the person lay on the right side with the pillow under the liver area after a liver biopsy, and have him lay with the pillow under the appropriate costovertebral angle for kidney biopsy)

Nursing Observations

Inspect for bleeding
Inspect for hemorrhage

Monitor blood studies for abnormal clotting mechanism (increased bleeding, clotting, prothrombin, or partial thromboplastin time)

Monitor blood studies for abnormal hematology (decreased blood antihemophiliac factor, fibrinogen, hematocrit, hemoglobin or platelet count)

Health Teaching

Describe those symptoms that should be reported (bleeding)

Advise against pulling off scabs

Inform that coughing should be avoided
> AND

Inform that elimination straining should be avoided
> AND

Inform that heavy lifting should be avoided (for potential internal bleeding)

Advise not to stand for prolonged periods (for potential bleeding after childbirth, excessive menstrual flow, or rectal bleeding)

Instruct to change position gradually

Explain the need to avoid mechanical trauma

Instruct to carefully move the injured body part

Instruct to use a soft, new toothbrush and to apply only mild toothbrush pressure (for potential gum or oral bleeding)

Explain why the potential problem could become actual (the potential for bleeding increases when there is a blood coagulation defect in liver or bone marrow disorders, when drugs form an antithrombin that prevents blood coagulation by inhibiting prothrombin conversion to thrombin, when malignant cells invade tissue and arteries, when tissue is not completely healed, when there is pressure on tissue from edema, tumors, etc.)

Explain the reason for and intended effect of the preventive therapy

EVALUATION

Record actual outcome

POTENTIAL FOR BLOOD TRANSFUSION REACTION[26,73,399]

ASSESSMENT

Data Collection

Subjective Data
• There are no actual symptoms of a blood transfusion reaction

Objective Data
• There are no actual signs of a blood transfusion reaction

Related Data
• There are one or more stressors present that increase the possibility that a blood transfusion reaction will occur

HEALTH CARE FACTORS: *Medical therapy:* Blood transfusion(s), rapid or excessive blood transfusion(s)

Data Analysis

Nursing Diagnosis
POTENTIAL FOR BLOOD TRANSFUSION REACTION: The presence of stressors that increase the possibility of the actual occurrence of an adverse reaction to a blood transfusion

PLANNING

Unmet Needs

Protection from physical harm, increased learning

Expected Outcome

No signs or symptoms of blood transfusion reaction will occur
    OR
If signs and symptoms occur, they will be promptly recognized as an actual problem and
    will be treated appropriately

NURSING INTERVENTIONS

Nursing Treatments

Attend the patient constantly (while the first 50 cc of blood is being administered)
Do not give blood unrefrigerated for more than 1 hour
Do not give blood that is more than 3 weeks old
Administer isotonic saline intravenous fluid between the blood transfusion and glucose
    infusion
Do not inject drugs into a blood transfusion
Provide frequent contact with the person
Restrict the blood transfusion rate to 500 cc every 2–4 hours
Discontinue the blood transfusion (immediately at the very first sign that a reaction
    might be about to occur)

Nursing Observations

Check the label on the blood container for correct patient identification
Observe for a blood transfusion reaction (fever, rash, tachycardia, dyspnea, decreased
    blood pressure, anxiety, chest tightness, back pain)

Health Teaching

Describe those symptoms that should be reported (immediate symptoms of chills, itch-
    ing, dyspnea, rash, back or chest pain; delayed symptoms of hepatitis or malaria that
    could occur within weeks or months after the transfusion)
Explain why the potential problem could become actual (any foreign object introduced
    into the body raises the potential for an adverse reaction)
Explain the reason for and intended effect of the preventive therapy

EVALUATION

Record actual outcome

POTENTIAL FOR DYSRHYTHMIA[339,443,469]

ASSESSMENT

Data Collection

Subjective Data
• There are no actual symptoms of dysrhythmia

Objective Data
• There are no actual signs of dysrhythmia

Related Data
• There are one or more stressors present that increase the possibility that a
    dysrhythmia will occur
BIRTH DEFECTS: Aortic insufficiency or stenosis, atrial septal defect, tetralogy of Fallot
DISEASES: Anemia, arteriosclerotic heart disease, congestive heart failure, endocarditis,

hemorrhage, hypertension, hypoglycemia, hypotension, mitral stenosis, mitral valve prolapse, myocardial infarction, myocarditis, pericarditis, rheumatic heart disease, thyrotoxicosis

SIGNS AND SYMPTOMS: Fever, hyperkalemia, hypokalemia, hypoxia

PSYCHOSOCIAL FACTORS: Excess of emotional excitement, threat of real or imagined danger

HEALTH CARE FACTORS: *Drug therapy:* Adverse effects of belladonna, digitalis, procainamide, propantheline, quinidine. *Surgical therapy:* Anesthesia

LIFESTYLE: Overvigorous exercise, high caffeine intake, high nicotine intake, marijuana smoking

Data Analysis

Nursing Diagnosis

POTENTIAL FOR DYSRHYTHMIA: The presence of stressors that increase the possibility of the actual occurrence of an abnormal heart rhythm

PLANNING

Unmet Needs

Protection from physical harm, increased learning

Expected Outcome

No signs or symptoms of dysrhythmia will occur
    OR
If signs and symptoms occur, they will be promptly recognized as an actual problem and will be treated appropriately

NURSING INTERVENTIONS

Nursing Treatments

In Critical Care Situation
Connect the person to an ECG monitor
Provide standby equipment and drugs (oxygen, defibrillator)

General Measures
Encourage adequate rest
Discourage the intake of oral stimulants (caffeine)
Discourage smoking

Nursing Observations

Check the monitor electrodes for placement periodically
Monitor the cardiogram
Auscultate the apical heartbeat for rate and rhythm
Monitor the blood pressure
Monitor blood studies for abnormal cardiac enzymes, abnormal electrolytes, arterial blood gases

Health Teaching

Advise that highly emotional situations be avoided
Explain the need to avoid overexertion
Instruct to use vagal stimulation methods to terminate dysrhythmias
Instruct to report any serious symptoms immediately (pain, dyspnea)
Recommend methods for achieving total relaxation (to control anxiety-produced dysrhythmias through controlled breathing, listening to soft music, etc.)
Explain why the potential problem could become actual (drugs, metabolic changes, or impaired myocardial circulation affect the electrical, i.e., pacemaker, function of the heart)
Explain the reason for and intended effect of the preventive therapy

EVALUATION

Record actual outcome

POTENTIAL FOR EPISTAXIS[42,399]

ASSESSMENT

Data Collection

Subjective Data
• There are no actual symptoms of epistaxis

Objective Data
• There are no actual signs of epistaxis

Related Data
• There are one or more stressors present that increase the possibility that epistaxis will occur

DISEASES: Aplastic anemia, hemophilia, Hodgkin's disease, hypertension, leukemia, malaria, purpura, rhinitis, scarlet fever, scurvy, sinusitis (chronic), telangiectasis (hemorrhagic), typhoid fever

INJURIES: Contusion of nose, foreign body in nose, nasal fracture

HEALTH CARE FACTORS: *Medical therapy:* Nasal packing. *Drug therapy:* Anticoagulant therapy, large doses of aspirin

ENVIRONMENTAL FACTORS: *Altitude:* High. *Chemical substances:* Inhalation of chemical substances. *Humidity:* Dry climate

Data Analysis

Nursing Diagnosis
POTENTIAL FOR EPISTAXIS: The presence of stressors that increase the possibility of the actual occurrence of bleeding from the nose

PLANNING

Unmet Needs

Protection from physical harm, increased learning

Expected Outcome

No signs or symptoms of epistaxis will occur
OR
If signs and symptoms occur, they will be promptly recognized as an actual problem and will be treated appropriately
Person verbalizes an understanding of and practices preventive methods

NURSING INTERVENTIONS

Nursing Treatments

Apply an ice pack
OR
Apply manual pressure over the potential bleeding area (if there has been a contusion to the nose)
Do not place in the flat position
Elevate the head
Maintain adequate atmospheric humidity (especially in a dry climate or high altitude)
Administer vaporized air (if the internal nares are dry)

Nursing Observations

Inspect the nose for epistaxis

Health Teaching

Explain how to prevent sneezing (by placing pressure against the upper lip, if there is a high potential for epistaxis)
Inform that coughing should be avoided (temporarily)
Inform that elimination straining should be avoided (temporarily)

Instruct not to blow the nose (temporarily)
Instruct not to pick the nose
Instruct not to insert foreign objects into body orifices
Instruct to change position gradually
Explain why the potential problem could become actual (blood vessels within the nares may rupture when subjected to pressure or irritation)
Explain the reason for and intended effect of the preventive therapy (to keep nasal pressure and irritation at a minimum)

EVALUATION
Record actual outcome

POTENTIAL FOR FAT EMBOLUS[116,616,629]

ASSESSMENT
Data Collection
Subjective Data
• There are no actual symptoms of a fat embolus
Objective Data
• There are no actual signs of a fat embolus
Related Data
• There are one or more stressors present that increase the possibility that a fat embolus will occur
DISEASE: Alcoholism, diabetes mellitus, pancreatitis, sickle cell anemia
INJURIES: Bone fracture (of the long bones, pelvis, and ribs), burn wound (severe second- or third-degree), poisoning, crushing injury (of adipose tissue)
SIGNS AND SYMPTOMS: Dehydration
HEALTH CARE FACTORS: *Surgical procedures:* Abdominal surgery (on any obese person), cardiopulmonary bypass, transplantation of kidney
DEVELOPMENTAL PHASES: Young adulthood, old age
Data Analysis
Nursing Diagnosis
POTENTIAL FOR FAT EMBOLUS: The presence of stressors that increase the possibility of the actual occurrence of a fat embolus in the circulatory system

PLANNING
Unmet Needs
Protection from physical harm, increased learning
Expected Outcome
No signs or symptoms of fat embolus will occur
    OR
If signs and symptoms occur, they will be promptly recognized as an actual problem and will be treated appropriately

NURSING INTERVENTIONS
Nursing Treatments
Immobilize the fractured body part (as early as possible, after injury)
Handle gently (the fracture site)
Provide frequent contact with the person
Consult with the physician (if signs of fat embolus occur)

Nursing Observations

Early Signs of Fat Embolus
Observe for confusion, restlessness (within first 48 hours after trauma)
Palpate the pulse for rate, rhythm, and volume (for tachycardia)
Monitor the oral temperature (for fever)

Later Signs of Fat Embolus
Inspect the chest for respiratory rate and rhythm (for tachypnea)
Auscultate the chest for adventitious sounds
Observe for cyanosis, dyspnea
Monitor the blood pressure (for decreasing blood pressure leading to shock)
Inspect the skin for petechiae (over the anterior chest and anterior axillary fold)
Measure the intake and output (report fluid loss)
Observe the urine for abnormal content (fat globules in the urine)

Health Teaching

Inform that coughing should be avoided
AND
Inform that elimination straining should be avoided
AND
Instruct to avoid the Valsalva maneuver (all of which strain the cardiovascular system)
Explain why the potential problem could become actual (if appropriate to the situation; explain that during trauma fat is released from the bone marrow and can enter the circulation and affect vital organs)
Explain the reason for and intended effect of the preventive therapy

EVALUATION

Record actual outcome

POTENTIAL FOR IMPAIRED PERIPHERAL CIRCULATION[73,371,451]

ASSESSMENT

Data Collection

Subjective Data
• There are no actual symptoms of impaired peripheral circulation

Objective Data
• There are no actual signs of impaired peripheral circulation

Related Data
• There are one or more stressors present that increase the possibility that impaired peripheral circulation will occur
DISEASES: Arteriosclerosis, cerebrovascular accident, congestive heart failure, diabetes mellitus, obesity
INJURIES: Bone fracture, joint injury
HUMAN BODY: *Body state:* Pregnancy
HEALTH CARE FACTORS: *Diagnostic procedures:* Angiography, cardiac catheterization. *Medical or surgical therapy:* Adverse effects, such as circulatory constriction from a cast, elastic bandage, or dressing. *Medical therapy:* Prolonged bed rest. *Surgical therapy:* Arterial by-pass surgery, lumbar sympathectomy

Data Analysis

Nursing Diagnosis

POTENTIAL FOR IMPAIRED PERIPHERAL CIRCULATION (POTENTIAL FOR VENOUS STASIS) (POTENTIAL FOR BLOOD POOLING): The presence of stressors that increase the possibility of the actual occurrence of blood flowing sluggishly through the circulatory system, resulting in inadequate tissue oxygenation

PLANNING

Unmet Needs

Protection from physical harm, increased learning

Expected Outcome

No signs or symptoms of impaired peripheral circulation will occur
    OR
If signs and symptoms occur, they will be promptly recognized as an actual problem and will be treated appropriately
Person verbalizes an understanding of and practices preventive methods

NURSING INTERVENTIONS

Nursing Treatments

Ambulate the patient (as much as possible)
Apply an elastic bandage ⎤
    OR   ⎬ To the legs
Apply elastic stockings ⎦
Change the patient's position frequently
Exercise in range of motion
Increase fluid intake to about 2,000 cc daily (during periods of immobility)
Refrain from elevating the bed at the knee gatch
Refrain from placing a pillow under the knee
Refrain from tight bandaging
Remove constrictive clothing
Discourage smoking

Nursing Observations

Inspect the extremity for inadequate circulation (cold skin, cyanosis, pallor, absence of pulse, poor capillary refill)
Inspect for edema
Inspect the skin for color (redness)

Health Teaching

Describe those symptoms that should be reported (cold skin, blueness, pallor, swelling, numbness and tingling, skin ulceration, absence of extremity pulse)
Advise that positions that impair circulation be avoided (prolonged knee bending or standing, crossing the legs, dangling the legs so that there is pressure behind the knees)
Instruct to change position frequently
Instruct that pillows, blankets, or trochanter rolls not be placed under the knee (pressure from such impairs circulation)
Advise against wearing constrictive clothing (such as girdles, garters, tight wrist bands)
Explain how to apply elastic stockings or an elastic bandage (to the legs, which supports return of venous flow to the heart)
Emphasize the danger of excessive body weight (which increases the circulatory workload)
Recommend activities that improve circulation (brisk walking, running, bicycling, rocking in a chair, swimming)
Teach how to do isometric exercises (moving the foot up and down and opening and closing the hands)
Explain why the potential problem could become actual (immobility, insufficient exer-

cise, or weakened vessel walls prevent normal blood flow, with resulting blood pooling and/or clot formation; pressure on veins or arteries in the pelvic area reduces
circulation; a failing heart is unable to pump blood adequately)
Explain the reason for and intended effect of the preventive therapy

EVALUATION
Record actual outcome

POTENTIAL FOR RECTAL BLEEDING[73,278]

ASSESSMENT
Data Collection
Subjective Data
• There are no actual symptoms of rectal bleeding

Objective Data
• There are no actual signs of rectal bleeding

Related Data
• There are one or more stressors present that increase the possibility that rectal
   bleeding will occur
DISEASES: Anal fissure, carcinoma of the rectum, hemorrhoids
INJURIES: Foreign body in rectum, anal tear
SIGNS AND SYMPTOMS: Constipation, diarrhea (prolonged)
HEALTH CARE FACTORS: *Diagnostic procedures:* Anoscopy, colonoscopy, proctoscopy, proctosig-
   moidoscopy. *Surgical procedures:* Hemorrhoidectomy

Data Analysis
Nursing Diagnosis
POTENTIAL FOR RECTAL BLEEDING: The presence of stressors that increase the possibility of the
   actual occurrence of bleeding from the rectum

PLANNING
Unmet Needs
Protection from physical harm, increased learning

Expected Outcome
No signs or symptoms of rectal bleeding will occur
   OR
If signs and symptoms occur, they will be promptly recognized as an actual problem and
   will be treated appropriately
Person verbalizes an understanding of and practices preventive methods

NURSING INTERVENTIONS
Nursing Treatments
Refrain from giving enemas, from giving laxatives
Refrain from inserting a rectal tube
Refrain from taking rectal temperatures
Give nonprescription drug (stool softener)

Nursing Observations
Inspect for bleeding

Health Teaching
Advise not to stand for prolonged periods
Instruct to respond immediately to the elimination reflex
Explain the need for scheduled bowel elimination (which prevents the irritation of con-
   stipated stool)

Inform that elimination straining should be avoided

Teach how to adjust the diet (to control stool consistency)

Explain why the potential problem could become actual (pressure or irritation to the rectal area could cause bleeding)

Explain the reason for and intended effect of the preventive therapy

EVALUATION

Record actual outcome

POTENTIAL FOR SHOCK[42,72,278,399]

ASSESSMENT

Data Collection

Subjective Data

• There are no actual symptoms of shock

Objective Data

• There are no actual signs of shock

Related Data

• There are one or more stressors present that increase the possibility that shock will occur

DISEASES: Addison's disease, bacteremia, carcinoma (metastatic), diabetes insipidus, hemorrhage, hepatic failure, intestinal obstruction, Laennec's cirrhosis, malnutrition, myocardial infarction, pancreatitis (acute), peritonitis

INJURIES: Trauma (severe), bone fracture, burn wound, insect bite or sting, poisoning

SIGNS AND SYMPTOMS: Ascites, dehydration, diarrhea (severe), pain (severe)

HEALTH CARE FACTORS: *Diagnostic procedures:* Radiographic contrast dyes used in diagnostic procedures. *Medical procedures:* Hemodialysis, radiation therapy, therapeutic apheresis. *Drug therapy:* Adverse effects of drugs such as antibiotics (especially penicillin), antihypertensive drugs, immunization therapy, immunosuppressive therapy with corticosteroids. *Surgical therapy:* Anesthesia, any. *Surgical procedure:* Any

ENVIRONMENTAL FACTORS: *Biological agents:* Exposure to bacteria, viruses, protozoa

Data Analysis

Nursing Diagnosis

POTENTIAL FOR SHOCK: The presence of stressors that increase the possibility of the actual occurrence of insufficient blood flow to peripheral tissues to maintain life

PLANNING

Unmet Needs

Protection from physical harm, increased learning

Expected Outcome

No signs or symptoms of shock will occur

OR

If signs and symptoms occur, they will be promptly recognized as an actual problem and will be treated appropriately

NURSING INTERVENTIONS

Nursing Treatments

Provide standby equipment and drugs (oxygen, tracheostomy tray, etc.)

Attend the patient constantly (for an impending threat of shock)

Place on complete bed rest

OR

Encourage adequate rest

Give warm fluids (when there is a blood volume deficit, and no contraindication to oral fluids)

Provide quiet

Cover with lightweight blankets

Handle gently

Maintain a warm room temperature (not hot)

Nursing Observations

Inspect the chest for respiratory rate and rhythm (rapid respirations)

Monitor the blood pressure (for decreased blood pressure)

Palpate the pulse for rate, rhythm, and volume (for rapid, weak pulse)

Measure the intake and output

Observe for restlessness

Observe for complaints of anxiety

Health Teaching

Explain the importance of wearing a Medic Alert tag (for allergic disorders)

Recommend methods for achieving total relaxation (in conditions such as Addison's disease, in which emotional stress can precipitate shock)

Explain why the potential problem could become actual (foreign protein or bacterial toxins in the blood, insufficient blood volume, or impaired cardiac capacity to pump blood can prevent adequate circulation to body parts, resulting in shock)

Explain the reason for and intended effect of the preventive therapy

EVALUATION

Record actual outcome

POTENTIAL FOR THROMBUS DISPLACEMENT[73,451]

ASSESSMENT

Data Collection

Subjective Data

• There are no actual symptoms of thrombus displacement

Objective Data

• There are no actual signs of thrombus displacement

Related Data

• There are one or more stressors present that increase the possibility that thrombus displacement will occur

DISEASES: Phlebitis, phlebothrombosis, thrombophlebitis

HUMAN ERROR: Massaging a hot, tender, reddened calf area, walking on a thrombosed leg

Data Analysis

Nursing Diagnosis

POTENTIAL FOR THROMBUS DISPLACEMENT: The presence of stressors that increase the possibility of the actual occurrence of an existing thrombus being dislodged from its position

PLANNING

Unmet Needs

Protection from physical harm, increased learning

Expected Outcome

No signs or symptoms of thrombus displacement will occur
    OR

If signs and symptoms occur, such will be promptly recognized as an actual problem and will be treated appropriately

Person verbalizes an understanding of and practices preventive methods

NURSING INTERVENTIONS

Nursing Treatments

Do not massage (the leg)
Elevate the extremity
Elevate the foot of the bed (on 6-inch blocks)
Encourage adequate rest (of the limb)
Handle gently
Place on complete bed rest
Refrain from elevating the bed at the knee gatch
Refrain from placing a pillow under the knee

Nursing Observations

Inspect (the extremity) for impaired circulation (cold skin, cyanosis, pallor, swelling, absence of pulse, poor capillary refill)
Observe for complaints of (chest) pain
Observe for coughing, cyanosis, dyspnea, hemoptosis
Observe for shock

Health Teaching

Emphasize the danger of massaging a painful calf
Instruct not to dangle the legs
Instruct to avoid the Valsalva maneuver (which could dislodge the clot)
Explain why the potential problem could become actual (rubbing or irritating an existing thrombus or sudden changes in vascular pressure can release it from a vessel wall and cause it to move to a vital organ)
Explain the reason for and intended effect of the preventive therapy

EVALUATION

Record actual outcome

POTENTIAL FOR THROMBUS FORMATION[278]

ASSESSMENT

Data Collection

Subjective Data
• There are no actual symptoms of a thrombus

Objective Data
• There are no actual signs of a thrombus

Related Data
• There are one or more stressors present that increase the possibility of a thrombus occurring
DISEASES: Arteriosclerosis, cancer (especially pancreatic and bronchogenic), heart failure, infection (acute and chronic), polycythemia, varicose veins
INJURIES: Bone fracture, burn wound, contusion, vascular damage, major trauma of any kind
SIGNS AND SYMPTOMS: Dehydration, shock
HUMAN BODY: *Natural body function:* Childbirth
HEALTH CARE FACTORS: *Diagnostic procedures:* Angiography. *Medical therapy:* Prolonged bed rest, intravenous fluids and medications (especially in foot/leg veins). *Surgical procedures:* Arterial bypass surgery, arterioplasty, any major surgery (especially splenectomy). *Drug therapy:* Thrombus formation from estrogen contraceptives. *History of:* Previous thrombus
HUMAN ERROR: Prolonged impairment of venous flow by garters, girdles, elastic-topped stockings, sitting with legs crossed or with pressure on backs of knees/thighs

Data Analysis

Nursing Diagnosis

POTENTIAL FOR THROMBUS FORMATION: The presence of stressors that increase the possibility of the actual occurrence of a blood clot in a vein

PLANNING

Unmet Needs

Protection from physical harm, increased learning

Expected Outcome

No signs or symptoms of thrombus formation will occur
    OR
If signs and symptoms occur, they will be promptly recognized as an actual problem and will be treated appropriately
Person verbalizes an understanding of and practices preventive methods

NURSING INTERVENTIONS

Nursing Treatments

Ambulate the patient (as much as possible)
Apply an elastic bandage ⎤
    OR   ⎬ To the legs, especially while the
Apply elastic stockings ⎦ person is in bed
Change the patient's position frequently
Exercise in range of motion
Increase fluid intake to about 2,000 cc daily (during periods of immobility)
Refrain from elevating the bed at the knee gatch
Refrain from placing a pillow under the knee
Refrain from tight bandaging
Remove constrictive clothing

Nursing Observations

Inspect for inflammation (redness, heat, swelling, or pain in an extremity)
Measure the circumference of the calves (for one increasing in size)
Palpate for tenderness (in the calf and pain on dorsiflexion of foot)
Monitor blood studies for abnormal hematology (for elevated hematocrit suggesting dehydration, as the hemoconcentration of cells makes the person highly susceptible to thrombus formation)

Health Teaching

Describe those symptoms that should be reported (redness, heat, swelling, pain)
Advise that positions that impair circulation be avoided (prolonged knee bending or standing, crossing the legs, dangling the legs so there is pressure behind the knees)
Instruct to change position frequently
Instruct that pillows, blankets, or trochanter rolls not be placed under the knee (pressure from such impairs circulation)
Advise against wearing constrictive clothing (such as girdles and garters)
Recommend activities that improve circulation (brisk walking, running, swimming, bicycling, rocking in a chair)
Teach how to do isometric exercises (moving the foot up and down, opening and closing the hands)
Explain why the potential problem could become actual (immobility and lack of exercise or pressure on veins and arteries prevent normal blood flow, which can result in clot formation)
Explain the reason for and intended effect of the preventive therapy

EVALUATION

Record actual outcome

Potential Threats to Cognition Homeostasis

POTENTIAL FOR CONFUSION[42,358,476]

ASSESSMENT

Data Collection

Subjective Data
- There are no actual symptoms of confusion

Objective Data
- There are no actual signs of confusion

Related Data
- There are one or more stressors present that increase the possibility that confusion will occur

DISEASES: Alcoholism, arteriosclerosis, brain tumor, congestive heart failure, emphysema, hepatic failure, hypoglycemia

INJURIES: Burn wound, concussion

SIGNS AND SYMPTOMS: High fever, pain

PSYCHOSOCIAL FACTORS: Threat of severe stress

HEALTH CARE FACTORS: *Health care environment:* Coronary care unit, intensive care unit. *Medical therapy:* Recovery from electroconvulsive therapy, hemodialysis, prolonged intermittent positive-pressure breathing, placement in therapeutic isolation, alcohol or drug withdrawal, radiation therapy. *Drug therapy:* Adverse effects of drugs, especially hypnotics, narcotics sedatives. *Surgical therapy:* Recovery from anesthesia

DEVELOPMENTAL PHASES: Advanced old age (age 70 or above)

LIFESTYLE: Drug abuse, including marijuana, lysergic acid diethylamide (LSD), and phencyclidine (PCP)

Data Analysis

Nursing Diagnosis
POTENTIAL FOR CONFUSION: The presence of stressors that increase the possibility of the actual occurrence of a state of mental disorganization

PLANNING

Unmet Needs
Protection from physical harm, increased learning

Expected Outcome
No signs or symptoms of confusion will occur
OR
If signs and symptoms occur, they will be promptly recognized as an actual problem and will be treated appropriately

NURSING INTERVENTIONS

Nursing Treatments
Approach unhurriedly
Provide frequent contact with the person
Arrange orderly surroundings
Arrange a structured environment (the same daily routine every day)
Illuminate the room adequately
Provide quiet (quiet reduces the potential for confusion)
Maintain consistent staff behavior (and consistent assignment of personnel, whenever possible)

Give one direction at a time

Encourage attentive patient listening (so that messages from others are correctly perceived)

Present change gradually

Do not allow unpleasant surprise situations (prepare the person before treatments, etc.)

Encourage quiet diversional activities

Use the person's name frequently

Nursing Observations

Observe for confusion (bewildered or perplexed)

Determine the degree of insight the person has about his potential for confusion

Health Teaching

Recommend the pursuit of only one activity at a time

Explain (to families) that persons with limited attention span require message repetition

Explain the reason for and intended effect of the preventive therapy

EVALUATION

Record actual outcome

POTENTIAL FOR DISORIENTATION[471,476]

ASSESSMENT

Data Collection

Subjective Data

• There are no actual symptoms of disorientation

Objective Data

• There are no actual signs of disorientation

Related Data

• There are one or more stressors present that increase the possibility that disorientation will occur

DISEASES: Alcoholism, arteriosclerosis, brain tumor

INJURIES: Concussion

SIGNS AND SYMPTOMS: High fever, pain

PSYCHOSOCIAL FACTORS: Threat of severe stress

HEALTH CARE FACTORS: *Health care environment*: Coronary care unit, intensive care unit. *Medical therapy*: Recovery from electroconvulsive therapy, placement in therapeutic isolation, alcohol or drug withdrawal. *Drug therapy*: Adverse effects of drugs, especially hypnotics, narcotics, and sedatives. *Surgical therapy*: Recovery from anesthesia

DEVELOPMENTAL PHASES: Advanced old age (age 70 or above)

LIFESTYLE: Drug abuse, including marijuana, lysergic acid diethylamide (LSD), phencyclidine (PCP)

Data Analysis

Nursing Diagnosis

POTENTIAL FOR DISORIENTATION: The presence of stressors that increase the possibility of the actual occurrence of being unable to determine time, place, or the identity of persons

PLANNING

Unmet Needs

Protection from physical harm, increased learning

Expected Outcome

No signs or symptoms of disorientation will occur

OR

If signs and symptoms occur, they will be promptly recognized as an actual problem and will be treated appropriately

NURSING INTERVENTIONS

Nursing Treatments

Approach unhurriedly

Provide frequent contact with the person

Relate the time, day, place, and events occurring (as often as needed to prevent disorientation)

Use the person's name frequently

Place by a window (so he can determine night from day)

Provide a clock

Provide a calendar

Involve the family (by encouraging a family member to stay with the person)

Nursing Observations

Observe for disorientation

Health Teaching

Explain the reason for and intended effect of the preventive therapy (to the patient and/or family)

EVALUATION

Record actual outcome

Potential Threats to Electrolyte Homeostasis

POTENTIAL FOR HYPERCALCEMIA[371,399]

ASSESSMENT

Data Collection

Subjective Data

• There are no actual symptoms of hypercalcemia

Objective Data

• There are no actual signs of hypercalcemia

Related Data

• There are one or more stressors present that increase the possibility that hypercalcemia will occur

DISEASES: Adrenal insufficiency, hyperparathyroidism, hypervitaminosis, milk-alkali syndrome, multiple myeloma, sarcoidosis, nephritis

INJURIES: Bone fractures (multiple)

SIGNS AND SYMPTOMS: Dehydration

HEALTH CARE FACTORS: *Medical therapy:* Prolonged bed rest. *Drug therapy:* Adverse effects of thiazide diuretics, prolonged antacid therapy

HUMAN ERROR: Excess intake of vitamin D

Data Analysis

Nursing Diagnosis

POTENTIAL FOR HYPERCALCEMIA: The presence of stressors that increase the possibility of the actual occurrence of a serum calcium level above 5.5 mEq/liter

PLANNING

Unmet Needs

Protection from physical harm, increased learning

Expected Outcome

No signs or symptoms of hypercalcemia will occur
   OR
If signs and symptoms occur, they will be promptly recognized as an actual problem and
   will be treated appropriately
Person verbalizes an understanding of and practices preventive methods

NURSING INTERVENTIONS

Nursing Treatments

Encourage decreased calcium-food intake (avoid meat and poultry, dark leafy green vegetables, sardines, clams, oysters, yogurt)
Give low-calcium fluids orally (avoid drinks containing milk)

Nursing Observations

Monitor blood studies for abnormal electrolytes (increased calcium)
Observe for complaints of constipation, headache, nausea, thirst, weakness, pain (bone)
Observe for lethargy, irritability, confusion
Monitor blood pressure (for increase)
Measure the intake and output (for polydipsia)
Monitor the ECG (for heart block)
Observe the urine for abnormal content (visible precipitates such as calcium particles or
   bacteria)

Health Teaching

Explain why the potential problem could become actual (excessive alkali intake inhibits
   renal excretion of calcium, blood saturation with calcium cations contained in milk
   and alkalis prevents normal serum concentrations)
Teach how to adjust the diet (for decreased calcium intake and absorption)
Advise not to take any drug (containing vitamin D)
Explain the reason for and intended effects of the preventive therapy

EVALUATION

Record actual outcome

POTENTIAL FOR HYPOCALCEMIA[371,399]

ASSESSMENT

Data Collection

Subjective Data
• There are no actual symptoms of hypocalcemia

Objective Data
• There are no actual signs of hypocalcemia

Related Data
• There are one or more stressors present that increase the possibility that hypocalcemia
   will occur
BIRTH STATUS: Premature infant
DISEASES: Cushing's syndrome, hypoparathyroidism, Laennec's cirrhosis, nephrotic syn-
   drome, pancreatitis, renal failure (chronic), sprue (causing malabsorption of calcium)
INJURIES: Burn wounds

SIGNS AND SYMPTOMS: Severe diarrhea, obstructive jaundice (in which there is malabsorption of calcium)

HEALTH CARE FACTORS: *Medical therapy*: Blood transfusion (multiple), surgery, thyroidectomy (damage to parathyroids), therapeutic apheresis. *Drug therapy* : Adverse effects of corticosteroids, glucagon, and mithramycin; excessive use of bicarbonates to correct acidosis, resulting in alkalosis, a state in which calcium is bound, thereby reducing the functional amount of calcium

HUMAN ERROR: Excessive intake of laxatives

Data Analysis

Nursing Diagnosis

POTENTIAL FOR HYPOCALCEMIA: The presence of stressors that increase the possibility of the actual occurrence of a serum calcium level below 4.5 mEq/liter and/or a disproportionate amount of the calcium in the protein-bound state

PLANNING

Unmet Needs

Protection from physical harm, increased learning

Expected Outcome

No signs or symptoms of hypocalcemia will occur
   OR
If signs and symptoms occur, they will be promptly recognized as an actual problem and will be treated appropriately

Person verbalizes an understanding of and practices preventive methods

NURSING INTERVENTIONS

Nursing Treatments

Give high-calcium fluids orally (milk, malts, cocoa, and milk punch, with a 1-quart limit per day of milk)

Encourage increased calcium-food intake (broccoli, turnip greens, watercress, almonds, mackerel, baked beans with molasses, dried brewer's yeast, yogurt, cheddar cheese)

Give nonprescription drug (aluminum hydroxide gel before each meal, which decreases phosphorus absorption; when the phosphorus level decreases, the calcium level increases; this treatment is primarily applicable to persons who are unable to eat high-calcium foods such as milk)

Nursing Observations

Monitor the blood pressure (for hypotension)

Monitor blood studies for abnormal electrolytes (decreased calcium, decreased serum albumin)

Observe for complaints of numbness and tingling, of pain (abdominal or muscle cramps)

Observe for irritability, muscle twitching

Auscultate the apical heartbeat for rate and rhythm (dysrhythmias)

Auscultate the abdomen for abnormal bowel sounds (increased peristalsis)

Test for Chvostek's sign (when taping the face just below the temple, twitching occurs)

Test for a positive Trousseau's sign (when a blood pressure cuff is applied to the upper arm and inflated, the hand will bend downward between the systolic and diastolic readings)

Health Teaching

Explain why the potential problem could become actual (calcium levels can be reduced from calcium loss through feces, from kidney retention of phosphate, which increases calcium excretion, from chemical binding by the citrate in transfused blood, and from excessive binding by serum albumin during alkalosis)

Teach how to adjust the diet (for increased calcium intake and absorption)

Explain the reason for and intended effect of the preventive therapy

EVALUATION

Record actual outcome

POTENTIAL FOR HYPERKALEMIA[371,399]

ASSESSMENT

Data Collection

Subjective Data
• There are no actual symptoms of hyperkalemia

Objective Data
• There are no actual signs of hyperkalemia

Related Data
• There are one or more stressors present that increase the possibility that hyperkalemia will occur
DISEASES: Addison's disease, metabolic (diabetic) acidosis, myocardial infarction, renal insufficiency or failure
INJURIES: Burn wound, crushing injury
SIGNS AND SYMPTOMS: Dehydration, shock (hemorrhagic)
HEALTH CARE FACTORS: *Adverse effects of drug therapy*: Diuretics (potassium-sparing diuretics such as triamterene and spironolactone), bicarbonates used for rapid correction of acidosis. *Medical therapy*: Intravenous infusions with large doses of potassium, large doses (10 million units) of potassium penicillin G, blood transfusion with rapid transfusion of a large volume of blood

Data Analysis

Nursing Diagnosis
POTENTIAL FOR HYPERKALEMIA: The presence of stressors that increase the possibility of the actual occurrence of a serum potassium level above 5.5 mEq/liter

PLANNING

Unmet Needs

Protection from physical harm, increased learning

Expected Outcome

No signs or symptoms of hyperkalemia will occur
   OR
If signs and symptoms occur, they will be promptly recognized as an actual problem and will be treated appropriately
Person verbalizes an understanding of and practices preventive methods

NURSING INTERVENTIONS

Nursing Treatments

Give low-potassium fluids orally (cranberry juice, ginger ale, root beer, 7-Up, Pepsi Cola)
Refrain from giving potassium-containing drugs and solutions (penicillin G potassium, blood from the blood bank)
Encourage decreased potassium food intake (avoiding high-potassium foods such as bananas, oranges, chocolate candy, raisins, nuts, ice cream)
Restrict the intravenous potassium to 20 mEq/hour or 200 mEq/24 hour

Nursing Observations

Monitor blood studies for abnormal electrolytes (increased potassium)
Observe for complaints of numbness and tingling, weakness, nausea, pain (abdominal cramps), apprehension, diarrhea
Measure the intake and output (for anuria, oliguria)
Palpate the pulse for rate, rhythm, and volume (tachycardia or bradycardia)
Monitor the ECG (for prolonged P-R internal, widened QRS, depressed S-T segment, heightened T-wave)
Test for abnormal deep-reflex responses (for hyperactive response)

Health Teaching

Explain why the potential problem could become actual (in impaired kidney function, the kidneys do not excrete potassium adequately; certain diuretics cause retention of potassium; large intravenous doses of potassium can saturate the blood beyond the normal level)

Teach how to adjust the diet (for decreased potassium intake; explain that a low-potassium, high-carbohydrate diet will help prevent hyperkalemia if intake is limited to 40 mEq or less daily; high-potassium foods to avoid include chocolate, coffee, cocoa, tea, dried fruits, dried peas or beans, ice cream or sherbet, milk desserts, molasses, nuts; provide a list of other foods, showing the amount of potassium per serving; when preparing foods that are relatively high in potassium, such as potatoes, chicken, turkey, and broccoli, the amount of potassium can be approximately halved by boiling the food and discarding the water; canned foods are higher in potassium than are fresh foods; decrease the potassium content by at least one-third by discarding the fluid in the can and rinsing the food when possible; never use a salt substitute)

Explain the reason for and intended effect of the preventive therapy

EVALUATION

Record actual outcome

POTENTIAL FOR HYPOKALEMIA[306,399]

ASSESSMENT

Data Collection

Subjective Data
• There are no actual symptoms of hypokalemia

Objective Data
• There are no actual signs of hypokalemia

Related Data
• There are one or more stressors present that increase the possibility that hypokalemia will occur

DISEASES: Aldosteronism, alkalosis, congestive heart failure, Cushing's syndrome, hyperglycemia, renal tubular acidosis, ulcerative colitis

INJURIES: Burn wound (healing stage), crushing injury (healing stage)

SIGNS AND SYMPTOMS: Anorexia, dehydration, diaphoresis, diarrhea, vomiting

HUMAN BODY: *Body states*: Excessive lactation

HEALTH CARE FACTORS: *Medical therapy*: Dextrose infusion without potassium (less than 30 mEq of potassium replaced daily), prolonged normal saline infusions, nasogastric suction, T-tube drainage, therapeutic apheresis. *Drug therapy*: Adverse effects of corticosteroids, diuretics, carbenicillin, gentamycin, testosterone; rapid correction of acidosis when glucose is given with insulin to diabetics in ketoacidosis. *Surgical procedures*: Colostomy, ileostomy, ureteroileostomy

SITUATIONAL FACTORS: Chronic or severe stress

HUMAN ERROR: Excess intake of antacids (bicarbonates), laxatives and/or licorice, chronic use of enemas

Data Analysis

Nursing Diagnosis

POTENTIAL FOR HYPOKALEMIA: The presence of stressors that increase the possibility of the actual occurrence of a serum potassium level below 3.5 mEq/liter

PLANNING

Unmet Needs

Protection from physical harm, increased learning

Expected Outcome

No signs or symptoms of hypokalemia will occur
OR
If signs and symptoms occur, they will be promptly recognized as an actual problem and
will be treated appropriately

Person verbalizes an understanding of and practices preventive methods

NURSING INTERVENTIONS

Nursing Treatments

Encourage increased potassium-food intake (meat, poultry, nuts, whole-grain cereals,
dried peas and beans, fresh fruits)

Give high-potassium fluids orally (orange juice, prune juice, chocolate drinks)

Refrain from giving enemas (which further deplete potassium levels)

Nursing Observations

Monitor blood studies for abnormal electrolytes (decreased potassium)

Monitor the blood pressure (for decrease)

Palpate the pulse for rate, rhythm, and volume (tachycardia, weak, irregular pulse)

Observe for complaints of anorexia, nausea, weakness, pain (leg cramps), dizziness

Observe for depression, irritability, vomiting

Inspect the abdomen for distention

Measure the intake and output (for polyuria)

Monitor the ECG (for S-T segment depression, flattened T-wave, prominent U-wave; if
hypokalemia should become severe, ventricular fibrillation could occur)

Test for abnormal deep-reflex responses (for decreased knee/patella reflex)

Health Teaching

Explain why the potential problem could become actual (in the average 1,500-cc daily
urine output, 50–150 mEq of potassium are excreted; under the stress of illness, the
potassium output reaches 60–200 mEq; the loss of 1,000 cc of liquid stool results in
an approximate potassium loss of 18 mEq; 1,000-cc ileostomy drainage results in a
potassium loss of 18 mEq; 1,000 cc of lost gastric juices results in an approximate potassium loss of 10 mEq; in diuresis, fluid reabsorption from the renal tubules is prevented with a loss of potassium in the urine, causing potassium depletion; 5%
dextrose in water does not contain potassium; large volumes of nonelectrolyte dextrose in water dilute the body's concentration of potassium)

Teach how to adjust the diet (for increased potassium intake)

Explain the reason for and intended effect of the preventive therapy

EVALUATION

Record actual outcome

POTENTIAL FOR HYPERMAGNESEMIA[371,399]

ASSESSMENT

Data Collection

Subjective Data

• There are no actual symptoms of hypermagnesemia

Objective Data
• There are no actual signs of hypermagnesemia

Related Data
• There are one or more stressors present that increase the possibility that hyper-magnesemia will occur
DISEASES: Chronic renal insufficiency, diabetic acidosis (with severe dehydration)
SIGNS AND SYMPTOMS: Severe dehydration, diaphoresis
HUMAN ERROR: Chronic use of laxatives containing magnesium, such as milk of magnesia, magnesium citrate, or sulfate; chronic use of antacids containing magnesium in renal insufficiency or failure; chronic use of magnesium sulfate enemas; insufficient fluid intake

Data Analysis

Nursing Diagnosis
POTENTIAL FOR HYPERMAGNESEMIA: The presence of stressors that increase the possibility of the actual occurrence of a serum magnesium level above 2.5 mEq/liter

PLANNING

Unmet Needs
Protection from physical harm, increased learning

Expected Outcome
No signs or symptoms of hypermagnesemia will occur
    OR
If signs and symptoms occur, they will be promptly recognized as an actual problem and will be treated appropriately
Person verbalizes an understanding of and practices preventive methods

NURSING INTERVENTIONS

Nursing Treatments
Give low-magnesium fluids orally (water, cranberry juice, ginger ale, root beer, etc.; and avoid liquids such as milk, fruit juice, cocoa, chocolate)
Refrain from giving magnesium laxatives, antacids, and enemas

Nursing Observations
Monitor blood studies for abnormal electrolytes (increased magnesium)
Observe for complaints of weakness, warmth (peripheral dilatation), thirst, nausea
Observe for confusion, dyspnea, lethargy, vomiting
Palpate the pulse for rate, rhythm, and volume (for bradycardia or weak pulse)
Monitor blood pressure (for decrease)
Monitor the ECG (for heart block or sinus arrest)
Test for abnormal deep-reflex responses (for decreased response)

Health Teaching
Explain why the potential problem could become actual (dehydration increases the concentration of magnesium in the blood; impaired kidney function reduces the amount of magnesium normally excreted)
Teach how to adjust the diet (for decreased magnesium intake, avoid high-magnesium foods such as nuts, cereals, green vegetables, legumes, fruits, peanut butter, and chocolate and take small portions of meat, milk, eggs, cheese)
Explain the reason for and intended effect of the preventive therapy

EVALUATION
Record actual outcome

POTENTIAL FOR HYPOMAGNESEMIA[371,399]

ASSESSMENT

Data Collection

Subjective Data
• There are no actual symptoms of hypomagnesemia

Objective Data
• There are no actual signs of hypomagnesemia

Related Data
• There are one or more stressors present that increase the possibility that hypomagnesemia will occur
DISEASES: Alcoholism, aldosteronism, hyper- or hypoparathyroidism, malabsorption syndrome, malnutrition, metabolic (diabetic) acidosis
INJURIES: Starvation
SIGNS AND SYMTOMS: Severe dehydration, chronic diarrhea, steatorrhea
HEALTH CARE FACTORS: *Medical therapy*: Dextrose infusion without potassium, prolonged normal saline infusion, nasogastric suction. *Drug Therapy*: Adverse effects of diuretics. *Post-operative period*: First 24 hours after major surgery

Data Analysis

Nursing Diagnosis
POTENTIAL FOR HYPOMAGNESEMIA: The presence of stressors that increase the possibility of the actual occurrence of a serum magnesium level below 1.5 mEq/liter

PLANNING

Unmet Needs
Protection from physical harm, increased learning

Expected Outcome
No signs or symptoms of hypomagnesemia
    OR
If signs and symptoms occur, they will be promptly recognized as an *actual* problem and will be treated appropriately
Person verbalizes an understanding of and practices preventive methods

NURSING INTERVENTIONS

Nursing Treatments
Give high-magnesium fluids orally (cocoa, chocolate, prune juice, fruit juices)
Give high-magnesium snacks (nuts, bananas, oranges, chocolate, peanut butter, ice cream)

Nursing Observations
Monitor blood studies for abnormal electrolytes (decreased magnesium)
Monitor the blood pressure (for increase or decrease)
Observe for complaints of pain (cramping or paresthesia of feet and legs, painful cold feet or hands)
Observe for confusion, irritability, tremors, and convulsions
Test for abnormal deep-reflex responses (for increased response, clonus, presence of Babinski sign)

Health Teaching
Explain why the potential problem could become actual (5% dextrose in water does not contain magnesium, large volumes of nonelectrolyte dextrose in water dilute the body's concentration of magnesium, loss of liquid feces depletes the body of magnesium)

Teach how to adjust the diet (for increased magnesium intake and absorption)
Explain the reason for and intended effect of the preventive therapy

EVALUATION

Record actual outcome

POTENTIAL FOR HYPERNATREMIA[371,399]

ASSESSMENT

Data Collection

Subjective Data
• There are no actual symptoms of hypernatremia

Objective Data
• There are no actual signs of hypernatremia

Related Data
• There are one or more stressors present that increase the possibility that
  hypernatremia will occur
DISEASES: Cushing's syndrome, diabetes insipidus
SIGNS AND SYMPTOMS: Dehydration
HEALTH CARE FACTORS: *Medical therapy*: Prolonged normal saline infusions. *Drug therapy*:
  Corticosteroids
LIFESTYLE: High-salt/sodium intake
HUMAN ERROR: Insufficient fluid intake, excessive ingestion of solutes such as nasogastric
  feedings, intake of milk and cream for peptic ulcer, diet very high in carbohydrates

Data Analysis

Nursing Diagnosis
POTENTIAL FOR HYPERNATREMIA: The presence of stressors that increase the possibility of the
  actual occurrence of a serum sodium level above 145 mEq/liter

PLANNING

Unmet Needs

Protection from physical harm, increased learning

Expected Outcome

No signs or symptoms of hypernatremia will occur
  OR
If signs and symptoms occur, they will be promptly recognized as an actual problem and
  will be treated appropriately
Person verbalizes an understanding of and practices preventive methods

NURSING INTERVENTIONS

Nursing Treatments

Encourage decreased sodium-food intake
Give low-sodium fluids orally (water, orange juice, pineapple juice, apple juice, cranber-
  ry juice, lemonade, ginger ale; ensure adequate water with high-solute gastric feed-
  ings)
Refrain from giving saline laxatives
Refrain from giving table salt
Substitute artificial salt

Nursing Observations

Monitor blood studies for abnormal electrolytes (increased sodium)
Observe for complaints of thirst, weakness

Observe for restlessness
Inspect for edema
Monitor the oral temperature (for fever)
Monitor the blood pressure (for increase)
Palpate the pulse for rate, rhythm, and volume (tachycardia)
Inspect the skin for color (flushing)

Health Teaching

Explain why the potential problem could become actual (a loss of water in excess of salt
loss, or an intake of salt in excess of water intake can lead to hypernatremia; Corticosteroids increase the renal tubular reabsorption of sodium; large volumes of infused
saline increases the serum level of sodium)
Teach how to adjust the diet (for decreased sodium intake and retention)
Explain the reason for and intended effect of the preventive therapy

EVALUATION

Record actual outcome

POTENTIAL FOR HYPONATREMIA[73,376,399,451,]

ASSESSMENT

Data Collection

Subjective Data
• There are no actual symptoms of hyponatremia

Objective Data
• There are no actual signs of hyponatremia

Related Data
• There are one or more stressors present that increase the possibility that
hyponatremia will occur
DISEASES: Addison's disease, cerebrovascular accident, carcinoma (neoplasm), congestive
heart failure, fistula, hypoaldosteronism, Laennec's cirrhosis, malnutrition, renal fail-
ure
INJURIES: Burn wound, starvation, trauma (in which there is inappropriate secretion of
antidiuretic hormone)
SIGNS AND SYMPTOMS: Diaphoresis, diarrhea, high fever, vomiting
HEALTH CARE FACTORS: *Medical therapy*: Prolonged dextrose infusion, paracentesis,
nasogastric suction, T-tube drainage, wound drainage. *Drug therapy*: Adverse effects of
diuretics. *Surgical procedures*: Colostomy, ileostomy, ureteroileostomy
LIFESTYLE: Low-sodium intake
ENVIRONMENTAL FACTORS: *Environmental heat*: High environmental temperature
HUMAN ERROR: Chronic use of tap-water enemas, excessive water intake

Data Analysis

Nursing Diagnosis
POTENTIAL FOR HYPONATREMIA: The presence of stressors that increase the possibility of the
actual occurrence of a serum sodium level below 135 mEq/liter

PLANNING

Unmet Needs

Protection from physical harm, increased learning

Expected Outcome

No signs or symptoms of hyponatremia will occur
OR

If signs and symptoms occur, they will be promptly recognized as an actual problem and will be treated appropriately

Person verbalizes an understanding of and practices preventive methods

NURSING INTERVENTIONS

Nursing Treatments

Encourage increased sodium-food intake (salted crackers and chips, bacon, sausage)

Give high-sodium fluids orally (salted tomato juice, bouillon)

Give a salt–soda solution orally (Moyer's solution, Gatorade, if person is exposed to high environmental temperature; solution consists of 1 quart water, 1 level teaspoon of salt, 1/2 teaspoon baking soda; add lemon or orange juice to taste)

Irrigate the gastric tube with (normal) saline (instead of water)

Nursing Observations

Monitor blood studies for abnormal electrolytes (decreased sodium)

Monitor the blood pressure (for decrease)

Palpate the pulse for rate, rhythm, and volume (for tachycardia, weak pulse)

Observe for complaints of headache, weakness, nausea, and pain (abdominal and muscle cramps)

Observe for muscle twitching, vomiting

Observe for apathy and confusion

Measure the intake and output (for anuria, oliguria)

Health Teaching

Explain why the potential problem could become actual (in the average 1,500-cc daily urine output, 6–15 grams or 100 mEq of sodium are excreted; the loss of 1,000 cc of liquid stool results in an approximate sodium loss of 15 mEq; 1,000 cc of ileostomy drainage results in a sodium loss of 125 mEq; 1,000 cc of lost gastric juices results in an approximate sodium loss of 55 mEq; in diuresis, fluid reabsorption from the renal tubules is prevented with a loss of sodium in the urine; if diuresis continues after a normal blood sodium has been reached, sodium depletion will occur; 5% dextrose in water does not contain sodium; large volumes of nonelectrolyte dextrose in water dilute the body's concentration of sodium; 1,000 cc of perspiration results in an approximate sodium loss of 82 mEq and a chloride loss of 12 mEq)

Teach how to adjust the diet (for increased sodium intake, for example; add salt to food on plate rather than while cooking)

Explain the reason for and intended effects of the preventive therapy

EVALUATION

Record actual outcome

Potential Threats to Endocrine Homeostasis

POTENTIAL FOR HYPERGLYCEMIA[42,278]

ASSESSMENT

Data Collection

Subjective Data

• There are no actual symptoms of hyperglycemia

Objective Data
• There are no actual signs of hyperglycemia

Related Data
• There are one or more stressors present that increase the possibility that hyperglycemia will occur

DISEASES: Diabetes mellitus
HEALTH CARE FACTORS: *Medical therapy*: 10% dextrose infusions
LIFESTYLE: Marked decrease in exercise or activity (of diabetic)
HUMAN ERROR: Improper dosage of (or failure to give) insulin, diabetic eating high-carbohydrate meals or snacks

Data Analysis

Nursing Diagnosis
POTENTIAL FOR HYPERGLYCEMIA: The presence of stressors that increase the possibility of the actual occurrence of a serum sugar level above 130 mg/100 ml in the young and middle-aged, or about 140 mg/100 ml in the elderly

PLANNING

Unmet Needs
Protection from physical harm, increased learning

Expected Outcome
No signs or symptoms of hyperglycemia will occur
   OR
If signs and symptoms occur, they will be promptly recognized as an actual problem and will be treated appropriately
Person verbalizes an understanding of and practices preventive methods

NURSING INTERVENTIONS

Nursing Treatments
Provide standby equipment and drugs (IV saline, insulin)
Encourage decreased carbohydrate intake
Encourage moderate physical exercise, moderate activity (and to avoid fluctuations of activity and inactivity if diabetic)

Nursing Observations
Monitor blood studies for abnormal glucose (for an increase)
Test the urine for sugar (note glucosuria)
Observe for complaints of nausea, fatigue, (abdominal) pain and tenderness
Observe for vomiting
Measure the intake and output (note excessive output)

Health Teaching
Instruct (diabetics) to eat only prescribed foods and amounts of foods
Teach how to test the urine for sugar and acetone
Explain why the potential problem could become actual (10% dextrose infusion, because of its high sugar content, can elevate the blood sugar; a diabetic's intake of more nutrients than allowed, especially carbohydrates, or failure to take insulin will increase blood sugar)
Instruct to increase fluid intake (at first signs of polyuria, glycosuria, fatigue, to prevent dehydration)
Explain the reason for and intended effect of the preventive therapy

EVALUATION
Record actual outcome

POTENTIAL FOR HYPOGLYCEMIA[26,42,73,278]

ASSESSMENT

Data Collection

Subjective Data
• There are no actual symptoms of hypoglycemia

Objective Data
• There are no actual signs of hypoglycemia

Related Data
• There are one or more stressors present that increase the possibility that hypoglycemia will occur

BIRTH STATUS: Premature infant

INHERITED FACTORS: Familial tendency, infant has a diabetic mother

DISEASES: Addison's disease, alcoholism, extrapancreatic tumor, erythroblastosis, hepatic
failure, hypopituitarism, ketotic hypoglycemia (age 18 months through 5 years), leukemia, malabsorption syndrome, malnutrition, myxedema, pancreatic tumor, renal glucosuria

INJURIES: Starvation

SIGNS AND SYMPTOMS: Fever

HUMAN BODY: *Body state*: Pregnancy

HEALTH CARE FACTORS: *Drug therapy*: Adverse effects of drugs (insulin therapy). *Medical Therapy*: Blood exchange on newborn

LIFESTYLE: Overvigorous exercise

HUMAN ERROR: Improper dosage of insulin, exposure of premature infant to the cold

Data Analysis

Nursing Diagnosis

POTENTIAL FOR HYPOGLYCEMIA (POTENTIAL FOR INSULIN SHOCK): The presence of stressors that increase the possibility of the actual occurrence of a serum sugar level below 60
mg/100 ml in adults or below 40 mg/100 ml in premature and newborn infants

PLANNING

Unmet Needs

Protection from physical harm, increased learning

Expected Outcome

No signs or symptoms of hypoglycemia will occur
OR
If signs and symptoms occur, they will be promptly recognized as an actual problem and
will be treated appropriately
Person verbalizes an understanding of and practices preventive methods

NURSING INTERVENTIONS

Nursing Treatments

Provide standby equipment and drugs (IV glucose, orange juice, sugar)
Encourage decreased carbohydrate intake (carbohydrates stimulate release of additional
insulin, causing a backlash hypoglycemia)
Encourage increased protein-food intake, fatty-food intake (both are converted slowly to
glycogen, causing less fluctuation of the blood glucose)
Give small, frequent feedings

Specific to Infants

Reduce infant handling to a minimum (to reduce stress, which can lower the infant's
glucose level)
Feed by bottle (or gavage if appropriate)
OR

Start infant on breast feedings (1–2 hours after birth)
Decrease the time interval between infant feedings
Place the infant in an incubator (where there is a neutral thermal environment, to reduce energy needs)

Nursing Observations
Monitor blood studies for abnormal glucose (decreased)
Observe for complaints of nervousness, weakness
Observe for tremors
Inspect the skin for abnormal perspiration (profuse sweating)
Palpate the pulse for rate, rhythm, and volume (tachycardia)
Test the blood for glucose level (with a Dextrostix, especially after intravenous glucose is stopped, which is when the serum glucose level could decrease)
Test the urine for ketones (in ketotic hypoglycemia)

Specific to Infants
Test the blood for glucose level (with a Dextrostix within 1 hour of birth, then every 1–2 hours for 6–8 hours, then every 4–6 hours until 24 hours old, or until stabilized)
Observe for tremors, convulsions, cyanosis (in an infant; also observe for jitteriness, hypotonia, refusal to suck, apnea, and abnormal eye movements)
Observe the characteristics of the child's cry (note a weak high-pitched cry)

Health Teaching
Describe those symptoms that should be reported (weakness trembling, sweating, nervousness, tachycardia, palpitations)
Explain why the potential problem could become actual (oversecretion or injection of insulin will decrease blood glucose; lack of nutritional intake will prevent normal glucose levels)
Teach how to adjust the diet (to maintain a normal blood glucose)
Recommend that a high glucose source be carried at all times
Explain the importance of wearing a Medic-Alert tag
Explain the reason for and intended effect of the preventive therapy

EVALUATION
Record actual outcome

POTENTIAL FOR ADRENAL CRISIS[42,73]

ASSESSMENT
Data Collection

Subjective Data
• There are no actual symptoms of adrenal crisis

Objective Data
• There are no actual signs of adrenal crisis

Related Data
• There are one or more stressors present that increase the possibility of adrenal crisis occurring
DISEASES: Septicemia or any infection in a person with Addison's disease
INJURIES: Trauma of any kind to a person with Addison's disease, especially trauma to the adrenal gland

PSYCHOSOCIAL FACTORS: Threat of severe stress

HEALTH CARE FACTORS: *Drug therapy*: Anticoagulant therapy, withdrawal of corticosteroids, effects of thyroid preparations on insulin in persons having panhypopituitarism. *Medical therapy*: Prolonged absence of food intake (for therapeutic or diagnostic reasons). *Surgical procedures*: Any, especially adrenalectomy

ENVIRONMENTAL FACTORS: *Environmental heat*: High external temperature. *Environmental cold*: Low external temperature (in Addison's disease)

HUMAN ERROR: Not taking maintenance dosages of corticosteroids

Data Analysis

Nursing Diagnosis

POTENTIAL FOR ADRENAL CRISIS: The presence of stressors that increase the possibility of the actual occurrence of a rapidly overwhelming insufficiency of adrenocortical hormones, usually in a person with chronic adrenal insufficiency

PLANNING

Unmet Needs

Protection from physical harm, increased learning

Expected Outcome

No signs or symptoms of adrenal crisis will occur
   OR
If signs and symptoms occur, such will be promptly recognized as an actual problem and will be treated appropriately
Person verbalizes an understanding of and practices preventive methods

NURSING INTERVENTIONS

Nursing Treatments

Provide standby equipment and drugs (saline IV fluids, oxygen, Solu-Cortef or cortisone acetate, epinephrine)
Maintain a normal room temperature (to avoid environmental extremes)
Provide quiet (prohibit noise stressors)
Encourage adequate rest
Refrain from performing nonessential procedures (which increase stress)
Encourage increased carbohydrate intake, increased protein-food intake

Nursing Observations

Monitor blood studies for abnormal adrenal function (decreased cortisol level, decreased sodium and glucose, increased potassium)
Observe for complaints of pain (abdominal, lower back, or leg pain), weakness, headache, nausea, weakness
Observe for restlessness, vomiting, diarrhea, lethargy
Monitor the blood pressure (for hypotension)
Palpate the pulse for rate, rhythm, and volume (tachycardia, weak pulse)
Monitor the oral temperature (for fever)

Health Teaching

Explain the need to recognize highly stressful situations (and to avoid them)
Explain that fatigue should be recognized as a stress factor
Instruct to increase fluid intake (and sodium intake)
Recommend methods for achieving total relaxation (for coping with daily stressors)
Explain why the potential problem could become actual (the stress of infection, trauma, everyday living, etc., taxes an already poorly functioning adrenal gland)
Explain the reason for and intended effect of the preventive therapy

EVALUATION

Record actual outcome

POTENTIAL FOR THYROID CRISIS [26,42,73,278]

ASSESSMENT
Data Collection
Subjective Data
• There are no actual symptoms of thyroid crisis

Objective Data
• There are no actual signs of thyroid crisis

Related Data
• There are one or more stressors present that increase the possibility that thyroid crisis will occur
DISEASES: Any infection in a person having thyrotoxicosis (hyperthyroidism)
PSYCHOSOCIAL FACTORS: Threat of severe stress
INJURIES: Any major trauma (to a person having hyperthyroidism)
HUMAN BODY: *Natural body function:* Labor of childbirth
HEALTH CARE FACTORS: *Medical therapy:* Radioactive iodine therapy administered to a person with hyperthyroidism. *Surgical procedure:* Any, especially thyroidectomy

Data Analysis
Nursing Diagnosis
POTENTIAL FOR THYROID CRISIS (POTENTIAL FOR THYROID STORM): The presence of stressors that increase the possibility of the actual occurrence of an acute onset of signs and symptoms of severe thyrotoxicosis

PLANNING
Unmet Needs
Protection from physical harm, increased learning

Expected Outcome
No signs or symptoms of thyroid crisis will occur
   OR
If signs and symptoms occur, they will be promptly recognized as an actual problem and will be treated appropriately

NURSING INTERVENTIONS
Nursing Treatments
Provide standby equipment and drugs (oxygen, sedatives, propranolol, propylthiouracil, corticosteroids, hypothermia blanket, hypertonic IV fluids, injectable vitamins B-complex and thiamine)
Provide quiet
Encourage adequate rest
Refrain from giving oral stimulants (coffee, tea, soft drinks containing caffeine)
Refrain from performing nonessential procedures (which increase stress)
Limit visitors
Withhold all drugs (stimulants, such as epinephrine and norepinephrine)

Nursing Observations
Monitor blood studies for abnormal thyroid function (increased level)
Monitor the oral temperature (for fever about 100° F)
Palpate the pulse for rate, rhythm, and volume (tachycardia above 120 beats/minute)
Observe for irritability, restlessness, confusion, delirium
Monitor the blood pressure (for hypotension)

Health Teaching
Explain the need to recognize highly stressful situations
Explain that fatigue should be recognized as a stress factor

Explain why the potential problem could become actual (when the thyroid gland is handled in surgery or damaged by trauma, the gland releases a large amount of thyroxine, resulting in thyroid crisis)

Instruct to avoid direct contact with infected persons (and other stressors while being treated with antithyroid drugs; as long as the person is in a hyperthyroid state, stress could precipitate a crisis)

Explain the reason for and intended effect of the preventive therapy

EVALUATION

Record actual outcome

Potential Threats to Fluid Homeostasis

POTENTIAL FOR FLUID DEPLETION[26,73,451]

ASSESSMENT

Data Collection

Subjective Data
• There are no actual symptoms of fluid depletion

Objective Data
• There are no actual signs of fluid depletion

Related Data
• There are one or more stressors present that increase the possibility that fluid depletion will occur

DISEASES: Diabetes mellitus, diabetes insipidus, hemorrhage, hyperparathyroidism

INJURIES: Burn wound

SIGNS AND SYMPTOMS: Diaphoresis, diarrhea, fever, polyuria, vomiting

HEALTH CARE FACTORS: *Medical therapy:* Gastrostomy, jejunostomy, nasogastric feeding, gastrointestinal suction/drainage. *Drug therapy:* Adverse effects of diuretics

ENVIRONMENTAL FACTORS: *Environmental heat:* High external temperature

HUMAN ERROR: Chronic use of saline enemas, excessive intake of laxatives, fluid intake of less than 1,200–1,500 cc daily

Data Analysis

Nursing Diagnosis
POTENTIAL FOR FLUID DEPLETION: The presence of stressors that increase the possibility of the actual occurrence of the loss of large amounts of body fluids without adequate replacement

PLANNING

Unmet Needs

Protection from physical harm, increased learning

Expected Outcome

No signs or symptoms of fluid depletion will occur
   OR

If signs and symptoms occur, they will be promptly recognized as an actual problem and
will be treated appropriately

Person verbalizes an understanding of and practices preventive methods

NURSING INTERVENTIONS

Nursing Treatments

Balance fluid intake to equal output

Give small, frequent drinks (if needed, to maintain intake)

Nursing Observations

Measure the intake and output

Inspect for dehydration

Monitor the flow rate of the intravenous fluids (to prevent delayed administration of the
day's fluid order)

Health Teaching

Explain that fluid intake and output should be balanced

Instruct to increase fluid intake (to the specific amount needed)

Explain why the potential problem could become actual (excess fluid loss without equal
replacement results in fluid depletion)

Explain the reason for and intended effect of the preventive therapy

EVALUATION

Record actual outcome

POTENTIAL FOR FLUID OVERLOAD[26,72,371]

ASSESSMENT

Data Collection

Subjective Data

• There are no actual symptoms of fluid overload

Objective Data

• There are no actual signs of fluid overload

Related Data

• There are one or more stressors present that increase the possibility of fluid overload
occurring

DISEASES: Acute infection, congestive heart failure, myocardial infarction, renal insufficiency or failure

HEALTH CARE FACTORS: *Medical therapy:* Overload of intravenous infusion. *Drug therapy:* Adverse effects of corticosteroids

HUMAN ERROR: Multiple tap-water enemas

Data Analysis

Nursing Diagnosis

**POTENTIAL FOR FLUID OVERLOAD (POTENTIAL FOR OVERHYDRATION, POTENTIAL FOR WATER INTOXICATION, PO-
TENTIAL FOR DILUTION SYNDROME):** The presence of stressors that increase the possibility of
the actual occurrence of fluid intake in excess of the amount the kidneys can excrete

PLANNING

Unmet Needs

Protection from physical harm, increased learning

Expected Outcome

No signs or symptoms of fluid overload will occur
  OR
If signs and symptoms occur, they will be promptly recognized as an actual problem and
  will be treated appropriately

NURSING INTERVENTIONS

Nursing Treatments

Balance fluid intake to equal output
Slow the intravenous infusion or blood transfusion flow rate (so that overload does not
  occur)

Nursing Observations

Monitor blood studies for abnormal electrolytes (decreased sodium)
Measure the intake and output (for a normal output that exceeds 50 cc/per hour or an
  abnormal output below 30 cc/hour)
Monitor the flow rate of the intravenous fluids (including blood transfusions to prevent
  excessive speed of flow)
Observe for dyspnea, coughing, cyanosis, confusion, vomiting
Observe for complaints of headache, weakness, malaise, anorexia, nausea
Palpate the pulse for rate, rhythm, and volume (tachycardia)
Palpate the skin for temperature (warmth, flushing, and slight moisture)
Inspect for edema
Inspect the arms and hands for venous distention
Inspect the neck veins for distention
Monitor the central venous pressure (for an increase)
Measure the body weight (and check for sudden weight gain)

Health Teaching

Explain why the potential problem could become actual (fluid intake, when in excess of
  the cardiovascular or renal capacity to handle the fluid, results in fluid overload)
Explain the reason for and intended effect of the preventive therapy

EVALUATION

Record actual outcome

POTENTIAL FOR LOCALIZED EDEMA [42,73,371]

ASSESSMENT

Data Collection

Subjective Data
• There are no actual symptoms of edema

Objective Data
• There are no actual signs of edema

Related Data
• There are one or more stressors present that increase the possibility that edema will
  occur

DISEASES: Abscess, cellulitis, filiariasis, Milroy's disease, rheumatoid arthritis
INJURIES: Bone fracture, burn wound, contusion, joint sprain, insect bite or sting
HEALTH CARE FACTORS: *Surgical procedures:* Any surgery

Data Analysis

Nursing Diagnosis
POTENTIAL FOR LOCALIZED EDEMA: The presence of stressors that increase the possibility of the actual occurrence of fluid accumulation confined to specific body tissues and not extending throughout the entire body

PLANNING

Unmet Needs
Protection from physical harm, increased learning

Expected Outcome
No signs or symptoms of localized edema will occur
   OR
If signs and symptoms occur, they will be promptly recognized as an actual problem and will be treated appropriately
Person verbalizes an understanding of and practices preventive methods

NURSING INTERVENTIONS

Nursing Treatments
Apply a cold, moist compress
   OR
Apply an ice pack (immediately to the injured site)
   OR
Apply a warm, moist compress (to infected, inflammed site)
Elevate the affected body part
Give nonprescription drugs (antihistamines for an allergic response)
Massage gently
   AND
Exercise in range of motion (for lymph obstruction)
Remove constrictive clothing (around extremities)
Refrain from tight bandaging
Refrain from giving intravenous or intramuscular injections (in a limb susceptible to lymphedema)

Nursing Observations
Inspect for edema
Measure the circumference of the body part (for early signs of edema)

Health Teaching
Describe those symptoms that should be reported (skin tightness, pain)
Instruct to elevate the body part (after trauma)
Advise not to stand for prolonged periods (if there is a potential for leg or ankle edema)
Explain why the potential problem could become actual (inflammation, trauma, lymphatic obstruction, or allergic reactions cause fluid to accumulate within body tissues as a result of injury to the tissue)
Explain the reason for and intended effect of the preventive therapy

EVALUATION

Record actual outcome

Potential Threats to Gastrointestinal Homeostasis

POTENTIAL FOR ABDOMINAL DISTENTION[73,371]

ASSESSMENT

Data Collection

Subjective Data
• There are no actual symptoms of abdominal distention

Objective Data
• There are no actual signs of abdominal distention

Related Data
• There are one or more stressors present that increase the possibility of abdominal distention occurring

DISEASES: Hemorrhage (intraperitoneal), hernia, intestinal obstruction, pneumonia
INJURIES: Abdominal trauma
SIGNS AND SYMPTOMS: Air swallowing, hypokalemia
HEALTH CARE FACTORS: *Medical therapy:* Prolonged intermittent positive-pressure breathing. *Surgical therapy:* Anesthesia. *Surgical procedure:* Any abdominal surgery. *Drug therapy:* Adverse effect of anticholinergics. *Therapeutic equipment:* Malfunctioning nasogastric suction

Data Analysis

Nursing Diagnosis
POTENTIAL FOR ABDOMINAL DISTENTION: The presence of stressors that increase the possibility of the actual occurrence of swelling and pressure within the abdominal cavity

PLANNING

Unmet Needs
Protection from physical harm, increased learning

Expected Outcome
No signs or symptoms of abdominal distention will occur
    OR
If signs and symptoms occur, they will be promptly recognized as an actual problem and will be treated appropriately

NURSING INTERVENTIONS

Nursing Treatments
Change the person's position frequently
Ambulate the person (as much as possible)
Give warm liquids (if there are no fluid restrictions)
Encourage decreased gas-forming food intake

Nursing Observations
Inspect the abdomen for distention
    OR
Measure the circumference of the abdomen (periodically; if the person is on IPPB treatment or continuous respirator, he is susceptible to distention)
Auscultate the abdomen for abnormal bowel sounds (high-pitched gurgling sounds gradually decreasing to cessation of bowel sounds; or for decreased bowel sounds postoperatively)
Percuss the abdomen for abnormal resonance (tympany)
Check the (nasogastric) tube for patency

Health Teaching

Describe those symptoms that should be reported (abdominal fullness, tightness, pain)

Explain why the potential problem could become actual (the accumulation of gas or fluid in the intestines results in abdominal distention; when the intestinal contents do not move through the intestines because of metabolic changes, spasm, trauma, or chemical irritation, distention occurs)

Explain the reason for and intended effect of the preventive therapy

EVALUATION

Record actual outcome

POTENTIAL FOR CONSTIPATION/FECAL IMPACTION[42,73,399]

ASSESSMENT

Data Collection

Subjective Data

• There are no actual symptoms of constipation or fecal impaction

Objective Data

• There are no actual signs of constipation or fecal impaction

Related Data

• There are one or more stressors present that increase the possibility that constipation or fecal impaction will occur

DISEASES: Hyperparathyroidism, hypothyroidism (myxedema), megacolon, paralytic ileus

INJURIES: Fracture and compression of the spinal cord

SIGNS AND SYMPTOMS: Immobility, weakness

PSYCHOSOCIAL FACTORS: Threat of chronic stress

HEALTH CARE FACTORS: *Diagnostic procedures:* Barium enema. *Medical therapy:* Prolonged bed rest. *Surgical therapy:* Anesthesia. *Drug therapy:* Adverse effects of antacids

DEVELOPMENTAL PHASES: Old age

LIFESTYLE: Low-bulk diet, lack of exercise

HUMAN ERROR: Insufficient fluid intake, inattention to the defecation reflex

Data Analysis

Nursing Diagnosis

POTENTIAL FOR CONSTIPATION/FECAL IMPACTION: The presence of stressors that increase the possibility of the actual occurrence of dry, hard stools with decreased frequency of bowel elimination

PLANNING

Unmet Needs

Protection from physical harm, increased learning

Expected Outcome

No signs or symptoms of constipation or fecal impaction will occur
OR
If signs and symptoms occur, they will be promptly recognized as an actual problem and will be treated appropriately

Person verbalizes an understanding of and practices preventive methods

NURSING INTERVENTIONS

Nursing Treatments

Ambulate the person (frequently)

Encourage moderate physical exercise
Encourage increased residue-food intake
Give fresh fruits (daily)
OR
Give prune juice (daily)
Give hot coffee
Increase fluid intake to about 2,000 cc daily
Give nonprescription drugs (stool softeners, laxatives)

Nursing Observations
Observe for complaints of constipation

Health Teaching
Describe those symptoms that should be reported (abdominal or rectal fullness, pain)
Explain the need for scheduled bowel elimination
Instruct to respond immediately to the elimination reflex
Instruct to increase fluid intake
Teach how to adjust the diet (to control bowel elimination)
Explain why the potential problem could become actual (constipation can result from such factors as excessive water absorption from the stool by the colon, inattention to the defecation reflex, sigmoid spasms, altered daily schedule, decreased digestive juices and slowed peristalsis with aging, lack of energy to evacuate the bowel, emotional tension)
Explain the reason for and intended effect of the preventive therapy

EVALUATION

Record actual outcome

POTENTIAL FOR DIARRHEA [42,399]

ASSESSMENT

Data Collection

Subjective Data
• There are no actual symptoms of diarrhea

Objective Data
• There are no actual signs of diarrhea

Related Data
• There are one or more stressors present that increase the possibility that diarrhea will occur
DISEASES: Addison's disease, allergic disorder (food), malabsorption syndrome, malnutrition
PSYCHOSOCIAL FACTORS: Threat of severe stress
HEALTH CARE FACTORS: *Medical therapy:* Gastrostomy, jejunostomy, or nasogastric feeding, alcohol or drug withdrawal. *Surgical therapy:* Colostomy, ileostomy. *Drug therapy:* Adverse effects of chemotherapy, antacids containing magnesium, antibiotics, laxatives
LIFESTYLE: Foreign travel
ENVIRONMENTAL FACTORS: Food substances contaminated by bacteria or toxic agents

Data Analysis

Nursing Diagnosis
POTENTIAL FOR DIARRHEA: The presence of stressors that increase the possibility of the actu-

al occurrence of unformed stools in abnormal frequency

PLANNING

Unmet Needs

Protection from physical harm, increased learning

Expected Outcome

No signs or symptoms of diarrhea will occur
> OR

If signs and symptoms occur, they will be promptly recognized as an actual problem and will be treated appropriately

Person verbalizes an understanding of and practices preventive methods

NURSING INTERVENTIONS

Nursing Treatments

Encourage decreased residue-food intake

Refrain from giving hot liquids, iced liquids, oral stimulants

Refrain from giving enemas, laxatives, inserting a rectal tube, or taking rectal temperatures (which could stimulate peristalsis)

Withhold drugs (that might cause intestinal irritation)

Give nonprescription drugs (antidiarrheal drugs to take on trips, etc.)

Nursing Observations

Observe for diarrhea

Health Teaching

Recommend eating only well-cooked meat and vegetables in foreign countries

Advise against using ice cubes made from potentially unsafe water

Explain that teeth should not be brushed with potentially unsafe water

Emphasize that potentially unsafe water should be boiled for 10 minutes

Inform that halazone tablets should be added to potentially unsafe water

Explain why the potential problem could become actual (diarrhea can occur when there is mechanical, biological, or chemical irritation of the intestinal mucosa)

Explain the reason for and intended effects of the preventive therapy

EVALUATION

Record actual outcome

POTENTIAL FOR GASTROENTERITIS[164,278]

ASSESSMENT

Data Collection

Subjective Data
• There are no actual symptoms of gastroenteritis

Objective Data
• There are no actual signs of gastroenteritis

Related Data
• There are one or more stressors present that increase the possibility that gastroenteritis will occur

DISEASES: Alcoholism

HEALTH CARE FACTORS: *Adverse effects of drugs:* Gastric irritation from antibiotics, vitamins, aspirin, potassium chloride, salt tablets

LIFESTYLE: Spicy food intake
SITUATIONAL FACTORS: Foreign travel
ENVIRONMENTAL FACTORS: *Food:* Inadequate food storage or refrigeration

Data Analysis

Nursing Diagnosis
POTENTIAL FOR GASTROENTERITIS: The presence of stressors that increase the possibility of the actual occurrence of the stomach and intestinal mucosa becoming painful and inflamed

PLANNING

Unmet Needs
Protection from physical harm, increased learning

Expected Outcome
No signs or symptoms of gastritis will occur
   OR
If signs and symptoms occur, they will be promptly recognized as an actual problem and will be treated appropriately
Person verbalizes an understanding of and practices preventive methods

NURSING INTERVENTIONS

Nursing Treatments
Specific to Drug Effects
Dilute the medication
   OR
Give enteric-coated medications
   OR
Give the medication by injection or in liquid form instead of pills
   OR
Give milk with medications
   OR
Give nonprescription drugs (an antacid with the irritating medication, provided the antacid does not decrease the drug's effectiveness)

Nursing Observations
Inspect the abdomen for distention
Observe for complaints of (cramping) pain, anorexia, nausea
Observe for diarrhea, vomiting

Health Teaching
Describe those symptoms that should be reported (anorexia, nausea, vomiting, generalized epigastric discomfort, chills, fever, diarrhea)
Recommend adequate food refrigeration (to prevent food spoilage)
Recommend eating only well-cooked meat and vegetables in foreign countries
Advise against using ice cubes made from potentially unsafe water
Explain that teeth should not be brushed with potentially unsafe water
Emphasize that potentially unsafe water should be boiled for 10 minutes
Inform that halazone tablets should be added to potentially unsafe water
Teach how to adjust the diet (by avoiding highly spiced foods, especially hot peppers and other irritants)
Explain why the potential problem could become actual (the ingestion of irritating foods or chemicals causes inflammation of the gastric mucosa)
Explain the reason for and intended effects of the preventive therapy

EVALUATION
Record actual outcome

POTENTIAL FOR STOMATITIS[26,42]

ASSESSMENT

Data Collection

Subjective Data
• There are no actual symptoms of stomatitis

Objective Data
• There are no actual signs of stomatitis

Related Data
• There are one or more stressors present that increase the possibility that stomatitis will occur

DISEASES: Alcoholism, celiac disease (sprue), diabetes mellitus, infectious mononucleosis, iron deficiency anemia, leukemia, measles, pellagra, pernicious anemia, scurvy

SIGNS AND SYMPTOMS: Mouth breathing, fever

HEALTH CARE FACTORS: *Drug therapy*: Adverse effects of chemotherapy. *Medical therapy*: Adverse effects of oral radiation therapy. *Therapeutic devices*: Poor-fitting or plastic dentures, nursing bottle with a hard nipple

LIFESTYLE: Tobacco smoking or chewing, spicy food intake

ENVIRONMENTAL FACTORS: *Biological agents*: Viruses, bacteria. *Chemical substances*: Sensitivity to toothpaste or mouthwash

Data Analysis

Nursing Diagnosis
POTENTIAL FOR STOMATITIS: The presence of stressors that increase the possibility of the actual occurrence of inflammation of the mouth

PLANNING

Unmet Needs

Protection from physical harm, increased learning

Expected Outcome

No signs or symptoms of stomatitis will occur
OR
If signs and symptoms occur, they will be promptly recognized as an actual problem and will be treated appropriately
Person verbalizes an understanding of and practices preventive methods

NURSING INTERVENTIONS

Nursing Treatments

Brush and floss the teeth
Rinse the mouth with diluted hydrogen peroxide
OR
Swab the mouth with diluted glycerine (or with milk of magnesia substrate)
Give bland foods (to avoid mouth irritation)
Refrain from giving hot liquids, iced liquids (which could irritate mucosa)
Discourage the intake of oral stimulants (such as alcohol, caffeine, and nicotine)

Nursing Observations

Inspect the (oral) mucous membranes for abnormalities (lesions, inflammation, dryness)

Health Teaching

Recommend the use of a mouthwash (warm normal saline for a dry mouth or when receiving oral radiation therapy, include instructions in oral hygiene)
Explain why the potential problem could become actual (chemical or bacterial irritation of the oral mucosa can destroy mouth tissue)
Teach how to adjust the diet (avoiding highly spiced and irritating foods)
Explain the reason for and intended effects of the preventive therapy

EVALUATION
Record actual outcome

POTENTIAL FOR STRESS ULCER[42,446,561]

ASSESSMENT
Data Collection
Subjective Data
• There are no actual symptoms of a stress ulcer

Objective Data
• There are no actual signs of a stress ulcer

Related Data
• There are one or more stressors present that increase the possibility that a stress ulcer will occur
DISEASES: Any serious infection, cerebrovascular accident
INJURIES: Extensive second- or third-degree burn wound (ulcer will most likely occur 3–10 days or within 30 days after injury), fracture and compression of the spinal cord
SIGNS AND SYMPTOMS: Shock
PSYCHOSOCIAL FACTORS: Threat of chronic severe stress
HEALTH CARE FACTORS: *Health care environment*: Intensive care unit. *Drug therapy*: Corticosteroids. *Surgical therapy*: Multiple surgeries

Data Analysis
Nursing Diagnosis
POTENTIAL FOR STRESS ULCER: The presence of stressors that increase the possibility of the actual occurrence of gastric ulcerations after serious injury, surgery, illness, or other threatening conditions

PLANNING
Unmet Needs
Protection from physical harm, increased learning

Expected Outcome
No signs or symptoms of stress ulcer will occur
  OR
If signs and symptoms occur, they will be promptly recognized as an actual problem and will be treated appropriately

NURSING INTERVENTIONS
Nursing Treatments
Approach unhurriedly
Provide quiet
Encourage adequate rest
Reduce the demands placed on the person
Refrain from performing nonessential procedures
Do not allow unpleasant surprise situations (which cause fear, or stress)
Encourage increased protein-food intake (in small, frequent meals)
Give nonprescription drugs (give antacids prophylactically)

Nursing Observations
Monitor blood studies for evidence of gastric ulceration (increased serum amylase and lipase, decreased hematocrit from bleeding)
Observe for complaints of (epigastric or abdominal) pain, nausea

Observe for vomiting (coffee-ground fluid, bright blood)

Inspect for stool abnormalities (such as tarry stools, and note stool examination reports of occult blood)

Health Teaching

Describe those symptoms that should be reported (pain, rectal bleeding, dark stools, hematemesis)

Explain why the potential problem could become actual (stress ulcers can occur from the effects of acid hypersecretion, endotoxins, microemboli, and steroids or from rapid loss of protein; decreased blood supply to the mucosa increases the likelihood of ulceration; the stomach mucous cells undergo tissue breakdown and fail to duplicate themselves normally; resulting in erosion of the stomach's superficial mucosa and causes ulceration)

Explain the reason for and intended effect of the preventive therapy

EVALUATION

Record actual outcome

POTENTIAL FOR VOMITING[42,371]

ASSESSMENT

Data Collection

Subjective Data

• There are no actual symptoms of vomiting

Objective Data

• There are no actual signs of vomiting

Related Data

• There are one or more stressors present that increase the possibility that vomiting will occur

DISEASES: Alcoholism, brain tumor, carcinoma, chronic indigestion, gastritis, gastric hemorrhage, hepatitis, infectious mononucleosis, labyrinthitis, migraine headache

INJURIES: Cerebral concussion

SIGNS AND SYMPTOMS: Severe pain

PSYCHOSOCIAL FACTORS: Threat of severe or chronic stress

HUMAN BODY: *Body state*: Pregnancy

HEALTH CARE FACTORS: *Diagnostic procedures*: Angiography, bronchoscopy, gastric analysis, gastroscopy. *Medical therapy*: Prolonged intermittent positive-pressure breathing, ear irrigation (with cold water), radiation therapy, alcohol or drug withdrawal. *Drug therapy*: Adverse effects of chemotherapy. *Surgical therapy*: Recovery from anesthesia. *Surgical procedure*: Any surgery but especially abdominal surgery

ENVIRONMENTAL FACTORS: Inhalation of chemical substances

Data Analysis

Nursing Diagnosis

POTENTIAL FOR VOMITING: The presence of stressors that increase the possibility of the actual occurrence of the forceful ejection of stomach contents through the mouth

PLANNING

Unmet Needs

Protection from physical harm, increased learning

Expected Outcome

No signs or symptoms of vomiting will occur
> OR

If signs and symptoms occur, they will be promptly recognized as an actual problem and
will be treated appropriately

Person verbalizes understanding of and practices preventive methods

NURSING INTERVENTIONS

Nursing Treatments

Apply a cool, damp cloth to the face
Apply an ice collar
Elevate the head
Encourage deep breathing (through the mouth)   } If vomiting seems imminent
Feed slowly
Give bland foods
> OR

Give clear-liquid foods (or ice chips)
> OR

Give full-liquid foods
> OR

Withhold food until the patient requests it
> OR

Restrict the intake to nothing by mouth
Give small, frequent feedings
Limit IPPB treatments to short periods (and avoid giving treatments near mealtimes)
Refresh with a mouthwash (to reduce offensive mouth order which in itself stimulates
vomiting)
Subdue the room lighting (especially for migraine headaches or concussion)
Control offensive odors by removing the source
Give nonprescription drugs (for pain or nausea)

Nursing Observations

Observe for vomiting (and gagging)

Health Teaching

Explain why the potential problem could become actual (vomiting can occur when there
is gastric irritation or inflammation, increased intracranial pressure, or toxicity)
Explain the reason for and intended effects of the preventive therapy

EVALUATION
Record actual outcome

Potential Threats to Genitourinary Homeostasis

POTENTIAL FOR URINARY TRACT INFECTION[73,520]

ASSESSMENT

Data Collection

Subjective Data
• There are no actual symptoms of genitourinary infection

Objective Data
• There are no actual signs of genitourinary infection

Related Data
• There are one or more stressors present that increase the possibility that a genitourinary infection will occur

DISEASES: Gonorrhea, pharyngitis, renal insufficiency, syphilis, urinary tract obstruction, vesicoureteral reflux

INJURIES: Fracture and compression of the spinal cord

SIGNS AND SYMPTOMS: Alkaline urine (pH above 6.5), immobility, residual urine

HEALTH CARE FACTORS: *Diagnostic procedures*: Kidney biopsy, cystoscopy, cystourethrography, retrograde pylogram or urethrography, urinary catheterization. *Medical therapy*: Genitourinary drainage, bladder irrigation, prolonged bed rest. *Surgical procedures*: Nephrectomy, nephrostomy, nephrotomy, ureterostomy, ureterotomy

DEVELOPMENT PHASES: Old age (age 60 years and above)

LIFESTYLE: Insufficient sleep and rest, engaging in sexual intercourse

HUMAN ERROR: Insufficient fluid intake, inadequate or incorrect hygiene methods of toileting, use of bubble bath and fragrances in bath water

Data Analysis

Nursing Diagnosis

POTENTIAL FOR GENITOURINARY INFECTION: The presence of stressors that increase the possibility of the actual occurrence of the invasion of pathogenic organisms into the kidneys, ureters, bladder, or urethra

PLANNING

Unmet Needs
Protection from physical harm, increased learning

Expected Outcome
No signs or symptoms of urinary tract infection will occur
   OR
If signs and symptoms occur, they will be promptly recognized as an actual problem and will be treated appropriately
Person verbalizes an understanding of and practices preventive methods

NURSING INTERVENTIONS

Nursing Treatments
Ambulate the person (as much as possible)
Change the person's position frequently
Give urine-acidifying juices orally (four times daily)
Increase fluid intake to about 2,000 cc daily (if there are no fluid restrictions)
Sterilize the bedpan after each use
Change the urinary drainage apparatus (frequently)
Keep the drainage container below bladder level
Use sterile technique (when disconnecting urinary drainage system)
Clean the urinary catheter externally at the meatus (or around an ostomy tube)

Nursing Observations
Monitor the oral temperature (for fever)
Monitor urine studies for evidence of urinary tract infection (for bacteria count above 100,000)
   OR
Test the urine by Dipstik (for positive nitrite, and blood)
Test the urine for pH (urine acidity reduces the potential for infection)
Observe the urine for abnormal color, content, and odor (cloudiness, blood, foul odor)

Health Teaching
Describe those symptoms that should be reported (frequency, dysuria, chills, fever)
Instruct to increase fluid intake (to about 2,000 cc daily)

Explain how to use toilet tissue correctly by cleansing from front to back (which prevents fecal contamination of the urinary meatus)

Advise voiding every 4 hours during waking hours

Recommend voiding after sexual intercourse

Explain why the potential problem could become actual (urinary tract infection results from the external introduction of microorganisms into the genitourinary tract from inadequate or incorrect hygiene methods, from use of bubble bath, etc.; urine stagnation also causes infection when there is infrequent voiding, residual urine, etc.)

Explain the reason for and intended effect of the preventive therapy

EVALUATION

Record actual outcome

POTENTIAL FOR VOIDING DIFFICULTY[26]

ASSESSMENT

Data Collection

Subjective Data
• There are no actual symptoms of voiding difficulty

Objective Data
• There are no actual signs of voiding difficulty

Related Data
• There are one or more stressors present that increase the possibility that voiding difficulty will occur

DISEASES: Benign prostatic hypertrophy, meatal stenosis, multiple sclerosis, prostatitis

HEALTH CARE FACTORS: *Drug therapy*: Adverse effects of anticholenergic drugs. *Surgical therapy*: Anesthesia

DEVELOPMENTAL PHASES: Old age

Data Analysis

Nursing Diagnosis
POTENTIAL FOR VOIDING DIFFICULTY: The presence of stressors that increase the possibility of the actual occurrence of difficulty urinating

PLANNING

Unmet Needs

Protection from physical harm, increased learning

Expected Outcome

No signs or symptoms of voiding difficulty will occur
OR
If signs and symptoms occur, they will be promptly recognized as an actual problem and will be treated appropriately

NURSING INTERVENTIONS

Nursing Treatments

Ambulate the person (as much as possible)

Change the person's position frequently

Use methods for stimulating urination (help a man stand up and a woman assume the sitting position, provide the sound of nearby running water, pour water over the perineum, or sit the person in a tub of warm water, if such is not contraindicated)

Nursing Observations
Measure the intake and output
Palpate the bladder for distention
Observe for urinary frequency and incontinence (and complaints of hesitancy)

Health Teaching
Instruct to increase fluid intake
Explain why the potential problem could become actual (certain drugs prevent normal nerve stimulation to void; in old age, reduced bladder elasticity affects the voiding reflex; an enlarged prostate exerts pressure against the urethra, which can make voiding difficult)
Explain the reason for and intended effect of the preventive therapy

EVALUATION
Record actual outcome

Potential Threats to Hematopoietic Homeostasis

POTENTIAL FOR SPLEEN RUPTURE[26,125,522]

ASSESSMENT

Data Collection

Subjective Data
• There are no actual symptoms of spleen rupture

Objective Data
• There are no actual signs of spleen rupture

Related Data
• There are one or more stressors present that increase the possibility that a ruptured spleen will occur
DISEASES: Infectious mononucleosis, chronic malaria, typhoid fever
INJURIES: Trauma to the spleen, subcapsular hemorrhage

Data Analysis

Nursing Diagnosis
POTENTIAL FOR SPLEEN RUPTURE: The presence of stressors that increase the possibility of the actual occurrence of the splitting open of the splenic capsule due to internal pressure or damage to the capsule

PLANNING

Unmet Needs
Protection from physical harm, increased learning

Expected Outcome
No signs or symptoms of spleen rupture will occur
  OR
If signs and symptoms occur, they will be promptly recognized as an actual problem and will be treated appropriately

NURSING INTERVENTIONS

Nursing Treatments

Handle gently

Place on complete bed rest

Position comfortably

Refrain from giving enemas

Remove constrictive clothing

Refrain from applying pressure to the body part (such as palpating the abdomen, placing a pillow across the abdomen)

Nursing Observations

Monitor the blood pressure (for hypotension)

Monitor the oral temperature (for a decrease)

Observe for complaints of pain (severe abdominal pain or pain in the left scapular region)

Health Teaching

Instruct to avoid the Valsalva maneuver

Inform that coughing should be avoided

Inform that elimination straining should be avoided (to prevent pressure on the spleen)

Explain the need to avoid trauma (to the spleen from heavy lifting, sports activities, etc.)

Explain why the potential problem could become actual (pressure on a swollen, injured spleen could cause the spleen to rupture)

Explain the reason for and intended effect of the preventive therapy

EVALUATION

Record actual outcome

Potential Threats to Immunologic Homeostasis

POTENTIAL FOR INFECTION[26,278,371]

ASSESSMENT

Data Collection

Subjective Data

• There are no actual symptoms of infection

Objective Data

• There are no actual signs of infection

Related Data

• There are one or more stressors present that increase the possibility that infection will occur

BIRTH STATUS: Premature infant

DISEASES: Acquired immune deficiency syndrome (AIDs), aplastic anemia, diabetes mellitus, leukemia, chronic glomerulonephritis, malnutrition, nephrotic syndrome, sickle cell disease

INJURY: Any injury

SIGNS AND SYMPTOMS: Dehydration, fatigue

HEALTH CARE FACTORS: *Medical therapy*: Hyperalimentation infusion, therapeutic apheresis, urinary catheterization. *Drug therapy*: Chemotherapy, immunosuppressive therapy. *Surgical procedures*: Any but especially splenectomy

DEVELOPMENTAL PHASES: Infancy (early), old age

LIFESTYLE: Insufficient or unbalanced diet, insufficient sleep or rest, lack of hygiene

LIFESTYLE: Insufficient or unbalanced diet, insufficient sleep or rest, lack of hygiene

ENVIRONMENTAL FACTORS: *Chemical substances*: Toxic gases from tobacco smoking or from being around persons who smoke

Data Analysis

Nursing Diagnosis

POTENTIAL FOR INFECTION: The presence of stressors that increase the possibility of the actual occurrence of the development of a generalized body infection in a noninfected person

PLANNING

Unmet Needs

Protection from physical harm, increased learning

Expected Outcome

No signs or symptoms of infection will occur

OR

If signs and symptoms occur, they will be promptly recognized as an actual problem and will be treated appropriately

Person verbalizes an understanding of and practices preventive methods

NURSING INTERVENTIONS

Nursing Treatments

Encourage adequate rest

Encourage increased protein-food intake (in a well-balanced diet)

Maintain a clean environment

Maintain reverse isolation (when needed)

Nursing Observations

Monitor blood studies for evidence of infection (increased white blood count, neutrophils, lymphocytes, monocytes)

Health Teaching

Advise adherence to the immunization schedule (if the person is traveling, if a child is attending school)

Explain how to prevent cross-infection

Advise against exposure to inclement weather

Advise against mingling in crowds

Inform that cleanliness is essential to infection prevention

Teach the principles of good nutrition

Advise against exposure to airborne irritants (especially smoke from cigarettes, etc., which is of special concern when small children are present)

Explain why the potential problem could become actual (a potential for infection can result from the following: a general state of poor health causes lowered body resistance, drugs such as Imuran, (azathioprine), prednisone, and actinomycin C cause immunologic suppression; in leukemia, there are increased white blood cells that are immature and unable to protect against infection; a reduction in white blood cells fails to protect the body against infection; in acquired immune deficiency syndrome, sexual contact, needle injection from drug abuse, etc., are believed to be the sources of infection)

Explain the reason for and intended effect of the preventive therapy

EVALUATION

Record actual outcome

POTENTIAL FOR TRANSMITTING INFECTION [42,73,84,278,406,451]

ASSESSMENT

Data Collection

Subjective Data
• There are no actual symptoms of infection (except in the infectious person)

Objective Data
• There are no actual signs of infection (except in the infectious person)

Related Data
• There are one or more stressors present that increase the possibility that the infected person will transmit the infection

DISEASES: Anthrax, bronchiectasis, bronchitis, bronchopneumonia, cholera, diphtheria, dysentery, encephalitis, gonorrhea, hepatitis, hookworm, influenza, leprosy, measles, meningitis, mumps, nasopharyngitis, pertussis, pneumonia, poliomyelitis, scarlet fever, syphilis, tuberculosis, typhoid fever

HEALTH CARE FACTORS: *Therapeutic equipment*: Use of the same hemodialyzer or intermittent positive-pressure breathing machine by more than one person, blood transfusions

LIFESTYLE: Lack of hygiene (for self and home environment)

ENVIRONMENTAL FACTORS: *Human*: Exposure to infected persons. *Biological agents*: Exposure to insects and infected animals. *Food substances*: Contaminated by bacteria or toxic agents. *Water*: Exposure to contaminated water. *Waste disposal*: Substandard

HUMAN ERROR: Using contaminated needles to inject drugs, failure to wash hands after toileting

Data Analysis

Nursing Diagnosis
POTENTIAL FOR TRANSMITTING INFECTION: The presence of stressors that increase the possibility of the actual occurrence of an infected person transmitting pathologic organisms to another

PLANNING

Unmet Needs
Protection from physical harm, increased learning

Expected Outcome
No signs or symptoms of infection transmission will occur
   OR
If signs and symptoms occur, they will be promptly recognized as an actual problem and the resulting infection will be treated appropriately
Person verbalizes an understanding of and practices preventive methods

NURSING INTERVENTIONS

Nursing Treatments
Maintain a clean environment
Disinfect contaminated articles
Provide disposable tissue
Provide a paper bag for tissue disposal
Provide a sputum container
Encourage adequate rest
Isolate infected persons
Isolate persons exposed to communicable disease
Take nasal and oral secretion precautions (for diphtheria, hepatitis, influenza, meningi-

tis, mumps, poliomyelitis, pneumonia, scarlet fever, smallpox, tuberculosis, whooping cough)

Take needle-syringe precautions (for hepatitis, syphilis)

Take skin-contact precautions (for gonorrhea, leprosy, smallpox, syphilis, tuberculosis)

Take sputum precautions (for diphtheria, influenza, pneumonia, tuberculosis, whooping cough)

Take stool precautions (for cholera, dysentery, hepatitis, hookworm, poliomyelitis, tuberculosis, typhoid fever)

Take urine precautions (for typhoid fever, hepatitis)

Cover the bed with netting (when windows are unscreened against mosquitos in malaria and encephalitis and for flies in meningitis, poliomyelitis, typhoid fever)

Use sterile technique (as appropriate, and especially with dialysis and ventilation equipment)

Detect communicable disease cases

Make a referral (to the local health department)

Nursing Observations

Inspect the mucous membranes for abnormalities (mouth, nose, and throat)

Inspect the skin for infectious lesions

Monitor blood studies for evidence of infection (increased white blood count, neutrophils, lymphocytes, monocytes)

Monitor blood studies for abnormal liver function (do a serum hepatitis-associated antigen (HAA), Australia antigen (Au antigen) or hepatitis B surface antigen (HBs) on all persons coming into the dialysis program and then periodically; staff personnel and persons donating blood for transfusions should also be screened)

Monitor the oral temperature (for fever)

Observe for complaints of headache, malaise, weakness, chills

Observe for irritability

Obtain a bacterial culture (of blood and body discharges)

Health Teaching

Describe those symptoms that should be reported (fever, chills, malaise)

Inform that cleanliness is essential to infection prevention

Advise handwashing after elimination

Explain the need to avoid contaminated soil (for hookworm and pinworm)

Explain how to dispose of infectious expectoration (burn or dispose via the sewer system)

Recommend the use of double-thickness tissue for infected sputum

Explain how to prevent cross-infection (handwashing, cleaning contaminated articles)

Explain how to prevent the common cold (good nutrition, adequate rest, etc.)

Explain that the common cold is contagious for 48 hours after symptom onset

Instruct to cover the mouth when coughing

Instruct to cover the nose when sneezing

Explain how veneral disease is transmitted (sexual contact)

Inform that immunity does not occur with veneral infection

Instruct to limit direct contact with infected persons

Explain how to sterilize contaminated dishes

Recommend the use of disposable dishes for contagious diseases

Recommend the use of individual dishes, utensils, and drinking glasses

Recommend the use of individual towels and washcloths

Explain why the potential problem could become actual (infectious organisms are easily transferred from one person to another)

Explain the reason for and intended effect of the preventive therapy

EVALUATION

Record actual outcome

POTENTIAL FOR REJECTION OF TRANSPLANTED ORGAN[72,73,451,486]

ASSESSMENT

Data Collection

Subjective Data
- There are no actual symptoms of organ rejection

Objective Data
- There are no actual signs of organ rejection

Related Data
- There are one or more stressors present that increase the possibility that an organ rejection will occur

HEALTH CARE FACTORS: *Surgical procedures*: Transplantation of bone, cornea, heart, kidney, lung, liver, or skin

Data Analysis

Nursing Diagnosis
POTENTIAL FOR REJECTION OF TRANSPLANTED ORGAN: The presence of stressors that increase the possibility of the actual occurrence of the body rejecting a transplanted organ

PLANNING

Unmet Needs

Protection from physical harm, increased learning

Expected Outcome

No signs or symptoms of rejection of a transplanted organ will occur
OR
If signs and symptoms occur, they will be promptly recognized as an actual problem and will be treated appropriately

NURSING INTERVENTIONS

Nursing Treatments

Attend the patient constantly (during the early postoperative days)
Provide frequent contact with the person (after hospital discharge)

Nursing Observations

Specific for Kidney Transplant
Inspect for edema
Measure the body weight (daily)
Measure the intake and output (for decreased output)
Monitor the blood pressure (for increase)
Monitor the oral temperature (for fever)
Monitor blood studies for abnormal renal function (elevated BUN and creatinine, decreased renal clearance of creatinine, and decreased serum protein)
Test the urine for protein
Palpate for tenderness (and swelling over the kidney transplant area)
Observe for complaints of pain (over that area)
Obtain a bacterial culture (of blood, stool, urine, respiratory secretions, and wounds if fever occurs during the first 3 postsurgical days)

Specific for Corneal Transplant
Monitor the oral temperature (for fever)
Observe for complaints of severe eye pain
Observe for complaints of visual disturbance (in delayed rejection)

Specific for Skin Transplant

Inspect for signs of infection (necrosis, drainage, or inflammation of the skin)

Specific for Heart Transplant

Monitor the oral temperature (for fever)

Monitor blood studies for abnormal cardiac enzymes (increased levels of transaminases SGOT, LDH, and SHBD indicate damage to the cardiac muscle)

Observe for heart failure (dyspnea on exertion, neck vein distention, nonproductive cough, rales at the base of the lungs)

Specific for Liver Transplant

Monitor the oral temperature (for fever)

Monitor blood studies for abnormal liver function (increased serum levels of bilirubin, alkaline phosphatase, and SGOT and decreased albumin indicate hepatic failure)

Specific for Lung Transplant

Monitor the oral temperature (for fever)

Monitor blood studies for arterial blood gases (decreased ventilation and gas exchange indicate pulmonary failure)

Observe for dyspnea, cyanosis

Health Teaching

Describe those symptoms that should be reported (fever, decreased urine output, edema, pain, weight gain)

Advise to observe for signs of infection (around the wound such as heat, redness, swelling)

Instruct to immediately report all symptoms

Explain how to measure the intake and output

Teach how to test the urine for pH, protein, sugar-acetone

Teach how to take and accurately read a temperature

Explain the importance of continuing (immunosuppressive) therapy

Explain the need to avoid trauma (to the transplant site)

Explain why the potential problem could become actual (the body's immunologic system rejects all foreign matter; when the kidney becomes infiltrated with lymphocytes, they attempt to destroy the foreign kidney, as a result of the inflammation, the renal tubule epithelium develops necrosis and small blood vessel thrombosis occurs in the kidney, resulting in rejection)

Explain the reason for and intended effect of the preventive therapy

EVALUATION

Record actual outcome

Potential Threats to Integument Homeostasis

POTENTIAL FOR DELAYED WOUND HEALING[676]

ASSESSMENT

Data Collection

Subjective Data

• There are no actual symptoms of delayed wound healing

Objective Data
- There are no actual signs of delayed wound healing

Related Data
- There are one or more stressors present that increase the possibility that delayed wound healing will occur

DISEASES: Anemia (hemoglobin less than 10 gm/100 ml), diabetes mellitus, infection, leukemia, malnutrition, obesity, peripheral vascular disease, renal insufficiency or failure

SIGNS AND SYMPTOMS: Cachexia from cancer

HEALTH CARE FACTORS: *Medical therapy:* Adverse effects of radiation to the specific area *Adverse effects of Drug therapy:* Corticosteroids

HUMAN ERROR: Inadequate cleaning of a wound (in which debris such as dead cells, exudate, grease, foreign bodies, etc., remain in the wound), placing tension on a wound (and preventing the approximation of the wound edges)

Data Analysis

Nursing Diagnosis
POTENTIAL FOR DELAYED WOUND HEALING: The presence of stressors that increase the possibility of the actual occurrence of a wound healing slowly or not at all

PLANNING

Unmet Needs
Protection from physical harm, increased learning

Expected Outcome
No signs or symptoms of delayed wound healing will occur
 OR
If signs and symptoms occur, they will be promptly recognized as an actual problem and will be treated appropriately
Person verbalizes understanding of and practices preventive methods

NURSING INTERVENTIONS

Nursing Treatments
Encourage increased protein-food intake (which promotes healing)
Give citrus fruit juices (vitamin C will promote healing)
Restrict the intake to nothing by mouth (until the possibility of vomiting, which puts pressure on an incision, subsides)
Irrigate the wound (and clean out all debri)
Change the dressing frequently (to reduce bacterial contamination)
Avoid placing tension on the wound
Encourage deep breathing (which promotes tissue oxygenation)
Change the person's position frequently (for improved circulation)
Splint the incisional area (with a pillow whenever there is a potential for pressure on the wound)
Apply an abdominal support garment (if appropriate)

Nursing Observations
Inspect (the wound) for signs of infection (heat, redness, swelling)
Inspect the wound dressing frequently (for blood, pus, or other drainage)

Health Teaching
Inform that coughing should be avoided
Inform that elimination straining be avoided (to prevent pressure on the wound)
Explain how to splint an incision (with a pillow)
Explain why the potential problem could become actual (steroid drugs suppress capillary formation and fibrogenesis; cancerous disorders cause reduced immunocompetence; radiation causes vasculitis and fibrosis in connective tissue, which interferes with normal nutrient and oxygen delivery; diabetes causes microangiopathy (small blood vessel disease), which results in poor tissue perfusion; when the hemoglobin is

less than 10 g/100 ml, the decreased tissue oxygenation impairs healing. When the serum albumin (protein) is less than 3.2 g/100 ml, the skin is deficient in nutrients needed for healing)
Explain the reason for and intended effect of the preventive therapy

EVALUATION

Record actual outcome

POTENTIAL FOR SKIN BREAKDOWN[42,72]

ASSESSMENT

Data Collection

Subjective Data
• There are no actual symptoms of skin breakdown

Objective Data
• There are no actual signs of skin breakdown

Related Data
• There are one or more stressors present that increase the possibility that skin breakdown will occur
BIRTH STATUS: Premature infant
DISEASES: Advanced cancer, Cushing's disease, diabetes mellitus, malnutrition
SIGNS AND SYMPTOMS: Ascites (striae), cachexia, chronic diarrhea, edema, immobility, incontinence, paralysis, rapid weight gain (striae), weight loss
HUMAN BODY: *Body states*: Pregnancy (striae)
HEALTH CARE FACTORS: *Medical therapy*: Prolonged bed rest, wound drainage, radiation therapy, intravenous infusions containing drugs. *Surgical procedures*: Colostomy, cystostomy, gastrostomy, ileostomy, nephrostomy, ureterocolostomy, ureteroileostomy, ureterotomy. *Medical therapy*: Adverse effects, such as circulatory constriction or pressure from a cast, immobility from traction. *Therapeutic equipment or devices*: Artificial limb, brace, or crutches, rotating tourniquets, safety restraints
DEVELOPMENTAL PHASES: Old age
ENVIRONMENTAL FACTORS: *Chemical substances*: Excessive powdering of the skin. *Environmental heat*: High external temperature. *Water*: Prolonged exposure to water
HUMAN ERROR: Infrequent changing of soiled diapers or sheets, infrequent relief of pressure on skin surfaces, inadequate cleansing of skin surfaces

Data Analysis

Nursing Diagnosis
POTENTIAL FOR SKIN BREAKDOWN: The presence of stressors that increase the possibility of the actual occurrence of skin undergoing tissue destruction from injury, irritation, or hypoxia

PLANNING

Unmet Needs

Protection from physical harm, increased learning

Expected Outcome

No signs or symptoms of skin breakdown will occur
OR
If signs and symptoms occur, they will be promptly recognized as an actual problem and will be treated appropriately
Person verbalizes an understanding of and practices preventive methods

NURSING INTERVENTIONS

Nursing Treatments

Ambulate the person (as much as possible)
Change the person's position frequently
Cleanse with castile or lanolin soap (and rinse thoroughly)
    OR
Cleanse with surgical soap
Refrain from using an alkaline soap on the skin
Maintain dry skin
Change the wet diaper immediately
Avoid using rough-textured bed linens
Maintain dry, clean linen
Maintain wrinkle-free sheets
Refrain from pulling the person across the sheets
Massage bony prominences
Pad the bony prominences
Pad the bedpan
Place on an alternating pressure mattress
    OR
Place on a CircOlectric bed
    OR
Place on a flotation mattress
    OR
Place on a Stryker frame
Place on a sheepskin
    OR
Place on a silicone pad
    OR
Place on a split-foam mattress
    OR
Place on a polyurethane foam pad
Place a pillow between the knees (to prevent knee-on-knee pressure)
Lubricate the skin with baby oil, bath oil, or body lotion
Lubricate the skin (breasts, abdomen, thighs) with cocoa butter, glycerine, lanolin, min-
    eral oil, or olive oil (to prevent skin striae during pregnancy or severe obesity)
Refrain from simulanteously powdering and lubricating the skin (powder for hot, humid
    conditions and lubricate for dry, cool conditions)
Apply cornstarch to the skin (each time rotating tourniquets are removed, as tourni-
    quets place severe pressure on the skin)
Do not allow overlapping skin surfaces to touch
Refrain from tight bandaging
Use paper or transparent tape instead of adhesive on the skin

Nursing Observations

Inspect the skin for breakdown (redness, tissue thinness, blistering, petechiae, or necrosis)

Health Teaching

Instruct to maintain skin cleanliness
Instruct to inspect the skin
Instruct to lubricate the skin
Instruct to maintain skin dryness
Advise limited use of powder on the infant's skin
Advise against prolonged skin exposure to the water or to the sun
Inform that the skin should be protected from windburn
Advise against scratching (the skin)
Explain the importance of testing cosmetics for skin irritation

Explain how to pad bony prominences
Explain how to massage (to improve skin circulation)
Instruct not to use rubber rings and doughnuts (which put pressure on the skin)
Recommend the use of a sheepskin
Instruct to do wheelchair pushups
Explain how to wash diapers correctly
Describe those symptoms that should be reported (skin redness, irritation, blisters)
Explain why the potential problem could become actual (prolonged pressure on tissue, impaired circulation, or chemical injury cause skin breakdown)
Explain the reason for and intended effect of the preventive therapy

EVALUATION

Record actual outcome

POTENTIAL FOR WOUND DEHISCENCE[73,391]

ASSESSMENT

Data Collection

Subjective Data
• There are no actual symptoms of a wound dehiscence

Objective Data
• There are no actual signs of a wound dehiscence

Related Data
• There are one or more stressors present that increase the possibility that a wound dehiscence will occur
DISEASES: Wound infection
SIGNS and SYMPTOMS: Abdominal distention, malnutrition, obesity, persistent coughing, severe edema
HEALTH CARE FACTORS: *Medical therapy*: Radiation therapy to the area
HUMAN ERROR: Excessive straining at stool, heavy lifting, using incorrect lifting methods

Data Analysis

Nursing Diagnosis
POTENTIAL FOR WOUND DEHISCENCE: The presence of stressors that increase the possibility of the actual occurrence of a disruption of wound closure from severe tension or devitalized tissue failing to support sutures

PLANNING

Unmet Needs

Protection from physical harm, increased learning

Expected Outcome

No signs or symptoms of wound dehiscence will occur
OR
If signs and symptoms occur, they will be promptly recognized as an actual problem and will be treated appropriately

NURSING INTERVENTIONS

Nursing Treatments

Handle gently
Approach unhurriedly
Avoid placing tension on the wound
Change the person's position gradually
Refrain from jarring the bed

Elevate the head

AND

Do not place in the flat position $\Big\}$ For abdominal incisions

Ambulate the person (as much as possible to reduce abdominal distention)

Refrain from giving enemas (when abdominal wounds exist)

Apply a supportive splint (to extremity wounds)

Nursing Observations

Observe for dehiscence (pulling apart of the wound edges)

Observe for complaints of pain

Inspect for signs of infection

Health Teaching

Instruct to change position gradually (and how to avoid strain against the wound)

Inform that coughing should be avoided

Inform that elimination straining should be avoided

Inform that heavy lifting should be avoided

Explain why the potential problem could become actual (tension and injury to or infection of a wound can cause the wound edges to tear apart)

Explain the reason for and intended effect of the preventive therapy

EVALUATION

Record actual outcome

POTENTIAL FOR WOUND INFECTION [73,371,451,536]

ASSESSMENT

Data Collection

Subjective Data

• There are no actual symptoms of a wound infection

Objective Data

• There are no actual signs of a wound infection

Related Data

• There are one or more stressors present that increase the possibility that a wound infection will occur

DISEASES: Cushing's syndrome, diabetes mellitus

INJURIES: Any traumatic wound, burn wound

HEALTH CARE FACTORS: *Medical therapy*: Continuous ambulatory peritoneal dialysis, hyperalimentation. *Surgical incision*: Any

LIFESTYLE: Unclean clothing (coming in contact with a wound)

ENVIRONMENTAL FACTORS: *Objects*: Dirt, dust, oil, metal, wood, or glass particles in the wound

HUMAN ERROR: Infrequent dressing changes, unclean dressings, wet, unsterile dressing, airtight dressing

Data Analysis

Nursing Diagnosis

POTENTIAL FOR WOUND INFECTION (POTENTIAL FOR SURGICAL INCISION INFECTION): The presence of stressors that increase the possibility of the actual occurrence of pathogenic organisms infecting a break in the skin

PLANNING

Unmet Needs

Protection from physical harm, increased learning

Expected Outcome

No signs or symptoms of wound infection will occur
> OR

If signs and symptoms occur, they will be promptly recognized as an actual problem and will be treated appropriately

Person verbalizes an understanding of and practices preventive methods

NURSING INTERVENTIONS

Nursing Treatments

Specific for Nonburn Wounds
Clean with antiseptic solution
> OR

Clean with hydrogen peroxide
> OR

Clean with surgical soap
Irrigate the wound (if appropriate)
Position to promote drainage of the infected area
Apply an antibiotic ointment
Apply a sterile dressing
Change the dressing frequently
Use sterile technique

Specific for Burn Wounds
Clean with hydrogen peroxide
> OR

Clean with surgical soap
Maintain a clean environment
Maintain reverse isolation
Place on sterile linens
Apply a sterile dressing
Change the dressing frequently
Use sterile technique

Specific for a Wound Under a Cast
Palpate the skin for temperature (feel under the cast and over the wound for increased warmth)
Observe the cast for odor (foul odor from drainage)
Observe for complaints of pain

Nursing Observations

Inspect the skin for infectious lesions
Inspect for inflammation
Obtain a bacterial culture (of the wound)

Health Teaching

Describe those symptoms that should be reported (purulent drainage)
Advise against pulling off scabs
Teach how to clean and dress a wound
Teach how to irrigate a wound
Inform that cleanliness is essential to infection prevention
Explain why the potential problem could become actual (bacteria entering a wound will multiply and attack tissue)
Explain the reason for and intended effect of the preventive therapy

EVALUATION

Record actual outcome

Potential Threats to Musculoskeletal Homeostasis

POTENTIAL FOR BONE DEFORMITY[73,371]

ASSESSMENT

Data Collection

Subjective Data
• There are no actual symptoms of bone deformity present

Objective Data
• There are no actual signs of bone deformity present

Related Data
• There are one or more stressors present that increase the possibility that bone deformity will occur

DISEASES: Rickets, osteomyelitis, Perthes's disease

INJURIES: Bone fracture

SIGNS AND SYMPTOMS: Immobility

HEALTH CARE FACTORS: *Medical therapy*: Prolonged bed rest. *Medical therapy*: Adverse effects such as nonaligned healing of a bone when a cast is indented, incorrectly applied; radiation therapy (in children)

HUMAN ERROR: Failure to have bone fractures treated, as in child abuse

Data Analysis

Nursing Diagnosis

POTENTIAL FOR BONE DEFORMITY: The presence of stressors that increase the possibility of the actual occurrence of distorted bone alignment

PLANNING

Unmet Needs

Protection from physical harm, increased learning

Expected Outcome

No signs or symptoms of bone deformity will occur
    OR
If signs and symptoms occur, they will be promptly recognized as an actual problem and will be treated appropriately

Person verbalizes an understanding of and practices preventive methods

NURSING INTERVENTIONS

Nursing Treatments

Maintain body alignment

Exercise in range of motion (after immobilization by a cast or traction)

Place a trochanter roll for positioning
    OR
Position with pillows
    OR
Position with sandbags

Encourage normal use of the involved limb

Consult with the physician (regarding a new cast if the current one is indented or nonsupportive, or if traction force is disaligned)

Nursing Observations

Inspect for body alignment (of the fractured body part and determine whether the cast is adequately supporting the part)

OR

Check the traction ropes and pulleys for alignment (so that the traction force is sufficient to prevent deformity)

Health Teaching

Explain how to maintain body alignment

Advise not to move or use joints immediately distal and proximal to the fracture (until the fracture is sufficiently immobilized by a cast or traction)

Advise against weight-bearing (on the fractured bone until it is sufficiently immobilized or healed; healing time varies with different bones and is affected by the person's age and nutritional status)

Teach how to do range of motion exercises (after the bone is immobilized by a cast or traction)

Explain why the potential problem could become actual (bone deformity can occur from poor body alignment; when a wet cast becomes indented or deformed and then hardens, its irregular formation will cause the bone to heal in a non-aligned position)

Explain the reason for and intended effect of the preventive therapy

Medical Treatments Performed by Nurses

Apply the prescribed preventive splint

Apply the prescribed traction

EVALUATION

Record actual outcome

POTENTIAL FOR BONE DEMINERALIZATION[35,522]

ASSESSMENT

Data Collection

Subjective Data
• There are no actual symptoms of bone demineralization

Objective Data
• There are no actual signs of bone demineralization

Related Data
• There are one or more stressors present that increase the possibility that bone demineralization will occur

DISEASES: Acidosis, acromegaly, Cushing's syndrome, hyperparathyroidism, hyperthyroidism, hypothyroidism, scurvy

SIGNS AND SYMPTOMS: Prolonged immobility

HUMAN BODY: *Body state*: Pregnancy, lactation

HEALTH CARE FACTORS: *Medical therapy*: Prolonged bed rest

DEVELOPMENTAL PHASES: Middle age (decreased estrogen, androgen secretion), old age

LIFESTYLE: Low protein, calcium, phosphorus, or vitamin D intake/diet, inactivity

Data Analysis

Nursing Diagnosis
POTENTIAL FOR BONE DEMINERALIZATION (POTENTIAL FOR DISUSE OSTEOPOROSIS): The presence of stressors that increase the possibility of the actual occurrence of lime salts being withdrawn from the bones and causing decreased bone density

PLANNING

Unmet Needs

Protection from physical harm, increased learning

Expected Outcome

No signs or symptoms of bone demineralization will occur
> OR

If signs and symptoms occur, they will be promptly recognized as an actual problem and
will be treated appropriately

NURSING INTERVENTIONS

Nursing Treatments

Ambulate the person (as much as possible)
Change the person's position frequently
Exercise in range of motion
Encourage moderate physical exercise (within the person's capability)
Encourage increased calcium-food intake, increased protein-food intake, increased high-
vitamin-food intake (vitamin D)

Nursing Observations

Measure the body weight (periodically for weight loss, which indicates bone loss)
Measure the girth of the bone (for atrophy)
Observe for complaints of pain

Health Teaching

Instruct to change position frequently
Teach how to do range-of-motion exercises
Teach the principles of good nutrition
Explain why the potential problem could become actual (bone demineralization is due
to bone atrophy from lack of exercise and weight bearing, resulting from a failure of
the bone matrix to form and an increase of bone reabsorption)
Explain the reason for and intended effect of the preventive therapy

EVALUATION

Record actual outcome

POTENTIAL FOR JOINT CONTRACTURE [35,108,451]

ASSESSMENT

Data Collection

Subjective Data
• There are no actual symptoms of joint contracture

Objective Data
• There are no actual signs of joint contracture

Related Data
• There are one or more stressors present that increase the possibility that joint
contracture will occur
DISEASES: Arthritis, bursitis, cerebrovascular accident, muscular dystrophy, multiple scle-
rosis, sickle cell anemia
INJURIES: Burn wound, fracture and compression of the spinal cord, joint injuries, tendon
or ligament damage
SIGNS AND SYMPTOMS: Pain (joint), prolonged immobility, paralysis

Data Analysis

Nursing Diagnosis
POTENTIAL FOR JOINT CONTRACTURE: The presence of stressors that increase the possibility of
the actual occurrence of a muscle becoming so flexible that it will prevent normal
functional movement of the joint

PLANNING

Unmet Needs

Protection from physical harm, increased learning

Expected Outcome

No signs or symptoms of joint contracture will occur
>OR

If signs and symptoms occur, they will be promptly recognized as an actual problem and will be treated appropriately

Person verbalizes an understanding of and practices preventive methods

NURSING INTERVENTIONS

Nursing Treatments

Maintain body alignment

Change the patient's position frequently

Exercise in range of motion (in warm water when range of motion is painful)

Massage gently

Place a footboard at the feet

Place a hand roll under the fingers

Elevate the affected body part (elevate the forearm on the chest if the elbow or shoulder is affected)

Encourage normal use of the involved limb

Encourage active diversional activities (which support needed exercise, such as croquet, playing a musical instrument, swimming, etc.)

Specific for the Inflamed Joint (Arthritis, Bursitis, Sickle Cell Crisis)

Immobilize the joint (with support, during acute inflammatory process)

Exercise in range of motion (gently, gradually, after inflammation is diminished)

Specific to Potential Wrist Contracture

Maintain body alignment

Exercise in range of motion

Place a hand roll under the fingers

Place in the functional position (moderate dorsiflexion of hand)

Encourage normal use of the involved limb

Specific to Potential Foot Contracture

Maintain body alignment

Apply a bed cradle

Cover with lightweight blankets

Provide loose bedding with toe pleats

Exercise in range of motion

Place in the functional position

Place the feet in hard-soled ankle-top shoes
>OR

Place a footboard at the feet

Position with pillows
>OR

Position with sandbags

Nursing Observations

Inspect the joints for impending contractures (gradual resistance of the muscle to stretching)

Health Teaching

Explain how to maintain body alignment

Teach how to apply preventive splints

Teach how to do range-of-motion exercises

Explain why the potential problem could become actual (plantar flexion can occur when there is Achilles tendon shortening, resulting in gastrocnemius and soleus muscle contraction; palmar flexion can occur when there is cervical or radial nerve injury or

paralysis of wrist and hand extensor muscles; poor body alignment and muscle spasm can result in contracture)
Explain the reason for and intended effect of the preventive therapy

Medical Treatments Performed by Nurses
Apply the prescribed preventive splint

EVALUATION
Record actual outcome

POTENTIAL FOR MUSCLE SPASMS[72,451]

ASSESSMENT

Data Collection

Subjective Data
• There are no actual symptoms of a muscle spasm

Objective Data
• There are no actual signs of a muscle spasm

Related Data
• There are one or more stressors present that increase the possibility that a muscle spasm will occur
DISEASES: Addison's disease, hypocalcemia, hypoparathyroidism, hypothyroidism, tetanus, Thomsen's disease
INJURIES: Fracture and compression of the spinal cord (with paralysis)
SIGNS AND SYMPTOMS: Ischemia (of the muscle)
PSYCHOSOCIAL FACTORS: Threat of chronic or severe stress
HEALTH CARE FACTORS: *Medical therapy*: Hemodialysis.
HUMAN ERROR: Heavy lifting, using incorrect lifting methods, inadequate exercise (stretching) of gastrocnemius muscles

Data Analysis

Nursing Diagnosis
POTENTIAL FOR MUSCLE SPASMS: The presence of stressors that increase the possibility of the actual occurrence of sudden, painful contraction and tightness of muscle tissue

PLANNING

Unmet Needs
Protection from physical harm, increased learning

Expected Outcome
No signs or symptoms of muscle spasm will occur
  OR
If signs and symptoms occur, they will be promptly recognized as an actual problem and will be treated appropriately
Person verbalizes an understanding of and practices preventive methods

NURSING INTERVENTIONS

Nursing Treatments
Handle gently (but with firm, full-hand pressure when touching spastic parts)
Change the person's position gradually
Remove constrictive clothing
Apply a bed cradle (to prevent the bed clothes from stimulating spasms)
Drape for warmth

Place only warm hands and objects on the patient
Decrease drafts (cold air can stimulate spasms)
Maintain a warm room temperature
Apply a heating pad
    AND
Massage gently (the area in which spasms have a potential for occurring)
Refrain from giving local cold applications
Refrain from jarring the bed (or wheelchair)
Refrain from performing nonessential procedures (which could stimulate spasms)
Give high-calcium fluids orally
    AND   }If the blood calcium is low
Encourage increased calcium-food intake
Encourage moderate physical exercise (with gentle stretching exercises to spastic muscles, except in tetanus or meningitis)

Nursing Observations
Observe for complaints of (muscle spasm) pain

Health Teaching
Explain why the potential problem can become actual (muscle spasms can occur when there is repetitive activation of efferent nerve fibers carrying motor impulses to muscle fibers before relaxation can occur or when there is ischemia to muscles)
Explain the reason for and intended effect of the preventive therapy

EVALUATION

Record actual outcome

POTENTIAL FOR MUSCLE WEAKNESS[73,125]

ASSESSMENT

Data Collection

Subjective Data
• There are no actual symptoms of muscle weakness present

Objective Data
• There are no actual signs of muscle weakness present

Related Data
• There are one or more stressors present that increase the possibility that muscle weakness will occur
DISEASES: Major depression, myasthenia gravis
SIGNS AND SYMPTOMS: Prolonged immobility, hyperkalemia, hypokalemia, hyponatremia
HEALTH CARE FACTORS: *Medical therapy*: Prolonged bed rest
DEVELOPMENTAL PHASES: Old age
LIFESTYLE: Insufficient or unbalanced diet, lack of exercise

Data Analysis

Nursing Diagnosis
POTENTIAL FOR MUSCLE WEAKNESS: The presence of stressors that increase the possibility of the actual occurrence of muscle losing strength and functioning capacity

PLANNING

Unmet Needs
Protection from physical harm, increased learning

Expected Outcome

No signs or symptoms of muscle weakness will occur
OR
If signs and symptoms occur, they will be promptly recognized as an actual problem and will be treated appropriately
Person verbalizes an understanding of and practices preventive methods

NURSING INTERVENTIONS

Nursing Treatments

Ambulate the person (as much as possible)
Encourage moderate physical exercise
Exercise in range of motion
Massage (the muscles) vigorously
Encourage alternate rest and activity
Provide a balanced nutritional diet (to meet the need for decreased potassium, increased potassium or sodium, improved nutrition)

Nursing Observations

Test for the degree of muscle strength (periodically)

Health Teaching

Teach muscle strengthening exercises (resistive exercises, in which the person uses various muscles against pressure exerted by the nurse, against weights, or against his own weight, as in pushups)
Explain why the potential problem could become actual (muscle degenerative diseases, electrolyte imbalance, nutritional deficit, and lack of use can result in muscle weakness)
Explain the reason for and intended effect of the preventive therapy

EVALUATION

Record actual outcome

Potential Threats to Neurologic Homeostasis

POTENTIAL FOR CENTRAL NERVOUS SYSTEM DEPRESSION [72,73,399,451]

ASSESSMENT

Data Collection

Subjective Data
• There are no actual symptoms of central nervous system depression

Objective Data
• There are no actual signs of central nervous system depression

Related Data
• There are one or more stressors present that increase the possibility of central nervous system depression occurring
DISEASES: Alcoholism, cerebrovascular accident, metabolic alkalosis
INJURIES: Cerebral concussion, poisoning

HEALTH CARE FACTORS: *Drug therapy*: Adverse effects of hypnotics, narcotics, sedatives. *Surgical therapy*: Anesthesia

LIFESTYLE: Alcohol intake, drug abuse

Data Analysis

Nursing Diagnosis

POTENTIAL FOR CENTRAL NERVOUS SYSTEM DEPRESSION: The presence of stressors that increase the possibility of the actual occurrence of decreased functioning of the brain and spinal cord

PLANNING

Unmet Needs

Protection from physical harm, increased learning

Expected Outcome

No signs or symptoms of central nervous system depression will occur
 OR
If signs and symptoms occur, they will be promptly recognized as an actual problem and will be treated appropriately

NURSING INTERVENTIONS

Nursing Treatments

Provide frequent contact with the person
Stimulate by movement, touch, sternal pressure, or speech (periodically)
Give hot coffee
 OR
Give hot tea
Ambulate the person (as much as possible, if there are no contraindications for ambulation)

Nursing Observations

Inspect the eyes for pupil size, equality, and response to light
Inspect the chest for respiratory rate, depth, and rhythm
Test for motor function
Test for abnormal deep-reflex responses
Observe the level of consciousness
Observe for confusion and lethargy

Health Teaching

Explain why the potential problem could become actual (whenever the central nervous system is subject to decreased excitation, there is a potential for central nervous system depression)
Explain the reason for and intended effect of the preventive therapy

EVALUATION

Record actual outcome

POTENTIAL FOR HEADACHE[72,451]

ASSESSMENT

Data Collection

Subjective Data
• There are no actual symptoms of headache

Objective Data
• There are no actual signs of headache

Related Data

• There are one or more stressors present that increase the possibility that headache will occur

INHERITED FACTORS: Familial tendency to migraine headaches

DISEASES: Hypertension

INJURIES: Cerebral concussion

PSYCHOSOCIAL FACTORS: Threat of chronic or severe stress

HEALTH CARE FACTORS: *Diagnostic procedures*: Angiography, lumbar puncture, pneumoenceph-alogram, ventriculogram. *Medical therapy*: Hemodialysis, alcohol or drug withdrawal. *Drug therapy*: Adverse effects of drugs

Data Analysis

Nursing Diagnosis

POTENTIAL FOR HEADACHE: The presence of stressors that increase the possibility of the actual occurrence of pain in the cerebral area

PLANNING

Unmet Needs

Protection from physical harm, increased learning

Expected Outcome

No signs or symptoms of headache will occur

OR

If signs and symptoms occur, they will be promptly recognized as an actual problem and will be treated appropriately

Person verbalizes an understanding of and practices preventive methods

NURSING INTERVENTIONS

Nursing Treatments

Encourage adequate rest

Elevate the head

OR

Place in the flat position (12–24 hours after spinal puncture)

Position comfortably

Change the patient's position gradually

Massage gently (the neck and shoulders if in spasm)

Provide quiet

Subdue the room lighting

Refrain from jarring the bed

Discourage the intake of oral stimulants

Discourage smoking

Give nonprescription drugs (analgesics, if the headache is threatening)

Nursing Observations

Observe for complaints of headache

Health Teaching

Advise not to take hot baths

Advise that highly emotional situations be avoided

Recommend methods for achieving total relaxation (for controlling emotional stress)

Inform that coughing should be avoided

Inform that elimination straining should be avoided

Explain why the potential problem could become actual (headache can result from increased intracranial pressure, inflammation, brain tissue irritation, or physiochemical disturbance)

Explain the reason for and intended effect of the preventive therapy

EVALUATION

Record actual outcome

POTENTIAL FOR INCREASED INTRACRANIAL PRESSURE[35,72]

ASSESSMENT

Data Collection

Subjective Data
• There are no actual symptoms of increased intracranial pressure

Objective Data
• There are no actual signs of increased intracranial pressure

Related Data
• There are one or more stressors present that increase the possibility that increased intracranial pressure will occur
DISEASES: Brain tumor, encephalitis, hydrocephalus, hypertension, hypertensive encephalopathy, leaking or ruptured cerebral aneurysm, meningitis, subarachnoid hemorrhage, subdural hematoma
INJURIES: Cerebral concussion or contusion, skull fracture, lead poisoning
SIGNS AND SYMPTOMS: Hypoventilation (hypercapnia), hypoxia
HEALTH CARE FACTORS: *Medical therapy*: Radiation therapy (to the head), rapid IV flow (water intoxication), hemodialysis (disequilibrium phenomenon). *Surgical therapy*: Brain surgery

Data Analysis

Nursing Diagnosis
POTENTIAL FOR INCREASED INTRACRANIAL PRESSURE: The presence of stressors that increase the possibility of the actual occurrence of pressure within the cranial cavity increasing to an abnormal and dangerous level

PLANNING

Unmet Needs

Protection from physical harm, increased learning

Expected Outcome

No signs or symptoms of increased intracranial pressure will occur
  OR
If signs and symptoms occur, they will be promptly recognized as an actual problem and will be treated appropriately

NURSING INTERVENTIONS

Nursing Treatments

Provide standby equipment and drugs (tracheostomy tray, suction equipment, intravenous steroids, and mannitol)
Place on complete bed rest
Provide quiet
Subdue the room lighting
Elevate the head
Do not place in the flat position
Change the patient's position gradually
Discourage the intake of oral stimulants
Handle (the head) gently
Maintain a steady intravenous infusion flow rate (so that circulatory volume does not increase pressure)
Limit infant crying by feeding on schedule and immediately changing soiled diapers
Refrain from jarring the bed
Refrain from performing nonessential procedures
Refrain from giving enemas

Nursing Observations

Observe the level of consciousness (alertness)

Observe for confusion, lethargy, restlessness

Inspect the chest for respiratory rate and rhythm (slow, irregular respirations)

Palpate the pulse for rate (tachycardia or bradycardia), rhythm, and volume (bounding)

Monitor the blood pressure (for decreased diastolic pressure)

Monitor the pulse pressure (for widening)

Monitor the oral or rectal temperature (for slow temperature rise)

Inspect the eyes for pupil size, equality, and response to light

Inspect the eyes for papilledema

Inspect the ears and nose for cerebrospinal fluid leakage (if it occurs, verify the presence of spinal fluid by testing with Clinistix for a positive sugar)

OR

Observe for a halo sign (when spinal fluid drains on linen, it leaves a blood-tinged center spot surrounded by a lighter-colored ring)

Observe for complaints of headache, nausea

Observe for vomiting

Health Teaching

Describe those symptoms that should be reported (headache, nausea, bounding pulse beat, dyspnea, inappropriate drowsiness)

Instruct to change position gradually

Advise gentle nose blowing

Inform that coughing should be avoided

Inform that elimination straining should be avoided

Advise not to take enemas

Explain why the potential problem could become actual (increased intracranial pressure could occur from intracranial bleeding, edema, tumor, abscess or increased spinal fluid within the cranial ventricles)

Explain the reason for and intended effect of the preventive therapy

EVALUATION

Record actual outcome

POTENTIAL FOR NERVE INJURY[72,451]

ASSESSMENT

Data Collection

Subjective Data

• There are no actual symptoms of nerve injury

Objective Data

• There are no actual signs of nerve injury

Related Data

• There are one or more stressors present that increase the possibility that nerve injury will occur

INJURIES: Bone fracture, burn (deep), laceration (deep), puncture wound (gunshot wound near a nerve)

HEALTH CARE FACTORS: *Diagnostic procedures*: Angiography. *Surgical procedures*: Lumbar sympathectomy. *Medical therapy*: Adverse effects, such as circulatory constriction from a cast or elastic bandage or stockings, disrupted traction

HUMAN ERROR: Nonaligned positioning, prolonged pressure on a nerve, incorrect use of crutches

Data Analysis

Nursing Diagnosis
POTENTIAL FOR NERVE INJURY: The presence of stressors that increase the possibility of the actual occurrence of damage to vital nerves

PLANNING

Unmet Needs
Protection from physical harm, increased learning

Expected Outcome
No signs or symptoms of nerve injury will occur
> OR

If signs and symptoms occur, they will be promptly recognized as an actual problem and will be treated appropriately

Person verbalizes an understanding of and practices preventive methods

NURSING INTERVENTIONS

Nursing Treatments
Handle gently (to prevent further injury)

Immobilize the affected body part (until the fracture can be treated or until disrupted traction can be reapplied properly)

Maintain body alignment

Position comfortably (to relieve pressure on nerves)

Nursing Observations
Observe for complaints of numbness and tingling (in the affected area)

Test for motor function (by applying counterpressure in the flexion, extension, and lateral position against an injured finger or limb)

Test for range of motion (decreased active range of motion)

Inspect for edema

Palpate the (peripheral) pulses for rate, rhythm, and volume

Check the traction ropes and pulleys for alignment

Health Teaching
Explain why the potential problem could become actual (the sharp edges of a fractured bone, other injury, or pressure can damage a nerve)

Teach good crutch-walking posture (and technique to avoid axillary pressure from the crutches)

Explain the reason for and intended effect of the preventive therapy

EVALUATION

Record actual outcome

POTENTIAL FOR SEIZURES [42,278,522]

ASSESSMENT

Data Collection

Subjective Data
• There are no actual symptoms of seizures

Objective Data
• There are no actual signs of seizures

Related Data

• There are one or more stressors present that increase the possibility that seizures will occur

DISEASES: Brain tumor, cerebrovascular accident, eclampsia (toxemia of pregnancy), encephalitis, epilepsy, acute hypoglycemia, malaria, meningitis, tetanus

INJURIES: Cerebral concussion, poisoning

SIGNS AND SYMPTOMS: Acute hypoxia, high fever

PSYCHOSOCIAL FACTORS: Threat of severe stress (for persons likely to have seizures)

HEALTH CARE FACTORS: *Medical therapy*: Hemodialysis

Data Analysis

Nursing Diagnosis

POTENTIAL FOR SEIZURES: The presence of stressors that increase the possibility of the actual occurrence of convulsions

PLANNING

Unmet Needs

Protection from physical harm, increased learning

Expected Outcome

No signs or symptoms of seizure(s) will occur

   OR

If signs and symptoms occur, they will be promptly recognized as an actual problem and will be treated appropriately

Person verbalizes an understanding of and practices preventive methods

NURSING INTERVENTIONS

Nursing Treatments

Provide standby equipment and drugs (oral airway, padded tongue blade, Dilantin)

Provide quiet (prevent sudden noises)

Subdue the room lighting

Refrain from jarring the bed

Refrain from performing nonessential procedures (which could stimulate seizures)

Place only warm hands and objects on the person (use firm full-hand pressure rather than fingertip touching; cold hands and objects may act as a seizure stimuli)

Nursing Observations

Observe for convulsions

Observe for muscle jerking (reflective muscle jerking when the person is touched or jerking that occurs from other stimuli, indicating that seizures are imminent)

Health Teaching

Describe the manifestations of an impending seizure (seeing bright lights, hearing unusual noises, smelling strange odors)

Inform of those conditions that precipitate seizures (lack of rest, fever, infection, flashing light patterns, emotional excitement)

Explain how to manage seizure episodes (have the person lie down in a safe place at the first sign of an impending seizure, patient's clothing should be loosened, a soft object should be placed between the jaw teeth on one side, the patient should be protected from injury)

Explain the importance of continuing (drug) therapy

Explain why the potential problem could become actual (disease, toxicity, or irritation of cerebral cortex can result in a seizure)

Explain the reason for and intended effect of the preventive therapy

EVALUATION

Record actual outcome

Potential Threats to Reproductive System Homeostasis

POTENTIAL FOR COMPLICATED PREGNANCY[133,527]

ASSESSMENT

Data Collection

Subjective Data
• There are no actual symptoms of a complicated pregnancy

Objective Data
• There are no actual signs of a complicated pregnancy

Related Data
• There are one or more stressors present that increase the possibility that a complicated pregnancy will occur

BIRTH DEFECTS: Maternal congenital heart disease

DISEASES: *Maternal*: Cardiovascular disease, cystitis, diabetes mellitus, glomerulonephritis, gonorrhea, herpes simplex, hypertension, obesity (weight above 200 lb), malaria, nephrotic syndrome, polycystic kidney disease, pyelonephritis, rubella, sickle cell anemia, syphilis, thyrotoxicosis, toxoplasmosis, tuberculosis

INJURIES: *Maternal*: Trauma of any kind

HUMAN BODY: *Anatomic abnormalities*: Incompetent cervix

HEALTH CARE FACTORS: *History*: Preeclampsia, eclampsia. *Diagnostic procedures*: X-ray (during the first trimester of pregnancy). *Medical therapy*: Radiation therapy, radioisotope therapy. *Drug therapy*: Any drugs or immunizations (when not prescribed by a physician)

DEVELOPMENTAL FACTORS: Adolescence (under 16 years old), early adulthood (when over age 35)

LIFESTYLE: Alcohol intake, insufficient or unbalanced diet, drug abuse or dependence, high caffeine intake, cigarette or tobacco smoking

Data Analysis

Nursing Diagnosis

POTENTIAL FOR COMPLICATED PREGNANCY (POTENTIAL FOR HIGH-RISK PREGNANCY): The presence of stressors that increase the possibility of the actual occurrence of injury to the unborn fetus or the pregnant woman

PLANNING

Unmet Needs

Protection from physical harm, increased learning

Expected Outcome

No signs or symptoms of a complicated pregnancy will occur
    OR
If signs and symptoms occur, they will be promptly recognized as an actual problem and will be treated appropriately
Person verbalizes an understanding of and practices preventive methods

NURSING INTERVENTIONS

Nursing Treatments

Provide a balanced nutritional diet
Encourage moderate physical exercise
Encourage adequate rest
Discourage the intake of oral stimulants

Discourage smoking
Withhold all drugs (unless prescribed by a physician)

Nursing Observations

Specific to the Initial Visit
Measure the pelvic size
Monitor blood studies for blood type
Monitor blood studies for Rh factor
Monitor blood studies for positive VDRL
Monitor the Pap smear study for positive findings
Obtain a bacterial culture (to screen for gonorrhea)

Initial and Follow-up Visits
Monitor the fetal heart sounds
Palpate the uterus for fundus height
Inspect the breasts for abnormalities
Inspect for edema and bleeding
Inspect the vagina for discharge (especially bleeding)
Measure the body weight
Monitor the blood pressure
Monitor blood studies for abnormal hematology (especially for anemia or infection)
Observe for complaints of constipation, backache, and (vaginal) itching
Test the urine for protein
Test the urine for sugar and acetone

Health Teaching

Recommend that self-medication be avoided
Teach the principles of good nutrition
Explain how to control weight gain during pregnancy
Inform that heavy lifting should be avoided
Emphasize the danger of x-ray exposure during early pregnancy
Describe the danger signs of pregnancy (persistent headache, nausea or vomiting, dizziness, edema, vaginal bleeding or fluid, abdominal pain, absence of fetal movement after the fourth month, acute illness)
Instruct to report any serious symptoms immediately
Explain why the potential problem could become actual (existing disease or conditions can dangerously affect both mother and fetus)
Explain the reason for and intended effect of the preventive therapy

EVALUATION

Record actual outcome

POTENTIAL FOR COMPLICATED LABOR AND DELIVERY[133,527]

ASSESSMENT

Data Collection

Subjective Data
• There are no actual symptoms of a complicated labor and delivery

Objective Data
• There are no actual signs of a complicated labor and delivery

Related Data
• There are one or more stressors present that increase the possibility that a complicated labor and delivery will occur
HEALTH CARE FACTORS: *Complications*: Complicated pregnancy, previous complicated labor and delivery
SITUATIONAL FACTORS: Maternal chronic illness, multiple pregnancy (twins, triplets, etc.), beyond-term pregnancy status
HUMAN BODY: *Anatomic abnormalities*: Small pelvis
HEALTH CARE FACTORS: *History of*: Cesarean section, prolonged labor, eclampsia, hemorrhage, abnormal fetal position

Data Analysis

Nursing Diagnosis
POTENTIAL FOR COMPLICATED LABOR AND DELIVERY: The presence of stressors that increase the possibility of the actual occurrence of an abnormal process of childbirth

PLANNING

Unmet Needs
Protection from physical harm, increased learning

Expected Outcome
No signs or symptoms of a complicated labor or delivery will occur
OR
If signs and symptoms occur, they will be promptly recognized as an actual problem and will be treated appropriately

NURSING INTERVENTIONS

Nursing Treatments
Attend the patient constantly
OR
Provide frequent contact with the person
Reassure verbally

Nursing Observations

First-Stage Labor
Monitor the fetal heart sounds
Palpate the cervix for dilatation
Palpate the uterus for contraction quality
Time the uterine contractions
Monitor the blood pressure (every hour)
Monitor the oral temperature
Palpate the pulse for rate, rhythm, and volume
Inspect the chest for respiratory rate and rhythm
Observe for uterine membrane rupture
Inspect the amniotic fluid for meconium
Inspect the vagina for a prolapsed umbilical cord
Observe for complaints of pain and fatigue
Test the urine for protein
Test the urine for sugar and acetone

Second-Stage Labor
Monitor the fetal heart sounds (until birth occurs)

Third-Stage Labor
Inspect for bleeding
Inspect the placenta for abnormalities
Inspect the umbilical cord for abnormalities
Palpate the uterus for firmness

Monitor the blood pressure

Palpate the pulse for rate, rhythm, and volume

Health Teaching

Describe those symptoms that should be reported (contractions, membrane rupture, pink "show," bleeding)

Explain why the potential problem could become actual (existing disease or conditions can have an adverse effect on labor and delivery)

EVALUATION

Record actual outcome

POTENTIAL FOR COMPLICATED PUERPERIUM [55,133,291,405,496,527]

ASSESSMENT

Data Collection

Subjective Data

• There are no actual symptoms of a complicated puerperium

Objective Data

• There are no actual signs of a complicated puerperium

Related Data

• There are one or more stressors present that increase the possibility that a complicated puerperium will occur

HEALTH CARE FACTORS: *Complications*: Complicated pregnancy or delivery. *History of*: Thrombophlebitis, hemorrhage, exposure to infection

Data Analysis

Nursing Diagnosis

POTENTIAL FOR COMPLICATED PUERPERIUM: The presence of stressors that increase the possibility of the actual occurrence of an abnormal postpartal period

PLANNING

Unmet Needs

Protection from physical harm, increased learning

Expected Outcome

No signs or symptoms of a complicated puerperium will occur

  OR

If signs and symptoms occur, they will be promptly recognized as an actual problem and will be treated appropriately

NURSING INTERVENTIONS

Nursing Treatments

Encourage adequate rest

Cover with warm blankets

Give warm liquids

Provide quiet

Massage the uterine fundus (if it becomes relaxed)

Ambulate the patient (as soon as possible if there are no contraindications)

Nursing Observations

Inspect for bleeding

Inspect the skin for perspiration abnormality (profuse perspiration)

Measure the intake and output (if there have been pregnancy complications)
Monitor the blood pressure
Monitor the oral temperature (for fever)
Inspect for edema, inflammation, bleeding (of the incision site if an episiotomy is done)
Inspect the vagina for discharge
Observe for complaints of thirst
Palpate the uterus for firmness (every 15 minutes after delivery)
Palpate the bladder for distention
Palpate the pulse for rate, rhythm, and volume
Monitor blood studies for evidence of infection

Health Teaching

Describe those symptoms that should be reported (bleeding, pain, etc.)
Explain why the potential problem could become actual (the exposure of the uterine endometrium, pelvis, and peritoneum during childbirth increases the possibility of *Streptococcus* and *Staphlococcus* invasion; infection of organs proximal to the uterus or the retention of placenta fragments can cause puerperal infection)
Teach how to do postpartum exercises (when the woman feels ready for such)
Explain the reason for and intended effect of the preventive therapy

EVALUATION

Record actual outcome

Potential Threats to Respiratory Homeostasis

POTENTIAL FOR AIRWAY OBSTRUCTION[35,339,371]

ASSESSMENT

Data Collection

Subjective Data
• There are no actual symptoms of airway obstruction

Objective Data
• There are no actual signs of airway obstruction

Related Data
• There are one or more stressors present that increase the possibility that airway obstruction will occur

BIRTH DEFECTS: Cystic fibrosis
DISEASES: Alcoholism, asthma, cerebrovascular accident, epilepsy, esophageal stricture, Guillain-Barré syndrome, multiple sclerosis, myasthenia gravis, rabies
INJURIES: Foreign body in nose, mouth, or upper airways, nasal fracture
SIGNS AND SYMPTOMS: Vomiting, unconsciousness
HEALTH CARE FACTORS: *Medical therapy*: Electroconvulsive therapy, nasal packing, nasogastric suction, endotracheal intubation. *Surgical therapy*: Anesthesia, recovery from anesthesia. *Surgical procedures*: Glossectomy, laryngectomy, rhinoplasty, thyroidectomy, tonsilectomy, tracheostomy
DEVELOPMENTAL PHASE: Toddler
SITUATIONAL FACTORS: Impending death

HUMAN ERROR: Rapid eating or drinking, laughing or talking while eating or drinking

Data Analysis

Nursing Diagnosis

POTENTIAL FOR AIRWAY OBSTRUCTION: The presence of stressors that increase the possibility of the actual occurrence of air being unable to pass through the respiratory tract

PLANNING

Unmet Needs

Protection from physical harm, increased learning

Expected Outcome

No signs or symptoms of airway obstruction will occur
    OR
If signs and symptoms occur, they will be promptly recognized as an actual problem and will be treated appropriately
Person verbalizes an understanding of and practices preventive methods

NURSING INTERVENTIONS

Nursing Treatments

Administer vaporized air (for thick secretions)
Increase fluid intake to about 2,000 cc daily (if secretions are thick)
Insert an oral airway (as needed)
Suction the airway (as needed)
Elevate the head (especially while eating)
Feed unhurriedly
Inflate the airway tube cuff (before feeding)
Discourage talking while eating
Refrain from distracting the patient while he swallows
Restrict the intake to nothing by mouth (when there is cerebral impairment)
Place in the side-lying (Sim's) position (during coma, after a seizure or anesthesia)
Encourage coughing
    AND
Encourage deep breathing
Clear nasal secretions
Refrain from using a cotton-filled gauze tracheostomy dressing
Drain the condensation from the nebulizer tubing periodically
Provide standby equipment (suction machine, airway tube, tracheostomy tray, wire cutters)

Nursing Observations

Inspect the chest for respiratory rate and rhythm
Inspect the chest for symmetrical expansion
Auscultate the chest for abnormal breath sounds
Auscultate the chest for lung aeration
Inspect for foreign bodies
Observe for cyanosis, dyspnea, mouth breathing, nasal flare
Observe for complaints of nasal congestion
Monitor blood studies for arterial blood gases

Health Teaching

Explain that fluids should not be given to persons unable to swallow
Inform that airway noise indicates obstruction
Recommend that bones be removed from foods before eating
Recommend thorough food chewing
Instruct not to insert foreign objects into the mouth or nose
Describe those symptoms that should be reported (dyspnea, choking)
Explain why the potential problem could become actual (airway obstruction can result from poor control of respiratory secretions, impairment of respiratory or swallowing

reflexes, structural abnormality of a respiratory organ, weakness or paralysis that prevents clearing of one's own airway)

Explain the reason for and intended effect of the preventive therapy

EVALUATION

Record actual outcome

POTENTIAL FOR ASPIRATION[26,371]

ASSESSMENT

Data Collection

Subjective Data

• There are no actual symptoms of aspiration

Objective Data

• There are no actual signs of aspiration

Related Data

• There are one or more stressors present that increase the possibility that aspiration will occur

BIRTH STATUS: Newborn

DISEASES: Cerebrovascular accident, Guillain-Barré syndrome, multiple sclerosis, myasthenia gravis

INJURIES: Foreign body in mouth

SIGNS AND SYMPTOMS: Vomiting, somnolence, hemiplegia

HUMAN BODY: *Natural body function*: Childbirth

HEALTH CARE FACTORS: *Medical therapy*: Gavage feedings (if the tube becomes displaced). *Surgical therapy*: General anesthesia, local anesthesia (for bronchoscopy, etc.), recovery from anesthesia, partial laryngectomy, tracheostomy

DEVELOPMENTAL PHASE: Toddler

SITUATIONAL FACTORS: Impending death

HUMAN ERROR: Rapid eating or drinking, laughing or talking while eating

Data Analysis

Nursing Diagnosis

POTENTIAL FOR ASPIRATION: The presence of stressors that increase the possibility of the actual occurrence of fluid or objects entering the lungs during inspiration

PLANNING

Unmet Needs

Protection from physical harm, increased learning

Expected Outcome

No signs or symptoms of aspiration will occur
  OR
If signs and symptoms occur, they will be promptly recognized as an actual problem and will be treated appropriately

Person verbalizes an understanding of and practices preventive methods

NURSING INTERVENTIONS

Nursing Treatments

Elevate the head (while eating; while giving gavage feedings)

Feed unhurriedly

Inflate the airway tube cuff (before feeding)

Discourage talking while eating

Nursing Observations
Observe for coughing, cyanosis, dyspnea
Inspect the chest for symmetrical expansion (chest retraction occurs in aspiration with obstruction)
Inspect the chest for respiratory rate and rhythm

Health Teaching
Explain that fluids should not be given to persons unable to swallow (and that fluids are not given until the gag reflex returns after local anesthesia)
Recommend thorough food chewing
Instruct not to insert foreign objects into the mouth
Explain why the potential problem could become actual (food or foreign objects could be inhaled into the lungs)
Explain the reason for and intended effect of the preventive therapy

EVALUATION

Record actual outcome

POTENTIAL FOR ATELECTASIS[32,35,399]

ASSESSMENT

Data Collection

Subjective Data
• There are no actual symptoms of atelectasis

Objective Data
• There are no actual signs of atelectasis

Related Data
• There are one or more stressors present that increase the possibility that atelectasis will occur
BIRTH DEFECTS: Cystic fibrosis
DISEASES: Asthma, bronchitis, cerebrovascular accident, emphysema, Guillain-Barré syndrome, myasthenia gravis, multiple sclerosis, thoracic tumor
INJURIES: Fracture and compression of the spinal cord, rib or sternal fracture, pneumothorax
SIGNS AND SYMPTOMS: Immobility, pain, weakness
HEALTH CARE FACTORS: *Medical therapy*: Prolonged bed rest. *Drug therapy*: Adverse effects of hypnotics, narcotics, sedatives. *Surgical therapy*: Anesthesia, recovery from anesthesia

Data Analysis

Nursing Diagnosis
POTENTIAL FOR ATELECTASIS (POTENTIAL FOR INADEQUATE PULMONARY VENTILATION): The presence of stressors that increase the possibility of the actual occurrence of incomplete expansion of portions of a lung or one or both lungs with air

PLANNING

Unmet Needs
Protection from physical harm, increased learning

Expected Outcome
No signs or symptoms of atelectasis will occur
   OR
If signs and symptoms occur, they will be promptly recognized as an actual problem and will be treated appropriately

NURSING INTERVENTIONS

Nursing Treatments

Ambulate the person (as much and as soon as possible)

Change the person's position frequently

Suction the airway (periodically)

Encourage coughing

OR

Encourage deep breathing

Encourage alternate rest and activity

Withhold the (sedatives) drugs (or give analgesics judiciously when they cause hypoventilation)

Nursing Observations

Inspect the chest for respiratory rate and rhythm

Inspect the chest for symmetrical expansion

Auscultate the chest for lung aeration

Monitor blood studies for arterial blood gases

Observe for complaints of (chest) pain, cyanosis, dyspnea, fatigue

Observe for restlessness (especially in semiconscious states)

Palpate the pulse for rate (tachycardia), rhythm, and volume

Health Teaching

Explain why the potential problem could become actual (inadequate pulmonary ventilation can occur from decreased respiratory muscle strength, pain-inhibited normal respiratory depth, severe abdominal pressure causing pressure on the diaphragm, drug-depressed respirations, thoracic tumor, excessively enlarged heart, a fluid-distended pericardium compressing the lung)

Teach how to do bronchopulmonary hygiene measures (to persons with chronic pulmonary problems)

Explain the reason for and intended effect of the preventive therapy

EVALUATION

Record actual outcome

POTENTIAL FOR HYPEROXIA [42,451]

ASSESSMENT

Data Collection

Subjective Data

• There are no actual symptoms of hyperoxia

Objective Data

• There are no actual signs of hyperoxia

Related Data

• There are one or more stressors present that increase the possibility that hyperoxia will occur

DISEASES: Guillain-Barré syndrome, myasthenia gravis, poliomyelitis, respiratory distress syndrome

HEALTH CARE FACTORS *Medical therapy*: The administration of high concentrations of oxygen

Data Analysis

Nursing Diagnosis

POTENTIAL FOR HYPEROXIA (POTENTIAL FOR OXYGEN TOXICITY): The presence of stressors that increase the possibility of the actual occurrence of an above normal increase in oxygen content, tension, or concentration

PLANNING

Unmet Needs
Protection from physical harm, increased learning

Expected Outcome
No signs or symptoms of hyperoxia will occur
 OR
If signs and symptoms occur, they will be promptly recognized as an actual problem and will be treated appropriately

NURSING INTERVENTIONS

Nursing Treatments
Limit the therapeutic oxygen concentrations to below 40% (for long-term oxygen administration)

Nursing Observations
Inspect the chest for respiratory rate and rhythm
Inspect the chest for symmetrical expansion
Auscultate the chest for lung aeration
Inspect the skin for color (rosy, pink)
Monitor blood studies for arterial blood gases (increased O_2 saturation)

Specific to Acute Hyperoxia (Oxygen Toxicity)
Observe for complaints of nausea, dizziness, visual disturbances, numbness and tingling
Observe for muscle twitching, restlessness, irritability, convulsions

Specific to Chronic Hyperoxia (Oxygen Toxicity)
Auscultate the chest for rales (indicating pulmonary congestion)
Inspect for edema

Health Teaching
Explain why the potential problem could become actual (breathing high levels of oxygen has a respiratory depressing effect in conditions with inadequate gas exchange and damages tissue cells, especially those of the airways)
Explain the reason for and intended effect of the preventive therapy

EVALUATION

Record actual outcome

POTENTIAL FOR HYPOXIA[42,339]

ASSESSMENT

Data Collection

Subjective Data
• There are no actual symptoms of hypoxia

Objective Data
• There are no actual signs of hypoxia

Related Data
• There are one or more stressors present that increase the possibility that hypoxia will occur
DISEASES: Anemia, arteriosclerotic heart disease, cerebrovascular accident, chronic obstructive pulmonary disease, leukemia, myocardial infarction, pneumonia
INJURIES: Carbon monoxide poisoning, fractured neck, pneumothorax
SIGNS AND SYMPTOMS: Shock
HEALTH CARE FACTORS: *Surgical therapy*: Anesthesia, recovery from anesthesia
SITUATIONAL FACTORS: Impending death

Data Analysis

Nursing Diagnosis

POTENTIAL FOR HYPOXIA (POTENTIAL FOR OXYGEN INSUFFICIENCY): The presence of stressors that increase the possibility of the actual occurrence of inadequate amounts of oxygen being available to body cells

PLANNING

Unmet Needs

Protection from physical harm, increased learning

Expected Outcome

No signs or symptoms of hypoxia will occur
> OR

If signs and symptoms occur, they will be promptly recognized as an actual problem and will be treated appropriately

NURSING INTERVENTIONS

Nursing Treatments

Provide standby equipment (oxygen)
Place in the sitting position (for full chest expansion)
Encourage coughing
> AND

Encourage deep breathing
Discourage smoking
Encourage adequate rest
Encourage alternate rest and activity
Discourage strenuous activities (if the person has returned to normal daily living)

Nursing Observations

Inspect the chest for respiratory rate and rhythm
Inspect the chest for symmetrical expansion
Auscultate the chest for lung aeration
Monitor the blood pressure (for decrease)
Monitor blood studies for arterial blood gases (decreased O_2 saturation)
Observe for complaints of headache, difficulty concentrating, apprehension
Observe for restlessness, confusion, lethargy
Observe the level of consciousness (and any changes occurring)
Palpate the pulse for rate (bradycardia or tachycardia), rhythm, and volume

Specific to Cardiogenic Hypoxia
Observe for complaints of nausea
Observe for cyanosis, dyspnea, vomiting

Health Teaching

Describe those symptoms that should be reported (headache, nausea, confusion, cyanosis, dyspnea, lethargy, restlessness, vomiting)
Explain the need to avoid overexertion
Recommend that high altitudes be avoided (after cardiac damage)
Emphasize the need to fly in pressurized airplanes
Teach how to give oxygen therapy
Teach the principles of good nutrition (with special emphasis on protein- and iron-containing foods)
Explain why the potential problem could become actual (oxygen insufficiency can result from the inability of the red blood cells to transport oxygen to body organs, inability of the heart to pump adequate blood for the oxygenation of body cells, and impaired circulation in one or more body areas)
Explain the reason for and intended effect of the preventive therapy

EVALUATION

Record actual outcome

POTENTIAL FOR INFANT APNEA[9,39,577]

ASSESSMENT

Data Collection

Subjective Data
• There are no actual symptoms of infant apnea

Objective Data
• There are no actual signs of infant apnea

Related Data
• There are one or more stressors present that increase the possibility that infant apnea
  will occur
BIRTH DEFECT: Hyaline membrane disease
INHERITED FACTORS: *Sex*: Greater incidence in males than in females. *Race*: Greater in non-
  Caucasions
BIRTH STATUS: Premature infant or low-birth-weight infant
SIGNS AND SYMPTOMS: Seizures associated with apnea episodes
HEALTH CARE FACTORS: *History of*: Respiratory infection, previous apnea for more than 20
  seconds, family history of brothers or sisters with sudden infant death syndrome
DEVELOPMENTAL PHASE: Babyhood (between ages 1–6 months)
ENVIRONMENTAL FACTORS: *Months of the year*: More prevalent in November, December, Janu-
  ary, and February

Data Analysis

Nursing Diagnosis
POTENTIAL FOR INFANT APNEA: The presence of stressors that increase the possibility of the
  actual occurrence of the cessation of an infant's respirations

PLANNING

Unmet Needs
Protection from physical harm, increased learning

Expected Outcome
If signs and symptoms of infant apnea occur, such will be detected and treated within
  seconds of onset

NURSING INTERVENTIONS

Nursing Treatments
Change the infant's position frequently
Maintain adequate atmospheric humidity
Provide frequent contact with the infant
Make a follow-up evaluation
Place the infant on an apnea pad (for constant monitoring)
Stimulate by touch (gentle, light touch when the infant is apneic or having bradycardia)

Nursing Observations
Inspect the chest for respiratory rate and rhythm
Inspect the chest for symmetrical expansion
Auscultate the chest for lung aeration
Monitor the infant for apnea
Monitor the ECG (for bradycardia)
    AND
Auscultate the apical pulse for rate and rhythm (bradycardia)
Observe for cyanosis, dyspnea, mouth breathing, nasal flare

Health Teaching
Describe those symptoms that should be reported (periods of apnea, a respiratory infection)

Explain how to observe respirations (by home apnea monitor, by chest/abdomen movement)

Instruct how to keep a daily apnea chart

Explain that premature infants require at-home supervision

Inform that airway noise indicates obstruction

Instruct to change (the child's) position frequently

Instruct to immediately report any early symptoms (and to use light tactile stimulation if apnea persists longer than 15–20 seconds)

Teach measures to prevent apnea (avoid cooling or overheating of the infant; avoid distention of the stomach from overfeeding or failure to burp properly; avoid dehydration from inadequate fluids, especially during fever, in a warm environment, and during activity; avoid positions that lead to airway congestion and obstruction with mucus)

Explain why the potential problem could become actual (research verifies that certain stressors predispose to infant apnea)

Explain the reason for and intended effects of the preventive methods

EVALUATION

Record actual outcome

POTENTIAL FOR PNEUMOTHORAX[26,73,219,451]

ASSESSMENT

Data Collection

Subjective Data
• There are no actual symptoms of pneumothorax

Objective Data
• There are no actual signs of pneumothorax

Related Data
• There are one or more stressors present that increase the possibility that pneumothorax will occur

DISEASES: Chronic obstructive pulmonary disease, emphysema, pertussis, pneumonia, tuberculosis

INJURIES: Any chest trauma

SIGNS AND SYMPTOMS: *Diagnostic procedures*: Biopsy of the lung, bronchoscopy, gastroscopy. *Medical therapy*: Interrupted closed-chest drainage

Data Analysis

Nursing Diagnosis

POTENTIAL FOR PNEUMOTHORAX (POTENTIAL FOR INCREASED INTRAPLEURAL PRESSURE): The presence of stressors that increase the possibility of the actual occurrence of increased pressure within the pleural cavity resulting in collapse of the lung

PLANNING

Unmet Needs

Protection from physical harm, increased learning

Expected Outcome

No signs or symptoms of pneumothorax will occur
OR
If signs and symptoms occur, they will be promptly recognized as an actual problem and will be treated appropriately

NURSING INTERVENTIONS

Nursing Treatments

Specific for Chest Trauma

Cover the sucking wound immediately (with a sterile dressing or the palm of a clean hand)

Encourage deep breathing (forceful inhalation and exhalation as the sterile dressing is applied)

Position comfortably

Place in the slight sitting (semi-Fowler's) position

Place on the affected side

Place on complete bed rest

Attend the patient constantly

Specific for Disrupted Closed-Chest Drainage

Cover the sucking wound immediately (if the tube slips from the chest)

Clamp the chest tube, but only for a short time (immediately if the water-seal pressure is lost or the container is elevated above the chest level)

Attach the chest tube to a water-seal drainage (if a new tube is inserted)

Strip the chest tubing (if drainage ceases)

Specific for Prevention of Spontaneous Pneumothorax

Increase fluid intake to about 2,000 cc daily (to loosen secretions)

Change the person's position frequently (to promote drainage)

Give nonprescription drugs (expectorant)

Suction the airway (as needed)

Administer vaporized air (if the environment is dry)

Nursing Observations

Inspect the chest for respiratory rate and rhythm (shallow or rapid respirations)

Inspect the chest for symmetrical expansion (asymmetrical expansion indicates pneumo-thorax

Auscultate the chest for abnormal (absent) breath sounds

Monitor the blood pressure

Palpate the pulse for rate, rhythm, and volume

Observe for complaints of pain (upon movement)

Observe for cyanosis, dyspnea, cough, restlessness

Inspect the skin for pallor

Specific for Disrupted Closed-Chest Drainage

Check the drainage system for leakage (and replace if leakage exits)

Check the tube for patency

Check for fluctuation of the fluid level in the water-seal container

Health Teaching

Explain why the potential problem could become actual (whenever air collects in the thorax, the resulting pressure can collapse the lung)

Explain the reason for and intended effect of the preventive therapy

EVALUATION

Record actual outcome

POTENTIAL FOR PULMONARY CONGESTION[125,476]

ASSESSMENT

Data Collection

Subjective Data

• There are no actual symptoms of pulmonary congestion

Objective Data
• There are no actual signs of pulmonary congestion

Related Data
• There are one or more stressors present that increase the possibility that pulmonary congestion will occur
DISEASES: Influenza, nasopharyngitis (which has moved to the chest)
SIGNS AND SYMPTOMS: Hypoventilation, immobility, weakness
HEALTH CARE FACTORS: *Drug therapy*: Adverse effects of drugs such as hypnotics, narcotics, sedatives, decongestants. *Surgical therapy*: Anesthesia, recovery from anesthesia

Data Analysis

Nursing Diagnosis
POTENTIAL FOR PULMONARY CONGESTION: The presence of stressors that increase the possibility of the actual occurrence of collected exudate developing in the lungs

PLANNING

Unmet Needs

Protection from physical harm, increased learning

Expected Outcome

No signs or symptoms of pulmonary congestion will occur
OR
If signs and symptoms occur, they will be promptly recognized as an actual problem and will be treated appropriately
Person verbalizes an understanding of and practices preventive methods

NURSING INTERVENTIONS

Nursing Treatments

Ambulate the person (as much and as soon as possible)
Change the person's position frequently (every 2 hours)
Encourage coughing
AND
Encourage deep breathing
Suction the airway (as needed)
Discourage smoking

Nursing Observations

Inspect the chest for respiratory rate and rhythm
Inspect the chest for symmetrical expansion
Auscultate the chest for lung aeration
Auscultate the chest for rales and rhonchi
Monitor the oral temperature (for fever)
Observe for (productive) coughing

Health Teaching

Instruct to change position frequently
Instruct to increase fluid intake (to thin secretions for ease of elimination through coughing)
Describe those symptoms that should be reported (fever, cough, fatigue)
Explain why the potential problem could become actual (pulmonary congestion can result from inadequate lung ventilation or from insufficient use of the cough reflex to clear secretions in the respiratory system)
Explain the reason for and intended effect of the preventive therapy

EVALUATION

Record actual outcome

POTENTIAL FOR PULMONARY EDEMA[35,73,125]

ASSESSMENT

Data Collection

Subjective Data
• There are no actual symptoms of pulmonary edema

Objective Data
• There are no actual signs of pulmonary edema

Related Data
• There are one or more stressors present that increase the possibility that pulmonary edema will occur

DISEASES: Arteriosclerotic heart disease, congestive heart failure, myocardial infarction, renal insufficiency or failure

INJURIES: Burn wounds (second- and third-degree burns between the second and fifth postburn day), near drowning (in fresh water)

HEALTH CARE FACTORS: *Medical therapy*: Overload of intravenous infusion. *Surgical therapy*: Anesthesia

ENVIRONMENTAL FACTORS: *Blast/explosion*: Exposure to blast or explosion. *Chemical substances*: Inhalation of chemicals, especially ammonia

Data Analysis

Nursing Diagnosis
POTENTIAL FOR PULMONARY EDEMA: The presence of stressors that increase the possibility of the actual occurrence of fluid accumulation in the extravascular spaces of the lung

PLANNING

Unmet Needs

Protection from physical harm, increased learning

Expected Outcome

No signs or symptoms of pulmonary edema will occur
OR
If signs and symptoms occur, they will be promptly recognized as an actual problem and will be treated appropriately

NURSING INTERVENTIONS

Nursing Treatments

Change the patient's position frequently (unless contraindicated in severe cardiac disease)
Elevate the head (put the head of the bed on a 10-inch block while the patient is sleeping)
Encourage adequate rest
Encourage decreased sodium-food intake (in cardiac disease)
Restrict the fluid intake according to the weight gain
Maintain a steady intravenous infusion flow rate (to prevent overhydration)
Provide standby equipment and drugs (oxygen, morphine, cedilanid D, intravenous diuretics, rotating tourniquets, IPPB machine, surface-active aerosol drug)
Give light foods (for the evening meal to decrease the cardiac workload)

Nursing Observations

Auscultate the chest for abnormal breath sounds (wheezing)
Auscultate the chest for rales (bubbling)
Auscultate the apical heartbeat for rate and rhythm (for dysrhythmias, gallop)
Inspect the sputum for characteristics (frothy pink)
Measure the body weight (daily, for gain due to fluid retention)
Monitor the central venous pressure (for elevation)

Observe for coughing, cyanosis, dyspnea, orthopnea, restlessness
Palpate the pulse for rate (tachycardia), rhythm, and volume
Inspect the neck veins for distention

Health Teaching

Describe those symptoms that should be reported (orthopnea, dyspnea, coughing, frothy pink sputum, rapid pulse)

Explain why the potential problem could become actual (pulmonary edema can occur when the left ventricle is unable to pump blood away from the lungs into the circulation, causing the lungs to become engorged with fluid; from damage to the alveolar–capillary membrane, allowing fluid to leak into the alveoli)

Explain the reason for and intended effect of the preventive therapy

EVALUATION

Record actual outcome

POTENTIAL FOR RESPIRATORY DEPRESSION/ARREST[42,249]

ASSESSMENT

Data Collection

Subjective Data
• There are no actual symptoms of respiratory depression or arrest

Objective Data
• There are no actual signs of respiratory depression or arrest occurring

Related Data
• There are one or more stressors present that increase the possibility that respiratory depression/arrest will occur

BIRTH DEFECTS: Hyaline membrane disease

BIRTH STATUS: Premature infant

DISEASES: Alcoholism, asthma, brain abscess, brain tumor, cerebrovascular accident, drug addiction, emphysema, encephalitis, Guillain-Barré syndrome, multiple sclerosis, myasthenia gravis, myocardial infarction, poliomyelitis, pulmonary edema, pulmonary embolus, subarachnoid hemorrhage

INJURIES: Burn wound (severe), cerebral concussion, near drowning, electric shock, flail chest, foreign body in larynx, penetrating or puncture wound of the chest, poisoning, venomous snakebite

SIGNS AND SYMPTOMS: Coma, dyspnea, hypoxia, laryngeal edema or spasm, paralysis, weakness (severe)

HEALTH CARE FACTORS: *Diagnostic Procedures:* Bronchoscopy. *Medical therapy:* Chest tube drainage, interrupted closed-chest drainage, electroconvulsive therapy, prolonged intermittent positive-pressure breathing, the administration of high concentrations of oxygen, carbon dioxide therapy. *Drug therapy:* Adverse effects of anticonvulsants, antidepressants, barbiturates, hypnotics, narcotics, sedatives, tranquilizers. *Surgical therapy:* Anesthesia. *Surgical procedures:* Pneumonectomy

DEVELOPMENTAL PHASES: Newborn

LIFESTYLE: Drug abuse

ENVIRONMENTAL FACTORS: *Chemical substances:* Exposure to toxic gases

Data Analysis

Nursing Diagnosis
POTENTIAL FOR RESPIRATORY DEPRESSION (POTENTIAL FOR RESPIRATORY ARREST): The presence of

stressors that increase the possibility of the actual occurrence of a severely impaired respiratory drive or ventilatory response

PLANNING

Unmet Needs

Protection from physical harm, increased learning

Expected Outcome

No signs or symptoms of respiratory depression or arrest will occur
  OR
If signs and symptoms occur, they will be promptly recognized as an actual problem and will be treated appropriately

NURSING INTERVENTIONS

Nursing Treatments

Suction the airway (as needed)
Encourage coughing
  AND
Encourage deep breathing
Withhold the drugs (respiratory depressants such as morphine)
Withhold the oxygen therapy (if the blood O_2 is elevated)
Provide frequent contact with the patient
Provide standby equipment and drugs (suction machine, oxygen, airway tube, stimulant drugs)
Stimulate by touch or voice (so the person will resume breathing or breathe faster or deeper)

Nursing Observations

Inspect the chest for respiratory rate and rhythm
Inspect the chest for symmetrical expansion
Auscultate the chest for lung aeration (periodically)
Monitor blood studies for arterial blood gases
Observe for complaints of respiratory muscle weakness
Observe for cyanosis, dyspnea
Check the respirator for proper functioning
Monitor the infant for apnea (with an apnea monitor)

Health Teaching

Describe those symptoms that should be reported (dyspnea, weakness)
Explain why the potential problem could become actual (respiratory depression or arrest occurs when the respiratory reflex is inhibited by brain center damage or by drug or neurologic effects)
Explain the reason for and intended effect of the preventive therapy

EVALUATION

Record actual outcome

POTENTIAL FOR RESPIRATORY INFECTION[73,371,451]

ASSESSMENT

Data Collection

Subjective Data
• There are no actual symptoms of respiratory infection

Objective Data
• There are no actual signs of respiratory infection

Related Data
- There are one or more stressors present that increase the possibility that a respiratory infection will occur

BIRTH DEFECTS: Cystic fibrosis

BIRTH STATUS: Premature infant

DISEASES: Alcoholism, asthma, atelectasis, cancer, chronic obstructive pulmonary disease, malnutrition, respiratory distress syndrome, respiratory allergic disorder

SIGNS AND SYMPTOMS: Immobility

PSYCHOSOCIAL FACTORS: Chronic and/or severe stress

HEALTH CARE FACTORS: *History of:* Exposure to infected persons. *Drug therapy:* Immunosuppressive therapy. *Surgical therapy:* Anesthesia. *Surgical procedure:* Tracheostomy

DEVELOPMENTAL PHASE: Old age

LIFESTYLE: Cigarette or tobacco smoking

SITUATIONAL FACTORS: Chronic illness

ENVIRONMENTAL FACTORS: *Chemicals:* Inhalation of toxic gases

Data Analysis

Nursing Diagnosis
POTENTIAL FOR RESPIRATORY INFECTION: The presence of stressors that increase the possibility of the actual occurrence of an infection of the respiratory system

PLANNING

Unmet Needs
Protection from physical harm, increased learning

Expected Outcome
No signs or symptoms of respiratory infection will occur
> OR

If signs and symptoms occur, they will be promptly recognized as an actual problem and will be treated appropriately

Person verbalizes an understanding of and practices preventive methods

NURSING INTERVENTIONS

Nursing Treatments
Ambulate the person (as much as possible)

Change the person's position frequently

Encourage adequate rest

Encourage coughing
> AND

Encourage deep breathing

Provide a balanced nutritional diet

Discourage smoking

Nursing Observations
Inspect the chest for respiratory rate and rhythm

Auscultate the chest for lung aeration

Auscultate the chest for rales and rhonchi

Monitor the oral temperature (for fever)

Observe for coughing, dyspnea

Observe for complaints of pain (sore throat, chest pain)

Palpate the pulse for rate, rhythm, and volume

Health Teaching
Describe those symptoms that should be reported (fever, chills, sore throat, cough, malaise)

Explain how to prevent cross-infection (hand washing, sterilizing dishes, disposal of tissues and sputum, etc.)

Instruct that premature infants require protection against infection

Instruct to avoid direct contact with infected persons

Advise against mingling in crowds

Teach the principles of good nutrition

Instruct to increase fluid intake

Explain why the potential problem could become actual (respiratory infection is more likely to occur with decreased vital lung capacity, diminished cough reflex, debilitation, or drug therapy, causing lowered resistance to infection)

Explain the reason for and intended effect of the preventive therapy

EVALUATION

Record actual outcome

Potential Threats to Sensory Homeostasis

POTENTIAL FOR INCREASED INTRAOCULAR PRESSURE[35,253,371]

ASSESSMENT

Data Collection

Subjective Data

• There are no actual symptoms of increased intraocular pressure

Objective Data

• There are no actual signs of increased intraocular pressure

Related Data

• There are one or more stressors present that increase the possibility that increased intraocular pressure will occur

INJURIES: Contusion to the eye

SURGICAL PROCEDURES: Any on the eye

Data Analysis

Nursing Diagnosis

POTENTIAL FOR INCREASED INTRAOCULAR PRESSURE: The presence of stressors that increase the possibility of the actual occurrence of increased pressure within the eye

PLANNING

Unmet Needs

Protection from physical harm, increased learning

Expected Outcome

No signs or symptoms of increased intraocular pressure will occur

    OR

If signs and symptoms occur, they will be promptly recognized as an actual problem and will be treated appropriately

Person verbalizes an understanding of and practices preventive methods

NURSING INTERVENTIONS

Nursing Treatments

Change the patient's position gradually

Elevate the head (slightly)

Do not place in the flat position

Refrain from jarring the bed
Encourage adequate rest
Subdue the room lighting
Discourage the intake of oral stimulants
Discourage smoking

Nursing Observations

Observe for complaints of (eye) pain

Health Teaching

Advise gentle nose blowing
Inform that coughing should be avoided and that elimination straining should be avoided
Inform that stooping or lowering the head should be avoided and that heavy lifting should be avoided
Instruct to avoid rubbing the eyes
Instruct to change position gradually
Advise that highly emotional situations be avoided
Explain why the potential problem could become actual (if bleeding or edema occur within the eye tissue, the tension within the eyeball will increase)
Explain the reason for and intended effect of the preventive therapy

EVALUATION

Record actual outcome

POTENTIAL FOR SENSORY DEPRIVATION[13,14,529]

ASSESSMENT

Data Collection

Subjective Data
• There are no actual symptoms of sensory deprivation

Objective Data
• There are no actual signs of sensory deprivation

Related Data
• There are one or more stressors present that increase the possibility that sensory deprivation will occur
DISEASES: Blindness, deafness
INJURIES: Fracture and compression of the spinal cord
PSYCHOSOCIAL FACTORS: Lack of communication with others, lack of touch contact with others
HEALTH CARE FACTORS: *Health care environment*: Absence of natural light and dark in the health care environment such as in intensive care, isolation unit
LIFESTYLE: Lack of exercise
SITUATIONAL FACTORS: Chronic illness
ENVIRONMENTAL FACTORS: *Color*: Dull environmental color *Food*: Plain, poorly seasoned food. *Light*: Inadequate environmental light. *Odors*: Absence of a variety of odors. *Quiet*: Excessive quiet. *Windows*: Absence of windows

Data Analysis

Nursing Diagnosis
POTENTIAL FOR SENSORY DEPRIVATION: The presence of stressors that increase the possibility of the actual occurrence of being without externally stimulated sensory experience

PLANNING

Unmet Needs

Protection from physical harm, increased learning

Expected Outcome

No signs or symptoms of sensory deprivation will occur
  OR
If signs and symptoms occur, they will be promptly recognized as an actual problem and will be treated appropriately

NURSING INTERVENTIONS

Nursing Treatments

Allow unlimited visitors
Dress in colorful clothing
Illuminate the room adequately
Keep the person's door open
Place by a window
Provide an attractive meal tray
Provide radio, television and reading material for diversion
Encourage active diversional activities
Sit with the person
Talk with the person
Provide frequent contact with the person
Touch the patient judiciously
Offer environmental stimulation through contact with varied personnel, environmental change, and variety in the daily routine

Specific for Children
Place in an infant seat
Stimulate the infant with a mobile

Nursing Observations

Observe for irritability, restlessness, confusion, disorientation
Observe for complaints of fatigue

Health Teaching

Describe those symptoms that should be reported (boredom, depression, anxiety, fatigue, restlessness)
Recommend methods for increasing sensory stimulation (use of bright colors, viewing television, listening to the radio, mingling in crowds, exciting entertainment, living in a big city, etc.)
Explain why the potential problem could become actual (sensory deprivation can occur when the person receives little or no external input)
Explain the reason for and intended effect of the preventive therapy

EVALUATION

Record actual outcome

POTENTIAL FOR SENSORY OVERLOAD[471]

ASSESSMENT

Data Collection

Subjective Data
• There are no actual symptoms of sensory overload

Objective Data
• There are no actual signs of sensory overload

Related Data
• There are one or more stressors present that increase the possibility that sensory overload will occur

SIGNS AND SYMPTOMS: Pain

PSYCHOSOCIAL FACTORS: Exhaustion of adaptive reserves, threat of severe or chronic stress

HEALTH CARE FACTORS: *Health care environment*: Noise and crowding in the health care environment, exposure to intense human suffering of persons in the health care environment, lack of privacy, intensive care unit. *Diagnostic procedures*: Frequent diagnostic procedures. *Health therapy*: Frequent and/or prolonged health therapy

LIFESTYLE: Involvement in too many activities above the person's comfort level; insufficient relaxation, rest, and sleep; overwork

SITUATIONAL FACTORS: Multiple crisis situations

ENVIRONMENTAL FACTORS: *Housing*: Overcrowded. *Noise*: Prolonged exposure to loud noise. *Sights*: Obnoxious

Data Analysis

Nursing Diagnosis

POTENTIAL FOR SENSORY OVERLOAD: The presence of stressors that increase the possibility of the actual occurrence of an excessive stimulation of the senses

PLANNING

Unmet Needs

Protection from physical harm, increased learning

Expected Outcome

No signs or symptoms of sensory overload will occur
  OR
If signs and symptoms occur, they will be promptly recognized as an actual problem and will be treated appropriately

NURSING INTERVENTIONS

Nursing Treatments

Arrange orderly surroundings, pleasant surroundings
Arrange a structured environment
Provide quiet
Encourage adequate rest
Encourage quiet diversional activities
Keep the person's door closed
Plan undisturbed periods for the person
Reduce the demands placed on the person
Refrain from performing nonessential procedures
Avoid causing intense emotional situations
Restrict unwanted visitors

Nursing Observations

Observe for irritability, confusion, tremors
Observe for complaints of nervousness, fatigue

Health Teaching

Describe the behavioral pattern indicating overstimulation (fatigue, insomnia, irritability, confusion, tremors, palpitations, panicky feeling)
Recommend methods for reducing sensory stimulation (avoiding crowds, working in a small office, avoiding competitive work or games, traveling to familiar places, etc.)
Explain why the potential problem could become actual (sensory overload can occur whenever the person receives excessive external input)
Explain the reason for and intended effects of the preventive therapy

EVALUATION

Record actual outcome

Potential Threats of Pain During Illness

POTENTIAL FOR PAIN[362,371]

ASSESSMENT
Data Collection
Subjective Data
- There are no actual symptoms of pain

Objective
- There are no actual signs of pain

Related Data
- There are one or more stressors present that increase the possibility that pain will occur

DISEASES: Any

INJURIES: Any

PSYCHOSOCIAL FACTORS: Threat of real or imagined danger

HUMAN BODY: *Natural body function*: Childbirth. *Body states*: Menses

HEALTH CARE FACTORS: *Diagnostic procedures*: Any diagnostic procedure. *Medical therapy*: Ambulation, cardioversion, coughing and deep breathing, removal of dressings, removal of a cast, enemas, therapeutic exercise, hemodialysis, hyperalimentation or intravenous infusion, needle injection, irrigations (bladder, colonic, ear), nasal packing, paracentesis, peritoneal dialysis, phlebotomy, physical therapy, painful positioning, Thoracentesis, traction, therapeutic turning, urinary catheterization. *Surgical procedure*: Any surgical procedure, positioning during surgery. *Therapeutic devices*: Use of an artificial limb, brace, cardiac pacemaker

Data Analysis
Nursing Diagnosis
POTENTIAL FOR PAIN: The presence of stressors that increase the possibility of the actual occurrence of a distressful hurting

PLANNING
Unmet Needs
Protection from physical harm, increased learning

Expected Outcome
No signs or symptoms of pain will occur
    OR
If signs and symptoms occur, they will be promptly recognized as an actual problem and will be treated appropriately

NURSING INTERVENTIONS
Nursing Treatments
Approach unhurriedly
Handle gently
Position comfortably
Prepare the patient for a painful experience

Nursing Observations
Observe for complaints of pain
Observe for nonverbal communication of pain

Health Teaching

Explain how to describe pain (cramping, stabbing, constricting, etc.)

Explain that it is acceptable to admit the existence of pain (if it should occur)

Explain why the potential problem could become actual (certain physiologic changes or therapeutic treatments unavoidably will stimulate pain)

Explain the reason for and intended effect of the preventive therapy

EVALUATION

Record actual outcome

Potential Threats to Physical Strength and Strength Restoration

POTENTIAL FOR GENERALIZED WEAKNESS[371,396,451]

ASSESSMENT

Data Collection

Subjective Data
• There are no actual symptoms of generalized weakness

Objective Data
• There are no actual signs of generalized weakness

Related Data
• There are one or more stressors present that increase the possibility that generalized weakness will occur

DISEASES: Any

INJURIES: Any

SIGNS AND SYMPTOMS: Fever

HUMAN BODY: *Natural body function*: Childbirth.

HEALTH CARE FACTORS: *Diagnostic procedures*: Frequent diagnostic procedures. *Health therapy*: Frequent or painful medical or surgical therapy. *Drug therapy*: Cathartics or purgatives, chemotherapy, sedatives. *Medical therapy*: Prolonged bed rest

DEVELOPMENTAL PHASES: Old age

LIFESYTLE: Insufficient or unbalanced diet, lack of exercise or overvigorous exercise, insufficient sleep and rest

Data Analysis

Nursing Diagnosis

POTENTIAL FOR GENERALIZED WEAKNESS: The presence of stressors that increase the possibility of the actual occurrence of a loss of normal physical strength

PLANNING

Unmet Needs

Protection from physical harm, increased learning

Expected Outcome

No signs or symptoms of generalized weakness will occur
> OR

If signs and symptoms occur, they will be promptly recognized as an actual problem and will be treated appropriately

Person verbalizes an understanding of and practices preventive methods

NURSING INTERVENTIONS

Nursing Treatments

Ambulate the person (as much as possible)
> OR

Sit the person in an armchair

Encourage moderate physical exercise

Encourage adequate rest

Encourage alternate rest and activity

Encourage self-performance (whenever possible)

Exercise in range of motion (and resistive exercise)

Provide a balanced nutritional diet

Encourage increased protein-food intake

Nursing Observations

Observe for complaints of weakness

Observe for conditions indicating a need for increased nutritional requirements (fever, childhood growth, pregnancy, weight loss)

Health Teaching

Describe those symptoms that should be reported (weakness, which includes a desire to lie down, clumsy body movements, rapid breathing, feeling hot, being unable to deal with complex problems)

Advise a gradual return to activity (as a means of conserving strength)

Explain why the potential problem could become actual (weakness can occur with diseased body musculature, impaired circulation, stress-related energy depletion, severe metabolic changes)

Explain the reason for and intended effect of the preventive therapy

EVALUATION

Record actual outcome

POTENTIAL FOR INADEQUATE SLEEP/REST[72,451]

ASSESSMENT

Data Collection

Subjective Data
- There are no actual symptoms of inadequate sleep or rest

Objective Data
- There are no actual signs of inadequate sleep or rest

Related Data
- There are one or more stressors present that increase the possibility that inadequate sleep or rest will occur

DISEASES: Any
INJURIES: Any
SIGNS AND SYMPTOMS: Dyspnea, fever, pain, polyuria
PSYCHOSOCIAL FACTORS: Threat of severe or chronic stress
HUMAN BODY: *Natural body function*: Breast-feeding an infant. *Body states*: Pregnancy
HEALTH CARE FACTORS: *Health care environment*: Excessive stimuli in the health care environment. *Hospitalization*: Hospitalization of self or significant other. *Patients*: Disruptive patients. *Visitors*: Disturbing visitors. *Diagnostic procedure*: Prediagnostic preparation, frequent diagnostic procedures. *Health therapy*: Frequent medical therapy. *Surgical therapy*: Presurgical preparation, painful surgical incision
LIFESTYLE: Involvement in too many activities above the person's comfort level
SITUATIONAL FACTORS: Child rearing, acute or chronic illness of significant other, impending death of significant other, situation crisis

Data Analysis

Nursing Diagnosis
POTENTIAL FOR INADEQUATE SLEEP/REST: The presence of stressors that increase the possibility of the actual occurrence of a person obtaining insufficient sleep or rest

PLANNING

Unmet Needs
Protection from physical harm, increased learning

Expected Outcome
No signs or symptoms of inadequate sleep or rest will occur
  OR
If signs and symptoms occur, they will be promptly recognized as an actual problem and will be treated appropriately
Person verbalizes an understanding of and practices preventive methods

NURSING INTERVENTIONS

Nursing Treatments
Encourage adequate rest
Encourage alternate rest and activity
Plan undisturbed periods for the patient
Provide quiet

Nursing Observations
Observe the pattern of sleep (the sleep schedule)
Observe for the quantity (number of hours) and inquire about the quality of sleep (light, deep, interrupted, or uninterrupted sleep)

Health Teaching
Describe those symptoms that should be reported (lack of sleep)
Inform of the recommended minimum hours of sleep (infants 10–20 hours, children 10–14 hours, adults 7–9 hours, aging persons 5–7 hours, ill persons require additional sleep)
Inform that underweight persons require additional sleep
Recommend a regular sleeping schedule
Explain why the potential problem could become actual (a person could fail to obtain adequate sleep if the body needs additional rest, in excess of normal requirements, to restore cell energy depleted by activity, healing, or stress)
Explain the reason for and intended effect of the preventive therapy

EVALUATION
Record actual outcome

Potential Threats to Communication During Illness

POTENTIAL FOR IMPAIRED VERBAL COMMUNICATIONS[362,371,451]

ASSESSMENT
Data Collection
Subjective Data
• There are no actual symptoms of impaired communications

Objective Data
• There are no actual signs of impaired communications

Related Data
• There are one or more stressors present that increase the possibility that impaired communications will occur

HEALTH CARE FACTORS: *Surgical procedure*: Scheduled glossectomy, laryngectomy, tracheostomy, wiring of mandible fracture, endotracheal intubation

Data Analysis
Nursing Diagnosis
POTENTIAL FOR IMPAIRED VERBAL COMMUNICATIONS: The presence of stressors that increase the possibility of the actual occurrence of a person being unable to verbally communicate

PLANNING
Unmet Needs
Protection from physical harm, increased learning

Expected Outcome
Person will be prepared for communication impairment that can potentially occur from illness or therapy
Person will express satisfaction with alternate communication methods offered in preparation for the potential loss

NURSING INTERVENTIONS
Nursing Treatments
Approach unhurriedly
Arrange geographic placement (so the person can see the nurses)
Encourage the person to ask questions (about the potential communication loss)
Reassure verbally (that the nurse will anticipate the person's needs and will provide communication methods)
Encourage simple signal language during impaired communication

Nursing Observations
Observe for an excessive stress level (about the potential loss of speech)

Health Teaching
Explain that questions need to be phrased for yes and no answers when there is impaired speech delivery
Recommend communication by gesture
Inform that the tracheostomy must be covered in order to speak
Inform that artificial larynxes are available
Inform that esophageal speech therapy is available
Explain why the potential problem could become actual (disease or removal of speech organs often result in loss of verbal communication)
Explain the reason for and intended effect of the assistive therapy

EVALUATION
Record actual outcome

Potential Threats from Drug Therapy

POTENTIAL FOR ADVERSE RESPONSE RELATED TO DRUG INTAKE[299,386]

ASSESSMENT
Data Collection
Subjective Data
• There are no actual symptoms of an adverse drug effect

Objective Data
• There are no actual signs of an adverse drug effect

Related Data
• There are one or more stressors present that increase the possibility that an adverse drug effect will occur
BIRTH DEFECTS: Cretinism
BIRTH STATUS: Premature infant
INHERITED FACTORS: Familial tendency for allergies
DISEASES: Addison's disease, allergic rhinitis, asthma, cachexia, eczema, hepatic insufficiency or failure, malnutrition, renal insufficiency or failure, thyrotoxicosis
SIGNS AND SYMPTOMS: Dehydration, low weight
HEALTH CARE FACTORS: *Drug therapy*: Known sensitivity to or intolerance for a drug(s), prolonged drug therapy
DEVELOPMENTAL PHASE: Infancy, old age
HUMAN ERROR: Duplication of drugs, taking an incorrect drug dosage

Data Analysis
Nursing Diagnosis
POTENTIAL FOR ADVERSE DRUG EFFECT: The presence of stressors that increase the possibility of the actual occurrence of an undesirable or exaggerated reaction to a drug

PLANNING
Unmet Needs
Protection from physical harm, increased learning
Expected Outcome
No signs or symptoms of adverse response to drug intake will occur
   OR
If signs and symptoms occur, they will be promptly recognized as an actual problem and will be treated appropriately

NURSING INTERVENTIONS
Nursing Treatments
Provide standby equipment and drugs (intravenous fluids, oxygen, epinephrine)
Obtain a complete present and past history
Provide frequent contact with the person (every 5 minutes for 30 minutes after the drug is administered)
   OR
Attend the patient constantly (if appropriate)

Administer a drug sensitivity test (if appropriate)
Withhold the drug (if the person's drug intolerance is known to exist)

Nursing Observations
Measure the body weight
Inspect the chest for respiratory rate and rhythm
Monitor the blood pressure
Palpate the pulse for rate, rhythm, and volume
Observe for complaints of dizziness, headache, nausea, numbness and tingling, weakness, headache, tinnitus, nervousness, nasal congestion
Observe for dyspnea, irritability, confusion, restlessness, tetany, vomiting

Health Teaching
Describe those symptoms which should be reported (adverse symptoms of the specific drug)
Explain the importance of wearing a Medic Alert tag (if the intolerance is known)
Recommend that self-medication be avoided
Explain why the potential problem could become actual (an exaggerated reaction to a drug can occur when there is excessively rapid drug absorption, when the dose is too large for body weight, or when impaired circulation or excretion causes cumulative effects)
Explain the reason for and intended effect of the preventive therapy

EVALUATION

Record actual outcome

POTENTIAL FOR ADVERSE RESPONSE RELATED TO DRUG INTERACTIONS[212,299]

ASSESSMENT

Data Collection

Subjective Data
• There are no actual symptoms of an adverse drug interaction

Objective Data
• There are no actual signs of an adverse drug interaction

Related Data
• There are one or more stressors present that increase the possibility that an adverse drug interaction will occur
HEALTH CARE FACTORS: *Drug therapy:* The intake of multiple drugs, the intake of foods that alter the chemical components of the drug

Data Analysis

Nursing Diagnosis
POTENTIAL FOR ADVERSE RESPONSE RELATED TO DRUG INTERACTIONS: The presence of stressors that increase the possibility of the actual occurrence of an undesired drug effect resulting from the drug's chemical interaction with another drug or food substance

PLANNING

Unmet Needs
Protection from physical harm, increased learning

Expected Outcome
No signs or symptoms of adverse response to drug interactions will occur

OR

If signs and symptoms occur, they will be promptly recognized as an actual problem and will be treated appropriately

Person verbalizes an understanding of and practices preventive methods

NURSING INTERVENTIONS

Nursing Treatments

Obtain a complete present and past history (regarding illnesses, problems with drugs, etc.)

Provide standby equipment and drugs (intravenous fluids, oxygen, drug antidotes, etc.)

Consult with the physician (about possible adverse responses to drug or food interactions)

Nursing Observations

Inspect the chest for respiratory rate and rhythm

Monitor the blood pressure

Palpate the pulse for rate, rhythm, and volume

Observe for complaints of dizziness, headache, nausea, numbness and tingling, weakness, tinnitus, nervousness, nasal congestion

Observe for dyspnea, irritability, confusion, restlessness, tetany, vomiting

Health Teaching

Describe those symptoms that should be reported (adverse symptoms of the specific drug or food interactions)

Recommend that self-medication be avoided

Explain which drugs and foods have adverse interactions (look up this intervention in Part Four for details of the most common adverse interactions)

Explain the importance of learning and practicing health principles

Explain why the potential problem could become actual (the chemical properties of foods and drugs have the capacity to interact adversely)

Explain the reason for and intended effects of the preventive methods

EVALUATION

Record actual outcome

Potential Threats to Psychosocial Homeostasis

POTENTIAL FOR ANXIETY/FEAR[105,471]

ASSESSMENT

Data Collection

Subjective Data
• There are no actual symptoms of anxiety or fear

Objective Data
• There are no actual signs of anxiety or fear

Related Data
• There are one or more stressors present that increase the possibility that anxiety or fear will occur

BIRTH DEFECTS: Giving birth to an imperfect infant

DISEASES: Any

INJURIES: Any

SIGNS AND SYMPTOMS: Any but especially pain, hypoxia

PSYCHOSOCIAL FACTORS: A possible threat of real or imagined danger

HUMAN BODY: *Natural body function:* Childbirth. *Body states:* Menses, pregnancy, menepause, male climacteric

HEALTH CARE FACTORS: *Health care costs:* High. *Health care environment:* Contact with sick persons in the health care environment; admittance to a coronary, intensive care, or isolation unit or to a locked psychiatric unit or emergency room; exposure to intense human suffering of persons in the health care environment; unfamiliar health care environment. *Health care provider:* Absence of or lack of a health care provider. *Hospitalization or institutionalization of self or significant other:* Separation from significant other during hospitalization. *Visiting hours:* Limited and restrictive visiting hours. *Diagnostic procedures:* Any. *Medical diagnosis:* Impending, inconclusive, or unfavorable. *Health therapy:* Unfamiliar or termination of health therapy. *Medical therapy:* Impending or any medical therapy. *Drug therapy:* Impending or any drug therapy, especially stimulant drugs such as amphetamines, corticosteroids, epinephrine, etc. *Surgical therapy:* Impending or any surgery, anesthesia. *Therapeutic equipment or devices:* Any. *Follow-up evaluation:* Impending

LIFESTYLE: High caffeine or sugar intake, alcohol or drug abuse

DEVELOPMENTAL PHASES: Any but especially adolescence, old age

SITUATIONAL FACTORS: Any impending situational crisis or stress, especially impending death of self or significant other

ENVIRONMENTAL FACTORS: *Cataclysm:* Flood, hurricane, etc. *Darkness:* In the patient's room or at night. *Sights:* Obnoxious. *Television:* Frightening or violent films

Data Analysis

Nursing Diagnosis

POTENTIAL FOR ANXIETY/FEAR: The presence of stressors that increase the possibility of the actual occurrence of nonspecific or specific perceptions of threat or danger

PLANNING

Unmet Needs

Protection from psychologic threat, increased learning

Expected Outcome

No signs or symptoms of anxiety or fear will occur
> OR

If signs and symptoms occur, they will be promptly recognized as an actual problem and will be treated appropriately

NURSING INTERVENTIONS

Nursing Treatments

Approach unhurriedly

Reassure verbally

Demonstrate calmness

Provide an atmosphere of acceptance

Attend the patient constantly (during potentially anxiety-provoking procedures, etc.)
> AND

Provide frequent contact with the person (at other times)

Encourage the expression of feelings

Listen attentively
> AND

Talk with the person

Encourage the person to ask questions (about the situation)

Provide reliable information

Arrange situations that encourage the person's autonomy

Avoid causing embarrassing situations, causing intense emotional situations

Do not allow unpleasant surprise situations
Encourage gradual mastery of a situation
Ensure the person's feeling of safety before introducing any unpleasantness
Introduce one anxiety-provoking situation at a time
Present change gradually
Avoid forcing the person into rapid adaptation to change by accepting the person's unique pattern of adjustment
Provide objects that symbolize safeness (a child's favorite toy, an adult's special pillow)
Reduce the demands placed on the patient
Refrain from performing nonessential procedures
Introduce to persons who have successfully undergone the same experience
Give the patient a tour through the health care facility
Touch the patient judiciously
Involve the family (as much as possible)

Nursing Observations

Observe for complaints of anxiety or fear (restlessness, irritability, impaired functioning)
Identify disturbing conversation topics

Health Teaching

Describe those symptoms that should be reported (anxiety, fear)
Recommend methods for achieving total relaxation (such as controlled breathing, listening to soft music)
Explain why the potential problem could become actual (any perception of threat results in anxiety or fear)
Explain the reason for and intended effect of the preventive therapy

EVALUATION

Record actual outcome

POTENTIAL FOR ASSAULTIVE/VIOLENT BEHAVIOR[338,481,656]

ASSESSMENT

Data Collection

Subjective Data
• There are no actual symptoms of assaultive or violent behavior

Objective Data
• There are no actual signs of assaultive or violent behavior

Related Data
• There are one or more stressors present that increase the possibility that assaultive or violent behavior will occur
DISEASES: Alcoholism, drug addiction, manic–depressive psychosis, paranoid state, schizophrenia
PSYCHOSOCIAL FACTORS: Lack of affection, nonachievement of developmental conscience, lack of impulse and emotional control, threat of real or imagined danger, incorrect early learning that aggression is a normal response to threat, threat of frustration, lack of fear of punishment, lack of training in self-discipline, exposure to parental aggression, threat of lack of control of a life situation, history of aggression, lack of training in social skills, lack of or threat to self-esteem, threat of having needs unfulfilled through constructive behavior (which results in negative or destructive behavior), lack of motivation toward standards of high performance
LIFESTYLE: Alcohol or drug abuse

Data Analysis

Nursing Diagnosis

POTENTIAL FOR ASSAULTIVE/VIOLENT BEHAVIOR: The presence of stressors that increase the possibility of the actual occurrence of a person becoming actively aggressive toward others

PLANNING

Unmet Needs

Protection from physical harm and psychologic threat, increased learning

Expected Outcome

No signs or symptoms of assaultive or violent behavior will occur
>OR

If signs and symptoms occur, they will be promptly recognized as an actual problem and will be treated appropriately

NURSING INTERVENTIONS

Nursing Treatments

Approach unhurriedly
Demonstrate calmness (do not express or display any anxiety)
Provide an atmosphere of acceptance
Encourage the expression of feelings (ask the person why he is angry)
Listen attentively
>AND

Talk with the patient
Provide whatever the person needs to use his usual coping mechanisms (provided the coping mechanisms are normal)
Encourage mutual problem solving
Explore with the patient the effects of his behavior on others
Encourage respect for the rights of others
Encourage role-playing to develop sensitivity
Encourage participation in therapeutic group interaction
Encourage the acceptance of partial goal satisfaction (if frustration precipitates aggression)
Encourage noncompetitive activities (if competition precipitates aggression)
Support a realistic assessment of the situation (if misperception precipitates aggression)
Hold the person responsible for his behavior (do not allow the person to blame others)
Suggest more appropriate means of need gratification (if pleasure is gained from hurting others)
Set limits on unacceptable behavior (violence is not acceptable)
Remove the stimulus for the emotion (of anger)
Arrange geographic placement (in a room near the nurses' station)
Arrange orderly surroundings (to reduce confusion, which can precipitate violence)
Keep the person's door open (so the nurse has an exit available if acute violence occurs)
Provide seclusion (if needed)
Reduce the demands placed on the person
Refrain from arguing, from negatively criticizing
Refrain from using punitive measures (in exercising authority)
Involve the family (and accept what they relate causes violence in the person)
Consult with the physician (about medications to be given early before violence occurs)

Nursing Observations

Determine the degree of insight that the person has
Evaluate the person's relatedness with others
Evaluate the significance of emotional distress mannerisms, of nonverbal communication
Identify abnormal perceptions (illusions, hallucinations)
Identify abnormal thought content (delusions, obsessive thoughts)

Observe for impaired conceptual thinking (irrational thought)
Observe for incoherent thinking (disorganized thought processes)
Identify disturbing conversation topics and emotion-stimulating events
Identify the current dominant emotion (anger, and note its severity)
Identify inappropriate emotional responses (increasing agitation or irritability, refusal to cooperate)
Identify potentially destructive behavior (threats of assault or violence)
Determine the extent of group pressure conformity (in relationship to potential destructive behavior)
Identify life values significant to the person (that favor nonviolence)
Identify the appropriate use of defense mechanisms, the inappropriate use of defense mechanisms
Observe for evidence that the person is reaching out for emotional support
Observe for an excessive stress level (such as exaggerated sensitivity to noise or activity)

Health Teaching

Advise against causing defensive responses in others
Explain what is considered justifiable aggression (defending oneself)
Advise that highly emotional situations be avoided
Advise that negative responses from others be regarded with minimum significance (even though there are feelings about such responses)
Advise that significant persons express caring for one another
Explain how to channel emotional energy and obtain release from stress (running, chopping wood, creative activities, talking things over, laughing)
Recommend things to do when the person begins to feel out of control (wash the hands and face with cold water, withdraw from the situation, etc.)
Teach how to use the problem-solving method
Explain why persons should maintain self-control (out of respect for others, to obtain social acceptance)
Recommend that behavioral limits be set (by the family)
Explain how to set behaviorial limits
Advise that discipline be consistent
Explain why the potential problem could become actual (the perception of threat and lack of impulse control can lead to assaultive or violent behavior)
Explain the reason for and intended effect of the preventive therapy

EVALUATION

Record actual outcome

POTENTIAL FOR DISTRUST[105,471]

ASSESSMENT

Data Collection

Subjective Data
• There are no actual symptoms of distrust

Objective Data
• There are no actual signs of distrust

Related Data
• There are one or more stressors present that increase the possibility that distrust will occur
DISEASES: Paranoia, schizophrenia

PSYCHOSOCIAL FACTORS: Lack of communication with others, threat of deception by a significant other or health care provider

HEALTH CARE FACTORS: *Health care delivery*: Low-quality health care delivery. *Health care provider*: The suggestion by a health care provider that symptoms are not real. *Medical diagnosis*: Inconclusive medical diagnosis, differing opinions of the medical diagnosis. *Health therapy*: Delayed or unsuccessful medical, drug, or surgical therapy. *Drug therapy*: Use of placebos

Data Analysis

Nursing Diagnosis

POTENTIAL FOR DISTRUST: The presence of stressors that increase the possibility of the actual occurrence of a trusting person developing a sense of distrust toward others

PLANNING

Unmet Needs

Protection from psychologic threat, increased learning

Expected Outcome

No signs or symptoms of distrust will occur

OR

If signs and symptoms occur, they will be promptly recognized as an actual problem and will be treated appropriately

NURSING INTERVENTIONS

Nursing Treatments

Approach unhurriedly

Provide an atmosphere of acceptance

Demonstrate calmness

Touch the person judiciously

Arrange situations that encourage the person's autonomy

Ensure the person's feeling of safety before introducing unpleasantness

Maintain consistent staff behavior

Follow through on promises

OR

Refrain from making promises

Maintain social formality or informality (whichever is most suitable to the patient)

Provide emotionally safe experiences

Talk with the person

Encourage the person to ask questions

Listen attentively

Provide reliable information

Provide frequent contact with the person

Refrain from negatively criticizing

Refrain from performing nonessential procedures

Involve the family (as much as possible)

Nursing Observations

Identify disturbing conversation topics (indicating distrust)

Evaluate the significance of nonverbal communication (such as hiding things, which suggests distrust)

Health Teaching

Explain why the potential problem could become actual (previous deception by others and learned distrust can result in disturbing behavior)

Explain the reason for and intended effect of the preventive therapy

EVALUATION

Record actual outcome

POTENTIAL FOR EMOTIONAL DEPRIVATION[105,471]

ASSESSMENT

Data Collection

Subjective Data
• There are no actual symptoms of emotional deprivation

Objective Data
• There are no actual signs of emotional deprivation

Related Data
• There are one or more stressors present that increase the possibility that emotional deprivation will occur
BIRTH STATUS: Premature infant (in an isolette)
PSYCHOSOCIAL FACTORS: Use of passive–aggressive behavior
HEALTH CARE FACTORS: *Hospitalization or institutionalization*: Of self or significant other. *Health care environment*: Intensive care, isolation unit, locked psychiatric unit
DEVELOPMENTAL FACTORS: Old age
LIFESTYLE: Little or no socialization
SITUATIONAL FACTORS: Chronic illness, neglect of child or elderly parent

Data Analysis

Nursing Diagnosis
POTENTIAL FOR EMOTIONAL DEPRIVATION: The presence of stressors that increase the possibility of the actual occurrence of being without externally stimulated emotional experience

PLANNING

Unmet Needs
Protection from psychologic threat, increased learning

Expected Outcome
No signs or symptoms of emotional deprivation will occur
OR
If signs and symptoms occur, they will be promptly recognized as an actual problem and will be treated appropriately

NURSING INTERVENTIONS

Nursing Treatments
Approach unhurriedly
Reassure verbally (that the nurse cares about the person)
Touch the person frequently
Provide frequent contact with the person
Involve the family (as much as possible)
Encourage visiting by significant others (who can relate caring)

Nursing Observations
Observe for lethargy, apathy
Observe for complaints of fatigue
Observe for impaired self-attitude
Observe for evidence that the person is reaching out for emotional support (through frequent complaints and requests)

Health Teaching
Advise that significant persons express caring for one another
Recommend the person have a pet (if there are no friends or relatives available)
Explain why the potential problem could become actual (persons who receive little or no positive emotional responses from social contacts can become emotionally deprived)
Explain the reason for and intended effect of the preventive therapy

EVALUATION
Record actual outcome

POTENTIAL FOR DELAYED MATERNAL–INFANT BONDING[313,527]

ASSESSMENT

Data Collection

Subjective Data
• There are no actual symptoms of delayed bonding

Objective Data
• There are no actual signs of delayed bonding

Related Data
• There are one or more stressors present that increase the possibility that delayed bonding will occur
BIRTH STATUS: Premature infant, sick newborn
HEALTH CARE FACTORS: *Surgical procedures*: Cesarean section
SITUATIONAL FACTORS: Illness of mother or infant

Data Analysis

Nursing Diagnosis
POTENTIAL FOR DELAYED MATERNAL–INFANT BONDING: The presence of stressors that increase the possibility of the actual occurrence of a delayed attachment between a mother and child

PLANNING

Unmet Needs
Comfort, protection from psychologic threat, caring and communicating relationships, increased learning

Expected Outcome
Mother will express warm, caring feelings about and toward the infant
Infant will respond positively to the mother

NURSING INTERVENTIONS

Nursing Treatments
Encourage the mother to see and touch the newborn immediately after birth (by placing the infant on the mother's abdomen or in her arms if possible or by allowing her to touch the infant in the incubator)
Encourage the mother to explore the newborn (to unwrap the infant, to look at and feel the infant's body as soon as possible after birth)
Encourage the expression of feelings (about the child)
Offer feedback of the mother's expressed feelings
Involve the mother (in the infant's care, feeding, and therapy as much as possible)
Set an example by role modeling (show how to care for and relate to the infant by your example)
Provide rooming-in (if appropriate to the situation)

Nursing Observations
Observe for evidence of a favorable response to therapy (bonding between mother and child)

Health Teaching

Explain about the unique personality of each child (that even if the child is not what was expected, the mother can give to and receive love from the child)

Explain the reason for and intended effect of the methods used

EVALUATION

Record actual outcome

POTENTIAL FOR PSYCHOLOGIC DECOMPENSATION[105,471]

ASSESSMENT

Data Collection

Subjective Data
• There are no actual symptoms of psychologic decompensation

Objective Data
• There are no actual signs of psychologic decompensation

Related Data
• There are one or more stressors present that increase the possibility that psychologic decompensation will occur

DISEASES: Paranoia, major depression, manic–depressive psychosis, schizophrenia

PSYCHOSOCIAL FACTORS: Lack of competency in using effective coping mechanisms

HEALTH CARE FACTORS: *History of*: Previous decompensation

SITUATIONAL FACTORS: Acute or chronic illness, maturational crisis or stress, multiple crisis situations, situational crisis or stress

Data Analysis

Nursing Diagnosis

POTENTIAL FOR PSYCHOLOGIC DECOMPENSATION: The presence of stressors that increase the possibility of the actual occurrence of a recurrence of nonadaptive thoughts and behaviors resulting in possible psychosis

PLANNING

Unmet Needs

Protection from psychologic threat, increased learning

Expected Outcome

No signs or symptoms of psychologic decompensation will occur
   OR
If signs and symptoms occur, they will be promptly recognized as an actual problem and will be treated appropriately

Person verbalizes an understanding of and practices preventive methods

NURSING INTERVENTIONS

Nursing Treatments

Approach unhurriedly

Reassure verbally (that the nurse is available whenever needed)

Encourage the expression of feelings (during the early stages of stress buildup, before stress becomes overwhelming)

Listen attentively
   AND
Talk with the patient

Provide meetings with supportive persons or groups
Support a realistic assessment of the situation
Encourage the use of normal coping mechanisms
Make a follow-up evaluation (at frequent, periodic intervals)

Nursing Observations

Determine the degree of insight that the person has (into recognizing high stress levels and abnormal coping)
Evaluate the significance of emotional distress mannerisms (which indicate increased stress or decreased functioning ability)
Identify abnormal perceptions (illusions, hallucinations)
Identify abnormal thought content (delusions, obsessive thoughts)
Observe for impaired conceptual thinking (irrational thinking)
Observe for incoherent thinking (disorganized thought process)
Identify disturbing conversation topics (such as expressions of fears, topics that arouse strong emotion, that the person does not feel like himself or that something strange is happening)
Observe for an excessive stress level (exhibited by very active or withdrawn behavior)
Observe for emotional instability (unstable behaviors that become more pronounced)
Observe personal hygiene habits (and determine whether there is decreased ability to care for self)
Observe for requests for increased drug dosage (or for demands for excessive or inappropriate treatment)

Health Teaching

Describe those symptoms that should be reported (depression, anxiety, violence or symptoms specific to the person's problem)
Instruct to report any early symptoms immediately
Explain the importance of persons offering emotional support to one another (to prevent decompensation)
Emphasize the importance of recognizing tension within oneself
Explain that some tension is normal
Explain how to channel emotional energy and obtain release from stress (running, creative activities, talking things over, laughing)
Teach how to use the problem-solving method
Advise that significant others express caring for one another (which provides support and reduces the potential for decompensation)
Explain why the potential problem could become actual (excessive life stresses could cause an inability to continue to function, and the mind escapes from what cannot be dealt with)
Explain the reason for and intended effect of the preventive therapy (to help the patient function at the highest level possible)

EVALUATION

Record actual outcome

12 Nursing Diagnoses of SELF-RESTORATIVE DEFICITS

Domain of Nursing Expertise: Self-Restorative Deficits

This chapter covers that sphere of nursing knowledge and skill related to the individual's incapacity to promote sleep in the manner to which his body is accustomed to falling asleep. It involves substituting the nurse as a sleep-supporting agent. The focus also includes knowledge of energy conservation in dealing with the limited energy resources of illness.

Views of Nursing Leaders That Support This Domain of Nursing Expertise

Components of basic nursing include assisting the patient with . . . sleep and rest. . . .

Virginia Henderson[220:12]

Nursing's object is not only to cure the sick and heal the wounded, but to bring health and ease, rest and comfort to mind and body. . . .

Bertha Harmer[379:67]

As a comprehensive service, nursing includes . . . The promotion of optimal rest and sleep.

Faye Abdellah[187:107 & 111]

Self-Care Deficits in Sleep/Rest

INCAPACITY TO PROMOTE SLEEP READINESS[362,371]

ASSESSMENT

Data Collection

Subjective Data
- Person may or may not relate being unable to attain those environmental and personal factors that help him sleep

  May request special lighting, certain pillows, and blankets, soft music, glass of warm milk, etc.

Objective Data
- Person exhibits behavior such as minimal, ineffective, or no body movement and makes no attempt to prepare for sleep

Data Analysis

Nursing Diagnosis

INCAPACITY TO PROMOTE SLEEP READINESS: Being incapable of carrying out those sleep rituals that one usually carries out in preparation for sleep

Common Etiology (Stressors)

BIRTH DEFECTS: Cerebral palsy, developmental deficit, Duchenne's muscular dystrophy

DISEASES: Brain tumor, carcinoma, cerebrovascular accident, congestive heart failure, diabetic ketoacidosis, encephalitis, Friedreich's ataxia, Guillain-Barré syndrome, Hodgkin's disease, Laennec's cirrhosis, leukemia, major depression, meningitis, multiple sclerosis, myasthenia gravis, myocardial infarction, organic brain syndrome, osteoarthritis, Parkinson's disease, posterolateral sclerosis, psychosis, renal failure, retinal detachment, rheumatoid arthritis, senility, subarachnoid hemorrhage, subdural hematoma, Sydenham's chorea

INJURIES: Burn wound, cerebral concussion, drug overdose, fracture, fracture and compression of the spinal cord, herniated intervertebral disc, traumatic amputation

SIGNS AND SYMPTOMS: Difficulty concentrating, confusion, dizziness, dyspnea, joint swelling, hallucinations, memory loss, pain, paralysis, vertigo, weakness

HEALTH CARE FACTORS: *Medical therapy*: Casting, traction. *Surgical therapy*: Surgery of any kind. *Surgical procedures*: Amputation, replantation of digits, tenoplasty of hand. *Surgical incision*: Painful surgical incision

DEVELOPMENTAL PHASES: Old age

MAJOR PATHOPHYSIOLOGIC FACTORS CAUSING THE PROBLEM: Incapacity to perform activities of daily living can result from any of the following: decreased cardiac output, impaired oxygenation of tissue cells, organ degeneration or damage, impaired transmission of impulses from nerves to muscles, accumulation of toxic metabolic by-products, disrupted cerebral chemical/neuronal balance, tissue function impaired by the inflammatory process, brain cell damage or deficient development

PLANNING

Unmet Needs
Sleep, rest, comfort, dependence, increased learning

Expected Outcome
A nonstimulating environment of quiet and minimal light
Person verbalizes feelings of comfort and relaxation
Person verbalizes readiness for sleep

NURSING INTERVENTIONS

Nursing Treatments
Anticipate needs

Arrange pleasant surroundings
Provide quiet
Maintain a normal room temperature (comfortable to the person)
Darken the room (before sleep)
   OR
Provide a night light
Change the patient's clothing at bedtime
Refresh the patient before sleep (by washing his hands and face, combing his hair, etc.)
Encourage bladder emptying before rest
Massage (the back) gently (before sleep)
Position comfortably
Maintain the person's usual bedtime rituals

Nursing Observations
Observe for evidence of a favorable response to therapy (restful sleep)

Health Teaching
Recommend methods for achieving total relaxation (controlled breathing, soft music)
Explain the reason for and intended effect of the therapy (restful sleep)

EVALUATION

Record actual outcome

PARTIAL INCAPACITY TO PROMOTE SLEEP READINESS[362,371]

ASSESSMENT

Data Collection

Subjective Data
• Person relates his attempt to provide those environmental and personal factors that
   help him sleep
• Requests assistance
   May relate a need for special lighting, certain pillows and blankets, soft music, glass of
   warm milk, etc.

Objective Data
• Person exhibits behavior such as struggling to retrieve desired sleep-inducing object,
   restlessness

Data Analysis

Nursing Diagnosis
PARTIAL INCAPACITY TO PROMOTE SLEEP READINESS: Being capable of but needing assistance with
   carrying out those sleep rituals that one usually carries out in preparation for sleep

Common Etiology (Stressors)
BIRTH DEFECTS: Blindness, cerebral palsy, developmental deficit, Down's syndrome, Duchenne's muscular dystrophy
DISEASES: Aortic insufficiency, aortic stenosis, aplastic anemia, blindness, bursitis, cachexia, carcinoma, cataracts, cerebrovascular accident, congestive heart failure, diplopia,
   encephalitis, Friedreich's ataxia, Guillain-Barré syndrome, Hodgkin's disease, Laennec's cirrhosis, leukemia, major depression, manic–depressive psychosis, multiple sclerosis, myasthenia gravis, myocardial infarction, organic brain syndrome, osteoarthritis,
   Parkinson's disease, posterolateral sclerosis, psychosis, retinal detachment, rheumatoid arthritis, senility, Sydenham's chorea
INJURIES: Back strain, burn wound, cerebral concussion, dislocation, drug overdose, fracture, fracture and compression of the spinal cord, herniated intervertebral disc, traumatic amputation, whiplash injury
SIGNS AND SYMPTOMS: Blurred vision, difficulty concentrating, confusion, diplopia, dizziness, dyspnea, joint swelling, memory loss, pain, vertigo, weakness

HEALTH CARE FACTORS: *Drugs*: Narcotics, sedatives, tranquilizers. *Medical therapy*: Blood transfusion, casting, intravenous infusion, traction. *Surgical therapy*: Surgery of any kind. *Surgical procedures*: Amputation, replantation of digits, tenoplasty of hand. *Surgical incision*: Painful surgical incision

DEVELOPMENTAL PHASES: Old age

MAJOR PATHOPHYSIOLOGIC FACTORS CAUSING THE PROBLEM: Partial incapacity to perform activities of daily living can result from any of the following: decreased cardiac output, impaired oxygenation of tissue cells, organ degeneration or damage, impaired transmission of impulses from nerves to muscles, accumulation of toxic metabloic byproducts, disrupted cerebral chemical/neuronal balance, tissue function impaired by the inflammatory process, brain cell damage or deficient development

PLANNING

Unmet Needs

Sleep, rest, comfort, dependence, increased learning

Expected Outcome

A nonstimulating environment of quiet and minimal light
Person verbalizes feelings of comfort and relaxation
Person verbalizes readiness for sleep

NURSING INTERVENTIONS

Nursing Treatments

Anticipate needs (for assistance)
Arrange pleasant surroundings
Provide quiet
Maintain a normal room temperature (comfortable for the person)
Darken the room (before sleep)
   OR
Provide a night light
Change the patient's clothing at bedtime
Refresh the patient before sleep (by washing hands and face, combing hair, etc.)
Encourage bladder emptying before rest
Massage (the back) gently (before sleep)
Position comfortably
Maintain the person's usual bedtime rituals

Nursing Observations

Observe for evidence of a favorable response to therapy (restful sleep)

Health Teaching

Recommend methods for achieving total relaxation (controlled breathing, soft music)
Explain the reason for and intended effect of the therapy (restful sleep)

EVALUATION

Record actual outcome

Self-Care Deficits in Energy Needs

UNSKILLED AT CONSERVING PHYSICAL ENERGY[108,735]

ASSESSMENT

Data Collection

Subjective Data

• Person's discussion or questions indicate a need for additional information,

clarification, or validation of information about performing the task of conserving physical energy
OR
- Person's lack of questions or comments indicates not wanting information or not knowing enough to seek information about performing the task of conserving physical energy

Person may not know:
Which activities tend to deplete energy reserves
Methods that can be employed to ease the workload

Objective Data
- Person cannot correctly demonstrate how to perform tasks in an energy-conserving way

Related Data

Commonly Associated Conditions
Aging, postoperative convalescence

Commonly Related Diseases or Injuries
Any disease or injury that weakens the body

Data Analysis

Nursing Diagnosis
UNSKILLED AT CONSERVING PHYSICAL ENERGY: Being nonproficient, with or without knowledge, in the performance of the specific methods used to conserve human energy as it relates to the person's state of health

Common Etiology (Stressors)
HEALTH CARE FACTORS: Lack of health instruction, lack of health-skill experience

PLANNING

Unmet Needs
Comfort, protection from physical harm, dependence, independence, increased learning

Expected Outcome
Correct verbal feedback of the information taught
Behavior modification of using energy-conserving methods

NURSING INTERVENTIONS

Nursing Treatments
Encourage adequate rest
Encourage alternate rest and activity
Encourage the person to ask questions

Nursing Observations
Observe performance level and problems involved in completing the task
Determine teaching effectiveness by verbal feedback

Health Teaching
Explain that socialization depletes the ill person's energy
Explain the need to avoid overexertion (especially when feeling reasonably well)
Recommend adherence to a pace of living with which one is comfortable
Recommend work methods for decreasing human energy consumption (such as eliminating unnecessary work; combining work activities by making two cakes at one time, washing dishes only once a day, etc.; dividing one's time between high-energy- and low-energy-consuming activities by washing the dishes and then sitting down to sew, vacuuming and then preparing a menu; distributing heavy tasks throughout the week by splitting heavy washloads into two days or cleaning one shelf of a large closet each day; duplicating equipment in work areas by keeping one mop upstairs and another downstairs; putting salt and pepper shakers on both the stove and the table; using a cannister or self-propelled vacuum; using a rolling table on which to move things; using lightweight household items such as a travel iron instead of a regular iron, an

electric broom instead of a vacuum cleaner, and plastic mixing bowels instead of glass ones; installing push-bar windows and electric garage doors; living in a single-level ground-floor dwelling to avoid the use of stairs; consistently planning easy meals that include dishes such as casseroles, salads, baked potatoes, frozen cakes or pies, frozen vegetables, brown-and-serve rolls, instant puddings, and premixed foods; doing all the housework in each room instead of moving from room to room doing single tasks; napping whenever possible)

Recommend energy-conserving methods for lifting and moving objects (pushing or pulling should be done with the entire body weight, objects should be lifted with the arms close to the body)

Recommend the pursuit of only one activity at a time

Inform that heavy lifting should be avoided
   AND
Instruct to avoid pushing and pulling activities (in severe energy depletion)

Teach good body mechanics (for ease of movement)

Instruct to sit down whenever possible

EVALUATION

Record actual outcome

13 Nursing Diagnoses of SELF-THERAPY DEFICITS

Domain of Nursing Expertise: Self-Therapy Deficits

This chapter covers that sphere of nursing knowledge and skill related to a person's nonexpertise in performing prescribed therapy for himself. It includes knowledge of treatment methods and methods of bringing the person to the capability of performing his own therapy. It also involves being a substitute agent for those who cannot achieve therapy independence.

Views of Nursing Leaders That Support This Domain of Nursing Expertise

Modern medical advances require nurses to be well-grounded in . . . various medical technologies if they are to effectively assist individuals with health deviation self-care . . . such as effectively carrying out medically prescribed therapeutic measures.

Dorothea Orem[380:50]

It should be made clear that the nurse's function in helping the patient to learn . . . is interpreted here as reinforcing and following the physician's plan of therapy. . . . The nurse's constant purpose should be kept in mind—to restore the patient's independence if this is possible, to help him live as effectively as he can with his inescapable limitations.

Virginia Henderson[220:47&49]

Self-Care Deficits in Managing/Performing Health Therapy

INCAPACITY TO MANAGE HEALTH THERAPY (NAME SPECIFIC THERAPY)[73,278,380]

ASSESSMENT

Data Collection

Subjective Data
- Person may or may not relate being unable to carry out health therapy
  May express feelings of frustration, anger, helplessness

Note: No subjective data in person with an unconscious, immature, or infirmed mental state

Objective Data
- Person exhibits behavior such as minimal, ineffective, or no body movement and makes no visible attempt toward performing the prescribed therapy

Data Analysis

Nursing Diagnosis
INCAPACITY TO MANAGE HEALTH THERAPY: Being incapable of managing the procedures and methods used in prescribed health therapy

Common Etiology (Stressors)
BIRTH DEFECTS: Developmental deficit, Down's syndrome, hydrocephalus
DISEASES: Autism, blindness, cachexia, carcinoma, cerebrovascular accident, congestive heart failure, eclampsia, encephalitis, Friedreich's ataxia, Guillain-Barré syndrome, Hodgkin's disease, Laennec's cirrhosis, leukemia, major depression, manic-depressive psychosis, multiple sclerosis, myasthenia gravis, myocardial infarction, organic brain syndrome, osteoarthritis, Parkinson's disease, posterolateral sclerosis, psychosis, renal failure, rheumatoid arthritis, senility, subarachnoid hemorrhage, subdural hematoma, Sydenham's chorea
INJURIES: Burn wound, cerebral concussion, bone fracture, fracture and compression of the spinal cord, herniated intervertebral disc, poisoning, traumatic amputation
SIGNS AND SYMPTOMS: Difficulty concentrating, confusion, convulsions, dyspnea, hallucinations, memory loss, pain, paralysis, joint swelling, vertigo, weakness
HEALTH CARE FACTORS: *Medical therapy*: Casting, traction. *Surgical therapy*: Surgery of any kind. *Surgical procedures*: Amputation. *Surgical incision*: Painful surgical incision
DEVELOPMENTAL PHASES: Infancy, toddler, childhood, old age
MAJOR PATHOPHYSIOLOGIC FACTORS CAUSING THE PROBLEM: Incapacity to manage health therapy can result from any of the following: decreased cardiac output, impaired oxygenation of tissue cells, organ degeneration or damage, impaired transmission of impulses from nerves to muscles, accumulation of toxic metabolic by-products, disrupted cerebral chemical/neuronal balance, tissue function impaired by the inflammatory process, brain cell damage or deficient development

PLANNING

Unmet Needs
Comfort, protection from physical harm, dependence, increased learning

Expected Outcome
Person receives therapy according to standard procedure at stated times and by prescribed amounts
No evidence of physical injury
Improved health status resulting from therapy

NURSING INTERVENTIONS

Nursing Treatments

Acknowledge dependency

Anticipate needs

Provide and manage the health therapy

Note: The appropriate nursing interventions for *Incapacity to manage (a specific health therapy)* are the same as those listed under *Unskilled at (a specific health therapy)*. For example, the nursing interventions for *Unskilled at amputation stump care* can be used for the diagnosis of *Incapacity to manage amputation stump care*.

Nursing Observations

Observe for side effects of therapy

Observe for evidence of a favorable response to therapy

Observe for readiness to assume self-care

Health Teaching

Explain the reason for and intended effect of the therapy

EVALUATION

Record actual outcome

PARTIAL INCAPACITY TO MANAGE HEALTH THERAPY (NAME SPECIFIC THERAPY)[73,278,380]

ASSESSMENT

Data Collection

Subjective Data

• Person relates attempts at carrying out health therapy

• Requests assistance to complete self-care

  May express feelings of frustration or anger

  May complain of fatigue before completing health therapy

Objective Data

• Person exhibits behaviors such as initiating action toward performing the prescribed therapy

Data Analysis

Nursing Diagnosis

PARTIAL INCAPACITY TO MANAGE HEALTH THERAPY: Being capable of but needing assistance with the procedures and methods used in the prescribed health therapy

Common Etiology (Stressors)

BIRTH DEFECTS: Cerebral palsy, developmental deficit, Down's syndrome, hydrocephalus, Duchenne's muscular dystrophy

DISEASES: Autism, blindness, cachexia, carcinoma, cerebrovascular accident, congestive heart failure, Friedreich's ataxia, Guillain-Barré syndrome, Hodgkin's disease, Laennec's cirrhosis, leukemia, major depression, manic-depressive psychosis, multiple sclerosis, myasthenia gravis, myocardial infarction, organic brain syndrome, osteoarthritis, Parkinson's disease, posterolateral sclerosis, renal failure, retinal detachment, rheumatoid arthritis, senility, Sydenham's chorea

INJURIES: Burn wound, bone fracture, fracture and compression of the spinal cord

SIGNS AND SYMPTOMS: Difficulty concentrating, confusion, diplopia, dizziness, dyspnea, fatigue, memory loss, pain, joint swelling, vertigo, weakness

HEALTH CARE FACTORS: *Drug therapy*: Narcotics, sedatives, tranquilizers. *Medical therapy*: Casting, intravenous infusion, traction, blood transfusion. *Surgical therapy*: Surgery of any kind. *Surgical procedures*: Amputation. *Surgical incision*: Painful surgical incision

DEVELOPMENTAL PHASES: Childhood, old age.

MAJOR PATHOPHYSIOLOGIC FACTORS CAUSING THE PROBLEM: Partial incapacity to manage health therapy can result from any of the following: decreased cardiac output, impaired oxygenation of tissue cells, organ degeneration or damage, impaired transmission of impulses from nerves to muscles, accumulation of toxic metabolic by-products, disrupted cerebral chemical/neuronal balance, tissue function impaired by the inflammatory process, brain cell damage or deficient development

PLANNING

Unmet Needs

Comfort, protection from physical harm, dependence, independence, increased learning

Expected Outcome

Person receives therapy according to standard procedure at stated times and by the prescribed amounts

No evidence of physical injury

Improved health status resulting from therapy

Person performs at an expected level of independent self-care

NURSING INTERVENTIONS

Nursing Treatments

Provide assistance until the person is fully able to assume self-care

Anticipate needs (for assistance)

Provide and manage the health therapy (as needed)

Encourage self-performance

Note: The appropriate nursing interventions for *Partial incapacity to manage (a specific health therapy)* are the same as those listed under *Unskilled at (a specific health therapy).* For example, the nursing interventions for *Unskilled at amputation stump care* can be used for the diagnosis of *Partial incapacity to manage amputation stump care.*

Nursing Observations

Observe for side effects of therapy

Observe for evidence of a favorable response to therapy

Observe performance level and problems involved in completing the tasks

Health Teaching

Explain the reason for and intended effect of the therapy

EVALUATION

Record actual outcome

UNSKILLED AT AMPUTATION STUMP CARE[73,451]

ASSESSMENT

Data Collection

Subjective Data

• Person's discussion or questions indicate a need for additional information, clarification, or validation of information about performing the task of caring for an amputation stump

  OR

• Person's lack of questions or comments indicates not wanting information or not knowing enough to seek information about performing the task of caring for an amputation stump

  Person may not know:

    When and how to change the dressing

Correct stump positioning
Specific exercises
What preparations are necessary for wearing a prosthesis

Objective Data
• Person cannot correctly demonstrate how to:
Clean the site
Wrap or bandage the stump for shaping or molding it
Apply a stump sock
Percuss the stump
Do therapeutic exercises
Properly position the stump

Related Data
Commonly Related Diseases
Arteriosclerosis, Buerger's disease, carcinoma, diabetes mellitus, Raynaud's disease

Commonly Related Injuries
Crush injury, frostbite

Data Analysis

Nursing Diagnosis
UNSKILLED AT AMPUTATION STUMP CARE: Being nonproficient, with or without knowledge, in the performance of the specific task of cleansing and caring for an amputation stump and preparing the stump for a prosthesis

Common Etiology (Stressors)
HEALTH CARE FACTORS: Lack of health instruction, lack of health-skill experience

PLANNING

Unmet Needs
Exercise, comfort, cleanliness, protection from physical harm, dependence, mastery and competence in skills, independence, increased learning

Expected Outcome
Clean amputation stump and dressing
Routine stump exercising and percussing
Correct stump shaping and positioning
Correct verbal feedback of the information taught
Correct return demonstration of how to clean and bandage the amputation stump, apply a stump sock, exercise, percuss and position the stump

NURSING INTERVENTIONS

Nursing Treatments
Provide temporary assistance until the skill is learned
Anticipate needs (for assistance)
Change the dressing frequently
Clean (stump) with surgical soap
Wrap the amputation stump
Place the amputation stump in the extension position
Do not place the amputation stump in the flexion position
Exercise in range of motion
Place a bedboard under the mattress
Percuss the amputation stump to increase firmness
Apply a stump sock
Encourage the person to ask questions
Encourage self-performance

Nursing Observations
Observe for signs of healing (closure of wound edges, no inflammation or drainage)
Inspect for bleeding

Observe the amputation stump for odor
Determine if the prosthesis is effective
Inspect for signs of (skin) irritation (from the prosthesis)
Observe for readiness to assume self-care
Determine teaching effectiveness by testing, verbal feedback, and return demonstration

Health Teaching

Explain the need for maintaining a firm surface under the hip of an amputated leg
Instruct to lie in the prone position (several times each day and night)
Instruct that the flexion stump position be avoided, that pillows not be placed under the
  knees, that the amputation stump should not be rested on the crutch handrail
Instruct to place a pillow between the thighs in below-knee amputation
Teach how to apply a stump sock
Instruct to frequently wash the stump sock
Instruct that several stump socks should not be worn simultaneously
Instruct to gradually increase the wearing time of the prosthesis
Teach good posture when walking with a leg prosthesis
Instruct to avoid hiking the shoulder when walking with a leg prosthesis
Teach how to use a temporary prosthesis, how to do above-knee stump exercises, how
  to do below-knee stump exercises, how to percuss the amputation stump, how to
  wrap an amputation stump, how to do range-of-motion exercises
Explain the reason for and the intended effect of the therapy

EVALUATION

Record actual outcome

UNSKILLED AT ARTERIOVENOUS SHUNT CARE[72,73,451]

ASSESSMENT

Data Collection

Subjective Data

• Person's discussion or questions indicate a need for additional information,
  clarification, or validation of information about performing the task of caring for an
  arteriovenous (AV) shunt
    OR
• Person's lack of questions or comments indicates not wanting information or not
  knowing enough to seek information about performing the task of caring for an AV
  shunt
  Person may not know:
    The methods of cleaning and handling the shunt
    The precautions to be taken to prevent injury and hemorrhage
    The signs and symptoms that should be reported

Objective Data

• Person cannot correctly demonstrate how to:
    Maintain sterile technique
    Clean the cannula
    Clean the dressing
    Maintain shunt patency for use in hemodialysis

Related Data
Commonly Related Diseases
Renal failure

Data Analysis

Nursing Diagnosis
UNSKILLED AT ARTERIOVENOUS SHUNT CARE: Being nonproficient, with or without knowledge, in the performance of the specific task of maintaining proper care and functioning of tubing surgically placed in an artery and vein for the purpose of hemodialysis

Common Etiology (Stressors)
HEALTH CARE FACTORS: Lack of health instruction, lack of health-skill experience

PLANNING

Unmet Needs
Comfort, cleanliness, protection from physical harm, dependence, mastery and competence in skills, independence, increased learning

Expected Outcome
Clean, patent, noninfected AV shunt
Correct verbal feedback of the information taught
Correct return demonstration of how to clean the cannula and maintain patency and sterile technique

NURSING INTERVENTIONS

Nursing Treatments
Provide and manage the health therapy
    OR
Provide temporary assistance until the skill is learned
Anticipate needs (for assistance)
Handle gently
Clean with surgical soap (around the cannula)
Apply an antibiotic ointment
Apply a sterile dressing
Change the dressing frequently
Refrain from giving local cold applications
Refrain from tight bandaging
Encourage the person to ask questions
Encourage self-performance

Nursing Observations
Auscultate and palpate the AV shunt for patency
Inspect for edema, for inflammation, for drainage
Monitor the oral temperature (for fever)
Obtain a bacterial culture (of any exudate)
Observe for readiness to assume self-care
Determine teaching effectiveness by testing, verbal feedback, and return demonstration

Health Teaching
Teach how to care for an AV shunt (clean the shunt and surrounding skin, change the dressing daily, observe for joint kinks and slipping of joint rings)
Explain the need to avoid sudden movements of an extremity having an AV shunt
Instruct to maintain skin dryness (on the extremity with the AV shunt)
Instruct that it is essential to carry an AV shunt clamp
Describe those symptoms that should be reported (pain, inflammation)
Explain the reason for and intended effect of the therapy

EVALUATION

Record actual outcome

UNSKILLED AT BANDAGING[138,662]

ASSESSMENT

Data Collection

Subjective Data
- Person's discussion or questions indicate a need for additional information, clarification, or validation of information about performing the task of applying a bandage
   OR
- Person's lack of questions or comments indicates not wanting information or not knowing enough to seek information about performing the task of applying a bandage
  Person may not know:
    Different types of bandages
    Purposes of bandaging
    Precautions to be taken when bandaging

Objective Data
- Person cannot correctly demonstrate how to:
    Apply and remove a bandage

Data Analysis

Nursing Diagnosis
UNSKILLED AT BANDAGING: Being nonproficient, with or without knowledge, in the performance of the specific task of applying a comfortable and effective bandage to a body part

Common Etiology (Stressors)
HEALTH CARE FACTORS: Lack of health instruction, lack of health-skill experience

PLANNING

Unmet Needs
Comfort, cleanliness, protection from physical harm, dependence, mastery and competence in skills, independence, increased learning

Expected Outcome
Clean, nonconstrictive but securely anchored bandage
Correct verbal feedback of the information taught
Correct return demonstration of how to apply and remove a bandage

NURSING INTERVENTIONS

Nursing Treatments
Provide temporary assistance until the skill is learned
Apply a sterile dressing (before applying the clean bandage)
Refrain from tight bandaging (over the dressing)
Encourage the person or family to ask questions
Encourage self-performance

Nursing Observations
Observe for readiness to assume self-care
Determine teaching effectiveness by testing, verbal feedback, and return demonstration

Health Teaching
Teach the types of bandages to be used (ace bandage for support, gauze for molding, flannel for warmth)
Teach the specific procedure of how to apply bandages (of all types such as circular, spiral, figure-eight, etc.)
Teach the precautions to be taken in bandaging (avoid constriction of circulation, joint nonalignment)

Explain the reason for and intended effect of the therapy (for skin cleanliness, to limit body movement, to secure dressings in place, to provide support, to maintain pressure, to aid circulation)

EVALUATION

Record actual outcome

UNSKILLED AT BURN WOUND CARE[26,42,73,219,451,768]

ASSESSMENT

Data Collection

Subjective Data

- Person's discussion or questions indicate a need for additional information, clarification, or validation of information about performing the task of caring for a burn wound

  OR

- Person's lack of questions or comments indicates not wanting information or not knowing enough to seek information about performing the task of caring for a burn wound

  Person may not know:

  The precautions to be taken to reduce burn wound complications

  The signs of burn wound infection

Objective Data

- Person cannot correctly demonstrate how to:

  Bathe and debride a burn wound

  Apply prescribed medication

  Change the dressing

  Do the prescribed exercises

Related Data

Commonly Related Injury

Second-degree (partial thickness) or third-degree (full thickness) burn

Data Analysis

Nursing Diagnosis

UNSKILLED AT BURN WOUND CARE: Being nonproficient, with or without knowledge, in the performance of the specific task of maintaining proper care of a wound resulting from a burn injury

Common Etiology (Stressors)

HEALTH CARE FACTORS: Lack of health instruction, lack of health-skill experience

PLANNING

Unmet Needs

Comfort, cleanliness, protection from physical harm, dependence, mastery and competence in skills, independence, increased learning

Expected Outcome

Healing or healed noninfected burn wound

Correct verbal feedback of the information taught

Correct return demonstration of how to change the dressing, apply medication, etc.

NURSING INTERVENTIONS

Nursing Treatments

Provide temporary assistance until the skill is learned

Anticipate needs (for assistance)

Handle gently

Soak in a germicidal solution (Betadine for cleaning and debridement of the wound)

Do not allow burned skin surfaces to touch

Apply fine mesh gauze (between the burned fingers and toes)

Apply a sterile dressing (fine mesh gauze on the burned surface, anchor lightly with Kling, Kerlix, or Surgiflex)

OR

Apply an occlusive dressing (closed method with medication)

OR

Expose the burn wound to air (open method)

Maintain body alignment (place the fingers in slight flexion around a gauze ball, place the wrist and elbow in straight extension; for an axillary burn, place the elbow at a 90-degree angle to the body)

Exercise (burned joints) in range-of-motion (unless contraindicated by infection, new graft, or inadequate healing of fingers)

Immobilize the graft site (for the first 5–7 days)

Moisten the dressing before removal (if the dressing removal is not intended for debridement)

Bathe in a shower

OR

Bathe in a tub (submerge the patient in water for closed wounds)

} To remove the prescribed topical agent before reapplication of the agent

Apply a bed cradle (if the trunk and legs are burned)

Cover with lightweight blankets (unless a heat lamp is used)

Maintain a warm room temperature (about 80° F or a temperature comfortable to the patient)

OR

Apply a heat cradle or heat lamp

Maintain adequate atmospheric humidity (40–50% or a percentage comfortable to the patient)

Maintain a clean environment

Maintain reverse isolation (if the burn covers a large area)

Maintain dry, clean linen

OR

Place on sterile linens (if the burn covers a large area)

Encourage increased protein-food intake, increased calorie intake

Encourage self-performance

Nursing Observations

Monitor the body temperature (for fever caused by systemic sepsis)

Palpate the pulse for rate, rhythm, and volume

Inspect the chest for respiratory rate and rhythm

Auscultate the chest for abnormal breath sounds

Inspect for signs of (wound) infection

Inspect for impaired circulation (from circumferential burns)

Observe for signs of healing (decreased inflammation, no purulent drainage, evidence of granulation tissue)

Observe for delayed healing (taking longer than 4–7 days)

Obtain a bacterial culture (of the burned surface)

Monitor blood studies for arterial blood gases, for abnormal renal function

Health Teaching

Teach sterile technique

Teach how to clean and dress a (burn) wound

Teach how to apply the prescribed topical ointment

Teach how to do range-of-motion exercises (to maintain joint function)

Instruct to increase fluid intake

Describe those symptoms that should be reported (fever, wound inflammation, purulent drainage)

Explain the reason for and intended effect of the therapy (promote healing, prevent infection)

Medical Treatments Performed by Nurses

Pain Relief

Apply the prescribed topical agent (silver sulfadiazine)

Give the prescribed drugs (small doses of narcotics intravenously)

Fluid Resuscitation

Administer intravenous fluids

Administer a blood transfusion

Infection Prevention and Wound Care

Apply the prescribed topical agent

Apply a biologic dressing (heterograft or xenograph for partial thickness injuries)

Apply a medicated dressing (*Wet-wet dressing*: a thick dressing that has been saturated with a prescribed solution; wet the dressing with the solution every 4 hours and change the dressing every 8 hours; this dressing is not intended for debridement. *Wet-dry dressing*: apply the dressing as above; remove the dry dressing every 4 hours and reapply for debridement purposes)

Give the prescribed drugs (antibiotics, tetanus toxoid, antacids)

EVALUATION

Record actual outcome

UNSKILLED AT CAST CARE[72,451]

ASSESSMENT

Data Collection

Subjective Data

• Person's discussion or questions indicate a need for additional information, clarification, or validation of information about performing the task of caring for a cast

    OR

• Person's lack of questions or comments indicates not wanting information or not knowing enough to seek information about performing the task of caring for a cast

Person may not know:

    When the cast is ready for weight-bearing

    The significance of cast odor or bleeding

    Important symptoms to report

Objective Data

• Person cannot correctly demonstrate how to:

    Wrap a cast to keep it dry

    Pad the cast's rough edges

    Do isometric exercises

Related Data

Commonly Related Diseases

Ankylosing spondylitis, osteogenesis imperfecta

Commonly Related Injury

Fracture

Data Analysis

Nursing Diagnosis

UNSKILLED AT CAST CARE: Being nonproficient, with or without knowledge, in the performance of the specific task of caring for a cast and the casted body part

Common Etiology (Stressors)

HEALTH CARE FACTORS: Lack of health instruction, lack of health-skill experience

PLANNING

Unmet Needs

Comfort, protection from physical harm, dependence, mastery and competence in skills, independence, increased learning

Expected Outcome

Properly aligned, clean, dry and intact cast

No evidence of extremity or skin injury from the cast

Correct verbal feedback of the information taught

Correct return demonstration of how to wrap a cast for dryness, pad cast edges, do isometric exercises, protect a cast

NURSING INTERVENTIONS

Nursing Treatments

Provide temporary assistance until the skill is learned

Elevate the affected body part (in the cast)

Expose the drying cast to air

Fully support the drying cast on pillows

Avoid misshaping the wet cast (lift the cast with the palms of your hand, support the full length of the cast, move the entire cast as a single unit, do not turn the person on the casted side until the cast is dry)

Pad the rough cast edges (with petal padding after the cast is completely dry)

Consult with the physician (about a new cast if the current one has an unpleasant odor or loses its firmness from being wet)

Bivalve and spread the cast to relieve pressure (ET) (if there are indications of existing or potential tissue damage)

Encourage the person to ask questions

Encourage self-performance

Nursing Observations

Inspect the cast for tightness

Inspect for signs of (skin) irritation (around the cast edges)

Observe the cast for an expanding bleeding area (make an outline of the bleeding area at regular intervals)

Observe the cast for odor

Observe for cyanosis (of the casted extremity)

Palpate the skin for temperature (report coldness)

Determine teaching effectiveness by verbal feedback and return demonstration

Health Teaching

Instruct to elevate the body part (put the casted upper extremity in a sling or put the casted lower extremity on pillows first 2–3 days)

Instruct to allow the cast to dry 2–3 days before approved weight-bearing

Instruct to keep the cast dry with a plastic wrap when bathing

Explain how to pad rough cast edges

Instruct not to pull out cast padding

Instruct not to use a scratching device under the cast (instead, hold a hand hair dryer, direct its cool air toward the skin under the cast to relieve itching and remove debris)

Teach how to do isometric exercises (when in an extremity cast)

Teach good body mechanics (for easier mobility)

Explain that a cast should not be painted with nonporous paint (since it macerates the skin)

Teach how to clean a soiled cast with a moist cloth and Bon Ami cleanser

Instruct to bring crutches when the leg cast is removed (since walking is postponed for some time after cast removal)

Teach skin care following cast removal (apply vegetable or mineral oil to the casted area, leave it on for several hours, then gently wash it off with mild soap and water)

Describe those symptoms that should be reported (swelling, blueness, coldness, localized pain, impaired finger/toe movement, cast odor, warm spots, or fresh blood)

Explain the reason for and the intended effect of the care

EVALUATION

Record actual outcome

UNSKILLED AT CIRCUMCISION CARE[313,527]

ASSESSMENT

Data Collection

Subjective Data
- Person's discussion or questions indicate a need for additional information, clarification, or validation of information about performing the task of caring for a circumcision wound
  OR
- Person's lack of questions or comments indicates not wanting information or not knowing enough to seek information about performing that task of caring for a circumcision wound
  Person may not know:
    Important symptoms to report

Objective Data
- Person cannot correctly demonstrate how to:
    Clean the area of circumcision
    Do periodic dressing changes

Data Analysis

Nursing Diagnosis
UNSKILLED AT CIRCUMCISION CARE: Being nonproficient, with or without knowledge, in the performance of the specific task of cleaning and caring for a circumcision wound

Common Etiology (Stressors)
HEALTH CARE FACTORS: Lack of health instruction, lack of health-skill experience

PLANNING

Unmet Needs

Comfort, cleanliness, protection from physical harm, dependence, mastery and competence is skills, independence, increased learning

Expected Outcome

Clean, uninfected, healed circumcision wound

Correct verbal feedback of information taught

Correct return demonstration of how to clean and change the dressing on a circumcision wound

NURSING INTERVENTIONS

Nursing Treatments

Provide temporary assistance until the skill is learned

Bathe locally (with each diaper change)

Retract and clean the foreskin

Apply sterile petrolatum gauze (with each diaper change for 24 hours after surgery)

Apply an antibiotic ointment

Avoid forceful removal of the yellowish-white exudate at the circumcision site

Handle gently

Apply diapers loosely (to prevent friction)

Encourage self-performance (usually by the mother)

Nursing Observations

Inspect for bleeding, for edema, for inflammation, for (purulent) drainage, for necrosis

Determine teaching effectiveness by verbal feedback and return demonstration

Health Teaching

Advise daily bathing (of the circumcision area)

Teach the specific procedure (of cleansing and applying petrolatum gauze for the first 24 hours, cleansing and gentle care thereafter)

Describe those symptoms that should be reported (bleeding, edema, inflammation, purulent drainage)

Explain the reason for and intended effect of the care (promote healing, prevent infection)

EVALUATION

Record actual outcome

UNSKILLED AT COLOSTOMY/ILEOSTOMY CARE[72,451]

ASSESSMENT

Data Collection

Subjective Data

• Person's discussion or questions indicate a need for additional information, clarification, or validation of information about performing the task of caring for a colostomy or ileostomy

  OR

• Person's lack of questions or comments indicates not wanting information or not knowing enough to seek information about performing the task of caring for a colostomy or ileostomy

  Person may not know:

  About the changes in anatomic structure and physiologic function by the ostomy

  The importance of ostomy cleanliness

  The appropriate diet to support ostomy control

  Those symptoms that should be reported

Objective Data

• Person cannot correctly demonstrate how to:

  Clean and irrigate the ostomy

  Clean the skin around the ostomy

  Apply and remove the ostomy appliance

  Control ostomy odor

Related Data

Commonly Related Diseases
Carcinoma, enteritis, intussusception, paralytic ileus, ulcerative colitis, volvulus

Commonly Related Injuries
Gunshot wound of abdomen

Data Analysis

Nursing Diagnosis
UNSKILLED AT COLOSTOMY/ILEOSTOMY CARE: Being nonproficient, with or without knowledge, in the performance of the specific task of caring for a colostomy or ileostomy

Common Etiology (Stressors)
HEALTH CARE FACTORS: Lack of health instruction, lack of health-skill experience

PLANNING

Unmet Needs
Waste elimination of food residue, comfort. Cleanliness, protection from physical harm, dependence, mastery and competence in skills, independence, increased learning

Expected Outcome
A consistently clean ostomy and ostomy appliance
Clean, nonirritated skin around the ostomy
Correct verbal feedback of the information taught
Correct return demonstration of how to clean and irrigate the ostomy and protect surrounding skin; how to attach, remove, and clean the ostomy appliance; methods of odor control

NURSING INTERVENTIONS

Nursing Treatments
Provide temporary assistance until the skill is learned
Introduce irrigating solutions slowly
Clean (the skin) with surgical soap (around the ostomy)
Apply aluminum paste to the skin or zinc oxide to the skin (around a colostomy)
Apply milk of magnesia to the skin or apply karaya powder to the skin (around the ileostomy)
Apply ostomy adhesive (Stomahesive, Rebiaseal) and then an ostomy appliance
Empty the collection appliance (as needed)
Change the ostomy appliance as needed
Encourage decreased gas-forming food intake
Refrain from giving laxatives (or laxative-type foods)
Provide needed supplies
Introduce to persons who have successfully undergone the same experience
Make a referral (to local United Ostomy Association)
Encourage the person to ask questions
Encourage self-performance

Nursing Observations
Inspect for signs of (skin) irritation
Inspect for (excess) drainage
Observe for readiness to assume self-care
Determine teaching effectiveness by testing, verbal feedback, and return demonstration

Health Teaching
Explain the body alterations associated with the surgical procedure
Teach how and when to irrigate a colostomy
Teach how to control ileostomy–colostomy odor by deodorization
Instruct to avoid foods having strong odors
Teach the specific procedure (of regulating colostomy function with irrigations and diet)

Explain how to maintain ileostomy or colostomy cleanliness

Instruct how to maintain skin cleanliness (and protect the skin from fecal drainage)

Teach how to apply and remove the ostomy appliance

Explain how to maintain cleanliness of the ostomy appliance

Recommend that two ostomy appliances be alternately used

Explain how to obtain therapeutic supplies

Recommend that extra therapeutic supplies be carried

Describe those symptoms that should be reported (excessive drainage, skin irrigation, pain)

Explain the reason for and intended effect of the therapy (cleanliness and maintenance of bowel function)

Medical Treatments Performed by Nurses

Irrigate the ostomy

EVALUATION

Record actual outcome

UNSKILLED AT CONTINUOUS AMBULATORY PERITONEAL DIALYSIS[71,725]

ASSESSMENT

Data Collection

Subjective Data

• Person's discussion or questions indicate a need for additional information, clarification, or validation of information about performing the task of continuous ambulatory peritoneal dialysis
  OR

• Person's lack of questions or comments indicates not wanting information or not knowing enough to seek information about performing the task of continuous ambulatory peritoneal dialysis

  Person may not know:

    The purpose of continuous ambulatory peritoneal dialysis

    The physiologic effects of such

    The precautions to be taken to avoid dangerous side effects

Objective Data

• Person cannot correctly demonstrate how to:

    Maintain sterile technique

    Instill and drain the dialysate solution

    Cap, uncap, and secure the peritoneal catheter

Related Data

Commonly Related Diseases

Renal failure

Data Analysis

Nursing Diagnosis

UNSKILLED AT CONTINUOUS AMBULATORY PERITONEAL DIALYSIS: Being nonproficient, with or without knowledge, in the performance of the specific task of managing the continuous, everyday, presence of dialysis fluid in the the peritoneal cavity with intermittent drainage and instillation, for the purpose of removing chemical wastes and excesses from the blood

Common Etiology (Stressors)
HEALTH CARE FACTORS: Lack of health instruction, lack of health-skill experience

PLANNING

Unmet Needs
Waste elimination of nitrogenous substances, comfort, cleanliness, protection from physical harm, dependence, mastery and competence in skills, independence, increased learning

Expected Outcome
To restore serum electrolytes and nitrogenous substances (urea and creatinine) to acceptable levels
A clean, uninfected peritoneal catheter site
No evidence of infection or fluid imbalance
Correct verbal feedback of the information taught
Correct return demonstration of how to assemble the dialysis equipment, instill dialysate into the peritoneal cavity (inflow), manage the fluid while it is in the cavity (dwell-time), drain the dialysate from the peritoneal cavity (outflow), keep a flow record, monitor the vital signs, clean and dress the peritoneal catheter site

NURSING INTERVENTIONS

Nursing Treatments
Provide temporary assistance until the skill is learned
Encourage the person to ask questions
Encourage self-performance
Introduce to persons who have successfully undergone the same experience

Nursing Observations
Observe for readiness to assume self-care
Determine teaching effectiveness by testing, verbal feedback, and return demonstration

Health Teaching
Explain how to obtain therapeutic supplies (dialysate fluid, tubing)
Exlain normal organ (kidney) function (the kidney produces urine, reabsorbs water and chemicals, filters body wastes, maintains blood pressure, controls the rate of the red blood cells made by the bone marrow)
Teach sterile technique (which is extremely important)
Teach how to take a temperature and accurately read a thermometer
Teach how to locate and count a pulse
Teach how to take a blood pressure, how to weigh (daily)
Explain how to measure the intake and output (of the dialysate fluid during inflow and outflow)
Instruct the patient to empty his bladder before the (instillation) procedure
Familiarize the person with the component parts of the equipment (peritoneal catheter, bags of dialysate fluid, tubing, clamps)
Explain how the (dialysis) equipment works (dialysate fluid is instilled in the peritoneal cavity where metabolic wastes move into the dialysate by filtration, osmosis, and diffusion after which the fluid is drained from the peritoneal cavity)
Teach the specific procedure (continuous ambulatory peritoneal dialysis):
  Have the person place himself in the sitting position
  Check the peritoneal dialysis catheter for leakage or displacement
  Warm the dialysis fluid before instillation (at 98.6° F or at environmental temperature if preferred)
  Take a new bag of dialysate solution, remove the plastic covering, and check the bag for leaks
  Attach the dialysis tubing to the bag of dialysate solution; do not allow air into the tubing

Using sterile technique, specifically prescribed, remove the cap from the peritoneal dialysis catheter

Connect the dialysis solution and tubing to the peritoneal dialysis catheter

Instill the fresh solution by gravity. This should take about 10 minutes

Using sterile technique, specifically prescribed, disconnect the bag and tubing from the peritoneal catheter. Recap the external end of the peritoneal catheter, and hold it to the skin with a sterile dressing and gauze

OR

Clamp the solution bag, fold, and attach to the waist so that the bag can be used later for drainage

At the specified time (usually 4 hours later), again using prescribed sterile technique, reattach the bag and tubing to the peritoneal catheter and drain

OR

Remove the bag from the waist, drop it to the floor and drain the fluid by gravity for 15–20 minutes

Instill fresh solution by gravity as before

Encourage increased protein-food intake (to offset the protein lost in the dialysate solution)

Describe those symptoms that should be reported (fever, cloudy dialysate solution, retention of dialysate solution, abdominal tenderness, nausea, vomiting, ankle edema, rapid pulse or respirations, inflammation or drainage around the catheter site)

Advise how to integrate the dialysis procedure into the daily routine

Emphasize the importance of follow-up care (for blood studies, especially BUN and creatinine, bacterial culture of peritoneal catheter tip, etc.)

EVALUATION

Record actual outcome

UNSKILLED AT DIABETIC INSULIN THERAPY[26,73,376]

ASSESSMENT

Data Collection

Subjective Data

• Person's discussion or questions indicate a need for additional information, clarification, or validation of information about performing the task of giving prescribed insulin dosages

OR

• Person's lack of questions or comments indicates not wanting information or not knowing enough to seek information about performing the task of giving prescribed insulin dosages

Person may not know:

The types of insulin and their varying effects

The correct calibration of insulin syringe and needle to use

The proper injection sites

The correct time to give insulin

Objective Data

• Person cannot correctly demonstrate how to:

Maintain sterile technique

Rotate the insulin bottle when mixing the solution

Draw up a correct insulin dose into a syringe

Administer insulin into the tissue

Related Data
Commonly Related Diseases
Diabetes mellitus

Data Analysis

Nursing Diagnosis
UNSKILLED AT DIABETIC INSULIN THERAPY: Being nonproficient, with or without knowledge, in the performance of the specific task of administering insulin for control of diabetes

Common Etiology (Stressors)
HEALTH CARE FACTORS: Lack of health instruction, lack of health-skill experience

PLANNING

Unmet Needs
Comfort, protection from physical harm, dependence, mastery and competence in skills, independence, increased learning

Expected Outcome
Consistent administration of correct doses of insulin at appropriate times, in correct sites
Correct verbal feedback of the information taught
Correct return demonstration of how to draw up the insulin dosage, select the correct site, and administer the insulin

NURSING INTERVENTIONS

Nursing Treatments
Provide temporary assistance until the skill is learned
Encourage the person to ask questions
Encourage self-performance

Nursing Observations
Observe for side effects of drug
Observe for readiness to assume self-care
Determine teaching effectiveness by testing, verbal feedback, and return demonstration

Health Teaching
Teach sterile technique
Explain the various types of insulin and their effects (regular and semilente are short-acting; NPH, globin, and lente are intermediate-acting; PZI and ultralente are long-acting)
Explain that proper storage of insulin ensures drug potency
Instruct to avoid storing insulin in a syringe
Explain the importance of giving insulin on schedule
Teach the specific procedure:
    Explain how to correctly mix the cloudy insulins
    Explain correct selection and rotation of site, using tissues with good circulation: upper arms, thighs, anterior abdomen, subscapular, and buttocks
    Explain how to draw insulin into the syringe
    Explain the importance of using correct calibration of insulin syringe
    Instruct to give insulin deep subcutaneously
    Instruct to record each injection on a diagram to ensure proper site rotation
Teach how to test the urine for sugar-acetone
Teach how to test the blood for glucose using the finger-stick method
Describe those problems that should be reported (allergy to insulin, hypoglycemia, excess sugar in urine, blood or acetone in urine)
Teach the specific procedure (of emergency measures for insulin overdose and/or hypoglycemia)
Explain how to manage insulin therapy on sick days (take usual insulin dose, test urine

four times daily, call the doctor if urine glucose is high, increase fluid intake, keep a record of fluid intake, glucose level, and insulin dosage)

EVALUATION

Record actual outcome

UNSKILLED AT DIABETIC SKIN/FOOT/NAIL CARE[26,73,376]

ASSESSMENT

Data Collection

Subjective Data
• Person's discussion or questions indicate a need for additional information, clarification, or validation of information about performing the task of caring for a diabetic's skin, feet, and nails
  OR
• Person's lack of questions or comments indicates not wanting information or not knowing enough to seek information about performing the task of caring for a diabetic's skin, feet, and nails
  Person may not know:
  Of the sensitivity of diabetic skin
  The dangers of pressure on or trauma to the skin
  That constant observation for diabetic skin/nail problems is essential

Objective Data
• Person cannot correctly demonstrate how to:
  Properly clean the diabetic's skin/nails
  Lubricate the skin/nails
  Treat the diabetic's hands and feet
  Take special precautions for diabetics

Related Data
Commonly Related Diseases
Diabetes mellitus

Data Analysis

Nursing Diagnosis
UNSKILLED AT DIABETIC SKIN/FOOT/NAIL CARE: Being nonproficient, with or without knowledge, in the performance of the specific task of caring for the skin and nails of persons with diabetes

Common Etiology (Stressors)
HEALTH CARE FACTORS: Lack of health instruction, lack of health-skill experience

PLANNING

Unmet Needs

Comfort, cleanliness, protection from physical harm, dependence, mastery and competence in skills, independence, increased learning

Expected Outcome
Clean, intact, moisturized skin
No evidence of injury or infection
Clean, shaped, trimmed nails
Unbroken, smooth cuticles
Correct verbal feedback of the information taught
Correct return demonstration of how to clean and lubricate the skin/nails

NURSING INTERVENTIONS

Nursing Treatments
Provide temporary assistance until the skill is learned
Bathe daily (unless the person is aged or has a skin disorder)
Maintain dry, clean skin
Clean the nails (of the feet daily, filing instead of cutting the toenails)
Lubricate the skin with cocoa butter, glycerine, lanolin, mineral oil, or olive oil
Encourage the person to ask questions
Encourage self-performance
Make a referral (to the local chapter of the American Diabetes Association for informational programs and literature)

Nursing Observations
Inspect the nails for abnormalities (clubbing, splitting, discoloration, inflammed borders)
Inspect the skin for breakdown, for infectious lesions, for color
Inspect for signs of irritation
Observe for evidence of pressure on the skin
Test the skin for impaired feeling perception
Palpate the skin for temperature
Observe for readiness to assume self-care
Determine teaching effectiveness by testing, verbal feedback, and return demonstration

Health Teaching
Teach diabetic foot care by providing a written guide that includes the following:
Wash the skin gently in warm water (test the water temperature with the elbow), pat dry the entire skin area, including between the toes
Apply a light coating of lanolin immediately after drying the skin if the skin needs lubricating, do not use the lanolin too frequently
Apply a mild foot powder between the toes and to the socks and shoes if the feet perspire heavily
Lightly rub the feet with alcohol instead of lanolin if perspiration is extreme
Lightly rub callouses and corns with a towel after bathing; do not trim them with a razor blade, pocket knife, etc., or apply corn removers
Do not walk barefoot
Do not wear shoes without socks
Alternate shoes and socks daily to allow thorough drying
Wear warm wool or cotton socks in cold weather, avoid polyester socks
Instruct to wear well-fitting shoes (with sturdy toes and low heels)
Advise against wearing constrictive clothing (garters or constrictive hose)
Instruct to avoid heat applications (to the feet, such as a hot water bottle or heating pad, an electric blanket, or electric socks)
Teach diabetic nail care (by providing a written guide that includes the following:
Wash the feet thoroughly in warm, soapy water
Clean the nails with a softened orange stick
File the nails frequently to keep them smooth and short
File the toenails straight across, keeping their length even with the end of the toe
Apply lanolin to brittle nails and dry cuticles immediately after soaking them in warm water and patting them dry)

Instruct to maintain skin cleanliness, to lubricate the skin, to inspect the skin

Explain the need to avoid mechanical trauma (to the diabetic's skin by avoiding sunburn and windburn, by testing cosmetics for a skin reaction before using the cosmetics, and by avoiding the squeezing or piercing of pimples)

Explain the reasons for and intended effect of the therapy (to maintain intact, healthy skin and nails and to promote healing of injuries or lesions)

Medical Treatments Performed by Nurses

Encourage the prescribed (Buerger–Allen) exercises (to help develop collateral circulation)

EVALUATION

Record actual outcome

UNSKILLED AT ESOPHAGOSTOMY FEEDING[362]

ASSESSMENT

Data Collection

Subjective Data

• Person's discussion or questions indicate a need for additional information, clarification, or validation of information about performing the task of feeding through an esophagostomy

OR

• Person's lack of questions or comments indicates not wanting information or not knowing enough to seek information about performing the task of feeding through an esophagostomy

Person may not know:

The amounts and kinds of feeding to be used

Methods for preventing complications

The symptoms that should be reported

Objective Data

• Person cannot correctly demonstrate how to:

Insert and remove the esophagostomy tube for each feeding after the healing of the channel or opening is complete

Care for the stoma

Prepare and administer tube feeding

Related Data

Commonly Related Diseases

Dysphagia

Data Analysis

Nursing Diagnosis

UNSKILLED AT ESOPHAGOSTOMY FEEDING: Being nonproficient, with or without knowledge, in the performance of the specific task of providing nutritional feedings through a tube inserted into a cervical esophagostomy stoma into the stomach

Common Etiology (Stressors)

HEALTH CARE FACTORS: Lack of health instruction, lack of health-skill experience

PLANNING

Unmet Needs

Fluid and electrolyte balance, nutritional balance, comfort, cleanliness, protection from physical harm, dependence, mastery and competence in skills, independence, increased learning

Expected Outcome

Daily adequate calorie intake

Daily intake of 1,500–3,000 cc of fluid including the tube feeding formula

Correct verbal feedback of the information taught

Correct return demonstration of how to prepare and administer the tube feeding formula

NURSING INTERVENTIONS

Nursing Treatments

Provide temporary assistance (with tube feeding) until the skill is learned

Estimate the required daily calories

Position comfortably

Place in a sitting position (before, during, and for one hour after feeding)

Refrain from giving cold liquids

Feed slowly (average feeding time is 30–40 minutes)

Balance fluid intake to equal output

Encourage patient questions

Encourage self-performance

Nursing Observations

Check the tube's placement before giving the tube feeding

Inspect the abdomen for distention

Measure the intake and the output

Observe for complaints of nausea

Observe for diarrhea, for diet intolerance, for conditions indicating a need for increased nutritional requirements (fever, tissue damage, weight loss, etc.)

Observe for readiness to assume self-care

Determine teaching effectiveness by testing, verbal feedback, and return demonstration

Health Teaching

Explain how to obtain therapeutic supplies

Teach how to prepare a formula (for tube feeding)

Recommend a regular feeding schedule

Teach how to administer tube feeding (lubricate the tip of the feeding tube and gently insert it into the channel and the stomach; check for residual food in the stomach before each feeding by aspirating the stomach contents, measuring the residual, and returning it to the stomach; adjust the feeding/fluid intake according to the residual; when the residual is 150 ml, subtract that amount from the total to be given; for fever of 1° C, increase the water intake by 10–15% of the usual total; administer the tube feeding according to the basic need of 35 ml per kg of body weight; the person must receive a minimum of 7 cc of water per 1 g of protein in the formula; for fever states, increase the water by 10–15% per 1° C of fever; if receiving 150 g of protein or more per day, observe for hypertonic dehydration; provide after-feeding tube care by pinching and removing the tube and clearing the tube with water)

Describe those symptoms that should be reported (nausea, diarrhea)

Explain the reason for and intended effect of the therapy (to maintain nutrition to cells)

Medical Treatments Performed by Nurses

Give the prescribed tube feeding

EVALUATION

Record actual outcome

UNSKILLED AT GASTROSTOMY FEEDING[72,362,451]

ASSESSMENT

Data Collection

Subjective Data
- Person's discussion or questions indicate a need for additional information, clarification, or validation of information about performing the task of feeding through a gastrostomy
  OR
- Person's lack of questions or comments indicates not wanting information or not knowing enough to seek information about performing the task of feeding through a gastrostomy

  Person may not know:
  The amounts and kinds of feeding to be used
  Methods for preventing complications
  The symptoms that should be reported

Objective Data
- Person cannot correctly demonstrate how to:
  Properly position for the feeding
  Insert the gastrostomy tube
  Prepare and administer the feeding
  Clamp and remove the tube at appropriate times
  Properly care for the retention tube in order to prevent gastric distention and leakage
  Dress the gastrostomy
  Maintain clean technique

Related Data
Commonly Related Diseases
Esophageal carcinoma, cerebrovascular accident, esophageal stricture

Data Analysis

Nursing Diagnosis
UNSKILLED AT GASTROSTOMY FEEDING: Being nonproficient, with or without knowledge, in the performance of the specific task of providing nutritional feedings through a surgical opening through the abdominal wall into the stomach

Common Etiology (Stressors)
HEALTH CARE FACTORS: Lack of health instruction, lack of health-skill experience

PLANNING

Unmet Needs
Fluid and electrolyte balance, nutritional balance, comfort, cleanliness, protection from physical harm, dependence, mastery and competence in skills, independence, increased learning

Expected Outcome
Daily adequate calorie intake
Daily intake of 1,500–3,000 cc of fluid including tube feeding formula
Clean, nonirritated skin around the gastrostomy
Correct verbal feedback of the information taught
Correct return demonstration of how to prepare and administer tube feeding formula and how to apply dressing to the gastrostomy

NURSING INTERVENTIONS

Nursing Treatments
Provide temporary assistance until the skill is learned

Estimate the required daily calories (nine calories per pound of body weight; for gain or
  loss of weight, determine the desired weight and multiply by 9 calories per pound)
Place in a sitting position (before, during, and for about 30 minutes after feeding)
Refrain from giving cold liquids (which stimulate peristalsis and cause diarrhea)
Feed slowly (the average feeding time is 30–40 minutes, or by giving continuous drip
  over 24 hours)
Provide frequent patient contact (during the feeding)
Refrain from sealing the feeding tube with a heavy clamp (to avoid dislodging the tube)
Apply a sterile dressing (after the feeding)
Balance fluid intake to equal output
Encourage the person or family to ask questions

Nursing Observations
Inspect the abdomen for distention
Inspect for signs of (skin) irritation and infection
Measure the intake and output
Observe for complaints of nausea or pain
Observe for diarrhea, for diet intolerance, for conditions indicating a need for increased
  nutritional requirements (fever, tissue damage, weight loss, etc.)
Observe for readiness to assume self-care
Determine teaching effectiveness by testing, verbal feedback, and return demonstration

Health Teaching
Explain how to obtain therapeutic supplies
Teach how to prepare a formula (for tube feeding)
Recommend a regular feeding schedule
Teach how to administer tube feeding (have the person check for residual feed in the
  stomach before each feeding by aspirating the stomach contents, measuring the residual and returning it to the stomach; adjust feeding/fluid intake according to the residual; when the residual is 150 ml or more, subtract that amount from the total feeding
  to be given; for fever of 1° C, increase the water intake by 10–15% of the usual total;
  administer the tube feeding according to basic need of 35 ml per kg body weight; the
  person must receive a minimum of 7 cc of water per 1 g of protein in the formula; for
  fever states, increase the water by 10–15% per 1° C of fever; if receiving 150 g of protein or more per day, observe for hypertonic dehydration. Provide after-feeding tube
  care; for the retention tube, either clamp or leave the tube open as needed for decompression; use gentle traction on a balloon type tube; for an intermittent tube,
  clamp and remove the tube and apply a sterile dressing)
Describe those symptoms that should be reported (nausea, diarrhea)
Explain the reason for and intended effect of the therapy (to maintain nutrition to cells)

Medical Treatments Performed by Nurses
Give the prescribed tube feeding

EVALUATION

Record actual outcome

UNSKILLED AT HEMODIALYSIS[71,201,578]

ASSESSMENT

Data Collection

Subjective Data
• Person's discussion or questions indicates a need for additional information,
  clarification, or validation of information about performing the task of hemodialysis
  OR

- Persons lack of questions or comments indicates not wanting information or not knowing enough to seek information about performing the task of hemodialysis

  Person may not know:

  The purpose and desired effects of hemodialysis

  Which supplies are needed or the source of the supplies

  The danger signs associated with dialysis

  The best way to fit dialysis into the daily living schedule

Objective Data
- Person cannot correctly demonstrate how to:

  Maintain sterile technique

  Take a blood pressure

  Administer medications

  Assemble the artificial kidney

  Mix the hemodialysis fluid

  Prepare, operate, and clean the machine

  Do blood sampling

Related Data
Commonly Related Diseases
Renal failure

Data Analysis

Nursing Diagnosis
UNSKILLED AT HEMODIALYSIS: Being nonproficient, with or without knowledge, in the performance of the specific task of managing hemodialysis therapy

Common Etiology (Stressors)
HEALTH CARE FACTORS: Lack of health instruction, lack of health-skill experience

PLANNING

Unmet Needs

Fluid and electrolyte balance, waste elimination of nitrogenous substances, comfort, cleanliness, protection from physical harm, dependence, mastery and competence in skills, independence, increased learning

Expected Outcome

To restore serum electrolytes and nitrogenous substances (urea and creatinine) to acceptable levels

A clean, uninfected cannula site

No evidence of infection, hemorrhage, or fluid imbalance

Correct verbal feedback of the information taught

Correct return demonstration of how to assemble the artificial kidney, mix the hemodialysis fluid, prepare, operate, and clean the machine, administer medications, monitor vital signs, do blood sampling

NURSING INTERVENTIONS

Nursing Treatments

Provide temporary assistance until the skill is learned

Attend the patient constantly

Change the patient's position frequently

Place in the flat position (if the blood pressure drops)

Refrain from jarring the bed

Refrain from giving intravenous or intramuscular injections (postdialysis)

Encourage the person or family to ask questions

Encourage self-performance

Introduce to persons who have successfully undergone the same experience

Nursing Observations

Auscultate the apical heartbeat for rate and rhythm

Check the dialysis circuit for leakage

Check the hemodialysis AV shunt for cleanliness and patency
Check the hemodialysis equipment for mechanical breakdown
Inspect the chest for respiratory rate and rhythm
Inspect for bleeding (around dressings, in stools, gastric drainage, gums, nose)
Inspect the skin for perspiration abnormality (profuse perspiration)
Measure the body weight (before and after dialysis)
Monitor the blood pressure (before and at the start of dialysis, then every 15 minutes to 1 hour)
Observe for complaints of headache, itching, nausea, pain (muscle cramps or chest pain), weakness
Observe for shock, vomiting
Monitor blood studies for abnormal clotting mechanism (decreased clotting time due to heparin)
Monitor blood studies for abnormal electrolytes (before and after dialysis)
Monitor blood studies for abnormal hematology (hematocrit)
Monitor blood studies for abnormal renal function (urea and creatinine before and after dialysis)
Monitor the oral temperature (for fever)
Observe for readiness to assume self-care
Determine teaching effectiveness by testing, verbal feedback, and return demonstration

Health Teaching

For Home Hemodialysis
Recommend home adaptations appropriate to the health problem (plumbing and electrical changes, auxilliary electrical power, waterproofing the floor, readily available telephone, hemodialysis machine in a separate room)
Teach how to obtain therapeutic supplies
Explain normal organ (kidney) function (the kidney produces urine, reabsorbs water and chemicals, filters body wastes, maintains blood pressure, controls the rate the red blood cells are made by the bone marrow)
Explain how the (dialysis) equipment works (the person's blood circulates through the dialysis machine between cellophane sheets or tubes and through a cleansing solution; then the blood returns to the person free of harmful body wastes)
Teach sterile technique (this is extremely important)
Teach how to take a temperature, accurately read a thermometer, how to locate and count a pulse
Explain how to observe respirations
Teach how to take a blood pressure, how to weigh
Teach how to do blood sampling (to measure the hematocrit)
Explain how to measure the intake and output
Familiarize the person with the component parts of the equipment (dialyzer, dialysate circuit, pressure gauges, blood pump, access tubing, etc.)
Teach how to do home dialysis (to prepare, operate, and clean the equipment, prepare dialysis solution, etc., specific to the type of dialyzer used and the institutional procedure)
Teach how and when to administer medications (such as heparin, etc.)
Teach how to care for an arteriovenous shunt (inspection and cleaning of the site, applying a sterile dressing)
Describe those symptoms that should be reported (weakness, pain, headache, edema, nausea, twitching, convulsions, any acute illness between dialysis)
Advise how to integrate the dialysis procedure into the daily routine

Medical Treatments Performed by Nurses

Administer the hemodialysis treatment (as prescribed by physician or institutional policy, until the person and his partner become skilled at the procedure)
Give the prescribed drugs (heparin, protamine sulfate, dialysate fluid)

EVALUATION
Record actual outcome

UNSKILLED AT HYPERALIMENTATION INFUSION[26,73,593]

ASSESSMENT

Data Collection

Subjective Data
- Person's discussion or questions indicate a need for additional information, clarification, or validation of information about performing the task of providing nutrients by hyperalimentation

  OR

- Person's lack of questions or comments indicates not wanting information or not knowing enough to seek information about performing the task of providing nutrients by hyperalimentation

  Person may not know:

  The physiologic effects of hyperalimentation

  The methods of the procedure

  How to avoid dangerous side effects

  The symptoms that should be reported

Objective Data
- Person cannot correctly demonstrate how to:

  Clean the catheter insertion site

  Change the hyperalimentation tubing

  Keep the tubing patent

  Change the dressing

  Maintain sterile technique

Related Data

Commonly Related Diseases

Cachexia, carcinoma, cerebrovascular accident, ileus, malabsorption syndrome

Commonly Related Injuries

Burn wound

Data Analysis

Nursing Diagnosis

UNSKILLED AT HYPERALIMENTATION INFUSION: Being nonproficient, with or without knowledge, in the performance of the specific task of providing feeding through a venous catheter with a concentrated nutrient solution of calories (2,000–4,000 daily), protein, dextrose, electrolytes, vitamins, and trace elements

Common Etiology (Stressors)

HEALTH CARE FACTORS: Lack of health instruction, lack of health-skill experience

PLANNING

Unmet Needs

Fluid and electrolyte balance, nutritional balance, comfort, cleanliness, protection from physical harm, dependence, mastery and competence in skills, independence, increased learning

Expected Outcome

A consistently clean, noninfected catheter insertion site

Daily prescribed intake of the concentrated nutrient solution

Correct verbal feedback of the information taught

Correct return demonstration of how to administer the concentrated nutrient solution, clean the catheter site, change the dressing, maintain sterile technique, and record the intake and output

NURSING INTERVENTIONS

Nursing Treatments
Provide temporary assistance until the skill is learned
Position comfortably
Change the patient's position gradually
Clean (the skin around the catheter insertion site) with surgical soap
Apply providone-iodine sponges around the tubing connections
Apply a sterile dressing
Wear sterile gloves (during a dressing change)
Change the dressing frequently (three or four times a week)
Change the hyperalimentation tubing with each dressing change
Use separate hyperalimentation infusion sets for incompatible solutions
Keep the hyperalimentation tube patent with 5% dextrose in water
Refrain from drawing blood studies via the hyperalimentation catheter
Do not give a blood transfusion of medications via the hyperalimentation catheter
Refrain from rapidly replacing lagging hyperalimentation solution
Remove the therapeutic tube when the treatment is terminated
Provide frequent patient contact (during the hyperalimentation procedure)
Encourage the person or family to ask questions
Encourage self-performance (when appropriate)

Nursing Observations
Check the (hyperalimentation) tube for patency
Check the (hyperalimentation) solution for cloudiness and precipitation
Check the (hyperalimentation) solution for flow rate, check for infiltration of the solution
Inspect the arms and hands for venous distention
Inspect the chest for respiratory rate and rhythm
Inspect the neck veins for distention
Inspect for edema (around the neck and face)
Measure the body weight (daily)
Measure the intake and output (for excessive urine output if rapid infusion occurs)
Monitor the blood pressure
Monitor blood studies for abnormal (decreased) glucose (if the infusion slows down)
Monitor the oral temperature (for fever)
Observe for complaints of headache ⎤
Observe for confusion, for lethargy ⎟ If rapid infusion
Observe the level of consciousness ⎟ occurs
Observe for complaints of nausea ⎦
Obtain a bacterial culture (of the catheter tip and bottle if fever occurs)
Test the urine for sugar and acetone
Observe for readiness to assume self-care
Determine teaching effectiveness by testing, verbal feedback, and return demonstration

Health Teaching
Explain how to obtain therapeutic supplies
Teach sterile technique
Teach the specific procedure (of checking the tube for patency, checking the solution for cloudiness and precipitation, administering the solution, checking the flow rate, inspecting for venous distention, cleaning and dressing the catheter site)
Explain how to measure the intake and output
Teach how to take a blood pressure, how to take a temperature and accurately read a thermometer
Teach how to test the urine for sugar-acetone
Describe those symptoms that should be reported (nausea, fever, confusion, inflammation of the infusion site)

Explain the reason for and intended effect of the therapy (the maintenance of or increased nutritional intake)

Medical Treatments Performed by Nurses
Give the prescribed hyperalimentation feeding

EVALUATION
Record actual outcome

UNSKILLED AT INTRAVENOUS INFUSION[72,451]

ASSESSMENT

Data Collection

Subjective Data
- Person's discussion or questions indicate a need for additional information, clarification, or validation of information about performing the task of infusing fluids intravenously

   OR
- Person's lack of questions or comments indicates not wanting information or not knowing enough to seek information about performing the task of infusing fluids intravenously

   Person may not know:

   The physiologic effects of the intravenous infusion

   The methods of the procedure

   How to avoid dangerous side effects

   The symptoms that should be reported

Objective Data
- Person cannot correctly demonstrate how to:

   Start or connect an intravenous infusion

   Correctly administer the fluid

   Manage drugs to be put in the fluid

   Make dressing changes

   Maintain sterile technique

Data Analysis

Nursing Diagnosis

UNSKILLED AT INTRAVENOUS INFUSION MANAGEMENT: Being nonproficient, with or without knowledge, in the performance of the specific task of administering intravenous fluids

Common Etiology (Stressors)

HEALTH CARE FACTORS: Lack of health instruction, lack of health-skill experience

PLANNING

Unmet Needs
Fluid and electrolyte balance, comfort, cleanliness, protection from physical harm, dependence, mastery and competence in skills, independence, increased learning

Expected Outcome
Correct, on-time administration of intravenous fluids

Clean, noninfected insertion site

No symptoms of fluid overload

Correct verbal feedback of the information taught

Correct return demonstration of how to insert the infusion needle or tubing, attach bottle or bags, regulate the flow rate, change the dressing, maintain sterile technique, and record intake and output

NURSING INTERVENTIONS

Nursing Treatments

Provide temporary assistance until the skill is learned

Distribute the intravenous fluid infusion over 12–24 hours

Restrict the glucose intravenous solution rate according to the weight (0.5 g of glucose hourly per kilogram of body weight)

Restrict the hypertonic intravenous solution rate to 200 cc per hour (solutions containing more than 0.9% salt or more than 5% sugar in water)

Restrict the hypotonic intravenous solution rate to 400 cc per hour (solutions containing less than 0.9% salt or less than 5% sugar in water)

Restrict the isotonic intravenous solution rate to 600 cc per hour (solutions containing 0.9% salt or 5% sugar in water)

Position (the arm) comfortably

Anchor the tubing securely

Provide sufficiently long tubing to allow freedom of movement

Apply a sterile dressing (over the injection site)

Encourage the person or family to ask questions

Encourage self-performance

Nursing Observations

Check the (intravenous) tube for patency

Check the (intravenous) solution for flow rate

Check the infiltration of the solution

Inspect for inflammation (of the infusion site)

Measure the intake and output

Monitor the blood pressure

Observe for water intoxication (*rapid onset*: strange behavior, confusion, sleepiness, delirium, weakness. *slow onset*: apathy, sleepiness, nausea, vomiting, weakness. *late onset*: convulsions)

Palpate the pulse for rate, rhythm, and volume

Observe for readiness to assume self-care

Determine teaching effectiveness by testing, verbal feedback, and return demonstration

Health Teaching

Explain how to obtain therapeutic supplies

Teach sterile technique

Teach the specific procedure (of setting up tubing, bags or bottles, removing air from the tubing, inserting and anchoring the infusion needle or tubing, administering the solution, applying and changing the dressing, checking the flow rate, and checking for infiltration)

Explain how to measure the intake and output

Describe those symptoms that should be reported (confusion, dyspnea, edema, inflammation of the infusion site)

Explain the reason for and intended effect of the therapy (the maintenance of fluid intake)

Medical Treatments Performed by Nurses

Administer intravenous fluids

Give the prescribed drugs (intravenously)

EVALUATION

Record actual outcome

UNSKILLED AT JEJUNOSTOMY FEEDING[72,362,451]

ASSESSMENT

Data Collection

Subjective Data
- Person's discussion or questions indicate a need for additional information, clarification, or validation of information about performing the task of feeding through a jejunostomy
  OR
- Person's lack of questions or comments indicates not wanting information or not knowing enough to seek information about performing the task of feeding through a jejunostomy
  Person may not know:
    The amounts and kinds of feeding to be used
    Methods for preventing complications
    The symptoms that should be reported

Objective Data
- Person cannot correctly demonstrate how to:
    Properly position for feeding
    Prepare and administer the feeding
    Dress the jejunostomy site
    Maintain sterile technique

Related Data
Commonly Related Diseases
Duodneal, esophageal, and gastric carcinoma

Data Analysis

Nursing Diagnosis
UNSKILLED AT JEJUNOSTOMY FEEDING: Being nonproficient, with or without knowledge, in the performance of the specific task of providing nutritional feedings through a surgical opening through the abdominal wall into the jejunum

Common Etiology (Stressors)
HEALTH CARE FACTORS: Lack of health instruction, lack of health-skill experience

PLANNING

Unmet Needs
Fluid and electrolyte balance, nutritional balance, comfort, cleanliness, protection from physical harm, dependence, mastery and competence in skills, independence, increased learning

Expected Outcome
Daily adequate calorie intake
Daily intake of 1,500–3,000 cc of fluid, including tube feeding formula
Clean, nonirritated skin around the jejunostomy
Correct verbal feedback of the information taught
Correct return demonstration of how to prepare and administer the tube feeding formula, how to apply the dressing to the jejunostomy site

NURSING INTERVENTIONS

Nursing Treatments
Provide temporary assistance until the skill is learned
Estimate the required daily calories (9 calories per pound of body weight; for gain or loss of weight, determine the desired weight and multiply by 9 calories per pound)
Position comfortably

Place in a sitting position (before, during, and for about 30 minutes after feeding)

Refrain from giving cold liquids (which stimulate peristalsis and causes diarrhea)

Feed slowly (the average feeding time is 30–40 minutes or by continuous drip over 24 hours)

Provide frequent patient contact (during the feeding)

Refrain from sealing the feeding tube with a heavy clamp (to avoid dislodging the tube)

Apply a sterile dressing (after the feeding)

Balance fluid intake to equal output

Encourage the person to ask questions

Nursing Observations

Inspect the abdomen for distention

Inspect for signs of infection

Measure the intake and output

Observe for complaints of nausea, pain

Observe for diarrhea, for diet intolerance, for conditions indicating a need for increased nutritional requirements (fever, tissue damage, weight loss, etc.)

Observe for readiness to assume self-care

Determine teaching effectiveness by testing, verbal feedback, and return demonstration

Health Teaching

Explain how to prepare a formula (for tube feeding)

Recommend a regular feeding schedule

Teach how to adminster tube feeding (have the person check for residual food in the stomach before each feeding by aspirating the stomach contents, measuring the residual, and returning it to the stomach; adjust the feeding/fluid intake according to the residual; when the residual is 150 ml or above, subtract that amount from the total feeding to be given; for a fever of 1° C, increase the water intake by 10–15% of the usual total; administer the tube feeding according to the basic need of 35 ml per kg body weight; the person requires a minimum of 7 cc of water per 1 g of protein in the formula; for fever states, increase the water by 10–15% per 1° C of fever; if receiving 150 g of protein or more per day, observe for hypertonic dehydration; provide after-feeding tube care; for a retention tube, either clamp or leave the tube open as needed for decompression; for an intermittent tube, clamp and remove the tube and apply a sterile dressing)

Describe those symptoms that should be reported (nausea, diarrhea)

Explain the reason for and intended effect of the therapy (to maintain nutrition to cells)

Medical Treatments Performed by Nurses

Give the prescribed tube feeding

EVALUATION

Record actual outcome

UNSKILLED AT LARYNGECTOMY CARE [451,620,705,706,707]

ASSESSMENT

Data Collection

Subjective Data

• Person's discussion or questions indicate a need for additional information, clarification, or validation of information about performing the task of caring for a laryngectomy

   OR

• Person's lack of questions or comments indicates not wanting information or not knowing enough to seek information about performing the task of caring for a laryngectomy

Person may not know:
The purpose of the laryngectomy
Of the clothing adjustments necessary
Precautions for avoiding complications
Those symptoms that should be reported

Objective Data
• Person cannot correctly demonstrate how to:
Keep the stoma and inner cannula clean
Suction the airway
Lubricate the stoma
Administer vaporized air

Related Data
Commonly Related Diseases
Laryngeal carcinoma

Data Analysis

Nursing Diagnosis
UNSKILLED AT LARYNGECTOMY CARE: Being nonproficient, with or without knowledge, in the performance of the specific task of caring for an opening surgically placed in the anterior neck and joined to the trachea following removal of the larynx

Common Etiology (Stressors)
HEALTH CARE FACTORS: Lack of health instruction, lack of health-skill experience

PLANNING

Unmet Needs
Oxygen, comfort, cleanliness, protection from physical harm, dependence, mastery and competence in skills, independence, increased learning

Expected Outcome
A consistently clean and humidified stoma
A clean and patent cannula
Correct verbal feedback of the information taught
Correct return demonstration of how to clean the stoma and cannula and suction and humidify the airway

NURSING INTERVENTIONS

Nursing Treatments
Provide temporary assistance until the skill is learned
Anticipate needs
Defer speech communication for 72 hours after a partial laryngectomy
Clean the laryngectomy tube inner cannula
Suction the airway (as needed)
Administer vaporized air
Shield the laryngectomy stoma from water
Rinse the mouth with diluted hydrogen peroxide
OR
Swab the mouth with diluted glycerine
OR
Refresh with a mouthwash
Provide an alternative method of communication appropriate to the person's specific needs and abilities (such as a writing pad and pencil)
Make a referral (to the Lost Cord Club)
Encourage the person or family to ask questions
Encourage self-performance

Nursing Observations

Check the (laryngectomy) tube for patency

Inspect the chest for respiratory rate and rhythm; for symmetrical expansion

Auscultate the chest for lung aeration

Observe for coughing, for airway obstruction (indicating the need to suction)

Inspect for bleeding (around the laryngectomy site)

Observe for readiness to assume self-care

Determine teaching effectiveness by testing, verbal feedback, and return demonstration

Health Teaching

Teach the specific procedure (of laryngectomy care)

Inform that handwashing is essential before touching the laryngectomy stoma

Teach how to clean a laryngectomy tube (the removable inner cannula is cleaned with hydrogen peroxide or saline)

Instruct that soap should not be used on the laryngectomy stoma

Instruct to protect the laryngectomy opening from water

Instruct to use a water-based lubricant around the laryngectomy stoma

Recommend the use of a laryngectomy bib

Instruct to maintain a moist laryngectomy bib

Teach how to suction an airway, how to give vaporized-solution inhalation

Instruct to apply a warm, moist, nonobstructive compress to the laryngectomy stoma for dyspnea

Advise against exposure to airborne irritants

Inform that the laryngectomy stoma should be protected against sunburning

Recommend that the tongue be brushed (to prevent mouth odor)

Inform that heavy lifting should be avoided (to prevent increased intrathoracic pressure and dyspnea)

Explain how to adjust clothing to meet health problems (using high-necked clothing and scarves)

Explain the importance of wearing a Medic Alert tag

Describe those symptoms that should be reported (respiratory distress)

Explain the reason for and intended effect of the therapy (to maintain a clean, patent airway)

EVALUATION

Record actual outcome

UNSKILLED AT MANAGING DRUGS[299]

ASSESSMENT

Data Collection

Subjective Data

• Person's discussion or questions indicate a need for additional information, clarification, or validation of information about performing the task of drug management

    OR

• Person's lack of questions or comments indicates not wanting information or not knowing enough to seek information about performing the task of drug management

  Person may not know:

    The purpose of the drug(s)

    The drug(s) side effects

    What the body's response should be in relation to the intended effect of the drug(s)

Objective Data
- Person cannot correctly demonstrate how to:
    Administer drug(s) in correct doses at the appropriate times
  Drugs have been professionally prescribed

Data Analysis

Nursing Diagnosis

UNSKILLED AT MANAGING DRUGS: Being nonproficient, with or without knowledge, in the performance of the specific task of providing the correct drugs, in appropriate doses, at required times

Common Etiology (Stressors)

HEALTH CARE FACTORS: Lack of health instruction, lack of health-skill experience

PLANNING

Unmet Needs

Protection from physical harm, dependence, mastery and competence in skills, independence, increased learning

Expected Outcome

Correct, on-time administration of therapeutic drugs
Correct verbal feedback of the information taught
Correct return demonstration of how to administer correct doses at appropriate times

NURSING INTERVENTIONS

Nursing Treatments

Provide temporary assistance (with drug management) until the skill is learned
Encourage the person to ask questions
Encourage self-performance

Nursing Observations

Observe for side effects of drugs
Observe for readiness to assume self-care
Determine teaching effectiveness by testing, verbal feedback, and return demonstration

Health Teaching

Teach how and when to administer medications
Teach how to remember to take medications (take drugs with routine activities such as meals, going to bed; place a written reminder on the mirror, refrigerator, etc.; set the alarm on a clock or wristwatch)
Teach which drugs and foods have potential adverse interactions (tetracycline, Ecotrin, etc., should not be taken with dairy products; sulfonamide antibiotics and Benemid should be taken with a full glass of water; anticholinergic drugs should be taken before meals; spinach and turnip greens should not be eaten when on anticoagulants, etc.)
Explain how to give medications to children
Describe those symptoms that should be reported (specific to the side effect of the drug
Explain how to obtain therapeutic supplies (drugs, syringes, etc.)
Emphasize that outdated drugs should be discarded (flushed into the sewage system)
Emphasize the danger of mixing drugs and alcohol, of sharing drugs between persons
Teach which drugs and chemicals have the potential for habituation
Recommend that self-medication be avoided
Explain the reason for and intended effect of the (drug) therapy

Medical Treatments Performed by Nurses

Give the prescribed drugs

EVALUATION

Record actual outcome

UNSKILLED AT MONITORING BLOOD PRESSURE[362,451]

ASSESSMENT

Data Collection

Subjective Data

- Person's discussion or questions indicate a need for additional information, clarification, or validation of information about performing the task of monitoring blood pressure
  OR
- Person's lack of questions or comments indicates not wanting information or not knowing enough to seek information about performing the task of monitoring a blood pressure

  Person may not know:
  The best position for taking a blood pressure
  Normal and abnormal blood pressure levels
  When to notify the physician

Objective Data

- Person cannot correctly demonstrate how to:
  Apply the blood pressure cuff
  Determine the blood pressure reading
  Record the blood pressure

Related Data

Commonly Related Diseases

Hypertension, aldosteronism, arteriosclerosis, patent ductus arteriosus, polycythemia, renal insufficiency, renal failure, thyrotoxicosis

Data Analysis

Nursing Diagnosis

UNSKILLED AT MONITORING BLOOD PRESSURE: Being nonproficient, with or without knowledge, in the performance of the specific task of taking a blood pressure reading

Common Etiology (Stressors)

HEALTH CARE FACTORS: Lack of health instruction, lack of health-skill experience

PLANNING

Unmet Needs

Comfort, protection from physical harm, dependence, mastery and competence in skills, independence, increased learning

Expected Outcome

Correct verbal feedback of the information taught
Correct return demonstration of how to take a blood pressure

NURSING INTERVENTIONS

Nursing Treatments

Provide temporary assistance until the skill is learned
Position comfortably
Place in the sitting position
Encourage the person to ask questions
Encourage self-performance

Nursing Observations

Monitor the blood pressure (for normal and abnormal levels)

Observe for readiness to assume self-care

Determine teaching effectiveness by testing, verbal feedback, and return demonstration

Health Teaching

Teach how to take a blood pressure (positioning, cuff application, reading and recording the blood pressure level)

Explain the reason for and intended effect of the procedure (to identify and control blood pressure levels)

Describe those symptoms that should be reported (*Adults*: diastolic of 90 mm Hg or above, or below 60 mm Hg. *Under 35 years of age*: systolic over 150 mm Hg. *Over 60 years of age*: systolic over 180 mm Hg)

Explain when to perform the procedure (blood pressure checks specific to the individual)

EVALUATION

Record actual outcome

UNSKILLED AT MONITORING BLOOD/URINE GLUCOSE[362,376]

ASSESSMENT

Data Collection

Subjective Data

• Person's discussion or questions indicate a need for additional information, clarification, or validation of information about performing the task of monitoring blood/urine glucose

    OR

• Person's lack of questions or comments indicates not wanting information or not knowing enough to seek information about performing the task of monitoring blood/urine glucose

Person may not know:

    Why blood and urine glucose is done

    When it should be done

Objective Data

• Person cannot correctly demonstrate how to:

    Obtain the needed specimen

    Perform the specific glucose test

Related Data

Commonly Related Diseases

Diabetes mellitus

Data Analysis

Nursing Diagnosis

UNSKILLED AT MONITORING BLOOD/URINE GLUCOSE: Being nonproficient, with or without knowledge, in the performance of the specific task of reading levels of glucose in blood and/or urine

Common Etiology (Stressors)
HEALTH CARE FACTORS: Lack of health instruction, lack of health-skill experience

PLANNING

Unmet Needs
Comfort, protection from physical harm, dependence, mastery and competence in skills, independence, increased learning

Expected Outcome
Correct verbal feedback of the information taught
Correct return demonstration of how to do a blood and/or urine glucose

NURSING INTERVENTIONS

Nursing Treatments
Provide temporary assistance until the skill is learned
Encourage the person to ask questions
Encourage self-performance

Nursing Observations
Test the urine for sugar, the blood for glucose level
Observe for readiness to assume self-care
Determine teaching effectiveness by testing, verbal feedback, and return demonstration

Health Teaching
Explain when to perform the procedure (before mealtime and bedtime)
Teach how to test the blood for glucose using the finger-stick method
Explain how to collect a (urine) specimen (empty the bladder and collect the urine 30 minutes later)
Teach how to test the urine for sugar-acetone (and to read urine glucose in terms of percentage because of plus-value differences)
Explain the reason for and intended effect of the procedure (to identify glucose levels, regulate insulin dosages)
Describe those symptoms that should be reported (elevated glucose levels)
Teach the common factors that will cause a false-positive or inaccurate glucose reading (certain antibiotics such as cephalothins, excessive salicylate ingestion, shaking the solution during processing)

EVALUATION

Record actual outcome

UNSKILLED AT MONITORING PULSE[362,423]

ASSESSMENT

Data Collection

Subjective Data
• Person's discussion or questions indicate a need for additional information, clarification, or validation of information about performing the task of monitoring the pulse
  OR

- Person's lack of questions or comments indicates not wanting information or not knowing enough to seek information about performing the task of monitoring the pulse

Person may not know:
    Why the pulse should be taken
    How long the pulse should be counted
    When to take the pulse

Objective Data
- Person cannot correctly demonstrate how to:
    Locate the pulse
    Apply appropriate finger pressure to the pulse site

Related Data
Commonly Related Diseases
Congestive heart failure, myocardial infarction, paroxysmal atrial tachycardia, peripheral vascular insufficiency

Data Analysis

Nursing Diagnosis
UNSKILLED AT MONITORING PULSE: Being nonproficient, with or without knowledge, in the performance of the specific task of locating and counting a pulse rate

Common Etiology (Stressors)
HEALTH CARE FACTORS: Lack of health instruction, lack of health-skill experience

PLANNING

Unmet Needs
Comfort, protection from physical harm, dependence, mastery and competence in skills, independence, increased learning

Expected Outcome
Correct verbal feedback of the information taught
Correct return demonstration of how to count a pulse

NURSING INTERVENTIONS

Nursing Treatments
Provide temporary assistance until the skill is learned
Encourage the person to ask questions
Encourage self-performance

Nursing Observations
Palpate the pulse for rate, rhythm, and volume
Observe for readiness to assume self-care
Determine teaching effectiveness by testing, verbal feedback, and return demonstration

Health Teaching
Teach how to locate and count a pulse (*Location specific to patient's condition*: pedal pulse for casted leg, apical pulse for child or person on digitalis therapy. *Counting*: light but firm forefinger pressure, count one full minute)
Explain the reason for and intended effect of the procedure (to identify pulse rate, regulate the pulse with medication, identify abnormalities)
Describe those symptoms that should be reported (irregular, fast, slow pulse, absent peripheral pulse)
Explain when to perform the procedure (check the pulse when the person is at rest, preferably before getting out of bed in the morning; immediately before giving digitalis preparation)

EVALUATION
Record actual outcome

UNSKILLED AT MONITORING TEMPERATURE[362,423]

ASSESSMENT

Data Collection

Subjective Data
- Person's discussion or questions indicate a need for additional information, clarification, or validation of information about performing the task of monitoring the body temperature
  OR
- Person's lack of questions or comments indicates not wanting information or not knowing enough to seek information about performing the task of monitoring the body temperature

  Person may not know:
  Why the temperature should be taken
  When to take the temperature
  How long to keep the thermometer in place

Objective Data
- Person cannot correctly demonstrate how to:
  Insert the thermometer
  Determine the thermometer reading
  Clean the thermometer, if nondisposable

Related Data
Commonly Related Diseases
Childhood diseases, infectious mononucleosis, influenza, nasopharyngitis, sinusitis, any disease in which there is fever

Data Analysis

Nursing Diagnosis
UNSKILLED AT MONITORING TEMPERATURE: Being nonproficient, with or without knowledge, in the performance of the specific task of taking a body temperature reading

Common Etiology (Stressors)
HEALTH CARE FACTORS: Lack of health instruction, lack of health-skill experience

PLANNING

Unmet Needs
Comfort, protection from physical harm, dependence, mastery and competence in skills, independence, increased learning

Expected Outcome
Correct verbal feedback of the information taught
Correct return demonstration of how to take a temperature

NURSING INTERVENTIONS

Nursing Treatments
Provide temporary assistance until the skill is learned
Encourage the person to ask questions
Encourage self-performance

Nursing Observations
Monitor the axillary temperature, the oral temperature, or the rectal temperature
Observe for readiness to assume self-care
Determine teaching effectiveness by testing, verbal feedback, and return demonstration

Health Teaching
Describe the signs and symptoms that indicate the need for taking the temperature (hot and dry skin, flushed face, malaise, rash, respiratory distress)

Teach how to take a temperature and accurately read a thermometer (according to the type of temperature needed and the type of thermometer to be used)

Teach how to clean a nondisposable thermometer

Explain the reason for and intended effect of the procedure (to determine excessive body heat production or heat loss)

Describe those signs that should be reported (a temperature above 101° F or below 97° F)

Explain when to perform the procedure (check the temperature every 4–8 hours as needed)

Teach the specific procedure (of emergency measures for very high fever such as removing unneeded clothing, sponging with tepid but not cold water, giving aspirin)

EVALUATION

Record actual outcome

UNSKILLED AT NASOGASTRIC FEEDING[73,362,451]

ASSESSMENT

Data Collection

Subjective Data
- Person's discussion or questions indicate a need for additional information, clarification, or validation of information about performing the task of feeding through a nasogastric tube
  OR
- Person's lack of questions or comments indicates not wanting information or not knowing enough to seek information about performing the task of feeding through a nasogastric tube
  Person may not know:
  The amounts and kinds of feeding to be used
  Methods for preventing complications
  The symptoms that should be reported

Objective Data
- Person cannot correctly demonstrate how to:
  Insert the nasogastric tube
  Test for correct placement of the tube
  Properly position the person for a feeding
  Prepare and administer the tube feeding
  Clamp and remove the tube after the feeding
  Care for an indwelling nasogastric tube

Related Data
Commonly Related Diseases
Laryngeal carcinoma, cerebrovascular accident

Data Analysis

Nursing Diagnosis
UNSKILLED AT NASOGASTRIC FEEDING: Being nonproficient, with or without knowledge, in the performance of the specific task of providing nutritional feedings through a tube inserted through the nose into the stomach

Common Etiology (Stressors)
HEALTH CARE FACTORS: Lack of health instruction, lack of health-skill experience

PLANNING

Unmet Needs

Fluid and electrolyte balance, nutritional balance, comfort, cleanliness, protection from physical harm, dependence, mastery and competence in skills, independence, increased learning

Expected Outcome

Daily adequate calorie intake

Daily intake of 1,500–3,000 cc of fluid including the tube feeding formula

Correct verbal feedback of the information taught

Correct return demonstration of how to prepare and administer tube feeding formula

NURSING INTERVENTIONS

Nursing Treatments

Provide temporary assistance (with tube feeding) until the skill is learned

Estimate the required daily calories

Position comfortably

Place in a sitting position (before, during, and for 30 minutes after the feeding)

Refrain from giving cold liquids

Feed slowly (the average feeding time is 30–40 minutes or by continuous drip over 24 hours)

Attend the patient constantly (during the feeding)

Refrain from sealing the feeding tube with a heavy clamp (to avoid dislodging the tube)

Balance fluid intake to equal output

Encourage self-performance

Nursing Observations

Check the tube's placement before giving the tube feeding

Inspect the abdomen for distention

Measure the intake and output

Observe for complaints of nausea

Observe for diarrhea, for diet intolerance, for conditions indicating a need for increased nutritional requirements (fever, tissue damage, weight loss, etc.)

Observe for readiness to assume self-care

Determine teaching effectiveness by testing, verbal feedback, and return demonstration

Health Teaching

Explain how to obtain therapeutic supplies

Teach how to prepare a formula (for tube feeding)

Recommend a regular feeding schedule

Teach how to administer the tube feeding (how to insert the nasogastric tube and check for residual food in the stomach before each feeding by aspirating the stomach contents, measuring the residual and returning it to the stomach, and how to adjust the feeding/fluid intake according to the residual; when the residual is 150 ml or more, subtract that amount from the total fluid to be given; for fever of 1° C, increase the water intake by 10–15% of the usual total; administer the tube feeding according to basic need of 35 ml per kg of body weight; the person requires a minimum of 7 cc water per 1 g of protein in the formula; for fever states, increase the water by 10–15% per 1° C fever; if the person is receiving 150 g or more protein per day, observe for hypertonic dehydration; provide after-feeding tube care; for a retention tube, either clamp or leave the tube open as needed for decompression; use gentle traction to the balloon type tube. For an intermittent tube, clamp and remove the tube and apply a sterile dressing)

Describe those symptoms that should be reported (nausea, diarrhea)

Explain the reason for and intended effect of the therapy (to maintain nutrition to cells)

Medical Treatments Performed by Nurses

Give the prescribed tube feeding

EVALUATION

Record actual outcome

UNSKILLED AT PERITONEAL DIALYSIS[71,201,451]

ASSESSMENT

Data Collection

Subjective Data

• Person's discussion or questions indicate a need for additional information, clarification, or validation of information about performing the task of peritoneal dialysis

OR

• Person's lack of questions or comments indicates not wanting information or not knowing enough to seek information about performing the task of peritoneal dialysis

Person may not know:

The purpose of peritoneal dialysis by gravity or machine

The physiologic effects of such

The precautions to be taken to avoid dangerous side effects

Objective Data

• Person cannot correctly demonstrate how to:

Maintain sterile technique

Use the peritoneal dialysis machine if such is being used

Instill and drain the dialysate solution

Clean and dress the peritoneal catheter site

Related Data

Commonly Related Diseases

Renal failure

Data Analysis

Nursing Diagnosis

UNSKILLED AT PERITONEAL DIALYSIS: Being nonproficient, with or without knowledge, in the performance of the specific task of administering peritoneal dialysis by machine or gravity for the purpose of removing chemical wastes and excesses from the blood

Common Etiology (Stressors)

HEALTH CARE FACTORS: Lack of health instruction, lack of health-skill experience

PLANNING

Unmet Needs

Waste elimination of nitrogenous substances, comfort, cleanliness, protection from physical harm, dependence, mastery and competence in skills, independence, increased learning

Expected Outcome

To restore serum electrolytes and nitrogenous substances (urea and creatinine) to acceptable levels

A clean, uninfected peritoneal catheter site

No evidence of infection or fluid imbalance

Correct verbal feedback of the information taught

Correct return demonstration of how to assemble the dialysis equipment, instill dialysate into the peritoneal cavity (inflow), manage the fluid while it is in the cavity (dwell-time), drain the dialysate from the peritoneal cavity (outflow), keep a flow record, monitor the vital signs, clean and dress the peritoneal catheter site

NURSING INTERVENTIONS

Nursing Treatments

Provide temporary assistance until the skill is learned
Attend the patient constantly (during the procedure)
Place in the flat position
  OR
Place in the slight sitting position
Warm the dialysate fluid before instillation (98.6° F)
Do not allow air into the dialysate instillation tubing
Elevate the head
  OR ⎤
Change the patient's position ⎬ If the dialysis fluid does not drain adequately
  frequently (from side to side) ⎦
Refrain from giving enemas (while the dialysis fluid is in the peritoneum)
Refrain from giving intravenous or intramuscular injections (postdialysis)
Refrain from jarring the bed
Change the dressing frequently (around the catheter)
Apply a sterile dressing (after the dialysis is completed)
Encourage the person or family to ask questions
Encourage self-performance
Introduce to persons who have successfully undergone the same experience

Nursing Observations

Auscultate the apical heartbeat for rate and rhythm (specifically for arrythmias)
Check the dialysis circuit for leakage
Check the peritoneal dialysis catheter for leakage or displacement
Check the peritoneal dialysis fluid for bloody or cloudy return
Check (dialysis) solution for flow rate (2,000 cc per 10–15 minutes)
Check the peritoneal dialysis fluid for retention or drainage in excess of 500 cc
Inspect the chest for respiratory rate and rhythm (drain the fluid from the peritoneum
  immediately if there is severe respiratory distress)
Inspect for bleeding (around the catheter)
Keep a dialysis flow sheet
Measure the body weight (before and after dialysis)
Measure the intake and output
Monitor the blood pressure (every 15 minutes for the first 2 hours, then every hour)
Monitor the oral temperature (every 4 hours)
Monitor blood studies for abnormal renal function (urea and creatinine before and dur-
  ing dialysis)
Observe for complaints of pain (severe abdominal pain, especially during fluid drainage)
Observe for complaints of pain radiation (to the left shoulder during instillation)
Observe for complaints of fatigue
Observe for shock
Obtain a bacterial culture (from the catheter tip and the last bottle of fluid drained)
Observe for readiness to assume self-care
Determine teaching effectiveness by testing, verbal feedback, and return demonstration

Health Teaching

Recommend home adaptations appropriate to the health problem (plumbing for sterile,
  deionized water; auxillary electrical power)
Teach how to obtain therapeutic supplies
Explain normal organ (kidney) function (the kidney produces urine, reabsorbs water and
  chemicals, filters body wastes, maintains blood pressure, controls the rate the red
  blood cells are made by the bone marrow)
Explain how the (dialysis) equipment works (dialysate fluid is instilled into the peritoneal cavity where metabolic wastes move into dialysate by filtration, osmosis, and diffusion after which the fluid is drained from the peritoneal cavity)

Teach sterile technique (this is extremely important)
Teach how to take a temperature and accurately read a thermometer
Teach how to locate and count a pulse
Explain how to observe respirations
Teach how to take a blood pressure
Teach how to weigh (before dialysate instillation and after dialysate drainage)
Explain how to measure the intake and output
Instruct the patient to empty his bladder before the procedure
Familiarize the person with the component parts of the equipment (peritoneal catheter, bags of dialysate fluid, Y connector, etc.)
Teach how to do home dialysis (how to prepare, operate, and clean the equipment specific to the prescribed procedure; how to regulate the dialysate flow cycle and warm the dialysate fluid; how to clean and dress the peritoneal catheter site, etc.)
Teach how to test the urine for glucosuria (after dialysate outflow)
Encourage increased protein-food intake (to offset protein lost in the dialysate)
Describe those symptoms that should be reported (left shoulder pain, fever, cloudy dialysate, dyspnea, severe abdominal discomfort, nausea, vomiting, inflammation or drainage around the catheter site, rapid respirations or pulse, confusion or disorientation)
Advise how to integrate the dialysis procedure into the daily routine
Explain the reason for and intended effect of the therapy (to remove body wastes)

Medical Treatments Performed by Nurses
Instill dialysate into the peritoneum (10–15 minutes), allow it to remain in the abdomen (30–35 minutes), then drain dialysate (10–15 minutes)
Give the prescribed number of peritoneal dialysis exchanges
Give the prescribed drugs (heparin, potassium, antibiotics)

EVALUATION
Record actual outcome

UNSKILLED AT POSTMASTECTOMY CARE[73,451]

ASSESSMENT
Data Collection
Subjective Data
• Person's discussion or questions indicate a need for additional information, clarification, or validation of information about performing the task of breast care following a mastectomy
  OR
• Person's lack of questions or comments indicates not wanting information or not knowing enough to seek information about performing the task of breast care following a mastectomy
  Woman may not know:
    Of the need to support the unamputated breast
    Of the need for careful, periodic examination of the remaining breast
    About breast prosthesis

Objective Data
• Person cannot correctly demonstrate how to:
    Do postmastectomy range-of-motion exercises

Care for the healing site following a mastectomy

Related Data
Commonly Related Diseases
Fibrosarcoma, hemangiosarcoma, lymphosarcoma

Data Analysis

Nursing Diagnosis
UNSKILLED AT POSTMASTECTOMY CARE: Being nonproficient, with or without knowledge, in the performance of the specific task of caring for the healing site and remaining breast following a mastectomy

Common Etiology (Stressors)
HEALTH CARE FACTORS: Lack of health instruction, lack of health-skill experience

PLANNING

Unmet Needs
Exercise, comfort, protection from physical harm, dependence, mastery and competence in skills, independence, increased learning

Expected Outcome
Correct verbal feedback of the information taught
Correct return demonstration of how to do self-breast examination and postmastectomy exercises

NURSING INTERVENTIONS

Nursing Treatments
Provide temporary assistance until the skill is learned (with prosthesis, range-of-motion exercises, self-breast examination)
Encourage the person to ask questions
Encourage self-care
Make a referral (to the local Reach-to-Recovery Program of the American Cancer Society)

Nursing Observations
Inspect for inflammation, drainage, edema (lymphedema of the arm)
Test for range of motion (of the arm and hand)
Observe for readiness to assume self-care
Determine teaching effectiveness by testing, verbal feedback, and return demonstration

Health Teaching
Teach how to clean and dress the surgical site
Instruct to lubricate the skin (at the healed surgical site)
Recommend the use of a brassiere for breast support (of the unamputated breast)
Recommend an appropriate breast prosthesis (soft padding shortly after surgery, with professional fitting later)
Teach how to do postmastectomy exercises
Explain the importance of periodic breast inspection
Inform of when to do the breast examination (1–2 days after completion of menstruation; after menopause, same time, once a month)
Demonstrate how to do the breast examination (over all breast areas)
Explain the reasons for and intended effect of the therapy (range-of-motion exercises promote circulation, joint mobility, and strengthen muscle tone)
Emphasize the importance of follow-up care
Describe those symptoms that should be reported (inflammation, drainage, new masses, increasing lymphedema of the arm)

EVALUATION

Record actual outcome

UNSKILLED AT POSTPARTUM PERINEAL CARE[286,527]

ASSESSMENT

Data Collection

Subjective Data
- Person's discussion or questions indicate a need for additional information, clarification, or validation of information about performing the task of perineal care following childbirth

  OR
- Person's lack of questions or comments indicates not wanting information or not knowing enough to seek information about performing the task of perineal care following childbirth

  Woman may not know:

  The importance of episiotomy care

  The methods of preventing infection

  The symptoms that should be reported

  The comfort measures to use

Objective Data
- Person cannot correctly demonstrate how to:

  Cleanse the perineal area

  Properly dry the sutured region

  Apply warmth to the area

Related Data

Commonly Related Conditions

Childbirth

Data Analysis

Nursing Diagnosis

UNSKILLED AT POSTPARTUM PERINEAL CARE/EPISIOTOMY CARE: Being nonproficient, with or without knowledge, in the performance of the specific task of cleansing and promoting healing of a surgical incision in perineal tissue

Common Etiology (Stressors)

HEALTH CARE FACTORS: Lack of health instruction, lack of health-care experience

PLANNING

Unmet Needs

Comfort, cleanliness, protection from physical harm, dependence, mastery and competence in skills, independence, increased learning

Expected Outcome

A clean perineal area

A dry suture area

No inflammation or edema at the time of suture removal

Correct verbal feedback of the information taught

Correct return demonstration of how to do perineal care

NURSING INTERVENTIONS

Nursing Treatments

Provide temporary assistance until the skill is learned

Apply an ice bag (to the perineum immediately after delivery to reduce edema formation)

Apply a heat lamp (2–3 times daily after 24 hours)

Soak in a sitz bath (2–3 times daily)

Apply an analgesic ointment or spray

Give perineal care (wash the vulva, perineum, and groin with soap and water. Pour warm water over the area and dry)

Change the sanitary pads frequently (after each voiding and defecation)

Encourage self-performance

Encourage the person to ask questions

Nursing Observations

Inspect for bleeding, edema, inflammation, drainage

Obtain a bacterial culture (of any drainage)

Observe for readiness to assume self-care

Determine teaching effectiveness by testing, verbal feedback, and return demonstration

Health Teaching

Teach how to do perineal care

Teach how to apply heat therapy

Explain how to use toilet tissue correctly by cleansing from front to back

Advise frequent sanitary pad change (after each voiding and defecation)

Describe those symptoms that should be reported (fever, bleeding, inflammation)

Explain the reason for and intended effect of the therapy (to promote comfort and healing and to prevent infection)

EVALUATION

Record actual outcome

UNSKILLED AT RETRAINING IN ELIMINATION CONTROL [41,72,108]

ASSESSMENT

Data Collection

Subjective Data

• Person's discussion or questions indicate a need for additional information, clarification, or validation of information about performing the task of regaining control of elimination

  OR

• Person's lack of questions or comments indicates not wanting information or not knowing enough to seek information about performing the task of regaining control of elimination

  Person may not know:

  The importance of high fluid intake, proper positioning, and exercise

  About scheduled toileting

  Of the need to avoid enemas and laxatives

Objective Data

• Person cannot correctly demonstrate how to:

  Stimulate the reflex bladder and bowel

  Insert a suppository rectally

  Person has involuntary voiding and bowel movements

Related Data

Commonly Related Conditions

Neurogenic bladder

Commonly Related Diseases

Cerebrovascular accident, multiple sclerosis, posterolateral sclerosis

Commonly Related Injuries
Fracture and compression of the spinal cord

Data Analysis

Nursing Diagnosis
UNSKILLED AT RETRAINING IN ELIMINATION CONTROL: Being nonproficient, with or without knowledge, in the performance of the specific task of reestablishing bowel and/or bladder control following the loss of such from disease or injury

Common Etiology (Stressors)
HEALTH CARE FACTORS: Lack of health instruction, lack of health-skill experience

PLANNING

Unmet Needs
Comfort, protection from physical harm, dependence, mastery and competence in skills, independence, increased learning

Expected Outcome
Scheduled control of voiding and bowel elimination
Correct verbal feedback of the information taught
Correct return demonstration of how to clamp an indwelling catheter, stimulate the reflex bowel and bladder, insert a suppository

NURSING INTERVENTIONS

Nursing Treatments
Provide temporary assistance until the skill is learned
Encourage the person to ask questions

General Measures
Place in the sitting position (for elimination)
Encourage the use of the bathroom
> OR
Provide a bedside commode
> OR
Provide a bedpan (placed on a chair)
Encourage moderate physical exercise

Bladder Training
Give small, frequent drinks
Increase fluid intake to about 2,000 cc daily
Clamp the indwelling urinary catheter intermittently (release the clamp every 1–2 hours, progressing to 3–4 hours)
Schedule toileting (at regular intervals of every 2 hours, progressing to 3–4 hours; if a catheter has recently been removed, schedule toileting every hour)
Stimulate the reflex bladder by applying cold to the abdomen, stroking the inner thigh, or running water
Restrict the intake to nothing by mouth (no fluids after the evening meal)
Refrain from giving oral stimulants (until just before the scheduled toileting)
Respond immediately to the patient's call (for assistance with toileting)
Dress in personal clothing

Bowel Training
Schedule toileting (at the same time every day, preferably after a scheduled meal)
Provide a balanced nutritional diet
Increase fluid intake to about 3,000 cc daily
Give nonprescription drugs (glycerine suppository rectally 30 minutes before scheduled toileting)
Give prune juice (daily in the morning)
Stimulate the reflex bowel by abdominal stroking and anal stimulation
Refrain from giving enemas, from giving laxatives

Nursing Observations
Measure the intake and output
Measure the residual urine (if urine retention is suspected)
Observe for readiness to assume self-care
Determine teaching effectiveness by testing, verbal feedback, and return demonstration

Health Teaching
Teach the specific procedure (for elimination control)
Explain the reason for and intended effect of the methods used

EVALUATION
Record actual outcome

UNSKILLED AT THERAPEUTIC TRACTION [72,451]

ASSESSMENT
Data Collection

Subjective Data
• Person's discussion or questions indicate a need for additional information, clarification, or validation of information about performing the task of therapeutic traction
    OR
• Person's lack of questions or comments indicates not wanting information or not knowing enough to seek information about performing the task of therapeutic traction
  Person may not know:
    The purpose or physical effects of traction
    The precautions that should be taken

Objective Data
• Person cannot correctly demonstrate how to:
    Set up the traction apparatus
    Maintain correct body alignment
    Maintain traction alignment
    Cleanse the traction pin or tong sites
    Prevent ropes, halter, or tape irritation

Related Data
Commonly Related Injuries
Bone fracture, fracture and compression of spinal cord, whiplash

Data Analysis

Nursing Diagnosis
UNSKILLED AT THERAPEUTIC TRACTION: Being nonproficient, with or without knowledge, in the performance of the specific task of managing an applied, weighted, pulling device on bones and muscles

Common Etiology (Stressors)
HEALTH CARE FACTORS: Lack of health instruction, lack of health-skill experience

PLANNING
Unmet Needs
Comfort, protection from physical harm, dependence, mastery and competence in skills, independence, increased learning

Expected Outcome

Cleanliness of the pin or tong sites

No skin irritation from ropes, tape, or halters

Correct verbal feedback of the information taught

Correct return demonstration of how to apply and remove intermittent traction, maintain alignment, prevent skin irritation, manage pin care

NURSING INTERVENTIONS

Nursing Treatments

Provide temporary assistance (with traction) until the skill is learned

Maintain body alignment

Change the patient's position gradually (when in traction)

Provide orthopedic pin care (gently clean around the pin with a sterile cotton-tipped applicator soaked in hydrogen peroxide, then clean the area with normal saline; apply a nonocclusive antibacterial agent, Betadine Halafoam, and allow to air dry)

Maintain countertraction force

Place a bedboard under the mattress

Provide a firm mattress

Position comfortably

Refrain from jarring the bed

Encourage the person to ask questions

Encourage self-performance

Nursing Observations

Check that the traction weights are hanging free

Check the traction ropes and pulleys for alignment

Inspect the skin for breakdown

Inspect the orthopedic pin site (for position, cleanliness, tension, redness, and drainage)

Observe for cyanosis (of the area in traction)

Observe for readiness to assume self-care

Determine teaching effectiveness by testing, verbal feedback, and return demonstration

Health Teaching

Teach the specific procedure (for managing traction such as applying intermittent Buck's extension, correct positioning and alignment, pin care, how to protect external fixation devices and halo traction from damage or disruption, how to ambulate with such devices)

Teach how to do range-of-motion exercises

Explain how to adjust clothing to meet the health needs (for ease of dressing with traction, for covering the devices)

Explain the reason for and intended effect of the therapy (to promote aligned healing)

Medical Treatments Performed by Nurses

Apply the prescribed traction

EVALUATION

Record actual outcome

UNSKILLED AT TRACHEOSTOMY CARE[73,451]

ASSESSMENT

Data Collection

Subjective Data

• Person's discussion or questions indicate a need for additional information,

clarification, or validation of information about performing the task of caring for a tracheostomy

OR

• Person's lack of questions or comments indicates not wanting information or not knowing enough to seek information about performing the task of caring for a tracheostomy

Person may not know:

The purpose of a tracheostomy

The precautions that should be taken

Objective Data

• Person cannot correctly demonstrate how to:

Suction the tracheostomy

Clean the inner and outer cannula

Change the tracheostomy dressing

Maintain aseptic technique

Humidify the tracheostomy

Related Data

Commonly Related Diseases

Laryngeal carcinoma, cerebrovascular accident, diphtheria, Guillain-Barré syndrome

Commonly Related Injuries

Fracture and compression of spinal cord

Data Analysis

Nursing Diagnosis

UNSKILLED AT TRACHEOSTOMY CARE: Being nonproficient, with or without knowledge, in the performance of the specific task of caring for and cleansing a tracheostomy airway

Common Etiology (Stressors)

HEALTH CARE FACTORS: Lack of health instruction, lack of health-skill experience

PLANNING

Unmet Needs

Oxygen, comfort, cleanliness, protection from physical harm, dependence, mastery and competence in skills, independence, increased learning

Expected Outcome

A clean, patent tracheostomy inner and outer cannula and dressing

A humidified tracheostomy

Correct verbal feedback of the information taught

Correct return demonstration of how to suction and clean the tracheostomy tube, change the dressing, humidify the tracheostomy, maintain sterile or clean technique

NURSING INTERVENTIONS

Nursing Treatments

Provide temporary assistance until the skill is learned

Administer vaporized air (by tracheostomy collar)

Maintain adequate atmospheric humidity

Maintain a warm room temperature (80° F)

Suction the airway (as needed)

Change the catheter each time the airway is suctioned

Wear a mask when suctioning

Wear sterile gloves (when suctioning)

Change the dressing frequently

Change the tracheostomy tube (only if the trach site is well healed and the tube change is approved by the physician)

Clean the tracheostomy tube inner cannula (every 4 hours)

Clean (the skin around the tracheostomy site) with surgical soap

Shield the tracheostomy from water
Encourage coughing
Encourage deep breathing
Inflate the airway-tube cuff
Deflate the airway-tube cuff periodically
Place in the sitting position (unless contraindicated)
Rinse the mouth with dilute hydrogen peroxide
   OR
Swab the mouth with diluted glycerine
   OR
Refresh with a mouthwash
Brush and floss the teeth
Encourage the person to ask questions
Encourage self-performance

Nursing Observations
Check the (tracheostomy) tube for patency and cleanliness
Inspect for bleeding (around the tracheostomy site)
Inspect the chest for respiratory rate and rhythm; for symmetrical expansion
Auscultate the chest for lung aeration
Monitor blood studies for arterial blood gases
Observe for cyanosis, for dyspnea
Observe for readiness to assume self-care
Determine teaching effectiveness by testing, verbal feedback, and return demonstration

Health Teaching
Advise against exposure to airborne irritants and inclement weather
Describe those symptoms that should be reported (dyspnea, severe coughing, bleeding
  around the tracheostomy site, purulent mucus)
Emphasize the danger of breathing cold air
Inform that the tracheostomy must be covered in order to speak
Inform that airway noise indicates obstruction
Instruct to protect the tracheostomy from water
Teach how to clean a tracheostomy, how to inflate and deflate an airway cuff, how to
  suction an airway, and how to give vaporized-solution inhalation
Explain the reason for and intended effect of the therapy

Medical Treatments Performed by Nurses
Administer humidified oxygen

EVALUATION

Record actual outcome

UNSKILLED AT URETEROILEOSTOMY CARE[72,451]

ASSESSMENT

Data Collection

Subjective Data
• Person's discussion or questions indicate a need for additional information,
  clarification, or validation of information about performing the task of caring for a
  ureteroileostomy
   OR
• Person's lack of questions or comments indicates not wanting information or not
  knowing enough to seek information about performing the task of caring for a
  ureteroileostomy

Person may not know:
    The foods that should be avoided
    The need to increase fluids
    Methods of odor control
    The precautions that should be taken
    Those symptoms that should be reported

Objective Data
• Person cannot correctly demonstrate how to:
    Clean and protect the skin around the ureteroileostomy stoma
    Dilate the stoma with a catheter
    Apply, remove, and empty the collection container
    Maintain sterile and clean technique

Related Data
Commonly Related Diseases
Carcinoma of the bladder

Data Analysis

Nursing Diagnosis
UNSKILLED AT URETEROILEOSTOMY CARE (UNSKILLED AT IDEAL CONDUIT CARE) (UNSKILLED AT BRICKER PROCE-DURE CARE)   Being nonproficient, with or without knowledge, in the performance of the specific task of managing the care of an artificial opening in which the ureter has been surgically implanted into a loop of the ileum, with urine flowing externally from stomas or buds

Common Etiology (Stressors)
HEALTH CARE FACTORS: Lack of health instruction, lack of health-skill experience

PLANNING

Unmet Needs
Fluid and electrolyte balance, acid-base balance, waste elimination of urine, comfort, cleanliness, protection from physical harm, dependence, mastery and competence in skills, independence, increased learning

Expected Outcome
A consistently clean stoma, surrounding the skin and collection container
A urine output of 1,500–3,000 cc daily or equivalent to the intake
A urine pH of 4.8–8.0
Less than 100,000 bacteria per cubic mm on urine culture
Correct verbal feedback of the information taught
Correct return demonstration of cleaning the stoma and surrounding skin; stoma dilatation; attaching, removing, and emptying the drainage system; maintaining sterile technique

NURSING INTERVENTIONS

Nursing Treatments
Provide temporary assistance until the skill is learned
Clean with surgical soap (around the ureteroileostomy)
Apply calamine lotion ⎤
    OR   ⎥
Apply milk of magnesia to the skin ⎬ Around the ureteroileostomy
    OR   ⎥
Lubricate the skin with petrolatum ⎦
Apply ostomy adhesive and then an ostomy appliance
Attach the collection appliance to straight drainage and a collection container (if preferred, in order to protect the incision from urine contamination)
Empty the collection appliance (every 2–3 hours or when it contains 100 cc of urine, if it is not attached to a straight drainage)
Change the ostomy appliance as needed
Give urine-acidifying juices orally (four times a day)

Increase fluid intake to about 2,000 cc daily

Introduce to persons who have successfully undergone the same experience (if the patient is anxious)

Make a referral (to the local United Ostomy Association)

Encourage the person to ask questions

Encourage self-performance

Nursing Observations

Check the drainage system for leakage

Inspect for signs of (skin) irritation

Measure the intake and output

Monitor urine studies for evidence of urinary tract infection

Observe for complaints of pain (in the lower abdomen)

Observe the urine for abnormal color, content, and odor

Inspect for bleeding (hematuria)

Obtain a bacterial culture (of the urine periodically)

Test the urine for pH

Observe for readiness to assume self-care

Determine teaching effectiveness by testing, verbal feedback, and return demonstration

Health Teaching

Teach how to clean and dress the surgical site

Teach how to dilate the stoma with a sterile catheter

Teach how to apply and remove the ostomy appliance

Explain how to attach the drainage system to the appliance

Recommend that two ostomy appliances be alternately used

Explain how to maintain cleanliness of the ostomy appliances

Instruct to avoid foods having strong odors

Instruct to increase fluid intake (to about 2,000 cc daily)

Explain how to keep the urine within the desired pH range (using acid-ash fluids, vitamin C)

Teach how to test urine pH

Explain how to obtain therapeutic supplies

Recommend that extra therapeutic supplies be carried (to assure comfort and cleanliness)

Describe those symptoms that should be reported (bleeding, abdominal pain, cloudy urine, malodorous urine, urine pH above 8.5)

Explain the reason for and intended effect of the therapy (to prevent infection, reduce skin irritation)

Medical Treatments Performed by Nurses

Irrigate the ostomy

EVALUATION

Record actual outcome

UNSKILLED AT URETEROSIGMOIDOSTOMY CARE [72,451]

ASSESSMENT

Data Collection

Subjective Data

• Person's discussion or questions indicate a need for additional information,

clarification, or validation of information about performing the task of caring for a ureterosigmoidostomy

OR

• Person's lack of questions or comments indicates not wanting information or not knowing enough to seek information about performing the task of caring for a ureterosigmoidostomy

Person may not know:

Of special foods to avoid

Of the need for frequent toileting

The importance of increasing oral fluids

Those symptoms that should be reported

Objective Data

• Person cannot correctly demonstrate how to:

Clean and protect the skin around a ureterosigmoidostomy

Insert and remove the colon tube

Attach the tube to a collection container

Related Data

Commonly Related Diseases

Prostate or bladder carcinoma, prostatic hypertrophy, urethral calculi

Data Analysis

Nursing Diagnosis

UNSKILLED AT URETEROSIGMOIDOSTOMY CARE: Being nonproficient, with or without knowledge, in the performance of the specific task of managing the care of a person with a surgical implantation of ureters in the sigmoid colon, which results in elimination of urine from the anus

Common Etiology (Stressors)

HEALTH CARE FACTORS: Lack of health instruction, lack of health-skill experience

PLANNING

Unmet Needs

Fluid and electrolyte balance, acid-base balance, waste elimination of urine, comfort, cleanliness, protection from physical harm, dependence, mastery and competence in skills, independence, increased learning

Expected Outcome

A consistently clean anal area and collection container

No evidence of systemic infection

Balanced serum electrolytes

Correct verbal feedback of the information taught

Correct return demonstration of how to insert and remove the colon tube, how to clean the anal area and collection container

NURSING INTERVENTIONS

Nursing Treatments

Provide temporary assistance until the skill is learned

Encourage decreased gas-forming-food intake (before and after surgery)

Toilet frequently (every 2–4 hours)

Remove the colon tube for bowel elimination and then reinsert about 4 inches (during the early postoperative period)

Anchor the (colon) tubing securely (to the buttocks)

Attach the tube to straight drainage and a collection container (during the night)

Increase fluid intake to about 3,000 cc daily

Refrain from giving enemas, from giving laxatives

Lubricate the skin with petrolatum (around the rectal area if it becomes irritated)

Apply a heat lamp (for skin irritation)

Protect with plastic pants

Introduce to persons who have successfully undergone the same experience (if the patient is anxious)

Make a referral (to the local United Ostomy Association)

Encourage the person to ask questions

Encourage self-performance

Nursing Observations

Check the (ureterosigmoidostomy) tube for patency

Inspect for signs of (skin) irritation

Measure the urine output hourly (for the first 24 hours after surgery)

Measure the intake

Measure the output (after the first 24 hours)

Monitor blood studies for abnormal electrolytes

Monitor urine studies for evidence of urinary tract infection

Monitor the oral temperature (for fever)

Observe for complaints of nausea, of pain

Observe for vomiting

Observe the urine for abnormal color, content, and odor

Inspect for bleeding (hematuria)

Obtain a bacterial culture (of the urine periodically)

Test the urine for pH

Observe for readiness to assume self-care

Determine teaching effectiveness by testing, verbal feedback, and return demonstration

Health Teaching

Teach how to clean and dress the surgical site

Instruct to toilet frequently (every 2–4 hours and to expell gas into the toilet to prevent soiling)

Instruct to increase fluid intake (to at least 3,000 cc daily)

Advise not to take enemas and laxatives

Teach the specific procedure (of using a colon tube at night, or sleeping in a semi-sitting position to avoid urinary reflux)

Explain how to attach the drainage system to the tube

Recommend the carrying of extra undergarments when away from home

Describe those symptoms that should be reported (fever, nausea, vomiting, pain, hematuria, skin irritation)

Explain the reason for and intended effect of the therapy (to maintain comfort and cleanliness, to reduce skin irritation)

EVALUATION

Record actual outcome

UNSKILLED AT URETEROSTOMY CARE[72,451]

ASSESSMENT

Data Collection

Subjective Data

• Person's discussion or questions indicate a need for additional information, clarification, or validation of information about performing the task of caring for a ureterostomy

 OR

• Person's lack of questions or comments indicates not wanting information of not knowing enough to seek information about performing the task of caring for a ureterostomy

Person may not know:

Methods of odor control

The importance of increasing fluids

The precautions that should be taken

Those symptoms that should be reported

Objective Data

• Person cannot correctly demonstrate how to:

Clean and protect the skin around the ureterostomy stoma

Dilate the stoma with a sterile catheter

Apply, remove, and empty the collection container

Maintain sterile and clean technique

Related Data

Commonly Related Diseases

Ureteral carcinoma, nephrolithiasis, rectocaval ureter, rectoperitoneal fibrosis, ureteral calculi

Data Analysis

Nursing Diagnosis

UNSKILLED AT URETEROSTOMY CARE: Being nonproficient, with or without knowledge, in the performance of the specific task of managing the care of an artificial opening in which the ureter(s) have been surgically implanted into the abdominal wall, with urine flowing from the stoma(s)

Common Etiology (Stressors)

HEALTH CARE FACTORS: Lack of health instruction, lack of health-skill experience

PLANNING

Unmet Needs

Fluid and electrolyte balance, acid-base balance, waste elimination of urine, comfort, cleanliness, protection from physical harm, dependence, mastery and competence in skills, independence, increased learning

Expected Outcome

A consistently clean stoma, surrounding skin, and collection container

A urine output of 1,500–3,000 cc daily or equivalent to the intake

A urine pH of 4.8–8.5

Less than 100,000 bacteria per cubic mm on urine culture

Correct verbal feedback of the information taught

Correct return demonstration of cleaning the stoma and surrounding skin; stoma dilatation; attaching, removing, and emptying the drainage system; maintaining sterile technique

NURSING INTERVENTIONS

Nursing Treatments

Provide temporary assistance until the skill is learned

First 5–10 Days When the Catheter Is in the Ureter

Apply a (sterile) saline compress (over the ureteral buds)

Apply a sterile dressing (over the saline compress)

Apply zinc oxide to the skin

OR

Apply aluminum paste to the skin (around the ureterostomy)

OR

Lubricate the skin with petrolatum

After the Ureter Catheter Is Removed

Apply an ostomy appliance

Empty the collection appliance (frequently during the day)
Attach the collection appliance to straight drainage and a collection container (during the night)
Change the ostomy appliance as needed (usually every 3–4 days)
Bathe locally (with soap and water when changing the appliance)
Apply tincture of benzoin (over the skin area covered by the appliance)
Give urine-acidifying juices orally (four times a day)
Increase fluid intake to about 2,000 cc daily
Introduce to persons who have successfully undergone the same experience (if the patient is anxious)
Make a referral (to the local United Ostomy Association)
Encourage the person to ask questions
Encourage self-performance

Nursing Observations
Check the ureterostomy tube for patency
Inspect for edema (of the stoma)
Inspect (the skin) for signs of irritation
Measure the intake and output
Observe for complaints of pain (backache indicates that drainage is not flowing)
Observe the urine for abnormal color, content, and odor
Obtain a bacterial culture (of the urine periodically)
Test the urine for pH
Observe for readiness to assume self-care
Determine teaching effectiveness by testing, verbal feedback, and return demonstration

Health Teaching
Teach how to clean and dress the surgical site
Teach how to dilate the stoma with a sterile catheter
Teach how to apply and remove the ostomy appliance
Explain how to attach the drainage system to the appliance
Recommend that two ostomy appliances be alternately used
Explain how to maintain cleanliness of the ostomy appliances
Instruct to avoid foods having strong odors
Explain how to keep the urine within the desired pH range (using acid-ash fluids, vitamin C)
Teach how to test the urine for pH
Instruct to increase fluid intake (to about 2,000 cc daily)
Explain how to obtain therapeutic supplies
Recommend that extra therapeutic supplies be carried (for comfort and cleanliness)
Describe those symptoms that should be reported (back pain, cloudy urine, hematuria, malodorous urine, urine pH over 8.5)
Explain the reason for and intended effect of the therapy (to prevent infection, to reduce skin irritation)

EVALUATION

Record actual outcome

UNSKILLED AT URINARY CATHETER CARE[73,451]

ASSESSMENT

Data Collection

Subjective Data
• Person's discussion or questions indicate a need for additional information,

clarification, or validation of information about performing the task of caring for a urinary catheter
OR
• Person's lack of questions or comments indicates not wanting information or not knowing enough to seek information about performing the task of caring for a urinary catheter
Person may not know:
The importance of increasing fluids
Methods of odor control
The precautions to be taken
Those symptoms that should be reported

Objective Data
• Person cannot correctly demonstrate how to:
Insert an indwelling catheter
Attach, remove, and empty a drainage system
Irrigate a catheter
Maintain sterile technique

Related Data
Commonly Related Diseases
Bladder or urethral calculi, carcinoma of the bladder, cerebrovascular accident, multiple sclerosis
Commonly Related Injuries
Fracture and compression of spinal cord

Data Analysis
Nursing Diagnosis
UNSKILLED AT URINARY CATHETER CARE: Being nonproficient, with or without knowledge, in the performance of the specific task of managing an indwelling urinary catheter and bladder drainage system

Common Etiology (Stressors)
HEALTH CARE FACTORS: Lack of health instruction, lack of health-skill experience

PLANNING

Unmet Needs
Fluid and electrolyte balance, acid-base balance, waste elimination of urine, comfort, cleanliness, protection from physical harm, dependence, mastery and competence in skills, independence, increased learning

Expected Outcome
A urine output of 1,500–3,000 cc daily, or equivalent to the intake
A consistently clean perineum, catheter, and drainage system
A urine pH of 4.8–8.5
Less than 100,000 bacteria per cubic mm on urine culture
Correct verbal feedback of the information taught
Correct return demonstration of how to insert, irrigate, and remove a catheter; attach, remove and empty the drainage system; maintain sterile technique; and record intake and output

NURSING INTERVENTIONS

Nursing Treatments
Provide temporary assistance until the skill is learned
Clean the urinary catheter externally at the meatus (daily)
Change the urinary catheter (as needed)
Irrigate the urinary catheter (periodically)
Tape the urinary catheter onto the abdomen (if the catheter is inserted for a prolonged period)

Provide sufficiently long tubing to allow freedom of movement
Attach the tube to straight drainage and a collection container
> OR

Attach the tube to a leg urinal
Keep the drainage container below bladder level
Change the urinary drainage apparatus (frequently)
Use sterile technique (when disconnecting the urinary drainage system)
Give urine-acidifying juices orally (four times daily)
Increase fluid intake to about 2,000 cc daily
Encourage the person to ask questions
Encourage self-performance

Nursing Observations

Check the drainage system for leakage
Check the tube (indwelling urinary catheter) for patency
Measure the intake and output
Monitor urine studies for evidence of urinary tract infection
Observe for complaints of pain
Observe the urine for abnormal color, content, and odor
Inspect for bleeding (hematuria)
Test the urine for pH
Observe for readiness to assume self-care
Determine teaching effectiveness by testing, verbal feedback, and return demonstration

Health Teaching

Teach how to do a catheterization, how to irrigate a urinary catheter, how to apply an external urinary catheter
Explain how to clean the external part of the indwelling urinary catheter (and the adjacent tissues)
Explain that the urinary catheter should be taped to the abdomen of males
Instruct to anchor the urinary catheter securely
Teach how to apply a urinary collection container
Instruct that the drainage container should be kept below the bladder level
Explain how to keep the urine within the desired pH range (using acid-ash fluids, vitamin C)
Teach how to test the urine for pH
Teach sterile techniques
Instruct to increase fluid intake
Explain how to obtain therapeutic supplies
Describe those symptoms that should be reported (pain, fever, cloudy urine)
Explain the reason for and intended effect of the therapy (drainage of urine, prevention of infection)

EVALUATION

Record actual outcome

UNSKILLED AT WOUND CARE[73,362,451]

ASSESSMENT

Data Collection

Subjective Data

• Person's discussion or questions indicate a need for additional information, clarification, or validation of information about performing the task of caring for a wound

OR
- Person's lack of questions or comments indicates not wanting information or not knowing enough to seek information about performing the task of caring for a wound

Person may not know:
   When to leave a wound open or to bandage it
   Those symptoms that should be reported
   The precautions to be taken

Objective Data
- Person cannot correctly demonstrate how to:
   Clean a wound
   Change a dressing
   Properly position the wounded body part
   Apply a protective splint
   Medicate a wound
   Maintain sterile technique

Related Data
Commonly Related Injuries
Abrasion wound, incisional wound, puncture wound, stab wound

Data Analysis

Nursing Diagnosis
UNSKILLED AT WOUND CARE: Being nonproficient, with or without knowledge, in the performance of the specific task of cleansing and caring for a wound

Common Etiology (Stressors)
HEALTH CARE FACTORS: Lack of health instruction, lack of health-skill experience

PLANNING

Unmet Needs
Comfort, cleanliness, protection from physical harm, dependence, mastery and competence in skills, independence, increased learning

Expected Outcome
A clean, dressed, healing wound with proper positioning and protection of the body part
Correct verbal feedback of the information taught
Correct return demonstration of how to clean and dress a wound, how to position and protect the body part properly, and how to maintain sterile technique

NURSING INTERVENTIONS

Nursing Treatments
Provide temporary assistance until the skill is learned
Sponge the wound clean
   OR
Irrigate the wound
   OR
Clean with hydrogen peroxide
   OR
Clean with surgical soap
   OR
Soak in providone-iodine solution
Apply an antibiotic ointment
Apply a sterile dressing
Refrain from tight bandaging
Change the dressing frequently
Moisten the dressing before removal (if adherent)
Avoid placing tension on the wound

Pack the draining wound with fine mesh gauze
 OR
Expose the wound to air
Maintain dry skin (around the wound)
Remove adhesive tape and adhesive debris (to prevent skin irritation)
Support the affected body part
Encourage the person to ask questions
Encourage self-performance

Nursing Observations

Inspect for bleeding, edema, foreign bodies, inflammation, drainage
Obtain a bacterial culture (of any drainage)
Observe for readiness to assume self-care
Determine teaching effectiveness by testing, verbal feedback, and return demonstration

Health Teaching

Teach how to clean and dress a wound
Teach sterile technique
Explain how to dispose of soiled dressings
Explain the need to avoid mechanical trauma
Instruct to move the injured body part carefully
Describe those symptoms that should be reported (fever, purulent drainage, increased inflammation, necrosis)
Explain the reason for and intended effect of the therapy (to prevent infection and promote healing)

EVALUATION

Record actual outcome

Family Self-Care Deficits in Providing Therapeutic Care

FAMILY INABILITY TO PROVIDE THERAPEUTIC CARE[775]

ASSESSMENT

Data Collection

Subjective Data
• Family relates being unable to carry out all prescribed treatments and procedures
• May or may not know of or have attempted solution methods
  May express feelings of frustration, anger, helplessness
  Family members may exhibit resentment or refuse to give care

Objective Data
• Family or ill member may exhibit behavior or signs indicating that care is not achieved; e.g., family may demonstrate the use of unsafe methods, the ill person may have an unresolved infection, glucosuria, unhealing wound, etc.

Data Analysis

Nursing Diagnosis
FAMILY INABILITY TO PROVIDE THERAPEUTIC CARE: Being ineffective in providing prescribed treatments and procedures for a family member who is unable to do so alone

Common Etiology (Stressors)

BIRTH DEFECTS: Developmental deficit of care provider

PSYCHOSOCIAL FACTORS: Lack of responsibility, lack of knowledge about role expectations

HEALTH CARE FACTORS: Lack of health instruction, lack of health-skill experience

SITUATIONAL FACTORS: Prolonged illness/injury or hospitalization of care provider; youth, old age, or death of care provider; employment of care provider; poverty

PLANNING

Unmet Needs

Protection from physical harm, dependence, group (family) unity, mastery and competence in skills, independence, increased learning

Expected Outcome

At least one, but preferably all, family members are actively responsible for the therapeutic care of the family member(s)

Family can correctly demonstrate procedural methods

Overt evidence exists indicating that treatments are being carried out (progressive wound healing, no glucosuria, etc.)

NURSING INTERVENTIONS

Nursing Treatments

Acknowledge dependency

Provide assistance until the family is fully able to assume self-care (as a unit)

Encourage self-performance (as a family unit)

Encourage acceptance of interdependency (among family members)

Explore with the family their strengths and resources

Encourage family-shared responsibility

Nursing Observations

Observe for (family) readiness to assume self-care

Make a follow-up evaluation (if and when the family assumes self-care)

Health Teaching

Explain how to perform the procedure (to all family members)

Explain the reason for and intended effect of the therapy

Explain the importance of persons offering emotional support to one another

Advise how to integrate the therapeutic procedure into the daily routine (so as to least disrupt the family routine)

EVALUATION

Record actual outcome

FAMILY DIFFICULTY PROVIDING THERAPEUTIC CARE[775]

ASSESSMENT

Data Collection

Subjective Data

• Family relates that it is hard to carry out the prescribed treatments and procedures

• Verbalizes unsuccessful methods attempted

 May express feelings of frustration or anger

 Family members may exhibit resentment and unnecessary anxiety

Objective Data

• Family has demonstrated repeated efforts to carry out therapeutic care

• Family or ill person may exhibit behavior or signs that methods attempted are partially but not completely effective; e.g., family demonstration of procedural methods is awkward and ineffective; ill persons's dressing is clean, but the wound is unclean; ill person dangles on the side of the bed with assistance but does not walk because the family cannot get the person out of bed

Data Analysis

Nursing Diagnosis

FAMILY DIFFICULTY PROVIDING THERAPEUTIC CARE: Family is only partially effective in providing prescribed treatments and procedures for a family member who is unable to do so alone

Common Etiology (Stressors)

BIRTH DEFECTS: Developmental deficit of care provider
PSYCHOSOCIAL FACTORS: Lack of responsibility, lack of knowledge about role expectations
HEALTH CARE FACTORS: Lack of health instruction, lack of health-skill experience
SITUATIONAL FACTORS: Prolonged illness/injury or hospitalization of care provider; youth, old age, or death of care provider; employment of care provider; poverty

PLANNING

Unmet Needs

Protection from physical harm, dependence, group (family) unity, mastery and competence in skills, independence, increased learning

Expected Outcome

At least one family member is actively responsible for the therapeutic care of the family member(s)
Can correctly demonstrate procedural methods
Overt evidence exists indicating that treatments are being carried out (progressive wound healing and clean dressing in place, etc.)

NURSING INTERVENTIONS

Nursing Treatments

Acknowledge dependency
Provide assistance until the family is fully able to resume self-care (as a unit)
Encourage self-performance (as a family unit)
Encourage acceptance of interdependency (among family members)
Explore with the family their strengths and resources
Encourage family-shared responsibility
Discuss priority setting (with family members who do not share in physical care)

Nursing Observations

Observe performance level and problems involved in completing the task
Make a follow-up evaluation (to determine if the situation has improved)
Observe for evidence of a favorable response to therapy (wound healing, no decubitus, etc.)

Health Teaching

Explain how to perform the procedure (to all family members)
Explain the reason for and intended effect of the therapy
Advise how to integrate the therapeutic procedure into the daily routine (so as to least disrupt the family routine)
Explain the importance of persons offering emotional support to one another

EVALUATION

Record actual outcome

14 Nursing Diagnoses of PSYCHOSOCIAL ADAPTATION

Domain of Nursing Expertise: Psychosocial Adaptation

This chapter covers that sphere of nursing knowledge and skill related to problems of adjustment to the experience of being ill, meeting life crisis, and developmental phases. Such responses include those that fall within the scope of normalcy and bring about effective personal growth.

Views of Nursing Leaders That Support This Domain of Nursing Expertise

The predominant focus of nursing is on the person who is ill, or threatened with illness, while the primary focus of medicine is on pathologic changes. . . . Nursing is involved with how the person perceives the illness, how it changes his usual behavior, his lifestyle, or self-concept. Nursing and medicine therefore compliment each other.

Dorothy Johnson[410:217 & 218]

Man is a system capable of intake of extrapersonal and interpersonal factors from the external environment. He interacts with this environment by adjusting himself to it or adjusting it to himself. By a process of interaction and adjustment, the individual maintains varying degrees of harmony and balance between his internal and external environment.

Betty Neuman[410:122]

Nurses must assist persons in learning to live with the effects of pathological conditions and states and the effects of medical diagnostic and treatment measures in a lifestyle that promotes continued personal development.

Dorothea Orem[380:50 & 51]

Fostering personality development in the direction of maturity is the function of nursing and nursing education. . . . Peplau defines nursing as an interpersonal process that focuses on the support processes or self-repair and self-renewal. . . . The patient is a person undergoing stress, whether of a biological or psychological origin. Stress creates tension and produces energy that can be used well or poorly. The nurse acts with the patient to help him define, understand, and deal productively with the problem at hand.

Hildegard Peplau[410:54 & 57]

Nursing is unique because it focuses on the patient as a person adapting to those stimuli present as a result of his position on the health-illness continuum. . . . The function of nursing, then, in this concept, is to support and promote patient adaptation.

Sister Callista Roy[410:139, 668:42]

The nurse assists an individual or family to cope with the experience of illness and suffering.

Joyce Travelbee[484:5 & 6]

403

Adaptive Responses of Emotion (Affect): Aloneness

ABANDONED FEELING RELATED TO AN ABSENT HEALTH CARE PROVIDER[105,524]

ASSESSMENT

Data Collection

Subjective Data
- Person verbalizes that he has been forsaken
- Expresses concern that the care provider will not return or will return too late
  Perceives the health care provider as a rescuer in his time of need

Objective Data
- May exhibit behavior such as anger, demanding care, withdrawal, refusing therapy until the health care provider arrives or returns

Data Analysis

Nursing Diagnosis
ABANDONED FEELING RELATED TO AN ABSENT HEALTH CARE PROVIDER: A feeling of having been deserted by a health care provider who is not available when expected to be, whether the desertion is real or imagined

Common Etiology (Stressors)
PSYCHOSOCIAL FACTORS: Absence of a significant other, lack of attention from a significant other
HEALTH CARE FACTORS: *Health care provider:* Loss of health care provider (who has moved, changed jobs, become ill, or died). *Patient overload:* Limiting the health care provider's availability. *Physicians and physician visits:* The absence of physician contact immediately before surgery or during delivery, infrequent physician visits. *Follow-up evaluation:* Infrequent follow-up care

PLANNING

Unmet Needs

Comfort, protection from psychologic threat, caring and communicating relationships, high evaluation of self, increased learning, increased reality perception or problem-solving ability

Expected Outcome

Person verbalizes an expression of feelings
Acknowledges unfounded feelings of abandonment
Accepts and plans for alternative support systems
Calm, contented facial expression

NURSING INTERVENTIONS

Nursing Treatments

Approach unhurriedly
Reassure verbally (that health care providers are available)
Provide an atmosphere of acceptance
Provide frequent contact with the person (to assure the person that the nurse is there)
Encourage the expression of feelings (about feeling abandoned)
Listen attentively
Offer feedback to the person's expressed feelings
Communicate nurse sensitivity to the person's problem

Support a realistic assessment of the situation (that the health care provider is interested and caring but also has other patients)

Provide reliable information (about when the health care provider will arrive, about a substitute person, or about decreased need for intense health supervision)

Call the person's physician (to the bedside)

Encourage telephone calls with significant persons (the health care provider)

Nursing Observations

Observe for an excessive stress level (resulting from feeling abandoned)

Observe for evidence of a favorable response to therapy (the person is satisfied with the attention given by the health care provider or a substitute person)

Health Teaching

Explain (to the family) that ill persons are often hypersensitive (about relationships)

EVALUATION

Record actual outcome

ABANDONED FEELING RELATED TO AN ABSENT SIGNIFICANT OTHER[105,524]

ASSESSMENT

Data Collection

Subjective Data

• Person verbalizes that he has been forsaken by a loved one
• Expresses concern that the significant other will not return or will return too late
  Experiences long, unfulfilled waiting periods

Objective Data

• Children may exhibit behavior such as crying, bed-wetting, thumb-sucking, returning to bottle-feeding; adults may become unusually quiet, exhibit anger, or become demanding

Data Analysis

Nursing Diagnosis

ABANDONED FEELING RELATED TO AN ABSENT SIGNIFICANT OTHER: A feeling of having been deserted by a significant other who is not available when expected to be, whether the desertion is real or imagined

Common Etiology (Stressors)

PSYCHOSOCIAL FACTORS: The absence of, loss of, lack of attention from, or separation from a significant other or the threat of desertion by a significant other

HEALTH CARE FACTORS: *Hospitalization:* Separation from a significant other during hospitalization. *Institutionalization:* Of self by a significant other

DEVELOPMENTAL PHASES: All ages but especially early childhood and old age

SITUATIONAL FACTORS: Death of a significant other, divorce of parents or from spouse, child being put up for adoption, frequent changes of foster parents, chronic or critical illness of significant other, extensive travel by a significant other, geographically distant family

PLANNING

Unmet Needs

Comfort, protection from psychologic threat, caring and communicating relationships, unity with loved ones, high evaluation of self, increased learning, increased reality perception or problem-solving ability

Expected Outcome

Person verbalizes an expression of feelings
Acknowledges unfounded feelings of abandonment
Accepts and plans for alternative support systems
Calm, contented facial expression

NURSING INTERVENTIONS

Nursing Treatments

Approach unhurriedly
Reassure verbally (that the significant other cares, if such is true)
Provide an atmosphere of acceptance
Provide frequent contact with the person (to assure the person that the nurse is there)
Encourage the expression of feelings (about being abandoned)
Listen attentively
Offer feedback to the person's expressed feelings
Communicate nurse sensitivity to the person's problem
Support a realistic assessment of the situation (that the significant other is caring but
   has other responsibilities, etc.)
Provide reliable information (about when the significant other is expected to come or
   why that person cannot be there)
Call the person's family (to the bedside)
Encourage telephone calls with significant persons
Allow unlimited visiting

Nursing Observations

Evaluate the person's relatedness with others (are relationships meaningful or superficial?)
Observe for an excessive stress level (resulting from feeling abandoned)
Observe for evidence of a favorable response to therapy (sense of unity with the significant other)

Health Teaching

Advise that significant persons express caring for one another
Explain (to the family) that ill persons are often hypersensitive (about relationships)

EVALUATION

Record actual outcome

LONELINESS/ISOLATED FEELING RELATED TO LOSS OF A SIGNIFICANT OTHER[105,168,215,471,525]

ASSESSMENT

Data Collection

Subjective Data

• Person relates a sense of distance from others
• May express a longing for human contact
• Feels there is no one with whom the patient can currently share
   Experiences a sense of emptiness
   Is preoccupied with thoughts of the significant other

Objective Data

• Reaching out behavior (makes excessive and repeated requests or demands, prolongs
      conversations, reaches out for physical contact such as hand-holding and hugging)
   May become tearful when thinking or talking about the significant other

Data Analysis

Nursing Diagnosis

LONELINESS/ISOLATED FEELING RELATED TO LOSS OF A SIGNIFICANT OTHER: A feeling of being separate and remote from others after being permanently parted from a significant other

Common Etiology (Stressors)

DISEASES: Natural abortion, stillbirth, sudden infant death

PSYCHOSOCIAL FACTORS: Lack of intimacy, lack of communication with others, an attempt to control others or a life situation

HEALTH CARE FACTORS: *Hospital discharge:* Without the expected infant

SITUATIONAL FACTORS: Placing a child up for adoption, child being put up for adoption, death of a significant other, divorce of parents or from spouse, retirement, frequent change of foster parents, giving up a foster child, holidays without a significant other, relocation of a home

PLANNING

Unmet Needs

Comfort, protection from psychologic threat, caring and communicating relationships, unity with loved one, group companionship, attention, increased learning, increased problem-solving ability

Expected Outcome

Person verbalizes feelings of loneliness
Verbalizes feelings of satisfaction from supportive human contact
Verbalizes plans for coping with chronic loneliness
Substitutes positive interrelatedness for attention-seeking behavior

NURSING INTERVENTIONS

Nursing Treatments

Approach unhurriedly
Provide an atmosphere of acceptance
Touch the person frequently (hold or pat his hand, etc.)
Reassure verbally (that the nurse is with him)
Attend the person constantly (until he feels sufficiently comfortable to be alone)
Provide frequent contact with the person (thereafter)
Provide a compatible room companion
Encourage the expression of feelings (about the loss)
Listen attentively
Offer feedback to the person's expressed feelings
Encourage mutual problem solving (about how to overcome loneliness)
Support a realistic assessment of the situation (that caring persons are nearby)
Call the person's family (to the bedside)
Encourage telephone calls with significant persons
Provide radio and television for diversion
Provide a night light (darkness increases the sense of aloneness and isolation)
Allow unlimited visiting
Encourage awareness of positive responses from others
Recommend the person have a pet

Specific to Chronic Loneliness

Encourage social and community activities
Encourage part-time employment
Encourage meaningful activity
Encourage relationships with persons with common interests and goals

Nursing Observations

Determine the degree of insight that the person has
Evaluate the person's relatedness with others
Observe for an excessive stress level (resulting from the loneliness)

Observe for impaired self-attitudes (which lead to loneliness)
Observe for evidence of a favorable response to therapy (satisfaction in relationships)

Health Teaching

Explain that the person's response is appropriate and commonly experienced (after the loss of a significant other)
Advise that significant persons express caring for one another (which reduces loneliness)
Explain (to the family) the importance of persons offering support to one another (especially after a loss)
Explain that ill persons are often hypersensitive (to being alone)

EVALUATION

Record actual outcome

LONELINESS/ISOLATED FEELING RELATED TO PHYSICAL LOSS[105,168,215,471,525]

ASSESSMENT

Data Collection

Subjective Data

- Person relates a sense of distance from others
- May express a longing for human contact
- Feels there is no one with whom he can currently share
  Is preoccupied with thoughts of ill health and self
  Experiences a sense of emptiness
  If ill, the person is aware that he must experience the illness by himself, that the experience is his alone and involves no other person

Objective Data

- Reaching out behavior (makes excessive and repeated requests or demands, prolongs conversations, reaches out for physical contact such as hand-holding and hugging)

Data Analysis

Nursing Diagnosis

LONELINESS/ISOLATED FEELING RELATED TO PHYSICAL LOSS: A feeling of being separate and remote from others following the loss of a positive, balanced state of health

Common Etiology (Stressors)

DISEASES: Any but especially aphasia, apraxia, blindness, deafness, major depression
INJURIES: Any
SIGNS AND SYMPTOMS: Confusion, immobility, memory loss, pain, paralysis, unconsciousness (intermittent), weakness
PSYCHOSOCIAL FACTORS: Lack of intimacy, lack of communication with others, the threat of rejection, lack of self-esteem
HEALTH CARE FACTORS: *Adverse effects of medical or surgical therapy:* Any but especially loss of speech through endotracheal intubation, glossectomy, laryngectomy, tracheostomy, vocal cordectomy (which causes isolation feelings)
DEVELOPMENTAL PHASES: Old age
SITUATIONAL FACTORS: Childlessness, illness (acute, chronic, terminal), the experience of dying

PLANNING
Unmet Needs
Comfort, protection from psychologic threat, caring and communicating relationships, unity with loved one, group companionship, attention, increased learning, increased problem-solving ability

Expected Outcome
Person verbalizes feelings of loneliness
Verbalizes feelings of satisfaction from supportive human contact
Verbalizes plans for coping with chronic loneliness
Substitutes positive interrelatedness for attention-seeking behavior

NURSING INTERVENTIONS

Nursing Treatments
Approach unhurriedly
Provide an atmosphere of acceptance
Touch the person frequently (hold or pat his hand etc., especially important when the person cannot respond verbally)
Reassure verbally (that the nurse is with him)
Attend the person constantly (until he feels sufficiently comfortable to be alone)
Provide frequent contact with the person (thereafter)
Arrange geographic placement (so the person can see the nurse and other people)
Keep the person's door open (if it does not disturb privacy)
Provide a compatible room companion
Encourage the expression of feelings (about the physical loss)
Listen attentively
Talk with the person (especially if the person feels isolated by aphasia, semicoma, etc., even if he cannot respond verbally)
Offer feedback to the person's expressed feelings
Encourage mutual problem solving (about how to overcome chronic loneliness)
Support a realistic assessment of the situation (that loneliness can be minimized)
Call the person's family (to the bedside)
Encourage telephone calls with significant persons
Encourage volunteers to visit the sick and lonely
Provide radio and television for diversion
Provide a night light (darkness increases the sense of aloneness and isolation)
Allow unlimited visiting
Encourage awareness of positive responses from others

Specific to Chronic Loneliness
Encourage social and community activities (whenever possible)
Encourage meaningful activity
Encourage relationships with persons with common interests and goals

Nursing Observations
Determine the degree of insight that the person has
Evaluate the person's relatedness with others
Observe for an excessive stress level (resulting from the loneliness)
Observe for impaired self-attitudes (which lead to loneliness)
Observe for evidence of a favorable response to therapy (satisfaction in relationships)

Health Teaching
Explain that the person's response is appropriate and commonly experienced
Advise that significant persons express caring for one another (which reduces loneliness)
Explain (to families) the importance of persons offering support to one another (especially during illness)
Explain that ill and aged persons are often hypersensitive (to being alone)

EVALUATION

Record actual outcome

LONELINESS/ISOLATED FEELING RELATED TO SEPARATION FROM A SIGNIFICANT OTHER [105,168,215,471,525]

ASSESSMENT

Data Collection

Subjective Data
• Person relates a sense of distance from others
• May express a longing for human contact
• Relates there is no one with whom he can currently share
  Feels cut off from others
  Is often preoccupied with thoughts of the significant other
  Awaits the loved one's return
  Experiences a sense of emptiness

Objective Data
• May exhibit behavior such as making repeated requests or demands, prolonging conversations, frequent telephoning, reaching for another's hand or avoiding contacts, overactivity

Data Analysis

Nursing Diagnosis
LONELINESS/ISOLATED FEELING RELATED TO SEPARATION FROM A SIGNIFICANT OTHER: A feeling of being separate and remote from others while being temporarily apart from a significant other

Common Etiology (Stressors)
PSYCHOSOCIAL FACTORS: Lack of intimacy, lack of communication with others
HEALTH CARE FACTORS: *Health care environment:* Locked psychiatric unit; intensive care, coronary care, or isolation unit; lack of or limited phone privileges. *Hospitalization or institutionalization:* Of self or significant other. *Visitors:* Restriction of. *Diagnostic procedure:* Any. *Medical diagnosis:* Unfavorable. *Medical therapy:* Any. *Convalescence:* Reduced human contact during convalescence. *Surgical therapy:* Induction of or recovery from anesthesia (both cause isolation feelings). *Surgical procedures:* Any. *Adverse effects of drug therapy:* Heavy drug sedation from sedatives (causes isolation feelings)
SITUATIONAL FACTORS: Confinement in prison, marital separation from spouse or of parents, launching grown children, geographically distant family, holidays without a significant other, military service, extensive travel by a significant other, change of school, living alone

PLANNING

Unmet Needs
Comfort, protection from psychologic threat, caring and communicating relationships,

unity with loved one, group companionship, attention, increased learning, increased problem-solving ability

Expected Outcome
Person verbalizes expressions of loneliness
Verbalizes feelings of satisfaction from supportive human contact
Verbalizes plans for coping with chronic loneliness (if the separation is long-term)
Substitutes positive interrelatedness for attention-seeking behavior

NURSING INTERVENTIONS

Nursing Treatments
Approach unhurriedly
Provide an atmosphere of acceptance
Touch the person frequently (hold or pat his hand, etc., especially important when the person cannot respond verbally)
Reassure verbally (that the nurse is with him)
Attend the person constantly (until he feels sufficiently comfortable to be alone)
Provide frequent contact with the person (thereafter)
Arrange geographic placement (so the person can see the nurse and other people)
Keep the person's door open (if it does not disturb privacy)
Provide a compatible room companion
Encourage the expression of feelings
Listen attentively
Talk with the person (especially if the person feels isolated by drug depression, etc., even if he cannot respond verbally)
Offer feedback to the person's expressed feelings
Encourage mutual problem solving (about how to overcome chronic loneliness)
Support a realistic assessment of the situation (that caring health care providers are nearby)
Call the person's family (to the bedside)
Encourage telephone calls with significant persons
Provide radio and television for diversion
Provide a night light (darkness increases the sense of aloneness and isolation)
Allow unlimited visiting
Encourage awareness of positive responses from others
Recommend the person have a pet

Specific to Chronic Loneliness
Encourage social and community activities
Encourage meaningful activity
Encourage relationships with persons with common interests and goals

Nursing Observations
Observe for an excessive stress level (resulting from loneliness)
Observe for impaired self-attitudes (which lead to loneliness)
Observe for evidence of a favorable response to therapy (satisfaction with supportive human contact)

Health Teaching
Explain that the person's response is appropriate and commonly experienced
Explain (to families) the importance of persons offering support to one another (when one family member is separated from the group)
Explain that ill and aged persons are often hypersensitive (to being alone)

EVALUATION
Record actual outcome

Adaptive Responses of Emotion (Affect): Ambivalence

AMBIVALENCE RELATED TO HEALTH CARE TERMINATION[432,471,524]

ASSESSMENT
Data Collection
Subjective Data
- Person relates being troubled by opposing emotions
- Verbalizes both positive and negative feelings or is unable to state feelings clearly
  Feels anxious or uneasy about no longer having supervised health care
  May doubt his ability to maintain his health on termination of care
  Often perceives the termination of care as a permanent break with the health care provider
  Feels that his invested trust and a favorable relationship are lost
  Verbalizes that he wished the physician or nurse would continue to see him
  May openly reject the idea of new health personnel taking the place of others
  May ask permission at the time of termination to visit at a later date if he should desire to
  Wants to go home and be self-directed

Objective Data
- May exhibit contradictory behavior such as anger and kindness, dependent and independent behavior

Data Analysis
Nursing Diagnosis
AMBIVALENCE RELATED TO HEALTH CARE TERMINATION: The existence of two or more opposing emotions at the conclusion of a therapeutic relationship that has been perceived as highly favorable

Common Etiology (Stressors)
PSYCHOSOCIAL FACTORS: The threat of powerful and opposing simultaneous emotions, an attempt to maintain the present status and to avoid moving forward
HEALTH CARE FACTORS: *Health care provider:* The security of having a dependable health care provider. *Health therapy:* Successful therapy. *Hospital or medical discharge:* Termination of supervised health care. *Recovery from illness:* Successful recovery.

PLANNING
Unmet Needs
Comfort, protection from psychologic threat, acceptance, caring and communicating relationships, sense of adequacy, independence, increased learning, increased reality perception and problem-solving ability.

Expected Outcome
Person verbalizes opposing emotions
Acknowledges the existence of such emotion
Allows one of the two opposing emotions to dominate the other
Substitutes positive behavior for contradictory behavior

NURSING INTERVENTIONS
Nursing Treatments
Approach unhurriedly
Provide an atmosphere of acceptance

Reassure verbally (that he is capable of self-care or of progressing to another health care provider)

Encourage the expression of feelings (of both positive and negative feelings)

Listen attentively

Offer feedback to the person's expressed feelings

Reveal the person's ambivalent feelings (directly, so that he knows what is psychologically occurring)

Provide prior notification of an impending separation

Offer assurance that return visits are acceptable despite termination of the therapeutic relationship

Introduce the patient to replacement personnel before an impending separation

Avoid forcing the person into rapid adaptation to change by accepting the person's unique pattern of adjustment

Refrain from negatively criticizing

Support a realistic assessment of the situation (that health care must be terminated)

Involve the family (as a support system)

Nursing Observations

Determine the degree of insight that the person has

Evaluate the significance of emotional distress mannerisms and nonverbal communication

Identify disturbing conversation topics

Identify the current dominant emotions (positive and negative emotions)

Observe for an excessive stress level (resulting from the health care termination)

Observe for evidence that the person is reaching out for emotional support

Observe for evidence of a favorable response to therapy (dominance of the positive emotion)

Health Teaching

Explain that the peron's response is appropriate and commonly experienced

Explain the causes of the problem (that the opposing feelings prevent the person from moving forward to self-care or to another health care provider)

Explain the importance of maintaining a positive self-attitude (regarding the person's ability to maintain his own health or relate to a substitute provider)

EVALUATION

Record actual outcome

AMBIVALENCE RELATED TO RECOVERY FROM ILLNESS[432,471,524]

ASSESSMENT

Data Collection

Subjective Data

• Person relates being troubled by opposing emotions

• Verbalizes both positive and negative feelings or is unable to state feelings clearly

  Wants to get well but recognizes that wellness requires resumption of previous or new responsibilities

  Does not yet feel well enough to assume those responsibilities

  Is no longer sick enough to be unconcerned about responsibilities

May express concern about resuming activities too soon
May associate wellness with the loss of special privileges or advantages

Objective Data
- May exhibit contradictory behavior such as attempting responsible behavior that he finds he cannot perform and so reverts temporarily to dependent behavior

Data Analysis

Nursing Diagnosis
AMBIVALENCE RELATED TO RECOVERY FROM ILLNESS: The existence of two or more opposing emotions during the period of adjustment from illness to wellness

Common Etiology (Stressors)
PSYCHOSOCIAL FACTORS: The threat of powerful and opposing simultaneous emotions, an attempt to maintain the present status and to avoid moving forward
HEALTH CARE FACTORS: *Health therapy:* Successful. *Drug therapy:* Curative or controlling effects of drug therapy. *Convalescence:* Naturally slow recovery during convalescence

PLANNING

Unmet Needs
Comfort, protection from psychologic threat, acceptance, caring and communicating relationships, sense of adequacy, independence, increased learning, increased reality perception and problem-solving ability

Expected Outcome
Person verbalizes opposing emotions
Acknowledges the existence of such emotion
Allows one of the two opposing emotions to dominate the other
Substitutes positive behavior for contradictory behavior
As health improves, the person gradually becomes more self-directed and confident in self-responsibility

NURSING INTERVENTIONS

Nursing Treatments
Approach unhurriedly
Provide an atmosphere of acceptance
Reassure verbally (that independence increases with higher levels of wellness)
Encourage the expression of feelings (of both positive and negative feelings)
Listen attentively
Offer feedback to the person's expressed feelings
Reveal the person's ambivalent feelings (directly, so that he knows what is psychologically occurring)

Nursing Observations
Determine the degree of insight that the person has
Identify the current dominant emotions (positive and negative emotions)
Observe for an excessive stress level (resulting from recovery from illness)
Observe for evidence that the person is reaching out for emotional support
Observe for evidence of a favorable response to therapy (dominance of the positive emotion)

Health Teaching
Explain that the person's response is appropriate and commonly experienced (when recovering from illness)
Explain the causes of the problem (that the opposing feelings prevent the person from moving forward from illness to wellness)
Explain the importance of maintaining a positive self-attitude (regarding the ability to move forward toward wellness)

EVALUATION
Record actual outcome

AMBIVALENCE RELATED TO REMOVAL OF LIFE-SUPPORT SYSTEMS[432,471,524]

ASSESSMENT

Data Collection

Subjective Data
- Person relates being troubled by opposing emotions
- Verbalizes both positive and negative feelings or is unable to state feelings clearly
  Is intensely aware that his existence has been maintained by a life-supporting device
  Wants the security of relying on dependable assistive methods
  Wants to be self-directed
  May frequently call for the health or therapeutic device, or drug, even though such is not needed

Objective Data
- May exhibit contradictory behavior such as sighing with relief that the life-support system has been removed, then asking for it shortly after

Data Analysis

Nursing Diagnosis
AMBIVALENCE RELATED TO REMOVAL OF LIFE-SUPPORT SYSTEMS: The existence of two or more opposing emotions of dependence and independence as the person relinquishes a life-supportive device that is no longer needed

Common Etiology (Stressors)
PSYCHOSOCIAL FACTORS: The threat of powerful and opposing simultaneous emotions (the desire to be well, opposed by the security of being dependent on reliable equipment), lack of confidence in the body's ability to sustain itself, an attempt to maintain the present status and to avoid moving forward

HEALTH CARE FACTORS: *Drug therapy:* Cardiac drugs, corticosteroids. *Medical therapy:* Hemodialysis, hyperalimentation infusion, intermittent positive-pressure breathing, oxygen therapy, peritoneal dialysis, blood transfusions. *Therapeutic equipment:* Use of a cardiac pacemaker or respirator, defibrillator, monitoring equipment

SITUATIONAL FACTORS: Recovery from illness

PLANNING

Unmet Needs
Comfort, protection from psychologic threat, acceptance, caring and communicating relationships, sense of adequacy, independence, increased learning, increased reality perception and problem-solving ability

Expected Outcome
Person verbalizes opposing emotions
Acknowledges the existence of such emotion
Allows one of the two opposing emotions to dominate the other
Substitutes positive behavior for contradictory behavior
As health improves, the person gradually becomes more self-directed and confident in the body's ability to maintain life unaided

NURSING INTERVENTIONS

Nursing Treatments
Approach unhurriedly
Reassure verbally (that the person is safe without the life-support system)
Demonstrate calmness
Provide an atmosphere of acceptance
Encourage the expression of feelings (both positive and negative feelings)
Listen attentively

Offer feedback to the person's expressed feelings

Reveal the person's ambivalent feelings (directly, so that he knows what is psychologically occurring)

Attend the person constantly (during the initial withdrawal)

Respond immediately to the person's call (especially during the withdrawal period)

Increase the weaning time off the therapeutic devices gradually

Place the equipment within sight (until the person feels more secure)

Encourage gradual mastery of the situation

Provide radio and television for diversion (during the withdrawal period)

Avoid forcing the person into rapid adaptation to change by accepting the person's unique pattern of adjustment

Support a realistic assessment of the situation (that the body is now able to maintain itself)

Nursing Observations

Determine the degree of insight that the person has

Evaluate the significance of emotional distress mannerisms, of nonverbal communication

Identify disturbing conversation topics

Identify the current dominant emotions (positive and negative emotions)

Observe for an excessive stress level (from the removal of life-support system)

Observe for evidence that the person is reaching out for emotional support

Observe for evidence of a favorable response to therapy (dominance of the positive emotion)

Health Teaching

Explain that the person's response is appropriate and commonly experienced

Explain the causes of the problem (that the opposing feelings prevent the person from making the decision to try living without the support system)

Explain the importance of maintaining a positive self-attitude (about the body's ability to maintain itself)

Describe those symptoms that should be reported (during the withdrawal)

EVALUATION

Record actual outcome

AMBIVALENCE RELATED TO A SIGNIFICANT OTHER[432,471,524]

ASSESSMENT

Data Collection

Subjective Data

• Person relates being troubled by opposing emotions

• Verbalizes both positive and negative feelings or is unable to state feelings clearly

  May be indecisive about plans concerning the significant other

Objective Data

• May exhibit contradictory behavior such as anger and loving behavior, dependent and independent behavior

Data Analysis

Nursing Diagnosis

AMBIVALENCE RELATED TO A SIGNIFICANT OTHER: The existence of two or more opposing emotions directed toward a significant other

Common Etiology (Stressors)
BIRTH DEFECTS: Imperfect infant or child
DISEASES: Of self or significant other
INJURIES: Of self or significant other
SIGNS AND SYMPTOMS: Of self or significant other such as confusion, immobility, incontinence, irritability, memory loss, pain, weakness
PSYCHOSOCIAL FACTORS: The threat of frustration, the threat of powerful and opposing simultaneous emotions, an attempt to maintain the present status and to avoid moving forward
HEALTH CARE FACTORS: *Natural body states:* Pregnancy. *Health care decisions for significant other:* Having to make decisions for a significant other. *Health care procedures for significant other:* Having to perform procedures for a significant other. *Hospitalization of significant other:* Prolonged. *Wellness of significant other:* When the person himself is ill. *Health therapy of significant other:* Prolonged, time-consuming health therapy of a significant other
DEVELOPMENTAL PHASES: Adolescence, old age
LIFESTYLE OF SIGNIFICANT OTHER: Nonconformity to cultural mores, excess time and effort at employment, changes in sexual activity/performance or response, drug abuse, cigarette smoking
SITUATIONAL FACTORS: Adoption of a child, impending death of significant other, divorce from a spouse, launching grown children, child rearing, attempted suicide by a significant other, widowhood

PLANNING

Unmet Needs
Comfort, protection from psychologic threat, acceptance, caring and communicating relationships, sense of adequacy, independence, increased learning, increased reality perception and problem-solving ability

Expected Outcome
Person verbalizes opposing emotions
Acknowledges the existence of such emotion
Allows one of the two opposing emotions to dominate the other
Substitutes positive behavior for contradictory behavior

NURSING INTERVENTIONS

Nursing Treatments
Approach unhurriedly
Provide an atmosphere of acceptance
Reassure verbally (that the nurse will help the person)
Encourage the expression of feelings (of both positive and negative feelings)
Listen attentively
Offer feedback to the person's expressed feelings
Reveal the person's ambivalent feelings (directly, so that he knows what is psychologically occurring)

Nursing Observations
Determine the degree of insight that the person has
Evaluate the significance of emotional distress mannerisms, of nonverbal communication
Identify disturbing conversation topics
Identify the current dominant emotions (positive and negative emotions)
Observe for an excessive stress level
Observe for evidence that the person is reaching out for emotional support
Observe for evidence of a favorable response to therapy (dominance of the positive emotion)

Health Teaching
Explain that the person's response is appropriate and commonly experienced

Explain the causes of the problem (that the opposing feelings prevent the relationship from moving to a more open or intimate level)

Advise that significant persons express caring for one another (whenever possible)

Explain (to families) the importance of persons offering support to one another (especially during crisis)

EVALUATION

Record actual outcome

Adaptive Responses of Emotion (Affect): Anger

ANGER RELATED TO APPROACHING DEATH[105,432,471,525]

ASSESSMENT

Data Collection

Subjective Data
- Person relates experiencing frustration
- May or may not verbalize or openly express anger
- When expressing anger, verbalizations reveal hostility or resentment
  Is aware that his health or the health of a significant other is deteriorating
  No longer denies the approaching death but feels angry about it
  Quick to blame others
  Complains chronically

Objective Data
- Manifests physical findings such as facial flushing or pallor, rapid or deep respirations, rapid or bounding pulse, increased blood pressure, perspiration, trembling
- May exhibit behavior such as demanding and controlling behavior that evokes negative responses from others, may withdraw by not returning to the doctor who made the diagnosis or who gave unsuccessful therapy, may tell the nurses to "go away and leave me alone," may refuse to allow friends to visit, may reject spouse, may avoid persons who are well

Data Analysis

Nursing Diagnosis

ANGER RELATED TO APPROACHING DEATH: A feeling of resentment or hostility resulting from a person's awareness that his life or the life of a significant other is soon to end

Common Etiology (Stressors)

DISEASES: Any

INJURIES: Any

PSYCHOSOCIAL FACTORS: The threat of lack of or loss of control of a life situation, the threat of loss of self-esteem

HEALTH CARE FACTORS: *Medical diagnosis:* An unfavorable medical diagnosis for self or significant other. *Health therapy:* Unsuccessful or ineffective medical, drug, or surgical therapy. *Prognosis:* An unfavorable prognosis

SITUATIONAL FACTORS: Terminal illness of self or significant other, the experience of dying

PLANNING

Unmet Needs

Comfort, protection from psychologic threat, acceptance, caring and communicating re-

lationships, personal growth and maturity, increased learning, increased reality perception and problem-solving ability

Expected Outcome
Person verbalizes feelings of anger
Verbalizes specific problem-solving methods for overcoming the source of anger
Uses constructive outlets for angry feelings
Uses assertive rather than attacking behavior

NURSING INTERVENTIONS

Nursing Treatments
Approach unhurriedly
Reassure verbally (that the nurse will be available whenever needed)
Demonstrate calmness
Provide an atmosphere of acceptance
Encourage the expression of feelings (about the anger and approaching death)
   BUT
Terminate emotionally threatening conversation immediately
Listen attentively
Communicate that the nurse feels comfortable with the person's discussion of death
Offer feedback to the person's expressed feelings
Communicate nurse sensitivity to the person's problem
Relate to the person on an adult–adult level, not on a parent–child level (which could increase anger)
Ask the person to identify the problem
Ask for specifics, not generalizations, about the problem
Reveal the person's angry feelings (if he is unaware of them)
Explore with the person his strengths and resources (to cope with death and dying)
Provide meetings with a supportive person or group (minister, etc.)
Encourage gradual mastery of the situation ⎤ During the
Encourage planned one-day-at-a-time living ⎬ early stages
Encourage meaningful activity ⎦ of dying
Reduce the demands placed on the person (so that more energy is available for coping)
Suggest more appropriate means of emotional expression (assertive rather than aggressive behavior)
Touch the person judiciously (angry persons often prefer not to be touched)
Refrain from arguing, from negatively criticizing, from teasing (all of which increase anger)
Explore with the person the (negative) effects of his behavior on others

Nursing Observations
Determine the degree of insight that the person has (into the response of anger)
Observe for an excessive stress level (resulting from the anger)
Observe for evidence that the person is reaching out for emotional support
Observe for evidence of a favorable response to therapy (acceptance of death, decreased anger)

Health Teaching
Explain that the person's response is appropriate and commonly experienced
Explain and offer hope that the emotional pain will decrease with time
Explain how to channel emotional energy and obtain release from stress (laughing, talking things over)

EVALUATION
Record actual outcome

ANGER RELATED TO FAMILY BURDENS [105,432,442,471,525]

ASSESSMENT

Data Collection

Subjective Data
- Person relates experiencing frustration
- May or may not verbalize or openly express anger about imposed hardships
- When expressing anger, verbalizations reveal hostility and resentment
  Family relates:
  - Feeling obligated to care for the ill or dependent person
  - That they can no longer indulge in life's extras
  - That they are barely able to make financial ends meet
  - That someone must remain at home to care for the ill or dependent person
  - That social activities are curtailed, both in the home and away from home

Objective Data
- Manifests physical findings such as facial flushing or pallor, rapid or deep respirations, rapid or bounding pulse, increased blood pressure, perspiration, trembling
- May exhibit behavior such as demanding and controlling behavior, clenching the jaw or fist, shouting, throwing or slamming objects, unusual quietness, avoiding persons or situations, somatic complaints

Data Analysis

Nursing Diagnosis
ANGER RELATED TO FAMILY BURDENS: A feeling of resentment or hostility about the hardships imposed on a family because of the illness or dependency of one member

Common Etiology (Stressors)
BIRTH DEFECTS: Imperfect child (mentally or physically)
PSYCHOSOCIAL FACTORS: The threat of frustration or delayed goal achievement, the threat of lack of or loss of control of a life situation, lack of emotional control
DEVELOPMENTAL PHASES: Old age of a significant other
SITUATIONAL FACTORS: Acute, chronic, disabling, or terminal illness of or injury to a significant other

PLANNING

Unmet Needs
Comfort, protection from psychologic threat, acceptance, caring and communicating relationships, personal growth and maturity, increased learning, increased reality perception and problem-solving ability

Expected Outcome
Person verbalizes feelings of anger
Verbalizes specific problem-solving methods for overcoming the source of anger
Uses constructive outlets for angry feelings
Uses assertive rather than attacking behavior

NURSING INTERVENTIONS

Nursing Treatments
Approach unhurriedly
Reassure verbally (that the nurse will help the person solve his problem, if possible)
Demonstrate calmness
Provide an atmosphere of acceptance
Encourage the expression of feelings (about the source of the anger)
Listen attentively

Offer feedback to the person's expressed feelings
Communicate nurse sensitivity to the person's problem
Relate to the person on an adult–adult level, not on a parent–child level (which could increase anger)
Ask the person to identify the problem
Ask for specifics, not generalizations, about the problem
Provide reliable information (which often reduces anger)
Reveal the person's angry feelings (if he is unaware of them)
Encourage mutual problem solving (for ways to minimize the burden)
Explore with the person his strengths and resources (to overcome the problem)
Touch the person judiciously (angry persons often prefer not to be touched)
Refrain from arguing, from negatively criticizing, from teasing (which increase anger)
Explore with the person the (negative) effects of his behavior on other family members
Make a referral (to agencies that can assist the family)

Nursing Observations

Determine the degree of insight that the person has (into the response of anger)
Observe for an excessive stress level (resulting from the anger)
Observe for evidence that the person is reaching out for emotional support
Observe for evidence of a favorable response to therapy (resolution of the problem, decreased anger)

Health Teaching

Explain that the person's response is appropriate and commonly experienced (when caring for ill family members)
Explain and offer hope that the emotional pain will decrease with time
Explain how to channel emotional energy and obtain release from stress (running, swimming, other sports, creative activities, hobbies, work, laughing, talking things over, hitting a punching bag or pillow)
Recommend new options for effective methods of coping (assertive rather than aggressive behavior)

EVALUATION

Record actual outcome

ANGER RELATED TO HEALTH CARE DELIVERY[105,432,471,525]

ASSESSMENT

Data Collection

Subjective Data
• Person relates experiencing frustration
• May or may not verbalize or openly express anger
• When expressing anger, verbalizations reveal hostility and resentment
  Expectations for health care are greater than care received
  Complains about the quality of care, the facilities, health care providers, the inefficient or restrictive system, other patients, visitors, health care costs, etc.

Objective Data
• Manifests physical findings such as facial flushing or pallor, rapid or deep respirations,

rapid or bounding pulse, increased blood pressure, perspiration, trembling
• May exhibit behavior such as demanding and controlling behavior, clenching the jaw
  or fist, shouting, throwing or slamming objects, unusual quietness, avoiding persons
  or situations in which health care delivery was unsatisfactory

Data Analysis

Nursing Diagnosis
ANGER RELATED TO HEALTH CARE DELIVERY: A feeling of resentment or hostility about the quality of health care services being received

Common Etiology (Stressors)
PSYCHOSOCIAL FACTORS: The threat of frustration or delayed goal achievement, the threat
  of loss of self-esteem, the threat of lack of or loss of control of a life situation, the
  threat of having needs unfulfilled through constructive behavior (which results in destructive behavior), lack of emotional control
HEALTH CARE FACTORS: *Health care costs:* High. *Health care delivery:* Low quality. *Health care environment:* Unsuitable health care facilities, crowding, noise, uncleanliness of the health
  care environment. *Health care provider:* Lack of health care provider(s). *Health care system:* Delayed entry into the health care system, an ineffective or rigid health care system *Health information:* Lack of health information *Patients:* Disruptive. *Visitors:*
  Disturbing. *Welfare/Human resources services:* Inadequate or dehumanizing services
SITUATIONAL FACTORS: Restrictions and limitations on insurance coverage

PLANNING

Unmet Needs
Comfort, protection from psychologic threat, acceptance, caring and communicating relationships, personal growth and maturity, increased learning, increased reality perception and problem-solving ability

Expected Outcome
Person verbalizes feelings of anger
Verbalizes specific problem-solving methods for overcoming the source of anger
Uses constructive outlets for angry feelings
Uses assertive rather than attacking behavior

NURSING INTERVENTIONS

Nursing Treatments
Approach unhurriedly
Reassure verbally (that the nurse will help the person solve his problem, if possible)
Demonstrate calmness
Provide an atmosphere of acceptance
Encourage the expression of feelings (about the source of the anger)
Listen attentively
Offer feedback to the person's expressed feelings
Communicate nurse sensitivity to the person's problem
Relate to the person on an adult–adult level, not on a parent–child level (which could
  increase anger)
Ask the person to identify the problem
Ask for specifics, not generalizations, about the problem
Provide reliable information (about what can realistically be expected from the health
  care system)
Reveal the person's angry feelings (if he is unaware of them)
Encourage mutual problem solving
Explore with the person his strengths and resources (to overcome the problem)
Reduce the demands placed on the person (so that more energy is available for coping)
Touch the person judiciously (angry persons often prefer not to be touched)

Refrain from arguing, from negatively criticizing, from teasing (all of which increase anger)

Explore with the person the (negative) effects of his behavior on others

Make a referral (to persons who can provide the desired health care or solve the problem of inadequate facilities, etc.)

Nursing Observations

Determine the degree of insight that the person has (into the response of anger)

Observe for an excessive stress level (resulting from the anger)

Observe for evidence that the person is reaching out for emotional support

Observe for evidence of a favorable response to therapy (resolution of the problem, decreased anger)

Health Teaching

Explain that the person's response is appropriate and commonly experienced

Recommend new options for effective methods of coping (assertive rather than aggressive behavior)

Explain how to channel emotional energy and obtain release from stress (talking things over)

EVALUATION

Record actual outcome

ANGER RELATED TO INFLICTED PHYSICAL PAIN[105,432,471,525]

ASSESSMENT

Data Collection

Subjective Data

- Person relates experiencing frustration
- May or may not verbalize or openly express anger
- When expressing anger, verbalizations reveal hostility and resentment
  Person focuses on the pain instead of the intended helping effect of treatment, etc.
  If pregnant, may perceive the partner or fetus as responsible for the pain

Objective Data

- Manifests physical findings such as facial flushing or pallor, rapid or deep respirations, rapid or bounding pulse, increased blood pressure, perspiration, trembling
- May exhibit behavior such as demanding and controlling behavior, shouting, unusual quietness, avoiding persons who inflict the pain

Data Analysis

Nursing Diagnosis

ANGER RELATED TO INFLICTED PHYSICAL PAIN: A feeling of resentment or hostility about pain imposed on the individual by others

Common Etiology (Stressors)

PSYCHOSOCIAL FACTORS: The threat of frustration, the threat of loss of self-esteem, the threat of lack of or loss of control of a life situation, lack of emotional control

HUMAN BODY: Pregnancy, the pain of childbirth

HEALTH CARE FACTORS: *Painful diagnostic procedures:* Such as angiography, barium enema, bone marrow, lumbar puncture, Pap smear, proctosigmoidiscopy, withdrawing blood samples. *Painful medical therapy:* Such as therapeutic exercise, hemodialysis, intravenous infusions, paracentesis, rehabilitation therapy, traction. *Painful surgical procedures:* Any surgery. *Therapeutic devices:* Safety restraints

PLANNING

Unmet Needs

Comfort, protection from physical and psychologic threat, acceptance, caring and communicating relationships, personal growth and maturity, increased learning, increased reality perception and problem-solving ability .

Expected Outcome

Person verbalizes feelings of anger
Verbalizes specific problem-solving methods for overcoming the source of anger
Uses constructive outlets for angry feelings
Uses assertive rather than attacking behavior

NURSING INTERVENTIONS

Nursing Treatments

Approach unhurriedly
Reassure verbally (that the pain will be kept to a minimum)
Demonstrate calmness
Provide an atmosphere of acceptance
Encourage the expression of feelings (about the pain and anger)
Listen attentively
Offer feedback to the person's expressed feelings
Communicate nurse sensitivity to the person's problem
Relate to the person on an adult–adult level, not on a parent–child level (which could increase anger)
Ask the person to identify the problem (the procedure causing the pain)
Support a realistic assessment of the situation (Is it really as painful as he perceives it? Is it necessary to endure pain in order to regain health?)
Provide reliable information (about how long the pain will last)
Reveal the person's angry feelings (if he is unaware of them)
Encourage mutual problem solving (about ways to reduce the pain)
Reduce the demands placed on the person (so that more energy is available for coping with the anger and the pain)
Touch the person judiciously (angry persons often prefer not to be touched)
Refrain from arguing, from negatively criticizing, from teasing (which increase anger)
Do not allow unpleasant, surprise situations

Nursing Observations

Determine the degree of insight that the person has (into the responses of anger)
Observe for evidence of a favorable response to therapy (pain reduction, decreased anger)

Health Teaching

Explain that the person's response is appropriate and commonly experienced
Explain how to channel emotional energy and obtain release from stress (talking things over, hitting a pillow)
Recommend methods for achieving total relaxation (such as deep breathing, which will reduce the pain)
Recommend new options for effective methods of coping (assertive rather than aggressive behavior)

EVALUATION

Record actual outcome

ANGER RELATED TO LOSS OF PERSONAL FREEDOM [105,432,471,525]

ASSESSMENT

Data Collection

Subjective Data
- Person relates experiencing frustration
- May or may not verbalize or openly express anger
- When expressing anger, verbalizations reveal hostility and resentment
  Person feels trapped and enslaved by therapy schedules
  Resents activity limitations imposed by dependent loved ones
  Wants more freedom and decision-making for self

Objective Data
- Manifests physical findings such as facial flushing or pallor, rapid or deep breathing, rapid or bounding pulse, increased blood pressure
- May exhibit behavior such as demanding and controlling behavior, clenching the jaw or fist, shouting, throwing or slamming objects, unusual quietness, avoiding persons or situations, somatic complaints

Data Analysis

Nursing Diagnosis
ANGER RELATED TO LOSS OF PERSONAL FREEDOM: A feeling of resentment or hostility about time limitations, decreased opportunity for decision making, and limitations on moving about freely

Common Etiology (Stressors)
PSYCHOSOCIAL FACTORS: The threat of frustration or delayed goal achievement, the threat of loss of self-esteem, the threat of lack of or loss of control of a life situation, the threat of having needs unfulfilled through constructive behavior (which results in destructive behavior), lack of emotional control

HUMAN BODY: *Natural body function:* Breast feeding an infant.

HEALTH CARE FACTORS: *Health care environment:* Locked psychiatric unit; isolation, intensive care, or coronary care unit; lack of phone privileges; lack of food/kitchen privileges. *Institutional policies:* Restrictive. *Institutional routine:* Inflexible. *Visitors:* Restriction of. *Hospitalization:* Prolonged. *Hospitalization of significant other:* Any. *Drug therapy:* Chemotherapy. *Medical therapy:* Prolonged bed rest, body casting, therapeutic diet, drainage by tube(s), hemodialysis, hyperalimentation and intravenous infusion, inhalation therapy, radiation, physical or rehabilitation therapy, speech therapy, traction. *Therapeutic devices:* Safety restraints, Stryker frame

DEVELOPMENTAL PHASES: Old age of self or significant other

LIFESTYLE: Loss of preillness lifestyle, overwork

SITUATIONAL FACTORS: Employment, illness of or injury to self or significant other, the curtailment of a parent's activities and freedom during the child-rearing years

PLANNING

Unmet Needs
Comfort, protection from psychologic threat, acceptance, caring and communicating relationships, personal growth and maturity, increased learning, increased reality perception and problem-solving ability

Expected Outcome
Person verbalizes feelings of anger
Verbalizes specific problem-solving methods for overcoming the source of anger
Uses constructive outlets for angry feelings
Uses assertive rather than attacking behavior

NURSING INTERVENTIONS

Nursing Treatments

Approach unhurriedly

Reassure verbally (that the nurse will help the person solve the problem)

Demonstrate calmness

Provide an atmosphere of acceptance

Encourage the expression of feelings (about the source of the anger)

Listen attentively

Offer feedback to the person's expressed feelings

Communicate nurse sensitivity to the person's problem

Relate to the person on an adult–adult level, not on a parent–child level (which could increase anger)

Ask the person to identify the problem

Ask for specifics, not generalizations, about the problem

Reveal the person's angry feelings (if he is unaware of them)

Encourage mutual problem solving (to help the person gain more freedom through improved scheduling of therapy, increasing inpatient privileges, finding care providers for children, etc.)

Touch the person judiciously (angry persons often prefer not to be touched)

Refrain from arguing, from negatively criticizing, from teasing (which increase anger)

Explore with the person the (negative) effects of his behavior on others

Nursing Observations

Determine the degree of insight that the person has (into the response of anger)

Observe for an excessive stress level (resulting from the anger)

Observe for evidence that the person is reaching out for emotional support

Observe for evidence of a favorable response to therapy (resolution of the problem, decreased anger)

Health Teaching

Explain that the person's response is appropriate and commonly experienced (that it is okay not to want to be with your children or a loved one all the time)

Explain how to channel emotional energy and obtain release from stress (running, swimming, other sports, creative activities, laughing, talking things over, hitting a punching bag or pillow, working)

Recommend new options for effective methods of coping (assertive rather than aggressive behavior)

EVALUATION

Record actual outcome

ANGER RELATED TO LOSS OF A SIGNIFICANT OTHER [105,432,471,525]

ASSESSMENT

Data Collection

Subjective Data

• Person relates experiencing frustration

• May or may not verbalize or openly express anger toward the person who is gone or at persons who failed to prevent the loss such as health care providers, etc.

• When expressing anger, verbalizations reveal hostility and resentment

Person perceives that the loss of the loved one has left him alone and without the support he needs

May experience guilt for feeling angry

Objective Data
- Manifests physical findings such as facial flushing or pallor, rapid or deep respirations, rapid or bounding pulse, increased blood pressure, perspiration, trembling
- May exhibit behavior such as demanding and controlling behavior, clenching the jaw or fist, shouting, throwing or slamming objects, unusual quietness, avoiding persons or situations, somatic complaints

Data Analysis

Nursing Diagnosis
ANGER RELATED TO LOSS OF A SIGNIFICANT OTHER: A feeling of resentment or hostility about being permanently parted from a significant other

Common Etiology (Stressors)
BIRTH DEFECTS: Giving birth to an imperfect child (loss of a perfect child)
DISEASES: Natural abortion, stillbirth, sudden infant death
PSYCHOSOCIAL FACTORS: The threat of frustration or delayed goal achievement, the threat of loss of self-esteem, the threat of lack of or loss of control of a life situation, the threat of having needs unfulfilled through constructive behavior (which results in destructive behavior), lack of emotional control
HEALTH CARE FACTORS: *Hospital discharge:* Without the expected infant
SITUATIONAL FACTORS: Placing a child up for adoption, child being put up for adoption, death of a significant other, divorce of parents or from spouse, frequent change of foster parents, giving up a foster child

PLANNING

Unmet Needs
Comfort, protection from psychologic threat, acceptance, caring and communicating relationship, personal growth and maturity, increased learning, increased reality perception and problem-solving ability

Expected Outcome
Person verbalizes feelings of anger
Verbalizes specific problem-solving methods for overcoming the source of anger
Uses constructive outlets for angry feelings
Uses assertive rather than attacking behavior

NURSING INTERVENTIONS

Nursing Treatments
Approach unhurriedly
Reassure verbally (that the nurse will be available when needed)
Demonstrate calmness
Provide an atmosphere of acceptance
Encourage the experession of feelings (about the anger and the loss)
Listen attentively
Offer feedback to the person's expressed feelings
Communicate nurse sensitivity to the person's problem
Relate to the person on an adult–adult level, not on a parent–child level (which could increase anger)
Ask the person to identify the problem
Ask for specifics, not generalizations, about the problem
Reveal the person's angry feelings (if he is unaware of them)
Encourage mutual problem solving
Explore with the person his strenghs and resources (to adjust to the loss)
Reduce the demands placed on the person (so that more energy is available for coping)
Touch the person judiciously (angry persons often prefer not to be touched)
Refrain from arguing, from negatively criticizing, from teasing (which increase anger)
Explore with the person the (negative) effects of his behavior on others

Nursing Observations
Determine the degree of insight that the person has (into the response of anger)

Observe for evidence that the person is reaching out for emotional support
Observe for evidence of a favorable response to therapy (decreased anger and effective coping with the loss)

Health Teaching

Explain that the person's response is appropriate and commonly experienced (following loss of a significant other)
Explain and offer hope that the emotional pain will decrease with time
Explain how to channel emotional energy and obtain release from stress (running, swimming, other sports, creative activities, laughing, talking things over, hitting a punching bag or pillow)

EVALUATION

Record actual outcome

ANGER RELATED TO MATERIAL LOSS [105,432,471,525]

ASSESSMENT

Data Collection

Subjective Data
• Person relates experiencing frustration
• May or may not verbalize or openly express anger
• When expressing anger, verbalizations reveal hostility and resentment
  Is concerned about home, financial security, or personal objects
  Is worried about replacing the loss

Objective Data
• Manifests physical findings such as facial flushing or pallor, rapid or deep respirations, rapid or bounding pulse, increased blood pressure, perspiration, trembling
• May exhibit behavior such as demanding and controlling behavior, clenching the jaw or fist, shouting, throwing or slamming objects, unusual quietness, avoiding persons or situations, somatic complaints

Data Analysis

Nursing Diagnosis
ANGER RELATED TO MATERIAL LOSS: A feeling of resentment or hostility about the loss of tangible, valued objects

Common Etiology (Stressors)
PSYCHOSOCIAL FACTORS: The threat of frustration or delayed goal achievement, the threat of loss of self-esteem, the threat of lack of or loss of control of a life situation, lack of emotional control
HEALTH CARE FACTORS: *Health care provider*: Misplacing the patient's personal property
SITUATIONAL FACTORS: Accident, loss of or relocation of a home, loss of employment, lack of finances, insufficient or lack of insurance coverage, loss of property through illness or injury, unfavorable economic factors, arson, theft
ENVIRONMENTAL FACTORS: *Cataclysm*: Cyclone, earthquake, flood, hailstorm, hurricane, volcanic eruption *Environmental heat*: Fire

PLANNING

Unmet Needs

Comfort, protection from psychologic threat, acceptance, caring and communicating relationships, personal growth and maturity, increased learning, increased reality perception and problem-solving ability

Expected Outcome
Person verbalizes feelings of anger
Verbalizes specific problem-solving methods for overcoming the source of anger
Uses constructive outlets for angry feelings
Uses assertive rather than attacking behavior

NURSING INTERVENTIONS

Nursing Treatments
Approach unhurriedly
Reassure verbally (that the nurse will help the person solve the problem)
Demonstrate calmness
Provide an atmosphere of acceptance
Encourage the expression of feelings (about the source of the anger)
Listen attentively
Offer feedback to the person's expressed feelings
Communicate nurse sensitivity to the person's problem
Relate to the person on an adult–adult level, not on a parent–child level (which could increase anger)
Ask the person to identify the problem
Ask for specifics, not generalizations, about the problem
Provide reliable information (about resources that can be used)
Reveal the person's angry feelings (if he is unaware of them)
Explore with the person his strengths and resources (to restore the loss and prevent further loss)
Reduce the demands placed on the person (so that more energy is available for coping)
Touch the person judiciously (angry persons often prefer not to be touched)
Refrain from arguing, from negatively criticizing, from teasing (which increase anger)
Explore with the person the (negative) effects of his behavior on others

Nursing Observations
Determine the degree of insight that the person has (into the response of anger)
Observe for evidence that the person is reaching out for emotional support
Observe for evidence of a favorable response to therapy (resolution of the problem, decreased anger)

Health Teaching
Explain that the person's response is appropriate and commonly experienced
Explain and offer hope that the emotional pain will decrease with time
Explain how to channel emotional energy and obtain release from stress (running, swimming, or other sports, creative activities, laughing, talking things over, hitting a punching bag or pillow)
Recommend new options for effective methods of coping (assertive rather than aggressive behavior)

EVALUATION

Record actual outcome

ANGER RELATED TO PHYSICAL LOSS[105,338,432,471,525]

ASSESSMENT

Data Collection

Subjective Data
• Person relates experiencing frustration
• May or may not verbalize or openly express anger

- When experiencing anger, verbalizations reveal hostility and resentment
  Feels bitter that the illness happened to him
  Feels resentment and hostility toward those who are well
  Wonders "Why me?" "What did I ever do to deserve this?"
  Perceives that others are involved in life's trivia while he is struggling to function or survive

Objective Data
- Manifests physical findings such as facial flushing or pallor, rapid or deep respirations, rapid or bounding pulse, increased blood pressure
- May exhibit behavior such as demanding and controlling behavior, shouting, throwing or slamming objects, unusual quietness, avoiding persons involved in the physical loss or persons who are well

Data Analysis

Nursing Diagnosis
ANGER RELATED TO PHYSICAL LOSS: A feeling of resentment or hostility about the loss of a positive, balanced state of health

Common Etiology (Stressors)
DISEASES: Any
INJURIES: Any
SIGNS AND SYMPTOMS: Immobility, memory loss, pain, paralysis, weakness
PSYCHOSOCIAL FACTORS: The threat of frustration or delayed goal achievement, the threat of loss of self-esteem, the threat of lack of or loss of control of a life situation, lack of emotional control
HUMAN BODY: *Body appearance*: Changes in body appearance, disfigured body. *Body function*: Loss of body function. *Body part*: Loss of a body part. *Body state*: Loss of the prepregnancy body
DEVELOPMENTAL PHASES: Middle age, old age
SITUATIONAL FACTORS: Childlessness, acute or chronic illness

PLANNING

Unmet Needs

Comfort, protection from psychologic threat, acceptance, caring and communicating relationships, personal growth and maturity, increased learning, increased reality perception and problem-solving ability

Expected Outcome

Person verbalizes feelings of anger
Verbalizes specific problem-solving methods for overcoming the source of anger
Uses constructive outlets for angry feelings
Uses assertive rather than attacking behavior

NURSING INTERVENTIONS

Nursing Treatments

Approach unhurriedly
Demonstrate calmness
Provide an atmosphere of acceptance
Encourage the expression of feelings (about the source of the anger)
Listen attentively
Offer feedback to the person's expressed feelings
Communicate nurse sensitivity to the person's problem
Relate to the person on an adult–adult level, not on a parent–child level (which could increase anger)
Ask the person to identify the problem

Ask for specifics, not generalizations, about the problem

Provide reliable information (about the physical status; this often reduces anger)

Reveal the person's angry feelings (if he is unaware of them)

Encourage mutual problem solving

Explore with the person his strengths and resources (to overcome the problem)

Reduce the demands placed on the person (so that more energy is available for coping)

Suggest appropriate means of emotional expression (assertive rather than aggressive behavior)

Touch the person judiciously (angry persons often prefer not to be touched)

Refrain from arguing, from negatively criticizing, from teasing (all of which increase anger)

Explore with the person the (negative) effects of his behavior on others

Nursing Observations

Determine the degree of insight that the person has (into the response of anger)

Observe for evidence that the person is reaching out for emotional support

Observe for evidence of a favorable response to therapy (decreased anger)

Health Teaching

Explain that the person's response is appropriate and commonly experienced (during illness)

Explain and offer hope that the emotional pain will decrease with time

Explain how to channel emotional energy and obtain release from stress (through creative activities, laughing, talking things over, hitting a punching bag or pillow)

Recommend new options for effective methods of coping (assertive rather than aggressive behavior)

EVALUATION

Record actual outcome

ANGER RELATED TO ROLE LOSS[105,130,432,471,525]

ASSESSMENT

Data Collection

Subjective Data

• Person relates experiencing frustration

• May or may not verbalize or openly express anger

• When expressing anger, verbalizations reveal hostility and resentment

Husband may relate that his wife now supports the family, although he had previously done so

Person no longer assumes previous responsibilities, which remain unattended to, are divided or are assigned to others

May feel he was unfairly forced from his role by persons or circumstances

Objective Data

• Manifests physical findings such as facial flushing or pallor, rapid or deep respirations, rapid or bounding pulse, increased blood pressure, perspiration, trembling

• May exhibit behavior such as demanding and controlling behavior, clenching the jaw or fist, shouting, throwing or slamming objects, unusual quietness, avoiding persons or situations, somatic complaints

Data Analysis

Nursing Diagnosis

ANGER RELATED TO ROLE LOSS: A feeling of resentment or hostility about losing a position, situation, or responsibility in life and being unable to perform the associated, expected behaviors

Common Etiology (Stressors)

DISEASES: Any

INJURIES: Any

SIGNS AND SYMPTOMS: Immobility, pain, weakness

PSYCHOSOCIAL FACTORS: The threat of frustration or delayed goal achievement, the threat of loss of self-esteem, the threat of lack of or loss of control of a life situation, lack of emotional control

DEVELOPMENTAL PHASES: Adolescence, middle age, old age

SITUATIONAL FACTORS: Death of a significant other, divorce, loss of employment, launching grown children, illness of or injury to self or significant other, marriage, parenthood, retirement, the end of school

PLANNING

Unmet Needs

Comfort, protection from psychologic threat, acceptance, caring and communicating relationships, personal growth and maturity, increased learning, increased reality perception and problem-solving ability

Expected Outcome

Person verbalizes feelings of anger
Verbalizes specific problem-solving methods for overcoming the source of anger
Uses constructive outlets for angry feelings
Uses assertive rather than attacking behavior

NURSING INTERVENTIONS

Nursing Treatments

Approach unhurriedly
Reassure verbally (that the nurse will help the person solve his problem, if possible)
Demonstrate calmness
Provide an atmosphere of acceptance
Encourage the expression of feelings (about the source of the anger)
Listen attentively
Offer feedback to the person's expressed feelings
Communicate nurse sensitivity to the person's problem
Relate to the person on an adult–adult level, not on a parent–child level (which could increase anger)
Ask the person to identify the problem
Ask for specifics, not generalizations, about the problem
Support a realistic assessment of the situation (Is the role loss permanent or temporary?)
Reveal the person's angry feelings (if he is unaware of them)
Encourage mutual problem solving
Explore with the person his strengths and resources (for adjusting to the new role)
Reduce the demands placed on the person (so that more energy is available for coping)
Touch the person judiciously (angry persons often prefer not to be touched)
Refrain from arguing, from negatively criticizing, from teasing (which increase anger)
Explore with the person the (negative) effects of his behavior on others

Nursing Observations

Determine the degree of insight that the person has (into the response of anger)

Observe for evidence that the person is reaching out for emotional support

Observe for evidence of a favorable response to therapy (adjustment to the role change, decreased anger)

Health Teaching

Explain that the person's response is appropriate and commonly experienced (when role loss occurs)

Explain and offer hope that the emotional pain will decrease with time

Explain how to channel emotional energy and obtain release from stress (running, swimming, other sports, creative activities, laughing, talking things over, hitting a punching bag or pillow)

Recommend new options for effective methods of coping (assertive rather than aggressive behavior)

EVALUATION

Record actual outcome

ANGER RELATED TO SEPARATION FROM A SIGNIFICANT OTHER[105,432,471,525]

ASSESSMENT

Data Collection

Subjective Data

• Person relates experiencing frustration

• May or may not verbalize or openly express anger about the separation and toward persons responsible for the separation

• When expressing anger, verbalizations reveal hostility and resentment

Objective Data

• Manifests physical findings such as facial flushing or pallor, rapid or deep respirations, rapid or bounding pulse, increased blood pressure, trembling

• May exhibit behavior such as demanding and controlling behavior, shouting, unusual quietness, avoiding persons or situations, somatic complaints

Data Analysis

Nursing Diagnosis

ANGER RELATED TO SEPARATION FROM A SIGNIFICANT OTHER: A feeling of resentment or hostility about being temporarily apart from a significant other

Common Etiology (Stressors)

PSYCHOSOCIAL FACTORS: The threat of frustration or delayed goal achievement, the threat of loss of self-esteem, the threat of lack of or loss of control of a life situation, the threat of having needs unfulfilled through constructive behavior (which results in destructive behavior), lack of emotional control

HEALTH CARE FACTORS: *Health care environment*: Coronary care, intensive care, or isolation unit, locked psychiatric unit. *Hospitalization or institutionalization*: Of self or significant other. *Visitors*: Restriction of

DEVELOPMENTAL PHASES: Toddler (ages 1–3)

SITUATIONAL FACTORS: Confinement in prison, marital separation from spouse or of parents, geographically distant family, military service

PLANNING

Unmet Needs

Comfort, protection from psychologic threat, acceptance, caring and communicating relationships, personal growth and maturity, increased learning, increased reality perception and problem-solving ability

Expected Outcome

Person verbalizes feelings of anger
Verbalizes specific problem-solving methods for overcoming the source of anger
Uses constructive outlets for angry feelings
Uses assertive rather than attacking behavior

NURSING INTERVENTIONS

Nursing Treatments

Approach unhurriedly
Reassure verbally (that the nurse will help the person solve the problem, if possible)
Demonstrate calmness
Provide an atmosphere of acceptance
Encourage the expression of feelings (about the source of the anger)
Listen attentively
Offer feedback to the person's expressed feelings
Communicate nurse sensitivity to the person's problem
Relate to the person on an adult–adult level, not on a parent–child level (which could increase anger)
Ask the person to identify the problem
Ask for specifics, not generalizations, about the problem
Provide reliable information (about visiting hours, about the length of separation due to hospitalization, etc.)
Reveal the person's angry feelings (if he is unaware of them)
Encourage mutual problem solving (about how to bring the persons together or find supportive groups)
Provide meetings with supportive persons or groups (if the separation is due to military service, confinement in jail, or the like)
Explore with the person his strengths and resources (such as being able to make long-distance calls to the loved one)
Reduce the demands placed on the person (so that more energy is available for coping)
Touch the person judiciously (angry persons often prefer not to be touched)
Refrain from arguing, from negatively criticizing, from teasing
Explore with the person the (negative) effects of his behavior on others

Nursing Observations

Determine the degree of insight that the person has (into the response of anger)
Observe for evidence that the person is reaching out for emotional support
Observe for evidence of a favorable response to therapy (decreased anger despite the separation)

Health Teaching

Explain that the person's response is appropriate and commonly experienced (during separation from a significant other)
Explain and offer hope that the emotional pain will decrease with time
Recommend new options for effective methods of coping (assertive rather than aggressive behavior)
Explain how to channel emotional energy and obtain release from stress (running, swimming, other sports, creative activities, laughing, talking things over, hitting a punching bag or pillow)

EVALUATION

Record actual outcome

Adaptive Responses of Emotion (Affect): Anxiety

ANXIETY RELATED TO UNDEFINED THREAT[105,432,471,525]

ASSESSMENT
Data Collection

Subjective Data
• Person relates experiencing feelings of threat or danger to self or others
• Is unable to identify or describe what causes the feeling
• Usually verbalizes "I don't know why I'm upset," "I don't understand what's bothering me"

Mild Anxiety
Minimum focus on self
Increased awareness and alertness
Preoccupied with the anxiety
Maintains some interest in the external environment
Nervousness

Moderate Anxiety
Narrowed sensory perception
Unaware of peripheral activities
Considerable fatigue
Preoccupied with the anxiety
Poor or increased appetite
Insomnia

Severe Anxiety
Greatly narrowed perception
Focuses on details
Unable to distinguish between safe and harmful stimuli
Temporarily unable to learn
Preoccupied with the anxiety
Poor or increased appetite
Somatic complaints such as insomnia, nausea, palpitations

Objective Data
• Manifests physical findings such as facial flushing or pallor, rapid or deep respirations, rapid or bounding pulse, increased blood pressure, sweating, trembeling
• May exhibit behavior such as:

Mild Anxiety
Demonstrates some interest in the external environment
Talkative or verbally very quiet
Mood swings
May take direct action

Moderate Anxiety
Voice tremors
Selective inattention
Difficulty performing poorly developed or recently acquired skills
Easily performs long-established skills
Avoids persons or situations

Severe Anxiety
Is easily distracted, makes poor judgments

Unusual quietness
Forgetfulness
Irritability
Poorly organized behavior
Rapid speech
Avoids persons or situations

Data Analysis

Nursing Diagnosis
ANXIETY RELATED TO UNDEFINED THREAT: A vague, ill-defined feeling of apprehension and uneasiness

Common Etiology (Stressors)
DISEASES: Any
INJURIES: Any
SIGNS AND SYMPTOMS: Any
PSYCHOSOCIAL FACTORS: The threat of a danger not clearly identified or perceived
HEALTH CARE FACTORS: *Health care decisions*: For self or significant other. *Health care environment*: Any. *Hospitalization or institutionalization*: Of self or significant other. *Diagnostic procedures*: Any. *Medical diagnosis*: For self or significant other. *Medical therapy*: Any. *Surgical procedures*: Any. *Therapeutic equipment or devices*: Any
DEVELOPMENTAL PHASES: Any
SITUATIONAL FACTORS: Any

PLANNING

Unmet Needs

Comfort, protection from psychologic threat, predictable and orderly world, acceptance, caring and communicating relationships, high evaluation of self, sense of adequacy, personal growth and maturity, increased learning, spiritual and philosophic satisfaction, increased reality perception and problem-solving ability

Expected Outcome

Person verbalizes feelings of anxiety
Converts vague anxiety feelings into a specifically identified fear
Calm, relaxed facial expression, body movements, and behavior

NURSING INTERVENTIONS

Nursing Treatments

General Interventions
Approach unhurriedly
Demonstrate calmness
Provide an atmosphere of acceptance
Touch the person judiciously
Reassure verbally (that the nurse will help the person solve his own problem)
Attend the person constantly (until he feels sufficiently comfortable to be alone)
Provide frequent contact with the person (thereafter)
Encourage the expression of feelings
Listen attentively
Offer feedback to the person's expressed feelings
Communicate nurse sensitivity to the person's problem
Relate to the person on an adult–adult level, not on a parent–child level (which could increase anxiety)
Ask for specifics, not generalizations, about the problem
Support a realistic assessment of the situation
Provide reliable information (which may ease the anxiety)
Assist the person to convert the anxiety into a specifically identified fear (so the problem can be recognized and dealt with)

Encourage the person to face the anxiety (avoidance increases anxiety)
Encourage the use of normal coping mechanisms
Reduce the demands placed on the person (so that more energy is available for coping)
Do not allow unpleasant surprise situations (which increase anxiety)
Avoid placing the person on enforced inactivity (which heightens anxiety)
Massage gently
  OR
Bathe in warm water (for the relaxation effect)
Call the person's family (to the bedside)
Encourage telephone calls with significant persons

Specific to High-Level Anxiety
Arrange a structured environment (with routines that are familiar to the person)
Arrange orderly surroundings
Provide quiet
Acknowledge dependency (if dependency is increased by high-level anxiety)
Restrict unwanted visitors

Specific to Chronic Anxiety
Explore with the person the reasons for recurring problems (related to the anxiety)
Encourage the identification of specific life values (if poorly defined values are precipitating the anxiety)
Encourage active diversional activities (to promote periods of rest from anxiety)
Encourage gradual mastery of a situation (causing the anxiety)
Encourage planned one-day-at-a-time living
Encourage the sharing of common problems with others

Nursing Observations
Determine the degree of insight that the person has
Determine the precipitating factors, the relieving factors
Evaluate the significance of emotional distress mannerisms, of nonverbal communication
Identify disturbing conversation topics
Identify the appropriate use of defense mechanisms, the inappropriate use of defense mechanisms
Observe for side effects of drugs (such as caffeine or epinephrine) ⎤
Monitor blood studies for abnormal (decreased) glucose
Monitor blood studies for abnormal (decreased) parathyroid function ⎬ Indicating the anxiety is of physical origin
Monitor blood studies for arterial blood gases (decreased O_2 level)
Monitor blood studies for abnormal (increased) adrenal function
Monitor blood studies for increased lactic acid ⎦
Observe for evidence of a favorable response to therapy (reduced anxiety, identified fear)

Health Teaching
Explain that the person's response is appropriate and commonly experienced
Explain and offer hope that the emotional pain will decrease with time
Explain the importance of recognizing tension within oneself
Explain that fatigue should be recognized as a stress factor (causing anxiety)
Explain the need to recognize highly stressful situations
Explain how to channel emotional energy and obtain release from stress (through running, swimming and other sports, creative activities, laughing, talking things over)
Advise against fighting anxiety (this reinforces the emotion)
Explain the difference between freedom from anxiety and freedom from problems
Explain the importance of persons' offering support to one another

Recommend methods for achieving total relaxation (controlled breathing, quietly listening to music, doing nothing)
Recommend a habitual, positive mental attitude
Teach how to use the problem-solving method

EVALUATION

Record actual outcome

ANXIETY RELATED TO PHYSIOLOGIC IMBALANCE [105,278,432,455,471,525]

ASSESSMENT
Data Collection
Subjective Data
• Person relates experiencing feelings of threat or danger to self
• Is unable to identify or describe what causes the feeling
• Usually verbalizes, "I don't know why I'm upset," "I don't understand what's bothering me"

Mild Anxiety
Minimum focus on self
Increased awareness and alertness
Preoccupied with the anxiety
Maintains some interest in the external environment
Nervousness

Moderate Anxiety
Narrowed sensory perception
Unaware of peripheral activities
Considerable fatigue
Internal shaking or trembling
Preoccupied with the anxiety
Poor appetite or increased appetite
Insomnia

Severe Anxiety
Greatly narrowed perception
Focuses on details
Unable to distinguish between safe and harmful stimuli
Temporarily unable to learn
Preoccupied with the anxiety
Poor appetite or increased appetite
Somatic complaints such as insomnia, nausea, palpitations

Objective Data
• Manifests physical findings such as facial flushing or pallor, rapid or deep respirations, rapid or bounding pulse, increased or decreased blood pressure, sweating, trembling
Decreased serum glucose
  OR
Decreased serum O_2 level
  OR
Increased serum lactic acid

OR

Decreased serum calcium and increased serum phosphate (abnormal parathyroid function)

OR

Increased serum cortisol, sodium, glucose (abnormal adrenal function)
• May exhibit behavior such as:

Mild Anxiety
Demonstrates some interest in the external environment
Talkative or verbally very quiet
Mood swings

Moderate Anxiety
Voice tremors
Selective inattention
Difficulty performing poorly developed or recently acquired skills
Easily performs long-established skills
Avoids persons or situations

Severe Anxiety
Is easily distracted, makes poor judgments
Unusual quietness
Forgetfulness
Irritability
Poorly organized behavior
Rapid speech
Avoids persons or situations

Data Analysis

Nursing Diagnosis
ANXIETY RELATED TO PHYSIOLOGIC IMBALANCE: A vague, ill-defined feeling of apprehension and uneasiness due to the body system conveying there is a physiologic threat

Common Etiology (Stressors)
BIRTH DEFECTS: Cystic fibrosis
DISEASES: Asthma, emphysema, hyperthyroidism, thyrotoxicosis, hypoglycemia, hypocalcemia, hypoparathyroidism, mitral valve prolapse, myocardial infarction, pancreatitis, paroxysmal atrial tachycardia, pheochromocytoma, thrombophlebitis, thyrotoxicosis
SIGNS AND SYMPTOMS: Anoxia, bleeding (internal), breathing difficulty, pain
HUMAN BODY: *Body states*: Climacteric, menopause, menstruation
HEALTH CARE FACTORS: *Drug therapy*: Adverse effects of amphetamines, broncodilators, corticosteroids, epinephrine, L-dopa, psychotropic drugs (such as thorazine, stelazine, novene, hadol), thyroid preparations, tricyclic antidepressents. *Medical therapy*: Withdrawal from alcohol, drugs, tobacco
DEVELOPMENTAL PHASES: Puberty, adolescence, middle age
LIFESTYLE: High caffeine intake (50–200 mg of caffeine will cause anxiety, one cup coffee contains 100–150 mg caffeine, one glass of cola contains 40–60 mg caffeine), drug abuse, especially marijuana, lysergic acid diethylamide (LSD), phencyclidine (PCP), excessive alcohol intake
MAJOR PATHOPHYSIOLOGIC FACTORS CAUSING THE PROBLEM: Certain physiologic reactions produce anxiety; inadequate tissue oxygenation reduces circulation to the brain; increased lactic acid blood levels bind calcium, making it inaccessible to the nerve endings; decreased blood glucose stimulates the adrenal gland to secrete epinephrine (adrenalin) for the purpose of elevating the blood sugar; tumors of the adrenal gland or adjacent kidney also stimulate adrenalin, and the increased epinephrine level causes physiologic anxiety; increased levels of thyroid and pain cause nervous system irritability and hypersensitivity to nerve fibers that mimic anxiety; hormonal changes in which the body undergoes considerable physiologic stress cause sensations interpreted as anxiety

PLANNING

Unmet Needs

Comfort, protection from physical and psychologic threat, predictable and orderly world, acceptance, caring and communicating relationships, high evaluation of self, sense of adequacy, personal growth and maturity, increased learning, spiritual-philosophic satisfaction, increased reality perception and problem-solving ability

Expected Outcome

Person verbalizes feelings of anxiety
Converts vague anxiety feelings into a specifically identified fear
Calm, relaxed facial expression, body movements, and behavior

NURSING INTERVENTIONS

Nursing Treatments

General Interventions
Approach unhurriedly
Demonstrate calmness
Provide an atmosphere of acceptance
Touch the person judiciously
Reassure verbally (that the nurse will do everything possible to relieve the anxiety)
Attend the person constantly (until he feels sufficiently comfortable to be alone)
Provide frequent contact with the person (thereafter)
Encourage the expression of feelings
Listen attentively
Offer feedback to the person's expressed feelings
Communicate nurse sensitivity to the person's problem
Relate to the person on an adult–adult level, not on a parent–child level (which could increase anxiety)
Support a realistic assessment of the situation
Provide reliable information (explain the physiologic reason for body sensations that mimic anxiety)
Encourage the use of normal coping mechanisms
Reduce the demands placed on the person (so that more energy is available for coping)
Do not allow unpleasant surprise situations (which increase anxiety)
Avoid placing the person on enforced inactivity (which heightens anxiety)
Massage gently
    OR
Bathe in warm water (for the relaxation effect)
Administer heated humidified oxygen (after ensuring air passages are clear of obstructions, if oxygenation is poor)
Give high-glucose fluids orally (if the glucose level is below normal)
Withhold drugs (such as epinephrine, bronchodilators, thyroid preparations, etc.)
Refrain from giving oral stimulants (cola, coffee, tea, alcohol, nicotine)
Discourage strenuous activity (if the person has a problem with lactic acid accumulation)
Call the person's family (to the bedside if it increases comfort)
Encourage telephone calls with significant persons

Specific to High-Level Anxiety
Arrange a structured environment (with routines that are familiar to the patient)
Arrange orderly surroundings
Provide quiet
Acknowledge dependency (if dependency is increased by high-level anxiety)
Restrict unwanted visitors

Specific to Chronic Anxiety
Encourage active diversional activities (to promote periods of rest from anxiety)
Encourage planned one-day-at-a-time living

Nursing Observations

Determine the precipitating factors, the relieving factors (so they can be altered to reduce the anxiety)

Observe for side effects of drugs (such as caffeine or epinephrine)

Monitor blood studies for abnormal (decreased) glucose

Monitor blood studies for abnormal (decreased) parathyroid function

Monitor blood studies for arterial blood gases (decreased O_2 level)

Monitor blood studies for abnormal (increased) adrenal function

Monitor blood studies for increased lactic acid

So the physiologic abnormalities can be altered to reduce the anxiety

Observe for evidence of a favorable response to therapy (reduced anxiety)

Health Teaching

Explain that the person's response is appropriate and commonly experienced

Explain and offer hope that the emotional pain will decrease with time

Explain that fatigue should be recognized as a stress factor (causing anxiety)

Explain the importance of persons' offering support to one another

Recommend methods for achieving total relaxation (controlled breathing, quietly listening to music, doing nothing)

Recommend a habitual, positive mental attitude

EVALUATION

Record actual outcome

Adaptive Responses of Emotion (Affect): Conflict

CONFLICT RELATED TO DIFFERENCES BETWEEN SIGNIFICANT OTHERS [13,105,432,471,525]

ASSESSMENT

Data Collection

Subjective Data

• Person relates thinking about a choice of options
• Discusses the pros and cons and that the choices are both acceptable and unacceptable
• Prolongs making a decision

Health Decisions

Person's choice of treatment may be different than what family members want for him

Person may desire to die naturally, but family members may want him to use every method available to continue living

Some family members may want a dependent loved one institutionalized, while others do not

Person who is expected to care for a dependent loved one may refuse to do so

Family members may argue over who will pay the bills
Some family members may want to prohibit visits and decisions by other family member(s)

Life-Situation Decisions
Persons may disagree on how to raise children
Parent and adolescent may be in conflict over the adolescent's companions, late hours, etc.
One spouse may make a choice, on any subject, that is not acceptable to the other spouse
Individuals may seek the advice of persons outside the family

Objective Data
• May exhibit behavior such as restlessness, heavy smoking, anger, unusual quietness, seeking others' opinions, not taking decisive action, becoming tearful when asked for a decision

Data Analysis

Nursing Diagnosis
CONFLICT RELATED TO DIFFERENCES BETWEEN SIGNIFICANT OTHERS: A conscious or unconscious struggle between opposing persons who are significant in each other's lives

Common Etiology (Stressors)
DISEASES: Any disease
INJURIES: Any injury
PSYCHOSOCIAL FACTORS: The threat of frustration regardless of the course chosen, the threat and arousal of two or more incompatible choices requiring a decision, differences between the essential needs of the persons involved
HEALTH CARE FACTORS: *Health care costs*: High. *Health care decisions for self*: Decision about the choice of treatment options, to continue or discontinue therapy, to die naturally, to donate a body organ, to donate blood, to donate the body to science, to seek diagnosis and treatment; decisions made independently of a significant other. *Health care decision for significant other*: Decision to donate a significant other's body organ, to institutionalize a significant other, to prolong life mechanically, to seek diagnosis and treatment for a significant other, to withdraw life-support systems. *Hospitalization or institutionalization*: Of self or significant other. *Diagnostic Procedures*: Any *Medical therapy*: Any *Surgical procedures*: Any
DEVELOPMENTAL PHASES: Any but especially adolescence
LIFESTYLE: Lack of conformity of a significant other to cultural mores, poverty
SITUATIONAL FACTORS: Adoption of a child, placing a child up for adoption, impending death or death of a significant other, divorce, child-parent difficulties, illness or injury to self or significant other, child rearing, marriage of a significant other

PLANNING

Unmet Needs
Comfort, protection from psychologic threat, caring and communicating relationships, sense of adequacy, personal growth and maturity, increased learning, increased reality perception and problem-solving ability

Expected Outcome
Person verbalizes about the choice of options
Relates a specific problem-solving approach to coping with the choices
Verbalizes satisfaction with the choice
Takes decisive action

NURSING INTERVENTIONS

Nursing Treatments
Approach unhurriedly
Demonstrate calmness

Provide an atmosphere of acceptance
Encourage the expression of feelings (by all persons involved)
Listen attentively
Offer feedback to the person's expressed feelings
Communicate nurse sensitivity to the person's problem
Ask the person to identify the problem
Ask for specifics, not generalizations, about the problem
Provide reliable information (about the subject of the conflict)
Introduce to persons who have successfully undergone the same experience
Explore with the person his strengths and resources (to solve the problem)
Encourage mutual problem solving (among persons significant in the conflict)
Encourage decision making (to resolve the conflict)

Nursing Observations
Determine the degree of insight that the persons have (about the conflict)
Observe for an excessive stress level (as a result of the conflict)
Observe for evidence that the person is reaching out for emotional support
Observe for evidence of a favorable response to therapy (resolution of the conflict)

Health Teaching
Explain that the person's response is appropriate and commonly experienced
Recommend new options for effective methods of coping (such as dealing with the feel-
ings that cause the conflict, such as anger, rejection, and threatened self-esteem, by
having the persons involved list the pros and cons of making a decision)
Teach how to use the problem-solving method (to reach satisfactory decisions)

EVALUATION
Record actual outcome

CONFLICT RELATED TO HEALTH DECISIONS FOR SELF[105,432,471,525]

ASSESSMENT
Data Collection
Subjective Data
• Person relates thinking about a choice of options
• Discusses the pros and cons and that the choices are both acceptable and unacceptable
• Prolongs making a decision
  May vascillate between seeking treatment and ignoring symptoms
  May perceive treatment as a step toward health but also as expensive and time-con-
    suming
  May desire health, but wants to avoid pain and dependency
  May desire health care but be concerned about the effects on family members
  May want to donate blood or an organ but be concerned about the consequences
  Often seeks the advice of others

Objective Data
• May exhibit behavior such as restlessness, pacing, sleeplessness, unusual quietness,
  seeking others' opinions, not taking decisive action

Data Analysis
Nursing Diagnosis
CONFLICT RELATED TO HEALTH DECISIONS FOR SELF: A conscious or unconscious struggle between
  opposing choices regarding the person's own health care or health situation

Common Etiology (Stressors)

PSYCHOSOCIAL FACTORS: The threat and arousal of two or more incompatible choices requiring a decision, the threat of frustration regardless of the course chosen, the threat of failure to make the right choice

HEALTH CARE FACTORS: *Health care decisions for self*: Decision about the choice of treatment options, to continue or discontinue health therapy, to die naturally, to donate a body organ, to donate blood, to donate the body to science, to seek diagnosis and treatment. *Health therapy*: Irreversible medical or surgical therapy such as radiation, blood transfusion, amputation, fallopian tube ligation, mastectomy, vasectomy. *Medical therapy*: Withdrawal from alcohol, drugs, tobacco

SITUATIONAL FACTORS: Adoption of a child

PLANNING

Unmet Needs

Comfort, protection from psychologic threat, caring and communicating relationships, sense of adequacy, personal growth and maturity, increased learning, increased reality perception and problem-solving ability

Expected Outcome

Person verbalizes about the choice of options

Relates a specific problem-solving approach to coping with the choices

Verbalizes satisfaction with the choice

Takes decisive action

NURSING INTERVENTIONS

Nursing Treatments

Approach unhurriedly

Demonstrate calmness

Provide an atmosphere of acceptance

Encourage the expression of feelings (about the conflict)

Listen attentively

Offer feedback to the person's expressed feelings

Communicate nurse sensitivity to the person's problem

Ask the person to identify the problem

Ask for specifics, not generalizations, about the problem

Provide reliable information (about the subject of the conflict)

Introduce to persons who have successfully undergone the same experience (if appropriate)

Explore with the person his strengths and resources (to solve the problem)

Encourage mutual problem solving (among persons significant in the conflict)

Encourage decision making (to resolve the conflict)

Nursing Observations

Determine the degree of insight that the person has (about the conflict)

Observe for an excessive stress level (as a result of the conflict)

Observe for evidence that the person is reaching out for emotional support

Observe for evidence of a favorable response to therapy (resolution of the conflict)

Health Teaching

Explain that the person's response is appropriate and commonly experienced

Recommend new options for effective methods of coping (such as dealing with the feelings that are causing the conflict, such as fear of physical injury and fear of the unknown, by having the person list the pros and cons of making a decision)

Teach how to use the problem-solving method (to reach satisfactory health care decisions)

EVALUATION

Record actual outcome

CONFLICT RELATED TO HEALTH DECISIONS FOR A SIGNIFICANT OTHER[13,105,432,471,525]

ASSESSMENT
Data Collection
Subjective Data
- Person relates thinking about a choice of options
- Discusses the pros and cons and that the choices are both acceptable and unacceptable
- Prolongs making a decision
  May be preoccupied with:
    Whether certain treatments should be performed on a loved one
    Whether the loved one should be cared for at home or in a nursing home
    Whether the loved one should be committed to a mental institution or drug or alcohol center
    Wanting to remove the loved one from the hospital against medical advice
    Seeking the advice of others, frequently of family members

Objective Data
- May exhibit behavior such as restlessness, pacing, heavy smoking, seeking others' opinions, unusual quietness, anger toward the staff, not taking decisive action, becoming tearful when asked for a decision

Data Analysis
Nursing Diagnosis
CONFLICT RELATED TO HEALTH DECISIONS FOR A SIGNIFICANT OTHER: A conscious or unconscious struggle between opposing choices in which the person cannot decide about the health care to be approved of or instigated for a loved one

Common Etiology (Stressors)
PSYCHOSOCIAL FACTORS: The threat and arousal of two or more incompatible choices requiring a decision, the threat of frustration regardless of the course chosen, the threat of failure to make the right choice
HEALTH CARE FACTORS: *Health care decisions for significant other*: Decision to donate a significant other's body organ, to institutionalize a significant other, to prolong life mechanically, to seek diagnosis and treatment for a significant other, to withdraw life-support systems
SITUATIONAL FACTORS: Placing a child up for adoption

PLANNING
Unmet Needs
Comfort, protection from psychologic threat, caring and communicating relationships, sense of adequacy, personal growth and maturity, increased learning, increased reality perception and problem-solving ability

Expected Outcome
Person verbalizes about the choice of options
Relates a specific problem-solving approach to coping with the choice
Verbalizes satisfaction with the choice
Takes decisive action

NURSING INTERVENTIONS
Nursing Treatments
Approach unhurriedly
Demonstrate calmness
Provide an atmosphere of acceptance
Encourage the expression of feelings (about the decisions to be made)

Listen attentively

Offer feedback of the person's expressed feelings

Communicate nurse sensitivity to the person's problem

Ask the person to identify the problem

Ask for specifics, not generalizations, about the problem

Provide reliable information (about the subject of the conflict)

Introduce to persons who have successfully undergone the same experience (if appropriate)

Explore with the person his strengths and resources (to solve the problem)

Encourage mutual problem solving (among persons significant in the conflict)

Encourage decision making (to resolve the conflict)

Nursing Observations

Determine the degree of insight that the person has (about the conflict)

Observe for an excessive stress level (as a result of the conflict)

Observe for evidence that the person is reaching out for emotional support

Observe for evidence of a favorable response to therapy (resolution of the conflict)

Health Teaching

Explain that the person's response is appropriate and commonly experienced

Recommend new options for effective methods of coping (such as dealing with the feelings that are causing the conflict, such as guilt about institutionalizing a significant other, by having the person list the pros and cons of making a decision)

Teach how to use the problem-solving method (to reach satisfactory health care decisions)

EVALUATION

Record actual outcome

Adaptive Responses of Emotion (Affect): Dependency Feelings

DEPENDENCY FEELINGS RELATED TO LIFE-SUPPORT SYSTEMS [105,471,525]

ASSESSMENT

Data Collection

Subjective Data
• Person verbalizes a need for protection
• Requests help from others
• Relates concern with matters of self
  Is intensely aware that his existence is being maintained by a life-supporting method

Objective Data
• May exhibit behavior such as being helpless, seeking reassurance, demanding help, trying to do more than he is able to counteract the dependency feeling

Data Analysis

Nursing Diagnosis
DEPENDENCY FEELINGS RELATED TO LIFE-SUPPORT SYSTEMS: Feeling the need to rely on supportive

and assistive methods that maintain life and without which life would cease or be seriously threatened

Common Etiology (Stressors)

PSYCHOSOCIAL FACTORS: The threat of being unable to meet own needs, lack of resources to achieve a goal, loss of physiologic independence, the threat of lack of control of a life situation

HEALTH CARE FACTORS: *Drug therapy:* Cardiac drugs, chemotherapy, insulin, anticonvulsants, corticosteroids, immunosuppressant therapy. *Medical therapy:* Hemodialysis, hyperalimentation infusion, intermittent positive-pressure breathing, oxygen therapy, peritoneal dialysis, blood transfusion. *Therapeutic equipment:* Use of a cardiac pacemaker, respirator, defibrillator, monitoring equipment

PLANNING

Unmet Needs

Comfort, protection from psychologic threat, dependence, acceptance, caring and communicating relationships, high evaluation of self, independence, dignity, personal growth and maturity, increased learning, increased reality perception and problem-solving ability

Expected Outcome

Person verbalizes about feelings of dependency
Relates receiving needed support from others
Verbalizes self-satisfaction in accepting support
Assumes as much self-directed behavior as possible

NURSING INTERVENTIONS

Nursing Treatments

Approach unhurriedly
Reassure verbally (that the life-support systems are available whenever needed)
Demonstrate calmness
Provide an atmosphere of acceptance
Encourage the expression of feelings (about the dependency)
Listen attentively
Offer feedback to the person's expressed feelings
Communicate nurse sensitivity to the person's problem
Relate to the person on an adult–adult level, not on a parent–child level (which would increase dependency feelings)
Acknowledge dependency (as a consequence of severe illness)
Arrange situations that encourage the person's autonomy (give him some control over the use of the equipment)
Encourage decision making (by the dependent person)
Explore with the person his strengths and resources (especially as he improves physiologically; stress the body's ability to function independently)
Support a realistic assessment of the situation (he may be less dependent than he perceives himself to be)
Respond immediately to the person's call (waiting for others to meet needs increases dependency feelings)
Encourage family-shared responsibility (if the person is chronically dependent on a life-support system, discuss how much responsibility. should be assumed by the patient and how much by the family)

Nursing Observations

Determine the degree of insight that the person has
Observe for an excessive stress level (about being dependent)
Observe for evidence that the person is reaching out for emotional support
Observe for evidence of a favorable response to therapy (maximum independence attainable, increased comfort feelings)

Health Teaching

Explain that the person's response is appropriate and commonly experienced (by others using life-support systems)

Explain (to the family) that ill or aged persons are often hypersensitive (about their dependence)

Recommend a habitual, positive mental attitude (if the use of life-support systems is long term)

EVALUATION

Record actual outcome

DEPENDENCY FEELINGS RELATED TO NATURAL BODY CHANGES[105,471,525]

ASSESSMENT

Data Collection

Subjective Data

• Person verbalizes a need for protection
• Requests help from others
• Relates concern with matters of self

Pregnant woman feels that her body and her fetus are vulnerable, and toward the end of pregnancy, she feels a need for assistance with tasks

Adolescents may feel a need for help in coping with menses or other body changes

Persons may feel a need for help in coping with physiologic changes of menopause and climacteric

Objective Data

• May exhibit behavior such as helplessness, seeking reassurance, demanding help, or appearing uninterested in body changes

Data Analysis

Nursing Diagnosis

DEPENDENCY FEELINGS RELATED TO NATURAL BODY CHANGES: Feeling the need to rely on others for support during periods of life in which the body naturally changes

Common Etiology (Stressors)

PSYCHOSOCIAL FACTORS: The threat of being unable to meet own needs, the threat of being unable to manage independently, lack of self-confidence, lack of resources to achieve a goal, the threat of lack of control of a life situation, an attempt by a significant other to reinforce the illness role of another

HUMAN BODY: *Body state*: Pregnancy, onset of menstruation, menopause, male climacteric

DEVELOPMENTAL PHASES: Puberty, middle age

PLANNING

Unmet Needs

Comfort, protection from psychologic threat, dependence, acceptance, caring and communicating relationships, high evaluation of self, independence, dignity, personal growth and maturity, increased learning, increased reality perception and problem-solving ability

Expected Outcome

Person verbalizes about feelings of dependency

Relates receiving needed support from other

Verbalizes self-satisfaction in accepting support
Assumes as much self-directed behavior as possible

NURSING INTERVENTIONS

Nursing Treatments

Approach unhurriedly
Reassure verbally (that the person's dependent needs will be met)
Demonstrate calmness
Provide an atmosphere of acceptance
Encourage the expression of feelings (about feeling dependent)
Listen attentively
Offer feedback to the person's expressed feelings
Communicate nurse sensitivity to the person's problem
Relate to the person on an adult–adult level, not on a parent–child level (which would increase dependency feelings)
Acknowledge dependency (as sometimes necessary to reach wellness)
Arrange situations that encourage the person's autonomy
Encourage decision making (by the dependent person)
Explore with the person his strengths and resources
Support a realistic assessment of the situation (is the need for dependency as great as it is perceived to be?)
Respond immediately to the person's call (waiting for others to meet needs increases dependency feelings)

Nursing Observations

Determine the degree of insight that the person has
Evaluate the person's relatedness with others (in regard to dependence–independence)
Observe for an excessive stress level (about being dependent)
Observe for impaired self-attitudes
Observe for evidence that the person is reaching out for emotional support
Observe for evidence of a favorable response to therapy (maximum independence attainable, increased comfort feelings)

Health Teaching

Explain that the person's response is appropriate and commonly experienced (by others during natural body changes)
Provide information (about the body changes and what the person can expect)
Recommend a habitual, positive mental attitude (despite feeling dependent)

EVALUATION

Record actual outcome

DEPENDENCY FEELINGS RELATED TO PHYSICAL LOSS [105,471,525]

ASSESSMENT

Data Collection

Subjective Data

• Person verbalizes a need for protection
• Requests help from others
• Relates concern with matters of self
  Is aware of his physical limitations

Recognizes the strengths of others
Feels secure when receiving help

Objective Data
• May exhibit behavior such as being helpless, seeking reassurance, demanding help, difficulty with decision making, trying to do more than he is able to, or appearing uninterested to counteract the dependency feeling

Data Analysis

Nursing Diagnosis
DEPENDENCY FEELINGS RELATED TO PHYSICAL LOSS: Feeling the need to rely on others for support following the loss of a positive, balanced state of health

Common Etiology (Stressors)
DISEASES: Any severe
INJURIES: Any severe
SIGNS AND SYMPTOMS: Confusion, immobility, memory loss, pain, paralysis, weakness
PSYCHOSOCIAL FACTORS: The threat of being unable to meet own needs, the threat of being unable to manage independently, lack of self-confidence, lack of resources to achieve a goal, loss of physiologic independence, the threat of lack of control of a life situation, an attempt by a significant other to reinforce the illness role of another
HUMAN BODY: *Body function*: Loss of body function. *Body part*: Loss of body part
HEALTH CARE FACTORS: *Adverse effects of medical, drug, or surgical therapy*: Loss of a body part from amputation, cholecystectomy, enucleation or evisceration of eyeball, gastrectomy, hemipelvectomy, hysterectomy, ileostomy, lobectomy of the brain, liver, or lungs, mastectomy, nephrectomy, prostatectomy, spleenectomy, thryoidectomy, tonsillectomy; loss of mobility from traction; loss of natural elimination and elimination control from colostomy, ileocolostomy, ileostomy, ureterocolostomy, ureteroileostomy, ureterosigmoidostomy, ureterostomy, ureterotomy; loss of normal food intake from esophagectomy; loss of reproductive ability from fallopian tube ligation, hysterectomy, oophorectomy, orchidectomy, prostatectomy, salpingectomy, vasectomy; loss of speech from glossectomy, laryngectomy, tracheostomy, vocal cordectomy; loss of vision from enucleation or evisceration of eyeball
DEVELOPMENTAL PHASES: Old age
SITUATIONAL FACTORS: Illness of or injury to self

PLANNING

Unmet Needs
Comfort, protection from psychologic threat, dependence, acceptance, caring and communicating relationships, high evaluation of self, independence, dignity, personal growth and maturity, increased learning, increased reality perception and problem-solving ability

Expected Outcome
Person verbalizes about feelings of dependency
Relates receiving needed support from others
Verbalizes self-satisfaction in accepting support
Assumes as much self-directed behavior as possible

NURSING INTERVENTIONS

Nursing Treatments
Approach unhurriedly
Reassure verbally (that the person's dependent needs will be met)
Demonstrate calmness
Provide an atmosphere of acceptance
Encourage the expression of feelings (about dependency)
Listen attentively
Offer feedback to the person's expressed feelings

Communicate nurse sensitivity to the person's problem

Relate to the person on an adult–adult level, not on a parent–child level (which would increase dependency feelings)

Acknowledge dependency (as necessary to regain health or as a consequence of failing health)

Arrange situations that encourage the person's autonomy

Encourage decision making (by the dependent person)

Explore with the person his strengths and resources (which allow as much independence as possible)

Support a realistic assessment of the situation (he may be less dependent than he perceives himself to be)

Respond immediately to the person's call (waiting for others to meet needs increases dependency feelings)

Nursing Observations

Determine the degree of insight that the person has

Evaluate the person's relatedness with others (in regard to dependence–independence)

Observe for an excessive stress level (about being dependent)

Observe for impaired self-attitudes

Observe for evidence that the person is reaching out for emotional support

Observe for evidence of a favorable response to therapy (maximum independence attainable, increased comfort feelings)

Health Teaching

Explain that the person's response is appropriate and commonly experienced (by others during illness)

Explain (to the family) that ill or aged persons are often hypersensitive (about their dependence)

Recommend a habitual, positive mental attitude

EVALUATION

Record actual outcome

Adaptive Response of Emotion (Affect): Depression

DEPRESSION RELATED TO APPROACHING DEATH[90,105,471]

ASSESSMENT

Data Collection

Subjective Data

• Person states feeling moody and sad
• Is preoccupied with the approaching loss of life
• Expresses the wish that the loss be restored
• Complains of lack of energy, nervousness, early morning insomnia, fretful or excessive sleep, appetite changes

Mild Depression

Let-down feeling occurs as the end of life is perceived

Feelings of moodiness disappear when and if there are moments of hope
Somatic complaints involve multiple body systems

Moderate Depression
Let-down feeling lasts more than several weeks
Difficulty concentrating
Feels tense
Mental rumination about the person's past life
Preoccupied with body function involving multiple body systems

Objective Data
• May exhibit behavior such as slowed body movements, overactivity, restlessness, and indifferent attitude

Mild Depression
Saddened facial expression, tearfulness

Moderate Depression
Unkempt appearance, poor posture, irritability, forgetfulness, difficulty making decisions, decreased involvement in usual interests

Data Analysis
Nursing Diagnosis
DEPRESSION RELATED TO APPROACHING DEATH: A mental state of gloom and sadness about the ending of one's life

Common Etiology (Stressors)
DISEASES: Any
INJURIES Any
PSYCHOSOCIAL FACTORS: The threat of loss of control of a life situation, loss of a significant other (the self), lack of or loss of emotional support (positive reinforcement) from others, exhaustion of adaptive reserves
HEALTH CARE FACTORS: *Medical diagnosis:* Unfavorable medical diagnosis for self. *Health therapy:* Unsuccessful or ineffective medical, drug or surgical therapy. *Prognosis:* Unfavorable prognosis
SITUATIONAL FACTORS: Terminal illness of self, the experience of dying

PLANNING
Unmet Needs
Comfort, stimulation, protection from psychologic threat, acceptance, caring and communicating relationships, sense of adequacy, high evaluation of self, endurance, personal growth and maturity, increased learning, increased pleasantness

Expected Outcome
Person verbalizes feelings of moodiness, sadness
Acknowledges that the loss cannot be restored

NURSING INTERVENTIONS
Nursing Treatments
Approach unhurriedly
Reassure verbally (that the nurse will help the person overcome the depression)
Demonstrate calmness
Provide an atmosphere of acceptance
Encourage the expression of feelings (of moodiness, sadness)
Listen attentively
Talk with the person and family
Offer feedback to the person's expressed feelings
Communicate that the nurse feels comfortable with the person's discussion of death
Relate to the person on an adult–adult level, not on a parent–child level (which could increase depression)
Reveal the person's depressed feelings (if he is unaware of them)

Encourage awareness of positive responses from others (that others are offering love and support, that by allowing others to do this for him, he is helping others meet their needs to love him)

Explore with the person his strengths and resources (to overcome depression; to cope with dying)

Encourage planned one-day-at-a-time living

Encourage pride in appearance (despite the depression)

Reduce the demands placed on the person (so that more energy is available for coping)

Refrain from negatively criticizing

Encourage telephone calls with significant persons (who can be supportive)

Touch the person frequently

Provide frequent patient contact (share as much time with the person as possible)

Avoid attempting to cheer up the depressed person (the inability to respond cheerfully makes the depressed person more depressed)

Nursing Observations

Determine the degree of insight that the person has (into the depression)

Evaluate the person's relatedness with others (and its effect on the depression)

Observe for an excessive stress level

Observe for evidence of a favorable response to therapy (decreased moodiness, sadness, improved functioning ability)

Health Teaching

Explain that the person's response is appropriate and commonly experienced

Describe the factors associated with the occurrence of the problem (explain that complaints such as insomnia, tiredness, wanting to sleep excessively, etc. are normal parts of depression)

Explain and offer hope that the emotional pain will decrease with time (that acceptance will eventually come, despite the present discomfort)

Advise that significant persons express acceptance of one another, express caring for one another

Explain the importance of persons offering support to one another

Explain the importance of maintaining a positive self-attitude

Advise that negative responses from others be regarded with minimum significance (even though there are feelings about such responses)

Describe those symptoms that should be reported (severe depression in which the person considers suicide)

EVALUATION

Record actual outcome

DEPRESSION RELATED TO LOSS OF A SIGNIFICANT OTHER[105,471]

ASSESSMENT DATA

Data Collection

Subjective Data

- Person states feeling moody and sad
- Is preoccupied with the loss of a significant loved one
- Expresses the wish that the loss be restored
- Complains of lack of energy, nervousness, early morning insomnia, fretful or excessive sleep, appetite changes
  Feels that no one else could ever measure up to the lost person

May discuss how the loss will cause changes in the person's life
May express angry feelings

Mild Depression
Let-down feeling occurs when an event ends (after the divorce, funeral, adoption proceedings, etc.)
Feelings of moodiness disappear when something new is planned
Somatic complaints involving multiple body systems

Moderate Depression
Let-down feeling lasts more than several weeks
Difficulty concentrating
Feels tense
Mental rumination
Preoccupied with body function involving multiple body systems

Objective Data
• May exhibit behaviors such as slowed body movements, overactivity, restlessness, indifferent attitude

Mild Depression
Saddened facial expression, tearfulness

Moderate Depression
Unkempt appearance, poor posture, irritability, forgetfulness, difficulty making decisions, decreased involvement in usual interests

Data Analysis

Nursing Diagnosis
DEPRESSION RELATED TO LOSS OF A SIGNIFICANT OTHER: A mental state of gloom and sadness about being permanently parted from a significant other

Common Etiology (Stressors)
BIRTH DEFECTS: Giving birth to an imperfect infant (loss of the perfect child)
DISEASES: Natural abortion, stillbirth, sudden infant death
PSYCHOSOCIAL FACTORS: Loss of a significant other, the threat of loss of self-esteem, loss of an ideal or imagined relationship, the threat of loss of security, the threat of loss of control of a life situation, lack of or loss of emotional support (positive reinforcement) from others, exhaustion of adaptive reserves
HEALTH CARE FACTORS: *Hospital discharge:* Without the expected infant
SITUATIONAL FACTORS: Placing a child up for adoption, child being put up for adoption, death of a significant other, divorce of parents, divorce from spouse, frequent change of foster parents, giving up a foster child, holidays without a significant other

PLANNING

Unmet Needs
Comfort, stimulation, protection from psychologic threat, acceptance, caring and communicating relationships, sense of usefulness and adequacy, high evaluation of self, endurance, personal growth and maturity, increased learning, increased reality perception and problem-solving ability, increased pleasantness

Expected Outcome
Person verbalizes feelings of moodiness, sadness
Acknowledges that the loss cannot be restored
   OR
Accepts and plans for restoring reversible losses
Verbalizes an increased energy level
Person's body activity is at a level normal for the individual

NURSING INTERVENTIONS

Nursing Treatments
Approach unhurriedly

Reassure verbally (that the nurse will help the person overcome his depression)
Demonstrate calmness
Provide an atmosphere of acceptance
Encourage the expression of feelings (of moodiness, sadness, helplessness)
Listen attentively
Offer feedback to the person's expressed feelings
Communicate nurse sensitivity to the person's problems
Relate to the person on an adult–adult level, not on a parent–child level (which could increase depression)
Ask the person to identify the problem
Ask for specifics, not generalizations, about the problem
Support a realistic assessment of the situation (that the loss cannot be restored)
Provide reliable information (which often reduces depression)
Reveal the person's depressed feelings (if he is unaware of them)
Encourage the sharing of common problems with others
Encourage awareness of positive responses from others (that others are offering love and support)
Explore with the person the reasons for self-criticism (which reinforces depression)
Explore with the person his strengths and resources (to overcome depression)
Encourage involvement in helping others, involvement in totally new interests
Encourage meaningful activity, a full day of activities, active diversional activities (all of which divert the person's attention from depression and focuses attention on the external)
Encourage planned one-day-at-a-time living
Encourage pride in appearance (despite the depression)
Introduce to persons who have successfully undergone the same experience
Avoid forcing the person into rapid adaptation to change by accepting the person's unique pattern of adjustment
Reduce the demands placed on the person (so that more energy is available for coping)
Refrain from negatively criticizing
Encourage telephone calls with significant persons (who can be supportive)
Touch the person judiciously
Provide frequent contact with the person (share as much time with the patient as possible)
Arrange a structured environment (suitable to the person)
Arrange pleasant surroundings
Avoid attempting to cheer up the depressed person (the inability to respond cheerfully makes the depressed person more depressed)

Nursing Observations
Determine the degree of insight that the person has
Determine the precipitating factors, the relieving factors (of the depression)
Evaluate the person's relatedness with others (and its effect on the depression)
Observe for an excessive stress level
Observe for evidence of a favorable response to therapy (decreased moodiness, sadness, improved functioning ability)

Health Teaching
Explain that the person's response is appropriate and commonly experienced (that depression is normal after a loss)
Explain that the situation is temporary (that the depression is difficult but will subside)
Describe the factors associated with the occurrence of the problem (explain the complaints such as insomnia, tiredness, wanting to sleep excessively, etc., are normal parts of depression)
Explain and offer hope that the emotional pain will decrease with time (that the depression will eventually end, despite the present discomfort)
Advise that significant persons express acceptance of one another, express caring for one another

Explain the importance of persons offering support to one another

Explain the importance of maintaining a positive self-attitude

Advise that negative responses from others be regarded with minimum significance (even though there are feelings about such responses)

Emphasize the importance of recognizing internal tension

Explain the need to recognize highly stressful situations

Describe those symptoms that should be reported (severe depression in which the person cannot function or considers suicide)

Teach how to use the problem-solving method (to overcome problems that contribute to the depression or result from the loss)

EVALUATION

Record actual outcome

DEPRESSION RELATED TO MATERIAL LOSS[105,471]

ASSESSMENT

Data Collection

Subjective Data
- Person states feeling moody and sad
- Is preoccupied with the loss of a valued object
- Expresses the wish that the loss be restored
- Complains of lack of energy, nervousness, early morning insomnia, fretful or excessive sleep, appetite changes

Acknowledges that the lost object was very valuable to the person, that there is sentimental attachment, that it met an important human need

May express anger

Mild Depression
Let-down feeling occurs when the event ends (the theft, fire, tornado, sale of home, etc.)

Feelings of moodiness disappear when something new is planned

Somatic complaints involving multiple body systems

Moderate Depression
Let-down feeling lasts more than several weeks

Difficulty concentrating

Feels tense

Mental rumination

Preoccupied with body function involving multiple body systems

Objective Data
- May exhibit behavior such as slowed body movements, overactivity, restlessness, and indifferent attitude

Mild Depression
Saddened facial expression, tearfulness

Moderate Depression
Unkempt appearance, poor posture, irritability, forgetfulness, difficulty making decisions, decreased involvement in usual interests

Data Analysis

Nursing Diagnosis

DEPRESSION RELATED TO MATERIAL LOSS: A mental state of gloom and sadness about the loss of tangible, valued objects

Common Etiology (Stressors)

PSYCHOSOCIAL FACTORS: Loss of a significant or valued object, the threat of loss of self-esteem, the threat of loss of security, the threat of loss of control of a life situation, lack of or loss of emotional support (positive reinforcement) from others, nonachievement of unrealistic or unattainable goals, exhaustion of adaptive reserves

HEALTH CARE FACTORS: *Health care costs:* High

SITUATIONAL FACTORS: Accident, loss of or relocation of a home, loss of employment, lack of finances, lack of insurance coverage, loss of property through illness or injury, natural disaster, arson, theft

ENVIRONMENTAL FACTORS: *Cataclysm:* Cyclone, earthquake, flood, hailstorm, hurricane, volcanic eruption *Environmental heat:* Fire

PLANNING

Unmet Needs

Comfort, stimulation, protection from psychologic threat, acceptance, caring and communicating relationships, sense of usefulness and adequacy, high evaluation of self, endurance, personal growth and maturity, increased learning, increased reality perception and problem-solving ability, increased pleasantness

Expected Outcome

Person verbalizes feelings of moodiness, sadness
Acknowledges that the loss cannot be restored
　OR
Accepts and plans for restoring reversible losses
Verbalizes an increased energy level
Person's body activity is at a level normal for the individual

NURSING INTERVENTIONS

Nursing Treatments

Approach unhurriedly
Reassure verbally (that the nurse will help the person overcome his depression)
Demonstrate calmness
Provide an atmosphere of acceptance
Encourage the expression of feelings (of moodiness, sadness, helplessness)
Listen attentively
Offer feedback to the person's expressed feelings
Communicate nurse sensitivity to the person's problem
Relate to the person on an adult–adult level, not on a parent–child level (which could increase depression)
Ask the person to identify the problem
Ask for specifics, not generalizations, about the problem
Support a realistic assessment of the situation (that it may be possible to rebuild or replace the object)
Reveal the person's depressed feelings (if he is unaware of them)
Encourage the sharing of common problems with others
Encourage awareness of positive responses from others (that others are offering to help restore the loss)
Explore with the person the reasons for self-criticism (which reinforces depression)
Explore with the person his strengths and resources (to overcome depression)
Encourage meaningful activity, a full day of activities, active diversional activities (all of which divert attention from depression and focus attention on the external)
Encourage planned one-day-at-a-time living
Encourage pride in appearance (despite the depression)
Introduce to persons who have successfully undergone the same experience
Avoid forcing the person into rapid adaptation to change be accepting the person's unique pattern of adjustment
Reduce the demands placed on the person (so that more energy is available for coping)

Refrain from negatively criticizing
Encourage telephone calls with significant persons (who can be supportive)
Touch the person frequently
Provide frequent patient contact (share as much time with the person as possible)
Arrange a structured environment (suitable to the person)
Arrange pleasant surroundings
Avoid attempting to cheer up the depressed person (the inability to respond cheerfully makes the depressed person more depressed)

Nursing Observations
Determine the degree of insight that the person has
Determine the precipitating factors, the relieving factors (of the depression)
Observe for an excessive stress level
Observe for evidence of a favorable response to therapy (decreased moodiness, sadness, improved functioning ability)

Health Teaching
Explain that the person's response is appropriate and commonly experienced (that it is normal after a loss)
Explain that the situation is temporary (that the depression is difficult but will subside)
Describe the factors associated with the occurrence of the problem (explain that complaints such as insomnia, tiredness, wanting to sleep excessively, etc., are normal parts of depression)
Explain and offer hope that the emotional pain will decrease with time (that the depression will eventually end, despite the present discomfort)
Advise that significant persons express acceptance of one another, express caring for one another
Explain the importance of persons' offering support to one another
Explain the importance of maintaining a positive self-attitude
Advise that negative responses from others be regarded with minimum significance (even though there are feelings about such responses)
Emphasize the importance of recognizing tension
Explain the need to recognize highly stressful situations
Describe those symptoms that should be reported (severe depression in which the person cannot function or considers suicide)
Teach how to use the problem-solving method (to overcome problems that contribute to the depression or result from the loss)

EVALUATION

Record actual outcome

DEPRESSION RELATED TO PHYSICAL LOSS[105,471]

ASSESSMENT

Data Collection

Subjective Data
• Person states feeling moody and sad
• Is preoccupied with the loss of health
• Expresses the wish that the loss be restored
• Complains of lack of energy, nervousness, early morning insomnia, fretful or excessive sleep, appetite changes
  Acknowledges that the physical loss has brought about unwanted changes
  May feel he does not deserve such a loss
  May express anger

Mild Depression
Let-down feeling occurs when an event ends (when the acute illness phase is over)
Feelings of moodiness disappear when something new is planned
Somatic complaints involving multiple body systems

Moderate Depression
Let-down feeling lasts more than several weeks
Difficulty concentrating
Feels tense
Mental rumination
Preoccupied with body function involving multiple body systems

Objective Data
• May exhibit behavior such as slowed body movements, overactivity, restlessness, indifferent attitude

Mild Depression
Saddened facial expression, tearfulness

Moderate Depression
Unkempt appearance, poor posture, irritability, forgetfulness, difficulty making decisions, decreased involvement in usual interests

Data Analysis
Nursing Diagnosis
DEPRESSION RELATED TO PHYSICAL LOSS: A mental state of gloom and sadness about the loss of a positive, balanced state of health

Common Etiology (Stressors)
DISEASES: Any
INJURIES: Any
SIGNS AND SYMPTOMS: Confusion, immobility, memory loss, pain, paralysis, weakness
PSYCHOSOCIAL FACTORS: The threat of loss of self-esteem, the threat of loss of security, the threat of loss of control of a life situation, lack of or loss of emotional support (positive reinforcement) from others, lack of achievement of unrealistic or unattainable goals, exhaustion of adaptive reserves
HUMAN BODY: *Body appearance*: Changes in body appearance, disfigured body. *Body Function*: Loss of body function. *Natural body function*: Loss of fetus from the maternal body at childbirth. *Body part*: Loss of a body part. *Body states*: Loss of the prepregnancy body·
HEALTH CARE FACTORS: *Adverse effects of medical, drug or surgical therapy*: Loss of a body part from amputation, cholecystectomy, enucleation or evisceration of eyeball, gastrectomy, hemipelvectomy, hysterectomy, or ileotomy; lobectomy of the brain, liver, or lungs; mastectomy, nephrectomy, prostatectomy, spleenectomy, thyroidectomy, or tonsillectomy; loss of the fetus due to a therapeutic abortion; loss of hair from chemotherapy or radiation therapy; loss of mobility from traction; loss of natural elimination control from colostomy, ileocolostomy, ileostomy, ureterocolostomy, ureteroileostomy, ureterosigmoidostomy, ureterostomy, or ureterotomy; loss of normal food intake from esophagectomy; loss of the reproductive ability from fallopian tube ligation, hysterectomy, oophorectomy, orchidectomy, prostatectomy, salpingectomy, or vasectomy; loss of speech from glossectomy, laryngectomy, tracheostomy, or vocal cordectomy; loss of vision from enucleation or evisceration of· eyeball. *Therapeutic equipment*: Use of a cardiac pacemaker, brace, cane, crutches, hemodializer, respirator, walker, or wheelchair
DEVELOPMENTAL PHASES: Middle age, old age
SITUATIONAL FACTORS: Childlessness, illness (acute, chronic, terminal)

PLANNING
Unmet Needs
Comfort, stimulation, protection from psychologic threat, acceptance, caring and communicating relationships, sense of usefulness and adequacy, high evaluation of self,

endurance, personal growth and maturity, increased learning, increased reality perception and problem-solving ability, increased pleasantness

Expected Outcome
Person verbalizes feelings of moodiness, sadness
Acknowledges that the loss cannot be restored
   OR
Accepts and plans for restoring reversible losses
Verbalizes an increased energy level
Person's body activity is at a level attainable by the individual

NURSING INTERVENTIONS

Nursing Treatments
Approach unhurriedly
Reassure verbally (that the nurse will help the person overcome his depression)
Demonstrate calmness
Provide an atmosphere of acceptance
Encourage the expression of feelings (of moodiness, sadness, helplessness)
Listen attentively
Offer feedback to the person's expressed feelings
Communicate nurse sensitivity to the person's problem
Relate to the person on an adult–adult level, not on a parent–child level (which could increase depression)
Ask the person to identify the problem
Ask for specifics, not generalizations, about the problem
Provide reliable information (that the physical loss may not be as severe as perceived, that the physical loss may improve, that the loss will require adjustment)
Reveal the person's depressed feelings (if he is unaware of them)
Encourage the sharing of common problems with others
Encourage the acceptance of self-limitations (if nonacceptance of physical limitations is causing the depression)
Encourage awareness of positive responses from others (that others are offering love and support)
Explore with the person the reasons for self-criticism (which reinforces depression)
Explore with the person his strengths and resources (to overcome depression)
Encourage involvement in helping others, involvement in totally new interests
Encourage meaningful activity, a full day of activities, active diversional activities (all of which divert attention from depression and focus attention on the external)
Encourage planned one-day-at-a-time living
Encourage pride in appearance (despite the depression)
Introduce to persons who have successfully undergone the same experience
Avoid forcing the person into rapid adaptation to change by accepting the person's unique pattern of adjustment
Reduce the demands placed on the person (so that more energy is available for coping)
Refrain from negatively criticizing
Call the person's family to the bedside (if the person desires such)
Encourage telephone calls with significant persons (who can be supportive)
Touch the person frequently
Provide frequent contact with the person (share as much time with the person as possible)
Arrange a structured environment (suitable to the person)
Arrange pleasant surroundings
Avoid attempting to cheer up the depressed person (the inability to respond cheerfully makes the depressed person more depressed)

Nursing Observations
Determine the degree of insight that the person has

Determine the precipitating factors, the relieving factors (of the depression)

Observe for an excessive stress level

Monitor blood studies for abnormal (decreased) adrenal function

Monitor blood studies for abnormal (decreased) glucose

Monitor blood studies for (increased) dexamethasone suppression level (DST)

} If there is suspicion that the depression is of a physical origin

Observe for evidence of a favorable response to therapy (decreased moodiness, sadness, improved functioning ability)

Health Teaching

Explain that the person's response is appropriate and commonly experienced (that it is normal after a loss)

Explain that the situation is temporary (that the depression is difficult but will subside)

Describe the factors associated with the occurrence of the problem (explain that complaints such as insomnia, tiredness, wanting to sleep excessively, etc., are normal parts of depression)

Explain and offer hope that the emotional pain will decrease with time (that the depression will eventually end, despite the present discomfort)

Advise that significant persons express acceptance of one another, express caring for one another

Explain the importance of persons offering support to one another

Explain the importance of maintaining a positive self-attitude

Advise that negative responses from others be regarded with minimum significance (even though there are feelings about such responses)

Emphasize the importance of recognizing tension within oneself

Explain the need to recognize highly stressful situations

Describe those symptoms that should be reported (severe depression in which the person cannot function or considers suicide)

Teach how to use the problem-solving method (to overcome the physical limitations and the depression)

EVALUATION

Record actual outcome

DEPRESSION RELATED TO ROLE LOSS[105,471]

ASSESSMENT

Data Collection

Subjective Data
- Person states feeling moody and sad
- Is preoccupied with a loss of a role important to the person
- Expresses the wish that the loss be restored
- Complains of lack of energy, nervousness, early morning insomnia, fretful or excessive sleep, appetite changes

  May frequently relate the joys of the former role

  May discuss the new role in negative terms

Mild Depression

Let-down feeling occurs when an era ends (retirement, children off to college, etc.)

Feelings of moodiness disappear when something new is planned

Somatic complaints involving multiple body systems

Moderate Depression
Let-down feeling lasts more than several weeks
Difficulty concentrating
Feels tense
Mental rumination
Preoccupied with body function involving multiple body systems

Objective Data
• May exhibit behavior such as slowed body movements, overactivity, restlessness, indifferent attitude

Mild Depression
Saddened facial expression, tearfulness

Moderate Depression
Unkempt appearance, poor posture, irritability, forgetfulness, difficulty making decisions, decreased involvement in usual interests

Data Analysis
Nursing Diagnosis
DEPRESSION RELATED TO ROLE LOSS: A mental state of gloom and sadness about losing a position, situation, or responsibility in life and being unable to perform the associated, expected behaviors

Common Etiology (Stressors)
DISEASES: Any
INJURIES: Any
SIGNS AND SYMPTOMS: Immobility, pain, weakness
PSYCHOSOCIAL FACTORS: Loss of or separation from a significant or valued situation, loss of a valued concept, the threat of loss of self-esteem, loss of an ideal or imagined relationship, the threat of loss of security, the threat of loss of control of a life situation, lack of or loss of emotional support (positive reinforcement) from others, lack of achievement of unrealistic or unattainable goals, exhaustion of adaptive reserves
DEVELOPMENTAL PHASES: Adolescence, middle age, old age
SITUATIONAL FACTORS: Death of a significant other, divorce, loss of employment, launching grown children, illness of or injury to self or significant other, marriage, parenthood, retirement, the end of school
PLANNING

Unmet Needs
Comfort, stimulation, protection from psychologic threat, acceptance, caring and communicating relationships, sense of usefulness and adequacy, high evaluation of self, endurance, personal growth and maturity, increased learning, increased reality perception and problem-solving ability, increased pleasantness

Expected Outcome
Person verbalizes feelings of moodiness, sadness
Acknowledges that the loss cannot be restored
   OR
Accepts and plans for restoring reversible losses
Verbalizes an increased energy level
Person's body activity is at a level normal for the individual
NURSING INTERVENTIONS

Nursing Treatments
Approach unhurriedly
Reassure verbally (that the nurse will help the person overcome his depression)
Demonstrate calmness
Provide an atmosphere of acceptance
Encourage the expression of feelings (of moodiness, sadness, helplessness)
Listen attentively

Offer feedback to the person's expressed feelings

Communicate nurse sensitivity to the person's problem

Relate to the person on an adult–adult level, not on a parent–child level (which could increase depression)

Ask the person to identify the problem

Ask for specifics, not generalizations, about the problem

Support a realistic assessment of the situation (that the new role has advantages, that the loss will require adjustment)

Reveal the person's depressed feelings (if he is unaware of them)

Encourage the sharing of common problems with others

Encourage awareness of positive responses from others (about the role change)

Explore with the person the reasons for self-criticism (which reinforces depression)

Explore with the person his strengths and resources (to overcome depression)

Encourage involvement in helping others, involvement in totally new interests

Encourage meaningful activity, a full day of activities, active diversional activities (all of which divert attention from depression and focus attention on the external)

Encourage planned one-day-at-a-time living

Encourage pride in appearance (despite the depression)

Introduce to persons who have successfully undergone the same experience

Avoid forcing the person into rapid adaptation to change by accepting the person's unique pattern of adjustment

Reduce the demands placed on the person (so that more energy is available for coping)

Refrain from negatively criticizing

Encourage telephone calls with significant persons (who can be supportive)

Touch the person frequently

Provide frequent contact with the person (share as much time with the person as possible)

Arrange a structured environment (suitable to the person)

Arrange pleasant surroundings

Avoid attempting to cheer up the depressed person (the inability to respond cheerfully makes the depressed person more depressed)

Nursing Observations

Determine the degree of insight that the person has

Determine the precipitating factors, the relieving factors

Evaluate the person's relatedness with others (and its effect on the depression)

Observe for an excessive stress level

Monitor blood studies for abnormal (decreased) adrenal function

Monitor blood studies for abnormal (decreased) glucose

Monitor blood studies for (increased) dexamethasone suppression level (DST)

⎫ If there is suspicion
⎬ that the depression
⎭ is of physical origin

Observe for evidence of a favorable response to therapy (decreased moodiness, sadness)

Health Teaching

Explain that the person's response is appropriate and commonly experienced (that it is normal after a loss)

Explain that the situation is temporary (that the depression is difficult but will subside)

Describe the factors associated with the occurrence of the problem (explain that complaints such as insomnia, tiredness, wanting to sleep excessively, etc., are normal parts of depression)

Explain and offer hope that the emotional pain will decrease with time (that the depression will eventually end, despite the present discomfort)

Advise that significant persons express acceptance of one another, express caring for one another

Explain the importance of persons offering support to one another

Explain the importance of maintaining a positive self-attitude

Advise that negative responses from others be regarded with minimum significance (even though there are feelings about such responses)

Emphasize the importance of recognizing tension

Explain the need to recognize highly stressful situations

Describe those symptoms that should be reported (severe depression in which the person cannot function or considers suicide)

Teach how to use the problem-solving method (to adjust to a new role and overcome depression)

EVALUATION

Record actual outcome

DEPRESSION RELATED TO SEPARATION FROM A SIGNIFICANT OTHER[105,471]

ASSESSMENT

Data Collection

Subjective Data

- Person states feeling moody and sad
- Is preoccupied with the separation from a loved one
- Expresses the wish that the loss be restored
- Complains of a lack of energy, nervousness, early morning insomnia, fretful or excessive sleep, appetite changes
  May discuss how the separation will cause changes in the person's life
  Is concerned with the length of separation
  Consoles self with the hope for being reunited later

Mild Depression

Let-down feeling occurs when an event ends (after the separation begins)

Feelings of moodiness disappear when something new is planned

Somatic complaints involving multiple body systems

Moderate Depression

Let-down feeling lasts more than several weeks

Difficulty concentrating

Feels tense

Mental rumination

Preoccupied with body function involving multiple body systems

Objective Data

- May exhibit behavior such as slowed body movements, overactivity, restlessness, indifferent attitude

Mild Depression

Saddened facial expression, tearfulness

Moderate Depression

Unkempt appearance, poor posture, irritability, forgetfulness, difficulty making decisions, decreased involvement in usual interests

Data Analysis

Nursing Diagnosis

DEPRESSION RELATED TO SEPARATION FROM A SIGNIFICANT OTHER: A mental state of gloom and sadness about being temporarily apart from a significant other

Common Etiology (Stressors)

PSYCHOSOCIAL FACTORS: Loss of an ideal or imagined relationship, the threat of loss of security, the threat of loss of control of a life situation, lack of or loss of emotional support (positive reinforcement) from others, exhaustion of adaptive reserves

HEALTH CARE FACTORS: *Health care environment*: Coronary care, intensive care, or isolation unit; locked psychiatric unit. *Hospitalization or institutionalization*: Of self or significant other. *Visitors*: Restriction of. *Convalescence*: Reduced human contact during convalescence

SITUATIONAL FACTORS: Confinement in prison, marital separation from spouse or of parents, launching grown children, geographically distant family, holidays without a significant other, military service, retirement

PLANNING

Unmet Needs

Comfort, stimulation, protection from psychologic threat, acceptance, caring and communicating relationships, sense of usefulness and adequacy, high evaluation of self, endurance, personal growth and maturity, increased learning, increased reality perception and problem-solving ability, increased pleasantness

Expected Outcome

Person verbalizes feelings of moodiness, sadness

Accepts and plans for restoring reversible losses

Verbalizes an increased energy level

Person's body activity is at a level normal for the individual

NURSING INTERVENTIONS

Nursing Treatments

Approach unhurriedly

Reassure verbally (that the nurse will help the person overcome his depression)

Demonstrate calmness

Provide an atmosphere of acceptance

Encourage the expression of feelings (of moodiness, sadness, helplessness)

Listen attentively

Offer feedback to the person's expressed feelings

Communicate nurse sensitivity to the person's problem

Relate to the person on an adult–adult level, not on a parent–child level (which could increase depression)

Ask the person to identify the problem

Ask for specifics, not generalizations, about the problem

Support a realistic assessment of the situation (that the separation is temporary)

Reveal the person's depressed feelings (if he is unaware of them)

Encourage the sharing of common problems with others

Encourage awareness of positive responses from others (who are offering love and support)

Explore with the person the reasons for self-criticism (which reinforces depression)

Explore with the person his strengths and resources (to overcome the depression)

Encourage involvement in helping others, involvement in totally new interests

Encourage meaningful activity, a full day of activities, active diversional activities (all of which divert attention from depression and focus attention on the external)

Encourage planned one-day-at-a-time living

Encourage pride in appearance (despite the depression)

Introduce to persons who have successfully undergone the same experience

Avoid forcing the person into rapid adaptation to change by accepting the person's unique pattern of adjustment

Reduce the demands placed on the person (so that more energy is available for coping)

Refrain from negatively criticizing

Encourage telephone calls with significant persons (the separated person or others who can be supportive)

Touch the person frequently

Provide frequent contact with the person (share as much time with the person as possible)

Arrange a structured environment (suitable to the person)

Arrange pleasant surroundings

Avoid attempting to cheer up the depressed person (the inability to respond cheerfully makes the depressed person more depressed)

Nursing Observations

Determine the degree of insight that the person has

Determine the precipitating factors, the relieving factors

Evaluate the person's relatedness with others (and its effect on the depression)

Observe for evidence of an excessive stress level

Observe for evidence of a favorable response to therapy (decreased moodiness, sadness)

Health Teaching

Explain that the person's response is appropriate and commonly experienced (that it is normal during a separation)

Explain that the situation is temporary (that the depression is difficult but will subside)

Describe the factors associated with the occurrence of the problem (explain that complaints such as insomnia, tiredness, wanting to sleep excessively, etc., are normal parts of depression)

Explain and offer hope that the emotional pain will decrease with time (that the depression will eventually end, despite the present discomfort)

Advise that significant persons express acceptance of one another, express caring for one another

Explain the importance of persons offering support to one another

Explain the importance of maintaining a positive self-attitude

Advise that negative responses from others be regarded with minimum significance (even though there are feelings about such responses)

Emphasize the importance of recognizing tension

Explain the need to recognize highly stressful situations

Describe those symptoms that should be reported (severe depression in which the person cannot function or considers suicide)

Teach how to use the problem-solving method (to overcome depression and reduce the separation, if possible)

EVALUATION

Record actual outcome

DEPRESSION RELATED TO PHYSIOLOGIC IMBALANCE[105,471,596]

ASSESSMENT

Data Collection

Subjective Data

- Person states feeling moody and sad
- Is preoccupied with a loss of well-being
- Expresses the wish that the loss be restored
- Complains of lack of energy, nervousness, early morning insomnia, fretful or excessive sleep, appetite changes

May relate that there is nothing in the person's life to be depressed about, that life is normal and going well

Mild Depression
Let-down feeling occurs when a task is completed or an event ends
Feelings of moodiness disappear when something new is planned
Somatic complaints involving multiple body systems

Moderate Depression
Let-down feeling lasts more than several weeks
Difficulty concentrating
Feels tense
Mental rumination
Preoccupied with body function involving multiple body systems

Objective Data
• Manifests blood analysis findings of:
　Positive DST (dexamethasone suppression test) for depression
　　OR
　Decreased serum glucose
　　OR
　Decreased adrenal function
• May exhibit behavior such as slowed body movements, overactivity, restlessness, indifferent attitude

Mild Depression
Saddened facial expression, tearfulness

Moderate Depression
Unkempt appearance, poor posture, irritability, forgetfulness, difficulty making decisions, decreased involvement in usual interests

Data Analysis

Nursing Diagnosis
DEPRESSION RELATED TO PHYSIOLOGIC IMBALANCE: A mental state of gloom and sadness due to the body system conveying a lack of physiologic balance (homeostasis)

Common Etiology (Stressors)
DISEASES: Alcoholism, anemia, brain abscess or tumor, carcinoma of the pancreas, diabetic ketoacidosis, encephalitis, hyperbilirubinemia, hypoglycemia, hypothyroidism (myxedema), manic-depressive psychosis (genetic transmission), meningitis, Parkinson's disease
INJURIES: Cerebral concussion
SIGNS AND SYMPTOMS: Hyperkalemia, hypokalemia, hypoxia
HUMAN BODY: *Natural body function*: Maternal energy depletion after childbirth
HEALTH CARE FACTORS: *Drug therapy*: Adverse effects of antianxiety agents (meprobamate, tybamate, Valium), antibiotics (Chloromycetin, gentamicin), anticonvulsants (dilantin), antiemetics (Dramamine, Marezine, Tigan), antihistamines (Benadryl, Chlor-Trimeton, Phenergan), antihypertensive agents (Aldomet, Apresoline, Catapres, guanethidine or Ismelin, propranolol or Inderal, reserpine or Serpasil, antineoplastic agents (Nolvadex), barbiturates (Ambobarbital, phenobarbital, secobarbital), estrogen agents (diethylstilbesterol, estradiol), muscle relaxants (Dantrium, Flexeril, Lioresal, Soma), narcotics (codeine, demerol, morphine, Talwin), oral contraceptives (Enovid, Ortho-Novum, Ovulen); depression is more likely to occur at the initiation or termination of dosage. *Medical therapy*: Withdrawal from alcohol, drugs, tobacco. *Surgical therapy*: Energy depletion following surgery, recovery from anesthesia. *Surgical procedures*: Adrenalectomy, lobectomy of the brain, lobotomy, thyroidectomy
DEVELOPMENTAL PHASES: Puberty, adolescence, middle age
LIFESTYLE: High sugar intake, insufficient or unbalanced diet, insufficient sleep and rest
SITUATIONAL FACTORS: Energy depletion following illness or injury

ENVIRONMENTAL FACTORS: *Chemical substances*: Toxic gases or vapors

MAJOR PATHOPHYSIOLOGIC FACTORS CAUSING THE PROBLEM: Physiologic depression can result from the following: decreased norephinephrine or blood glucose level, central nervous system depression, impaired transmission of electrical components between neuroreceptors in the brain, energy depletion following severe physiologic stress, physiologic hormone changes during puberty, menopause, climacteric, or pregnancy

PLANNING

Unmet Needs

Comfort, stimulation, protection from physical and psychologic threat, acceptance, caring and communicating relationships, sense of usefulness and adequacy, high evaluation of self, endurance, personal growth and maturity, increased learning, increased reality perception and problem-solving ability, increased pleasantness

Expected Outcome

Person verbalizes feelings of moodiness, sadness
Verbalizes an increased energy level
Person's body activity is at a level normal for the individual

NURSING INTERVENTIONS

Nursing Treatments

Approach unhurriedly
Reassure verbally (that the nurse will help the person overcome his depression)
Demonstrate calmness
Provide an atmosphere of acceptance
Encourage the expression of feelings (of moodiness, sadness, helplessness)
Listen attentively
Offer feedback to the person's expressed feelings
Communicate nurse sensitivity to the person's problem
Relate to the person on an adult–adult level, not on a parent–child level (which could increase depression)
Provide reliable information (explain that the depression results from chemical body changes)
Reveal the person's depressed feelings (if he is unaware of them)
Explore with the person his strengths and resources (to overcome depression)
Encourage meaningful activity, a full day of activities, active diversional activities (all of which divert attention from depression and focus attention on the external)
Reduce the demands placed on the person (so that more energy is available for coping)
Touch the person frequently
Provide frequent patient contact (share as much time with the person as possible)
Avoid attempting to cheer up the depressed person (the inability to respond cheerfully makes the depressed person more depressed)
Encourage decreased carbohydrate (high sugar) intake
Withhold the drugs (causing the depression)
Make a referral (to a physician for antidepressant drugs)

Nursing Observations

Determine the degree of insight that the person has
Determine the precipitating factors, the relieving factors (of the depression)
Observe for an excessive stress level
Monitor blood studies for dexamethasone suppression level (DSM) ⎫
Monitor blood studies for normal glucose. ⎬ To determine if or when the blood studies return to normal levels
Observe for evidence of a favorable response to therapy (decreased moodiness, sadness)

Health Teaching

Explain that the person's response is appropriate and commonly experienced (during physiologic, chemical imbalance)

Explain that the situation is temporary (that the depression is difficult but will subside)

Describe the factors associated with the occurrence of the problem (explain that complaints such as insomnia, tiredness, wanting to sleep excessively, etc., are normal parts of depression)

Explain and offer hope that the emotional pain will decrease with time (that the depression will eventually end as the physiologic status improves)

Explain the importance of persons offering support to one another

Explain the importance of maintaining a positive self-attitude (despite the depression)

Recommend a regular sleeping schedule (to reduce fatigue that causes depression)

Explain the need to recognize highly stressful situations (which increase depression)

Describe those symptoms that should be reported (severe depression in which the person cannot function or considers suicide)

Teach how to use the problem-solving method (in determining the physiologic cause and in finding ways to reduce depression, such as avoiding alcohol, drugs, fatigue, high sugar intake, toxic gases, stress)

EVALUATION

Record actual outcome

Adaptive Responses of Emotion (Affect): Embarrassment

EMBARRASSMENT RELATED TO BODY EXPOSURE [471,480,524]

ASSESSMENT

Data Collection

Subjective Data

• Person may or may not relate experiencing self-consciousness

• Acknowledges feeling threatened with humiliation or indignity

Person relates feeling uncomfortable undressing or being undressed in front of others

Verbalizes objections to being bathed, treated, or clinically viewed by others

May refuse to assume positions necessary for examination or treatment

May request that curtains be pulled around the bed, the door be closed, or a screen put up

Objective Data

• May manifest physical findings such as facial flushing

• May exhibit behavior such as drooping the shoulders, holding the head downward, inappropriate laughter, flustered speech, hiding the face, crying, angry outbursts, avoiding embarrassing discussions or situations, clinging to clothing or sheets when undressed in front of another, undressing only partially or not at all, bathing under the sheets

Data Analysis

Nursing Diagnosis

EMBARRASSMENT RELATED TO BODY EXPOSURE: A state of self-conscious uneasiness and noncomposure about having the unclothed body visible to others while undergoing health examinations or procedures

Common Etiology (Stressors)

PSYCHOSOCIAL FACTORS: The threat of loss or loss of self-esteem

HEALTH CARE FACTORS: *Health care environment*: Lack of privacy in the health care environment, hospital or clinic gowns. *Diagnostic procedures*: Anoscopy, barium enema, breast examination, colonoscopy, culdoscopy, cystoscopy, cystourethrography, dilatation and curettage (D and C), mammography, hysterosalpingography, pap smear, physical examination, pelvic examination, proctoscopy, proctosigmoidoscopy, rectal examination, retrograde pylogram or urethrography, urinary catheterization for specimens. *Health therapy*: Undignified positioning for health therapy. *Drug therapy*: Rectal instillations, vaginal inserts, injections in the buttocks. *Medical/nursing therapy*: Bed bath, therapeutic dressing changes, douches, enemas, body exposure for hygiene, bladder or colonic irrigations, delivery procedure, perineal care, peritoneal dialysis, urinary catheterization. *Surgical therapy*: Presurgical prep (abdominal, bowel, cranial, or genital). *Surgical procedures*: Circumcision, colostomy, cystostomy, dilation and curettage (D and C), hemorrhoidectomy, ileostomy, mastectomy, proctectomy, proctotomy, prostatectomy, ureterocolostomy, ureterotomy, vasectomy

DEVELOPMENTAL PHASES: Any but especially early school-age (age 6–9) and adolescence

SITUATIONAL FACTORS: Lack of privacy in the home

PLANNING

Unmet Needs

Comfort, protection from psychologic threat, caring and communicating relationships, dignity, increased learning

Expected Outcome

Person verbalizes feelings

Relates an improved level of comfort with the embarrassing situation

Calm, composed appearance

NURSING INTERVENTIONS

Nursing Treatments

Approach unhurriedly

Reassure verbally (that the person will be protected from unnecessary embarrassment)

Demonstrate calmness

Provide an atmosphere of acceptance

Encourage the expression of feelings (about the embarrassment)

Listen attentively

Talk with the person (as a diversion during examination or procedures)

Communicate nurse sensitivity to the person's problem

Avoid causing embarrassing situations (by knocking before entering, by exposing the body for short periods only, etc.)

Provide privacy (by screening the person, placing him in a private room, keeping the door closed, etc.)

Dress in personal clothing (if this reduces embarrassment)

Drape modestly (keeping as much of the body covered as possible at all times)

Encourage self-performance (of bathing, dressing, procedures, etc., if the person is able)

Restrict unwanted visitors (during bath time, etc.)

Nursing Observations

Observe for an excessive stress level (resulting from embarrassment)

Observe for evidence that the person is reaching out for emotional support

Observe for evidence of a favorable response to therapy (an increased comfort level)

Health Teaching

Explain that the person's response is appropriate and commonly experienced (during examinations, procedures, etc.)

Explain how to adjust clothing to meet health needs (which will reduce exposure of the body or body impairments)

EVALUATION

Record actual outcome

EMBARRASSMENT RELATED TO HEALTH DEVICES[471,524]

ASSESSMENT

Data Collection

Subjective Data
- Person may or may not relate experiencing self-consciousness
- Acknowledges feeling threatened with humiliation or indignity
  Feels that the health devices make him less acceptable
  Is sensitive to the comments of others
  Does not want the device seen by others

Objective Data
- Facial blushing
- Flustered speech
  May attempt to cover the device with clothing, hide it under a sheet or towel or in a drawer or closet
  Device may be therapeutic, prosthetic, or assistive in nature
  May refuse to leave the bed (or room) because others may see the device

Data Analysis

Nursing Diagnosis
EMBARRASSMENT RELATED TO HEALTH DEVICES: A sense of uneasiness or noncomposure about having devices visible to others that are used to replace a body part, improve body function, or assist the person to function more completely or easily

Common Etiology (Stressors)
PSYCHOSOCIAL FACTORS: The threat of loss, or loss of self-esteem
HEALTH CARE FACTORS: *Health care environment*: Lack of privacy in the health care environment. *Therapeutic equipment*: Therapeutic devices (cannula for hemodialysis; cardiac pacemaker; chest tube, genitourinary tube, nasogastric tube, and drainage apparatus for each; tracheostomy or laryngectomy tube), prosthetic devices (artificial eye or limb, breast prosthesis, dental bridge, dentures, assistive devices (bedpan, bedside commode, brace, cane, crutches, eyeglasses, hearing aid, urinal, walker, wheelchair). *Surgical Therapy:* Removal of a prosthesis before surgery

PLANNING

Unmet Needs

Comfort, protection from psychologic threat, caring and communicating relationships, dignity, increased learning

Expected Outcome

Person verbalizes feelings
Relates an improved level of comfort with the embarrassing situation
Calm, composed appearance

NURSING INTERVENTIONS

Nursing Treatments

Approach unhurriedly

Reassure verbally (that the person will be protected from unnecessary embarrassment)

Demonstrate calmness

Provide an atomosphere of acceptance

Encourage the expression of feelings (about the embarrassing device)

Listen attentively

Communicate nurse sensitivity to the person's problem

Avoid causing embarrassing situations (by not allowing the person to be viewed by others while he is using certain devices)

Support a realistic assessment of the situation (some devices are essential for independent functioning)

Keep treatment equipment (drainage systems, bedside commodes, artificial limbs, etc.) out of sight (when not in use)

Sit the person in an armchair (if he prefers that visitors not see him in a wheelchair)

Remove the dentures (and other prosthesis just before giving the preoperative medication to reduce the person's time without them; do this in privacy)

Restrict unwanted visitors (when devices are being applied, adjusted, etc.)

Nursing Observations

Determine the degree of insight that the person has

Observe for an excessive stress level (resulting from embarrassment)

Observe for evidence that the person is reaching out for emotional support

Observe for evidence of a favorable response to therapy (an increased comfort level)

Health Teaching

Explain that the person's response is appropriate and commonly experienced

Advise that negative responses from others be regarded with minimum significance (even though there are feelings about such responses)

Explain the importance of maintaining a positive self-attitude

Explain how to adjust clothing to meet health needs (long sleeves to cover a hemodialysis cannula or shunt, a high neck or scarf to cover a tracheostomy, long pants to cover an artificial leg, full skirts to hide a clostomy dressing, etc.)

EVALUATION

Record actual outcome

EMBARRASSMENT RELATED TO NATURAL BODY FUNCTION[471,524]

ASSESSMENT

Data Collection

Subjective Data

• Person may or may not relate experiencing self-consciousness

• Acknowledges feelings threatened with humiliation or indignity
  May refuse to use the bedpan, urinal, or bedside commode, or to breast feed with others in the room

Objective Data
- May manifest physical findings of constipation or inadequate hydration from avoiding or attempting to decrease the use of the bedpan or urinal
- May exhibit behavior such as inappropriate laughter, flustered speech, hiding the face, crying, angry outbursts

Data Analysis

Nursing Diagnosis
EMBARRASSMENT RELATED TO NATURAL BODY FUNCTION: A state of self-conscious uneasiness and noncomposure about body functions that occur as a normal process

Common Etiology (Stressors)
PSYCHOSOCIAL FACTORS: The threat of loss or loss of self-esteem

HUMAN BODY: *Body function*: Changes in body function. *Natural body function*: Defecation, voiding, membrane rupture before or during childbirth, childbirth, breast feeding an infant, discussions about sexual activity. *Body states*: Lactation, menstruation

HEALTH CARE FACTORS: *Diagnostic studies*: Specimen collection for diagnostic studies, especially when using 24-hour urine and stool container, etc.

PLANNING

Unmet Needs
Comfort, protection from psychologic threat, caring and communicating relationships, dignity, increased learning

Expected Outcome
Person verbalizes feelings
Relates an improved level of comfort with the embarrassing situation
Calm, composed appearance

NURSING INTERVENTIONS

Nursing Treatments
Approach unhurriedly
Reassure verbally (that the person will be protected from unnecessary embarrassment)
Demonstrate calmness
Provide an atmosphere of acceptance
Encourage the expression of feelings (about the embarrassment)
Listen attentively
Talk with the person (as a diversion during natural function)
Communicate nurse sensitivity to the person's problem
Support a realistic assessment of the situation (that natural body processes are normal and expected)
Provide privacy (by screening the person, placing him in a private room, keeping the door closed, etc.)
Drape modestly (if such is appropriate)
Encourage self-performance (of toileting, etc.)
Keep collection equipment out of sight (such as urine or stool specimen containers, etc.)

Nursing Observations
Observe for an excessive stress level (resulting from embarrassment)
Observe for evidence that the person is reaching out for emotional support
Observe for evidence of a favorable response to therapy (an increased comfort level)

Health Teaching
Explain that the person's response is appropriate and commonly experienced
Advise that negative responses from others be regarded with minimum significance (even though there are feelings about such responses)
Explain the importance of maintaining a positive self-attitude

EVALUATION

Record actual outcome

Adaptive Responses of Emotion (Affect): Fear

FEAR OF ABANDONMENT[105,471,525]

ASSESSMENT

Data Collection

Subjective Data
- Person experiences feelings of threat or danger
- Can describe or identify the threat or danger
  Expresses a strong need for a particular person, concerned that the person will leave him in his time of need
  Seeks assurance of the person's commitment to him

Objective Data
- May manifest physical findings such as facial flushing or pallor, rapid or deep respirations, rapid or bounding pulse, increased blood pressure, sweating, trembling
- May exhibit behavior such as restlessness, sleep disturbances, change in eating habits, irritability, short attention span, making poor judgments, forgetfulness, rapid speech, demanding and controlling behavior, crying, avoiding persons or situations

Data Analysis

Nursing Diagnosis
FEAR OF ABANDONMENT: A feeling of alarm and fright about losing a protective, concerned relationship with another

Common Etiology (Stressors)
DISEASES: Any disease but especially incapacitating diseases such as alcoholism, blindness, carcinoma, cerebovascular accident, drug addiction, Guillain-Barre syndrome, Hansen's disease, Hodgkin's disease, leukemia, multiple sclerosis, myocardial infarction, organic brain syndrome, Parkinson's disease, renal failure
INJURIES: Any injury but especially an incapacitating and disfiguring injury such as severe burn wounds, fracture and compression of the spinal cord, flail chest, etc.
SIGNS AND SYMPTOMS: Memory loss, pain, paralysis, weakness
PSYCHOSOCIAL FACTORS: The threat of a specific and clearly identified danger, the threat of real or imagined danger, separation from a significant other
HEALTH CARE FACTORS: *Health care delivery*: Low-quality health care delivery. *Hospitalization* Any
DEVELOPMENTAL PHASES: Toddler (age 1–3), preschooler (age 3–6), old age
SITUATIONAL FACTORS: Confinement in prison, being a foster child, chronic or terminal illness, death of one parent, divorce, marital separation of parents

PLANNING

Unmet Needs

Comfort, protection from psychologic threat, acceptance, caring and communicating relationships, high evaluation of self, sense of adequacy, personal growth and maturity, increased learning, increased reality perception and problem-solving ability

Expected Outcome

Person verbalizes fears
Verbalizes feelings of adequacy and competence in meeting the fear-creating experience
Verbalizes self-satisfaction and growth in having coped with the fear-creating experience
Calm, relaxed facial expression, body movements, and behavior

NURSING INTERVENTIONS

Nursing Treatments

Approach unhurriedly
Reassure verbally (that the nurse will help the person solve his problem)
Demonstrate calmness
Provide an atmosphere of acceptance
Encourage the expression of feelings (about the fear of abandonment)
Listen attentively
Offer feedback to the person's expressed feelings
Communicate nurse sensitivity to the person's problem
Relate to the person on an adult–adult level, not on a parent–child level (which could increase fear)
Attend the person constantly (until he feels sufficiently comfortable to be alone)
Provide frequent contact with the person (thereafter)
Ask the person to identify the problem
Ask for specifics, not generalizations, about the problem
Support a realistic assessment of the situation (is he being abandoned or is the family attending to other responsibilities?)
Ask how the person normally copes with fear (what does he usually do when fearful that reduces fear?)
Provide whatever the person needs to use his usual coping mechanisms (if he wants to talk out the problem, the nurse listens; if he wants to cry, the nurse provides privacy, etc.)
Explore with the person his strengths and resources (if abandonment is likely)
Provide emotionally safe experiences (whenever possible)
Provide objects that symbolize safeness
Do not allow unpleasant surprise situations (which increase fear)
Call the person's family (to the bedside)
Encourage telephone calls between significant persons
Avoid placing the person on enforced inactivity (which heightens fear)
Reduce the demands placed on the person (so that more energy is available for coping)

Nursing Observations

Observe for an excessive stress level (resulting from the fear)
Determine the degree of insight that the person has
Observe for evidence of a favorable response to therapy (reduced fear and increased comfort)

Health Teaching

Explain that the person's response is appropriate and commonly experienced (when persons are ill, aged, hospitalized, etc.)
Explain that fatigue should be recognized as a stress factor (which heightens fear)
Explain the need to recognize highly stressful situations (if they actually exist)
Explain how to channel emotional energy and obtain release from stress (through laughing, talking things over)
Recommend methods for achieving total relaxation (controlled breathing, quietly listening to music, doing nothing, which reduces fear)
Recommend a habitual, positive mental attitude

EVALUATION

Record actual outcome

FEAR OF ABNORMAL CHILD DEVELOPMENT[105,251,471,525]

ASSESSMENT

Data Collection

Subjective Data
- Person experiences feelings of threat or danger
- Can describe or identify the threat or danger
  Relates doubt that the child is normal
  Seeks information about normal development
  Relates past contacts with abnormal children and the difficulties resulting from such
  May express anger or guilt

Objective Data
- May manifest physical findings such as facial flushing or pallor, rapid or deep respirations, rapid or bounding pulse, increased blood pressure, sweating, trembling
- May exhibit behavior such as restlessness, sleep disturbances, change in eating habits, irritability, short attention span, making poor judgments, forgetfulness, rapid speech, demanding and controlling behavior, crying
  May avoid visiting the hospitalized infant, may make frequent calls or clinic visits to gain reassurance of the child's normalcy

Data Analysis

Nursing Diagnosis
FEAR OF ABNORMAL CHILD DEVELOPMENT: A feeling of alarm and fright that an infant's growth and development might not be within normal limits

Common Etiology (Stressors)
BIRTH STATUS: *Infant*: Premature
DEVELOPMENTAL PHASE: Puberty
PSYCHOSOCIAL FACTORS: The threat of a specific and clearly identified danger, the threat of real or imagined danger

PLANNING

Unmet Needs

Comfort, protection from psychologic threat, acceptance, caring and communicating relationships, high evaluation of self, sense of adequacy, personal growth and maturity, increased learning, increased reality perception and problem-solving ability

Expected Outcome

Person verbalizes fears
Verbalizes feelings of adequacy and competence in meeting the fear-creating experience
Verbalizes self-satisfaction and growth in having coped with the fear-creating experience
Calm, relaxed facial expression, body movements, and behavior

NURSING INTERVENTIONS

Nursing Treatments

Approach unhurriedly
Reassure verbally (that the nurse will help the person solve his problem)
Demonstrate calmness
Provide an atmosphere of acceptance
Encourage the expression of feelings (about the fear)
Listen attentively
Offer feedback to the person's expressed feelings
Communicate nurse sensitivity to the person's problem
Relate to the person on an adult–adult level, not on a parent–child level (which could increase fear)
Attend the person constantly (until he feels sufficiently comfortable to be alone)

Provide frequent contact with the person (thereafter)

Ask the person to identify the problem

Ask for specifics, not generalizations, about the problem

Provide reliable information (about the child's normal responses to the parent, that premature infants are normal, that parents will be informed if their child has an abnormality and will receive assistance with coping)

Ask how the person normally copes with fear (what does he usually do when fearful that reduces the fear?)

Provide whatever the person needs to use his usual coping mechanisms (if he wants to talk out the problem, the nurse listens; if he wants to cry, the nurse provides privacy, etc.)

Encourage the person to face the fear (it will reduce the fear if he visits the infant and sees how normal the child is)

Explore with the person his strengths and resources (to overcome any fear)

Do not allow unpleasant surprise situations (such as seeing the infant with tubes, etc., without first being informed)

Reduce the demands placed on the person (so that more energy is available for coping)

Introduce to persons who have undergone the same experience (such as having a premature infant)

Make a referral (to a supportive group or professional specialist)

Nursing Observations

Observe for an excessive stress level (resulting from the fear)

Determine the degree of insight that the person has (into the fear)

Observe for evidence of a favorable response to therapy (reduced fear and increased comfort)

Health Teaching

Explain that the person's response is appropriate and commonly experienced (especially by new mothers)

Advise against fighting fear (this reinforces the emotion)

Explain the importance of recognizing tension within oneself

Explain that fatigue should be recognized as a stress factor (which heightens fear)

Explain how to channel emotional energy and obtain release from stress (running, swimming, and other sports, creative activities, laughing, talking things over)

Recommend methods for achieving total relaxation (controlled breathing, quietly listening to music, doing nothing, which reduces fear)

Recommend a habitual, positive mental attitude (about self and the infant)

EVALUATION

Record actual outcome

FEAR OF ADVERSE DRUG EFFECTS [105,471,525]

ASSESSMENT

Data Collection

Subjective Data

• Person experiences feeling of threat or danger

• Can describe or identify the threat or danger

• Relates side effects he knows will occur or asks about side effects he has heard about

 States he will take the drug later or does not need the drug

 May refuse the drug

 May express fearful thoughts

Objective Data
- May manifest physical findings such as facial flushing or pallor, rapid or deep respirations, rapid or bounding pulse, increased blood pressure, sweating, trembling
- May exhibit behavior such as restlessness, sleep disturbances, change in eating habits, irritability, short attention span, making poor judgments, forgetfulness, rapid speech, demanding and controlling behavior, crying, avoiding situations, such as being unavailable at medication time

Data Analysis

Nursing Diagnosis

FEAR OF ADVERSE DRUG EFFECTS: A feeling of alarm and fright about the possibility of a drug or drugs having unfavorable side effects

Common Etiology (Stressors)

PSYCHOSOCIAL FACTORS: The threat of a specific and clearly identified danger, the threat of real or imagined danger

HEALTH CARE FACTORS: *Diagnostic studies*: Dyes used in diagnostic studies. *Drug therapy*: Adverse effects and adverse interactions of drugs, chemotherapy, immunization therapy, specific drugs (antihypertensive drugs, contraceptive drugs, corticosteroids, hormone drugs, phenothiazine, etc.). *Surgical therapy*: Anesthesia

PLANNING

Unmet Needs

Comfort, protection from psychologic threat, acceptance, caring and communicating relationships, high evaluation of self, sense of adequacy, personal growth and maturity, increased learning, increased reality perception and problem-solving ability

Expected Outcome

Person verbalizes fears
Verbalizes feelings of adequacy and competence in meeting the fear-creating experience
Verbalizes self-satisfaction and growth in having coped with the fear-creating experience
Calm, relaxed facial expression, body movements, and behavior
Person takes the drug(s) as prescribed

NURSING INTERVENTIONS

Nursing Treatments

Approach unhurriedly
Reassure verbally (that the drugs are therapeutic)
Demonstrate calmness
Provide an atmosphere of acceptance
Encourage the expression of feelings (about the fear)
Listen attentively
Offer feedback to the person's expressed feelings
Communicate nurse sensitivity to the person's problem
Relate to the person on an adult–adult level, not on a parent–child level (which could increase fear)
Attend the person constantly (until he feels sufficiently comfortable to be alone)
Provide frequent contact with the person (thereafter)
Obtain a complete present and past history (of drug effects on the person and family members)
Ask the person to identify the problem
Ask for specifics, not generalizations, about the problem
Provide reliable information (if side effects are expected, what they are, action to take to prevent them, that all drugs have potential side effects but the favorable effects outweigh the possibility of harmful effects)
Ask how the person normally copes with fear (what does he usually do when fearful that reduces the fear?)

Provide whatever the person needs to use his usual coping mechanisms (if he wants to talk out the problem, the nurse listens; if he wants to be observed after taking the drug, the nurse checks him frequently)

Provide emotionally safe experiences (give drugs with the least potential side effect)

Do not allow unpleasant surprise situations (avoid giving drugs without warning, or explanation of the drug's purpose, effects, etc.)

Introduce to persons who have undergone the same experience (if appropriate)

Nursing Observations

Observe for an excessive stress level (resulting from the fear)

Determine the degree of insight that the person has (into the fear)

Observe for evidence of a favorable response to therapy (reduced fear and increased comfort)

Health Teaching

Explain that the person's response is appropriate and commonly experienced (especially if the person has experienced previous drug side effects)

Teach how to use the problem-solving method (to control drug intake; the person may prefer to take a small initial dose, gradually increasing it until he is assured it is not harmful)

EVALUATION

Record actual outcome

FEAR OF ALONENESS/ISOLATION [105,471,525]

ASSESSMENT

Data Collection

Subjective Data
- Person experiences feelings of threat or danger
- Can describe or identify the threat or danger
  Feels heightened fear when without companionship
  Is unsure that he can cope with himself or external situations without assistance from another

Objective Data
- May manifest physical findings such as facial flushing or pallor, rapid or deep respirations, rapid or bounding pulse, increased blood pressure, sweating, trembling
- May exhibit behavior such as restlessness, sleep disturbances, change in eating habits, irritability, frequent call-light signaling, frequent phone calling or visiting others, prolonging conversations, reaching out to touch others or comforting objects, demanding and controlling behavior, crying

Data Analysis

Nursing Diagnosis
FEAR OF ALONENESS/ISOLATION: A feeling of alarm and fright about being alone for a period of time

Common Etiology (Stressors)
DISEASES: Any
INJURY: Any
SIGNS AND SYMPTOMS: Confusion, immobility, memory loss, pain, vertigo, vision loss, weakness

PSYCHOSOCIAL FACTORS: The threat of a specific and clearly identified danger, the threat of real or imagined danger, loss of or separation from a significant other

HEALTH CARE FACTORS: *Hospitalization*: Hospitalization of significant other. *Visitors*: Restriction of. *Diagnostic procedures*: Any. *Medical or surgical therapy*: Any. *Hospital discharge*: Impending. *Convalescence:* Reduced human contact during convalescence

DEVELOPMENTAL PHASES: Toddler (age 1–3), preschooler (age 3–6), old age

SITUATIONAL FACTORS: Childbirth, the experience of dying, impending death of a significant other, divorce, launching grown children, marital separation from spouse, retirement

ENVIORNMENTAL FACTORS: Darkness

PLANNING

Unmet Needs

Comfort, protection from psychologic threat, acceptance, caring and communicating relationships, high evaluation of self, sense of adequacy, personal growth and maturity, increased learning, increased reality perception and problem-solving ability

Expected Outcome

Person verbalizes fears

Verbalizes feelings of adequacy and competence in meeting the fear-creating experience

Verbalizes self-satisfaction and growth in having coped with the fear-creating experience

Calm, relaxed facial expression, body movements, and behavior

NURSING INTERVENTIONS

Nursing Treatments

Approach unhurriedly

Reassure verbally (that the nurse will be available whenever needed)

Demonstrate calmness

Provide an atmosphere of acceptance

Encourage the expression of feelings (about the fear of being alone)

Listen attentively

Offer feedback to the person's expressed feelings

Communicate nurse sensitivity to the person's problem

Relate to the person on an adult–adult level, not on a parent–child level (which could increase fear)

Attend the patient constantly (until he feels sufficiently comfortable to be alone)

Provide frequent contact with the person (thereafter)

Ask the person to identify the problem

Ask for specifics, not generalizations, about the problem

Provide reliable information (that he is not alone, that someone is close by)

Ask how the person normally copes with fear (what does he usually do when fearful that reduces the fear?)

Provide whatever the person needs to use his usual coping mechanisms (if he wants to talk out the problem, the nurse listens; if he wants to turn on the television, the nurse will do so, etc.)

Provide a compatible room companion

Provide radio and television for diversion

Allow unlimited visiting (of family, friends, and pets if the pet is vitally significant)

Provide a night light (darkness increases the sense of aloneness)

Encourage the person to face the fear (when able, to reduce the fear)

Provide objects that symbolize safeness (a favorite picture, blanket, etc.)

Avoid placing the person on enforced inactivity (which heightens feelings of aloneness)

Reduce the demands placed on the person (so that more energy is available for coping)

Introduce to persons who have undergone the same experience (if appropriate)

Encourage social activities (with friends when lonely)

Encourage involvement in helping others

Encourage relationships with persons with common interests and goals

Nursing Observations

Observe for an excessive stress level (resulting from the fear)

Determine the degree of insight that the person has

Observe for evidence of a favorable response to therapy (reduced fear and increased comfort)

Health Teaching

Explain that the person's response is appropriate and commonly experienced (during illness, old age)

Explain that fatigue should be recognized as a stress factor (which heightens fear of aloneness)

Recommend a habitual, positive mental attitude

Recommend the person have a pet

Teach how to use the problem-solving method (to assure himself that he will not be alone for prolonged periods)

EVALUATION

Record actual outcome

FEAR OF BEARING A CHILD WITH A BIRTH DEFECT[105,471,525]

ASSESSMENT

Data Collection

Subjective Data

• Person experiences feelings of threat or danger

• Can describe or identify the threat or danger

Is aware that not all children are born perfect

Wonders if her child will be normal

May or may not have previously had a child with a birth defect

Quick to inquire about the child's normalcy at birth

Objective Data

• May manifest physical findings such as facial flushing or pallor, rapid or deep respirations, rapid or bounding pulse, increased blood pressure, sweating, trembling, especially when discussing the subject

May exhibit behavior such as restlessness, sleep disturbances, change in eating habits, irritability, short attention span, making poor judgments, forgetfulness, rapid speech, demanding and controlling behavior, engaging in superstitous practices to ensure a perfect child

Data Analysis

Nursing Diagnosis

FEAR OF BEARING A CHILD WITH A BIRTH DEFECT: A feeling of alarm and fright about possibly producing a child with physical or mental birth defects

Common Etiology (Stressors)

BIRTH DEFECTS: Previous birth of an imperfect child, previously having given birth to an imperfect child

INHERITED FACTORS: Familial history of birth defects, known genetic chromosomal abnormality in the person or spouse

DISEASES: Viral diseases such as measles or rubella during pregnancy

PSYCHOSOCIAL FACTORS: The threat of a specific and clearly identified danger, the threat of real or imagined danger

HUMAN BODY: *Body State*: Pregnancy
HEALTH CARE FACTORS: *Complications*: Previous or current complicated pregnancy or delivery
DEVELOPMENTAL PHASES: Middle age (being over age 35 during the first pregnancy)
HUMAN ERROR: Drug ingestion during the first trimester of pregnancy

PLANNING

Unmet Needs

Comfort, protection from psychologic threat, acceptance, caring, and communicating relationships, high evaluation of self, sense of adequacy, personal growth and maturity, increased learning, increased reality perception and problem-solving ability

Expected Outcome

Person verbalizes fears
Verbalizes feelings of adequacy and competence in meeting the fear-creating experience
Verbalizes self-satisfaction and growth in having coped with the fear-creating experience
Calm, relaxed facial expression, body movements, and behavior

NURSING INTERVENTIONS

Nursing Treatments

Approach unhurriedly
Reassure verbally (that everything is being done to ensure the birth of a normal infant)
Demonstrate calmness
Provide an atmosphere of acceptance
Encourage the expression of feelings (about the fear)
Listen attentively
Offer feedback to the person's expressed feelings
Communicate nurse sensitivity to the person's problem
Relate to the person on an adult–adult level, not on a parent–child level (which could increase fear)
Obtain a complete present and past history (of birth defects in the family)
Support a realistic assessment of the situation (if there is reason to believe the infant could be abnormal)
Provide reliable information (that the mother is healthy, that prenatal examinations reveal a healthy fetus)
Ask how the person normally copes with fear (what does she usually do when fearful that reduces the fear?)
Provide whatever the person needs to use her usual coping mechanisms (if she wants to talk about the problem, the nurse listens, etc.)
Make a referral (to the appropriate specialist to determine the probability of a birth defect, if there is a probability)

Nursing Observations

Observe for an excessive stress level (resulting from the fear)
Determine the degree of insight that the person has
Observe for evidence of a favorable response to therapy (reduced fear and increased comfort)

Health Teaching

Explain that the person's response is appropriate and commonly experienced (among expecting parents)
Explain that fatigue should be recognized as a stress factor (which heightens fear)
Explain how to channel emotional energy and obtain release from stress (during the pregnancy waiting period by diverting attention through creative activities, interests, etc.)
Recommend methods for achieving total relaxation (controlled breathing, quietly listening to music, doing nothing, which reduces fear)
Recommend a habitual, positive mental attitude

EVALUATION

Record actual outcome

FEAR OF BECOMING ILL[105,471,525]

ASSESSMENT

Data Collection

Subjective Data
- Person experiences feelings of threat or danger
- Can describe or identify the threat or danger
  Relates that illness is unacceptable
  Is preoccupied with excessive health foods, vitamins, exercise

Objective Data
- May manifest physical findings such as facial flushing or pallor, rapid or deep respirations, rapid or bounding pulse, increased blood pressure, sweating, trembling
- May exhibit behavior such as restlessness, sleep disturbances, change in eating habits, irritability, rapid speech, demanding and controlling behavior, crying, avoiding visiting sick persons

Data Analysis

Nursing Diagnosis
FEAR OF BECOMING ILL: A feeling of alarm and fright that one's present state of health will be lost

Common Etiology (Stressors)
INHERITED FACTORS: Familial tendency to disease or disorder
PSYCHOSOCIAL FACTORS: The threat of a specific and clearly identified danger, the threat of real or imagined danger
HEALTH CARE FACTORS: *Health care environment*: Contact with sick or very sick persons in the health care environment, exposure to the intense human suffering of persons in the health care environment. *Diagnostic procedures*: Any. *Medical therapy*: Any, such as amniocentesis, blood transfusion, hemodialysis, intravenous infusion, inhalation therapy, paracentesis, phlebotomy, radiation therapy, thoracentesis, urinary catheterization. *Surgical Therapy*: Any
DEVELOPMENTAL PHASES: Any beyond toddler age, especially old age
ENVIRONMENTAL FACTORS: *Chemical substances*: Exposure to pollution, toxic gases. *Environmental Radiation*: Exposure to radiation

PLANNING

Unmet Needs

Comfort, protection from psychologic threat, acceptance, caring and communicating relationships, high evaluation of self, sense of adequacy, personal growth and maturity, increased learning, increased reality perception and problem-solving ability

Expected Outcome

Person verbalizes his fears
Verbalizes feelings of adequacy and competence in meeting the fear-creating experience
Verbalizes self-satisfaction and growth in having coped with the fear-creating experience
Calm, relaxed facial expression, body movements, and behavior

NURSING INTERVENTIONS

Nursing Treatments

Approach unhurriedly
Reassure verbally
Demonstrate calmness
Provide an atmosphere of acceptance
Encourage the expression of feelings (about the fear)
Listen attentively
Offer feedback to the person's expressed feelings

Communicate nurse sensitivity to the person's problem

Relate to the person on an adult–adult level, not on a parent–child level (which could increase fear)

Attend the person constantly (if there is a likelihood that he will become ill immediately; e.g., vomiting during radiation therapy or hemodialysis)

Provide frequent contact with the person (thereafter)

Ask the person to identify the problem (if the fear relates to the possible onset or recurrence of disease)

Ask for specifics, not generalizations, about the problem

Support a realistic assessment of the situation (that illness is a part of life that eventually touches everyone)

Provide reliable information (about methods of promoting wellness and preventing illness)

Ask how the person normally copes with fear (what does he usually do when fearful that reduces the fear?)

Provide whatever the person needs to use his usual coping mechanisms (if he wants to talk about the problem, the nurse listens; if he wants to take realistic precautions against contact with ill persons, the nurse provides needed assistance, etc.)

Explore with the person his strengths and resources (to overcome fear and to maintain health practices)

Do not allow unpleasant surprise situations (such as exposure to ill persons without previous warning)

Make a referral (to a psychiatric nurse specialist, psychiatrist, etc. if the fear affects daily functioning)

Nursing Observations

Observe for an excessive stress level (resulting from the fear)

Determine the degree of insight that the person has

Observe for evidence of a favorable response to therapy (reduced fear and increased comfort)

Health Teaching

Explain that the person's response is appropriate and commonly experienced (especially if the person has experienced a serious illness or frequent, less serious illnesses)

Explain the importance of recognizing tension within oneself (tension increases fear)

Explain that fatigue should be recognized as a stress factor (which heightens fear)

Explain the need to recognize highly stressful situations

Explain how to channel emotional energy and obtain release from stress (running, swimming, other sports, creative activities, laughing, talking things over)

Recommend methods for achieving total relaxation (controlled breathing, quietly listening to music, doing nothing, which reduces fear)

Recommend a habitual, positive mental attitude (which supports wellness)

EVALUATION

Recommend actual outcome

FEAR OF BECOMING INFECTED [105,471,525]

ASSESSMENT

Data Collection

Subjective Data

- Person experiences feelings of threat or danger
- Can describe or identify the threat or danger

Is aware of his vulnerability to infection
Feels unable to protect self against infection
Inquires about preventive methods

Objective Data
• May manifest physical findings such as facial flushing or pallor, rapid or deep respirations, rapid or bounding pulse, increased blood pressure, sweating, trembling
• May exhibit behavior such as restlessness, irritability, rapid speech, demanding and controlling behavior, avoiding persons or crowds
  May be seen washing the hands, changing linens, etc.

Data Analysis

Nursing Diagnosis
FEAR OF BECOMING INFECTED: A feeling of alarm and fright about pathogenic agents invading the body

Common Etiology (Stressors)
SIGNS AND SYMPTOMS: Weakness
PSYCHOSOCIAL FACTORS: The threat of a specific and clearly identified danger, the threat of real or imagined danger
HEALTH CARE FACTORS: *Health care environment*: Isolation unit. *Diagnostic procedures*: Cardiac catheterization, cystoscopy. *Drug therapy*: Immunosuppressant therapy. *Medical therapy*: Blood transfusion, continuous ambulatory peritoneal dialysis, hemodialysis, urinary catheterization. *Surgical procedure*: Surgery of any kind
DEVELOPMENTAL PHASES: Old age
SITUATIONAL FACTORS: Illness, illness of a significant other or other persons, foreign travel

PLANNING

Unmet Needs
Comfort, protection from psychologic threat, acceptance, caring and communicating relationships, high evaluation of self, sense of adequacy, personal growth and maturity, increased learning, increased reality perception and problem-solving ability

Expected Outcome
Person verbalizes fears
Verbalizes feelings of adequacy and competence in meeting the fear-creating experience
Verbalizes self-satisfaction and growth in having coped with the fear-creating experience
Calm, relaxed facial expression, body movements, and behavior

NURSING INTERVENTIONS

Nursing Treatments
Approach unhurriedly
Reassure verbally (that the nurse will help the person avoid becoming infected)
Demonstrate calmness
Provide an atmosphere of acceptance
Encourage the expression of feelings (about the fear)
Listen attentively
Offer feedback to the person's expressed feelings
Communicate nurse sensitivity to the person's problem
Relate to the person on an adult–adult level, not on a parent–child level (which could increase fear)
Attend the person constantly (until he feels sufficiently comfortable to be alone)
Provide frequent contact with the person (thereafter)
Ask the person to identify the problem
Ask for specifics, not generalizations, about the problem
Provide reliable information (about the probability of becoming infected)
Ask how the person normally copes with fear (what does he usually do when fearful that reduces the fear?)

Provide whatever the person needs to use his usual coping mechanisms

Provide objects that symbolize safeness (cleansing supplies, needed sterile items, face mask if appropriate, etc.)

Nursing Observations

Observe for an excessive stress level (resulting from the fear)

Determine the degree of insight that the person has (into the fear)

Observe for evidence of a favorable response to therapy (reduced fear and increased comfort)

Health Teaching

Explain that the person's response is appropriate and commonly experienced

Explain how to prevent cross-infection (hand-washing, use of sterile technique, etc.)

Instruct to avoid direct contact with infected persons

Teach proper care of equipment (indwelling urinary or peritoneal dialysis catheter, arteriovenous shunt, etc.)

FEAR OF BRAIN DAMAGE[105,471,525]

ASSESSMENT

Data Collection

Subjective Data

• Person experiences feelings of threat or danger

• Can describe or identify the threat or danger

Is overwhelmed by the thought of loss of mental faculties

Asks for details about the threatening disease or procedure

Relates previous experience with brain-damaged persons

May refuse to submit to therapy with a risk of brain damage

Objective Data

• May manifest physical findings such as facial flushing or pallor, rapid or deep respirations, rapid or bounding pulse, increased blood pressure, sweating, trembling

• May exhibit behavior such as restlessness, sleep disturbances, change in eating habits, irritability, short attention span, making poor judgments, forgetfulness, rapid speech, demanding and controlling behavior, crying, avoiding persons or situations, frequent call-light signaling, prolonging conversations

Data Analysis

Nursing Diagnosis

FEAR OF BRAIN DAMAGE: A feeling of alarm and fright about losing all or part of one's mental capacities, cerebral or cerebral-controlled neurologic function

Common Etiology (Stressors)

DISEASES: Cerebrovascular accident, diabetic ketoacidosis, drug addiction, encephalitis, epilepsy, malaria, malignant hypertension, meningitis, typhoid fever

INJURIES: Cerebral concussion, drowning, electric shock, heat stroke

SIGNS AND SYMPTOMS: Convulsions, fever

PSYCHOSOCIAL FACTORS: The threat of a specific and clearly identified danger, the threat of real or imagined danger

HEALTH CARE FACTORS: *Diagnostic procedures*: Angiography, pneumoencephalogram. *Medical therapy*: Electroconvulsive shock therapy, hemodialysis, radiation therapy. *Surgical therapy*: Anesthesia, arterial bypass, cranioplasty, craniotomy, lobectomy of the brain

ENVIRONMENTAL FACTORS: *Chemical substances*: Inhalation of chemical substances

PLANNING

Unmet Needs

Comfort, protection from psychologic threat, acceptance, caring and communicating re-

lationships, high evaluation of self, sense of adequacy, personal growth and maturity, increased learning, increased reality perception and problem-solving ability

Expected Outcome

Person verbalizes fears
Verbalizes feelings of adequacy and competence in meeting the fear-creating experience
Verbalizes self-satisfaction and growth in having coped with the fear-creating experience
Calm, relaxed facial expression, body movements, and behavior

NURSING INTERVENTIONS

Nursing Treatments

Approach unhurriedly
Reassure verbally (that the nurse will be available whenever needed)
Demonstrate calmness
Provide an atmosphere of acceptance
Encourage the expression of feelings (about the fear)
Listen attentively
Talk with the person (and concerned family)
Offer feedback to the person's expressed feelings
Communicate nurse sensitivity to the person's problem
Relate to the person on an adult–adult level, not on a parent–child level (which could increase fear)
Attend the person constantly (until he feels sufficiently comfortable to be alone)
Provide frequent contact with the person (thereafter)
Ask the person to identify the problem
Ask for specifics, not generalizations, about the problem
Provide reliable information (about the feared object, that modern medicine takes every precaution to avoid patient injury, that long-term drug addiction will cause brain damage, etc.)
Ask how the person normally copes with fear (what does he usually do when fearful that reduces the fear?)
Provide whatever the person needs to use his usual coping mechanisms
Explore with the person his strengths and resources (to overcome the fear)
Do not allow unpleasant surprise situations (such as surgery performed earlier than scheduled)
Consult with the physician (giving anesthesia or performing a procedure, so he is aware of the person's fears)
Reduce the demands placed on the person (so that more energy is available for coping)
Introduce to persons who have undergone the same experience (if appropriate)

Nursing Observations

Observe for an excessive stress level (resulting from the fear)
Determine the degree of insight that the person has
Observe for evidence of a favorable response to therapy (reduced fear and increased comfort)

Health Teaching

Explain how the equipment works (such as a bypass machine, hemodialyzer, etc.)
Explain that the person's response is appropriate and commonly experienced (during illness)
Explain how to channel emotional energy and obtain release from stress (laughing, talking things over, diverting attention into creative activities or work)
Recommend methods for achieving total relaxation (controlled breathing, quietly listening to music, doing nothing)
Recommend a habitual, positive mental attitude (that all will go well)

EVALUATION

Record actual outcome

FEAR OF BURDENING OTHERS[105,471,525]

ASSESSMENT

Data Collection

Subjective Data
- Person experiences feelings of threat or danger
- Can describe or identify the threat or danger
  Concerned with being unable to carry out personal responsibilities
  Feels the other person already has enough responsibility
  Verbalizes the difficulties ahead for the person assuming the added burden

Objective Data
- May manifest physical findings such as facial flushing or pallor, rapid or deep respirations, rapid or bounding pusle, increased blood pressure, sweating, trembling
- May exhibit behavior such as restlessness, sleep disturbances, change in eating habits, rapid speech, crying, avoiding requests for legitimate needs

Data Analysis

Nursing Diagnosis
FEAR OF BURDENING OTHERS: A feeling of alarm and fright about placing additional responsibility on another person

Common Etiology (Stressors)
DISEASES: Any
INJURIES: Any
SIGNS AND SYMPTOMS: Immobility, pain, weakness
PSYCHOSOCIAL FACTORS: The threat of a specific, clearly identified danger, the threat of real or imagined danger, role changes with a significant other
HUMAN BODY: *Body function*: Loss of body function. *Body part*: Loss of a body part
DEVELOPMENTAL PHASES: Any beyond toddler age, but especially old age
SITUATIONAL FACTORS: Acute, chronic, or terminal illness or injury

PLANNING

Unmet Needs
Comfort, protection from psychologic threat, acceptance, caring and communicating relationships, high evaluation of self, sense of adequacy, personal growth and maturity, increased learning, increased reality perception and problem-solving ability

Expected Outcome
Person verbalizes fears
Verbalizes feelings of adequacy and competence in meeting the fear-creating experience
Relates acceptance of the situation
Verbalizes self-satisfaction and growth in having coped with the fear-creating experience
Calm, relaxed facial expression, body movements, and behavior

NURSING INTERVENTIONS

Nursing Treatments
Approach unhurriedly
Reassure verbally (that the nurse will help the person solve his problem)
Demonstrate calmness
Provide an atmosphere of acceptance
Encourage the expression of feelings (about the fear)
Listen attentively
Talk with the person (and significant others involved)
Offer feedback to the person's expressed feelings
Communicate nurse sensitivity to the person's problem
Relate to the person on an adult–adult level, not on a parent–child level (which could increase fear)

Ask the person to identify the problem

Ask for specifics, not generalizations, about the problem

Support a realistic assessment of the situation (that the ill or aged person has limitations, certain responsibilities must be assumed by others, that family members are willing to take the responsibility)

Ask how the person normally copes with fear (what does he usually do when fearful, that reduces the fear?)

Provide whatever the person needs to use his usual coping mechanisms

Reduce the demand placed on the person (so that more energy is available for coping)

Nursing Observations

Observe for an excessive stress level (resulting from the fear)

Determine the degree of insight that the person has (into the problem)

Obseve for evidence of a favorable response to therapy (reduced fear and increased comfort)

Health Teaching

Explain that the person's response is appropriate and commonly experienced (during illness and aging)

Recommend a habitual, positive mental attitude

Teach how to use the problem-solving method (to minimize the burden on others, to help the patient maintain autonomy)

EVALUATION

Record actual outcome

FEAR OF BURN INJURY[105,471,525]

ASSESSMENT

Data Collection

Subjective Data

• Person experiences feelings of threat or danger

• Can describe or identify the threat or danger

Directly or indirectly relates concern about being burned

May relate previous experience with a burn injury to self or significant other

May refuse the procedure or therapy

Objective Data

• May manifest physical findings such as facial flushing or pallor, rapid or deep respirations, rapid or bounding pulse, increased blood pressure, sweating, trembling

• May exhibit behavior such as cautiously touching the heated object to determine the degree of heat, removing a device providing therapeutic heat such as a heated vaporizer or oxygen mask

Data Analysis

Nursing Diagnosis

FEAR OF BURN INJURY: A feeling of alarm and fright that one might be harmed by heat or heat-producing therapy

Common Etiology (Stressors)

PSYCHOSOCIAL FACTORS: The threat of a specific and clearly identified danger, the threat of real or imagined danger

HEALTH CARE FACTORS: *Diagnostic procedures*: X-ray of any kind. *Medical therapy*: Application of heat (hot packs, heating pad, etc.), diathermy, heated mist inhalation therapy, radiation or radioisotope therapy. *Surgical procedure*: Cauterization by electrocautery, cryosurgery

PLANNING

Unmet Needs

Comfort, protection from psychologic threat, acceptance, caring and communicating relationships, high evaluation of self, sense of adequacy, personal growth and maturity, increased learning, increased reality perception and problem-solving ability

Expected Outcome

Person verbalizes fears

Verbalizes feelings of adequacy and competence in meeting the fear-creating experience

Verbalizes self-satisfaction and growth in having coped with the fear-creating experience

Calm, relaxed facial expression, body movements, and behavior

NURSING INTERVENTIONS

Nursing Treatments

Approach unhurriedly

Reassure verbally (that the nurse will be available whenever needed)

Demonstrate calmness

Provide an atmosphere of acceptance

Encourage the expression of feelings (about the fear)

Listen attentively

Offer feedback to the person's expressed feelings

Communicate nurse sensitivity to the person's problem

Relate to the person on an adult–adult level, not on a parent–child level (which could increase fear)

Attend the person constantly (until he feels sufficiently comfortable to be alone)

Provide frequent contact with the person (thereafter)

Ask the person to identify the problem

Ask for specifics, not generalizations, about the problem

Provide reliable information (about prevention of burns, that modern medicine takes every precaution to avoid injury)

Ask how the person normally copes with fear (what does he usually do when fearful that reduces the fear?)

Provide whatever the person needs to use his usual coping mechanisms

Encourage the person to face the fear (when able, and especially if there is a high probability of success with the therapy)

Do not allow unpleasant surprise situations (such as therapy given without prior explanation)

Avoid placing the person on enforced inactivity (which heightens fear)

Reduce the demands placed on the person (so that more energy is available for coping

Introduce to persons who have undergone the same experience (if appropriate)

Nursing Observations

Observe for an excessive stress level (resulting from the fear)

Determine the degree of insight that the person has (into the fear)

Observe for evidence of a favorable response to therapy (reduced fear and increased comfort)

Health Teaching

Describe those symtoms that should be reported (excessive heat, tissue breakdown after radiation therapy, etc.)

Explain that the person's response is appropriate and commonly experienced (during certain therapy)

Explain how to channel emotional energy and obtain release from stress (talking things over, diverting one's attention during therapy)

Recommend methods for achieving total relaxation (controlled breathing)

Recommend a habitual, positive mental attitude (to overcome fear)

EVALUATION

Record actual outcome

FEAR OF CASTRATION[105,471,525]

ASSESSMENT
Data Collection
Subjective Data
- Person experiences feelings of threat or danger
- Can describe or identify the threat or danger
  Relates concern about the effects of disease, procedures, etc., on male genitalia
  May refuse the procedure or therapy

Objective Data
- May manifest physical findings such as facial flushing or pallor, rapid or deep respirations, rapid or bounding pulse, increased blood pressure, sweating, trembling
- May exhibit behavior such as restlessness, sleep disturbances, change in eating habits, irritability, short attention span, making poor judgments, forgetfulness, rapid speech, demanding, and controlling behavior, touching or inspecting the genitalia for evidence of injury

Data Analysis
Nursing Diagnosis
FEAR OF CASTRATION: A feeling of alarm and fright about losing the male genitalia

Common Etiology (Stressors)
DISEASES: Cancer, gonorrhea, mumps, syphilis
INJURIES: Any injury to the genitalia
PSYCHOSOCIAL FACTORS: The threat of a specific and clearly identified danger, the threat of real or imagined danger
HEALTH CARE FACTORS: *Diagnostic procedures*: Cystometry, cystoscopy, cystourethrography, retrograde pyleogram or urethrography. *Medical therapy*: Bladder irrigation, radiation therapy to the genitalia, urinary catheterization. *Drug therapy*: Contraceptive medication for men. *Surgical procedures*: Circumcision after infancy, cystectomy of bladder, cystostomy, orchiectomy (unilateral), prostatectomy, ureterocolostomy, ureteroileostomy, ureterosigmoidostomy, ureterostomy, ureterotomy, vasectomy
DEVELOPMENTAL PHASE: Preschooler (age 2–6)
LIFESTYLE: Promiscuous sexual activity (which leads to infection), participation in sports or exposure to occupational hazards that lead to injury of the genitalia

PLANNING
Unmet Needs
Comfort, protection from psychologic threat, acceptance, caring and communicating relationships, high evaluation of self, sense of adequacy, personal growth and maturity, increased learning, increased reality perception and problem-solving ability

Expected Outcome
Person verbalizes his fears
Verbalizes feelings of adequacy and comptence in meeting the fear-creating experience
Verbalizes self-satisfaction and growth in having coped with the fear-creating experience
Calm, relaxed facial expression, body movements, and behavior

NURSING INTERVENTIONS
Nursing Treatments
Approach unhurriedly
Reassure verbally
Demonstrate calmness
Provide an atmosphere of acceptance
Encourage the expression of feelings (about the fear)
Listen attentively
Offer feedback to the person's expressed feelings

Communicate nurse sensitivity to the person's problem

Relate to the person on an adult–adult level, not on a parent–child level (which could increase fear)

Attend the patient constantly (until he feels sufficiently comfortable to be alone)

Provide frequent contact with the person (thereafter)

Ask the person to identify the problem

Ask for specifics, not generalizations, about the problem

Provide reliable information (about the specifics of procedures or therapy, about how to be protected against sports and occupational hazards, that castration will not occur)

Ask how the person normally copes with fear (what does he usually do when fearful that reduces the fear?)

Provide whatever the person needs to use his usual coping mechanisms

Do not allow unpleasant surprise situations (such as unexplained procedures or therapy)

Reduce the demands placed on the person (so that more energy is available for coping)

Introduce to persons who have undergone the same experience (if appropriate)

Nursing Observations

Observe for an excessive stress level (resulting from the fear)

Determine the degree of insight that the person has (into the fear)

Observe for evidence of a favorable response to therapy (reduced fear and increased comfort)

Health Teaching

Explain that the person's response is appropriate and commonly experienced

EVALUATION

Record actual outcome

FEAR OF CONFINEMENT[105,471,525]

ASSESSMENT

Data Collection

Subjective Data
- Person experiences feelings of threat or danger
- Can describe or identify the threat or danger

  Requests or demands that restrictions on movement be lifted

  Is intensely frustrated if confined

  May refuse to be admitted to a locked psychiatric unit or to continue traction or cast therapy, etc.

Objective Data
- May manifest physical findings such as facial flushing or pallor, rapid or deep respirations, rapid or bounding pulse, increased blood pressure, sweating, trembling
- May exhibit behavior such as restlessness, sleep disturbances, change in eating habits, irritability; rapid speech, demanding and controlling behavior, crying, calling for help, attempting to remove self from the restricting area, device, or situation

Data Analysis

Nursing Diagnosis
FEAR OF CONFINEMENT: A feeling of alarm and fright about restrictions on freedom of movement

Common Etiology (Stressors)
DISEASES: Any severe or infectious disease, emotional disorder
INJURIES: Any serious injury (especially fractures)

SIGNS AND SYMPTOMS: Confusion, weakness

PSYCHOSOCIAL FACTORS: The threat of a specific, clearly identified danger, the threat of real or imagined danger

HUMAN BODY: Loss of body function (which may reduce body movement)

HEALTH CARE FACTORS: *Health care environment*: Coronary or intensive care units (lack of windows may make the person feel walled in), locked psychiatric unit (may be perceived as a prison). *Hospitalization*: Any (may feel confined to one room). *Diagnostic equipment*: Audiometer booth (confined to a small space), CAT scanner (confined by the machine hovering over). *Medical therapy*: Prolonged bed rest (confined to bed space), body casting, especially with hip spica cast (confined body movement, with an inability to get away from the cast), preventive, protective, or psychiatric isolation (may be perceived as a prison), traction (the inability to see a clear space through the traction apparatus, and the unorganized sequence of rope and traction hardware lends itself to feelings of confinement and environmental confusion), intravenous infusion (limits body movement), hemodialysis (confines the person to a bed or chair with little body movement for 4–6 hours at a time). *Therapeutic equipment or devices*: CircOlectric or Stryker frame (when sandwiched between the turning frames, the person feels severely confined), respirator or oxygen tent (confines body movement to a small area), safety restraints (may be perceived as hand or leg cuffs, confines body movement to a very small space), side rails (may be perceived as barriers that cannot be overcome)

DEVELOPMENTAL PHASES: Old age (often confines the person to the home)

SITUATIONAL FACTORS: Illness of significant other, childrearing (both confine the person to the home)

PLANNING

Unmet Needs

Comfort, protection from psychologic threat, acceptance, caring and communicating relationships, high evaluation of self, sense of adequacy, personal growth and maturity, increased learning, increased reality perception and problem-solving ability

Expected Outcome

Person verbalizes fears

Verbalizes feelings of adequacy and competence in meeting the fear-creating experience

Verbalizes self-satisfaction and growth in having coped with the fear-creating experience

Calm, relaxed facial expression, body movements, and behavior

NURSING INTERVENTIONS

Nursing Treatments

Approach unhurriedly

Reassure verbally (that the nurse will help the person solve his problem, be available whenever needed, that the confinement is only temporary)

Demonstrate calmness

Provide an atmosphere of acceptance

Arrange pleasant surroundings (placing the person in a large, uncrowded room with windows or reducing clutter in a small room will reduce the confined feeling)

Encourage the expression of feelings (about the fear)

Listen attentively

Offer feedback to the person's expressed feelings

Communicate nurse sensitivity to the person's problem

Relate to the person on an adult–adult level, not on a parent–child level (which could

Attend the person constantly (until he feels sufficiently comfortable to be alone)

Provide frequent contact with the person (thereafter)

Ask the person to identify the problem

Ask for specifics, not generalizations, about the problem

Support a realistic assessment of the situation (certain procedures must be done for the person's benefit)

Provide reliable information (about how long the situation will exist, what can be done to change it)

Ask how the person normally copes with fear (what does he usually do when fearful that reduces the fear)

Provide whatever the person needs to use his usual coping mechanisms

Encourage the person to face the fear (when able, if the therapy is essential)

Provide emotionally safe experiences (whenever possible)

Provide objects that symbolize safeness (to the person)

Do not allow unpleasant surprise situations (of unexpected or increased confinement)

Walk with the person (out in the halls, even outside the hospital, if he feels confined to the bed, room, unit, or hospital)

Use a chest restraint (instead of hand and leg restraints to increase freedom of movement)

Provide radio and television for diversion

Place by a window (looking out into an open sky gives a sense of freedom and space)

Avoid placing the person on enforced inactivity (which heightens fear)

Reduce the demands placed on the person (so that more energy is available for coping)

Introduce to persons who have undergone the same experience (such as being in a body cast or under a CAT scanner)

Nursing Observations

Observe for an excessive stress level (resulting from the fear)

Determine the degree of insight that the person has (into the fear)

Observe for evidence of a favorable response to therapy (reduced fear and increased comfort)

Health Teaching

Explain that the person's response is appropriate and commonly experienced

Advise against fighting fear (this reinforces the emotion)

Explain the importance of recognizing tension within oneself

Explain the importance of persons offering support to one another (such as relieving those confined to the home by dependent others)

Recommend methods for achieving total relaxation (such as controlled breathing before and during confining procedures)

EVALUATION

Record actual outcome

FEAR OF CONFISCATION OF PERSONAL BELONGINGS[105,471,525]

ASSESSMENT

Data Collection

Subjective Data

• Person experiences feelings of threat or danger
• Can describe or identify the threat or danger
  Relates that specific objects are important to him
  Feels involvement or identity with the objects
  May deny possessing them
  Is disturbed about removal of personal items (for safe keeping)

Objective Data
- May manifest physical findings such as facial flushing or pallor, rapid or deep respirations, rapid or bounding pulse, increased blood pressure, sweating, trembling
- May exhibit behavior such as restlessness, sleep disturbances, change in eating habits, irritability, rapid speech, demanding and controlling behavior, insisting that personal belongings not be touched, concealing or carrying significant objects that could be confiscated

Data Analysis

Nursing Diagnosis
FEAR OF CONFISCATION OF PERSONAL BELONGINGS: A feeling of alarm and fright about other persons taking away material objects perceived as important to the person

Common Etiology (Stressors)
PSYCHOSOCIAL FACTORS: The threat of a specific and clearly identified danger, the threat of real or imagined danger, loss of independence
HEALTH CARE FACTORS: *Hospitalization:* Any. *Institutional policies:* Restrictive
DEVELOPMENTAL PHASES: Toddler (around age 2), preschooler (age 2–6), old age
LIFESTYLE: Lack of finances to replace material possessions

PLANNING

Unmet Needs
Comfort, protection from psychologic threat, acceptance, caring and communicating relationships, high evaluation of self, sense of adequacy, personal growth and maturity, increased learning, increased reality perception and problem-solving ability

Expected Outcome
Person verbalizes fears
Verbalizes feelings of adequacy and competence in meeting the fear-creating experience
Verbalizes self-satisfaction and growth in having coped with the fear-creating experience
Calm, relaxed facial expression, body movements, and behavior

NURSING INTERVENTIONS

Nursing Treatments
Approach unhurriedly
Reassure verbally (that the nurse will not confiscate, but will protect the person's valued belongings)
Demonstrate calmness
Provide an atmosphere of acceptance
Encourage the expression of feelings (about the fear)
Listen attentively
Offer feedback to the person's expressed feelings
Communicate nurse sensitivity to the person's problem
Relate to the person on an adult–adult level, not on a parent–child level (which could increase fear)
Ask the person to identify the problem
Ask for specifics, not generalizations, about the problem
Provide reliable information (about facilities for safe-keeping valued articles)
Encourage mutual problem-solving (to ensure safety of the person's belongings)
Safeguard the person's personal belongings
Do not allow unpleasant surprise situations (such as taking the person to therapy before he has time to place his belongings safely)

Nursing Observations
Observe for an excessive stress level (resulting from the fear)
Determine the degree of insight that the person has (into the fear)
Observe for evidence of a favorable response to therapy (reduced fear and increased comfort)

Health Teaching

Explain that the person's response is appropriate and commonly experienced (especially among the aged)

EVALUATION

Record actual outcome

FEAR OF DEATH[90,105,195,279,471,525]

ASSESSMENT

Data Collection

Subjective Data
• Person experiences feelings of threat or danger
• Can describe or identify the threat or danger
  May ask if he is going to die
  May initiate or avoid discussion of death
  May seek frequent reassurance that hope still exists

Specific to the Nondying Person
May compare his symptoms to those of another person who died
May have misinterpreted information or medical terms (may think *tumor* means *cancer*, etc.)
May attribute unwarranted significance to physical symptoms (may think that a "racing heart" is dangerous, that lightheadedness from hyperventilation is illness, etc.)

Specific to the Dying Person
Relates an awareness that life is ending
Perceives decreased physical strength
Is concerned about the experience of death, when it will occur, if it will be painful, if he will be at home or hospitalized, etc.
May want to talk about life experiences

Objective Data
• May manifest physical findings such as facial flushing or pallor, rapid or deep respirations, rapid or bounding pulse, increased blood pressure, sweating, trembling
• May exhibit behavior such as restlessness, sleep disturbances, change in eating habits, irritability, short attention span, making poor judgments, forgetfulness, rapid speech, demanding and controlling behavior, crying, avoiding persons or stiuations, frequent call-light signaling, prolonging conversations, reaching out to touch persons

Data Analysis

Nursing Diagnosis
FEAR OF DEATH: A feeling of alarm and fright about the thought of cessation of life

Common Etiology (Stressors)
DISEASES: Any serious disease
INJURIES: Any serious injury
SIGNS AND SYMPTOMS: Dyspnea, pain, weakness
PSYCHOSOCIAL FACTORS: The threat of a specific and clearly identified danger, the threat of real or imagined danger
HUMAN BODY: *Body function*: Loss of body function. *Natural body function*: Childbirth. *Body states*: Pregnancy (a woman may feel that by being closer to birth, she is closer to death)

HEALTH CARE FACTORS: *Health care decision*: Decision to donate a body organ, decision about the choice of high-risk treatment options. *Health care environment*: Crisis-oriented health care environment such as an emergency room or intensive care unit. *Diagnostic procedure*: High-risk diagnostic procedures such as angiography, cardiac catheterization. *Medical diagnosis*: Unfavorable. *Drug therapy*: Adverse effects or interactions of drugs. *Medical therapy*: Electroconvulsive therapy, hemodialysis, radiation therapy, blood transfusion, exchange blood transfusion, withdrawal from alcohol or drugs. *Surgical therapy*: Impending surgery and anesthesia. *Therapeutic equipment or devices*: Use of or failure of a cardiac pacemaker, respirator, or hemodialyzer; incorrect patient interpretation of monitor readouts. *Prognosis*: Unfavorable

DEVELOPMENTAL PHASES: Middle age, old age

SITUATIONAL FACTORS: Death of a significant other (especially parents or friends), life-threatening or terminal illness

ENVIRONMENTAL FACTORS: *Cataclysm*: Cyclone, earthquake, flood, hurricane, etc. *Darkness*: In the patient's room

PLANNING

Unmet Needs

Comfort, protection from psychologic threat, acceptance, caring and communicating relationships, high evaluation of self, sense of adequacy, personal growth and maturity, increased learning, increased reality perception and problem-solving ability

Expected Outcome

Person verbalizes fears
Verbalizes feelings of adequacy and competence in meeting the fear-creating experience
Verbalizes self-satisfaction and growth in having coped with the fear-creating experience
Calm, relaxed facial expression, body movements, and behavior

NURSING INTERVENTIONS

Nursing Treatments

Approach unhurriedly
Reassure verbally (that the nurse is available whenever needed)
Demonstrate calmness
Provide an atmosphere of acceptance
Arrange pleasant surroundings
Encourage the expression of feelings (about the fear)
Listen attentively
Offer feedback to the person's expressed feelings
Communicate nurse sensitivity to the person's problem
Relate to the person on an adult–adult level, not on a parent–child level (which could increase fear)
Attend the person constantly (until he feels sufficiently comfortable to be alone)
Provide frequent contact with the person (thereafter)
Touch the person frequently
Ask the person to identify the problem
Ask for specifics, not generalizations, about the problem
Provide reliable information (if death is not likely, communicate such; relate that every effort will be made to protect the person)
Ask how the person normally copes with fear (what does he usually do when fearful that reduces the fear)
Provide whatever the person needs to use his usual coping mechanisms (if he wants to talk out the problem, the nurse listens; if he wants to cry, the nurse provides privacy, etc.)
Encourage the person to face the fear (when able, to reduce the fear)
Explore with the person his strengths and resources (to overcome the fear)
Provide emotionally safe experiences (nonthreatening experiences)

Provide objects that symbolize safeness

Do not allow unpleasant surprise situations (which increase fear)

Place the patient in a room with a person having a favorable prognosis (instead of in a room with a critically ill person)

Avoid placing the person on enforced inactivity (which heightens fear)

Reduce the demands placed on the person (so more energy is available for coping)

Introduce to persons who have undergone the same experience (such as surgery, hemodialysis, etc.)

Provide a night light (darkness heightens fear)

Specific to the Dying Person

Suggest that one relative remain with the dying person

Nursing Observations

Observe for an excessive stress level (resulting from the fear)

Determine the degree of insight that the person has (into the fear)

Observe for evidence of a favorable response to therapy (reduced fear and increased comfort)

Health Teaching

Explain that the person's response is appropriate and commonly experienced (by ill, aged persons)

Advise against fighting fear (this reinforces the emotion)

Explain how to channel emotional energy and obtain release from stress (through creative efforts, helping others, talking things over, conscious acceptance of death)

Recommend methods for achieving total relaxation (controlled breathing, quietly listening to music, doing nothing, which reduces fear)

Specific to the Dying Person

Explain the causes of the fear of death (the unknown, the loss of life, self, time, and pleasure)

Recommend new options for effective methods of coping (viewing death as peace, sleep, release from suffering, reunion with loved ones)

Advise that significant persons express caring for one another

EVALUATION

Record actual outcome

FEAR OF DEATH OF A SIGNIFICANT OTHER[105,471,525]

ASSESSMENT

Data Collection

Subjective Data

▪ Person experiences feelings of threat or danger

• Can describe or identify the threat or danger

Asks frequently about significant other's condition or does not inquire at all

May deny seriousness of significant other's illness

May have never seen anyone die

May not know what to expect during impending death

Objective Data

• May manifest physical findings such as facial flushing or pallor, rapid or deep respirations, rapid or bounding pulse, increased blood pressure, sweating, trembling

• May exhibit behavior such as restlessness, sleep disturbances, change in eating habits, irritability, short attention span, making poor judgments, forgetfulness, rapid speech, demanding and controlling behavior, crying, avoiding or constantly being near the ill person, making frequent phone calls to seek reassurance of the person's condition

Family members gather if they fear imminent death

Data Analysis

Nursing Diagnosis

FEAR OF DEATH OF A SIGNIFICANT OTHER: A feeling of alarm and fright that the life of a significant other will cease

Common Etiology (Stressors)

BIRTH STATUS: Premature infant

DISEASES: Any severe disease

INJURIES: Any severe injury

SIGNS AND SYMPTOMS (OF SIGNIFICANT OTHER): Bleeding, breathing difficulty, choking, convulsions, fever, pain, weakness

PSYCHOSOCIAL FACTORS: The threat of a specific and clearly identified danger, the threat of real or imagined danger

HUMAN BODY: *Natural body function*: Childbirth. *Body states*: Pregnancy (of significant other)

HEALTH CARE FACTORS: *Health care decision*: Decision about the choice of high-risk treatment options. *Health care environment*: Crisis-oriented health care environment such as an emergency room or intensive care unit. *Diagnostic procedure*: High-risk diagnostic procedures such as angiography, cardiac catheterization. *Medical diagnosis*: Unfavorable. *Drug therapy*: Adverse effects and interactions of drugs. *Medical therapy*: Electroconvulsive therapy, hemodialysis, radiation therapy, blood transfusion, exchange blood transfusion, withdrawal from alcohol or drugs. *Surgical therapy*: Impending surgery or anesthesia. *Therapeutic equipment or devices*: Use of or failure of a cardiac pacemaker, respirator, or hemodialyzer, incorrect family interpretation of monitor readouts. *Prognosis*: Unfavorable

DEVELOPMENTAL PHASES: Old age

SITUATIONAL FACTORS: Death of one parent, life-threatening or terminal illness

ENVIRONMENTAL FACTORS: *Cataclysm*: Cyclone, earthquake, flood, hurricane, etc.

PLANNING

Unmet Needs

Comfort, protection from psychologic threat, acceptance, caring and communicating relationships, high evaluation of self, sense of adequacy, personal growth and maturity, increased learning, increased reality perception and problem-solving ability

Expected Outcome

Person verbalizes fears

Verbalizes feelings of adequacy and competence in meeting the fear-creating experience

Verbalizes self-satisfaction and growth in having coped with the fear-creating experience

Calm, relaxed facial expression, body movements, and behavior

NURSING INTERVENTIONS

Nursing Treatments

Approach unhurriedly

Reassure verbally (that the nurse will be available whenever needed)

Demonstrate calmness

Provide an atmosphere of acceptance

Encourage the expression of feelings (about the fear)

Listen attentively

Offer feedback to the person's expressed feelings

Communicate nurse sensitivity to the person's problem

Relate to the person on an adult–adult level, not on a parent–child level (which could increase fear)

Attend the person constantly (until he feels sufficiently comfortable to be alone)

Provide frequent contact with the person (thereafter)

Ask the person to identify the problem

Ask for specifics, not generalizations, about the problem

Support a realistic assessment of the situation (about whether or not the fear is justified)

Provide reliable information (about the patient's condition, intermittently)

Ask how the person normally copes with fear (what does he usually do when fearful that reduces the fear?)

Provide whatever the person needs to use his usual coping mechanisms

Do not allow unpleasant surprise situations (such as misleading reports of improvement with a sudden critical change)

Nursing Observations

Observe for an excessive stress level (resulting from the fear)

Determine the degree of insight that the person has (into the fear)

Observe for evidence of a favorable response to therapy (reduced fear and increased comfort)

Health Teaching

Explain that the person's response is appropriate and commonly experienced (when a loved one is ill or dying)

Explain that fatigue should be recognized as a stress factor (which heightens fear, especially when family members become fatigued while caring for a loved one)

Explain how to channel emotional energy and obtain release from stress (talking things over, participation in sports, creative activities)

Recommend methods for achieving total relaxation (controlled breathing, quietly listening to music, doing nothing, which reduces fear)

Recommend a habitual, positive mental attitude (about the person's ability to cope)

EVALUATION

Record actual outcome

FEAR OF DEPENDENCY[105,471,525]

ASSESSMENT

Data Collection

Subjective Data

• Person experiences feelings of threat or danger

• Can describe or identify the threat or danger

   Wants to take care of himself and meet his own needs

   Feels that dependency on others is unacceptable

   Is concerned that others will not meet his needs adequately

   Feels threatened with less control over his life

Objective Data

• May manifest physical findings such as facial flushing or pallor, rapid or deep respirations, rapid or bounding pulse, increased blood pressure, sweating, trembling

• May exhibit behavior such as restlessness, sleep disturbances, change in eating habits, irritability, rapid speech, demanding and controlling behavior toward persons who offer to help, avoiding persons or situations that may lead to dependency

   May attempt activities beyond his capabilities

Data Analysis

Nursing Diagnosis

FEAR OF DEPENDENCY: A feeling of alarm and fright about losing the ability to meet one's own needs

Common Etiology (Stressors)
DISEASES: Any
INJURIES: Any
SIGNS AND SYMPTOMS: Immobility, pain, paralysis, weakness
PHYCHOSOCIAL FACTORS: The threat of a specific and clearly identified danger, the threat of real or imagined danger, nonachievement of developmental trust
HUMAN BODY: *Body function*: Loss of body function *Natural body function*: Childbirth. *Body part*: Loss of a body part
HEALTH CARE FACTORS: *Health care costs*: High. *Hospitalization:* Any. *Institutionalization:* Any. *Diagnostic procedures*: Especially high-risk diagnostic procedures. *Medical therapy*: Hemodialysis, oxygen therapy. *Surgical procedures*: Impending surgery, surgery of any kind
DEVELOPMENTAL PHASES: Old age
SITUATIONAL FACTORS: Acute, chronic or terminal illness; loss of or uncertain employment; poverty; lack of finances

PLANNING
Unmet Needs
Comfort, protection from psychologic threat, acceptance, caring and communicating relationships, high evaluation of self, sense of adequacy, personal growth and maturity, increased learning, increased reality perception and problem-solving ability

Expected Outcome
Person verbalizes fears
Verbalizes feelings of adequacy and competence in meeting the fear-creating experience
Verbalizes self-satisfaction and growth in having coped with the fear-creating experience
Calm, relaxed facial expression, body movements, and behavior

NURSING INTERVENTIONS
Nursing Treatments
Approach unhurriedly
Reassure verbally (that the person will be given every opportunity to be independent)
Demonstrate calmness
Provide an atmosphere of acceptance
Encourage the expression of feelings (about the fear)
Listen attentively
Offer feedback to the person's expressed feelings
Communicate nurse sensitivity to the person's problem
Relate to the person on an adult–adult level, not on a parent–child level (which could increase fear)
Ask the person to identify the problem
Ask for specifics, not generalizations, about the problem
Support a realistic assessment of the situation (about the level of his independence)
Provide reliable information (whether or not the illness causes dependency)
Ask how the person normally copes with fear (what does he usually do when fearful that reduces the fear?)
Provide whatever the person needs to use his usual coping mechanisms
Arrange situations that encourage the person's autonomy
Do not allow unpleasnat situations (such as sudden situations of dependency)
Reduce the demands placed on the person (so that more energy is available for coping)
Introduce to persons who have undergone the same experience (if dependency occurs)

Nursing Observations
Observe for an excessive stress level (resulting from the fear)
Determine the degree of insight that the person has
Observe for evidence of a favorable response to therapy (reduced fear and increased comfort)

Health Teaching
Explain that the person's response is appropriate and commonly experienced (during illness, aging)

Explain the need to recognize highly stressful situations (since high stress levels tend to increase dependency behaviors)

Recommend methods for achieving total relaxation (controlled breathing, quietly listening to music, doing nothing)

Recommend a habitual, positive mental attitude (even if dependency exists)

Teach how to use the problem-solving method (to reduce dependency on others)

EVALUATION
Record actual outcome

FEAR OF DISFIGUREMENT[105,471,525]

ASSESSMENT

Data Collection

Subjective Data
• Person experiences feelings of threat or danger
• Can describe or identify the threat or danger
  Is concerned with personal appearance
  Is worried about the effects of disease, injury, or therapy on his looks
  Requests a time frame in which a return to normal appearance can be expected

Objective Data
• May manifest physical findings such as facial flushing or pallor, rapid or deep respirations, rapid or bounding pulse, increased blood pressure, sweating, trembling
• May exhibit behavior such as restlessness, sleep disturbances, change in eating habits, irritability, rapid speech, demanding and controlling behavior, crying
  Avoids being seen by anyone but close family or friends
  If disfigurement has occurred, the person may frequently view himself in a mirror to determine progression toward normal appearance or may refuse to look in a mirror

Data Analysis

Nursing Diagnosis
FEAR OF DISFIGUREMENT: A feeling of alarm and fright that one's beauty or external appearance is or might be marred

Common Etiology (Stressors)
DISEASES: Acne vulgaris, carcinoma, discoid lupus, Hansen's disease, herpes zoster, Horner's syndrome, Parkinson's disease, poison ivy, poison oak, psoriasis

INJURIES: Abrasion, burn wound, laceration wound

SIGNS AND SYMPTOMS: Edema, rash, spasms, tremors

PSYCHOSOCIAL FACTORS: The threat of a specific, clearly identified danger; the threat of real or imagined danger

HUMAN BODY: *Body states*: Pregnancy

HEALTH CARE: *Adverse effects of medical therapy*: Loss of hair from radiation therapy. *Drug therapy*: Loss of hair from chemotherapy, edema from corticosteroids, jerking and involuntary movements from levodopa and antipsychotic drugs. *Surgical therapy*: Disfigurement from surgery

PLANNING

Unmet Needs
Comfort, protection from psychologic threat, acceptance, caring and communicating relationships, high evaluation of self, sense of adequacy, personal growth and maturity, increased learning, increased reality perception and problem-solving ability

Expected Outcome
Person verbalizes fears

Verbalizes feelings of adequacy and competence in meeting the fear-creating experience
Verbalizes self-satisfaction and growth in having coped with the fear-creating experience
Calm, relaxed facial expression, body movements, and behavior

NURSING INTERVENTIONS

Nursing Treatments
Approach unhurriedly
Reassure verbally (that the nurse is available whenever needed)
Demonstrate calmness
Provide an atmosphere of acceptance
Encourage the expression of feelings (about the fear)
Listen attentively
Offer feedback to the person's expressed feelings
Communicate nurse sensitivity to the person's problem
Relate to the person on an adult–adult level, not on a parent–child level (which could increase fear)
Attend the person constantly (until he feels sufficiently comfortable to be alone)
Provide frequent contact with the person (thereafter)
Ask the person to identify the problem
Ask for specifics, not generalizations, about the problem
Provide reliable information (about whether or not there will be disfigurement, about the length of and degree of expected disfigurement)
Ask how the person normally copes with fear (what does he usually do when fearful that reduces the fear?)
Provide whatever the person needs to use his usual coping mechanism s
Explore with the person his strengths and resources (to overcome the fear)
Do not allow unpleasant surprise situations (such as the person looking into the mirror before being warned of disfigurement or having bandages removed before being warned)
Encourage mutual problem solving (to reduce the potential for disfigurement or to cover or reduce the disfigurement)

Nursing Observations
Observe for an excessive stress level (resulting from the fear)
Determine the degree of insight that the person has (into the fear)
Observe for evidence of a favorable response to therapy (reduced fear and increased comfort)

Health Teaching
Explain that the person's response is appropriate and commonly experienced (when ill, injured, or pregnant)
Recommend a habitual, positive mental attitude (even if disfigured)

EVALUATION
Record actual outcome

FEAR OF DISRUPTION OF PERSONAL/FAMILY/LIFE PLANS[105,471,525]

ASSESSMENT

Data Collection

Subjective Data
• Person experiences feelings of threat or danger
• Can describe or identify the threat or danger

Relates the original, intended plans
Anticipates how the original plans will be changed
Is concerned with the effects of change on the person's life

Objective Data
- May manifest physical findings such as facial flushing or pallor, rapid or deep respirations, rapid or bounding pulse, increased blood pressure, sweating, trembling
- May exhibit behavior such as restlessness, sleep disturbances, change in eating habits, irritability, short attention span, making poor judgments, forgetfulness, rapid speech, demanding and controlling behavior, crying, avoiding persons or situations that could cause the disruption

Data Analysis

Nursing Diagnosis
FEAR OF DISRUPTION OF PERSONAL/FAMILY/LIFE PLANS: A feeling of alarm and fright about unwanted changes in personal, family, or life plans brought about by unexpected events

Common Etiology (Stressors)
DISEASES: Any
INJURIES: Any
PSYCHOSOCIAL FACTORS: The threat of a specific and clearly identified danger, the threat of real or imagined danger
HUMAN BODY: *Body states*: Pregnancy
HEALTH CARE FACTORS: *Hospitalization*: Recommendation for hospitalization. *Recovery from illness*: Delayed recovery from illness
SITUATIONAL FACTORS: Acute or chronic illness of self or significant other, parenthood

PLANNING

Unmet Needs
Comfort, protection from psychologic threat, acceptance, caring and communicating relationships, high evaluation of self, sense of adequacy, personal growth and maturity, increased learning, increased reality perception and problem-solving ability

Expected Outcome
Person verbalizes fears
Verbalizes feelings of adequacy and competence in meeting the fear-creating experience
Verbalizes self-satisfaction and growth in having coped with the fear-creating experience
Calm, relaxed facial expression, body movements, and behavior

NURSING INTERVENTIONS

Nursing Treatments
Approach unhurriedly
Reassure verbally
Demonstrate calmness
Provide an atmosphere of acceptance
Encourage the expression of feelings (about the fear)
Listen attentively
Offer feedback to the person's expressed feelings
Communicate nurse sensitivity to the person's problem
Relate to the person on an adult–adult level, not on a parent–child level (which could increase fear)
Ask the person to identify the problem
Ask for specifics, not generalizations, about the problem
Provide reliable information (about the effects of the illness or injury; about whether the disruption will be severe, short-term; etc.; about what combinations of stress factors could cause a disruption)
Ask how the person normally copes with fear (what does he usually do when fearful that reduces the fear?)

Provide whatever the person needs to use his usual coping mechanisms

Explore with the person his strengths and resources (to continue the pursuit of life plans)

Do not allow unpleasant surprise situations (of therapy schedules, etc., which will disrupt plans even more)

Avoid placing the person on enforced inactivity (which heightens fear)

Introduce to persons who have undergone the same experience (and have successfully readjusted their lives)

Nursing Observations

Observe for an excessive stress level (resulting from the fear)

Determine the degree of insight that the person has (into the fear)

Observe for evidence of a favorable response to therapy (reduced fear and increased comfort)

Health Teaching

Explain that the person's response is appropriate and commonly experienced (during illness and pregnancy)

Advise against fighting fear (this reinforces the emotion)

Recommend methods for achieving total relaxation (controlled breathing, quietly listening to music, doing nothing)

Recommend a habitual, positive mental attitude (toward achieving plans, even if some adjustment is required)

Teach how to use the problem-solving method (to cause the least disruption of plans)

EVALUATION

Record actual outcome

FEAR OF DISTURBING IDEATION [105,471,525]

ASSESSMENT

Data Collection

Subjective Data

• Person experiences feelings of threat or danger
• Can describe or identify the threat or danger
  Relates details of the unwanted ideas
  Verbalizes about their disturbing effect
  Is concerned that coping methods have not alleviated the ideas

Objective Data

• May manifest physical findings such as facial flushing or pallor, rapid or deep respirations, rapid or bounding pulse, increased blood pressure, sweating, trembling
• May exhibit behavior such as restlessness, sleep disturbances, change in eating habits; irritability, short attention span, making poor judgments, forgetfulness, rapid speech, demanding and controlling behavior, crying, avoiding persons or situations that might stimulate the ideation

Data Analysis

Nursing Diagnosis

FEAR OF DISTURBING IDEATION: A feeling of alarm and fright about unwanted ideas that emerge into consciousness and cannot be controlled

Common Etiology (Stressors)

DISEASES: Alcoholism, drug addiction, paranoid state
SIGNS AND SYMPTOMS: Delusions, obsessive thoughts

PSYCHOSOCIAL FACTORS: The threat of a specific and clearly identified danger, the threat of real or imagined danger

HEALTH CARE FACTORS: *Adverse effects of drugs*: Amphetamines, antihistamines, bromides, caffeine, ketamine (as an anesthetic), narcotics

LIFESTYLE: Drug use

PLANNING

Unmet Needs
Comfort, protection from psychologic threat, acceptance, caring and communicating relationships, high evaluation of self, sense of adequacy, personal growth and maturity, increased learning, increased reality perception and problem-solving ability

Expected Outcome
Person verbalizes fears
Verbalizes feelings of adequacy and competence in meeting the fear-creating experience
Verbalizes self-satisfaction and growth in having coped with the fear-creating experience
Calm, relaxed facial expression, body movements, and behavior

NURSING INTERVENTIONS

Nursing Treatments
Approach unhurriedly
Reassure verbally (that the disturbing ideas have no basis in reality)
Demonstrate calmness
Provide an atmosphere of acceptance
Encourage the expression of feelings (about the fear)
Listen attentively
Offer feedback to the person's expressed feelings
Communicate nurse sensitivity to the person's problem
Relate to the person on an adult–adult level, not on a parent–child level (which could increase fear)
Attend the person constantly (until he feels sufficiently comfortable to be alone)
Provide frequent contact with the person (thereafter)
Ask the person to identify the problem
Ask for specifics, not generalizations, about the problem
Support a realistic assessment of the situation (that delusions do not exist in reality, even though they seem real)
Refrain from supporting the person's delusions
Ask how the person normally copes with fear (what does he usually do when fearful that reduces the fear?)
Provide whatever the person needs to use his usual coping mechanisms
Encourage the person to face the fear (when able, to reduce the fear)
Avoid placing the person on enforced inactivity (which heightens fear)
Encourage active diversional activities (solitude promotes ideation)
Withhold the drugs (if ideation is drug-induced)
Provide quiet (if ketamine-induced, reduce all stimuli to an absolute minimum)
Make a referral (for psychiatric evaluation, if the person has not obtained help)

Nursing Observations
Observe for an excessive stress level (resulting from the fear)
Determine the degree of insight that the person has (into the fear)
Observe for evidence of a favorable response to therapy (reduced fear and increased comfort)

Health Teaching
Explain that the person's response is appropriate and commonly experienced (from alcoholism, drug addiction, drug side effects)
Advise against fighting fear (it is better to ignore the ideation)
Explain how to use the stop-and-think technique (the person shouts "stop" to himself, then thinks a new thought)

Explain the need to recognize highly stressful situations (which might precipitate the i-deation)

Explain how to channel emotional energy and obtain release from stress (through running, swimming, other sports, creative activities, laughing, talking things over)

Recommend methods for achieving total relaxation (controlled breathing, quietly listening to music, which reduces fear)

Recommend a habitual, positive mental attitude (despite the fear or ideation)

EVALUATION

Record actual outcome

FEAR OF DRUG DEPENDENCY[105,471,525]

ASSESSMENT

Data Collection

Subjective Data
• Person experiences feelings of threat or danger
• Can describe or identify the threat or danger
  Is concerned that drug therapy has been recommended
  Is worried that dependency on the drug might occur
  Exhibits resistance or refusal to take the drug
  May not request drug (analgesic) even though pain is severe

Objective Data
• May manifest physical findings such as facial flushing or pallor, rapid or deep respirations, rapid or bounding pulse, increased blood pressure, sweating, trembling
• May exhibit behavior such as restlessness, sleep disturbances, change in eating habits, irritability, forgetting to take the drug, rapid speech, demanding and controlling behavior, crying, being unavailable at medication time

Data Analysis

Nursing Diagnosis
FEAR OF DRUG DEPENDENCY: A feeling of alarm and fright about becoming physically or emotionally reliant on a particular drug

Common Etiology (Stressors)
SIGNS AND SYMPTOMS: Pain
PSYCHOSOCIAL FACTORS The threat of a specific, clearly identified danger, the threat of real or imagined danger
HEALTH CARE FACTORS: *Drug therapy*: Any drug but especially antidepressants, barbiturates, narcotics, sedatives, tranquilizers

PLANNING

Unmet Needs

Comfort, protection from psychologic threat, acceptance, caring and communicating relationships, high evaluation of self, sense of adequacy, personal growth and maturity, increased learning, increased reality perception and problem-solving ability

Expected Outcome

Person verbalizes fears
Verbalizes feelings of adequacy and competence in meeting the fear-creating experience
Verbalizes self-satisfaction and growth in having coped with the fear-creating experience
Calm, relaxed facial expression, body movements, and behavior

NURSING INTERVENTIONS

Nursing Treatments

Approach unhurriedly

Reassure verbally (that the nurse will help the person avoid drug dependency)

Demonstrate calmness

Provide an atmosphere of acceptance

Encourage the expression of feelings (about the fear)

Listen attentively

Offer feedback to the person's expressed feelings

Communicate nurse sensitivity to the person's problem

Relate to the person on an adult–adult level, not on a parent–child level (which could increase fear)

Ask the person to identify the problem

Ask for specifics, not generalizations, about the problem

Provide reliable information (about which drugs do or do not cause dependency, about the probability of becoming dependent)

Ask how the person normally copes with fear (what does he usually do when fearful that reduces the fear?)

Provide whatever the person needs to use his usual coping mechanisms

Do not allow unpleasant surprise situations (such as giving drugs that the person fears without his consent)

Consult with the physician (about a substitute drug)

Nursing Observations

Observe for an excessive stress level (resulting from the fear)

Determine the degree of insight that the person has (into the fear)

Observe for evidence of a favorable response to therapy (reduced fear and increased comfort)

Health Teaching

Explain that the person's response is appropriate and commonly experienced (during illness)

EVALUATION

Record actual outcome

FEAR OF DYSFUNCTION OF AN INTERNAL PROSTHESIS[105,471,525]

ASSESSMENT

Data Collection

Subjective Data

• Person experiences feelings of threat or danger

• Can describe or identify the threat or danger

Believes he can feel the prosthesis

Feels it is not as good as the natural body part

Waits for it to rupture or stop functioning

Questions the reliability of the prosthesis

Anticipates repeated surgery if the prosthesis fails

Objective Data

• May manifest physical findings such as facial flushing or pallor, rapid or deep respirations, rapid or bounding pulse, increased blood pressure, sweating, trembling

• May exhibit behavior such as restlessness, sleep disturbances, irritability, rapid speech, demanding and controlling behavior, frequent call-light signaling, seeking reassurance, unusual quietness

Data Analysis

Nursing Diagnosis

FEAR OF DYSFUNCTION OF AN INTERNAL PROSTHESIS: A feeling of alarm and fright about possible malfunction of a replacement body part that has been surgically implanted

Common Etiology (Stressors)

PSYCHOSOCIAL FACTORS: The threat of a specific and clearly identified danger, the threat of real or imagined danger

HEALTH CARE FACTORS: *Surgical procedures*: Arterioplasty, mammoplasty, valvuloplasty. *Therapeutic devices*: Arterial, hip, knee, or penile internal prosthesis

PLANNING

Unmet Needs

Comfort, protection from phychologic threat, acceptance, caring and communicating relationships, high evaluation of self, sense of adequacy, personal growth and maturity, increased learning, increased reality perception and problem-solving ability

Expected Outcome

Person verbalizes fears
Verbalizes feelings of adequacy and competence in meeting the fear-creating experience
Verbalizes self-satisfaction and growth in having coped with the fear-creating experience
Calm, relaxed facial expression, body movements, and behavior

NURSING INTERVENTIONS

Nursing Treatments

Approach unhurriedly
Reassure verbally
Demonstrate calmness
Provide an atmosphere of acceptance
Encourage the expression of feelings (about the fear)
Listen attentively
Offer feedback to the person's expressed feelings
Communicate nurse sensitivity to the person's problem
Relate to the person on an adult–adult level, not on a parent–child level (which could increase fear)
Attend the person constantly (until he feels sufficiently comfortable to be alone)
Provide frequent contact with the person (thereafter)
Ask the person to identify the problem
Ask for specifics, not generalizations, about the problem
Provide reliable information (about the reliability of the prosthesis)
Ask how the person normally copes with fear (what does he usually do when fearful that reduces the fear?)
Provide whatever the person needs to use his usual coping mechanisms
Explore with the person his strengths and resources (to cope with the fear)
Reduce the demands placed on the person (so that more energy is available for coping)
Introduce to persons who have undergone the same experience (if appropriate)

Nursing Observations

Observe for an excessive stress level (resulting from the fear)
Determine the degree of insight that the person has (into the fear)
Observe for evidence of a favorable response to therapy (reduced fear and increased comfort)

Health Teaching

Explain that the person's response is appropriate and commonly experienced
Recommend a habitual, positive mental attitude (toward the prosthesis)
Explain how the equipment works (show the person a similar prosthesis)

EVALUATION

Record actual outcome

FEAR OF DYSFUNCTION OF A LIFE-SUPPORT SYSTEM [105,471,525]

ASSESSMENT

Data Collection

Subjective Data
- Person experiences feelings of threat or danger
- Can describe or identify the threat or danger
  Questions the reliability of the support system
  Inquires about how it works
  Is concerned with the outcome should the system fail
  Wonders if there is a back-up system
  Fears being alone

Objective Data
- May manifest physical findings such as facial flushing or pallor, rapid or deep respirations, rapid or bounding pulse, increased blood pressure, sweating, trembling
- May exhibit behavior such as restlessness, sleep disturbances, change in eating habits, irritability, rapid speech, demanding and controlling behavior, frequent call-light signaling, seeking reassurance, unusual quietness

Data Analysis

Nursing Diagnosis
FEAR OF DYSFUNCTION OF LIFE-SUPPORT SYSTEM: A feeling of alarm and fright about possible malfunction of a mechanical system used as a substitute for life-supporting vital functions

Common Etiology (Stressors)
PSYCHOSOCIAL FACTORS: The threat of a specific, clearly identified danger, the threat of real or imagined danger
HEALTH CARE FACTORS: *Therapeutic equipment*: Bypass machine (cardiopulmonary), cannula for hemodialysis (previous or potential loss of the cannula site, or cannula clotting), cardiac pacemaker, defibrillator, hemodialyzer, respirator

PLANNING

Unmet Needs
Comfort, protection from psychologic threat, acceptance, caring and communicating relationships, high evaluation of self, sense of adequacy, personal growth and maturity, increased learning, increased reality perception and problem-solving ability

Expected Outcome
Person expresses fears
Verbalizes feelings of adequacy and competence in meeting the fear-creating experience
Verbalizes self-satisfaction and growth in having coped with the fear-creating experience
Calm, relaxed facial expression, body movements, and behavior

NURSING INTERVENTIONS

Nursing Treatments
Approach unhurriedly
Reassure verbally (that the nurse is available whenever needed)
Demonstrate calmness
Provide an atmosphere of acceptance
Encourage the expression of feelings (about the fear)
Listen attentively
Offer feedback to the person's expressed feelings

Communicate nurse sensitivity to the person's problems

Relate to the person on an adult–adult level, not on a parent–child level (which could increase fear)

Attend the person constantly (until he feels sufficiently comfortable to be alone)

Provide frequent contact with the person (thereafter)

Ask the person to identify the problem

Ask for specifics, not generalizations, about the problem

Provide reliable information (about the reliability of the support system, that there are back-up systems)

Ask how the person normally copes with fear (what does he usually do when fearful that reduces the fear?)

Provide whatever the person needs to use his usual coping mechanisms

Do not allow unpleasant surprise situations (such as malfunctioning equipment)

Nursing Observations

Observe for an excessive stress level (resulting from the fear)

Determine the degree of insight that the person has (into the fear)

Observe for evidence of a favorable response to therapy (reduced fear and increased comfort)

Health Teaching

Explain that the person's response is appropriate and commonly experienced (that it is normal to be fearful of that which is new to the person)

Explain how the equipment works (show its safety devices)

EVALUATION

Record actual outcome

FEAR OF ELECTROCUTION [105,471,525]

ASSESSMENT

Data Collection

Subjective Data
• Person experiences feelings of threat or danger
• Can describe or identify the threat or danger
  Makes direct or indirect references to being electrocuted
  May perceive electrical currents, jolts, lights, or alarms as painful or fatal
  May or may not be familiar with the procedure or equipment

Objective Data
• May manifest physical findings such as facial flushing or pallor, rapid or deep respirations, rapid or bounding pulse, increased blood pressure, sweating; trembling
• May exhibit behavior such as restlessness, sleep disturbances, change in eating habits, irritability, short attention span, making poor judgments, forgetfulness, rapid speech, demanding and controlling behavior, crying, avoiding any form of electrical therapy, quietly observing the equipment

Data Analysis

Nursing Diagnosis
FEAR OF ELECTROCUTION: A feeling of alarm and fright about being harmed or killed by procedures or therapy performed with electrical devices

Common Etiology (Stressors)

PSYCHOSOCIAL FACTORS: The threat of a specific and clearly identified danger, the threat of real or imagined danger

HEALTH CARE FACTORS: *Diagnostic procedures*: Electrocardiogram, electroencephalogram, electromyogram. *Medical therapy*: Electroconvulsive therapy. *Surgical therapy*: Cauterization by electrocautery. *Therapeutic equipment*: Cardiac pacemaker, defibrillator, monitoring equipment

PLANNING

Unmet Needs

Comfort, protection from psychologic threat, acceptance, caring and communicating relationships, high evaluation of self, sense of adequacy, personal growth and maturity, increased learning, increased reality perception and problem-solving ability

Expected Outcome

Person verbalizes fears
Verbalizes feelings of adequacy and competence in meeting the fear-creating experience
Verbalizes self-satisfaction and growth in having coped with the fear-creating experience
Calm, relaxed facial expression, body movements, and behavior

NURSING INTERVENTIONS

Nursing Treatments

Approach unhurriedly
Reassure verbally (that the procedures are safe)
Demonstrate calmness
Provide an atmosphere of acceptance
Encourage the expression of feelings (about the fear)
Listen attentively
Offer feedback to the person's expressed feelings
Communicate nurse sensitivity to the person's problem
Relate to the person on an adult–adult level, not on a parent–child level (which could increase fear)
Attend the person constantly (until he feels sufficiently comfortable to be alone)
Provide frequent contact with the person (thereafter)
Ask the person to identify the problem
Ask for specifics, not generalizations, about the problem
Provide reliable information (about the safety of the equipment, that there is no danger because of safety precautions)
Ask how the person normally copes with fear (what does he usually do when fearful that reduces the fear?)
Provide whatever the person needs to use his usual coping mechanisms
Do not allow unpleasant surprise situations (such as electric stimulation without previous warning and explanation)
Introduce to persons who have undergone the same experience (if appropriate)

Nursing Observations

Observe for an excessive stress level (resulting from the fear)
Determine the degree of insight that the person has (into the fear)
Observe for evidence of a favorable response to therapy (reduced fear and increased comfort)

Health Teaching

Explain that the person's response is appropriate and commonly experienced (that it is normal to be fearful of that which is new to the person)
Explain how the equipment works (its purpose, safety features, intended effects)

EVALUATION

Record actual outcome

FEAR OF EMOTIONAL PAIN[105,471,525]

ASSESSMENT

Data Collection

Subjective Data
• Person experiences feelings of threat or danger
• Can describe or identify the threat or danger
  Circumvents the emotional topic in conversation
  Refuses to discuss emotional feelings or situations
  Relates a pattern of avoiding relationships

Objective Data
• May manifest physical findings such as facial flushing or pallor, rapid or deep
  respirations, rapid or bounding pulse, increased blood pressure, sweating, trembling
• May exhibit behavior such as restlessness, sleep disturbances, change in eating habits,
  irritability, short attention span, forgetfulness, rapid speech, demanding and
  controlling behavior, crying, being unavailable for scheduled psychotherapy during
  family crisis, etc.

Data Analysis

Nursing Diagnosis
FEAR OF EMOTIONAL PAIN: A feeling of alarm and fright that severe mental anguish will
  emerge into consciousness

Common Etiology (Stressors)
DISEASES: Major depression
PSYCHOSOCIAL FACTORS: The threat of a specific and clearly identified danger, the threat of
  real or imagined danger
HEALTH CARE FACTORS: *Medical therapy*: Psychotherapy
SITUATIONAL FACTORS: Situational crises such as death of a significant other, divorce, etc.

PLANNING

Unmet Needs

Comfort, protection from psychologic threat, acceptance, caring and communicating relationships, high evaluation of self, sense of adequacy, personal growth and maturity,
  increased learning, increased reality perception and problem-solving ability

Expected Outcome

Person verbalizes fears
Verbalizes feelings of adequacy and competence in meeting the fear-creating experience
Verbalizes self-satisfaction and growth in having coped with the fear-creating experience
Calm, relaxed facial expression, body movements, and behavior

NURSING INTERVENTIONS

Nursing Treatments

Approach unhurriedly
Reassure verbally (that the nurse is available during times of emotional pain)
Demonstrate calmness
Provide an atmosphere of acceptance
Encourage the expression of feelings (about the fear)
Listen attentively
Offer feedback to the person's expressed feelings
Communicate nurse sensitivity to the person's problem
Relate to the person on an adult–adult level, not on a parent–child level (which could
  increase fear)
Attend the person constantly (until he feels sufficiently comfortable to be alone)
Provide frequent contact with the person (thereafter)

Ask the person to identify the problem

Ask for specifics, not generalizations, about the problem

Support a realistic assessment of the situation (that emotional pain is a reality of life)

Ask how the person normally copes with fear (what does he usually do when fearful that reduces the fear?)

Provide whatever the person needs to use his usual coping mechanisms

Encourage the person to face the fear (when able, to reduce the fear)

Explore with the person his strengths and resources (to cope with the fear and the pain)

Encourage awareness of positive responses from others (and focus on positive relationships)

Provide emotionally safe experiences (whenever possible)

Do not allow unpleasant surprise situations (such as discussing very painful subjects without gradual introduction of the subject)

Reduce the demands placed on the person (so that more energy is available for coping)

Introduce to persons who have undergone the same experience (if appropriate)

Nursing Observations

Observe for an excessive stress level (resulting from the fear)

Determine the degree of insight that the person has (into the fear)

Observe for evidence of a favorable response to therapy (reduced fear and increased comfort)

Health Teaching

Explain that the person's response is appropriate and commonly experienced

Advise against fighting fear (this reinforced the emotion)

Explain the importance of recognizing tension within oneself

Explain that fatigue should be recognized as a stress factor (which heightens fear)

Explain the need to recognize highly stressful situations

Explain how to channel emotional energy and obtain release from stress (running, swimming, other sports, creative activities, laughing, talking things over, divert energy into work)

Recommend methods for achieving total relaxation (controlling breathing, quietly listening to music, doing nothing, which reduces fear)

Recommend a habitual, positive mental attitude (about self worth)

Teach how to use the problem-solving method (to reduce emotional pain)

EVALUATION

Record actual outcome

FEAR OF EXSANGUINATION[105,471,525]

ASSESSMENT

Data Collection

Subjective Data

• Person experiences feelings of threat or danger

• Can describe or identify the threat or danger

Is concerned that blood is being drawn from and leaving the body

Wonders if the remaining blood supply is sufficient to sustain him

Inquiries about how the blood will replace itself or be replaced

Fears that if there is mechanical failure of the equipment such as a hemodialyzer, a fatal blood loss will occur

Objective Data

• May manifest physical findings such as facial flushing or pallor, rapid or deep respirations, rapid or bounding pulse, increased blood pressure, sweating, trembling

• May exhibit behavior such as restlessness, sleep disturbances, change in eating habits, irritability, rapid speech, demanding and controlling behavior, crying, avoiding blood donations and blood sampling, fainting at the sight of his own blood

Data Analysis

Nursing Diagnosis
FEAR OF EXSANGUINATION: A feeling of alarm and fright about having blood taken from the body

Common Etiology (Stressors)
PSYCHOSOCIAL FACTORS: The threat of a specific and clearly identified danger, the threat of real or imagined danger.
HEALTH CARE FACTORS: *Health care decisions*: Decision to donate blood. *Diagnostic procedures*: Withdrawing blood samples. *Medical therapy*: Blood exchange on a newborn, hemodialysis, phlebotomy, plasmapheresis, therapeutic apheresis. *Therapeutic equipment*: Extracorporeal circulation by bypass machine

PLANNING

Unmet Needs

Comfort, protection from psychologic threat, acceptance, caring and communicating relationships, high evaluation of self, sense of adequacy, personal growth and maturity, increased learning, increased reality perception and problem-solving ability

Expected Outcome

Person verbalizes fears
Verbalizes feelings of adequacy and competence in meeting the fear-creating experience
Verbalizes self-satisfaction and growth in having coped with the fear-creating experience
Calm, relaxed facial expression, body movements, and behavior

NURSING INTERVENTIONS

Nursing Treatments

Approach unhurriedly
Reassure verbally (that the nurse will not allow the person to be harmed)
Demonstrate calmness
Provide an atmosphere of acceptance
Encourage the expression of feelings (about the fear)
Listen attentively
Offer feedback to the person's expressed feelings
Communicate nurse sensitivity to the person's problem
Relate to the person on an adult–adult level, not on a parent–child level (which could increase fear)
Attend the person constantly (until he feels sufficiently comfortable to be alone)
Provide frequent contact with the person (thereafter)
Ask the person to identify the problem
Ask for specifics, not generalizations, about the problem
Provide reliable information (about the physiologic effects of the procedure)
Ask how the person normally copes with fear (what does he usually do when fearful that reduces the fear?)
Provide whatever the person needs to use his usual coping mechanisms
Explore with the person his strengths and resources (to cope with the fear)
Do not allow unpleasant surprise situations (such as therapy without preparation)
Reduce the demands placed on the person (so that more energy is available for coping)
Introduce to persons who have undergone the same experience (if appropriate)

Nursing Observations

Observe for an excessive stress level (resulting from the fear)
Determine the degree of insight (into the fear)
Observe for evidence of a favorable response to therapy (reduced fear and increased comfort)

Health Teaching
Explain that the person's response is appropriate and commonly experienced

Recommend a habitual, positive mental attitude (that the hemodializer, though often an object of fear and dependence, is primarily a source of improved health)

Explain how the equipment works (the anticipated loss of blood and replacement time, the equipment's positive and safety features)

EVALUATION
Record actual outcome

FEAR OF FAILURE[105,471,525]

ASSESSMENT
Data Collection
Subjective Data
- Person experiences feelings of threat or danger
- Can describe or identify the threat or danger

  Relates an intended goal

  Perceives obstacles to the goal

  Person doubts that he can achieve it, despite wanting to

  Feels threatened by the possibility of nonachievement

  May want to pursue new life endeavors but is concerned that illness might curtail their successful completion

Objective Data
- May manifest physical findings such as facial flushing or pallor, rapid or deep respirations, rapid or bounding pulse, increased blood pressure, sweating, trembling
- May exhibit behavior such as restlessness, sleep disturbances, change in eating habits, irritability, short attention span, making poor judgments, forgetfulness, rapid speech, demanding and controlling behavior, crying, avoiding situations in which failure is possible, seeking reassurance

Data Analysis
Nursing Diagnosis

FEAR OF FAILURE: A feeling of alarm and fright about not being able to achieve an expected or anticipated goal

Common Etiology (Stressors)

SIGNS AND SYMPTOMS: Pain, weakness

PSYCHOSOCIAL FACTORS: The threat of a specific and clearly identified danger; the threat of real or imagined danger; unrealistic expectations of self, or significant other; repeated failure to achieve; lack of emotional support; the threat of delayed goal achievement; lack of training in self-discipline

HUMAN BODY: *Natural body function*: Attempts at conception of a child, childbirth, breastfeeding. *Body state*: Pregnancy

HEALTH CARE FACTORS: *Medical therapy*: Rehabilitation therapy, withdrawal from alcohol, drugs, tobacco *Recovery from illness or injury*: Any. *Hospital leave*: Trial hospital leave

DEVELOPMENTAL PHASES: Childhood, adolescence, early adulthood, adulthood, middle ages, old age

SITUATIONAL FACTORS: Marriage, child rearing

PLANNING

Unmet Needs

Comfort, protection from psychologic threat, acceptance, caring and communicating relationships, high evaluation of self, sense of adequacy, personal growth and maturity, increased learning, increased reality perception and problem-solving ability

Expected Outcome

Person verbalizes fears
Verbalizes feelings of adequacy and competence in meeting the fear-creating experience
Verbalizes self-satisfaction and growth in having coped with the fear-creating experience
Calm, relaxed facial expression, body movements, and behavior

NURSING INTERVENTIONS

Nursing Treatments

Approach unhurriedly
Reassure verbally (that the nurse will help the person to succeed)
Demonstrate calmness
Provide an atmosphere of acceptance
Encourage the expression of feelings (about the fear)
Listen attentively
Offer feedback to the person's expressed feelings
Communicate nurse sensitivity to the person's problem
Relate to the person on an adult–adult level, not on a parent–child level (which could increase fear)
Ask the person to identify the problem
Ask for specifics, not generalizations, about the problem
Provide reliable information (which will reduce the probability of failure)
Ask how the person normally copes with fear (what does he usually do when fearful that reduces the fear?)
Provide whatever the person needs to use his usual coping mechanisms
Encourage the person to face the fear (when able, to reduce the fear)
Explore with the person his strengths and resources (to bring about success rather than failure)
Introduce to persons who have undergone the same experience (if appropriate)

Nursing Observations

Observe for an excessive stress level (resulting from the fear)
Determine the degree of insight that the person has (into the fear)
Observe for evidence of a favorable response to therapy (reduced fear and increased comfort)

Health Teaching

Explain that the person's response is appropriate and commonly experienced
Explain that fatigue should be recognized as a stress factor (which heightens fear)
Explain the need to recognize highly stressful situations
Explain how to channel emotional energy and obtain release from stress (sports, creative activities, laughing, talking things over)
Recommend methods for achieving total relaxation (controlled breathing, quietly listening to music, doing nothing, which reduces fear)
Recommend a habitual, positive mental attitude (toward the endeavor)
Teach how to use the problem-solving method (include setting short-term, readily attainable goals to avoid failure)

EVALUATION

Record actual outcome

FEAR OF FALLING [105,471,525]

ASSESSMENT

Data Collection

Subjective Data
- Person experiences feelings of threat or danger
- Can describe or identify the threat or danger
  Feels unsteady
  Prefers not to be rushed
  May refuse to attempt body movement

Objective Data
- May manifest physical findings such as facial flushing or pallor, rapid or deep respirations, rapid or bounding pulse, increased blood pressure, sweating, trembling
- May exhibit behavior such as restlessness, rapid speech, demanding and controlling behavior, crying, avoiding situations in which he might fall, holding onto another person or stable objects

Data Analysis

Nursing Diagnosis
FEAR OF FALLING: A feeling of alarm and fright about losing one's balance or support and dropping to the ground or floor

Common Etiology (Stressors)
BIRTH DEFECTS: Cerebral palsy, club foot, congenital hip dislocation, Duchenne's muscular dystrophy
DISEASES: Cerebrovascular disease, epilepsy, glaucoma, labyrinthitis, Meniere's disease, multiple sclerosis, myasthenia gravis, Parkinson's disease, rheumatoid arthritis
INJURIES: Bone fracture
SIGNS AND SYMPTOMS: Ataxia, dizziness, weakness, vertigo
PSYCHOSOCIAL FACTORS: The threat of a specific and clearly identified danger, the threat of real or imagined danger
HUMAN BODY: *Body States*: Pregnancy
HEALTH CARE FACTORS: *Health care environment*: Hospital bed, stretcher. *Diagnostic equipment*: Tilt table or somersault chair used in x-ray. *Medical therapy*: Tilt table for physical therapy. *Surgical therapy*: Recovery from anesthesia. *Drug therapy*: Adverse effects of heavy drug sedation from sedatives. *Therapeutic equipment*: CircOlectic bed, Stryker frame. *Therapeutic devices*: Use of a brace, cane, crutches, leg/foot prosthesis, walker
DEVELOPMENTAL PHASES: Infancy, old age

PLANNING

Unmet Needs
Comfort, protection from psychologic threat, acceptance, caring and communicating relationships, high evaluation of self, sense of adequacy, personal growth and maturity, increased learning, increased reality perception and problem-solving ability

Expected Outcome
Person verbalizes fears
Verbalizes feelings of adequacy and competence in meeting the fear-creating experience
Verbalizes self-satisfaction and growth in having coped with the fear-creating experience
Calm, relaxed facial expression, body movements, and behavior

NURSING INTERVENTIONS

Nursing Treatments
Approach unhurriedly
Reassure verbally (that the nurse will safeguard the person)
Demonstrate calmness
Provide an atmosphere of acceptance

Encourage the expression of feelings (about the fear)

Listen attentively

Offer feedback to the person's expressed feelings

Communicate nurse sensitivity to the person's problem

Assist with mobility

Attend the person constantly (until he can walk steadily)

Provide reliable information (about the safety of the equipment or devices from which he thinks he might fall)

Do not allow unpleasant surprise situations (such as turning the person on a Stryker frame without warning)

Encourage mutual problem solving (in determining methods to avoid falling)

Nursing Observations

Observe for an excessive stress level (resulting from the fear)

Observe for evidence of a favorable response to therapy (reduced fear and increased comfort)

Health Teaching

Explain that the person's response is appropriate and commonly experienced

EVALUATION

Record actual outcome

FEAR OF FETAL INJURY[105,471,525]

ASSESSMENT

Data Collection

Subjective Data

• Person experiences feelings of threat or danger

• Can describe or identify the threat or danger

  Is concerned about the unborn fetus

  Desires to protect the child

  Questions the effect of procedures, disease, etc., on the fetus

  May refuse certain procedures or therapy

  May relate the practice of superstitious rituals to protect the fetus

Objective Data

• May manifest physical findings such as facial flushing or pallor, rapid or deep respirations, rapid or bounding pulse, increased blood pressure, sweating, trembling

• May exhibit behavior such as restlessness, sleep disturbances, change in eating habits, irritability, demanding and controlling behavior, crying, seeking reassurance

Data Analysis

Nursing Diagnosis

FEAR OF FETAL INJURY: A feeling of alarm and fright that an external force might injure the unborn child

Common Etiology (Stressors)

DISEASES (MATERNAL): Alcoholism, drug addiction, measles, rubella

INJURIES: Trauma of any kind

PSYCHOSOCIAL FACTORS: The threat of a specific, clearly identified danger; the threat of real or imagined danger

HEALTH CARE FACTORS: *Diagnostic procedures*: Amniocentesis, exposure to x-ray. *Drug therapy*: Adverse effects of or adverse interactions of drugs. *Surgical therapy*: Anesthesia, cesarean section, forceps delivery

LIFESTYLE: *Cultural*: Superstitions. *Smoking*: High nicotine intake (of mother)

SITUATIONAL FACTORS: Mother victimized by sexual assault
ENVIRONMENTAL FACTORS: *Chemical substances*: Inhalation or ingestion of chemical substances.
Environmental radiation: Overexposure to

PLANNING

Unmet Needs

Comfort, protection from psychologic threat, acceptance, caring and communicating relationships, high evaluation of self, sense of adequacy, personal growth and maturity
increased learning, increased reality perception and problem-solving ability

Expected Outcome

Person verbalizes fears
Verbalizes feelings of adequacy and competence in meeting the fear-creating experience
Verbalizes self-satisfaction and growth in having coped with the fear-creating experience
Calm, relaxed facial expression, body movements, and behavior

NURSING INTERVENTIONS

Nursing Treatments

Approach unhurriedly
Reassure verbally (that the nurse will help protect the fetus)
Demonstrate calmness
Provide an atmosphere of acceptance
Encourage the expression of feelings (about the fear)
Listen attentively
Offer feedback to the person's expressed feelings
Communicate nurse sensitivity to the person's problem
Attend the person constantly (until she feels assured of the fetus' safety)
Ask the person to identify the problem
Ask for specifics, not generalizations, about the problem
Provide reliable information (about procedures and their safeness)
Ask how the person normally copes with fear (what does she usually do when fearful
that reduces the fear?)
Provide whatever the person needs to use her usual coping mechanisms
Do not allow unpleasant surprise situations (such as procedures that might threaten the
fetus without prior explanation)
Introduce to persons who have undergone the same experience (if appropriate)

Nursing Observations

Observe for an excessive stress level (resulting from the fear)
Determine the degree of insight that the person has (into the fear)
Observe for evidence of a favorable response to therapy (reduced fear and increased
comfort)

Health Teaching

Explain that the person's response is appropriate and commonly experienced

EVALUATION

Record actual outcome

FEAR OF FINANCIAL LOSS [105,471,525]

ASSESSMENT

Data Collection

Subjective Data
• Person experiences feelings of threat or danger

- Can describe or identify the threat or danger
  Is concerned with personal money matters
  Indicates that funds will be wiped out or that funds are insufficient to meet the situation
  May be concerned with obtaining assistance
  May describe feeling helpless

Objective Data
- May manifest physical findings such as facial flushing or pallor, rapid or deep respirations, rapid or bounding pulse, increased blood pressure, sweating, trembling
- May exhibit behavior such as restlessness, sleep disturbances, change in eating habits, irritability, demanding and controlling behavior, not keeping health care appointments because of worry about costs

Data Analysis

Nursing Diagnosis
FEAR OF FINANCIAL LOSS: A feeling of alarm and fright about losing financial reserves or being plunged into debt

Common Etiology (Stressors)
PSYCHOSOCIAL FACTORS: The threat of a specific and clearly identified danger, the threat of real or imagined danger
HEALTH CARE FACTORS: *Health Care Costs*: High
SITUATIONAL FACTORS: Natural or man-made disaster, illness (acute or chronic), loss of or uncertain employment, insufficient or lack of insurance coverage

PLANNING

Unmet Needs

Comfort, protection from psychologic threat, acceptance, caring and communicating relationships, high evaluation of self, sense of adequacy, personal growth and maturity, increased learning, increased reality perception and problem-solving ability

Expected Outcome

Person verbalizes fears
Verbalizes feelings of adequacy and competence in meeting the fear-creating experience
Verbalizes self-satisfaction and growth in having coped with the fear-creating experience
Calm, relaxed facial expression, body movements, and behavior

NURSING INTERVENTIONS

Nursing Treatments

Approach unhurriedly
Reassure verbally (that the nurse will help the person as much as possible)
Demonstrate calmness
Provide an atmosphere of acceptance
Encourage the expression of feelings (about the fear)
Listen attentively
Offer feedback to the person's expressed feelings
Communicate nurse sensitivity to the person's problem
Ask the person to identify the problem
Ask for specifics, not generalizations, about the problem
Provide reliable information (about financial resources available)
Ask how the person normally copes with fear (what does he usually do when fearful that reduces the fear?)
Provide whatever the person needs to use his usual coping mechanisms
Explore with the person his strengths and resources
Do not allow unpleasant surprise situations (such as unexpected health care bills)
Make a referral (for financial counseling or to other appropriate agencies)

Nursing Observations

Observe for an excessive stress level (resulting from the fear)

Observe for evidence of a favorable response to therapy (reduced fear and increased comfort)

Health Teaching
Explain that the person's response is appropriate and commonly experienced
Teach how to use the problem-solving method (to prevent or diminish financial loss)

EVALUATION
Record actual outcome

FEAR OF HARMING ANOTHER[105,471,525]

ASSESSMENT
Data Collection
Subjective Data
• Person experiences feelings of threat or danger
• Can describe or identify the threat or danger
  Is concerned that his actions might result in another's suffering
  Questions what the effects of his actions will be
  Recognizes limitations within himself
  Verbalizes fear of losing control

Objective Data
• May manifest physical findings such as facial flushing or pallor, rapid or deep respirations, rapid or bounding pulse, increased blood pressure, sweating, trembling
• May exhibit behavior such as restlessness, sleep disturbances, change in eating habits, irritability, demanding and controlling behavior, crying, avoiding being with or doing things for the other person, showing excessive concern for the person he fears harming

Data Analysis
Nursing Diagnosis
FEAR OF HARMING ANOTHER: A feeling of alarm and fright about being the cause of physical injury, emotional pain, or other untoward effects to another person

Common Etiology (Stressors)
DISEASES: Alcoholism, drug addiction, major depression
INJURIES: Child, parent, or spouse abuse
PSYCHOSOCIAL FACTORS: The threat of a specific and clearly identified danger, the threat of real or imagined danger, lack of emotional control, the threat of compelling thoughts
HEALTH CARE FACTORS: *Health care procedures for a significant other*: Having to perform health care procedures for a significant other
SITUATIONAL FACTORS: First experience with child rearing

PLANNING
Unmet Needs
Comfort, protection from psychologic threat, acceptance, caring and communicating relationships, high evaluation of self, sense of adequacy, personal growth and maturity, increased learning, increased reality perception and problem-solving ability

Expected Outcome
Person verbalizes fears
Verbalizes feelings of adequacy and competence in meeting the fear-creating experience
Verbalizes self-satisfaction and growth in having coped with the fear-creating experience
Calm, relaxed facial expression, body movements, and behavior

NURSING INTERVENTIONS

Nursing Treatments

Approach unhurriedly

Reassure verbally (that the nurse will help the person so that he will not harm others)

Demonstrate calmness

Provide an atmosphere of acceptance

Obtain a complete present and past history

Encourage the expression of feelings (about the fear)

Listen attentively

Offer feedback to the person's expressed feelings

Communicate nurse sensitivity to the person's problem

Relate to the person on an adult–adult level, not on a parent–child level (which could increase fear)

Attend the person constantly (until he feels sufficiently sure that he will not harm another person)

Provide frequent contact with the person (thereafter)

Ask the person to identify the problem

Ask for specifics, not generalizations, about the problem

Support a realistic assessment of the situation (of the probability of harming another)

Ask how the person normally copes with fear (what does he usually do when fearful that reduces the fear?)

Provide whatever the person needs to use his usual coping mechanisms

Encourage the person to face the fear (when able, to reduce the fear)

Nursing Observations

Observe for an excessive stress level (resulting from the fear)

Determine the degree of insight that the person has (into the fear)

Observe for evidence of a favorable response to therapy (reduced fear and increased comfort)

Health Teaching

Explain that the person's response is appropriate and commonly experienced

Explain the importance of recognizing tension within oneself (to aid impulse control)

Explain why persons should maintain self-control (out of self-respect for others, because of the harmful effect that noncontrol has on others, because such behavior is often futile in attaining goals)

Explain the need to recognize highly stressful situations (such as family discord, etc.)

Explain how to channel emotional energy and obtain release from stress (through sports, work, creative activities, laughing, talking things over)

Recommend things to to when the person begins to feel out of control (temporary withdrawal from the situation, deep breathing to promote relaxation, washing the face and hands in cold water)

Explain the reason for and intended effect of the methods used (to prevent the person from harming others; include an explanation of nursing's legal responsibility to prevent a person from harming himself or others)

EVALUATION

Record actual outcome

FEAR OF HEARING LOSS[105,471,525]

ASSESSMENT

Data Collection

Subjective Data

• Person experiences feelings of threat or danger

• Can describe or identify the threat or danger
  Relates concern about hearing perception
  May be experiencing diminished hearing
  Contemplates the unfavorable effects of hearing loss

Objective Data
• May manifest physical findings such as facial flushing or pallor, rapid or deep respirations, rapid or bounding pulse, increased blood pressure, sweating, trembling
• May exhibit behavior such as restlessness, sleep disturbances, change in eating habits, irritability, rapid speech, demanding and controlling behavior, accusing others of not speaking clearly, avoiding drugs, surgery, etc., guessing at what is being said if hearing is impaired

Data Analysis

Nursing Diagnosis
FEAR OF HEARING LOSS: A feeling of alarm and fright that hearing might be or become impaired

Common Etiology (Stressors)
DISEASES: Acoustic nerve tumor, mastoiditis, otitis media, otoscleroris, serous otitis media
INJURIES: Contusion of ear, foreign body in ear
SIGNS AND SYMPTOMS: Earache, tinnitus
PSYCHOSOCIAL FACTORS: The threat of a specific and clearly identified danger, the threat of real or imagined danger
HEALTH CARE FACTORS: *Drug therapy*: Adverse effects of gentamicin, streptomycin. *Surgical procedures*: Tympanoplasty
DEVELOPMENTAL PHASES: Old age
ENVIRONMENTAL FACTORS: *Blast or explosion*: Exposure to blast. *Noise*: Prolonged exposure to loud noise or music

PLANNING

Unmet Needs

Comfort, protection from psychologic threat, acceptance, caring and communicating relationships, high evaluation of self, sense of adequacy, personal growth and maturity, increased learning, increased reality perception and problem-solving ability

Expected Outcome

Person verbalizes fears
Verbalizes feelings of adequacy and competence in meeting the fear-creating experience
Verbalizes self-satisfaction and growth in having coped with the fear-creating experience
Calm, relaxed facial expression, body movements, and behavior

NURSING INTERVENTIONS

Nursing Treatments

Approach unhurriedly
Reassure verbally (that the nurse will help the person as much as possible)
Demonstrate calmness
Provide an atmosphere of acceptance
Encourage the expression of feelings (about the fear)
Listen attentively
Offer feedback to the person's expressed feelings
Communicate nurse sensitivity to the person's problem
Ask the person to identify the problem
Ask for specifics, not generalizations, about the problem
Support a realistic assessment of the situation (about the probability of hearing loss occurring)
Provide reliable information (about procedures, environmental noise, etc.)

Ask how the person normally copes with fear (what does he usually do when fearful that reduces the fear?)

Provide whatever the person needs to use his usual coping mechanisms

Make a referral (to a physician if hearing is diminished)

Nursing Observations

Observe for an excessive stress level (resulting from the fear)

Observe for evidence of a favorable response to therapy (reduced fear and increased comfort)

Health Teaching

Explain that the person's response is appropriate and commonly experienced (after trauma or before impending ear surgery)

Recommend a habitual, positive mental attitude (toward surgery, procedures, and preventive noise reduction)

EVALUATION

Record actual outcome

FEAR OF IMPOTENCE[105,471,525]

ASSESSMENT

Data Collection

Subjective Data

• Person experiences feelings of threat or danger

• Can describe or identify the threat or danger

Verbalizes fear that certain diseases, drugs, or procedures will affect his ability to engage in sexual intercourse

Relates that sexual limitations are unacceptable

May relate avoiding sexual activity for fear of discovering limitations

May relate over-engaging in sexual activity to prove the absence of impotence

Objective Data

• May manifest physical findings such as facial flushing or pallor, rapid or deep respirations, rapid or bounding pulse, increased blood pressure, sweating, trembling

• May exhibit behavior such as restlessness, sleep disturbances, change in eating habits, irritability, short attention span, making poor judgments, forgetfulness, rapid speech, demanding and controlling behavior, frequent call-light signaling, seeking reassurance, making sexual advances to nurses

Data Analysis

Nursing Diagnosis

FEAR OF IMPOTENCE: A feeling of alarm and fright about a man's being unable to engage in sexual intercourse

Common Etiology (Stressors)

DISEASES: Cancer of or near the reproductive organs, diabetes mellitus, infection of the reproductive organs, sickle cell anemia

INJURIES: Any injury to the genitalia, compression and fracture of the spinal cord

SIGNS AND SYMPTOMS: Priapism

PSYCHOSOCIAL FACTORS: The threat of a specific and clearly identified danger, the threat of real or imagined danger

HEALTH CARE FACTORS: *Diagnostic procedures*: Cystometry, cystoscopy, cystourethrography, retrograde pyleogram or urethrography. *Drug therapy*: Chemotherapy, antihypertensive drugs, antidepressants, Tagamet, major tranquilizers. *Medical therapy*: Bladder irrigation, radiation therapy of the genitalia, urinary catheterization. *Surgical procedures*: Cystectomy, cystostomy, orchiectomy, prostatectomy, ureterocolostomy, ureteroileostomy, ureterosigmoidostomy, ureterostomy, ureterotomy, vasectomy

PLANNING

Unmet Needs

Comfort, protection from psychologic threat, acceptance, caring and communicating relationships, high evaluation of self, sense of adequacy, personal growth and maturity, increased learning, spiritual-philosophic satisfaction, increased reality perception and problem-solving ability

Expected Outcome

Person verbalizes fears
Verbalizes feelings of adequacy and competence in meeting the fear-creating experience
Verbalizes self-satisfaction and growth in having coped with the fear-creating experience
Calm, relaxed facial expression, body movements, and behavior

NURSING INTERVENTIONS

Nursing Treatments

Approach unhurriedly
Reassure verbally (that the nurse will help the person as much as possible)
Demonstate calmness
Provide an atmosphere of acceptance
Encourage the expression of feelings (about the fear)
Listen attentively
Offer feedback to the person's expressed feelings
Communicate that the nurse feels comfortable with the person's discussions of sex
Relates to the person on an adult–adult level, not on a parent–child level (which could increase fear)
Ask the person to identify the problem
Ask for specifics, not generalizations, about the problem
Provide reliable information (about procedures, drugs, and diseases, about the probability of impotence, about how to attain returned sexual function or make adaptations for satisfying sexual relations)
Ask how the person normally copes with fear (what does he usually do when fearful that reduces the fear)
Provide whatever the person needs to use his usual coping mechanisms
Introduce to persons who have undergone the same experience (if appropriate)

Nursing Observations

Observe for an excessive stress level (resulting from the fear)
Determine the degree of insight that the person has (into the fear)
Observe for evidence of a favorable response to therapy (reduced fear and increased comfort)

Health Teaching

Explain that the person's response is appropriate and commonly experienced
Explain that sexual function may be slow to return (such as following a prostatectomy when erection is difficult for a few weeks, but sexual function does return to normal)

EVALUATION

Record actual outcome

FEAR OF INCISION RUPTURE[105,471,525]

ASSESSMENT
Data Collection

Subjective Data
- Person experiences feelings of threat or danger
- Can describe or identify the threat or danger
  Frequently discusses or visualizes the incision
  Perceives the incision as a weakened body area
  May ask if the incision will break apart
  May refuse certain treatments

Objective Data
- May manifest physical findings such as facial flushing or pallor, rapid or deep respirations, rapid or bounding pulse, increased blood pressure, sweating, trembling
- May exhibit behavior such as restlessness, sleep disturbances, change in eating habits, irritability, rapid speech, demanding and controlling behavior, guarding the incision, seeking reassurance

Data Analysis

Nursing Diagnosis
FEAR OF INCISION RUPTURE: A feeling of alarm and fright that a surgical or traumatic incision might break open

Common Etiology (Stressors)
DISEASES: Obesity
INJURIES: Any trauma
SIGNS AND SYMPTOMS: Ascites, edema
PSYCHOSOCIAL FACTORS: The threat of a specific and clearly identified danger, the threat of real or imagined danger
HEALTH CARE FACTORS: *Medical therapy*: Ambulation, coughing and deep breathing, enemas, exercise, intermittent positive pressure breathing, bladder or colonic irrigations, therapeutic turning. *Surgical procedures*: Removal of sutures
LIFESTYLES: Employment requiring heavy lifting

PLANNING
Unmet Needs
Comfort, protection from psychologic threat, acceptance, caring and communicating relationships, high evaluation of self, sense of adequacy, personal growth and maturity, increased learning, increased reality perception and problem-solving ability

Expected Outcome
Person verbalizes fears
Verbalizes feelings of adequacy and competence in meeting fear-creating experience
Verbalizes self-satisfaction and growth in having coped with the fear-creating experience
Calm, relaxed facial expression, body movements, and behavior

NURSING INTERVENTIONS
Nursing Treatments
Approach unhurriedly
Reasurre verbally (that the incision will not rupture)
Support a realistic assessment of the situation (that incision rupture rarely occurs, but if it does, it will be repaired)
Demonstrate calmness
Provide an atmosphere of acceptance
Encourage the expression of feelings (about the fear)

Listen attentively

Offer feedback to the person's expressed feelings

Communicate nurse sensitivity to the person's problems

Relate to the person on an adult–adult level, not on a parent–child level (which could increase fear)

Ask the person to identify the problem

Ask for specifics, not generalizations, about the problem

Provide reliable information (that the sutures are strong and resist tension, that they are not removed until healing has occurred)

Ask how the person normally copes with fear (what does he usually do when fearful that reduces the fear?)

Provide whatever the person needs to use his usual coping mechanisms

Nursing Observations

Observe for an excessive stress level (resulting from the fear)

Determine the degree of insight that the person has (into the fear)

Observe for evidence of a favorable response to therapy (reduced fear and increased comfort)

Health Teaching

Explain that the person's response is appropriate and commonly experienced

Teach the specific procedures (of coughing and deep breathing, turning, ambulation, etc., so there is minimal tension on the incision)

EVALUATION

Record actual outcome

FEAR OF INTERNAL ORGAN INJURY[105,471,525]

ASSESSMENT

Data Collection

Subjective Data

• Person experiences feelings of threat or danger
• Can describe or identify the threat or danger
  Relates concern about organs within the body
  May focus on a specific organ
  Inquires about possible harm to the organ
  May refuse invasive procedures

Objective Data

• May manifest physical findings such as facial flushing or pallor, rapid or deep respirations, rapid or bounding pulse, increased blood pressure, sweating, trembling
• May exhibit behavior such as restlessness, sleep disturbances, change in eating habits, irritability, demanding and controlling behavior, crying, avoiding activity or being unavailable for invasive procedures, seeking reassurance

Data Analysis

Nursing Diagnosis

FEAR OF INTERNAL ORGAN INJURY: A feeling of alarm and fright about injury occurring to organs within the body

Common Etiology (Stressors)

INJURIES: Contusion, electric shock, penetrating wound, poisoning

PSYCHOSOCIAL FACTORS: The threat of a specific and clearly identified danger, the threat of real or imagined danger

HEALTH CARE FACTORS: *Diagnostic procedures*: Barium enema, biopsy (kidney, liver, lung), broncoscopy, cardiac catheterization, colonscopy, gastroscopy, proctoscopy. *Medical therapy*: Chest tubes and drainage, coughing and deep breathing, enemas, intermittent positive-pressure breathing, irrigation (bladder, colonic, ear), paracentesis, radiation therapy, thoracentesis, urinary catheterization. *Therapeutic equipment*: Cardiac pacemaker

PLANNING

Unmet Needs

Comfort, protection from psychologic threat, acceptance, caring and communicating relationships, high evaluation of self, sense of adequacy, personal growth and maturity, increased learning, increased reality perception and problem-solving abiity

Expected Outcome

Person verbalizes fears

Verbalizes feelings of adequacy and competence in meeting the fear-creating experience

Verbalizes self-satisfaction and growth in having coped with the fear-creating experience

Calm, relaxed facial expression, body movements, and behavior

NURSING INTERVENTIONS

Nursing Treatments

Approach unhurriedly

Reassure verbally (that the nurse will help the person as much as possible)

Demonstrate calmness

Provide an atmosphere of acceptance

Encourage the expression of feelings (about the fear)

Listen attentively

Offer feedback to the person's expressed feelings

Communicate nurse sensitivity to the person's problem

Relate to the person on an adult–adult level, not on a parent–child level (which could increase fear)

Ask the person to identify the problem

Ask for specifics, not generalizations, about the problem

Provide reliable information (about the effects of specific procedures, about the probability of internal organ injury)

Ask how the person normally copes with fear (what does he usually do when fearful that reduces the fear?)

Provide whatever the person needs to use his usual coping mechanisms

Do not allow unpleasant surprise situations (such as performing procedures without prior information)

Introduce to persons who have undergone the same experience (if appropriate)

Nursing Observations

Observe for an excessive stress level (resulting from the fear)

Determine the degree of insight that the person has (into the fear)

Observe for evidence of a favorable response to therapy (reduced fear and increased comfort)

Health Teaching

Explain that the person's response is appropriate and commonly experienced

Teach the specific methods (that can prevent injury of internal organs, such as correct positioning, proper support, specified immobility, etc.)

EVALUATION

Record actual outcome

FEAR OF INVOLUNTARY INSTITUTIONALIZATION[105,471,525]

ASSESSMENT

Data Collection

Subjective Data
- Person experiences feelings of threat or danger
- Can describe or identify the threat or danger
  Is concerned about being placed in a hospital, nursing home, rehabilitation center, etc.
  Feels such placement is unacceptable
  Verbalizes preference for other choices
  May plead or beg not to be forced into an institution
  May refuse to be institutionalized or threaten those involved in the proceedings

Objective Data
- May manifest physical findings such as facial flushing or pallor, rapid or deep respirations, rapid or bounding pulse, increased blood pressure, sweating, trembling
- May exhibit behavior such as restlessness, sleep disturbances, change in eating habits, irritability, rapid speech, demanding and controlling behavior, crying, avoiding persons who could institutionalize him, running away

Data Analysis

Nursing Diagnosis
FEAR OF INVOLUNTARY INSTITUTIONALIZATION: A feeling of alarm and fright about being placed in an institution against one's will or without one's permission

Common Etiology (Stressors)
BIRTH DEFECTS: Cerebral palsy, developmental deficit, Down's syndrome
DISEASES: Alcoholism, carcinoma, cerebrovascular accident, drug addiction, multiple sclerosis, myasthenia gravis, organic brain syndrome, Parkinson's disease, schizophrenia
INJURIES: Fracture and compression of the spinal cord
SIGNS AND SYMPTOMS: Immobility, weakness, psychosis
PSYCHOSOCIAL FACTORS: The threat of a specific and clearly identified danger, the threat of real or imagined danger, loss of independence, lack of a care-providing significant other
DEVELOPMENTAL PHASES: Old age
SITUATIONAL FACTORS: Being a foster child, death of a significant other, loss of home, lack of finances, geographically distant family

PLANNING

Unmet Needs

Comfort, protection from psychologic threat, acceptance, caring and communicating relationships, high evaluation of self, sense of adequacy, personal growth and maturity, increased learning, increased reality perception and problem-solving ability

Expected Outcome

Person verbalizes fears
Verbalizes feelings of adequacy and competence in meeting the fear-creating experience
Verbalizes self-satisfaction and growth in having coped with the fear-creating experience
Calm, relaxed facial expression, body movements, and behavior

NURSING INTERVENTIONS

Nursing Treatments

Approach unhurriedly
Reassure verbally (that the nurse will help the person as much as possible)
Demonstrate calmness

Provide an atmosphere of acceptance
Encourage the expression of feelings (about the fear)
Listen attentively
Offer feedback to the person's expressed feelings
Communicate nurse sensitivity to the person's problem
Relate to the person on an adult–adult level, not on a parent–child level (which could increase fear)
Ask the person to identify the problem
Ask for specifics, not generalizations, about the problem
Support a realistic assessment of the situation (if institutionalization is the only safe choice)
Provide reliable information (about other choices, about the benefits of some institutions)
Ask how the person normally copes with fear (what does he usually do when fearful that reduces the fear?)
Provide whatever the person needs to use his usual coping mechanisms
Do not allow unpleasant surprise situations (such as unexpected moves to a nursing home or institution)
Introduce to persons who have undergone the same experience (if appropriate)

Nursing Observations
Observe for an excessive stress level (resulting from the fear)
Observe for evidence of a favorable response to therapy (reduced fear and increased comfort)

Health Teaching
Explain that the person's response is appropriate and commonly experienced
Recommend a preadmission visit to a nursing home or institution
Recommend a trial period before making a final decision (many persons find that they prefer a rehabilitation center to a hospital after they become acquainted with and begin the program)

EVALUATION
Record actual outcome

FEAR OF LOSS OF THE ABILITY TO COMMUNICATE[105,471,525]

ASSESSMENT
Data Collection
Subjective Data
• Person experiences feelings of threat or danger
• Can describe or identify the threat or danger
  Relates concern about not being able to communicate
  May seek agreement on signals for communicating
  Is concerned that impairment may be permanent

Objective Data
• May manifest physical findings such as facial flushing or pallor, rapid or deep respirations, rapid or bounding pulse, increased blood pressure, sweating, trembling
• May exhibit behavior such as restlessness, sleep disturbances, change in eating habits, irritability, demanding and controlling behavior, crying, avoiding threatening situations such as surgery, frequent call-light signaling, unusual quietness

Data Analysis

Nursing Diagnosis

FEAR OF LOSS OF THE ABILITY TO COMMUNICATE: A feeling of alarm and fright about being unable to verbally relate to another one's needs or desires

Common Etiology (Stressors)

DISEASES: Carcinoma (of larynx, tongue, mouth), cerebral vascular accident, subarachnoid hemorrhage, subdural hematoma

SIGNS AND SYMPTOMS: Laryngeal edema

PSYCHOSOCIAL FACTORS: The threat of a specific and clearly identified danger, the threat of real or imagined danger

HEALTH CARE FACTORS: *Diagnostic procedures*: Broncoscopy, gastroscopy. *Medical therapy*: Heated mist inhalation therapy, continuous or intermittent positive-pressure breathing, endotracheal intubation. *Surgical therapy*: Anesthesia. *Surgical procedure*: Gingivectomy, gingivoplasty, laryngotomy, thyroidectomy, wiring of mandible fracture (or other oral surgery). *Adverse effects of drug or surgical therapy*: Heavy drug sedation from sedatives, loss of speech from glossectomy, laryngectomy, tracheostomy, vocal cordectomy

PLANNING

Unmet Needs

Comfort, protection from psychologic threat, acceptance, caring and communicating relationships, high evaluation of self, sense of adequacy, personal growth and maturity, increased learning, increased reality perception and problem-solving ability

Expected Outcome

Person verbalizes fear

Verbalizes feelings of adequacy and competence in meeting the fear-creating experience

Verbalizes self-satisfaction and growth in having coped with the fear-creating experince

Calm, relaxed facial expression, body movements, and behavior

NURSING INTERVENTIONS

Nursing Treatments

Approach unhurriedly

Reassure verbally (that the nurse will help the person as much as possible)

Demonstrate calmness

Provide an atmosphere of acceptance

Encourage the expression of feelings (about the fear)

Listen attentively

Offer feedback to the person's expressed feelings

Communicate nurse sensitivity to the person's problem

Relate to the person on an adult–adult level, not on a parent–child level (which could increase fear)

Ask the person to identify the problem

Ask for specifics, not generalizations, about the problem

Provide reliable information (about the degree of communication impairment to expect)

Attend the person constantly (until he appears satisfied that he will be able to communicate)

Ask how the person normally copes with fear (what does he usually do when fearful that reduces the fear?

Provide whatever the person needs to use his usual coping mechanisms

Explore with the person his strengths and resources (to cope with the loss of communication ability)

Provide an alternative method of communication appropriate to the person's specific needs and abilities (such as paper and pencil, magic slate, hand and eye signals, words and phrases cards, picture cards of objects, alphabet letters for word composition, computerized devices)

Respond immediately to the person's call (if he has a problem communicating)
Avoid placing the person on enforced inactivity (which heightens fear)
Reduce the demands placed on the person (so more energy is available for coping)
Introduce to persons who have undergone the same experience (if appropriate)

Nursing Observations
Observe for an excessive stress level (resulting from the fear)
Observe for evidence of a favorable response to therapy (reduced fear and increased comfort)

Health Teaching
Explain that the person's response is appropriate and commonly experienced
Recommend a habitual, positive mental attitude (nonverbal communication can be very effective)

EVALUATION
Record actual outcome

FEAR OF LOSS OF BODY FUNCTION[105,471,525]

ASSESSMENT
Data Collection
Subjective Data
• Person experiences feelings of threat or danger
• Can describe or identify the threat or danger
  Focuses on a certain body function associated with a specific organ(s)
  Discusses the disease or injury associated with the loss of function
  Is concerned with the effects of such loss
  Feels the threat of unwholeness

Objective Data
• May manifest physical findings such as facial flushing or pallor, rapid or deep respirations, rapid or bounding pulse, increased blood pressure, sweating, trembling
• May exhibit behavior such as restlessness, sleep disturbances, change in eating habits, irritability, forgetfulness, rapid speech, demanding and controlling behavior, crying, unusual quietness, self-imposed inactivity, frequent call-light signaling, seeking reassurance

Data Analysis
Nursing Diagnosis
FEAR OF LOSS OF BODY FUNCTION: A feeling of alarm and fright about the possible loss of normal body activity that maintains body systems

Common Etiology (Stressors)
DISEASES: Addison's disease, carcinoma, cataracts, cerebrovascular accident, congestive heart failure, diabetes mellitus, epilepsy, glaucoma, Guillian-Barré syndrome, hepatitis, Hodgkin's disease, leukemia, multiple sclerosis, myasthenia gravis, myocardial infarction, organic brain syndrome, Parkinson's disease, posterolateral sclerosis, renal insufficiency or failure, bilateral salpingitis
INJURIES: Bone fracture, herniated intervertebral disc, splenic fracture/tear
SIGNS AND SYMPTOMS: Confusion, pain, memory loss, weakness

PSYCHOSOCIAL FACTORS: The threat of a specific and clearly identified danger, the threat of real or imagined danger

HEALTH CARE FACTORS: *Drug therapy:* Antihypertensive drugs, contraceptive drugs. *Medical therapy:* Gastrostomy or jejunostomy feeding, hyperalimentation infusion. *Surgical procedures:* Adrenalectomy, cesarean section, esophagogastrectomy, glossectomy, ileostomy, jejunostomy, laryngectomy, lobectomy of the lung, nephrectomy, oophorectomy, orchiectomy, salpingectomy, thyroidectomy, ureterocolostomy, ureteroileostomy, ureterosigmoidistomy, ureterostomy, ureterotomy, vasectomy

DEVELOPMENTAL PHASES: Old age

PLANNING

Unmet Needs

Comfort, protection from psychologic threat, acceptance, caring and communicating relationships, high evaluation of self, sense of adequacy, personal growth and maturity, increased learning, increased reality perception and problem-solving ability

Expected Outcome

Person verbalizes fears
Verbalizes feelings of adequacy and competence in meeting the fear-creating experience
Verbalizes self-satisfaction and growth in having coped with the fear-creating experience
Calm, relaxed facial expression, body movements, and behavior

NURSING INTERVENTIONS

Nursing Treatments

Approach unhurriedly
Reassure verbally (that the nurse will help the person as much as possible)
Demonstrate calmness
Provide an atmosphere of acceptance
Encourage the expression of feelings (about the fear)
Listen attentively
Offer feedback to the person's expressed feelings
Communicate nurse sensitivity to the person's problem
Relate to the person on an adult–adult level, not on a parent–child level (which could increase fear)
Ask the person to identify the problem
Ask for specifics, not generalizations, about the problem
Provide reliable information (about the probability of the loss of body function, about treatment to restore body function or adaptations for the loss)
Ask how the person normally copes with fear (what does he usually do when fearful that reduces the fear?)
Provide whatever the person needs to use his usual coping mechanisms
Introduce to persons who have undergone the same experiences (if appropriate)

Nursing Observations

Observe for an excessive stress level (resulting from the fear)
Determine the degree of insight that the person has (into the fear)
Observe for evidence of a favorable response to therapy (reduced fear and increased comfort)

Health Teaching

Explain that the person's response is appropriate and commonly experienced
Explain how to channel emotional energy and obtain release from stress (through walking, sports, creative activities, laughing, talking things over)
Recommend methods for achieving total relaxation (controlled breathing, quietly listening to music, doing nothing, which reduces fear)
Recommend a habitual, positive mental attitude (about the remaining body function)

EVALUATION

Record actual outcome

FEAR OF LOSS OF A BODY PART[105,471,525]

ASSESSMENT

Data Collection

Subjective Data
• Person experiences feelings of threat or danger
• Can describe or identify the threat or danger
  Focuses on the endangered body part
  Is concerned with the effects of such a loss on daily life
  Feels the threat of unwholeness

Objective Data
• May manifest physical findings such as facial flushing or pallor, rapid or deep respirations, rapid or bounding pulse, increased blood pressure, sweating, trembling
• May exhibit behavior such as restlessness, sleep disturbances, change in eating habits, irritability, short attention span, making poor judgments, forgetfulness, rapid speech, demanding and controlling behavior, crying, unusual quietness, frequent call-light signaling, touching others

Data Analysis

Nursing Diagnosis
FEAR OF LOSS OF A BODY PART: A feeling of alarm and fright about the loss of a specific body organ or extremity

Common Etiology (Stressors)
DISEASES: Carcinoma, arteriosclerosis, Buerger's disease, gangrene, Hansen's disease, Raynaud's disease
INJURIES: Burn (chemical, electrical, thermal), frostbite, laceration wound, traumatic amputation
SIGNS AND SYMPTOMS: Pain, paresthesia
PSYCHOSOCIAL FACTORS: The threat of a specific and clearly identified danger, the threat of real or imagined danger
HEALTH CARE FACTORS: *Adverse effects of surgical therapy*: Loss of a body part from amputation, cholecystectomy, enucleation or evisceration of the eyeball, gastrectomy, glossectomy, hemipelvectomy, hysterectomy, ileotomy, laryngectomy, lobectomy of the brain, liver or lungs, mastectomy, nephrectomy, prostatectomy, splenectomy, thyroidectomy, tonsillectomy

PLANNING

Unmet Needs
Comfort, protection from psychologic threat, acceptance, caring and communicating relationships, high evaluation of self, sense of adequacy, personal growth and maturity, increased learning, increased reality perception and problem-solving ability

Expected Outcome
Person verbalizes fears
Verbalizes feelings of adequacy and competence in meeting the fear-creating experience
Verbalizes self-satisfaction and growth in having coped with the fear-creating experience
Calm, relaxed facial expression, body movements, and behavior

NURSING INTERVENTIONS

Nursing Treatments
Approach unhurriedly
Reassure verbally (that the nurse will help the person as much as possible)
Demonstrate calmness
Provide an atmosphere of acceptance
Encourage the expression of feelings (about the fear)

Listen attentively

Offer feedback to the person's expressed feelings

Communicate nurse sensitivity to the person's problem

Relate to the person on an adult–adult level, not on a parent–child level (which could increase fear)

Ask the person to identify the problem

Ask for specifics, not generalizations, about the problem

Provide reliable information (about the probability of loss of a body part, about the effects of the loss, about available prosthesis)

Ask how the person normally copes with fear (what does he usually do when fearful that reduces the fear?)

Provide whatever the person needs to use his usual coping mechanisms

Do not allow unpleasant surprise situations (such as unexpected surgery, viewing the damaged body part without preparation)

Avoid placing the person on enforced inactivity (which heightens fear)

Reduce the demands placed on the person (so that more energy is available for coping)

Introduce to persons who have undergone the same experience (if appropriate)

Nursing Observations

Observe for an excessive stress level (resulting from the fear)

Determine the degree of insight that the person has (into the fear)

Observe for evidence of a favorable response to therapy (reduced fear and increased comfort)

Health Teaching

Explain that the person's response is appropriate and commonly experienced

Recommend methods for achieving total relaxation (controlled breathing, quietly listening to music, doing nothing, which reduces fear)

EVALUATION

Record actual outcome

FEAR OF LOSS OF CONSCIOUSNESS[105,471,525]

ASSESSMENT

Data Collection

Subjective Data

• Person experiences feelings of threat or danger

• Can describe or identify the threat or danger

 May relate having previously lost consciousness

 May perceive unconsciousness as being out of control or like death

 Is concerned with injury to self or others

 Inquires about prevention of episodes

 May refuse surgery requiring general anesthesia

Objective Data

• May manifest physical findings such as facial flushing or pallor, rapid or deep respirations, rapid or bounding pulse, increased blood pressure, sweating, trembling

• May exhibit behavior such as restlessness, sleep disturbances, change in eating habits, irritability, demanding and controlling behavior, crying, unusual quietness, frequent call-light signaling, seeking reassurance

Data Analysis

Nursing Diagnosis

FEAR OF LOSS OF CONSCIOUSNESS: A feeling of alarm and fright about losing one's state of awareness and comprehension of external reality

Common Etiology (Stressors)

DISEASES: Carotid atherosclerosis, brain tumor, cerebral aneurysm, epilepsy

INJURIES: Cerebral concussion, severe trauma of any kind

SIGNS AND SYMPTOMS: Syncope

PSYCHOSOCIAL FACTORS: The threat of a specific and clearly identified danger, the threat of real or imagined danger

HEALTH CARE FACTORS: *Drug therapy*: Barbiturates, insulin, narcotics, sedatives, tranquilizers. *Medical therapy*: Electroconvulsive shock therapy. *Surgical anesthesia*: Any

PLANNING

Unmet Needs

Comfort, protection from psychologic threat, acceptance, caring and communicating relationships, high evaluation of self, sense of adequacy, personal growth and maturity, increased learning, increased reality perception and problem-solving ability

Expected Outcome

Person verabilizes fears

Verbalizes feelings of adequacy and competence in meeting the fear-creating experience

Verbalizes self-satisfaction and growth in having coped with the fear-creating experience

Calm, relaxed facial expression, body movements, and behavior

NURSING INTERVENTIONS

Nursing Treatments

Approach unhurriedly

Reassure verbally (that the nurse will help the person as much as possible)

Demonstrate calmness

Provide an atmosphere of acceptance

Encourage the expression of feelings (feelings about the fear, feelings of loss of control, feelings related to comparing unconsciousness to death)

Listen attentively

Offer feedback to the person's expressed feelings

Communicate nurse sensitivity to the person's problem

Relate to the person on an adult–adult level, not on a parent–child level (which could increase fear)

Ask the person to identify the problem

Ask for specifics, not generalizations, about the problem

Provide reliable information (about the probability of losing consciousness, about how long the person will be unconscious, methods used for protecting the unconscious person, the aftereffects, etc.)

Ask how the person normally copes with fear (what does he usually do when fearful that reduces the fear?)

Provide whatever the person needs to use his usual coping mechanisms

Explore with the person his strengths and resources (to cope with the fear)

Provide objects that symbolize safeness (side rails, padded tongue depressor, orange juice or candy, ventilator, etc.)

Avoid placing the person on enforced inactivity (which heightens fear)

Introduce to persons who have undergone the same experience (if appropriate)

Nursing Observations

Observe for an excessive stress level (resulting from the fear)

Determine the degree of insight that the person has (into the fear)

Observe for evidence of a favorable response to therapy (reduced fear and increased comfort)

Health Teaching

Explain that the person's response is appropriate and commonly experienced

Recommend methods for achieving total relaxation (controlled breathing, quietly listening to music, doing nothing, which reduces fear)

Inform of those conditions that precipitate seizures (excitement, fatigue, flashing light patterns, fever)

Explain how to manage seizure episodes (to lie down in a safe place at the first sign of an impending seizure)

Recommend that a glucose source be carried at all times (and be taken promptly at the first sign of an insulin reaction)

EVALUATION

Record actual outcome

FEAR OF LOSS OF CONTROL OF BODY FUNCTION[105,471,476,525]

ASSESSMENT

Data Collection

Subjective Data

• Person experiences feelings of threat or danger
• Can describe or identify the threat or danger

Focuses on body function over which the person has some control such as voiding, defecation, cerebral function, breathing, motor control

Is concerned that autonomous (self) control of function has been or will be interrupted

Feels helpless and/or frustrated

May feel guilty and feel that he should be able to control body function

May express shame (about possible incontinence, impaired motor control, etc.)

Objective Data

• May manifest physical findings such as facial flushing or pallor, rapid or deep respiration, rapid or bounding pulse, increased blood pressure, sweating, trembling
• May exhibit behavior such as restlessness, sleep disturbances, irritability, rapid speech, demanding and controlling behavior, unusual quietness, seeking reassurance

May cry, especially if some loss of control occurs

Data Analysis

Nursing Diagnosis

FEAR OF LOSS OF CONTROL OF BODY FUNCTION: A feeling of alarm and fright about loss of control of those body activities over which a person normally has some control

Common Etiology (Stressors)

DISEASES: Asthma, emphysema, esophageal stricture, multiple sclerosis, myasthenia gravis, Parkinson's disease

SIGNS AND SYMPTOMS: Breathing difficulty, convulsions, diarrhea, dizziness, immobility, incontinence, pain, paralysis, weakness

PSYCHOSOCIAL FACTORS: The threat of a specific and clearly identified danger, the threat of real or imagined danger

HUMAN BODY: *Natural body function*: Childbirth. *Body state*: Pregnancy

HEALTH CARE FACTORS: *Drug therapy*: Barbiturates, narcotics, sedatives, tranquilizers. *Medical therapy*: Gastrostomy feeding, genitourinary drainage, hyperalimentation infusion, jejunostomy feeding. *Surigical therapy*: Anesthesia. *Surgical procedures*: Colostomy, ileostomy, ureterocolostomy, ureteroileostomy, ureterotomy. *Therapeutic equipment*: Respirator
DEVELOPMENTAL PHASES: Old age

PLANNING
Unmet Needs
Comfort, protection from psychologic threat, acceptance, caring and communicating relationships, high evaluation of self, sense of adequacy, personal growth and maturity, increased learning, increased reality perception and problem-solving ability

Expected Outcome
Person verbalizes fears
Verbalizes feelings of adequacy and competence in meeting the fear-creating experience
Verbalizes self-satisfaction and growth in having coped with the fear-creating experience
Calm, relaxed facial expression, body movements, and behavior

NURSING INTERVENTIONS
Nursing Treatments
Approach unhurriedly
Reassure verbally (that the nurse will help the person as much as possible)
Demonstrate calmness
Provide an atmosphere of acceptance
Encourage the expression of feelings (about the fear)
Listen attentively
Offer feedback to the person's expressed feelings
Communicate nurse sensitivity to the person's problem
Relate to the person on an adult–adult level, not on a parent–child level (which could increase fear)
Ask the person to identify the problem
Ask for specifics, not generalizations, about the problem
Provide reliable information (about the probability of the loss of control of body function, about methods to control body function, about ways to adapt to the loss)
Ask how the person normally copes with fear (what does he usually do when fearful that reduces the fear?)
Provide whatever the person needs to use his usual coping mechanisms
Arrange situations that encourage the person's autonomy (which will increase a sense of control)
Avoid placing the person on enforced inactivity (which heightens fear)
Reduce the demands placed on the person (so that more energy is available for coping)

Nursing Observations
Observe for an excessive stress level (resulting from the fear)
Determine the degree of insight that the person has (into the fear)
Observe for evidence of a favorable response to therapy (reduced fear and increased comfort)

Health Teaching
Explain that the person's response is appropriate and commonly experienced
Explain how to channel emotional energy and obtain release from stress (through creative activities, laughing, talking things over)
Recommend methods for achieving total relaxation (controlled breathing, quietly listening to music, doing nothing, which reduces stress)

EVALUATION
Record actual outcome

FEAR OF LOSS OF DECISIONAL CONTROL[105,471,525]

ASSESSMENT
Data Collection

Subjective Data
- Person experiences feelings of threat or danger
- Can describe or identify the threat or danger
  Is concerned that others will be making decisions on his behalf
  Wonders if the decisions will be favorable or appropriate
  Does not want others to control decision making
  May verbalize anger

Objective Data
- May manifest physical findings such as facial flushing or pallor, rapid or deep respirations, rapid or bounding pulse, increased blood pressure, sweating, trembling
- May exhibit behavior such as restlessness, sleep disturbances, change in eating habits, irritability, rapid speech, demanding and controlling behavior, avoiding or leaving the situation

Data Analysis

Nursing Diagnosis
FEAR OF LOSS OF DECISIONAL CONTROL: A feeling of alarm and fright about having little or no control over decisions regarding oneself or significant others

Common Etiology (Stressors)
SIGNS AND SYMPTOMS: Confusion, memory loss, pain
PSYCHOSOCIAL FACTORS: The threat of a specific and clearly identified danger, the threat of real or imagined danger, loss of independence, the threat of being overly controlled or dominated
HEALTH CARE FACTORS: *Health care consent forms*: Signing health care consent forms. *Health care environment*: Intensive care, isolation, or locked psychiatric unit. *Health care system*: Entry into the health care system. *Institutional policies*: Restrictive. *Institutional routine*: Inflexible. *Adverse effects of drug or surgical therapy*: Heavy drug sedation from sedatives; unconsciousness from anesthesia
DEVELOPMENTAL PHASES: Old age
SITUATIONAL FACTORS: Illness of or injury to self; poverty

PLANNING
Unmet Needs
Comfort, protection from psychologic threat, acceptance, caring and communicating relationships, high evaluation of self, sense of adequacy, personal growth and maturity, increased learning, increased reality perception and problem-solving ability

Expected Outcome
Person verbalizes fears
Verbalizes feelings of adequacy and competence in meeting the fear-creating experience
Calm, relaxed facial expression, body movements, and behavior

NURSING INTERVENTIONS
Nursing Treatments
Approach unhurriedly
Reassure verbally (that the nurse will help the person maintain control of decisions)
Demonstrate calmness
Provide an atmosphere of acceptance
Encourage the expression of feelings (about the fear)
Listen attentively
Offer feedback to the person's expressed feelings

Communicate nurse sensitivity to the person's problem

Relate to the person on an adult–adult level, not on a parent–child level (which could increase fear)

Ask the person to identify the problem

Ask for specifics, not generalizations, about the problem

Support a realistic assessment of the situation (that the physician and nurses can provide expert information, but that the person must make the actual decision about his health care, unless, of course, the person is unable to make decisions)

Provide reliable information (about the situation so that the person can make wise decisions)

Ask how the person normally copes with fear (what does he usually do when fearful that reduces the fear?)

Provide whatever the person needs to use his usual coping mechanisms

Explore with the person his strengths and resources (to cope with the fear and make wise decisions)

Do not allow unpleasant surprise situations (over which the person has no control)

Arrange situations that encourage the person's autonomy (which will increase a sense of control and help the person feel involved in the decision-making process)

Introduce to persons who have undergone the same experience (if appropriate)

Nursing Observations

Observe for an excessive stress level (resulting from the fear)

Determine the degree of insight that the person has (into the fear)

Observe for evidence of a favorable response to therapy (reduced fear and increased comfort)

Health Teaching

Explain that the person's response is appropriate and commonly experienced

Teach how to use the problem-solving method (to maintain control over decisions for self)

EVALUATION

Record actual outcome

FEAR OF LOSS OF EMOTIONAL CONTROL [105,471,525]

ASSESSMENT

Data Collection

Subjective Data

• Person experiences feelings of threat or danger
• Can describe or identify the threat or danger
    Doubts about ability to maintain self-control
    May feel on the brink of losing control

Objective Data

• May manifest physical findings such as facial flushing or pallor, rapid or deep respirations, rapid or bounding pulse, increased blood pressure, sweating, trembling
• May exhibit behavior such as restlessness, sleep disturbances, demanding and controlling behavior, avoiding persons with whom and situations in which emotions might become uncontrolled

Data Analysis

Nursing Diagnosis

FEAR OF LOSS OF EMOTIONAL CONTROL: A feeling of alarm and fright about being unable to control an emotional response to stress

Common Etiology (Stressors)

DISEASES: Alcoholism, drug addiction, major depression, schizophrenia

SIGNS AND SYMPTOMS: Fatigue, irritability, pain

PSYCHOSOCIAL FACTORS: The threat of a specific and clearly identified danger, the threat of real or imagined danger, the threat of abuse from a significant other, the threat of severe stress, loss of or separation from a significant other, lack of training in self-discipline

HUMAN BODY: *Natural body function:* Childbirth

HEALTH CARE FACTORS: *Medical diagnosis:* Unfavorable *Drug therapy:* Amphetamines, barbiturates, epinephrine, narcotics, sedatives, tranquilizers, chemotherapy *Medical therapy:* Psychotherapy, withdrawal from alcohol, drugs, tobacco. *Surgical therapy:* Recovery from anesthesia

SITUATIONAL FACTORS: The threat of loss, death of a significant other, natural disaster, illness or injury, childrearing.

PLANNING

Unmet Needs

Comfort, protection from psychologic threat, acceptance, caring and communicating relationships, high evaluation of self, sense of adequacy, personal growth and maturity, increased learning, increased reality perception and problem-solving ability

Expected Outcome

Person verbalizes fears

Verbalizes feelings of adequacy and competence in meeting the fear-creating experience

Verbalizes self-satisfaction and growth in having coped with the fear-creating experience

Calm, relaxed facial expression, body movement, and behavior

NURSING INTERVENTIONS

Nursing Treatments

Approach unhurriedly

Reassure verbally (that the nurse will help the person as much as possible)

Demonstrate calmness

Provide an atmosphere of acceptance

Encourage the expression of feelings (about the fear)

Listen attentively

Offer feedback to the person's expressed feelings

Communicate nurse sensitivity to the person's problem

Relate to the person on an adult–adult level, not on a parent–child level (which could increase fear)

Attend the person constantly (until he feels sufficiently confortable to be alone)

Provide frequent patient contact (thereafter)

Ask the person to identify the problem

Ask for specifics, not generalizations, about the problem

Ask how the person normally copes with fear (what does he usually do when fearful that reduces the fear?)

Provide whatever the person needs to use his usual coping mechanisms

Encourage the person to face the fear (when able, to reduce the fear)

Explore with the person his strengths and resources (to cope with the fear and maintain control)

Provide emotionally safe experiences (whenever possible, if the person is in poor control)

Do not allow unpleasant surprise situations (which may cause loss of emotional control)

Reduce the demands placed on the person (so that more energy is available for coping)

Nursing Observations

Determine the degree of insight that the person has (into the fear)

Observe for evidence of a favorable response to therapy (reduced fear and increased comfort)

Health Teaching

Explain that the person's response is appropriate and commonly experienced

Explain how emotional responses occur (a situation is perceived in terms of its significance to the individual, an emotional response is experienced, physiologic changes accompany the response)

Advise against fighting fear (this reinforces the emotion)

Explain the importance of recognizing tension within oneself (high levels of tension can lead to loss of emotional control)

Explain that fatigue should be recognized as a stress factor (which heightens fear and loss of control)

Explain the need to recognize highly stressful situations

Explain how to channel emotional energy and obtain release from stress (through running, swimming, other sports, creative activities, laughing, talking things over)

Recommend things to do when a person begins to feel out of control (such as washing the face and hands in cold water, taking deep breaths, counting to 500, to give the person something to do besides feel)

Explain why persons should maintain self-control (out of respect for others, because of the harmful effect that noncontrol has on others, because such behavior is often futile in attaining goals)

Recommend a habitual, positive mental attitude (that the person has maintained control so far, that temporary loss of control can be overcome by increased effort)

Explain the importance of maintaining a positive self-attitude (if the person believes he is capable of self-control, he will succeed; if he is unsure, he is likely to lose control)

EVALUATION

Record actual outcome

FEAR OF LOSS OF EMPLOYMENT[105,315,471,525]

ASSESSMENT

Data Collection

Subjective Data
• Person experiences feelings of threat or danger
• Can describe or identify the threat or danger
 Is concerned about a present job position remaining available
 May discuss his ability to fulfill employment requirements
 Is concerned about the alternatives and consequences if loss of employment occurs

Objective Data
• May manifest physical findings such as facial flushing or pallor, rapid or deep respirations, rapid or bounding pulse, increased blood pressure, sweating, trembling
• May exhibit behavior such as restlessness, sleep disturbances, change in eating habits, irritability, demanding and controlling behavior, frequently calling the employer or asking the nurse to call, seeking reassurance

Data Analysis

Nursing Diagnosis
FEAR OF LOSS OF EMPLOYMENT: A feeling of alarm and fright about losing a job or occupation

Common Etiology (Stressors)
DISEASES: Any but especially alcoholism, drug addiction, schizophrenia, syphilis, tuberculosis
INJURY: Any severe injury

SIGNS AND SYMPTOMS: Hearing, vision, or voice loss; pain; weakness

PSYCHOSOCIAL FACTORS: The threat of a specific and clearly identified danger, the threat of real or imagined danger

HUMAN BODY: *Body appearance*: A disfigured body. *Body function*: Loss of body function. *Body part*: Loss of a body part. *Body state*: Pregnancy

HEALTH CARE FACTORS: *Hospitalization*: Of self or significant other. *Medical diagnosis*: An unfavorable medical diagnosis for self. *Health therapy*: Loss of on-the-job time because of therapy (chemotherapy, radiation, rehabilitation therapy, hemodialysis, psychotherapy). *Hospital discharge*: Delayed. *Recovery*: Delayed recovery from illness

DEVELOPMENTAL PHASES: Middle age, old age

LIFESTYLE: Lack of education

SITUATIONAL FACTORS: Illness of or injury to self or significant other, disclosure of illness, unfavorable economic factors, attempted suicide

PLANNING

Unmet Needs

Comfort, protection from psychologic threat, acceptance, caring and communicating relationships, high evaluation of self, sense of adequacy, personal growth and maturity, increased learning, increased reality perception and problem-solving ability

Expected Outcome

Person verbalizes fears

Verbalizes feelings of adequacy and competence in meeting the fear-creating experience

Verbalizes self-satisfaction and growth in having coped with the fear-creating experience

Calm, relaxed facial expression, body movements, and behavior

NURSING INTERVENTIONS

Nursing Treatments

Approach unhurriedly

Reassure verbally (that the nurse will help the person as much as possible)

Demonstrate calmness

Provide an atmosphere of acceptance

Encourage the expression of feelings (about the fear)

Listen attentively

Offer feedback to the person's expressed feelings

Communicate nurse sensitivity to the person's problem

Relate to the person on an adult–adult level, not on a parent–child level (which could increase fear)

Ask the person to identify the problem

Ask for specifics, not generalizations, about the problem

Support a realistic assessment of the situation (reality reduces fear; support assessment of why the person believes the job is in jeopardy, whether he has performed well in the past, and which of his abilities or limitations affect the job situation)

Ask how the person normally copes with fear (what does he usually do when fearful that reduces the fear?)

Provide whatever the person needs to use his usual coping mechanisms

Encourage the person to face the fear (when able, to reduce the fear)

Explore with the person his strengths and resources (to cope with the fear and the employment situation; discuss all the possibilities a person has to earn money, such as temporarily assuming a less strenuous position, taking several part-time jobs, etc.)

Make a referral (to a physician, if a letter from a physician will ensure employment)

Introduce to persons who have undergone the same experience (if appropriate)

Nursing Observations

Observe for an excessive stress level (resulting from the fear)

Determine the degree of insight that the person has (into the fear)

Observe for evidence of a favorable response to therapy (reduced fear and increased comfort)

Health Teaching

Explain that the person's response is appropriate and commonly experienced

Explain how to channel emotional energy and obtain release from stress (through creative activities, laughing, talking things over)

Recommend methods for achieving total relaxation (controlled breathing, quietly listening to music, doing nothing, which reduces stress)

Recommend a habitual, positive mental attitude (about the person's capabilities)

Teach how to use the problem-solving method (to keep the present job or adjust the current work to the person's limitations)

EVALUATION

Record actual outcome

FEAR OF LOSS OF LIFESTYLE[105,471,525]

ASSESSMENT

Data Collection

Subjective Data
• Person experiences feelings of threat or danger
• Can describe or identify the threat or danger
  Relates that he is aware that his habits of living may require change
  Conveys dissatisfaction with the change
  Wants the daily routine and habits to remain the same

Objective Data
• May manifest physical findings such as facial flushing or pallor, rapid or deep respirations, rapid or bounding pulse, increased blood pressure, sweating, trembling
• May exhibit behavior such as restlessness, sleep disturbances, change in eating habits, irritability, rapid speech, demanding and controlling behavior, attempting activities beyond his capabilities in an effort to maintain lifestyle

Data Analysis

Nursing Diagnosis
FEAR OF LOSS OF LIFESTYLE: A feeling of alarm and fright about losing the habits and pleasures of daily living

Common Etiology (Stressors)
BIRTH DEFECTS: Birth of an imperfect child
DISEASES: Any
INJURIES: Any
SIGNS AND SYMPTOMS: Immobility, pain, paralysis, weakness
PSYCHOSOCIAL FACTORS: The threat of a specific and clearly identified danger, the threat of real or imagined danger, loss of independence, loss of role performance
HEALTH CARE FACTORS: *Hospitalization:* Any. *Institutionalization.* Any. *Drug Therapy:* Chemotherapy. *Medical therapy:* Hemodialysis, frequent radiation or rehabilitation therapy. *Surgical procedures:* Colostomy, ileostomy, ureterocolostomy, ureteroileostomy
SITUATIONAL FACTORS: The death of a significant other, divorce, marital separation, illness of or injury to self or a significant other, a new baby, retirement

PLANNING

Unmet Needs

Comfort, protection from psychologic threat, acceptance, caring and communicating relationships, high evaluation of self, sense of adequacy, personal growth and maturity, increased learning, increased reality perception and problem-solving ability

Expected Outcome

Person verbalizes fears
Verbalizes feelings of adequacy and competence in meeting the fear-creating experience
Verbalizes self-satisfaction and growth in having coped with the fear-creating experience
Calm, relaxed facial expression, body movement, and behavior

NURSING INTERVENTIONS

Nursing Treatments

Approach unhurriedly
Reassure verbally
Demonstrate calmness
Provide an atmosphere of acceptance
Encourage the expression of feelings (about the fear)
Listen attentively
Offer feedback to the person's expressed feelings
Communicate nurse sensitivity to the person's problem
Relate to the person on an adult–adult level, not on a parent–child level (which could increase fear)
Ask the person to identify the problem
Ask for specifics, not generalizations, about the problem
Provide reliable information (about the probability of such a loss, about the limitations imposed by the illness or situation)
Ask how the person normally copes with fear (what does he usually do when fearful that reduces the fear?)
Provide whatever the person needs to use his usual coping mechanisms
Assist the person to restructure his lifestyle (by setting up new daily schedules, maintaining as many pleasurable situations as possible)
Introduce to persons who have undergone the same experience (if appropriate)

Nursing Observations

Observe for an excessive stress level (resulting from the fear)
Determine the degree of insight that the person has (into the fear)
Observe for evidence of a favorable response to therapy (reduced fear and increased comfort)

Health Teaching

Explain that the person's response is appropriate and commonly experienced
Explain how to channel emotional energy and obtain release from stress (through running, swimming, other sports, creative activities, laughing, talking things over)
Recommend a habitual, positive mental attitude (toward his ability to cope)
Teach how to use the problem-solving method (to retain as much of the former lifestyle as possible

EVALUATION

Record actual outcome

FEAR OF LOSS OF MARITAL INTEGRITY WITH SPOUSE[105,471,525]

ASSESSMENT

Data Collection

Subjective Data
• Person experiences feelings of threat or danger

- Can describe or identify the threat or danger
  Focuses on the marital spouse
  Is concerned about the unity of their relationship
  Is worried about the partner's being alone, being without the ill spouse
  Concerned about a possible change in their intimate relationship

Objective Data
- May manifest physical findings such as facial flushing or pallor, rapid or deep respirations, rapid or bounding pulse, increased blood pressure, sweating, trembling
- May exhibit behavior such as restlessness, sleep disturbances, change in eating habits, irritability, crying, avoiding unpleasant situations with the spouse, seeking reassurance

Data Analysis

Nursing Diagnosis
FEAR OF LOSS OF MARITAL INTEGRITY WITH SPOUSE: A feeling of alarm and fright that one might lose marital unity with one's marriage partner

Common Etiology (Stressors)
BIRTH DEFECTS: Giving birth to an imperfect child
DISEASES: Any severe, prolonged disease
INJURIES: Any severe injury
SIGNS AND SYMPTOMS: Immobility, pain, weakness
PSYCHOSOCIAL FACTORS: The threat of a specific and clearly identified danger, the threat of real or imagined danger
HUMAN BODY: *Body appearance*: Body distortion during pregnancy, a disfigured body. *Body function*: Loss of body function. *Body part*: Loss of a body part. *Body state*: Pregnancy
HEALTH CARE FACTORS: *Health care decisions for self*: Decisions made independently of a significant other. *Hospitalization or institutionalization*: Of self or a significant other. *Adverse effects of medical, drug, surgical therapy*: Loss of hair from radiation and chemotherapy; loss of libido from antihypertensive drugs, tagament, hemodialysis; loss of reproductive ability from fallopian tube ligation, hysterectomy, oophorectomy, orchiectomy, prostatectomy, salpingectomy, vasectomy. *Recovery*: Delayed recovery from illness
DEVELOPMENTAL PHASES: Middle age, old age
LIFESTYLE: Alcohol or drug abuse
SITUATIONAL FACTORS: Childlessness, a newborn infant, confinement in prison, loss of employment, lack of finances, illness of or injury to self or a significant other, attempted suicide

PLANNING

Unmet Needs
Comfort, protection from psychologic threat, acceptance, caring and communicating relationships, high evaluation of self, sense of adequacy, personal growth and maturity, increased learning, increased reality perception and problem-solving ability

Expected Outcome
Person verbalizes fears
Verbalizes feelings of adequacy and competence in meeting the fear-creating experience
Verbalizes self-satisfaction and growth in having coped with the fear-creating experience
Calm, relaxed facial expression, body movements, and behavior

NURSING INTERVENTIONS

Nursing Treatments
Approach unhurriedly
Reassure verbally (that the nurse will help the person as much as possible)
Demonstrate calmness
Provide an atmosphere of acceptance
Encourage the expression of feelings (about the fear; encourage the person to express openly his needs to the significant other)

Listen attentively

Offer feedback to the person's expressed feelings

Communicate nurse sensitivity to the person's problem

Relate to the person on an adult–adult level, not on a parent–child level (which could increase fear)

Ask the person to identify the problem

Ask for specifics, not generalizations, about the problem

Support a realistic assessment of the situation (about the probability of such occurring: has the couple been in a previous, similar situation; if so, did they maintain unity; if not, what was the problem?)

Ask how the person normally copes with fear (what does he usually do when fearful that reduces the fear?)

Provide whatever the person needs to use his usual coping mechanisms

Explore with the person his strengths and resources (to cope with the situation)

Allow unlimited visiting (of the spouse)

Encourage telephone calls with significant persons

Nursing Observations

Determine the degree of insight that the person has (into the fear)

Observe for evidence of a favorable response to therapy (reduced fear and increased comfort)

Health Teaching

Explain that the person's response is appropriate and commonly experienced

Recommend a habitual, positive mental attitude (toward himself even when ill, avoid making degrading comments about himself to the spouse)

Advise that significant persons express caring for one another (encourage closeness of family and friends, especially if the overt expression of such has been withheld)

Explain (to the couple) the importance of persons offering support to one another

Explain that ill persons are often hypersensitive (to responses from significant others)

EVALUATION

Record actual outcome

FEAR OF LOSS OF PARENTAL CONTROL OF CHILDREN[26,105,471,525]

ASSESSMENT

Data Collection

Subjective Data

• Person experiences feelings of threat or danger

• Can describe or identify the threat or danger

 Is concerned that the children are without adequate supervision

 Is worried about where they are, what they are doing, whom they are with

 Is concerned that it will be difficult to reestablish control later

Objective Data

• May manifest physical findings such as facial flushing or pallor, rapid or deep respirations, rapid or bounding pulse, increased blood pressure, sweating, trembling

• May exhibit behavior such as restlessness, sleep disturbances, change in eating habits, irritability, demanding and controlling behavior, crying, frequent telephoning to check on the children

Data Analysis

Nursing Diagnosis

FEAR OF LOSS OF PARENTAL CONTROL OF CHILDREN: A feeling of alarm and fright about possibly losing control over one's children's activities and behavior

Common Etiology (Stressors)

DISEASES: Any severe or prolonged disease

INJURIES: Any severe injury

SIGNS AND SYMPTOMS: Immobility, pain, weakness

PSYCHOSOCIAL FACTORS: The threat of a specific and clearly identified danger, the threat of real or imagined danger, parental loss of independence, loss of role performance, conflicting parental and community values

HEALTH CARE FACTORS: *Health care environment*: The admittance of a parent or child to an intensive care, isolation, or locked psychiatric unit. *Hospitalization or instituionalization*: Of self or a significant other (child). *Health therapy*: Time-consuming therapy. *Recovery*: Delayed recovery from illness

DEVELOPMENTAL PHASES: Adolescence or young adulthood of the child

LIFESTYLE: Excess (parental) time and effort at employment

SITUATIONAL FACTORS: Confinement in prison, death of a significant other (spouse), divorce, illness of or injury to self or a child, launching grown children, extensive travel by a parent

PLANNING

Unmet Needs

Comfort, protection from psychologic threat, acceptance, caring and communicating relationships, high evaluation of self, sense of adequacy, personal growth and maturity, increased learning, increased reality perception and problem-solving ability

Expected Outcome

Person verbalizes fears

Verbalizes feelings of adequacy and competence in meeting the fear-creating experience

Verbalizes self-satisfaction and growth in having coped with the fear-creating experience

Calm, relaxed facial expression, body movements, and behavior

NURSING INTERVENTIONS

Nursing Treatments

Approach unhurriedly

Reassure verbally

Demonstrate calmness

Provide an atmosphere of acceptance

Encourage the expression of feelings (about the fear, and the expression of the current need to family and friends who can help)

Listen attentively

Offer feedback to the person's expressed feelings

Communicate nurse sensitivity to the person's problem

Relate to the person on an adult–adult level, not on a parent–child level (which could increase fear)

Ask the person to identify the problem

Ask for specifics, not generalizations, about the problem

Support a realistic assessment of the situation (that other family members can guide the children during the parent's absence)

Provide reliable information (about what the children are doing)

Ask how the person normally copes with fear (what does he usually do when fearful that reduces the fear?)

Provide whatever the person needs to use his usual coping mechanisms

Explore with the person his strengths and resources (to cope with the problem)

Do not allow unpleasant surprise situations (which undisciplined children might cause)

Avoid placing the person on enforced inactivity (which heightens fear)
Encourage telehone calls between parent and children
Allow unlimited visiting (between parent and children)

Nursing Observations

Observe for an excessive stress level (resulting from the fear)
Determine the degree of insight that the person has (into the fear)
Observe for evidence of a favorable response to therapy (reduced fear and increased comfort)

Health Teaching

Explain that the person's response is appropriate and commonly experienced
Explain how to channel emotional energy and obtain release from stress (through laughing, talking things over)
Recommend methods for achieving total relaxation (controlled breathing, quietly listening to music, doing nothing, which reduces fear)
Recommend a habitual, positive mental attitude (toward the parent–child relationship)
Teach how to use the problem-solving method (to maintain a worthwhile parent–child relationship, to promote acceptance of responsibility by the child, which is a primary parental task)

EVALUATION

Record actual outcome

FEAR OF LOSS OF PARENTAL INTEGRITY WITH CHILDREN [26,105,471,525]

ASSESSMENT

Data Collection

Subjective Data
• Person experiences feelings of threat or danger
• Can describe or identify the threat or danger
Focuses concern on his children
Is worried about the unity of the parent–child relationship
Is concerned that the children may feel unloved or unwanted when parents approve of unpleasant medical therapy
Wonders if the children will know and recognize the parent after a long absence
May feel the child has lost interest in the family, especially during adolescence
May verbalize anger or frustration with the situation

Objective Data
• May manifest physical findings such as facial flushing or pallor, rapid or deep respirations, rapid or bounding pulse, increased blood pressure, sweating, trembling
• May exhibit behavior such as restlessness, sleep disturbances, change in eating habits, irritability, crying, avoiding unpleasant situations with the children, seeking reassurance

Data Analysis

Nursing Diagnosis
FEAR OF LOSS OF PARENTAL INTEGRITY WITH CHILDREN: A feeling of alarm and fright about losing unity with one's children

Common Etiology (Stressors)
DISEASES: Any severe or prolonged disease of parent or child
INJURIES: Any severe injury

SIGNS AND SYMPTOMS: Weakness

PSYCHOSOCIAL FACTORS: The threat of a specific and clearly identified danger, the threat of real or imagined danger, loss of independence (of the parent), loss of role performance, role change with a significant other (child), conflicting parental and community values or conflicting parental and children's values

HEALTH CARE FACTORS: *Health care environment*: Intensive care unit, isolation unit, locked psychiatric unit. *Hospitalization*: Of self or a significant other (child)

LIFESTYLE: Alcohol or drug abuse, gambling

SITUATIONAL FACTORS: Confinement in prison, loss of employment, lack of finances, divorce, marital separation from a spouse who has child custody, illness of or injury to self or a significant other, extensive travel by a parent

PLANNING

Unmet Needs

Comfort, protection from psychologic threat, acceptance, caring and communicating relationships, high evaluation of self, sense of adequacy, personal growth and maturity, increased learning, increased reality perception and problem-solving ability

Expected Outcome

Person verbalizes fears

Verbalizes feelings of adequacy and competence in meeting the fear-creating experience

Verbalizes self-satisfaction and growth in having coped with the fear-creating experience

Calm, relaxed facial expression, body movements, and behavior

NURSING INTERVENTIONS

Nursing Treatments

Approach unhurriedly

Reassure verbally (that the nurse will help the person as much as possible)

Demonstrate calmness

Provide an atmosphere of acceptance

Encourage the expression of feelings (about the fear)

Listen attentively

Talk with the person (and with the children about the situation)

Offer feedback to the person's expressed feelings

Communicate nurse sensitivity to the person's problem

Relate to the person on an adult–adult level, not on a parent–child level (which could increase fear)

Ask the person to identify the problem

Ask for specifics, not generalizations, about the problem

Support a realistic assessment of the situation (about the probability of such occurring: is the child–parent relationship sound; if not, what is the problem?)

Ask how the person normally copes with fear (what does he usually do when fearful that reduces the fear?)

Provide whatever the person needs to use his usual coping mechanisms

Explore with the person his strengths and resources (to cope with the fear and the changed or changing parent role)

Provide emotionally safe experiences (whenever possible, between parent and child; have the parent do things for the sick child, while the nurse performs the painful treatments, etc.)

Allow unlimited visiting (of parents or children, depending on who is ill)

Encourage telephone calls with significant persons

Nursing Observations

Observe for an excessive stress level (resulting from the fear)

Determine the degree of insight that the person has (into the fear)

Observe for evidence of a favorable response to therapy (reduced fear and increased comfort)

Health Teaching

Explain that the person's response is appropriate and commonly experienced

Advise (parents and children) that significant persons express caring for one another

Explain that ill persons are often hypersensitive (to responses from significant others)

EVALUATION

Record actual outcome

FEAR OF LOSS OF PERSONAL IDENTITY[105,471,525]

ASSESSMENT

Data Collection

Subjective Data
* Person experiences feelings of threat or danger
* Can describe or identify the threat or danger
  Is concerned that he will be perceived as merely part of a group
  Is worried that individual desires or needs will be ignored
  Is aware of being identified by number or disease entity
  Perceives certain personal items as important to self identity

Objective Data
* May manifest physical findings such as facial flushing or pallor, rapid or deep respirations, rapid or bounding pulse, increased blood pressure, sweating, trembling
* May exhibit behavior such as restlessness, irritability, rapid speech, demanding and controlling behavior

Data Analysis

Nursing Diagnosis
FEAR OF LOSS OF PERSONAL IDENTITY: A feeling of alarm and fright about losing one's separateness, distinct characteristics, and needs, as distinguished from those of another

Common Etiology (Stressors)
PSYCHOSOCIAL FACTORS: The threat of a specific and clearly identified danger, the threat of real or imagined danger
HEALTH CARE FACTORS: *Health care environment*: Lack of privacy. *Health care provider*: Preoccupation of the health care provider with equipment, routine, treatment, pathology. *Hospitalization or institutionalization*: Of self. *Institutional policies*: Restrictive. *Institutional routine*: Inflexible. *Welfare or human resource services*: Dehumanizing welfare services
DEVELOPMENTAL PHASES: Old age
LIFESTYLE: Communal living
SITUATIONAL FACTORS: Being adopted or available for adoption, illness or injury, confinement in prison

PLANNING

Unmet Needs

Comfort, protection from psychologic threat, acceptance, caring and communicating relationships, high evaluation of self, sense of adequacy, personal growth and maturity, increased learning, increased reality perception and problem-solving ability

Expected Outcome

Person verbalizes fears

Verbalizes feelings of adequacy and competence in meeting the fear-creating experience

Verbalizes self-satisfaction and growth in having coped with the fear-creating experience
Calm, relaxed facial expression, body movements, and behavior

NURSING INTERVENTIONS

Nursing Treatments

Approach unhurriedly
Reassure verbally (that the nurse will help maintain the person's individuality)
Demonstrate calmness
Provide an atmosphere of acceptance
Encourage the expression of feelings (about the fear)
Listen attentively
Offer feedback to the person's expressed feelings
Communicate nurse sensitivity to the person's problem
Ask for specifics, not generalizations, about the problem
Provide privacy (as much as possible)
Grant special requests (and allow to retain selected personal items)
Explore with the person his value as an individual
Use the person's name frequently

Nursing Observations

Determine the degree of insight that the person has (into the fear)
Observe for evidence of a favorable response to therapy (reduced fear and increased
   comfort)

Health Teaching

Explain that the person's response is appropriate and commonly experienced
Recommend a habitual, positive mental attitude (toward self)

EVALUATION

Record actual outcome

FEAR OF LOSS OF SEXUALITY[105,471,525]

ASSESSMENT

Data Collection

Subjective Data
• Person experiences feelings of threat or danger
• Can describe or identify the threat or danger
  May relate a decreased interest or changes in patterns of sexual functioning
  Is concerned about not being attractive to the opposite sex
  May feel that others do not perceive him or her as wholly male or female, as in the
  past

Objective Data
• May manifest physical findings such as facial flushing or pallor, rapid or deep respirations, rapid or bounding pulse, increased blood pressure, sweating, trembling
• May exhibit behavior such as restlessness, sleep disturbances, change in eating habits,
  irritability, demanding and controlling behavior, crying, seeking reassurance

Data Analysis

Nursing Diagnosis
FEAR OF LOSS OF SEXUALITY: A feeling of alarm and fright about losing physical or social
   qualities that make a person distinctly male or female

Common Etiology (Stressors)

DISEASES: Cachexia, carcinoma, cerebrovascular accident, diabetes mellitus, Hansen's disease, hirsutism (female), major depression, multiple sclerosis, myocardial infarction, Parkinson's disease, rheumatoid arthritis

INJURIES: Burn wound, fracture and compression of the spinal cord, traumatic amputation or disfigurement

SIGNS AND SYMPTOMS: Edema, fatigue, jaundice, pain, rash, weakness

PSYCHOSOCIAL FACTORS: The threat of a specific and clearly identified danger, the threat of real or imagined danger, loss of independence, role change with a significant other, loss of role performance

HUMAN BODY: *Body appearance*: A disfigured body. *Body function*: Loss of body function. *Body part*: Loss of a body part. *Body states*: Climacteric, menopause

HEALTH CARE FACTORS: *Diagnostic procedures*: Exposure to x-ray, cystoscopy (men), dilation and curettage (women). *Adverse effects of medical, drug, or surgical therapy*: Loss of hair from radiation or chemotherapy; loss of libido from antihypertensive drugs, tagamet, hemiodialysis; loss of reproductive ability from fallopian tube ligation, hysterectomy, oophorectomy, orchiectomy, prostatectomy, salpingectomy, vasectomy

DEVELOPMENTAL PHASES: Middle age, old age

SITUATIONAL FACTORS: Childlessness

PLANNING

Unmet Needs

Comfort, protection from psychologic threat, acceptance, caring and communicating relationships, high evaluation of self, sense of adequacy, personal growth and maturity, increased learning, increased reality perception and problem-solving ability

Expected Outcome

Person verbalizes fears

Verbalizes feelings of adequacy and competence in meeting the fear-creating experience

Verbalizes self-satisfaction and growth in having coped with the fear-creating experience

Calm, relaxed facial expression, body movements, and behavior

NURSING INTERVENTIONS

Nursing Treatments

Approach unhurriedly

Reassure verbally (that the nurse will help the person as much as possible)

Demonstrate calmness

Provide an atmosphere of acceptance

Encourage the expression of feelings (about the fear)

Listen attentively

Offer feedback to the person's expressed feelings

Communicate nurse sensitivity to the person's problem

Communicate that the nurse feels comfortable with the person's discussion of sexuality

Relate to the person on an adult–adult level, not on a parent–child level (which could increase fear)

Ask the person to identify the problem

Ask for specifics, not generalizations, about the problem

Provide reliable information (about the probability of loss of sexuality, about the effects of drugs, procedures, etc.)

Ask how the person normally copes with fear (what does he usually do when fearful that reduces the fear?)

Provide whatever the person needs to use his usual coping mechanisms

Explore with the person his strengths and resources (to overcome the situation)

Explore with the person his individual characteristics (besides those related to sexuality)

Provide objects that symbolize sex identity (such as a pipe, fishing hat, perfume, needlework)

Do not allow unpleasant surprise situations (such as unexpected procedure that might be perceived as threatening sexuality or a visit from a person of the opposite sex without opportunity to prepare for the visit)

Reduce the demands placed on the person (so that more energy is available for coping)

Introduce to persons who have undergone the same experience (if appropriate)

Nursing Observations

Observe for an excessive stress level (resulting from the fear)

Determine the degree of insight that the person has (into the fear)

Observe for evidence of a favorable response to therapy (reduced fear and increased comfort)

Health Teaching

Explain that the person's response is appropriate and commonly experienced

Explain that sexuality is but one part of human development (and that the whole of the person is equally important)

Explain how to channel emotional energy and obtain release from stress (through running, swimming, other sports, creative activities, laughing, talking things over)

Recommend a habitual, positive mental attitude (toward the person's sexuality)

EVALUATION

Record actual outcome

FEAR OF LOSS OF SOCIAL INTEGRITY WITH FRIENDS [105,471,525]

ASSESSMENT

Data Collection

Subjective Data
• Person experiences feelings of threat or danger
• Can describe or identify the threat or danger
  Is concerned about keeping friends
  Wonders if friends will show continued interest
  Is worried that his place in the group will be taken by someone else
  Expects friends to be loyal, but realistically knows that time and distance separate people

Objective Data
• May manifest physical findings such as facial flushing or pallor, rapid or deep respirations, rapid or bounding pulse, increased blood pressure, sweating, trembling
• May exhibit behavior such as restlessness, sleep disturbances, change in eating habits, irritability, crying, making frequent phone calls to friends

Data Analysis

Nursing Diagnosis
FEAR OF LOSS OF SOCIAL INTEGRITY WITH FRIENDS: A feeling of alarm and fright about losing unity with friends

Common Etiology (Stressors)
DISEASES: Any severe or prolonged disease
INJURIES: Any severe injury, especially disfigurement
SIGNS AND SYMPTOMS: Immobility, pain, weakness
PSYCHOSOCIAL FACTORS: The threat of a specific and clearly identified danger, the threat of real or imagined danger, loss of independence, repeated failure to achieve, lack of emotional control, lack of responsibility, loss of role performance

HUMAN BODY: *Body appearance*: Body changes that seem different than changes in the bodies of peers, a disfigured body. *Body function*: Loss of body function. *Body part*: Loss of a body part. *Body size*: Delayed body growth

HEALTH CARE FACTORS: *Hospitalization or institutionalization*: Of self. *Adverse effects of medical, drug, or surgical therapy*: Loss of body part from amputation, loss of hair from radiation and chemotherapy. *Recovery*: Delayed recovery from illness

LIFESTYLE: Alcohol or drug abuse, gambling

SITUATIONAL FACTORS: Childlessness, marital separation, divorce, retirement

PLANNING

Unmet Needs

Comfort, protection from psychologic threat, acceptance, caring and communicating relationships, high evaluation of self, sense of adequacy, personal growth and maturity, increased learning, increased reality perception and problem-solving ability

Expected Outcome

Person verbalizes fears

Verbalizes feelings of adequacy and competence in meeting the fear-creating experience

Verbalizes self-satisfaction and growth in having coped with the fear-creating experience

Calm, relaxed facial expression, body movements, and behavior

NURSING INTERVENTIONS

Nursing Treatments

Approach unhurriedly

Reassure verbally

Demonstrate calmness

Provide an atmosphere of acceptance

Encourage the expression of feelings (about the fear and the expression of the need for friendship to friends)

Listen attentively

Offer feedback to the person's expressed feelings

Communicate nurse sensitivity to the person's problems

Ask the person to identify the problem

Ask for specifics, not generalizations, about the problem

Support a realistic assessment of the situation (that with life's changes, some people who have been friends will no longer be friends; a person constantly meets new people and makes new friends throughout life)

Provide reliable information (about the friends who inquire and send messages)

Ask how the person normally copes with fear (what does he usually do when fearful that reduces the fear?)

Provide whatever the person needs to use his usual coping mechanisms)

Encourage awareness of positive responses from others (such as cards, calls, visits, flowers)

Encourage telephone calls with significant persons

Allow unlimited visitors (friends)

Nursing Observations

Determine the degree of insight that the person has (into the fear)

Observe for evidence of a favorable response to therapy (reduced fear and satisfaction with the relationships of friends)

Health Teaching

Explain that the person's response is appropriate and commonly experienced

Explain (to family and friends) that ill or aged persons are hypersensitive (to relatedness)

Recommend a habitual, positive mental attitude (about maintaining unity with friends)

EVALUATION

Record actual outcome

FEAR OF MUTILATION[105,471,525]

ASSESSMENT

Data Collection

Subjective Data
- Person experiences feelings of threat or danger to the self
- Can describe or identify the threat or danger
  Is intensely concerned about his body parts being cut off, cut up, or radically altered
  Finds the thought intolerable

Objective Data
- May manifest physical findings such as facial flushing or pallor, rapid or deep respirations, rapid or bounding pulse, increased blood pressure, sweating, trembling
- May exhibit behavior such as restlessness, sleep disturbances, change in eating habits, irritability, short attention span, making poor judgments, forgetfulness, rapid speech, demanding and controlling behavior; crying

Data Analysis

Nursing Diagnosis
FEAR OF MUTILATION: A feeling of alarm or fright about the removal or destruction of a visible part of the body

Common Etiology (Stressors)
PSYCHOSOCIAL FACTORS: The threat of a specific and clearly identified danger, the threat of real or imagined danger
HEALTH CARE FACTORS: *Diagnostic procedure*: A biopsy, especially a facial biopsy. *Surgical procedures*: Surgery of any kind, but especially amputation, glossectomy, hemipelvectomy, mastectomy; enucleation or evisceration of an eyeball; neck or skin tumor resection

PLANNING

Unmet Needs

Comfort, protection from psychologic threat, acceptance, caring and communicating relationships, high evaluation of self, sense of adequacy, personal growth and maturity, increased learning, increased reality perception and problem-solving ability

Expected Outcome

Person verbalizes fears
Verbalizes feelings of adequacy and competence in meeting the fear-creating experience
Verbalizes self-satisfaction and growth in having coped with the fear-creating experience
Calm, relaxed facial expression, body movements, and behavior

NURSING INTERVENTIONS

Nursing Treatments

Approach unhurriedly
Reassure verbally (that the nurse will help the person as much as possible)
Demonstrate calmness
Provide an atmosphere of acceptance
Encourage the expression of feelings (about the fear, not only to the nurse, but also to the physician)
Listen attentively
Offer feedback to the person's expressed feelings
Communicate nurse sensitivity to the person's problem
Relate to the person on an adult–adult level, not on a parent–child level (which could increase fear)
Attend the person constantly (until he feels sufficiently comfortable to be alone)
Provide frequent contact with the person (thereafter)
Ask the person to identify the problem

Ask for specifics, not generalizations, about the problem

Provide reliable information (about the procedure or surgery, about the invasive process of malignant cells, etc.)

Ask how the person normally copes with fear (what does he usually do when fearful that reduces the fear?)

Provide whatever the person needs to use his usual coping mechanisms

Explore with the person his positive characteristics (and avoid focusing primarily on the body change)

Explore with the person his strengths and resources (to cope with the situation)

Do not allow unpleasant surprise situations (such as unexpected or unexplained procedures)

Offer assurance that decisions are revokable (if the person has changed his former decision about surgery)

Avoid placing the person on enforced inactivity (which heightens fear)

Reduce the demands placed on the person (so that more energy is available for coping)

Introduce to persons who have undergone the same experience (if appropriate)

Nursing Observations

Determine the degree of insight that the person has (into the fear)

Observe for evidence of a favorable response to therapy (reduced fear and increased comfort)

Health Teaching

Explain that the person's response is appropriate and commonly experienced

Recommend methods for achieving total relaxation (controlled breathing, quietly listening to music, doing nothing, which reduces fear)

Teach the specific methods (for disguising disfigured areas of body parts with prosthesis, cosmetics, clothing, etc.)

EVALUATION

Record actual outcome

FEAR OF PAIN [105,471,525,543,663]

ASSESSMENT

Data Collection

Subjective Data

• Person experiences feelings of threat or danger

• Can describe or identify the threat or danger

Relates a dread of pain

Anticipates pain before it occurs

Desires to withdraw from the experience perceived as painful

May seek drug relief before or as soon as pain occurs

Feels irritable

Objective Data

• May manifest physical findings such as facial flushing or pallor, rapid or deep respirations, rapid or bounding pulse, increased blood pressure, sweating, trembling

• May exhibit behavior such as restlessness, sleep disturbances, change in eating habits, irritability, rapid speech, demanding and controlling behavior, crying, avoiding persons (such as nurses and doctors) associated with pain, being unavailable at the scheduled time of a painful experience, touching or holding out arms to comforting persons

Data Analysis

Nursing Diagnosis

FEAR OF PAIN: A feeling of alarm and fright about the perception of distressful hurting

Common Etiology (Stressors)

DISEASES: Any

INJURIES: Any

SIGNS AND SYMPTOMS: Pain

PSYCHOSOCIAL FACTORS: The threat of a specific, clearly identified danger; the threat of real or imagined danger

HUMAN BODY: *Natural body function*: Childbirth. *Body states*: Menstruation

HEALTH CARE FACTORS: *Diagnostic procedures*: Any, such as barium enema, bone marrow aspiration, cardiac catheterization, cisternal puncture, lumbar puncture, Pap smear, physical examination, proctoscopy. *Drug therapy*: Such as chemotherapy, tissue irritation from drug therapy. *Medical therapy*: Therapeutic ambulation, breast pump therapy, cardioversion, coughing and deep breathing, dressing changes, enemas, therapeutic and postmastectomy exercise, venipuncture for hemodialysis, hyperalimentation or intravenous infusion, needle injections, nerve block, irrigations, paracentesis, peritoneal dialysis, phlebotomy, painful positioning, rehabilitation therapy, therapeutic apheresis, thoracentesis, traction, therapeutic turning, urinary catheterization, withdrawal from alcohol or drugs *Surgical procedures*: Any, such as appendectomy, cauterization, cesarean section, hemorrhoidectomy, lobectomy of lung, etc. *Surgical incision*: Painful

DEVELOPMENTAL PHASES: Preschooler (age 3–6 years)

SITUATIONAL FACTORS: Impending death, terminal illness

PLANNING

Unmet Needs

Comfort, protection from psychologic threat, acceptance, caring and communicating relationships, high evaluation of self, sense of adequacy, personal growth and maturity, increased learning, increased reality perception and problem-solving ability

Expected Outcome

Person verbalizes fears

Verbalizes feelings of adequacy and competence in meeting the fear-creating experience

Verbalizes self-satisfaction and growth in having coped with the fear-creating experience

Calm, relaxed facial expression, body movements, and behavior

NURSING INTERVENTIONS

Nursing Treatments

Approach unhurriedly

Reassure verbally (that the nurse will stay with the person during the painful experience)

Demonstrate calmness

Provide an atmosphere of acceptance

Arrange pleasant surroundings

Encourage the expression of feelings (about the fear)

Listen attentively

Offer feedback to the person's expressed feelings

Communicate nurse sensitivity to the person's problem

Relate to the person on an adult–adult level, not on a parent–child level (which could increase fear)

Attend the person constantly (until he feels sufficiently comfortable to be alone and during the painful experience)

Ask for specifics, not generalizations, about the problem

Support a realistic assessment of the situation (that pain is often necessary to achieve health)

Provide reliable information (about the painful procedure, illness, etc.)

Ask how the person normally copes with fear (what does he usually do when fearful that reduces the fear?)

Provide whatever the person needs to use his usual coping mechanisms

Prepare the person for the painful experience

Explore with the person his strengths and resources (to cope with the fear and the pain)

Explore with the person previous displays of courage (in stressful situations)

Provide emotionally safe experiences (whenever possible, such as scheduling nonpainful procedures first)

Provide objects that symbolize safeness (a child's favorite doll, a blanket, etc.)

Do not allow unpleasant surprise situations (such as unexpected, unexplained procedures)

Refrain from forcing the treatment

Refrain from performing nonessential procedures

Avoid placing the person on enforced inactivity (which heightens fear)

Reduce the demands placed on the person (so that more energy is available for coping)

Introduce to persons who have undergone the same experience (if appropriate)

Involve the family (if the family can comfort the person)

Nursing Observations

Determine the degree of insight that the person has

Observe for evidence of a favorable response to therapy (reduced fear and increased comfort)

Health Teaching

Explain that the person's response is appropriate and commonly experienced

Explain that it is acceptable to admit the existence of pain (to cry, to request pain medication)

Recommend methods for achieving total relaxation (since fear increases the pain intensity. Suggest controlled breathing, which reduces fear)

Explain how to channel emotional energy and obtain release from stress (by talking things over)

Explain the causes of fear of pain (past unpleasant experiences, the threat to self)

EVALUATION

Record actual outcome

FEAR OF PARALYSIS [105,471,525]

ASSESSMENT

Data Collection

Subjective Data

• Person experiences feelings of threat or danger

• Can describe or identify the threat or danger

Relates having heard that paralysis has occurred to someone else in a similar situation

Questions in detail the possible effects of the threatening disease, injury, or procedures

May complain of muscle weakness or paraesthesias

Objective Data

• May manifest physical findings such as facial flushing or pallor, rapid or deep respirations, rapid or bounding pulse, increased blood pressure, sweating, trembling

• May exhibit behavior such as restlessness, sleep disturbances, irritability, demanding and controlling behavior, seeking reassurance

Data Analysis

Nursing Diagnosis

FEAR OF PARALYSIS: A feeling of alarm and fright about the loss of voluntary body motion and sensation

Common Etiology (Stressors)

INJURIES: Fracture and compression of the spinal cord

SIGNS AND SYMPTOMS: Numbness, stiffness, weakness

PSYCHOSOCIAL FACTORS: The threat of a specific and clearly identified danger, the threat of real or imagined danger

HEALTH CARE FACTORS: *Diagnostic procedures*: Lumbar puncture, myelography, pneumoen-cephalogram. *Medical therapy*: Nerve block, disrupted spinal traction. *Surgical therapy*: Spinal anesthesia. *Surgical procedures*: Craiotomy, decompression of the spinal cord, laminectomy, laminotomy

PLANNING

Unmet Needs

Comfort, protection from psychologic threat, acceptance, caring and communicating relationships, high evaluation of self, sense of adequacy, personal growth and maturity, increased learning, increased reality perception and problem-solving ability

Expected Outcome

Person verbalizes fears

Verbalizes feelings of adequacy and competence in meeting the fear-creating experience

Verbalizes self-satisfaction and growth in having coped with the fear-creating experience

Calm, relaxed facial expression, body movements, and behavior

NURSING INTERVENTIONS

Nursing Treatments

Approach unhurriedly

Reassure verbally (that the nurse will help the person as much as possible)

Demonstrate calmness

Provide an atmosphere of acceptance

Encourage the expression of feelings (about the fear)

Listen attentively

Offer feedback to the person's expressed feelings

Communicate nurse sensitivity to the person's problem

Relate to the person on an adult–adult level, not on a parent–child level (which could increase fear)

Attend the person constantly (until he feels sufficiently comfortable to be alone)

Ask the person to identify the problem

Ask for specifics, not generalizations, about the problem

Provide reliable information (about the probability of paralysis; about the procedure, injury, illness, body sensations)

Ask how the person normally copes with fear (what does he usually do when fearful that reduces the fear?)

Provide whatever the person needs to use his usual coping mechanisms

Provide emotionally safe experiences (whenever possible, such as skillful nursing care and handling of the spinal traction equipment, etc.)

Do not allow unpleasant surprise situations (such as unexpected, unexplained procedures)

Reduce the demands placed on the person (so that more energy is available for coping)

Introduce to persons who have undergone the same experience (if appropriate)

Nursing Observations

Determine the degree of insight that the person has (into the fear)

Observe for evidence of a favorable response to therapy (reduced fear and increased comfort)

Health Teaching

Explain that the person's response is appropriate and commonly experienced

Explain how to channel emotional energy and obtain release from stress (by talking things over)

Recommend methods for achieving total relaxation (controlled breathing, quietly listening to music, doing nothing, which reduces fear)

Recommend a habitual, positive mental attitude

EVALUATION

Record actual outcome

FEAR OF PHYSICAL INJURY[105,471,525]

ASSESSMENT

Data Collection

Subjective Data

- Person experiences feelings of threat or danger
- Can describe or identify the threat or danger

  Verbalizes concern that he will be harmed

  Focuses on a threatening person, procedure, or event

  May anticipate injury such as bone fracture, accidental wounds, or assault by others

Objective Data

- May manifest physical findings such as facial flushing or pallor, rapid or deep respirations, rapid or bounding pulse, increased blood pressure, sweating, trembling
- May exhibit behavior such as restlessness, sleep disturbances, change in eating habits, irritability, demanding and controlling behavior, crying, avoiding threatening persons and situations, seeking reassurance

Data Analysis

Nursing Diagnosis

FEAR OF PHYSICAL INJURY: A feeling of alarm and fright about being physically harmed in some way

Common Etiology (Stressors)

DISEASES: Paranoid state

SIGNS AND SYMPTOMS: Convulsions

PSYCHOSOCIAL FACTORS: The threat of a specific and clearly identified danger, the threat of real or imagined danger, loss of independence, the threat of abuse from a significant other

HEALTH CARE FACTORS: *Health care decision*: To donate a body organ, to donate blood. *Health care delivery*: Low quality

HUMAN BODY: *Natural body function*: Childbirth. *Body state*: Pregnancy. *Health care environment*: Locked psychiatric unit. *Hospitalization:* Any. *Institutionalization:* Any. *Diagnostic procedures*: Any. *Health therapy*: Delayed, painful, or experimental health therapy. *Medical therapy*: Bivalve of a cast, intermittent positive pressure breathing, intravenous infusion, blood transfusion. *Recovery*: Renewed physical activity or sexual activity after recovery. *Surgical therapy*: Anesthesia. *Surgical procedures*: Any. *Therapeutic equipment*: Cardiac pacemaker, CircOlectric bed, defibrillator, monitoring equipment, Stryker frame

DEVELOPMENTAL PHASES: Preschooler (age 2–6 years), old age

ENVIRONMENTAL FACTORS: *Environmental radiation*: Exposure to damaging microwaves

PLANNING

Unmet Needs

Comfort, protection from psychologic threat, acceptance, caring and communicating relationships, high evaluation of self, sense of adequacy, personal growth and maturity, increased learning, increased reality perception and problem-solving ability

Expected Outcome

Person verbalizes fears
Verbalizes feelings of adequacy and competence in meeting the fear-creating experience
Verbalizes self-satisfaction and growth in having coped with the fear-creating experience
Calm, relaxed facial expression, body movements, and behavior

NURSING INTERVENTIONS

Nursing Treatments

Approach unhurriedly
Reassure verbally (that the nurse will help the person as much as possible)
Demonstrate calmness
Provide an atmosphere of acceptance
Encourage the expression of feelings (about the fear)
Listen attentively
Offer feedback to the person's expressed feelings
Communicate nurse sensitivity to the person's problem
Relate to the person on an adult–adult level, not on a parent–child level (which could increase fear)
Attend the person constantly (until he feels sufficiently comfortable to be alone)
Provide frequent contact with the person (thereafter)
Ask the person to identify the problem
Ask for specifics, not generalizations, about the problem
Provide reliable information (about the probability of physical harm; about the condition, illness, procedures, equipment)
Ask how the person normally copes with fear (what does he usually do when fearful that reduces the fear?)
Provide whatever the person needs to use his usual coping mechanisms
Provide objects that symbolize safeness (person's religious medallion, bed rails, etc.)
Do not allow unpleasant surprise situations (such as unexpected, unexplained procedures)
Avoid placing the person on enforced inactivity (which heightens fear)
Reduce the demands placed on the person (so that more energy is available for coping)
Introduce to persons who have undergone the same experience (if appropriate)

Nursing Observations

Observe for an excessive stress level (resulting from the fear)
Determine the degree of insight that the person has (into the fear)
Observe for evidence of a favorable response to therapy (reduced fear and increased comfort)

Health Teaching

Explain that the person's response is appropriate and commonly experienced
Explain that fatigue should be recognized as a stress factor (which heightens fear)
Explain how to channel emotional energy and obtain release from stress (by talking things over, laughing)
Recommend methods for achieving total relaxation (controlled breathing, quietly listening to music, doing nothing, which reduces fear)
Recommend a habitual, positive mental attitude
Teach how to use the problem-solving method (to prevent physical injury of any kind)

EVALUATION

Record actual outcome

FEAR OF PREGNANCY[105,471,525]

ASSESSMENT

Data Collection

Subjective Data
- Person experiences feelings of threat or danger
- Can describe or identify the threat or danger
  Relates concern that the woman might be or might become pregnant
  Is concerned with the effects of the pregnancy on self or others
  Requests immediate pregnancy-test results

Objective Data
- May manifest physical findings such as facial flushing or pallor, rapid or deep respirations, rapid or bounding pulse, increased blood pressure, sweating, trembling
- May exhibit behavior such as sleep disturbances, irritability, controlling behavior, crying, avoiding sexual relations

Data Analysis

Nursing Diagnosis
FEAR OF PREGNANCY: A feeling of alarm and fright about the possibility of a woman becoming pregnant

Common Etiology (Stressors)
PSYCHOSOCIAL FACTORS: The threat of a specific and clearly identified danger, the threat of real or imagined danger, the threat of a deteriorating relationship with spouse
HEALTH CARE FACTORS: A previous complicated pregnancy or delivery (that endangered the woman's or fetal life)
DEVELOPMENTAL PHASES: Adolescence, middle age, menopause
LIFESTYLE: Cultural superstitions
SITUATIONAL FACTORS: Lack of finances, loss of or threat of loss of employment, having been victimized by sexual assault

PLANNING

Unmet Needs
Comfort, protection from psychologic threat, acceptance, caring and communicating relationships, high evaluation of self, sense of adequacy, personal growth and maturity, increased learning, increased reality perception and problem-solving ability

Expected Outcome
Person verbalizes feelings
Verbalizes feelings of adequacy and competence in meeting the fear-creating experience
Verbalizes self-satisfaction and growth in having coped with the fear-creating experience
Calm, relaxed facial expression, body movements, and behavior

NURSING INTERVENTIONS

Nursing Treatments
Approach unhurriedly
Reassure verbally (that the nurse will help the person as much as possible)
Demonstrate calmness
Provide an atmosphere of acceptance
Encourage the expression of feelings (about the fear)
Listen attentively
Offer feedback to the person's expressed feelings
Communicate nurse sensitivity to the person's problem
Relate to the person on an adult–adult level, not on a parent–child level (which could increase fear)
Ask the person to identify the problem

Ask for specifics, not generalizations, about the problem

Provide reliable information (about the effects of pregnancy on specific diseases, about the probability of a successful uncomplicated pregnancy)

Perform a pregnancy test (to determine if the woman is pregnant)

Ask how the person normally copes with fear (what does she usually do when fearful that reduces the fear?)

Provide whatever the person needs to use her usual coping mechanisms

Explore with the person her strengths and resources (to cope with a pregnancy if she is pregnant)

Nursing Observations

Observe for an excessive stress level (resulting from the fear)

Determine the degree of insight that the person has (into the fear)

Observe for evidence of a favorable response to therapy (reduced fear and increased comfort)

Health Teaching

Explain that the person's response is appropriate and commonly experienced

Explain the options available for family planning (considering the person's religious and cultural beliefs and practices)

Recommend a habitual, positive mental attitude (toward herself and the pregnancy, if the woman is pregnant)

EVALUATION

Record actual outcome

FEAR OF RECURRENCE OF AN ILLNESS[105,471,525]

ASSESSMENT

Data Collection

Subjective Data
- Person experiences feelings of threat or danger
- Can describe or identify the threat or danger
  Relates having had a previous, life-threatening, or severe health problem or one causing severe limitations
  Is preoccupied with the possibility of the illness returning
  May medicate self with megavitamins, frequently checks for signs and symptoms, etc.
  Fears the worst but hopes for the best

Objective Data
- May manifest physical findings such as facial flushing or pallor, rapid or deep respirations, rapid or bounding pulse, increased blood pressure, sweating, trembling
- May exhibit behavior such as restlessness, sleep disturbances, irritability, controlling behavior, crying, frequent call-light signaling, seeking reassurance

Data Analysis

Nursing Diagnosis
FEAR OF RECURRENCE OF AN ILLNESS: A feeling of alarm and fright that a disease or condition that has been in remission might occur again

Common Etiology (Stressors)
DISEASES: Any but especially carcinoma, Guillian-Barré syndrome, Hodgkin's disease, leukemia, myocardial infarction, tuberculosis
PSYCHOSOCIAL FACTORS: The threat of a specific and clearly identified danger, the threat of real or imagined danger
HEALTH CARE FACTORS: *Follow-up evaluation*: An impending or ongoing follow-up evaluation

PLANNING

Unmet Needs

Comfort, protection from psychologic threat, acceptance, caring and communicating relationships, high evaluation of self, sense of adequacy, personal growth and maturity, increased learning, increased reality perception and problem-solving ability

Expected Outcome

Person verbalizes fears

Verbalizes feelings of adequacy and competence in meeting the fear-creating experience

Verbalizes self-satisfaction and growth in having coped with the fear-creating experience

Calm, relaxed facial expression, body movements, and behavior

NURSING INTERVENTIONS

Nursing Treatments

Approach unhurriedly

Reassure verbally (that the nurse will help the person as much as possible)

Demonstrate calmness

Provide an atmosphere of acceptance

Encourage the expression of feelings (about the fear)

Listen attentively

Offer feedback to the person's expressed feelings

Communicate nurse sensitivity to the person's problem

Relate to the person on an adult–adult level, not on a parent–child level (which could increase fear)

Ask the person to identify the problem

Ask for specifics, not generalizations, about the problem

Provide reliable information (about the probability of the illness recurring, about how to prevent a recurrence of the illness)

Ask how the person normally copes with fear (what does he usually do when fearful that reduces the fear?)

Provide whatever the person needs to use his usual coping mechanisms

Explore with the person his strengths and resources (to cope with the fear, to prevent a recurrence, and to cope with the illness should it recur)

Nursing Observations

Determine the degree of insight that the person has (into the fear)

Observe for evidence of a favorable response to therapy (reduced fear and increased comfort)

Health Teaching

Explain that the person's response is appropriate and commonly experienced

Explain that fatigue should be recognized as a stress factor (which heightens fear)

Explain how to channel emotional energy and obtain release from stress (by running, swimming, other sports, creative activities, laughing, talking things over)

Recommend a habitual, positive mental attitude (toward himself and his health)

EVALUATION

Record actual outcome

FEAR OF REJECTION [105,471,525]

ASSESSMENT

Data Collection

Subjective Data

• Person experiences feelings of threat or danger

- Can describe or identify the threat or danger
  Has reason to believe that another might disapprove of him
  May want to relate overtly to that person but fears a negative response

Objective Data
- May manifest physical findings such as facial flushing or pallor, rapid or deep respirations, rapid or bounding pulse, increased blood pressure, sweating, trembling
- May exhibit behavior such as restlessness, controlling behavior, crying, overattentiveness to the person, seeking reassurance

Data Analysis

Nursing Diagnosis
FEAR OF REJECTION: A feeling of alarm and fright that one might be refused or unaccepted by another

Common Etiology (Stressors)
BIRTH DEFECTS: Any, such as cleft lip, club foot or hand, dwarfism
DISEASES: Any, such as acne vulgaris, alcoholism, blindness, carcinoma, cerebrovascular accident, dermatitis, drug addiction, gonorrhea, Hansen's disease, multiple sclerosis, obesity, Parkinson's disease, renal failure, schizophrenia, syphilis
INJURIES: Any, such as burn wound, fracture and compression of the spinal cord, traumatic amputation or disfigurement
SIGNS AND SYMPTOMS: Edema, hair loss, incontinence, jaundice, memory loss, paralysis, rash, tremor, weakness
PSYCHOSOCIAL FACTORS: The threat of a specific and clearly identified danger, the threat of real or imagined danger, loss of independence, the threat of repeated failure to achieve, lack of achievement of developmental intimacy (young adulthood), the threat of previous rejection by a significant other
HUMAN BODY: *Body appearance*: A disfigured body. *Body function*: Loss of body function. *Body part*: Loss of a body part. *Body state*: Pregnancy, menopause
HEALTH CARE FACTORS: *Health care provider*: The suggestion by a health care provider that symptoms are not real. *Medical therapy*: Psychotherapy. *Surgical therapy*: Disfigurement from surgery. *Adverse effects of medical, drug, or surgical therapy*: Loss of hair from radiation, chemotherapy, or presurgical cranial preparation, edema from corticosteroids; loss of natural elimination and elimination control from colostomy, ileocolostomy, ileostomy, ureterocolostomy, ureteroileostomy, ureterosigmoidostomy, ureterostomy, ureterotomy; loss of normal food intake from esophagectomy; loss of reproductive ability from fallopian tube ligation, hysterectomy, oophorectomy, orchidectomy, prostatectomy, salpingectomy, vasectomy; loss of speech from glossectomy, laryngectomy, tracheostomy, vocal cordectomy; loss of vision from enucleation or evisceration of an eyeball; loss of libido from antihypertensive drugs, tagamet, hemodialysis.
DEVELOPMENTAL PHASES: Any but especially adolescence, old age
LIFESTYLE: Lack of conformity (by self) to cultural mores
SITUATIONAL FACTORS: Being a foster child, confinement in prison, poverty

PLANNING

Unmet Needs
Comfort, protection from psychologic threat, acceptance, caring and communicating relationships, high evaluation of self, sense of adequacy, personal growth and maturity, increased learning, increased reality perception and problem-solving ability

Expected Outcome
Person verbalizes fears
Verbalizes feelings of adequacy and competence in meeting the fear-creating experience
Verbalizes self-satisfaction and growth in having coped with the fear-creating experience
Calm, relaxed facial expression, body movements, and behavior

NURSING INTERVENTIONS

Nursing Treatments
Approach unhurriedly

Reassure verbally (that the nurse will not reject the person)
Demonstrate calmness
Provide an atmosphere of acceptance
Encourage the expression of feelings (about the fear)
Listen attentively
Offer feedback to the person's expressed feelings
Communicate nurse sensitivity to the person's problem
Touch the person judiciously
Relate to the person on an adult–adult level, not on a parent–child level
Ask the person to identify the problem
Ask for specifics, not generalizations, about the problem
Support a realistic assessment of the situation (is there true rejection or misperceived rejection?)
Ask how the person normally copes with fear (what does he usually do when fearful that reduces the fear?)
Provide whatever the person needs to use his usual coping mechanisms
Encourage the person to face the fear (when able, to reduce the fear)
Explore with the person his strengths and resources (to promote positive interrelated-ness and to help the person focus on his assets)
Provide emotionally safe experiences (whenever possible, especially with the persons who the patient thinks might reject him)
Encourage awareness of positive responses from others

Nursing Observations
Determine the degree of insight that the person has (into the fear)
Observe for evidence of a favorable response to therapy (reduced fear and increased comfort)

Health Teaching
Explain that the person's response is appropriate and commonly experienced
Explain (to families) the importance of persons offering emotional support to one an-other
Explain (to families) that ill and aged persons are hypersensitive (to rejection)
Recommend a habitual positive mental attitude (about self worth, even if rejection does occur)

EVALUATION

Record actual outcome

FEAR OF RETALIATION [105,471,525]

ASSESSMENT

Data Collection

Subjective Data
• Person experiences feelings of threat or danger
• Can describe or identify the threat or danger
  Feels dependent on another
  Relates distrust of the integrity of the person(s) involved
  Is concerned with avoiding any ill-will toward the person on whom he depends
  Fears he will be subject to mistreatment

Objective Data
- May manifest physical findings such as facial flushing or pallor, rapid or deep respirations, rapid or bounding pulse, increased blood pressure, sweating, trembling
- May exhibit behavior such as restlessness, sleep disturbances, change in eating habits, irritability, short attention span, making poor judgments, forgetfulness, rapid speech, crying, being completely nonresistant to the threatening person

Data Analysis

Nursing Diagnosis
FEAR OF RETALIATION: A feeling of alarm and fright that one might be punished or neglected by others who wish to make reprisals

Common Etiology (Stressors)
SIGNS AND SYMPTOMS: Confusion, weakness
PSYCHOSOCIAL FACTORS: The threat of a specific and clearly identified danger, the threat of real or imagined danger, loss of independence, separation from a significant other (who was protective or abusive)
HEALTH CARE FACTORS: *Health care provider*: Unfavored by a health care provider
DEVELOPMENTAL PHASES: Old age
LIFESTYLE: Lack of conformity (by self) to cultural mores

PLANNING

Unmet Needs
Comfort, protection from psychologic threat, acceptance, caring and communicating relationships, high evaluation of self, sense of adequacy, personal growth and maturity, increased learning, increased reality perception and problem-solving ability

Expected Outcome
Person verbalizes fears
Verbalizes feelings of adequacy and competence in meeting the fear-creating experience
Verbalizes self-satisfaction and growth in having coped with the fear-creating experience
Calm, relaxed facial expression, body movements, and behavior

NURSING INTERVENTIONS

Nursing Treatments
Approach unhurriedly
Reassure verbally (that the nurse will help the person as much as possible)
Demonstrate calmness
Provide an atmosphere of acceptance
Encourage the expression of feelings (about the fear)
Listen attentively
Offer feedback to the person's expressed feelings
Communicate nurse sensitivity to the person's problem
Relate to the person on an adult–adult level, not on a parent–child level (which could increase fear)
Attend the person constantly (until he feels sufficiently comfortable to be alone)
Provide frequent contact with the person (thereafter)
Ask the person to identify the problem
Ask for specifics, not generalizations, about the problem
Support a realistic assessment of the situation (about the probability of reprisal)
Provide reliable information (to significant others or authorities if the fear of reprisal is valid)
Ask how the person normally copes with fear (what does he usually do when fearful that reduces the fear?)
Provide whatever the person needs to use his usual coping mechanisms
Explore with the person his strengths and resources (to cope with such persons, to protect himself from retaliation)

Limit visitors (whom the patient perceives as threatening)

Provide objects that symbolize safeness (put the signal button within easy reach, etc.)

Nursing Observations

Observe for an excessive stress level (resulting from the fear)

Determine the degree of insight that the person has (into the fear)

Observe for evidence of a favorable response to therapy (reduced fear and increased comfort)

Health Teaching

Explain that the person's response is appropriate and commonly experienced (especially among the ill and aged)

Explain (to the family) that ill or aged persons are hypersensitive (and may perceive as reprisal, statements or actions not intended as such)

EVALUATION

Record actual outcome

FEAR OF ROLE LOSS[105,251,471,525]

ASSESSMENT

Data Collection

Subjective Data

• Person experiences feelings of threat or danger

• Can describe or identify the threat or danger

Strongly identifies with a particular role

Is concerned about performing the role responsibilities

Is worried that someone else may assume his role

Is concerned that he may be forced into an unacceptable role

Objective Data

• May manifest physical findings such as facial flushing or pallor, rapid or deep respirations, rapid or bounding pulse, increased blood pressure, sweating, trembling

• May exhibit behavior such as restlessness, sleep disturbances, change in eating habits, irritability, demanding and controlling behavior, seeking reassurance

Data Analysis

Nursing Diagnosis

FEAR OF ROLE LOSS: A feeling of alarm and fright about being unable to perform a sequence of activities that interact with the actions of another person to accomplish goals of the social group

Common Etiology (Stressors)

DISEASES: Any

INJURIES: Any

SIGNS AND SYMPTOMS: Immobility, pain, weakness

PSYCHOSOCIAL FACTORS: The threat of a specific and clearly identified danger, the threat of real or imagined danger

HUMAN BODY: *Body function*: Loss of body function. *Body part*: Loss of a body part

HEALTH CARE FACTORS: *Hospitalization*: Of self or a significant other. *Health therapy*: Loss of on-the-job time because of health therapy

DEVELOPMENTAL PHASES: Old age

SITUATIONAL FACTORS: Death of a significant other, divorce, separation, loss of employment, illness of or injury to self or a significant other, launching grown children

PLANNING

Unmet Needs

Comfort, protection from psychologic threat, acceptance, caring and communicating relationships, high evaluation of self, sense of adequacy, personal growth and maturity, increased learning, increased reality perception and problem-solving ability

Expected Outcome

Person verbalizes fears

Verbalizes feelings of adequacy and competence in meeting the fear-creating experience
Verbalizes self-satisfaction and growth in having coped with the fear-creating experience
Calm, relaxed facial expression, body movements, and behavior

NURSING INTERVENTIONS

Nursing Treatments

Approach unhurriedly
Reassure verbally (that the nurse will help the person as much as possible)
Demonstrate calmness
Provide an atmosphere of acceptance
Encourage the expression of feelings (about the fear)
Listen attentively
Offer feedback to the person's expressed feelings
Communicate nurse sensitivity to the person's problem
Relate to the person on an adult–adult level, not on a parent–child level (which could increase fear)
Ask the person to identify the problem
Ask for specifics, not generalizations, about the problem
Provide reliable information (to the patient, family, employer, etc. about the effects of the disease or injury on role performance; discuss the probability of role loss with the patient)
Ask how the person normally copes with fear (what does he usually do when fearful that reduces the fear?)
Provide whatever the person needs to use his usual coping mechanisms
Explore with the person his strengths and resources (to overcome fear, maintain the desired role or adjust to a new role)
Encourage recognition of his various roles in life (and that even with one role change, other roles remain stable)
Introduce to persons who have undergone the same experience (if appropriate)

Nursing Observations

Determine the degree of insight that the person has (into the fear)
Observe for evidence of a favorable response to therapy (reduced fear and increased comfort)

Health Teaching

Explain that the person's response is appropriate and commonly experienced
Explain how to channel emotional energy and obtain release from stress (by talking things over, laughing, etc.)
Recommend a habitual, positive mental attitude (toward himself and toward former and current roles)

EVALUATION

Record actual outcome

FEAR OF SEPARATION FROM A SIGNIFICANT OTHER[105,471,525]

ASSESSMENT

Data Collection

Subjective Data
- Person experiences feelings of threat or danger
- Can describe or identify the threat or danger
  Wants to be near a significant other
  Cannot tolerate the thought of being apart
  Feels nervous and uneasy at the thought or reality of being apart from a loved one
  Feels more secure when with the person

Objective Data
- May manifest physical findings such as facial flushing or pallor, rapid or deep respirations, rapid or bounding pulse, increased blood pressure, sweating, trembling
- May exhibit behavior such as restlessness, sleep disturbances, change in eating habits, irritability, controlling behavior, crying, touching, caressing the significant other

Data Analysis

Nursing Diagnosis
FEAR OF SEPARATION FROM A SIGNIFICANT OTHER: A feeling of alarm and fright about being apart from a significant other

Common Etiology (Stressors)
DISEASES: Any
INJURIES: Any
PSYCHOSOCIAL FACTORS: The threat of a specific and clearly identified danger, the threat of real or imagined danger
HEALTH CARE FACTORS: *Health care environment*: Locked psychiatric unit, intensive care unit, coronary care unit, isolation unit. *Hospitalization or institutionalization*: Of self or a significant other. *Visitors*: Restriction of. *Surgical procedures*: Any
DEVELOPMENTAL PHASES: Infancy (6 months), toddler (age 1–3), preschooler (age 3–6), old age
SITUATIONAL FACTORS: Childbirth, confinement in prison, impending death of a significant other, launching grown children, entry into school, military service, travel, war

PLANNING

Unmet Needs
Comfort, protection from psychologic threat, acceptance, caring and communicating relationships, high evaluation of self, sense of adequacy, personal growth and maturity, increased learning, increased reality perception and problem-solving ability

Expected Outcome
Person verbalizes fears
Verbalizes feelings of adequacy and competence in meeting the fear-creating experience
Verbalizes self-satisfaction and growth in having coped with the fear-creating experience
Calm, relaxed facial expression, body movements, and behavior

NURSING INTERVENTIONS

Nursing Treatments
Approach unhurriedly
Reassure verbally (that the nurse will help the person as much as possible)
Demonstrate calmness
Provide an atmosphere of acceptance
Encourage the expression of feelings (about the fear)

Listen attentively

Offer feedback to the person's expressed feelings

Communicate nurse sensitivity to the person's problem

Relate to the person on an adult–adult level, not on a parent–child level (which could increase fear)

Attend the person constantly (until he feels sufficiently comfortable to be alone)

Ask the person to identify the problem

Ask for specifics, not generalizations, about the problem

Support a realistic assessment of the situation (that health care does require some separation)

Provide reliable information (about the length of separation, about alternatives to separation)

Ask how the person normally copes with fear (what does he usually do when fearful that reduces the fear?)

Provide whatever the person needs to use his usual coping mechanisms

Encourage the person to face the fear (when able, to reduce the fear)

Explore with the person his strengths and resources (to cope with the fear and the separation, to limit the length of separation)

Do not allow unpleasant surprise situations (give the person time to adjust before the separation)

Avoid placing the person on enforced inactivity (which heightens fear)

Reduce the demands placed on the person (so that more energy is available for coping)

Encourage telephone calls between significant persons (who are separated)

Allow unlimited visiting

Nursing Observations

Observe for an excessive stress level (resulting from the fear and the impending or actual separation)

Determine the degree of insight that the person has (into the fear)

Observe for evidence of a favorable response to therapy (reduced fear and increased comfort)

Health Teaching

Explain that the person's response is appropriate and commonly experienced

Explain that fatigue should be recognized as a stress factor (which heightens fear)

EVALUATION

Record actual outcome

FEAR OF SEXUAL ASSAULT[105,471,525]

ASSESSMENT

Data Collection

Subjective Data

• Person experiences feelings of threat or danger

• Can describe or identify the threat or danger

  May relate previous assaults on self or reported assaults on others

  May feel uncomfortable around a particular person

  May relate misinterpreted intentions of innocent persons during diagnostic or therapeutic procedures

Objective Data

• May manifest physical findings such as facial flushing or pallor, rapid or deep respirations, rapid or bounding pulse, increased blood pressure, sweating, trembling

• May exhibit behavior such as restlessness, sleep disturbances, change in eating habits, irritability, rapid speech, demanding and controlling behavior, crying

Data Analysis

Nursing Diagnosis

FEAR OF SEXUAL ASSAULT: A feeling of alarm and fright about being a victim of unwanted sexual activity or advances

Common Etiology (Stressors)

SIGNS AND SYMPTOMS: Weakness

PSYCHOSOCIAL FACTORS: The threat of a specific and clearly identified danger, the threat of real or imagined danger

HEALTH CARE AND FACTORS: *Patients*: Sexually provocative patients. *Diagnostic procedures*: Breast examination, Pap smear, pelvic examination. *Medical/nursing therapy*: Back rub, bed bath, urinary catheterization

SITUATIONAL FACTORS: Victimized by sexual assault previously, living alone, working night shifts

PLANNING

Unmet Needs

Comfort, protection from psychologic threat, acceptance, caring and communicating relationships, high evaluation of self, sense of adequacy, personal growth and maturity, increased learning, increased reality perception and problem-solving ability

Expected Outcome

Person verbalizes fears
Verbalizes feelings of adequacy and competence in meeting the fear-creating experience
Verbalizes self-satisfaction and growth in having coped with the fear-creating experience
Calm, relaxed facial expression, body movements, and behavior

NURSING INTERVENTIONS

Nursing Treatments

Approach unhurriedly
Reassure verbally (that the nurse will stay with the person during procedures and will help the person as much as possible)
Demonstrate calmness
Provide an atmosphere of acceptance
Encourage the expression of feelings (about the fear)
Listen attentively
Offer feedback to the person's expressed feelings
Communicate nurse sensitivity to the person's problem
Relate to the person on an adult–adult level, not on a parent–child level (which could increase fear)
Attend the person constantly (until she feels sufficiently comfortable to be alone)
Provide frequent patient contact (thereafter)
Ask the person to identify the problem
Ask for specifics, not generalizations, about the problem
Provide reliable information (about the feared procedure)
Ask how the person normally copes with fear (what does she usually do when fearful that reduces the fear)
Provide whatever the person needs to use her usual coping mechanisms
Explore with the person her strengths and resources (to overcome fear, to protect herself from assault)
Provide emotionally safe experiences (whenever possible)
Provide objects that symbolize safeness (personal clothing, adequate draping)
Do not allow unpleasant surprise situations (such as unexpected procedures)
Avoid placing the person on enforced inactivity (which heightens fear)

Reduce the demands placed on the person (so that more energy is available for coping)

Make a referral (to self-defense or safety programs if the fear is due to weakness, aging, etc.)

Nursing Observations

Determine the degree of insight that the person has (into the fear)

Observe for evidence of a favorable response to therapy (reduced fear, increased comfort, and increased ability to protect herself)

Health Teaching

Explain that the person's response is appropriate and commonly experienced

Explain the importance of recognizing tension within oneself (from previous experiences)

Recommend methods for achieving total relaxation (such as controlled breathing, quietly listening to music, doing nothing, which reduces fear)

Recommend a habitual, positive mental attitude (about being able to protect herself)

EVALUATION

Record actual outcome

FEAR OF SOCIAL STIGMA[105,471,525]

ASSESSMENT

Data Collection

Subjective Data
- Person experiences feelings of threat or danger
- Can describe or identify the threat or danger
  Knows that the illness or behavior does not fit into society's positive value system
  Is inclined to secrecy about the stigmatizing disease, injury, or condition

Objective Data
- May manifest physical findings such as facial flushing or pallor, rapid or deep respirations, rapid or bounding pulse, increased blood pressure, sweating, trembling
- May exhibit behavior such as restlessness, sleep disturbances, irritability, demanding and controlling behavior, seeking reassurance

Data Analysis

Nursing Diagnosis
FEAR OF SOCIAL STIGMA: A feeling of alarm and fright about being looked on with shame or discredit by society in general because of a particular health problem

Common Etiology (Stressors)
DISEASES: Alcoholism, carcinoma, drug addiction, eczema, epilepsy, gonorrhea, Hansen's disease, herpes genitalia, homosexuality, impotence, Parkinson's disease, psoriasis, schizophrenia, senility, syphilis, tuberculosis
INJURIES: Traumatic disfigurement
SIGNS AND SYMTOMS: Paralysis, rash, tremor
PSYCHOSOCIAL FACTORS: The threat of a specific and clearly identified danger, the threat of real or imagined danger, role changes with a significant other
HUMAN BODY: *Body appearance*: A disfigured body. *Body function*: Loss of body function. *Body part*: Loss of a body part

HEALTH CARE FACTORS: *Medical therapy*: Preventive isolation, psychotherapy. *Adverse effects of surgical therapy*: Loss of natural elimination and elimination control from a colostomy, ileocolostomy, ileostomy, ureterocolostomy, ureteroileostomy, ureterosigmoidostomy, ureterostomy, ureterotomy

DEVELOPMENTAL PHASES: Old Age

SITUATIONAL FACTORS: Confinement in prison, being a foster or adopted child, divorce, marital separation, attempted suicide, victimized by sexual assault, unwed parents

PLANNING

Unmet Needs
Comfort, protection from psychologic threat, acceptance, caring and communicating relationships, high evaluation of self, sense of adequacy, personal growth and maturity, increased learning, increased reality perception and problem-solving ability

Expected Outcome
Person verbalizes fears
Verbalizes feelings of adequacy and competence in meeting the fear-creating experience
Verbalizes self-satisfaction and growth in having coped with the fear-creating experience
Calm, relaxed facial expression, body movements, and behavior

NURSING INTERVENTIONS

Nursing Treatments
Approach unhurriedly
Reassure verbally (that the nurse will help the person as much as possible)
Demonstrate calmness
Provide an atmosphere of acceptance
Encourage the expression of feelings (about the fear)
Listen attentively
Offer feedback to the person's expressed feelings
Communicate nurse sensitivity to the person's problem
Relate to the person on an adult–adult level, not on a parent–child level (which could increase fear)
Ask the person to identify the problem
Ask for specifics, not generalizations, about the problem
Support a realistic assessment of the situation (about the probability of social stigma)
Ask how the person normally copes with fear (what does he usually do when fearful that reduces the fear?)
Provide whatever the person needs to use his usual coping mechanisms
Encourage the person to face the fear (when able, to reduce the fear)
Explore with the person his strengths and resources (to overcome the fear, to cope with the stigmatizing persons)
Explore with the person his value as an individual (despite social stigma)
Encourage an awareness of positive responses from others

Nursing Observations
Determine the degree of insight that the person has (into the fear)
Observe for evidence of a favorable response to therapy (reduced fear and increased comfort)

Health Teaching
Explain that the person's response is appropriate and commonly experienced
Advise that negative responses from others be regarded with minimum significance (even though there are feelings about such responses)
Recommend a habitual, positive mental attitude

EVALUATION
Record actual outcome

FEAR OF A STRANGE ENVIRONMENT[105,471,525]

ASSESSMENT

Data Collection

Subjective Data
- Person experiences feelings of threat or danger
- Can describe or identify the threat or danger
  Has not previously been in the environment
  Asks questions about where things are
  Feels uncomfortable

Objective Data
- May manifest physical findings such as facial flushing or pallor, rapid or deep respirations, rapid or bounding pulse, increased blood pressure; sweating, trembling
- May exhibit behavior such as restlessness, irritability, demanding and controlling behavior, not venturing far from the room, frequent call-light signaling, detaining the nurse, crying, looking around, surveying the premises

Data Analysis

Nursing Diagnosis
FEAR OF A STRANGE ENVIRONMENT: A feeling of alarm and fright about an unfamiliar environment

Common Etiology (Stressors)
PSYCHOSOCIAL FACTORS: The threat of a specific and clearly identified danger, the threat of real or imagined danger
HEALTH CARE FACTORS: *Health care environment*: Intensive care, coronary care, isolation or locked psychiatric unit, emergency room, radiology, surgical suite. *Hospitalization/Institutionalization*: Any
DEVELOPMENTAL PHASES: Toddler (age 1–3), preschooler (age 3–6), old age
SITUATIONAL FACTORS: Confinement in prison, relocation of home, entry into school, travel

PLANNING

Unmet Needs

Comfort, protection from psychologic threat, acceptance, caring and communicating relationships, high evaluation of self, sense of adequacy, personal growth and maturity, increased learning, increased reality perception and problem-solving ability

Expected Outcome

Person verbalizes fears
Verbalizes feelings of adequacy and competence in meeting the fear-creating experience
Verbalizes self-satisfaction and growth in having coped with the fear-creating experience
Calm, relaxed facial expression, body movements, and behavior

NURSING INTERVENTIONS

Nursing Treatments

Approach unhurriedly
Reassure verbally (that the nurse will familiarize the person with the environment and that the person is safe)
Demonstrate calmness
Provide an atmosphere of acceptance
Arrange pleasant surroundings, orderly surroundings
Encourage the expression of feelings (about the fear)
Listen attentively
Offer feedback to the person's expressed feelings
Communicate nurse sensitivity to the person's problem

Relate to the person on an adult–adult level, not on a parent–child level (which could increase fear)

Attend the person constantly (until he feels sufficiently comfortable to be alone)

Provide frequent patient contact (thereafter)

Ask the person to identify the problem

Ask for specifics, not generalizations, about the problem

Ask how the person normally copes with fear (what does he usually do when fearful that reduces the fear?)

Provide whatever the person needs to use his usual coping mechanisms

Provide objects that symbolize safeness (for a small child, a security blanket or favorite toy will increase feelings of safeness)

Provide reliable information (about the environment and explain where things are)

Tour the health care facility with the person

Provide a night-light (until the person is familiar with the environment)

Nursing Observations

Observe for an excessive stress level (resulting from the fear)

Observe for evidence of a favorable response to therapy (reduced fear and increased comfort)

Health Teaching

Explain that the person's response is appropriate and commonly experienced (especially when hospitalized or institutionalized)

EVALUATION

Record actual outcome

FEAR OF STRANGE EQUIPMENT[105,471,525]

ASSESSMENT

Data Collection

Subjective Data

• Person experiences feelings of threat or danger

• Can describe or identify the threat or danger

　Has not previously come in contact with the equipment

　Questions what it is for and how it works

　May perceive it as a monsterlike figure

　A small child may believe that if the equipment moves it is alive

　May refuse to have the testing done

Objective Data

• May manifest physical findings such as facial flushing or pallor, rapid or deep respirations, rapid or bounding pulse, increased blood pressure, sweating, trembling

• May exhibit behavior such as restlessness, irritability, rapid speech, demanding and controlling behavior, crying, looking or pointing at the equipment, avoids going near the equipment

Data Analysis

Nursing Diagnosis

FEAR OF STRANGE EQUIPMENT: A feeling of alarm and fright about unfamiliar equipment

Common Etiology (Stressors)

PSYCHOSOCIAL FACTORS: The threat of a specific and clearly identified danger, the threat of real or imagined danger

HEALTH CARE FACTORS: Diagnostic equipment: X-ray machine, CAT scanner, stethoscope, otoscope, ophthalmoscope, sphygmomanometer. *Therapeutic equipment*: Apheresis equipment, cardiac pacemaker, defibrillator, electroconvulsive shock equipment, hemodialyzer, intermittent positive pressure breathing machine, Isolette, oxygen mask, cannula, tent, Stryker frame, crutches, braces, walker, wheelchair, safety restraints, suction apparatus, therapeutic tubes

DEVELOPMENTAL PHASES: Any but especially preschooler (age 3–6)

PLANNING

Unmet Needs

Comfort, protection from psychologic threat, acceptance, caring and communicating relationships, high evaluation of self, sense of adequacy, personal growth and maturity, increased learning, increased reality perception and problem-solving ability

Expected Outcome

Person verbalizes fears
Verbalizes feelings of adequacy and competence in meeting the fear-creating experience
Verbalizes self-satisfaction and growth in having coped with the fear-creating experience
Calm, relaxed facial expression, body movements, and behavior

NURSING INTERVENTIONS

Nursing Treatments

Approach unhurriedly
Reassure verbally (that the equipment will not harm the person)
Demonstrate calmness
Provide an atmosphere of acceptance
Encourage the expression of feelings (about the fear)
Listen attentively
Offer feedback to the person's expressed feelings
Communicate nurse sensitivity to the person's problem
Relate to the person on an adult–adult level, not on a parent–child level (which could increase fear)
Attend the person constantly (until he feels sufficiently comfortable with the equipment)
Provide frequent contact with the person (thereafter)
Ask the person to identify the problem
Ask for specifics, not generalizations, about the problem
Provide reliable information (about the feared equipment)
Ask how the person normally copes with fear (what does he usually do when fearful that reduces the fear?)
Provide whatever the person needs to use his usual coping mechanisms
Do not allow unpleasant surprise situations (which involve equipment)
Keep the equipment out of sight (if the fear persists)

Nursing Observations

Observe for an excessive stress level (resulting from the fear)
Determine the degree of insight that the person has (into the fear)
Observe for evidence of a favorable response to therapy (reduced fear and increased comfort)

Health Teaching

Explain that the person's response is appropriate and commonly experienced (especially by children)
Explain how the equipment works (and let the person touch it; when possible, demonstrate its function and safety)

EVALUATION

Record actual outcome

FEAR OF STRANGERS [105,471,525]

ASSESSMENT

Data Collection

Subjective Data
- Person experiences feelings of threat or danger
- Can describe or identify the threat or danger
  Feels uncomfortable in a stranger's presence
  Withholds information from strangers

Objective Data
- May manifest physical findings such as facial flushing or pallor, rapid or deep respirations, rapid or bounding pulse, increased blood pressure, sweating, trembling
- May exhibit behavior such as restlessness, irritability, rapid speech, demanding and controlling behavior, cautiously approaching and keeping a distance from strangers; a child will cling to a familiar person and cry when strangers approach

Data Analysis

Nursing Diagnosis
FEAR OF STRANGERS: A feeling of alarm and fright about meeting unfamiliar persons

Common Etiology (Stressors)
DISEASES: Psychosis
PSYCHOSOCIAL FACTORS: The threat of a specific and clearly identified danger, the threat of real or imagined danger
HEALTH CARE FACTORS: *Health care provider*: Unfamiliar
DEVELOPMENTAL PHASES: Infancy (age 6 months), toddler (age 1–3)
LIFESTYLE: Little or no socialization
SITUATIONAL FACTORS: Entry into school

PLANNING

Unmet Needs
Comfort, protection from psychologic threat, acceptance, caring and communicating relationships, high evaluation of self, sense of adequacy, personal growth and maturity, increased learning, increased reality perception and problem-solving ability

Expected Outcome
Person verbalizes fears
Verbalizes feelings of adequacy and competence in meeting the fear-creating experience
Verbalizes self-satisfaction and growth in having coped with the fear-creating experience
Calm, relaxed facial expression, body movements, and behavior

NURSING INTERVENTIONS

Nursing Treatments
Approach unhurriedly (if the person is a small child, approach the parent first, to allow the child enough time to conquer the fear)
Reassure verbally (that the nurse is not threatening; a smile is reassuring)
Demonstrate calmness
Provide an atmosphere of acceptance
Encourage the expression of feelings (about the fear of strangers)
Listen attentively
Offer feedback to the person's expressed feelings
Communicate nurse sensitivity to the person's problem
Relate to the person on an adult–adult level, not on a parent–child level (which could increase fear)

Touch the person judiciously (until he feels safe with the nurse)

Provide frequent contact with the person (so the person can better know the nurse)

Attend the person constantly (if the person feels safe with the nurse, but unsafe with other strangers such as physicians, x-ray personnel, etc.)

Do not allow unpleasant surprise situations (involving strangers)

Nursing Observations

Observe for an excessive stress level (resulting from the fear)

Observe for evidence of a favorable response to therapy (reduced fear and increased comfort)

Health Teaching

Explain that the person's response is appropriate and commonly experienced

EVALUATION

Record actual outcome

FEAR OF SUFFOCATION[105,471,525]

ASSESSMENT

Data Collection

Subjective Data

• Person experiences feelings of threat or danger

• Can describe or identify the threat or danger

May be experiencing or has previously experienced air hunger

Fears his air intake will be insufficient

May refuse threatening procedure(s)

Objective Data

• May manifest physical findings such as facial flushing or pallor, rapid or deep respirations, rapid or bounding pulse, increased blood pressure, sweating, trembling

• May exhibit behavior such as restlessness, irritability, demanding and controlling behavior, seeking reassurance

Data Analysis

Nursing Diagnosis

FEAR OF SUFFOCATION: A feeling of alarm and fright about being without sufficient air intake

Common Etiology (Stressors)

DISEASES: Asthma, emphysema, pneumonia, pneumothorax, pulmonary edema, pulmonary embolus

INJURIES: Flail chest

SIGNS AND SYMPTOMS: Breathing difficulty, chest tightness, laryngeal edema or spasms, nasal congestion,

PSYCHOSOCIAL FACTORS: The threat of a specific and clearly identified danger, the threat of real or imagined danger

HEALTH CARE FACTORS: *Diagnostic procedures*: Broncoscopy, gastroscopy, vital capacity and residual capacity pulmonary function tests (when done with a mask or nose clip). *Medical therapy*: Airway suctioning, mask application (during oxygen inhalation, heated-mist inhalation therapy, intermittent positive pressure breathing), nasal packing, nasogastric or endotracheal intubation. *Surgical therapy*: Induction of general anesthesia (by mask). *Surgical procedures*: Rhinoplasty, wiring of a mandible fracture, oral surgery. *Therapeutic equipment*: Use of an oxygen tent.

ENVIRONMENTAL FACTORS: *Altitude*: High. *Cataclysm*: Debri from a volcanic eruption, dust storm. *Chemical substances*: Inhalation of

PLANNING

Unmet Needs

Comfort, protection from psychologic threat, acceptance, caring and communicating relationships, high evaluation of self, sense of adequacy, personal growth and maturity, increased learning, increased reality perception and problem-solving ability

Expected Outcome

Person verbalizes fears
Verbalizes feelings of adequacy and competence in meeting the fear-creating experience
Verbalizes self-satisfaction and growth in having coped with the fear-creating experience
Calm, relaxed facial expression, body movements, and behavior

NURSING INTERVENTIONS

Nursing Treatments

Approach unhurriedly
Reassure verbally (that the nurse will do everything possible to make breathing easier)
Demonstrate calmness
Provide an atmosphere of acceptance
Encourage the expression of feelings (about the fear)
Listen attentively
Offer feedback to the person's expressed feelings
Communicate nurse sensitivity to the person's problem
Relate to the person on an adult–adult level, not on a parent–child level (which could increase fear)
Attend the person constantly (until he feels sufficiently comfortable to be alone)
Provide frequent contact with the person (thereafter)
Ask the person to identify the problem
Ask for specifics, not generalizations, about the problem
Provide reliable information (about the effects of diseases, procedures, and environmental factors on breathing ability)
Place in the sitting position (if the person feels more comfortable)
Limit IPPB treatments to short periods (while the person learns to use it)
Refrain from strapping the ventilator mask in place (or substitute a mouthpiece)
Refrain from using a ventilator nose clip
Arrange situations that encourage the person's autonomy (so there is patient control over breathing)

Nursing Observations

Observe for an excessive stress level (resulting from the fear)
Determine the degree of insight that the person has (into the fear)
Observe for evidence of a favorable response to therapy (reduced fear and increased comfort)

Health Teaching

Explain that the person's response is appropriate and commonly experienced
Teach the specific method (of coughing and deep breathing to help keep the airway clear)
Recommend methods for achieving total relaxation (when possible, such as allowing the ventilator to do the work of breathing)

EVALUATION

Record actual outcome

FEAR OF TERMINATION OF LIFE-SUPPORT SYSTEMS [105,451,472,525]

ASSESSMENT

Data Collection

Subjective Data
* Person experiences feelings of threat or danger
* Can describe or identify the threat or danger
  Intense awareness that the person's existence has been maintained by a life-supporting device or drug
  Frequently calls for the therapeutic device or drugs, even though they are not needed
  Verbally resists removal of the device
  Asks to have the device within sight

Objective Data
* May manifest physical findings such as facial flushing or pallor, rapid or deep respirations, rapid or bounding pulse, increased blood pressure, sweating, trembling
* May exhibit behavior such as restlessness, sleep disturbances, change in eating habits, irritability, demanding and controlling behavior, unusual quietness, seeking reassurance, frequent call-light signaling

Data Analysis

Nursing Diagnosis
FEAR OF TERMINATION OF LIFE-SUPPORT SYSTEMS: A feeling of alarm and fright about relinquishing reliance on life-support systems and reestablishing confidence in the body's ability to maintain life unaided

Common Etiology (Stressors)
PSYCHOSOCIAL FACTORS: The threat of a specific and clearly identified danger, the threat of real or imagined danger
HEALTH CARE FACTORS: *Drug therapy*: Life-maintenance drugs such as insulin, digoxin, corticosteroids, etc. *Therapeutic equipment or devices*: Cardiac pacemaker, defibrillator, hemodialyzer, hyperalimentation setup, intermittent positive pressure breathing machine, Isolette, oxygen (by mask, cannula, tent), respirator

PLANNING

Unmet Needs
Comfort, protection from psychologic threat, acceptance, caring and communicating relationships, high evaluation of self, sense of adequacy, personal growth and maturity, increased learning, increased reality perception and problem-solving ability

Expected Outcome
Person verbalizes fears
Verbalizes feelings of adequacy and competence in meeting the fear-creating experience
Verbalizes self-satisfaction and growth in having coped with the fear-creating experience
Calm, relaxed facial expression, body movements, and behavior

NURSING INTERVENTIONS

Nursing Treatments
Approach unhurriedly
Reassure verbally (that the person is safe without the life-support system, if such is true)
Demonstrate calmness
Provide an atmosphere of acceptance
Arrange pleasant surroundings
Encourage the expression of feelings (about the fear)
Listen attentively

Talk with the person (about what would happen if the support systems were terminated)

Offer feedback to the person's expressed feelings

Communicate nurse sensitivity to the person's problems

Relate to the person on an adult–adult level, not on a parent–child level (which could increase fear)

Attend the person constantly (at the initial withdrawal of the life-support system)

Provide frequent contact with the person (thereafter)

Respond immediately to the person's call (especially during the withdrawal periods)

Increase the weaning time off the therapeutic devices gradually

Place equipment within sight (until the person feels more secure)

Provide reliable information (about the person's improved condition)

Ask how the person normally copes with fear (what does he usually do when fearful that reduces the fear?)

Provide whatever the person needs to use his usual coping mechanisms

Encourage gradual mastery of the situation

Provide radio and television for diversion (during the withdrawal periods)

Avoid forcing the person into rapid adaptation to change by accepting the person's unique pattern of adjustment

Do not allow unpleasant surprise situations (such as the sudden termination of a life support system)

Nursing Observations

Observe for an excessive stress level (resulting from the fear)

Determine the degree of insight that the person has (into the fear)

Observe for evidence of a favorable response to therapy (reduced fear and increased comfort)

Health Teaching

Explain that the person's response is appropriate and commonly experienced

Describe those symptoms that should be reported (during the withdrawal)

Recommend methods for achieving total relaxation (controlled breathing, which will reduce the fear)

Recommend a habitual, positive mental attitude

EVALUATION

Record actual outcome

FEAR OF THE UNAVAILABILITY OF PRESCRIBED DRUGS [105,471,525]

ASSESSMENT

Data Collection

Subjective Data
• Person experiences feelings of threat or danger
• Can describe or identify the threat or danger
  Is aware that he requires certain maintenance drugs
  Is quick to imagine what could happen if the drugs were not available
  Has intense dependency feelings
  Is concerned if a scheduled dose is missed or late
  Experiences heightened fear if there is any problem with refilling a prescription

Objective Data
• May manifest physical findings such as facial flushing or pallor, rapid or deep respirations, rapid or bounding pulse, increased blood pressure, sweating, trembling

• May exhibit behavior such as irritability, demanding and controlling behavior, stocking up on drugs, seeking reassurance that drugs are available, frequently checking to be sure he has the drug(s)

Related Data
Person is taking drugs such as Prostigmin (neostigmine) for myasthenia gravis, cortisone for Addison's disease, insulin for diabetes, antidepressants for a depressive reaction

Data Analysis

Nursing Diagnosis
FEAR OF THE UNAVAILABILITY OF PRESCRIBED DRUGS: A feeling of alarm and fright about not being able to obtain essential drugs prescribed by the physician for control of a chronic disease

Common Etiology (Stressors)
DISEASES: Addison's disease, asthma, congestive heart failure, diabetes mellitus, emphysema, epilepsy, malignant or essential hypertension, major depression, myasthenia gravis, Parkinson's disease, rheumatoid arthritis, schizophrenia

PSYCHOSOCIAL FACTORS: The threat of a specific and clearly identified danger, the threat of real or imagined danger

HEALTH CARE FACTORS: *Follow-up care*: Delayed

SITUATIONAL FACTORS: Pharmacy closure on holidays, lack of finances to purchase medicine, foreign travel, war

PLANNING

Unmet Needs
Comfort, protection from psychologic threat, acceptance, caring and communicating relationships, high evaluation of self, sense of adequacy, personal growth and maturity, increased learning, increased reality perception and problem-solving ability

Expected Outcome
Person verbalizes fears
Verbalizes feelings of adequacy and competence in meeting the fear-creating experience
Verbalizes self-satisfaction and growth in having coped with the fear-creating experience
Calm, relaxed facial expression, body movements, and behavior

NURSING INTERVENTIONS

Nursing Treatments
Approach unhurriedly
Reassure verbally (that the drug is available)
Demonstrate calmness
Provide an atmosphere of acceptance
Encourage the expression of feelings (about the fear)
Listen attentively
Talk with the person
Offer feedback to the person's expressed feelings
Communicate nurse sensitivity to the person's problem
Relate to the person on an adult–adult level, not on a parent–child level (which could increase fear)
Ask the person to identify the problem
Ask for specifics, not generalizations, about the problem
Provide reliable information (about how long the dosage can be withheld before adverse effects occur)
Encourage early replacement of dwindling therapeutic drugs
Make a referral (to Social Services, if financially unable to obtain drugs)

Nursing Observations
Observe for an excessive stress level (resulting from the fear)
Identify disturbing conversation topics (about the drug)

Observe for evidence of a favorable response to therapy (reduced fear and increased comfort)

Health Teaching

Explain that the person's response is appropriate and commonly experienced

Explain how to obtain therapeutic drugs

Recommend that extra therapeutic drugs be carried (especially on trips, etc.)

EVALUATION

Record actual outcome

FEAR OF THE UNCERTAIN DIAGNOSIS [105,471,525]

ASSESSMENT

Data Collection

Subjective Data

- Person experiences feelings of threat or danger
- Can describe or identify the threat or danger

  Relates that a diagnosis has not been made

  May have reason to suspect an unfavorable diagnosis

  Both individuals and families find the waiting difficult

  Hopes for a favorable diagnosis

Objective Data

- May manifest physical findings such as facial flushing or pallor, rapid or deep respirations, rapid or bounding pulse, increased blood pressure, sweating, trembling
- May exhibit behavior such as restlessness, sleep disturbances, change in eating habits, irritability, short attention span, rapid speech, avoiding threatening visits from the doctor, seeking reassurance that there are no unfavorable reports

Data Analysis

Nursing Diagnosis

FEAR OF THE UNCERTAIN DIAGNOSIS: A feeling of alarm and fright about not knowing if an impending diagnosis will be favorable or unfavorable

Common Etiology (Stressors)

PSYCHOSOCIAL FACTORS: The threat of a specific and clearly identified danger, the threat of real or imagined danger

HEALTH CARE FACTORS: *Medical diagnosis of self or a significant other*: Impending or inconclusive diagnosis

PLANNING

Unmet Needs

Comfort, protection from psychologic threat, acceptance, caring and communicating relationships, high evaluation of self, sense of adequacy, personal growth and maturity, increased learning, increased reality perception and problem-solving ability

Expected Outcome

Person verbalizes fears

Verbalizes feelings of adequacy and competence in meeting the fear-creating experience

Verbalizes self-satisfaction and growth in having coped with the fear-creating experience

Calm, relaxed facial expression, body movements, and behavior

NURSING INTERVENTIONS

Nursing Treatments

Approach unhurriedly

Reassure verbally (that the nurse will be available whenever needed)
Demonstrate calmness
Provide an atmosphere of acceptance
Encourage the expression of feelings (about the fear)
Listen attentively
Offer feedback to the person's expressed feelings
Communicate nurse sensitivity to the person's problem
Relate to the person on an adult–adult level, not on a parent–child level (which could increase fear)
Attend the person constantly (until he feels sufficiently comfortable to be alone)
Provide frequent contact with the person (thereafter)
Ask the person to identify the problem
Ask for specifics, not generalizations, about the problem
Support a realistic assessment of the situation (about the probability of it being favorable or unfavorable)
Ask how the person normally copes with fear (what does he usually do when fearful that reduces the fear?)
Provide whatever the person needs to use his usual coping mechanisms
Explore with the person his strengths and resources (to cope with the fear and the diagnosis)

Nursing Observations
Observe for an excessive stress level (resulting from the fear)
Observe for evidence of a favorable response to therapy (reduced fear and increased comfort)

Health Teaching
Explain that the person's response is appropriate and commonly experienced
Explain the meaning of the diagnostic reports (as is appropriate)
Explain the importance of persons offering emotional support to one another (during such times of stress)

EVALUATION

Record actual outcome

FEAR OF THE UNCERTAIN OUTCOME OF A PROCEDURE/THERAPY[105,471,525]

ASSESSMENT

Data Collection

Subjective Data
• Person experiences feelings of threat or danger
• Can describe or identify the threat or danger
  Relates that the outcome of a procedure/therapy is not assured
  Is concerned that the outcome is often known to be unfavorable
  Finds the waiting difficult
  Hopes for the best

Objective Data
• May manifest physical findings such as facial flushing or pallor, rapid or deep respirations, rapid or bounding pulse, increased blood pressure, sweating, trembling
• May exhibit behavior such as restlessness, sleep disturbances, irritability, avoiding threatening visits to the doctor, seeking reassurance about the outcome

Data Analysis

Nursing Diagnosis

FEAR OF THE UNCERTAIN OUTCOME OF A PROCEDURE/THERAPY: A feeling of alarm and fright about the doubtful results of a medical or surgical procedure or therapy

Common Etiology (Stressors)

PSYCHOSOCIAL FACTORS: The threat of a specific and clearly identified danger, the threat of real or imagined danger

HEALTH CARE FACTORS: *Drug therapy*: Any drug therapy but especially chemotherapy. *Medical therapy*: Any medical therapy but especially therapy such as radiation or rehabilitation. *Surgical therapy*: Any surgery. *Follow-up evaluation*: Impending

PLANNING

Unmet Needs

Comfort, protection from psychologic threat, acceptance, caring and communicating relationships, high evaluation of self, sense of adequacy, personal growth and maturity, increased learning, increased reality perception and problem-solving ability

Expected Outcome

Person verbalizes fears

Verbalizes feelings of adequacy and competence in meeting the fear-creating experience

Verbalizes self-satisfaction and growth in having coped with the fear-creating experience

Calm, relaxed facial expression, body movements, and behavior

NURSING INTERVENTIONS

Nursing Treatments

Approach unhurriedly

Reassure verbally (that the nurse will be available whenever needed)

Demonstrate calmness

Provide an atmosphere of acceptance

Encourage the expression of feelings (about the fear)

Listen attentively

Offer feedback to the person's expressed feelings

Communicate nurse sensitivity to the person's problem

Relate to the person on an adult–adult level, not on a parent–child level (which could increase fear)

Attend the person constantly (until he feels sufficiently comfortable to be alone)

Ask the person to identify the problem

Ask for specifics, not generalizations, about the problem

Provide reliable information (about the probability of it being favorable or unfavorable, about the procedure or therapy)

Ask how the person normally copes with fear (what does he usually do when fearful that reduces the fear?)

Provide whatever the person needs to use his usual coping mechanisms

Explore with the person his strengths and resources (to cope with the fear and the outcome)

Introduce to persons who have undergone the same experience (if appropriate)

Nursing Observations

Observe for an excessive stress level (resulting from the fear)

Observe for evidence of a favorable response to therapy (reduced fear and increased comfort)

Health Teaching

Explain that the person's response is appropriate and commonly experienced

Explain the importance of persons offering emotional support to one another (during such times of stress)

EVALUATION

Record actual outcome

FEAR OF THE UNKNOWN HEALTH CARE ROUTINE[105,471,525]

ASSESSMENT

Data Collection

Subjective Data
• Person experiences feelings of threat or danger
• Can describe or identify the threat or danger
  Relates being unfamiliar with the routine of the health care system
  Asks questions about what to expect
  Is concerned that the unknown routine will disrupt the person's valued routine
  May resist the routine if it varies greatly from the person's daily life routine

Objective Data
• May manifest physical findings such as facial flushing or pallor, rapid or deep respirations, rapid or bounding pulse, increased blood pressure, sweating, trembling
• May exhibit behavior such as restlessness, irritability, demanding and controlling behavior, doing things in familiar ways avoiding the unknown routine

Data Analysis

Nursing Diagnosis
FEAR OF THE UNKNOWN HEALTH CARE ROUTINE: A feeling of alarm and fright about the daily schedule of activities in a hospital or institution

Common Etiology (Stressors)
PSYCHOSOCIAL FACTORS: The threat of a specific and clearly identified danger, the threat of real or imagined danger
HEALTH CARE FACTORS: *Hospitalization/Institutionalization*: Any. *Medical therapy*: Rehabilitation therapy

PLANNING

Unmet Needs

Comfort, protection from psychologic threat, acceptance, caring and communicating relationships, high evaluation of self, sense of adequacy, personal growth and maturity, increased learning, increased reality perception and problem-solving ability

Expected Outcome

Person verbalizes fears
Verbalizes feelings of adequacy and competence in meeting the fear-creating experience
Verbalizes self-satisfaction and growth in having coped with the fear-creating experience
Calm, relaxed facial expression, body movements, and behavior

NURSING INTERVENTIONS

Nursing Treatments

Approach unhurriedly
Reassure verbally (that the nurse will acquaint the person with the routine)
Demonstrate calmness
Provide an atmosphere of acceptance
Encourage the expression of feelings (about the fear)
Listen attentively
Offer feedback to the person's expressed feelings
Communicate nurse sensitivity to the person's problem
Relate to the person on an adult–adult level, not on a parent–child level (which could increase fear)
Ask the person to identify the problem
Ask for specifics, not generalizations, about the problem

Support a realistic assessment of the situation (that some established routine is essential in any institution)

Provide reliable information (about the established routine and its purpose)

Arrange situations that encourage the person's autonomy (so that the person can fit his routine into the established routine and still feel comfortable)

Grant special requests

Ask how the person normally copes with fear (what does he usually do when fearful that reduces the fear?)

Provide whatever the person needs to use his usual coping mechanisms

Do not allow unpleasant surprise situations (such as unexpected, unexplained changes in routine)

Nursing Observations

Observe for an excessive stress level (resulting from the fear)

Observe for evidence of a favorable response to therapy (reduced fear and increased comfort)

Health Teaching

Explain that the person's response is appropriate and commonly experienced

Explain that ill or aged persons and small children are often hypersensitive (to change)

EVALUATION

Record actual outcome

FEAR OF THE UNKNOWN HEALTH PROCEDURE/THERAPY[105,471,525]

ASSESSMENT

Data Collection

Subjective Data

• Person experiences feelings of threat or danger

• Can describe or identify the threat or danger

Questions what the procedure/therapy will be like

Is reluctant to accept it, yet desires to get it over with

Objective Data

• May manifest physical findings such as facial flushing or pallor, rapid or deep respirations, rapid or bounding pulse, increased blood pressure, sweating, trembling

• May exhibit behavior such as restlessness, irritability, rapid speech, demanding and controlling behavior, crying, canceling appointments or being unavailable for the procedure/therapy

Data Analysis

Nursing Diagnosis

FEAR OF THE UNKNOWN HEALTH PROCEDURE/THERAPY: A feeling of alarm and fright about the methods and performance of procedures or therapy that the person seeking health

Common Etiology (Stressors)

PSYCHOSOCIAL FACTORS: The threat of a specific and clearly identified danger, the threat of real or imagined danger

HEALTH CARE FACTORS: *Health therapy*: Delayed, experimental, painful, unfamiliar, health therapy, or unscheduled therapy (such as organ transplant or emergency surgery). *Diagnostic procedure*: Any. *Medical, drug, or surgical therapy*: Any

PLANNING

Unmet Needs

Comfort, protection from psychologic threat, acceptance, caring and communicating relationships, high evaluation of self, sense of adequacy, personal growth and maturity, increased learning, increased reality perception and problem-solving ability

Expected Outcome

Person verbalizes fears

Verbalizes feelings of adequacy and competence in meeting the fear-creating experience

Verbalizes self-satisfaction and growth in having coped with the fear-creating experience

Calm, relaxed facial expression, body movements, and behavior

NURSING INTERVENTIONS

Nursing Treatments

Approach unhurriedly

Reassure verbally (that the nurse will be with the person during the procedure or therapy)

Demonstrate calmness

Provide an atmosphere of acceptance

Encourage the expression of feelings (about the fear)

Listen attentively

Offer feedback to the person's expressed feelings

Communicate nurse sensitivity to the person's problem

Relate to the person on an adult–adult level, not on a parent–child level (which could increase fear)

Attend the person constantly (until he feels sufficiently comfortable with the procedure)

Provide frequent contact with the person (thereafter)

Ask the person to identify the problem

Ask for specifics, not generalizations, about the problem

Provide reliable information (about the procedure or therapy)

Ask how the person normally copes with fear (what does he usually do when fearful that reduces the fear?)

Provide whatever the person needs to use his usual coping mechanisms

Encourage the person to face the fear (when able. This will reduce the fear)

Explore with the person his strengths and resources (to overcome the fear and to become comfortable with the therapy)

Provide emotionally safe experiences (whenever possible)

Do not allow unpleasant surprise situations (such as unexpected or unexplained procedures or therapy)

Prepare the patient for a painful experience (if such is going to occur)

Reduce the demands placed on the person (so that more energy is available for coping)

Introduce to persons who have undergone the same experience (if appropriate)

Nursing Observations

Observe for an excessive stress level (resulting from the fear)

Determine the degree of insight (into the fear)

Observe for evidence of a favorable response to therapy (reduced fear and increased comfort)

Health Teaching

Explain that the person's response is appropriate and commonly experienced

Explain the importance of recognizing tension within oneself (which increases the fear of the therapy, which, in turn, enhances the negative perception of the therapy)

Recommend methods for achieving total relaxation (controlled breathing, which reduces the fear)

EVALUATION

Record actual outcome

FEAR OF TRANSMITTING DISEASE BY CONTACT[105,471,525]

ASSESSMENT

Data Collection

Subjective Data
- Person experiences feelings of threat or danger
- Can describe or identify the threat or danger
  Knows that he can transmit disease by contact
  Is concerned that others may contact the disease
  May inquire as to methods of and prevention of transmission
  Expresses anger over having the disease

Objective Data
- May manifest physical findings such as facial flushing or pallor, rapid or deep respirations, rapid or bounding pulse, increased blood pressure, sweating, trembling
- May exhibit behavior such as restlessness, avoiding persons who are likely to contract the disease, seeking reassurance that he is taking the right precautions

Data Analysis

Nursing Diagnosis
FEAR OF TRANSMITTING DISEASE BY CONTACT: A feeling of alarm and fright about passing a particular disease to another person by contact

Common Etiology (Stressors)
DISEASES: Acquired immune deficiency syndrome (AIDS), gonorrhea, Hansen's disease, hepatitis, herpes genitalia, measles, pheumonia, scarlet fever, syphilis, tuberculosis, thrush, trench mouth
PSYCHOSOCIAL FACTORS: The threat of a specific and clearly identified danger, the threat of real or imagined danger

PLANNING

Unmet Needs
Comfort, protection from psychologic threat, acceptance, caring and communicating relationships, high evaluation of self, sense of adequacy, personal growth and maturity, increased learning, increased reality perception and problem-solving ability

Expected Outcome
Person verbalizes fears
Verbalizes feelings of adequacy and competence in meeting the fear-creating experience
Verbalizes self-satisfaction and growth in having coped with the fear-creating experience
Calm, relaxed facial expression, body movements, and behavior

NURSING INTERVENTIONS

Nursing Treatments
Approach unhurriedly
Reassure verbally (that the nurse will help the person as much as possible)
Demonstrate calmness
Provide an atmosphere of acceptance
Encourage the expression of feelings (about the fear)
Listen attentively
Offer feedback to the person's expressed feelings
Communicate nurse sensitivity to the person's problem
Relate to the person on an adult–adult level, not on a parent–child level (which could increase fear)

Ask the person to identify the problem

Ask for specifics, not generalizations, about the problem

Provide reliable information (about the probability of transmitting the disease, about modes of transmission and methods of prevention)

Ask how the person normally copes with fear (what does he usually do when fearful that reduces the fear?)

Provide whatever the person needs to use his usual coping mechanisms

Nursing Observations

Observe for an excessive stress level (resulting from the fear)

Observe for evidence of a favorable response to therapy (reduced fear, increased comfort, and the practice of preventive methods)

Health Teaching

Explain that the person's response is appropriate and commonly experienced

Explain how to prevent cross-infection (limiting human contact, hand washing, etc.)

Describe those signs/symptoms that should be reported (both in self and significant other, those that are specific to the disease)

Instruct to report early signs/symptoms (since early recognition and treatment will reduce the danger)

EVALUATION

Record actual outcome

FEAR OF TRANSMITTING FAMILIAL DISEASE[105,471,525]

ASSESSMENT

Data Collection

Subjective Data

• Person experiences feelings of threat or danger

• Can describe or identify the threat or danger

Relates a family history of a specific disease or condition other than a birth defect

Inquires about the probability of transmission of the disease or condition

Objective Data

• May manifest physical findings such as facial flushing or pallor, rapid or deep respirations, rapid or bounding pulse, increased blood pressure, sweating, trembling

• May exhibit behavior such as restlessness, sleep disturbances, avoiding sexual activity that might result in pregnancy, expressing anger at having the problem

Data Analysis

Nursing Diagnosis

FEAR OF TRANSMITTING FAMILIAL DISEASE: A feeling of alarm and fright about passing on to offspring a disease or condition known to be present in family members

Common Etiology (Stressors)

INHERITED FACTORS: Familial tendency to disease

DISEASES: Alcoholism, carcinoma, diabetes mellitus, epilepsy, Hodgkin's disease, Huntington's chorea, malignant or essential hypertension, leukemia, myocardial infarction, Raynaud's disease, schizophrenia, sickle cell anemia or trait

PSYCHOSOCIAL FACTORS: The threat of a specific and clearly identified danger, the threat of real or imagined danger

PLANNING

Unmet Needs

Comfort, protection from psychologic threat, acceptance, caring and communicating relationships, high evaluation of self, sense of adequacy, personal growth and maturity, increased learning, increased reality perception and problem-solving ability

Expected Outcome

Person verbalizes fears
Verbalizes feelings of adequacy and competence in meeting the fear-creating experience
Verbalizes self-satisfaction and growth in having coped with the fear-creating experience
Calm, relaxed facial expression, body movements, and behavior

NURSING INTERVENTIONS

Nursing Treatments

Approach unhurriedly
Reassure verbally (that the nurse will help the person as much as possible)
Demonstrate calmness
Provide an atmosphere of acceptance
Encourage the expression of feelings (about the fear)
Listen attentively
Offer feedback to the person's expressed feelings
Communicate nurse sensitivity to the person's problem
Relate to the person on and adult–adult level, not on a parent–child level (which could increase fear)
Ask the person to identify the problem
Ask for specifics, not generalizations, about the problem
Support a realistic assessment of the situation (that there is a risk)
Provide reliable information (about the probability of a child having or developing the disease, the cures or controls available for the disease)
Ask how the person normally copes with fear (what does he usually do when fearful that reduces the fear?)
Provide whatever the person needs to use his usual coping mechanisms
Explore with the person his strengths and resources (to overcome the fear and to cope with the familial disease should it occur)

Nursing Observations

Observe for an excessive stress level (resulting from the fear)
Determine the degree of insight that the person has (into the fear)
Observe for evidence of a favorable response to therapy (reduced fear and increased comfort)

Health Teaching

Explain that the person's response is appropriate and commonly experienced
Explain the high-risk factors and how to reduce them
Explain how to channel emotional energy and obtain release from stress (through running, swimming, other sports, creative activities, laughing, talking things over)
Recommend methods for achieving total relaxation (controlled breathing, quietly listening to music, which reduces fear)
Recommend a habitual, positive mental attitude (toward himself, despite the familial disease)
Teach how to use the problem-solving method (to deal with the difficulty should the familial disease occur)

EVALUATION

Record actual outcome

FEAR OF UNFAMILIAR DEVELOPMENTAL CHANGES[105,471,525]

ASSESSMENT

Data Collection

Subjective Data
- Person experiences feelings of threat or danger
- Can describe or identify the threat or danger
  Is aware that the body is changing
  Is concerned about the meaning of the changes
  Feels unfamiliar with the new body
  May experience unfamiliar emotions accompanying body changes
  May be concerned about the variation in physical maturation as compared to that of his peers

Objective Data
- May manifest physical findings such as facial flushing or pallor, rapid or deep respirations, rapid or bounding pulse, increased blood pressure, sweating, trembling
- May exhibit behavior such as restlessness, sleep disturbances, change in eating habits, irritability, demanding and controlling behavior, crying, unusual quietness
  May attempt to handle the problem with clothing changes

Data Analysis

Nursing Diagnosis
FEAR OF UNFAMILIAR DEVELOPMENTAL CHANGES: A feeling of alarm and fright about physical changes that normally occur as the individual moves through life's developmental phases

Common Etiology (Stressors)
PSYCHOSOCIAL FACTORS: The threat of a specific and clearly identified danger, the threat of real or imagined danger
HUMAN BODY: *Body states*: Male climacteric, menopause, menstruation
DEVELOPMENTAL PHASES: Puberty, adolescence, ongoing aging

PLANNING

Unmet Needs

Comfort, protection from psychologic threat, acceptance, caring and communicating relationships, high evaluation of self, sense of adequacy, personal growth and maturity, increased learning, increased reality perception and problem-solving ability

Expected Outcome

Person verbalizes fears
Verbalizes feelings of adequacy and competence in meeting the fear-creating experience
Verbalizes self-satisfaction and growth in having coped with the fear-creating experience
Calm, relaxed facial expression, body movements, and behavior

NURSING INTERVENTIONS

Nursing Treatments

Approach unhurriedly
Reassure verbally (that the nurse will help the person as much as possible)
Demonstrate calmness
Provide an atmosphere of acceptance
Encourage the expression of feelings (about the fear)
Listen attentively
Offer feedback to the person's expressed feelings
Communicate nurse sensitivity to the person's problem

Relate to the person on an adult–adult level, not on a parent–child level (which could increase fear)

Ask the person to identify the problem

Ask for specifics, not generalizations, about the problem

Provide reliable information (about normal developmental changes)

Ask how the person normally copes with fear (what does he usually do when fearful that reduces the fear?)

Provide whatever the person needs to use his usual coping mechanisms

Explore with the person his strengths and resources (in using the changes to enhance self-identity, function, personality, and appearance)

Nursing Observations

Observe for an excessive stress level (resulting from the fear)

Determine the degree of insight that the person has (into the fear)

Observe for evidence of a favorable response to therapy (reduced fear and increased comfort)

Health Teaching

Explain that the person's response is appropriate and commonly experienced

Recommend a habitual, positive mental attitude (toward himself)

EVALUATION

Record actual outcome

FEAR OF UNFAMILIAR/UNEXPECTED BODY SENSATIONS[105,471,525]

ASSESSMENT

Data Collection

Subjective Data

• Person experiences feelings of threat or danger
• Can describe or identify the threat or danger
  Is concerned about body sensations never before experienced
  Questions the meaning of such sensations
  Fears that the sensations may have negative physical implications

Objective Data

• May manifest physical findings such as facial flushing or pallor, rapid or deep respirations, rapid or bounding pulse, increased blood pressure, sweating, trembling
• May exhibit behavior such as restlessness, sleep disturbances, change in eating habits, irritability, demanding and controlling behavior, unusual quietness

Data Analysis

Nursing Diagnosis

FEAR OF UNFAMILIAR/UNEXPECTED BODY SENSATIONS: A feeling of alarm and fright about body sensations that the person has never experienced before or that the person did not anticipate

Common Etiology (Stressors)

DISEASES: Air sickness (hot, weak feeling), aneurysm (pumping sensation near the skin surface), aplastic anemia (weakness), angina pectoris (pain), cataracts (blurred vision), diabetes mellitus (thirst), gastric ulcer (gnawing sensation), Guillain-Barré syndrome (weakness), essential or malignant hypertension (irritability), Meniere's disease (dizziness), myasthenia gravis (intermittent weakness), retinal detachment (stabbing pain), rheumatoid arthritis (stiffness, pain), thyrotoxicosis (irritability, energetic restlessness), Buerger's disease, cerebrovascular accident, Hansen's disease, multiple sclerosis (sensation loss)

INJURIES: Fracture and compression of the spinal cord (numbness, paralysis), frostbite (numbness), tick bite of the neck (paralysis)

PSYCHOSOCIAL FACTORS: The threat of a specific and clearly identified danger, the threat of real or imagined danger

HUMAN BODY: *Natural body function*: Breast feeding an infant (pleasurable sexual sensations, pulling sensation), childbirth (pain, pressure). *Body state*: Pregnancy (pressure, shortness of breath, fatigue, fetal movement, lightning)

HEALTH CARE FACTORS: *Diagnostic procedures*: Angiography, cardiac catheterization, cystoscopy, urinary catheterization (burning sensation); anoscopy, barium enema, cisternal puncture, colonoscopy, proctoscopy, proctosigmoidoscopy (pressure sensation); bone marrow aspiration, Pap smear (pain); broncoscopy, gastroscopy, vital capacity pulmonary function test (shortness of breath); electromyogram (stinging sensation). *Drug therapy*: Anticholinergics (mouth dryness); antihistamines, antihypertensive drugs, tranquilizers, barbiturates, narcotics (drowsiness); chemotherapy (nausea, vomiting); corticosteroids (edema, tightness, restlessness); diuretics (urinary urgency); laxatives, purgatives (cramping); hormones, antidepressants (feeling of well-being); decongestants, amphetamines (tachycardia); Ophthaine optic solution (sensation loss). *Medical therapy*: Cardioversion (jolting sensation); therapeutic dressings, enemas, intermittent positive pressure breathing, irrigations, nasal packing, peritoneal dialysis (pressure sensation); hemodialysis (nausea, headache); inhalation mist therapy (facial wetness); rehabilitation therapy (aching, stiffness); nerve block (sensation loss); traction (pulling sensation); nasogastric or endotracheal intubation (sore throat); withdrawal from alcohol, drugs, tobacco (nervousness, irritability, anxiety). *Surgical therapy*: Local or spinal anesthesia (sensation loss). *Surgical incision*: Any (degrees of pain)

SITUATIONAL FACTORS: The experience of dying (hot, weak feeling)

PLANNING

Unmet Needs

Comfort, protection from psychologic threat, acceptance, caring and communicating relationships, high evaluation of self, sense of adequacy, personal growth and maturity, increased learning, increased reality perception and problem-solving ability

Expected Outcome

Person verbalizes fears

Verbalizes feelings of adequacy and competence in meeting the fear-creating experience

Verbalizes self-satisfaction and growth in having coped with the fear-creating experience

Calm, relaxed facial expression, body movements, and behavior

NURSING INTERVENTIONS

Nursing Treatments

Approach unhurriedly

Reassure verbally (that the nurse will help the person as much as possible)

Demonstrate calmness

Provide an atmosphere of acceptance

Encourage the expression of feelings (about the fear)

Listen attentively

Offer feedback to the person's expressed feelings

Communicate nurse sensitivity to the person's problem

Relate to the person on an adult–adult level, not on a parent–child level (which could increase fear)

Attend the person constantly (until he feels sufficiently comfortable with the sensation to be alone)

Provide frequent contact with the person (thereafter, until the sensation subsides)

Ask the person to identify the problem

Ask for specifics, not generalizations, about the problem

Provide reliable information (about the effects of the disease, injury, or procedures; the duration of the unfamiliar sensation and the expected time the sensation will subside or return)

Ask how the person normally copes with fear (what does he usually do when fearful that reduces the fear?)

Provide whatever the person needs to use the usual coping mechanisms

Do not allow unpleasant surprise situations (such as unexpected or unexplained procedures that cause unfamiliar sensations)

Avoid placing the person on enforced inactivity (which heightens fear)

Introduce to persons who have undergone the same experience (if appropriate)

Nursing Observations

Observe for an excessive stress level (resulting from the fear)

Determine the degree of insight that the person has (into the fear)

Observe for evidence of a favorable response to therapy (reduced fear and increased comfort)

Health Teaching

Explain that the person's response is appropriate and commonly experienced

Recommend methods for achieving total relaxation (such as controlled breathing, which will reduce the fear)

EVALUATION

Record actual outcome

FEAR OF UNREAL IMAGES/VOICES[105,471,525]

ASSESSMENT

Data Collection

Subjective Data
- Person experiences feelings of threat or danger
- Can describe or identify the threat or danger

Perceives sights and sounds that are unreal

Desperately wants the perceptions to cease

May be afraid to verbalize about the images or voices because of concern about how others will respond to information about his perceptions

Objective Data
- May manifest physical findings such as facial flushing or pallor, rapid or deep respirations, rapid or bounding pulse, increased blood pressure, sweating, trembling
- May exhibit behavior such as restlessness, sleep disturbances, change in eating habits, irritability, short attention span, making poor judgments, forgetfulness, rapid speech, demanding and controlling behavior, crying, avoiding persons or situations that stimulate images or voices, frequent call-light signaling, detaining the nurse

May respond by speech or action to the unreal voices

Data Analysis

Nursing Diagnosis
FEAR OF UNREAL IMAGES/VOICES: A feeling of alarm and fright about the perception of visions or voices that the person knows are not real

Common Etiology (Stressors)
DISEASES: Alcoholism (delirium tremens), brain tumor, major depression, organic brain syndrome, schizophrenia

SIGNS AND SYMPTOMS: Delusions, hallucinations, high fever

PSYCHOSOCIAL FACTORS: The threat of a specific and clearly identified danger, the threat of real or imagined danger, the threat of sensory deprivation or sensory overload

HEALTH CARE FACTORS: *Adverse effects of drugs*: Hallucinogenic drugs (images perceived after drug ingestion). *Medical therapy*: Alcohol or drug withdrawal

LIFESTYLE: Drug abuse, prolonged lack of sleep

ENVIRONMENTAL FACTORS: *Chemical substances*: Exposure to toxic gases or vapors

PLANNING

Unmet Needs

Comfort, protection from psychologic threat, acceptance, caring and communicating relationships, high evaluation of self, sense of adequacy, personal growth and maturity, increased learning, increased reality perception and problem-solving ability

Expected Outcome

Person verbalizes fears

Verbalizes feelings of adequacy and competence in meeting the fear-creating experience

Verbalizes self-satisfaction and growth in having coped with the fear-creating experience

Calm, relaxed facial expression, body movements, and behavior

NURSING INTERVENTIONS

Nursing Treatments

Approach unhurriedly

Reassure verbally (that the nurse will help the person as much as possible)

Demonstrate calmness

Provide an atmosphere of acceptance

Arrange pleasant surroundings

Encourage the expression of feelings (about the visions or voices)

Listen attentively

Offer feedback to the person's expressed feelings

Communicate nurse sensitivity to the person's problem

Relate to the person on an adult–adult level, not on a parent–child level (which could increase fear)

Attend the person constantly (until he feels sufficiently comfortable to be alone)

Provide frequent contact with the person (thereafter)

Ask the person to identify the problem

Ask for specifics, not generalizations, about the problem (encourage him to describe the experiences)

Refrain from supporting the person's hallucinations or illusions (and do not indulge or appease the person)

Ask how the person normally copes with fear (what does he usually do when fearful that reduces the fear?)

Provide whatever the person needs to use his usual coping mechanisms

Encourage the person to face the fear (when able. This will reduce the fear)

Explore with the person his strengths and resources (to cope with the fear)

Increase environmental stimulants (if there is sensory deprivation, provide more visitors, radio/TV, mobiles above the bed, a wide mirror for enlarging the field of vision)

Decrease environmental stimulants (if there is sensory overload, provide minimal light and noise, limited visitors for specified rest and sleep periods)

Avoid placing the person on enforced inactivity (which heightens fear)

Reduce the demands placed on the person (so that more energy is available for coping)

Nursing Observations

Observe for an excessive stress level (resulting from the fear)

Determine the degree of insight that the person has (into the fear)

Observe for evidence of a favorable response to therapy (reduced fear and increased comfort)

Health Teaching

Explain that the person's response is appropriate and commonly experienced (when a person experiences perceptions that he knows are not real)

Explain the causes of the health problem (if induced by fever, drugs, toxic chemicals, sensory alteration, etc.)

EVALUATION

Record actual outcome

FEAR OF VISION LOSS [105,471,525]

ASSESSMENT

Data Collection

Subjective Data

• Person experiences feelings of threat or danger
• Can describe or identify the threat or danger
  Suddenly places a heightened value on the sense of sight
  Relates concern about visual perception
  May enumerate the unfavorable effects of vision loss

Objective Data

• May manifest physical findings such as facial flushing or pallor, rapid or deep respirations, rapid or bounding pulse, increased blood pressure, sweating, trembling
• May exhibit behavior such as restlessness, sleep disturbances, change in eating habits, irritability, rapid speech, demanding and controlling behavior, crying, unusual quietness, frequent call-light signaling, seeking reassurance

Data Analysis

Nursing Diagnosis

FEAR OF VISION LOSS: A feeling of alarm and fright that one's vision might be or become impaired

Common Etiology (Stressors)

DISEASES: Brain tumor, cataracts, cerebrovascular accident, conjunctivitis, diabetes mellitus, glaucoma, keratitis, multiple sclerosis, retinal detachment, retinitis

INJURIES: Burns (chemical, ultraviolet), contusion of the eye, corneal abrasion, a foreign body in the eye

SIGNS AND SYMPTOMS: Blurred vision, diplopia, eye swelling, photophobia, tunnel vision

PSYCHOSOCIAL FACTORS: The threat of a specific and clearly indentified danger, the threat of real or imagined danger

HEALTH CARE FACTORS: *Diagnostic procedures*: Gonioscopy, tonometry. *Drug therapy*: Belladonna or atropine optic solution. *Medical therapy*: Eye irrigation or patching, phototherapy. *Surgical procedures*: Enucleation or evisceration of eyeball, cataract extraction, photocoagulation (for retinal reattachment), scleral buckling, sclerotomy

PLANNING

Unmet Needs

Comfort, protection from psychologic threat, acceptance, caring and communicating relationships, high evaluation of self, sense of adequacy, personal growth and maturity, increased learning, increased reality perception and problem-solving ability

Expected Outcome

Person verbalizes fears

Verbalizes feelings of adequacy and competence in meeting the fear-creating experience

Verbalizes self-satisfaction and growth in having coped with the fear-creating experience

Calm, relaxed facial expression, body movements, and behavior

NURSING INTERVENTIONS

Nursing Treatments

Approach unhurriedly

Reassure verbally (that the nurse will help the person as much as possible)

Demonstrate calmness

Provide an atmosphere of acceptance

Encourage the expression of feelings (about the fear)

Listen attentively

Offer feedback to the person's expressed feelings

Communicate nurse sensitivity to the person's problem

Relate to the person on an adult–adult level, not on a parent–child level (which could increase fear)

Attend the person constantly (until he feels sufficiently comfortable to be alone)

Provide frequent contact with the person (thereafter)

Ask the person to identify the problem

Ask for specifics, not generalizations, about the problem

Provide reliable information (about the probability of vision loss; about procedures, diseases, injuries, etc. related to vision)

Ask how the person normally copes with fear (what does he usually do when fearful that reduces the fear?)

Provide whatever the person needs to use his usual coping mechanisms

Do not allow unpleasant surprise situations (such as unexpected or unexplained procedures that cause impaired vision)

Introduce to persons who have undergone the same experience (if appropriate)

Nursing Observations

Observe for an excessive stress level (resulting from the fear)

Determine the degree of insight that the person has (into the fear)

Observe for evidence of a favorable response to therapy (reduced fear and increased comfort)

Health Teaching

Explain that the person's response is appropriate and commonly experienced

Recommend a habitual, positive mental attitude (toward himself and his ability to cope)

Teach the specific methods (for decreasing the chance of vision loss, such as minimizing intraoccular pressure following eye surgery, using good light when there are cataracts)

EVALUATION

Record actual outcome

Adaptive Responses of Emotion (Affect): Frustration

FRUSTRATION RELATED TO A DEPENDENT SIGNIFICANT OTHER [105,317,432,471,525]

ASSESSMENT

Data Collection

Subjective Data

• Person relates that a desired goal is delayed or unattainable

• Verbalizes irritability toward the significant other causing the delay

Person feels internal tension when the significant other attempts activities that take a long time

Prefers to do the activity himself rather than watch the significant other struggle with it

Wonders how long he can tolerate the situation

May want to forsake responsibility for the significant other

Objective Data
- May exhibit behavior such as heavy sighing, frowning, shaking the head, clenching the hands

Data Analysis

Nursing Diagnosis

FRUSTRATION RELATED TO A DEPENDENT SIGNIFICANT OTHER: Feelings of irritation and tension when a desired personal goal is blocked because of having to care for a dependent loved one

Common Etiology (Stressors)

BIRTH DEFECTS: Any

INJURIES: Any

SIGNS AND SYMPTOMS (OF A SIGNIFICANT OTHER): Fatigue, immobility, limping, memory loss, pain, paralysis, tremor, vision loss, weakness

PSYCHOSOCIAL FACTORS: The threat of delayed goal achievement, lack of resources to achieve a goal, the threat of failure to achieve

HUMAN BODY (OF A SIGNIFICANT OTHER): *Body function*: Loss of body function. *Body part*: Loss of a body part

DEVELOPMENTAL PHASE (OF A SIGNIFICANT OTHER): Toddler, childhood, old age

PLANNING

Unmet Needs

Comfort, protection from psychologic threat, acceptance, caring and communicating relationships, sense of adequacy, goal achievement, endurance, personal growth and maturity, increased learning, increased reality perception and problem-solving ability

Expected Outcome

Person verbalizes feelings of tension

Relates constructive outlets for tension release

Verbalizes specific problem-solving methods for overcoming the source of frustration

Takes specific action to overcome the frustration

NURSING INTERVENTIONS

Nursing Treatments

Approach unhurriedly

Reassure verbally (that the nurse will help the person with the problem)

Demonstrate calmness

Provide an atmosphere of acceptance

Encourage the expression of feelings (about the frustration)

Listen attentively

Offer feedback to the person's expressed feelings

Communicate nurse sensitivity to the person's problem

Discourage the setting of time limits (which increases frustration)

Encourage striving toward realistic goals

Suggest substitute means of goal attainment (ways to accomplish care more quickly)

Encourage the acceptance of partial goal satisfaction

Encourage laughter (to relieve the tension of frustration)

Encourage planned one-day-at-a-time living

Encourage the sharing of common problems with others (who have dependent loved ones)

Explore with the person his strengths and resources (to overcome the frustration and cope with the dependent person)

Offer praise (for the care the person gives)

Nursing Observations

Determine the precipitating factors, the relieving factors (of frustration)

Observe for an excessive stress level (resulting from the frustration)

Observe for evidence of a favorable response to therapy (reduced frustration, goal achievement)

Health Teaching

Explain that the person's response is appropriate and commonly experienced (when caring for a dependent person)

Explain the importance of persons offering support to one another (when one family member is dependent)

Explain the importance of meeting his own needs as well as those of a significant other (disregarding his own needs reduces his competency to help others; it is important for the care giver to maintain planned recreation and relaxation, to obtain relief from the situation for periods of time)

Emphasize the importance of recognizing tension within oneself

Explain that fatigue should be recognized as a stress factor (makes him more vulnerable to frustration)

Explain how to channel emotional energy and obtain release from stress (through talking things out, creative activities, exercise, etc.)

Explain the importance of maintaining a positive self-attitude

EVALUATION

Record actual outcome

FRUSTRATION RELATED TO PHYSICAL LIMITATIONS[105,317,432,471,525]

ASSESSMENT

Data Collection

Subjective Data

• Person relates a desired goal is delayed or unattainable
• Verbalizes irritability
  Expresses experiencing internal tension
  Relates feeling thwarted when tasks take longer than they used to
  Verbalizes that diminished strength is hard to believe
  Relates that the mind races ahead of the body's capabilities

Objective Data

• May exhibit behavior such as heavy sighing, frowning, shaking the head, clenching the hands
  May attempt to establish a wellness routine on his own, but soon returns to limited activity, may decrease involvement in usual interests

Data Analysis

Nursing Diagnosis

FRUSTRATION RELATED TO PHYSICAL LIMITATIONS: Feelings of irritation and tension when a desired goal is blocked by acitivty limitations imposed by the body

Common Etiology (Stressors)

BIRTH DEFECTS: Any
DISEASES: Any
INJURIES: Any
SIGNS AND SYMPTOMS: Aphasia, fatigue, immobility, limping, memory loss, pain, paralysis, tremor, vision loss, weakness

PSYCHOSOCIAL FACTORS: The threat of delayed goal achievement, lack of resources to achieve a goal, any kind of loss that deprives the person of need gratification, the threat of failure to achieve

HUMAN BODY: *Body adjustment*: As the body strives toward wellness, it reaches a plateau, and from that point progress toward greater health is very slow

HEALTH CARE FACTORS: *Surgical procedures*: Any *Therapeutic equipment/devices*: Use of an artificial limb, eyeglasses, cane, crutches, brace, walker, wheelchair. *Convalescence*: Slow recovery during convalescence. *Complications*: Unforseen health complications

DEVELOPMENTAL PHASES: Old age

SITUATIONAL FACTORS: Illness of or injury to self or significant other

PLANNING
Unmet Needs
Comfort, protection from psychologic threat, acceptance, caring and communicating relationships, sense of adequacy, goal achievement, endurance, personal growth and maturity, increased learning, increased reality perception and problem-solving ability

Expected Outcome
Person verbalizes feelings of tension
Relates constructive outlets for tension release
Verbalizes specific problem-solving methods for overcoming the source of frustration
Takes specific action to overcome the frustration

NURSING INTERVENTIONS
Nursing Treatments
Approach unhurriedly
Reassure verbally (that the nurse will help the person with the problem)
Demonstrate calmness
Provide an atmosphere of acceptance
Encourage the expression of feelings (about the frustration)
Listen attentively
Offer feedback to the person's expressed feelings
Communicate nurse sensitivity to the person's problem
Discourage the setting of time limits (to achieve tasks, which increases frustration)
Encourage striving toward realistic goals (unrealistic goals cause unresolvable frustration)
Suggest substitute means of goal attainment (easier ways to achieve tasks)
Encourage the acceptance of partial goal satisfaction
Encourage the person to seek one goal at a time (multiple goals, simultaneously pursued, heighten frustration)
Encourage both long- and short-term goals
Encourage gradual mastery of a situation
Encourage laughter (to relieve the tension of frustration)
Encourage patience in illness adjustment
Encourage planned one-day-at-a-time living
Explore with the person his strengths and resources (to overcome the frustration)
Verbalize daily the person's successful progress
Offer praise (for even small progress)
Introduce to persons who have successfully undergone the same experience
Reduce the demands placed on the person (so that more energy is available for coping)
Refrain from teasing (this heightens the frustration of the person who is struggling with physical limitations)

Nursing Observations
Determine the degree of insight that the person has
Determine the precipitating factors, the relieving factors (of the frustration)
Observe for evidence that the person is reaching out for emotional support
Observe for evidence of a favorable response to therapy (reduced frustration, goal achievement)

Health Teaching

Explain that the person's response is appropriate and commonly experienced

Explain the importance of persons offering support to one another

Emphasize the importance of recognizing tension within oneself

Explain that fatigue should be recognized as a stress factor (making the person more vulnerable to frustration)

Explain how to channel emotional energy and obtain release from stress (by talking things out, exercising)

Explain the importance of maintaining a positive self-attitude

Explain that ill or aged persons are often hypersensitive (to frustration)

EVALUATION

Record actual outcome

Adaptive Responses of Emotion (Affect): Grief (Mourning)

GRIEF REACTION RELATED TO ANTICIPATORY LOSS [105,197,471,525,568]

ASSESSMENT

Data Collection

Subjective Data
- Person relates an initial feeling of shock and disbelief
- Later expresses anger
- Then acknowledges the loss and that the loss will not be restored
- Relates feeling unsettled, vaguely confused, and intensely sad
  Is preoccupied with the impending loss
  Complains of feelings of weakness, anorexia, sleeplessness, or fretful sleep
  Feels as though the loss has already occurred

Objective Data
- May exhibit grieving behavior such as weeping, saddened facial expression, decreased participation in external interests

Data Analysis

Nursing Diagnosis
GRIEF REACTION RELATED TO ANTICIPATORY LOSS: Feelings of deep sorrow and distress about a loss that will soon occur but has not yet occurred

Common Etiology (Stressors)
PSYCHOSOCIAL FACTORS: Impending loss of or separation from a significant other or from a significant or valued situation or object, impending loss of a normal attachment
DEVELOPMENTAL PHASES: Old age of a significant other
SITUATIONAL FACTORS: Impending death of self or a significant other, placing a child up for adoption, a child being put up for adoption, an impending divorce or marital separation, the launching of grown children, a frequent change of foster parents, the change of or end of school, selling a home, being relocated in a distant city

PLANNING

Unmet Needs

Comfort, protection from psychologic threat, acceptance, caring and communicating relationships, unity with loved ones, personal growth and maturity, increased learning, spiritual–philosophic satisfaction

Expected Outcome

Person verbalizes feelings of sadness
Relates feeling adequate and competent to move through the grief process
Acknowledges the experience as a potential for personal growth
Relates gradual, increased concern for external interests

NURSING INTERVENTIONS

Nursing Treatments

Approach unhurriedly
Reassure verbally (that the nurse is available if needed)
Demonstrate calmness
Provide an atmosphere of acceptance
Encourage the expression of feelings (about the loss)
Listen attentively
Offer feedback to the person's expressed feelings
Communicate nurse sensitivity to the person's problem
Touch the person frequently
Attend the person constantly (until he feels sufficiently comfortable to be alone)
Provide frequent contact with the person (thereafter)
Explore with the person his strengths and resources (to cope with the impending loss)
Reduce the demands placed on the person (so that more energy is available for coping)
Provide objects that symbolize safeness (a picture of a loved one, the person's own blanket, etc.)
Call the person's family (to the bedside if supportive family members are needed)
Encourage telephone calls between significant persons (who can support each other)
Assist the family to prepare for life changes that will occur after the loved one's death
Encourage planned one-day-at-a-time living
Encourage the use of spiritual resources
Avoid forcing the person into rapid adaptation to change by accepting the person's unique pattern of adjustment
Provide privacy (for grieving)
Allow unlimited visiting (of the persons the patient wants to see)
Avoid attempting to cheer up the grieving person (the inability to respond cheerfully makes the grieving person think less of himself)

Nursing Observations

Determine the degree of insight that the person has (into his feelings and the grief process)
Observe for the stages of grief
Observe for an excessive stress level (resulting from the grief)
Observe for evidence of a favorable response to therapy (tension relief by grieving, control of the grief, acceptance of the impending loss)

Health Teaching

Explain that the person's response is appropriate and commonly experienced
Explain and offer hope that the emotional pain will decrease with time
Advise that significant persons express caring for one another (especially at the time of loss)
Explain the importance of persons offering support to one another

EVALUATION

Record actual outcome

GRIEF REACTION RELATED TO APPROACHING DEATH[90,105,471,525,568]

ASSESSMENT

Data Collection

Subjective Data
- Person relates an initial feeling of shock and disbelief
- Later expresses anger
- Then acknowledges the approaching loss of life and that the loss will not be restored
- Relates feeling unsettled, vaguely confused, and intensely sad
  Perceives with great sadness his loss of past and future meaningful persons, objects, and situations
  May verbalize angry feelings

Objective Data
- May exhibit grieving behavior such as weeping, saddened facial expression, withdrawal from persons or situations

Data Analysis

Nursing Diagnosis
GRIEF REACTION RELATED TO APPROACHING DEATH: Feelings of deep sorrow and distress from an awareness that one's life is soon to come to an end

Common Etiology (Stressors)
DISEASES: Any
INJURIES: Any
PSYCHOSOCIAL FACTORS: Loss of or separation from a significant other or from significant or valued situation(s) or object(s)
HEALTH CARE FACTORS: *Medical diagnosis*: An unfavorable medical diagnosis for self. *Health therapy*: Unsuccessful or ineffective medical, drug, or surgical therapy. *Prognosis*: An unfavorable prognosis
SITUATIONAL FACTORS: Terminal illness of self, the experience of dying

PLANNING

Unmet Needs

Comfort, protection from psychologic threat, acceptance, caring and communicating relationships, unity with loved ones, personal growth and maturity, increased learning, spiritual–philosophic satisfaction

Expected Outcome

Person verbalizes feelings of sadness at the loss of his own life
Relates feeling adequate and competent to move through the grief process
Acknowleges the experience as an opportunity for personal growth

NURSING INTERVENTIONS

Nursing Treatments

Approach unhurriedly
Reassure verbally (that the nurse is available whenever needed)
Demonstrate calmness
Provide an atomosphere of acceptance
Encourage the expression of feelings (about the loss)
Listen attentively
Talk with the person and the family
Offer feedback to the person's expressed feelings
Communicate that the nurse feels comfortable with the person's discussion of death (the nurse can best support the patient when the nurse is in touch with her own feelings about death and dying)

Touch the person judiciously

Sit with the person

Attend the person constantly (until he feels sufficiently comfortable to be alone)

Provide frequent contact with the person (thereafter)

Explore with the person his strengths and resources (to cope with his approaching death)

Reduce the demands placed on the person (so that more energy is available for coping)

Refrain from performing nonessential procedures

Provide objects that symbolize safeness (a picture of a loved one, the person's own blanket, etc.)

Call the person's family (to the bedside if he desires such)

Encourage telephone calls between significant persons (who can support each other)

Assist the dying person with unfinished business

Assist the family to prepare for life changes that will occur after the loved one's death

Encourage planned one-day-at-a-time living

Encourage the use of spiritual resources

Provide privacy (so the person can express and explore his feelings)

Allow unlimited visiting (of the persons the patient wants to see)

Avoid attempting to cheer up the grieving person (the inability to respond cheerfully makes the grieving person think less of himself)

Nursing Observations

Determine the degree of insight that the person has (into his feelings and the grief process)

Observe for the stages of grief

Observe for an excessive stress level (resulting from the grief)

Observe for evidence of a favorable response to therapy (tension relief by grieving, control of the grief, acceptance of the loss)

Determine the extent of the child's comprehension of death (if children are involved)

Health Teaching

Explain that the person's response is appropriate and commonly experienced

Explain and offer hope that the emotional pain will decrease with time (as acceptance begins to occur)

Advise that significant persons express caring for one another (especially when a loved one is dying)

Advise that children participate in grief-related activities

Explain the importance of persons offering support to one another

EVALUATION

Record actual outcome

GRIEF REACTION RELATED TO LOSS OF A SIGNIFICANT OTHER[105,471,525,568]

ASSESSMENT

Data Collection

Subjective Data

• Person relates an initial feeling of shock and disbelief

• Later expresses anger

• Then acknowledges the loss of the significant other and that the loss will not be restored

• Relates feeling unsettled, vaguely confused, and intensely sad

Is preoccupied with thoughts of the lost loved one
Focuses on the loved one's finer qualities
May engage in self-recrimination about neglect or misdeeds toward the loved one
Complains of feelings of weakness, anorexia, sleeplessness, or fretful sleep
May verbalize angry feelings
Feels that a part of his self has been lost

Objective Data
• May exhibit grieving behavior such as weeping, saddened facial expression, decreased participation in external interests, withdrawal from persons or situations

Data Analysis

Nursing Diagnosis
GRIEF REACTION RELATED TO LOSS OF A SIGNIFICANT OTHER: Feelings of deep sorrow and distress about being permanently parted from a significant other

Common Etiology (Stressors)
BIRTH DEFECTS: Giving birth to an imperfect infant
DISEASES: Natural abortion, stillbirth, sudden infant death
PSYCHOSOCIAL FACTORS: Loss of a significant other, loss of a normal attachment
HEALTH CARE FACTORS: *Hospital discharge*: Without the expected infant
SITUATIONAL FACTORS: Placing a child up for adoption, a child's being put up for adoption, death of a significant other, divorce of parents or from a spouse, the frequent change of foster parents, giving up a foster child, holidays without a significant other

PLANNING

Unmet Needs
Comfort, protection from psychologic threat, acceptance, caring and communicating relationships, unity with loved ones, personal growth and maturity, increased learning, spiritual–philosophic satisfaction

Expected Outcome
Person verbalizes feelings of sadness
Relates feeling adequate and competent to move through the grief process
Acknowledges the experience as a potential for personal growth
Relates gradual, increased concern for external interests

NURSING INTERVENTIONS

Nursing Treatments
Approach unhurriedly
Reassure verbally (that the nurse is available whenever needed)
Demonstrate calmness
Provide an atmosphere of acceptance
Encourage the expression of feelings (about the loss)
Listen attentively
Offer feedback to the person's expressed feelings
Communicate nurse sensitivity to the person's problem
Touch the person frequently
Attend the person constantly (until he feels sufficiently comfortable to be alone)
Provide frequent contact with the person (thereafter)
Explore with the person his strengths and resources (to cope with the loss)
Reduce the demands placed on the person (so that more energy is available for coping)
Refrain from performing nonessential procedures
Encourage telephone calls between significant persons (who can support each other)
Assist the family to prepare for life changes that will occur after the loved one's death
Encourage planned one-day-at-a-time living
Encourage the use of spiritual resources
Avoid forcing the person into rapid adaptation to change by accepting the person's unique pattern of adjustment

Provide privacy (for grieving)

Allow unlimited visiting (between persons involved in the loss)

Avoid attempting to cheer up the grieving person (the inability to respond cheerfully makes the grieving person think less of himself)

Nursing Observations

Determine the degree of insight that the person has (into his feelings and the grief process)

Observe for the stages of grief

Observe for an excessive stress level (resulting from the grief)

Observe for evidence of a favorable response to therapy (tension relief by grieving, control of the grief, acceptance of the loss)

Health Teaching

Explain that the person's response is appropriate and commonly experienced

Explain and offer hope that the emotional pain will decrease with time (as acceptance of the loss occurs)

Advise that significant persons express caring for one another (especially at the time of loss)

Explain the importance of persons offering support to one another

Advise that children participate in grief-related activities

Advise against correlating God's love and death to children

EVALUATION

Record actual outcome

GRIEF REACTION RELATED TO MATERIAL LOSS [13,105,432,471,525]

ASSESSMENT

Data Collection

Subjective Data

• Person relates an initial feeling of shock and disbelief

• Later expresses anger

• Then acknowledges the loss of the valued object and that the loss will not be restored

• Relates feeling unsettled, vaguely confused, and intensely sad

 Is preoccupied with the loss of home, financial security, or a personal object

 Complains of feelings of weakness, sleeplessness, or fretful sleep

 May verbalize angry feelings

Objective Data

• May exhibit grieving behavior such as weeping, saddened facial expression, decreased participation in external interests, seeking a substitute for the lost object

Data Analysis

Nursing Diagnosis

GRIEF REACTION RELATED TO MATERIAL LOSS: Feelings of deep sorrow and distress about the loss of tangible, valued objects

Common Etiology (Stressors)

PSYCHOSOCIAL FACTORS: Loss of or separation from a significant or valued object, loss of a normal attachment

HEALTH CARE FACTORS: High health care costs

SITUATIONAL FACTORS: Accident, loss of or relocation of a home, loss of employment, lack of finances, insufficient or lack of insurance coverage, loss of property through illness or injury, unfavorable economic factors, arson, theft

ENVIRONMENTAL FACTORS: *Cataclysm*: Cyclone, earthquake, flood, hailstorm, hurricane, volcanic eruption. *Environmental*: Fire

PLANNING

Unmet Needs

Comfort, protection from psychologic threat, acceptance, caring and communicating relationships, unity with loved ones, personal growth and maturity, increased learning, spiritual–philosophic satisfaction

Expected Outcome

Person verbalizes feelings of sadness

Relates feeling adequate and competent to move through the grief process

Acknowledges the experience as a potential for personal growth

Relates gradual, increased concern for external interests

NURSING INTERVENTIONS

Nursing Treatments

Approach unhurriedly

Reassure verbally (that the nurse is available whenever needed)

Demonstrate calmness

Provide an atmosphere of acceptance

Encourage the expression of feelings (about the loss)

Listen attentively

Offer feedback to the person's expressed feelings

Communicate nurse sensitivity to the person's problem

Touch the person frequently

Attend the person constantly (until he feels sufficiently comfortable to be alone)

Provide frequent patient contact (thereafter)

Explore with the person his strengths and resources (to cope with the loss)

Reduce the demands placed on the person (so that more energy is available for coping)

Call the person's family (to the bedside if the person desires such)

Encourage telephone calls between significant persons (who can support each other through the loss)

Encourage planned one-day-at-a-time living

Encourage the use of spiritual resources

Avoid forcing the person into rapid adaptation to change by accepting the person's unique pattern of adjustment

Provide privacy (for grieving)

Allow unlimited visiting (of the persons the patient wants to see)

Avoid attempting to cheer up the grieving person (the inability to respond cheerfully makes the grieving person think less of himself)

Nursing Observations

Determine the degree of insight that the person has (into his feelings and the grief process)

Observe for the stages of grief

Observe for an excessive stress level (resulting from the grief)

Observe for evidence of a favorable response to therapy (tension relief by grieving, control of the grief, acceptance of the loss)

Health Teaching

Explain that the person's response is appropriate and commonly experienced

Explain and offer hope that the emotional pain will decrease with time (as acceptance occurs)

Advise that significant persons express caring for one another (especially at the time of loss)

Explain the importance of persons offering support to one another

EVALUATION

Record actual outcome

GRIEF REACTION RELATED TO PHYSICAL LOSS[105,471,525,568]

ASSESSMENT

Data Collection

Subjective Data
• Person relates an initial feeling of shock and disbelief
• Later expresses anger
• Then acknowledges the loss of health and that the loss will not be restored
• Relates feeling unsettled, vaguely confused, and intensely sad
  Is preoccupied with the illness
  Relates an awakened appreciation for past good health
  Complains of feelings of weakness, anorexia, sleeplessness, or fretful sleep

Objective Data
• May exhibit grieving behavior such as weeping, saddened facial expression, decreased participation in external interests, withdrawal from persons or situations

Data Analysis

Nursing Diagnosis
GRIEF REACTION RELATED TO PHYSICAL LOSS: Feelings of deep sorrow and distress about the loss of a positive, balanced state of health

Common Etiology (Stressors)
DISEASES: Any
INJURIES: Any
SIGNS AND SYMPTOMS: Confusion, immobility, memory loss, pain, paralysis, weakness
PSYCHOSOCIAL FACTORS: Loss of a normal attachment (to self as formerly perceived)
HUMAN BODY: *Body appearance*: Changes in body appearance, disfigured body. *Body function*: Loss of body function. *Natural body function*: Loss of the fetus from the maternal body at childbirth. *Body part*: Loss of a body part. *Body states*: Loss of the prepregnancy body
HEALTH CARE FACTORS: *Health care decisions*: To donate a body organ, to donate blood. *Health therapy*: Unsuccessful or ineffective therapy. *Adverse effects of medical, drug, or surgical therapy*: Loss of a body part (from amputation, cholecystectomy, enucleation or evisceration of an eyeball, gastrectomy, hemipelvectomy, hysterectomy, ileotomy, lobectomy of the brain, liver, or lungs, mastectomy, nephrectomy, prostatectomy, splenectomy, thyroidectomy, tonsillectomy), loss of hair (from chemotherapy and radiation therapy), loss of natural elimination and elimination control (from a colostomy, ileocolostomy, ileostomy, ureterocolostomy, ureteroileostomy, ureterosigmoidostomy, ureterostomy, ureterotomy), loss of normal food intake (from an esophagectomy), loss of reproductive ability (from a fallopian tube ligation, hysterectomy, oophorectomy, orchidectomy, prostatectomy, salpingectomy, vasectomy), loss of speech (from a glossectomy, laryngectomy, tracheostomy, vocal cordectomy), loss of vision (from an enucleation or evisceration of an eyeball), edema (from corticosteroids), loss of libido (from antihypertensive drugs). *Therapeutic equipment*: Use of a brace, cane, cardiac pacemaker, crutches, hemodialyzer, respirator, walker, wheelchair
DEVELOPMENTAL PHASES: Middle age, old age
SITUATIONAL FACTORS: Childlessness, illness (acute, chronic, terminal)

PLANNING

Unmet Needs

Comfort, protection from psychologic threat, acceptance, caring and communicating relationships, unity with loved ones, personal growth and maturity, increased learning, spiritual–philosophic satisfaction

Expected Outcome

Person verbalizes feelings of sadness
Relates feeling adequate and competent to move through the grief process
Acknowledges the experience as a potential for personal growth
Relates gradual, increased concern for external interests

NURSING INTERVENTIONS

Nursing Treatments

Approach unhurriedly
Reassure verbally (that the nurse is available whenever needed)
Demonstrate calmness
Provide an atmosphere of acceptance
Encourage the expression of feelings (about the loss)
Listen attentively
Offer feedback to the person's expressed feelings
Communicate nurse sensitivity to the person's problem
Touch the person frequently
Attend the person constantly (until he feels sufficiently comfortable to be alone)
Provide frequent contact with the person (thereafter)
Explore with the person his strengths and resources (to cope with the physical loss)
Reduce the demands placed on the person (so that more energy is available for coping)
Call the person's family (to the bedside if the person desires such)
Encourage telephone calls between significant persons (who can support each other)
Encourage planned one-day-at-a-time living (at least u ntil adjustment to the loss occurs)
Encourage the use of spiritual resources
Avoid forcing the person into rapid adaptation to change by accepting the person's unique pattern of adjustment
Provide privacy (for grieving)
Allow unlimited visiting (of the persons the patient wants to see)
Avoid attempting to cheer up the grieving person (the inability to respond cheerfully makes the grieving person think less of himself)

Nursing Observations

Determine the degree of insight that the person has (into his feelings and the grief process)
Observe for the stages of grief
Observe for an excessive stress level (resulting from the grief)
Observe for evidence of a favorable response to therapy (tension relief by grieving, control of the grief, acceptance of the loss)

Health Teaching

Explain that the person's response is appropriate and commonly experienced (following physical loss)
Explain and offer hope that the emotional pain will decrease with time (when acceptance occurs)
Advise that a poor prognosis be shared with significant others
Explain that significant persons express caring for one another (especially at the time of loss)
Explain the importance of persons offering support to one another

EVALUATION

Record actual outcome

GRIEF REACTION RELATED TO ROLE LOSS[105,471,525,568]

ASSESSMENT
Data Collection
Subjective Data
- Person relates an initial feeling of shock and disbelief
- Later expresses anger
- Then acknowledges the loss of the role and that the loss will not be restored
- Relates feeling unsettled, vaguely confused, and intensely sad
  Is preoccupied with thoughts of the past role
  Complains of feelings of weakness, anorexia, sleeplessness, or fretful sleep
  May verbalize angry feelings

Objective Data
- May exhibit grieving behavior such as weeping, saddened facial expression, decreased participation in external interests, withdrawal from persons or situations

Data Analysis
Nursing Diagnosis
GRIEF REACTION RELATED TO ROLE LOSS: Feelings of deep sorrow and distress about losing a position, situation, or responsibility in life and being unable to perform the associated, expected behavior

Common Etiology (Stressors)
DISEASES: Any
INJURIES: Any
SIGNS AND SYMPTOMS: Immobility, pain, weakness
PSYCHOSOCIAL FACTORS: Loss of or separation from a significant other, loss of or separation from a significant or valued situation, loss of a normal attachment
DEVELOPMENTAL PHASES: Adolescence, middle age, old age
SITUATIONAL FACTORS: Death of a significant other, divorce, marital separation, loss of employment, launching grown children, illness of or injury to self or a significant other, marriage, parenthood, retirement, the end of school

PLANNING
Unmet Needs
Comfort, protection from psychologic threat, acceptance, caring and communicating relationships, unity with loved ones, personal growth and maturity, increased learning, spiritual–philosophic satisfaction

Expected Outcome
Person verbalizes feelings of sadness
Relates feeling adequate and competent to move through the grief process
Acknowledges the experience as a potential for personal growth
Relates gradual, increased concern for external interests

NURSING INTERVENTIONS
Nursing Treatments
Approach unhurriedly
Reassure verbally (that the nurse is available whenever needed)
Demonstrate calmness
Provide an atmosphere of acceptance
Encourage the expression of feelings (about the loss)
Listen attentively
Offer feedback to the person's expressed feelings
Communicate nurse sensitivity to the person's problem
Touch the person frequently

Explore with the person his strengths and resources (to cope with the role loss)

Reduce the demands placed on the person (so that more energy is available for coping)

Call the person's family (to the bedside if such is desired)

Encourage telephone calls between significant persons (who can support each other)

Encourage planned one-day-at-a-time living

Encourage the use of spiritual resources

Avoid forcing the person into rapid adaptation to change by accepting the person's unique pattern of adjustment

Provide privacy (for grieving)

Allow unlimited visiting (of the persons the patient wants to see)

Avoid a up the grieving person (the inability to respond cheerfully makes the grieving person think less of himself)

Nursing Observations

Determine the degree of insight that the person has (into his feelings and the grief process)

Observe for the stages of grief

Observe for an excessive stress level (resulting from the grief)

Observe for evidence of a favorable response to therapy (tension relief by grieving, control of the grief, acceptance of the loss)

Health Teaching

Explain that the person's response is appropriate and commonly experienced

Explain and offer hope that the emotional pain will decrease with time (when acceptance occurs)

Advise that significant persons express caring for one another (especially at the time of loss)

Explain the importance of persons offering support to one another

EVALUATION

Record actual outcome

Adaptive Responses of Emotion (Affect): Guilt

GUILT RELATED TO BEING A SURVIVOR [105,269,464,471,525]

ASSESSMENT

Data Collection

Subjective Data

• Person may or may not verbalize regret and remorse

• Blames self for causing a recent or past situation

  Feels that others, especially the young, should have survived

  Verbalizes things he could have done to have saved those lost

  Contemplates over and over the meaning of his survival, why he has lived when others have died

  May expect reproach from those who are grieving for the lost ones

Objective Data

• May exhibit behavior such as being overactive, using self-punishing behavior, projecting blame for loss of the nonsurvivors, being overly attentive to the nonsurvivors' relatives

Data Analysis

Nursing Diagnosis

GUILT RELATERD TO BEING A SURVIVOR: Blaming oneself for having continued to live while others in the same situation have died

Common Etiology (Stressors)

DISEASES: Epidemic diseases such as cholera, influenza, Legionnaire's disease, malaria, typhoid

INJURIES: Multiperson trauma (see "Environmental Factors")

PSYCHOSOCIAL FACTORS: Failure to live up to one's ethical and moral values (of allowing others to survive first)

SITUATIONAL FACTORS: Being a survivor of an accident or disaster, war

ENVIRONMENTAL FACTORS: *Blast or explosion*: Any. *Cataclysm*: Earthquake, flood, tidal wave, tornado, volcanic eruption. *Crushing*: By cave-in, building collapse. *Environmental cold or heat*: Freezing or high external temperature, burning building or home. *Moving vehicle accident*: Involvement in

PLANNING

Unmet Needs

Comfort, protection from psychologic threat, acceptance, caring and communicating relationships, personal growth and maturity, increased learning, increased reality perception and problem-solving ability

Expected Outcome

Person verbalizes feelings of guilt

Relates having learned from the guilt-producing behavior

Acknowledges unfounded guilt

Sets the guilt aside and moves forward with positive behavior

NURSING INTERVENTIONS

Nursing Treatments

Approach unhurriedly

Reassure verbally (that the nurse is available whenever needed)

Provide an atmosphere of acceptance

Encourage the expression of feelings (about the guilt)

Listen attentively

Offer feedback to the person's expressed feelings

Communicate nurse sensitivity to the person's problem

Relate to the person on an adult–adult level, not on a parent–child level (which could increase guilt feelings)

Ask the person to identify the problem (causing the guilt)

Ask for specifics, not generalizations, about the problem

Support a realistic assessment of the situation (that the possibility of nonsurvival is a reality)

Provide reliable information (which may clarify facts and reduce the guilt)

Explore with the person the reasons for self-criticism

Encourage the acceptance of forgiveness offered by others (if forgiveness is appropriate)

Nursing Observations

Evaluate the significance of emotional distress mannerisms

Identify disturbing conversation topics

Identify life values significant to the person (which may reinforce the guilt)

Observe for evidence that the person is reaching out for emotional support

Observe for evidence of a favorable response to therapy (the acceptance of forgiveness and reduced guilt feelings)

Health Teaching

Explain that the person's response is appropriate and commonly experienced

Explain and offer hope that the emotional pain will decrease with time

Recommend new options for effective methods of coping (such as reassessment of his purpose in life, new life direction, etc.)

Explain how to channel emotional energy and obtain release from stress (through running, swimming, other sports, creative activities, laughing, talking things over)

Advise that negative responses from others be regarded with minimum significance (even though there are feelings about such responses)

Advise that significant persons express acceptance of one another

Advise that significant persons express caring for one another (especially when one person feels guilty)

Explain the importance of persons offering support to one another

Explain the importance of maintaining a positive self-attitude

EVALUATION

Record actual outcome

GUILT RELATED TO THE BIRTH OF AN IMPERFECT CHILD [36,105,269,464,471,525]

ASSESSMENT

Data Collection

Subjective Data
- Person may or may not verbalize regret and remorse
- Blames self for causing a recent or past situation
  Relates having parented a child with some physical or mental defect

Objective Data
- May exhibit behavior such as projecting blame, using self-punishing behavior, being overactive, being overattentive to the child

Data Analysis

Nursing Diagnosis
GUILT RELATED TO THE BIRTH OF AN IMPERFECT CHILD: Blaming oneself for having transmitted to a child defective hereditary characteristics resulting in the child's physical or mental weakness

Common Etiology (Stressors)
BIRTH DEFECTS: *Infant*: Imperfect. *Birth defects*: Acrocephaly, cleft lip or palate, cretinism, cystic fibrosis, Down's syndrome, dwarfism, hemophilia, hemangioma, sickle cell anemia, spinal bifida, tetralogy of Fallot, etc.

PSYCHOSOCIAL FACTORS: Failure to live up to one's ethical and moral values (that one's children must be perfect)

PLANNING

Unmet Needs
Comfort, protection from psychologic threat, acceptance, caring and communicating relationships, personal growth and maturity, increased learning, increased reality perception and problem-solving ability

Expected Outcome
Person verbalizes feelings of guilt
Relates having learned from the guilt-producing behavior
Acknowledges unfounded guilt
Sets the guilt aside and moves forward with positive behavior

NURSING INTERVENTIONS

Nursing Treatments

Approach unhurriedly

Reassure verbally (that the nurse is available whenever needed)

Provide an atmosphere of acceptance

Encourage the expression of feelings (about the guilt)

Listen attentively

Offer feedback to the person's expressed feelings

Communicate nurse sensitivity to the person's problem

Relate to the person on an adult–adult level, not on a parent–child level (which could increase guilt feelings)

Ask the person to identify the problem (causing the guilt)

Ask for specifics, not generalizations, about the problem

Support a realistic assessment of the situation (that there is no control of genetic factors)

Provide reliable information (which may clarify facts and reduce guilt)

Explore with the person the reasons for self-criticism

Encourage the acceptance of forgiveness offered by others

Make a referral (for genetic counseling, if appropriate, and to support groups of other persons with imperfect children)

Nursing Observations

Evaluate the significance of emotional distress mannerisms

Identify disturbing conversation topics

Identify life values significant to the person (which may reinforce guilt)

Observe for evidence that the person is reaching out for emotional support

Observe for evidence of a favorable response to therapy (acceptance or forgiveness and reduced guilt feelings)

Health Teaching

Explain that the person's response is appropriate and commonly experienced (after an imperfect child is born into a family)

Explain and offer hope that the emotional pain will decrease with time

Recommend new options for effective methods of coping (specific to the situation)

Explain how to channel emotional energy and obtain release from stress (through running, swimming, other sports, creative activities, laughing, talking things over)

Advise that negative responses from others be regarded with minimum significance (even though there are feelings about such responses)

Advise that significant persons express acceptance of one another

Advise that significant persons express caring for one another (especially when one person feels guilty)

Explain the importance of maintaining a positive self-attitude

EVALUATION

Record actual outcome

GUILT RELATED TO HARM INFLICTED ON SELF/OTHERS [36,105,269,471,525]

ASSESSMENT

Data Collection

Subjective Data

• Person may or may not verbalize regret and remorse

- Blames self for causing a recent or past situation
Aware that past behavior has hurt self or another
Contemplates how things could have been different had he acted differently
If a loved one has died, the person realizes that the opportunity to express feelings to the significant other is lost forever, that harm done cannot be changed or repaired
If the person himself is dying, he realizes that he has not done all he wanted to do for those he is leaving behind or that his own behavior has resulted in his present ill health

Objective Data
- May exhibit behavior such as attempting to correct an error, doing nothing about the situation, being overly attentive, overactive, projecting blame, making excuses, engaging in self-punishing behavior

Data Analysis

Nursing Diagnosis
GUILT RELATED TO HARM INFLICTED ON SELF/OTHERS: Blaming oneself for having physically, mentally, or emotionally injured oneself or another

Common Etiology (Stressors)
Harm Inflicted on Self
INJURIES: Any self-inflicted trauma
PSYCHOSOCIAL FACTORS: Failure to live up to one's ethical and moral values, failure to follow one's conscience by not doing what should be done, the threat of violating one's conscience by doing wrong
HEALTH CARE FACTORS: *Health therapy*: Lack of compliance to prescribed therapy
LIFESTYLE: Fad dieting, high caffeine, calorie, sugar, fat, or cholesterol intake; lack of exercise; lack of hygiene; nonallocation of leisure time; promiscuous sexual activity; high nicotine intake; drug or alcohol abuse
SITUATIONAL FACTORS: Dropping out of school, attempted suicide
HUMAN ERROR: Overeating

Harm Inflicted on Others
DISEASE: Having transmitted disease to others, alcoholism
INJURIES: Any trauma inflicted on or occurring to others; child, parent, or spouse abuse
PSYCHOSOCIAL FACTORS: Failure to live up to one's ethical and moral values, failure to follow one's conscience by not doing what should be done, the threat of violating one's conscience by doing wrong
HEALTH CARE FACTORS: *Drug or medical therapy*: Incorrectly administering drugs to or performing a health procedure for a significant other. *Surgical procedures*: Therapeutic abortion
LIFESTYLE: alcohol or drug abuse, sexual promiscuity
SITUATIONAL FACTORS: Divorce and its effect on children, the use of violence
ENVIRONMENTAL FACTORS: *Chemical substances*: Lack of prevention of ingestion of chemical substances. *Moving vehicle accident*: Involvement in a moving vehicle accident

PLANNING

Unmet Needs
Comfort, protection from psychologic threat, acceptance, caring and communicating relationships, personal growth and maturity, increased learning, increased reality perception and problem-solving ability

Expected Outcome
Person verbalizes feelings of guilt
Relates having learned from the guilt-producing behavior
Verbalizes the intention of correcting the behavior
Acknowledges unfounded guilt
Sets the guilt aside and moves forward with positive behavior

NURSING INTERVENTIONS

Nursing Treatments

Approach unhurriedly

Reassure verbally (that the nurse is available whenever needed)

Provide an atmosphere of acceptance

Encourage the expression of feelings (about the guilt)

Listen attentively

Offer feedback to the person's expressed feelings

Communicate nurse sensitivity to the person's problem

Relate to the person on an adult–adult level, not on a parent–child level (which could increase guilt feelings)

Ask the person to identify the problem (causing the guilt)

Ask for specifics, not generalizations, about the problem

Provide reliable information (which may clarify facts and reduce guilt)

Encourage the admission of wrongdoing (which often reduces guilt)

Explore with the person the reasons for self-criticism

Suggest that reparation will diminish guilt (if the person feels he can offer reparation)

Encourage the acceptance of forgiveness offered by others

Nursing Observations

Evaluate the significance of emotional distress mannerisms

Identify disturbing conversation topics

Identify life values significant to the person (which may reinforce guilt)

Observe for evidence that the person is reaching out for emotional support

Observe for evidence of a favorable response to therapy (the acceptance of forgiveness and reduced guilt feelings)

Health Teaching

Explain that the person's response is appropriate and commonly experienced

Explain and offer hope that the emotional pain will decrease with time

Recommend new options for effective methods of coping (specific to the situation)

Advise that negative responses from others be regarded with minimum significance (even though there are feelings about such responses)

Advise that significant persons express acceptance of one another

Advise that significant persons express caring for one another (especially when one person feels guilty)

Explain the importance of maintaining a positive self-attitude

Explain how to channel emotional energy and obtain release from stress (through running, swimming and other sports, creative activities, laughing, talking things over)

Teach how to use the problem-solving method (to decide on positive action to reduce the guilt)

EVALUATION

Record actual outcome

GUILT RELATED TO THE BURDEN PLACED ON OTHERS [36,105,269,464,471,525]

ASSESSMENT

Data Collection

Subjective Data

• Person may or may not verbalize regret and remorse

• Blames self for causing a recent or past situation

Person perceives that his illness or old age has brought hardship and sorrow to others

Is preoccupied with the effect of his illness or old age on others and how things might have been had he not become ill or infirmed

Wonders about his worthiness of love

Wonders if the family feels unexpressed anger toward him

Senses the weariness of others who wait on him and their decreased resistance to exposure to illness

Feels that he deserves some reproach for having become a burden to others

Apologizes for being ill or infirmed

Objective Data

• May exhibit behavior such as projecting blame, making excuses, trying to assume responsibilities before being physically able, using self-punishing behavior

Data Analysis

Nursing Diagnosis

GUILT RELATED TO THE BURDEN PLACED ON OTHERS: Blaming oneself for the hardship and suffering that one's illness or reduced role responsibility places on significant others

Common Etiology (Stressors)

DISEASES: Any

INJURIES: Any

SIGNS AND SYMPTOMS: Immobility, pain, weakness

PSYCHOSOCIAL FACTORS: Failure to live up to one's ethical and moral values, failure to follow one's conscience by not doing what should be done

DEVELOPMENTAL PHASES: Old age

SITUATIONAL FACTORS: Acute, chronic, disabling, or terminal illness or injury

PLANNING

Unmet Needs

Comfort, protection from psychologic threat, acceptance, caring and communicating relationships, personal growth and maturity, increased learning, increased reality perception and problem-solving ability

Expected Outcome

Person verbalizes feelings of guilt

Relates having learned from the guilt-producing behavior

Acknowledges unfounded guilt

Sets the guilt aside and moves forward with positive behavior

NURSING INTERVENTIONS

Nursing Treatments

Approach unhurriedly

Reassure verbally (that the nurse is available whenever needed)

Provide an atmosphere of acceptance

Encourage the expression of feelings (about the guilt)

Listen attentively

Offer feedback to the person's expressed feelings

Communicate nurse sensitivity to the person's problem

Relate to the person on an adult–adult level, not on a parent–child level (which would increase guilt feelings)

Ask the person to identify the problem (causing the guilt)

Ask for specifics, not generalizations, about the problem

Support a realistic assessment of the situation (that well persons expect to care for the ill and aged; have the person recount all the people he has aided in his lifetime)

Explore with the person the reasons for self-criticism

Nursing Observations

Evaluate the significance of emotional distress mannerisms

Identify disturbing conversation topics
Identify life values significant to the person (which may reinforce the guilt)
Observe for evidence that the person is reaching out for emotional support
Observe for evidence of a favorable response to therapy (acceptance of forgiveness)

Health Teaching

Explain that the person's response is appropriate and commonly experienced
Explain and offer hope that the emotional pain will decrease with time
Recommend new options for effective methods of coping (with the guilt)
Explain how to channel emotional energy and obtain release from stress (by laughing, talking things over)
Advise that negative responses from others be regarded with minimum significance (even though there are feelings about such responses)
Advise that significant persons express acceptance of one another
Advise that significant persons express caring for one another (especially when one person feels guilty)
Explain the importance of maintaining a positive self-attitude
Teach how to use the problem-solving method (to decrease the burden on others)

EVALUATION

Record actual outcome

GUILT RELATED TO UNACCEPTABLE THOUGHTS/EMOTIONS/BEHAVIOR[105,471,525]

ASSESSMENT

Data Collection

Subjective Data
• Person may or may not verbalize regret and remorse about certain thoughts, emotions, or behavior
• Blames self for causing a recent or past situation
  Has thoughts, feelings, or acts out in a way that he considers to be wrong
  Would prefer that others not know about such
  May believe that his wishes or fantasies actually cause troublesome events to occur

Objective Data
• May exhibit behavior such as being overactive, using self-punishing behavior, attempting to correct an error, projecting blame

Data Analysis

Nursing Diagnosis
GUILT RELATED TO UNACCEPTABLE THOUGHTS/EMOTIONS/BEHAVIOR: Blaming oneself for thoughts, feelings, or actions engaged in

Common Etiology (Stressors)
PSYCHOSOCIAL FACTORS: Failure to live up to one's ethical and moral values, the threat of violating one's conscience by doing wrong
DEVELOPMENTAL PHASES: Any developmental phase but especially preschooler (age 3–6) and adolescence
SITUATIONAL FACTORS: Dying or death of a significant other, illness of or injury to a significant other, childrearing

PLANNING

Unmet Needs

Comfort, protection from psychologic threat, acceptance, caring and communicating relationships, personal growth and maturity, increased learning, increased reality perception and problem-solving ability

Expected Outcome

Person verbalizes feelings of guilt
Relates having learned from the guilt-producing behavior
Verbalizes the intention of correcting the thoughts, emotions, or behavior
Acknowledges unfounded guilt
Sets the guilt aside and moves forward with positive behavior

NURSING INTERVENTIONS

Nursing Treatments

Approach unhurriedly
Reassure verbally (that the nurse is available whenever needed)
Provide an atmosphere of acceptance
Encourage the expression of feelings (about the guilt)
Listen attentively
Offer feedback to the person's expressed feelings
Communicate nurse sensitivity to the person's problem
Relate to the person on an adult–adult level, not on a parent–child level (which could
increase guilt feelings)
Ask the person to identify the problem (causing the guilt)
Ask for specifics, not generalizations, about the problem
Support a realistic assessment of the situation (that unacceptable thoughts and feelings
are normal and can be controlled)
Encourage the admission of wrongdoing (if behavior has been inappropriate)
Explore with the person the reasons for self-criticism
Suggest that reparation will diminish guilt (if the person feels he can offer reparation)
Encourage the acceptance of forgiveness offered by others

Nursing Observations

Evaluate the significance of emotional distress mannerisms
Identify disturbing conversation topics
Identify life values significant to the person (which may reinforce the guilt)
Observe for evidence that the person is reaching out for emotional support
Observe for evidence of a favorable response to therapy (the acceptance of forgiveness,
reduced guilt feelings)

Health Teaching

Explain that the person's response is appropriate and commonly experienced
Explain and offer hope that the emotional pain will decrease with time
Recommend new options for effective methods of coping (to ignore unacceptable
thoughts and feelings, to change behavior)
Explain how to channel emotional energy and obtain release from stress (through run-
ning, swimming, other sports, creative activities, laughing, talking things over)
Advise that negative responses from others be regarded with minimum significance
(even though there are feelings about such responses)
Advise that significant persons express acceptance of one another
Advise that significant persons express caring for one another (especially when one per-
son feels guilty)
Explain the importance of maintaining a positive self-attitude

EVALUATION

Record actual outcome

GUILT RELATED TO UNINTENTIONAL NEGLECT OF OTHERS [36,105,269,464,471,525]

ASSESSMENT

Data Collection

Subjective Data
- Person may or may not verbalize regret and remorse
- Blames self for causing a recent or past situation
  May relate not having given enough time and attention to a sick family member while attending to the needs of healthy family members or neglecting healthy family members while attending the sick
  While hospitalized, the person may verbalizes that he should be home caring for his family

Objective Data
- May exhibit behavior such as being overly attentive, using self-punishing behavior, projecting blame, making excuses

Data Analysis

Nursing Diagnosis
GUILT RELATED TO UNINTENTIONAL NEGLECT OF OTHERS: Blaming oneself for not doing all that one thinks one should have done for specific persons

Common Etiology (Stressors)
PSYCHOSOCIAL FACTORS: Failure to live up to one's ethical and moral values, failure to follow one's conscience by not doing what should be done
HEALTH CARE FACTORS: *Institutionalization*: Of a significant other. *Institutional policies*: Enforced exclusion from the care of a significant other
LIFESTYLE: Excessive time and effort at employment, excessive socialization
SITUATIONAL FACTORS: Geographically distant family, the stress of the illness or injury of a significant other, lack of time, significant other dying alone, runaway parent or adolescent, placing a child up for adoption, financial needs requiring maternal employment, illness of or injury to a significant other

PLANNING

Unmet Needs
Comfort, protection from psychologic threat, acceptance, caring and communicating relationships, personal growth and maturity, increased learning, increased reality perception and problem-solving ability

Expected Outcome
Person verbalizes feelings of guilt
Relates having learned from the guilt-producing behavior
Verbalizes the intention of correcting the behavior
Acknowledges unfounded guilt
Sets the guilt aside and moves forward with positive behavior

NURSING INTERVENTIONS

Nursing Treatments
Approach unhurriedly
Reassure verbally (that the nurse is available whenever needed)
Provide an atmosphere of acceptance
Encourage the expression of feelings (about the guilt)
Listen attentively
Offer feedback to the person's expressed feelings
Communicate nurse sensitivity to the person's problem

Relate to the person on an adult–adult level, not on a parent–child level (which could increase guilt feelings)

Ask the person to identify the problem (causing the guilt)

Ask for specifics, not generalizations, about the problem

Support a realistic assessment of the situation (that everyone has time limitations, that illness reduces the ability to assume responsibilities)

Encourage the admission of wrongdoing (if such exists)

Explore with the person the reasons for self-criticism

Suggest that reparation will diminish guilt (if the person feels he can offer reparation)

Encourage the acceptance of forgiveness offered by others

Nursing Observations

Evaluate the significance of emotional distress mannerisms

Identify disturbing conversation topics

Identify life values significant to the person (which may reinforce the guilt)

Observe for evidence that the person is reaching out for emotional support

Observe for evidence of a favorable response to therapy (the acceptance of forgiveness, reduced guilt feelings)

Health Teaching

Explain that the person's response is appropriate and commonly experienced

Explain and offer hope that the emotional pain will decrease with time

Recommend new options for effective methods of coping (transferring responsibility to others, etc.)

Explain how to channel emotional energy and obtain release from stress (by talking things over)

Advise that negative responses from others be regarded with minimum significance (even though there are feelings about such responses)

Advise that significant persons express acceptance of one another

Advise that significant persons express caring for one another (especially when one person feels guilty)

Explain the importance of maintaining a positive self-attitude

EVALUATION

Record actual outcome

GUILT RELATED TO UNSANCTIONED HEALTH THERAPY[36,105,269,471,525]

ASSESSMENT

Data Collection

Subjective Data

• Person may or may not verbalize regret and remorse

• Blames self for causing a recent or past situation

Person is aware that seeking certain health therapy is not approved of by significant others, his church, or culture

Seeks a specific therapy despite such disapproval

May expect reproach from others

Objective Data

• May exhibit behavior such as being overactive, attempting to correct an error by not following recommended therapy, projecting blame, using self-punishing behavior

Data Analysis

Nursing Diagnosis

GUILT RELATED TO UNSANCTIONED HEALTH THERAPY: Blaming oneself for seeking health therapy when such is not approved of by one's family, church, or culture

Common Etiology (Stressors)

PSYCHOSOCIAL FACTORS: Failure to live up to one's ethical and moral values, failure to follow one's conscience by not doing what should be done, the threat of violating one's conscience by doing wrong

HEALTH CARE FACTORS: *Health care decision*: To seek diagnois and treatment. *Drug therapy*: Any. *Medical therapy*: Any but especially such therapy as acupuncture, biofeedback, blood transfusions, intravenous infusions, psychotherapy, radiation therapy. *Surgical therapy*: Any but especially therapeutic abortion, amputations, fallopian tube ligation, vasectomy

LIFESTYLE: Cultural traditions or prohibitions, religious beliefs

PLANNING

Unmet Needs

Comfort, protection from psychologic threat, acceptance, caring and communicating relationships, personal growth and maturity, increased learning, increased reality perception and problem-solving ability

Expected Outcome

Person verbalizes feelings of guilt

Relates having learned from the guilt-producing behavior

Verbalizes the intention of correcting the behavior, if appropriate

Acknowledges unfounded guilt

Sets the guilt aside and moves forward with positive behavior

NURSING INTERVENTIONS

Nursing Treatments

Approach unhurriedly

Reassure verbally (that the nurse is available whenever needed)

Provide an atmosphere of acceptance

Encourage the expression of feelings (about the guilt)

Listen attentively

Offer feedback to the person's expressed feelings

Communicate nurse sensitivity to the person's problem

Relate to the person on an adult–adult level, not on a parent–child level (which could increase guilt feelings)

Ask the person to identify the problem (causing the guilt)

Ask for specifics, not generalizations, about the problem

Support a realistic assessment of the situation (certain health therapy is essential to the maintenance of life, the ultimate choice of therapy is the patient's)

Encourage the admission of wrongdoing (if such is appropriate)

Explore with the person the reasons for self-criticism

Encourage the acceptance of forgiveness offered by others

Refrain from negatively criticizing

Nursing Observations

Evaluate the significance of emotional distress mannerisms

Identify disturbing conversation topics

Identify life values significant to the person (which may reinforce the guilt)

Observe for evidence that the person is reaching out for emotional support

Observe for evidence of a favorable response to therapy (the acceptance of forgiveness, reduced guilt feelings)

Health Teaching

Explain that the person's response is appropriate and commonly experienced

Explain and offer hope that the emotional pain will decrease with time

Recommend new options for effective methods of coping (specific to the situation)

Explain how to channel emotional energy and obtain release from stress (by talking things over, through creative activities)

Advise that negtive responses from others be regarded with minimum significance (even though there are feelings about such responses)

Advise that significant persons express acceptance of one another

Advise that significant persons express caring for one another (especially when one person feels guilty)

Explain the importance of maintaining a positive self-attitude

EVALUATION

Record actual outcome

Adaptive Responses of Emotion (Affect): Helplessness

HELPLESSNESS RELATED TO HEALTH CARE/HEALTH THERAPY[213,471,525]

ASSESSMENT

Data Collection

Subjective Data
- Person verbalizes that he has little control over a situation
- Relates being unable to handle the situation alone
- Expects others to aid him to cope effectively

    Relates he has no control over his health care, the procedures being performed on him, their effect on him

    May verbalize anger

Objective Data
- May exhibit behavior such as seeking answers by talking to others, reading, acting out, crying, making somatic complaints

Data Analysis

Nursing Diagnosis

HELPLESSNESS RELATED TO HEALTH CARE/HEALTH THERAPY: Feeling the one has no power or resources to control his health care or specific types of therapy and is unable to manage the situation alone

Common Etiology (Stressors)

PSYCHOSOCIAL FACTORS: Lack of or loss of control of a situation, the threat of forced adaptation to change, loss of autonomy or freedom in self-direction

HEALTH CARE FACTORS: *Health care consent forms*: Signing health care consent forms. *Health care delivery*: Low-quality health care delivery. *Health care environment*: Locked psychiatric unit, intensive care unit, coronary care unit, isolation unit, lack of or limited phone privileges. *Health care system*: Delayed entry into the health care system.

Hospitalization/institutionalization: Any. *Institutional policies*: Restrictive institutional policies, enforced exclusion from the care of a significant other. *Welfare or human resources services*: Inadequate welfare services. *Diagnostic procedures*: Any diagnostic procedure, but especially the high-risk or painful procedures. *Health therapy*: Unsuccessful or ineffective medical, drug, or surgical therapy. *Medical therapy*: Any but especially cardioversion, electroconvulsive therapy, gastrostomy or jejunostomy feeding, hemodialysis, phlebotomy, radiation therapy, traction, blood transfusion. *Drug therapy*: The need to use life maintenance drugs (insulin, cortisone, thyroid, cardiac drugs). *Surgical therapy*: Induction of anesthesia, recovery from anesthesia. *Surgical procedures*: Any surgical procedure. *Adverse effects of medical, drug, or surgical therapy*: Any but especially the loss of speech (from endotracheal intubation, glossectomy, laryngectomy, tracheostomy, vocal cordectomy), hair loss (from chemotherapy), heavy drug sedation (from sedatives). *Therapeutic equipment and devices*: Cardiac pacemaker, enforced confinement with safety restraints, respirator, prone positioning on a CircOlectric bed or Stryker frame

PLANNING

Unmet Needs
Comfort, protection from psychologic threat, predictable and orderly world, acceptance, caring and communicating relationships, sense of adequacy, self-reliance, control over others or situations, personal growth and maturity, increased learning, increased reality perception and problem-solving ability

Expected Outcome
Person verbalizes feelings of helplessness
Relates having gained at least some control of the situation
Takes specific action to exert control

NURSING INTERVENTIONS

Nursing Treatments
Approach unhurriedly
Reassure verbally (that the nurse will consult the person before all health care or therapy)
Demonstrate calmness
Provide an atmosphere of acceptance
Encourage the expression of feelings (about the helplessness)
Listen attentively
Offer feedback to the person's expressed feelings
Communicate nurse sensitivity to the person's problem
Support a realistic assessment of the situation (that health care and procedures do involve routine, but that the person has choices in what he wants done)
Offer assurance that decisions are revokable (signed operative or procedural consent forms can be revoked before the scheduled time, etc.)
Arrange situations that encourage the person's autonomy (so he can make decisions on his own behalf)
Explore with the person his strengths and resources (which increase his sense of control)
Encourage self-performance (of whatever the person desires to do)
Relate to the person on an adult–adult level, not on a parent–child level (which would increase feelings of helplessness)
Offer hope
Make a referral (to the appropriate persons or agencies who can help the person gain a sense of control)

Nursing Observations
Observe for an excessive stress level
Observe for impaired self-attitudes (which increase a sense of helplessness)
Observe for a favorable response to therapy (that the person feels in control of the situation)

Health Teaching

Describe those factors that intensify helplessness (allowing others to make decisions for him, physical limitations, dominating significant others)

Explain the importance of maintaining a positive self-attitude

Emphasize the need to develop self-reliance

Explain how to set behavioral limits (for significant others who over-control)

Explain the need to predict and plan for change (occurring during health care; this gives the person more control)

Recommend new options for effective methods of coping (taking control of his life or a situation)

Explain the importance of persons offering support to one another (to reduce a sense of helplessness)

Teach how to use the problem-solving method (to cope effectively with health care)

Explain that the situation is temporary (and, if possible, give an estimated time of how long it will last)

EVALUATION

Record actual outcome

HELPLESSNESS RELATED TO A LIFE SITUATION[213,471,525]

ASSESSMENT

Data Collection

Subjective Data
- Person verbalizes that he has little control over a situation
- Relates being unable to handle the situation alone
- Expects others to aid him to cope effective
  Is involved in a situation specific to the person's life state
  May express anger

Objective Data
- May exhibit behavior such as seeking answers by talking to others, reading, acting out, crying, making somatic complaints

Data Analysis

Nursing Diagnosis
HELPLESSNESS RELATED TO A LIFE SITUATION: Feeling that one has no power or resources to control a specific life situation and is unable to manage the situation alone

Common Etiology (Stressors)
BIRTH DEFECTS: Giving birth to an imperfect child
PSYCHOSOCIAL FACTORS: Lack of or loss of control of a life situation, the threat of forced adaptation to change, the threat of being overly controlled, the threat of ineffective problem-solving efforts
DEVELOPMENTAL PHASES: Any
LIFESTYLE: Unacceptable cultural changes, loss of preillness or preretirement lifestyle, loss of quality of life
SITUATIONAL FACTORS: Runaway adolescent or parent, loss of property (by arson, disaster, theft), giving up a foster child, child–parent difficulties, confinement in prison, death of or dying significant other, divorce from a spouse or of parents, unfavorable economic factors, loss of employment, lack of finances, loss of a home, legal termination of parental rights, military service, poverty, entry into school, marital separation from a spouse or of parents, having been victimized by violence

PLANNING

Unmet Needs

Comfort, protection from psychologic threat, predictable and orderly world, acceptance, caring and communicating relationships, sense of adequacy, self-reliance, control over others or situations, personal growth and maturity, increased learning, increased reality perception and problem-solving ability

Expected Outcome

Person verbalizes feelings of helplessness

Relates having gained at least some control of the situation

Takes specific action to exert control

NURSING INTERVENTIONS

Nursing Treatments

Approach unhurriedly

Reassure verbally (that the nurse is available whenever needed)

Demonstrate calmness

Provide an atmosphere of acceptance

Encourage the expression of feelings (about the helplessness)

Listen attentively

Offer feedback to the person's expressed feelings

Communicate nurse sensitivity to the person's problem

Support a realistic assessment of the situation (that the person may not be as helpless as he perceives himself to be)

Arrange situations that encourage the person's autonomy (so that he can make decisions on his own behalf)

Explore with the person his strengths and resources (which can increase his sense of control)

Encourage self-performance (of whatever the person desires to do)

Relate to the person on an adult–adult level, not on a parent–child level (which could increase feelings of helplessness)

Offer hope

Make a referral (to the appropriate persons or agencies who can help the person gain a sense of control)

Nursing Observations

Observe for impaired self-attitudes (which support feelings of helplessness)

Observe for a favorable response to therapy (that the person feels in control of the situation)

Health Teaching

Describe those factors that intensify helplessness (allowing others to make decisions for him, physical limitations, dominating significant others)

Explain the importance of maintaining a positive self-attitude

Emphasize the need to develop self-reliance

Explain how to set behavioral limits (for significant others who over-control)

Explain the need to predict and plan for change (which gives the person control)

Recommend new options for effective methods of coping (taking control of his life or a situation)

Explain the importance of persons offering support to one another (to reduce a sense of helplessness)

Teach how to use the problem-solving method (to cope effectively with the life situation)

Explain that the situation is temporary (and, if possible, give an estimated time of how long it will last)

EVALUATION

Record actual outcome

HELPLESSNESS RELATED TO NATURAL BODY FUNCTION[213,471,525]

ASSESSMENT

Data Collection

Subjective Data
- Person verbalizes that he has little control over a situation
- Relates being unable to handle the situation
- Expects others to aid him to cope effectively
  The pregnant woman feels helpless to control fetal development, her own body changes, or the sex of the child
  During childbirth, the woman feels helpless to stop, slow, or hasten the birth process
  The adolescent feels helpless to alter rapidly changing body size, contour, and sensations
  May express anger

Objective Data
- May exhibit behavior such as seeking answers by talking to others, reading, acting out, crying, making somatic complaints

Data Analysis

Nursing Diagnosis
HELPLESSNESS RELATED TO NATURAL BODY FUNCTION: Feeling that one has no power to control certain natural body functions and is unable to manage them alone

Common Etiology (Stressors)
PSYCHOSOCIAL FACTORS: Lack of or loss of control of a situation, the threat of forced adaptation to change
HUMAN BODY: *Natural body function*: Childbirth. *Body states*: Pregnancy, menstruation

PLANNING

Unmet Needs
Comfort, protection from psychologic threat, predictable and orderly world, acceptance, caring and communicating relationships, sense of adequacy, self-reliance, control over the situation, personal growth and maturity, increased learning, increased reality perception and problem-solving ability

Expected Outcome
Person verbalizes feelings of helplessness
Relates having gained at least some control of the situation
Takes specific action to exert control

NURSING INTERVENTIONS

Nursing Treatments
Approach unhurriedly
Reassure verbally (that the nurse is available whenever needed)
Demonstrate calmness
Provide an atmosphere of acceptance
Encourage the expression of feelings (about the helplessness)
Listen attentively
Offer feedback to the person's expressed feelings
Communicate nurse sensitivity to the person's problem
Support a realistic assessment of the situation (that the person may not be as helpless as he perceives himself to be, that knowledge of how to cope with natural body changes puts the person in control)
Arrange situations that encourage the person's autonomy (so that he can make decisions on his own behalf)

Relate to the person on an adult–adult level, not on a parent–child level (which could increase feelings of helplessness)

Nursing Observations

Observe for an excessive stress level

Observe for impaired self-attitudes (which increase a sense of helplessness)

Observe for a favorable response to therapy (that the person feels in control of the situation)

Health Teaching

Describe those factors that intensify helplessness (allowing others to make decisions regarding how the natural changes will be dealt with)

Explain the importance of maintaining a positive self-attitude

Explain the need to predict and plan for change (occurring during pregnancy, delivery, adolescence, etc., to give the person more control)

Explain the importance of persons offering support to one another (to reduce a sense of helplessness)

Explain that the situation is temporary (and, if possible, give an estimated time of how long it will last)

EVALUATION

Record actual outcome

HELPLESSNESS RELATED TO PHYSICAL LOSS[213,471,525]

ASSESSMENT

Data Collection

Subjective Data
- Person verbalizes that he has little control over a situation
- Relates being unable to handle the situation alone
- Expects others to aid him to cope effectively
  Relates having experienced a loss of body function or part that he cannot control
  May verbalize anger

Objective Data
- May exhibit behavior such as seeking answers by talking to others, reading, acting out, crying, avoiding persons or situations, somatic complaints

Data Analysis

Nursing Diagnosis

HELPLESSNESS RELATED TO PHYSICAL LOSS: Feeling that one has no power or resources to control the loss of a positive, balanced state of health and is unable to manage alone

Common Etiology (Stressors)

DISEASES: Any

INJURIES: Any

SIGNS AND SYMPTOMS: Breathing difficulty, blurred vision, confusion, immobility, memory loss, pain, weakness, lack of energy

PSYCHOSOCIAL FACTORS: Lack of or loss of control of a situation, the threat of forced adaptation to change, the threat of being overly controlled, loss of physiologic independence, the threat of not being able to preserve oneself, the threat of ineffective problem-solving efforts

HUMAN BODY: *Body function*: Loss of body function. *Body part*: Loss of body part. *Body states*: Menopause, male climacteric

HEALTH CARE FACTORS: *Medical diagnosis*: Unfavorable
DEVELOPMENTAL PHASES: Old age
SITUATIONAL FACTORS: Childlessness

PLANNING

Unmet Needs

Comfort, protection from psychologic threat, predictable and orderly world, acceptance, caring and communicating relationships, sense of adequacy, self-reliance, control over others or situations, personal growth and maturity, increased learning, increased reality perception and problem-solving ability

Expected Outcome

Person verbalizes feelings of helplessness
Relates having gained at least some control of the situation
Takes specific action to exert control

NURSING INTERVENTIONS

Nursing Treatments

Approach unhurriedly
Reassure verbally (that the nurse is available whenever needed)
Demonstrate calmness
Provide an atmosphere of acceptance
Encourage the expression of feelings (about the helplessness)
Listen attentively
Offer feedback to the person's expressed feelings
Communicate nurse sensitivity to the person's problem
Support a realistic assessment of the situation (that the person may not be as helpless as he perceives himself to be)
Arrange situations that encourage the person's autonomy (so he can make decisions on his own behalf)
Explore with the person his strengths and resources (which can increase his sense of control)
Encourage self-performance (of whatever the person desires to do)
Relate to the person on an adult–adult level, not on a parent–child level (which could increase feelings of helplessness)
Make a referral (to the appropriate persons or agencies who can help the person gain a sense of control such as rehabilitation and financial-assisting agencies)

Nursing Observations

Observe for an excessive stress level
Observe for impaired self-attitudes (which support feelings of helplessness)
Observe for a favorable response to therapy (that the person feels in control of the situation)

Health Teaching

Describe those factors that intensify helplessness (allowing others to make decisions for him, not using assistive devices that can reduce physical limitations)
Explain the importance of maintaining a positive self-attitude
Explain the need to predict and plan for change (which gives the person control)
Recommend new options for effective methods of coping (taking control of his life or a situation)
Explain the importance of persons offering support to one another (to reduce a sense of helplessness)
Teach how to use the problem-solving method (to cope effectively with the physical loss)

EVALUATION

Record actual outcome

Adaptive Responses of Emotion (Affect): Hopelessness

HOPELESSNESS RELATED TO A LIFE SITUATION[213,471]

ASSESSMENT
Data Collection

Subjective Data
- Person verbalizes that efforts toward resolving a life situation are futile
- Expresses feelings of extreme discouragement and negative expectations
- Relates having given up trying
  Is experiencing a difficult life situation
  Has tried all the ways he knows to resolve or improve it
  Perceives that the situation remains relatively unchanged
  May have thoughts of failure and worthlessness
  May continuously think about the situation
  May wonder if life is worth living

Objective Data
- May exhibit behavior such as crying, saddened facial expression, indifferent attitude, unusual quietness, ceasing any further effort

Data Analysis

Nursing Diagnosis
HOPELESSNESS RELATED TO A LIFE SITUATION: The feeling that efforts are useless and ineffective in trying to resolve or improve a life situation

Common Etiology (Stressors)
PSYCHOSOCIAL FACTORS: The threat of repeated failure to achieve a goal, loss of control of a life situation, the threat of ineffective problem-solving efforts
DEVELOPMENTAL PHASES: Adolescence, old age
SITUATIONAL FACTORS: Runaway adolescent or parent, loss of property (by arson, disaster, theft), childlessness, child–parent difficulties, confinement in prison, death of or dying significant other, divorce from a spouse or of parents, loss of employment, lack of finances, loss of a home, legal termination of parental rights, poverty, marital separation from a spouse or of parents, mental illness of self or a significant other

PLANNING
Unmet Needs
Comfort, protection from psychologic threat, acceptance, caring and communicating relationships, endurance, personal growth and maturity, increased learning, spiritual–philosophic satisfaction, increased reality perception and problem-solving ability

Expected Outcome
Person verbalizes feelings of hopelessness
Acknowledges the hopelessness, if such is true
Relates feeling adequate and competent to accept and adjust to a hopeless situation
Relates a specific problem-solving approach if, realistically, there is hope for overcoming the problem

NURSING INTERVENTIONS
Nursing Treatments
Approach unhurriedly
Reassure verbally (that the nurse is available whenever needed)
Demonstrate calmness

Provide an atmosphere of acceptance
Encourage the expression of feelings (about the hopelessness)
Listen attentively
Offer feedback to the person's expressed feelings
Communicate nurse sensitivity to the person's problem
Ask the person to identify the problem
Ask for specifics, not generalizations, about the problem
Support a realistic assessment of the situation (regarding the reality of the hopelessness)
Provide reliable information (specific to the situation)
Explore with the person his strengths and resources (to cope with the problem)
Offer hope (if hope actually exists)
Do not encourage or reinforce hope (if there is little or no hope)
Encourage the use of spiritual resources
Make a referral (to appropriate persons or agencies who can help resolve the problem)

Nursing Observations
Observe for an excessive stress level
Determine the degree of insight that the person has (into the problem)
Observe for evidence of a favorable response to therapy (resolution of the problem, a feeling of hope)

Health Teaching
Explain that the person's response is appropriate and commonly experienced
Recommend a habitual, positive mental attitude
Explain that the situation is temporary
Explain the importance of persons offering support to one another (to reduce feelings of hopelessness)
Teach how to use the problem-solving method (to resolve the hopeless situation)

EVALUATION

Record actual outcome

HOPELESSNESS RELATED TO APPROACHING DEATH[90,154,213,471]

ASSESSMENT

Data Collection

Subjective Data
• Person verbalizes that efforts toward reversing approaching death are futile
• Expresses feelings of extreme discouragement and negative expectations
• Relates having given up trying
  Loses interest in all normal activities
  Relates that his health or the health of a significant other is deteriorating
  Relates having given up the will to live
  Sees no future
  May secretly bargain with God for health and time, as a last flicker of hope

Objective Data
• May exhibit behavior such as crying, saddened facial expression, indifferent attitude, unusual quietness, ceasing any further effort

Data Analysis

Nursing Diagnosis
HOPELESSNESS RELATED TO APPROACHING DEATH: The feeling that efforts toward regaining

health are useless and ineffective when a person becomes aware that his life or the life of a significant other is soon to come to an end

Common Etiology (Stressors)

DISEASES: Any

INJURIES: Any

PSYCHOSOCIAL FACTORS: The threat of repeated failure to achieve a goal, loss of control of a life situation

HEALTH CARE FACTORS: *Medical diagnosis:* Unfavorable medical diagnosis for self or a significant other. *Health therapy:* Unsuccessful or ineffective, medical, drug, or surgical therapy. *Prognosis:* An unfavorable prognosis

SITUATIONAL FACTORS: Terminal illness of self or a significant other, the experience of dying

PLANNING

Unmet Needs

Comfort, protection from psychologic threat, acceptance, caring and communicating relationships, endurance, personal growth and maturity, increased learning, spiritual–philosophic satisfaction, increased reality perception and problem-solving ability

Expected Outcome

Person verbalizes feelings of hopelessness

Acknowledges the hopelessness, if such is true

Relates feeling adequate and competent to accept and cope with approaching death

Exhibits a peaceful, calm facial expression

NURSING INTERVENTIONS

Nursing Treatments

Approach unhurriedly

Reassure verbally (that the nurse will be with the person when needed, that death may not come as soon as expected, that death can be peaceful when it does come)

Demonstrate calmness

Provide an atmosphere of acceptance

Encourage the expression of feelings (about the hopelessness)

Listen attentively

Talk with the person and family

Offer feedback to the person's expressed feelings (about feeling hopeless)

Communicate nurse sensitivity to the person's problem

Sit with the person (if it brings comfort)

Touch the person judiciously

Provide reliable information (when the person asks for it)

Explore with the person his strengths and resources (to face death peacefully)

Offer hope (if hope actually exists)

Do not encourage or reinforce hope (after the person has accepted the reality of approaching death)

Encourage the use of spiritual resources

Refrain from making a specific length-of-life estimate

Reinforce concern throughout the entire illness

Nursing Observations

Observe for an excessive stress level

Determine the degree of insight that the person has (into the nearness of death)

Observe for evidence of a favorable response to therapy (feelings of hope or the peaceful acceptance of death)

Health Teaching

Explain that the person's response is appropriate and commonly experienced

Explain the importance of persons offering support to one another (to reduce feelings of hopelessness)

Advise that significant persons express caring for one another (until death occurs)

EVALUATION

Record actual outcome

HOPELESSNESS RELATED TO PHYSICAL LOSS[213,471]

ASSESSMENT
Data Collection
Subjective Data
- Person verbalizes that efforts toward health restoration are futile
- Expresses feelings of extreme discouragement and negative expectations
- Relates having given up trying
  Has been ill for some time
  Has tried multiple treatment methods
  Relates little or no improvement in the health state
  May continuously think about the situation
  May feel life is not worth living

Objective Data
- May exhibit behavior such as crying, saddened facial expression, indifferent attitude, unusual quietness, ceasing any further effort

Data Analysis
Nursing Diagnosis
HOPELESSNESS RELATED TO PHYSICAL LOSS: The feeling that efforts are useless and ineffective toward reestablishing or improving the state of health

Common Etiology (Stressors)
BIRTH DEFECTS: Of infant

DISEASES: Any disease such as carcinoma, cerebrovascular accident, Guillan-Barré syndrome, Hodgkin's disease, leukemia, multiple sclerosis, myasthenia gravis, myocardial infarction, organic brain syndrome, Parkinson's disease, renal failure, subarachnoid hemorrhage, etc.

INJURIES: Severe injuries such as burn wounds, poisoning, etc.

SIGNS AND SYMPTOMS: Pain, paralysis, tremor, weakness

PSYCHOSOCIAL FACTORS: The threat of repeated failure to achieve a goal, loss of control of a life situation

HEALTH CARE FACTORS: *Health therapy*: Unsuccessful or ineffective health therapy, the uncertain outcome of health therapy, long-term health therapy. *Convalescence*: Slow recovery during convalescence. *Prognosis*: Unfavorable. *Hospital discharge*: Delayed. *Complications*: Unforseen health complications

SITUATIONAL FACTORS: Critical, chronic, disabling, or terminal illness of self or a significant other

PLANNING
Unmet Needs
Comfort, protection from psychologic threat, acceptance, caring and communicating relationships, endurance, personal growth and maturity, increased learning, spiritual–philosophic satisfaction, increased reality perception and problem-solving ability

Expected Outcome
Person verbalizes feelings of hopelessness
Acknowledges the hopelessness, if such is true
Relates feeling adequate and competent to cope with and adjust to the physical loss

Relates a specific problem-solving approach if, realistically, there is hope for improved physical health

NURSING INTERVENTIONS

Nursing Treatments
Approach unhurriedly
Reassure verbally (that the nurse is available whenever needed)
Demonstrate calmness
Provide an atmosphere of acceptance
Encourage the expression of feelings (about the hopelessness)
Listen attentively
Offer feedback to the person's expressed feelings
Communicate nurse sensitivity to the person's problem
Ask the person to identify the problem
Ask for specifics, not generalizations, about the problem
Provide reliable information (about the current status of treating certain diseases)
Explore with the person his strengths and resources (to cope with the problem)
Offer hope (if hope actually exists)
Do not encourage or reinforce hope (if there is little or no hope of a cure)
Encourage the use of spiritual resources
Make a referral (to the appropriate persons or agencies who can maximize the person's potential despite the physical loss)

Nursing Observations
Observe for an excessive stress level
Determine the degree of insight that the person has (into the problem)
Observe for evidence of a favorable response to therapy (effective coping with the problem, a feeling of hope)

Health Teaching
Explain that the person's response is appropriate and commonly experienced
Recommend a habitual, positive mental attitude
Explain the importance of persons offering support to one another (to reduce feelings of hopelessness)
Teach how to use the problem-solving method (to cope in the most effective manner with the hopeless situation)

EVALUATION
Record actual outcome

Adaptive Responses of Emotion (Affect): Rejection Feelings

FEELING REJECTED RELATED TO A LIFE SITUATION[105]

ASSESSMENT

Data Collection

Subjective Data
• Person expresses feelings that others do not care about or approve of him
• Verbalizes thoughts that others do not see him as a person of worth

Is keenly aware of a changed relationship
Wants love and affection that has been withheld
Feels anxious and insecure
May verbalize anger at persons or situations
May relate the changes required by others for him to achieve acceptance

Objective Data
• May exhibit behavior such as acting out, somatic complaints, avoiding the person, unusual quietness, crying

Data Analysis

Nursing Diagnosis
FEELING REJECTED RELATED TO A LIFE SITUATION: Feeling that one is not acceptable to others during a difficult life situation

Common Etiology (Stressors)
PSYCHOSOCIAL FACTORS: Lack of affection and respect from a significant other; lack of interest shown by a significant other; the threat of being overly controlled or restricted; the threat of hostility, disapproval, or ridicule from others; lack of emotional support (positive reinforcement) from others; failure to achieve unrealistic expectations of a significant other; lack of guidance from and control by parents
LIFESTYLE: Nonconformity (of self) to cultural mores, changes in sexual responses of a significant other
SITUATIONAL FACTORS: A child's being put up for adoption, the frequent change of foster parents, divorce or marital separation from a spouse or of parents

PLANNING

Unmet Needs
Comfort, protection from psychologic threat, acceptance, caring and communicating relationships, high evaluation of self, sense of adequacy, personal growth and maturity, increased learning, increased reality perception and problem-solving ability

Expected Outcome
Person verbalizes about feeling rejected by others
Relates the feeling that others accept him
Verbalizes specific problem-solving methods for improved interrelatedness
Takes specific action toward positive interrelatedness

NURSING INTERVENTIONS

Nursing Treatments
Approach unhurriedly
Reassure verbally (that the nurse is available whenever needed)
Provide an atmosphere of acceptance
Encourage the expression of feelings (about feeling rejected)
Relate to the person on an adult–adult level, not on a parent–child level (which increases a sense of rejection)
Listen attentively
Offer feedback to the person's expressed feelings
Communicate nurse sensitivity to the person's problem (by stating that the nurse does care and is concerned)
Ask the person to identify the problem
Ask for specifics, not generalizations, about the problem
Support a realistic assessment of the situation (about whether the sense of rejection is real or imagined, about the need to accept the human aspect of others)
Explore with the person the reasons for recurring problems (in the life situation)
Refrain from negatively criticizing (which increases feelings of rejection)
Encourage an awareness of positive responses from others

Nursing Observations
Observe for an excessive stress level
Determine the degree of insight that the person has (into the feelings of rejection)

Evaluate the person's relatedness with others (and its effect on the life situation)

Observe for evidence that the person is reaching out for emotional support

Observe for evidence of a favorable response to therapy (improved relations between persons, feeling accepted by others)

Health Teaching

Explain that the person's response is appropriate and commonly experienced

Explain the need for realistic expectations of others

Advise that negative responses from others be regarded with minimum significance (even though there are feelings about such responses)

Explain the importance of maintaining a positive self-attitude (which increases positive perceptions)

Teach how to use the problem-solving method (to meet his needs)

EVALUATION

Record actual outcome

FEELING REJECTED RELATED TO PHYSICAL LOSS[105]

ASSESSMENT

Data Collection

Subjective Data

- Person expresses feelings that others do not care about or approve of him
- Verbalizes thoughts that others do not see him as a person of worth

  Relates some physical loss and feels that others are very aware of it

  Feels anxious and insecure

Objective Data

- May exhibit behavior such as acting out, somatic complaints, crying, unusual quietness

Data Analysis

Nursing Diagnosis

FEELING REJECTED RELATED TO PHYSICAL LOSS: Feeling that one is not acceptable to others due to the loss of a balanced state of health

Common Etiology (Stressors)

BIRTH DEFECTS: Any such as a cleft lip, cleft palate, cerebral palsy, Down's syndrome, dwarfism

DISEASES: Acne vulgaris, alcoholism, cerebrovascular accident, drug addiction, elephantiasis, gonorrhea, Hansen's disease, hepatitis, Huntington's chorea, organic brain syndrome, Parkinson's disease, schizophrenia, syphilis

INJURIES: Traumatic disfigurement, burn wounds, facial lacerations

PSYCHOSOCIAL FACTORS: Lack of affection and respect from a significant other; lack of interest shown by a significant other; the threat of being overly controlled or restricted; the threat of hostility, disapproval, or ridicule from others; lack of emotional support (positive reinforcement) from others; failure to achieve unrealistic expectations of a significant other; lack of guidance from and control by parents

DEVELOPMENTAL PHASES: Old age

PLANNING

Unmet Needs

Comfort, protection from psychologic threat, acceptance, caring and communicating relationships, high evaluation of self, sense of adequacy, personal growth and maturity, increased learning, increased reality perception and problem-solving ability

Expected Outcome

Person verbalizes about feeling rejected by others

Relates the feeling that others accept him
Verbalizes specific problem-solving methods for improved interrelatedness
Takes specific action toward positive interrelatedness

NURSING INTERVENTIONS

Nursing Treatments
Approach unhurriedly
Reassure verbally (that the person is worthy and productive)
Provide an atmosphere of acceptance
Encourage the expression of feelings (about feeling rejected)
Relate to the person on an adult–adult level, not on a parent–child level (which increases a sense of rejection)
Listen attentively
Offer feedback to the person's expressed feelings
Communicate nurse sensitivity to the person's problem
Ask the person to identify the problem
Ask for specifics, not generalizations, about the problem
Support a realistic assessment of the situation (about whether the sense of rejection is real or imagined, about the need to accept the human aspect of others)
Explore with the person the reasons for recurring problems (in relatedness)
Encourage an awareness of positive responses from others
Encourage visiting by significant others (who have positive attitudes toward the person)

Nursing Observations
Observe for an excessive stress level
Determine the degree of insight that the person has (into the feelings of rejection)
Evaluate the person's relatedness with others
Observe for evidence that the person is reaching out for emotional support
Observe for evidence of a favorable response to therapy (improved relations between persons, feeling accepted by others)

Health Teaching
Explain that the person's response is appropriate and commonly experienced
Advise that significant persons express acceptance of one another, express caring for one another
Explain the importance of persons offering support to one another
Explain the need for realistic expectations of others
Advise that negative responses from others be regarded with minimum significance (even though there are feelings about such responses)
Explain the importance of maintaining a positive self-attitude
Teach how to use the problem-solving method (specific to the situation)

EVALUATION

Record actual outcome

REJECTION OF A SIGNIFICANT OTHER RELATED TO PHYSICAL LOSS[105]

ASSESSMENT

Data Collection

Subjective Data
• Person relates that a significant other has not met his expectations
• Expresses feelings of anger, disapproval, lack of interest
  May feel that the significant other is no longer physically attractive or acceptable

Verbalizes that the person's behavior is intolerable
May refuse to live with the other person's limitations
May relate the changes required for him to accept the other person

Objective Data
• May exhibit behavior such as spending less time with the person, refraining from caressing, failing to fulfill his expected role, intimidating, ridiculing, or abusing the other person

Data Analysis

Nursing Diagnosis
REJECTION OF A SIGNIFICANT OTHER RELATED TO PHYSICAL LOSS: Feeling that a loved one is no longer acceptable to a person following loss of a balanced state of health

Common Etiology (Stressors)
BIRTH DEFECTS: Imperfect infant or child
DISEASES: Any
INJURIES: Any
PSYCHOSOCIAL FACTORS: Lack of enjoyment of a particular role with another person, failure of one person to meet the expectations of another, an attempt to lessen one's attachment to another, the threat of burdens placed on one person by another, the threat of termination of a relationship by another, the threat of being unable to meet one's own needs
HUMAN BODY: *Body appearance*: A disfigured body, body distortion during pregnancy
HEALTH CARE FACTORS: *Adverse effects of medical, drug, or surgical therapy*: Loss of a body part (from an amputation, enucleation or evisceration of an eyeball, hemipelvectomy, ileotomy, mastectomy), loss of hair (from chemotherapy and radiation therapy), loss of natural elimination and elimination control (from a colostomy, ileocolostomy, ileostomy, ureterocolostomy, ureteroileostomy, ureterosigmoidostomy, ureterostomy, ureterotomy), edema (from corticosteroids), decreased sexual arousal of a significant other (from antihypertensive drugs or tagamet). *Surgical incision*: Disfiguring
DEVELOPMENTAL PHASES (OF A SIGNIFICANT OTHER): Middle age, old age
SITUATIONAL FACTORS: A dying significant other, chronic or terminal illness of or injury to a significant other, unplanned or unwanted pregnancy

PLANNING

Unmet Needs
Comfort, protection from psychologic threat, acceptance, caring and communicating relationships, personal growth and maturity, increased learning, increased reality perception and problem-solving ability

Expected Outcome
Person verbalizes feelings about the significant other whom he is rejecting
Relates sensitivity to the effect of such behavior on the other person
Relates a problem-solving approach toward improving the interpersonal interrelatedness
Takes positive action toward improving relations regardless of the outcome

NURSING INTERVENTIONS

Nursing Treatments
Approach unhurriedly
Reassure verbally (that the nurse will help the person)
Provide an atmosphere of acceptance
Encourage the expression of feelings (about the rejected loved one)
Relate to the person on an adult–adult level, not on a parent–child level (which could increase negative feelings)
Listen attentively
Talk with the person and the significant other
Offer feedback to the person's expressed feelings
Communicate nurse sensitivity to the person's problem
Ask the person to identify the problem

Ask for specifics, not generalizations, about the problem

Support a realistic assessment of the situation (from both parties' perspective)

Encourage a realistic perception of others (their needs, their limitations)

Explore with the person his strengths and resources (to cope with the unpleasant situation in which the significant other is involved)

Explore with the person the reasons for criticism of others

Explore with the person the reasons for recurring problems (in relatedness)

Refrain from negatively criticizing

Nursing Observations

Observe for an excessive stress level

Determine the degree of insight that the person has (into such feelings)

Evaluate the person's relatedness with others (other than the person being rejected)

Observe for evidence that the person is reaching out for emotional support

Observe for evidence of a favorable response to therapy (improved relations between the persons involved)

Health Teaching

Explain that the person's response is appropriate and commonly experienced

Advise that significant persons express acceptance of one another, express caring for one another

Explain the importance of persons offering support to one another

Explain the need for realistic expectations of others

Explain the importance of maintaining a positive self-attitude (which increases positive relatedness)

Teach how to use the problem-solving method (specific to the situation)

EVALUATION

Record actual outcome

Adaptive Ego Defense Responses

DENIAL OF A LIFE SITUATION[471,525,680]

ASSESSMENT

Data Collection

Subjective Data

• Person verbally rejects the occurring life situation

    OR

• Ignores references made regarding the reality

• If confronted, does not want to discuss the issue openly

  Refuses to admit that the life situation exists

  Will not recognize the relationship of facts to the situation

Objective Data

• May exhibit unrealistic behavior such as making excuses for an abusing spouse, spending large sums of money when in financial distress, laughing or joking about the life situation

Data Analysis

Nursing Diagnosis

DENIAL OF A LIFE SITUATION: Being unable to admit the existence of a difficult, significant life experience

Common Etiology (Stressors)

PSYCHOSOCIAL FACTORS: The threat of an unpleasant reality

LIFESTYLE: Alcohol or drug abuse

SITUATIONAL FACTORS: Accident, natural or manmade disaster, lack of finances, unwanted or unplanned pregnancy, failure in school, having been victimized by violence, war, physical abuse by a significant other

PLANNING

Unmet Needs

Comfort, protection from psychologic threat, acceptance, caring and communicating relationships, sense of adequacy, personal growth and maturity, increased learning, increased reality perception and problem-solving ability

Expected Outcome

Person verbalizes feelings about the situation

Relates sufficient insight to substitute more growth-oriented coping mechanisms for the denial

Verbalizes feelings of satisfaction for having achieved self-growth

NURSING INTERVENTIONS

Nursing Treatments

Approach unhurriedly

Reassure verbally (that the nurse is available whenever needed)

Provide an atmosphere of acceptance

Support the use of appropriate defense mechanisms (do not oppose or attack the denial if it is the person's most effective defense against overwhelming anxiety)

Avoid forcing the person into rapid adaptation to change by accepting the person's unique pattern of adjustment (wait for the person to show readiness to face the life situation, after the denial is no longer completely effective)

When the Person Is Ready to Work Through the Denial

Encourage the expression of feelings (about the life situation)

Listen attentively

Talk with the person

Periodically verbalize the denied reality

Offer feedback to the person's expressed feelings

Communicate nurse sensitivity to the person's problems

Provide reliable information (giving small amounts of information at a time, amounts the person indicates he can handle)

Ask the person to identify the problem

Ask for specifics, not generalizations, about the problem (specifics may penetrate the denial)

Support a realistic assessment of the situation (that reality may not be as threatening as perceived and is less painful when faced promptly)

Do not encourage or reinforce the denial (by giving false information or reassurance or by diverting attention from the life situation)

Ask questions that encourage answers that reflect reality perception (straightforward questions such as "When did the situation become intolerable? What do you think will improve the situation?")

Ensure the person's feeling of safety before introducing unpleasantness (if the person feels unsafe, denial may be reinforced)

Explore with the person his strengths and resources (to cope with the life situation, since awareness of his own strength may reduce the need for denial)

Nursing Observations

Determine whether the denial is adaptive or nonadaptive (is it an adaptive response to crisis or a nonadaptive escape mechanism?)

Determine the need that the denial is serving (is it an attempt to maintain emotional stability or an escape from reality, responsibility, and personal growth)

Determine the degree of insight that the person has (into the denial)

Evaluate the significance of emotional distress mannerisms

Identify cues indicating some acceptance of reality (statements such as "I know that the situation has to be dealt with sooner or later")

Observe for an excessive stress level (talkativeness, pacing, nervousness, heavy smoking)

Observe for evidence that the person is reaching out for emotional support

Observe for evidence of a favorable response to therapy (acceptance of and dealing with the life situation)

Health Teaching

Explain that the person's response is appropriate and commonly experienced

Teach how to use the problem-solving method (to improve the situation)

Explain (to the family) that persons must make adjustments at their own pace

EVALUATION

Record actual outcome

DENIAL OF APPROACHING DEATH[90,471,525,680]

ASSESSMENT
Data Collection
Subjective Data
• Person verbally rejects the approaching death
   OR
• Ignores references made regarding the reality
• If confronted, does not want to discuss the issue openly
   Relates in conversation that he refuses to accept that his health or the health of a significant other is worsening
   Refuses to discuss the possibility of death
   May perceive the symptoms to be the consequences of treatment rather than from the disease
   May discuss what he will do when he or the significant other gets well
   May pursue expanded business activities
   May avoid making a will or providing financially for the family
   May refuse therapy or avoid follow-up appointments
   May verbalize that the loved one cannot die because he cannot go on without her
   Feels that the thought of the dying self or significant other is impossible to endure

Objective Data
• May exhibit unrealistic behavior such as purchasing objects to wear or use after getting well, planning a trip a year ahead, laughing or joking about the situation, functioning well

Data Analysis
Nursing Diagnosis
DENIAL OF APPROACHING DEATH: Being unable to admit the existence of the fact that one's life or the life of a significant other is soon to end

Common Etiology (Stressors)
DISEASES: Any

INJURIES: Any

PSYCHOSOCIAL FACTORS: The threat of unpleasant reality

HEALTH CARE FACTORS: *Medical Diagnosis*: An unfavorable medical diagnosis for oneself or a significant other. *Health therapy*: Unsuccessful or ineffective medical, drug, or surgical therapy. *Prognosis*: An unfavorable prognosis

SITUATIONAL FACTORS: The terminal illness of oneself or a significant other, the experience of dying

PLANNING

Unmet Needs

Comfort, protection from psychologic threat, acceptance, caring and communicating relationships, sense of adequacy, personal growth and maturity, increased learning, increased reality perception and problem-solving ability

Expected Outcome

Person verbalizes feelings about the situation

Relates sufficient insight to substitute more growth-oriented coping mechanisms for the denial

Verbalizes feelings of satisfaction for having achieved self-growth

NURSING INTERVENTIONS

Nursing Treatments

Approach unhurriedly

Reassure verbally (that the nurse is available whenever needed)

Provide an atmosphere of acceptance

Support the use of appropriate defense mechanisms (do not oppose or attack the denial if it is the person's most effective defense against overwhelming anxiety)

Avoid forcing the person into rapid adaptation to change by accepting the person's unique pattern of adjustment (wait for the person to show readiness to face reality, after the denial is no longer completely effective)

When the Person Is Ready to Work Through the Denial

Encourage the expression of feelings (about the approaching death)

Listen attentively

Periodically verbalize the denied reality

Offer feedback to the person's expressed feelings

Communicate nurse sensitivity to the person's problems

Provide reliable information (giving small amounts of information at a time, amounts the person indicates he can handle)

Support a realistic assessment of the situation

Do not encourage or reinforce the denial (by giving false information or reassurance or by diverting attention from the reality)

Ask questions that encourage answers that reflect reality perception (straightforward questions such as "Do you think you are sick? Do you think your wife will die?")

Ensure the person's feeling of safety before introducing unpleasantness (if the person feels unsafe, denial may be reinforced)

Explore with the person his strengths and resources (to cope with the problem, since awareness of his own strength may reduce the need for denial)

Nursing Observations

Determine whether the denial is adaptive or nonadaptive (is it an adaptive response to crisis or a nonadaptive escape mechanism?)

Determine the need that the denial is serving (is it an attempt to maintain emotional stability or an escape from reality and personal growth?)

Determine the degree of insight that the person has (into the denial)

Evaluate the significance of emotional distress mannerisms

Identify cues indicating some acceptance of reality (statements such as "Everyone in my family has had cancer, why shouldn't I have it?")

Observe for an excessive stress level (talkativeness, pacing, nervousness, heavy smoking)

Observe for evidence that the person is reaching out for emotional support

Observe for evidence of a favorable response to therapy (acceptance of the approaching death)

Health Teaching

Explain that the person's response is appropriate and commonly experienced

Explain (to the family) that persons must make adjustments at their own pace

EVALUATION

Record actual outcome

DENIAL OF EMOTIONS[471,525,680]

ASSESSMENT

Data Collection

Subjective Data
- Person verbally rejects the occurring emotions
     OR
- Ignores references made regarding the reality
- If confronted, does not want to discuss the issue openly
  Will not become involved in emotion-arousing discussions
  May quickly change the subject, if the topic becomes emotional

Objective Data
- May exhibit unrealistic behavior such as failing to confront an out-of-control child when feeling angry toward the child, may rationalize or laugh about a situation that usually arouses sadness

Data Analysis

Nursing Diagnosis
DENIAL OF EMOTIONS: Being unable to admit the existence of the fact that one has intense emotional feelings

Common Etiology (Stressors)
PSYCHOSOCIAL FACTORS: The threat of unpleasant reality, the threat of upsetting a significant other
HEALTH CARE FACTORS: *Health therapy*: The threat of unwanted health therapy such as psychotherapy
LIFESTYLE: Cultural prohibitions (against expressing feelings)

PLANNING

Unmet Needs

Comfort, protection from psychologic threat, acceptance, caring and communicating relationships, sense of adequacy, personal growth and maturity, increased learning, increased reality perception and problem-solving ability

Expected Outcome

Person verbalizes feelings about the situation

Relates sufficient insight to substitute more growth-oriented coping mechanisms for the denial

Verbalizes feelings of satisfaction for having achieved self-growth

NURSING INTERVENTIONS

Nursing Treatments

Approach unhurriedly

Reassure verbally (that the nurse is available whenever needed)

Provide an atmosphere of acceptance

Support the use of appropriate defense mechanisms (do not oppose or attack the denial if it is the person's most effective defense against overwhelming anxiety)

Avoid forcing the person into rapid adaptation to change by accepting the person's unique pattern of adjustment (wait for the person to show readiness to face the life situation, after the denial is no longer completely effective)

When the Person Is Ready to Work Through the Denial

Encourage the expression of feelings (about the life situation)

Listen attentively

Talk with the person

Periodically verbalize the denied reality

Offer feedback to the person's expressed feelings

Communicate nurse sensitivity to the person's problems

Provide reliable information (giving small amounts of information at a time, amounts the person indicates he can handle)

Ask the person to identify the problem

Ask for specifics, not generalizations, about the problem (specifics may penetrate the denial)

Support a realistic assessment of the situation (that reality may not be as threatening as perceived and is less painful when faced promptly)

Do not encourage or reinforce the denial (by giving false information or reassurance or by diverting attention from the life situation)

Ask questions that encourage answers that reflect reality perception (straightforward questions such as "When did the situation become intolerable? What do you think will improve the situation?")

Ensure the person's feeling of safety before introducing unpleasantness (if the person feels unsafe, denial may be reinforced)

Explore with the person his strengths and resources (to cope with the life situation, since awareness of his own strength may reduce the need for denial)

Nursing Observations

Determine whether the denial is adaptive or nonadaptive (is it an adaptive response to crisis or a nonadaptive escape mechanism?)

Determine the need that the denial is serving (is it an attempt to maintain emotional stability or an escape from reality, responsibility, and personal growth?)

Determine the degree of insight that the person has (into the denial)

Identify disturbing conversation topics (which reveal emotions)

Evaluate the significance of emotional distress mannerisms

Identify cues indicating some acceptance of reality (statements such as "I'm so lonely since my husband died" or "The children make me so angry when they . . . ")

Observe for an excessive stress level (talkativeness, pacing, nervousness, heavy smoking)

Observe for evidence that the person is reaching out for emotional support

Observe for evidence of a favorable response to therapy (acceptance of and expression of feeling)

Health Teaching

Explain that the person's response is appropriate and commonly experienced

Teach how to use the problem-solving method (if appropriate)

Explain (to the family) that persons must make adjustments at their own pace

EVALUATION
Record actual outcome

DENIAL OF HABITUATION [224,300,471,525,680]

ASSESSMENT
Data Collection
Subjective Data
- Person verbally rejects that he frequently uses chemical substances
  OR
- Ignores references made regarding the reality
- If confronted, does not want to discuss the issue openly
  Insists that drinking, smoking, or drug abuse can be stopped whenever the abuser desires to do so
  States that he simply does not want to stop
  Terminates the habit for a short period in order to establish self-assurance of nondependence, then returns to the habit because of the dependence
  If the habituation is alcohol, there is failure to recognize that the gradual increase in the amount and frequency of alcohol use, the poor dietary intake, slackened personal appearance, and nonattendance to responsibilities are related to the alcohol dependence
  If the habituation is smoking, there is failure to recognize that the breathlessness, chronic productive cough, elevated blood pressure, lessened sense of taste and smell, poor appetite, and tachycardia are related to the smoking dependence
  If the habituation is narcotic or barbiturate drug abuse, there is failure to recognize that gradual increase in drug dosage, guarding of personal possessions, inability to complete goals, wearing of long-sleeved clothing and sunglasses, and painful body sensations if the drug dosage is decreased are related to drug dependence

Objective Data
- May exhibit unrealistic behavior such as continuing to smoke, drink, or take drugs, refusing to seek help, laughing and joking about the situation

Data Analysis
Nursing Diagnosis
DENIAL OF HABITUATION: Being unable to admit the existence of the fact of a habitual need for the intake of chemical products as a source of pleasure and strength

Common Etiology (Stressors)
PSYCHOSOCIAL FACTORS: The threat of unpleasant reality
LIFESTYLE: Alcohol abuse, drug abuse, excessive gambling, high caffeine or nicotine intake

PLANNING
Unmet Needs
Comfort, protection from psychologic threat, acceptance, caring and communicating relationships, sense of adequacy, personal growth and maturity, increased learning, increased reality perception and problem-solving ability

Expected Outcome
Person verbalizes feelings about the situation
Relates sufficient insight to substitute more growth-oriented coping mechanisms for the denial
Decreases or discontinues the use of the chemical substance
Verbalizes feelings of satisfaction for having achieved self-growth

NURSING INTERVENTIONS
Nursing Treatments

Approach unhurriedly
Reassure verbally (that the nurse is available whenever needed)
Provide an atmosphere of acceptance
Support the use of appropriate defense mechanisms (do not oppose or attack the denial
  if it is the person's most effective defense against overwhelming anxiety)
Avoid forcing the person into rapid adaptation to change by accepting the person's
  unique pattern of adjustment (wait for the person to show readiness to face the habit-
  uation, after the denial is no longer completely effective)

When the Person Is Ready to Work Through the Denial
Encourage the expression of feelings (about the habituation)
Listen attentively
Periodically verbalize the denied reality
Offer feedback to the person's expressed feelings
Communicate nurse sensitivity to the person's problems
Provide reliable information (giving small amounts of information at a time, amounts
  the person indicates he can handle)
Ask the person to identify the problem
Ask for specifics, not generalizations, about the problem (specifics may penetrate the
  denial)
Support a realistic assessment of the situation (how often, how much, and in what situa-
  tions is the substance taken)
Do not encourage or reinforce the denial (by giving false information or reassurance or
  by diverting attention from the habituation problem)
Ask questions that encourage answers that reflect reality perception (straightforward
  questions such as "Do you think you are dependent on drugs, alcohol, etc.?")
Ensure the person's feelings of safety before introducing unpleasantness (if the person
  feels unsafe, denial may be reinforced)
Explore with the person his strengths and resources (to cope with the habituation problem, since awareness of his own strength may reduce the need for denial)

Nursing Observations

Determine whether the denial is adaptive or nonadaptive (is it an adaptive response to
  crisis or a nonadaptive escape mechanism?)
Determine the need that the denial is serving (is it an attempt to maintain emotional
  stability or an escape from reality, responsibility, and personal growth?)
Determine the degree of insight that the person has (into the denial)
Identify disturbing conversation topics (about the habituation)
Evaluate the significance of emotional distress mannerisms
Identify cues indicating some acceptance of reality (statements such as "I can't get
  through the evening without a drink?" and "I've been drinking since I was twelve
  years old")
Observe for an excessive stress level (talkativeness, pacing, nervousness, heavy smoking)
Observe for evidence that the person is reaching out for emotional support
Observe for evidence of a favorable response to therapy (acceptance of and treatment
  for the habituation)

Health Teaching

Explain that the person's response is appropriate and commonly experienced
Advise early correction of problems
Explain (to the family) that persons must make adjustments at their own pace

EVALUATION

Record actual outcome

DENIAL OF LOSS OF A SIGNIFICANT OTHER[471,525,680]

ASSESSMENT
Data Collection
Subjective Data
- Person verbally rejects the loss of a significant other
  OR
- Ignores references made regarding the reality
- If confronted, does not want to discuss the issue openly
  Relates waiting for the lost person to return
  May talk about the person as if he were there

Objective Data
- May exhibit unrealistic behavior such as keeping the room in order, washing clothes, or planning an outing for a lost significant other

Data Analysis
Nursing Diagnosis
DENIAL OF LOSS OF A SIGNIFICANT OTHER: Being unable to admit the existence of the fact that one is permanently parted from a significant other

Common Etiology (Stressors)
BIRTH DEFECTS: Giving birth to an imperfect infant
DISEASES: Natural abortion, stillbirth, sudden infant death
PSYCHOSOCIAL FACTORS: The threat of unpleasant reality
HEALTH CARE FACTORS: *Hospital discharge*: Without the expected infant
SITUATIONAL FACTORS: Placing a child up for adoption, a child's being put up for adoption, death of a significant other, divorce from a spouse or of parents, the frequent change of foster parents, giving up a foster child

PLANNING
Unmet Needs
Comfort, protection from psychologic threat, acceptance, caring and communicating relationships, sense of adequacy, personal growth and maturity, increased learning, increased reality perception and problem-solving ability

Expected Outcome
Person verbalizes feelings about the situation
Relates sufficient insight to substitute more growth-oriented coping mechanisms for the denial
Verbalizes feelings of satisfaction for having achieved self-growth

NURSING INTERVENTIONS
Nursing Treatments
Approach unhurriedly
Reassure verbally (that the nurse is available whenever needed)
Provide an atmosphere of acceptance
Support the use of appropriate defense mechanisms (do not oppose or attack the denial if it is the person's most effective defense against overwhelming anxiety)
Avoid forcing the person into rapid adaptation to change by accepting the person's unique pattern of adjustment (wait for the person to show readiness to face reality, after the denial is no longer completely effective)

When the Person Is Ready to Work Through the Denial
Encourage the expression of feelings (about the loss)
Listen attentively
Periodically verbalize the denied reality
Offer feedback to the person's expressed feelings

Communicate nurse sensitivity to the person's problem

Provide reliable information (giving small amounts of information at a time, amounts the person indicates he can handle)

Support a realistic assessment of the situation (that the reality of the loss may be less threatening than perceived)

Do not encourage or reinforce the denial (by giving false information or reassurance or by diverting attention from the loss)

Ask questions that encourage answers that reflect reality perception (straightforward questions such as "Did your loved one die peacefully?" "It is frightening being divorced after so many years of marriage, isn't it?")

Ensure the person's feeling of safety before introducing unpleasantness (if the person feels unsafe, denial may be reinforced)

Explore with the person his strengths and resources (to cope with the problem, since awareness of his own strength may reduce the need for denial)

Nursing Observations

Determine whether the denial is adaptive or nonadaptive (is it an adaptive response to crisis or a nonadaptive escape mechanism?)

Determine the need that the denial is serving (is it an attempt to maintain emotional stability or an escape from reality, responsibility, and personal growth?)

Determine the degree of insight that the person has (into the denial)

Evaluate the significance of emotional distress mannerisms

Identify cues indicating some acceptance of reality (statements such as "I'm so glad I was with him when he died")

Observe for an excessive stress level (talkativeness, pacing, nervousness, heavy smoking)

Observe for evidence that the person is reaching out for emotional support

Observe for evidence of a favorable response to therapy (acceptance of the loss of a significant other)

Health Teaching

Explain that the person's response is appropriate and commonly experienced (following loss of a significant other)

Teach how to use the problem-solving method (if appropriate)

Explain (to the family) that persons must make adjustments at their own pace

EVALUATION

Record actual outcome

DENIAL OF PAIN [471,525,626,680]

ASSESSMENT

Data Collection

Subjective Data

• Person verbally rejects the occurring pain
  OR
• Ignores references made regarding the reality
• If confronted, does not want to discuss the issue openly
  Refuses to admit that he feels pain
  Rejects offers for pain relief
  May complain of fatigue
  May request increased privacy or time alone

Objective Data

• May exhibit unrealistic behavior such as smiling, laughing, attempting activities difficult to endure when in pain; may exhibit sudden facial expressions of pain but quickly regain self-control; only evidence of pain may be a tightened hand or tearfulness

Data Analysis

Nursing Diagnosis
DENIAL OF PAIN: Being unable to admit the existence of the fact that one is experiencing distressful hurting

Common Etiology (Stressors)
PSYCHOSOCIAL FACTORS: The threat of unpleasant reality, the threat of upsetting a significant other, an attempt to maintain a favorable self-concept, the valued concept of self-control, the threat of rejection (from others who have questioned the validity of the pain), the threat of real danger (such as dreaded diseases of cancer, heart attack, etc.)

HEALTH CARE FACTORS: *Hospitalization*: The threat of hospitalization. *Drug therapy*: The threat of the adverse effects of pain-relief drugs. *Health therapy*: The threat of unwanted health therapy

LIFESTYLE: Cultural prohibitions (against expressing pain, the idea that good patients do not express pain)

SITUATIONAL FACTORS: The threat of loss of employment

PLANNING

Unmet Needs
Comfort, protection from physical and physiologic threat, acceptance, caring and communicating relationships, sense of adequacy, personal growth and maturity, increased learning, increased reality perception and problem-solving ability

Expected Outcome
Person verbalizes feelings about the situation

Relates sufficient insight to substitute more growth-oriented coping mechanisms for the denial

Verbalizes feelings of satisfaction for having achieved self-growth

Accepts therapy for the relief or control of pain, as needed

NURSING INTERVENTIONS

Nursing Treatments
Approach unhurriedly

Reassure verbally (that the nurse is available whenever needed)

Provide an atmosphere of acceptance

Support the use of appropriate defense mechanisms (do not oppose or attack the denial if it is the person's most effective defense against overwhelming anxiety)

Avoid forcing the person into rapid adaptation to change by accepting the person's unique pattern of adjustment (wait for the person to show readiness to face the reality of pain, after the denial is no longer completely effective)

When the Person Is Ready to Work Through the Denial

Encourage the expression of feelings (about the pain)

Listen attentively

Periodically verbalize the denied reality

Offer feedback to the person's expressed feelings

Communicate nurse sensitivity to the person's problems

Encourage the person to ask questions (which indicate what the person wants to know about the significance of the pain)

Provide reliable information (giving small amounts of information at a time, amounts the person indicates he can handle, especially if the pain indicates serious illness)

Support a realistic assessment of the situation (that it is acceptable to admit pain, that pain is a warning symptom)

Do not encourage or reinforce the denial (by giving false information or reassurance or by diverting attention from the pain)

Ask questions that encourage answers that reflect reality perception (straightforward questions such as "Do you think you need pain relief?")

Ensure the person's feeling of safety before introducing unpleasantness (if the person feels unsafe, denial may be reinforced)

Explore with the person his strengths and resources (to cope with the problem, since awareness of his own strength may reduce the need for denial)

Nursing Observations

Determine whether the denial is adaptive or nonadaptive (is it an adaptive response to crisis or a nonadaptive escape mechanism?)

Determine the need that the denial is serving (is it an attempt to maintain emotional stability, an escape from reality, or a response to cultural expectations)

Determine the degree of insight that the person has (into the denial)

Evaluate the significance of emotional distress mannerisms

Identify cues indicating some acceptance of reality (statements such as "My abdomen feels like it is going to split in half," "I don't know how much more of this I can take")

Observe for an excessive stress level (talkativeness, pacing, nervousness, restlessness, fist clenching)

Observe for evidence that the person is reaching out for emotional support

Observe for evidence of a favorable response to therapy (acceptance of pain relief and relief of pain)

Health Teaching

Explain that the person's response is appropriate and commonly experienced

Recommend new options for effective methods of coping (admitting pain increases control over it)

Explain (to the family) that persons must make adjustments at their own pace (if the pain is chronic)

EVALUATION

Record actual outcome

DENIAL OF PHYSICAL LOSS [471,525,680]

ASSESSMENT

Data Collection

Subjective Data

- Person verbally rejects the physical loss
  OR
- Ignores references made regarding the reality
- If confronted, does not want to discuss the issue openly
  Exclaims "No, it can't be. It isn't true."
  Claims that x-rays or test results are incorrect
  Relates traveling from physician to physician seeking to refute the truth
  Resorts to faith healers, sometimes
  Still seeks treatment, despite the denial
  May refuse to participate in self-care
  May refuse to admit that he cannot work as hard or as long, that he is unable to perform strenuous physical activity, that his responses are slower, that he has difficulty learning new things, or that his memory is less reliable

Objective Data

- May exhibit unrealistic behavior such as refusing to seek medical help, attempting difficult physical or mental tasks beyond his limitations, laughing or joking about the situation

Data Analysis
Nursing Diagnosis
DENIAL OF PHYSICAL LOSS: Being unable to admit the existence of the fact that one has lost a positive, balanced state of health, a body part, or body function

Common Etiology (Stressors)
DISEASES: Any
INJURIES: Any
SIGNS AND SYMPTOMS: Confusion, immobility, memory loss, paralysis, weakness
PSYCHOSOCIAL FACTORS: The threat of unpleasant reality
HUMAN BODY: *Body appearance*: Changes in body appearance, disfigured body. *Body function*: Loss of body function. *Body part*: Loss of a body part
HEALTH CARE FACTORS: *Drug therapy*: The need to use life maintenance drugs. *Adverse effects of medical, drug, or surgical therapy*: Loss of a body part (from an amputation, cholecystectomy, enucleation or evisceration of an eyeball, gastrectomy, hemipelvectomy, hysterectomy, ileotomy, laryngectomy, lobectomy of the brain, liver, lungs, mastectomy, nephrectomy, prostatectomy, splenectomy, thyroidectomy, tonsillectomy), loss of the fetus (from a therapeutic abortion), loss of libido (from antihypertensive drugs, Tagamet, hemodialysis), loss of natural elimination and elimination control (from a colostomy, ileocolostomy, ileostomy, ureterocolostomy, ureteroileostomy, ureterosigmoidostomy, ureterostomy, ureterotomy), loss of normal food intake (from an esophagectomy), loss of the reproductive ability (from a fallopian tube ligation, hysterectomy, oophorectomy, orchidectomy, prostatectomy, salpingectomy, vasectomy), loss of vision (from enucleation or evisceration of an eyeball). *Prognosis*: An unfavorable prognosis. *Therapeutic equipment*: The need to use a cardiac pacemaker, brace, cane, crutches, hemodialyzer, respirator, walker, wheelchair
DEVELOPMENTAL PHASES: Middle age, old age
LIFESTYLE: Cultural expectations of personal independence
SITUATIONAL FACTORS: Childlessness, acute or chronic illness

PLANNING
Unmet Needs
Comfort, protection from psychologic threat, acceptance, caring and communicating relationships, sense of adequacy, personal growth and maturity, increased learning, increased reality perception and problem-solving ability

Expected Outcome
Person verbalizes feelings about the situation
Relates sufficient insight to substitute more growth-oriented coping mechanisms for the denial
Verbalizes feelings of satisfaction for having achieved self-growth

NURSING INTERVENTIONS
Nursing Treatments
Approach unhurriedly
Reassure verbally (that the nurse is available whenever needed)
Provide an atmosphere of acceptance
Support the use of appropriate defense mechanisms (do not oppose or attack the denial if it is the person's most effective defense against overwhelming anxiety)
Avoid forcing the person into rapid adaptation to change by accepting the person's unique pattern of adjustment (wait for the person to show readiness to face the physical loss, after the denial is no longer completely effective)

When the Person Is Ready to Work Through the Denial
Encourage the expression of feelings (about the physical loss)
Listen attentively
Periodically verbalize the denied reality
Offer feedback to the person's expressed feelings

Communicate nurse sensitivity to the person's problems

Encourage the person to ask questions (which indicate what the person wants to know about the physical loss)

Provide reliable information (giving small amounts of information at a time, amounts the person indicates he can handle)

Support a realistic assessment of the situation (about how the body adapts to the physical loss, how the therapy is effective)

Do not encourage or reinforce the denial (by giving false information or reassurance or by diverting attention from the physical loss)

Ask questions that encourage answers that reflect reality perception (straightforward questions such as "Do you think you are sick?" "How long do you think you will need to convalesce?")

Ensure the person's feeling of safety before introducing unpleasantness (if the person feels unsafe, denial may be reinforced)

Explore with the person his strengths and resources (to cope with the loss, since awareness of his own strength may reduce the need for denial)

Nursing Observations

Determine whether the denial is adaptive or nonadaptive (is it an adaptive response to crisis or a nonadaptive escape mechanism?)

Determine the need that the denial is serving (is it an attempt to maintain emotional stability or an escape from reality, responsibility, and personal growth)

Determine the degree of insight that the person has (into the denial)

Evaluate the significance of emotional distress mannerisms

Identify cues indicating some acceptance of reality (statements such as "I'm only half a person now," "Who wants to look at a person like me?")

Observe for an excessive stress level (talkativeness, pacing, nervousness, heavy smoking)

Observe for evidence that the person is reaching out for emotional support

Observe for evidence of a favorable response to therapy (acceptance of the physical loss)

Health Teaching

Explain that the person's response is appropriate and commonly experienced (following physical loss)

Teach how to use the problem-solving method (if appropriate)

Explain (to the family) that persons must make adjustments at their own pace

EVALUATION

Record actual outcome

DENIAL OF ROLE LOSS[471,525,680]

ASSESSMENT

Data Collection

Subjective Data
- Person verbally rejects the loss of a role
    OR
- Ignores references made regarding the reality
- If confronted, does not want to discuss the issue openly
    Talks and fantasizes about the role as if he currently fulfills it

Objective Data
- May exhibit unrealistic behavior such as responding angrily toward anyone who attempts to assume his role, refusing to let children go when grown, refusing to retire

Data Analysis

Nursing Diagnosis

DENIAL OF ROLE LOSS: Being unable to admit the existence of the fact that one has lost one's position, situation, or responsibility in life and can no longer perform the associated, expected behavior

Common Etiology (Stressors)

DISEASES: Any

INJURIES: Any

SIGNS AND SYMPTOMS: Immobility, pain, weakness

PSYCHOSOCIAL FACTORS: The threat of unpleasant reality

DEVELOPMENTAL PHASES: Adolescence, middle age, old age

SITUATIONAL FACTORS: Death of a significant other, divorce, marital separation, loss of employment, launching grown children, illness of or injury to self or a significant other, marriage, parenthood, retirement, the end of school

PLANNING

Unmet Needs

Comfort, protection from psychologic threat, acceptance, caring and communicating relationships, sense of adequacy, personal growth and maturity, increased learning, increased reality perception and problem-solving ability

Expected Outcome

Person verbalizes feelings about the situation

Relates sufficient insight to substitute with more growth-oriented coping mechanisms for the denial

Verbalizes feelings of satisfaction for having achieved self-growth

NURSING INTERVENTIONS

Nursing Treatments

Approach unhurriedly

Reassure verbally (that the nurse is available whenever needed)

Provide an atmosphere of acceptance

Support the use of appropriate defense mechanisms (do not oppose or attack the denial if it is the person's most effective defense against overwhelming anxiety)

Avoid forcing the person into rapid adaptation to change by accepting the person's unique pattern of adjustment (wait for the person to show readiness to face the role loss, after the denial is no longer completely effective)

When the Person Is Ready to Work Through the Denial

Encourage the expression of feelings (about the role loss)

Listen attentively

Periodically verbalize the denied reality

Offer feedback to the person's expressed feelings

Communicate nurse sensitivity to the person's problem

Provide reliable information (giving small amounts of information at a time and in amounts the person indicates he can handle)

Ask the person to identify the problem

Ask for specifics, not generalizations, about the problem (specifics may penetrate the denial)

Support a realistic assessment of the situation (that new roles are valuable)

Do not encourage or reinforce denial (by giving false information or reassurance or by diverting attention from the role loss)

Ask questions that encourage answers that reflect reality perception (straightforward questions such as "What do you like about your new role?")

Ensure the person's feelings of safety before introducing unpleasantness (if the person feels unsafe, denial may be reinforced)

Explore with the person his strength and resources (to cope with the problem, since awareness of his own strength may reduce the need for denial)

Nursing Observations

Determine whether the denial is adaptive or nonadaptive (is it an adaptive response to crisis or a nonadaptive escape mechanism?)

Determine the need that the denial is serving (is it an attempt to maintain emotional stability or an escape from reality, responsibility, and personal growth?)

Determine the degree of insight that the person has (into the denial)

Evaluate the significance of emotional distress mannerisms

Identify cues indicating some acceptance of reality (statements such as "When I used to farm, I . . ." "Before my retirement, I . . .")

Observe for an excessive stress level (talkativeness, pacing, nervousness, heavy smoking)

Observe for evidence that the person is reaching out for emotional support

Observe for evidence of a favorable response to therapy (acceptance of the role loss)

Health Teaching

Explain that the person's response is appropriate and commonly experienced (following a role loss)

Teach how to use the problem-solving method (if appropriate)

Explain (to the family) that persons must make adjustments at their own pace

EVALUATION

Record actual outcome

REGRESSION RELATED TO PHYSICAL LOSS[105,432,471,525]

ASSESSMENT

Data Collection

Subjective Data

- Person relates feeling that the past was safe and that the present and future are unsafe
- Verbalizes primarily about self

  Has difficulty appreciating the needs of others

  Expresses concern with trifling matters

  May discuss the health problem in detail and for a prolonged period

Objective Data

- May exhibit behavior such as unquestioning compliance, accepting assistance, seeking reassurance, approval, and physical closeness, and relinquishing responsibility to others; children often return to earlier behavior patterns such as bed-wetting, thumb-sucking, bottle-feeding, temper tantrums, and baby talk

Data Analysis

Nursing Diagnosis

REGRESSION RELATED TO PHYSICAL LOSS: An attempt to protect the self by using coping behavior appropriate at an earlier developmental level during the loss of a balanced state of health

Common Etiology (Stressors)

DISEASES: Any

INJURIES: Any

PSYCHOSOCIAL FACTORS: The threat of real or imagined danger, the use of previously successful defense mechanism behavior, an attempt to reduce present life responsibilities and assume a less demanding personal status, the threat of severe stress, the threat of loss of control of a life situation

HEALTH CARE FACTORS: *Health care environment*: Locked psychiatric unit, intensive care unit, coronary care unit, isolation unit. *Hospitalization/institutionalization*: Any. *Diagnostic procedure*: Any. *Medical diagnosis*: An unfavorable diagnosis. *Medical therapy*: Any. *Surgical therapy*: Any

DEVELOPMENTAL PHASES: Any but especially old age

PLANNING

Unmet Needs

Comfort, protection from physical or psychologic threat, dependence, acceptance, caring and communicating relationships, high evaluation of self, dignity, personal growth and maturity, increased learning

Expected Outcome

Person verbalizes about feeling unsafe

As health and energy level increases or stress is reduced, the person gradually assumes previous responsibilities and becomes a functioning, independent person

As the child adjusts to the threatening or fearful situation, he gradually returns to his previous developmental level

NURSING INTERVENTIONS

Nursing Treatments

Approach unhurriedly

Reassure verbally (that the nurse is available whenever needed)

Provide an atmosphere of acceptance

Encourage the expression of feelings

Listen attentively

Offer feedback to the person's expressed feelings

Communicate nurse sensitivity to the person's problem

Communicate with the person on an adult–adult level, not on a parent–child level (which could increase regression)

Ask the person to identify the problem

Ask for specifics, not generalizations, about the problem

Support a realistic assessment of the situation (regression allows for more energy to be available for healing and coping, but it also is a way of escaping responsibility)

Explore with the person his strengths and resources (awareness of his strength may reduce the need for regression)

Ensure the person's feeling of safety before introducing unpleasantness (feeling safe reduces the need for regression)

Support the use of appropriate defense mechanisms (by supporting the regression if it is the person's most effective defense mechanism)

Avoid forcing the person into rapid adaptation to change by accepting the person's unique pattern of adjustment

Nursing Observations

Determine the degree of insight that the person has (into the regression)

Identify disturbing conversation topics (that worsen regression)

Evaluate the significance of emotional distress mannerisms

Observe for an excessive stress level (severely regressive behavior)

Observe for evidence that the person is reaching out for emotional support

Observe for evidence of a favorable response to therapy (a return to the person's former developmental level)

Health Teaching

Explain that the person's response is appropriate and commonly experienced

Recommend new options for effective methods of coping (learning new techniques of self-care, learning new social or job skills)

Explain (to the family) the significance of regressive behavior in illness (parents often punish children for regressive behavior because they do not understand that it is a normal response to severe stress; some families also find it very embarrassing)

Explain (to the family) that persons must make adjustments at their own pace

EVALUATION

Record actual outcome

WITHDRAWAL FROM A LIFE SITUATION[105,432,471,525]

ASSESSMENT

Data Collection

Subjective Data
- Person relates the perception of a threatening person or situation
- Expresses a need to move away from or avoid the threat
  Relates involvement in an unpleasant or unresolvable situation
  Feels overcome by the situation

Objective Data
- May physically or emotionally remove himself by exhibiting behaviors such as resigning employment, not keeping appointments for health care, running away from home

Data Analysis

Nursing Diagnosis
WITHDRAWAL FROM A LIFE SITUATION: Moving away from a difficult or unwanted situation

Common Etiology (Stressors)
PSYCHOSOCIAL FACTORS: The threat of real or imagined danger, the threat of failure to achieve, the threat of severe stress, an attempt to control a life situation or resist control by others
SITUATIONAL FACTORS: Situational crisis or stress, an intolerable situation

PLANNING

Unmet Needs

Comfort, protection from psychologic threat, acceptance, caring and communicating relationships, high evaluation of self, sense of adequacy, control over others or situations, personal growth and maturity, increased learning, increased reality perception and problem-solving ability

Expected Outcome

Person verbalizes feelings about the threat
Continues to use withdrawal, if it is the person's most effective coping method
  OR
Relates a problem-solving approach that could be more effective than withdrawal
Takes specific action to overcome the threat
Verbalizes feelings of satisfaction for achieving self-growth

NURSING INTERVENTIONS

Nursing Treatments

Approach unhurriedly
Reassure verbally (that the nurse is available whenever needed)
Provide an atmosphere of acceptance
Encourage the expression of feelings (about the situation precipitating the withdrawal)
Listen attentively
Offer feedback to the person's expressed feelings
Communicate nurse sensitivity to the person's problem

Ask the person to identify the problem

Ask for specifics, not generalizations, about the problem

Support a realistic assessment of the situation (that the reality may not be as threatening as perceived)

Explore with the person his strengths and resources (which will help him move forward)

Ensure the person's feeling of safety before introducing unpleasantness (which has caused the withdrawal)

Encourage gradual mastery of a situation

Avoid forcing the person into rapid adaptation to change by accepting the person's unique pattern of adjustment

Nursing Observations

Observe for evidence of a favorable response to therapy (reduced withdrawal)

Health Teaching

Recommend new options for effective methods of coping (such as confronting the situation, reassessing the situation)

Explain the importance of maintaining a positive self-attitude

Explain (to the family) that persons must make adjustments at their own pace

Teach how to use the problem-solving method (to cope with the situation)

EVALUATION

Record actual outcome

WITHDRAWAL FROM A SIGNIFICANT OTHER[105,432,471,525]

ASSESSMENT

Data Collection

Subjective Data
- Person relates the perception of a threatening person
- Expresses a need to move away from or avoid the threat

  Perceives an impending loss of or unfavorable relationship with a significant other

  Feels unable to cope with the significant other

Objective Data
- May physically or emotionally remove himself by exhibiting behaviors such as excessive sleeping, extended silence, turning away, pretending not to hear, avoiding eye contact, refusing to talk, avoiding association with the person

Data Analysis

Nursing Diagnosis

WITHDRAWAL FROM A SIGNIFICANT OTHER: Moving away from interaction with a significant person when such interaction presents relationship difficulties

Common Etiology (Stressors)

BIRTH DEFECTS: Of a child

PSYCHOSOCIAL FACTORS: The threat of real or imagined danger, an attempt to change the direction of one's life, the threat of severe stress, the threat of an unpleasant reality, an attempt to lessen one's attachment to another, the threat of intimacy, an attempt to control a life situation or resist control by others, an attempt to control emotions

LIFESTYLE: Lack of conformity (of a significant other) to cultural mores

SITUATIONAL FACTORS: Placing a child up for adoption, the impending death of a significant other, the impending separation or divorce from a spouse or of parents, marriage of a significant other, chronic or terminal illness or injury of a significant other, impending retirement

PLANNING

Unmet Needs

Comfort, protection from psychologic threat, acceptance, caring and communicating relationships, high evaluation of self, sense of adequacy, control over others or situations, personal growth and maturity, increased learning, increased reality perception and problem-solving ability

Expected Outcome

Person verbalizes feelings about the threat

Continues to use withdrawal, if it is the person's most effective coping method
    OR
Relates a problem-solving approach that could be more effective than withdrawal

Takes specific action to overcome the threat

Verbalizes feelings of satisfaction for achieving self-growth

NURSING INTERVENTIONS

Nursing Treatments

Approach unhurriedly

Reassure verbally (that the nurse is available whenever needed)

Provide an atmosphere of acceptance

Encourage the expression of feelings (about the difficult significant other)

Listen attentively

Offer feedback to the person's expressed feelings

Communicate nurse sensitivity to the person's problem

Ask the person to identify the problem

Ask for specifics, not generalizations, about the problem

Support a realistic assessment of the situation (that withdrawal from the significant other widens the communication gap)

Explore with the person his strengths and resources (which will help him move forward)

Ensure the person's feeling of safety before introducing unpleasantness (which could cause further withdrawal)

Encourage gradual mastery of a situation

Avoid forcing the person into rapid adaptation to change by accepting the person's unique pattern of adjustment

Nursing Observations

Observe for evidence of a favorable response to therapy (reduced withdrawal)

Health Teaching

Recommend new options for effective methods of coping (improved communications with the significant person)

Explain the importance of maintaining a positive self-attitude

Explain (to the family) that persons must make adjustments at their own pace

Teach how to use the problem-solving method (to cope with the significant other)

EVALUATION

Record actual outcome

WITHDRAWAL FROM SOCIALIZATION [105,432,471,525]

ASSESSMENT

Data Collection

Subjective Data

• Person relates the perception of a threatening group of persons

• Expresses a need to move away from or avoid the threat

  Does not want to be seen by others

  Does not want to participate in social activities with others

Objective Data
• May physically or emotionally remove self by exhibiting behaviors such as refusing or canceling invitations, failing to call friends, staying in his room with the door closed

Data Analysis

Nursing Diagnosis
WITHDRAWAL FROM SOCIALIZATION: Moving away from interaction with others when such interaction poses a threat

Common Etiology (Stressors)
BIRTH DEFECTS: Being a person with a birth defect
DISEASES: Any but especially disfiguring or communicable diseases, disorders that affect communications such as aphasia
INJURIES: Any but especially disfiguring injuries
SIGNS AND SYMPTOMS: Edema, immobility, incontinence, jaundice, rash, seizures, tremor
PSYCHOSOCIAL FACTORS: The threat of real or imagined danger, the threat of failure to achieve, the threat of severe stress, an attempt to control a life situation or resist control by others, an attempt to control painful emotions
HUMAN BODY: *Body appearance*: Changes in body appearance, a disfigured body. *Body function*: Loss of control of body function. *Body part*: Loss of a body part. *Body size*: Delayed body growth. *Body states*: Pregnancy
HEALTH CARE FACTORS: *Hospitalization or institutionalization*: Prolonged. *Medical therapy*: Therapeutic diet limitations visible when eating outside the home, hemodialysis and rehabilitation therapy (which leaves little time for socializing). *Surgical incision*: A disfiguring incision. *Adverse effects of medical, drug or, surgical therapy*: Loss of a visible body part (from an amputation, enucleation or evisceration of an eyeball), loss of hair (from chemotherapy and radiation therapy), loss of mobility (from traction), loss of natural elimination and elimination control (from a colostomy, ileocolostomy, ileostomy, ureterocolostomy, ureteroileostomy, ureterosigmoidostomy, ureterostomy, ureterotomy), loss of normal food intake (from an esophagectomy), loss of speech (from a glossectomy, laryngectomy, tracheostomy, vocal cordectomy), loss of vision (from an enucleation or evisceration of an eyeball), edema (from corticosteroids). *Therapeutic equipment*: The use of an artificial eye or limb, brace, breast prosthesis, cane, cannula for hemodialysis, urinary catheter, crutches, dentures, hearing aid, therapeutic tubes, walker, wheelchair. *Prognosis*: An unfavorable prognosis. *Convalescence*: Slow recovery during convalescence.
LIFESTYLE: Alcohol or drug abuse
SITUATIONAL FACTORS: The death of a significant other or an old friend, divorce from a spouse, lack of finances, illness of a significant other (acute, chronic, terminal), relocation of a home

PLANNING

Unmet Needs
Comfort, protection from psychologic threat, acceptance, caring and communicating relationships, high evaluation of self, sense of adequacy, control over others or situations, personal growth and maturity, increased learning, increased reality perception and problem-solving ability

Expected Outcome
Person verbalizes feelings about the threat
Continues to use withdrawal, if it is the person's most effective coping method
  OR
Relates a problem-solving approach that could be more effective than withdrawal
Takes specific action to overcome the threat
Verbalizes feelings of satisfaction for achieving self-growth

NURSING INTERVENTIONS

Nursing Treatments
Approach unhurriedly

Reassure verbally (that the nurse is available whenever needed)
Provide an atmosphere of acceptance
Encourage the expression of feelings (about the situation precipitating the withdrawal)
Listen attentively
Offer feedback to the person's expressed feelings
Communicate nurse sensitivity to the person's problem
Ask the person to identify the problem
Ask for specifics, not generalizations, about the problem
Support a realistic assessment of the situation (that social withdrawal increases a sense of isolation and aloneness)
Explore with the person his strengths and resources (which will help him socialize comfortably)
Encourage gradual mastery of a situation (initially socialize with a few caring friends)
Avoid forcing the person into rapid adaptation to change by accepting the person's unique pattern of adjustment
Encourage visiting by significant others (if the hospitalization is long-term)

Nursing Observations
Observe for evidence of a favorable response to therapy (reduced withdrawal)

Health Teaching
Recommend new options for effective methods of coping (such as compensation in which the person develops a skill or characteristic that is socially valued and gives self-gratification)
Explain the importance of maintaining a positive self-attitude
Explain (to the family) that persons must make adjustments at their own pace
Teach how to use the problem-solving method (such as how to use make-up and clothing to cover a disfigurement, how to choose a therapeutic diet in a restaurant without revealing it to others, how to protect oneself if incontinent, etc.)

EVALUATION

Record actual outcome

Adaptive Responses Involving Attachment

BONDING INTERRUPTION RELATED TO HEALTH CARE/HEALTH THERAPY[207,251,313,414]

ASSESSMENT

Data Collection

Subjective Data
• Person verbalizes a strong attachment for another
• Relates wanting to enter into the feelings of and share intimately the experience of the loved one
• Expresses a desire to make his resources of strength, time, thought, etc. available to the loved one
• Relates feeling cut off from expressing care, concern, and responsibility for the loved one
  May express frustration or anger
  May relate feelings of having deserted the loved one
  Wonders how the loved one is and what is being done to him

Objective Data
- May exhibit behavior such as very frequent phone calls, visiting at unauthorized times, prolonging allowed visiting, sitting long hours in the waiting room, crying, attempting to assist with and/or supervise physical needs

Data Analysis

Nursing Diagnosis

BONDING INTERRUPTION RELATED TO HEALTH CARE/HEALTH THERAPY: Feeling cut off from relating to a significant other expressions of emotional closeness and caring during health care or therapy

Common Etiology (Stressors)

PSYCHOSOCIAL FACTORS: Separation from or absence of a significant other

HEALTH CARE FACTORS: *Health care environment*: Locked psychiatric unit, intensive care, coronary care, isolation unit. *Hospitalization/institutionalization*: Separation from a significant other during hospitalization or institutionalization. *Institutional policies*: Enforced exclusion from the care of a significant other. *Visiting hours*: Limited and restrictive visiting hours

PLANNING

Unmet Needs

Comfort, protection from psychologic threat, acceptance, caring and communicating relationships, unity with loved one(s), sense of usefulness (to the loved one), increased learning

Expected Outcome

Person verbalizes his feelings about the situation
Relates a feeling of unity and sharing of the illness experience with the loved one
Expresses that the experience has been one of personal growth

NURSING INTERVENTIONS

Nursing Treatments

Approach unhurriedly
Reassure verbally (that the loved one will be allowed to participate in the patient's care)
Provide an atmosphere of acceptance
Encourage the expression of feelings (about the interruption)
Listen attentively
Communicate nurse sensitivity to the person's problem
Involve the significant other (in the patient's care and therapy as much as possible, communicate what is to be done and what the person can do to make him feel that he is an important part of the patient's care)
Encourage significant other's questions (about the patient's condition)
Provide reliable information (about the patient's condition at frequent intervals)
Allow a significant other to sit quietly at the bedside (most of the time)
Allow unlimited visiting
Encourage telephone calls with significant persons
Support a realistic assessment of the situation (that some bonding interruption will occur because of certain therapy, but that the interruption will be kept to a minimum)

Nursing Observations

Observe for evidence of a favorable response to therapy (satisfaction with being able to share the experience with the loved one)

Health Teaching

Explain that the person's response is appropriate and commonly experienced

EVALUATION

Record actual outcome

BONDING INTERRUPTION RELATED TO A LIFE SITUATION [207,251,313,414]

ASSESSMENT

Data Collection

Subjective Data
- Person verbalizes a strong attachment for another
- Relates wanting to enter into the feelings of and share intimately the experience of the loved one
- Expresses a desire to make his resources of strength, time, thought, etc., available to the loved one
- Relates feeling cut off from expressing care, concern, and responsibility for the loved one

  Wonders how the loved one is and what he is doing

  Is preoccupied with thoughts of the loved one

  May express frustration and anger

Objective Data
- May exhibit behavior such as very frequent phone calls, crying, sitting looking at the loved one's picture

Data Analysis

Nursing Diagnosis
BONDING INTERRUPTION RELATED TO A LIFE SITUATION: Feeling cut off from relating to a significant other expressions of emotional closeness and caring during a specific life situation

Common Etiology (Stressors)
PSYCHOSOCIAL FACTORS: Separation from or absence of a significant other

SITUATIONAL FACTORS: Marital separation or divorce of parents or from a spouse, legal termination of parental rights, one-parent custody of a child, limited visitation rights of a child, relocation of a home, a geographically distant family, retirement, the end of school, extensive travel by a significant other, military service, confinement in prison

PLANNING

Unmet Needs
Comfort, protection from psychologic threat, acceptance, caring and communicating relationships, unity with loved one(s), sense of usefulness (to the loved one), increased learning

Expected Outcome
Person verbalizes feelings about the situation

Relates a feeling of unity and sharing with the loved one

Expresses that the experience has been one of personal growth

NURSING INTERVENTIONS

Nursing Treatments
Approach unhurriedly

Reassure verbally (that love can exist and be communicated even though persons are separated)

Provide an atmosphere of acceptance

Encourage the expression of feelings (about the interruption)

Listen attentively

Communicate nurse sensitivity to the person's problem

Encourage telephone calls with significant persons

Support a realistic assessment of the situation (that some bonding interruption will occur in certain life situations, that the interruption is temporary or permanent, short- or long-term)

Nursing Observations
Observe for evidence of a favorable response to therapy (that the bonding interruption be minimized, that the person is satisfied with the amount of sharing possible)

Health Teaching
Explain that the person's response is appropriate and commonly experienced
Advise that significant persons express caring for one another (through letters, gifts, etc.)

EVALUATION
Record actual outcome

DISENGAGEMENT/DETACHMENT RELATED TO APPROACHING DEATH[90,154,525]

ASSESSMENT
Data Collection
Subjective Data
- Person acknowledges that his involvement with life itself is ending
- Expresses feelings of decreased interest
  Person relates experiencing decreased vitality
  Focuses his remaining energy primarily on himself
  Person relates that he does not want life prolonged
  Wishes to die in peace
  Perceives that death would be a relief
  Relates preoccupation with a life review
  Prefers not to be bothered but to be left alone

Objective Data
- May exhibit behaviors such as frequent sleeping or lying still, passively ceasing all efforts, talking very little to visitors or nurses, ignoring the presence of other persons

Data Analysis

Nursing Diagnosis
DISENGAGEMENT/DETACHMENT RELATED TO APPROACHING DEATH: An attempt to release oneself from personal attachments after one becomes aware that one's life will soon end

Common Etiology (Stressors)
DISEASES: Any
INJURIES: Any
PSYCHOSOCIAL FACTORS: The exhaustion of adaptive reserves
HEALTH CARE FACTORS: *Health therapy*: Unsuccessful or ineffective medical, drug, or surgical therapy
SITUATIONAL FACTORS: The terminal illness of oneself, the experience of dying

PLANNING

Unmet Needs
Comfort, protection from psychologic threat, acceptance, caring and communicating relationships, less rigid conventiality

Expected Outcome
Person relates an acceptance of his own decreased interaction with others
Family members relate an understanding of the adaptive nature of the detachment behaviors

NURSING INTERVENTIONS

Nursing Treatments

Approach unhurriedly

Reassure verbally (that even though the person prefers not to be bothered, the nurse is available whenever needed)

Provide an atmosphere of acceptance

Encourage the expression of feelings (about disengaging)

Touch the person frequently

Provide frequent contact with the person (so he knows that the nurse is there)

Relate to the person on an adult–adult level, not on a parent–child level

Reduce the demands placed on the person (do not insist he eat, drink fluid, bathe, etc.)

Refrain from performing nonessential procedures

Suggest that one relative remain with the dying person

Encourage family support of the person's acceptance of dying

Provide conditions that the person desires for peaceful dying

Reinforce concern throughout the entire illness

Assist the dying person with detachment from life (if the person wishes, turn off the television or radio, provide quiet time)

Restrict unwanted visitors

Nursing Observations

Observe for evidence of a favorable response to therapy (that both the person and family feel comfortable with the normal disengagement as death approaches)

Health Teaching

Explain (to the family) that the person's response is appropriate and commonly experienced

Advise that significant persons express caring for one another (until the end)

EVALUATION

Record actual outcome

DISENGAGEMENT/DETACHMENT RELATED TO PHYSICAL LOSS[525]

ASSESSMENT

Data Collection

Subjective Data

• Person acknowledges that his involvement with the everyday activities of the world has lost significance

• Expresses feelings of decreased interest

  The ill or aged person relates less concern with social obligations

  Acknowledges increased concern with himself and his problems

Objective Data

• May exhibit behaviors such as sleeping, having a contemplative appearance, not making phone calls, appearing disinterested when others relate their problems

Data Analysis

Nursing Diagnosis

DISENGAGEMENT/DETACHMENT RELATED TO PHYSICAL LOSS: An attempt to release oneself from personal attachments when one is ill or aged

Common Etiology (Stressors)

DISEASES: Any serious

INJURIES: Any serious
SIGNS AND SYMPTOMS: Confusion, fatigue, memory loss, pain, vision loss, weakness
PSYCHOSOCIAL FACTORS: The exhaustion of adaptive reserves, the threat of deprivation of essential needs, the threat of severe (physiologic) stress, changes in needs
HEALTH CARE FACTORS: *Medical diagnosis*: An unfavorable medical diagnosis for oneself
DEVELOPMENTAL PHASES: Old age

PLANNING

Unmet Needs

Comfort, protection from psychologic threat, acceptance, caring and communicating relationships, less rigid conventiality

Expected Outcome

Person relates acceptance of his own disengagement behavior
Reengages when the level of wellness makes increased involvement possible

NURSING INTERVENTIONS

Nursing Treatments

Approach unhurriedly
Reassure verbally (that the nurse is available if needed)
Provide an atmosphere of acceptance
Encourage the expression of feelings (about the physical loss, about the decreased interest in the outside world, and the focus on himself)
Provide frequent contact with the person (so the person knows that the nurse is there)
Relate to the person on an adult–adult level, not on a parent–child level
Reduce the demands placed on the person (as much as possible)
Provide quiet (turn off the television and radio, if the person wishes such)
Restrict unwanted visitors (until the person is ready for visitors)

Nursing Observations

Observe for evidence of a favorable response to therapy (reengagement as health is restored)

Health Teaching

Explain (to the significant others) that the person's response is appropriate and commonly experienced

EVALUATION
Record actual outcome

Adaptive Responses to Role Relationships

ROLE CONFLICT RELATED TO A DEVELOPMENTAL PHASE [105,251,424,471,525]

ASSESSMENT

Data Collection

Subjective Data
• Person relates certain behaviors that are expected of a particular role by himself, others, or society
• Relates that the expected role behaviors are difficult to achieve or are not compatible with his needs

The adolescent relates the behavior he expects of himself as different from the behavior his parents expect of him

Grown children admit to expecting different behavior of an aged parent than the parent expects of himself

Objective Data

• May exhibit behavior such as avoiding or refusing to fulfill the role or trying to assume the role despite the conflict

The adolescent does not look for a job though his parents expect him to

The aged parent continues to work when the grown children think the parent should retire

Data Analysis

Nursing Diagnosis

ROLE CONFLICT RELATED TO A DEVELOPMENTAL PHASE: A difference between what individuals perceive their behavior should be at varying life stages

Common Etiology (Stressors)

PSYCHOSOCIAL FACTORS: Loss of a role, a threat to the person's self-concept, differences in the expected role behavior between two or more people, lack of knowledge about role expectations, lack of resources for role performance, differences in personal and social or cultural role expectations

DEVELOPMENTAL PHASES: Childhood, puberty, adolescence, young adulthood, middle age, old age

PLANNING

Unmet Needs

Comfort, protection from psychologic threat, acceptance, caring and communicating relationships, sense of adequacy, high evaluation of self, personal growth and maturity, increased learning, increased problem-solving ability

Expected Outcome

Person verbalizes feelings about the expected role behavior

Relates having arrived at a consistent set of expected role behaviors

Relates satisfaction as the person moves toward role modification

NURSING INTERVENTIONS

Nursing Treatments

Approach unhurriedly

Reassure verbally (that the nurse will assist the persons involved)

Provide an atmosphere of acceptance

Encourage the expression of feelings (about the role conflict)

Listen attentively

Offer feedback to the person's expressed feelings (to help the person recognize and deal with the conflict)

Communicate nurse sensitivity to the person's problem

Explore with the person his strengths and resources (for role achievement)

Encourage striving toward realistic goals (toward role responsibilities that one can achieve)

Encourage mutual problem solving (between persons involved in the role conflict)

Encourage decision making (about chosing one set of role behaviors over the other or about compromising the expected role behaviors with other persons involved)

Nursing Observations

Determine the degree of insight that the person has (into the role conflict)

Observe for an excessive stress level

Observe for evidence of a favorable response to therapy (consistentcy in defining the expected role behavior)

Health Teaching

Explain that the person's response is appropriate and commonly experienced

Explain the cause of the problem (different needs and expectations of the persons involved, individual limitations, circumstances)

Teach how to use the problem-solving method (to overcome the role conflict and move toward role modification)

EVALUATION

Record actual outcome

ROLE CONFLICT RELATED TO LOSS/GAIN OF A SIGNIFICANT OTHER[105,251,424,471,525]

ASSESSMENT

Data Collection

Subjective Data
- Person relates certain behaviors that are expected of a particular role by either himself, others, or society
- Relates that the expected role behaviors are difficult to achieve or are not compatible with his needs

  The new mother states that since her child's birth, her husband should help her with child care if he is to be a good father

  The recently widowed woman wants to begin actively socializing while her children want her to wait a year

Objective Data
- May exhibit behavior such as avoiding or refusing to fulfill the role or trying to assume the role despite the conflict

  The husband, and new father, will not participate in child care, but instead acts out his fatherhood by providing financial resources

  The recently widowed woman immediately begins socializing with male companions

Data Analysis

Nursing Diagnosis
ROLE CONFLICT RELATED TO LOSS/GAIN OF A SIGNIFICANT OTHER: A difference between what various individuals perceive their behavior should be when there is a role change because of the loss or gain of a significant other

Common Etiology (Stressors)
PSYCHOSOCIAL FACTORS: Loss of a role, a threat to the person's self-concept, differences in the expected role behavior between two or more people, lack of knowledge about role expectations, lack of resources for role performance

SITUATIONAL FACTORS: *Loss of a significant other*: Placing a child up for adoption, the death of a significant other, divorce of parents or from a spouse, launching grown children, retirement, separation from a significant other, the frequent change of foster parents, giving up a foster child. *Gain of a significant other*: Marriage, adoption of a child, childbirth, grandparenthood, a new family member (other than the above)

PLANNING

Unmet Needs

Comfort, protection from psychologic threat, acceptance, caring and communicating relationships, approval from others, sense of usefulness and adequacy, control over others or situations, personal growth and maturity, increased learning, increased reality perception and problem-solving ability

Expected Outcome

Person verbalizes feelings about the expected role behavior

Relates having arrived at a consistent set of expected role behaviors

Relates satisfaction as the person moves toward role modification

NURSING INTERVENTIONS

Nursing Treatments

Approach unhurriedly

Reassure verbally (that the nurse will assist whenever possible)

Provide an atmosphere of acceptance

Encourage the expression of feelings (about the role conflict)

Listen attentively

Offer feedback to the person's expressed feelings (to help the person recognize and deal with the conflict)

Communicate nurse sensitivity to the person's problem

Explore with the person his strengths and resources (for role achievement)

Encourage striving toward realistic goals (toward role responsibilities that he can achieve)

Encourage mutual problem solving (between persons involved in the role conflict)

Encourage decision making (about choosing one set of role behaviors over the other or about compromising the expected role behaviors with others persons involved)

Nursing Observations

Determine the degree of insight that the person has (into the role conflict)

Observe for an excessive stress level

Observe for evidence of a favorable response to therapy (consistency in defining the expected role behaviors)

Health Teaching

Explain that the person's response is appropriate and commonly experienced

Explain the cause of the problem (different needs and expectations of the persons involved, individual limitations and strengths)

Teach how to use the problem-solving method (to overcome the role conflict and move toward role modification)

EVALUATION

Record actual outcome

ROLE CONFLICT RELATED TO PHYSICAL LOSS/GAIN[105,251,424,471,525]

ASSESSMENT

Data Collection

Subjective Data

• Person relates certain behaviors that are expected of a particular role by either himself, others, or society

• Relates that the expected role behaviors are difficult to achieve or are not compatible with his needs

Person may state his physical limitations or the qualities of his renewed health

May relate that significant others expect him to assume responsibilities that he cannot or does not want to assume

May express concern about being expected to care for a significant other who has become ill

Objective Data

• May exhibit behavior such as avoiding or refusing to fulfill the role or trying to assume the role despite the conflict

A high school student who has had a cardiac valve disorder may not attend school full-time even though the heart has been repaired

A nurse who is hospitalized for an illness may be seen feeding the patient in the next bed

The spouse of an ill person may continually call the nurse to come and care for the ill person, when the spouse is expected to assume that responsibility

Data Analysis

Nursing Diagnosis

ROLE CONFLICT RELATED TO PHYSICAL LOSS/GAIN: A difference between what others perceive and what a person perceives his behavior should be when there is a loss or gain of physical health by himself or a significant other

Common Etiology (Stressors)

DISEASES: Any

INJURIES: Any

SIGNS AND SYMPTOMS: Fatigue, immobility, pain, weakness

PSYCHOSOCIAL FACTORS: A threat to the person's selfconcept, differences in the expected role behavior between two or more people, the threat of incompatible role demands, lack of knowledge about role expectations, lack of resources for role performance

HUMAN BODY: *Body function*: Loss of body function. *Body part*: Loss of a body part. *Body state*: Complicated pregnancy

HEALTH CARE FACTORS: *Health therapy*: Long-term or time-consuming therapy. *Health care procedures*: Having to perform health care

PLANNING

Unmet Needs

Comfort, protection from psychologic threat, acceptance, caring and communicating relationships, sense of usefulness and adequacy, control over others or situations, personal growth and maturity, increased learning, increased reality perception and problem-solving ability

Expected Outcome

Person verbalizes feelings about the expected role behavior

Relates having arrived at a consistent set of expected role behaviors

Relates satisfaction as the person moves toward role modification

NURSING INTERVENTIONS

Nursing Treatments

Approach unhurriedly

Reassure verbally (that the nurse will assist the persons involved)

Provide an atmosphere of acceptance

Encourage the expression of feelings (about the role conflict)

Listen attentively

Offer feedback to the person's expressed feelings (to help the person recognize and deal with the conflict)

Communicate nurse sensitivity to the person's problem

Explore with the person his strengths and resources (for role achievement)

Encourage striving toward realistic goals (toward role responsibilities that he can achieve)

Encourage mutual problem solving (between persons involved in the role conflict)

Encourage decision making (about choosing one set of role behaviors over the other or about compromising the expected role behaviors with others persons involved)

Nursing Observations

Determine the degree of insight that the person has (into the role conflict)

Observe for an excessive stress level

Observe for evidence of a favorable response to therapy (consistency in defining the expected role behaviors)

Health Teaching

Explain that the person's response is appropriate and commonly experienced

Explain the cause of the problem (different needs and expectations of the persons involved, individual limitations and strengths)

Teach how to use the problem-solving method (to overcome the role conflict and move toward role modification)

EVALUATION

Record actual outcome

ROLE MODIFICATION RELATED TO A DEVELOPMENTAL PHASE[471,524]

ASSESSMENT

Data Collection

Subjective Data

- Person recognizes changes in self or significant other that indicates a need for a role change
- Identifies the expected behaviors of the new or changed role
- May express awkwardness, uncertainty, or relief with the new role
  May express satisfaction as the new role becomes familiar
  Person may discuss factors regarding entry into a new developmental phase

Objective Data

- May exhibit behaviors such as learning new skills and abilities, performing new role behaviors, assuming new responsibilities as in adolescence and young adulthood, releasing responsibilities as in illness or old age

Data Analysis

Nursing Diagnosis

ROLE MODIFICATION RELATED TO A DEVELOPMENTAL PHASE: Adjusting to changes in the expected role behaviors specific to a person's responsibilities, position, or situation in life during stages of development through life

Common Etiology (Stressors)

PSYCHOSOCIAL FACTORS: An attempt to adjust to change

DEVELOPMENTAL PHASES: Puberty, adolescence, young adulthood, middle age, old age

PLANNING

Unmet Needs

Comfort, protection from psychologic threat, acceptance, caring and communicating relationships, approval from others, sense of usefulness and adequacy, high evaluation of self, mastery and competence in skills, personal growth and maturity, increased learning, increased problem-solving ability

Expected Outcome

Person verbalizes feelings about the role changes

Relates feeling comfortable with the new role

Successfully demonstrates new role skills and abilities

NURSING INTERVENTIONS

Nursing Treatments

Approach unhurriedly

Reassure verbally (that the nurse will assist whenever possible)

Provide an atmosphere of acceptance

Encourage the expression of feelings (about the new role)

Listen attentively

Offer feedback to the person's expressed feelings

Communicate nurse sensitivity to the person's problem

Encourage recognition of the person's various roles in life

Arrange situations that encourage patient autonomy (in choosing and performing the new role)

Encourage new skill development (appropriate to the role)

Provide temporary assistance until the skill is learned

Offer praise (for new skill development and role responsibility)

Explore with the person his strengths and resources (which make role modification easier)

Avoid forcing the person into rapid adaptation to change by accepting the person's unique pattern of adjustment

Encourage striving toward realistic goals

Introduce to persons who have successfully undergone the same experience (if appropriate)

Nursing Observations

Determine the degree of insight that the person has

Identify disturbing conversation topics (which might indicate the person is having difficulty modifying his role)

Observe for evidence that the person is reaching out for emotional support (frequent help-seeking, asking questions, seeking reassurance)

Observe for evidence of a favorable response to therapy (satisfaction with a new role)

Health Teaching

Explain that the person's response is appropriate and commonly experienced

Teach how to use the problem-solving method (specific to the situation)

Explain (to the family) that persons must make adjustments at their own pace

EVALUATION

Record actual outcome

ROLE MODIFICATION RELATED TO LOSS/GAIN OF A SIGNIFICANT OTHER[471,524]

ASSESSMENT

Data Collection

Subjective Data

• Person recognizes changes of loss or gain in significant others that indicate a need for a role change

• Identifies the expected behaviors of the new or changed role

• May express awkwardness, uncertainty, or relief with the new role

 May relate having more or less responsibility than previously

 The widow relates difficulty with the loss of the role of a spouse and the gain of the role of a single person

 The retired person conveys feelings about the loss of employment and the gain of a more sedentary role

The married woman relates adjustments to becoming a mother with the birth of a child

Person may express feelings of fear, anger, frustration or pleasure about the new situation

Objective Data

• May exhibit behavior such as learning new skills and abilities, performing new role behaviors

Data Analysis

Nursing Diagnosis

ROLE MODIFICATION RELATED TO LOSS/GAIN OF A SIGNIFICANT OTHER: Adjusting to changes in the expected role behaviors specific to a person's responsibilities, position, or situation in life after he has been parted from or has added another person to the significant persons in his life

Common Etiology (Stressors)

PSYCHOSOCIAL FACTORS: An attempt to adjust to change, change of a vital life role

SITUATIONAL FACTORS: *Loss of a significant other*: Placing a child up for adoption, the death of a significant other, divorce of parents or from a spouse, launching grown children, retirement, separation from a significant other, the frequent change of foster parents, giving up a foster child. *Gain of a significant other*: Marriage, adoption of a child, childbirth, grandparenthood, a new family member (other than the above)

PLANNING

Unmet Needs

Comfort, protection from psychologic threat, acceptance, caring and communicating relationships, approval from others, sense of usefulness and adequacy, high evaluation of self, mastery and competence in skills, personal growth and maturity, increased learning, increased problem-solving ability

Expected Outcome

Person verbalizes feelings about the role changes

Relates feeling comfortable with the new role

Successfully demonstrates new role skills and abilities

NURSING INTERVENTIONS

Nursing Treatments

Approach unhurriedly

Reassure verbally (that the nurse will assist whenever possible)

Provide an atmosphere of acceptance

Encourage the expression of feelings (about the new role)

Listen attentively

Offer feedback to the person's expressed feelings

Communicate nurse sensitively to the person's problem

Encourage recognition of the persons various roles in life

Arrange situations that encourage the person's autonomy (in the new role)

Encourage new skills development (appropriate to the role)

Provide temporary assistance until the skill is learned

Offer praise (for new skill development and role responsibility)

Explore with the person his strengths and resources (which are available to help him modify the role)

Avoid forcing the person into rapid adaptation to change by accepting the person's unique pattern of adjustment

Encourage striving toward realistic goals

Introduce to persons who have successfully undergone the same experience (if appropriate)

Nursing Observations

Determine the degree of insight that the person has

Identify disturbing conversation topics

Observe for evidence that the person is reaching out for emotional support (frequent help seeking, asking questions, seeking reassurance)

Observe for evidence of a favorable response to therapy (satisfaction with the new role)

Health Teaching

Explain that the person's response is appropriate and commonly experienced

Teach how to use the problem-solving method (specific to the situation)

Explain (to the family) that persons must make adjustments at their own pace

EVALUATION

Record actual outcome

ROLE MODIFICATION RELATED TO PHYSICAL LOSS/GAIN[471,524]

ASSESSMENT

Data Collection

Subjective Data

• Person recognizes physical changes in self or significant other that indicate a need for a role change

• Identifies the expected behaviors of the new or changed role

• May express awkwardness, uncertainty, or relief with the new role

  Acknowledges that with physical loss, responsibilities are usually decreased and with physical gain, the expected responsibilities are increased

  May express feelings of anger, frustration, or fear about the new situation

Objective Data

• May exhibit behavior such as learning new skills and abilities, performing new role behaviors, assuming new responsibilities, releasing responsibilities

Data Analysis

Nursing Diagnosis

ROLE MODIFICATION RELATED TO PHYSICAL LOSS/GAIN: Adjusting to changes in the expected role behaviors specific to a persons responsibilities, position, or situation in life following the loss or gain of a balanced state of health by the person or a significant other

Common Etiology (Stressors)

Physical Loss

DISEASES: Any

INJURIES: Any

SIGNS AND SYMPTOMS: Immobility, pain, weakness

PSYCHOSOCIAL FACTORS: Loss of a role, an attempt to adjust to change, loss of independence or self-sufficiency

HUMAN BODY: *Body function*: Loss of body function. *Body part*: Loss of body part

HEALTH CARE FACTORS: *Health therapy*: Frequent, long-term or time-consuming therapy. *Medical therapy*: Hemodialysis, radiation therapy, rehabilitation therapy. *Drug therapy*: Chemotherapy. *Adverse effects of medical, drug, or surgical therapy*: Loss of a body part (from an amputation, enucleation or evisceration of an eyeball, hemipelvectomy, hysterectomy, ileotomy, prostatectomy), loss of natural elimination and elimination control (from colostomy, ileocolostomy, ileostomy, ureterocolostomy, ureteroileostomy, ureterosigmoidostomy, ureterostomy, ureterotomy), loss of normal food intake (from esophagectomy), loss of reproductive ability (from fallopian tube ligation, hysterectomy, oophorectomy, orchidectomy, prostatectomy, salpingectomy, vasectomy), loss of speech from glossectomy, laryngectomy, tracheostomy, vocal cordectomy), loss of vision (from enucleation or evisceration of eyeball). *Therapeutic equipment*: Use of a wheelchair, walker, or pacemaker (which may limit places the person can go), brace, cane, crutches, hemodialyzer (limits personal freedom), respirator

SITUATIONAL FACTORS: Acute, chronic, or terminal illness

Physical Gain

PSYCHOSOCIAL FACTORS: An attempt to adjust to change, the threat of forced adaptation to change from a dependent to an independent role (e.g., repaired cardiac defect) or from being socially undesirable to desirable (e.g., plastic reconstruction or repair)

HEALTH CARE FACTORS: *Health therapy*: Successful. *Drug therapy*: Curative or controlling effects of drug therapy. *Medical therapy*: Psychotherapy, rehabilitation therapy, speech therapy, withdrawal from alcohol, drugs, or tobacco. *Surgical procedures*: Arterial bypass, cosmetic operation, craniofacial surgery, reconstruction procedure, transplantation of bone, cornea, hair, kidney, liver, heart, muscle

PLANNING

Unmet Needs

Comfort, protection from psychologic threat, acceptance, caring and communicating relationships, approval from others, sense of usefulness and adequacy, high evaluation of self, mastery and competence in skills, personal growth and maturity, increased learning, increased problem-solving ability

Expected Outcome

Person verbalizes feelings about the role changes
Relates feeling comfortable with the new role
Successfully demonstrates the new role skills and abilities

NURSING INTERVENTIONS

Nursing Treatments

Approach unhurriedly
Reassure verbally (that the nurse will assist whenever possible)
Provide an atmosphere of acceptance
Encourage the expression of feelings (about the new role)
Listen attentively
Offer feedback to the person's expressed feelings
Communicate nurse sensitivity to the person's problem
Encourage recognition of the person's various roles in life
Arrange situations that encourage the person's autonomy (in developing the new role)
Encourage the acceptance of interdependency, the acceptance of self-limitations (if the role results from a physical loss)
Encourage new skill development (appropriate to the role)
Provide temporary assistance until the skill is learned
Offer praise (for new skill development and role responsibility)
Explore with the person his strengths and resources (available to help him modify the role)
Avoid forcing the person into rapid adaptation to change by accepting the person's unique pattern of adjustment
Encourage striving toward realistic goals
Introduce to persons who have successfully undergone the same experience (if appropriate)

Nursing Observations

Determine the degree of insight that the person has

Identify disturbing conversation topics (which might indicate the person is having difficulty modifying his role)

Observe for evidence that the person is reaching out for emotional support (frequent
help seeking, asking questions, seeking reassurance)

Observe for evidence of a favorable response to therapy (satisfactory role modification)

Health Teaching

Explain that the person's response is appropriate and commonly experienced

Teach how to use the problem-solving method (specific to the situation)

Explain (to the family) that persons must make adjustments at their own pace

EVALUATION

Record actual outcome

FAMILY ROLE MODIFICATION RELATED TO A DISRUPTED LIFESTYLE[471,524]

ASSESSMENT

Data Collection

Subjective Data

• Family recognizes changes in a significant other that indicate a need for a role change

• Identifies the expected behaviors of the new or changed role

• Family members may express awkwardness, uncertainty, or relief with the new role
  May complain that some family members are duplicating or omitting expected behaviors
  Family relates that the disrupted usual life routine is difficult

Objective Data

• Family members may exhibit behavior such as learning new skills and abilities, performing new role behaviors

Data Analysis

Nursing Diagnosis

FAMILY ROLE MODIFICATION RELATED TO A DISRUPTED LIFESTYLE: Adjusting to changes in the
expected role behaviors specific to a family's responsibilities, position, or situation in
life after the normal life routine has been thrown into disarray

Common Etiology (Stressors)

BIRTH DEFECTS: Premature or imperfect infant, any birth defect of a new infant

DISEASE: Any disease of a family member

INJURIES: Any injury of a family member

PSYCHOSOCIAL FACTORS: An attempt to adjust to change

HEALTH CARE FACTORS: *Health care procedures for significant other*: Having to perform health
care procedures for a significant other. *Hospitalization*: Of significant other. *Health therapy*: Long-term or time-consuming therapy, transporting a significant other to health
therapy. *Visiting hours*: Limited and restrictive visiting hours

LIFESTYLE: A change of social status, changes that occur when a mother becomes
employed

SITUATIONAL FACTORS: The death of a significant other, marital separation or divorce from
a spouse or of parents, a new family member, illness of or injury to a significant other, reconciliation of a marriage, retirement of a family member, extensive travel by a
significant other

PLANNING

Unmet Needs

Comfort, protection from psychologic threat, acceptance, caring and communicating relationships, approval from others, sense of usefulness and adequacy, high evaluation of self, mastery and competence in skills, personal growth and maturity, increased learning, increased problem-solving ability

Expected Outcome

Family verbalizes feelings about the role change
Family relates feeling comfortable with the new role
Family succesfully demonstrates new role skills and abilities

NURSING INTERVENTIONS

Nursing Treatments

Approach unhurriedly
Reassure verbally (that the nurse will assist whenever possible)
Provide an atmosphere of acceptance
Encourage the expression of feelings (about the new role)
Listen attentively
Talk with the family
Offer feedback to the person's expressed feelings
Communicate nurse sensitivity to the person's problem
Encourage recognition of everyone's various roles in life
Arrange situations that encourage family autonomy (in the new role)
Encourage the acceptance of interdependency, the acceptance of self-limitations (among family members)
Encourage new skill development (appropriate to the role)
Provide temporary assistance until the skill is learned
Assist the family to restructure their lifestyle
Offer praise (for new skill development and role responsibility)
Explore with the family their strengths and resources (which are available to help them modify the roles)
Avoid forcing the family into rapid adaptation to change by accepting the family's unique pattern of adjustment
Encourage striving toward realistic goals
Encourage family-shared responsibilities
Introduce to persons who have successfully undergone the same experience (if appropriate)

Nursing Observations

Determine the degree of insight that the family has
Identify disturbing conversation topics
Observe for evidence that the family is reaching out for emotional support (frequent help seeking, asking questions, seeking reassurance)
Observe for evidence of a favorable response to therapy (successful adaptation to the new role)

Health Teaching

Explain that the family's response is appropriate and commonly experienced
Recommend new options for effective methods of coping (reassessment of the roles of family members)
Teach how to use the problem-solving method (specific to the situation)
Explain (to the family) that persons must make adjustments at their own pace

EVALUATION

Record actual outcome

Adaptive Responses in Self-Esteem (Self-Worth, Self-Ideal)

LOW SELF-ESTEEM RELATED TO ADAPTIVE BEHAVIOR CHANGE[105,471]

ASSESSMENT

Data Collection

Subjective Data
• Person relates certain unfulfilled expectations of self regarding behavior
• Makes self-depreciating remarks or is highly critical of others
Relates a current life crisis or illness
Is aware that his behavior is unusual for him
Relates preoccupation with self, indulgence in self-pity, moodiness, calling for help, giving less time and concern to significant others, releasing responsibility to others
May ask "What's wrong with me?"

Objective Data
• May exhibit behavior such as avoiding interaction with others, apologizing for adaptive behavior, unusual quietness

Data Analysis

Nursing Diagnosis
LOW SELF-ESTEEM RELATED TO ADAPTIVE BEHAVIOR CHANGE: Having feelings of negative self-worth when one exhibits behavior that would be considered acceptable during periods of adjustment to life crises or illness but would be considered unacceptable under normal circumstances

Common Etiology (Stressors)
DISEASES: Any
INJURIES: Any
SIGNS AND SYMPTOMS: Any but especially pain, weakness
PSYCHOSOCIAL FACTORS: The threat of inadequacy, failure to achieve unreasonable expectations of self or a significant other
HUMAN BODY: *Body appearance*: A disfigured body. *Body function*: Loss of body function. *Body part*: Loss of a body part. *Body states*: Climacteric, menopause, menstruation, pregnancy
HEALTH CARE FACTORS: *Diagnostic procedures*: Extensive or painful diagnostic procedures. *Medical diagnosis*: An unfavorable diagnosis. *Medical therapy*: Painful or prolonged therapy. *Surgical procedures*: Painful or frequent surgical procedures. *Adverse effects of medical or drug therapy*: Loss of libido from antihypertensive drugs, Tagamet, and hemodialysis, irritability from epinephrine and thyroid preparations, moodiness and weeping from hormone therapy. *Hospital discharge*: Any. *Convalescence*: Any
DEVELOPMENTAL PHASES: Puberty, adolescence, old age
SITUATIONAL FACTORS: Multiple crisis situations, the death of a significant other, the experience of dying, divorce or marital separation from a spouse or of parents, illness of or injury to self or a significant other, multiple births (twins, triplets, etc.)

PLANNING

Unmet Needs

Comfort, protection from psychologic threat, acceptance, caring and communicating relationships, high evaluation of self, sense of adequacy, personal growth and maturity, increased learning, increased reality perception and problem-solving ability

Expected Outcome

Person verbalizes feelings about self

Sets realistic expectations for self

Expresses satisfaction with having met the realistic expectations

Speaks of self in positive terms

NURSING INTERVENTIONS

Nursing Treatments

Approach unhurriedly

Reassure verbally (that the behavior is normal and to be expected)

Provide an atmosphere of acceptance

Encourage the expression of feelings (about his low self-esteem)

Listen attentively

Offer feedback to the person's expressed feelings

Communicate nurse sensitivity to the person's problem

Relate to the person on an adult–adult level, not on a parent–child level (which could reduce self-esteem)

Explore with the person his value as an individual

Explore with the person his positive characteristics

Encourage the acceptance of self-limitations

Encourage an awareness of positive responses from others

Explore with the person his strengths and resources

Explore with the person the reasons for self-criticism

Support a realistic assessment of the situation (that severe stress changes his usual behavioral responses)

Nursing Observations

Determine the degree of insight that the person has

Evaluate the person's relatedness with others (which may reflect his feelings about himself)

Identify disturbing conversation topics

Identify life values significant to the person (which could affect self-esteem)

Observe for evidence that the person is reaching out for emotional support

Observe for evidence of a favorable response to therapy (positive self-attitudes)

Health Teaching

Explain that the person's reponse is appropriate and commonly experienced

Advise that negative responses from others be regarded with minimum significance (even though there are feelings about such responses)

Instruct to avoid self-defeating thoughts (such as failing to forgive oneself for being human, thinking negatively about one's worth)

Advise that significant persons express acceptance of one another (despite changes in behavior)

Explain the importance of person's offering support to one another

Explain the importance of maintaining a positive self-attitude

Relate ways the person can enhance his self-image (making decisions and being responsible for self, accepting all of his feelings as part of the self)

Explain that ill persons are often hypersensitive

EVALUATION

Record actual outcome

LOW SELF-ESTEEM RELATED TO HEALTH CARE/THERAPY/DEVICES[105,207,471]

ASSESSMENT

Data Collection

Subjective Data
* Person relates certain unfilled expectations of self
* Makes self-depreciating remarks or is highly critical of others
  Relates feeling that the health care or therapy has in some way lessened his worth
  May verbalize negatively about the care or therapy

Objective Data
* May exhibit behavior such as avoiding interaction with others, avoiding participation in care or therapy, avoiding the use of devices, crying, angry outbursts, demanding and controlling behavior

Data Analysis

Nursing Diagnosis
LOW SELF-ESTEEM RELATED TO HEALTH CARE/THERAPY/DEVICES: Having feelings of negative self-worth resulting from the effects of or attitudes about health care or specific types of therapy

Common Etiology (Stressors)
PSYCHOSOCIAL FACTORS: The threat of inadequacy, loss of a valued concept of self, the threat of being overly controlled or restricted, failure to achieve unreasonable expectations of self or a significant other

HEALTH CARE FACTORS: *Health care environment*: Locked psychiatric unit, isolation unit, lack of privacy, *Health care provider*: Nonprivate discussion of health care matters by the health care provider, suggestion by a health care provider that symptoms are not real or that the condition is the result of the person's inadequacy. *Hospitalization/institutionalization*: Any. *Institutional policies*: Restrictive institutional policies. *Welfare or human resources services*: Dehumanizing welfare services. *Diagnostic procedures*: Undignified positioning for diagnostic procedure, prediagnostic bowel preparation with purgatives or cathartics that cause incontinence, specific procedures such as barium enema, colonoscopy, cystoscopy, voiding cystourethrography, Pap smear, pelvic examinations, proctoscopy, proctosigmoidoscopy, or urinary catheterization. *Health therapy*: Unsuccessful or ineffective medical, drug, or surgical therapy. *Medical therapy*: Therapeutic diet limitations that are visible when eating outside the home, enemas, gastrostomy or jejunostomy feedings, psychotherapy. *Drug therapy*: The need to use life-maintenance drugs such as insulin, cortisone, thyroid drugs, or cardiac drugs or the use of pain medication. *Surgical therapy*: Anesthesia for childbirth. *Surgical procedures*: Many, including cesarean section. *Adverse effects of medical, drug, or surgical therapy*: Loss of a body part (from an amputation, enucleation or evisceration of an eyeball, hemipelvectomy, hysterectomy, ileotomy, mastectomy, prostatectomy), loss of hair (from chemotherapy and radiation therapy), loss of natural elimination and elimination control (from a colostomy, ileocolostomy, ileostomy, ureterocolostomy, ureteroileostomy, ureterosigmoidostomy, ureterostomy, ureterotomy), loss of normal food intake (from an esophagectomy), loss of the reproductive ability (from a fallopian tube ligation, hysterectomy, oophorectomy, orchidectomy, prostatectomy, salpingectomy, vasectomy), loss of speech (from a glossectomy, laryngectomy, tracheostomy, vocal cordectomy), loss of vision (from an enucleation or evisceration of an eyeball), loss of libido (from antihypertensive drugs), hesitancy of urination (from anticholenergic drugs). *Therapeutic equipment*: Use of an artificial eye or limb, bedpan, bedside commode, brace, breast prosthesis, cane, cannula for hemodialysis, cardiac pacemaker, urinary catheter, crutches, dentures, dental bridge, eyeglasses, hearing aid, hemodialyzer, therapeutic tubes, urinal, walker, or wheelchair

PLANNING

Unmet Needs
Comfort, protection from psychologic threat, acceptance, caring and communicating relationships, high evaluation of self, sense of adequacy, personal growth and maturity, increased learning, increased reality perception and problem-solving ability

Expected Outcome
Person verbalizes feelings about self
Sets realistic expectations for self
Expresses satisfaction with having met the realistic expectations
Speaks of self in positive terms

NURSING INTERVENTIONS

Nursing Treatments
Approach unhurriedly
Reassure verbally (that the nurse will treat the person with dignity)
Provide an atmosphere of acceptance
Encourage the expression of feelings (about the person's low self-esteem)
Listen attentively
Offer feedback to the person's expressed feelings
Communicate nurse sensitivity to the person's problem
Relate to the person on an adult–adult level, not on a parent–child level (which could reduce self-esteem)
Explore with the person his value as an individual
Explore with the person his positive characteristics
Encourage the acceptance of self-limitations
Encourage an awareness of positive responses from others
Explore with the person his strengths and resources
Explore with the person the reasons for self-criticism
Support a realistic assessment of the situation (that therapy, though unpleasant, is offered because the individual is a person of worth)
Avoid forcing the person into rapid adaptation to change by accepting the person's unique pattern of adjustment
Provide privacy (in situations that tend to reduce self-esteem)

Nursing Observations
Determine the degree of insight that the person has
Evaluate the person's relatedness with others (which may affect self-esteem)
Identify disturbing conversation topics
Identify life values significant to the person (which affect the level of esteem)
Observe for impaired self-attitudes (which lead to loss of self-esteem)
Observe for evidence that the person is reaching out for emotional support
Observe for evidence of a favorable response to therapy (positive self-attitudes)

Health Teaching
Explain that the person's response is appropriate and commonly experienced
Advise that negative responses from others be regarded with minimum significance (even though there are feelings about such responses)
Instruct to avoid self-defeating thoughts (such as thinking negatively about one's worth, thinking of oneself as "poor me")
Advise that significant persons express acceptance of one another
Explain the importance of persons offering support to one another
Explain the importance of maintaining a positive self-attitude
Relate ways the person can enhance his self-image (making decisions for self, assuming responsibility for his actions, being as independent as possible during therapy)

Explain that ill persons are often hypersensitive (to comments that they interpret as criticism, resulting in lowered self-esteem)

EVALUATION

Record actual outcome

LOW SELF-ESTEEM RELATED TO LOSS OF EMOTIONAL CONTROL[105,471]

ASSESSMENT

Data Collection

Subjective Data
- Person relates certain unfulfilled expectations of self regarding emotional control
- Makes self-depreciating remarks or is highly critical of others
  Relates being consumed with intense feelings
  Relates having openly expressed feelings of anger, grief, anxiety, fear, helplessness, etc.

Objective Data
- May exhibit behavior such as avoiding interaction with others, apologizing for loss of emotional control, unusual quietness

Data Analysis

Nursing Diagnosis
LOW SELF-ESTEEM RELATED TO LOSS OF EMOTIONAL CONTROL: Having feelings of negative self-worth for allowing oneself to give in to impulse and for being unable to control the expression of intense feelings .

Common Etiology (Stressors)
DISEASES: Any but especially alcoholism, drug addiction
INJURIES: Any
SIGNS AND SYMPTOMS: Pain, weakness
PSYCHOSOCIAL FACTORS: Failure to achieve unreasonable expectations of self or a significant other
HUMAN BODY: *Natural body function*: Pain of childbirth. *Body states*: Pregnancy
HEALTH CARE FACTORS: *Diagnostic procedures*: Extensive or painful. *Medical Diagnosis*: An unfavorable medical diagnosis. *Medical therapy*: Painful or prolonged. *Surgical procedures*: Painful or frequent
SITUATIONAL FACTORS: Multiple crisis situations, the death of a significant other, the experience of dying, divorce or marital separation from a spouse or of parents, illness of or injury to self or a significant other, child rearing

PLANNING

Unmet Needs
Comfort, protection from psychologic threat, acceptance, caring and communicating relationships, high evaluation of self, sense of adequacy, personal growth and maturity, increased learning, increased reality perception and problem-solving ability

Expected Outcome
Person verbalizes feelings about self
Sets realistic expectations for self
Expresses satisfaction with having met the realistic expectations
Speaks of self in positive terms

NURSING INTERVENTIONS

Nursing Treatments

Approach unhurriedly

Reassure verbally (that the behavior is normal)

Provide an atmosphere of acceptance

Encourage the expression of feelings (about the person's low self-esteem)

Listen attentively

Offer feedback to the person's expressed feelings

Communicate nurse sensitivity to the person's problem

Relate to the person on an adult–adult level, not on a parent–child level (which could reduce self-esteem)

Explore with the person his value as an individual

Explore with the person his positive characteristics

Encourage the acceptance of self-limitations

Encourage an awareness of positive responses from others

Explore with the person his strengths and resources

Explore with the person the reasons for self-criticism

Support a realistic assessment of the situation (that stress can cause loss of emotional control)

Nursing Observations

Determine the degree of insight that the person has

Evaluate the person's relatedness with others (which may affect self-esteem)

Identify disturbing conversation topics

Identify life values significant to the person

Observe for impaired self-attitudes (which lead to loss of self-esteem)

Observe for evidence that the person is reaching out for emotional support

Observe for evidence of a favorable response to therapy (positive self-attitudes)

Health Teaching

Explain that the person's response is appropriate and commonly experienced

Instruct to avoid self-defeating thoughts (such as failing to forgive oneself for human error)

Advise that negative responses from others be regarded with minimum significance (even though there are feelings about such responses)

Advise that significant persons express acceptance of one another (despite the loss of emotional control)

Explain the importance of persons offering support to one another

Explain the importance of maintaining a positive self-attitude

Relate ways the person can enhance self-image (accepting all of his feelings as part of the self and maintaining control of feelings, which heightens the ego)

EVALUATION

Record actual outcome

LOW SELF-ESTEEM RELATED TO NATURAL BODY CHANGES[105,471]

ASSESSMENT

Data Collection

Subjective Data

• Person relates certain unfulfilled expectations of self

• Makes self-depreciating remarks or is highly critical of others

A youth or adult perceives his body as less than that of others

Relates perceiving body changes during growth as threatening

If body changes vary from the norm, the youth dislikes himself intensely

Middle-aged or older persons may relate discontent with a change in muscle tone, stature, hair color, etc.

Person is not experiencing an illness

Objective Data
• May exhibit behavior such as unkept appearance, poor posture, avoiding interaction with others, demanding and controlling behavior, underachieving, covering up a body part

Data Analysis

Nursing Diagnosis

LOW SELF-ESTEEM RELATED TO NATURAL BODY CHANGES: Having feelings of negative self-worth from body changes that normally occur during developmental stages and that change the body's external appearance

Common Etiology (Stressors)

PSYCHOSOCIAL FACTORS: A lack of affection or appreciation from significant others, failure to achieve unreasonable expectations of self or a significant other, the threat of inadequacy

HUMAN BODY: *Body appearance*: Appearance changes during puberty, body changes that seem different from changes in the bodies of peers. *Body size*: Changes in body size during growth. *Body states*: The onset of menstruation, menopause, climacteric

DEVELOPMENTAL PHASES: Puberty, adolescence, middle age, old age, nonoccurrence of or complications of developmental stages or changes

PLANNING

Unmet Needs

Comfort, protection from psychologic threat, acceptance, caring and communicating relationships, high evaluation of self, sense of adequacy, personal growth and maturity, increased learning, increased reality perception and problem-solving ability

Expected Outcome

Person verbalizes feelings about self

Sets realistic expectations for self

Expresses satisfaction with having met the realistic expectations

Speaks of self in positive terms

NURSING INTERVENTIONS

Nursing Treatments

Approach unhurriedly

Reassure verbally (that the body changes are normal and desirable)

Provide an atmosphere of acceptance

Encourage the expression of feelings (about the person's low self-esteem)

Listen attentively

Offer feedback to the person's expressed feelings

Communicate nurse sensitivity to the person's problem

Relate to the person on an adult–adult level, not on a parent–child level (which could reduce self-esteem)

Explore with the person his value as an individual

Explore with the person his normal characteristics (and that developmental changes are normal)

Encourage the acceptance of self-limitations

Encourage an awareness of positive responses from others

Explore with the person his strengths and resources

Explore with the person the reasons for self-criticism

Support a realistic assessment of the situation (that changes in body appearance do not affect self-worth)

Avoid forcing the person into rapid adaptation to change by accepting the person's unique pattern of adjustment

Nursing Observations

Determine the degree of insight that the person has

Evaluate the person's relatedness with others (which may affect self-esteem)

Identify disturbing conversation topics

Identify life values significant to the person

Observe for evidence that the person is reaching out for emotional support

Observe for evidence of a favorable response to therapy (positive self-attitudes)

Health Teaching

Explain that the person's response is appropriate and commonly experienced

Advise that negative responses from others be regarded with minimum significance (even though there are feelings about such responses)

Advise that significant persons express acceptance of one another

Explain the importance of persons offering support to one another

Explain the importance of maintaining a positive self-attitude

Instruct to avoid self-defeating thoughts (such as failing to forgive oneself for being human, thinking negatively about one's worth, thinking of oneself as "poor me")

Relate ways the person can enhance his self-image (accepting all of his physiologic changes or limitations as part of the self, being independent as much as possible)

Explain that adolescents, etc., are often hypersensitive (to comments or situations that might cause decreased self-esteem)

EVALUATION

Record actual outcome

LOW SELF-ESTEEM RELATED TO PHYSICAL LOSS

ASSESSMENT

Data Collection

Subjective Data

• Person relates certain unfulfilled expectations of self

• Makes self-depreciating remarks or is highly critical of others

Relates perceiving his sick body as no longer measuring up to the standards by which it can be considered an object of value

May relate that since his body is part of what makes up his total being, he is a person of less value than he was before the illness

May state that others perceive him with less respect because of his illness

Relates being sensitive to comments by others about the illness

Is quick to enumerate the strengths of others

Is preoccupied with his own weakness

Objective Data

• May exhibit behavior such as having an unkempt appearance, avoiding interaction with others, crying, demanding and controlling behavior, underachieving

Data Analysis

Nursing Diagnosis

LOW SELF-ESTEEM RELATED TO PHYSICAL LOSS: Having feelings of negative self-worth from the loss of a balanced state of health

Common Etiology (Stressors)
DISEASES: Any
INJURIES: Any
SIGNS AND SYMPTOMS: Belching (eructation), confusion, drooling, edema, immobility, incontinence, jaundice, memory loss, pain, paralysis, rash, tremors, weakness, weight loss or gain
PSYCHOSOCIAL FACTORS The threat of inadequacy, a lack of affection or appreciation from significant others, a lack of encouragement and motivation toward independence, the threat of being overly controlled or restricted, failure to achieve unreasonable expectations of self or a significant other, the threat of repeated failure to achieve
HUMAN BODY: *Body appearance*: Changes in body appearance, a disfigured body. *Body function*: Loss of body function. *Body part*: Loss of a body part. *Body states*: Loss of the prepregnancy body
DEVELOPMENTAL PHASES: Any but especially old age
SITUATIONAL FACTORS: Childlessness or acute, chronic, disabling, terminal, or socially unacceptable illness

PLANNING

Unmet Needs
Comfort, protection from phychologic threat, acceptance, caring and communicating relationships, high evaluation of self, sense of adequacy, personal growth and maturity, increased learning, increased reality perception and problem-solving ability

Expected Outcome
Person verbalizes feelings about self
Sets realistic expectations for self
Expresses satisfaction with having met the realistic expectations
Speaks of self in positive terms

NURSING INTERVENTIONS

Nursing Treatments
Approach unhurriedly
Reassure verbally (that illness does not change a person's worth)
Provide an atmosphere of acceptance
Encourage the expression of feelings (about the person's low self-esteem)
Listen attentively
Offer feedback to the person's expressed feelings
Communicate nurse sensitivity to the person's problem
Relate to the person on an adult–adult level, not on a parent–child level (which could reduce self-esteem)
Explore with the person his value as an individual
Explore with the person his positive characteristics
Encourage the acceptance of self-limitations
Encourage an awareness of positive responses from others
Explore with the person his strengths and resources
Explore with the person the reasons for self-criticism
Explore with the person the need for approval
Support a realistic assessment of the situation (that the individual is a person of worth because he is a human being)
Avoid forcing the person into rapid adaptation to change by accepting the person's unique pattern of adjustment

Nursing Observations
Determine the degree of insight that the person has
Evaluate the person's relatedness with others (which may affect self-esteem)
Identify disturbing conversation topics
Identify life values significant to the person

Observe for evidence that the person is reaching out for emotional support
Observe for evidence of a favorable response to therapy (positive self-attitudes)

Health Teaching

Explain that the person's response is appropriate and commonly experienced
Advise that negative responses from others be regarded with minimum significance (even though there are feelings about such responses)
Advise that significant persons express acceptance of one another
Explain the importance of persons offering support to one another
Explain the importance of maintaining a positive self-attitude
Instruct to avoid self-defeating thoughts (such as failing to forgive oneself for being human, thinking negatively about one's worth, thinking of oneself as "poor me")
Relate ways the person can enhance his self-image (making decisions for and being responsible for self, accepting all of his physical limitations as a part of the self)
Explain that ill persons are often hypersensitive (about the physical loss, resulting in decreased self-esteem)

EVALUATION

Record actual outcome

LOW SELF-ESTEEM RELATED TO UNATTAINED GOALS[105,279,471]

ASSESSMENT

Data Collection

Subjective Data
- Person relates certain unfulfilled expectations of self
- Makes self-depreciating remarks or is highly critical of others
  Relates having set health goals that were not reached, having had life dreams that were never realized
  May express feelings that opportunity is forever lost

Objective Data
- May exhibit behavior such as having an unkempt appearance, having poor posture, avoiding interaction with others, apologizing unnecessarily, demanding and controlling behavior, crying

Data Analysis

Nursing Diagnosis
LOW SELF-ESTEEM RELATED TO UNFULFILLED GOALS: Having feelings of negative self-worth for not having achieved goals set for oneself

Common Etiology (Stressors)
PSYCHOSOCIAL FACTORS: A lack of affection or appreciation from significant others, lack of encouragement and motivation toward independence, the threat of being overly controlled or restricted, failure to achieve unreasonable expectations of self or a significant other, the threat of an unusually successful significant other (usually siblings or parents), the threat of repeated failure to achieve, lack of meaning and purpose in one's life, lack of freedom in self-direction, exposure to negative attitudes of a significant other (usually parents), lack of self-reinforcement of positive self-attitudes

HEALTH CARE FACTORS: *Health therapy*: Unsuccessful or ineffective health therapy, controlling but not curative effects of therapy, lack of follow-through with prescribed therapy
DEVELOPMENTAL PHASES: Any but especially old age
SITUATIONAL FACTORS: Being unable to adopt a child, a divorce or marital separation from a spouse, retirement, failure in school, demotion or loss of employment

PLANNING

Unmet Needs
Comfort, protection from psychologic threat, acceptance, caring and communicating relationships, high evaluation of self, sense of adequacy, personal growth and maturity, increased learning, increased reality perception and problem-solving ability

Expected Outcome
Person verbalizes feelings about self
Sets realistic expectations for self
Expresses satisfaction with having met the realistic expectations
Speaks of self in positive terms

NURSING INTERVENTIONS

Nursing Treatments
Approach unhurriedly
Reassure verbally (that the nurse will help him set and reach realistic goals)
Provide an atmosphere of acceptance
Encourage the expression of feelings (about the person's low self-esteem)
Listen attentively
Offer feedback to the person's expressed feelings
Communicate nurse sensitivity to the person's problem
Relate to the person on an adult–adult level, not on a parent–child level (which could reduce self-esteem)
Explore with the person his value as an individual (that the individual is a person of worth because he is a human being, not because of goals attained)
Encourage the acceptance of self-limitations
Encourage an awareness of positive responses from others
Explore with the person his strength and resources
Explore with the person the reasons for self-criticism
Support a realistic assessment of the situation (that all goals are not attainable)
Encourage the acceptance of partial goal satisfaction

Nursing Observations
Determine the degree of insight that the person has
Evaluate the person's relatedness with others (which may affect self-esteem)
Identify disturbing conversation topics
Identify life values significant to the person
Observe for evidence that the person is reaching out for emotional support
Observe for evidence of a favorable response to therapy (positive self-attitudes)

Health Teaching
Explain that the person's response is appropriate and commonly experienced
Advise that negative responses from others be regarded with minimum significance (even though there are feelings about such responses)
Advise that significant persons express acceptance of one another
Explain the importance of persons offering support to one another
Explain the importance of maintaining a positive self-attitude
Instruct to avoid self-defeating thoughts (such as belittling oneself for nonaccomplishments)

Relate ways the person can enhance his self-image (assuming responsibility for his actions, accepting all of his limitations as part of the self)

EVALUATION

Record actual outcome

Adaptive Responses in Self-Identity/ Self-Image

THREATENED BODY IMAGE RELATED TO NATURAL BODY CHANGES[105,471,525,704]

ASSESSMENT

Data Collection

Subjective Data
- Person relates a change in body sensation, size, function, or appearance
- Verbalizes that the body is different than before
- Expresses feeling threatened by the change
  Person is not experiencing an illness
  May feel uncomfortable with body changes during puberty such as developing breasts and genitalia, appearance of body hair, etc.
  Experiences a sense of imbalance as the body heightens during periods of natural growth or enlarges during pregnancy

Objective Data
- Person has visible or verifiable body changes
- May exhibit behavior such as avoiding looking at or touching the body part, facial expressions of displeasure when viewing the body, attempting to cover up body changes by wearing loose blouses during breast development or using hair dyes for graying hair, etc.

Data Analysis

Nursing Diagnosis
THREATENED BODY IMAGE RELATED TO NATURAL BODY CHANGES: Feeling endangered by changes in the body that normally occur during life and developmental stages and that alter one's concept of the body

Common Etiology (Stressors)
PSYCHOSOCIAL FACTORS: The loss of a valued concept of the self (about body appearance and boundaries where the body leaves off and the environment begins)
HUMAN BODY: *Body Appearance*: Appearance changes during puberty, body changes that seem different than changes in the bodies of peers. *Body size*: Changes in body size during growth. *Body states*: Pregnancy, the onset of menstruation, menopause, male climacteric
DEVELOPMENTAL PHASES: Puberty, adolescence, middle age

PLANNING

Unmet Needs
Comfort, protection from psychologic threat, acceptance, caring and communicating re-

lationships, high evaluation of self, sense of adequacy, dignity, personal growth and maturity, increased learning, increased reality perception and problem-solving ability

Expected Outcome

Person verbalizes feelings about the unacceptable body image
Relates feeling less threatened and more comfortable with his body
Looks at, touches, and cares for his body
Verbalizes acceptance of the body

NURSING INTERVENTIONS

Nursing Treatments

Approach unhurriedly
Reassure verbally (that the nurse is available whenever needed)
Provide an atmosphere of acceptance (about the changed body)
Encourage the expression of feelings (about the person's body)
Listen attentively
Offer feedback to the person's expressed feelings
Communicate nurse sensitivity to the person's problem
Provide reliable information (about the expected body changes)
Explore with the person his normal characteristics
Explore with the person his strengths and resources (to cope with the body change)
Encourage the acceptance of self-limitations
Support a realistic assessment of the situation (is the threat as severe as perceived?)
Reduce the demands placed on the person (so that there is more energy for coping)
Refrain from performing nonessential procedures (which further threaten the body image)
Arrange situations that encourage the person's autonomy (autonomy reduces the sense of threat)
Ask how the person normally copes with stress
Provide whatever the person needs to use his usual coping mechanisms
Encourage pride in appearance (despite the body alterations)
Encourage an awareness of positive responses from others (such as complaints about appearance, offers of friendship, etc.)
Introduce to persons or groups who have successfully undergone the same experience

Nursing Observations

Determine the degree of insight that the person has (into the perceived threat)
Observe for evidence of a favorable response to therapy (that the person is ready for body-image modification)

Health Teaching

Explain that the person's response is appropriate and commonly experienced
Explain the importance of maintaining a positive self-attitude
Relate ways the person can enhance his self-image (accepting all of his physiologic changes as part of the self, being as independent as possible)
Advise that negative responses from others be regarded with minimum significance (even though there may be feelings about such responses)
Advise that significant persons express acceptance of one another (especially of the person who feels threatened)
Explain that adolescents, pregnant women, etc. are often hypersensitive (about their bodies)
Explain that persons must make adjustments at their own pace

EVALUATION

Record actual outcome

THREATENED BODY IMAGE RELATED TO PHYSICAL LOSS[105,471,525,704]

ASSESSMENT
Data Collection
Subjective Data
- Person relates a change in body sensation, size, function, or appearance
- Verbalizes that the body is different than before
- Expresses being threatened by the change
    Person may relate perceiving a change in the body's boundaries, such as a person on hemodialysis perceiving the machine as an extension of the body's boundaries if the body is to maintain renal function or a paralyzed person in a wheelchair perceiving the chair as an extension of the body's boundaries if mobility is to occur
    May experience a change of body function such as a colostomy changing the natural mode of elimination
    May verbalize about appearance changes such as after surgery, a burn, or a crushing injury

Objective Data
- Person has visible or verifiable body changes
- May exhibit behavior such as avoiding looking at or touching the body part, having facial expressions of displeasure when viewing the body, demanding that others care for him, covering up body parts

Data Analysis
Nursing Diagnosis
THREATENED BODY IMAGE RELATED TO PHYSICAL LOSS: Feeling endangered by changes in the body that result from the loss of a positive, balanced state of health and that alter one's concept of the body

Common Etiology (Stressors)
DISEASES: Any
INJURIES: Any
SIGNS AND SYMPTOMS: Edema, immobility, jaundice, memory loss, pain, paralysis, rash, tremor, weakness
PSYCHOSOCIAL FACTORS: The loss of a valued concept of self (about body appearance and boundaries where the body leaves off and the environment begins)
HUMAN BODY: *Body appearance*: Changes in body appearance, a disfigured body. *Body function*: Loss of body function. *Body part*: Loss of a body part
HEALTH CARE FACTORS: *Health therapy*: Unsuccessful or ineffective therapy. *Drug therapy*: Life-maintenance drug therapy. *Adverse effects of medical, drug, or surgical therapy*: Loss of a body part (from an amputation, cholecystectomy, enucleation or evisceration of an eyeball, gastrectomy, hemipelvectomy, hysterectomy, ileotomy, laryngectomy, lobectomy of the brain, liver, or lungs, mastectomy, nephrectomy, prostatectomy, splenectomy, thryoidectomy, tonsillectomy), loss of hair (from chemotherapy and radiation therapy), loss of mobility (from traction), loss of natural elimination and elimination control (from a colostomy, ileocolostomy, ileostomy, ureterocolostomy, ureteroileostomy, ureterosigmoidostomy, ureterostomy, ureterotomy), loss of normal food intake (from an esophagectomy), loss of reproductive ability (from a fallopian tube ligation, hysterectomy, oophorectomy, orchidectomy, prostatectomy, salpingectomy, vasectomy), loss of speech (from a glossectomy, laryngectomy, tracheostomy, vocal cordectomy), loss of vision (from enucleation or evisceration of an eyeball), loss of libido (from antihypertensive drugs and tagament), edema (from corticosteroids), hesitance of urination (from anticholenergic drugs). *Therapeutic equipment*: The use of an artificial eye or limb, brace, breast prosthesis, cane, cannula for hemodialysis, cardiac pacemaker, urinary catheter, crutches, dentures, dental bridge, eyeglasses, hearing aid, hemodialyzer, hyperalimentation set-up, respirator, therapeutic tubes, walker, or wheelchair

DEVELOPMENTAL PHASES: Middle age, old age
SITUATIONAL FACTORS: Childlessness, or acute, chronic or terminal illness

PLANNING

Unmet Needs

Comfort, protection from psychologic threat, acceptance, caring and communicating relationships, high evaluation of self, sense of adequacy, dignity, personal growth and maturity, increased learning, increased reality perception and problem-solving ability

Expected Outcome

Person verbalizes feelings about the unacceptable body image
Relates feeling less threatened and more comfortable with his body
Looks at, touches, and cares for his body
Verbalizes acceptance of the body

NURSING INTERVENTIONS

Nursing Treatments

Approach unhurriedly
Reassure verbally (that the nurse is available whenever needed)
Provide an atmosphere of acceptance (about the changed body)
Encourage the expression of feelings (about the person's body)
Listen attentively
Offer feedback to the person's expressed feelings
Communicate nurse sensitivity to the person's problem
Provide reliable information (about the body's health or state)
Explore with the person his normal characteristics
Explore with the person his strengths and resources (to cope with the body change)
Encourage the acceptance of self-limitations
Support a realistic assessment of the situation (is the threat as severe as perceived?)
Reduce the demands placed on the person (so that there is more energy for coping)
Refrain from performing nonessential procedures (which further threaten the body image)
Arrange situations that encourage the person's autonomy (autonomy reduces the sense of threat)
Ask how the person normally copes with stress
Provide whatever the person needs to use his usual coping mechanisms
Encourage pride in appearance (despite the body alterations)
Encourage an awareness of positive responses from others (such as compliments about appearance)
Introduce to persons or groups who have successfully undergone the same experience

Nursing Observations

Determine the degree of insight that the person has (into the perceived threat)
Observe for evidence of a favorable response to therapy (that the person is ready for body-image modification)

Health Teaching

Explain that the person's response is appropriate and commonly experienced
Explain the importance of developing or maintaining a positive self-attitude
Relate ways the person can enhance his self-image (accepting all his limitations as part of the self, being as independent as possible)
Advise that negative responses from others be regarded with minimum significance (even though there may be feelings about such responses)
Advise that significant persons express acceptance of one another (especially of the person who feels threatened)
Explain that ill persons are often hypersensitive (about their bodies)
Explain that persons must make adjustments at their own pace

EVALUATION

Record actual outcome

BODY-IMAGE MODIFICATION RELATED TO IMPROVED HEALTH STATUS[105,471]

ASSESSMENT

Data Collection

Subjective Data
- Person relates a change in body sensation, size, function or appearance
- Verbalizes that the body is different than before
- Relates a sense of gain
- Expresses a need to integrate the former body with the new body
  Person relates having previously experienced poor health that was successfully treated
  Previously felt ill but now feels well
  May have never known what it is like to feel well and is uncomfortable with the new feeling

Objective Data
- Person has visible or verifiable body changes (such as improved skin color, loss or gain of weight, more attractive appearance, etc.)
- May exhibit behavior such as looking at and touching the body part, caring for the body, cautiously attempting increased activity, showing off body changes

Data Analysis

Nursing Diagnosis
BODY-IMAGE MODIFICATION RELATED TO IMPROVED HEALTH STATUS: Adjusting one's concept of the body as a result of body changes that are an improvement over the previous health status

Common Etiology (Stressors)
PSYCHOSOCIAL FACTORS: The gain of a valued concept of self, an attempt to adjust to change
HEALTH CARE FACTORS: *Health therapy*: Successful. *Drug therapy*: Curative or controlling effects of drug therapy. *Medical therapy*: Psychotherapy, rehabilitation therapy, speech therapy, withdrawal from alcohol, drugs, or tobacco. *Surgical procedures*: Any but especially arterial bypass, cosmetic operation, craniofacial surgery, reconstruction procedure, and transplantation of bone, cornea, hair, kidney, liver, heart or muscle

PLANNING

Unmet Needs
Comfort, protection from psychologic threat, acceptance, caring and communicating relationships, high evaluation of self, sense of adequacy, dignity, personal growth and maturity, increased learning, increased reality perception and problem-solving ability

Expected Outcome
Person verbalizes feelings about body
Expresses how current body changes have been integrated with the former body
Relates feeling comfortable with current body

NURSING INTERVENTIONS

Nursing Treatments
Approach unhurriedly
Reassure verbally (that he will adjust to feeling well)
Provide an atmosphere of acceptance
Encourage the expression of feelings (about the new body and loss of the former body)
Listen attentively
Offer feedback to the person's expressed feelings
Communicate nurse sensitivity to the person's problem

Arrange situations that encourage the person's autonomy (to care for his own body)

Offer praise (for looking and feeling well)

Encourage pride in appearance

Explore with the person his strengths and resources (to adjust to change)

Encourage an awareness of positive responses from others (about his body)

Encourage striving toward realistic goals (appropriate to the body's capabilities)

Avoid forcing the person into rapid adaptation to change by accepting the person's unique pattern of adjustment

Nursing Observations

Observe for evidence that the person is reaching out for emotional support (frequent help seeking, asking questions, seeking reasssurance)

Observe for evidence of a favorable response to therapy (satisfaction with the new body image)

Health Teaching

Recommend new options for effective methods of coping (new ways to achieve maximum body function with the well body)

Explain the importance of maintaining a positive self-attitude (as he assumes a new image because of improved health)

Explain (to the family) that persons must make adjustments at their own pace

EVALUATION

Record actual outcome

BODY-IMAGE MODIFICATION RELATED TO NATURAL BODY CHANGES[105,471]

ASSESSMENT

Data Collection

Subjective Data

• Person relates a change in body sensation, size, function, or appearance

• Verbalizes that the body is different than before

• Relates a sense of loss or gain

• Expresses a need to integrate the former body with the new body

Youth may relate experiencing body changes during puberty such as developing breasts and genitalia, appearance of body hair, etc.

Middle-aged or older persons may relate changes in muscle tone, stature, hair color, etc.

Person is not experiencing an illness

Objective Data

• Person has visible or verifiable body changes

• May exhibit behavior such as looking at and touching the body part, changing clothing to accommodate body changes, showing off body changes

Data Analysis

Nursing Diagnosis

BODY-IMAGE MODIFICATION RELATED TO NATURAL BODY CHANGES: Adjusting one's concept of the body as a result of body changes that normally occur during developmental stages

Common Etiology (Stressors)

PSYCHOSOCIAL FACTORS: The loss of a valued concept of self, an attempt to adjust to change

HUMAN BODY: *Body appearance*: Appearance changes during puberty, body changes that seem different than changes in the bodies of peers. *Body size*: Change in body size during growth. *Body states*: Pregnancy, the onset of menstruation, menopause, male climacteric

DEVELOPMENTAL PHASES: Any but especially puberty, adolescence, middle age, old age

PLANNING

Unmet Needs

Comfort, protection from psychologic threat, acceptance, caring and communicating relationships, high evaluation of self, sense of adequacy, dignity, personal growth and maturity, increased learning, increased reality perception and problem-solving ability

Expected Outcome

Person verbalizes feelings about body

Expresses how current body changes have been integrated with the former body

Relates feeling comfortable with current body

NURSING INTERVENTIONS

Nursing Treatments

Approach unhurriedly

Reassure verbally (that the nurse is available whenever needed)

Provide an atmosphere of acceptance (about the changed body)

Encourage the expression of feelings (about the new body and the loss of the former body)

Listen attentively

Offer feedback to the person's expressed feelings

Communicate nurse sensitivity to the person's problem

Arrange situations that encourage the person's autonomy (to care for his own body)

Encourage new skill development (needed for self-care of the body)

Provide temporary assistance until the skill is learned

Offer praise (for new skill development)

Refrain from performing nonessential procedures (which might be perceived as threatening the body image)

Encourage pride in appearance (despite the body alterations, and when possible, cultivate a positive attitude about the body change)

Explore with the person his positive characteristics (including those that have not changed)

Explore with the person his strengths and resources (to cope with the change)

Encourage an awareness of positive responses from others (about his body)

Encourage striving toward realistic goals (appropriate to the body's capabilities)

Avoid forcing the person into rapid adaptation to change by accepting the person's unique pattern of adjustment

Nursing Observations

Observe for evidence that the person is reaching out for emotional support (frequent help seeking, asking questions, seeking reassurance)

Observe for evidence of a favorable response to therapy (satisfaction with the new body image)

Health Teaching

Recommend new options for effective methods of coping (new ways to achieve maximum body function despite body changes)

Explain the importance of maintaining a positive self-attitude

Explain (to the family) that persons must make adjustments at their own pace

Explain that adolescents, pregnant women, etc. are often hypersensitive (about their bodies)

EVALUATION

Record actual outcome

BODY-IMAGE MODIFICATION RELATED TO PHYSICAL LOSS[105,130,225,471,647,672]

ASSESSMENT

Data Collection

Subjective Data
- Person relates a change in body sensation, size, function, or appearance
- Verbalizes that the body is different than before
- Relates a sense of loss
- Expresses a need to integrate the former body with the new body

May relate perceiving a change in the body's boundaries such as a person with chronic obstructive pulmonary disease perceiving the IPPB machine as an extension of the body's boundaries if the body is to maintain adequate pulmonary ventilation or an unsteady person using a walker perceiving the walker as an extension of the body's boundary if mobility is to occur

May relate experiencing a change of body function such as a hysterectomy changing the woman's childbearing function

May verbalize about appearance changes occurring after an amputation, a burn, a surgical procedure

Objective Data
- Person has visible or verifiable body changes
- May exhibit behavior such as looking at and touching the body part, caring for the body, using devices needed for improved body function, appropriately decreasing activity

Data Analysis

Nursing Diagnosis

BODY-IMAGE MODIFICATION RELATED TO PHYSICAL LOSS: Adjusting one's concept of the body as a result of body changes that result from the loss of a balanced state of health

Common Etiology (Stressors)

DISEASES: Any

INJURIES: Any

SIGNS AND SYMPTOMS: Edema, immobility, memory loss, pain, paralysis, rash, tremor, weakness

PSYCHOSOCIAL FACTORS: The loss of a valued concept of self, an attempt to adjust to change

HUMAN BODY: *Body appearance*: Change in body appearance, a disfigured body. *Body function*: Loss of body function

HEALTH CARE FACTORS: *Health therapy*: Unsuccessful or ineffective therapy. *Drug therapy*: Life-maintenance drug therapy. *Adverse effects of medical, drug, or surgical therapy*: Loss of a body part (from an amputation, cholecystectomy, enucleation or evisceration of an eyeball, gastrectomy, hemipelvectomy, hysterectomy, ileotomy, laryngectomy, lobectomy of the brain, liver, or lungs, mastectomy, nephrectomy, prostatectomy, splenectomy, thyroidectomy, tonsillectomy), loss of hair (from chemotherapy and radiation therapy), loss of mobility (from traction), loss of natural elimination and elimination control (from a colostomy, ileocolostomy, ileostomy, ureterocolostomy, ureteroileostomy, ureterosigmoidostomy, ureterostomy, ureterotomy), loss of normal food intake (from an esophagectomy), loss of the reproductive ability (from a fallopian tube ligation, hysterectomy, oophorectomy, orchidectomy, prostatectomy, salpingectomy, vasectomy), loss of speech (from a glossectomy, laryngectomy, tracheostomy, vocal cordectomy), loss of vision (from an enucleation or evisceration of an eyeball), loss of libido (from antihypertensive drugs and tagamet), edema (from corticosteroids), hesitancy of urination (from anticholinergic drugs). *Therapeutic equipment*: The use of an artificial eye or limb, brace, breast prosthesis, cane, cannula for hemodialysis, cardiac pacemaker, urinary catheter, crutches, dentures, dental bridge, eyeglasses, hearing aid, hemodialyzer, hyperalimentary setup, respirator, therapeutic tubes, walker, wheel-chair

DEVELOPMENTAL PHASES: Middle age, old age
SITUATIONAL FACTORS: Childlessness, acute, chronic, or terminal illness

PLANNING

Unmet Needs

Comfort, protection from psychologic threat, acceptance, caring and communicating re-lationships, high evaluation of self, sense of adequacy, dignity, personal growth and maturity, increased learning, increased reality perception and problem-solving ability

Expected Outcome

Person verbalizes feelings about body
Expresses how current body changes have been integrated with the former body
Relates feeling comfortable with current body

NURSING INTERVENTIONS

Nursing Treatments

Approach unhurriedly
Reassure verbally (that the nurse is available whenever needed)
Provide an atmosphere of acceptance (about the changed body)
Encourage the expression of feelings (about the new body and loss of the former body)
Listen attentively
Offer feedback to the person's expressed feelings
Communicate nurse sensitivity to the person's problem
Arrange situations that encourage the person's autonomy (to care for his own body)
Encourage acceptance of interdependency, acceptance of self-limitations (if the modified body image results from physical loss)
Encourage new skill development (needed for self-care of the body)
Provide temporary assistance until the skill is learned
Offer praise (for new skill development)
Refrain from performing nonessential procedures (which might be perceived as threat-ening the body image)
Encourage pride in appearance (despite body alterations)
Explore with the person his individual characteristics (which are unchanged)
Explore with the person his strengths and resources (to cope with the change)
Encourage an awareness of positive responses from others (about his body)
Encourage striving toward realistic goals (appropriate to the body's capabilities)
Avoid forcing the person into rapid adaptation to change by accepting the person's unique pattern of adjustment
Introduce to persons or groups who have successfully undergone the same experience (if appropriate)

Nursing Observations

Observe for evidence that the person is reaching out for emotional support (frequent help seeking, asking questions, seeking reassurance)
Observe for evidence of a favorable response to therapy (satisfaction with the new body image)

Health Teaching

Recommend new options for effective methods of coping (new ways to achieve maxi-mum body function despite body changes)
Explain the importance of maintaining a positive self-attitude
Explain (to the family) that persons must make adjustments at their own pace
Explain that ill or aged perosns are often hypersensitive (about their bodies)

EVALUATION

Record actual outcome

SELF-IDENTITY MODIFICATION RELATED TO A DEVELOPMENTAL PHASE[105,432,471]

ASSESSMENT
Data Collection
Subjective Data
- Person has experienced a significant life change
- Relates perceiving self as different than before
- Expresses a need to integrate the former self with the new by asking: "Who am I?" (worth as a person), "What am I?" (qualities and characteristics), "Where am I?" (status as an individual in social groups), "Why am I?" (philosophy of life)

  Person relates feeling a vagueness about himself while moving through life phases such as adolescence, adulthood, old age

  Confirms gradually becoming comfortable with his self-concept until he moves into a new life phase

Objective Data
- May exhibit behavior such as changing appearance, associating with different social groups, advancing educational level

Data Analysis
Nursing Diagnosis
SELF-IDENTITY MODIFICATION RELATED TO A DEVELOPMENTAL PHASE: Adjusting the beliefs, attitudes, ideas, and feelings one has about oneself during the various developmental stages of life

Common Etiology (Stressors)
PSYCHOSOCIAL FACTORS: An attempt to adjust to change, an attempt to change the direction of one's life, the threat of loss of identity, changes in a vital life role
DEVELOPMENTAL PHASES: Any but especially puberty, adolescence, middle age, old age

PLANNING
Unmet Needs
Comfort, protection from psychologic threat, acceptance, caring and communicating relationships, high evaluation of self, sense of adequacy, personal growth and maturity, increased learning, full development of potential, identification of values, increased reality perception and problem-solving ability

Expected Outcome
Person verbalizes feelings about self-identity
Relates how current life changes have been integrated with the previous perception of self
Relates feeling comfortable with who he is, what he is, where he is, and why he is

NURSING INTERVENTIONS
Nursing Treatments
Approach unhurriedly
Assist the person to define consistent life standards
Reassure verbally (that there is worth in the new identity equal to the worth of the former identity)
Provide an atmosphere of acceptance
Encourage the expression of feelings (about the new self-identity)
Listen attentively
Offer feedback to the person's expressed feelings
Communicate nurse sensitivity to the person's problem
Explore with the person his worth as an individual (that because he is a human being, he is a person of worth, that worth is not based on performance)

Ask questions that encourage answers that reflect reality perception (about the person's worth, individual characteristics, group status, life philosophy)

Encourage the identification of specific life values, of values acquired from the person's own culture, of values in common with the values of others

Encourage the identification of success standards

Encourage the differentiation between self-ideal and actual self (the kind of person he would like to be, the kind of person he is)

Offer praise (for successful modification of self-identity)

Avoid forcing the person into rapid adaptation to change by accepting the person's unique pattern of adjustment

Nursing Observations

Determine the degree of insight that the person has (about his self-identity)

Observe for an excessive stress level

Observe for impaired self-attitudes (about the modified self)

Observe for evidence that the person is reaching out for emotional support

Observe for evidence of a favorable response to therapy (the person verbalizes satisfaction with the changed self)

Health Teaching

Recommend new options for effective methods of coping (new ways to perceive the person's characteristics, status among others, and life philosophy)

Explain the importance of maintaining a positive self-attitude

Advise that negative responses from others be regarded with minimum significance (even though there are feelings about such responses)

Explain (to the family) that persons must make adjustments at their own pace

Explain that adolescents and the aged are often hypersensitive (about themselves)

EVALUATION

Record actual outcome

SELF-IDENTITY MODIFICATION RELATED TO LOSS/GAIN OF A SIGNIFICANT OTHER[105,432,471]

ASSESSMENT

Data Collection

Subjective Data

• Person has experienced a significant life change
• Relates perceiving self as different than before
• Expresses a need to integrate the former self with the new by asking: "Who am I?" (worth as a person), "What am I?" (qualities and characteristics), "Where am I?" (status as an individual in social groups), "Why am I?" (philosophy of life)

If two persons have been emotionally close, the remaining person may complain of feeling incomplete, or lost, that part of his self is gone

May relate struggling with who he is without the significant other

May relate perceiving himself more clearly as an individual

If a significant other is gained, the person may relate feeling more complete

Relates gradually becoming more comfortable with his new self-concept

Objective Data

• May exhibit changed behavior such as a man who socialized primarily with couples before he lost his wife now socializing only with "the boys" or a person who has lost a child changing his life philosophy and becoming involved with unfortunate children

Data Analysis

Nursing Diagnosis

SELF-IDENTITY MODIFICATION RELATED TO LOSS/GAIN OF A SIGNIFICANT OTHER: Adjusting the beliefs, attitudes, ideas, and feelings one has about oneself when there has been a loss or gain of a significant other

Common Etiology (Stressors)

BIRTH DEFECTS: Giving birth to an imperfect infant

DISEASES: Natural abortion, stillbirth

PSYCHOSOCIAL FACTORS: An attempt to adjust to change, an attempt to change the direction of life, the threat of loss of identity, changes in vital life role

SITUATIONAL FACTORS: *Loss of a significant other*: Placing a child up for adoption, being adopted or available for adoption, the death of a significant other, marital separation or divorce of parents or from a spouse, launching grown children, retirement, the frequent change of foster parents, giving up a foster child. *Gain of a significant other*: Marriage, adoption of a child, childbirth, grandparenthood, a new family member (other than the above)

PLANNING

Unmet Needs

Comfort, protection from psychologic threat, acceptance, caring and communicating relationships, high evaluation of self, sense of adequacy, personal growth and maturity, increased learning, full development of potential, identification of values, increased reality perception and problem-solving ability

Expected Outcome

Person verbalizes feelings about self-identity

Relates how current life changes have been integrated with the previous perception of self

Relates feeling comfortable with who he is, what he is, where he is, and why he is

NURSING INTERVENTIONS

Nursing Treatments

Approach unhurriedly

Reassure verbally (that the person is capable of making the necessary modification)

Provide an atmosphere of acceptance

Encourage the expression of feelings (about the new self-identity)

Listen attentively

Offer feedback to the person's expressed feelings

Communicate nurse sensitivity to the person's problem

Explore with the person his worth as an individual (that because he is a human being, he is a person of worth, that worth is not based on relatedness with others)

Ask questions that encourage answers that reflect reality perception (about the person's worth, individual characteristics, group status, life philosophy)

Encourage the identification of specific life values, of values acquired from the person's own culture, of values in common with the values of others

Encourage the identification of success standards

Encourage the differentiation between self-ideal and actual self (the kind of person he would like to be, the kind of person he is)

Offer praise (for successful modification of self-identity)

Avoid forcing the person into rapid adaptation to change by accepting the person's unique pattern of adjustment

Nursing Observations

Determine the degree of insight that the person has (about his self-identity)

Observe for an excessive stress level

Observe for impaired self-attitudes (about the modified self)

Observe for evidence that the person is reaching out for emotional support

Observe for evidence of a favorable response to therapy (the person verbalizes satisfaction with the changed self)

Health Teaching
Recommend new options for effective methods of coping (new ways to perceive the person's characteristics, status among others, and life philosophy)
Explain the importance of maintaining a positive self-attitude
Advise that negative responses from others be regarded with minimum significance (even though there are feelings about such responses)
Explain (to the family) that persons must make adjustments at their own pace

EVALUATION
Record actual outcome

SELF-IDENTITY MODIFICATION RELATED TO PHYSICAL LOSS[105,432,471]

ASSESSMENT
Data Collection

Subjective Data
- Person has experienced a significant life change
- Relates perceiving self as different than before
- Expresses a need to integrate the former self with the new by asking: "Who am I?" (worth as a person), "What am I?" (qualities and characteristics), "Where am I?" (status as an individual in social groups), "Why am I?" (philosophy of life)

  Person relates feeling unsure of how the physical loss has changed his self

  Usually questions his value as a person if the physical loss is permanent

  May relate altering his philosophy of life after becoming aware of his vulnerability

  As the self-identity is modified, the person relates feeling comfortable with his new self-identity

Objective Data
- May exhibit behavior such as changing appearance, changing to a more appropriate job, becoming involved in an organization dedicated to conquering a specific disease

Data Analysis

Nursing Diagnosis
SELF-IDENTITY MODIFICATION RELATED TO PHYSICAL LOSS: Adjusting the beliefs, attitudes, ideas, and feelings one has about oneself when there is a loss of a balanced state of health

Common Etiology (Stressors)
DISEASES: Any disease
INJURIES: Any injury
SIGNS AND SYMPTOMS: Pain, weakness
PSYCHOSOCIAL FACTORS: An attempt to adjust to change, an attempt to change the direction of one's life, the threat of loss of identity, changes in a vital life role
SITUATIONAL FACTORS: Acute, critical, chronic, or terminal illness

PLANNING
Unmet Needs
Comfort, protection from psychologic threat, acceptance, caring and communicating relationships, high evaluation of self, sense of adequacy, personal growth and maturity, increased learning, full development of potential, identification of values, increased reality perception and problem-solving ability

Expected Outcome

Person verbalizes feelings about self-identity

Relates how current life changes have been integrated with the previous perception of self

Relates feeling comfortable with who he is, what he is, where he is, and why he is

NURSING INTERVENTIONS

Nursing Treatments

Approach unhurriedly

Reassure verbally (that there is worth in the new identity equal to the worth of the former identity)

Provide an atmosphere of acceptance

Encourage the expression of feelings (about the new self-identity)

Listen attentively

Offer feedback to the person's expressed feelings

Communicate nurse sensitivity to the person's problem

Explore with the person his worth as an individual (that because he is a human being, he is a person of worth, that worth is not based on physical or mental competence)

Ask questions that encourage answers that reflect reality perception (about the person's worth, individual characteristics, group status, life philosophy)

Encourage the identification of specific life values, of values acquired from the person's own culture, of values in common with the values of others

Encourage the identification of success standards

Encourage the differentiation between self-ideal and actual self (the kind of person he would like to be, the kind of person he is)

Offer praise (for successful modification of self-identity)

Avoid forcing the person into rapid adaptation to change by accepting the person's unique pattern of adjustment

Nursing Observations

Determine the degree of insight that the person has (about his self-identity)

Observe for an excessive stress level

Observe for impaired self-attitudes (about the modified self)

Observe for evidence that the person is reaching out for emotional support

Observe for evidence of a favorable response to therapy (the person verbalizes satisfaction with the changed self)

Health Teaching

Recommend new options for effective methods of coping (new ways to perceive the person's characteristics, status among others, and life philosophy)

Explain the importance of maintaining a positive self-attitude

Advise that negative responses from others be regarded with minimum significance (even though there are feelings about such responses)

Explain (to the family) that persons must make adjustments at their own pace

Explain that ill persons are often hypersensitive (about their selves)

EVALUATION

Record actual outcome

PART THREE
DUAL NURSING DIAGNOSES

Part Three covers that sphere of knowledge and skill related to health problems that professional nurses treat independently but that are also treated by physicians or allied health professionals, depending on who is available to diagnose the problem and provide the intervention. Dual diagnoses include problems of emergency conditions; minor illnesses, disorders, and conditions; symptoms; health maintenance risk factors; suspected disease factors; drug and nutrition problems; psychosocial nonadaptation; occupational, physical, and speech rehabilitation; spiritual care; wellness; and health care resources. The intervention approach for these problems may or may not be the same for each profession.

15 Nursing Diagnoses of EMERGENCY CONDITIONS

Dual Domain of Nursing Expertise: Emergency Conditions

This chapter covers thatsphere of nursing knowledge and skill related to problems involving unexpected, life-threatening conditions or injury that require immediate intervention for life-saving purposes. The stabilization of such problems so that the life-threatening factor is minimized is shared by the nurse, the physician, and emergency-allied health professionals.

Views of Nursing Leaders That Support This Domain of Nursing Expertise

In certain situations the nurse may find it necessary to assume the role of a physician . . . for instance, in emergencies.

Virginia Henderson[221:30]

Acute care functions for which nurses are now generally responsible are: Provision of emergency treatment as appropriate; e.g., in cardiac arrest, shock, hemorrhage, convulsions, and poisoning.

Faye Abdellah[3:127]

Nurses exist to serve people. Its direct and overriding responsibility is to society. Nursing has no dependent functions but, like all other professions, it has many collaborative ones. Health services to people require the concerted action of a range of disciplines if such services are to approach safety and adequacy.

Martha Rogers[419:122]

Neuman's total person approach to health care . . . was developed to demonstrate how all health professionals can utilize their own assessments to interact with one another in order to provide the level of care necessary to meet the demands of the consumer.

Betty Neuman[410:159]

Emergency Conditions of Acid–Base Balance

METABOLIC ACIDOSIS[219,247,371,528]

ASSESSMENT
Data Collection
Subjective Data
Malaise
Fatigue
Nausea and vomiting
Drowsiness

Objective Data
• Bicarbonate (HCO_3) concentration below 22 mEq/liter
• Base excess less than -2
• Reduced PCO_2 below 35 mm Hg
• Arterial pH below 7.35
  Increased serum potassium
  Confusion
  Coma
  Deep, rapid respirations (Kussmaul's)
  Hypotension
  Cardiac dysrrythmias

Data Analysis

Nursing Diagnosis
METABOLIC ACIDOSIS: An umbalanced chemical state of bicarbonate deficit in the extracellular fluid

Common Etiology (Stressors)
DISEASE: Diabetes, renal failure, draining fistula
INJURIES: Starvation
SIGNS AND SYMPTOMS: Diarrhea, shock
HEALTH CARE FACTORS: *Drug therapy*: Adverse effects of drugs (large doses of aspirin, the administration of carbonic anhydrase inhibitors). *Medical therapy*: Intravenous infusion (the rapid infusion of sodium chloride that does not contain HCO_3). *Surgical procedure*: Colostomy, ileostomy (pancreatic or small bowel surgery), ileal conduit
LIFESTYLE: High fat diet
HUMAN ERROR: Accidental or intentional overdose of drugs (salicylates), ingestion of acids (ammonium chloride, paraldehyde, methyl alcohol, ethanol intoxication)
MAJOR PATHOPHYSIOLOGIC FACTORS CAUSING THE PROBLEM: Acid accumulation can result from abnormal carbohydrate metabolism; low carbohydrate intake increases the amount of fat metabolized, which results in excess acid production; metabolism is also affected by high fever; in renal insufficiency, acid retention is evidenced by increased levels of urea nitrogen, creatinine, and uric acid; base or electrolyte loss from diarrhea, intestinal or biliary fistulas, ileostomy, or colostomy can cause acidosis since chloride is depleted

PLANNING

Unmet Needs
Fluid and electrolyte balance, acid–base balance, rest, comfort, protection from physical harm, increased learning

Expected Outcome

Serum bicarbonate (HCO_3) between 24–26 mEq/liter

Arterial pH between 7.35–7.45

NURSING INTERVENTIONS

Nursing Treatments

Administer intravenous fluids (ET)* (containing sodium bicarbonate)

Connect the person to an ECG monitor (especially if the serum potassium is elevated)

Obtain a blood (arterial) sample and send for analysis (electrolytes, arterial blood gases)

Obtain a urine sample and send for analysis (pH)

Provide standby equipment (nasogastric tube) and drugs (sodium bicarbonate)

Position comfortably (to facilitate respiratory efficiency)

Cover with warm blankets

Attend the person constantly

Consult with the physician (immediately after giving emergency treatment)

Obtain a complete present and past history

Nursing Observations

Observe the level of consciousness

Inspect the skin for color

Observe for cyanosis

Monitor blood studies for arterial blood gases and abnormal electrolytes

Monitor the blood pressure

Test the urine for pH (for acidosis)

Inspect the chest for respiratory rate and rhythm

Palpate the pulse for rate, rhythm, and volume

Auscultate the apical heartbeat for rate and rhythm (especially if the potassium is elevated)

Observe the ECG monitor (for cardiac abnormalities)

Measure the intake and output

Measure the body weight (daily)

Health Teaching

Explain the causes of the health problem (abnormal metabolism, loss of bicarbonate)

Explain the reason for and intended effect of the therapy (to reestablish acid–base balance)

Medical Treatments Performed by Nurses

Give the prescribed drugs (sodium bicarbonate to supplement loss and reestablish acid–base balance)

EVALUATION

Record actual outcome

METABOLIC ALKALOSIS[219,247,371,528]

ASSESSMENT

Data Collection

Subjective Data

Anxiety

Anorexia

Nausea and vomiting

Weakness

---

*Emergency treatment

Objective Data
- Bicarbonate (HCO_3) concentration above 26 mEq/liter
- Delta base above +2
- Increased PCO_2 above 45 mm Hg
- Arterial pH above 7.45
  Decreased serum chloride, potassium, calcium
  Tetany
  Shallow respirations
  Cardiac dysrhythmias
  Belligerent behavior
  Confusion
  Seizures
  Stupor
  Coma

Data Analysis

Nursing Diagnosis
METABOLIC ALKALOSIS: An imbalanced chemical state of bicarbonate excess in the extracellular fluid

Common Etiology (Stressors)
DISEASES: Cushing's syndrome, hyperaldosteronism
SIGNS AND SYMPTOMS: Diarrhea, vomiting
HEALTH CARE FACTORS: *Drug therapy*: Antacids such as bicarbonate of soda, corticosteroids, diuretics such as Lasix, Edecrin, excessive dosages of sodium bicarbonate IV. *Medical therapy*: Intravenous infusion (lactated Ringer's), nasogastric suction
HUMAN ERROR: Excessive ingestion of licorice
MAJOR PATHOPHYSIOLOGIC FACTORS CAUSING THE PROBLEM: Metabolic alkalosis occurs from an increase in the amount of base in the blood or from a decrease in the amount of acids; base may accumulate from excessive intake (sodium bicarbonate, lactate, or citrate); acids may be lost in large amounts in vomiting, diarrhea, diuresis, in which there is severe chloride and potassium depletion, or from excessive corticosteroid release or administration

PLANNING

Unmet Needs
Fluid and electrolyte balance, acid–base balance, rest, comfort, protection from physical harm, increased learning

Expected Outcome
Serum bicarbonate (HCO_3) between 22–26 mEq/liter
Arterial pH between 7.35–7.45

NURSING INTERVENTIONS

Nursing Treatments
Give high-potassium fluids orally (if on diuretics or adrenocorticosteroids, or if vomiting)
  OR
Give high-sodium fluids orally (such as salty bouillon, if person is dehydrated)
Refrain from giving bicarbonates
Administer intravenous fluids (ET) (isotonic saline, if the person is dehydrated or vomiting, in order to replace the extracellular fluid volume deficit)
Connect the person to an ECG monitor
Provide standby equipment (oxygen) and drugs (ammonium chloride, potassium chloride, calcium chloride)
Obtain a blood sample and send for analysis (electrolytes, arterial blood gases)
Place on complete bed rest
Cover with warm blankets

Attend the person constantly
Consult with the physician (immediately after giving emergency treatment)
Obtain a complete present and past history

Nursing Observations

Observe the level of consciousness
Monitor blood studies for arterial blood gases and abnormal electrolytes
Monitor the blood pressure
Test the urine for pH
Inspect the chest for respiratory rate and rhythm
Palpate the pulse for rate, rhythm, and volume
Observe the ECG monitor (for cardiac abnormalities)
Measure the intake and output
Measure the body weight (daily)

Health Teaching

Explain the causes of the health problem (increased bicarbonate in extracellular fluid)
Explain the reason for and intended effect of the therapy (to reestablish acid–base balance)
Recommend that alkalis be used conservatively

Medical Treatments Performed by Nurses

Give the prescribed drugs (ammonium chloride to counteract alkalosis and reestablish acid–base balance, potassium chloride to replace excessive potassium loss and chloride to promote bicarbonate excretion, calcium chloride to reduce tetany, carbonic anhydrase inhibitors to increase excretion of bicarbonate)

EVALUATION

Record actual outcome

KETOACIDOSIS [73,219,371,528]

ASSESSMENT

Data Collection

Subjective Data

Early Stage
• Malaise
  Excessive appetite

Midstage
• Severe thirst
• Polyuria
  Dizziness
  Nausea

Objective Data

Early Stage
• Fruity or acetone breath
• Urine glucose and acetone
  Restlessness

Midstage
• Deep, rapid respirations
• Acid urine with pH 4.6–5.2
• Blood glucose above 300 mg/100 ml
  Vomiting

Dry skin
Poor skin turgor
Sunken eyeballs
Decreased blood pressure

Data Analysis

Nursing Diagnosis

KETOACIDOSIS: An imbalanced chemical state of excess ketone bodies (ketoacids) in the blood with decreased bicarbonate in persons having impaired carbohydrate metabolism

Common Etiology (Stressors)

DISEASES: Diabetes mellitus, infection of any kind
SIGNS AND SYMPTOMS: Diarrhea, vomiting
HEALTH CARE FACTORS: *Surgical therapy:* Surgery of any kind
HUMAN ERROR: Improper dosage of insulin
MAJOR PATHOPHYSIOLOGIC FACTORS CAUSING THE PROBLEM: Persons with insufficient insulin develop "intracellular starvation"; because the cells are unable to use the supply of glucose/carbohydrates in the blood for metabolism, they must use fatty acids as a source of energy; ketones are the end product of this process and are not eliminated fast enough, resulting in high levels of ketones in the blood (ketonemia) and the urine (ketouria); the excess blood glucose causes osmotic diuresis and increased sodium loss, resulting in severe dehydration

PLANNING

Unmet Needs

Fluid and electrolyte balance, acid–base balance, rest, comfort, protection from physical harm, increased learning

Expected Outcome

Blood glucose between 80–120 mg/100 ml
Negative urine glucose and acetone
Urine pH between 4.8–8.5

NURSING INTERVENTIONS

Nursing Treatments

Give high-sodium fluids orally (specifically 8 oz of salty broth unless there is vomiting)
  OR
Administer intravenous fluids (ET) (5% glucose in saline or Ringer's lactate)
Catheterize with an indwelling urinary catheter (to facilitate urine testing)
Obtain a blood sample and send for analysis (glucose, electrolytes, arterial blood gases)
Obtain a urine sample and send for analysis (glucose, pH, acetone)
Provide standby drugs (crystalline insulin)
Place on complete bed rest
Cover with warm blankets
Attend the patient constantly
Make a referral
  OR
Consult with a physician (immediately after giving emergency treatment)
Obtain a complete present and past history

Nursing Observations

Measure the intake and output
Monitor the blood pressure
Monitor blood studies for abnormal (increased) glucose (every 2 hours) and electrolytes, for arterial blood gases
Test the urine for sugar and acetone (every 30 minutes)
Test the urine for pH

Inspect the chest for respiratory rate and rhythm
Palpate the pulse for rate, rhythm, and volume

Health Teaching
Explain the causes of the health problem (poorly regulated impaired carbohydrate metabolism)
Explain the reason for and intended effect of the therapy (to reestablish acid–base balance)

Medical Treatments Performed by Nurses
Give the prescribed drugs (fast-acting crystalline insulin, 50 units every 1–2 hours until the urine glucose reaches normal, if a sliding scale is not available)

EVALUATION
Record actual outcome

RESPIRATORY ACIDOSIS[73,247,528]

ASSESSMENT
Data Collection
Subjective Data
Weakness
Fatigue
Anxiety

Objective Data
• Serum PCO_2 above 45 mm Hg
• Normal or increased serum bicarbonate
• Arterial pH below 7.35
 Normal or increased sodium potassium
 Dull, slow mental responses
 Confusion or disorientation
 Decreased reflexes
 Flapping tremor
 Somnolence
 Coma

Data Analysis

Nursing Diagnosis
RESPIRATORY ACIDOSIS (CARBON DIOXIDE TOXICITY/NARCOSIS, HYPERCAPNIA, HYPERCARBIA): Excess carbon dioxide in the blood

Common Etiology (Stressors)
DISEASES: Acute pulmonary edema, bronchitis, chronic obstructive pulmonary disease (asthma, emphysema), Guillain-Barré syndrome, metabolic alkalosis, myasthenia gravis, obesity, pickwickian syndrome, pneumonia, pneumothorax
HEALTH CARE FACTORS: *Drug therapy:* Adverse effects of respiratory depressant drugs. *Medical therapy:* The administration of high concentrations of oxygen to persons with chronic obstructive pulmonary disease. *Surgical therapy:* Anesthesia
HUMAN ERROR: Accidental or intentional overdose of drugs
MAJOR PATHOPHYSIOLOGIC FACTORS CAUSING THE PROBLEM: With slowed and/or shallow breathing, there is insufficient elimination of carbon dioxide, so that it accumulates in the blood; persons with chronically high carbon dioxide levels lose their stimulus to breathe when their lowered oxygen level (hypoxia) is relieved by oxygen therapy

PLANNING

Unmet Needs

Acid–base balance, waste elimination of carbon dioxide, rest, stimulation, protection from physical harm, increased learning

Expected Outcome

Serum PCO_2 of 35–45 mm Hg
Arterial pH of 7.35–7.45

NURSING INTERVENTIONS

Nursing Treatments

Ventilate the person (ET) (if needed, using mouth-to-mouth breathing until spontaneous respirations occur or until the person can be intubated)
Initiate endotracheal intubation (ET) (if needed)
Administer intermittent positive-pressure breathing (ET) (with compressed air)
Suction the airway (as needed)
Withhold the oxygen therapy (high concentrations)
Withhold all drugs (that have a sedative effect and will further depress respirations)
Obtain a blood sample and send for analysis (CBC, electrolytes, arterial blood gases)
Provide standby equipment (endotracheal tube, tracheostomy tray, mechanical ventilators, and a bag-valve-mask unit, trade name AmbuBag)
Consult with the physician (immediately after giving emergency treatment)
Attend the patient constantly (until the episode subsides)
Obtain a complete present and past history

Nursing Observations

Observe the level of consciousness
Inspect the chest for respiratory rate and rhythm and symmetrical expansion
Auscultate the chest for abnormal breath sounds and lung aeration
Monitor blood studies for arterial blood gases, for abnormal electrolytes, and hematology
Observe for confusion
Palpate the pulse for rate (tachycardia), rhythm, and volume
Monitor the blood pressure

Health Teaching

Instruct to increase fluid intake (to thin respiratory secretions)
Teach how to do resistive breathing exercises (for emphysema)

Medical Treatments Performed by Nurses

Administer oxygen by Venturi mask
Give the prescribed drugs (antibiotics to combat infection)

EVALUATION

Record actual outcome

RESPIRATORY ALKALOSIS[42,278,528]

ASSESSMENT

Data Collection

Subjective Data

• Numbness and tingling of the nose, ears, fingertips, or lips
  Lightheadedness or vertigo
  Irritability
  Muscle cramps

Anxiety
Nervousness

Objective Data
- Decreased arterial P_{CO_2} below 35 mm Hg
- Increased arterial pH above 7.45

Decreased serum bicarbonate (HCO_3)
Hypotension
Cardiac dysrhythmias
Muscle twitching
Seizures

Data Analysis

Nursing Diagnosis
RESPIRATORY ALKALOSIS (CARBON DIOXIDE INSUFFICIENCY, HYPOCAPNIA, HYPOCARBIA): An imbalanced chemical state of carbonic acid deficit within the extracellular fluid

Common Etiology (Stressors)
DISEASES: Anemia, anxiety reaction, brain tumor, cirrhosis, congestive heart failure, encephalitis, gram-negative septicemia, meningitis, pneumonitis, pneumothorax, pulmonary edema, pulmonary embolus, thyrotoxicosis
INJURIES: Head injury, poisoning (alcohol or paraldehyde intoxication)
SIGNS AND SYMPTOMS: Fever, pain
HEALTH CARE FACTORS: *Drug therapy*: Adverse effects of respiratory stimulants, salicylate toxicity. *Medical therapy*: Hyperventilation from mechanical ventilation
ENVIRONMENTAL FACTORS: Environmental heat
HUMAN ERROR: Accidental or intentional overdose of drugs such as salicylates and alcohol
MAJOR PATHOPHYSIOLOGIC FACTORS CAUSING THE PROBLEM: Respiratory alkalosis is caused by the etiologic factors mentioned above that produce hyperventilation; the rapid breathing results in the exhalation of excessive amounts of carbon dioxide, which decreases the carbon dioxide reserves in the blood

PLANNING

Unmet Needs
Acid–base balance, protection from physical harm, increased learning

Expected Outcome
Arterial P_{CO_2} of 35–45 mm Hg
Arterial pH of 7.45
Cessation of deep, rapid breathing

NURSING INTERVENTIONS

Nursing Treatments
Attend the patient constantly (until the episode subsides)
Reassure verbally
Provide a paper bag for breathing (rebreathing exhaled carbon dioxide will relieve alkalosis)
Provide standby drugs (potassium)
Consult with a physician (if the condition persists)
Obtain a blood sample and send for analysis (arterial blood gases, electrolytes)
Obtain a complete present and past history

Nursing Observations
Observe the level of consciousness
Inspect the chest for respiratory rate and rhythm
Monitor the blood pressure
Monitor blood studies for arterial blood gases, for abnormal electrolytes
Observe for complaints of dizziness, pain, or respiratory muscle weakness
Observe for tetany

Health Teaching
Explain the causes of the health problem (overbreathing)
Explain how to use a paper bag to reduce hyperventilation
Teach how to do breath-holding (to prevent exhalation of carbon dioxide)
Explain the reason for and intended effect of the therapy (to reestablish acid–base balance)

Medical Treatments Performed by Nurses
Give prescribed drugs (potassium to supplement loss)

EVALUATION
Record actual outcome

Emergency Conditions of the Cardiovascular System

ACUTE CARDIAC ISCHEMIA[42,246,278]

ASSESSMENT
Data Collection
Subjective Data
- Severe precordial or substernal chest pain
- Crushing chest sensation
- Pain radiates to the left arm, shoulder, throat, jaw, or teeth
- Apprehension or a feeling of impending doom
  Nausea
  Weakness
  Dyspnea

Objective Data
- Pallor or cyanosis
- Cold, clammy skin
  Tachycardia
  Decreased blood pressure
  Vomiting
  Loss of consciousness

Data Analysis

Nursing Diagnosis
ACUTE CARDIAC ISCHEMIA: The sudden onset of a disruption of the blood supply to cardiac tissue

Common Etiology (Stressors)
DISEASES: Angina pectoris, arteriosclerotic heart disease, hypertension, myocardial infarction
PSYCHOSOCIAL FACTORS: The threat of cardiac or severe stress, excitement
LIFESTYLE: Cigarette smoking, high-fat diet, lack of exercise, excess time and effort at employment, heavy exertion
SITUATIONAL FACTORS: Situational crisis
ENVIRONMENTAL FACTORS: Excessive environmental cold
MAJOR PATHOPHYSIOLOGIC FACTORS CAUSING THE PROBLEM: The blood supply through the coronary arteries is compromised due to the narrowing of the vessel lumen from plaque

or spasm, and a disparity exists between the myocardial oxygen supply and demand

PLANNING

Unmet Needs

Tissue oxygenation or perfusion, rest, comfort, protection from physical harm, freedom from pain, increased learning

Expected Outcome

Warm, pink skin, nails, lips, earlobes
Blood pressure, pulse, respirations within normal limits
The person verbalizes the cessation of pain

NURSING INTERVENTIONS

Nursing Treatments

Place in the sitting position
Position comfortably (for maximum pain relief and respiratory efficiency)
Remove constrictive clothing
Refrain from giving hot and iced liquids
Give whiskey or brandy (1–2 ounces to promote circulation, if in an outpatient setting where medication is not available)
Administer humidified oxygen (ET) (if available)
Administer intravenous fluids (ET) (to provide an open line for drug administration)
Connect the person to an ECG monitor
Place on complete bed rest
Cover with lightweight blankets (if the environment is cold and if the person is not bordering on shock)
Refrain from giving oral stimulants (such as coffee and tea)
Reassure verbally (since the anxiety level is always high when a person experiences pain)
Obtain a blood sample and send for analysis (CBC, electrolytes, CPK, SGOT, SGPT, LDH, arterial blood gases)
Provide standby equipment (defibrillator) and drugs (morphine, lidocaine, nitroglycerine)
Consult with the physician (immediately after giving emergency treatment)
Obtain a complete present and past history

Nursing Observations

Auscultate the chest for abnormal heart sounds
Observe the ECG monitor (for dysrhythmias)
Monitor blood studies for abnormal hematology, electrolytes, cardiac enzymes, for arterial blood gases
Auscultate the chest for lung aeration (note any rales)
Inspect the neck veins for distention
Inspect the chest for respiratory rate and ryhthm (every 15 minutes)
Monitor the blood pressure (every 15 minutes)
Palpate the pulse for rate, rhythm, and volume (every 15 minutes)
Observe for complaints of (recurring) pain radiation

Health Teaching

Instruct to report immediately serious symptoms (of recurring chest pain)
Explain the causes of the pain (increased demands for oxygen by the heart)
Explain the reason for and intended effect of the therapy (to improve circulation resulting in pain relief)

Medical Treatments Performed by Nurses

Give the prescribed drugs (morphine to relieve pain, lidocaine drip to correct dysrhythmias, nitroglycerine to improve circulation)

EVALUATION

Record actual outcome

BLOOD TRANSFUSION REACTION[72,278,451]

ASSESSMENT

Data Collection

Subjective Data

Allergic Manifestations
• Itching
  Dyspnea

Hemolytic Manifestations
• Chills during a blood transfusion
• Sudden chest, back, or abdominal pain
• Head fullness sensation

Objective Data

Allergic Manifestations
• Facial flushing
• Urticaria (hives) or rash
  Wheezing breath sounds
  Laryngeal edema

Hemolytic Manifestations
• Fever during a blood transfusion
• Hemoglobinemia and hemoglobinuria
  Neck vein distention
  Tachycardia
  Increased respirations
  Decreased blood pressure
  Oliguria

Data Analysis

Nursing Diagnosis

BLOOD TRANSFUSION REACTION: An antigen–antibody reaction or an incompatibility of donor–recipient red blood cells during or following the administration of blood or blood components

Common Etiology (Stressors)

BIRTH DEFECTS: Atopy

HEALTH CARE FACTORS: *Medical therapy*: Blood transfusion, exchange blood transfusion

MAJOR PATHOPHYSIOLOGIC FACTORS CAUSING THE PROBLEM: A blood transfusion reaction is the result of the introduction of a foreign protein into the circulatory system; hemolysis of the donor red blood cells occurs when the ABO group and/or the Rh factors are incompatible, and allergic manifestations occur when the recipient has antibodies against food, drug, or other antigens in the donor blood

PLANNING

Unmet Needs

Rest, comfort, protection from physical harm, increased learning

Expected Outcome

Body temperature of 98.6° F (37° C)
Blood pressure, pulse, and respirations within normal limits
Urine output of at least 30 cc and preferably 60 cc per hour

NURSING INTERVENTIONS

Nursing Treatments

Discontinue the blood transfusion (immediately)
Administer intravenous fluids (ET) (saline solution to keep the line open in case shock

occurs, for emergency drug administration, and to prevent renal shutdown)

Cover with lightweight blankets (if the person is having a chill)

Consult with the physician (immediately following the emergency treatment)

Provide standby equipment (oxygen) and drugs (epinephrine, Benadryl, Levophed, mannitol, sodium bicarbonate)

Obtain a blood and urine sample and send for analysis (the presence of hemoglobin in the urine indicates intravascular hemolysis)

Send a blood sample for type and crossmatch (in case further transfusions are needed)

Return the blood to the blood bank after a reaction

Nursing Observations

Monitor the blood pressure (every 15 minutes)

Measure the urine output hourly

Monitor the oral temperature (for fever within the hour)

Inspect the chest for respiratory rate and rhythm

Palpate the pulse for rate, rhythm, and volume

Health Teaching

Explain the causes of the health problem (the presence of foreign protein in the circulatory system, the incompatibility of the red blood cells of the recipient and the donor)

Explain the reason for and intended effect of the therapy (to counteract the blood transfusion reaction)

Explain the importance of blood replacement after transfusion

Medical Treatments Performed by Nurses

Give the prescribed drugs (epinephrine to increase the blood pressure and myocardial contractility, Benadryl to prevent or minimize histamine release, Levophed to increase the blood pressure, mannitol to start diuresis, sodium bicarbonate to prevent hemoglobin precipitation in the renal tubules)

EVALUATION

Record actual outcome

CARDIAC ARREST [104,246,278,451,528,532]

ASSESSMENT

Data Collection

Subjective Data

None

Objective Data

• Unconsciousness and collapse

• Absent breathing

• Pulselessness

  Ventricular fibrillation or asystole

  Dilated pupils

  No audible blood pressure

  Cyanosis

  Grand mal seizue sometimes simultaneous with collapse

  Death within a few minutes if untreated

Data Analysis

Nursing Diagnosis

CARDIAC ARREST: The cessation of myocardial contraction and blood circulation

Common Etiology (Stressors)
DISEASES: Myocardial infarction
INJURIES: Electrical shock
HEALTH CARE FACTORS: *Drug therapy:* Narcotics
ENVIRONMENTAL FACTORS: *Electricity:* Exposure to ungrounded electrical currents, lightning
MAJOR PATHOPHYSIOLOGIC FACTORS CAUSING THE PROBLEM: During respirations, oxygen is inhaled into the lungs making a supply of oxygen available to the blood vessels and cardiac muscle; normally the heart perfuses the brain cells with oxygen, and the cardiac control center of the brain then sends signals to the heart to maintain cardiac functioning; the brain's oxygen supply can be cut off by respiratory or cardiac inefficiency; when this occurs, the heart does not receive the stimuli from the brain's cardiac control center and the heart stops (cardiac arrest)

PLANNING

Unmet Needs
Tissue oxygenation or perfusion, protection from physical harm

Expected Outcome
Immediately reestablished myocardial contractions and respirations
Eventual blood pressure, pulse, and respirations within normal limits
Consciousness without cerebral impairment

NURSING INTERVENTIONS

Nursing Treatments
Use either the head-tilt or jaw-thrust maneuver to maintain an airway
Ventilate the person (ET) (using mouth-to-mouth breathing or an AmbuBag until spontaneous respirations return, give four quick breaths initially, then one breath after every five chest compressions)
Ventilate the person mouth-to-stoma or bag-to-stoma when the patient has a laryngectomy/tracheostomy (ET)
Remove the foreign objects (from the airway if there is evidence of such)
Apply a precordial thump (ET) (if there is no carotid or femoral pulse, do this only once, do not do this on children)
Initiate external cardiac massage (ET) (if the heartbeat is not restored; slip a board under the person's back or place the person on a hard surface; apply chest compressions two finger breadths above the xyphoid process; single rescuer: 15 compressions to each two breaths, 80 compressions per minute; two rescuers: 60 compressions per minute; continue until spontaneous pulsations return)
Insert an oral airway
  OR
Initiate endotracheal intubation (ET)
Administer humidified oxygen (ET)
Administer intermittent positive-pressure breathing (ET) (or attach to another mechanical breathing device such as an AmbuBag or mechanical ventilator; do not use during external cardiac compression)
Suction the airway (as needed after respirations are reestablished)
Insert a nasogastric tube and attach to suction (ET) (if there is gastric distention and only after respirations are reestablished; do not interrupt cardiac compression to perform this procedure)
Connect the person to an ECG monitor
Defibrillate the heart muscle (ET) (after cardiac monitoring is established and if the person is in ventricular fibrillation; deliver countershock according to established procedure; to be done only by persons certified and experienced in this skill; observe precautionary methods against skin burns, myocardial damage, and electrical shock to the operator)
Administer intravenous fluids (ET) (to establish an open line for drug administration)

Nursing Observations

Observe the level of consciousness

Inspect the chest for respiratory rate and rhythm (note if the chest rises and falls and if the person's air on expiration can be heard and felt)

Inspect for foreign bodies in the airway (if there is not an immediate response to ventilation)

Observe the ECG monitor (for dysrhythmia detection)

Auscultate the apical heartbeat for rate and rhythm

Inspect the chest for respiratory rate and rhythm

Measure the intake

Measure the urine output hourly

Monitor the blood pressure

Palpate for arterial pulsations

Monitor blood studies for arterial blood gases

Health Teaching

Explain the causes of the health problem (after the episode)

Explain the reason for and intended effect of the therapy (after the episode)

Medical Treatments Performed by Nurses

Give the prescribed drugs:

Sodium bicarbonate intravenously for the purpose of combating metabolic acidosis and reestablishing acid–base balance

Epinephrine in a diluted intravenous solution for the purpose of restoring electrical activity

Atropine sulfate intravenously for the purpose of accelerating the cardiac rate

Lidocaine intravenously, since it has an antidysrhythmic effect, depressing ventricular irritability

Calcium chloride intravenously for the purpose of restoring electrical rhythm; do not administer sodium bicarbonate and calcium together, because they form a precipitate

EVALUATION

Record actual outcome

CIRCULATORY OVERLOAD[73,247]

ASSESSMENT

Data Collection

Subjective Data
- Pounding headache
  Dyspnea
  Anxiety

Objective Data
- Venous distention
- Increased blood pressure
- Increased venous pressure above 10 cm H_2O
- Increased pulmonary capillary wedge pressure
- Rapid pulse
- Flushed skin
  Coughing
  Rapid shallow breathing

Urine output exceeds 50 cc per hour
Decreased serum sodium
Decreased urine specific gravity
Rales

Data Analysis

Nursing Diagnosis
CIRCULATORY OVERLOAD (FLUID OVERLOAD): Excessive volume of fluid in the circulatory system

Common Etiology (Stressors)
DISEASES: Renal failure
HEALTH CARE FACTORS: *Medical therapy*: Intravenous infusion, blood transfusion, exchange blood transfusion
MAJOR PATHOPHYSIOLOGIC FACTORS CAUSING THE PROBLEM: Too rapid administration of intravenous fluids or blood produces a sudden increase in the blood volume, and the heart cannot hold and pump the excess blood volume, resulting in back pressure in the venous system and excessive work load on the myocardium

PLANNING

Unmet Needs
Tissue oxygenation and perfusion, fluid and electrolyte balance, rest, comfort, protection from physical harm

Expected Outcome
Central venous pressure of 4–10 cm H_2O
Pulmonary capillary wedge pressure of 4–12 mm Hg
Blood pressure, pulse, and respirations within normal limits
No venous distention
Warm, pink skin
No rales

NURSING INTERVENTIONS

Nursing Treatments
Attend the patient constantly
Discontinue the intravenous infusion or the blood transfusion
   OR
Slow the intravenous infusion or blood transfusion flow rate
Elevate the head
Place in the sitting position
Provide standby drugs
Consult with the physician (immediately after giving emergency treatment)

Nursing Observations
Measure the intake
Measure the urine output hourly
Monitor the blood pressure
Monitor the central venous pressure
Palpate the pulse for rate, rhythm, and volume
Inspect the chest for respiratory rate and rhythm
Auscultate the chest for rales

Health Teaching
Explain the causes of the health problem (excessive fluids)
Explain the reason for and intended effect of the therapy (to stabilize fluid volume)

Medical Treatments Performed by Nurses
Give the prescribed drugs

EVALUATION

Record actual outcome

HEAT EXHAUSTION [104,219,278]

ASSESSMENT

Data Collection

Subjective Data
- Weakness
  Extreme fatigue
  Headache
  Nausea
  Abdominal or extremity cramps, sometimes

Objective Data
- Pallor
- Profuse perspiration with cool, clammy skin
- Normal body temperature
- Weak, thready pulse
  Vomiting, sometimes

Data Analysis

Nursing Diagnosis
HEAT EXHAUSTION: The collapse of the peripheral circulatory system in response to fluid and salt depletion from exposure to intense environmental heat

Common Etiology (Stressors)
HEALTH CARE FACTORS: Lack of health instruction
ENVIRONMENTAL FACTORS: *Environmental heat*: High external temperature
HUMAN ERROR: Prolonged vigorous activity causing heavy perspiration without fluid and sodium replacement
MAJOR PATHOPHYSIOLOGIC FACTORS CAUSING THE PROBLEM: Heavy perspiration in a hot, humid environment leads to acute hypovolemia and salt depletion; blood pools beneath the skin in the blood vessels that are dilated to release heat; the inadequate return of blood to the heart triggers the generalized sympathetic nervous system into action, resulting in manifestations of hypovolemic shock

PLANNING

Unmet Needs
Fluid and electrolyte balance, normal temperature, sleep and rest, comfort, protection from physical harm, increased learning

Expected Outcome
Warm, slightly moist, pink skin
Blood pressure, pulse, respirations within normal limits
Gradual renewal of strength

NURSING INTERVENTIONS

Nursing Treatments
Give a salt-soda solution orally (one-half glass every 15 minutes for 1 hour of a mixture of 1 tsp salt and ½ tsp baking soda in 1 quart water, or give salty soups or bouillon)
  OR
Administer intravenous fluids (ET) (isotonic saline solution)
Bathe in cool water
Give iced liquids (iced coffee is preferable as a stimulant)
Place in the flat position (initially, with knees bent and feet elevated)
Place in the foot-elevated, head-lowered (Trendelenburg) position (if the patient fails to respond)
Increase drafts (with an electric fan)
Maintain a cool room temperature

Refrain from giving hot liquids

Provide standby equipment (oxygen, mechanical ventilator, ECG monitor) and drugs (Levophed, Aramine in case shock occurs)

Consult with a physician

OR

Make a referral (to a physicial immediately after giving emergency treatment)

Obtain a complete present and past history

Nursing Observations

Monitor the blood pressure

Monitor the rectal temperature (every 15 minutes)

Health Teaching

Advise against exposure to intense heat

Explain the reason for the intended effect of the therapy (to increase fluid volume and increase circulation)

Medical Treatments Performed by Nurses

Give the prescribed drugs (Levophed or Aramine to increase blood pressure if shock occurs)

EVALUATION

Record actual outcome

HEAT STROKE [26,73,104,219,278]

ASSESSMENT

Data Collection

Subjective Data
- Headache
- Dizziness
- Nausea

Objective Data
- Tachycardia
- Flushed, hot, dry skin with the absence of sweating
- Temperature elevation to or above 106° F (41.1° C)
  Decreased blood pressure
  Unconsciousness, sometimes

Related Data
  Persons aged 40 and over are most susceptible

Data Analysis

Nursing Diagnosis

HEAT STROKE: Impaired functioning of the body's heat regulating mechanism in response to exposure to intense environmental heat

Common Etiology (Stressors)

ENVIRONMENTAL FACTORS: *Environmental heat*: High external temperature

MAJOR PATHOPHYSIOLOGIC FACTORS CAUSING THE PROBLEM: A combined high or low environmental humidity, poor air circulation, and an excessively high environmental temperature prevent sufficient evaporation of perspiration for cooling the body, and dehydration and failure of the perspiration-regulating mechanism in the hypothalamus cause a rapid and extreme rise in the body temperature

PLANNING
Unmet Needs
Fluid and electrolyte balance, normal temperature, sleep and rest, comfort, protection from physical harm, increased learning

Expected Outcome
Immediate temperature reduction to 102° F (38.9° C) with gradual decrease to 98.6° F (37° C)
Blood pressure, pulse, respirations within normal limits
Warm, slightly moist, pink skin
Consciousness without cerebral impairment

NURSING INTERVENTIONS
Nursing Treatments
Administer mechanical ventilation (ET) (if there is respiratory distress)
Bathe in cool water (in a bathtub filled with ice water, until the person's temperature reaches 103° F (39.4° C)
> OR

Apply alcohol to the skin (if a cold tub bath is not available)
> OR

Apply an ice bag (around the torso, until the person's temperature reaches 103° F (39.4° C)
Administer an enema (cold, saline if the temperature remains elevated)
Massage gently (the entire body)
Administer intravenous fluids (ET) (give an isotonic solution only after the temperature is below 102° F, give slowly)
Provide standby equipment (oxygen, hypothermia blanket, endotracheal tube) and drugs (chlorpromazine, sedatives, isoproterenol)
Increase drafts (with an electric fan)
Maintain a cool room temperature
Refrain from giving hot liquids, from giving oral stimulants
Place on complete bed rest
Withhold the drugs (sedatives)
Consult with a physician
> OR

Make a referral (to a physician or emergency room immediately after giving emergency treatment)
Obtain a complete present and past history

Nursing Observations
Monitor the blood pressure
Monitor the rectal temperature (every 15 minutes)
Inspect the chest for respiratory rate and rhythm
Palpate the pulse for rate, rhythm, and volume
Inspect the eyes for pupil size, equality, and response to light
Measure the intake and output

Health Teaching
Explain the reason for and intended effect of the therapy (to bring the temperature to a normal level)
Describe those symptoms that should be reported (since faulty heat regulation and lowered heat tolerance may persist indefinitely)
Advise against exposure to intense heat

Medical Treatments Performed by Nurses
Place on a hypothermia blanket
Give the prescribed drugs

EVALUATION
Record actual outcome

HEMORRHAGE[73,104,246,278]

ASSESSMENT

Data Collection

Subjective Data
Generalized weakness
Anxiety
Dizziness
Nausea
Thirst

Objective Data
• Rapid, weak, irregular pulse
• Rapid, shallow respirations
• Extreme restlessness
• Pallor
• Cold, moist skin
  Decreased blood pressure
  Confusion
  Vomiting
  Progressive swelling and discoloration of soft tissue (from internal hemorrhage)

External Hemorrhage
Bright red blood from surface wounds

Internal Hemorrhage
Hematemesis (dark, red, black, or brown vomitus)
Tarry stools (black, sticky stools)
Severe hemoptysis (bright red, frothy sputum)
Severe hematuria (bright red blood in the urine)
Postpartum hemorrhage (bright red blood from the vagina within 48 hours following delivery)

Data Analysis

Nursing Diagnosis
HEMORRHAGE: The abnormal internal or external loss of blood from the body

Common Etiology (Stressors)
BIRTH DEFECTS: Hemophilia
DISEASES: Natural abortion, carcinoma, disseminated intravascular coagulation, esophageal varices, peptic ulcer, tuberculosis
INJURIES: Avulsion wound, bone fracture, fracture of the liver and/or spleen, incision wound, laceration wound, penetrating wound, puncture wound, ruptured aorta, sucking chest wound, traumatic amputation
HUMAN BODY: *Body state*: Pregnancy, childbirth
HEALTH CARE FACTORS: *Diagnostic procedure*: Angiography, biopsy. *Drug therapy*: Anticoagulant therapy. *Medical therapy*: Hemodialysis, radiation therapy. *Surgical therapy*: Surgery of any kind
ENVIRONMENTAL FACTORS: *Blast/explosion*: Exposure to. *Cataclysm*: Exposure to. *Chemical substances*: Ingestion of. *Crushing*: By cave-in, building collapse, falling object. *Foreign body*: Propelled. *Motor vehicles*: Impact or collision of. *Objects*: Pointed, sharp. *Tools*: Powered and nonpowered. *Weapons*: Gun, knife
MAJOR PATHOPHYSIOLOGIC FACTORS CAUSING THE PROBLEM: Abnormalities of the blood vessel walls can be caused by trauma or disease, allowing the blood to escape the blood vessels, to accumulate in the tissues or body spaces, or to drain from the body through wounds or orifices; abnormalities of the clotting mechanism, either hereditary or acquired, permit spontaneous hemorrhage and hemorrhage from minor vascular injury

PLANNING

Unmet Needs

Tissue oxygenation or perfusion, fluid and electrolyte balance, sleep and rest, comfort, protection from physical harm, increased learning

Expected Outcome

Cessation of hemorrhage
Blood pressure, pulse, respirations within normal limits
Warm, slightly moist, pink skin
Consciousness without cerebral impairment

NURSING INTERVENTIONS

Nursing Treatments

Cover with lightweight blankets
Handle gently (to prevent further injury)
Place on complete bed rest
Position comfortably
Refrain from giving hot liquids, oral stimulants, and local heat applications

Specific to External Hemorrhage

Apply manual pressure over the bleeding area
Apply an ice bag (to the bleeding area)
Apply a pressure dressing
Apply a tourniquet between the extremity wound and the body (only if other methods fail)
Elevate the extremity
Immobilize the affected body part
Give water orally (if the person is able to drink; give as much as the person can comfortably tolerate)

Specific to Internal Hemorrhage

Hematemesis or tarry stools:
    Restrict the intake to nothing by mouth
    Place in the flat position
    Refrain from inserting objects into a bleeding orifice
Hematuria:
    Place in the flat position
    Refrain from inserting objects into a bleeding orifice
Severe hemoptysis:
    Place in the slight sitting (semi-Fowler's, semirecumbent) position
    Place on the affected side
    Refrain from giving positive-pressure breathing
Administer humidified oxygen (ET)
Administer intravenous fluids (ET)
Catheterize with an indwelling urinary catheter (for accurate output)
Obtain a blood sample and send for analysis (CBC, electrolytes)
Send a blood sample for type and crossmatch
Provide standby equipment (suturing material, central venous pressure equipment, nasogastric tube and suction, airway suction), drugs, whole blood
Consult with the physician (immediately after giving emergency treatment)
Obtain a complete present and past history

Nursing Observations

Estimate the blood volume loss
Inspect the chest for respiratory rate and rhythm
Observe for dyspnea, for cyanosis
Palpate the pulse for rate, rhythm, and volume (compare pulses bilaterally)
Monitor the blood pressure (compare the blood pressure bilaterally (left and right sides), take every 10–15 minutes)

Palpate the skin for temperature (cold and warmth)
Inspect the skin for color (changes)
Inspect for edema
Observe for complaints of pain
Monitor blood studies for abnormal hematology and abnormal electrolytes
Measure the intake and output

Health Teaching
Explain the causes of the health problem (disruption of circulatory intactness)
Explain the reason for and intended effect of the therapy (to maintain blood perfusion
  to tissues)

Medical Treatments Performed by Nurses
Administer a blood transfusion
Give the prescribed drugs

EVALUATION

Record actual outcome

ANAPHYLACTIC SHOCK[20,56,104,219,246]

ASSESSMENT
Data Collection
Subjective Data
Weakness
Nausea
Choking sensation
Anxiety
Itching
Paresthesia
Thirst

Objective Data
• Decreased or absent blood pressure
• Rapid, weak pulse
• Wheezing respirations and dyspnea
• Cold, clammy skin
• Pallor or cyanosis
• Urticaria, angioedema, or erythema
• Onset from within seconds to 30 minutes of drug injection or insect bite
  Pupil dilatation (in late shock)
  Incontinence
  Unconsciousness sometimes

Data Analysis
Nursing Diagnosis
ANAPHYLACTIC SHOCK (ALLERGIC SHOCK): Sudden circulatory collapse resulting from foreign
  protein entering the blood of a sensitized person

Common Etiology (Stressors)
BIRTH DEFECTS: Atopy
HEALTH CARE FACTORS: *Drug therapy*: Adverse effects of drugs
ENVIRONMENTAL FACTORS: *Biologic agents*: Bites of insects
MAJOR PATHOPHYSIOLOGIC FACTORS CAUSING THE PROBLEM: The second or subsequent exposure
  of a sensitized person to an allergen produces an antigen-antibody (IgE) reaction that

results in profound bronchoconstriction, prolonged dilatation, and increased permeability of small blood vessels; the latter causes a decreased venous blood return to the heart, resulting in decreased cardiac output and inadequate tissue perfusion

PLANNING

Unmet Needs

Tissue oxygenation or perfusion, fluid and electrolyte balance, Acid–base balance, rest, comfort, protection from physical harm, increased learning

Expected Outcome

Blood pressure, pulse, respirations within normal limits
Warm, slightly moist, pink skin
Consciousness without cerebral impairment

NURSING INTERVENTIONS

Nursing Treatments

Insert an oral airway (if needed)
Ventilate the person (if there is respiratory distress, using mouth-to-mouth breathing until spontaneous respirations occur)
Give prescription drugs (use epinephrine in cold compounds or by inhaler if epinephrine is not available for subcutaneous administration, give an oral antihistamine if the person is able to swallow)
Place on complete bed rest
Place in the foot-elevated head-lowered (Trendelenburg) position
Cover with lightweight blankets
Administer humidified oxygen (ET) (if needed)
Administer intermittent positive-pressure breathing (ET) (if needed)
Administer intravenous fluids (ET) (lactated Ringer's or physiologic saline, immediately)
Apply a tourniquet between the extremity wound and the body (if shock is due to an insect bite)
Catheterize with an indwelling urinary catheter (for measuring the output)
Connect the person to an ECG monitor
Consult with a physician (immediately after giving emergency treatment)
Obtain a blood sample and send for analysis (CBC, electrolytes, arterial blood gases)
Provide standby equipment (oral airway, tracheostomy tube, oxygen, mechanical ventilator) and drugs (epinephrine, Benadryl, Levophed, dopamine, aminophyllin, dextran)
Obtain a complete present and past history
Make a referral (to an allergist for desensitization therapy, as part of discharge planning)

Nursing Observations

Palpate the pulse for rate, rhythm, and volume (every 15 minutes)
Inspect the chest for respiratory rate and rhythm (every 15 minutes)
Monitor the blood pressure (every 15 minutes)
Auscultate the apical heartbeat for rate and rhythm
Observe the ECG monitor
Measure the intake
Measure the urine output hourly (for an output of at least 30 cc per hour)

Health Teaching

Explain the importance of wearing a Medic Alert tag
Explain how to take allergy precautions (to carry an anaphylaxis kit)

Medical Treatments Performed by Nurses

Give the prescribed drugs (epinephrine to increase blood pressure and cardiac contractility, Benadryl to prevent or minimize histamine release, Levophed or dopamine to increase blood pressure, aminophylline to reduce bronchospasms)

EVALUATION

Record actual outcome

BACTEREMIC SHOCK [56,104,246,278,339]

ASSESSMENT

Data Collection

Subjective Data
Anxiety
Weakness
Nausea
Thirst

Objective Data
• Chills
• Decreased blood pressure
• Rapid bounding pulse
• Rapid respirations
• Cold, clammy skin following warm, flushed, dry skin
• Fever
• Elevated white blood count
• Pupil dilatation (in late shock)

Data Analysis

Nursing Diagnosis
BACTEREMIC SHOCK (SEPTIC SHOCK, ENDOTOXIC SHOCK, EXOTOXIC SHOCK): Circulatory collapse resulting from bacterial invastion into the bloodstream

Common Etiology (Stressors)
DISEASES: Carcinoma, diabetes mellitus, gastritis, glomerulonephritis, Laennec's cirrhosis, leukemia, peritonitis, pyelonephritis
INJURIES: Burn wound, intestinal perforation, laceration wound, penetrating wound, puncture wound, self-inflicted abortion
HEALTH CARE FACTORS: *Drug therapy*: Immunosuppressant therapy. *Surgical therapy*: Surgery of the genitourinary tract. *Therapeutic products*: Urinary and intravenous catheters, use of vaginal tampons
ENVIRONMENTAL FACTORS: *Biologic agents*: Exposure to infectious agents (bacteria)
MAJOR PATHOPHYSIOLOGIC FACTORS CAUSING THE PROBLEM: Overwhelming bacterial invasion of the bloodstream results in the release of toxins that precipitate shock by affecting vascular quality, causing pooling and stagnation of blood, and depressing cardiac function

PLANNING

Unmet Needs

Tissue oxygenation or perfusion, fluid and electrolyte balance, acid–base balance, rest, comfort, protection from physical harm, increased learning

Expected Outcome

Blood pressure, pulse, and respirations within normal limits
Temperature of 98.6° F (37° C)
Warm, slightly moist, pink skin
Consciousness without cerebral impairment

NURSING INTERVENTIONS

Nursing Treatments

Ventilate the person (if necessary, using mouth-to-mouth breathing until spontaneous respirations occur)
   OR
Administer mechanical ventilation (ET) (if needed)
Administer intravenous fluids (ET) (lactated Ringer's or isotonic saline solution, immediately)

Administer humidified oxygen (ET)
Connect the person to an ECG monitor
Catheterize with an indwelling urinary catheter (for measuring the output)
Place in the flat position
   OR
Place in the foot-elevated head-lowered (Trendelenburg) position
Place on complete bed rest
Cover with lightweight blankets
Maintain a warm room temperature
Consult with a physician (immediately after giving emergency treatment)
Obtain a blood sample and send for analysis (CBC, electrolytes, arterial blood gases)
Provide standby equipment (endotracheal tube, central venous pressure) and drugs

Nursing Observations
Palpate the pulse for rate, rhythm, and volume (every 15 minutes)
Inspect the chest for respiratory rate and rhythm (every 15 minutes)
Monitor the blood pressure (every 15 minutes)
Auscultate the apical heartbeat for rate and rhythm
Observe the ECG monitor
Measure the intake
Measure the urine output hourly (for an output of at least 30 cc per hour)
Monitor blood studies for abnormal hematology (increased WBC)
Monitor the central venous pressure
Monitor the rectal temperature

Health Teaching
Explain the causes of the health problem (bacteria in the bloodstream)
Explain the reason for and intended effect of the therapy (to reduce infection and restore adequate circulation)

Medical Treatments Performed by Nurses
Give the prescribed drugs

EVALUATION
Record actual outcome

CARDIOGENIC SHOCK [56,104,246,278,339]

ASSESSMENT
Data Collection
Subjective Data
Anxiety
Weakness
Nausea
Thirst

Objective Data
• Decreased blood pressure (systolic pressure is usually less than 90 mm Hg)
• Rapid, weak pulse
• Rapid, shallow respirations
• Cold, clammy skin
• Pallor or cyanosis
• Engorged neck veins
• Decreased urinary output
  Confusion to unconsciousness

Data Analysis

Nursing Diagnosis

CARDIOGENIC SHOCK: Primary dysfunction of the left ventricle resulting in inadequate forward blood flow

Common Etiology (Stressors)

DISEASES: Myocardial infarction

MAJOR PATHOPHYSIOLOGIC FACTORS CAUSING THE PROBLEM: The heart is unable to pump sufficient blood to all body parts, despite normal blood volume, resulting in inadequate peripheral circulation

PLANNING

Unmet Needs

Tissue oxygenation or perfusion, fluid and electrolyte balance, acid–base balance, rest, comfort, protection from physical harm

Expected Outcome

Normal sinus rhythm, if possible
Blood pressure, pulse, and respirations within normal limits
No venous distention
Urine output of at least 30 cc per hour
Warm, slightly moist, pink skin
Consciousness without cerebral impairment

NURSING INTERVENTIONS

Nursing Treatments

Ventilate the person (if there is respiratory distress, use mouth-to-mouth breathing until spontaneous respirations occur)
Insert an oral airway (if available)
Administer humidified oxygen (ET)
Administer intravenous fluids (ET) (to provide an open line for drug administration)
Connect the person to an ECG monitor
Catheterize with an indwelling urinary catheter (for measuring the output)
Elevate the head (30 degrees)
Place on complete bed rest
Cover with lightweight blankets
Maintain a warm room temperature
Consult with a physician (immediately after giving emergency treatment)
Obtain a blood sample and send for analysis (CBC, electrolytes, arterial blood gases)
Send a blood sample for type and crossmatch
Provide standby equipment (central venous pressure, Swan-Ganz catheter, intra-aortic balloon pump) and drugs (dopamine, Levophed, Isuprel, digitalis)
Obtain a complete present and past history

Nursing Observations

Palpate the pulse for rate, rhythm, and volume (every 15 minutes)
Inspect the chest for respiratory rate and rhythm (every 15 minutes)
Monitor the blood pressure (every 15 minutes)
Observe the ECG monitor (for cardiac abnormalities)
Auscultate the apical heartbeat for rate and rhythm
Measure the intake
Measure the urine output hourly (for an output of at least 30 cc per hour)
Monitor blood studies for arterial blood gases
Monitor the central venous pressure
Monitor the pulmonary artery (PA) pressure and pulmonary capillary wedge (PCWP) pressure by Swan-Ganz catheter
Monitor the internal counterpulsation intra-aortic balloon apparatus

Health Teaching

Explain the causes of the health problem (left ventricular dysfunction results in inadequate peripheral circulation)

Explain the reason for and intended effect of the therapy (to reestablish adequate cardiac output and circulation)

Medical Treatments Performed by Nurses

Give the prescribed drugs

EVALUATION

Record actual outcome

ELECTRICAL SHOCK[42,572]

ASSESSMENT

Date Collection

Subjective Data

Notification that a person has had contact with an electrical current

Objective Data

- Decreased or absent blood pressure
- Rapid, weak, or absent pulse
- Rapid or absent respirations
- Cold skin
- Pallor or cyanosis
- Ventricular fibrillation or absent pulse
- Momentary or prolonged unconsciousness
  Electrical burn may be evident on the skin
  Person may be frozen to an electrical source and in a rigid position

Data Analysis

Nursing Diagnosis

ELECTRICAL SHOCK: Cardiovascular collapse when ventricular fibrillation results from contact with an electric current

Common Etiology (Stressors)

ENVIRONMENTAL FACTORS: *Electricity*: Exposure to ungrounded electrical currents. *Lightning*: Exposure to

MAJOR PATHOPHYSIOLOGIC FACTORS CAUSING THE PROBLEM: When a low or moderate electric current hits the heart at the end of repolarization (T-wave), the heart may go into ventricular fibrillation; prolonged respiratory paralysis results from depression of the respiratory center by higher voltage electrical shock; moisture decreases the skin's resistance to an electrical current and permits better conduction with greater potential for tissue injury

PLANNING

Unmet Needs

Tissue oxygenation or perfusion, acid–base balance, rest, comfort, protection from physical harm, increased learning

Expected Outcome

Normal sinus rhythm

Blood pressure, pulse and respirations within normal limits

Urine output of at least 30 cc per hour

Warm, slightly moist, pink skin
Consciousness without cerebral impairment

NURSING INTERVENTIONS

Nursing Treatments

Cut off the electrical power source causing the injury
Remove the person from the electrocuting source with a nonconducting material
Ventilate the person (ET) (using mouth-to-mouth breathing until spontaneous respirations occur)
Initiate external cardiac massage (ET) (as needed)
Administer humidified oxygen (ET)
Administer intravenous fluids (ET)
Defibrillate the heart muscle (ET) (if needed)
Connect the person to an ECG monitor
Insert a gastric tube and attach to suction (ET) (to prevent vomiting)
Catheterize with an indwelling urinary catheter (for measuring the output)
Place in the flat position
Cover with lightweight blankets
Consult with a physician (immediately after giving emergency treatment)
Obtain a blood sample and send for analysis (CBC, electrolytes, arterial blood gases)
Send a blood sample for type and crossmatch
Provide standby equipment (central venous pressure) and drugs
Obtain a complete present and past history

Nursing Observations

Palpate the pulse for rate, rhythm, and volume (every 5 minutes)
Inspect the chest for respiratory rtae and rhythm (every 15 minutes)
Monitor the blood pressure (every 15 minutes)
Auscultate the apical heartbeat for rate and rhythm
Observe the ECG monitor
Measure the intake
Measure the urine output hourly (for an output of at least 30 cc per hour)
Monitor blood studies for arterial blood gases, for abnormal hematology, and abnormal electrolytes
Monitor the central venous pressure

Health Teaching

Explain the causes of the health problem (especially that of failing to turn off electricity before working on equipment)
Explain the importance of standing on dry surfaces and wearing insulated rubber gloves and rubber-soled shoes when working with electricity
Explain the importance of using grounded electrical equipment and appliances

Medical Treatments Performed by Nurses

Give the prescribed drugs

EVALUATION

Record actual outcome

HYPOVOLEMIC SHOCK[73,104,246,278,476]

ASSESSMENT

Data Collection

Subjective Data
• Thirst
  Anxiety

Dizziness
Weakness
Nausea

Objective Data
- Decreased blood pressure
- Rapid, weak pulse
- Rapid, shallow respirations
- Cold, clammy skin
- Pallor or cyanosis
  Decreased urinary output
  Unconsciousness

Data Analysis

Nursing Diagnosis

HYPOVOLEMIC SHOCK (HEMORRHAGIC SHOCK, HEMATOGENIC SHOCK, SURGICAL SHOCK, TRAUMATIC SHOCK, OLIGEMIC SHOCK): Circulatory collapse resulting from fluid or blood loss causing an inadequate circulating blood volume with impaired tissue perfusion

Common Etiology (Stressors)

BIRTH DEFECTS: Hemophelia

DISEASES: Natural abortion, carcinoma, disseminated intravascular coagulation, esophageal varices, hemorrhage, nephrotic syndrome, peptic ulcer, peritonitis

INJURIES: Avulsion wound, bone fracture, burn wound, fracture of liver and/or spleen, incision wound, laceration wound, penetrating wound, puncture wound, self-inflicted abortion, sucking chest wound, traumatic amputation

SIGNS AND SYMPTOMS: Dehydration, diarrhea

HUMAN BODY: *Body state*: Pregnancy

HEALTH CARE FACTORS: *Diagnostic procedures*: Angiography, biopsy. *Drug therapy*: Anticoagulant therapy. *Medical therapy*: Hemodialysis, radiation therapy. *Surgical therapy*: Surgery of any kind

ENVIRONMENTAL FACTORS: *Blast/explosion*: Exposure to. *Cataclysm*: Exposure to. *Chemical substances*: Ingestion of. *Crushing*: By cave-in, building collapse, falling object. *Foreign body*: Propelled. *Motor vehilces*: Impact or collision of. *Objects*: Pointed and sharp. *Tools*: Powered and nonpowered. *Weapons*: Guns

MAJOR PATHOPHYSIOLOGIC FACTORS CAUSING THE PROBLEM: Excessive fluid or blood loss causes reduced circulating blood volume with blood pressure reduction leading to shock

PLANNING

Unmet Needs
Tissue oxygenation or perfusion, fluid and electrolyte balance, acid–base balance, rest, comfort, protection from physical harm, increased learning

Expected Outcome
Cessation of hemorrhage or fluid loss
Blood pressure, pulse and respirations within normal limits
Urine output of at least 30 cc per hour
Warm, slightly moist, pink skin
Consciousness without cerebral impairment

NURSING INTERVENTIONS

Nursing Treatments
Ventilate the person (if there is respiratory distress, using mouth-to-mouth breathing until spontaneous respirations occur)
  OR
Administer mechanical ventilation (ET) (if needed)
Give a salt-soda solution orally (½ tsp baking soda and 1 tsp salt in 1 quart water)
  OR
Give water orally (as much as the patient can tolerate up to one quart)
  OR

Administer intravenous fluids (ET) (lactated Ringer's or isotonic saline, immediately)
Administer humidified oxygen (ET)
Connect the person to an ECG monitor
Catheterize with an indwelling urinary catheter (for measuring the output)
Place in the flat position
> OR

Place in the foot-elevated, head-lowered (Trendelenburg) position
Place on complete bed rest
Cover with lightweight blankets
Maintain a warm room temperature
Refrain from giving oral stimulants
Consult with a physician (immediately after giving emergency treatment)
Obtain a blood sample and send for analysis (CBC, electrolytes, arterial blood gases)
Send a blood sample for type and crossmatch
Provide standby equipment (central venous pressure, Swan-Ganz catheter) and drugs
Obtain a complete present and past history

Nursing Observations
Palpate the pulse for rate, rhythm, and volume (every 15 minutes)
Inspect the chest for respiratory rate and rhythm (every 15 minutes)
Monitor the blood pressure (every 15 minutes)
Auscultate the apical heartbeat for rate and rhythm
Observe the ECG monitor
Measure the intake
Measure the urine output hourly (for an output of at least 30 cc per hour)
Monitor blood studies for arterial blood gases
Monitor the central venous pressure
Monitor the pulmonary artery (PA) pressure and pulmonary capillary wedge (PCWP) pressure by Swan-Ganz catheter

Health Teaching
Explain the causes of the health problem (fluid and blood loss)
Explain the reason for and intended effect of the therapy (to reestablish adequate circulation)
Explain the importance of blood replacement after transfusion

Medical Treatments Performed by Nurses
Administer a blood transfusion (to replace the blood loss)
Give the prescribed drugs

EVALUATION
Record actual outcome

Emergency Conditions of the Endocrine System

ADRENAL SHOCK[72,451]

ASSESSMENT
Data Collection
Subjective Data
- Exhaustion
- Headache

- Nausea

Objective Data
- Decreased blood pressure
- Rapid, weak pulse
- Rapid breathing
- Cold, sweating skin
- Cyanosis of the extremities
- Vomiting
- Diarrhea
  Fever, high
  Costovertebral pain and tenderness on palpation
  Confusion
  Trembling

Data Analysis

Nursing Diagnosis
ADRENAL SHOCK (ADRENAL CRISIS, ADDISONIAN CRISIS): The acute onset of signs and symptoms indicating a severe inadequacy of the adrenocortical hormones glucocorticoids (hydrocortison/cortisol) and the mineralocorticoid (aldosterone)

Common Etiology (Stressors)
DISEASES: Addison's disease, infection of any kind
INJURIES: Severe trauma of any kind
HEALTH CARE FACTORS: *Surgical therapy*: Surgery of any kind
SITUATIONAL FACTORS: Situational stress or crisis
ENVIRONMENTAL FACTORS: *Environmental heat*: High external temperature
HUMAN ERROR: Not taking maintenance dose(s) of corticosteroids
MAJOR PATHOPHYSIOLOGIC FACTORS CAUSING THE PROBLEM: The inability of the adrenal glands to secrete adequate amounts of corticol hormones severly reduces the body's ability to adapt to stress, trauma, infection, and intense environmental heat, which can lead to adrenal shock

PLANNING

Unmet Needs
Tissue oxygenation or perfusion, fluid and electrolyte balance, acid–base balance, normal temperature, sleep and rest, comfort, protection from physical harm, increased learning

Expected Outcome
Blood pressure, pulse, respirations within normal limits
Temperature of 98.6° F (37° C)
Warm, slightly moist, pink skin
Consciousness without cerebral impairment

NURSING INTERVENTIONS

Nursing Treatments
Administer intravenous fluids (ET) (5% dextrose in normal saline)
Administer humidified oxygen (ET) (as needed)
Withhold the drugs (morphine or barbiturates until cortisone is given)
Place on complete bed rest (the patient must not turn or do anything for himself)
Cover with lightweight blankets
Maintain a normal room temperature
Provide quiet (eliminate all unnecessary stimuli)
Attend the patient constantly
Anticipate needs (so person will not move about)
Refrain from performing nonessential procedures
Maintain reverse isolation (if there is any potential for infection)
Consult with the physician (immediately after giving emergency treatment)
Obtain a blood sample and send for analysis (cortisol, sodium, glucose)

Provide standby drugs (hydrocortisone)
Obtain a complete present and past history

Nursing Observations
Auscultate the chest for abnormal heart sounds, for abnormal breath sounds
Measure the intake and output (save for a 24-hour period)
Monitor the blood pressure
Monitor blood studies for abnormal adrenal function
Monitor the oral temperature
Observe for shock
Inspect for signs of infection

Health Teaching
Explain the causes of the health problem (inadequate adrenal secretion of corticol hormones)
Explain the reason for and intended effect of the therapy (to improve and maintain adrenal function)

Medical Treatments Performed by Nurses
Give the prescribed drugs (hydrocortisone to supplement inadequate adrenal function)

EVALUATION

Record actual outcome

INSULIN SHOCK [35,72,73,339,371]

ASSESSMENT

Data Collection
Subjective Data
• Generalized weakness
  Nervousness
  Hunger
  Dizziness

Objective Data
• Pallor
• Sweating
• Shallow respirations
• Bounding, full pulse
  Tremors
  Restlessness
  Drowsiness or confusion
  Decreased blood glucose

Related Data

Commonly Related Diseases
Diabetes mellitus

Data Analysis
Nursing Diagnosis
INSULIN SHOCK (HYPOGLYCEMIC SHOCK): A critical decrease in the blood glucose of a diabetic receiving insulin therapy

Common Etiology (Stressors)

HEALTH CARE FACTORS: *Drug therapy*: Excessive insulin dosage. *Medical therapy*: Inappropriate therapeutic diet

HUMAN ERROR: Increased exercise without insulin or diet adjustment

MAJOR PATHOPHYSIOLOGIC FACTORS CAUSING THE PROBLEM: When exercise is increased, the need for insulin is decreased because glucose moves into the cells more efficiently causing the blood sugar to drop; the more efficient use of glucose by the cells requires an increase in dietary intake to prevent a severe drop in blood glucose; therefore, with increased exercise there is a decreased need for insulin and an increased need for food intake

PLANNING

Unmet Needs
Nutritional balance, rest, comfort, protection from physical harm, increased learning

Expected Outcome
Blood glucose between 80–120 mg/100 ml
Blood pressure, pulse, and respirations within normal limits
Consciousness without cerebral impairment

NURSING INTERVENTIONS

Nursing Treatments
Give hard candy (immediately)
    OR
Give high-glucose fluids orally (immediately)
Follow quick-acting glucose with long-acting carbohydrates and protein
    OR
Administer intravenous fluids (ET) (5% dextrose in water)
Place on complete bed rest
Cover with warm blankets
Maintain a warm room temperature
Refrain from giving insulin
Attend the patient constantly
Obtain a blood sample and send for analysis (glucose, electrolytes, arterial blood gases)
Consult with the physician (immediately after giving emergency treatment)
Provide standby drugs (50 cc of 50% glucose)
Obtain a complete present and past history

Nursing Observations
Monitor blood studies for abnormal glucose, electrolytes, and arterial blood gases
Test the urine for sugar and acetone
Monitor the blood pressure
Palpate the pulse for rate, rhythm, and volume
Inspect the chest for respiratory rate and rhythm
Observe the level of consciousness

Health Teaching
Explain the causes of the health problem (changes in the body's need for specific amounts of insulin)
Explain the reason for and intended effect of the therapy (to restore metabolic balance)

Medical Treatments Performed by Nurses
Give the prescribed drugs (50 cc of 50% glucose IV)

EVALUATION

Record actual outcome

THYROTOXIC SHOCK[35,42,73]

ASSESSMENT

Data Collection

Subjective Data
Weakness
Fatigue

Objective Data
• Tachycardia (140–200 beats each minute)
• Fever above 100° F
• Irritability
• Delirium or confusion
  Increased respirations
  Restlessness

Related Data
If related to a thyriodectomy, it occurs within 12 hours following surgery

Data Analysis

Nursing Diagnosis
THYROTOXIC SHOCK (THYROTOXIC STORM):   The presence of signs and symptoms indicating the onset of severe complications of thyrotoxicosis

Common Etiology (Stressors)
DISEASES: Infection of any kind, thyrotoxicosis
HEALTH CARE FACTORS: *Surgical therapy*: Surgery of any kind
SITUATIONAL FACTORS: Situational stress or crisis
MAJOR PATHOPHYSIOLOGIC FACTORS CAUSING THE PROBLEM: Increased amounts of thyroid hormones, suddenly released into the bloodstream of a person with thyrotoxicosis, causes a marked increase in metabolism, and elevation of body temperature above 106° F (hyperpyrexia) may develop as the body becomes unable to release the excessive heat of the increased metabolism

PLANNING

Nursing Treatments
Administer humidified oxygen (ET) (cool, not heated)
Administer intravenous fluids (ET) (10% dextrose in distilled water)
Connect the person to an ECG monitor
Place on complete bed rest
Maintain a cool room temperature
Provide quiet
Attend the patient constantly
Anticipate needs (so that the person does not move about)
Refrain from giving oral stimulants and hot liquids
Refrain from performing nonessential procedures
Consult with the physician (immediately after giving emergency treatment)
Obtain a blood sample and send for analysis (thryoid profile, electroytes)

Unmet Needs
Fluid and electrolyte balance, normal temperature, rest, comfort, protection from physical harm, increased learning

Expected Outcome
Reduced or no increase in blood pressure, pulse, or respirations
Temperature of 98.6° F (37° F)
Reduced restlessness

NURSING INTERVENTIONS

Provide standby equipment (nasogastric tube, hypothermia blanket) and drugs (antibiotics, propylthiouracil, sodium iodine, corticosteroids, Inderal, reserpine, or guanethidine)

Obtain a complete present and past history

Nursing Observations

Monitor the blood pressure (for decreased pressure)

Monitor the body temperature (for fever)

Observe for airway obstruction, for shock

Palpate the pulse for rate (tachycardia), rhythm, and volume

Inspect the chest for respiratory rate and rhythm

Observe the ECG monitor

Monitor blood studies for abnormal thyroid function and electrolytes

Health Teaching

Explain the causes of the health problem (a sudden increase in the production and release of thyroid hormone)

Explain the reason for and intended effect of the therapy (to reestablish balanced thyroid level)

Medical Treatments Performed by Nurses

Place on a hypothermia blanket

Give the prescribed drugs (antibiotics to reduce infection, propylthiouracil to supress thyroid hormone production, corticosteroids to supplement adrenocorticol insufficiency, Inderal, reserpine or guanethidine to block β-adrenergic receptors)

EVALUATION

Record actual outcome

Emergency Conditions of the Gastrointestinal System

ABDOMINAL EVISCERATION[73,451]

ASSESSMENT

Data Collection

Subjective Data

Person complains of a bursting abdominal sensation

Objective Data
- Dressing is wet with clear, pink drainage
- Abdominal wound edges are separated
- Abdominal contents protrude and are visible
- Surgical sutures break apart (or have pulled away from the abdominal tissue)

Data Analysis

Nursing Diagnosis

ABDOMINAL EVISCERATION (DEHISCENCE): The opening of an abdominal incision with the protrusion of intestinal contents outside the abdominal cavity

Common Etiology (Stressors)

HEALTH CARE FACTORS: *Medical therapy*: Coughing and deep breathing. *Surgical therapy*: Abdominal surgery

MAJOR PATHOPHYSIOLOGIC FACTORS CAUSING THE PROBLEM: Abdominal wound dehiscence occurs when pressure against the wound exceeds the strength of the sutures or the tissues; tissue strength is impaired in conditions such as obesity, disease (diabetes, infection), malnutrition, old age, and when sutures are removed too early; excessive pressure may result from abdominal distention and Valsalva maneuvers

PLANNING

Unmet Needs
Rest, comfort, cleanliness, protection from physical harm, increased learning

Expected Outcome
Blood pressure, pulse, and respirations within normal limits
No later evidence of wound inflammation, purulent drainage, or elevated temperature

NURSING INTERVENTIONS

Nursing Treatments
Apply a sterile dressing (soaked with warm sterile saline over the wound)
Cover with warm blankets
Place in the flat position (with legs flexed)
    OR
Place in the slight sitting position (low Fowler's)
Place on complete bed rest
Restrict the intake to nothing by mouth
Consult with the physician (immediately after giving emergency treatment)

Nursing Observations
Inspect the chest for respiratory rate and rhythm
Inspect for hemorrhage
Observe for shock
Monitor the blood pressure (for decreased pressure)
Palpate the pulse for rate, rhythm, and volume (for increased pulse)

Health Teaching
Explain the causes of the health problem (pressure against the wound)
Explain the reason for and intended effect of the therapy (to prevent infection and shock)

EVALUATION

Record actual outcome

ACUTE ABDOMINAL PAIN[104,113,246]

ASSESSMENT

Data Collection
Subjective Data
• Severe pain
• Nausea
  Anxious facial expression

Objective Data
• Tenderness on palpation of the abdomen
• Abdominal rigidity
• Vomiting
  Fever
  Abdominal distention

Data Analysis

Nursing Diagnosis

ACUTE ABDOMINAL PAIN (ACUTE ABDOMEN): The sudden onset of severe, persistent abdominal pain that involves one or more organs such as the lower esophagus, small or large intestines, liver, gallbladder, spleen, pancreas, bladder, or kidney

Common Etiology (Stressors)

DISEASES: Appendicitis, cholecystitis, pancreatitis, paralytic ileus, perforated appendix, perforated ulcer, strangulated hernia

MAJOR PATHOPHYSIOLOGIC FACTORS CAUSING THE PROBLEM: Distention or inflammation of abdominal organs or structures produces abdominal pain

PLANNING

Unmet Needs

Rest, comfort, protection from physical harm, increased learning

Expected Outcome

Blood pressure, pulse, and respirations within normal limits

Expressions of increased comfort

NURSING INTERVENTIONS

Nursing Treatments

Place on complete bed rest

Handle gently (moving the person as little as possible)

Cover with lightweight blankets

Restrict the intake to nothing by mouth

Administer intravenous fluids (ET) (to maintain an open line)

Obtain a blood sample and send for analysis (CBC, SMAC)

Obtain a urine sample and send for analysis (routine)

Send a blood sample for type and crossmatch (if blood will be needed)

Refrain from giving laxatives

Refrain from giving local heat applications

Provide standby equipment (nasogastric tube and suction, indwelling urinary catheter)

Consult with the physician (immediately, especially if there is a sudden cessation of pain)

Obtain a complete present and past history

Nursing Observations

Auscultate the abdomen for abnormal bowel sounds (absent or excessive sounds)

Inspect the abdomen for distention

Inspect the abdomen for visible peristalsis

Inspect for hemorrhage (under the abdominal surface, which indicates internal bleeding)

Monitor the oral temperature

Monitor the blood pressure

Inspect the chest for respiratory rate and rhythm

Palpate the pulse for rate, rhythm, and volume

Monitor blood studies for abnormal hematology, chemistry

Measure the intake and output

Health Teaching

Explain the reason for and intended effect of the therapy (to reduce the pain and its cause)

Medical Treatments Performed by Nurses

Give the prescribed drugs (analgesics to relieve the pain)

EVALUATION

Record actual outcome

ACUTE GASTRIC DILATATION[113,125,339]

ASSESSMENT
Data Collection

Subjective Data
- Continuous abdominal pain
  Anxiety

Objective Data
- Severe abdominal distention
- Abdominal tenderness
- Vomiting (overflow type)
- Diminished or absent bowel sounds
  Decreased blood pressure
  Rapid, weak pulse
  Cold, clammy skin
  Pallor

Data Analysis

Nursing Diagnosis
ACUTE GASTRIC DILATATION: Sudden, massive stomach distention with air and fluids that fail to pass through the gastrointestinal tract

Common Etiology (Stressors)
DISEASES: Paralytic ileus
HEALTH CARE FACTORS: *Medical therapy*: Prolonged intermittent positive-pressure breathing. *Surgical therapy*: Abdominal surgery. *Therapeutic device*: Hip spica cast
MAJOR PATHOPHYSIOLOGIC FACTORS CAUSING THE PROBLEM: Paralytic ileus prevents accumulated gas and liquid from leaving the stomach through the pylorus, and a feeling of fullness and vomiting develops; rapid distention of the stomach causes vagal stimulation and may result in shock

PLANNING
Unmet Needs
Fluid and electrolyte balance, rest, comfort, protection from physical harm, increased learning

Expected Outcome
None or decreased abdominal distention
Renewal of bowel sounds
Cessation of vomiting

NURSING INTERVENTIONS
Nursing Treatments
Administer intravenous fluids (ET) (lactated Ringer's isotonic saline solution)
Insert a nasogastric tube and attach to suction (ET)
Cover with lightweight blankets
Place in the slight sitting position
Place on complete bed rest
Restrict the intake to nothing by mouth
Withhold the drugs (sedatives)
Consult with the physician (immediately after giving emergency treatments)

Nursing Observations
Monitor the blood pressure
Palpate the pulse for rate, rhythm, and volume
Inspect the chest for respiratory rate and rhythm
Auscultate the abdomen for renewed bowel sounds
Check suction equipment for correct functioning

Health Teaching

Explain the causes of the health problem (fluid and gas accumulation in the intestines)

Explain the reason for and intended effect of the therapy (to reduce gastric distention)

EVALUATION

Record actual outcome

FOOD POISONING[20,22,42]

ASSESSMENT

Data Collection

Subjective Data

• Cramping abdominal pain soon after eating

• Nausea

• Diarrhea

• Vomiting

  Chills

  Dizziness, blurred vision, and muscle weakness only occur with botulism

  History of more than one person experiencing the symptoms

Objective Data

• No abdominal rigidity

  Fever

  Respiratory difficulty only occurs with botulism

Related Data

Onset in 2–4 hours indicates staphylococcus, onset in 6–48 hours indicates salmonella, onset in 15 hours indicates mushroom poisoning, onset in 18–48 hours indicates botulism

Data Analysis

Nursing Diagnosis

FOOD POISONING: A state of body toxicity following the intake of foods contaminated by bacteria or toxic substances

Common Etiology (Stressors)

ENVIRONMENTAL FACTORS: *Food substances*: Contaminated by bacteria or toxic agents

MAJOR PATHYPHYSIOLOGIC FACTORS CAUSING THE PROBLEM: Gastrointestinal mucosal damage and inflammation result from bacteria-contaminated food; most of the damage is caused by the toxins released by the bacteria; the toxins of botulism and the toxic chemicals of mushrooms cause central nervous system symptoms in addition to gastrointestinal disturbance

PLANNING

Unmet Needs

Fluid and electrolyte balance, rest, comfort, protection from physical harm, increased learning

Expected Outcome

Cessation of vomiting and diarrhea

Expressions of increased comfort

NURSING INTERVENTIONS

Nursing Treatments

Administer humidified oxygen (ET) (for respiratory distress)

Administer intravenous fluids (ET) (5% dextrose in water)

Lavage the stomach (ET)
Place on complete bed rest
Restrict the intake to nothing by mouth (until the nausea and vomiting subside)
Save the poison (food) container for content analysis
Consult with a physician (immediately after giving emergency treatment)
Obtain a blood sample and send for analysis (CBC, electrolytes)
Obtain a urine sample and send for analysis
Provide standby equipment (nasogastric tube with suction) and drugs (potassium, botulism antitoxin)
Obtain a complete present and past history

Nursing Observations
Inspect the chest for respiratory rate and rhythm
Palpate the pulse for rate, rhythm, and volume
Monitor the blood pressure
Monitor the oral temperature
Monitor blood studies for abnormal hematology and chemistry
Inspect for hemorrhage (gastrointestinal)
Measure the intake
Measure the output (for reduced urine output)

Health Teaching
Explain the causes of the health problem (contaminated food)
Explain the reason for and intended effect of the therapy (to reduce symptoms)

Medical Treatments Performed by Nurses
Give the prescribed drugs (botulism antitoxin, which counteracts the botulism agent *Clostridium botulinum*, potassium to replace electrolytes)

EVALUATION

Record actual outcome

INGESTION POISONING [42,72,246]

ASSESSMENT
Note: Each poison has specific signs and symptoms; those presented here are *generally* applicable to poisoning

Data Collection

Subjective Data
• Headache
• Nausea
  Blurred vision
  Dizziness
  Abdominal pain or cramping
  Thirst
  Weakness

Objective Data
• Pupil constriction or dilatation
• Slow, shallow or depressed respirations
• Rapid, weak pulse
• Decreased blood pressure
• Progressive drowsiness, stupor, and unconsciousness
  Particles of poison on or in the mouth
  Confusion

Restlessness
Vomiting
Convulsions
Cold, clammy, dry, or moist skin

Data Analysis

Nursing Diagnosis
INGESTION POISONING: A state of body toxicity following the intake of toxic substances into the gastrointestinal tract

Common Etiology (Stressors)
ENVIRONMENTAL FACTORS: *Chemical substances*: Drugs such as aspirin, cold and headache compounds, tranquilizers, antidepressants, barbiturates, etc.; noncaustic chemicals such as arsenic, benzene (gasoline, kerosene, naphtha lighter or cleaning fluid); bichloride of mercury, bromides, camphor, DDT, isopropyl (rubbing) alcohol, napthalene (moth balls), oil of wintergreen, phosphorous, sodium fluoride, strychnine, turpentine, pine oil; Corrosive chemicals such as corrosive acids, iodine, sulfuric acid, nitric acid, hydrochloric acid, acetic acid, phenol (carbolic acid), corrosive alkalis, lye (sodium hydroxide), ammonia, washing soda (sodium carbonate), household bleach (sodium hypochloride), potassium hydroxide (potash)
HUMAN ERROR: Accidental or intentional ingestion of substances
MAJOR PATHOPHYSIOLOGIC FACTORS CAUSING THE PROBLEM: The absorption of toxic chemicals into the body depresses the vital life centers of the brain, and respiratory and circulatory depression results, occasionally with pulmonary edema; the ingestion of a corrosive acid or alkali, burns and erodes the mucous membranes with which it comes in contact, and shock rapidly develops from the massive tissue trauma

PLANNING

Unmet Needs
Tissue oxygenation or perfusion, waste elimination of toxic substances, comfort, stimulation, protection from physical harm, increased learning

Expected Outcome
Vomiting of the stomach contents (except with the ingestion of corrosive poisons)
Blood pressure, pulse, and respirations within normal limits
Urine output of at least 30 cc per hour
Consciousness without cerebral impairment
Expressions of increased comfort

NURSING INTERVENTIONS

Nursing Treatments
Ventilate the person (ET) (if needed, using mouth-to-mouth breathing until spontaneous respirations occur)
OR
Administer mechanical ventilation (if needed)
Give water orally (*Age 1–5 years*: give 1–2 cups. *Age over 5 years*: give up to 1 quart)
OR
Give milk
OR
Give raw egg white orally
OR
Give a starch solution orally
⎫ To dilute the poison and slow absorption ⎬
Give an antidote as recommended on the poison container label
Induce vomiting immediately (one tablespoon Ipecac with one glass of water; *do not induce vomiting if the person is stuporous, unconscious, convulsing or has ingested a corrosive poison*)

Give a charcoal solution orally (one or 2 tablespoons of charcoal in a glass of water, only after the vomiting from the Ipecac has ceased, since charcoal inactivates Ipecac)
Do not induce vomiting (for corrosive poisons)
Refrain from giving bicarbonates (for acid corrosive poisons)
Refrain from giving laxatives (for corrosive poisons)
Restrict the intake (of food) to nothing by mouth (other than the antidote)
Administer humidified oxygen (ET) (for respiratory distress)
Administer intravenous fluids (ET) (5% dextrose in water)
Lavage the stomach (ET) (except with the ingestion of corrosive poisons)
Connect the person to an ECG monitor (if unconscious)
Cover with warm blankets
Stimulate by movement, touch, sternal pressure, or speech
Save the poison container for content analysis
Consult with a physician (immediately after giving emergency treatment)
Obtain a blood sample and send for analysis (CBC, electrolytes, arterial blood gases, toxic levels specific to the ingested substance)
Obtain a urine sample and send for analysis
Provide standby equipment (endotracheal tube, nasogastric tube, and suction) and drugs (sodium bicarbonate, Diamox or mannitol, potassium)
Obtain a complete present and past history

Nursing Observations
Inspect the chest for respiratory rate and rhythm
Observe for dyspnea
Palpate the pulse for rate, rhythm, and volume
Monitor the blood pressure
Monitor the oral temperature
Monitor blood studies for abnormal acid–base balance and chemistry
Observe the ECG monitor
Inspect for hemorrhage (gastrointestinal)
Measure the intake and output (for a reduced urine output)
Observe for complaints of pain (abdominal)
Observe for convulsions
Observe the level of consciousness

Health Teaching
Emphasize that dangerous products should be stored out of reach
Emphasize that medicine cabinets should be locked
Recommend that self-medication be avoided

Medical Treatments Performed by Nurses
Give the prescribed drugs (sodium bicarbonate to reverse the acidotic state and reestablish acid–base balance, Diamox or mannitol to promote diuresis, potassium to replace electrolytes)

EVALUATION

Record actual outcome

NONPENETRATING ABDOMINAL INJURY[20,104]

ASSESSMENT

Data Collection

Subjective Data
• History of an injury

- Pain
  Nausea

Objective Data
- No open abdominal wound
- Abdominal tenderness
- Muscle rigidity over a specific organ
  Abdominal distention
  Vomiting
  Fever

Data Analysis

Nursing Diagnosis

NONPENETRATING ABDOMINAL INJURY: An abdominal injury that has not opened the skin but has injured one or more of the underlying tissues and organs such as the esophagus, small or large intestines, liver, gallbladder, spleen, pancreas, bladder, or kidney

Common Etiology (Stressors)

ENVIRONMENTAL FACTORS: *Blast/explosion*: Exposure to. *Cataclysm*: Avalanche, cyclone, earthquake, hailstorm, tornado. *Crushing*: By cave-in, building collapse, falling object. *Foreign body*: Propelled. *Motor vehicles*: Impact or collision of. *Objects*: Blunt. *Tools*: Powered and nonpowered. *Weapons*: Club

HUMAN ERROR: Accidental falling

MAJOR PATHOPHYSIOLOGIC FACTORS CAUSING THE PROBLEM: Although the skin is not penetrated by the injuring object, the pressure of impact damages the tissues of the organs beneath the skin

PLANNING

Unmet Needs

Tissue oxygenation or perfusion, fluid and electrolyte balance, rest, comfort, protection from physical harm, increased learning

Expected Outcome

Blood pressure, pulse, and respirations within normal limits
Expressions of increased comfort

NURSING INTERVENTIONS

Nursing Treatments

Administer intravenous fluids (ET) (lactated Ringer's or isotonic saline solution)
Place on complete bed rest
Cover with lightweight blankets
Restrict the intake to nothing by mouth
Support (abdomen) with a binder
Obtain a blood sample and send for analysis (CBC, SMAC)
Obtain a urine sample and send for analysis (routine)
Send a blood sample for type and crossmatch
Provide standby equipment (nasogastric tube and suction, indwelling urinary catheter) and drugs
Consult with the physician (immediately after giving emergency treatment)
Obtain a complete present and past history

Nursing Observations

Monitor the blood pressure
Palpate the pulse for rate, rhythm, and volume
Inspect the chest for respiratory rate and rhythm
Monitor the oral temperature
Inspect for hemorrhage (from body orifices)
Monitor blood studies for abnormal hematology and chemistry
Auscultate the abdomen for abnormal bowel sounds (absent or excessive)

Palpate the abdomen for masses (which indicate hemorrhage or bladder injury)

Observe the urine for abnormal color, content, and odor (hematuria suggests kidney, bladder, ureter, or urethra injury)

Measure the urine output hourly (decreased output suggests kidney, bladder, ureter injury)

Health Teaching

Explain the reason for and intended effect of the therapy (to reduce tissue damage and prevent shock)

Medical Treatments Performed by Nurses

Give the prescribed drugs

EVALUATION

Record actual outcome

PENETRATING ABDOMINAL INJURY[20,104]

ASSESSMENT

Data Collection

Subjective Data
• History of an injury
• Severe pain
  Nausea

Objective Data
• Abdominal wound
• Bleeding or hemorrhage
• Abdominal rigidity
  Fever
  Elevated white blood count
  Vomiting

Data Analysis

Nursing Diagnosis

PENETRATING ABDOMINAL INJURY (INTERNAL ABDOMINAL INJURY): An abdominal injury that has opened the skin and resulted in injury to one or more abdominal organs such as the lower esophagus, small or large intestines, liver, gallbladder, spleen, pancreas, bladder, or kidney

Common Etiology (Stressors)

ENVIRONMENTAL FACTORS: *Blast/explosion*: Exposure to. *Cataclysm*: Exposure to. *Crushing*: By cave-in, building collapse, falling object. *Foreign body*: Propelled. *Moving Vehicles*: Impact or collision of. *Objects*: Pointed and sharp. *Tools*: Powered and nonpowered. *Weapons*: Gun, knife

HUMAN ERROR: Accidental falling

MAJOR PATHOPHYSIOLOGIC FACTORS CAUSING THE PROBLEM: The injuring object pierces the skin and damages the tissue of the organs beneath the skin

PLANNING

Unmet Needs

Tissue oxygenation or perfusion, fluid and electrolyte balance, rest, comfort, protection from physical harm, increased learning

Expected Outcome

Blood pressure, pulse, and respirations within normal limits

Expressions of increased comfort

No later evidence of wound inflammation, purulent drainage, or elevated temperature

NURSING INTERVENTIONS

Nursing Treatments

Administer intravenous fluids (ET) (lactated Ringer's or isotonic saline solution)

Place on complete bed rest

Place in the flat position

Restrict the intake to nothing by mouth

Support (abdomen) with a binder

Apply a sterile dressing (a clean cloth can be used if dressings are not available)

Cover with lightweight blankets

Obtain a blood sample and send for analysis (CBC, SMAC)

Obtain a urine sample and send for analysis (routine)

Send a blood sample for type and crossmatch

Provide standby equipment (nasogastric tube and suction, indwelling urinary catheter) and drugs

Consult with the physician (immediately after giving emergency treatment)

Obtain a complete present and past history

Nursing Observations

Monitor the blood pressure

Palpate the pulse for rate, rhythm, and volume

Inspect the chest for respiratory rate and rhythm

Inspect for hemorrhage

Monitor blood studies for abnormal hematology, chemistry

Auscultate the abdomen for abnormal bowel sounds (absent or excessive)

Palpate the abdomen for masses (which indicate hemorrhage or bladder injury)

Observe the urine for abnormal color, content, and odor (hematuria suggests kidney, bladder, ureter, or urethra injury)

Measure the urine output hourly (decreased output suggests kidney, bladder, or ureter injury)

Health Teaching

Explain the reason for and intended effect of the therapy (to reduce tissue damage and prevent shock)

Medical Treatments Performed by Nurses

Administer a blood transfusion

Give the prescribed drugs

EVALUATION

Record actual outcome

Emergency Conditions of the Integument

ANIMAL BITE[42]

ASSESSMENT

Data Collection

Subjective Data

- Pain
- History of a wound inflicted by a cat, dog, squirrel, mouse, rat, etc.

Objective Data
• Deep or superficial break in the skin
  Bleeding
  Teeth marks are frequently evident

Data Analysis

Nursing Diagnosis
ANIMAL BITE: A wound inflicted by an animal

Common Etiology (Stressors)
ENVIRONMENTAL FACTORS: *Biologic agents*: Animal bite
MAJOR PATHOPHYSIOLOGIC FACTORS CAUSING THE PROBLEM: Bacteria and viruses in the mouths
  of animals are transmitted through the open wound of an animal bite, causing soft-tissue damage and the potential for systemic disease or infection

PLANNING

Unmet Needs
Rest, comfort, cleanliness, protection from physical harm, freedom from pain, increased
  learning

Expected Outcome
Expressions of increased comfort
No later evidence of wound inflammation, purulent drainage, or elevated temperature
Closure of wound edges with granulation tissue formation between wound edges

NURSING INTERVENTIONS

Nursing Treatments
Apply an ice bag or cold pack (to the wound)
Soak in providane-iodine (Betadine) solution
  OR
Clean with surgical soap
Apply an antibiotic ointment
Apply a sterile dressing
Encourage adequate rest
Give nonprescription drugs (analgesics)
Confine the animal suspected of being infected
Provide standby drugs (antirabies serum, tetanus toxoid)
Make a referral (to a physician immediately after giving emergency treatment)

Nursing Observations
Inspect for bleeding
Inspect for inflammation (increased redness or swelling)
Observe for complaints of pain
Monitor the oral temperature (for fever)

Health Teaching
Teach how to clean and dress a wound
Instruct not to kill animals suspected of being infected (so the animal can be observed
  for disease)
Explain the reason for and intended effect of the therapy (to prevent infection)

Medical Treatments Performed by Nurses
Give the prescribed drugs (antirabies serum to prevent rabies onset, tetanus toxoid to
  prevent tetanus)

EVALUATION
Record actual outcome

BURN INJURY [49,104,219,451,768]

ASSESSMENT

Data Collection

First-Degree Burn in Which the Injury Extends Only to the Outer Layer (Epidermis) of the Skin

Subjective Data
• Mild pain

Objective Data
• Dry skin surface
• Skin redness or flush
  Shedding of superficial epidermis

Second-Degree Burn (Partial-Thickness Burn)

Subjective Data
• Severe pain

Objective Data
• Erythema (redness)
• Weeping, moist wound with blister formation
  Skin feels soft on palpation
  Edema

Third-Degree Burn (Full-Thickness Burn)

Subjective Data
• Feels little or no pain

Objective Data

• Insensitive to pinprick
• Pearly white or charred appearance of all skin layers and often deeper tissue
• Dry skin surface
  Leathery, without moisture, or may have bullae from steam trapped in the dermis
  Thrombosed blood vessels
  Function may be lost if the injured area is over a joint
  Tissue sloughing
  Scarring

Severity of Second- or Third-Degree Burn

Minor (may be treated as an outpatient) covers an area of less than 10% in children and 15% in adults of the total body surface; a minor full-thickness wound covers an area of less than 2%, except for burns of the face, legs, feet, hands, genitalia, inhalation injury, fractures, or soft tissue injury

Moderate (treated in a general hospital) covers an area of from 10–15% in children and 15–25% in adults

Critical (treated in a burn unit) involves any patient with involvement of the face, eyes, feet, hands, genitalia, or evidence of inhalation injury, soft tissue injury, fractures, etc., or with greater than 15% burn in children and 25% burn in adults

Data Analysis

Nursing Diagnosis

BURN INJURY: Tissue injury resulting from body exposure to intense heat, irritating chemicals, electricity, or radioactive substances

Common Etiology (Stressors)

ENVIRONMENTAL FACTORS: *Blast/Explosion:* Exposure to. *Cataclysm:* Volcanic eruption. *Chemical substances:* acids, industrial chemicals or solvents. *Electricity:* Exposure to ungrounded electrical currents. *Environmental heat:* High external temperature, fire, and flames. *Hot objects*: Heaters, hot liquids, steam, stoves, torches. *Lightning*: Exposure to. *Radiation*: Ultraviolet light from the sun. *Wind*: High

MAJOR PATHOPHYSIOLOGIC FACTORS CAUSING THE PROBLEM: Skin and other tissues exposed to thermal energy receive burn damage at 44° C (111.2° F) and higher, and cells of the skin, blood, and capillary walls are completely destroyed (necrosis); fluid shifts rapidly from the blood into the burned tissue, causing edema; shock develops rapidly in severe burns

PLANNING

Unmet Needs

Tissue oxygenation or perfusion, fluid and electrolyte balance, comfort, cleanliness (of the wound), protection from physical harm

Expected Outcome

Expressions of increased comfort

No later evidence of wound inflammation, purulent drainage, or elevated temperature

Blood pressure, pulse, and respirations within normal limits

Urine output of at least 30 cc per hour

NURSING INTERVENTIONS

Nursing Treatments (Minor Burns)

(May be treated on an outpatient basis)

Apply a cold, moist compress
   OR   } For about 30 minutes
Bathe in cool water

Apply a sterile dressing

Make a referral (to a physician or the emergency room as needed, both for immediate care or follow-up)

Nursing Treatments (Moderate or Critical Burns)

Airway

Use either the head-tilt or jaw-thrust
  maneuver to maintain an airway } As needed
   OR
Place in the side-lying position

Provide standby equipment (endotracheal tube)

Insert a nasal airway
   OR   } As needed
Insert an oral airway

Administer humidified oxygen (ET) (as needed)

Encourage coughing, deep breathing (every 30 minutes)

Place in the slight sitting (semi-Fowler's) position (if cyanosis and dyspnea are present)

Connect the person to an ECG monitor

Obtain a blood sample and send for analysis (CBC, SMAC, arterial blood gases and obtain a hematocrit every 6 hours)

Obtain a urine sample for analysis

Provide standby equipment (endotracheal tube, tracheostomy tray, mechanical ventilator) and drugs (antibiotics, bronchodilators, corticosteroids, mannitol)

Fluid Resuscitation

Administer intravenous fluids (ET) (according to one of several formulas: crystalloid, Evans', Moore's, hypertonic, or Brooke's, if the burn size is greater than 20% of the total body surface. Crystalloid formula is calculated by the following equation: 4 cc Ringer's lactate × weight in kilograms × percent of burn = fluid for a 24-hour period postinjury. One-half of the calculated amount is given in the first 8 hours, one-fourth in the second 8 hours, and one-fourth in the third 8 hours)

Catheterize with an indwelling urinary catheter (to measure the output)

Restrict the intake to nothing by mouth

Insert a gastric tube and attach to suction (ET)

Pain Relief
Decrease drafts (in the room)
Maintain a warm room temperature (above 80° F or a degree comfortable to the patient)

Infection Prevention and Wound Care
Maintain a clean environment
Use sterile technique
Maintain dry, clean linen
 OR
Place on sterile linens
Irrigate the wound (gently with water or saline)
 AND
Clean with an antibacterial agent
Shave the hair surrounding the burned area
Remove the loose burned skin with a gauze pad and slight pressure
Remove the foreign objects from the skin
Remove blisters from the burned area (except those on the palms and soles)

Maintenance of Function
Elevate the (burned) extremities (above the level of the heart)
Elevate the head (if the head or neck are burned)
Exercise (the extremities) in range of motion (gently every 2 hours, except in severe burn of the hands or fingers)
Do not allow overlapping skin surfaces to touch (especially in areas of the groin, axilla, and neck, to prevent maceration of the wound)
Do not allow (burned) skin surfaces to touch (especially fingers and toes)

Nursing Observations
Observe for airway obstruction
Observe the level of consciousness
Measure the intake (intravenous fluids)
Measure the urine output hourly (which should be 50–70 cc per hour; immediately notify the physician of an abnormal increase or decrease)
Monitor the central venous pressure (and/or pulmonary artery pressures)
Monitor the cardiogram
Palpate the pulse for rate, rhythm, and volume
Observe for shock and cyanosis
Inspect the chest for respiratory rate and rhythm
Inspect the nose, mouth, and throat for evidence of burns (singed nasal hairs, reddened dry buccal mucosa, soot in the sputum)
Auscultate the chest for lung aeration
Monitor the blood pressure
Inspect for the percentage of burned area (on arrival at the hospital and again following wound cleansing)
Observe for restlessness (assess for hypoxia or pain)
Inspect the extremities for impaired circulation (especially full-thickness burned tissue, every 30 minutes)
Observe for complaints of pain (deep aching)
Test the skin for impaired feeling perception
Observe the extremities for motor function
Test the urine for sugar and acetone (every 4 hours)
Monitor blood studies for abnormal hematology, electrolytes, glucose, renal function (urea nitrogen), for arterial blood gases

Medical Treatments Performed by Nurses
Pain Relief
Apply the prescribed topical agent (silver sulfadiazine)
Give the prescribed drugs (small doses of narcotics intravenously for pain relief)

Fluid Resuscitation
Administer intravenous fluids
Administer a blood transfusion

Infection Prevention and Wound Care
Apply the prescribed topical agent
Apply a biologic dressing (heterograft or homograft for partial thickness injuries)
Give the prescribed drugs (antibiotics to prevent infection, tetanus toxoid to prevent tetanus, antacids to prevent stress ulcer, mannitol to support diuresis, corticosteroids to reduce the inflammatory process, bronchodilators to open the bronchus and ease respiratory distress)

EVALUATION
Record actual outcome

FROSTBITE[104,219,278]

ASSESSMENT
Data Collection
Subjective Data
• Tingling followed by numbness and anesthesia
  Itching
  Burning pain

Objective Data
• Skin redness followed by pallor
  Edema
  Blistering and peeling (second degree)
  Necrosis and gangrene (third degree)
  Hands and feet are primarily involved

Data Analysis
Nursing Diagnosis
FROSTBITE: Tissue injury as a result of skin exposure to intense cold

Common Etiology (Stressors)
ENVIRONMENTAL FACTORS: *Environmental cold*: Freezing external temperature
MAJOR PATHOPHYSIOLOGIC FACTORS CAUSING THE PROBLEM: Exposure to severe environmental cold constricts blood vessels to such a degree that severe circulatory impairment occurs, threatening the survival of surrounding soft tissue

PLANNING
Unmet Needs
Tissue oxygenation or perfusion, normal temperature, comfort, protection from physical harm, increased learning

Expected Outcome
Warm, slightly moist, pink skin
No numbness or anesthesia
Full range of motion of affected extremities

NURSING INTERVENTIONS
Nursing Treatments
Soak (extremity) in saline solution (at 103–107° F (39.4–41.9° C))
Give hot coffee
  OR
Give hot tea

Discourage smoking
Cover with warm blankets
Do not massage (the frostbitten area)
Exercise in range of motion (once the limb is warmed)

Nursing Observations
Inspect for bleeding and edema
Inspect for impaired circulation
Palpate for arterial pulsations
Test for range of motion
Monitor the blood pressure and oral temperature

Health Teaching
Advise against exposure to inclement weather
Recommend the use of warm clothing
Explain the reason for and intended effect of the therapy (to warm the tissue gradually and maintain circulation)

EVALUATION

Record actual outcome

HUMAN BITE[20,21]

ASSESSMENT

Data Collection

Subjective Data
• Pain
• History of a wound inflicted by a person

Objective Data
• Deep or superficial break in the skin
 Bleeding
 Teeth marks are frequently evident

Data Analysis

Nursing Diagnosis
HUMAN BITE: A wound inflicted by human teeth

Common Etiology (Stressors)
ENVIRONMENTAL FACTORS: *Humans*: Human bite, exposure to agitated persons
MAJOR PATHOPHYSIOLOGIC FACTORS CAUSING THE PROBLEM: Bacteria in the mouths of humans are transmitted through the open wound of a human bite, causing soft-tissue damage and the potential for systemic disease; very serious cellulitis often develops

PLANNING

Unmet Needs
Comfort, cleanliness, protection from physical harm, freedom from pain, increased learning

Expected Outcome
Expressions of increased comfort
No later evidence of wound inflammation, purulent drainage, or elevated temperature
Closure of wound edges with the formation of granulation tissue between the wound edges

NURSING INTERVENTIONS

Nursing Treatments
Apply on ice bag or cold pack (to the wound)

Soak in providone-iodine (Betadine) solution
   OR
Clean with surgical soap
Apply an antibiotic ointment
Apply a sterile dressing
Give nonprescription drugs (analgesics)
Make a referral (to a physician)

Nursing Observations
Inspect for bleeding and edema
Inspect for inflammation
Monitor the oral temperature (for fever)
Test the skin for impaired feeling perception
Obtain a bacterial culture (of the wound)

Health Teaching
Teach how to clean and dress a wound
Explain the reason for and intended effect of the therapy (to prevent infection)

Medical Treatments Performed by Nurses
Give the prescribed drugs (tetanus toxoid to prevent tetanus)

EVALUATION

Record actual outcome

LACERATION[20,104,476]

ASSESSMENT

Data Collection

Subjective Data
• Pain
  Weakness

Objective Data
• Jagged, irregular, or blunt break or tear in the soft tissue
• Bleeding
  Intact tendons indicated by full flexion and extension of the body part
  Intact nerves indicated by positive responses to a pinprick

Data Analysis

Nursing Diagnosis
LACERATION: An irregular tear or wound of the flesh

Common Etiology (Stressors)
ENVIRONMENTAL FACTORS: *Blast explosion*: Exposure to. *Cataclysm*: Exposure to. *Crushing*: By cave-in, building collapse, falling object. *Foreign body*: Propelled. *Moving vehicles*: Impact or collision of. *Objects*: Sharp. *Tools*: Powered and nonpowered. *Weapons*: Knife
MAJOR PATHOPHYSIOLOGIC FACTORS CAUSING THE PROBLEM: Sharp objects penetrate the skin surface damaging not only the skin, but underlying structures of muscle, tendons, nerves, and blood vessels

PLANNING

Unmet Needs
Tissue oxygenation or perfusion, comfort, cleanliness, protection from physical harm, increased learning

Expected Outcome

Cessation of bleeding

Expressions of increased comfort

No later evidence of wound inflammation, purulent drainage, or elevated temperature

Closure of wound edges with the formation of granulation tissue between the wound edges

NURSING INTERVENTIONS

Nursing Treatments

Apply an ice bag or cold pack (to the wound)

OR

Apply manual pressure over the bleeding area

Soak in providone-iodine (Betadine) solution

OR

Clean with hydrogen peroxide

OR

Clean with surgical soap

Remove the foreign objects or debris (from the wound)

Apply a butterfly bandage or closure strips

OR

Suture the wound (if authorized to do so)

Apply a sterile dressing

Give nonprescription drugs (analgesics for pain)

Make a referral (to a physician for severe wound, tendon involvement, sensation loss, impaired circulation or wound depth below subcutaneous tissue)

Remove the sutures (in 7–10 days)

Nursing Observations

Test the skin for impaired feeling perception (by pinprick)

Test motor function (by counter pressure in the flexion, extension, and lateral positions)

Inspect for impaired circulation

Palpate for arterial pulsations

Test for range of motion

Monitor the blood pressure

Health Teaching

Explain the reason for and intended effect of the therapy (to prevent infection and maintain range of motion)

Teach how to clean and dress a wound

Medical Treatments Performed by Nurses

Give the prescribed drugs (analgesics for pain)

EVALUATION

Record actual outcome

VENOMOUS SNAKEBITE[20,42,219]

ASSESSMENT

Data Collection

Subjective Data

• Immediate, intense, local parasthesia, numbness, and pain

- Nausea
- Thirst
- Dyspnea

Objective Data
- Profuse perspiration
- Vomiting
- Two or more small fang punctures on the skin
  Rows of scratches on the skin
  Swelling
  Erythema and discoloration
  Hemorrhagic blisters around the bite
  Bleeding
  Tachycardia
  Shock

Related Data
Coral snakes have broad rings of scarlet and black separated by narrow rings of yellow, and their snouts are black
Pit vipers have a deep depression located midway between (but below) the level of the eye and nostril on each side
Rattlesnakes have rattles on the tip of the tail
Copperheads have a coppery tinge on the head, with a pale pinkish or reddish brown body, marked with large bands of chestnut brown hourglass patterns
Cottonmouths (water moccasins) have a white mouth, with a dingy brown or olive colored body, marked with darker blotches

Data Analysis

Nursing Diagnosis
VENOMOUS SNAKEBITE (POISONOUS SNAKEBITE): A skin wound inflicted by a poisonous snake

Common Etiology (Stressors)
ENVIRONMENTAL FACTORS: *Biologic agents*: Bite of a snake, specifically the poisonous snake
MAJOR PATHOPHYSIOLOGIC FACTORS CAUSING THE PROBLEM: When the snake's fangs penetrate the surface of the skin, it injects venom into the body, and since snake venoms contain a variety of chemicals including proteases (which destroy the lining of blood and lymph vessels), phosphatidases (which cause hemolysis, destroy capillaries, and myelin sheath and nerve fibers), cholinesterases (which cause neurotoxic damage), and other toxic proteins, the combined effect of the chemicals is life threatening; the extent of the edema is a clue to the amount of venom injected

PLANNING

Unmet Needs
Waste elimination of toxic substances, rest, comfort, cleanliness, protection from physical harm, freedom from pain, increased learning

Expected Outcome
Reduced swelling at the site of the bite
Blood pressure, pulse, and respirations within normal limits
No later evidence of wound inflammation, purulent drainage, elevated temperature, or bleeding
Consciousness without cerebral impairment

NURSING INTERVENTIONS

Nursing Treatments
Immobilize the affected body part
Apply a tourniquet between the extremity wound and the body (above the first joint proximal to the bite and not occluding the arterial flow)
Suction the snake venom (begin within the first 30 minutes following the bite)
Position the affected limb lower than the rest of the body

Administer intravenous fluids (ET) (to maintain an open line for drug administration)
Administer humidified oxygen (ET) (if needed)
Clean with antiseptic solution
  OR
Clean with surgical soap
Apply an antibiotic ointment
Apply a sterile dressing
Apply a cool, moist compress (50–59° F)
Cover with lightweight blankets
Place on complete bed rest
Place in the flat position
Refrain from oral stimulants
Give tetanus toxoid (ET)
Consult with a physician (immediately after giving emergency treatment)
Provide standby equipment (incision tray, suction machine, endotracheal tube, mechanical ventilator) and drugs (antivenom serum, corticosteroids, antibiotics, barbiturates)

Nursing Observations
Monitor the blood pressure
Inspect the chest for respiratory rate and rhythm
Palpate the pulse for rate, rhythm, and volume
Monitor the oral temperature
Inspect for bleeding, edema, or inflammation
Observe for complaints of pain (severe)
Observe the level of consciousness
Observe for shock

Health Teaching
Explain the reason for and intended effect of the therapy

Medical Treatments Performed by Nurses
Give the prescribed drugs (antivenom serum to counteract the poisonous venom, corticosteriods to reduce the inflammatory process, antibiotics to prevent infection, barbiturates to promote sedation)

EVALUATION
Record actual outcome

VENOMOUS SPIDER BITE[20,42,104,219]

ASSESSMENT
Data Collection
Subjective Data
• Severe abdominal and muscle cramping
• Absence of nausea
• Slight local pain
• Dyspnea
  Headache
  Numbness of the hands and feet
  Chills

Objective Data
Within 24–48 Hours
• Absence of vomiting

Fever
Rash sometimes
Sweating
Hyperactive reflexes
Twitching
Rigid abdomen
Local tissue necrosis
Two small puncture marks on the skin (black widow spider)
A black spot on the skin (brown recluse spider)

Related Data (Spider or Scorpion)
Black widow spider is coal black with a red hourglass design on the underside
Red-legged widow spider is black with red legs
Tarantula is brown and hairy, with a legspread of about 4.5 inches
Brown recluse spider is brown, with legs about 1.5 inches long
Scorpion has crablike feet and a tail

Data Analysis

Nursing Diagnosis
VENOMOUS SPIDER BITE (POISONOUS SPIDER BITE): A skin wound inflicted by a poisonous arachnid

Common Etiology (Stressors)
ENVIRONMENTAL FACTORS: *Biologic agents*: Bite of an insect, specifically a poisonous spider
MAJOR PATHOPHYSIOLOGIC FACTORS CAUSING THE PROBLEM: When the insect penetrates the surface of the skin, it injects venom into the body, and with toxic venom, systemic effects can be life threatening

PLANNING

Unmet Needs
Waste elimination of toxic substances, comfort, cleanliness, protection from physical harm, freedom from pain, increased learning

Expected Outcome
Reduced swelling at the site of the bite
Blood pressure, pulse, and respirations within normal limits
No later evidence of wound inflammation, purulent drainage, or elevated temperature
Expressions of increased comfort

NURSING INTERVENTIONS

Nursing Treatments
Apply a cold, moist compress
    OR
Apply an ice bag or ice pack
Apply a tourniquet between the extremity wound and the body
Suction the spider venom
Position the affected limb lower than the rest of the body
Administer intravenous fluids (ET) (to keep an open line for drug administration)
Clean with antiseptic solution
    OR
Clean with hydrogen peroxide
    OR
Clean with surgical soap
Apply sodium bicarbonate (baking soda) to the skin
    OR
Apply calamine lotion
Consult with a physician (immediately after giving emergency treatment)
Provide standby equipment (incision tray, suction machine) and drugs (specific antiserum, corticosteroids, or calcium gluconate)

Nursing Observations

Monitor the blood pressure

Inspect the chest for respiratory rate and rhythm

Palpate the pulse for rate, rhythm, and volume

Monitor the oral temperature

Inspect for bleeding, edema, and inflammation

Observe for shock

Observe for complaints of pain

Health Teaching

Explain the reason for and intended effect of the therapy (to relieve pain and counteract the venom)

Medical Treatments Performed by Nurses

Give the prescribed drugs (antivenom serum to counteract the spider's venom, cortico-steroids to reduce the inflammatory process, calcium gluconate for spasm relief)

EVALUATION

Record actual outcome

BONE FRACTURE[20,73,104,219,476]

ASSESSMENT

Data Collection

Subjective Data

- Acute pain at the site of injury
- Complains of being unable to use the injured area
  May have heard or felt the bone snap or pop
  Numbness at the injury site, sometimes

Objective Data

- Deformity evident by abnormal alignment
- Loss of or very limited range of motion
- Crepitus (an audible or palpable grating sound if the bone is moved)
- Swelling
- Localized tenderness
- Severe muscle spasm at the site of injury
- Subcutaneous bruising
  Bone penetration through the skin, sometimes
  X-ray film confirmation of the fracture

Related Data

Commonly Related Types of Bone Fracture

Closed fracture, compound fracture, extracapsular fracture, intracapsular fracture, com-muted fracture, longitudinal fracture, greenstick fracture, depressed fracture, impact-ed fracture, pathologic fracture, spiral fracture, oblique fracture, transverse fracture, skull fracture, cervical spine fracture, mandible fracture, clavicle fracture, rib fracture, humerus fracture, pelvis fracture, femur fracture, tibia fracture, fibula fracture, patella fracture, phalanx fracture, metatarsal fracture

Data Analysis
Nursing Diagnosis
BONE FRACTURE: The breaking of a bone

Common Etiology (Stressors)
BIRTH DEFECTS: Osteogenesis imperfecta

DISEASES: Bone cancer, osteomalacia, osteomyelitis, osteoporosis, syphilis

ENVIRONMENTAL FACTORS: *Blast/explosion*: Exposure to. *Cataclysm*: Exposure to. *Crushing*: By cave-in, building collapse, falling object. *Electricity*: Exposure to ungrounded electrical currents. *Foreign body*: Propelled. *Moving vehicles*: Impact or collision of. *Objects*: Blunt. *Tools*: Powered and nonpowered. *Weapons*: Club, gun

HUMAN ERROR: Accidental falling

MAJOR PATHOPHYSIOLOGIC FACTORS CAUSING THE PROBLEM: Force applied to a bone either directly or indirectly will fracture a bone, and sudden, violent muscle contractions will also cause a fracture

PLANNING
Unmet Needs
Tissue oxygenation or perfusion, comfort, protection from physical harm, increased learning

Expected Outcome
No additional soft-tissue or nerve injury beyond that which has traumatically occurred
Blood pressure, pulse, and respirations within or near normal limits
Cessation of hemorrhage, if present
Expressions of increased comfort

NURSING INTERVENTIONS
Nursing Treatments
Handle gently
Immobilize the affected body part
Apply a supportive splint, or
Apply an arm sling
Maintain body alignment
Administer intravenous fluids (ET) (lactated Ringer's solution)
Administer humidified oxygen (ET) (if there is respiratory distress)
Remove constrictive clothing
Consult with a physician (immediately after giving emergency treatment)
Provide standby equipment (for casting the fracture) and drugs (analgesics)
Obtain a blood sample and send for analysis (CBC, SMAC)
Obtain a urine sample and send for analysis
Obtain a complete present and past history

Nursing Observations
Observe for complaints of numbness and tingling, for complaints of pain
Palpate for arterial pulsations (in the injured area)
Monitor the blood pressure
Palpate the pulse for rate, rhythm, and volume
Inspect the chest for respiratory rate and rhythm
Observe for shock
Inspect for hemorrhage

Health Teaching
Explain the reason for and intended effect of the therapy (to minimize tissue injury)

Medical Treatments Performed by Nurses
Give the prescribed drugs (analgesics for pain relief)

EVALUATION
Record actual outcome

CERVICAL INJURY[20,22,73]

ASSESSMENT

Data Collection

Subjective Data
• Pain or spasm of the neck muscles
  Weakness, numbness below the injury level

Objective Data
• Neck flexion is painful
  Loss of motor function (if the injury is severe)
  Respiratory distress

Data Analysis

Nursing Diagnosis
CERVICAL INJURY (SPINAL CORD INJURY): Injury to the cervical vertebrae with the possibility of paralysis

Common Etiology (Stressors)
ENVIRONMENTAL FACTORS: *Blast/explosion*: Exposure to. *Cataclysm*: Exposure to. *Crushing*: By cave-in, building collapse, falling object. *Foreign body*: Propelled. *Moving vehicles*: Propulsion of the body into the air following the collision of moving vehicles, especially motorcycles and larger vehicles, or whiplash neck movements during the collision of moving vehicles. *Weapons*: Club, gun, knife
HUMAN ERROR: Nonuse of safety helmets or hard hats
MAJOR PATHOPHYSIOLOGIC FACTORS CAUSING THE PROBLEM: Fractured vertebrae have the potential for squeezing or tearing spinal cord tissue and, if this occurs, paralysis results

PLANNING

Unmet Needs

Tissue oxygenation or perfusion, comfort, protection from physical harm, increased learning

Expected Outcome

No additional nerve injury beyond that which has traumatically occurred
Blood pressure, pulse, and respirations within or near normal limits
Expressions of increased comfort, if conscious

NURSING INTERVENTIONS

Nursing Treatments

Ventilate the person (ET) (if needed, using mouth-to-mouth breathing until spontaneous respirations return)
Initiate endotracheal intubation (ET) (if needed)
Administer humidified oxygen (ET) (if needed)
Administer intermittent positive-pressure breathing (ET) (if needed)
Administer intravenous fluids (ET) (to maintain an open line for drug administration)
Position with sandbags (to assure immobility)
Maintain body alignment
Place in the flat position
Place in the face-upward (supine) position (in cervical vertebrae injury)
Place on complete bed rest
Move the entire body as a single unit (using a board to support the body)
Consult with a physician (immediately after giving emergency nursing treatment)
Provide standby equipment (endotracheal tube, tracheostomy tray, suction machine, mechanical respirator, nasogastric tube and suction, urinary catheter) and drugs
Obtain a blood sample and send for analysis (CBC, SMAC)
Obtain a complete present and past history

Nursing Observations

Inspect the chest for respiratory rate and rhythm (dyspnea, diaphragmatic breathing, respiratory failure)

Test motor function

Observe for complaints of numbness and tingling

Inspect for hemorrhage

Measure the intake and output (noting any urinary retention)

Inspect the abdomen for distention

Monitor the blood pressure

Palpate the pulse for rate, rhythm, and volume

Health Teaching

Explain the reason for and intended effect of the therapy (to prevent neurologic damage)

Medical Treatments Performed by Nurses

Give the prescribed drugs

EVALUATION

Record actual outcome

DISLOCATION [20,104]

ASSESSMENT

Data Collection

Subjective Data
• Pain at the site of injury
• Complaints of being unable to use the injured body area

Objective Data
• Obvious deformity
• Tenderness on slight palpation
• Loss of range of motion
• No crepitus
  Swelling
  Impaired circulation to the extremity may be present

Data Analysis

Nursing Diagnosis
DISLOCATION: The displacement of a bone from the joint

Common Etiology (Stressors)
ENVIRONMENTAL FACTORS: *Blast/explosion*: Exposure to. *Cataclysm*: Exposure to. *Crushing*: By cave-in, building collapse, falling object. *Electricity*: Exposure to ungrounded electrical currents. *Moving vehicles*: Impact or collision of. *Pressure*: Air. *Tools*: Powered and nonpowered

HUMAN ERROR: Accidental falling

MAJOR PATHOPHYSIOLOGIC FACTORS CAUSING THE PROBLEM: Force exerted against a joint causes the head of the bone to be displaced from the joint, resulting in dislocation

PLANNING

Unmet Needs

Comfort, protection from physical harm, increased learning

Expected Outcome

No additional soft-tissue or nerve injury beyond that which has traumatically occurred
Blood pressure, pulse, and respirations within normal limits
Expressions of increased comfort

NURSING INTERVENTIONS

Nursing Treatments

Apply a supportive splint
Handle gently
Immobilize the affected body part (and do not straighten or realign the joint)
Make a referral to a physician (immediately after giving emergency treatment)
Give nonprescription drug (analgesic for pain)

Nursing Observations

Palpate for arterial pulsations (distal to the injury)

Health Teaching

Explain the reason for and intended effect of the therapy (to prevent further injury)

EVALUATION

Record actual outcome

INTRACRANIAL INJURY[20,476]

ASSESSMENT

Data Collection

Subjective Data
• Headache (if conscious)
  Dizziness

Objective Data
• Loss of consciousness
• Unequal pupils (in increased intracranial pressure)
  Fleeting or prolonged loss of extremity function
  Speech disturbance
  Vomiting
  Blood or blood-tinged cerebrospinal fluid draining from the ear, nose, or mouth (in a
    basilar skull fracture)

Data Analysis

Nursing Diagnosis
INTRACRANIAL INJURY (BRAIN TISSUE INJURY): Concussion, contusion, or laceration of the brain
  tissue as a result of trauma

Common Etiology (Stressors)
ENVIRONMENTAL FACTORS: *Blast/explosion*: Exposure to. *Cataclysm*: Exposure to. *Crushing*: By
  cave-in, building collapse, falling object. *Foreign body*: Propelled. *Moving vehicles*: Impact of. *Objects*: Hard surfaced, pointed, sharp
HUMAN ERROR: Accidental falling, nonuse of safety helmets or hard hats
MAJOR PATHOPHYSIOLOGIC FACTORS CAUSING THE PROBLEM: Brain-tissue injury may be direct, as
  from a penetrating object that lacerates the tissue, or may be the result of the brain
  bouncing against the enclosing skull, as from a blow to the head; varying degrees of

damage may result with tissue swelling and possible hemorrhage contributing to increasing intracranial pressure; basilar skull fractures often allow cerebrospinal fluid to drain from the ears and nose

PLANNING

Unmet Needs

Tissue oxygenation or perfusion, rest, comfort, cleanliness, protection from physical harm, increased learning

Expected Outcome

Respirations within normal limits through an open airway

Cessation of bleeding at the injury site

Blood pressure and pulse within or near normal limits

No additional soft-tissue injury beyond that which has traumatically occurred

NURSING INTERVENTIONS

Nursing Treatments

Ventilate the person (ET) (if needed, using mouth-to-mouth breathing until spontaneous respirations return)

Insert an oral airway (if needed)

Initiate endotracheal intubation (ET) (if needed)

Administer humidified oxygen (ET) (if needed)

Administer intermittent positive-pressure breathing (ET) (if needed)

Administer intravenous fluids (ET) (to maintain an open line for drug administration)

Apply manual pressure over the bleeding area (using gentle pressure to prevent additional injury)

Apply a sterile dressing (over the wound)

Elevate the head (slightly, at about 30 degrees to control edema formation)

Remove constrictive clothing (around the neck)

Restrict the intake to nothing by mouth

Cover with lightweight blankets

Place on complete bed rest

Handle gently (to prevent further injury)

Withhold all drugs (that cause vital sign depression)

Connect the person to an ECG monitor

Consult with a physician (immediately after giving emergency treatment)

Provide standby equipment (endotracheal tube, tracheostomy tray, suction machine) and drugs

Obtain a blood sample and send for analysis (CBC, SMAC)

Obtain a complete present and past history

Nursing Observations

Observe the level of consciousness

Monitor the blood pressure

Palpate the pulse for rate, rhythm, and volume

Observe the ECG monitor

Inspect the chest for respiratory rate and rhythm

Inspect the eyes for pupil size, equality, and response to light

Test motor function

Inspect for hemorrhage

Health Teaching

Explain the reason for and intended effect of the therapy (to stabilize the condition and prevent further damage)

Medical Treatments Performed by Nurses

Give the prescribed drugs

EVALUATION

Record actual outcome

SCALP INJURY[20]

ASSESSMENT

Data Collection

Subjective Data
• Pain or headache

Objective Data
• Profuse bleeding from a scalp wound
  May be bone fragments in the wound

Data Analysis

Nursing Diagnosis
SCALP INJURY: An open wound into the subcutaneous and muscle tissues of the skull

Common Etiology (Stressors)
ENVIRONMENTAL FACTORS: *Blast/explosion*: Exposure to. *Cataclysm*: Exposure to. *Crushing*: By cave-in, building collapse, falling object. *Foreign body*: Propelled. *Moving vehicles*: Impact of. *Objects*: Hard surfaced, pointed, sharp
HUMAN ERROR: Accidental falling, nonuse of safety helmets or hard hats
MAJOR PATHOPHYSIOLOGIC FACTORS CAUSING THE PROBLEM: Trauma causing an open wound in the highly vascular scalp tissue will result in profuse bleeding, and strong enough force will fracture the bone underneath the scalp wound, resulting in a depressed fracture of bone particles in the wound

PLANNING

Unmet Needs

Rest, comfort, cleanliness, protection from physical harm, increased learning

Expected Outcome

Cessation of bleeding
Blood pressure, pulse, and respirations within normal limits
No later evidence of wound inflammation, purulent drainage, or elevated temperature
Expressions of increased comfort

NURSING INTERVENTIONS

Nursing Treatments

Elevate the head (if there is bleeding and no neck injury)
Apply manual pressure over the bleeding area (using gentle pressure in case the skull is fractured)
Clean with surgical soap (only after x-ray film results have ruled out a skull fracture)
Remove the foreign objects or debri (from the scalp *only* if the objects are loose; do not remove objects imbedded in the scalp)
Apply a sterile dressing (loosely over the wound and any imbedded object)
Consult with a physician (immediately after giving emergency treatment)

Nursing Observations

Observe the level of consciousness
Monitor the blood pressure
Palpate the pulse for rate, rhythm, and volume
Inspect the chest for respiratory rate and rhythm
Inspect the eyes for pupil size, equality, and response to light
Observe for complaints of numbness and tingling (of the extremities)
Inspect the wound dressing frequently (for fresh bleeding)

Health Teaching

Explain the reason for and intended effect of the therapy
Instruct to change position gradually (to reduce head pain)

EVALUATION
Record actual outcome

Emergency Conditions of a Psychiatric Nature

EMOTIONAL CRISIS[248,471]

ASSESSMENT
Data Collection
Subjective Data
- Person perceives an event, having occurred within the past two weeks, as very stressful
- Experiences severe tension
- Unsuccessfully attempts to cope with the tension
- Extreme mental preoccupation with the problem
- Feels very helpless
- Requests immediate help
- Unable to function effectively at his usual level (unable to manage the house, job, and usual responsibilities)

Objective Data
- Constant talking about the crisis subject
  Rapid or loud speech
  Excessive gesturing
  Pacing or sitting rigidly
  Demanding behavior
  Short attention span
  Possible use of profanity
  Possible use of negative coping mechanisms such as alcohol intoxication or suicide attempts

Data Analysis
Nursing Diagnosis
EMOTIONAL CRISIS: A state of critical emotional instability in which the person is emotionally unable to cope with a problem

Common Etiology (Stressors)
DISEASES: Any
INJURIES: Any
PSYCHOSOCIAL FACTORS: The threat of real or imagined danger, the threat of loss of control of a life situation, the threat of deprivation of essential needs, lack of realistic perception, a change in a vital life role, the threat of loss of self-esteem, the threat of not being able to preserve himself, the threat of chronic or severe stress
HUMAN BODY: Loss of body function, loss of a body part
HEALTH CARE FACTORS: *Hospitalization*: Of self or a significant other. *Diagnostic procedure*: Any. *Medical diagnosis*: An unfavorable medical diagnosis. *Medical or nursing therapy*: Any. *Surgical therapy*: Any. *Prognosis*: An unfavorable prognosis
DEVELOPMENTAL PHASES: Any but especially puberty and adolescence
SITUATIONAL FACTORS: The death of a significant other (especially an unexpected death), natural or man-made disaster, divorce, loss of employment, the stress of the holidays, loss of or relocation of a home, illness or injury to self or a significant other, legal termination of parental rights, marriage, unwanted or unplanned pregnancy, retirement, separation from a significant other, having been victimized by violence

PLANNING

Unmet Needs

Comfort, protection from psychologic threat, personal growth and maturity, increased reality perception and problem-solving ability

Expected Outcome

Person is able to function effectively at his usual level
Verbalizes self-confidence in being able to cope with the situation
Feels a sense of restored balance

NURSING INTERVENTIONS

Nursing Treatments

Attend the person constantly
Approach unhurriedly
Reassure verbally (that the nurse will help the person solve the problem)
Demonstrate calmness
Provide privacy
Provide quiet
Give explicit directions (such as sit down, stop screaming)
Encourage the expression of feelings (about the problem)
Listen attentively
Offer feedback to the person's expressed feelings
Ask the person to identify the problem
Ask for specifics, not generalizations, about the problem (if a person complains of being abused, ask for details of the abuse)
Support a realistic assessment of the situation (help the person see how it really is, not how he currently perceives it to be)
Ask how the person normally copes with stress (what does the person usually do when feeling extremely tense?)
Ask when the coping mechanism failed (at what point did the emotion become overwhelming?)
Encourage mutual problem solving (between the person and the nurse)
Explore with the person his strengths and resources (supportive friends or relatives, his church, financial resources, etc.)
Call the person's family (if he desires such)
Use the person's name frequently (to demonstrate caring)
Refrain from negatively criticizing
Touch the person judiciously
Remove harmful objects from the environment (if necessary to ensure the person's safety)
Make a referral (to a psychiatric nurse specialist, psychiatrist, or psychologist if the person's response is poor, if the person is out of touch with reality, or if he is suicidal)

Nursing Observations

Identify disturbing conversation topics
Determine the degree of insight that the person has (into the problem)
Observe for suicidal threats
Observe for contradictory verbal and nonverbal messages (may verbalize feeling calm but is pacing up and down)

Health Teaching

Recommend new options for effective methods of coping (new ways to solve the problem)
Explain the importance of persons offering support to one another

Medical Treatments Performed by Nurses

Give the prescribed drugs

EVALUATION

Record actual outcome

Emergency Conditions of the Reproductive System

ABNORMAL VAGINAL BLEEDING[246,527]

ASSESSMENT

Data Collection

Subjective Data
- Abdominal cramping or pain
- Backache
  Weakness
  Dizziness
  Anxiety

Objective Data
- Bright red vaginal bleeding
- Decreased blood pressure
- Rapid pulse
  Expulsion of tissue through the vagina

Data Analysis

Nursing Diagnosis
ABNORMAL VAGINAL BLEEDING: The unnatural loss of blood from the vagina

Common Etiology (Stressors)
DISEASES: Abruptio placentae, ectopic pregnancy, natural abortion, ovarian cyst, placenta previa
INJURIES: Self-inflicted abortion
MAJOR PATHOPHYSIOLOGIC FACTORS CAUSING THE PROBLEM: The interruption of a pregnancy causes bleeding as the uterine contents tear away from the uterine wall and are expelled through the vagina; also rupture of the fallopian tube from an ectopic pregnancy causes bleeding

PLANNING

Unmet Needs

Tissue oxygenation or perfusion, fluid and electrolyte balance, sleep and rest, comfort, protection from physical harm, increased learning

Expected Outcome

Cessation of the vaginal bleeding
Blood pressure, pulse, and respirations within normal limits
Warm, slightly moist, pink skin
Consciousness without cerebral impairment

NURSING INTERVENTIONS

Nursing Treatments

Administer humidified oxygen (ET) (if needed)
Administer intravenous fluids (ET) (to maintain an open line for drug administration)
Place on complete bed rest
Place in the foot-elevated, head-lowered (Trendelenburg) position
Cover with lightweight blankets
Restrict the intake to nothing by mouth

Refrain from doing a rectal or vaginal examination
Massage the uterine fundus (for postpartum hemorrhage)
Obtain a blood sample and send for analysis (CBC, electrolytes)
Send a blood sample for type and crossmatch
Consult with the physician (immediately after giving emergency treatment)
Obtain a complete present and past history

Nursing Observations

Estimate the blood volume loss (and save large clots or tissue for inspection)
Inspect the chest for respiratory rate and rhythm
Palpate the pulse for rate, rhythm, and volume
Monitor the blood pressure (every 10–15 minutes)
Palpate the skin for temperature
Inspect the skin for color (changes)
Observe for complaints of pain (especially shoulder pain which indicates a ruptured cyst or fallopian tube)
Monitor the fetal heart sounds (if appropriate)
Monitor the oral temperature (for fever)
Monitor blood studies for abnormal hematology and electrolytes
Measure the intake and output
Count the number of sanitary pads used

Health Teaching

Explain the causes of the health problem (the tearing of uterine contents from the uterine wall, rupture of a fallopian tube)
Explain the reason for and intended effect of the therapy (to terminate the bleeding)

Medical Treatments Performed by Nurses

Administer a blood transfusion
Give the prescribed drugs

EVALUATION

Record actual outcome

EMERGENCY CHILDBIRTH [20,241,384]

ASSESSMENT

Data Collection

Subjective Data
Woman is crying out in pain
Woman warns of impending birth

Objective Data
• Uterine contractions are about 2 minutes apart
• Woman is straining or pushing down with each contraction

Data Analysis

Nursing Diagnosis
EMERGENCY CHILDBIRTH: The delivery of a child at an unexpected and unprepared-for time

Common Etiology (Stressors)
SITUATIONAL FACTORS: *Pregnancy*: Termination of pregnancy
HUMAN ERROR: Miscalculation of the stage of the pregnancy or childbirth in process

MAJOR PATHOPHYSIOLOGIC FACTORS CAUSING THE PAIN: The normal process of childbirth, which continues until completion, regardless of the mother's environmental setting

PLANNING

Unmet Needs
Cleanliness, comfort, protection from physical harm, increased learning

Expected Outcome
Infant respirations and tissue oxygenation are within normal limits
There is no unusual maternal bleeding
There is no later evidence of maternal infection

NURSING INTERVENTIONS

Nursing Treatments

Specific to the Mother
Attend the mother constantly
Reassure verbally
Demonstrate calmness
Provide privacy (however possible)
Place in the lithotomy position (with newspapers or absorbent material under the pelvis)
Drape modestly (with clean cloths or clothing)
Refrain from giving oral stimulants
Withhold all drugs
Facilitate the delivery by gently guiding the infant through the vulva
Tie off and cut the umbilical cord (4–6 inches from the infant's navel and 8–10 inches from the navel, and cut between the ties)
Await delivery of the placenta
Refrain from pulling the umbilical cord during expulsion of the placenta
Refrain from removing the placenta except during uterine contraction
Massage the uterine fundus (if it fails to contract)

Specific to the Infant
Suction the (infant's) airway (with a bulb syringe)
    OR
Place the infant in the foot-elevated, head-lowered position (to facilitate removal of secretions)
Stimulate the infant with back stroking or spanking (if the infant does not cry at birth)
Cover with warm blankets (or a cloth)
Make a referral (of mother and infant to a hospital)

Nursing Observations

Specific to the Mother
Observe for uterine membrane rupture
Inspect the amniotic fluid for meconium
Inspect the vagina for a prolapsed umbilical cord
Inspect the placenta for abnormalities (placenta separation, atrophy, incompleteness)
Palpate the uterus for firmness

Specific to the Infant
Monitor the fetal heart sounds
Inspect the umbilical cord for abnormalities (the absence of the usual one vein and two arteries)

Health Teaching
Teach how to control breathing to aid the labor process (panting during contractions)
Inform that bearing down (during contractions) aids the process of second-stage labor

EVALUATION
Record actual outcome

RAPE-TRAUMA SYNDROME[209,278]

ASSESSMENT

Data Collection

Subjective Data
• Verbalization of forced sexual relations

Objective Data
• Abrasions, contusions, or lacerations
  Torn, stained, or bloody clothing
  Tremor
  Crying
  Restlessness

Data Analysis

Nursing Diagnosis
RAPE-TRAUMA SYNDROME: Being a victim of sexual activity without one's consent

Common Etiology (Stressors)
ENVIRONMENTAL FACTORS: *Humans*: Exposure to a sexually aroused person
MAJOR PATHOPHYSIOLOGIC FACTORS CAUSING THE PROBLEM: Forced sexual participation may result in tissue injury, such as vaginal/perineal tears, abrasions of the legs and back (from struggles), and vaginal infection

PLANNING

Unmet Needs
Comfort, protection from psychologic threat

Expected Outcome
Expressions of increased comfort
Woman obtains emotional support from the nurse and significant others

NURSING INTERVENTIONS

Nursing Treatments
Attend the woman constantly
Demonstrate calmness
Reassure verbally
Provide privacy
Provide quiet
Encourage the expression of feelings
Refrain from negatively criticizing
Perform the specific procedure of collecting legal evidence:
  Place each article of evidence in a separate container labeled with the woman's name, the date, the anatomic location of evidence, and the physician's name
  Inspect all garments and the examination sheets for blood or seminal fluid stains; place in separate paper, not plastic, bags
  If the victim has not bathed, cut a few pubic hairs and place them in a separate envelope
  If the victim scratched the assailant, cut her fingernails and place them in an envelope
  Remove stains from the body with a saline swab
  Assist the physician with aspiration and swabbing of material from the vulva, vagina, urethra, or cervix.
  Assist with preparation of a wet-mount slide to be examined for sperm
  Place the rest of the fluid or the swab in a test tube for other tests
  Safeguard the evidence material by giving it to the police, forensic pathologist, or locking it up
Make a referral (to a physician or counseling service, as needed)

Nursing Observations

Inspect for bleeding (and lacerations)

Inspect the skin for discoloration (bruising)

Health Teaching

Teach the specific procedure (of not changing clothing or bathing until after the physician has seen the woman)

Explain the reason for and intended effect of the procedure (to secure legal evidence)

EVALUATION

Record actual outcome

Emergency Conditions of the Respiratory System

ACUTE PULMONARY EDEMA [42,73,246,451]

ASSESSMENT

Data Collection

Subjective Data

• Dyspnea

• Intense anxiety

Objective Data

• Rapid, labored respirations

• Cyanosis

• Neck vein distention

• Cough with pink-tinged frothy sputum

Breath sounds (bilateral rales)

Tachycardia

Elevated blood pressure

Restlessness

Data Analysis

Nursing Diagnosis

ACUTE PULMONARY EDEMA: Excessive amounts of fluid initially collect in the interstitial tissue of the lungs and later in the alveoli causing respiratory distress

Common Etiology (Stressors)

DISEASES: Aortic stenosis, cirrhosis, congestive heart failure, emphysema, hypertension, mitral stenosis, myocardial infarction, pulmonary embolus

INJURIES: Burn wound, drowning, poisoning, (heroin overdose), pulmonary contusion

HEALTH CARE FACTORS: *Medical therapy*: Overload of intravenous infusion

ENVIRONMENTAL FACTORS: *Chemical substances*: Toxic gases, especially ammonia

MAJOR PATHOPHYSIOLOGIC FACTORS CAUSING THE PROBLEM: Pulmonary edema is an excessive accumulation of serous fluid in the alveoli precipitated by increased blood pressure in the pulmonary capillaries, by decreased albumin in the blood, causing a drop in osmotic pressure, or by damage to the capillary walls; pulmonary edema is most frequently the result of left ventricular failure

PLANNING

Unmet Needs

Tissue oxygenation or perfusion, fluid and electrolyte balance, rest, comfort, protection from physical harm, increased learning

Expected Outcome

Expressions of reduced respiratory distress

Blood pressure, pulse, and respirations within or near normal limits

Warm, slightly moist, pink skin

NURSING INTERVENTIONS

Nursing Treatments

Administer humidified oxygen (ET)

Administer intermittent positive-pressure breathing (ET) (if the respiratory distress does not improve with the administration of oxygen)

Apply rotating tourniquets (ET) (if the oxygen and IPPB fail to improve respirations)

Administer intravenous fluids (ET) (at a slow rate)

OR

Slow the intravenous infusion rate (if an IV is being infused)

Connect the person to an ECG monitor

Place in the sitting position

Provide standby equipment (endotracheal intubation tray) and drugs (aminophylline, digoxin, Lasix, morphine)

Obtain a blood sample and send for analysis (CBC, electrolytes, arterial blood gases)

Consult with the physician (immediately after giving emergency treatment)

Obtain a complete present and past history

Nursing Observation

Inspect the chest for respiratory rate (increased), rhythm, and symmetrical expansion

Auscultate the chest for lung aeration, rales, and rhonchi

Monitor the blood pressure

Palpate the pulse for rate, rhythm, and volume

Auscultate the apical heartbeat for rate and rhythm

Observe the ECG monitor (for evidence of cardiac damage)

Monitor blood studies for abnormal hematology, electrolytes, and arterial blood gases)

Measure the intake and output

Health Teaching

Explain the causes of the health problem (fluid collection in the lungs)

Explain the reason for and intended effect of the therapy (to improve circulation and ventilation)

Medical Treatments Performed by Nurses

Give the prescribed drugs (aminophylline to improve ventilation, digoxin to support cardiac function, Lasix to promote diuresis and reduce the fluid overload, morphine to ease respiratory distress and anxiety)

Administer intermittent positive-pressure breathing by expiratory positive-pressure mask (in pulmonary edema due to salt-water drowning)

EVALUATION

Record actual outcome

AIRWAY OBSTRUCTION [104,246]

ASSESSMENT
Data Collection
Subjective Data
• Intense facial anxiety
  Air hunger

Objective Data
• Coughing, gagging, choking
• Wheezing, snoring, grunting, or stridor respirations
  Mouth breathing
  Nasal flare
  Cyanosis
  Absent or decreased breath sounds
  Restlessness

Data Analysis
Nursing Diagnosis
AIRWAY OBSTRUCTION: The inability of air to pass through the respiratory passages

Common Etiology (Stressors)
DISEASES: Asthma, bronchitis, cerebrovascular accident, emphysema, epilepsy
INJURIES: Drowning, foreign body in nose or pharynx
SIGNS AND SYMPTOMS: Laryngeal spasm, stridor, unconsciousness
HEALTH CARE FACTORS: *Surgical therapy*: Anesthesia. *Therapeutic devices*: Dentures
ENVIRONMENTAL FACTORS: *Foreign body*: Food, drink. *Objects*: Wood, metal, glass, dirt parti-
  cles. *Water*: Submersion and drowning in
HUMAN ERROR: Rapid ingestion of liquid or food, swallowing food whole
MAJOR PATHOPHYSIOLOGIC FACTORS CAUSING THE PROBLEM: When objects, human secretions, or
  paralyzed or spastic tissue structures, obstruct the air passes, air cannot flow through
  the respiratory system, and oxygenation of tissues ceases or is severely impaired, presenting a life-threatening situation

PLANNING
Unmet Needs
Tissue oxygenation or perfusion, waste elimination of carbon dioxide, acid–base balance, comfort, protection from physical harm, increased learning

Expected Outcome
Unimpaired ventilation through a patent airway
Warm, slightly moist, pink skin
Expressions of increased comfort

NURSING INTERVENTIONS
Nursing Treatments
Remove all foreign objects (from the airway)
Use either the head-tilt or jaw-thrust maneuver to maintain an airway
  OR
Apply the Heimlich maneuver
Ventilate the person (if needed)
Insert an oral airway
  OR
Initiate endotracheal intubation (ET) (if unable to obtain an open airway)
Suction the airway (as needed)
Perform a tracheostomy (ET) (as a last resort)
Administer humidified oxygen (ET) (once the airway is cleared)

Encourage deep breathing (once the airway is cleared)

Place in the sitting position (with pillow or bed support)

Remove constrictive clothing (around the neck and the chest)

Administer intravenous fluids (ET) (to maintain an open line for drug administration)

Insert a gastric tube and attach to suction (ET) (to remove swallowed air and fluid in case of drowning)

Obtain a blood sample and send for analysis (arterial blood gases)

Consult with the physician (immediately after giving emergency treatment)

Provide standby equipment (endotracheal tube, tracheostomy tray, mechanical respirator) and drugs

Nursing Observations

Inspect the chest for respiratory rate and rhythm (note if the chest rises and falls and if the person's air on expiration can be heard and felt)

Inspect the chest for symmetrical expansion

Auscultate the chest for abnormal breath sounds and for adventitious sounds

Auscultate the chest for lung aeration

Palpate the pulse for rate, rhythm, and volume

Monitor the blood pressure

Monitor blood studies for arterial blood gases

Health Teaching

Describe those symptoms that should be reported (dyspnea, pain)

Inform that airway noise indicates obstruction

Recommend that bones be removed from foods before eating

Recommend that food be cut into small bite sizes

Medical Treatments Performed by Nurses

Give the prescribed drugs (aminophylline as a bronchodilator, Solu-Cortef to reduce the inflammatory process, epinephrine to relax the bronchioles in spasm, sodium bicarbonate to reverse acidosis and reestablish acid–base balance)

EVALUATION

Record actual outcome

FLAIL CHEST[20,42,104,246]

ASSESSMENT

Data Collection

Subjective Data
- Local chest pain increased by motion
- Dyspnea

Objective Data
- Tenderness and crepitation on palpation of the rib area
- Affected chest area moves inward as the chest wall moves outward on inhalation
- Cyanosis
  Localized edema
  Bruising

Data Analysis

Nursing Diagnosis

FLAIL CHEST: An unsupported, freely moving chest wall resulting in severe respiratory distress

Common Etiology (Stressors)

INJURIES: Fracture of the rib or sternum

ENVIRONMENTAL FACTORS: *Blast/explosion*: Exposure to. *Cataclysm*: Exposure to. *Crushing*: By cave-in, building collapse, falling objects. *Electricity*: Exposure to ungrounded electrical currents. *Moving vehicles*: Impact or collision of

MAJOR PATHOPHYSIOLOGIC FACTORS CAUSING THE PROBLEM: Fracture of several ribs and/or the sternum prevents effective ventilation of the lungs, thus the blood and tissues are inadequately oxygenated, and carbon dioxide is retained; retention of bronchopulmonary secretions further reduces the effectiveness of respiratory function

PLANNING

Unmet Needs

Tissue oxygenation or perfusion, waste elimination of carbon dioxide, comfort, protection from physical harm, increased learning

Expected Outcome

Expressions of reduced respiratory distress and increased comfort
Respirations within or near normal limits
Warm, pink skin, earlobes, lips, nails

NURSING INTERVENTIONS

Nursing Treatments

Apply a pressure dressing (to stabilize the chest wall)
Apply an elastic bandage (to hold the dressing in place)
Place on the affected side (for greater aeration of the unaffected lung)
Ventilate the person (ET) (if needed, using mouth-to-mouth breathing until spontaneous respirations occur)
Initiate endotracheal intubation (ET)
Administer humidified oxygen (ET)
Administer mechanical ventilation (ET)
Administer intravenous fluids (ET) (to maintain an open line for drug administration)
Handle gently (to prevent the fractured rib from penetrating the lung)
Elevate the head (for easier breathing)
Provide standby equipment (endotracheal tube, suction machine, mechanical respirator, chest tubes and water-seal drainage apparatus) and drugs (analgesics)
Consult with a physician (immediately after giving emergency treatment)
Obtain a blood sample and send for analysis (CBC, electrolytes, arterial blood gases)
Send a blood sample for type and crossmatch

Nursing Observations

Inspect the chest for respiratory rate, rhythm, and symmetrical expansion
Auscultate the chest for lung aeration
Monitor the blood pressure
Palpate the pulse for rate, rhythm, and volume
Monitor blood studies for abnormal hematology, chemistry, for arterial blood gases

Health Teaching

Explain the reasons for and intended effect of the therapy (to stabilize the chest and ease respirations)

Medical Treatments Performed by Nurses

Give the prescribed drugs (analgesics for pain relief)

EVALUATION

Record actual outcome

HYPOXIA [42,339]

ASSESSMENT

Data Collection

Subjective Data
- Anxiety
- Dyspnea
  Nausea
  Headache

Objective Data
- Cyanosis
  Lethargy
  Confusion
  Vomiting
  Restlessness
  Rapid pulse in the early stage
  Slow pulse in the late stage
  Speaks in short, broken sentences
  Decreased blood pressure
  Decreased blood O_2 saturation

Data Analysis

Nursing Diagnosis

HYPOXIA (OXYGEN INSUFFICIENCY): Inadequate oxygen available to body cells

Common Etiology (Stressors)

DISEASES: Aortic stenosis, arteriosclerosis, atrial fibrillation, atrial flutter, cerebrovascular accident, congestive heart failure, iron-deficiency anemia, mitral stenosis, myocardial infarction, pneumonia, pneumothorax, pulmonary edema, pulmonary embolus

INJURIES: Drowning, electrical shock, flail chest, sucking chest wound

ENVIRONMENTAL FACTORS: *Altitude*: High. *Chemical substances*: Inhalation of. *Electricity*: Exposure to ungrounded electrical currents. *Water*: Submersion and drowning in

HUMAN ERROR: Crawling into and closing abandoned refrigerator, placing plastic bags over the face

MAJOR PATHOPHYSIOLOGIC FACTORS CAUSING THE PROBLEM: Oxygen supply to tissues is reduced when there is circulatory impairment, a reduced amount of hemoglobin to transport the oxygen, or reduced oxygen content or tension within the tissues

PLANNING

Unmet Needs

Tissue oxygenation or perfusion, rest, comfort, protection from physical harm, increased learning

Expected Outcome

Blood pressure, pulse, and respirations within normal limits
Warm, slightly moist, pink skin, earlobes, lips, and nails
Consciousness without cerebral impairment
Blood PO_2 between 75–100 mm Hg

NURSING INTERVENTIONS

Nursing Treatments

Administer heated humidified oxygen (ET)
    OR
Administer intermittent positive-pressure breathing (ET) if needed
Elevate the head
    OR
Place in the sitting position

Place on complete bed rest
Obtain a blood sample and send for analysis (CBC, arterial blood gases)
Provide standby equipment (endotracheal tube, mechanical respirator)
Withhold all drugs (causing respiratory depression)
Reassure verbally (since anxiety is high during respiratory distress)
Consult with a physician (immediately after giving emergency treatment)

Nursing Observations
Inspect the chest for respiratory rate, rhythm, and symmetrical expansion
Auscultate the chest for abnormal breath sounds, lung aeration, and adventitious sounds
Monitor the blood pressure
Monitor blood studies for arterial blood gases (decreased O_2 saturation)
Observe for confusion, cyanosis, and dyspnea
Palpate the pulse for rate, rhythm, and volume

Health Teaching
Explain the causes of the health problem (inadequate transport of oxygen)
Explain the reason for and intended effect of the therapy (to increase oxygenation and ease respiration)

Medical Treatments Performed by Nurses
Administer controlled positive-pressure breathing

EVALUATION

Record actual outcome

INHALATION POISONING[219,278,522]

ASSESSMENT
Data Collection
Subjective Data
• Throbbing headache
• Dizziness
• Visual disturbance
  Nausea
  Dyspnea
  Tinnitus
  Relates exposure to dangerous gases

Objective Data
• Coughing, choking
  Hoarseness
  Increased respiratory secretions
  Confusion
  Drowsiness
  Vomiting
  Twitching
  Cherry-red skin color, nail beds, and mucous membranes (specific to carbon monoxide poisoning)

Data Analysis
Nursing Diagnosis
INHALATION POISONING: The breathing in of dangerous gases that interfere with or irritate the respiratory system

Common Etiology (Stressors)

ENVIRONMENTAL FACTORS: *Chemical substances*: Inhalation of toxic gases such as smoke, smog, household gas, mine dust, insulation, chlorine, carbon dioxide, carbon monoxide, nitrogen dioxide, ammonia, hydrogen sulfide

HUMAN ERROR: Uncontrolled use of gases in industry, warming a motor vehicle in an unventilated area, improperly ventilating gas and wood stoves or furnaces

MAJOR PATHOPHYSIOLOGIC FACTORS CAUSING THE PROBLEM: Inhaled chemical agents irritate the respiratory mucosa, causing an inflammatory reaction, an increased production of mucus, depression or damage to the cilia, and sometimes bronchospasm; highly corrosive fumes may cause burn injury of the mucosa. Some inhaled chemical agents cause systemic toxic reactions (bone marrow depression, nervous system damage, etc.), which can eventually cause death; carbon monoxide, when inhaled, more readily attaches itself to the hemoglobin of red blood cells than does oxygen, preventing the formation of oxyhemoglobin and reducing the amount of oxygen carried by the blood to tissues; severe insufficient oxygenation of blood (hypoxemia) leads to cerebral edema and then to death

PLANNING

Unmet Needs

Tissue oxygenation or perfusion, stimulation, protection from physical harm, increased learning

Expected Outcome

Unimpaired ventilation through a patent airway
Blood pressure, pulse, and respirations within normal limits
Warm, slightly moist, pink skin
Expressions of reduced respiratory distress
Consciousness without cerebral impairment

NURSING INTERVENTIONS

Nursing Treatments

Remove immediately to a safe area
Ventilate the person (ET) (using mouth-to-mouth breathing until spontaneous respirations return)
Administer humidified oxygen (ET)
　OR
Administer intermittent positive-pressure breathing (ET)
Suction the airway (as needed after respirations are reestablished)
Encourage coughing and deep breathing (in an area away from the toxic gases)
Connect the person to an ECG monitor (if needed)
Elevate the head
　OR
Place in the sitting position
Give hot coffee ⎫
　OR　　　　⎬ If conscious
Give hot tea ⎭
Stimulate by movement, touch, sternal pressure, or speech
Remove constrictive clothing
Cover with warm blankets
Obtain a blood sample and send for analysis (CBC, arterial blood gases)
Consult with a physician (immediately after giving emergency treatment)
Provide standby equipment (oral airway, endotracheal tube, mechanical ventilators) and drugs

Nursing Observations

Inspect the chest for respiratory rate, rhythm, and symmetrical expansion
Auscultate the chest for abnormal breath sounds, lung aeration, and adventitious sounds

Palpate the pulse for rate, rhythm, and volume
Observe the ECG monitor
Monitor the blood pressure
Monitor the oral temperature (for fever)
Observe the level of consciousness
Observe for cyanosis, dyspnea, or shock
Monitor blood studies for abnormal hematology and arterial blood gases

Health Teaching
Advise against exposure to airborne irritants
Describe those symptoms that should be reported (dyspnea, dizziness, headache)
Recommend safety measures to prevent suffocation (that heaters should be vented to the outside, that a car should never be started in a closed garage)

EVALUATION
Record actual outcome

NEAR DROWNING[246,278,522]

ASSESSMENT
Data Collection
Subjective Data
Notified of drowning victim

Objective Data

Salt Water Drowning
- Unconsciousness
- Cyanosis
- Cold skin
- Barely perceptible or absent pulse
- Increased blood erythrocytes and sodium (hemoconcentration)
  Decreased blood pressure
  Pulmonary edema
  Decreased blood protein

Fresh Water Drowning
- Unconsciousness
- Cyanosis
- Cold skin
- Barely perceptible or absent pulse
- Decreased blood erythrocytes and sodium (hemodilution)
  Increased blood pressure
  Ventricular fibrillation

Data Analysis
Nursing Diagnosis
NEAR DROWNING (DROWNING): Asphyxia from laryngeal spasm or water in the lungs resulting from submersion in water

Common Etiology (Stressors)
DISEASES: Epileptic episode or myocardial infarction while swimming
INJURIES: Cerebral concussion while swimming
ENVIRONMENTAL FACTORS: *Water*: Submersion and drowning in
HUMAN ERROR: Disregarding water safety methods

MAJOR PATHOPHYSIOLOGIC FACTORS CAUSING THE PROBLEM: *Hypertonic sea (ocean) water*: contains about 3.5% NaCl; when it is aspirated into the alveoli of the lung, the high percentage of NaCl causes rapid movement of water from the blood into the alveoli, resulting in excess fluid in the alveoli (pulmonary edema), decreased circulating blood volume (hypovolemia), and an increase in the number of red blood cells as a result of the decreased circulating plasma volume (hemoconcentration). *Hypotonic fresh water*: from lakes, pools, streams, and other inland water; when it is aspirated into the alveoli of the lung, the water moves rapidly into the blood, resulting in high levels of circulating blood volume (dilutional hypervolemia) and the destruction of red blood cells (hemolysis); the impurities (bacteria, chemicals) in the hypotonic fresh water result in a pulmonary inflammatory response, and the loss of the protein substance surfactant in the lungs results in delayed pulmonary edema

PLANNING

Unmet Needs

Tissue oxygenation or perfusion, fluid and electrolyte balance, stimulation, protection from physical harm, increased learning

Expected Outcome

Unimpaired ventilation through a patent airway
Blood pressure, pulse, and respirations within normal limits
Warm, slightly moist, pink skin
Consciousness without cerebral impairment

NURSING INTERVENTIONS

Nursing Treatments

Remove all foreign objects (from the airway)
Use either the head-tilt of jaw-thrust maneuver to maintain an airway
Ventilate the person (ET) (using mouth-to-mouth breathing until spontaneous respirations begin)
Suction the airway (as needed)
Insert an oral airway
  OR
Initiate endotracheal intubation (ET) (if needed)
Administer humidified oxygen (ET) (at a low percentage)
Administer intermittent positive-pressure breathing (ET) (in fresh-water drowning)
Encourage deep breathing (once the airway is cleared and when the person is conscious)
Initiate external cardiac massage (ET) (as needed)
Administer intravenous fluids (ET) (lactated Ringer's solution, isotonic saline. *Note*: In salt-water drowning *do not* give normal saline solution; 5% dextrose in water is appropriate)
Insert a nasogastric tube and attach to suction (ET) (to remove swallowed air and water)
Connect the person to an ECG monitor
Place in the foot-elevated, head-lowered (Trendelenburg) position
Cover with warm blankets
Remove constrictive clothing
Stimulate by movement, touch, sternal pressure, or speech
Obtain a blood sample and send for analysis (CBC, electrolytes, arterial blood gases)
Provide standby equipment (endotracheal tube, tracheostomy tray, mechanical respirator) and drugs
Consult with a physician (immediately after giving emergency treatments)

Nursing Observations

Inspect the chest for respiratory rate, rhythm, and symmetrical expansion
Auscultate the chest for abnormal breath sounds (wheezing), lung aeration, rales (bubbling), and rhonchi

Monitor the blood pressure
Monitor blood studies for hematology, electrolytes, and arterial blood gases
Observe for cyanosis and dyspnea
Observe the level of consciousness
Palpate the pulse for rate (tachycardia), rhythm, and volume
Observe the ECG monitor

Health Teaching

Explain the reason for and intended effect of the therapy (to reestablish respiratory and cardiac function)

Medical Treatments Performed by Nurses

Give the prescribed drugs

EVALUATION

Record actual outcome

OPEN CHEST WOUND[73,384]

ASSESSMENT

Data Collection

Subjective Data
• Dyspnea
• Chest pain

Objective Data
• Air moving through the chest wound, during inspiration and expiration, is audible and may cause wound drainage to bubble
• Coughing

Data Analysis

Nursing Diagnosis
OPEN CHEST WOUND (SUCKING CHEST WOUND): An open chest wound causing a collapsed, air-less lung and resulting in severe respiratory distress

Common Etiology (Stressors)
INJURIES: Laceration wound, puncture wound
ENVIRONMENTAL FACTORS: *Blast/explosion*: Exposure to. *Cataclysm*: Exposure to. *Crushing*: By cave-in, building collapse, falling object. *Moving vehicles*: Impact or collision of. *Weapons*: Gun, knife
MAJOR PATHOPHYSIOLOGIC FACTORS CAUSING THE PROBLEM: When there is an opening in the chest wall, air rushes into the pleural space during inspiration; the resulting air pressure collapses the lung, and consequently there is partial or total loss of ventilation of that lung

PLANNING

Unmet Needs

Tissue oxygenation or perfusion, comfort, protection from physical harm, increased learning

Expected Outcome

Expressions of reduced respiratory distress and increased comfort
Respirations within or near normal limits
Warm, pink skin, ear lobes, lips, nails

NURSING INTERVENTIONS

Nursing Treatments

Cover the sucking wound immediately (at the end of expiration, tape or hold in place the cleanest material available, a cloth, your hand, etc.)

Ventilate the person (ET) (if needed, using mouth-to-mouth breathing until spontaneous respirations occur)

Elevate the head (for easier breathing)

Place the person on the affected side (for greater aeration of the unaffected lung)

Administer humidified oxygen (ET)

Administer intravenous fluids (ET) (to maintain an open line for drug administration)

Obtain a blood sample and send for analysis (arterial blood gases)

Provide standby equipment (chest tubes and water-seal drainage apparatus, mechanical respirator) and drugs (analgesics)

Consult with a physician (immediately after giving emergency treatment)

Obtain a complete present and past history

Nursing Observations

Inspect the chest for respiratory rate and rhythm

Auscultate the chest for lung aeration

Monitor the blood pressure

Observe the level of consciousness

Palpate the pulse for rate, rhythm, and volume

Monitor blood studies for arterial blood gases

Health Teaching

Explain the reason for and intended effect of the therapy (to reduce the potential for lung collapse and reinflate the lung if collapse occurs)

Medical Treatments Performed by Nurses

Give the prescribed drugs (analgesics to relieve pain)

EVALUATION

Record actual outcome

RESPIRATORY ARREST[42,72,104,219,451]

ASSESSMENT

Data Collection

Subjective Data
None

Objective Data
- Unconsciousness and collapse
- No visible chest movements
- Absent breath sounds
  Cyanosis
  Increased heart rate with gradual slowing
  Low blood pressure
  Eventual death if untreated

Data Analysis

Nursing Diagnosis
RESPIRATORY ARREST (FAILURE OF RESPIRATION): Acute cessation of respirations

Common Etiology (Stressors)

DISEASES: Cerebrovascular accident, congestive heart failure, Guillain-Barré syndrome, myasthenia gravis, myocardial infarction, poliomyelitis, subarachnoid hemorrhage, ventricular fibrillation

INJURIES: Drowning, electrical shock, fracture and compression of the cervical and/or thoracic spinal cord

SIGNS AND SYMPTOMS: Laryngeal edema, laryngeal spasm

HEALTH CARE FACTORS: *Drug therapy*: Adverse effects of drugs (respiratory depression)

ENVIRONMENTAL FACTORS: *Chemical substances*: Toxic gases. *Crushing*: By cave-in, building collapse, falling object. *Electricity*: Exposure to ungrounded electrical currents. *Water*: Submersion and drowning in

MAJOR PATHOPHYSIOLOGIC FACTORS CAUSING THE PROBLEM: Respirations cease when there is damage to the respiratory center in the brain, when circulation is severely impaired, or when there is prolonged obstruction to air passages

PLANNING

Unmet Needs

Tissue oxygenation or perfusion, waste elimination of carbon dioxide, stimulation, protection from physical harm, increased learning

Expected Outcome

Unimpaired ventilation through a patent airway

Blood pressure, pulse, and respirations within or near normal limits

Warm, slightly moist, pink skin

Consciousness without cerebral impairment

NURSING INTERVENTIONS

Nursing Treatments

Use either the head-tilt or jaw-thrust maneuver to maintain the airway

Ventilate the person (ET) (using mouth-to-mouth breathing until spontaneous respirations return)

Ventilate the person mouth-to-stoma or bag-to-stoma when the patient has a laryngectomy or tracheostomy (ET)

Remove all foreign objects (from the airway if there is evidence of such)

Insert an oral airway

    OR

Initiate endotracheal intubation (ET)

Administer humidified oxygen (ET)

Administer intermittent positive-pressure breathing (ET) (or attach to other mechanical breathing devices such as resuscitators or inhalators)

Suction the airway (as needed after respirations are reestablished)

Connect the person to an ECG monitor

Obtain a blood sample and send for analysis (CBC, SMAC, arterial blood gases)

Withhold all drugs (that cause respiratory depression such as morphine)

Consult with a physician (immediately after giving emergency treatment)

Provide standby equipment (tracheostomy tray, mechanical ventilators) and drugs

Nursing Observations

During Emergency

Inspect the chest for respiratory rate and rhythm (note if the chest rises and falls and if the person's air on expiration can be heard and felt)

Inspect for foreign bodies (in the airway if there is not immediate response to ventilation)

Postemergency

Inspect the chest for respiratory rate, rhythm, and symmetric expansion

Auscultate the chest for lung aeration

Monitor the blood pressure

Monitor blood studies for arterial blood gases, abnormal hematology, and abnormal chemistry

Observe the level of consciousness

Palpate the pulse for rate, rhythm, and volume

Auscultate the apical pulse for rate and rhythm

Observe the ECG monitor (for cardiac abnormalities)

Health Teaching

Explain the reason for and intended effect of the therapy (to the family)

Medical Treatments Performed by Nurses

Give the prescribed drugs

EVALUATION

Record actual outcome

Emergency Conditions of the Sensory Systems

FOREIGN BODY IN THE EAR[42,72,451]

ASSESSMENT

Data Collection

Subjective Data
• Earache
  Complaints of diminished hearing
  Buzzing in the ear when an insect is lodged in the ear

Objective Data
• Object or insect is visible inside the ear
  Ear canal swelling and inflammation
  Purulent and bloody ear drainage

Data Analysis

Nursing Diagnosis
FOREIGN BODY IN THE EAR: The presence of an unnatural object in the ear

Common Etiology (Stressors)
ENVIRONMENTAL FACTORS: *Biologic agents*: Exposure to flying and crawling insects
HUMAN ERROR: Accidental or intentional insertion of objects into body orifices
MAJOR PATHOPHYSIOLOGIC FACTORS CAUSING THE PROBLEM: When objects are inserted into the narrow orifice of the ear, the resulting pressure causes pain, swelling, inflammation, impaired hearing and sometimes tympanic membrane rupture

PLANNING

Unmet Needs

Comfort, protection from physical harm, increased learning

Expected Outcome

The foreign object in the ear will be removed

There will be no additional injury to tissue beyond that which has traumatically occurred

NURSING INTERVENTIONS

Nursing Treatments

Remove the foreign object (with tweezers or forceps)

Insert an oiled cotton pledget into the ear

   OR

Instill warm oil into the ear (which will kill an insect)

Irrigate the ear (foreign particle) with alcohol (instead of water if the object is a bean or something that will expand when in contact with water, since the alcohol will not cause the object to swell)

Make a referral (to a physician if ear injury has occurred)

Nursing Observations

Inspect the ears with an otoscope (for inflammation, edema, and punctured tympanic membrane)

Observe for complaints of pain

Health Teaching

Instruct not to insert foreign objects into body orifices

EVALUATION

Record actual outcome

FOREIGN BODY IN THE EYE[20,73,219]

ASSESSMENT

Data Collection

Subjective Data

• Pain

  Diminished vision

Objective Data

• Frequent blinking

  Redness

  Inflammation

  Excessive tearing

  Visible foreign object

Data Analysis

Nursing Diagnosis

FOREIGN BODY IN THE EYE: The presence of an injurious or harmful object in the eye

Common Etiology (Stressors)

ENVIRONMENTAL FACTORS: *Biologic agents*: Exposure to flying insects. *Blast/explosion*: Exposure to. *Cataclysm*: Exposure to. *Chemical substances*: Propelled and splashing. *Crushing*: By cave-in, building collapse. *Foreign Object*: Propelled. *Moving vehicles*: Impact or collision of. *Objects*: Dirt, dust, glass, metal, wood particles. *Wind*: Exposure to

HUMAN ERROR: Nonuse of safety eyeglasses

MAJOR PATHOPHYSIOLOGIC FACTORS CAUSING THE PROBLEM: Foreign bodies, on entering the eye, cause irritation of eye tissue that results in pain or discomfort, an inflammatory response, and possibly impaired vision

PLANNING

Unmet Needs

Comfort, protection from physical harm, increased learning

Expected Outcome

The foreign object in the eye will be removed

There will be no additional injury to tissue beyond that which has traumatically occurred

Visual acuity will remain equal to that before injury

NURSING INTERVENTIONS

Nursing Treatments

Evert the eyelid (to facilitate visualization of the foreign body)

Remove the foreign object (with a saline moistened, sterile gauze or cotton-tipped applicator)

Irrigate the eye (with saline, plain water, or Dacriose solution)

Handle gently (to prevent further injury)

Make a referral (to a physician if there is any eye damage)

Nursing Observations

Inspect for (eye) edema

Observe for complaints of pain or visual disturbance

Test the eye for visual acuity (with the Snellen chart after removal of the foreign body)

Health Teaching

Instruct to avoid rubbing the eyes

Describe those symptoms that should be reported (continued pain, inflammation, tearing, visual disturbance)

Explain the reason for and intended effect of the therapy

EVALUATION

Record actual outcome

FOREIGN BODY IN THE NOSE[26,42,73]

ASSESSMENT

Data Collection

Subjective Data

Pain

Some difficulty breathing

Objective Data

• Distention of the nare(s)

• Object visible inside the nares

  Foul-smelling, bloody or purulent, unilateral discharge

Data Analysis

Nursing Diagnosis

FOREIGN BODY IN THE NOSE: The presence of an injurious or harmful object in the nose

Common Etiology (Stressors)

HUMAN ERROR: Accidental or intentional insertion of objects into body orifices

MAJOR PATHOPHYSIOLOGIC FACTORS CAUSING THE PROBLEM: When objects are inserted into the narrow orifices of the nose, the resulting pressure causes pain, swelling, inflammation, and possible impaired breathing

PLANNING

Unmet Needs

Comfort, protection from physical harm, increased learning

Expected Outcome

The foreign body in the nose will be removed

There will be full air intake through the person's nares
There will be no additional injury to tissue beyond that which has traumatically occurred

NURSING INTERVENTIONS

Nursing Treatments
Remove the foreign object (with a tweezer or forceps)
Suction the airway (if appropriate)
Handle gently
Make a referral (to a physician if the object is far back into the nares)

Nursing Observations
Inspect the chest for respiratory rate and rhythm
Inspect for bleeding (from the nose)

Health Teaching
Instruct not to insert foreign objects into body orifices
Explain the reason for and intended effect of the therapy (to reestablish a patent nasal airway)

EVALUATION

Record actual outcome

CHEMICAL EYE BURN[20,21,73,219]

ASSESSMENT

Data Collection

Subjective Data
• Severe pain
• Impaired vision

Objective Data
• Eye redness
  Loss of normal eye epithelium, sometimes
  Drainage

Data Analysis

Nursing Diagnosis
CHEMICAL EYE BURN: Eye injury as a result of harsh chemical substances in contact with the eye

Common Etiology (Stressors)
ENVIROMNEMTAL FACTORS: *Chemical substances*: Splashing or propelled acids or alkali
HUMAN ERROR: Incorrect use of eye medications, nonuse of safety eyeglasses
MAJOR PATHOPHYSIOLOGIC FACTORS CAUSING THE PROBLEM: Chemical agents, such as acids or alkali, burn the sensitive eye tissues, causing considerable pain and inflammation, and corneal burns result in impaired vision that may become permanent due to scarring

PLANNING

Unmet Needs
Rest, comfort, protection from physical harm, increased learning

Expected Outcome
There will be no additional tissue injury beyond that which has traumatically occurred

NURSING INTERVENTIONS

Nursing Treatments
Do not neutralize the chemical injuring the eye

Irrigate the eye (with saline or plain water)

Apply a sterile dressing

Make a referral (to a physician immediately after giving emergency treatment)

Nursing Observations

Observe for complaints of pain

Health Teaching

Explain the reason for and intended effect of the therapy (to dilute the irritating chemical)

Instruct to avoid rubbing the eyes

EVALUATION

Record actual outcome

HEAT EYE BURN[20,21,219]

ASSESSMENT

Data Collection

Subjective Data
* Severe pain
  Impaired vision sometimes

Objective Data
* Burned eyelids, sclera, or cornea
* Unable to open the eyes voluntarily
  Eye redness
  Swelling
  Drainage

Data Analysis

Nursing Diagnosis

HEAT EYE BURN: Eye injury as a result of contact with intense heat or radiant energy

Common Etiology (Stressors)

ENVIRONMENTAL HEAT: *Blast/explosion*: Exposure to. *Electricity*: Exposure to ungrounded electrical currents. *Environmental heat*: Fire and flames. *Environmental objects*: Hot liquids, steam. *Environmental radiation*: Infrared rays, ultraviolet light

HUMAN ERROR: Nonuse of safety eyeglasses

MAJOR PATHOPHYSIOLOGIC FACTORS CAUSING THE PROBLEM: Heat and radiant energy burn the sensitive eye tissues, causing considerable pain and inflammation; ultraviolet rays cause injury according to the length of the rays rather than the degree of heat produced; the cornea is rarely scarred permanently by radiant energy; heat burns may leave permanent scars of the cornea and eyelids

PLANNING

Unmet Needs

Rest, comfort, protection from physical harm, increased learning

Expected Outcome

There will be no additional tissue injury beyond that which has traumatically occurred

NURSING INTERVENTIONS

Nursing Treatments

Apply a cold, moist compress (intermittently until the pain subsides)

Lubricate the eye globes (instill sterile mineral oil drops)

Apply a sterile dressing (over the eye)

Make a referral (to a physician immediately after giving emergency treatment)

Nursing Observations
Observe for complaints of pain

Health Teaching
Instruct to avoid rubbing the eyes
Explain the reason for and intended effect of the therapy (to reduce heat in the eye)

EVALUATION

Record actual outcome

16 Nursing Diagnoses of MINOR HEALTH PROBLEMS

Dual Domain of Nursing Expertise: Minor Health Problems

This chapter covers that sphere of nursing knowledge and skill related to problems of non–life-threatening illnesses or perceived body changes that are simple in nature. Such problems include minor illnesses, disorders, conditions, trauma, and symptoms. These problems are solved by many health care providers, such as nurses, physicians, dentists, pharmacists, and physicians' assistants.

Views of Nursing Leaders That Support This Domain of Nursing Expertise

The nurse may intervene at the secondary prevention level which deals with the system after an encounter with a stressor has occurred and is concerned with . . . treatment of symptoms.

The Neuman model lends itself to a multiprofessional method of assessing clients' needs; one profession can benefit from the assessment and services offered to the client by another. . . . Neuman states her belief that nursing and medicine are complimentary.

Betty Neuman[410:136&161]

Modern medical advances require nurses to be well-grounded in pathology and in various medical technologies if they are to effectively assist individuals with health-deviation self-care.

Dorothea Orem[380:30]

Nursing will continue to assist medicine in the fulfillment of medicine's mission both because of the intrinsic value of that mission and because doing so will facilitate the fulfillment of nursing's mission.

Dorothy Johnson[410:218]

Man has four modes of adaptation. The first involves his basic physiologic needs. As he responds to environmental changes, he will need to keep in balance his needs relating to circulation, body temperature, oxygen, fluids, sleep and activity, elimination, and the appetite system.

Sister Callista Roy[669:254]

Minor Health Problems Associated with Body-Temperature Regulation

CHILLS [42,476]

ASSESSMENT

Data Collection

Subjective Data
• Feels cold

Objective Data
• Shivering
• Skin pallor
  Chattering of teeth
  Gooseflesh

Data Analysis

Nursing Diagnosis
CHILLS: A cold sensation followed by an increased temperature

Common Etiology (Stressors)
DISEASES: Bacteremia, bacterial infection, influenza, malaria, pneumococcal pneumonia, viral infection
SIGNS AND SYMPTOMS: Fever
HEALTH CARE FACTORS: *Drug therapy*: Immunization therapy. *Medical therapy*: Blood-transfusion reaction
MAJOR PATHOPHYSIOLOGIC FACTORS CAUSING THE PROBLEM: Chills occur as a reaction to infectious agents or a response to a disturbance in the temperature-regulating system of the hypothalamus

PLANNING

Unmet Needs
Comfort, normal temperature, protection from physical harm, increased learning

Expected Outcome
Person verbalizes that he feels comfortably warm
Cessation of shivering
Body temperature of 96.8° F (36° C) to 99.5° F (37.5° C)

NURSING INTERVENTIONS

Nursing Treatments
Cover with warm blankets.
Dress in warm clothing
Maintain a warm room temperature
Decrease drafts
Give warm liquids (lemonade, cocoa)
  OR
Give hot coffee
  OR
Give hot tea
Refrain from giving iced liquids
Place only warm hands and objects on the patient

Nursing Observations
Monitor the oral temperature (after the teeth stop chattering and repeat in 30 minutes)

Observe for complaints of (recurring) chills

Health Teaching

Explain the causes of the health problem (infection, reaction to the immunization vaccine, etc.)

Explain the reason for and intended effect of the therapy (to reestablish normal temperature)

Teach how to take a temperature and read a thermometer accurately

Recommend the use of warm clothing (during viral or bacterial illness)

EVALUATION

Record actual outcome

FEVER [35,72,88,371]

ASSESSMENT

Data Collection

Subjective Data

Malaise

Headache over the forehead, in back of the head, or generalized

Internal feeling of warmth

Chills

Objective Data

• Body temperature more than 1° F above the normal temperature—usually above 99.5° F (37.5° C) orally or 100.5° F (38.0° C) rectally

• Increased pulse rate

• Increased respirations

Restlessness

Irritability

Warm or hot skin

Skin wetness or dryness

Data Analysis

Nursing Diagnosis

FEVER (PYREXIA, ELEVATED BODY TEMPERATURE): Increased body-heat production exceeding the amount of heat lost from the body

Common Etiology (Stressors)

DISEASES: Actinomycosis, amyloidosis, anthrax, bacterial endocarditis, bronchiectasis, brucellosis, bubonic plague, chickenpox, Colorado tick fever, dengue fever, dermatitis, diptheria, diverticulitis, dysentery, encephalitis, endometritis, epidemic louse-born typhus, epididymitis, gastritis, glomerolunephritis, gout, hepatitis, herpes zoster, histoplasmosis, Hodgkin's disease, infection of any kind, infectious mononucleosis, influenza, kala-azar, leukemia, lupus erythematosus, lymphadenitis, malaria, mammary abscess, mastoiditis, measles, mediastinitis, meningitis, metastatic carcinoma, miliaria, mumps, myocardial infarction, myocarditis, otitis media, nephritis, parathyroid fever, pericarditis, pertussis, pheochromocytoma, photodermatitis, pneumonia, poliomyelitis, polyarteritis nodosa, polymyocitis, pyogenic osteomyelitis, rabies, rat-bite fever, renal calculi, rheumatic fever, rheumatoid arthritis, rickettsialpox, Rocky Mountain spotted fever, roseola infantum, salmonella gastroenteritis, smallpox, streptococcal pharyngitis, tetanus, thryotoxicosis, tuberculosis, tularemia, typhoid, ulcerative colitis, undulent fever, Weil's disease, yellow fever

INJURIES: Foreign body in the ear or nose, heat stroke
SIGNS AND SYMPTOMS: Dehydration
PSYCHOSOCIAL FACTORS: Excessive emotional excitement
HEALTH CARE FACTORS: *Drug therapy*: Adverse effects of drugs. *Medical therapy*: Blood-transfusion reaction, urinary catheterization
ENVIRONMENTAL FACTORS: *Environmental heat*: High external temperature
MAJOR PATHOPHYSIOLOGIC FACTORS CAUSING THE PROBLEM: Hypothalmic disturbance, infection, increased metabolic rate, impaired circulation, central nervous system depression or damage, the absence of sweat glands, conditions of tissue destruction, fluid imbalance

PLANNING

Unmet Needs
Fluid and electrolyte balance, normal temperature, sleep and rest, comfort, protection from physical harm, increased learning

Expected Outcome
Body temperature of 96.8° F (36° C) to 99.5° F (37.5° C)
Pulse rate 60–80 beats/minute
Respiratory rate 12–20 breaths/minute
Skin coolness

NURSING INTERVENTIONS

Nursing Treatments
Apply a cool, damp cloth to the face
Bathe in cool water
  OR
Apply an ice bag (to the head and torso in very high fever)
  OR
Apply alcohol to the skin
Cover with lightweight blankets
Dress in lightweight clothing
Dress in minimum clothing
Maintain a cool room temperature
Increase drafts
Encourage adequate rest
Give nonprescription drugs (antipyretics)
Increase fluid intake to about 2,000 cc daily
Give iced liquids
Discourage the intake of oral stimulants
Refrain from giving hot liquids
Refrain from giving local heat applications
Make a referral (to a physician if the fever is above 102° F or if an infant with fever is less than 6 weeks old)

Nursing Observations
Measure the intake and output
Monitor the body temperature
Obtain a bacterial culture (of blood, urine, sputum, stools)

Health Teaching
Explain the causes of the health problem (infection, drug reaction, fluid imbalance)
Teach how to take a temperature and read a temperature accurately
Teach how to clean a nondisposable thermometer
Explain how to estimate temperature by touch
Explain the reason for and intended effect of the therapy (to reestablish a normal temperature)

EVALUATION

Record actual outcome

HYPOTHERMIA [35,72,371]

ASSESSMENT

Data Collection

Subjective Data
Feels cold
Numbness in extremities

Objective Data
• Body temperature below 96° F (35.6° C) orally or 97° F (36.1° C) rectally
• Slow pulse
• Slow respirations
  Gooseflesh
  Pallor
  Shivering, shaking
  Cool skin

Data Analysis

Nursing Diagnosis
HYPOTHERMIA (SUBNORMAL TEMPERATURE): Decreased body-heat production below the normal
  amount of body heat

Common Etiology (Stressors)
DISEASES: Arteriosclerosis, diabetes mellitus, hypothyroidism, pheochromocytoma, Sim-
  mond's disease
INJURIES: Burn wound
SIGNS AND SYMPTOMS: Shock, weight loss
LIFESTYLE: Insufficient, imbalanced diet
ENVIRONMENTAL FACTORS: *Environmental cold*: Freezing external temperature
MAJOR PATHOPHYSIOLOGIC FACTORS CAUSING THE PROBLEM: Increased heat loss, impaired circu-
  lation, lowered metabolic rate, inadequate nutrition, decreased body fat associated
  with aging

PLANNING

Unmet Needs
Tissue oxygenation or perfusion, nutritional balance, normal temperature, sleep and
  rest, comfort, protection from physical harm, increased learning

Expected Outcome
Body temperature of 96.8° F (36° C) to 99.5° F (37.5° C)
Pulse rate 60–80 beats/minute
Respiratory rate 12–20 breaths/minute
Skin warmth

NURSING INTERVENTIONS

Nursing Treatments
Cover with warm blankets
Dress in warm clothing
Decrease drafts
Maintain a warm room temperature
Apply a heat cradle
Give warm liquids
Refrain from giving iced liquids
Encourage increased protein-food intake (if the problem is chronic)
Encourage moderate physical exercise
Encourage adequate rest
Refrain from giving local cold applications
Place only warm hands and objects on the patient

Nursing Observations
Monitor the oral temperature

Health Teaching
Explain the causes of the health problem (heat loss, impaired circulation)
Explain the reason for and intended effect of the therapy (to reestablish normal temperature)
Advise against exposure to inclement weather
Recommend the use of warm clothing

EVALUATION

Record actual outcome

Knowledge Deficits Associated with Body Temperature Regulation

UNKNOWLEDGEABLE ABOUT COPING WITH ENVIRONMENTAL COLD[20,22]

ASSESSMENT

Data Collection

Subjective Data
- Person's discussion or questions indicate a need for additional information, clarification, or validation of information
  OR
- Person's lack of questions or comments indicates not wanting information or not knowing enough to seek information
- When questioned directly, the person's response or lack of response indicates that he does not know:
  The dangers of severe environmental cold
  The need to stay indoors whenever possible
  Methods for keeping warm
  Dangerous warming methods sometimes used

Objective Data
- May exhibit behavior such as staying out in severe cold for a prolonged time, wearing insufficient clothing for warmth, etc.

Data Analysis

Nursing Diagnosis
UNKNOWLEDGEABLE ABOUT COPING WITH ENVIRONMENTAL COLD: Being without sufficient information about methods for protection against very low environmental temperatures

Common Etiology (Stressors)
HEALTH CARE FACTORS: Lack of health instruction

PLANNING

Unmet Needs
Protection from physical harm, independence, increased learning

Expected Outcome
Correct verbal feedback of the information taught

NURSING INTERVENTIONS
Nursing Treatments
Approach unhurriedly
Encourage the person to ask questions
Discourage smoking (which causes vasoconstriction that reduces body heat)

Nursing Observations
Determine teaching effectiveness by verbal feedback

Health Teaching
Advise against exposure to inclement weather (especially exposure to high, cold winds)
Emphasize the danger of breathing cold air (to keep the nose and mouth covered with a scarf to prevent injury to respiratory tissue)
Recommend the use of warm clothing (suitable to the individual)
Encourage moderate physical exercise (strenuous exercise can cause cramping and perspiration that will chill the body further)
Instruct to increase (warm) fluid intake
Advise not to partake of very cold foods or drinks (do not eat snow, which causes body heat to drop dangerously low)
Advise against drinking alcohol for warmth (after causing vasodilation, which increases body heat, alcohol causes vasoconstriction, which reduces body heat)
Emphasize the danger of massaging frostbitten tissue (rubbing increases cellular damage)
Advise to warm numbed tissue by immersing the body part in warm water (at 100–105° F)
Describe those symptoms that should be reported (decreased feeling sensation, edema, pallor, or bluish red skin)

EVALUATION
Record actual outcome

UNKNOWLEDGEABLE ABOUT COPING WITH ENVIRONMENTAL HEAT[20,22]

ASSESSMENT
Data Collection
Subjective Data
• Person's discussion or questions indicate a need for additional information, clarification, or validation of information
    OR
• Person's lack of questions or comments indicates not wanting information or not knowing enough to seek information
• When questioned directly, the person's response or lack of response indicates that he does not know:
    The dangers of intense environmental heat
    The need to stay out of midafternoon heat
    That the living pace must be slowed down during intense heat
    That fluid and salt intake must be increased
    That heavy work and active sports should be postponed

Objective Data
• May exhibit behavior such as engaging in play, heavy work, active sports, or exercise in high environmental temperature, failing to replace fluids while perspiring heavily, etc.

Data Analysis

Nursing Diagnosis

UNKNOWLEDGEABLE ABOUT COPING WITH ENVIRONMENTAL HEAT: Being without sufficient information about methods for protection against high environmental temperatures

Common Etiology (Stressors)

HEALTH CARE FACTORS: Lack of health instruction

PLANNING

Unmet Needs

Protection from physical harm, independence, increased learning

Expected Outcome

Correct verbal feedback of the information taught

NURSING INTERVENTIONS

Nursing Treatments

Approach unhurriedly

Encourage the person to ask questions

Nursing Observations

Determine teaching effectiveness by verbal feedback

Health Teaching

Advise against exposure to intense heat (especially in the midafternoon, if the person is very young, aged, or ill)

Instruct to increase fluid intake (water or Gatorade)

Recommend adherence to a pace of living with which the person is comfortable (according to the person's age and occupation, especially during the hot months of the year)

Describe those symptoms that should be reported (tachycardia, skin flushing, headache, dizziness, nausea, high fever, extreme fatigue, abdominal cramps)

Explain the causes of the health problem (fluid loss from a high environmental temperature)

EVALUATION

Record actual outcome

UNKNOWLEDGEABLE ABOUT FEVER [35,72,88,371]

ASSESSMENT

Data Collection

Subjective Data

• Person's discussion or questions indicate a need for additional information, clarification, or validation of information
    OR

- Person's lack of questions or comments indicates not wanting information or not knowing enough to seek information
- When questioned directly, the person's response or lack of response indicates that he does not know:
  The level of fever that requires medical intervention
  Methods for treating fever

Objective Data
- May exhibit behavior such as not treating his own or a significant other's temperature elevation, practicing superstitious rituals to reduce fever, etc.

Data Analysis

Nursing Diagnosis
UNKNOWLEDGEABLE ABOUT FEVER: Being without sufficient information about causes, effects, and therapeutic care associated with fever

Common Etiology (Stressors)
HEALTH CARE FACTORS: Lack of health instruction

PLANNING

Unmet Needs
Comfort, protection from physical harm, independence, increased learning

Expected Outcome
Correct verbal feedback of the information taught

NURSING INTERVENTIONS

Nursing Treatments
Approach unhurriedly
Encourage the person to ask questions
Encourage adequate rest

Nursing Observations
Determine teaching effectiveness by verbal feedback

Health Teaching
Describe those symptoms that should be reported (fever over 102° F, delirium, etc.)
Teach how and when to administer medications (for fever above 100° F, give aspirin or acetaminophen orally)
Instruct to increase fluid intake (cool fluids)
Teach the specific procedure:
  Bathe in cool water
  Cover with lightweight blankets
  Recommend the use of lightweight clothing
  Maintain a cool room temperature
  Give iced liquids
  Discourage the intake of oral stimulants
  Refrain from giving hot liquids
  Refrain from giving local heat applications
Explain the reason for and intended effect of the therapy (to reestablish normal temperature)
Explain the causes of the health problem (infection, increased metabolic rate, impaired circulation, emotional excitement, drug reactions, conditions of tissue destruction, antigen–antibody reaction, fluid imbalance)

EVALUATION

Record actual outcome

Minor Health Problems Associated with the Cardiovascular System

ARTERIAL PERIPHERAL INSUFFICIENCY[42,73,371,451]

ASSESSMENT

Data Collection

Subjective Data
Limb coolness or coldness
Aching pain (soreness) (heaviness)

Objective Data
• When the legs or arms are dependent, the feet or hands are blue or purple
• When the legs or arms are elevated, the feet or hands are pale, and when the extremity is lowered, normal color does not return within 20 seconds
• Diminished arterial pulsations
  Shiny skin appearance
  Skin wrinkles when pinched
  Lack of lanugo hair on the feet, toes, back of the hands, or fingers
  Round scars are covered with atrophied skin
  Ulcerated or gangrenous tissue
  Slow-growing, dry, brittle, thick nails
  Cold skin

Data Analysis

Nursing Diagnosis
ARTERIAL PERIPHERAL INSUFFICIENCY: An inadequate supply of blood flowing into extremity tissues

Common Etiology (Stressors)
DISEASES: Arteriosclerosis, atherosclerosis, Buerger's disease, hemorrhage, mitral stenosis, myocardial infarction, pulmonary stenosis
INJURIES: Burn wound, bone fracture, laceration wound
HEALTH CARE FACTORS: *Adverse effects of medical or surgical therapy*: Circulatory constriction from a cast or elastic bandage
MAJOR PATHOPHYSIOLOGIC FACTORS CAUSING THE PROBLEM: Reduced cardiac output, vascular occlusion or constriction, excessive blood or fluid loss resulting in reduced blood volume to the skin surface

PLANNING

Unmet Needs

Tissue oxygenation or perfusion, rest, exercise, comfort, protection from physical harm, increased learning

Expected Outcome

Warm, moist, natural color to the skin and nails
Rapid capillary refilling when pressure is released from the nail bed
Strong peripheral pulses

NURSING INTERVENTIONS

Nursing Treatments

Place on complete bed rest
Place on the slight-sitting (semi-Fowler's) position (with the legs and hands resting at the level of the heart)
Maintain a warm room temperature

Dress in warm clothing (that fits loosely)
Bathe in warm water (never hot water)
Exercise in range of motion (passive)
Discourage smoking
Refrain from giving local heat applications, from giving local cold applications
Refrain from elevating the bed at the knee gatch
Refrain from placing a pillow under the knee
Refrain from tight bandaging
Remove constrictive clothing
Bivalve and spread the cast to relieve pressure (ET) (if cast pressure is the cause)
Make a referral (to a physician when circulatory insufficiency is severe as in Buerger's disease, hemorrhage, myocardial infarction)

Nursing Observations
Inspect for impaired circulation (cold, cyanotic skin)
Palpate for arterial pulsations (periodically)
Monitor blood studies for arterial blood gases and abnormal hematology

Health Teaching
Explain the causes of the health problem (fluid loss, reduced cardiac function, etc.)
Advise against wearing constrictive clothing
Explain the need to avoid mechanical trauma (such as handling cold objects, body contact with furniture)
Inform that the extremities should be kept warm when the circulation is impaired (with loose clothing)
Advise not to partake of very cold foods and drinks
Instruct not to dangle the legs (or place the hands in a prolonged dependent position)
Teach how to do isometric exercises (opening and closing the hand, pushing down with the foot)
Explain the reason for and intended effect of the therapy (to improve circulation)

Medical Treatments Performed by Nurses
Give the prescribed exercises (Buerger–Allen exercises)

EVALUATION
Record actual outcome

BLEEDING[73,88,371,451]

ASSESSMENT
Data Collection
Subjective Data
• Acute onset
  Weakness

Objective Data
• Skin, mucous membrane, or tissue is not intact
• Blood oozing externally
  Warm skin
  Blood pressure is normal or slightly hypotensive

Data Analysis
Nursing Diagnosis
BLEEDING: The slow loss of small amounts of blood

Common Etiology (Stressors)
DISEASES: Hemophilia, hemorrhoids, Hodgkin's disease, leukemia, malnutrition, scurvy

INJURIES: Abrasion wound, animal bite, human bite, incision wound, laceration wound, puncture wound

HEALTH CARE FACTORS: *Diagnostic procedures*: Angiography, biopsy of muscle or skin, blood sampling, bone marrow sampling, cisternal puncture. *Drug therapy*: Anticoagulant therapy. *Medical therapy*: Intravenous infusion, paracentesis, thoracentesis, blood transfusion. *Surgical therapy*: Any surgery. *Surgical incision*: Any

ENVIRONMENTAL FACTORS: *Biologic agents*: Animal bite, insect bite. *Foreign body*: Propelled foreign body. *Machinery*: Injury from machinery. *Moving vehicles*: Impact or collision of. *Objects*: Exposure to falling, hard, pointed, or sharp objects. *Tools*: Powered and nonpowered tools. *Weapons*: Injury by knife or club

MAJOR PATHOPHYSIOLOGIC FACTORS CAUSING THE PROBLEM: Bleeding results when there is a disruption in the integrity of blood vessels, usually the result of trauma; other causes include spontaneous blood-vessel rupture, platelet deficiency, and blood-clotting defects

PLANNING

Unmet Needs

Fluid and electrolyte balance, rest, comfort, cleanliness, protection from physical harm, increased learning

Expected Outcome

Cessation of the oozing blood from the wound or orifice
Blood pressure reading within the person's normal level
Pulse rate of 60–80 beats/minute

NURSING INTERVENTIONS

Nursing Treatments

Apply an ice bag
   OR
Apply manual pressure over the bleeding area
   OR
Apply a pressure dressing
Clean with surgical soap
   OR
Soak in providone-iodine (Betadine) solution
Apply a sterile dressing
Elevate the affected body part
Immobilize the affected body part
Handle gently
Refrain from giving local heat applications
Encourage adequate rest
Discourage smoking (until the episode subsides)
Discourage the intake of oral stimulants (until the episode subsides)

Nursing Observations

Estimate the blood volume loss
Monitor the blood pressure
Monitor blood studies for abnormal hematology
Palpate the pulse for rate, rhythm, and volume

Health Teaching

Explain the causes of the health problem (vessel injury, drug effects)
Explain the need to avoid mechanical trauma (to the injured area)
Instruct to move the injured body part carefully
Instruct to increase fluid intake (in proportion to the amount of bleeding)
Explain the reason for and intended effect of the therapy (to support coagulation)

EVALUATION

Record actual outcome

EPISTAXIS [125,278]

ASSESSMENT

Data Collection

Subjective Data
- Acute onset
  Person relates feeling blood trickling down the back of the throat
  May swallow the blood
  May be fearful

Objective Data
- Blood oozing externally from the nose
- Bleeding from the anterior nasal septum or inferior meatus
  May be multiple oozing points in the nasal mucosa

Data Analysis

Nursing Diagnosis
EPISTAXIS: Blood oozing or flowing from the nose

Common Etiology (Stressors)
DISEASES: Aortic coartation, arteriosclerosis, diphtheria, glomerulonephritis, hemophilia, hypertension, Laennec's cirrhosis, leukemia, measles, Rendu–Osler Weber disease, rheumatic fever, scarlet fever, scurvy, sickle cell anemia, sinusitis, syphilis, thrombocytopenia purpura, tuberculosis, typhoid, von Willebrand's disease, Wegener's granulomatosis, yellow fever

INJURIES: Bone fracture of the nose or foreign body in the nose

HUMAN BODY: *Body state*: Menstruation, pregnancy

HEALTH CARE FACTORS: *Drug therapy*: Anticoagulant therapy. *Medical therapy*: Nasogastric tube, unhumidified oxygen

ENVIRONMENTAL FACTORS: *Altitude*: High altitude. *Chemical substances*: Specific drugs (cocaine sniffing). *Environmental cold*: Freezing external temperature. *Objects*: Contact with hard objects

MAJOR PATHOPHYSIOLOGIC FACTORS CAUSING THE PROBLEM: The rupture or deterioration of blood vessels in the nasal mucosa cause bleeding

PLANNING

Unmet Needs
Rest, comfort, protection from physical harm, increased learning

Expected Outcome
Cessation of blood oozing from the nose
Blood pressure reading within the person's normal level
Pulse rate of 60–80 beats/minute

NURSING INTERVENTIONS

Nursing Treatments
Apply an ice bag (to the back of the neck, under the upper lip and bridge of the nose)
Apply manual pressure over the bleeding area (over the bridge of the nose and nostrils)
Change the person's position gradually
Do not place in the flat position (so that the blood is not swallowed)
Elevate the head
Encourage adequate rest
Withhold the drugs (if blood studies indicate that anticoagulants are the cause and the epistaxis is serious)
Make a referral (to a physician if the epistaxis is chronic, due to anticoagulants, or is not controlled by nursing treatment)

Nursing Observations

Estimate the blood volume loss

Monitor the blood pressure (if the bleeding is severe)

Monitor blood studies for abnormal clotting mechanism

Monitor blood studies for abnormal hematology

Health Teaching

Explain the causes of the health problem (trauma, high blood pressure)

Explain how to prevent sneezing (temporarily)

Inform that coughing should be avoided (temporarily)

Inform that elimination straining should be avoided

Instruct not to blow the nose (temporarily)

Instruct not to pick the nose

Instruct not to swallow blood during epistaxis (since it causes vomiting)

Instruct to change position gradually

Explain the reason for and intended effect of the therapy (to support coagulation)

EVALUATION

Record actual outcome

GUM BLEEDING[72,88,451]

ASSESSMENT

Data Collection

Subjective Data

• Acute onset of gum bleeding when pressure or stimulation is applied to the gums
  Unpleasant taste

Objective Data

• Blood oozing from the gum surface
  Hypertrophied (enlarged) gums
  Clot formation around the teeth

Data Analysis

Nursing Diagnosis

GUM BLEEDING: Blood oozing or flowing from the gums

Common Etiology (Stressors)

DISEASES: Aplastic anemia, hemophilia, Hodgkin's disease, leukemia, pellegra, periodontal disease, scurvy, syphilis, thrombocytopenia, trench mouth, yellow fever

INJURIES: *Poisoning*: Lead, arsenic, phosphorous, or mercury poisoning

HEALTH CARE FACTORS: *Drug therapy*: Adverse effects of aspirin, anticoagulant therapy, hydantoin (Dilantin) therapy. *Medical therapy*: Radiation therapy (to the head or neck). *Therapeutic devices*: Dentures

HUMAN ERROR: Disregarding dental prophylaxis

MAJOR PATHOPHYSIOLOGIC FACTORS CAUSING THE PROBLEM: Blood-clotting disorders, chemical or mechanical trauma causing tissue degeneration, infection, tartar (plaque) accumulation on the teeth, and radiation to the head or neck damaging blood vessels in the mouth resulting in gum bleeding

PLANNING

Unmet Needs

Comfort, cleanliness, protection from physical harm, increased learning

Expected Outcome
Cessation of blood oozing from the gums
Clean, firm gums

NURSING INTERVENTIONS

Nursing Treatments
Brush the teeth with a soft toothbrush
Give iced liquids
Refrain from giving hot liquids
Give soft foods (tender meats, mashed potatoes)
Refresh with a mouthwash
Swab the mouth with diluted glycerine
Make a referral (to a dentist if there is excessive plaque or gum disease)

Nursing Observations
Estimate the blood volume loss (if bleeding is severe)
Monitor the blood studies for abnormal clotting mechanism, abnormal hematology, or a
  positive VDRL

Health Teaching
Explain the causes of the health problem (trauma, disease)
Instruct to use a soft, new toothbrush and to apply only mild toothbrush pressure
Advise not to use a harsh dentrifice
Teach how to massage the gums (for gum disease, hyperplasia, or when on dilantin
  therapy)
Explain the reason for and intended effect of the therapy (to support coagulation)

EVALUATION

Record actual outcome

HEMATOMA [125]

ASSESSMENT

Data Collection

Subjective Data
Aching (soreness, tenderness)

Objective Data
• Skin surface discoloration
• Skin is intact
• Edema of the skin or mucosa

Data Analysis

Nursing Diagnosis
HEMATOMA (BRUISING): A localized accumulation of blood in the tissue spaces resulting
  from bleeding beneath the skin

Common Etiology (Stressors)
DISEASES: Aplastic anemia, hemophilia, leukemia, thrombocytopenia
INJURIES: Trauma of any kind
HEALTH CARE FACTORS: *Diagnostic procedures*: Angiography, biopsy, blood sampling. *Medical
  therapy*: Intravenous infusion, blood transfusion
ENVIRONMENTAL FACTORS: *Objects*: Contact with hard, pointed, or sharp objects
MAJOR PATHOPHYSIOLOGIC FACTORS CAUSING THE PROBLEM: Bleeding from traumatized blood

vessels under the skin, capillary rupture, deficiency of platelets or other clotting factors

PLANNING

Unmet Needs
Comfort, protection from physical harm, increased learning

Expected Outcome
No edema at the site of the hematoma
Normal skin coloration within 10 days

NURSING INTERVENTIONS

Nursing Treatments
Apply an ice bag
   OR
Apply manual pressure over the bleeding area
Elevate the affected body part
Handle gently

Nursing Observations
Monitor blood studies for abnormal clotting mechanism
Monitor blood studies for abnormal hematology

Health Teaching
Explain the causes of the health problem (trauma, platelet deficiency)
Explain the need to avoid mechanical trauma (body contact with furniture, etc.)

EVALUATION

Record actual outcome

HYPERTENSION* [35,255,278,491,748]

ASSESSMENT

Data Collection

Subjective Data
Headache
Dizziness
Fatigue

Objective Data
• Blood pressure readings above:[255]

3–6 years	110/70	18–44 years	140/90
7–10 years	120/80	45–64 years	150/95
11–17 years	130/80	65 years or older	160/95

• Blood pressure is above normal on multiple readings

Note: Although averages have been set for normal blood pressure, conclusions should be based on the person's baseline reading

Data Analysis

Nursing Diagnosis
HYPERTENSION (HIGH BLOOD PRESSURE): Systolic and diastolic blood pressure readings above normal limits

Common Etiology (Stressors)
BIRTH DEFECTS: Adrenal hyperplasia

---

*Not to be confused with hypertensive disease.

DISEASES: Acromegaly, aortic coarctation, aortic stenosis, arteriosclerosis, Cushing's syndrome, essential hypertension, glomerulonephritis, lupus erythematosus, malignant hypertension, obesity, pheochromacytoma, polyarteritis nodosa, primary aldosteronism, pyelonephritis, scleroderma, thyrotoxicosis, toxemia of pregnancy

SIGNS AND SYMPTOMS: Edema

PSYCHOSOCIAL FACTORS: Excessive emotional excitement, the threat of real or imagined danger or chronic stress

HEALTH CARE FACTORS: *Drug therapy*: Adverse effects of deoxycorticosterone therapy given for adrenal insufficiency and contraceptive drugs

MAJOR PATHOPHYSIOLOGIC FACTORS CAUSING THE PROBLEM: Changes in arterial elasticity, increased resistance by the arterial wall, increased ventricular force during ventricular contraction, increased fluid volume within the arteries, increased metabolic rate

PLANNING

Unmet Needs

Fluid and electrolyte balance, rest and relaxation, comfort, protection from physical harm, increased learning

Expected Outcome

Blood pressure readings within the person's normal level
Stable blood pressure measurements on multiple readings

NURSING INTERVENTIONS

Nursing Treatments

Change the person's position gradually
Elevate the head
Do not place in the flat position
Provide quiet
Encourage adequate rest
Discourage the intake of oral stimulants
Substitute caffeine-free coffee or tea
Encourage decreased sodium-food intake
Discourage smoking
Slow the intravenous infusion flow rate
Make a referral (to a physician if the condition persists after numerous readings)

Nursing Observations

Monitor the blood pressure (frequently)
Palpate the pulse for rate, rhythm, and volume

Health Teaching

Explain the causes of the health problem (factors that contribute to hypertension include obesity, increased sodium intake, smoking, etc.)
Advise that highly emotional situations be avoided
Emphasize the danger of excessive body weight
Advise against exposure to extreme cold (low environmental temperature increases blood pressure because of its vasoconstriction effect)
Inform that (intense) coughing should be avoided (it increases intravascular pressure)
Inform that elimination straining should be avoided (it increases intravascular pressure)
Explain the reason for and intended effect of the therapy (to maintain normal blood pressure)

Medical Treatments Performed by Nurses

Give the prescribed diet
Give the prescribed drugs

EVALUATION

Record actual outcome

HYPOTENSION[35,73]

ASSESSMENT

Data Collection

Subjective Data
Weakness
Dizziness
Fatigue

Objective Data
• A blood pressure below 90/60 in adults
• Blood pressure is below normal on multiple readings
  Tachycardia
  Faint pulse

Note: Although averages have been set for normal blood pressure, conclusions should be based on the person's baseline reading

Data Analysis

Nursing Diagnosis
HYPOTENSION (LOW BLOOD PRESSURE): Systolic and diastolic blood pressure readings below normal limits

Common Etiology (Stressors)
DISEASES: Addison's disease, anemia, cachexia, carcinoma, hemorrhage, hyperventilation, mitral stenosis, neurasthenia, Simmond's disease
INJURIES: Any severe trauma such as cerebral concussion or bone fracture
SIGNS AND SYMPTOMS: Hypoxia, syncope
HEALTH CARE FACTORS: *Drug therapy*: Adverse effects of antihypertensive drugs or diuretics
DEVELOPMENTAL PHASES: Old age
MAJOR PATHOPHYSIOLOGIC FACTORS CAUSING THE PROBLEM: Decreased cardiac output, blood loss, blood-flow obstruction, endocrine imbalance

PLANNING

Unmet Needs

Tissue oxygenation or perfusion, fluid and electrolyte balance, rest, comfort, protection from physical harm, increased learning

Expected Outcome

Blood pressure readings within the person's normal level
Stable blood pressure measurements on multiple readings

NURSING INTERVENTIONS

Nursing Treatments

Give hot coffee
  OR
Give hot tea
Place in the foot-elevated head-lowered (Trendelenburg) position
Encourage adequate rest
Change the person's position gradually
Cover with warm blankets
Maintain a warm room temperature
Apply an elastic bandage
  OR   } To the legs
Apply elastic stockings
Withhold the drugs (if they precipitate the episode)
Make a referral (to a physician if hypotension persists or evolves into shock)

Nursing Observations
Inspect for hemorrhage
Monitor the blood pressure (frequently)
Observe for shock (tachycardia, pallor, increased respirations, and give emergency treatment for shock if it occurs)

Health Teaching
Explain the causes of the health problem (bleeding, drug effects, etc.)
Instruct to change position gradually
Advise against exposure to intense heat
Advise not to take hot baths (vasodilatation causes further hypotension)
Explain how to apply elastic stockings or an elastic bandage (to the legs)
Explain the reason for and intended effect of the therapy (to maintain a normal blood pressure)

EVALUATION
Record actual outcome

LYMPHATIC EDEMA [73,278]

ASSESSMENT

Data Collection

Subjective Data
• Localized aching pain (soreness, heaviness)

Objective Data
• Extreme swelling of an extremity
• Nonpitting edema
  Coarse skin

Data Analysis

Nursing Diagnosis
LYMPATHIC EDEMA (LYMPHADEMA): Inadequate lymph drainage from localized tissues because of obstructed or damaged lymphatic vessels

Common Etiology (Stressors)
DISEASES: Carcinoma, elephantiasis, filariasis, lymphadenitis, Milroy's disease
HEALTH CARE FACTORS: *Surgical procedures*: Excision of lymphatics, mastectomy
MAJOR PATHOPHYSIOLOGIC FACTORS CAUSING THE PROBLEM: Obstructed lymph flow to a body area causes edema, resulting in decreased arterial blood supply and decreased tissue oxygenation, inflammation of subcutaneous lymph vessels, and bacterial infection

PLANNING

Unmet Needs
Tissue oxygenation or perfusion, fluid and electrolyte balance, sleep and rest, comfort, protection from physical harm, increased learning

Expected Outcome
None, or minimal, edema of the extremity tissue
Warm, moist, natural color to the skin
Person verbalizes the absence of pain

NURSING INTERVENTIONS

Nursing Treatments
Apply an elastic bandage (to the extremity)

Refrain from tight bandaging
Change the person's position frequently
Do not place in the flat position
Elevate the extremity
Handle gently
Massage gently
Do not start IVs or draw blood in the affected extremity
Lubricate the skin with cocoa butter, glycerine, lanolin, mineral oil, or olive oil

Nursing Observations
Monitor the blood pressure (on the nonaffected limb)
Inspect for impaired circulation (poor capillary refill, cold skin)
Observe for complaints of pain

Health Teaching
Explain the causes of the health problem (obstruction, inflammation, infection)
Explain the reason for and intended effect of the therapy (to reestablish lymph circulation)
Explain how to apply an elastic bandage
Teach how to do postmastectomy exercises

Medical Treatments Performed by Nurses
Give the prescribed drugs (diuretics and antibiotics)

EVALUATION

Record actual outcome

ORAL MUCOSA BLEEDING [26,362]

ASSESSMENT

Data Collection

Subjective Data
• Acute onset
  Unpleasant taste

Objective Data
• Blood oozing from the mouth
• Oral mucosa or structures are not intact
  Blood clots in the mouth

Data Analysis

Nursing Diagnosis
ORAL MUCOSA BLEEDING (MOUTH BLEEDING): Blood oozing or flowing from mouth tissue

Common Etiology (Stressors)
DISEASES: Hemophilia, infectious mononucleosis, leukemia, thrombocytopenia
INJURIES: Trauma of any kind to the mouth
HEALTH CARE FACTORS: *Medical therapy*: Radiation therapy (on the face or neck). *Surgical procedures*: Gingivectomy, gingivoplasty, reconstruction procedure for the mouth, a tooth extraction
MAJOR PATHOPHYSIOLOGIC FACTORS CAUSING THE PROBLEM: Blood-clotting disorders associated with certain diseases and the disruption of vascular structures result in bleeding from the oral mucosa

PLANNING

Unmet Needs
Comfort, cleanliness, protection from physical harm, increased learning

Expected Outcome

Cessation of blood oozing from the mouth
A clean mouth
Person verbalizes that he has a pleasant-tasting mouth

NURSING INTERVENTIONS

Nursing Treatments

Apply an ice bag (to the external cheek for inner cheek bleeding)
Moisten the mouth with cracked ice
Give iced liquids
Refrain from giving hot liquids
Give pureed foods (mashed foods of all kinds)
> OR

Give soft foods (tender meats, mashed potatoes)
Discourage smoking
Brush the teeth with a soft toothbrush
Remove the dentures (if they irritate the mouth)
Refresh with a mouthwash (applied with a padded tongue blade)

Nursing Observations

Estimate the blood volume loss
Inspect for renewed bleeding
Monitor the blood pressure
Monitor blood studies for abnormal clotting mechanism
Monitor blood studies for abnormal hematology

Health Teaching

Explain the causes of the health problem (trauma, therapy)
Explain the need to avoid mechanical trauma
Instruct not to rinse the mouth vigorously (if clots exist)
Instruct not to use a drinking straw (the pressure from sucking causes bleeding)
Instruct to use a soft, new toothbrush and to apply only mild toothbrush pressure (if the bleeding is in the gum area)
Explain the reason for and intended effect of the therapy (to support coagulation)

EVALUATION

Record actual outcome

PACEMAKER FAILURE[544,581]

ASSESSMENT

Data Collection

Subjective Data
Dizziness
Chest pain

Objective Data
• Dial needle fails to move immediately before a pulse beat
• Electrical stimulus is not simultaneous with each heartbeat; it may occur between heartbeats, or there may be more than one stimulus to one heartbeat
Generator light fails to falsh
Artifact fails to appear on the ECG strip before each QRS complex
Increased or decreased pulse rate
Loss of consciousness

Data Analysis

Nursing Diagnosis

PACEMAKER FAILURE: Nonfunctioning of the cardiac electrical device that supports rhythmic heartbeats through regular electrical stimulation of the cardiac muscle

Common Etiology (Stressors)

HEALTH CARE FACTORS: *Therapeutic devices*: Failure of the cardiac pacemaker

ENVIRONMENTAL FACTORS: *Environmental radiation*: Exposure to damaging microwaves

HUMAN ERROR: Improper maintenance or replacement of the pacemaker battery

PLANNING

Unmet Needs

Tissue oxygenation or perfusion, protection from physical harm, increased learning

Expected Outcome

The electrical stimulus of the pacemaker is simultaneous with each heartbeat
Pulse rate of 60–80 beats/minute with a regular rhythm

NURSING INTERVENTIONS

Nursing Treatments

Attend the person constantly (until the pacemaker is functioning)
Provide standby equipment (defibrillator, drugs)
Reassure verbally
Replace the pacemaker batteries (immediately)
Make a referral (to a physician if the pacemaker is damaged by microwaves)

Nursing Observations

Auscultate the apical heartbeat for rate and rhythm
Monitor the cardiogram (as needed)

Health Teaching

Explain the causes of the health problem (mechanical failure)
Instruct to check the pulse daily when wearing a pacemaker
Teach safety measures to be practiced when wearing a pacemaker (avoiding high-frequency signals such as microwaves, or using battery-operated appliances instead of electrical ones, etc.)

EVALUATION

Record actual outcome

POSTURAL HYPOTENSION[278,522]

ASSESSMENT

Data Collection

Subjective Data

• Faintness
• Onset during sudden change from a lying to a sitting position or from a sitting to a standing position, or when lying flat on the back during pregnancy
  Dizziness
  Lightheadedness

Objective Data

• Below-normal systolic and diastolic blood pressure readings
  Tachycardia
  Pallor

Data Analysis

Nursing Diagnosis

POSTURAL HYPOTENSION: Decreased blood pressure readings occurring with a sudden position change

Common Etiology (Stressors)

DISEASES: Peripheral neuropathy, Simmond's disease

HUMAN BODY: *Body state*: Pregnancy

HEALTH CARE FACTORS: *Drug therapy*: Adverse effects of antihypertensive drugs, diuretics

DEVELOPMENTAL PHASES: Old age

ENVIRONMENTAL FACTORS: *Environmental heat*: Sitting in a hot bath

MAJOR PATHOPHYSIOLOGIC FACTORS CAUSING THE PROBLEM: Blood pooling in the extremities or in the abdominopelvic region

PLANNING

Unmet Needs

Tissue oxygenation or perfusion, comfort, protection from physical harm, increased learning

Expected Outcome

Blood pressure readings within the person's normal level

Stable blood pressure measurements on multiple readings

Person verbalizes no or minimal discomfort during position change

NURSING INTERVENTIONS

Nursing Treatments

Apply an elastic bandage ⎱
   OR   ⎰ To the legs while in bed
Apply elastic stockings ⎰

Change the patient's position gradually

Do not place in the flat position (during pregnancy)

Place in the side-lying position (during pregnancy)

Give hot coffee ⎱
   OR   ⎰ While in bed
Give hot tea ⎰

Remove constrictive clothing

Make a referral (to a physician if the condition persists)

Nursing Observations

Monitor the blood pressure

Observe for syncope

Health Teaching

Explain the causes of the health problem (blood pooling, drug side effects)

Instruct to change position gradually

Advise against exposure to intense heat

Advise not to take hot baths

Advise against wearing constrictive clothing

Explain how to apply elastic stockings

Explain how to apply an elastic bandage (to the legs)

Teach how to take a blood pressure

Explain the reason for and intended effect of the therapy

Medical Treatments Performed by Nurses

Give the prescribed drugs (ephedrine sulfate)

EVALUATION

Record actual outcome

RECTAL BLEEDING[72,278]

ASSESSMENT

Data Collection

Subjective Data
• Acute onset
  Pain, sometimes

Objective Data
• Blood oozing externally from the rectum, blood in or on the stool
  Positive Guaiac test

Data Analysis

Nursing Diagnosis
RECTAL BLEEDING: Blood oozing from the rectum

Common Etiology (Stressors)
DISEASES: Anal fissure, anal fistula, carcinoma of the rectum, fecal impaction, hemor-
  rhoids, rectal polyps, ulcerative proctitis
INJURIES: Foreign body in the rectum
SIGNS AND SYMPTOMS: Constipation, diarrhea
HEALTH CARE FACTORS: *Diagnostic procedures*: Anoscopy, colonoscopy, proctoscopy,
  protosigmoidoscopy. *Drug therapy*: Tissue irritation from cathartics, laxatives, purgatives. *Medical therapy*: Coughing and deep breathing, enemas. *Surgical procedures*: Hemorrhoidectomy
HUMAN ERROR: Straining at stool
MAJOR PATHOPHYSIOLOGIC FACTORS CAUSING THE PROBLEM: Pressure on or irritation of existing
  hemorrhoids, or foreign objects that stretch anal/rectal tissue can cause bleeding; tumor invasion of tissue erodes blood vessels

PLANNING

Unmet Needs

Rest, comfort, protection from physical harm, increased learning

Expected Outcome

Cessation of oozing blood from the rectum
Blood pressure readings within the person's normal level
Pulse rate of 60–80 beats/minute

NURSING INTERVENTIONS

Nursing Treatments

Apply an ice bag (to the rectal area)
Change the person's position gradually
Cover with warm blankets
Place on complete bed rest (if the bleeding is severe)
Elevate the foot of the bed
Refrain from giving enemas or laxatives
Refrain from inserting a rectal tube, from taking rectal temperature
Give nonprescription drugs (a stool softener)
Make a referral (to a physician to correct the underlying cause)

Nursing Observations

Estimate the blood volume loss
Inspect for renewed bleeding
Monitor the blood pressure
Monitor blood studies for abnormal hematology

Health Teaching
Explain the causes of the health problem (trauma, pressure, disease)
Advise not to stand for prolonged periods
Inform that coughing should be avoided
Inform that elimination straining should be avoided
Explain the reason for and intended effect of the therapy (to support coagulation)

EVALUATION
Record actual outcome

SINUS TACHYCARDIA [42,88]

ASSESSMENT
Data Collection
Subjective Data
Awareness of a rapid rate or forceful contractions of the heart (palpitations)

Objective Data
• Pulse rate is faster than 100 beats/minute
• Regular pulse rhythm

Data Analysis
Nursing Diagnosis
SINUS TACHYCARDIA: An abnormally rapid heartbeat

Common Etiology (Stressors)
DISEASES: Anemia, drug abuse (marijuana), hemorrhage, hypoglycemia, infection of any kind, rheumatic fever, thyrotoxicosis, tuberculosis
SIGNS AND SYMPTOMS: Fever, hypoxia, shock, weakness
PSYCHOSOCIAL FACTORS: Excessive emotional excitement, the threat of chronic stress
HEALTH CARE FACTORS: *Drug therapy*: Adverse effects of epinephrine
LIFESTYLE: *Diet*: High-caffeine intake. *Smoking*: High-nicotine intake
ENVIRONMENTAL FACTORS: *Environmental heat*: High external temperature
MAJOR PATHOPHYSIOLOGIC FACTORS CAUSING THE PROBLEM: Tachycardia results from:
   Rapid impulses produced by a normal pacemaker secondary to other conditions
   Decreased response of the vagus nerve with release of smaller amounts of acetylcholine (an ester that aids in the transmission of nerve impulses)
   Increased response of the sympathetic nervous system with release of catecholamine in the sinus node
   Increased rate of stimuli from the sinoatrial node

PLANNING
Unmet Needs
Tissue oxygenation or perfusion, fluid and electrolyte balance, comfort, protection from physical harm, increased learning

Expected Outcome
Pulse rate of 60–80 beats/minute
Person verbalizes that the heart has quieted

NURSING INTERVENTIONS
Nursing Treatments
Encourage adequate rest (at the time of the episode and as a daily routine)
Discourage the intake of oral stimulants (coffee, tea, chocolate, amphetamines)
Substitute caffeine-free coffee or tea

Discourage smoking

Make a referral (to a physician if the condition persists)

Nursing Observations

Palpate the pulse for rate, rhythm, and volume (every 5 minutes until stable)

Monitor the blood pressure (frequently)

Observe for cyanosis

Health Teaching

Instruct to use vagal stimulation methods to terminate tachycardia (breath-holding, massage of the carotid sinus, stimulating the gag reflex, drinking ice water)

Advise that highly emotional situations should be avoided

Explain the causes of the health problem (stimulants, heat, hypoxia, etc.)

Explain the reason for and intended effect of the therapy (to reestablish a regular cardiac rhythm)

EVALUATION

Record actual outcome

VENOUS PERIPHERAL INSUFFICIENCY[35,451]

ASSESSMENT

Data Collection

Subjective Data

Numbness and tingling in an extremity

Extremity coldness

Deep aching pain, sometimes

Feeling of heaviness in the extremity, especially the leg(s)

Objective Data

• Cyanosis or pallor of an extremity

• Skin pigmentation

Ankle edema

Hardness of the extremity tissue

Data Analysis

Nursing Diagnosis

VENOUS PERIPHERAL INSUFFICIENCY: An inadequate flow rate of venous blood from the peripheral veins to the large central veins (vena cava)

Common Etiology (Stressors)

DISEASES: Diabetes mellitus, phlebitis, phlebothrombosis, varicose veins

HUMAN BODY: *Body state*: Pregnancy

HEALTH CARE FACTORS: *Surgical therapy*: Postoperative inactivity. *Medical or surgical therapy*: Adverse effects of circulatory constriction from a cast

DEVELOPMENTAL PHASES: Old age

LIFESTYLE: Lack of exercise (especially prolonged sitting), wearing constrictive clothing (garters, girdles)

MAJOR PATHOPHYSIOLOGIC FACTORS CAUSING THE PROBLEM: Valve incompetency of the veins, loss of venous tone resulting in blood pooling, sluggish blood flow through the veins

PLANNING

Unmet Needs

Tissue oxygenation or perfusion, activity and exercise, comfort, protection from physical harm, increased learning

Expected Outcome
Natural warmth, moisture, and color of the skin and nails
Rapid capillary refilling when pressure is released from the nail bed
Strong peripheral pulses

NURSING INTERVENTIONS

Nursing Treatments
Ambulate the person (as much as possible)
Apply elastic stockings
Change the person's position frequently
Discourage smoking
Elevate the extremity
Exercise in range of motion
Limit blood-pressure–cuff inflation to a few moments (30 seconds–1 minute)
Maintain a warm room temperature
Refrain from giving iced liquids
Refrain from elevating the bed at the knee gatch
Refrain from placing a pillow under the knee
Refrain from giving local cold applications
Refrain from tight bandaging
Remove constrictive clothing

Nursing Observations
Inspect for impaired circulation (cold, cyanotic skin)
Monitor blood studies for abnormal hematology
Palpate for arterial pulsations (periodically)

Health Teaching
Explain the causes of the health problem (blood pooling, no exercise, etc.)
Advise against wearing constrictive clothing
Advise not to stand for prolonged periods
Advise that positions that impair circulation be avoided (crossing the legs, prolonged
   knee bending)
Emphasize the danger of excessive body weight
Inform that the extremities should be kept warm when the circulation is impaired
Instruct not to dangle the legs
Instruct to change position frequently
Recommend activities that improve circulation (brisk walking, rocking in a chair)
Teach how to do isometric exercises (pushing down with the feet)
Explain the reason for and intended effect of the therapy (to improve circulation)

EVALUATION

Record actual outcome

UNKNOWLEDGEABLE ABOUT BLEEDING OR HEMORRHAGE[73,88,371,451]

ASSESSMENT

Data Collection

Subjective Data
• Person's discussion or questions indicate a need for additional information,
   clarification, or validation of information
   OR

- Person's lack of questions or comments indicates not wanting information or not knowing enough to seek information
- When questioned directly, the person's response or lack of response indicates that he does not know:
  How to prevent bleeding and hemorrhage
  How to manage it if it occurs
  Symptoms to be reported

Objective Data
- May exhibit behavior such as not seeking health care for chronic bleeding

Data Analysis

Nursing Diagnosis
UNKNOWLEDGEABLE ABOUT BLEEDING OR HEMORRHAGE: Being without sufficient information about blood loss through bleeding or hemorrhage

Common Etiology (Stressors)
HEALTH CARE FACTORS: Lack of health instruction, lack of health-skill experience

PLANNING

Unmet Needs
Protection from physical harm, independence, increased learning

Expected Outcome
Correct verbal feedback of the information taught

NURSING INTERVENTIONS

Nursing Treatments
Approach unhurriedly
Encourage the person to ask questions

Nursing Observations
Determine teaching effectiveness by verbal feedback

Health Teaching
Instruct to use ice applications to control bleeding
Instruct to change position gradually
   AND
Instruct to move the injured body part carefully (if bleeding is likely)
Explain the need to avoid mechanical trauma
Inform that coughing should be avoided, and
Inform that elimination straining should be avoided, and
Inform that heavy lifting should be avoided (if internal or rectal bleeding is likely)
Advise not to stand for prolonged periods (following childbirth, during excessive menstrual flow, or rectal bleeding)
Advise against pulling off scabs
Advise not to partake of very hot foods or drinks (which will stimulate mouth bleeding)
Instruct to use a soft, new toothbrush and to apply only mild toothbrush pressure, and
Instruct not to use a drinking straw (when there is a gum or oral bleeding for tooth extraction, oral surgery, etc.)
Instruct not to pick the nose, and
Advise gentle nose blowing (for epistaxis)
Describe those symptoms that should be reported (prolonged or profuse bleeding)
Explain the causes of the problem (bleeding results from blood coagulation defects, from drug effects, pressure on tissue, trauma to tissue, rupture of weakened blood vessels)

EVALUATION
Record actual outcome

UNKNOWLEDGEABLE ABOUT DYSRHYTHMIAS[41,73,249]

ASSESSMENT

Data Collection

Subjective Data

• Person's discussion or questions indicate a need for additional information, clarification, or validation of information

OR

• Person's lack of questions or comments indicates not wanting information or not knowing enough to seek information

• When questioned directly, the person's response or lack of response indicates that he does not know:

How to recognize or check for dysrhythmias

The causes of dysrhythmias

How to prevent and manage dysrhythmias

Symptoms to be reported

Objective Data

• May exhibit behavior such as continuing heavy work despite dysrhythmias or remaining unusually sedentary following a diagnosis of dysrhythmia

Data Analysis

Nursing Diagnosis

UNKNOWLEDGEABLE ABOUT DYSRHYTHMIAS: Being without sufficient information about an abnormal heart rhythm

Common Etiology (Stressors)

HEALTH CARE FACTORS: Lack of health instruction, lack of health-skill experience

PLANNING

Unmet Needs

Protection from physical harm, independence, increased learning

Expected Outcome

Correct verbal feedback of the information taught

NURSING INTERVENTIONS

Nursing Treatments

Approach unhurriedly

Encourage the person to ask questions

Encourage adequate rest

Discourage strenuous exercise

Discourage the intake of oral stimulants (caffeine, amphetamines, epinephrine in decongestants)

Discourage smoking

Nursing Observations

Determine teaching effectiveness by verbal feedback

Health Teaching

Teach how to locate and count a pulse (and recognize its rhythm and quality)

Describe those symptoms that should be reported (specific to the dysrhythmia; e.g., the sudden onset of a rapid and irregular pulse accompanied by sensations of palpitations and heart flutter, faintness, shortness of breath, and apprehension)

Explain the causes of the problem (malfunction of the electrical pacemaker of the heart)

Instruct to use vagal stimulation methods to terminate dysrhythmia (breath holding or bending forward, the use of finger pressure on the carotid sinuses can be taught to the patient with paroxysmal tachycardia)

Advise that highly emotional situations be avoided
Explain the need to avoid overexertion
Recommend adherence to a pace of living with which the person is comfortable

EVALUATION
Record actual outcome

Knowledge Deficits Associated with the Cardiovascular System

UNKNOWLEDGEABLE ABOUT HEALTH RESTRICTIONS ON AIR TRAVEL[580]

ASSESSMENT
Data Collection
Subjective Data
- Person's discussion or questions indicate a need for additional information, clarification, or validation of information
  OR
- Person's lack of questions or comments indicates not wanting information or not knowing enough to seek information
- When questioned directly, the person's response or lack of response indicates that he does not know:
  Air travel is unsuitable for persons with severe anemia, leukemia, sickle cell disease or trait, cardiac disease sufficiently severe to present discomfort after walking a city block or up a flight of stairs, respiratory disease, recent pneumothorax, recent (within 10 days) encephalography or ventriculography, a poorly regulated colostomy, a contagious disease, an extreme fear of flying, or who are highly emotionally disturbed
  When a woman is 8-months pregnant, she must have a physician's written permission to board a plane
  Infants less than 10-days old should not travel by plane

Objective Data
- May exhibit behavior such as getting ready to take a 3-day-old infant or a 9-month-pregnant woman on a plane

Data Analysis
Nursing Diagnosis
UNKNOWLEDGEABLE ABOUT HEALTH RESTRICTIONS ON AIR TRAVEL: Being without sufficient information about the inadvisability of air travel in certain illnesses and conditions

Common Etiology (Stressors)
HEALTH CARE FACTORS: Lack of health instruction

PLANNING
Unmet Needs
Protection from physical harm, independence, increased learning
Expected Outcome
Correct verbal feedback of the information taught

NURSING INTERVENTIONS

Nursing Treatments

Approach unhurriedly

Encourage modes of travel other than flying (train, bus, car)

Encourage the person to ask questions

Nursing Observations

Determine teaching effectiveness by verbal feedback

Health Teaching

Emphasize the need to fly in pressurized airplanes

Explain the causes of the health problem (alterations in atmospheric pressure during ascent and descent, decreased barometric pressure causing gas to be trapped in the hollow organs, decreased barometric pressure reducing the alveolar oxygen pressure in the lungs that would require oxygen therapy for persons with respiratory disorders)

EVALUATION

Record actual outcome

UNKNOWLEDGEABLE ABOUT HYPERTENSION [61,73,155,278,522]

ASSESSMENT

Data Collection

Subjective Data

• Person's discussion or questions indicate a need for additional information, clarification, or validation of information

   OR

• Person's lack of questions or comments indicates not wanting information or not knowing enough to seek information

• When questioned directly, the person's response or lack of response indicates that he does not know:

   What hypertension is

   The signs and symptoms of hypertension

   The causes of hypertension

   Those precautions that can be taken to control the disease

   The reason for and effects of treatment

Objective Data

• May exhibit behavior such as eating a high-salt diet despite a diagnosis of hypertension or not taking medications as prescribed

Data Analysis

Nursing Diagnosis

UNKNOWLEDGEABLE ABOUT HYPERTENSION: Being without sufficient information about the causes, effects, and therapeutic plan associated with hypertension

Common Etiology (Stressors)

HEALTH CARE FACTORS: Lack of health instruction

PLANNING

Unmet Needs

Protection from physical harm, independence, increased learning

Expected Outcome

Correct verbal feedback of the information taught

NURSING INTERVENTIONS

Nursing Treatments

Approach unhurriedly

Encourage the person to ask questions

Discourage the intake of oral stimulants

Discourage smoking

Encourage moderate physical exercise

Discourage strenuous activities

Encourage adequate rest

Encourage decreased fatty-food intake (to decrease excessive calorie intake and slow arteriosclerotic plaque build-up)

Encourage decreased sodium-food intake (to decrease circulating fluid volume)

Nursing Observations

Determine teaching effectiveness by verbal feedback

Health Teaching

Advise against exposure to intense heat ⎫ When on antihypertensive drugs,
Advise not to take hot baths   ⎬ exposure to heat may cause excessive
                                        ⎭ hypotension

Advise that highly emotional situations be avoided

Explain that fatigue should be recognized as a stress factor

Emphasize the danger of excessive body weight (it puts a strain on the circulatory system to oxygenate the excessive tissue)

Recommend eating and drinking in moderation

Recommend adherence to a pace of living with which the person is comfortable (not working excessive hours, avoid hurrying, etc.)

Recommend methods for achieving total relaxation (controlled breathing, listening to music)

Teach how and when to take medications (as prescribed)

Teach how to take a blood pressure

Inform that a predisposition to the illness exists (in all family members)

Explain the reason for and intended effect of the therapy (to reduce the blood pressure to normal)

Explain the causes of the health problem (the constriction of arteries and arterioles throughout the body, fluid retention causing increased fluid volume)

EVALUATION

Record actual outcome

UNKNOWLEDGEABLE ABOUT SICKLE CELL ANEMIA [73,278,522]

ASSESSMENT

Data Collection

Subjective Data

• Person's discussion or questions indicate a need for additional information, clarification, or validation of information

OR

- Person's lack of questions or comments indicates not wanting information or not knowing enough to seek information
- When questioned directly, the person's response or lack of response indicates that he does not know:
  The cause or effect of sickle cell anemia
  The factors to be avoided to prevent sickle cell crisis
  Of the need for immediate attention during an impending crisis

Objective Data
- May exhibit behavior such as participating in strenuous sports despite symptoms or not seeking health care for joint swelling or abdominal pain

Data Analysis

Nursing Diagnosis
UNKNOWLEDGEABLE ABOUT SICKLE CELL ANEMIA: Being without sufficient information about the causes, effects, and therapeutic plan associated with sickle cell anemia

Common Etiology (Stressors)
HEALTH CARE FACTORS: Lack of health instruction

PLANNING

Unmet Needs
Protection from physical harm, independence, increased learning

Expected Outcome
Correct verbal feedback of the information taught

NURSING INTERVENTIONS

Nursing Treatments
Approach unhurriedly
Encourage the person to ask questions
Discourage strenuous activities (especially sports)
Encourage moderate activity (on a regular basis)

Nursing Observations
Determine teaching effectiveness by verbal feedback

Health Teaching
Explain that fatigue should be recognized as a stress factor
Instruct to limit direct contact with infected persons
Explain the need to avoid trauma (to the body)
Recommend that high altitudes be avoided
Encourage modes of travel other than flying
Inform that a predisposition to the illness exists (mostly in black families)
Describe those symptoms that should be reported (anorexia, weakness, pallor, joint swelling, jaundice, fever, headache, and abdominal, leg or arm pain indicate sickle-cell crisis)
Instruct to report serious (crisis) symptoms immediately (listed above)
Instruct to increase fluid intake (especially water, at the onset of serious (crisis) symptoms)
Explain the causes of the health problem (the sickle-cell trait is an abnormal hemoglobin-S gene, and the sickle (crescent) shape of the erythrocytes causes occlusion of the small blood vessels, decreasing oxygenation)
Explain the reason for and intended effect of the therapy (to reduce physiologic stress)

EVALUATION
Record actual outcome

UNKNOWLEDGEABLE ABOUT VEIN VARICOSITIES[26,73,451]

ASSESSMENT

Data Collection

Subjective Data
- Person's discussion or questions indicate a need for additional information, clarification, or validation of information
  OR
- Person's lack of questions or comments indicates not wanting information or not knowing enough to seek information
- When questioned directly, the person's response or lack of response indicates that he does not know:
  The causes of varicosities
  Ways of preventing them
  Symptoms to be reported

Objective Data
- May exhibit behavior such as wearing garters or standing for prolonged periods despite varicose veins

Data Analysis

Nursing Diagnosis
UNKNOWLEDGEABLE ABOUT VEIN VARICOSITIES: Being without sufficient information about dilated, swollen leg veins

Common Etiology (Stressors)
HEALTH CARE FACTORS: Lack of health instruction, lack of health-skill experience

PLANNING

Unmet Needs
Protection from physical harm, independence, increased learning

Expected Outcome
Correct verbal feedback of the information taught

NURSING INTERVENTIONS

Nursing Treatments
Approach unhurriedly
Encourage the person to ask questions

Nursing Observations
Determine teaching effectiveness by verbal feedback

Health Teaching
Advise against wearing constrictive clothing (girdles, garters, etc.)
Emphasize the danger of excessive body weight (which puts pressure on the lower extremity blood vessels)
Instruct to elevate the body part (the extremities whenever possible)
Recommend activities that improve circulation (running, bicycling, rocking in a chair)
Explain how to apply elastic stockings or an elastic bandage (to the legs)
Advise that positions that impair circulation be avoided (prolonged knee bending or standing, crossing the legs, dangling the legs so that there is pressure behind the knees)

Instruct to change position frequently

Explain the causes of the problem (weakening the blood vessel wall by increasing venous pressure can result in varicose veins; tall stature increases hydrostatic stress; familial tendency for varicose veins; pressure on the veins from pregnancy, obesity, ascites)

Describe those symptoms that should be reported (aching legs, bulging blood vessels)

EVALUATION

Record actual outcome

UNSKILLED AT MANAGING A PACEMAKER[451,537,581]

ASSESSMENT

Data Collection

Subjective Data

• Person's discussion or questions indicate a need for additional information, clarification, or validation of information about performing the task of managing a pacemaker
   OR
• Person's lack of questions or comments indicates not wanting information or not knowing enough to seek information about performing the task of managing a pacemaker
   Person may not know:
      How the pacemaker functions
      How or when it is worn
      The dangers associated with a pacemaker

Objective Data

• Person cannot correctly demonstrate how to:
   Take his pulse
   Do range-of-motion exercises
   Apply sterile dressing

Related Data

Commonly Related Diseases

Atrial fibrillation, AV heart block with digitalis therapy, myocardial infarction, rheumatic heart disease, ventricular fibrillation

Data Analysis

Nursing Diagnosis

UNSKILLED AT MANAGING A PACEMAKER: Being nonproficient, with or without knowledge, in the performance of the specific task of using a portable cardiac pacemaker

Common Etiology (Stressors)

HEALTH CARE FACTORS: Lack of health instruction, lack of health-skill experience

PLANNING

Unmet Needs

Comfort, protection from physical harm, dependence, mastery and competence in skills, independence, increased learning

Expected Outcome

A well-functioning pacemaker

Correct verbal feedback of the information taught

Correct return demonstration of how to handle a pacemaker and how to take one's pulse

NURSING INTERVENTIONS

Nursing Treatments

Provide temporary assistance until the skill is learned

Position the pacemaker generator box comfortably

Tape the pacemaker wire to the patient

Replace the pacemaker batteries (as needed)

Apply a sterile dressing (over the insertion site)

Exercise (shoulders) in range of motion (to prevent "frozen shoulder")

Protect the person wearing a pacemaker by practicing safety measures (such as avoiding simultaneously touching electrical equipment and the person, not using multiple electrical machines around a pacemaker, not using extension cords, worn electrical cords, plugs, or outlets, disconnecting unused electrical equipment, insulating exposed pacemaker electrodes, placing the person on a nonelectric bed)

Encourage patient questions

Encourage self-performance

Nursing Observations

Auscultate the chest for abnormal heart sounds

Check the pacemaker for pacing rate (by counting the apical pulse or running an ECG)

Palpate the pulse for rate, rhythm, and volume (at least once daily)

Observe for readiness to assume self-care

Determine teaching effectiveness by testing, verbal feedback, and return demonstration

Health Teaching

Explain normal organ (heart) function (the heart pumps blood through the arteries to oxygenate body cells)

Explain how the (pacemaker) equipment works (it stimulates the heartbeat when the rate is slow)

Explain the effects of the specific type pacemaker (asynchronous, synchronous, or demand pacemaker)

Explain how to detect pacemaker failure (by increased or decreased pulse rate, dizziness, and chest pain)

Explain that the pacemaker's electrical current is not strong enough to electrocute (it only stimulates the heartbeat)

Inform that bathing is permitted when wearing a pacemaker

Recommend the use of a pacemaker shirt (with a pocket to hold the pacemaker)

Teach safety measures to be practiced when wearing a pacemaker (teach the person to avoid high-frequency signals such as microwaves, to use battery-operated appliances instead of those that plug in, to avoid the use of ungrounded electrical equipment, and to avoid using worn electrical cords, plugs, or outlets)

Instruct to check the pulse daily when wearing a pacemaker

Teach how to locate and count a pulse

Teach how to do range-of-motion exercises

Explain the importance of wearing a Medic Alert tag (if the pacemaker is permanent or implanted)

EVALUATION

Record actual outcome

Minor Health Problems Associated with the Ear, Nose, and Throat

IMPACTED CERUMEN[72,88,451]

ASSESSMENT

Data Collection

Subjective Data
- Ear feels plugged
- Diminished hearing
- Itching
  Tinnitus
  Dizziness

Objective Data
- Brown, hard earwax in the ear canal
  Nonvisible tympanic membrane

Data Analysis

Nursing Diagnosis
IMPACTED CERUMEN: An excessive collection of earwax

Common Etiology (Stressors)
LIFESTYLE: Lack of hygiene
MAJOR PATHOPHYSIOLOGIC FACTORS CAUSING THE PROBLEM: Excessive secretion of the ceruminous glands, narrowed ear canal

PLANNING

Unmet Needs
Comfort, cleanliness, protection from physical harm, increased learning

Expected Outcome
Clear visualization of the ear canal and tympanic membrane
Person verbalizes reduced pressure sensation within the ear canal
Verbalizes that his hearing has improved

NURSING INTERVENTIONS

Nursing Treatments
Soften and remove the earwax (soften by instilling mineral oil or hydrogen peroxide drops, remove the wax with a bulb syringe or cerumen spoon)
Irrigate the ear with water or saline (using a lukewarm solution)
Refrain from irrigating (when there is chronic otitis, pus in the ear, or a perforated tympanic membrane)
Give nonprescription drugs (Debrox drops in the ear)

Nursing Observations
Inspect the ears with an otoscope (several days later to be sure the ear canal is clean)

Health Teaching
Explain how to remove earwax (using oil, hydrogen peroxide, or a bulb syringe)
Instruct not to insert foreign objects into the ear (such as hair pins, to remove earwax)
Explain the causes of the health problem (ceruminous gland oversecretion)
Explain the reason for and intended effect of the therapy (to remove the ear canal obstruction)

EVALUATION

Record actual outcome

NASAL CONGESTION[88,125,371]

ASSESSMENT

Data Collection

Subjective Data
• Sensation of nasal stuffiness
• Difficult nasal breathing

Objective Data
• Edematous nasal mucosa
• Red nasal mucosa if due to infection, pale nasal mucosa if due to allergy
• Diminished air passage through one or both nares
• Mouth breathing
• Fever, sometimes

Data Analysis

Nursing Diagnosis
NASAL CONGESTION: Increased fluid accumulation in the nasal mucosa

Common Etiology (Stressors)
DISEASES: Allergic disorder, nasopharyngitis, rhinitis, sinusitis
HEALTH CARE FACTORS: *Drug therapy*: Adverse effects of drugs
ENVIRONMENTAL FACTORS: *Biological agents*: Micropores, pollen from such plants as ragweed, grass and trees. *Chemical substances*: Inhalation of chemical substances. *Food substances*: Adverse effects of poorly tolerated formula. *Objects*: Paricles of dirt or dust, dander from animals
MAJOR PATHOPHYSIOLOGIC FACTORS CAUSING THE PROBLEM: Increased blood volume within the nasal vessels and increased fluid in the nasal tissues results in mucosal swelling

PLANNING

Unmet Needs

Tissue oxygenation or perfusion, rest, comfort, cleanliness, protection from physical harm, increased learning

Expected Outcome

Pink, nonedematous nasal mucosa
Clear air passage through both nares
Person verbalizes decreased or absent nasal stuffiness

NURSING INTERVENTIONS

Nursing Treatments

Administer vaporized air
Elevate the head (to promote effective drainage)
Increase fluid intake to about 2,000 cc daily
Give warm liquids
Refrain from giving milk or milk products (give infants Prosobee instead of milk if the congestion is chronic)
Give nonprescription drugs (decongestants; do not give decongestants if the person has hypertension, asthma, or diabetes)
Maintain adequate atmospheric humidity
Maintain a warm room temperature
Discourage smoking

Nursing Observations

Inspect the chest for respiratory rate and rhythm
Auscultate the chest for lung aeration
Observe for cyanosis, dyspnea, for complaints of fatique

Health Teaching

Emphasize the danger of excessive use of nosedrops (erosion of the nasal mucosa, worsening of the obstruction)

Advise gentle nose blowing

Instruct to elevate the head (for effective drainage)

Explain the causes of the health problem (edema of the nasal mucosa)

Explain the reason for and intended effect of the therapy (to reduce nasal mucosa edema)

EVALUATION

Record actual outcome

PHARYNGITIS [88,278,476]

ASSESSMENT

Data Collection

Subjective Data
- Throat dryness
- Throat aching (soreness, tenderness)
- Malaise
- Increased pain when swallowing
- Thick mucus
- Cough

Objective Data
- Red, swollen pharyngeal mucosa
- Anterior cervical lymph node enlargement, tenderness
- Fever
- Hoarseness
- White patches of exudate

Data Analysis

Nursing Diagnosis
PHARYNGITIS: Inflammation of the pharynx

Common Etiology (Stressors)
DISEASES: Bacterial pharyngitis, Dengue fever, diphtheria, encephalitis, gonoccoccal pharyngitis, hookworm disease, infectious mononucleosis, measles, moniliasis or candidiasis (thrush), nasopharyngitis, poliomyelitis, Rocky Mountain spotted fever, scarlet fever, streptococcal pharyngitis, thyrotoxicosis, tonsillitis, typhoid, Vincent's angina, viral pharyngitis

MAJOR PATHOPHYSIOLOGIC FACTORS CAUSING THE PROBLEM: Viral or bacterial infection is the most common cause of pharyngitis; during swallowing, the throat tissues move and the mucosal surfaces touch or rub against one another, and when the tissues are inflamed, the movement and surface contacts cause pain; during swallowing there is movement and irritation of enlarged, inflamed lymph nodes that results in pain

PLANNING

Unmet Needs

Rest, comfort, protection from physical harm, freedom from pain, increased learning

Expected Outcome

Pink, noninflamed, nonedematous palate and oropharynx

Person verbalizes the absence of throat pain

NURSING INTERVENTIONS

Nursing Treatments

Encourage the use of a warm, saline gargle

Give nonprescription drugs (anesthetic lozenges such as Sucrets, Spec-T, etc., and analgesics such as aspirin, acetaminophen, etc.)

Give full-liquid foods (cream soups, custards, ice cream)
  OR
Give soft foods (tender meats, mashed potatoes)
  OR
Give bland foods (avoid spices)

Refrain from giving hot liquids

Encourage adequate rest

Make a referral (to a physician if the fever is high or for suspicion of serious disease; refer for antibiotics for signs of bacterial infection, such as an increased white blood count—neutrophils/Segs—or a positive bacterial culture)

Nursing Observations

Obtain a bacterial culture (if there is tonsillar exudate or anterior cervical lymphadenopathy)

Health Teaching

Describe those symptoms that should be reported (severe difficulty swallowing)

Instruct to increase fluid intake

Explain the reason for and intended effect of the therapy (to reduce pain)

Explain the cause of the pain (inflammation of the tissues involved in swallowing)

EVALUATION

Record actual outcome

RHINITIS [88,125,151]

ASSESSMENT

Data Collection

Subjective Data
• Clear, watery nasal discharge
  Malaise
  Itching of the eyes, nose, or palate
  Drainage down the back of the throat, sometimes

Objective Data
• Edematous nasal mucosa
• Red nasal mucosa if due to infection, pale nasal mucosa if due to an allergy
  Low-grade fever, sometimes
  Hacking
  Coughing

Data Analysis

Nursing Diagnosis
RHINITIS: Inflammation of the nasal mucosa with increased secretion of mucus

Common Etiology (Stressors)
DISEASES: Allergic rhinitis (hay fever), nasopharyngitis, vasomotor rhinitis
PSYCHOSOCIAL FACTORS: Threat of chronic stress
HEALTH CARE FACTORS: *Drug therapy*: Adverse effects of drugs
ENVIRONMENTAL FACTORS: *Biologic agents*: Microspores, pollen from such plants as ragweed,

grass, and trees. *Chemical substances*: Inhalation of chemical substances. *Environmental cold*: Low external temperature. *Food substances*: Adverse effect of food substances. *Objects*: Particles of dirt or dust, dander from animals

MAJOR PATHOPHYSIOLOGIC FACTORS CAUSING THE PROBLEM: Inflammation of the nasal mucosa due to bacterial and viral infection causes increased secretion production; the release of histamine constricts blood vessels and increases capillary permeability with fluid passing through and out of the tissues

PLANNING

Unmet Needs
Comfort, protection from physical harm, increased learning

Expected Outcome
Pink, nonedematous nasal mucosa
Person verbalizes the cessation of watery nasal discharge

NURSING INTERVENTIONS

Nursing Treatments
Give nonprescription drug (antihistamine; warn the person about possible drowsiness)
Discourage smoking
Make a referral (to a physician if the condition persists)

Nursing Observations
Make a follow-up evaluation (to determine the effectiveness of the therapy)

Health Teaching
Explain the causes of the health problem (infection, allergy)
Explain how to take allergy precautions (if this is the cause)
Explain how to prevent cross-infection
Advise to observe for signs of infection (purulent nasal drainage, fever)
Instruct to elevate the head (to promote effective drainage)
Advise against drawing secretions to the back of the throat
Advise gentle nose blowing
Advise against exposure to airborne irritants
Explain the reason for and intended effect of the therapy (to dry up the secretions)

EVALUATION

Record actual outcome

SEROUS OTITIS [42,88,125,253,278]

ASSESSMENT

Data Collection

Subjective Data
• Feeling of fullness or pressure in the ear
• Diminished hearing
  Sound of the person's own voice echoing in the involved ear
  Internal popping sound
  Mild, intermittent pain
  Onset usually following upper respiratory infection

Objective Data
• Normal or retracted tympanic membrane
• Serous fluid is seen as a dull or amber color in the lower half of the tympanic membrane

• Retraction of the handle of malleus
• Displacement of or diminished reflex
• Immobility of the tympanic membrane during Valsalva maneuver
• No fever, pus in the ear canal, hyperemic or outwardly bulging tympanic membrane
  Visible air bubbles sometimes

Data Analysis

Nursing Diagnosis
SEROUS OTITIS (EUSTACHIAN TUBE OBSTRUCTION): The accumulation of fluid (sterile serum) in the
  middle ear

Common Etiology (Stressors)
DISEASES: Adenoiditis, allergic disorder, pharyngitis
ENVIRONMENTAL FACTORS: *Altitude*: High altitude. *Pressure*: Changes in atmospheric pressure
HUMAN ERROR: Feeding an infant in the flat position
MAJOR PATHOPHYSIOLOGIC FACTORS CAUSING THE PROBLEM: Altitude changes may cause either
  air trapping or negative pressure in the middle ear; inflammation or overgrowth of
  pharyngeal tissues (especially adenoids) obstructs the eustachian tube outlet; when air
  is unable to pass freely in and out of the middle ear, serous fluid secretion is increased, and this causes a feeling of middle ear pressure

PLANNING

Unmet Needs
Comfort, protection from physical harm, increased learning

Expected Outcome
Visualization of a clear, taut tympanic membrane, a nonretracted handle of malleus and
  the umbo, with a bright cone of light seen at the 5-o'clock position in the right ear
  and at the 7-o'clock position in the left ear
No inflammation or drainage
Person verbalizes a reduced pressure sensation within the ear canal
Verbalizes improved hearing

NURSING INTERVENTIONS

Nursing Treatments
Give nonprescription drugs (decongestant; do not give decongestants if the person has
  hypertension, asthma, or diabetes, give an antihistamine if an allergy is causing the se-
  rous otitis)
Discourage smoking
Make a referral (to a physician if the condition persists)

Nursing Observations
Make a follow-up evaluation (to determine the effectiveness of the therapy)
Test the ears for hearing acuity (if the condition persists)

Health Teaching
Describe those symptoms that should be reported (persistent ear fullness or impaired
  hearing)
Explain that yawning and swallowing will equalize ear pressure
Advise gentle nose blowing
Instruct to position correctly (the infant being fed should be placed in a semiupright position)
Teach the specific procedure (for eustachian tube ventilation; have the person pinch the
  nostrils together firmly, close the lips tightly, and tighten the diaphragm, forcing air
  into the eustachian tubes; or have the person blow up a firm balloon; do the aerating
  exercise 2–4 times daily, but discontinue at the first sign of a cold, influenza, sore
  throat, etc.)
Explain the reason for and intended effect of the therapy (to provide regular mechanical

means for aerating and equalizing pressure in the middle ear in prolonged serous otitis media)

EVALUATION
Record actual outcome

SNEEZING [12,475]

ASSESSMENT
Data Collection
Subjective Data
- Irritating nasal sensation
- Frequently recurrent sneezing

Objective Data
- Forceful expelling of air through the nose
  Nasal secretions

Data Analysis
Nursing Diagnosis
SNEEZING: The uncontrollable expulsion of air through the nose

Common Etiology (Stressors)
DISEASES: Allergic disorders, nasopharyngitis, sinusitis
INJURIES: Foreign body in the nose
PSYCHOSOCIAL FACTORS: The threat of chronic or severe stress
HEALTH CARE FACTORS: *Drug therapy*: Adverse effects of drugs
ENVIRONMENTAL FACTORS: *Biologic agents*: Microspores, pollen from such plants as ragweed, grass, and trees. *Chemical substances*: Inhalation of chemical substances. *Food substances*: Adverse effects of food substances. *Objects*: Particles of dirt or dust, dander of animals
MAJOR PATHOPHYSIOLOGIC FACTORS CAUSING THE PROBLEM: Spasmodic contraction of expiratory muscles, an attempt to clear the nasal passage of irritating substances

PLANNING
Unmet Needs
Comfort, cleanliness, protection from physical harm, increased learning

Expected Outcome
Cessation of uncontrollable sneezing

NURSING INTERVENTIONS
Nursing Treatments
Clear nasal secretions
Discourage smoking
Encourage adequate rest
Give nonprescription drugs (antihistamines; warn the person about possible drowsiness)
Maintain a cool room temperature
Maintain adequate atmospheric humidity

Nursing Observations
Inspect the nasal turbinates for abnormalities
Inspect the nose for asymmetry
Inspect the nose for polyps
Inspect for foreign bodies

Health Teaching

Advise against exposure to airborne irritants

Advise gentle nose blowing

Explain how to prevent sneezing (pressure under the nose, breathing through the mouth)

Explain the causes of the health problem (infection, allergy, stress)

Explain the reason for and intended effect of the therapy (to prevent sneezing)

EVALUATION

Record actual outcome

SORE THROAT[73,88]

ASSESSMENT

Data Collection

Subjective Data
- Acute onset
- Throat aching (soreness tenderness)
  Pain increased with swallowing

Objective Data
- No inflammation of pharyngeal mucosa
  Edema, sometimes
  No lymph node tenderness or swelling
  No pharyngeal exudate

Data Analysis

Nursing Diagnosis
SORE THROAT: A distressful hurting of the throat

Common Etiology (Stressors)
INJURIES: Foreign body in pharynx
HEALTH CARE FACTORS: *Diagnostic procedures*: Broncoscopy, gastric analysis, gastroscopy, upper GI endoscopy. *Drug therapy*: Adverse effects of bone marrow suppressing drugs. *Medical therapy*: Nasogastric or endotracheal tubes. *Surgical procedures*: Tonsillectomy
MAJOR PATHOPHYSIOLOGIC FACTORS CAUSING THE PROBLEM: The friction of foreign objects irritates the throat tissue, causing pain or soreness, surgical cutting of the throat tissue causes pain

PLANNING

Unmet Needs

Comfort, protection from physical harm, freedom from pain, increased learning

Expected Outcome

Person verbalizes that the throat pain has subsided or is decreased

NURSING INTERVENTIONS

Nursing Treatments

Encourage the use of a warm, saline gargle (be sure the gag reflex has returned following a local anesthetic)

Give nonprescription drugs (anesthetic lozenges, such as Sucrets, Spec-T, etc.)

Moisten the mouth with cracked ice

Apply an ice bag (to the throat if the person cannot have cracked ice)

Give full-liquid foods (cream soups, custards, ice cream)
    OR
Give soft foods (tender meats, mashed potatoes)
    OR
Give bland foods (avoid spices)
Refrain from giving hot liquids
Give iced liquids

Nursing Observations
Observe for evidence of a favorable response to therapy

Health Teaching
Describe those symptoms that should be reported (increased pain, difficulty swallowing)
Explain the reason for and intended effect of the therapy (to reduce the pain)
Explain the cause of the pain (irritation of the throat tissue)

EVALUATION
Record actual outcome

TINNITUS [125,522]

ASSESSMENT
Data Collection
Subjective Data
• Complains of buzzing, clicking, rumbling, ringing, thumping, hissing, rushing water, whistling, or roaring sounds heard in one or both ears
• Some hearing loss
  Tinnitus seems louder at night
  Ear sounds may pulsate with the heartbeat
  Continuous or intermittent

Objective Data
Tinnitus sound may be heard by the examiner when the stethoscope diaphragm is placed over the person's ear

Common Etiology (Stressors)
DISEASES: Acoustic nerve tumor, alcoholism, allergic disorders, anemia, aortic coarctation, aortic regurgitation, arteriosclerosis, diabetes mellitus, hypertension, labyinthitis, meningitis, Meniere's disease, nasopharyngitis, otitis media, otosclerosis, polycythemia vera, serous otitis media, syphilis, thyrotoxicosis
INJURIES: Basal skull fracture, cerebral concussion, foreign body in the ear
PSYCHOSOCIAL FACTORS: The threat of chronic or severe stress
HEALTH CARE FACTORS: *Drug therapy*: Adverse effects of antibiotics, diuretics, quinine, salicylates, streptomycin
ENVIRONMENTAL FACTORS: *Blast/Explosion*: Exposure to a blast or explosion. *Noise*: Prolonged exposure to noise, loud music
MAJOR PATHOPHYSIOLOGIC FACTORS CAUSING THE PROBLEM: Abnormal noises in the ear result from irritation or pressure on the nerve endings in the cochlea

PLANNING
Unmet Needs
Comfort, protection from physical harm, increased learning

Expected Outcome
Person verbalizes a reduced awareness of the tinnitus

NURSING INTERVENTIONS

Nursing Treatments

Place on the unaffected side

Provide radio and television for diversion (the radio, on low volume, is an effective diversion at night)

Withhold the drugs (salicylates, quinine, streptomycin)

Reassure verbally (that the condition is not serious as some persons might suspect a brain tumor, etc.)

Make a referral (to a physician, if there is pathology, or for a tinnitus masker, if the condition is severe)

Nursing Observations

Inspect the ears with an otoscope (for impacted cerumen, infection, perforated eardrum)

Monitor the blood pressure (for hypertension)

Health Teaching

Explain the causes of the health problem (infection, drug side effect, pressure within the ear)

Explain the reason for and intended effect of the therapy (to minimize tinnitus)

EVALUATION

Record actual outcome

Knowledge Deficits Associated with the Ears, Nose, and Throat

UNKNOWLEDGEABLE ABOUT OTITIS EXTERNA[42,88]

ASSESSMENT

Data Collection

Subjective Data

• Person's discussion or questions indicate a need for additional information, clarification, or validation of information
  OR
• Person's lack of questions or comments indicates not wanting information or not knowing enough to seek information
• When questioned directly, the person's response or lack of response indicates that he does not know:
  The causes of otitis externa
  When to seek treatment

Objective Data

• May exhibit behavior such as swimming while the ear is infected

Data Analysis

Nursing Diagnosis

UNKNOWLEDGEABLE ABOUT OTITIS EXTERNA: Being without sufficient information about the cause, effects and therapeutic plan associated with an infection of the ear canal

Common Etiology (Stressors)

HEALTH CARE FACTORS: Lack of health instruction

PLANNING

Unmet Needs

Protection from physical harm, independence, increased learning

Expected Outcome

Correct verbal feedback of the information taught

NURSING INTERVENTIONS

Nursing Treatments

Approach unhurriedly

Encourage the person to ask questions

Nursing Observations

Determine teaching effectiveness by verbal feedback

Health Teaching

Inform that water should be kept out of the ears (and the ears should be kept dry by instilling a few drops of alcohol in the ears daily)

Teach how and when to administer medications (ear drops or ointment)

Explain the causes of the health problem (bacteria such as *Pseudomonas*, staphylococci, and streptococci and sometimes fungi, water entering the ear canal causes cerumen to swell and occlude the canal, which sets up an environment for bacterial and fungal growth)

Explain the reason for and intended effect of the therapy (to reduce infection)

EVALUATION

Record actual outcome

Minor Health Problems Associated with the Endocrine System

SIMPLE GOITER[35,72,371]

ASSESSMENT

Data Collection

Subjective Data

• History of using noniodized salt

Feeling of throat fullness

Person lives in the Pacific Northwest or Great Lakes region

Objective Data

• Palpable thyroid enlargement

Data Analysis

Nursing Diagnosis

SIMPLE GOITER: Enlargement of the thyroid gland specific to low-iodine intake

Common Etiology (Stressors)

HUMAN BODY: *Body state*: Pregnancy

DEVELOPMENTAL PHASES: Adolescence

LIFESTYLE: *Diet*: Insufficient iodine intake

ENVIRONMENTAL FACTORS: *Geographical location*: Living in a region of the Pacific northwest or Great Lakes, including the upper Mississippi Valley, Minnesota, and the Dakotas

MAJOR PATHOPHYSIOLOGIC FACTORS CAUSING THE PROBLEM: Iodine is essential for the normal function of the thyroid gland, the absence of iodine impairs thyroxin production and causes the gland to enlarge in an effort to produce adequate amounts of hormone

PLANNING

Unmet Needs
Protection from physical harm, increased learning

Expected Outcome
Nonpalpable thyroid lobes
Person verbalizes that he uses iodized salt

NURSING INTERVENTIONS

Nursing Treatments
Give iodized salt (if the person is unable to obtain iodized salt for himself)
Encourage increased high-iodine–food intake (seafood, especially halibut or cod)
Make a referral (to a physician if the condition persists after the diet change)

Nursing Observations
Observe for evidence of a favorable response to therapy (deceased thyroid enlargement)

Health Teaching
Teach the principles of good nutrition (the basic food groups)
Recommend the use of iodized salt
Describe those symptoms that should be reported (wheezing, difficulty swallowing)
Explain the causes of the health problem (since there is little or no iodine in the soil of these regions, the food contains no iodine; persons who do not use salt or iodized salt do not have a sufficient iodine intake)
Explain the reason for and intended effect of the therapy (to reduce the thyroid enlargement)

Medical Treatments Performed by Nurses
Give the prescribed drug (Lugol's solution)

EVALUATION
Record actual outcome

Knowledge Deficits Associated with the Endocrine System

UNKNOWLEDGEABLE ABOUT DIABETES MELLITUS [73,202,376]

ASSESSMENT

Data Collection

Subjective Data
• Person's discussion or questions indicate a need for additional information, clarification, or validation of information
  OR
• Person's lack of questions or comments indicates not wanting information or not knowing enough to seek information

- When questioned directly, the person's response or lack of response indicates that he does not know:
  What diabetes is
  What causes diabetes
  That there is a hereditary predisposition to diabetes
  How to follow the prescribed diabetic regimen
  The possible complications associated with diabetes

Objective Data
- May exhibit behavior such as eating foods not on the prescribed diet or partaking in strenuous exercise without adjusting the insulin dosage, etc.

Data Analysis

Nursing Diagnosis
UNKNOWLEDGEABLE ABOUT DIABETES MELLITUS: Being without sufficient information about the causes, effects, and therapeutic plan associated with diabetes mellitus

Common Etiology (Stessors)
HEALTH CARE FACTORS: Lack of health instruction

PLANNING

Unmet Needs
Protection from physical harm, independence, increased learning

Expected Outcome
Correct verbal feedback of the information taught

NURSING INTERVENTIONS

Nursing Treatments
Approach unhurriedly
Encourage the person to ask questions
Encourage adequate rest
Encourage moderate physical exercise

Nursing Observations
Determine teaching effectiveness by verbal feedback

Health Teaching
Explain normal organ function (the pancreas normally excretes insulin in order to metabolize food; in diabetes, the reduced amount of insulin present may be due to decreased insulin secretion, insulin resistance in which the body blocks the use of the available insulin, or destruction of the insulin within the body; therapy is required to maintain metabolism)
Describe the characteristics of controlled diabetes (maintenance of body weight, negative urine tests, normal blood sugar and acetone)
Describe the manifestations of impending diabetic coma (thirst, polyuria, weakness, flushing and dry skin)
Describe the manifestations of impending insulin shock (sweating, dizziness, palpitations, shallow breathing, blurred vision)
Explain how impending insulin shock can be interrupted (by consuming fruit juice, sugar, candy, or carbonated beverage followed by regular meal or some high-protein food)
Recommend that a high-glucose source be carried at all times (candy, sugar)
Teach how and when to give medications (insulin)
Teach how to test the urine for sugar-acetone (using Clinitest, Diastix, or Tes-Tape)
Teach how to test the blood for glucose using the finger-stick method
Teach the common factors that will cause a false-positive or inaccurate glucose reading (taking antibiotics, salicylates, or large doses of vitamin C or vigorously shaking the urine during testing)
Inform that a predisposition to the illness exists (among family members)

Describe those symptoms that should be reported (dizziness, headache, nausea, thirst, weakness, malaise)

Explain the causes of the health problem (the inadequate production of insulin prevents normal food metabolism)

EVALUATION

Record actual outcome

Minor Health Problems Associated with Fluid Balance

FLUID VOLUME DEPLETION[35,371,451,638]

ASSESSMENT

Data Collection

Subjective Data
- Intense thirst (except in the aged who have diminished thirst sensation)
- Weakness
  Salty perspiration, sometimes

Objective Data
- Poor skin turgor (pinched skin, when released, remains raised for more than a few seconds)
- Decreased blood pressure (postural hypotension in the early stage, supine hypotension in the later stage)
- Low volume of urine output
- Increased specific gravity above 1.030
- Increased hematocrit and red blood count
  Tachycardia
  Acute weight loss of more than 3% of the total body weight
  Dry axilla and groins (indicates a deficit of at least 1,500 cc)
  Flat neck veins when the person is in the supine position
  Longitudinal furrows in the tongue

Data Analysis

Nursing Diagnosis
FLUID VOLUME DEPLETION: A condition in which the normal volume of body fluid is decreased

Common Etiology (Stressors)
DISEASES: Diabetes insipidus, hemorrhage
INJURIES: Burn wound
SIGNS AND SYMPTOMS: Dehydration, diarrhea, difficulty swallowing, fever, polyuria, sweating (diaphoresis), vomiting, weakness
HEALTH CARE FACTORS: *Drug therapy*: Adverse effects of diuretics. *Medical therapy*: Gastrostomy, jejunostomy, or nasogastric feeding. *Surgical procedures*: Colostomy, ileostomy, ureterocolostomy, ureteroileostomy
ENVIRONMENTAL FACTORS: *Water*: Inaccessibility of water/fluid
HUMAN ERROR: Refusal to drink fluids, fluid intake of less than 1,200–1,500 cc daily, incorrect use of diuretics
MAJOR PATHOPHYSIOLOGIC FACTORS CAUSING THE PROBLEM: Esophageal stricture or loss of the

swallowing reflex results in difficult fluid intake; loss of large amounts of body fluid depletes fluid within the cells, which causes weakness that impairs the person's ability to replace oral fluids

PLANNING

Unmet Needs

Fluid and electrolyte balance, comfort, protection from physical harm, increased learning

Expected Outcome

Good skin turgor
Fluid intake and output from 1,500–3,600 cc daily
Urine specific gravity 1.010–1.030
Person verbalizes the absence of intense thirst

NURSING INTERVENTIONS

Nursing Treatments

Increase fluid intake to about 2,000 cc daily (if there are no fluid restrictions)
Provide fresh drinking water
Provide fluid selection
Give small, frequent drinks
Make a referral (to a physician for fluid deficit from intractable vomiting or diarrhea, bloody diarrhea, presence of diseases such as diabetes or Addison's disease, extremes of age such as infancy or old age, or acute loss of 5% body weight)

Nursing Observations

Measure the intake and output
Measure the body weight (daily)

Health Teaching

Explain the reason for and intended effect of the therapy (to balance the body's fluid level)
Instruct to increase fluid intake

Medical Treatments Performed by Nurses

Administer intravenous fluids

EVALUATION

Record actual outcome

LOCALIZED EDEMA [42,371,522]

ASSESSMENT

Data Collection

Subjective Data

• Skin tightness and heaviness
  Sensory loss in severely edematous tissue

Objective Data

• Localized swelling
  Coolness
  Glossy skin
  Heat (with inflammation)
  Impaired mobility
  Pallor
  Redness (with inflammation)

Data Analysis

Nursing Diagnosis
LOCALIZED EDEMA: Fluid accumulation restricted to tissues in one body area

Common Etiology (Stressors)
DISEASES: Abscess, allergic disorders, cellulitis rheumatoid arthritis, thrombophlebitis
INJURY: Animal bite, bruising or hematoma, burn wound, dislocation, bone fracture, human bite, incision wound, insect bite, laceration wound, sprain
HEALTH CARE FACTORS: *Diagnostic procedures*: Angiography. *Drug therapy*: Adverse effects of drugs. *Medical therapy*: Intravenous infusion. *Surgical procedures*: Episiotomy, mastectomy
ENVIRONMENTAL FACTORS: *Chemical substances*: Contact with chemical substances. *Objects*: Contact with blunt, falling, hard, pointed, or sharp objects
MAJOR PATHOPHYSIOLOGIC FACTORS CAUSING THE PROBLEM: Lymphatic obstruction; inflammation that dilates blood vessels and increases blood flow to the area, thus increasing capillary pressure and causing the escape of fluid into the tissues; the presence of histamines in an allergic response causing the escape of fluid from the capillaries into the tissues

PLANNING

Unmet Needs
Fluid balance, rest, comfort, protection from physical harm, increased learning

Expected Outcome
No edema accumulation in the tissues
Person verbalizes the absence of the feeling of skin tightness

NURSING INTERVENTIONS

Nursing Treatments

Apply an ice bag or cold pack (intermittently to the edematous site) OR Apply a cold or cool, moist compress	During the first 24 hours following trauma
Apply a heat lamp (intermittently to the edematous site) OR Apply a heat cradle OR Apply a hot water bottle or hot pack OR Apply a warm, moist compress Elevate the affected body part	After the first 24 hours following trauma

Apply an elastic bandage
Massage gently
AND
Exercise in range of motion (for lymph obstruction)
Remove constrictive clothing
Give nonprescription drugs (antihistamines for an allergic response)
Handle gently
Lubricate the skin with cocoa butter, glycerine, lanolin, mineral oil, or olive oil (if the skin is intact)

Nursing Observations
Observe for complaints of pain
Observe for evidence of a favorable response to therapy (decreased edema)

Health Teaching
Describe those symptoms that should be reported (increased edema, pain)
Explain the causes of the health problem (fluid accumulation)

Explain the reason for and intended effect of the therapy (to reduce the edema)
Instruct to elevate the body part
Advise against wearing constrictive clothing
Teach how to apply cold therapy
Teach how to apply heat therapy (to avoid burning oneself)
Instruct to avoid heat applications (if diabetic)

EVALUATION
Record actual outcome

Knowledge Deficits Associated with Fluid and Electrolyte Balance

UNKOWLEDGEABLE ABOUT FLUID BALANCE[371,638]

ASSESSMENT
Data Collection
Subjective Data
• Person's discussion or questions indicate a need for additional information, clarification, or validation of information
    OR
• Person's lack of questions or comments indicates not wanting information or not knowing enough to seek information
• When questioned directly, the person's response or lack of response indicates that he does not know:
    How much fluid to drink daily
    The effects of fluid on the body
    Special needs for extra fluid intake
Objective Data
• May exhibit behavior such as consuming inadequate amounts of fluid
Data Analysis
Nursing Diagnosis
UNKNOWLEDGEABLE ABOUT FLUID BALANCE: Being without sufficient information about the causes, effects, and therapeutic plan associated with maintaining fluid balance and treating the imbalance

Common Etiology (Stressors)
HEALTH CARE FACTORS: Lack of health instruction

PLANNING
Unmet Needs
Protection from physical harm, independence, increased learning
Expected Outcome
Correct verbal feedback of the information taught

NURSING INTERVENTIONS
Nursing Treatments
Approach unhurriedly
Encourage the person to ask questions

Nursing Observations
Determine teaching effectiveness by verbal feedback

Health Teaching
Instruct to maintain fluid intake (at between 2,000–3,000 cc daily, provided there are no fluid restrictions)

Teach the specific procedure of:

Increasing fluid intake to 2,000 cc daily during fever, excessive perspiration, dehydration from vomiting, or diarrhea

Increasing fluid intake to 3,000 cc during urinary infection or calculi

Distributing the fluid intake over 24 hours to meet thirst needs, when on a restricted fluid intake

Explain normal body function (water flows to body tissues and is reabsorbed into the circulation; fluid provides nutrients for organs, maintains body temperature, and removes wastes)

Describe those symptoms that should be reported (unusual thirst, edema, absent or diminished urine output)

Explain the reason for and intended effect of the therapy (to hydrate body tissues)

EVALUATION
Record actual outcome

UNKNOWLEDGEABLE ABOUT ELECTROLYTE BALANCE[371,638]

ASSESSMENT
Data Collection
Subjective Data
• Person's discussion or questions indicate a need for additional information, clarification, or validation of information
  OR
• Person's lack of questions or comments indicates not wanting information or not knowing enough to seek information
• When questioned directly, the person's response or lack of response indicates that he does not know:
  What electrolytes are
  Their effects on the body
  Illnesses, conditions, drugs, etc. that can affect electrolyte balance
  Signs and symptoms of imbalance
  Methods for preventing and treating an imbalance

Objective Data
• May exhibit behavior such as drinking large, unneeded quantities of Gatorade® or overrestricting salt intake

Data Analysis
Nursing Diagnosis
UNKNOWLEDGEABLE ABOUT ELECTROLYTE BALANCE: Being without sufficient information about the causes, effects, and therapeutic plan associated with maintaining electrolyte balance and treating the imbalance

Common Etiology (Stressors)
HEALTH CARE FACTORS: Lack of health instruction

PLANNING
Unmet Needs
Protection from physical harm, independence, increased learning

Expected Outcome
Correct verbal feedback of the information taught

NURSING INTERVENTIONS

Nursing Treatments
Approach unhurriedly
Encourage increased sodium-food/fluid intake (ham, bacon, salted nuts, potato chips, bullion, tomato juice, after vomiting or diarrhea has subsided, during diaphoresis, or fistula drainage)
Encourage increased potassium-food/fluid intake (whole-grain cereals; fresh fruit; nuts; orange, grape, tomato, or prune juice; tea; coffee; chocolate; or meat broth while taking diuretics or after vomiting or diarrhea subsides)
Encourage increased calcium-food/fluid intake (meat, poultry, dark leafy green vegetables, milk, and milk products when taking large doses of antacids or vitamin D)
Encourage the person to ask questions

Nursing Observations
Determine teaching effectiveness by verbal feedback

Health Teaching
Teach the principles of good nutrition (so that the electrolyte intake is adequate)
Instruct to maintain fluid intake (at between 1,500–3,000 cc daily so the electrolytes will be in normal solution)
Explain normal body function (there are chemicals in the body fluids that are electrically charged, thus attracting one another to form a variety of substances, such as acids and salts, that help regulate the acid–base balance and maintain cellular and tissue function)
Describe those symptoms that should be reported (*Low sodium*: Weakness, muscle cramps, vomiting, diarrhea. *Low potassium*: Muscle weakness, arrhythmias, confusion, abdominal distention. *Low calcium*: Muscle twitching, extremity numbness. *Excess potassium*: Abdominal cramps, apathy, confusion, extremity numbness. *Excess calcium*: Polyuria and thirst, weakness)
Explain the causes of the health problem (electrolyte imbalance results from fluid loss through diuresis, fistula drainage, diarrhea, vomiting, gastric suction, excessive salt intake, malnutrition, etc.)
Explain the reason for and intended effect of the therapy (to maintain fluid and electrolyte balance)

EVALUATION
Record actual outcome

Minor Health Problems Associated with the Gastrointestinal System

ANOREXIA [72,451]

ASSESSMENT

Data Collection

Subjective Data
• No enthusiasm for food
• Unconcerned about the poor appetite

Objective Data
• Consumes only small amounts of food

Data Analysis

Nursing Diagnosis

ANOREXIA: Little or no desire for food

Common Etiology (Stressors)

DISEASES: Bacterial endocarditis, brucellosis, coccidioidomycosis, Colorado tick fever, fasciolopsiasis, gastritis, glomerulonephritis, hepatitis, hypothyroidism, infection of any kind, infectious mononucleosis, kwashiorkor, Laennec's cirrhosis, leukemia, metastatic carcinoma, pellagra, pernicious anemia, pheochromocytoma, rheumatic fever, sprue

INJURIES: Burn wound

SIGNS AND SYMPTOMS: Hypokalemia

PSYCHOSOCIAL FACTORS: Excessive emotional excitement, the threat of chronic or severe stress

HEALTH CARE FACTORS: *Drug therapy*: Adverse effects of drugs (such as digitalis intoxication)

DEVELOPMENTAL PHASE: Old age

LIFESTYLE: Cigarette smoking

ENVIRONMENTAL FACTORS: *Chemical substances*: Ingestion of or inhalation of chemical substances

MAJOR PATHOPHYSIOLOGIC FACTORS CAUSING THE PROBLEM: The discomforts and displeasurable feelings of illness or aging inhibit the normally pleasurable desire for food

PLANNING

Unmet Needs

Nutritional balance, comfort, protection from physical harm, increased learning

Expected Outcome

Renewed daily intake of the essential food groups

Renewed daily fluid intake of at least 2,000 cc if there are no fluid restrictions

NURSING INTERVENTIONS

Nursing Treatments

Approach unhurriedly

Arrange pleasant surroundings (during meals)

Provide an attractive meal tray

Postpone feeding when the patient is fatigued
 OR
Withhold food until the person requests it

Provide a balanced nutritional diet

Give small, frequent feedings

Provide food selection

Provide foods at their most appetizing temperature (cold foods cold, hot foods hot)

Encourage the bringing in of outside food (by the family)

Season the food for individual taste

Give high-potassium fluids orally (if the serum potassium is low, fluids such as grape, orange, prune, and tomato juice)

Discourage smoking

Nursing Observations

Measure the body weight (daily)

Observe and record the food intake

Observe for conditions indicating a need for increased nutritional requirements (for healing, growth, etc.)

Health Teaching

Explain the causes of the health problem (inhibited appetite from illness or aging)

Explain the need for pleasant mealtimes

Recommend that food servings be in proportion to the appetite (large amounts of food on the plate may discourage eating, small portions are preferable)

Teach the principles of good nutrition

EVALUATION

Record actual outcome

CONSTIPATION[73,371,451]

ASSESSMENT

Data Collection

Subjective Data
* Frequency of stool is less than the person's norm
* Abdominal fullness
* Hard, small, round masses of stool
  Alternating very large and very small stools
  Flatulence
  Headache
  Indigestion

Objective Data
Abdominal palpation may reveal hard fecal masses or tenderness in the right lower abdominal (cecum) area

Data Analysis

Nursing Diagnosis
CONSTIPATION: Decreased frequency of bowel elimination in relation to normal elimination

Common Etiology (Stressors)
DISEASES: Cerebrovascular accident, diverticulitis, hypercalcemia, hyperparathyroidism, hypothyroidism, rectocele, spastic colitis
INJURIES: Fracture and compression of the spinal cord
PSYCHOSOCIAL FACTORS: The threat of chronic or severe stress
HUMAN BODY: *Body state*: Pregnancy
HEALTH CARE FACTORS: *Diagnostic procedures*: Barium enema, upper GI series. *Drug therapy*: Adverse effects of antacids, anticholinergics, calcium, diuretics, iron compounds. *Medical therapy*: Prolonged bed rest, tobacco withdrawal
DEVELOPMENTAL PHASES: Old age
LIFESTYLE: High-nicotine intake. *Diet*: low-bulk diet
HUMAN ERROR: Insufficient fluid intake, inattention to the defecation reflex
MAJOR PATHOPHYSIOLOGIC FACTORS CAUSING THE PROBLEM: Immobility, low-bulk diet, and certain drugs result in reduced intestinal peristalsis, which slows the elimination of wastes; emotional stress prevents relaxation of intestinal musculature, inhibiting peristalsis; excessive water absorption from the stool in the colon hardens the stool

PLANNING

Unmet Needs
Fluid and electrolyte balance, waste elimination of food residue, exercise, comfort, protection from physical harm, increased learning

Expected Outcome
Soft, formed stools
Frequency of stools is within the person's norm

NURSING INTERVENTIONS

Nursing Treatments
Ambulate the person (frequently)
Encourage moderate physical exercise
Encourage increased residue-food intake (bran, raw vegetables, whole-grain bread)
Increase fluid intake to about 2,000 cc daily
Give fresh fruits (daily)
  OR
Give prune juice (daily)
Give hot coffee
  OR
Give iced liquids

OR

Give warm liquids (especially warm lemonade)
Place in the sitting position (for elimination)
Administer an enema (only if other treatments are ineffective)
Give nonprescription drugs (stool softeners, laxatives)

Nursing Observations

Measure the intake and output
Observe for evidence of a favorable response to therapy

Health Teaching

Advise not to take enemas and laxatives (chronically)
Explain that daily bowel elimination is not essential
Explain the need for scheduled bowel elimination
Instruct to respond immediately to the elimination reflex
Instruct to increase fluid intake
Inform that elimination straining should be avoided
Explain the causes of the health problem (low-fluid intake, tension, etc.)
Explain the reason for and intended effect of the therapy (adequate elimination)

EVALUATION

Record actual outcome

DIARRHEA[42,88,164]

ASSESSMENT

Data Collection

Subjective Data

• Watery or loose stools
• Cramping (spasmodic, colicky) pain along the colon area or referred to the umbilical area
  Flatulence

Objective Data

• Increased frequency and intensity of bowel sounds
  Slight abdominal distention
  Abdominal tympany

Data Analysis

Nursing Diagnosis
DIARRHEA: The passage of unformed stools at frequent, successive intervals

Common Etiology (Stressors)
DISEASES: Addison's disease, allergic disorder (food allergy), amyloidosis, appendicitis, carcinoma of the intestines, celiac disease (sprue), cholera, diabetes mellitus, diverticulitis, amoebic or bacillary dysentery, epidemic neuromyasthenia, gastritis, glomerulonephritis, hepatitis, histoplasmosis, kwashiorkor, lymphosarcoma, malaria, mesenteric vascular occlusion, pellagra, peptic ulcer, salmonella gastroenteritis, shigellosis, strongyloidiasis, thyrotoxicosis, trichinosis, trichuriasis, tuberculosis, typhoid, ulcerative colitis, Whipple's disease
INJURIES: Arsenic poisoning
PSYCHOSOCIAL FACTORS: Excessive emotional excitement, the threat of real or imagined danger
HEALTH CARE FACTORS: *Diagnostic procedures*: Prediagnostic bowel preparation. *Drug therapy*: Adverse effects of antibiotics, chemotherapy. *Medical therapy*: Radiation therapy, tobacco withdrawal. *Surgical procedures*: Gastrectomy

ENVIRONMENTAL FACTORS: *Biologic agents*: Virus or bacteria such as *Escherichia coli*, *Salmonella*, *Shigella*, *Entamoeba histolytica*. *Food substances*: Contaminated by bacteria or toxic agents
HUMAN ERROR: Overfeeding an infant
MAJOR PATHOPHYSIOLOGIC FACTORS CAUSING THE PROBLEM: Mechanical, chemical, or bacterial irritation of the intestinal mucosa causes rapid movement of feces through the intestinal tract; incompletely digested substances such as lactose (milk sugar) attract large amounts of fluid, causing (osmotic) diarrhea

PLANNING

Unmet Needs
Fluid and electrolyte balance, acid–base balance (if prolonged), rest, comfort, protection from physical harm, increased learning

Expected Outcome
Soft, formed stools
Frequency of stools is within the person's norm
Renewed intake of the essential food groups

NURSING INTERVENTIONS

Nursing Treatments
Balance fluid intake to equal output
Discourage the intake of oral stimulants (which increase peristalsis)
Encourage adequate rest
Encourage decreased residue-food intake (avoid vegetables, whole-grain cereals and breads, fresh fruit, etc.)
Give hot tea
  OR
Give carbonated beverages
  OR
Give clear liquid foods (broth, gelatin, fruit ices)
  OR
Give full-liquid foods (sherbert, noncream soups, thin wheat cereals)
  OR
Give rice cereal or rice water (gruel, most appropriate for children)
  OR
Give dry crackers
Refrain from giving milk or milk products (during diarrhea, the lactose in milk is not digested, and the undigested lactose pulls water into the intestines, increasing the diarrhea)
Encourage increased high-pectin–food intake (the pulp of an apple, pear, or ripe banana slows peristalsis by its soothing, emolient effect)
Refrain from giving hot liquids,
  iced liquids, oral stimulants,
  enemas, and laxatives; from } Which stimulate peristalsis
  inserting a rectal tube;
  and from taking rectal temperatures
Give nonprescription drugs (antidiarrheal drugs such as Rheaban, Kaopectate)
Make a referral (to a physician for intractable or bloody diarrhea)

Nursing Observations
Measure the body weight (daily)
Measure the intake and output
Monitor blood studies for abnormal acid–base, electrolytes (if the diarrhea persists)
Observe for complaints of pain
Obtain a bacterial culture (of the stool, if the condition persists)

Health Teaching
Explain the causes of the health problem (viruses, bacteria, stress)
Explain the reason for and intended effect of the therapy (to establish normal bowel elimination)

Medical Treatments Performed by Nurses
Give the prescribed drugs (antidiarrheal drugs)

EVALUATION
Record actual outcome

ERUCTATION[42,164]

ASSESSMENT
Data Collection
Subjective Data
• Feeling of stomach discomfort
• Frequently expels gas by mouth
• No pain or burning sensation
• Sense of relief following eructation
  Frequently occurs after meals

Objective Data
Increased bowel sounds
Gas expulsion may be audible

Data Analysis
Nursing Diagnosis
ERUCTATION (BELCHING): The expulsion of stomach gas through the mouth

Common Etiology (Stressors)
DISEASES: Cholecystitis, esophageal hernia
PSYCHOSOCIAL FACTORS: The threat of chronic or severe stress
LIFESTYLES: *Diet*: High intake of gas-forming foods
HUMAN ERROR: Swallowing large amounts of air, rapid eating
MAJOR PATHOPHYSIOLOGIC FACTORS CAUSING THE PROBLEMS: The person swallows air when eating food, drinking fluids, or swallowing saliva; relief is obtained by belching the air, but the air is swallowed again, setting up a cycle for eructation; air is also produced in the stomach by the fermentation of proteins and carbohydrates

PLANNING
Unmet Needs
Comfort, increased learning

Expected Outcome
Person verbalizes minimal or no eructation

NURSING INTERVENTIONS
Nursing Treatments
Discourage smoking (especially at mealtimes)
Encourage decreased gas-forming–food intake (avoid beans, cabbage, peas, onions, etc.)
Refrain from giving carbonated beverages
Give nonprescription drugs (Simethicone)
Encourage moderate physical exercise (especially after meals)

Nursing Observations
Observe for evidence of a favorable response to therapy

Health Teaching
Explain the causes of the health problem (air swallowing)
Advise against chewing gum

Instruct not to use a drinking straw (which pulls air into the stomach)
Recommend eating and drinking in moderation
Advise against gulping food and drink
Recommend thorough food chewing
Teach the specific method (of preventing air swallowing by exhaling when swallowing instead of inhaling)

EVALUATION

Record actual outcome

FECAL IMPACTION [73,125,371]

ASSESSMENT

Data Collection

Subjective Data
• No bowel movement for several days
  Abdominal and rectal discomfort

Objective Data
• Rectal distention
• Hard, palpable, fecal masses found on digital examination
  Oozing diarrhea around the fecal mass

Data Analysis

Nursing Diagnosis
FECAL IMPACTION: Hardened feces collected in the rectum or sigmoid

Common Etiology (Stressors)
DISEASES: Cerebrovascular accident, paralytic ileus
INJURIES: Fracture and compression of the spinal cord
SIGNS AND SYMPTOMS: Weakness
HEALTH CARE FACTORS: *Drug therapy*: Adverse effects of antacids, anticholinergics, calcium, diuretics, iron compounds. *Medical therapy*: Prolonged bed rest
DEVELOPMENTAL PHASE: Old age
HUMAN ERROR: Insufficient fluid intake
MAJOR PATHOPHYSIOLOGIC FACTORS CAUSING THE PROBLEM: Immobility, low-fluid intake; certain drugs result in reduced intestinal peristalsis, which slows the elimination of wastes; excessive reabsorption of water in the colon causes hard feces; weakness or nerve degeneration can result in loss of the elimination reflex

PLANNING

Unmet Needs

Fluid and electrolyte balance, waste elimination of food residue, exercise, comfort, protection from physical harm, increased learning

Expected Outcome

Soft, formed stools
Frequency of stools within the person's norm

NURSING INTERVENTIONS

Nursing Treatments

Remove the fecal impaction manually
Administer an (oil) enema
Encourage increased residue-food intake (bran, raw vegetables, whole-grain breads and cereals)

Encourage moderate physical exercise
Increase fluid intake to about 2,000 cc daily
Give nonprescription drugs (stool softener)

Nursing Observations
Inspect for bleeding (rectal)
Measure the intake and output
Observe for complaints of pain (rectal)

Health Teaching
Explain the causes of the health problem (low-fluid intake, drug effects, etc.)
Explain the need for scheduled bowel elimination
Instruct to respond immediately to the elimination reflex
Instruct to increase fluid intake
Explain the reason for and intended effect of the therapy (adequate elimination)

EVALUATION

Record actual outcome

FLATULENCE [42,164,278]

ASSESSMENT

Data Collection

Subjective Data
• Feeling of fullness
  Cramping (spasmodic, colicky) pain, sometimes

Objective Data
• Gurgling bowel sounds
• Generalized abdominal tympany on percussion
  Abdominal distention

Data Analysis

Nursing Diagnosis
FLATULENCE: Excessive gas accumulation in the intestinal tract

Common Etiology (Stressors)
DISEASES: Cholelithiasis, spastic colitis, sprue
PSYCHOSOCIAL FACTORS: The threat of chronic or severe stress
HEALTH CARE FACTORS: *Diagnostic procedures*: Barium enema. *Medical therapy*: Intermittent positive-pressure breathing. *Surgical procedures*: Abdominal surgery of any kind
LIFESTYLE: *Diet*: High intake of gas-forming foods
HUMAN ERROR: Rapid eating
MAJOR PATHOPHYSIOLOGIC FACTORS CAUSING THE PROBLEM: Gas is produced in the intestinal lumen by bacterial fermentative action on proteins and carbohydrates

PLANNING

Unmet Needs
Waste elimination of food residue, exercise, comfort, protection from physical harm, increased learning

Expected Outcome
Quieting of the bowel sounds

No abdominal tympany
Person verbalizes minimal or no flatus

NURSING INTERVENTIONS

Nursing Treatments

Change the patient's position frequently
Discourage smoking (especially at mealtime)
Encourage decreased gas-forming–food intake (avoid beans, cabbage, peas, onions, etc.)
Restrict fluids at mealtime
Give warm liquids after meals
Refrain from giving iced liquids
Refrain from giving carbonated beverages
Give nonprescription drugs (Simethicone)
Insert a colon tube (if the flatulence is severe)
Encourage moderate physical exercise

Nursing Observations

Observe for evidence of a favorable response to therapy

Health Teaching

Explain the causes of the health problem (rapid eating, bacterial fermentation)
Advise against chewing gum
Instruct not to use a drinking straw (which pulls air into the stomach)
Recommend eating and drinking in moderation
Advise against gulping food and drink
Recommend thorough food chewing
Explain the reason for and intended effect of the therapy (to reduce the flatulence)

EVALUATION

Record actual outcome

GASTROINTESTINAL IRRITATION [125,278,654]

ASSESSMENT

Data Collection

Subjective Data

• Nausea
• Mild abdominal churning or cramping
• Anorexia
  Diarrhea

Objective Data

Abdominal distention

Data Analysis

Nursing Diagnosis

GASTROINTESTINAL IRRITATION: Irritation of the digestive system by food or drugs

Common Etiology (Stressors)

DISEASES: Carcinoma of the stomach (meat intolerance), cholecystitis (fatty foods intolerance), enteritis (milk intolerance), sprue (gluten-containing grain intolerance)
HEALTH CARE FACTORS: *Drug therapy*: Adverse effects of drugs

MAJOR PATHOPHYSIOLOGIC FACTORS CAUSING THE PROBLEM: Milk intolerance is due to an inability of the stomach or intestines to digest and absorb milk or the absence of the intestinal enzyme needed for milk digestion; fatty food intolerance is due to insufficient bile available to aid digestion, and the lack of bile prevents fat breakdown into small globules, causing less effective digestion by intestinal enzymes; the chemical substances in some drugs irritates the intestinal mucosa; persons with gastric cancer have little or no hydrochloric acid production by gastric cells; hydrochloric acid is necessary for the first steps in the digestion of protein; the absence of hydrochloric acid prevents the meat from being digested, leading to indigestion, flatulence, steatorrhea, etc.; grain (wheat, rye, barley, oats) intolerance is due to complete breakdown of the protein gluten, resulting in a biproduct that damages the intestinal mucosa

PLANNING

Unmet Needs

Nutritional balance, comfort, protection from physical harm, increased learning

Expected Outcome

Person verbalizes cessation of nausea and/or abdominal cramping
Renewed intake of the essential food groups

NURSING INTERVENTIONS

Nursing Treatments

Specific to Foods
Boil the milk
   OR
Dilute the milk
   OR
Give a whole-milk substitute (for a milk intolerance; or add 10 drops of Lact Aid to 1 quart of milk and refrigerate for 1 day; this concentrated preparation of the enzyme lactase will decrease the level of lactose in the milk, which reduces gastric irritation)
Encourage decreased fatty-food intake (gravy, salad dressings, fried foods, heavy desserts for a fat intolerance)
Give bland foods (potatoes, tender meat, refined cereals for a gluten intolerance)
Provide food selection

Specific to Drugs
Dilute the medication
   OR
Give enteric-coated medications
   OR
Place drug tablets in a gelatin capsule
   OR
Give milk with medications
   OR
Give the medication by injection or in liquid form instead of pills (for a drug intolerance)

Nursing Observations

Observe for evidence of a favorable response to therapy

Health Teaching

Teach the principles of good nutrition (and how to plan a balanced diet while avoiding foods causing the irritation)
Instruct to take medications immediately after meals (provided there is no contraindication for such)
Explain the causes of the health problem (irritation of the stomach mucosa)
Explain the reason for and intended effect of the therapy (to reduce the irritation)

EVALUATION

Record actual outcome

GASTROINTESTINAL SPASMS[42,278,522]

ASSESSMENT

Data Collection

Subjective Data
- Localized abdominal pain
- Cramping (spasmodic, colicky) pain
- Intermittent pain
  Mild to severe pain

Objective Data
Hyperperistalsis heard on auscultation
Alternating diarrhea and constipation

Data Analysis

Nursing Diagnosis
GASTROINTESTINAL SPASMS: Painful, involuntary contraction of the smooth muscles of the gastrointestinal mucosa including the esophagus, stomach, or intestines

Common Etiology (Stressors)
DISEASES: Peptic ulcer, spastic colitis
PSYCHOSOCIAL FACTORS: Excessive emotional excitement, the threat of chronic or severe stress
LIFESTYLE: Insufficient relaxation
MAJOR PATHOPHYSIOLOGIC FACTORS CAUSING THE PROBLEM: Spasms of the gastrointestinal tract result from overstimulation of the vagus nerve

PLANNING

Unmet Needs
Fluid and electrolyte balance, waste elimination of food residue, rest and relaxation, comfort, protection from physical harm, freedom from pain, increased learning

Expected Outcome
Person verbalizes the cessation of abdominal cramping

NURSING INTERVENTIONS

Nursing Treatments
Apply a heating pad
   OR
Apply a hot water bottle
   OR
} To the abdomen

Give warm liquids
Refrain from giving hot liquids, from giving iced liquids
Massage gently (for the relaxation effect)
Give bland foods (potatoes, tender meat, refined cereals)
Encourage decreased gas-forming–food intake (avoid beans, cabbage, peas, onions, etc.)
Encourage decreased residue-food intake (avoid vegetables, whole-grain cereals and breads, fresh fruit, etc.)
Balance fluid intake to equal output
Refrain from giving enemas
Discourage the intake of oral stimulants
Discourage smoking
Encourage adequate rest
Give nonprescription drugs (antacids, stool softeners)

Nursing Observations
Observe for complaints of pain duration
Evaluate pain for intensity and quality
Evaluate the effectiveness of the pain-relief measures

Health Teaching
Explain the causes of pain (vagus nerve overstimulation)
Advise not to take enemas and laxatives
Inform that elimination straining should be avoided
Instruct to respond immediately to the elimination reflex
Instruct to increase fluid intake
Recommend thorough food chewing
Advise that highly emotional situations be avoided
Explain the reason for and intended effect of the therapy (to reduce spasms)

Medical Treatments Performed by Nurses
Give the prescribed drugs (antispasmodics)

EVALUATION
Record actual outcome

HEARTBURN [88,164,522]

ASSESSMENT
Data Collection
Subjective Data
• Burning (stinging) wavelike sensation slowly rising from the stomach to the throat, often extending into the neck or jaw
• Onset following heavy, spicy meals, hurried eating, or when lying down
  Increased salivation

Objective Data
May open the mouth during the episode

Data Analysis
Nursing Diagnosis
HEARTBURN (PYROSIS): A burning sensation in the midsternal area

Common Etiology (Stressors)
DISEASES: Duodenal ulcer, esophageal (hiatal) hernia, gastritis, peptic ulcer
HUMAN BODY: Body state: Pregnancy
LIFESTYLE: High-nicotine intake. Diet: Spicy-food intake.
HUMAN ERROR: Overeating, excessive alcohol intake
MAJOR PATHOPHYSIOLOGIC FACTORS CAUSING THE PROBLEM: The lower esophageal sphincter usually closes tightly to prevent food from the stomach entering the esophagus; in some instances, such as with the use of alcohol, or smoking, and during pregnancy, the lower esophageal sphincter relaxes, causing a gastroesophageal reflux (regurgitation of the gastric contents into the esophagus) with symptoms of heartburn; herniation of a portion of the stomach through the diaphragm (hiatus) results in gastroesophageal reflux

PLANNING
Unmet Needs
Comfort, increased learning

Expected Outcome
Person verbalizes the cessation of the burning esophageal sensation

NURSING INTERVENTIONS
Nursing Treatments
Discourage smoking (especially with meals)

Encourage decreased acid–food intake (avoid citrus fruits, vinegar pickles)
Encourage decreased gas-forming–food intake (avoid beans, cabbage, peas, onions)
Give bland foods (if the heartburn is chronic, give potatoes, tender meat, refined bread, etc.)
· Give carbonated beverages
Give nonprescription drugs (antacids, bicarbonates)

Nursing Observations
Observe for evidence of a favorable response to therapy

Health Teaching
Explain the causes of the health problem (food regurgitation)
Recommend eating and drinking in moderation
Recommend thorough food chewing
Advise against gulping food and drink
Instruct to elevate the head (recommend that the person remain in the upright position after meals; if the person has hiatal hernia, place blocks under the head of the bed to prevent nighttime esophageal reflux)
Explain the reason for and intended effect of the therapy (to promote comfort)

EVALUATION
Record actual outcome

HEMORRHOID PAIN [42,88,278,522]

ASSESSMENT

Data Collection

Subjective Data
• Burning (stinging, smarting) anal pain
  Anal itching

Objective Data
• Presence of small, round hemorrhoid masses
  Bleeding, sometimes

Data Analysis

Nursing Diagnosis
HEMORRHOID PAIN: Painful dilated and thrombosed rectal veins

Common Etiology (Stressors)
DISEASES: Portal hypertension
SIGNS AND SYMPTOMS: Ascites, constipation, diarrhea
HUMAN BODY: *Body state*: Pregnancy
LIFESTYLE: *Diet*: Spicy-food intake
HUMAN ERROR: Excessive straining at defecation
MAJOR PATHOPHYSIOLOGIC FACTORS CAUSING THE PROBLEM: Rectal pain results from increased intra-abdominal pressure, and portal hypertension causes congestion and weakening of the hemorrhoidal (rectal) veins; thrombosis of the veins causes swelling that is painful because of the nerve endings in the skin (external hemorrhoids)

PLANNING

Unmet Needs
Fluid and electrolyte balance, comfort, protection from physical harm, freedom from pain, increased learning

Expected Outcome
Person verbalizes cessation of the burning anal pain

NURSING INTERVENTIONS

Nursing Treatments

Apply a heating pad
   OR
Apply a hot water bottle
   OR   } To the anal area
Apply a warm, moist compress
   OR
Soak in a sitz bath
Arrange pillows comfortably (under the buttocks)
Place in the flat position (when hemorrhoids are severely dilated)
Refrain from giving enemas, from inserting a rectal tube, from taking rectal temperature, from performing a rectal examination
Increase fluid intake to about 2,000 cc daily
Encourage decreased residue-food intake (avoid vegtables, whole-grain cereals and breads, fresh fruits)
Ask the person what makes him comfortable
Discuss possible pain-reducing measures
Provide a pain-relief measure of the person's choice
Give nonprescription drugs (Nupercainal ointment, Anusol ointment or suppository, Wynoid suppository, and stool softeners)

Nursing Observations

Evaluate the effectiveness of the pain-relief measures

Health Teaching

Explain the causes of the pain (hard stools, pressure)
Describe those symptoms that should be reported (bleeding)
Advise not to stand for prolonged periods
Inform that coughing should be avoided
Inform that elimination straining should be avoided
Teach how to take a sitz bath
Explain the reason for and intended effect of the therapy (to reduce the pain)

Medical Treatments Performed by Nurses

Give the prescribed drugs (analgesics)

EVALUATION

Record actual outcome

HICCOUGH [35,125,278]

ASSESSMENT

Data Collection

Subjective Data

Nausea
Fatigue or exhaustion

Objective Data

• Persistent hiccough spasm
• Coarse "hic" sound every 1–2 minutes
  Vomiting, sometimes

Data Analysis

Nursing Diagnosis

HICCOUGH: The discomfort of spasmodic contractions of the diaphragm

Common Etiology (Stressors)

DISEASES: Alcoholism, cholera, conversion hysteria, encephalitis, esophageal hernia or stricture, glomerulonephritis, indigestion, meningitis, myocardial infarction, pancreatitis, peritonitis, pleurisy, splenic infarction, subdural hematoma

PSYCHOSOCIAL FACTORS: The threat of severe stress

LIFESTYLE: Cigarette smoking

MAJOR PATHOPHYSIOLOGIC FACTORS CAUSING THE PROBLEM: Contractions of the diaphragm are caused by irritation of the phrenic nerve, which controls the muscles separating the chest from the abdomen

PLANNING

Unmet Needs

Acid–base balance, rest, comfort, increased learning

Expected Outcome

Cessation of hiccough

NURSING INTERVENTIONS

Nursing Treatments

Give nonprescription drugs (antacids)
  OR
Give sugar (1–2 teaspoons, dry)
  OR
Give warm liquids
  OR
Provide a proper bag for breathing (3–5 minutes)

Nursing Observations

Inspect the abdomen for distention
Observe for complaints of fatigue (if the hiccough is prolonged)
Observe for evidence of a favorable response to therapy

Health Teaching

Explain the causes of the health problem (irritation of the phrenic nerve)
Teach how to do breath holding
Instruct to do the Valsalva maneuver (forcibly exhale with the nose and mouth closed)

Medical Treatments Performed by Nurses

Give the prescribed drugs (sedatives if other measures fail)

EVALUATION

Record actual outcome

INDIGESTION[164,522]

ASSESSMENT

Data Collection

Subjective Data

• Nausea
• Belching
• Flatulence
• Abdominal fullness
  Regurgitation
  Onset during a meal or several hours later

Objective Data

Mild abdominal distention, sometimes

Data Analysis

Nursing Diagnosis
INDIGESTION (DYSPEPSIA): A sense of fullness in the epigastrium

Common Etiology (Stressors)
DISEASES: Carcinoma (gastric), cholecystitis, cholelithiasis, enteritis, gastritis, glomerulo-nephritis, pancreatitis, peptic ulcer, sprue, tuberculosis
MAJOR PATHOPHYSIOLOGIC FACTORS CAUSING THE PROBLEM: Faulty enzyme functioning, gastric mucosa irritation or inflammation, liver distention resulting from impaired cardiac or circulatory function, difficulty in dissolving and breaking down food

PLANNING

Unmet Needs
Comfort, protection from physical harm, increased learning

Expected Outcome
Person verbalizes cessation of epigastric fullness

NURSING INTERVENTIONS

Nursing Treatments
Encourage decreased fatty-food intake (avoid gravy, salad dressings, heavy desserts, fried foods)
Encourage decreased gas-forming–food intake (avoid beans, cabbage, peas, onions)
Refrain from giving carbonated beverages
Give nonprescription drugs (antacids, Simethicone)

Nursing Observations
Observe for evidence of a favorable response to therapy

Health Teaching
Advise against gulping food and drink
Recommend thorough food chewing
Recommend eating and drinking in moderation
Explain the causes of the health problem (gastric irritation, food allergy, etc.)
Explain the reason for and intended effect of the therapy (to reduce the indigestion)

EVALUATION
Record actual outcome

MORNING SICKNESS[164,371]

ASSESSMENT

Data Collection

Subjective Data
• Nausea and vomiting
• Onset in the morning or evening
• Persistent over a prolonged period
  Headache
  Dizziness
  Weakness

Objective Data
Weight loss

Decreased serum chloride
Urine acetone
Vomiting

Data Analysis

Nursing Diagnosis
MORNING SICKNESS: Excessive vomiting occurring primarily in the morning or evening

Common Etiology (Stressors)
DISEASES: Carcinoma of the liver, gastritis, toxemia of pregnancy
HUMAN BODY: *Body state*: Pregnancy
MAJOR PATHOPHYSIOLOGIC FACTORS CAUSING THE PROBLEM: Severe vomiting can result from increased chorionic gonadotropin hormone blood level in pregnancy or endocrine or metabolic imbalance

PLANNING

Unmet Needs
Fluid and electrolyte balance, acid–base balance, rest, comfort, cleanliness, protection from physical harm, increased learning

Expected Outcome
Person verbalizes cessation of nausea and vomiting
Renewed intake of the essential food groups

NURSING INTERVENTIONS

Nursing Treatments
Restrict the intake to nothing by mouth (until the episode subsides)
Apply a cool, damp cloth to the face
Apply an ice collar
Balance fluid intake to equal output (after the vomiting subsides)
Moisten the mouth with cracked ice
Give hot tea
  OR
Give carbonated beverages
  OR
Give clear liquid foods (broth, clear juices, fruit ices)
  OR
Give full-liquid foods (clear soups, sherberts)
  OR
Give dry crackers
Give small, frequent feedings
Give nonprescription drugs (antiemetics, such as Marezine, Dramamine PO or by suppository, Emetrol)
Make a referral (to a physician, if the condition persists)

Nursing Observations
Measure the body weight (daily)
Measure the intake and output
Monitor blood studies for abnormal acid-base balance and for abnormal electrolytes (if the hyperemesis persists)

Health Teaching
Explain the causes of the health problem (hormone or metabolic imbalance)
Explain the reason for and intended effect of the therapy (to reduce the hyperemesis)

Medical Treatments Performed by Nurses
Give the prescribed drugs (antiemetics)

EVALUATION
Record actual outcome

NAUSEA [88,125,164]

ASSESSMENT

Data Collection

Subjective Data
- A queasy gastric sensation
- Stomach feels unsettled
  Difficulty eating
  Preference for liquids and soft foods

Objective Data
None

Data Analysis

Nursing Diagnosis
NAUSEA: A feeling that emesis is imminent

Common Etiology (Stressors)
DISEASES: Addison's disease, abdominal aneurysm, appendicitis, beriberi, gastric carcinoma, cerebrovascular accident, cholecystitis, cholelithiasis, Colorado tick fever, encephalitis, endometritis, gastric ulcer, gastritis, glomerulonephritis, hepatitis, Laennec's cirrhosis, lupus erythematosus, lymphocytic choriomeningitis, Meniere's disease, meningioma, mesenteric vascular occlusion, myocardial infarction, myocarditis, pancreatitis, pheochromocytoma, poliomyelitis, renal calculi, salmonella gastroenteritis, sinusitis, streptococcal pharyngitis, tularemia
INJURIES: Burn wound, cerebral concussion, poisoning
SIGNS AND SYMPTOMS: Dizziness, headache, pain, vertigo
PSYCHOSOCIAL FACTORS: Excessive emotional excitement, the threat of chronic or severe stress
HUMAN BODY: *Body state*: Pregnancy
HEALTH CARE FACTORS: *Diagnostic procedures*: Bronchoscopy, gastric analysis, gastroscopy. *Drug therapy*: Adverse effects of antibiotics, aspirin, digitalis, chemotherapy. *Medical therapy*: Hemodialysis, intermittent positive-pressure breathing, radiation therapy, nasogastric intubation. *Surgical therapy*: Anesthesia. *Surgical procedures*: Any
LIFESTYLE: High-nicotine intake. *Diet*: Spicy-food intake
ENVIRONMENTAL FACTORS: *Biologic agents*: Viruses *Chemical substances*: Ingestion or inhalation of chemical substances. *Environmental heat*: High external temperature. *Food substances* contaminated by bacteria or toxic agents. *Moving vehicles*: Riding in moving vehicles such as cars, boats, airplanes. *Odors*: Obnoxious odors. *Sights*: Obnoxious sights
MAJOR PATHOPHYSIOLOGIC FACTORS CAUSING THE PROBLEM: Nausea results from diminished gastric acid or enzyme activity, reduced motility of the duodenum and large intestines, a displaced stomach from an intraabdominal mass or pregnant uterus, equilibrium imbalance, impaired cardiac circulation, gastric irritation from foods and drugs, viral or bacterial infection, or failure of the body to excrete body wastes normally

PLANNING

Unmet Needs
Comfort, protection from physical harm, increased learning

Expected Outcome
Person verbalizes cessation of nausea
Renewed intake of the essential food groups

NURSING INTERVENTIONS

Nursing Treatments
Elevate the head
Encourage deep breathing

Give bland foods (tender meats, mashed potatoes)
  OR
Give carbonated beverages
  OR
Give hot tea
Give small, frequent feedings
Withhold food until the person requests it
Feed slowly
Give nonprescription drugs (Marezine, Dramamine PO or by suppository, Emetrol)
Make a referral (to a physician if the condition persists)

Nursing Observations
Observe for evidence of a favorable response to therapy

Health Teaching
Explain the causes of the health problem (viral or bacterial infection, acidosis, etc.)
Explain the reason for and intended effect of the therapy (to reduce the nausea)

Medical Treatments Performed by Nurses
Give the prescribed drugs

EVALUATION
Record actual outcome

PAINFUL DEFECATION[72,371,451]

ASSESSMENT
Data Collection
Subjective Data
• Localized rectal pain
• Burning (stinging) (smarting) pain
• Intermittent pain during and/or after elimination
  Person may delay bowel elimination in anticipation of pain

Objective Data
None

Data Analysis
Nursing Diagnosis
PAINFUL DEFECATION: A distressful hurting that occurs during or after bowel elimination

Common Etiology (Stressors)
DISEASES: Anal or rectal abscess, fissure, polyp, stricture, ulcer, carcinoma, endometriosis, hemorrhoids, metastic carcinoma, salpingitis
INJURIES: Foreign body in the rectum
SIGNS AND SYMPTOMS: Constipation, diarrhea
HEALTH CARE FACTORS: *Surgical procedures*: Fissurectomy (rectal), fistulectomy (rectal), hemorrhoidectomy
MAJOR PATHOPHYSIOLOGIC FACTORS CAUSING THE PROBLEM: Pressure from fecal bulk irritates the sensory nerve endings in an area of already existing sensitivity, lower bowel or rectal spasm, an obstructive growth

PLANNING
Unmet Needs
Waste elimination of food residue, comfort, protection from physical harm, freedom from pain, increased learning

Expected Outcome
Person verbalizes cessation of painful defecation

NURSING INTERVENTIONS

Nursing Treatments
Position comfortably
Apply a warm, moist compress (to the anal area)
    OR
Soak in a sitz bath
Increase fluid intake to about 2,000 cc daily
Encourage decreased residue-food intake (avoid vegetables, whole-grain cereals and bread, fresh fruits)
Give bland foods (avoid spices)
Ask the person what makes him comfortable
Discuss possible pain-reducing measures
Give nonprescription drugs (analgesics, stool softener)
Administer an (oil) enema (if needed)

Nursing Observations
Observe for complaints of pain duration
Evaluate the effectiveness of the pain-relief measures

Health Teaching
Inform that elimination straining should be avoided
Describe those symptoms that should be reported (bleeding)
Explain the causes of the pain (tissue inflammation, pressure)
Instruct to increase fluid intake
Teach how to take a sitz bath
Explain the reason for and intended effect of the therapy (to reduce the pain)

EVALUATION
Record actual outcome

PAROTITIS[278,522]

ASSESSMENT

Data Collection
Subjective Data
- Aching (soreness, tenderness) localized under the ears or chin
- Pain severity increases when opening the mouth or chewing
  Severe, continuous pain
  Earache

Objective Data
- Swelling around the jaw extending to the ear
- Test of eating acidic foods increases pain
  Fever

Data Analysis
Nursing Diagnosis
PAROTITIS: Painful swelling of the infected parotid gland

Common Etiology (Stressors)
DISEASES: Mumps
ENVIRONMENTAL FACTORS: *Biologic agents:* Viruses
MAJOR PATHOPHYSIOLOGIC FACTORS CAUSING THE PROBLEM: Inflammation of the parotid gland tissue results from infection by a filterable virus

PLANNING

Unmet Needs
Comfort, protection from physical harm, freedom from pain, increased learning

Expected Outcome
No edema around the jaw or ear
Eating acidic foods or chewing does not produce pain

NURSING INTERVENTIONS

Nursing Treatments
Apply an ice bag
   OR
Apply an ice collar   } To the side of the face
   OR
Apply a warm, moist compress
Give bland foods (avoid spices)
Encourage decreased acidic food intake (avoid citrus fruits, pickles, vinegar)
Encourage adequate rest (absolutely essential to prevent complications)
Ask the person what makes him comfortable
Provide a pain-relief measure of the patient's choice
Give nonprescription drugs (analgesics)

Nursing Observations
Observe for impaired judgment, incoherent thinking, memory impairment (which may indicate that the viral infection has spread to the brain)
Test the ears for hearing acuity (impaired hearing can be a complication of parotitis)
Inspect the genitalia for abnormalities (gonad or testes enlargement in males)
Evaluate the effectiveness of the pain-relief measures

Health Teaching
Explain the causes of the pain (virus, tissue inflammation)
Explain the reason for an intended effect of the therapy (to reduce the pain)

Medical Treatments Performed by Nurses
Give the prescribed drugs (analgesics)

EVALUATION
Record actual outcome

POSTMEAL DIARRHEA[72,278]

ASSESSMENT

Data Collection

Subjective Data
• Epigastric fullness and grumbling

- Liquid stools occur 20–30 minutes after each meal
  Nausea
  Acute onset

Objective Data
Pallor
Sweating
Tachycardia

Data Analysis

Nursing Diagnosis
POSTMEAL DIARRHEA (DUMPING SYNDROME): Liquid stools that occur shortly after ingestion of a meal and are sometimes accompanied by shocklike manifestations

Common Etiology (Stressors)
DISEASES: Malabsorption syndrome
HEALTH CARE FACTORS: *Surgical procedures*: Gastrectomy
MAJOR PATHOPHYSIOLOGIC FACTORS CAUSING THE PROBLEM: Postmeal diarrhea results form rapid gastric emptying of stomach contents into the jejunum with jejunal distention resulting in increased peristalsis; the highly acidic and hypertonic chyme (gastric contents) result in osmosis of water, producing liquid stools

PLANNING

Unmet Needs
Fluid and electrolyte balance, nutritional balance, rest, comfort, protection from physical harm, increased learning

Expected Outcome
Soft, formed stools
Frequency of stools within the person's norm
Stabilized body weight

NURSING INTERVENTIONS

Nursing Treatments
Encourage decreased carbohydrate intake (avoid sugar, jellies, honey, candy, pie, cakes, etc.)
Encourage increased fatty-food intake (meat, eggs, cheese, salad oils)
Encourage increased protein-food intake (meat, eggs, cheese, poultry, milk)
Feed slowly
Give small, frequent feedings
Place in the flat position (immediately after meals for about 30–45 minutes)
Refrain from giving hot liquids, from giving iced liquids (which stimulate peristalsis)
Restrict fluids at the mealtime
Make a referral (to a physician if the condition persists)

Nursing Observations
Measure the intake and output
Monitor the blood pressure
Monitor blood studies for abnormal electrolytes
Observe for evidence of a favorable response to therapy

Health Teaching
Explain the causes of the health problem (too rapid emptying of the stomach contents)
Explain the reason for and intended effect of the therapy (absence of diarrhea)

Medical Treatments Performed by Nurses
Give the prescribed drugs (tolbutamide)

EVALUATION

Record actual outcome

REGURGITATION, CHRONIC[371,451]

ASSESSMENT
Data Collection
Subjective Data
- Food is swallowed
- Returns to the mouth
- Is unintentionally swallowed again
  Person complains of a sour taste
  May occur only occasionally or after each meal

Objective Data
Episode can be observed, especially in children

Data Analysis
Nursing Diagnosis
CHRONIC REGURGITATION: The return of food into the mouth from the stomach following eating

Common Etiology (Stressors)
DISEASE: Esophageal carcinoma, esophageal stricture, pyloric stenosis
MAJOR PATHOPHYSIOLOGIC FACTORS CAUSING THE PROBLEM: Regurgitation results when stomach contents place pressure against the cardiac sphincter, causing stomach contractions that eject the food into the mouth; the vomiting mechanism is not involved

PLANNING
Unmet Needs
Comfort, cleanliness, protection from physical harm, increased learning
Expected Outcome
Food is chewed, swallowed, and retained in the stomach

NURSING INTERVENTIONS
Nursing Treatments
Feed slowly
Give small, frequent feedings
Place in the sitting position (during and after eating)
Refresh with a mouthwash (after regurgitation)
Nursing Observations
Observe for airway obstruction (from aspiration)
Health Teaching
Explain the causes of the health problem (pressure against the cardiac sphincter)
Explain the reason for and intended effect of the therapy (to reduce regurgitation)

EVALUATION
Record actual outcome

RUMINATION, CHRONIC[164]

ASSESSMENT
Data Collection
Subjective Data
- Food is swallowed

- Returns to the mouth
- Food is rechewed and reswallowed
- No abdominal pain or discomfort, heartburn, or nausea
  Onset 15–30 minutes after meals

Objective Data
Episode can be observed, especially in children

Data Analysis

Nursing Diagnosis
CHRONIC RUMINATION: The regurgitation, rechewing, and reswallowing of food

Common Etiology (Stressors)
PSYCHOSOCIAL FACTORS: An attempt to recreate the pleasurable experience of infant
    feeding
MAJOR PATHOPHYSIOLOGIC FACTORS CAUSING THE PROBLEM: The pressure of food against the
    cardiac sphincter causes stomach contractions that eject the food into the mouth

PLANNING

Unmet Needs
Comfort, cleanliness, protection from physical harm, increased learning

Expected Outcome
Food is chewed, swallowed, and retained in the stomach

NURSING INTERVENTIONS

Nursing Treatments
Feed (the infant) slowly
Give small, frequent feedings
Place in a sitting position (while feeding the infant)
Refresh with a mouthwash (after rumination)

Nursing Observations
Observe for airway obstruction (from aspiration)

Health Teaching
Recommend thorough food chewing (when food is first put into the mouth)
Advise against gulping food and drink
Recommend eating and drinking in moderation
Explain the causes of the health problem (pressure against cardiac sphincter results in
    stomach contractions)
Explain the reason for and intended effect of the therapy (to reduce rumination)

EVALUATION
Record actual outcome

SENSITIVE DENTIN[106]

ASSESSMENT

Data Collection

Subjective Data
- Aching (soreness, tenderness) generalized in all teeth, not in a single tooth

- Acute onset stimulated by hot, cold, or hard foods
  Mild to severe pain
  Occurs intermittently

Objective Data
- No evidence of dental caries
- No tenderness on palpation of sinuses
  Gums are sometimes receded from the teeth

Data Analysis

Nursing Diagnosis
SENSITIVE DENTIN (SENSITIVE TEETH): Teeth that hurt when exposed to cold, heat, sour, sweetness, or pressure

Common Etiology (Stressors)
DISEASES: Gingivitis, pyorrhea
HUMAN ERROR: Applying excessive friction or heavy abrasives when brushing the teeth
MAJOR PATHOPHYSIOLOGIC FACTORS CAUSING THE PROBLEM: Loss of enamel on the crown of the tooth, which can be caused by faulty brushing or abrasion; when gums recede below the neck of the tooth, the gums no longer protect the tooth; when nerves in the pulp of the tooth become exposed because of loss of the protective covering, pain is easily stimulated

PLANNING

Unmet Needs
Comfort, protection from physical harm, freedom from pain, increased learning

Expected Outcome
Person verbalizes cessation of tooth pain

NURSING INTERVENTIONS

Nursing Treatments
Reassure that the pain will subside
Give bland foods (tender meats, plain vegetables, and desserts, no spices or acids)
Give soft foods (tender meats, mild cheese, cooked fruits)
Refrain from giving carbonated beverages or hot or iced liquids
Encourage decreased acidic food intake (especially citrus fruits and juices)
Brush the teeth with a soft toothbrush
Discuss possible pain-reducing measures
Give nonprescription drugs (analgesics, strontium chloride toothpaste)
Make a referral (to a dentist if the pain persists)

Nursing Observations
Observe for complaints of pain duration
Evaluate pain for intensity and quality
Evaluate the effectiveness of the pain-relief measures

Health Teaching
Explain the causes of the pain (receding gums, nerve exposure around the tooth)
Advise against eating sweets
Advise not to partake of very hot or cold foods and drinks
Instruct to use a soft, new toothbrush and to apply only mild toothbrush pressure
Explain the reason for and intended effect of the therapy (to reduce the pain)

EVALUATION

Record actual outcome

SIMPLE GASTRITIS [88,125,164,278]

ASSESSMENT
Data Collection
Subjective Data
• Anorexia
• Nausea
• Vomiting
• Epigastric fullness, pressure, tenderness, or pain
  Weakness

Objective Data
• Epigastric palpation elicits tenderness
  Fever, sometimes
  Increased white blood cells, sometimes

Data Analysis
Nursing Diagnosis
SIMPLE GASTRITIS: Inflammation of the stomach

Common Etiology (Stressors)
DISEASES: Allergic disorder (to shellfish), hepatitis, influenza, measles, pneumonia, scarlet fever
INJURIES: Poisoning (food)
SIGNS AND SYMPTOMS: Uremia
ENVIRONMENTAL FACTORS: *Biologic agents*: Viruses, bacteria. *Food substances*: Contaminated by bacteria or toxic agents
HUMAN ERROR: Excessive alcohol intake
MAJOR PATHOPHYSIOLOGIC FACTORS CAUSING THE PROBLEM: Gastritis results from severe irritation of the gastric mucosa

PLANNING
Unmet Needs
Fluid and electrolyte balance, nutritional balance, comfort, protection from physical harm, increased learning

Expected Outcome
No epigastric tenderness
Person verbalizes cessation of nausea and vomiting
Renewed intake of the essential food groups

NURSING INTERVENTIONS
Nursing Treatments
Give nonprescription drugs (Marezine, Dramamine PO or by suppository, or Emetrol for vomiting, and Rheaban or Kaopectate for diarrhea)
Restrict the intake to nothing by mouth (until the vomiting subsides)
Moisten the mouth with cracked ice
Give clear liquid foods (such as carbonated beverages and broth for the first 24 hours)
Give soft foods (such as baked potato, creamed soup, sherbert, and vegetables without skins for the second 24 hours)
Give regular foods (thereafter)
Give small, frequent feedings (if preferred)
Encourage adequate rest

Nursing Observations
Make a follow-up evaluation (to determine if the condition has subsided)

Health Teaching
Explain the causes of the problem (virus, bacteria, chemical irritation such as alcohol)
Explain the reason for and intended effect of the therapy (to alleviate symptoms)

EVALUATION

Record actual outcome

TEETHING SYNDROME[106]

ASSESSMENT
Data Collection
Subjective Data
• Localized aching (soreness, tenderness) in the specific area of the erupting tooth
• Irritability
   Anorexia
Objective Data
• Drooling
• Appearance of teeth between age 6–9 months
   Crying
Data Analysis
Nursing Diagnosis
TEETHING SYNDROME: Pain occurring in the gums where teeth are budding through

Common Etiology (Stressors)
DEVELOPMENTAL PHASES: Infancy, childhood
MAJOR PATHOPHYSIOLOGIC FACTORS CAUSING THE PROBLEM: During normal teeth development, the budding tooth pushes through the gums, resulting in pain and discomfort

PLANNING
Unmet Needs
Sleep and rest, comfort, protection from physical harm, freedom from pain, increased learning
Expected Outcome
Cessation of irritability and crying

NURSING INTERVENTIONS
Nursing Treatments
Approach unhurriedly
Reassure (the mother) that the pain will subside (when the teeth are through)
Communicate nurse sensitivity to the infant's pain
Give the infant a chilled teething ring to chew
Massage the (infant's) gums
Give soft foods (strained vegetables, mashed potatoes)
Encourage adequate rest (to reduce irritability)
Give nonprescription drugs (mild analgesics such as Anbesol, acetaminophen)
Nursing Observations
Observe for complaints of pain duration
Evaluate the effectiveness of the pain-relief measures

Health Teaching

Explain the causes of the pain (rupture of the teeth through the gums)

Explain the reason for and intended effect of the therapy (to reduce the pain)

EVALUATION

Record actual outcome

THRUSH [42,88]

ASSESSMENT

Data Collection

Subjective Data

- Mouth dryness
- Onset of curds on the tongue and buccal mucosa, later spreading to the rest of the mouth

Objective Data

- White, slightly raised milk-curd patches on the tongue or buccal mucosa
- Removal of the curds causes bleeding
  Fever
  Lymphadenopathy
  Candida demonstrated by culture

Data Analysis

Nursing Diagnosis

THRUSH: A fungus infection of the mouth or throat

Common Etiology (Stressors)

ENVIRONMENTAL FACTORS: *Biologic agents*: Fungus and yeasts (*Candida/Monilia*)

MAJOR PATHOPHYSIOLOGIC FACTORS CAUSING THE PROBLEM: The mouth, being a warm, moist cavity, provides a desirable environment for fungus growth

PLANNING

Unmet Needs

Comfort, cleanliness, protection from physical harm, increased learning

Expected Outcome

Pink, noninflamed oral and pharyngeal structures

Negative culture for *Candida*

NURSING INTERVENTIONS

Nursing Treatments

Rinse the mouth with dilute hydrogen peroxide (for children, clean the mouth lesions with a cotton-tippd applicator soaked in hydrogen peroxide)
  OR
Give nonprescription drug (apply gentian violet to the mouth lesions)

Give soft foods (tender meats, cooked fruits)

Follow feedings with water (to cleanse milk and food from the mouth)

Make a referral (to a physician if the condition persists)

Nursing Observations

Observe for evidence of a favorable response to therapy

Health Teaching

Teach how to prepare formula (emphasizing the need to boil the nipples and bottles to prevent mouth infection and never to give formula contaminated or unrefrigerated for more than 1 hour)

Recommend the use of mouthwash (especially after meals)
Explain the cause of the health problem (a yeast-type fungus)
Explain the reason for and intended effects of the therapy (to deter fungus growth)

Medical Treatments Performed by Nurses
Give prescribed drugs (Myocostatin oral suspension)

EVALUATION
Record actual outcome

TOOTHACHE[106]

ASSESSMENT
Data Collection

Subjective Data
• Localized pain in the area surrounding the tooth
• Acute onset
• Throbbing (pounding) (pulsating) pain
  Inability to sleep

Objective Data
Evidence of dental caries, gum inflammation
Jaw swelling, sometimes

Data Analysis

Nursing Diagnosis
TOOTHACHE: Pain in the tooth and surrounding area

Common Etiology (Stressors)
DISEASES: Dental caries, gingivitis, pyorrhea
ENVIRONMENTAL FACTORS: *Biologic agents*: Bacteria
MAJOR PATHOPHYSIOLOGIC FACTORS CAUSING THE PROBLEM: Toothache results from bacterial invasion, causing decay and inflammation of the dental pulp and surrounding tissue

PLANNING
Unmet Needs
Rest, comfort, protection from physical harm, freedom from pain, increased learning

Expected Outcome
Person verbalizes cessation of tooth pain
Evidence that the dental caries or gum disorder has been treated

NURSING INTERVENTIONS
Nursing Treatments
Approach unhurriedly
Reassure that the pain will subside
Communicate nurse sensitivity to the person's pain
Give full-liquid foods (cream soups, custard, sherbert)
  OR
Give soft foods (tender meats, mild cheese, cooked fruits)
Refrain from giving hot liquids, from giving iced liquids (which stimulate pain)
Encourage decreased acidic food intake (especially citrus fruits and juices)
Encourage adequate rest
Ask the person what makes him comfortable
Discuss possible pain-reducing measures
Provide a pain-relief measure of the patient's choice

Give nonprescription drugs (analgesics such as aspirin, acetaminophen)
Make a referral (to a dentist) as needed

Nursing Observations
Observe for complaints of pain duration
Evaluate the effectiveness of the pain-relief measures

Health Teaching
Explain the causes of the pain (inflammation and infection)
Advise frequent and early dental attention
Advise not to partake of very hot or cold foods and drinks
Advise against eating sweets
Instruct to use a soft, new toothbrush and to apply only mild toothbrush pressure
Explain the reason for and intended effect of the therapy (to reduce the pain)

Medical Treatments Performed by Nurses
Give the prescribed drugs (analgesics)

EVALUATION
Record actual outcome

VOMITING [88,125,164,371]

ASSESSMENT

Data Collection

Subjective Data
• Nausea before the onset of vomiting
• Ejection of stomach contents
• Sour taste
  Weakness

Objective Data
Episode can be observed

Data Analysis

Nursing Diagnosis
VOMITING The involuntary ejection of stomach contents through the mouth

Common Etiology (Stressors)
DISEASES: Abdominal aneurysm, appendicitis, beriberi, gastric carcinoma, cerebrovascular accident, cholecystitis, cholelithiasis, cholera, Colorado tick fever, diabetes mellitus, diverticulitis, encephalitis, epidemic neuromyasthenia, ruptured esophageal abscess, gastric ulcer, gastritis, glomerulonephritis, hepatitis, hypertension, kwashiorkor, labyrinthitis, Laennec's cirrhosis, lupus erythematosus, Meniere's disease, meningioma, mesenteric vascular occlusion, myocardial infarction, myocarditis, pancreatitis, pheochromocytoma, pneumococcal pneumonia, poliomyelitis, pyloric stenosis, renal calculi, salmonella gastroenteritis, subdural hematoma, thrombophlebitis
INJURIES: Burn wound, cerebral concussion, poisoning
SIGNS AND SYMPTOMS: Dizziness, headache, pain, vertigo
PSYCHOSOCIAL FACTORS: The threat of chronic or severe stress
HUMAN BODY: *Body state*: Pregnancy
HEALTH CARE FACTORS: *Diagnostic procedures*: Broncoscopy, gastric analysis, gastroscopy. *Drug therapy*: Adverse effects of antibiotics, aspirin, chemotherapy, digitalis. *Medical therapy*: Intermittent positive-pressure breathing, radiation therapy, nasogastric intubation. *Surgical therapy*: Anesthesia. *Surgical procedures*: Any

ENVIRONMENTAL FACTORS: *Biologic agents*: Bacteria, viruses. *Chemical substances*: Ingestion or inhalation of chemical substances. *Environmental heat*: High external temperature. *Food substances*: Contaminated by bacteria or toxic agents

MAJOR PATHOPHYSIOLOGIC FACTORS CAUSING THE PROBLEM: Vomiting results from gastric and abdominal muscle contractions due to stimulation of the afferent impulses in the medulla

PLANNING

Unmet Needs

Fluid and electrolyte balance, nurtitional balance, rest, comfort, cleanliness, protection from physical harm, increased learning

Expected Outcome

Person verbalizes cessation of vomiting
Renewed intake of the essential food groups

NURSING INTERVENTIONS

Nursing Treatments

Give nonprescription drugs (Marezine, Dramamine PO or by suppository, Emetrol)
Restrict the intake to nothing by mouth (until the vomiting subsides)
Apply a cool, damp cloth to the face
Apply an ice collar
Moisten the mouth with cracked ice
Refresh with a mouthwash
Encourage adequate rest
Give hot tea
    OR
Give carbonated beverages — For the first 24 hours
    OR
Give clear liquid foods (broth, clear juices)
    OR
Give dry crackers
Give soft foods (such as baked potato, creamed soup, sherbert, and vegetables without skins for the second 24 hours)
Give regular foods (thereafter)
Give small, frequent feedings
Refrain from giving enemas
Make a referral (to a physician if vomiting persists or if there is severe abdominal pain or high fever)

Nursing Observations

Measure the intake and output
Monitor the blood pressure
Monitor blood studies for abnormal electrolytes
Observe for complaints of pain
Palpate the abdomen for tenderness, rigidity, and masses
Percuss the abdomen for abnormal resonance
Inspect the abdomen for distention
Observe for evidence of a favorable response to therapy

Health Teaching

Explain the causes of the health problem (virus, bacteria, chemical irritation such as alcohol)
Explain the reason for and intended effect of the therapy (to alleviate the symptoms)

Medical Treatments Performed by Nurses

Give the prescribed drugs (Compazine)

EVALUATION

Record actual outcome

Knowledge Deficits Associated with the Gastrointestinal System

UNKNOWLEDGEABLE ABOUT BOWEL ELIMINATION[88,362,371]

ASSESSMENT

Data Collection

Subjective Data
• Person's discussion or questions indicate a need for additional information, clarification, or validation of information
  OR
• Person's lack of questions or comments indicates not wanting information or not knowing enough to seek information
• When questioned directly, the person's response or lack of response indicates that he does not know:
  That daily bowel elimination is not essential
  The dangers of chronically taking laxatives and enemas
  The importance of responding to the elimination reflex immediately

Objective Data
None

Data Analysis

Nursing Diagnosis
UNKNOWLEDGEABLE ABOUT BOWEL ELIMINATION: Being without sufficient information about the regulation and maintenance of bowel elimination

Common Etiology (Stressors)
HEALTH CARE FACTORS: Lack of health information

PLANNING

Unmet Needs
Waste elimination of food residue, protection from physical harm, independence, increased learning

Expected Outcome
Correct verbal feedback of the information taught

NURSING INTERVENTIONS

Nursing Treatments
Approach unhurriedly
Encourage the person to ask questions
Encourage increased residue-food intake (whole-grain cereals and breads, high-fiber vegetables and fruits, prune juice)

Nursing Observations
Determine teaching effectiveness by verbal feedback

Health Teaching
Teach balanced nutrition (including foods and fluids which promote natural elimination)
Instruct to maintain fluid intake (at between 2,000–3,000 cc daily to aid elimination)
Advise not to take enemas and laxatives
Explain that daily bowel elimination is not essential (regular elimination is more important)

Explain the need for scheduled bowel elimination (same time of day for each elimination)
Inform that elimination straining should be avoided
Instruct to respond immediately to the elimination reflex (or it will become diminished)
Explain the reason for and intended effect of the therapy (to maintain elimination)

EVALUATION
Record actual outcome

Minor Health Problems Associated with the Genitourinary System

BLADDER SPASMS[72,371,451]

ASSESSMENT
Data Collection
Subjective Data
• Deep, lower midabdominal pain
• Intermittent cramping and colicky sensation

Objective Data
Urinary incontinence
Abdominal muscular contractions

Data Analysis
Nursing Diagnosis
BLADDER SPASMS: Colicky pain in the bladder area accompanied by muscular contraction

Common Etiology (Stressors)
DISEASES: Bladder calculus, prostatic carcinoma, prostatic hypertrophy
HEALTH CARE FACTORS: *Surgical procedures*: Prostatectomy
MAJOR PATHOPHYSIOLOGIC FACTORS CAUSING THE PROBLEM: Bladder spasms result from severe bladder contractions that are stimulated by a major irritant or obstructing lesion or object

PLANNING
Unmet Needs
Comfort, protection from physical harm, freedom from pain, increased learning

Expected Outcome
Person verbalizes increased comfort
Exhibits freedom of body movement

NURSING INTERVENTIONS
Nursing Treatments
Position comfortably
Apply a heating pad
  OR
Apply a hot water bottle (to the abdomen)
Give warm liquids
Refrain from giving iced liquids (which increase spasms)
Massage gently (the lumbar area)
Cover with warm blankets (to prevent chilling)
Place only warm hands and objects on the patient

Refrain from jarring the bed (which stimulates spasms)
Give nonprescription drugs (aspirin, acetaminophen)

Nursing Observations
Observe for a favorable response to therapy

Health Teaching
Explain the causes of the pain (contraction of the bladder muscles)
Explain the reason for and intended effect of the therapy (to relax bladder muscles)

Medical Treatments Performed by Nurses
Give the prescribed drugs (antispasmodics)

EVALUATION
Record actual outcome

DYSURIA [88,371,451]

ASSESSMENT

Data Collection

Subjective Data
• Pain localized in the area of the urinary meatus
• Intermittent, during or following voiding
• Burning (stinging, smarting) sensation
• Urinary frequency, urgency, hesitancy

Objective Data
Bacteriuria
Pyuria
Proteinuria
Urine may appear cloudy

Data Analysis

Nursing Diagnosis
DYSURIA (PAINFUL URINATION): Pain during or after urination

Common Etiology (Stressors)
DISEASES: Bladder calculus, cystitis, prostatic hypertrophy, prostatitis, urethral calculi, ureter or urethra stricture, urethritis
HEALTH CARE FACTORS: *Diagnostic procedures*: Cystoscopy
MAJOR PATHOPHYSIOLOGIC FACTORS CAUSING THE PROBLEM: Painful urination usually indicates the presence of a urinary tract infection that causes inflammation and sensitivity of the bladder mucosa; conditions that obstruct the flow of urine or damage the urinary tract mucosa promote infection and inflammation

PLANNING

Unmet Needs
Fluid and electrolyte balance, acid–base balance, comfort, cleanliness, protection from physical harm, freedom from pain, increased learning

Expected Outcome
Person verbalizes cessation of burning sensation during or after voiding
No bacteriuria

NURSING INTERVENTIONS

Nursing Treatments
Increase fluid intake to about 3,000 cc daily
Give urine-acidifying juices orally (apple, cranberry, plum or prune juice)

Give nonprescription drugs (Azo-Standard tablets)

Make a referral (to a physician if there is bacteriuria or hematuria)

Nursing Observations

Monitor the oral temperature (for fever)

Monitor urine studies for evidence of urinary tract infection (presence of red or white blood cells, hemoglobin, hyaline casts)

Observe for complaints of urinary frequency

Observe the urine for abnormal color, content, and odor (*Color*: Extremely yellow, black, blue, milky white, red, cloudy. *Content*: Albumin, mucus, fat, sugar, blood, foam. *Odor*: Ammonia, acetone, fecal, fishy)

Obtain a bacterial culture (of the urine)

Test the urine for pH (normal average is 7, below is increased acidity, above is increased alkalinity)

Health Teaching

Instruct to increase fluid intake (to about 2,500–3,000 cc daily)

Describe those symptoms that should be reported (hematuria, persistance of dysuria, pus in the urine)

EVALUATION

Record actual outcome

RETENTION OF URINE[72,371,451]

ASSESSMENT

Data Collection

Subjective Data
• Lower abdominal cramping pain or discomfort
• Sensation of bladder fullness

Objective Data
• Bladder distention evident by suprapubic swelling, which can extend to the umbilicus
• Little or no urine output
  Restlessness

Data Analysis

Nursing Diagnosis
RETENTION OF URINE: The collection of urine in the bladder because of the bladder's inability to expel urine

Common Etiology (Stressors)
DISEASES: Cystitis, prostatic hypertrophy, prostatitis, pyelonephritis, tabes dorsalis, urethral calculus or stricture
INJURIES: Fracture and compression of the spinal cord
HEALTH CARE FACTORS: *Drug therapy*: Anticholinergics, narcotics, sedatives, tranquilizers. *Medical therapy*: Prolonged bed rest, obstructed urinary catheter *Surgical therapy*: Anesthesia, postoperative inactivity
ENVIRONMENTAL FACTORS: *Environmental cold*: Low external temperature
MAJOR PATHOPHYSIOLOGIC FACTORS CAUSING THE PROBLEM: Urine retention results from decreased nerve stimulation to the bladder due to operative trauma or anesthesia, the reclining position fails to maintain normal bladder tone because of a lack of uniform hydrostatic pressure from the urine on all bladder surfaces that usually exists when there is normal ambulation, large amounts of rectal feces can cause sufficient pressure on the urethra to prevent urine flow, obstruction between the bladder and the urethra and loss of bladder muscle tone contribute to retention

PLANNING

Unmet Needs

Waste elimination of urine, comfort, protection from physical harm, increased learning

Expected Outcome

Person verbalizes the absence of abdominal discomfort and bladder fullness

A nonpalpable bladder

NURSING INTERVENTIONS

Nursing Treatments

Ambulate the person (as much as possible)

Apply a heating pad

    OR   } To the abdomen

Apply a hot water bottle

Catheterize with an indwelling urinary catheter (only if other measures fail)

Do not withdraw by catheter more than 1,000 cc of urine at one time

Increase fluid intake to about 2,000 cc daily

Stand the male patient for urination (if possible)

Irrigate the urinary catheter

    OR

Change the urinary catheter (if the catheter is obstructed)

Make a referral (to a physician if there are recurring episodes)

Nursing Observations

Inspect the abdomen for distention (periodically)

Palpate the bladder for distention

Measure the intake and output

Observe for complaints of pain

Check the tube (catheter) for patency (periodically)

Health Teaching

Instruct to increase fluid intake

Explain the causes of the health problem (anesthesia, obstructed catheter, decreased bladder tone)

EVALUATION

Record actual outcome

Knowledge Deficits Associated with the Genitourinary System

UNKNOWLEDGEABLE ABOUT JUVENILE ENURESIS[460,522]

ASSESSMENT

Data Collection

Subjective Data

• Person's discussion or questions indicate a need for additional information, clarification, or validation of information

    OR

• Person's lack of questions or comments indicates not wanting information or not knowing enough to seek information

- When questioned directly, the person's response or lack of response indicates that he does not know:
  How to prevent a child, over age 3, from wetting the bed
  What causes the problem

Objective Data
- May exhibit behavior such as a parent shaming the child in front of others

Data Analysis

Nursing Diagnosis
UNKNOWLEDGEABLE ABOUT JUVENILE ENURESIS: Being without sufficient information about managing the unintentional nocturnal voiding by children who have no urologic disorder

Common Etiology (Stressors)
HEALTH CARE FACTORS: Lack of health instruction

PLANNING

Unmet Needs
Comfort, independence, increased learning

Expected Outcome
Correct verbal feedback of the information taught

NURSING INTERVENTIONS

Nursing Treatments
Approach unhurriedly
Encourage the parents to ask questions

Nursing Observations
Monitor urine studies for evidence of urinary tract infection (positive nitrite, blood, protein, more than 2–5 red blood cells and white blood cells, and casts)
Determine teaching effectiveness by verbal feedback

Health Teaching
Advise that highly emotional situations be avoided (before sleep, such as rough play, watching thrilling movies on television, emotional encounters with peers or parents)
Describe those symptoms that should be reported (lack of urine control during the daytime or urine dribbling)
Explain that parental attitudes affect child development (teasing and punishment only make the child more tense)
Explain the causes of the health problem (excitement, tension, poor sphincter control)
Emphasize the need to develop self-reliance (in the child so that he can maintain control)
Instruct to toilet frequently (at night)
Recommend the use of warm clothing (when in bed)
Recommend fluid restriction (no fluids after 5 or 6 PM)

EVALUATION

Record actual outcome

UNKNOWLEDGEABLE ABOUT ORGAN DONATION[26,71,451]

ASSESSMENT

Data Collection

Subjective Data
- Person's discussion or questions indicate a need for additional information, clarification, or validation of information

OR
• Person's lack of questions or comments indicates not wanting information or not knowing enough to seek information
• When questioned directly, the person's response or lack of response indicates that he does not know:
How or where organs are donated
The procedure involved in organ donation
How it is determined if the person is a suitable donor
The state of health living donors can expect following donation of an organ

Objective Data
None

Data Analysis
Nursing Diagnosis
UNKNOWLEDGEABLE ABOUT ORGAN DONATION: Being without sufficient information about living or deceased persons giving an organ for transplant to another person

Common Etiology (Stressors)
HEALTH CARE FACTORS: Lack of health instruction

PLANNING

Unmet Needs
Comfort, independence, increased learning

Expected Outcome
Correct verbal feedback of the information taught

NURSING INTERVENTIONS

Nursing Treatments
Approach unhurriedly
Encourage the person to ask questions
Discuss the anticipated procedure (tests to determine organ compatibility and the organ transplant)
Introduce to persons who have successfully undergone the same experience

Nursing Observations
Determine teaching effectiveness by verbal feedback

Health Teaching
Explain the criteria for acceptance of an organ donor (compatible blood and tissue types; living donors must be in good health; deceased donors must donate a cornea, a kidney, a liver, a heart, or skin within a few hours, if the family gives permission)
Explain how and where organ donations are made (by surgical removal of a donor organ and surgical implantation; donor may be living or deceased)
Explain how the loss of an organ will affect the living donor's future health (most donors' health remains unchanged, but if their one remaining organ fails, they are at risk for illness)

EVALUATION
Record actual outcome

UNKNOWLEDGEABLE ABOUT CHRONIC RENAL DISEASE[26,71,85,371]

ASSESSMENT

Data Collection

Subjective Data
• Person's discussion or questions indicate a need for additional information, clarifi-

cation, or validation of information
OR
- Person's lack of questions or comments indicates not wanting information or not knowing enough to seek information
- When questioned directly, the person's response or lack of response indicates that he does not know:
  The cause of the renal disease
  The reason for and effects of treatment
  The precautions to be taken to control the disease
  The signs and symptoms to report
  The importance of follow-up care

Objective Data
- May exhibit behavior such as participating in very strenuous exercise, staying up until the early morning hours, consuming only small quantities of fluid instead of hydrating himself adequately

Data Analysis

Nursing Diagnosis
UNKNOWLEDGEABLE ABOUT CHRONIC RENAL DISEASE: Being without sufficient information about how to maintain maximum health and safeguard kidney function when one has chronic kidney disease

Common Etiology (Stressors)
HEALTH CARE FACTORS: Lack of health instruction

PLANNING

Unmet Needs
Protection from physical harm, independence, increased learning

Expected Outcome
Correct verbal feedback of the information taught

NURSING INTERVENTIONS

Nursing Treatments
Approach unhurriedly
Encourage the person to ask questions
Encourage adequate rest (8 hours of sleep each night with 1–2 hours rest during the day, additional rest is essential when the person has a respiratory infection)
Encourage moderate physical exercise (not overly strenuous exercise)

Nursing Observations
Determine teaching effectiveness by verbal feedback

Health Teaching
Instruct to increase fluid intake (to 2,000 cc daily if there is no fluid restriction)
Advise voiding every 4 hours while awake (stagnated urine supports the growth of bacteria)
Teach the principles of good nutrition (appropriate to the individual renal problem)
Explain that fatigue should be recognized as a stress factor
Recommend adherence to a pace of living with which the person is comfortable
Explain how to prevent cross-infection (hand washing, limiting direct human contact with infected persons)
Teach how to test the urine by Dipstick (for blood, nitrite, protein, pH)
Explain how to keep the urine within the desired pH range (with urine-acidifying juices that prevent bacterial growth, such as cranberry, plum, and prune juice)
Describe those symptoms that should be reported (hematuria, nausea, vomiting, respiratory infection, dysuria, urinary frequency, fever, edema)
Describe the specific dangerous effects of poor health practices (renal damage)
Explain the importance of continuing therapy (medications, etc.)
Explain the reason for and intended effect of the therapy (to improve or maintain renal function)

Emphasize the importance of follow-up care (to check the degree of renal function, to recognize and treat problems at their early stage)

Explain how to measure intake and output (as needed; include how to measure the ankles for edema)

Emphasize the need to avoid certain drugs and/or chemicals (*Nephrotoxic drugs*: Polymyxin B, Colistin, gentamicin, streptomycin, kanamycin, necomycin, cephaloridine, tetracycline, penicillin if hypersenstive to it thiazide diuretics, dilantin, Cytoxan, phenacetin, iodine contrast material. *Chemicals*: Carbon tetrachloride, chlorinated hydrocarbon and organophosphate insecticides; mercuric chloride, lead, arsenic, creosol)

Explain the causes of the problem (hereditary predisposition, the damaging effects of infection, usually streptococcus, and inflammation of the glomeruli, renal tubules, and/or vascular system of the kidneys; an allergic response to an infection located elsewhere in the body)

EVALUATION

Record actual outcome

UNKNOWLEDGEABLE ABOUT RENAL CALCULI [26,71,85,371]

ASSESSMENT

Data Collection

Subjective Data
- Person's discussion or questions indicate a need for additional information, clarification, or validation of information
  OR
- Person's lack of questions or comments indicates not wanting information or not knowing enough to seek information
- When questioned directly, the person's response or lack of response indicates that he does not know:
  How renal calculi are formed
  Methods for preventing their formation

Objective Data
- May exhibit behavior such as eating foods that could cause calculi or drinking inadequate amounts of fluid

Data Analysis

Nursing Diagnosis
UNKNOWLEDGEABLE ABOUT RENAL CALCULI: Being without sufficient information about kidney stones

Common Etiology (Stressors)
HEALTH CARE FACTORS: Lack of health instruction, lack of health-skill experience

PLANNING

Unmet Needs
Protection from physical harm, independence, increased learning

Expected Outcome
Correct verbal feedback of the information taught

NURSING INTERVENTIONS

Nursing Treatments

Approach unhurriedly

Encourage the person to ask questions

Encourage decreased calcium-food and fluid intake (for calcium calculi; no milk or milk products, dark leafy green vegatables, clams, oysters, yogurt)

Encourage decreased purine food intake (for uric acid calculi; no liver, kidney, poultry, fish, fried foods, spinach, mushrooms, alcohol)

Encourage decreased calorie intake, decreased fatty-food intake (for cystine or uric acid calculi)

Nursing Observations

Determine teaching effectiveness by verbal feedback

Health Teaching

Instruct to increase fluid intake (to 3,000 cc–4,000 cc daily)

Advise voiding every 4 hours while awake (stagnated urine supports the growth of bacteria, which serves as a nucleus around which the stone forms)

Teach how to test the urine by Dipstick (for urine pH)

Explain how to keep the urine within the desired pH range (with urine-acidifying juices for calcium calculi and struvite stones, with urine-alkalinizing juices for cystine or uric acid calculi)

Recommend that alkalis be used conservatively (for calcium calculi and struvite stones)

Emphasize the need to avoid certain drugs (such as Probenecid, which increases uric acid in the urine)

Explain how to strain urine (so that even small stones can be retrieved and analyzed)

Explain the cause of the problem (the collection of small chemical particles in the kidney, hereditary tendency)

Describe those symptoms that should be reported (flank pain, frequency, hematuria)

EVALUATION

Record actual outcome

UNKNOWLEDGEABLE ABOUT URINARY TRACT INFECTION[26,71,85,371]

ASSESSMENT

Data Collection

Subjective Data

- Person's discussion or questions indicate a need for additional information, clarification, or validation of information
    OR
- Person's lack of questions or comments indicates not wanting information or not knowing enough to seek information
- When questioned directly, the person's response or lack of response indicates that he does not know:
    How urinary tract infections occur
    Methods for preventing such infection
    Symptoms to be reported

Objective Data

- May exhibit behavior such as not seeking health care despite symptoms of urinary tract infection or voiding only every 8 hours

Data Analysis

Nursing Diagnosis

UNKNOWLEDGEABLE ABOUT URINARY TRACT INFECTION: Being without sufficient information about a condition of pathogenic organisms in the kidneys, ureters, bladder, or urethra

• Weakness

Common Etiology (Stressors)

HEALTH CARE FACTORS: Lack of health instruction, lack of health-skill experience

PLANNING

Unmet Needs

Protection from physical harm, independence, increased learning

Expected Outcome

Correct verbal feedback of the information taught

NURSING INTERVENTIONS

Nursing Treatments

Approach unhurriedly

Encourage the person to ask questions

Nursing Observations

Determine teaching effectiveness by verbal feedback

Health Teaching

Instruct to increase fluid intake (to about 2,000 cc daily)

Explain how to keep the urine within the desired pH range (with urine-acidifying juices that prevent bacterial growth, such as cranberry, plum, and prune juice)

Explain how to use toilet tissue correctly by cleansing from front to back (which prevents fecal contamination of the urinary meatus)

Recommend voiding after sexual intercourse (which flushes away bacteria that could enter the urinary meatus)

Advise voiding every 4 hours while awake (to reduce bacterial growth in retained urine)

Describe those symptoms that should be reported (fever, dysuria, nocturia, pain, cloudy and odorous urine)

Explain the cause of the health problem (microorganisms are externally introduced into the genitourinary tract where they multiply and infect specific urinary organs)

EVALUATION

Record actual outcome

Minor Health Problems Associated with the Immunologic System

EXTERNAL ABSCESS[35,371,522]

ASSESSMENT

Data Collection

Subjective Data

• Aching pain (soreness, tenderness)

Objective Data

• Inflammation (redness)

• Swelling

• Heat

- Purulent center in the lesion
- Well-defined borders
  Fever, sometimes

Data Analysis

Nursing Diagnosis
EXTERNAL ABSCESS: A local collection of pus anywhere on the body

Common Etiology (Stressors)
DISEASES: Acne vulgaris, boil (furuncle), carbuncle, diabetes mellitus
ENVIRONMENTAL FACTORS: *Biologic agents*: Bacteria
MAJOR PATHOPHYSIOLOGIC FACTORS CAUSING THE PROBLEM: Infectious microorganisms invade tissue and cause an inflammatory process that encloses the organisms within a small localized area

PLANNING

Unmet Needs
Rest, comfort, cleanliness, protection from physical harm, increased learning

Expected Outcome
Person verbalizes increased comfort
No observable inflammation, swelling, or heat in the abscess site
Full functional use of the affected area

NURSING INTERVENTIONS

Nursing Treatments
Clean with antiseptic solution
   OR
Clean with hydrogen peroxide
   OR
Clean with surgical soap
Soak in (warm) saline solution
   OR
Apply a warm, moist compress
Soak in a sitz bath (for a rectal or perineal abscess)
Apply an antibiotic ointment
Apply a sterile dressing
Change the dressing frequently
Give nonprescription drugs (analgesics for pain)
Encourage adequate rest
Make a referral (to a physician if there is delayed healing)

Nursing Observations
Monitor the oral temperature (for fever)
Obtain a bacterial culture (to identify the organisms)

Health Teaching
Explain the causes of the health problem (infection)
Advise against piercing lesions (which increases infection)
Teach how to apply heat therapy
Teach how to clean and dress a wound
Teach how to do therapeutic soaks
Explain the reason for and intended effect of the therapy (to decrease infection and promote healing)

Medical Treatments Performed by Nurses
Give the prescribed drugs
Soak in a medicated solution

EVALUATION

Record actual outcome

LIMITED CELLULITIS [35,104,371,522]

ASSESSMENT

Data Collection

Subjective Data
- Aching pain (soreness, tenderness)

Objective Data
- Inflammation (redness)
- Swelling
- Heat
- Poorly defined borders with spreading into tissue
  Fever, sometimes
  Impaired function of the affected area

Data Analysis

Nursing Diagnosis
LIMITED CELLULITIS: A diffuse or spreading inflammation with an infection of cellular or connective tissue that is limited to a small area

Common Etiology (Stressors)
INJURY: Trauma of any kind
ENVIRONMENTAL FACTORS: *Biologic agents*: Streptococci, staphylococci bacteria
MAJOR PATHOPHYSIOLOGIC FACTORS CAUSING THE PROBLEM: Infectious microorganisms, usually streptococci or staphylococci, invade soft tissue and spread too rapidly for the development of an abscess; however, the inflammatory process encloses the infection in a localized area; the bacteria can enter the tissues from the blood as well as from the skin

PLANNING

Unmet Needs
Rest, comfort, cleanliness, protection from physical harm, increased learning

Expected Outcome
Person verbalizes increased comfort
No observable inflammation, swelling, or heat in the cellulitis site
Full functional use of the affected area

NURSING INTERVENTIONS

Nursing Treatments
Apply a warm, moist compress
  OR
Apply a hot water bottle
  OR
Soak in (warm) saline solution
Clean with antiseptic solution
  OR
Clean with hydrogen peroxide
  OR
Clean with surgical soap
Apply an antibiotic ointment
Apply a sterile dressing (if the wound is open)
Change the dressing frequently
Elevate the extremity
Encourage adequate rest
Refrain from tight bandaging
Give nonprescription drugs (analgesics for pain)

Make a referral (to a physician if healing is delayed, cellulitis becomes extensive, or if the cellulitis is located on the face)

Nursing Observations

Monitor the oral temperature (for fever)

Obtain a bacterial culture (to identify the organisms)

Health Teaching

Teach how to apply heat therapy

Teach how to clean and dress a wound

Teach how to do therapeutic soaks

Describe those symptoms that should be reported (increased inflammation or drainage)

Explain the causes of the health problem (infectious microorganisms)

Explain the reason for and intended effect of the therapy (to decrease infection and promote healing)

Medical Treatments Performed by Nurses

Soak in a medicated solution

EVALUATION

Record actual outcome

Knowledge Deficits Associated with the Immunologic System

UNKNOWLEDGEABLE ABOUT INFECTION PREVENTION[42,73,278,371]

ASSESSMENT

Data Collection

Subjective Data

• Person's discussion or questions indicate a need for additional information, clarification, or validation of information
  OR
• Person's lack of questions or comments indicates not wanting information or not knowing enough to seek information
• When questioned directly, the person's response or lack of response indicates that he does not know:
  That cleanliness is essential to infection prevention
  The means by which infection is transmitted
  The proper methods of disinfecting
  How to avoid transmitting infection

Objective Data

• May exhibit behavior such as coughing or sneezing without covering the mouth and nose, hugging and kissing a baby when the person has a cold

Data Analysis

Nursing Diagnosis

UNKNOWLEDGEABLE ABOUT INFECTION PREVENTION: Being without sufficient information about the methods used for preventing infection and infection transmission

Common Etiology (Stressors)
HEALTH CARE FACTORS: Lack of health instruction

PLANNING

Unmet Needs
Protection from physical harm, independence, increased learning

Expected Outcome
Correct verbal feedback of the information taught

NURSING INTERVENTIONS

Nursing Treatments
Approach unhurriedly
Encourage the person to ask questions

Nursing Observations
Determine teaching effectiveness by verbal feedback

Health Teaching
Inform that cleanliness is essential to infection prevention
Instruct to avoid direct contact with infected persons (avoid kissing, hugging)
Instruct to cover the mouth when coughing
Instruct to cover the nose when sneezing
Explain how to dispose of infectious expectoration (use disposable tissue and place in a
    paper sack before discarding, place in an incinerator if available)
Explain how to dispose of soiled dressings (place in a paper or plastic sack, seal, burn
    or place in the garbage-collection container)
Explain how to handle contaminated linen (by boiling or burning)
Teach how to apply disinfecting solutions (such as Lysol)
Explain how to prevent cross-infection (wear a mask when caring for the sick, wash
    hands after each contact, keep infected person's dishes separate and either boil them
    or place them in a sterilizing dish washer)

EVALUATION

Record actual outcome

UNKNOWLEDGEABLE ABOUT DRUG ALLERGY[12,278,475,487]

ASSESSMENT

Data Collection

Subjective Data
• Person's discussion or questions indicate a need for additional information, clarifi-
    cation, or validation of information
    OR
• Person's lack of questions or comments indicates not wanting information or not
    knowing enough to seek information
• When questioned directly, the person's response or lack of response indicates that he
    does not know:
    The signs and symptoms of drug allergy
    What causes the problem
    How to avoid allergic responses
    The drugs with which allergy most frequently occurs

Objective Data
• May exhibit behavior such as continuing to take a drug when drug intake and onset of

a rash occurred at about the same time

Data Analysis

Nursing Diagnosis

UNKNOWLEDGEABLE ABOUT DRUG ALLERGY: Being without sufficient information about the cause, effects, and treatment of a hypersensitivity response to drugs

Common Etiology (Stressors)

HEALTH CARE FACTORS: Lack of health instruction

PLANNING

Unmet Needs

Protection from physical harm, independence, increased learning

Expected Outcome

Correct verbal feedback of the information taught

NURSING INTERVENTIONS

Nursing Treatments

Approach unhurriedly

Encourage the person to ask questions

Nursing Observations

Determine teaching effectiveness by verbal feedback

Health Teaching

Describe those symptoms that should be reported (itching, generalized weakness, joint pain, and signs such as respiratory difficulty, rash or hives, fever)

Explain the causes of the health problem (drug ingestion, inhalation, or injection produces a histamine response; the response does not occur with the initial drug dose; if on prolonged drug therapy, it will occur within 6-weeks of the initial dose and clears up within 2 days once the drug is stopped; the drugs with which it most frequently occurs are quinine, quinidine, antibiotics, tranquilizers, sulfonamides, antimalarial drugs, antihypertensive drugs, tetanus antitoxin)

Explain how to take allergy precautions (the person should inform health care personnel of any drug allergies)

Explain the importance of wearing a Medic Alert tag (which states the drug allergy)

Advise that the precipitating factor (the drug) should be avoided

Inform of the therapies available for the specific condition (antihistamines, antipruritics)

EVALUATION

Record actual outcome

UNKNOWLEDGEABLE ABOUT FOOD ALLERGY[12,42,278,475,487]

ASSESSMENT

Data Collection

Subjective Data

• Person's discussion or questions indicate a need for additional information, clarification, or validation of information
  OR

• Person's lack of questions or comments indicates not wanting information or not knowing enough to seek information

• When questioned directly, the person's response or lack of response indicates that he does not know:

The signs of food allergy (skin rash, hives, respiratory distress, nasal stuffiness, mouth and lip swelling, vomiting, diarrhea, slight fever)
The symptoms of food allergy (nausea, severe abdominal pain, headache, malaise)
The causes of food allergy
How to avoid allergic responses

Objective Data
• May exhibit behavior such as eating foods known to cause the specific allergic response being experienced

Data Analysis

Nursing Diagnosis
UNKNOWLEDGEABLE ABOUT FOOD ALLERGY: Being without sufficient information about the cause, effects, and treatment of antibody–antigen reactions to ingested foods

Common Etiology (Stressors)
HEALTH CARE FACTORS: Lack of health information

PLANNING

Unmet Needs
Protection from physical harm, independence, increased learning

Expected Outcome
Correct verbal feedback of the information taught

NURSING INTERVENTIONS

Nursing Treatments
Approach unhurriedly
Encourage the person to ask questions
Make a referral (to a physician for sensitivity testing and/or desensitizing)

Nursing Observations
Determine teaching effectiveness by verbal feedback

Health Teaching
Explain the causes of the health problem (an antigen–antibody reaction to ingested food)
Describe those symptoms that should be reported (vomiting, rash, edema, dyspnea)
Inform of the therapies available for the specific condition (antihistamines, desensitizing)
Inform that foods causing allergies fall into specific categories (dairy products, shellfish, fowl, etc.)
Advise that the precipitating factor (specific food) should be avoided
Explain how to interpret food contents listed on container labels (so foods causing the allergy can be avoided)

EVALUATION
Record actual outcome

UNKNOWLEDGEABLE ABOUT RESPIRATORY ALLERGY [12,42,278,475,487]

ASSESSMENT

Data Collection

Subjective Data
• Person's discussion or questions indicate a need for additional information, clarification, or validation of information

OR
- Person's lack of questions or comments indicates not wanting information or not knowing enough to seek information
- When questioned directly, the person's response or lack of response indicates that he does not know:
  The signs and symptoms of respiratory allergy
  What causes the problem
  How to avoid allergic responses

Objective Data
- May exhibit behavior such as keeping the windows open during an episode of respiratory allergy

Related Data

Commonly Related Diseases
Hay fever, rose fever, allergic rhinitis

Data Analysis

Nursing Diagnosis
UNKNOWLEDGEABLE ABOUT RESPIRATORY ALLERGY: Being without sufficient information about the cause, effects, and treatment of an antibody–antigen reaction to substances inhaled through the respiratory system

Common Etiology (Stressors)
HEALTH CARE FACTORS: Lack of health instruction

PLANNING

Unmet Needs
Protection from physical harm, independence, increased learning

Expected Outcome
Correct verbal feedback of the information taught

NURSING INTERVENTIONS

Nursing Treatments
Approach unhurriedly
Encourage the person to ask questions
Discourage smoking (which irritates the respiratory system)

Nursing Observations
Determine teaching effectiveness by verbal feedback

Health Teaching
Describe those symptoms that should be reported (malaise, headache, itching nose or eyes)
Explain the causes of the health problem (an allergic response is precipitated in early spring by exposure to tree pollen; in early summer, by exposure to grass or weed pollen; in early fall, by exposure to ragweed pollen; and at any time, exposure to animal fur, dust particles, or feathers may precipitate a response that is usually worse on windy days)
Explain how to take allergy precautions (avoid perfumes, scented cosmetics, swimming underwater, dust, short-haired animals, insecticides, etc.)
Advise that the precipitating factor (pollen, animal hair, etc.) should be avoided
Explain how to interpret product contents listed on container labels (so chemicals can be avoided)
Inform of the therapies available for the specific condition (antihistamines, sensitivity testing and/or desensitizing)
Explain the reason for and intended effect of the therapy (to alleviate the histamine response)

EVALUATION
Record actual outcome

UNKNOWLEDGEABLE ABOUT SKIN ALLERGY[12,278,475,487]

ASSESSMENT

Data Collection

Subjective Data
- Person's discussion or questions indicate a need for additional information, clarification, or validation of information
  OR
- Person's lack of questions or comments indicates not wanting information or not knowing enough to seek information
- When questioned directly, the person's response or lack of response indicates that he does not know:
  The signs and symptoms of skin allergy
  What causes the problem
  How to avoid allergic responses

Objective Data
- May exhibit behavior such as using a harsh detergent that irritates the skin, or not wearing gloves when working with certain chemicals

Data Analysis

Nursing Diagnosis
UNKNOWLEDGEABLE ABOUT SKIN ALLERGY: Being without sufficient information about the cause, effects, and treatments of an antigen–antibody reaction following skin contact with irritating substances

Common Etiology (Stressors)
HEALTH CARE FACTORS: Lack of health instruction

PLANNING

Unmet Needs
Protection from physical harm, independence, increased learning

Expected Outcome
Correct verbal feedback of the information taught

NURSING INTERVENTIONS

Nursing Treatments
Approach unhurriedly
Encourage the person to ask questions

Nursing Observations
Determine teaching effectiveness by verbal feedback

Health Teaching
Describe those symptoms that should be reported (burning, stinging, itching skin, and signs such as edema, hives, rash, redness, scaling, or peeling)
Explain the causes of the health problem (contact with and irritation from plants; metals, especially mercury; plastics; dyes; and soaps)
Explain how to take allergy precautions (avoid scented cosmetics, long-haired animals, fuzzy blankets and clothing, high environmental temperatures)
Explain how to interpret product contents listed on container labels (to avoid chemical skin irritation)
Advise that the precipitating factor should be avoided
Inform of the therapies available for the specific condition (antihistamines, antipruritics, sensitivity testing and/or desensitizing)
Explain the reason for and intended effect of the therapy (to alleviate the histamine response)

EVALUATION
Record actual outcome

UNKNOWLEDGEABLE ABOUT SEXUALLY TRANSMITTED DISEASES[88,371]

ASSESSMENT
Data Collection

Subjective Data
• Person's discussion or questions indicate a need for additional information, clarification, or validation of information
    OR
• Person's lack of questions or comments indicates not wanting information or not knowing enough to seek information
• When questioned directly, the person's response or lack of response indicates that he does not know:
    The signs and symptoms of the diseases
    What causes the problem
    Methods of treatment and prevention

Objective Data
None

Data Analysis

Nursing Diagnosis
UNKNOWLEDGEABLE ABOUT SEXUALLY TRANSMITTED DISEASES: Being without sufficient information about diseases that are transmitted by sexual activity

Common Etiology (Stressors)
HEALTH CARE FACTORS: Lack of health instruction

PLANNING
Unmet Needs
Protection from physical harm, independence, increased learning

Expected Outcome
Correct verbal feedback of the information taught

NURSING INTERVENTIONS
Nursing Treatments
Approach unhurriedly
Encourage the person to ask questions
Provide an atmosphere of acceptance

Nursing Observations
Determine teaching effectiveness by verbal feedback

Health Teaching
Describe those symptoms that should be reported (emphasize that sexually transmitted disease should be reported immediately during pregnancy. *Gonorrhea*: Painful urination, white or clear discharge 3–9 days after sexual contact, lower abdominal pain.

Syphilis: Painless chancre, or sore, on the genitalia or a rash that disappears after several weeks but recurs. *Herpes genitalia*: Painful blisters on the genitalia 3–6 weeks after sexual contact. *Venereal warts*: Painless lumps on the genitalia 1–3 months after sexual contact)

Explain how venereal disease is transmitted (by sexual contact, to the fetus through the placenta or the infected birth canal, by kissing if there are lip lesions; also explain that it is not transmitted by toilet seats and that one venereal disease cannot change into another)

Inform that immunity does not occur with venereal infection (and that contraceptives do not prevent it or cause immunity)

Instruct to avoid direct contact with infected persons (there should be no sexual contact until therapy is complete and all symptoms have subsided)

Inform of the therapies available for the specific condition (*Gonorrhea, syphilis*: Penicillin. *Herpes genitalia*: Currently no treatment, but a new antibiotic is on the horizon. *Venereal warts*: Cauterization, freezing or surgical or chemical removal)

EVALUATION
Record actual outcome

Minor Health Problems Associated with the Integument

CONTUSSION[20,42,73]

ASSESSMENT
Data Collection
Subjective Data
• Aching pain (soreness, tenderness)

Objective Data
• Edema
• Skin discoloration (bruise or ecchymosis)
• Skin is not broken

Data Analysis
Nursing Diagnosis
CONTUSSION: The presence of blood and fluid in subcutaneous tissues as a result of tissue injury

Common Etiology (Stressors)
ENVIRONMENTAL FACTORS: *Blast/Explosion*: Exposure to. *Cataclysm*: Exposure to. *Crushing*: By cave-in, building collapse, falling object. *Foreign body*: Propelled. *Moving vehicles*: Impact or collision of. *Objects*: Blunt. *Tools*: Powered and nonpowered. *Weapons*: Club

MAJOR PATHOPHYSIOLOGIC FACTORS CAUSING THE PROBLEM: Although the skin is not penetrated by the injuring object, tissues beneath the skin are damaged

PLANNING

Unmet Needs

Comfort, protection from physical harm, increased learning

Expected Outcome

Immediate reduction or absence of swelling

Later, reduction of discoloration until the injured site becomes the natural skin color

Expressions of increased comfort

NURSING INTERVENTIONS

Nursing Treatments

Elevate the affected body part

Apply an ice bag (intermittently for the first 24 hours)

Apply a pressure dressing

Apply a heating pad

   OR

Apply a hot water bottle or hot pack (after the first 24 hours)

Nursing Observations

Inspect for (increased) edema

Test the skin for impaired feeling perception

Test motor function (in the injured extremity, finger or toe, by testing counter pressure in the flexion, extension, and lateral positions)

Inspect for impaired circulation

Palpate for arterial pulsations

Test for range of motion

Health Teaching

Teach how to apply cold therapy

Teach how to apply heat therapy

Explain the reason for and intended effect of the therapy (to reduce edema and promote healing)

EVALUATION

Record actual outcome

DECUBITUS ULCER[42,73,451]

ASSESSMENT

Data Collection

Subjective Data

• Aching pain (soreness, tenderness)

Objective Data

• Small or large area of redness

• Located on the buttocks or bony prominences

Serous fluid, pus, or bleeding sometimes

Raw appearances when severe

Data Analysis

Nursing Diagnosis
DECUBITUS ULCER (SKIN BREAKDOWN, BEDSORE): An area of broken skin tissue

Common Etiology (Stressors)
DISEASES: Cerebrovascular accident; diabetes mellitus; Guillain-Barré syndrome, multiple sclerosis, subarachnoid hemorrhage, subdural hematoma
INJURIES: Bone fracture, fracture and compression of the spinal cord
SIGNS AND SYMPTOMS: Immobility and paralysis (resulting from the above-mentioned diseases and injuries)
HEALTH CARE FACTORS: *Medical therapy:* Prolonged bed rest
MAJOR PATHOPHYSIOLOGIC FACTORS CAUSING THE PROBLEM: Prolonged pressure on tissue, chemical irritation, friction, or oxygen deficiency to tissue causes progressive destruction of cutaneous and underlying tissue

PLANNING

Unmet Needs
Tissue oxygenation or perfusion comfort, cleanliness, protection from physical harm, increased learning

Expected Outcome
Warm, moist, intact, natural color skin

NURSING INTERVENTIONS

Nursing Treatments
Clean with hydrogen peroxide
  OR
Clean with surgical soap
Apply a saline compress
  OR
Soak in saline solution
  OR
Place in a whirlpool bath (to promote circulation)
Apply tincture of benzoin (to the tissue around the ulcer)
Massage vigorously (the tissue around the ulcer)
Apply a sterile dressing
  OR
Expose the decubitus wound to air
Apply a heat lamp
  OR
Apply a heat cradle
Change the person's position frequently
Place on an alternating pressure mattress
  OR
Place on a CircOlectric bed
  OR
Place on a flotation mattress
  OR
Place on a Stryker frame
Place on a sheepskin
  OR
Place on a silicone pad
  OR
Place on a split-foam mattress
  OR
Place on a polyurethane foam pad
Place on sterile linens (if the decubitus ulcer is infected)
Refrain from giving local cold applications
Make a referral (to a physician if the decubitus ulcer requires skin grafting, etc.)

Nursing Observations

Inspect the skin for further breakdown
Observe for evidence of a favorable response to therapy

Health Teaching

Instruct to maintain skin cleanliness
Teach decubitus ulcer care (skin cleansing, turning, use of healing agents)
Explain the causes of the health problem (pressure, impaired circulation, friction)
Explain the reason for and intended effect of the therapy (increase circulation, promote healing)

EVALUATION

Record actual outcome

DIAPER DERMATITIS[433,527]

ASSESSMENT

Data Collection

Subjective Data
Infant irritability

Objective Data
• Infant is wearing cloth or disposable diapers
• Diffuse buttocks redness
  Blisters or pustules, sometimes

Data Analysis

Nursing Diagnosis
DIAPER DERMATITIS: Inflammation of an infant's skin from diaper irritation

Common Etiology (Stressors)
ENVIRONMENTAL FACTORS: *Chemical substances*: Harsh detergents used for washing diapers, allergenic chemicals or substances in disposable diapers
HUMAN ERROR: Infrequent changing of soiled diapers
MAJOR PATHOPHYSIOLOGIC FACTORS CAUSING THE PROBLEM: The ammonia in decomposing urine and in harsh detergents irritates the infant's tender skin, causing inflammation; the plastic coating on disposable diapers keeps the skin warm and moist by decreasing air circulation, making it susceptible to breakdown

PLANNING

Unmet Needs

Comfort, cleanliness, protection from physical harm, increased learning

Expected Outcome

Warm, dry, natural color skin
No observable rash

NURSING INTERVENTIONS

Nursing Treatments

Bathe in warm water
Clean the skin with antibacterial soap (Dial soap, once daily)
Change the wet diapers immediately (after they are soiled)
Dust the skin with medicated powder
  OR

Lubricate the skin with a protective ointment or cream (Desitin or A&D ointment or cream)

Maintain dry, clean skin (with the exception of lubrication)

Refrain from simultaneously powdering and lubricating the skin

Nursing Observations

Inspect for skin breakdown

Observe for evidence of a favorable response to therapy

Health Teaching

Instruct to maintain skin cleanliness

Instruct to maintain skin dryness

Advise limited use of powder on the infant's skin

Instruct to change wet diapers immediately

Explain how to wash diapers correctly (use mild soap, double rinse)

EVALUATION

Record actual outcome

DIETARY CAROTENEMIA [125,476]

ASSESSMENT

Data Collection

Subjective Data
• Person relates prolonged, high intake of yellow vegetables
• No history of liver disease

Objective Data
• No yellow discoloration of the conjunctiva
• Yellowing of the skin
• Normal liver studies (bilirubin, SGPT)

Data Analysis

Nursing Diagnosis
DIETARY CAROTENEMIA: A yellowing of skin following the ingestion of yellow foods

Common Etiology (Stressors)
ENVIRONMENTAL FACTORS: *Food substances*: Adverse effects of vegetables containing carotene such as carrots, squash, corn, oranges, peaches, apricots, leafy vegetables
HUMAN ERROR: Excessive intake of vegetables containing carotene
MAJOR PATHOPHYSIOLOGIC FACTORS CAUSING THE PROBLEM: An excessive intake of foods containing high levels of carotene results in carotene infiltration into tissue with skin yellowing

PLANNING

Unmet Needs

Protection from physical harm, increased learning

Expected Outcome

Normal skin color

Person verbalizes decreased intake of yellow foods

NURSING INTERVENTIONS

Nursing Treatments

Encourage decreased yellow fruit and vegetable intake

Nursing Observations

Observe for evidence of a favorable response to therapy

Health Teaching

Explain the causes of the health problem (excessive intake of the carotene-coloring agent)

Explain the reason for and intended effect of the therapy (to reduce the amount of carotene stored in the tissue)

EVALUATION

Record actual outcome

FOREIGN BODY IN THE SKIN[42,278]

ASSESSMENT

Data Collection

Subjective Data
• Burning or stabbing pain if near the skin surface
• Aching (soreness, tenderness) if in the muscle

Objective Data
• Visible or palpable foreign object in the skin
  Inflammation, sometimes

Data Analysis

Nursing Diagnosis
FOREIGN BODY IN THE SKIN: The presence of an injurious or harmful object in the skin

Common Etiology (Stressors)
ENVIRONMENTAL FACTORS: *Blast/Explosion*: Exposure to. *Cataclysm*: Exposure to. *Foreign body*: Propelled objects, dirt, dust, glass, metal, or wood particles
MAJOR PATHOPHYSIOLOGIC FACTORS CAUSING THE PROBLEM Foreign bodies penetrate the skin surface and are imbedded in subcutaneous tissue, and infection and inflammation often result

PLANNING

Unmet Needs

Comfort, cleanliness, protection from physical harm, increased learning

Expected Outcome

The absence of a foreign body in the skin
No later evidence of inflammation, purulent drainage, or elevated temperature
Person verbalizes increased comfort

NURSING INTERVENTIONS

Nursing Treatments

Clean with alcohol
  OR
Clean with surgical soap
Remove the foreign object (with a sterile needle or tweezers)
Soak in providone-iodine (Betadine) solution (and scrub clean)
Apply an antibiotic ointment
Apply a sterile dressing (if needed)
Make a referral (to a physician if the foreign object cannot be retrieved)

Nursing Observations

Test the skin for impaired feeling perception
Inspect the skin for color

Health Teaching

Instruct to maintain skin cleanliness

Explain the reason for and intended effect of the therapy (to prevent skin infection)

EVALUATION

Record actual outcome

HERPES SIMPLEX [88,433]

ASSESSMENT

Data Collection

Subjective Data
- Burning (stinging, smarting) pain
- Itching
  Malaise
  History of fever, common cold, gastritis, trauma, exposure to the sun

Objective Data
- A single group of vesicles on an erythematous base
- Lesions are around the mouth, nose, or genitalia
  Lymph node swelling and tenderness

Data Analysis

Nursing Diagnosis

HERPES SIMPLEX: An acute local viral infection with vesticular manifestations

Common Etiology (Stressors)

ENVIRONMENTAL FACTORS: *Biologic agents*: Viruses (*Herpevirus hominis*)

MAJOR PATHOPHYSIOLOGIC FACTORS CAUSING THE PROBLEM: The invasion of viruses into tissue causes tissue inflammation and eruptions; the virus becomes dormant in the cells and is activated again during periods of physical and emotional stress

PLANNING

Unmet Needs

Comfort, cleanliness, protection from physical harm, increased learning

Expected Outcome

No observable vesicles

Absence of palpable lymph nodes

Person verbalizes increased comfort

NURSING INTERVENTIONS

Nursing Treatments

Apply alcohol to the lesion (every hour until the lesion is dried; warn the person that alcohol causes a burning sensation)

   OR

Apply camphor to the lesion (Blistex, Campho-Phenique liquid)

Make a referral (to a physician for lesions near the eye or genitalia or for multiple lesions)

Nursing Observations

Observe for evidence of a favorable response to therapy

Health Teaching

Advise against piercing or squeezing the lesions

Explain the cause of the health problem (viruses)

EVALUATION

Record actual outcome

HERPES ZOSTER[88,278]

ASSESSMENT

Data Collection

Subjective Data
• History of having had chickenpox
• Burning or stabbing pain along a nerve pathway
• Lesion eruption 48 hours following the onset of the pain

Objective Data
• Clusters of vesicular lesions
• Lesions are unilateral, usually on the face or trunk
• Tender lymph nodes
  Slight fever

Data Analysis

Nursing Diagnosis
HERPES ZOSTER (SHINGLES): An acute viral infection along the course of a nerve

Common Etiology (Stressors)
ENVIRONMENTAL FACTORS: *Biologic agents*: Varicella virus
MAJOR PATHOPHYSIOLOGIC FACTORS CAUSING THE PROBLEM: The varicella virus, dormant in the body from an earlier episode of chickenpox, becomes activated for an unknown reason

PLANNING

Unmet Needs
Comfort, protection from physical harm, freedom from pain, increased learning

Expected Outcome
No observable vesicles
Absence of palpable lymph nodes
Body temperature of 96.8° F (36° C) to 99.5° F (37.5° C)
Person verbalizes increased comfort

NURSING INTERVENTIONS

Nursing Treatments
Apply calamine lotion
  OR
Apply zinc oxide to the lesions (Anusol or zinc oxide ointment)
Apply fine mesh gauze (to allow drying of the lesion and protection from clothing)
Apply an antibiotic ointment (bacitracin after the lesions are crusted)
Give nonprescription drugs (aspirin, acetaminophen for pain)
Make a referral (to a physician immediately if near the eye or if in severe pain)

Nursing Observations
Observe for evidence of a favorable response to therapy

Health Teaching
Advise against piercing or squeezing the lesions
Explain the cause of the health problem (activation of the chicken pox virus)
Describe those symptoms that should be reported (severe pain or lesions near the eye that could cause blindness)

EVALUATION
Record actual outcome

IMPETIGO [88,433]

ASSESSMENT

Data Collection

Subjective Data
- Itching
- Spreads rapidly

Objective Data
- Small vesicles to large bullae
- Honey-colored serous drainage
- Crusting
  Usually on the face

Data Analysis

Nursing Diagnosis
IMPETIGO: A bacterial skin infection manifested by macules, vesicles, and pustules

Common Etiology (Stressors)
ENVIRONMENTAL FACTORS: *Biologic agents*: Streptococci and staphylococci bacteria
MAJOR PATHOPHYSIOLOGIC FACTORS CAUSING THE PROBLEM: Bacteria under the fingernails, which is transmitted to the skin, causes infectious impetigo

PLANNING

Unmet Needs

Comfort, cleanliness, protection from physical harm, increased learning

Expected Outcome

No observable lesions, drainage, or crusting
Person verbalizes cessation of itching

NURSING INTERVENTIONS

Nursing Treatments

Bathe in warm water
Clean the skin with antibacterial soap (use Dial soap and scrub to remove crusts), or
Clean with hydrogen peroxide (to loosen crusts), or
Apply cool, moist compresses (of Domeboro's solution, potassium permanganate, to soak the crusts and dry the lesions)
Apply an antibiotic ointment (Neopolycin ointment for three days or until the lesions disappear)
Make a referral (to a physician if fever exists or the lesions persist; fever increases the risk of glomerulonephritis, and antibiotics are needed)

Nursing Observations

Monitor the oral temperature (for fever)
Monitor urine studies for evidence of urinary tract infection (bacteriuria, proteinuria, hematuria)
Observe for evidence of a favorable response to therapy

Health Teaching

Inform that cleanliness is basic to health
Instruct to limit direct contact with infected persons
Recommend the use of individual towels and washcloths
Explain the cause of the health problem (bacteria)
Describe those symptoms that should be reported (fever)

EVALUATION

Record actual outcome

INCISIONAL PAIN[42,371,451,625,626]

ASSESSMENT

Data Collection

Subjective Data
• Localized stabbing (knifelike, piercing, cutting) pain around the incisional area
• Continuous for the first 48 hours, intermittent thereafter
• Very severe for the first 48 hours, especially following abdominal or thoracic surgery, felt even though the person sleeps; after the first 48 hours, pain may be mild, moderate, or severe; if infection exists, the pain will remain severe after the first 48 hours
• Increased anxiety

Objective Data
Crying
Moaning
Tendency to remain motionless from severe pain
Restless when attempting to find a comfortable position
Facial wincing
Complaints of pain
Flexes the kness (if the incision is abdominal)
Stoops the shoulders (when standing)

Data Analysis

Nursing Diagnosis
INCISIONAL PAIN: A distressful hurting occurring in an area where body tissues have been cut for reasons of surgical intervention or by accidental injury

Common Etiology (Stressors)
HEALTH CARE FACTORS: *Surgical incision*: Any
MAJOR PATHOPHYSIOLOGIC FACTORS CAUSING THE PROBLEM: Cutting into body tissues causes cell and tissue receptors to carry irritation stimuli by way of the nerves and spinal cord to the thalamus, the perception of pain occurs in the cerebral cortex; incisions across the muscle cause greater and more prolonged pain than incisions longitudinally in the muscle

PLANNING

Unmet Needs
Sleep, rest, relaxation, comfort, protection from physical harm, freedom from pain, increased learning

Expected Outcome
Person verbalizes increased comfort
No incisional inflammation

NURSING INTERVENTIONS

Nursing Treatments
Approach unhurriedly
Anticipate needs
Handle gently
Provide frequent contact with the person
Communicate nurse sensitivity to the person's pain
Reassure that the pain will subside or be relieved
Ask the person what makes him comfortable
Position comfortably
Change the person's position gradually
Place a pillow on the affected side (for support)
Splint the incisional area

Massage gently (for the relaxation effect)
   OR
Bathe in warm water
Discuss possible pain-reducing measures
Provide a pain-relief measure of the person's choice
Refrain from giving oral analgesics (the first 48 hours for abdominal incisions)
Give nonprescription drugs (when the pain intensity is less severe)
Offer assurance of other measures if the pain-relief method fails
Refrain from equating sleep with the absence of pain
Provide quiet
Encourage adequate rest
Refrain from performing nonessential procedures

Nursing Observations
Estimate the degree of pain experienced
Evaluate the pain for intensity and quality
Evaluate the effectiveness of the pain-relief measures
Observe for nonverbal communication of pain
Observe for evidence of a favorable response to therapy

Health Teaching
Describe those symptoms that should be reported (increased pain)
Explain that immobility related to pain causes increased pain
Explain that there are nondrug methods available for pain relief (such as heat, cold, positioning)
Explain the causes of the pain (tissue damage)
Explain the reason for the delay in giving a pain-relief drug (if a delay is necessary)

Medical Treatments Performed by Nurses
Give the prescribed drugs

EVALUATION

Record actual outcome

INFANTILE SEBORRHEIC DERMATITIS[88,433]

ASSESSMENT

Data Collection

Subjective Data
Scalp irritation

Objective Data
• Thick, yellow-crusted lesions on the scalp and behind the ears
• Scaling or shedding of the skin

Data Analysis

Nursing Diagnosis
INFANTILE SEBORRHEIC DERMATITIS (CRADLE CAP): A collection of vernix caseosa on the infant's scalp

Common Etiology (Stressors)
HUMAN ERROR: Withholding hygiene in order to avoid injuring the infant's soft spot (fontanelle)
MAJOR PATHOPHYSIOLOGIC FACTORS CAUSING THE PROBLEM: As oil collects on the scalp, it forms thick crusts and irritates the scalp

PLANNING

Unmet Needs
Comfort, cleanliness, protection from physical harm, increased learning

Expected Outcome
A clean, nonscaling infant scalp

NURSING INTERVENTIONS

Nursing Treatments
Shampoo the scalp (daily, with Fostex soap or Cradol shampoo)
Brush the infant's hair with a soft hairbrush

Nursing Observations
Observe for evidence of a favorable response to therapy

Health Teaching
Explain the causes of the health problem (poor hygiene, oil on the scalp)
Inform that cleanliness is basic to health
Explain how to shampoo the scalp
Advise frequent hair brushing
Explain the reason for and intended effect of the therapy (scalp cleanliness)

EVALUATION

Record actual outcome

INGROWING NAIL[362,433]

ASSESSMENT

Data Collection

Subjective Data
• Aching (soreness, tenderness) around the nail bed
  Painful walking if the ingrown nail is on the toe

Objective Data
• Nail margin penetrates the skin
• Redness
• Swelling

Data Analysis

Nursing Diagnosis
INGROWING NAIL: Nail tissue growing over its edges and pressing into soft skin tissue

Common Etiology (Stressors)
HUMAN ERROR: Wearing improperly fitting shoes, incorrect trimming of the nails
MAJOR PATHOPHYSIOLOGIC FACTORS CAUSING THE PROBLEM: Prolonged pressure on the nail distorts the direction of nail growth, particularly when the nail has been trimmed back into the nail corner

PLANNING

Unmet Needs
Comfort, cleanliness, protection from physical harm, increased learning

Expected Outcome
Normal skin color around the nail
Person verbalizes increased comfort

NURSING INTERVENTIONS

Nursing Treatments

Clean with hydrogen peroxide

OR

Clean with surgical soap

OR

Soak in saline solution

Apply an antibiotic ointment (Neopolycin, Mycitracin ointment)

Pack sterile cotton between the ingrown nail and the skin

Nursing Observations

Inspect for inflammation

Observe for evidence of a favorable response to therapy

Health Teaching

Explain the causes of the health problem (skin pressure on the nail)

Inform that cleanliness is basic to health

Instruct to cut the toenails straight across

Instruct to wear well-fitting shoes

Recommend closed shoes for foot protection

Describe those symptoms that should be reported (inflammation, severe pain)

EVALUATION

Record actual outcome

INSECT BITE[22,42]

ASSESSMENT

Data Collection

Subjective Data

• Burning (stinging, smarting) or stabbing (piercing, pricking) pain
  Itching

Objective Data

• Redness
• Swelling
  Single or clustered lesions

Related Data

• Bite was inflicted by a bee, wasp, yellor jacket, mosquito, or fly

Data Analysis

Nursing Diagnosis

INSECT BITE: A wound inflicted by a small invertebrate animal

Common Etiology (Stressors)

ENVIRONMENTAL FACTORS: *Biologic agents*: Bite of an insect

MAJOR PATHOPHYSIOLOGIC FACTORS CAUSING THE PROBLEM: Insect stings and bites release venom or enzymes into the skin; local reactions (urticarial-type lesions) are due to hypersensitivity to the proteins in the venom or enzymes

PLANNING

Unmet Needs

Comfort, cleanliness, protection from physical harm, freedom from pain, increased learning

Expected Outcome
Person expresses increased comfort
No later evidence of wound inflammation, purulent drainage, or elevated temperature

NURSING INTERVENTIONS

Nursing Treatments
Apply a cold, moist compress, or
Apply an ice bag or cold pack, or
Apply sodium bicarbonate (baking soda) to the skin (in paste form)
   OR
Apply a tenderizer paste to the lesion
Clean with alcohol
   OR
Clean with antiseptic solution
   OR
Clean with surgical soap
Elevate the extremity
Give nonprescription drugs (analgesics)
Remove the insect stinger (using a scraping motion)

Nursing Observations
Inspect for bleeding, edema and inflammation
Observe for complaints of itching
Observe for shock (anaphylactic shock)

Health Teaching
Explain the reason for and intended effect of the therapy (to promote comfort and prevent infection)

EVALUATION
Record actual outcome

JAUNDICE[42,499]

ASSESSMENT

Data Collection

Subjective Data
• Itching, often intense
• Dryness

Objective Data
• Yellow skin accompanied by yellow sclera
• Increased serum bilirubin
• Increased urine urobilinogen
  Scaling of the skin
  Scratch marks

Data Analysis

Nursing Diagnosis
JAUNDICE: A yellow condition of the skin in which bile pigment infiltrates and irritates the skin

Common Etiology (Stressors)
BIRTH DEFECTS: Premature infant
DISEASES: Cholecystitis, cholelithiasis, hemolytic jaundice, hepatitis

MAJOR PATHOPHYSIOLOGIC FACTORS CAUSING THE PROBLEM: Abnormally high-bilirubin pigments in the blood result from such conditions as liver dysfunction, excessive red blood cell destruction, ABO and Rh blood incompatibility, or biliary obstruction and cause yellow staining of the skin

PLANNING

Unmet Needs
Fluid and electrolyte balance, comfort, protection from physical harm, increased learning

Expected Outcome
Normal skin and sclera color
Normal serum bilirubin and urine urobilinogen

NURSING INTERVENTIONS

Nursing Treatments
Apply calamine lotion
   OR
Apply cornstarch to the skin
   OR
Apply sodium bicarbonate (baking soda) to the skin
Bathe in cool water
Lubricate the skin with baby oil, bath oil, or body lotion
Dress in minimum clothing
Increase fluid intake to about 2,000 cc daily
Maintain adequate atmospheric humidity (to minimize skin dryness)
Maintain a cool room temperature
Expose the skin to sunlight (which will decrease the yellow discoloration)

Nursing Observations
Observe for evidence of a favorable response to therapy

Health Teaching
Advise against scratching (which increases irritation)
Explain the causes of the health problem (high levels of bilirubin in the blood)

Medical Treatments Performed by Nurses
Administer phototherapy treatment

EVALUATION

Record actual outcome

MILIARIA [42,433]

ASSESSMENT

Data Collection

Subjective Data
• Itching
• Burning (stinging, smarting)

Objective Data
• Small, localized, pinpoint-sized vesicles or papules
• Distributed over the neck, back, chest, sides of the trunk, abdomen, and body folds
  Redness of the involved skin area

Data Analysis

Nursing Diagnosis

MILIARIA (PRICKLY HEAT): Obstruction of the sweat glands resulting in vesicles on the skin

Common Etiology (Stressors)

ENVIRONMENTAL FACTORS: *Environmental heat*: High external temperature. *Humidity*: High environmental humidity

HUMAN ERROR: Overdressing an infant in excessively warm clothing

MAJOR PATHOPHYSIOLOGIC FACTORS CAUSING THE PROBLEM: Excessive skin warmth combined with inadequate circulation of air cause increased amounts of perspiration and softening of skin oils, resulting in obstruction and inflammation of the sweat glands

PLANNING

Unmet Needs

Normal temperature, comfort, protection from physical harm, increased learning

Expected Outcome

No observable lesions on the body

Cessation of scratching

NURSING INTERVENTIONS

Nursing Treatments

Dress in lightweight clothing

Maintain a normal room temperature

OR

Maintain a cool room temperature

Dust the skin with medicated powder (small amounts of zinc oxide talcum powder)

OR

Apply calamine lotion

OR

Apply a cool, moist compress (of Burrow's solution or potassium permanganate, Domeboro's solution; these are astringents)

Do not allow skin surfaces to touch

Nursing Observations

Observe for evidence of a favorable response to therapy

Health Teaching

Recommend the use of lightweight clothing (for the infant instead of overdressing the infant for warmth)

Advise against (infant) exposure to intense heat

Advise against piercing or squeezing lesions

Advise limited use of powder on the infant's skin

Instruct to maintain skin dryness

EVALUATION

Record actual outcome

NONVENOMOUS SNAKEBITE[20,22,42,219]

ASSESSMENT

Data Collection

Subjective Data

• Stabbing (piercing, sharp) pain

Objective Data
* No fang marks on the skin
  Minimal swelling within 30 minutes
  Teeth marks, sometimes

Data Analysis

Nursing Diagnosis
NONVENOMOUS SNAKEBITE: A skin wound inflicted by a nonpoisonous snake

Common Etiology (Stressors)
ENVIRONMENTAL FACTORS: *Biologic agents*: Bite of a snake, specifically nonpoisonous snakes
MAJOR PATHOPHYSIOLOGIC FACTORS CAUSING THE PROBLEM: The bite of a nonpoisonous snake is similar to that of a small animal; no venom is injected into the wound, but a local inflammatory reaction occurs and sometimes a bacterial infection develops

PLANNING

Unmet Needs
Comfort, cleanliness, protection from physical harm, freedom from pain, increased learning

Expected Outcome
Reduced swelling at the site of the bite
No later evidence of wound inflammation, purulent drainage, or elevated temperature
Person verbalizes increased comfort

NURSING INTERVENTIONS

Nursing Treatments
Clean with alcohol
   OR
Clean with antiseptic solution
   OR
Clean with surgical soap
Apply an antibiotic ointment
Apply a sterile dressing
Encourage adequate rest
Give nonprescription drugs (analgesics)
Make a referral (to a physician)
   OR
Consult with a physician (if needed)

Nursing Observations
Monitor the blood pressure
Palpate the pulse for rate, rhythm, and volume
Inspect the chest for respiratory rate and rhythm
Monitor the oral temperature (for fever)
Inspect for inflammation
Observe for complaints of pain

Health Teaching
Explain the reason for and intended effect of the therapy

Medical Treatments Performed by Nurses
Give the prescribed drugs (antibiotics to prevent infection, tetanus toxoid to prevent tetanus)

EVALUATION
Record actual outcome

NONVENOMOUS SPIDER BITE[20,22,42,219]

ASSESSMENT

Data Collection

Subjective Data
• Stabbing (piercing, sharp) pain

Objective Data
• Local swelling
• Redness

Related Data
Spider may or may not be present

Data Analysis

Nursing Diagnosis
NONVENOMOUS SPIDER BITE: A skin wound inflicted by a nonpoisonous arachnid

Common Etiology (Stressors)
ENVIRONMENTAL FACTORS: *Biologic agents*: Bite of an insect, specifically the spider
MAJOR PATHOPHYSIOLOGIC FACTORS CAUSING THE PROBLEM: When the insect penetrates the surface of the skin, it injects venom into the body; with nontoxic venom, the effect is local, with mild inflammation

PLANNING

Unmet Needs
Comfort, cleanliness, protection from physical harm, freedom from pain, increased learning

Expected Outcome
Reduced swelling at the site of the bite
No later evidence of wound inflammation, purulent drainage, or elevated temperature
Person verbalizes increased comfort

NURSING INTERVENTIONS

Nursing Treatments
Apply a cold, moist compress
  OR
Apply an ice bag or ice pack
Clean with antiseptic solution
  OR
Clean with hydrogen peroxide
  OR
Clean with surgical soap
Apply sodium bicarbonate (baking soda) to the skin
  OR
Apply calamine lotion

Nursing Observations
Inspect for bleeding, edema, and inflammation
Observe for shock (anaphylactic shock)
Observe for complaints of pain

Health Teaching
Explain the reason for and intended effect of the therapy (to promote comfort and prevent infection)

EVALUATION
Record actual outcome

PEDICULOSIS[88,278,159]

ASSESSMENT

Data Collection

Subjective Data
• Itching

Objective Data
• Presence of small, crawling organisms (lice) on the body
• Presence of small white objects (nits) attached to the hair
• Found in the head, chest, axillary and genital hair and in the beard, eyebrows, and eyelashes
  Skin excoriation when scratching is intense

Data Analysis

Nursing Diagnosis
PEDICULOSIS: A parasitic infestation of the skin

Common Etiology (Stressors)
LIFESTYLE: Lack of hygiene
ENVIRONMENTAL FACTORS: *Biologic agents*: Exposure to lice. *Housing*: Overcrowding
MAJOR PATHOPHYSIOLOGIC FACTORS CAUSING THE PROBLEM: Following contact, the lice infest the hair and quickly multiply; they are then transmitted to others by contact with persons, linens, bathroom facilities

PLANNING

Unmet Needs
Comfort, cleanliness, protection from physical harm, increased learning

Expected Outcome
No observable parasites or nits on the body
Clean body hair
Person verbalizes increased comfort

NURSING INTERVENTIONS

Nursing Treatments
Apply nonprescription drugs (RID liquid pediculicide, A-200 Pyrinate liquid or liquid gel)
Shampoo the hair (frequently)
Brush and comb the hair (two or three times daily)
Maintain dry, clean linen (especially pillowcases)
Wash the brush and comb with a parasiticide

Nursing Observations
Observe for evidence of a favorable response to therapy
Inspect the hair for abnormalities (infestation, periodically)

Health Teaching
Explain the causes of the health problem (poor hygiene, lice)
Instruct to avoid direct contact with infested persons
Instruct to inspect the hair (if in contact with persons who are infested)
Explain how to remove hair lice (moistening the hair with warm vinegar and combing out the lice with a fine-tooth comb, shampooing, etc.)
Explain how to shampoo the hair (with a parasiticide)
Instruct to maintain scalp cleanliness
Explain the importance of individual use of a comb and brush
Recommend the use of individual towels and washcloths

Inform that clean linens are essential

Medical Treatments Performed by Nurses

Apply the prescribed drug (Kwell shampoo, a parasiticide)

EVALUATION

Record actual outcome

POISON IVY/POISON OAK DERMATITIS[42,278,476]

ASSESSMENT

Data Collection

Subjective Data
- Exposure to poison ivy or oak from several hours to days before onset
- Itching
  Burning (stinging, smarting) pain

Objective Data
- Small clusters of blisters surrounded by redness
  Oozing and crusting after the blisters rupture

Data Analysis

Nursing Diagnosis
POISON IVY/POISON OAK DERMATITIS: A skin irritation following contact with plants

Common Etiology (Stressors)
ENVIRONMENTAL FACTORS: *Plants*: Poison ivy, poison oak, poison sumac
MAJOR PATHOPHYSIOLOGIC FACTORS CAUSING THE PROBLEM: Resins of the poison ivy plant irritate the skin causing tissue injury

PLANNING

Unmet Needs
Comfort, protection from physical harm, increased learning

Expected Outcome
No observable blisters, inflammation, oozing or crusting
Person verbalizes increased comfort

NURSING INTERVENTIONS

Nursing Treatments
Bathe in warm water (washing the skin thoroughly with soap)
Expose the lesions to air
Apply cool, moist compress (of potassium permangenate, Domeboro's solution, intermittently)
  OR
Apply a cortisone ointment (Cortaid)
Make a referral (to a physician if the condition is severe or near the eyes)

Nursing Observations
Observe for evidence of a favorable response to therapy

Health Teaching
Emphasize that contaminated clothing should be changed immediately (and washed thoroughly to remove the oil from the poison ivy plant)

Advise against piercing or squeezing lesions

Advise against scratching (which irritates the skin and spreads the resin, creating new lesions)

Advise not to take hot baths (which stimulate itching)

Explain the cause of the health problem (irritation of the oil from the plant)

EVALUATION

Record actual outcome

PRURITIS [88,433]

ASSESSMENT

Data Collection

Subjective Data
* Itching
  Itching confined to the legs (winter pruritis)

Objective Data
* Skin feels dry
* Scratching
  Redness or excoriation
  Restlessness

Data Analysis

Nursing Diagnosis

PRURITIS: An itching skin sensation that induces scratching

Common Etiology (Stressors)

DISEASES: Allergic disorder, contact dermatitis, diabetes mellitus, Hodgkin's disease, Laennec's cirrhosis, leukemia, lymphoblastoma, mycosis fungoides, seborrhea dermatitis, tinea, urticaria

SIGNS AND SYMPTOMS: Dehydration, uremia

PSYCHOSOCIAL FACTORS: Excessive emotional excitement

HUMAN BODY: *Body state*: Pregnancy

HEALTH CARE FACTORS: *Drugs*: Adverse effects of drugs. *Medical therapy*: Casting. *Surgical therapy*: Ingrowing hair following presurgical prep

LIFESTYLE: Lack of hygiene

ENVIRONMENTAL FACTORS: *Biologic agents*: Exposure to animals, insects. *Chemical substances*: Disinfectants, household cleaning agents, industrial chemicals or solvents, paints or varnishes, pesticides. *Humidity*: Low environmental humidity

MAJOR PATHOPHYSIOLOGIC FACTORS CAUSING THE PROBLEM: Irritation to the epidermal nerve endings stimulates an itching sensation

PLANNING

Unmet Needs

Comfort, protection from physical harm, increased learning

Expected Outcome

Clean, moist, normal color skin

No observable scratching

Person verbalizes increased comfort

NURSING INTERVENTIONS

Nursing Treatments

General Interventions for Pruritis
Bathe in cool water
> OR

Apply a cold, moist compress
> OR

Bathe in warm water (to soften stubby hairs after a presurgical preparation)
Apply calamine lotion
> OR

Apply cornstarch to the skin
> OR

Apply sodium bicarbonate (baking soda) to the skin
> OR

Dust the skin with medicated powder
Do not allow skin surfaces to touch
Apply a bed cradle
Cover with lightweight blankets
Dress in lightweight clothing (made of soft material)
Dress in minimum clothing
Avoid using rough-textured bed linens
Decrease drafts
Lubricate the skin with baby oil, bath oil, or body lotion
> OR

Lubricate the skin with petrolatum
Maintain adequate admospheric humidity
Maintain a cool room temperature
Refrain from local heat applications
Use paper or transparent tape instead of adhesive on the skin
Refrain from using an alkaline soap on the skin
Give nonprescription drugs (an antihistamine)
Apply an analgesic ointment (if the itching is severe)
Apply a cortisone ointment (Cortaid)
Withhold any drugs (causing the pruritis)

Specific for Winter Pruritis
Bathe in warm (not hot) water
Clean with castile or lanolin soap (such as Dove, Ivory, Oilatum)
Lubricate the skin with baby oil, bath oil (Nivea, Alpha-Keri) or body lotion (Nivea skin
   oil or cream, Keri lotion, Nutraderm, Lubriderm)
> OR

Lubricate the skin with petrolatum
> OR

Apply a cortisone ointment (Cortaid)

Nursing Observations
Observe for evidence of a favorable response to therapy

Health Teaching
Advise not to take hot baths (which stimulates itching)
Instruct to decrease the frequency of bathing (to every second or third day for winter's
   itch or aging skin)
Advise against scratching (which stimulates itching)
Explain the causes of the health problem (skin irritation from foreign agents)

EVALUATION
Record actual outcome

SCABIES [88,278]

ASSESSMENT

Data Collection

Subjective Data
• Nocturnal itching
  Entire family may complain

Objective Data
• Generalized excoriations
• Vesicles and pustules on the sides of the fingers and heels of the palms
• Mites are visible microscopically

Data Analysis

Nursing Diagnosis
SCABIES: A mite infestation of the skin

Common Etiology (Stressors)
LIFESTYLE: Lack of hygiene
ENVIRONMENTAL FACTORS: *Biologic agents*: Mites
MAJOR PATHOPHYSIOLOGIC FACTORS CAUSING THE PROBLEM: Following contact, mites infest the
  skin and rapidly multiply

PLANNING

Unmet Needs
Comfort, cleanliness, protection from physical harm, increased learning

Expected Outcome
No mites on microscopic visualization of a skin scraping
No visible lesions on the skin
Person verbalizes increased comfort

NURSING INTERVENTIONS

Nursing Treatments
Provide clean clothing (for all family members)
Maintain dry, clean linen
Apply nonprescription drugs (Vleminckx solution)

Nursing Observations
Observe for evidence of a favorable response to therapy

Health Teaching
Inform that cleanliness is basic to health (for all family members)
Emphasize that contaminated clothing should be changed immediately (and boiled or
  discarded)
Instruct to limit direct contact with infested persons
Recommend the use of individual towels and washcloths
Inform that clean linens are essential

Medical Treatments Performed by Nurses
Apply the prescribed drug (Kwell or Eurax cream or lotion)

EVALUATION

Record actual outcome

SEBORRHEIC DERMATITIS[88,476]

ASSESSMENT

Data Collection

Subjective Data
• Itching
  Scalp irritation

Objective Data
• White, flaky, powdery scales scattered loosely in the hair (dry dandruff)
• Slightly yellow, sticky scales clinging to the scalp in patches (oily dandruff)
• Yellow-red scaling papules may appear at the hair line, behind the ears, in the external
  ear canal, or on the bridge of the nose

Data Analysis

Nursing Diagnosis
SEBORRHEIC DERMATITIS (DANDRUFF): A crust formation or scaling on the scalp

Common Etiology (Stressors)
DISEASES: Hypothyroidism
LIFESTYLE: High-fat or high-carbohydrate intake, lack of hygiene
ENVIRONMENTAL FACTORS: *Environmental cold*: Low external temperature
MAJOR PATHOPHYSIOLOGIC FACTORS CAUSING THE PROBLEM: The shedding of dry tissue from the
  epidermis causes scaling from the scalp

PLANNING

Unmet Needs
Comfort, stimulation, cleanliness, protection from physical harm, increased learning

Expected Outcome
A clean, nonscaling scalp
No observable scratching
Person verbalizes increased comfort

NURSING INTERVENTIONS

Nursing Treatments
Massage (the scalp) vigorously
Shampoo the hair (with DSH zinc dandruff shampoo)
Comb the dandruff up from the scalp

Nursing Observations
Inspect for dehydration
Observe for evidence of a favorable response to therapy

Health Teaching
Explain the causes of the health problem (poor hygiene, overproductive sebaceous
  glands)
Inform that cleanliness is basic to health
Advise against prolonged scalp exposure to the sun and the water
Advise against exposure to inclement (cold) weather (all of which cause scalp dryness)
Explain the importance of individual use of a comb and brush
Instruct to comb the dandruff up from the scalp
Teach the principles of good nutrition (fewer fats and carbohydrates)

EVALUATION

Record actual outcome

SKIN SLOUGHING[371,433]

ASSESSMENT

Data Collection

Subjective Data
• No sensation in the necrotic area
• Aching (tenderness, soreness) in tissue adjacent to the necrotic tissue

Objective Data
• Presence of necrotic tissue
• Skin cracks and separates from the wound edges, leaving skin patches in the middle

Data Analysis

Nursing Diagnosis
SKIN SLOUGHING: The separation of necrotic tissue from living tissue

Common Etiology (Stressors)
DISEASES: Phlebothrombosis
INJURIES: Burn wound
HEALTH CARE FACTORS: *Drug therapy*: Infiltration of drugs into tissue
MAJOR PATHOPHYSIOLOGIC FACTORS CAUSING THE PROBLEM: Tissue cell death results from severe injury, ischemia, infection, or inflammation; as the burned skin dries, a stiff skin-slough forms from coagulated protein; bacterial autolysis initiates the skin's separation from the wound

PLANNING

Unmet Needs

Comfort, cleanliness, protection from physical harm, increased learning

Expected Outcome

Healed, intact skin
Warm, moist, natural color skin

NURSING INTERVENTIONS

Nursing Treatments

Clean with hydrogen peroxide
    OR
Clean with surgical soap
Apply a saline compress
    OR
Soak in saline solution
    OR
Place in a whirlpool bath (to remove the necrotic tissue)
Apply an antibiotic ointment
Apply a sterile dressing
    OR
Expose the wound to air
Do not allow skin surfaces to touch
Maintain adequate atmospheric humidity (40–50% for burns)
Maintain a normal room temperature
Place on sterile linens
Refrain from giving local cold applications

Nursing Observations

Observe for evidence of a favorable response to therapy

Health Teaching

Advise against pulling off dead skin or scabs
Instruct to maintain skin cleanliness

Explain the causes of the health problem (ischemia, infection, inflammation)
Explain the reason for and intended effect of the therapy

EVALUATION

Record actual outcome

SKIN ULCER[42,433,451,499]

ASSESSMENT

Data Collection

Subjective Data
Burning (stinging, smarting) pain if the ulcer is superficial
Aching (soreness, tenderness) if the ulcer extends into the muscle

Objective Data
• Crater appearance
• Deep redness, raw appearance
• Drainage of serous fluid, pus, or blood

Data Analysis

Nursing Diagnosis
SKIN ULCER: The presence of an open sore on the skin tissue

Common Etiology (Stressors)
INJURY: Trauma of any kind that penetrates the skin
ENVIRONMENTAL FACTORS: *Biologic agents*: Viruses, bacteria, fungi. *Chemical substances*: Acids, alkalis
MAJOR PATHOPHYSIOLOGIC FACTORS CAUSING THE PROBLEM: Irritation or infection of the skin destroys tissue, causing ulceration

PLANNING

Unmet Needs
Comfort, cleanliness, protection from physical harm, increased learning

Expected Outcome
Healed, intact skin
Warm, moist, natural color skin
Person verbalizes increased comfort

NURSING INTERVENTIONS

Nursing Treatments
Clean with hydrogen peroxide
   OR
Clean with surgical soap
Apply a warm, moist compress
   OR
Soak in saline solution
Apply an antibiotic ointment
Apply a sterile dressing
   OR
Expose the wound to air

Nursing Observations
Observe for evidence of a favorable response to therapy

Health Teaching
Advise against pulling off scabs (as the healing occurs)
Explain the causes of the health problem (microorganisms or trauma)
Explain the reason for and intended efect of the therapy (to promote healing)

EVALUATION
Record actual outcome

STASIS ULCER[42,433]

ASSESSMENT
Data Collection
Subjective Data
* Aching (soreness, tenderness)
  OR
* Burning (stinging, smarting) in the early stages of ulceration
* Painless sensation in the late stages of ulceration
  Itching around the ulcer borders

Objective Data
* A deep crater appearance
* Black, cyanotic tissue
  Usually seen on the foot or leg
  Pus drainage
  Inflammation

Data Analysis
Nursing Diagnosis
STASIS ULCER: An open sore on a skin area having impaired circulation

Common Etiology (Stressors)
DISEASES: Arteriosclerosis, atherosclerosis, diabetes mellitus, Raynaud's disease, thrombo-phlebitis, varicose veins
INJURIES: Burn wound
SIGNS AND SYMPTOMS: Edema
ENVIRONMENTAL FACTORS: *Biologic agents*: Bacteria
MAJOR PATHOPHYSIOLOGIC FACTORS CAUSING THE PROBLEM: Tissue is destroyed by trauma, impaired blood flow to tissue, and infection that causes ulceration

PLANNING
Unmet Needs
Circulation, rest, comfort, cleanliness, protection from physical harm, increased learning

Expected Outcome
Healed, intact skin
Warm, moist, natural color skin
Person verbalizes increased comfort

NURSING INTERVENTIONS
Nursing Treatments
Clean with hydrogen peroxide
  OR
Clean with surgical soap
Apply a saline compress
  OR
Soak in saline solution

Apply an antibiotic ointment
Apply a sterile dressing
   OR
Expose the wound to air
Apply a heat lamp (if the arterial circulation is adequate)
   OR
Apply a heat cradle
Elevate the affected body part (and rest the involved extremity as much as possible)
Refrain from giving local cold applications

Nursing Observations
Observe for evidence of a favorable response to therapy

Health Teaching
Explain the need to avoid mechanical trauma
Inform that cleanliness is essential to infection prevention
Explain the causes of the health problem (ischemia, trauma)
Explain the reason for and intended effect of the therapy (to promote healing)

EVALUATION

Record actual outcome

SUBUNGUAL HEMORRHAGE[476]

ASSESSMENT

Data Collection

Subjective Data
• Throbbing (pounding, pulsating) nail pain

Objective Data
• Bluish nail color

Data Analysis

Nursing Diagnosis
SUBUNGUAL HEMORRHAGE: The presence of blood and fluid under the nail following tissue
   injury

Common Etiology (Stressors)
INJURIES: Contussion of the nail
ENVIRONMENTAL FACTORS: *Machinery*: Farm or industrial. *Tools*: Powered and nonpowered
HUMAN ERROR: Catching a finger in a door or tight place
MAJOR PATHOPHYSIOLOGIC FACTORS CAUSING THE PROBLEM: When severe pressure is placed on
   a finger or toe nail, the capillaries beneath the nail burst and the oozing blood cannot
   escape from beneath the nail; the increased pressure beneath the nail causes pain

PLANNING

Unmet Needs
Comfort, cleanliness, protection from physical harm, increased learning

Expected Outcome
Pink nail color
Person verbalizes increased comfort

NURSING INTERVENTIONS

Nursing Treatments
Clean (the nail) with alcohol
Pierce the nail with a nail drill and express the blood
Give nonprescription drugs (analgesics for pain)

Nursing Observations

Test for range of motion (of the finger)

Inspect for inflammation

Evaluate the effectiveness of the pain-relief measures

Health Teaching

Explain the reason for and intended effect of the therapy (to reduce the pressure under the fingernail)

Instruct to elevate the hand (if throbbing occurs)

EVALUATION

Record actual outcome

TICK BITE[42,278]

ASSESSMENT

Data Collection

Subjective Data

• Intense itching

• Painless

  Person is unaware of the burrowed tick, unless the person sees the tick

Objective Data

• Localized edema

  Ascending paralysis (if the bite is by an *Ixodidae pilosus* tick)

  Examination reveals the tick burrowed into the skin

Related Data

Commonly Related Diseases

Rocky Mountain spotted fever, tularemia

Data Analysis

Nursing Diagnosis

TICK BITE: A wound inflicted by a tick

Common Etiology (Stressors)

ENVIRONMENTAL FACTORS: *Biologic agents*: Bite of an insect (a tick)

MAJOR PATHOPHYSIOLOGIC FACTORS CAUSING THE PROBLEM: Ticks pierce the skin in order to feed on blood; many species introduce saliva, which causes a serious local irritation; the *Ixodidae pilosus* tick introduces saliva that produces an ascending paralysis; prompt removal of the tick usually results in recovery; respiratory paralysis may develop when the tick is allowed to remain in place; some ticks transmit Rocky Mountain spotted fever

PLANNING

Unmet Needs

Comfort, cleanliness, protection from physical harm, freedom from pain, increased learning

Expected Outcome

No portion of tick's head remains in the wound

Reduced swelling at the site of the bite

No later evidence of wound inflammation, purulent drainage, or elevated temperature

Person verbalizes increased comfort

NURSING INTERVENTIONS
Nursing Treatments
Apply a greasy substance over the tick
  OR
Place a smoldering match on the imbedded tick
Remove the tick with tweezers
Apply a cold, moist compress (to the wound)
Clean with antiseptic solution
  OR
Clean with surgical soap
Elevate the extremity

Nursing Observations
Observe for complaints of chills, headache, malaise, (muscle) weakness
Inspect for bleeding, edema, and inflammation
Monitor the oral temperature (for fever)
Inspect the chest for respiratory rate and rhythm

Health Teaching
Describe those symptoms that should be reported (chills, headache, malaise)

EVALUATION

Record actual outcome

TINEA [87,278,476]

ASSESSMENT
Data Collection
Subjective Data
• Itching

Objective Data
• Reddish or gray patches on the skin
• Small blisters may or may not ring the central lesion
• Fungus is microscopically visible
  May appear in the scalp, body, groin, or feet

Data Analysis
Nursing Diagnosis
TINEA (RINGWORM): A fungus infection of the skin

Common Etiology (Stressors)
LIFESTYLE: Lack of hygiene
ENVIRONMENTAL FACTORS: *Biologic agents*: Fungi
MAJOR PATHOPHYSIOLOGIC FACTORS CAUSING THE PROBLEM: Following contact, fungi invade the
  skin and cause infection

PLANNING
Unmet Needs
Comfort, cleanliness, protection from physical harm, increased learning

Expected Outcome
No fungus on microscopic visualization of the skin scraping
No observable skin lesions on scratching
Person verbalizes increased comfort

NURSING INTERVENTIONS

Nursing Treatments

Apply nonprescription drugs (tolnaftate, or Tinactin, solution or ointment or Whitfield's ointment to the lesions; Desenex powder to the feet; potassium permanganate soaks to the feet)

Make a referral (to a physician if the tinea is widespread, resistant to therapy, or of the nails)

Nursing Observations

Observe for evidence of a favorable response to therapy

Health Teaching

Instruct that cleanliness is basic to health

Recommend a daily change of clean clothing

Recommend the use of lightweight clothing (to prevent sweating)

Instruct to wear white socks (to prevent the dye from colored socks from irritating the lesions)

Medical Treatments Performed by Nurses

Give the prescribed drugs (Griseofulvin, for nail tinea)

EVALUATION

Record actual outcome

UREMIC FROST[451]

ASSESSMENT

Data Collection

Subjective Data
• Itching

Objective Data
• White, frosty, salty appearance of the skin
• Mostly on the face and hands, but can cover the entire body

Data Analysis

Nursing Diagnosis
UREMIC FROST: A condition in which urea is excreted by and crystallizes on the skin

Common Etiology (Stressors)
DISEASES: Renal failure
MAJOR PATHOPHYSIOLOGIC FACTORS CAUSING THE PROBLEM: In advanced kidney failure, some of the excess urea in the blood is excreted by the skin; the urea forms flaky white crystals on the skin that cause irritation and intense itching

PLANNING

Unmet Needs

Comfort, cleanliness, protection from physical harm, increased learning

Expected Outcome

No observable urea crystals on the skin

Person verbalizes increased comfort

NURSING INTERVENTIONS

Nursing Treatments

Bathe in vinegar water (to remove urate salts from the skin)

Lubricate the skin with baby oil, bath oil, or body lotion (after bathing in vinegar water)

Cover with lightweight blankets
Dress in lightweight clothing
Maintain a cool room temperature
Maintain dry skin

Nursing Observations
Observe for evidence of a favorable response to therapy

Health Teaching
Advise against scratching
Explain the causes of the health problem (retention of urea)

EVALUATION
Record actual outcome

URTICARIA [159,499]

ASSESSMENT

Data Collection

Subjective Data
• Itching

Objective Data
• Irregular or circular-shaped wheals in varied sizes
• Edema
  Localized or generalized
  White or pink edges

Data Analysis

Nursing Diagnosis
URTICARIA (HIVES): The presence of wheals on the skin

Common Etiology (Stressors)
DISEASES: Allergic disorders
INJURIES: Insect bites
PSYCHOSOCIAL FACTORS: Excessive emotional excitement
HEALTH CARE FACTORS: *Diagnostic procedure*: Dyes used in diagnostic studies. *Drug therapy*: Adverse effects of drugs. *Medical therapy*: Blood-transfusion reaction
ENVIRONMENTAL FACTORS: *Biologic agents*: Insects. *Chemical substances*: Disinfectants, household cleaning agents, paints or varnishes, pesticides, etc. *Food substances*: Adverse effect of food. *Plants*: Adverse effect of plants. *Pollen*: Ragweed, grass
MAJOR PATHOPHYSIOLOGIC FACTORS CAUSING THE PROBLEM: Urticaria is an eruptive response of the skin to irritating substances that trigger the body's hypersensitivity reaction

PLANNING

Unmet Needs
Comfort, cleanliness, protection from physical harm, increased learning

Expected Outcome
No observable lesions on the skin
Clean, moist, natural color skin
Person verbalizes increased comfort

NURSING INTERVENTIONS

Nursing Treatments
Apply a cold, moist compress
  OR

Bathe in cool water
Apply calamine lotion
Apply a bed cradle (if the lesions are widespread)
Cover with lightweight blankets
Dress in lightweight clothing
Give nonprescription drugs (antihistamine)
Maintain a cool room temperature

Nursing Observations
Observe for evidence of a favorable response to therapy

Health Teaching
Advise against scratching (which stimulates itching)
Explain the causes of the health problem (allergy)

EVALUATION

Record actual outcome

Knowledge Deficits Associated with the Integument

UNKNOWLEDGEABLE ABOUT SKIN CANCER[42,88,433,675]

ASSESSMENT

Data Collection

Subjective Data
• Person's discussion or questions indicate a need for additional information, clarification, or validation of information
    OR
• Person's lack of questions or comments indicates not wanting information or not knowing enough to seek information
• When questioned directly, the person's response or lack of response indicates that he does not know:
    The signs and symptoms of early skin cancer
    The factors associated with the occurrence of skin cancer
    The value of the prompt excision of suspected lesions

Objective Data
• May exhibit behavior such as ignoring a dangerous skin lesion

Related Data

Commonly Related Diseases
Basal cell carcinoma, melanoma, squamous cell carcinoma

Data Analysis

Nursing Diagnosis
UNKNOWLEDGEABLE ABOUT SKIN CANCER: Being without sufficient information about the signs, symptoms, causes, and treatment of skin cancer

Common Etiology (Stressors)
HEALTH CARE FACTORS: Lack of health information

PLANNING

Unmet Needs
Protection from physical harm, independence, increased learning

Expected Outcome

Correct verbal feedback of the information taught

NURSING INTERVENTIONS

Nursing Treatments

Approach unhurriedly

Encourage the person to ask questions

Discuss the anticipated procedure (biopsy, excision of the lesion)

Nursing Observations

Determine teaching effectiveness by verbal feedback

Health Teaching

Describe the factors associated with the occurrence of skin cancer (in the most common form of cancer, there is an increasing incidence with age; melanoma, a rare skin cancer, is most common in whites between age 40 and 70 years; other factors include frequent exposure to sunlight, radiation, arsenic; the presence of senile keratosis, moles, warts; chronic irritation of moles, warts, or of the skin by pressure, heat, etc.)

Describe those symptoms that should be reported (a painless lesion that does not heal, nodule or wartlike ulcer, changes in color or characteristics of a mole, itching of a mole or wart)

Instruct to report serious symptoms immediately (mentioned above)

Explain the causes of the health problem (chronic cellular damage from radiation or sunlight, or a familial tendency that can result in a disorganized proliferation of skin cell growth)

Explain the reason for and intended effect of the therapy (to remove the cancer and prevent metastasis)

EVALUATION

Record actual outcome

UNKNOWLEDGEABLE ABOUT SKIN PROTECTION[42,159,433]

ASSESSMENT

Data Collection

Subjective Data

• Person's discussion or questions indicate a need for additional information, clarification, or validation of information
    OR
• Person's lack of questions or comments indicates not wanting information or not knowing enough to seek information
• When questioned directly, the person's response or lack of response indicates that he does not know:
    About skin irritating factors
    Skin precautions to be taken
    Ways to clean the skin

Objective Data

• May exhibit behavior such as sunbathing for prolonged periods in intense environmental heat or swimming for excessive periods in skin-irritating water

Data Analysis

Nursing Diagnosis

UNKNOWLEDGEABLE ABOUT SKIN PROTECTION: Being without information about protecting the skin from irritation and damage

Common Etiology (Stressors)
HEALTH CARE FACTORS: Lack of health instruction

PLANNING
Unmet Needs
Comfort, protection from physical harm, independence, increased learning
Expected Outcome
Correct verbal feedback of the information taught

NURSING INTERVENTIONS
Nursing Treatments
Approach unhurriedly
Encourage the person to ask questions
Nursing Observations
Determine teaching effectiveness by verbal feedback
Health Teaching
Advise against prolonged skin exposure to the sun (especially if the person has a yellow-brown pregnancy mask, butterfly markings of lupus erythematosus, copper skin of Wilson's disease, white patches of vitiligo, white skin of albinism, brown markings of Addison's disease, strawberry or ruby or port-wine birthmarks, or very fair skin)
Recommend the use of sun-screening lotion (that contains palimate O and PABA, avoid lotions containing palimate A, which causes burns)
Advise against prolonged skin exposure to water (prolonged swimming or hands in water)
Advise against piercing or squeezing the skin
Emphasize the danger of cutting calloused skin (use a pumice stone instead)
Explain the importance of testing cosmetics for skin irritation
Inform that the skin should be protected from windburn
Instruct to maintain skin cleanliness (with nonirritating soap)
Instruct to lubricate the skin (daily to prevent dryness)
Instruct to inspect the skin (for abnormalities, periodically)
Explain how to adjust clothing to meet health problems (wear long sleeves, hats, and pants to cover sensitive skin)
Recommend that self-medication be avoided (if there are skin problems)

EVALUATION
Record actual outcome

Minor Health Problems Associated with the Musculoskeletal and Neurologic Systems

BONE PAIN[73,522]

ASSESSMENT
Data Collection
Subjective Data
• Pain localized in the bone area
• Severe aching (soreness, tenderness)

Objective Data
• Movement or weight-bearing increases pain
• No pain in muscles over the bone, on palpation
  Localized edema, sometimes

Data Analysis

Nursing Diagnosis
BONE PAIN: A distressful hurting felt within the bone itself

Common Etiology (Stressors)
DISEASES: Aplastic anemia, hyperparathyroidism, leukemia (pain over the tibia), multiple myeloma, osteoma, osteomyelitis, Paget's disease, syphilis, tuberculosis
INJURIES: Bone fracture
HEALTH CARE FACTORS: *Diagnostic procedures*: Bone marrow
MAJOR PATHOPHYSIOLOGIC FACTORS CAUSING THE PROBLEM: In leukemia, the bone marrow is infiltrated by large numbers of leukemic cells, resulting in bone marrow expansion; in aplastic anemia, increased destruction or decreased production of red blood cells results in compensatory bone-marrow expansion as the body attempts to offset the deficiency of RBCs and WBCs in the bone marrow; in bone fracture, there is pain from friction between the two pieces of separated bone

PLANNING

Unmet Needs
Rest, protection from physical harm, freedom from pain, increased learning

Expected Outcome
Person verbalizes increased comfort
Freedom of body movement

NURSING INTERVENTIONS

Nursing Treatments
Approach unhurriedly
Communicate nurse sensitivity to the person's pain
Handle gently
Position comfortably
Change the person's position gradually
Support the affected body part
Apply a warm, moist compress (to a localized area)
  OR
Apply a cold, moist compress (for inflammatory swelling or bone tumor)
  OR
Place in a whirlpool bath
Encourage adequate rest
Ask the person what makes him comfortable
Discuss possible pain-reducing measures
Provide a pain-relief measure of the person's choice
Give nonprescription drugs (analgesics)

Nursing Observations
Observe for complaints of pain duration
Evaluate the effectiveness of the pain-relief measures

Health Teaching
Explain the causes of pain (trauma, hyperplasia)
Explain the reason for and intended effect of the therapy (to promote comfort and healing)

Medical Treatments Performed by Nurses
Give the prescribed drugs (analgesics)

EVALUATION
Record actual outcome

DIZZINESS[88,125,278]

ASSESSMENT

Data Collection

Subjective Data
- Lightheadedness
- Feels unsteady, unbalanced
  Episodes are intermittent
  Constant dizziness is specific to functional disorders

Objective Data
Unsteady gait, sometimes

Data Analysis

Nursing Diagnosis
DIZZINESS: A sensation of unsteadiness of position

Common Etiology (Stressors)
DISEASES: Alcoholism, anemia, arrhythmias, arteriosclerosis, brain abscess or tumor, congestive heart failure, depression, encephalitis, hyperglycemia, hypertension, hyperventilation, hypochondriasis, hypoglycemia, meningitis, mitral stenosis, postrual hypotension, psychoneurosis, syphilis, tricuspid stenosis
INJURIES: Concussion
SIGNS AND SYMPTOMS: Hypoxia, uremia
PSYCHOSOCIAL FACTORS: Excessive emotional excitement, the threat of real or imagined danger
HEALTH CARE FACTORS: *Diagnostic procedures*: Angiography, pneumoencephalogram, vital capacity pulmonary function test. *Drug therapy*: Anticonvulsants, antihistamines, antihypertensive drugs, epinephrine, narcotics, sedatives, tranquilizers. *Medical therapy*: Intermittent positive-pressure breathing, ear irrigation. *Surgical therapy*: Anesthesia
ENVIRONMENTAL FACTORS: *Altitude*: High altitude. *Chemical Substances*: Inhalation of chemical substances such as disinfectants, paints, varnishes, toxic gases or vapors
MAJOR PATHOPHYSIOLOGIC FACTORS CAUSING THE PROBLEM: Dizziness can result from transient disturbances in circulation, oxygenation, or equilibrium

PLANNING

Unmet Needs
Rest, comfort, protection from harm, increased learning

Expected Outcome
Person verbalizes a feeling of steadiness and balance

NURSING INTERVENTIONS

Nursing Treatments
Sit the person in an armchair
  OR
Encourage adequate rest (until the episode subsides)
Give nonprescription drugs (Dramamine)
Withhold any drugs (causing dizziness such as antihistamines, tranquilizers, anticonvulsants, and notify the physician of the problem)
Make a referral (to a physician if the condition persists)

Nursing Observations
Monitor the blood pressure (in the supine, sitting, and standing position)
Auscultate the chest for abnormal heart sounds (arrhythmias)
Monitor the cardiogram (for abnormalities)
Palpate the pulse for rate, rhythm, and volume
Inspect the chest for respiratory rate and rhythm

Observe for emotional instability (severe anxiety or depression)

Monitor blood studies for abnormal electrolytes, glucose, hematology, liver function, renal function

Inspect the ears with an otoscope (for any abnormality)

Test the eyes for visual acuity

Health Teaching

Explain the causes of the health problem (rapid breathing, ear and cardiac disorders, hypotension)

Describe those symptoms that should be reported (increased or persistent dizziness, vomiting)

EVALUATION

Record actual outcome

FOOTDROP[35,73,451]

ASSESSMENT

Data Collection

Subjective Data
Person relates difficulty walking

Objective Data
• Sole of the foot falls downward
• Person cannot hold the foot in a normal position or in the dorsiflexion position
   Foot inversion may or may not occur
   Person drags the foot
   The heel fails to touch the ground if walking is attempted
   Person walks on his toes

Data Analysis

Nursing Diagnosis
FOOTDROP (PLANTAR FLEXION): Involuntary bending of the ankle in the direction of the sole of the foot

Common Etiology (Stressors)
DISEASES: Cerebrovascular accident
INJURIES: Fracture and compression of the spinal cord
SIGNS AND SYMPTOMS: Immobility, paralysis
HEALTH CARE FACTORS: *Medical therapy*: Prolonged bed rest
MAJOR PATHOPHYSIOLOGIC FACTORS CAUSING THE PROBLEM: Prolonged bed rest without proper alignment and joint exercise, pressure from heavy bed clothes on the foot, and paralysis of the ankle's flexion muscle produce a shortened Achilles' tendon

PLANNING

Unmet Needs

Protection from physical harm, increased learning

Expected Outcome

Optimum foot alignment and function attainable by the person

NURSING INTERVENTIONS

Nursing Treatments

Apply a bed cradle (to keep blankets off the feet)

Cover with lightweight blankets
Provide loose bedding with toe pleats
Exercise in range of motion
Place in a whirlpool bath (during exercise, if possible)
Place the feet in hard-soled ankle-top shoes
   OR
Place a footboard at the feet
Position with sandbags (to maintain alignment)

Nursing Observations

Observe for evidence of a favorable response to therapy

Health Teaching

Explain how to maintain body alignment (proper positioning)
Teach how to do range-of-motion exercises
Explain the causes of the health problem (poor body alignment, pressure against the foot, a shortened tendon)
Explain the reason for and intended effect of the therapy (to support the function of the foot)

Medical Treatments Performed by Nurses

Apply the prescribed preventive splint

EVALUATION

Record actual outcome

HEADACHE[42,88]

ASSESSMENT

Data Collection

Subjective Data
• Pain felt in the cranium, eye orbits, or nape of the neck
• Head pain lasts hours or days
  Localized or diffuse pain

Objective Data
Fever sometimes

Data Analysis

Nursing Diagnosis
HEADACHE: Pain located in the head

Common Etiology (Stressors)
DISEASES: Allergic disorder, aneurysm, brain tumor or abscess, encephalitis, farsightedness, hypertension, influenza, malaria, meningitis, renal insufficiency, renal failure, subarachnoid hemorrhage, subdural hematoma, toxemia of pregnancy, typhoid fever
INJURIES: Cerebral concussion, heat exhaustion, laceration wound of the head
SIGNS AND SYMPTOMS: Constipation, convulsions, edema, fatigue, fever
PSYCHOSOCIAL FACTORS: The threat of chronic or severe stress
HUMAN BODY: *Body state*: Menstruation, menopause
HEALTH CARE FACTORS: *Diagnostic procedures*: Angiography, lumbar puncture, myelography, pneumonencephalogram. *Drug therapy*: Adverse effects or interactions of drugs. *Surgi-*

cal therapy: Anesthesia. *Surgical procedures*: Cranioplasty, craniotomy

LIFESTYLE: Drug abuse, insufficient relaxation

ENVIRONMENTAL FACTORS: *Chemical substances*: Ingestion or inhalation of chemical substances. *Environmental cold*: Low external temperature. *Environmental heat*: High external temperature. *Noise*: Prolonged exposure to loud noise

MAJOR PATHOPHYSIOLOGIC FACTORS CAUSING THE PROBLEM: Tissue or artery inflammation, spasm, infection, cranial masses, or hemorrhage can cause pressure within or irritation of cranial tissue or nerves, resulting in a headache

PLANNING

Unmet Needs

Rest, comfort, protection from physical harm, freedom from pain, increased learning

Expected Outcome

Person verbalizes relief from head pain

Person returns to usual level of functioning

NURSING INTERVENTIONS

Nursing Treatments

Approach unhurriedly

Reassure that the pain will subside or be relieved

Position comfortably

Elevate the head

Apply a cool, moist compress (to the forehead)
    OR
Apply an ice bag or pack (to the head)

Massage (the neck and shoulders) gently

Provide quiet

Encourage adequate rest

Ask the person what makes him comfortable

Discuss possible pain-reducing measures

Provide a pain-relief measure of the person's choice

Give nonprescription drugs (analgesics)

Nursing Observations

Observe for a favorable response to therapy

Monitor the blood pressure

Inspect the eyes for pupil size, equality and response to light

Test the eyes for visual acuity (Snellen test)

Observe for a hypersensitivity response (eye tearing, rhinitis)

Auscultate the carotid arteries for bruit

Observe for complaints of dizziness, weakness

Palpate (the cranium) for tenderness

Test for range of motion (of the neck, note any stiffness)

Health Teaching

Explain the causes of the pain

Advise not to take hot baths (vasodilatation increases the headache)

Inform that coughing should be avoided

Inform that elimination straining should be avoided

Advise that highly emotional situations should be avoided (until the pain subsides)

Describe those symptoms that should be reported (vomiting, high fever, neck stiffness, visual disturbances)

Medical Treatments Performed by Nurses

Give the prescribed drugs (analgesics)

EVALUATION

Record actual outcome

CLUSTER HEADACHE[88,278,522]

ASSESSMENT

Data Collection

Subjective Data
- Severe pain localized, unilateral; located near the eye orbit, temple, or side of the face; sometimes radiates to the jaw and neck
- Constant, lasting about 1 hour; may occur each night for several nights, weeks, or months, but then disappears for a time
- Usually occurs several hours after falling asleep
- Throbbing (pounding, pulsating) pain

Objective Data
- Restlessness
- Rhinorrhea
- Tearing
  Red conjunctiva
  Sweating

Data Analysis

Nursing Diagnosis
CLUSTER HEADACHE: Headaches that occur consistently for a limited period and then disappear for a while

Common Etiology (Stressors)
DISEASES: Alcoholism, allergic disorder
PSYCHOSOCIAL FACTORS: The threat of severe or chronic stress
HEALTH CARE FACTORS: *Drug therapy*: Nitroglycerine
MAJOR PATHOPHYSIOLOGIC FACTORS CAUSING THE PROBLEM: Emotional stress, alcohol intake, nitroglycerine, and histamine cause vasodilatation of the cerebral blood vessels; it is recently believed that cluster headaches are due to a collection of carbon dioxide around the optic nerve, relieved by the intake of oxygen

PLANNING

Unmet Needs

Rest and relaxation, comfort, protection from physical harm, freedom from pain, increased learning

Expected Outcome

No observable conjunctiva redness, tearing, or rhinorrhea
Person verbalizes increased comfort

NURSING INTERVENTIONS

Nursing Treatments

Approach unhurriedly
Reassure that the pain will subside or be relieved
Communicate nurse sensitivity to the person's pain
Position comfortably
Change the person's position gradually
Elevate the head
Apply a cold, moist compress (to the forehead)
  OR
Apply an ice bag (to the head)
Massage gently (the neck and shoulders)
Subdue the room lighting
Provide quiet
Encourage adequate rest
Ask the person what makes him comfortable

Discuss possible pain-reducing measures
Provide the pain-relief measure of the person's choice
Give nonprescription drugs (analgesics, antihistamines)

Nursing Observations
Evaluate the effectiveness of the pain-relief measures

Health Teaching
Explain the causes of the pain (allergic response, CO_2 collection around the optic nerve)
Advise not to take hot baths (vasodilatation increases the headache)
Inform that coughing should be avoided
Inform that elimination straining should be avoided (pressure increases the headache)

Medical Treatments Performed by Nurses
Give prescribed drugs (analgesics)
Administer oxygen by mask

EVALUATION

Record actual outcome

HYPERTENSIVE HEADACHE[42,255,522]

ASSESSMENT

Data Collection

Subjective Data
• Throbbing (pounding, pulsating) pain
• Pain over the occipital lobe or the top of the head
• No preceding aura
• Vomiting, sometimes

Objective Data
• Elevated systolic pressure above 200 mm Hg
• Elevated diastolic pressure above 105 mm Hg
  Papilledema
  Epistaxis, sometimes

Data Analysis

Nursing Diagnosis
HYPERTENSIVE HEADACHE: Throbbing head pain associated with an elevated blood pressure

Common Etiology (Stressors)
DISEASES: Hypertension
MAJOR PATHOPHYSIOLOGIC FACTORS CAUSING THE PROBLEM: Increased intracranial pressure or cerebral vasodilatation; increased pressure within the brain when the person is in the flat position elevates the blood pressure

PLANNING

Unmet Needs
Rest and relaxation, comfort, protection from physical harm, freedom from pain, increased learning

Expected Outcome
Diastolic blood pressure below 105 mm Hg
Person verbalizes increased comfort

NURSING INTERVENTIONS

Nursing Treatments
Approach unhurriedly

Reassure that the pain will subside
Communicate nurse sensitivity to the person's pain
Position comfortably
Change the person's position gradually
Elevate the head
Apply a cold, moist compress (to the forehead)
   OR
Apply an ice bag (to the head)
Give hot coffee (black)
Massage gently (the neck and shoulders)
Subdue the room lighting
Provide quiet
Encourage adequate rest
Ask the person what makes him comfortable
Discuss possible pain-reducing measures
Provide a pain-relief measure of the person's choice
Give nonprescription drugs (acetylsalicyic acid simultaneously with coffee)
Consult with the physician (about increasing the dose of antihypertensive drugs)
Make a referral (to a physician, if the hypertension is untreated)

Nursing Observations
Evaluate the effectiveness of the pain-relief measures
Monitor the blood pressure

Health Teaching
Explain the causes of the pain (increased blood pressure)
Advise not to take hot baths (vasodilatation increases pain)
Advise that highly emotional situations should be avoided
Inform that coughing should be avoided
Inform that elimination straining should be avoided (pressure increases the pain)
Explain the reason for and intended effect of the therapy

Medical Treatments Performed by Nurses
Give the prescribed drugs (analgesics, antihypertensive drugs)

EVALUATION

Record actual outcome

MENINGEAL HEADACHE[42,522]

ASSESSMENT

Data Collection

Subjective Data
• Throbbing (pounding, pulsating) pain
• Pain is generalized, covering the entire head
• Especially severe at the base of the skull

Objective Data
• Neck stiffness
  Vomiting, sometimes
  Irritability
  Restlessness

Data Analysis

Nursing Diagnosis
MENINGEAL HEADACHE: Throbbing head pain associated with inflammation of the meninges

Common Etiology (Stressors)
DISEASES: Encephalitis, meningitis, subdural hematoma
MAJOR PATHOPHYSIOLOGIC FACTORS CAUSING THE PROBLEM: Headache results from chemical or inflammatory irritation of nerve fiber endings in the meninges

PLANNING

Unmet Needs
Rest and relaxation, comfort, protection from physical harm, freedom from pain, increased learning

Expected Outcome
Full range of motion of the neck
Person verbalizes increased comfort

NURSING INTERVENTIONS

Nursing Treatments
Approach unhurriedly
Reassure that the pain will subside or be relieved
Communicate nurse sensitivity to the person's pain
Position comfortably
Change the person's position gradually
Apply a cold, moist compress
    OR
Apply an ice bag (to the head)
Massage gently (the neck and shoulders)
Subdue the room lighting
Provide quiet
Encourage adequate rest
Refrain from jarring the bed (which increases the pain)
Refrain from performing nonessential procedures
Ask the person what makes him comfortable
Discuss possible pain-reducing measures
Provide a pain-relief measure of the person's choice
Give nonprescription drugs (analgesics)

Nursing Observations
Evaluate the effectiveness of the pain-relief measures

Health Teaching
Explain the causes of the pain (meningeal irritation)
Advise not to take hot baths (vasodilatation increases the pain)
Inform that coughing should be avoided
Inform that elimination straining should be avoided (pressure increases the pain)
Explain the reason for and intended effect of the therapy

Medical Treatments Performed by Nurses
Give the prescribed drugs (analgesics)

EVALUATION

Record actual outcome

MENSTRUAL–MIGRAINE HEADACHE[60,522]

ASSESSMENT

Data Collection

Subjective Data
• Severe pain usually confined to one side of the head, temporal or occipital

- Acute onset beginning several days before menstrual onset, reaching greatest intensity at the onset of flow
- Throbbing (pounding, pulsating) pain
  Irritability

Objective Data
Body edema

Data Analysis

Nursing Diagnosis
MENSTRUAL–MIGRAINE HEADACHE: A boring headache just before menstruation onset

Common Etiology (Stressors)
SIGNS AND SYMPTOMS: Edema
HUMAN BODY: *Body state*: Menstruation
MAJOR PATHOPHYSIOLOGIC FACTORS CAUSING THE PROBLEM: Excessive secretion of the follicle-stimulating hormone by the pituitary increases the estrogen secretion and inhibits the gonadotropic function of the pituitary, causing abnormal estrogen and gonadotropin excretion; allergy to a person's own hormones, fluid retention causing intermittent cranial edema

PLANNING

Unmet Needs
Fluid and electrolyte balance, rest and relaxation, comfort, protection from physical harm, freedom from pain, increased learning

Expected Outcome
Person verbalizes increased comfort
Menstruation onset without headache

NURSING INTERVENTIONS

Nursing Treatments
Approach unhurriedly
Reassure that the pain will subside or be relieved
Communicate nurse sensitivity to the person's pain
Position comfortably
Apply a cold, moist compress
  OR
Apply an ice bag
Provide quiet
Encourage adequate rest
Ask the person what makes her comfortable
Discuss possible pain-reducing measures
Provide a pain-relief measure of the person's choice
Give nonprescription drugs (analgesics)
Encourage decreased sodium-food intake (1 week before menstruation onset)

Nursing Observations
Observe for complaints of pain duration
Evaluate pain for intensity and quality
Evaluate the effectiveness of the pain-relief measures

Health Teaching
Advise not to take hot baths (vasodilatation increases the pain)
Inform that coughing should be avoided
Inform that elimination straining should be avoided (pressure increases the pain)
Describe those symptoms that should be reported (vomiting, impaired vision)
Explain the causes of the pain (fluid retention)
Explain the reason for and intended effect of the therapy (to promote comfort)

Medical Treatments Performed by Nurses
Give the prescribed drugs (analgesics)

EVALUATION
Record actual outcome

MIGRAINE HEADACHE [42,60,278,522]

ASSESSMENT
Data Collection
Subjective Data
- Before onset there is visualization of stars or zig-zag flashes of light of white, blue, yellow, or green color; person may then see only half of all objects; vision clears in 15–30 minutes, and the headache follows
- Throbbing (pounding, pulsating) pain
- Severe pain is unilateral or generalized
- Nausea
  Vomiting, sometimes
  Family history of migraine headaches

Objective Data
Eye squinting from light sensitivity

Data Analysis
Nursing Diagnosis
MIGRAINE HEADACHE: Extremely severe, constant head pain, following an aura

Common Etiology (Stressors)
DISEASES: Allergic disorder
HEALTH CARE FACTORS: *Drugs*: Contraceptive drugs
ENVIRONMENTAL FACTORS: *Food substances*: Adverse effect of specific food such as chocolate, nuts, dairy products
MAJOR PATHOPHYSIOLOGIC FACTORS CAUSING THE PROBLEM: The cause is uncertain at this time but is believed to be a histamine reaction or impaired cranial circulation that causes vasoconstriction followed by vasodilatation, which causes the pain

PLANNING
Unmet Needs
Sleep, rest, relaxation, comfort, protection from physical harm, freedom from pain, increased learning

Expected Outcome
Person verbalizes increased comfort

NURSING INTERVENTIONS
Nursing Treatments
Approach unhurriedly
Reassure that the pain will subside or be relieved
Communicate nurse sensitivity to the person's pain
Elevate the head
Position comfortably
Change the person's position gradually
Apply a cold, moist compress (to the forehead)
    OR
Apply an ice bag (to the head)
Massage gently (the neck and shoulders)
Subdue the room lighting
Provide quiet
Encourage adequate rest

Refrain from performing nonessential procedures
Ask the person what makes him comfortable
Discuss possible pain-reducing measures
Provide a pain-relief measure of the person's choice
Give nonprescription drugs (acetylsalicylic acid)
Encourage decreased sodium-food intake
Discourage the intake of oral stimulants (alcohol, caffeine in coffee, coke, chocolate)
Refrain from giving milk or milk products (cheese)
Make a referral (to a physician if a woman is taking birth control pills, which may precipitate migraine headaches)

Nursing Observations
Observe for complaints of pain duration
Evaluate the effectiveness of the pain-relief measures

Health Teaching
Advise not to take hot baths (vasodilatation increases the pain)
Describe those symptoms that should be reported (vomiting, vision problems)
Explain the causes of the pain (allergy, vasodilatation)
Inform that coughing should be avoided
Inform that elimination straining should be avoided (pressure increases the pain)

Medical Treatments Performed by Nurses
Give the prescribed drugs (Ergotamine)

EVALUATION

Record actual outcome

POSTSPINAL HEADACHE[522]

ASSESSMENT

Data Collection

Subjective Data
• Throbbing (pounding, pulsating) pain, shortly after a spinal puncture
• Generalized, occipital pain
• Severity increases when in the upright position and decreases when horizontal

Objective Data
None

Data Analysis

Nursing Diagnosis
POSTSPINAL HEADACHE: A severe headache occurring after a spinal puncture

Common Etiology (Stressors)
HEALTH CARE FACTORS: *Diagnostic procedure*: Lumbar puncture
MAJOR PATHOPHYSIOLOGIC FACTORS CAUSING THE PROBLEM: Following a spinal puncture, spinal fluid leaks through the puncture site and escapes from the spinal canal into surrounding tissues; this reduces the normal supply of spinal fluid to the brain, causing traction of the dural attachments to the venous sinuses, resulting in a headache

PLANNING

Unmet Needs
Rest and relaxation, comfort, protection from physical harm, freedom from pain, increased learning

Expected Outcome
Person verbalizes increased comfort

NURSING INTERVENTIONS

Nursing Treatments
Approach unhurriedly
Reassure that the pain will subside or be relieved
Communicate nurse sensitivity to the person's pain
Place in the flat position (12–24 hours after the spinal puncture)
Position comfortably
Apply a cold, moist compress
   OR
Apply an ice bag
Provide quiet
Subdue the room lighting
Encourage adequate rest
Refrain from performing nonessential procedures
Ask the person what makes him comfortable
Discuss possible pain-reducing measures
Provide a pain-relief measure of the person's choice
Give nonprescription drugs (analgesics)
Provide frequent contact with the person

Nursing Observations
Observe for complaints of pain duration
Estimate the degree of pain experienced
Evaluate the effectiveness of the pain-relief measures

Health Teaching
Explain the causes of the pain (decreased spinal fluid to the brain)
Explain the reason for and intended effect of the therapy

Medical Treatments Performed by Nurses
Give the prescribed drugs (analgesics)

EVALUATION

Record actual outcome

TENSION HEADACHE[42,278,522]

ASSESSMENT

Data Collection

Subjective Data
- Gradual onset, often associated with stress
- Pain at the back of the head, above both eyes, and on the top of the head
  Constrictive (squeezing, pressing) pain
  Head fullness, sensation of a band or vice around the head
  Nonthrobbing, dull, sometimes burning sensation, or a creeping sensation over the head
  Often occurs during both the day and night for several days
  Analgesics do not give complete pain relief

Objective Data
Patient may appear apathetic or tense and anxious

Data Analysis

Nursing Diagnosis
TENSION HEADACHE: A tight, viselike head pain

Common Etiology (Stressors)
PSYCHOSOCIAL FACTORS: Excessive emotional excitement, the threat of severe or prolonged stress

MAJOR PATHOPHYSIOLOGIC FACTORS CAUSING THE PROBLEM: Pain results from prolonged contraction of the head and neck muscles

PLANNING

Unmet Needs

Rest and relaxation, comfort, protection from physical harm, freedom from pain, increased learning

Expected Outcome

Person verbalizes increased comfort
Calm, relaxed appearance

NURSING INTERVENTIONS

Nursing Treatments

Approach unhurriedly
Reassure that the pain will subside or be relieved
Communicate nurse sensitivity to the person's pain
Elevate the head
Position comfortably
Change the person's position gradually
Apply a heating pad
    OR
Apply a hot water bottle   } To promote relaxation
Bathe in warm water
Massage gently (the neck and shoulders)
Subdue the room lighting
Provide quiet
Encourage adequate rest
Ask the person what makes him comfortable
Discuss possible pain-reducing measures
Provide a pain-relief measure of the person's choice
Give nonprescription drugs (analgesics)
Encourage the expression of feelings (about the current stress)
Reduce the demands placed on the person

Nursing Observations

Observe for complaints of pain duration
Evaluate pain for intensity and quality
Evaluate the effectiveness of the pain-relief measures
Monitor the blood pressure

Health Teaching

Explain the causes of the pain (stress)
Explain that fatigue should be recognized as a stress factor
Explain how to reduce muscular tension (stretching, yawning, allowing muscles to go limp)
Recommend adherence to a pace of living with which the person is comfortable

Medical Treatments Performed by Nurses

Give the prescribed drugs (analgesics, tranquilizers)

EVALUATION

Record actual outcome

INVOLUNTARY MUSCLE TWITCHING[298,522]

ASSESSMENT

Data Collection

Subjective Data

Person relates that the jerking interferes with sleep or rest

Objective Data

• Spontaneous and intermittent muscle jerking
• Twitching may be accentuated with voluntary movement or when at rest
  Twitching may involve any body area but usually the arm, leg, or head

Data Analysis

Nursing Diagnosis

INVOLUNTARY MUSCLE TWITCHING: Uncontrollable muscle contractions

Common Etiology (Stressors)

DISEASES: Amyotrophic lateral sclerosis, bulbar palsy, Huntington's chorea, hyperventilation, hypocalcemia, peripheral neuropathy, poliomyelitis, Syndeham's chorea

SIGNS AND SYMPTOMS: Uremia

MAJOR PATHOPHSIOLOGIC FACTORS CAUSING THE PROBLEM: Muscular twitching results from muscle depolarization before repolarization is complete, diseases of the basal ganglion, or decreased serum calcium level

PLANNING

Unmet Needs

Relaxation, comfort, protection from physical harm, increased learning

Expected Outcome

No observable muscle twitching
Person verbalizes cessation of jerking

NURSING INTERVENTIONS

Nursing Treatments

Apply a heating pad
  OR   } To the area
Apply a hot water bottle
  OR
Bathe in warm water
Cover with warm blankets
Maintain a warm room temperature
Decrease drafts
Handle gently
Massage gently
Refrain from jarring the bed (which may stimulate the twitching)
Encourage increased calcium-food intake
  AND   } If the serum calcium is low
Give high-calcium fluids orally

Nursing Observations

Monitor blood studies for abnormal electrolytes (decreased calcium)
Inspect for abnormal body movements (twitching)
Observe for evidence of a favorable response to therapy

Health Teaching

Teach how to apply heat therapy
Explain the causes of the health problem (low calcium, nerve disorders)

EVALUATION

Record actual outcome

IRRITABILITY[35,278,432,522]

ASSESSMENT

Data Collection

Subjective Data
- Easily angered
- Impatient
- Fatigue
  Uncooperative
  Quarrelsome
  Critical of others

Objective Data
- Startle response to minor stimuli
  Cries easily
  Overactivity

Related Data
  Manifestations are of recent origin

Data Analysis

Nursing Diagnosis
IRRITABILITY: A quick and excessive response to stimuli as a result of physical imbalance

Common Etiology (Stressors)
DISEASES: Addison's disease, arrhythmias, asthma, beriberi, eczema, epilepsy, hypertension, hypoglycemia, kwashiorkor, meningitis, milk alkali syndrome, scurvy, Sydenham's chorea, thyrotoxicoxis
SIGNS AND SYMPTOMS: Dehydration, edema, fatigue, fever, pain
HUMAN BODY: *Body state*: Menstruation, climacteric, menopause
HEALTH CARE FACTORS: *Drug therapy*: Corticosteroids, epinephrine
DEVELOPMENTAL PHASES: Puberty, adolescence
LIFESTYLE: High-caffeine intake, high-nicotine intake
ENVIRONMENTAL FACTORS: *Chemical substances*: Inhalation of chemical agents such as toxic gases or vapors
MAJOR PATHOPHYSIOLOGIC FACTORS CAUSING THE PROBLEM: Some physiologic changes, such as hormonal changes, metabolic hyperactivity, and cardiovascular disorders, cause increased internal body pressures resulting in irritability; prolonged nerve stimulation and sensitive nerve fibers result in an excessive response to stimulation

PLANNING

Unmet Needs
Sleep, rest, relaxation, comfort, protection from physical harm, acceptance, increased learning

Expected Outcome
Calm, relaxed appearance
No startle response to minor stimuli

NURSING INTERVENTIONS

Nursing Treatments
Approach unhurriedly
Provide an atmosphere of acceptance
Demonstrate calmness
Arrange orderly surroundings
Arrange pleasant surroundings
Arrange a structured daily routine
Provide quiet
Provide frequent contact with the person

Ensure the person's feeling of safety before introducing unpleasantness

Introduce one anxiety-producing situation at a time

Provide emotionally safe experiences

Reduce the demands placed on the person

Refrain from performing nonessential procedures

Encourage adequate rest

Massage gently
   OR   }   For the relaxing effect
Bathe in warm water

Nursing Observations

Observe for evidence of a favorable response to therapy

Health Teaching

Advise that highly emotional situations should be avoided

Describe the behavior pattern indicating overstimulation (fatigue, irritability, insomnia, panicky feeling)

Explain that fatigue should be recognized as a stress factor

Recommend methods for reducing sensory stimulation (involvement in quiet activities, have only a few visitors at a time)

Recommend methods for achieving total relaxation (deep breathing exercises, warm baths)

Explain the causes of the health problem (increased pressure within the body, hormonal changes)

Medical Treatments Performed by Nurses

Give the prescribed drugs

EVALUATION

Record actual outcome

JOINT CONTRACTURE[73,451]

ASSESSMENT

Data Collection

Subjective Data

• Relates loss of joint function

Objective Data

• Twisted position of the hand, finger, elbow, shoulder, hip, foot, knee, or toe
• Flexed (bent) position
  Limited movement ability
  Abnormal alignment

Data Analysis

Nursing Diagnosis

JOINT CONTRACTURE: Muscle and/or tendon shortening with impaired muscle and/or tendon use

Common Etiology (Stressors)

DISEASES: Cerebrovascular accident, multiple sclerosis, muscular dystrophy

INJURIES: Burn wounds, fracture and compression of the spinal cord

SIGNS AND SYMPTOMS: Immobility, paralysis

HEALTH CARE FACTORS: *Medical therapy*: Prolonged bed rest. *Adverse effects of medical or surgical therapy*: Knee flexion after prolonged use of a cast or corrective splint, hip flexion after an amputation

MAJOR PATHOPHYSIOLOGIC FACTORS CAUSING THE PROBLEM: Contractures result from the resistance of muscle tissue around joints caused by immobility or inflammation and infection

PLANNING

Unmet Needs
Activity and exercise, comfort, protection from physical harm, increased learning

Expected Outcome
Optimum joint alignment and function attainable by the person

NURSING INTERVENTIONS

Nursing Treatments
Ambulate the person (as much as possible)
Change the person's position frequently
Exercise in range of motion
Place in a whirlpool bath (during exercise, if possible)
 OR
Bathe in warm water
Massage gently
Place a footboard at the feet
Place a hand roll under the fingers
Place a trochanter roll for positioning
 OR
Position with sandbags (to maintain joint alignment)
Encourage normal use of the involved limb

Nursing Observations
Observe for evidence of a favorable response to therapy

Health Teaching
Explain the causes of the health problem (immobility, inflammation)
Explain how to maintain body alignment (proper positioning)
Teach how to apply preventive splints

Medical Treatments Performed by Nurses
Apply the prescribed preventive splint

EVALUATION
Record actual outcome

JOINT PAIN[278,371,522]

ASSESSMENT

Data Collection

Subjective Data
• Localized pain
• Aching (soreness, tenderness), often worse in the morning
• Increases with joint movement

Objective Data
• Limited range of motion of the joint

Data Analysis

Nursing Diagnosis
JOINT PAIN (ARTHRALGIA): A distressful hurting at the point of juncture between two bones

Common Etiology (Stressors)

DISEASES: Bursitis, fibromyositis, meningitis, rheumatoid arthritis, spondylitis, tuberculosis of the joint

SIGNS AND SYMPTOMS: Immobility

MAJOR PATHOPHYSIOLOGIC FACTORS CAUSING THE PROBLEM: Joint pain results from infection, inflammation, muscle rigidity, and spasm

PLANNING

Unmet Needs
Exercise, comfort, protection from physical harm, freedom from pain, increased learning

Expected Outcome
Optimum joint function attainable by the person
Person verbalizes increased comfort

NURSING INTERVENTIONS

Nursing Treatments
Approach unhurriedly
Reassure that the pain will subside or be relieved
Communicate nurse sensitivity to the person's pain
Handle gently
Position comfortably
Change the person's position gradually
Maintain body alignment
Support the affected body part
Apply a heating pad
  OR
Apply a hot water bottle
  OR
Apply a warm, moist compress
  OR
Apply mentholated ointment
  OR
Place in a whirlpool bath
Massage gently
Exercise in range of motion (gently)
Ask the person what makes him comfortable
Discuss possible pain-reducing measures
Provide a pain-relief measure of the person's choice
Give nonprescription drugs (analgesics)

Nursing Observations
Observe for complaints of pain duration
Evaluate the pain for intensity and quality
Evaluate the effectiveness of the pain-relief measures

Health Teaching
Explain the causes of the pain (immobility, trauma, inflammation)
Teach how to apply heat therapy
Explain how to maintain body alignment (positioning)
Explain that immobility related to pain causes increased pain
Teach how to do range-of-motion exercises
Explain the reason for and intended effect of the therapy (to promote comfort and joint function)

Medical Treatments Performed by Nurses
Give the prescribed drugs (analgesics, steroids)

EVALUATION

Record actual outcome

LUMBOSACRAL STRAIN[42,88,476]

ASSESSMENT
Data Collection
Subjective Data
• Aching (soreness, tenderness) back pain
• Onset 2–24 hours after strenuous exertion
• No numbness or tingling

Objective Data
• No increased pain following coughing, sneezing, straining
• No pain on straight-leg raising
• Limited range of motion of the back
• Palpable tenderness over the paravertebral muscles
• Deep-tendon reflexes (knee and ankle jerks) are present and symmetrical
• Normal sensory responses on examination
  Bruising if the muscle fibers are torn
  Stiff gait and stance
  Guarding (spine will be held out of alignment)

Data Analysis
Nursing Diagnosis
LUMBOSACRAL STRAIN: The overstretching and partial tearing of the muscle fibers in the area of the lumbar and/or sacral vertebrae

Common Etiology (Stressors)
ENVIRONMENTAL FACTORS: *Objects*: Heavy
HUMAN ERROR: Using incorrect lifting methods, heavy lifting, accidental falling
MAJOR PATHOPHYSIOLOGIC FACTORS CAUSING THE PROBLEM: Violent muscle contractions or excessive muscle stretching of the lumbosacral muscles injures the muscle fibers, resulting in a strain

PLANNING
Unmet Needs
Comfort, protection from physical harm, freedom from pain, increased learning

Expected Outcome
Full range of motion and ease of ambulation following healing
Person expresses increased comfort

NURSING INTERVENTIONS
Nursing Treatments
Apply a cold pack (intermittently for the first 24 hours)
Apply a heating pad
  OR
Apply a hot water bottle or hot pack (if no bleeding is present, after the first 24 hours)
Encourage rest
Place on a firm mattress
Give nonprescription drugs (muscle relaxant to relieve the spasm)
Make a referral (to a physician if there is no improvement within 24 hours)

Nursing Observations
Test for range of motion (as the condition improves)
Observe for evidence of a favorable response to therapy (ease of movement, pain relief)

Health Teaching
Inform that heavy lifting should be avoided
Teach good body mechanics
Teach how to apply heat therapy
Teach how to do back exercises

Medical Treatments Performed by Nurses

Give the prescribed drugs (muscle relaxants to relieve spasm, anti-inflammatory drugs to inhibit the inflammatory process)

EVALUATION

Record actual outcome

MOTION SICKNESS[278,522]

ASSESSMENT

Data Collection

Subjective Data
- Dizziness
- Nausea
- Vomiting
- Onset when in a moving vehicle

Objective Data
- Facial pallor
- Sweating

Data Analysis

Nursing Diagnosis
MOTION SICKNESS: A sensation of sickness occurring when in motion in a car, airplane, boat, or train

Common Etiology (Stressors)
ENVIRONMENTAL FACTORS: *Moving vehicles*: Riding in moving vehicles
MAJOR PATHOPHYSIOLOGIC FACTORS CAUSING THE PROBLEM: The labyrinth of the inner ear is stimulated by motion, which affects the vomiting center in the medulla of the brain

PLANNING

Unmet Needs

Rest, comfort, protection from physical harm, increased learning

Expected Outcome

Person verbalizes increased comfort

NURSING INTERVENTIONS

Nursing Treatments

Apply a cool, damp cloth to the face
Place in the slight-sitting position
Change the person's position gradually
Encourage adequate rest
Give nonprescription drugs (Dramamine, Marezine)
Make a referral (to a physician if the condition persists)

Nursing Observations

Observe for evidence of a favorable response to therapy

Health Teaching

Advise against reading or looking out the window while in a moving vehicle
Explain the causes of the health problem (stimulation of the inner ear by motion)
Explain the reason for and intended effect of the therapy (to promote comfort)

EVALUATION

Record actual outcome

MUSCLE SPASM[72,371,522]

ASSESSMENT

Data Collection

Subjective Data
- Sudden painful contractions
- Of short duration
- Cramping (twisting) pain

Objective Data
- Muscle soreness on palpation
- Muscle tightness on palpation
  Grasping or rubbing the area of spasm
  Decreased serum calcium, magnesium, and sodium levels
  Increased serum phosphorus level

Data Analysis

Nursing Diagnosis
MUSCLE SPASM: A continuous state of muscle contraction with intense pain

Common Etiology (Stressors)
DISEASES: Hyperventilation, hypocalcemia, hypoparathyroidism, tetanus
INJURIES: Fracture and compression of the spinal cord
SIGNS AND SYMPTOMS: Uremia
MAJOR PATHOPHYSIOLOGIC FACTORS CAUSING THE PROBLEM: Muscle spasms result from increased nervous and muscular excitability due to changes in serum calcium level and
  blood pH; repetitive activation of efferent nerve fibers carrying motor impulses to
  muscle fibers before relaxation can occur; inadequate muscle stretching (especially
  calf muscles) causes chronically short and tight muscles that are prone to nocturnal
  cramping

PLANNING

Unmet Needs

Fluid and electrolyte balance, relaxation, comfort, protection from physical harm, freedom from pain, increased learning

Expected Outcome

No soreness on muscle palpation
Person verbalizes cessation of cramping
Normal serum calcium, magnesium, and phosphorous levels

NURSING INTERVENTIONS

Nursing Treatments

Handle gently
Position comfortably
Change the person's position gradually
Remove constrictive clothing
Apply a heating pad
  OR
Apply a hot water bottle
  OR
Apply a warm, moist compress
  OR
Place in a whirlpool bath (for muscle relaxation)
Refrain from local cold applications
Massage gently (the area of spasm)
Cover with warm blankets

Maintain a warm room temperature (if the spasms are recurring)
Decrease drafts
Place only warm hands and objects on the patient
Place a footboard at the feet (to press against during the spasm)
Place a pillow between the knees (to prevent friction between spastic knees)
Refrain from jarring the bed (which may stimulate spasms)
Ask the person what makes him comfortable
Discuss possible pain-reducing measures
Provide a pain-relief measure of the person's choice
Give nonprescription drugs (analgesics, muscle relaxant)
Encourage increased calcim-food intake
    OR   } If the serum calcium level is low
Give high-calcium fluids orally
Give high-magnesium fluids orally (if the serum magnesium level is low)

Nursing Observations
Observe for complaints of pain duration
Evaluate the effectiveness of the pain-relief measures

Health Teaching
Explain the causes of the pain (muscle contraction)
Teach how to apply heat therapy
Explain the reason for and intended effect of the therapy (muscle relaxation)

Medical Treatments Performed by Nurses
Give the prescribed drugs (analgesics, antispasmodics)

EVALUATION

Record actual outcome

MUSCLE STRAIN [20,73,219,522]

ASSESSMENT

Data Collection

Subjective Data
• Aching (soreness, tenderness) pain along the distribution of the muscle
• Muscle feels like it is in a "knot"
  Stiffness

Objective Data
• Motion causes pain
• Muscle tenderness on palpation
  X-ray film reveals no valuable diagnostic information
  Bruising if the muscle fibers are torn

Data Analysis

Nursing Diagnosis
MUSCLE STRAIN: The overstretching and partial tearing of the muscle fibers

Common Etiology (Stressors)
ENVIRONMENTAL FACTORS: *Objects*: Heavy
HUMAN ERROR: Using incorrect lifting methods, heavy lifting, accidental falling
MAJOR PATHOPHYSIOLOGIC FACTORS CAUSING THE PROBLEM: Violent muscle contraction or exces-

sive muscle stretching injures the muscle fibers resulting in a strain

PLANNING

Unmet Needs

Comfort, protection from physical harm, freedom from pain, increased learning

Expected Outcome

Full range of motion and ambulation following healing
Person verbalizes increased comfort

NURSING INTERVENTIONS

Nursing Treatments

Apply a heating pad (if no bleeding is present)
    OR
Apply a hot water bottle or hot pack
Encourage rest
Give nonprescription drugs (a muscle relaxant to relieve the spasm)
Make a referral (to a physician if there is no improvement within 24 hours)

Nursing Observations

Test for range of motion
Observe for evidence of a favorable response to therapy (ease of movement, decreased
    pain)

Health Teaching

Inform that heavy lifting should be avoided
Teach good body mechanics
Teach how to apply heat therapy

Medical Treatments Performed by Nurses

Give the prescribed drugs (muscle relaxants to relieve the spasm, anti-inflammatory
    drugs to inhibit the inflammatory process)

EVALUATION

Record actual outcome

NEURALGIA [42,72,278,371]

ASSESSMENT

Data Collection

Subjective Data
- Stabbing (piercing, lancinating, cutting, knifelike) pain
- Severe pain
  Irritability

Objective Data
- Pain radiation follows the nerve pathway
  Restlessness

Data Analysis

Nursing Diagnosis
NEURALGIA: A warning sign of potential or existing tissue-cell damage manifested as se-
    vere, sharp pain radiating along a nerve pathway

Common Etiology (Stressors)

DISEASES: Herpes zoster, peripheral neuritis, polyarteritis nodosa, rheumatic fever, rheumatoid arthritis, tic doulourex, trigeminal neuritis

MAJOR PATHOPHYSIOLOGIC FACTORS CAUSING THE PROBLEM: Neuralgia results from inflammation of, trauma to, pressure on, or degeneration of nerves or nerve cells

PLANNING

Unmet Needs

Rest and relaxation, comfort, protection from physical harm, freedom from pain, increased learning

Expected Outcome

Person verbalizes increased comfort

NURSING INTERVENTIONS

Nursing Treatments

Approach unhurriedly
Reassure that the pain will subside or be relieved
Communicate nurse sensitivity to the person's pain
Handle gently
Position comfortably
Apply a heat lamp
    OR
Apply a heat cradle
    OR
Apply a heating pad
    OR
Apply a hot water bottle
    OR
Apply a warm, moist compress
    OR
Apply a cold, moist compress
    OR
Apply an ice bag
Massage gently (to relax tense muscles)
Refrain from tight bandaging
Remove constrictive clothing
Apply a bed cradle (to prevent blanket pressure on the nerves)
Cover with lightweight blankets
Decrease drafts
Refrain from jarring the bed
Ask the person what makes him comfortable
Discuss possible pain-reducing measures
Provide a pain-relief measure of the person's choice
Give nonprescription drugs (analgesics)
Encourage adequate rest

Nursing Observations

Observe for complaints of pain duration
Observe for complaints of pain radiation
Evaluate the effectiveness of the pain-relief measures

Health Teaching

Explain the causes of the pain (pressure, inflammation, trauma)
Teach how to apply cold therapy
Teach how to apply heat therapy

Medical Treatments Performed by Nurses

Give the prescribed drugs (analgesics, steroids, antibiotics)

EVALUATION

Record actual outcome

PHANTOM LIMB[35,451]

ASSESSMENT

Data Collection

Subjective Data

- Person feels sensation as if it were in the amputated body part
- Focuses attention on the amputated area

  May fear going insane because of awareness that, although the limb is not whole, the feeling is still perceived

Objective Data

- Amputated limb
- Often attempts to walk on the missing leg, but falls

Data Analysis

Nursing Diagnosis

PHANTOM LIMB: A feeling that a body part still exists even though the body part has been amputated

Common Etiology (Stressors)

HEALTH CARE FACTORS *Surgical procedure*: Surgical amputation

MAJOR PATHOPHYSIOLOGIC FACTORS CAUSING THE PROBLEM: The feeling that a body part still exists after it has been amputated is the result of stimulation from pressure on the ends of the severed afferent nerves

PLANNING

Unmet Needs

Activity and exercise, comfort, protection from psychologic threat, increased learning

Expected Outcome

Person verbalizes that he no longer feels the amputated body part

NURSING INTERVENTIONS

Nursing Treatments

Reassure verbally (that such sensations can be perceived)

Cover with lightweight blankets

Decrease drafts (which may stimulate sensation)

Handle gently

Encourage moderate physical exercise

Exercise in range of motion

Percuss the amputation stump to increase firmness

Wrap the amputation stump (with a pressure bandage)

Position comfortably

Nursing Observations

Observe for evidence of a favorable response to therapy

Health Teaching

Explain the causes of the health problem (autonomic nervous system response)

Teach how to percuss the amputation stump

Teach how to wrap an amputation stump

EVALUATION

Record actual outcome

PHANTOM PAIN [451,522]

ASSESSMENT

Data Collection

Subjective Data
• Pain localized in a body area where tissue no longer exists
• Onset following an amputation
• Burning (stinging, smarting) pain
  Fear of being labeled "crazy" for experiencing pain where there is no tissue
  Anxiety
  Nervousness

Objective Data
• Amputated limb

Data Analysis

PHANTOM PAIN: A distressful hurting felt in the amputated area of a limb

Common Etiology (Stressors)
HEALTH CARE FACTORS: *Surgical procedures*: Surgical amputation
MAJOR PATHOPHYSIOLOGIC FACTORS CAUSING THE PROBLEM: Phantom pain results from stimuli
  that continue to arise from severed sensory nerves; in some cases, a neuroma has
  formed at the end of the severed nerve

PLANNING

Unmet Needs

Comfort, protection from physical harm, freedom from pain, increased learning

Expected Outcome

Person verbalizes cessation of pain in the amputated body part

NURSING INTERVENTIONS

Nursing Treatments

Approach unhurriedly
Reassure that the pain will subside or be relieved
Communicate nurse sensitivity to the person's pain
Provide an atmosphere of acceptance
Handle gently
Position comfortably
Avoid placing tension on the wound
Support the affected body part
Refrain from tight bandaging
Ask the person what makes him comfortable
Provide a pain-relief measure of the person's choice
Give nonprescription drugs (analgesics)

Nursing Observations

Observe for complaints of pain duration
Evaluate the pain for intensity and quality
Evaluate the effectiveness of the pain-relief measures

Health Teaching

Explain that it is acceptable to admit the existence of pain
Explain the causes of the pain (sensory nerve stimuli)
Explain the reason for and intended effect of the therapy (to promote comfort)

Medical Treatments Performed by Nurses

Give the prescribed drugs (analgesics)

EVALUATION

Record actual outcome

RESTLESS LEG SYNDROME[201]

ASSESSMENT

Data Collection

Subjective Data
- Onset 15–30 minutes after sitting or lying down
- Prickly, creeping leg sensation associated with leg jerking
  Leg jerks only one or two times, or may last for hours
  Complaints of being awakened by the jerking limb
  Discomfort is intermittent, in that it occurs, then disappears for several months, then returns again
  Frequently associated with riding on trains or airplanes

Objective Data
- Constant leg activity
- Leg spasmodically and involuntarily kicks and jerks

Data Analysis

Nursing Diagnosis
RESTLESS LEG SYNDROME: A creeping, crawling, jerking leg sensation, occurring only when the limb is at rest

Common Etiology (Stressors)
DISEASES: Iron-deficiency anemia
SIGNS AND SYMPTOMS: Uremia
HUMAN BODY: *Body state*: Pregnancy
MAJOR PATHOPHYSIOLOGIC FACTORS CAUSING THE PROBLEM: The cause is unknown but is believed to be a disorder of the spinal cord or the affected limb, or nervous system excitement; in uremia, there is nerve irritation by toxic substances

PLANNING

Unmet Needs
Sleep, rest, relaxation, comfort, protection from physical harm, increased learning

Expected Outcome
No observable leg jerking
Person verbalizes the absence of the leg jerking

NURSING INTERVENTIONS

Nursing Treatments
Ambulate the person
Apply a heating pad (to the limb)
  OR
Bathe in warm water
  OR
Cover with warm blankets
Avoid the use of (leg) restraints (which intensifies the discomfort)
Maintain a warm room temperature (during the episode)
Give nonprescription drugs (aspirin)
Massage (the jerking limb) gently

Nursing Observations
Observe for evidence of a favorable response to therapy

Health Teaching
Explain the causes of the health problem (the cause is unknown but is believed to be nervous system excitement)
Teach how to apply heat therapy
Explain the reason for and intended effect of the therapy (to promote relaxation)

EVALUATION

Record actual outcome

SPRAIN[73,291,522]

ASSESSMENT

Data Collection

Subjective Data
• Painful joint
• Aching (soreness, tenderness)

Objective Data
• Rapid swelling of the joint
• Limited movement
• Joint heat
• Discoloration

Data Analysis

Nursing Diagnosis

SPRAIN: The stretching and tearing of ligaments, tendons, and blood vessels surrounding a joint

Common Etiology (Stressors)

ENVIRONMENTAL FACTORS: *Moving vehicles*: Whiplash neck movements during the collision of moving vehicles

HUMAN ERROR: Accidental falling (twisting)

MAJOR PATHOPHYSIOLOGIC FACTORS CAUSING THE PROBLEM: When a joint is moved or stretched beyond its normal range of motion, the ligaments and tendons are stretched and torn, resulting in a sprain

PLANNING

Unmet Needs

Comfort, protection from physical harm, freedom from pain, increased learning

Expected Outcome

Reduction of swelling
Person expresses increased comfort
Full range of motion and ambulation of the joint

NURSING INTERVENTIONS

Nursing Treatments

Elevate the affected body part
Apply an ice bag (at the time of injury and intermittently for the first 24 hours)
Apply a hot water bottle or hot pack (after 24 hours)
Apply an arm sling (for an upper extremity sprain)
Apply an elastic bandage
Mobilize with crutches (if unable to walk comfortably)
Give nonprescription drugs (analgesics to relieve pain, muscle relaxant to relieve the spasm)
Make a referral (to a physician if the injury is severe or there is no improvement within 24 hours)

Nursing Observations

Inspect for edema
Observe for evidence of a favorable response to therapy (ease of movement, decreased pain)

Health Teaching

Describe those symptoms that should be reported (severe pain)

Explain the causes of the health problem (tearing and stretching of tissue)

Instruct to elevate the body part

Teach that weight bearing should be done on the unaffected side (when the person is able to ambulate)

Explain the reason for and intended effect of the therapy (to promote healing and ease the pain)

EVALUATION

Record actual outcome

SYNCOPE [20,72,278]

ASSESSMENT

Data Collection

Subjective Data
- Lightheadedness
- Blurred vision

Objective Data
- Sudden loss of consciousness
- Systolic blood pressure below 70 mm Hg
- Pallor
- Consciousness regained on assuming the supine (flat on back) position
  Tachycardia
  Sweating

Data Analysis

Nursing Diagnosis

SYNCOPE: Loss of consciousness as a result of inadequate blood circulation to the brain tissue

Common Etiology (Stressors)

DISEASES: Anemia, aortic stenosis, hemorrhage, hypoglycemia, rheumatic heart disease, Stokes–Adams syndrome

INJURIES: Heat exhaustion

SIGNS AND SYMPTOMS: Dehydration, pain

PSYCHOSOCIAL FACTORS: Excessive emotional excitement, the threat of real or imagined danger

HEALTH CARE FACTORS: *Drug therapy*: Narcotics, sedatives (drugs causing respiratory depression)

MAJOR PATHOPHYSIOLOGIC FACTORS CAUSING THE PROBLEM: Syncope results from insufficient oxygenation of the brain

PLANNING

Unmet Needs

Tissue oxygenation or perfusion, rest, comfort, stimulation, protection from physical harm, increased learning

Expected Outcome

Pulse between 60–80 beats/minute

Systolic blood pressure above 100 mm Hg

Normal skin color and moisture

Full consciousness

Full ambulation

NURSING INTERVENTIONS

Nursing Treatments

Apply a cool, damp cloth to the face
Attend the person constantly
Change the person's position gradually
Cover with warm blankets
Discourage smoking (for some time after the episode)
Give hot coffee
   OR   } If conscious
Give hot tea
Give nonprescription drugs (ammonia spirits to inhale)
Place in the foot-elevated head-lowered (Trendelenburg) position
   OR
Place in the flat position
Place on complete bed rest (until the episode subsides)
Refrain from giving iced liquids
Remove constrictive clothing
Make a referral (to a physician if episodes persist)

Nursing Observations

Auscultate the apical heartbeat for rate and rhythm
Inspect for hemorrhage
Monitor the blood pressure (frequently, and in the sitting, standing, and lying position after the episode)
Monitor blood studies for abnormal glucose and hematology
Monitor the cardiogram (if there is evidence of impaired cardiac output)
Observe for an excessive stress level
Observe for shock

Health Teaching

Explain the causes of the health problem (impaired circulation, emotions, drugs, hunger)
Advise against exposure to intense heat
Advise against wearing constrictive clothing
Advise not to stand for prolonged periods
Advise that highly emotional situations be avoided
Advise that positions that impair circulation be avoided
Explain how to apply elastic stockings or an elastic bandage (to the legs if the episode is recurrent)
Instruct to change position gradually (if the episode is recurrent)

Medical Treatments Performed by Nurses

Give the prescribed drugs

EVALUATION

Record actual outcome

VERTIGO [42,88,522]

ASSESSMENT

Data Collection

Subjective Data
• Acute onset
• Intermittent attacks usually lasting only a few minutes

A sensation that the environment is whirling around, that the body is whirling around, or that the head is spinning

Tinnitus

Nausea

Vomiting

Objective Data

• Symptoms increased by head movement

Facial pallor

Unsteady gait, often falling to one side

Hearing acuity may be diminished

Unable to walk a straight line

Data Analysis

Nursing Diagnosis

VERTIGO: The sensation that the environment is whirling around the person or that the person is whirling around

Common Etiology (Stressors)

DISEASES: Encephalitis, labyrinthitis, Meniere's disease, otitis media

INJURIES: Cerebral concussion

ENVIRONMENTAL FACTORS: *Chemical substances*: Inhalation of chemical agents such as toxic gases or vapors, industrial chemicals, or solvents

MAJOR PATHOPHYSIOLOGIC FACTORS CAUSING THE PROBLEM: Vertigo results from middle ear imbalance, or transient ischemia from decreased cardiac output, or neoplastic lesions

PLANNING

Unmet Needs

Sleep and rest, comfort, protection from physical harm, increased learning

Expected Outcome

Person verbalizes cessation of the whirling sensation

Exhibits a steady gait

NURSING INTERVENTIONS

Nursing Treatments

Sit the person in an armchair

  OR

Place in the slight-sitting position (in bed)

  OR

Place in the flat position (if the vertigo is due to labyrinthitis)

Change the person's position gradually

Encourage adequate rest

Give nonprescription drugs (Dramamine, antihistamines)

Attend the patient constantly (until the episode subsides)

Refrain from jarring the bed

Withhold all drugs (such as streptomycin, salicylates, alcohol, if they are causing side effects)

Make a referral (to an ENT specialist if the person has impaired hearing or tinnitus, to a neurologist for neurologic abnormality, to a cardiologist for bruits in the carotid artery or other cardiac abnormalities)

Nursing Observations

Observe for evidence of a favorable response to therapy

Inspect the ears with an otoscope (for any abnormality)

Test the ears for hearing acuity

Test the eyes for visual acuity

Inspect the nasal turbinates for abnormalities

Palpate the sinuses for tenderness

Test the cranial nerves

Auscultate the carotid arteries for bruit
Auscultate the chest for abnormal heart sounds

Health Teaching
Explain the causes of the health problem (ischemia, drug toxicity)
Instruct to change position gradually
Explain the reason for and intended effect of the therapy (to promote comfort)

EVALUATION
Record actual outcome

WRISTDROP[72,451]

ASSESSMENT
Data Collection
Subjective Data
• Person relates difficulty with hand function

Objective Data
• Palm of the hand falls downward
• Hand cannot be extended at the wrist
• Limited range of motion

Data Analysis
Nursing Diagnosis
WRISTDROP: Bending of the wrist in a downward direction

Common Etiology (Stressors)
DISEASES: Cerebrovascular accident, multiple sclerosis, poliomyelitis
INJURIES: Fracture and compression of the spinal cord, poisoning from alcohol, arsenic, or lead
MAJOR PATHOPHYSIOLOGIC FACTORS CAUSING THE PROBLEM: Wristdrop results from radial or cervical nerve injury or from paralysis of the wrist and hand extensor muscles

PLANNING
Unmet Needs
Exercise, protection from physical harm, increased learning

Expected Outcome
Optimum wrist alignment and function attainable by the person

NURSING INTERVENTIONS
Nursing Treatments
Maintain body alignment
Apply a supportive splint
Exercise in range of motion
Place in a whirlpool bath (during exercise, if possible)
   OR
Bathe in warm water
Place a hand roll under the fingers
Encourage normal use of the involved limb

Nursing Observations
Observe for evidence of a favorable response to therapy

Health Teaching
Explain how to maintain body alignment (positioning)
Teach how to do range-of-motion exercises

Explain the causes of the health problem (muscle paralysis, nerve injury)
Explain the reason for and intended effect of the therapy (optimum function)

Medical Treatments Performed by Nurses
Apply the prescribed preventive splint

EVALUATION

Record actual outcome

Knowledge Deficits Associated with the Musculoskeletal and Neurologic Systems

UNKNOWLEDGEABLE ABOUT PHYSICAL GROWTH AND DEVELOPMENT[142,148,233,234]

ASSESSMENT

Data Collection

Subjective Data
• Person's discussion or questions indicate a need for additional information, clarification, or validation of information
  OR
• Person's lack of questions or comments indicates not wanting information or not knowing enough to seek information
• When questioned directly, the person's response or lack of response indicates that he does not know:
  The physical capabilities to expect of persons at a certain age
  If the present growth and body state is appropriate to the age

Objective Data
None

Data Analysis

Nursing Diagnosis
UNKNOWLEDGEABLE ABOUT PHYSICAL GROWTH AND DEVELOPMENT: Being without sufficient information about the orderly progression of physical growth and human development through the life stages from conception through senescence

Common Etiology (Stressors)
HEALTH CARE FACTORS: Lack of health instruction

PLANNING

Unmet Needs
Comfort, protection from physical harm, independence, increased learning

Expected Outcome
Correct verbal feedback of the information taught

NURSING INTERVENTIONS

Nursing Treatments
Approach unhurriedly
Encourage the parent or patient to ask questions

Nursing Observations
Determine teaching effectiveness by verbal feedback

Health Teaching

Explain the expected changes which occur during the developmental phases (*Prenatal period*: From conception to birth there is intrauterine physiologic growth. *Infancy*: From birth to 14 days of life there is a period of adjustment to the environment with little or no physical growth; the infant can perform simple reflex activities such as sucking, yawning, grunting, stretching, etc. *Babyhood*: From 14 days to 3 years body control is learned; skills are developed in self-feeding and -dressing, walking, talking, and playing; the child learns to trust and gradually develops some independence, the first physical growth cycle occurs. *Childhood*: From age 3 to puberty, which occurs between ages 11 and 13, the child learns to control the environment and make social adjustments; he begins to develop a conscience and becomes involved in work-life activities; the second physical growth cycle occurs. *Adolescence*: From puberty, between ages 11 and 13, to maturity, at age 21, a sense of identity is developed; the third growth cycle occurs, in which there is rapid physiologic development of secondary sex characteristics; the person gains independence from adults and becomes ready for the intimacy of marriage and for work responsibilities. *Young adulthood*: The person enters a lasting relationship in marriage, starts a home, a family, and a career. *Adulthood*: There is a mature interest in establishing and guiding the next generation; there is a gradual physical slowing; menopause and the climacteric occur; these are the most productive years. *Senescence*: The person begins to reach the end of life; there is an ego integrity and an acceptance of one's life for what it is; decreased physical strength and activity occur with adjustments to retirement, reduced income, and loss of spouse and friends)

Inform of the factors that affect growth and development (intelligence, sex, nutrition, presence or absence of injury or disease, endocrine gland function, race, and the position of the child in the family)

Explain that parental attitudes affect child development (positive attitudes support health)

Emphasize that children need guidance (children have only limited experience and knowledge on which to make judgments)

Advise early correction of problems (emphasizing that each child's growth and development occur at a consistent but often a more rapid or slower rate than others)

Inform of the resources available for health care (when growth and development at any age are not normal)

EVALUATION

Record actual outcome

UNKNOWLEDGEABLE ABOUT SEIZURES [42,73,522]

ASSESSMENT

Data Collection

Subjective Data

- Person's discussion or questions indicate a need for additional information, clarification, or validation of information
  OR
- Person's lack of questions or comments indicates not wanting information or not knowing enough to seek information
- When questioned directly, the person's response or lack of response indicates that he does not know:
  Why seizures occur
  How to handle impending seizures
  May believe in the traditional superstitions related to seizures

Objective Data
• May exhibit behavior such as not taking protective measures during an impending or ongoing seizure or not taking medication as prescribed

Related Data
Commonly Related Diseases
Epilepsy

Data Analysis
Nursing Diagnosis
UNKNOWLEDGEABLE ABOUT SEIZURES: Being without sufficient information about the cause, effects, and treatment of seizures
Common Etiology (Stressors)
HEALTH CARE FACTORS: Lack of health information

PLANNING
Unmet Needs
Comfort, protection from physical harm, independence, increased learning
Expected Outcome
Correct verbal feedback of the information taught

NURSING INTERVENTIONS
Nursing Treatments
Approach unhurriedly
Encourage the person to ask questions
Nursing Observations
Determine teaching effectiveness by verbal feedback
Health Teaching
Describe the manifestations of an impending seizure (confusion, lightheadedness, seeing bright lights, hearing strange noises, smelling unusual odors)
Explain how to manage seizure episodes (loosen clothing, place a soft object between the teeth on one side of the mouth, protect the person from injury, do not restrain the person)
Inform of those conditions that precipitate seizures (excessive food intake, excitement, fever, infection, insufficient rest, flashing-light patterns)
Inform that seizures are not contagious
Explain the causes of the health problem (abnormal electrical impulses in the brain)
Explain the reason for and intended effect of the therapy (to prevent or minimize seizures, to prevent injury)

EVALUATION
Record actual outcome

Minor Health Problems Associated with the Reproductive System

AFTERBIRTH PAIN[42,55,123]

ASSESSMENT
Data Collection
Subjective Data
• Localized abdominal pain

- Cramping (twisting, colicky) pain
- Usually occurs mostly during breast-feeding

Objective Data
- Palpable uterine contractions
  Restlessness

Related Data
Women who have had twin or multiple births are most prone to afterbirth pain

Data Analysis

Nursing Diagnosis
AFTERBIRTH PAIN: Spasmodic uterine pain following delivery

Common Etiology (Stressors)
HUMAN BODY: *Natural body function*: Breast-feeding following childbirth
MAJOR PATHOPHYSIOLOGIC FACTORS CAUSING THE PROBLEM: Afterbirth pain is caused by uterine retraction resulting from a gradual return of the uterus to normal size, from uterine contraction due to lochia discharge, or from breast-feeding stimulation

PLANNING

Unmet Needs
Rest and relaxation, comfort, protection from physical harm, freedom from pain, increased learning

Expected Outcome
Woman verbalizes increased comfort
Calm, contented, relaxed facial expression
Normal posture
Freedom of body movement

NURSING INTERVENTIONS

Nursing Treatments
Approach unhurriedly
Reassure that the pain will subside or be relieved
Communicate nurse sensitivity to the woman's pain
Handle gently
Position comfortably
Change the person's position gradually
Apply a heating pad ⎤
   OR   ⎬ To the abdomen
Apply a hot water bottle ⎦
   OR
Soak in a sitz bath (warm)
Give warm liquids
Refrain from giving iced liquids (which may stimulate contractions)
Massage gently (the lumbar area)
Refrain from giving enemas
Refrain from jarring the bed
Provide quiet
Encourage adequate rest
Refrain from performing nonessential procedures
Ask the person what makes her comfortable
Discuss possible pain-reducing measures
Provide a pain-relief measure of the person's choice
Give nonprescription drugs (analgesics)

Nursing Observations
Observe for complaints of pain duration
Evaluate the pain for intensity and quality
Evaluate the effectiveness of the pain-relief measures

Health Teaching
Explain the causes of the pain (uterine contractions)
Inform that afterbirth pains following delivery are normal
Teach how to apply heat therapy
Explain the reason for and intended effect of the therapy (to promote comfort)

Medical Treatments Performed by Nurses
Give the prescribed drugs (analgesics, antispasmodics)

EVALUATION

Record actual outcome

BREAST ENGORGEMENT[52,123,286,527]

ASSESSMENT

Data Collection

Subjective Data
• Breast fullness
• Throbbing (pounding, pulsating) pain in breasts
• Pain whenever the breasts are moved or touched

Objective Data
• Palpable breast hardness
• Breast distention with tight, shiny skin
  Skin redness
  Heat felt on palpation
  Visible distended veins
  Axillary node tenderness, sometimes

Data Analysis

Nursing Diagnosis
BREAST ENGORGEMENT: Painful fluid congestion in the breast

Common Etiology (Stressors)
HUMAN BODY: *Body state*: Lactation following childbirth
MAJOR PATHOPHYSIOLOGIC FACTORS CAUSING THE PROBLEM: Breast engorgement results from
  mammary gland oversecretion due to excessive estrogen and progesterone production, repeated breast stimulation, obstruction of mammary gland ducts, lymphatic and
  venous congestion

PLANNING

Unmet Needs
Rest, comfort, protection from physical harm, freedom from pain, increased learning

Expected Outcome
Woman verbalizes increased comfort
Palpable soft breast tissue with adequate milk flow

NURSING INTERVENTIONS

Nursing Treatments
Approach unhurriedly
Reassure that the pain will subside or be relieved
Communicate nurse sensitivity to the woman's pain
Handle gently
Position comfortably

Elevate the head
Apply a brassiere
  OR
Apply a breast binder
Apply an ice bag (to the breasts)
Apply hot packs to the breast before breast-feeding
Express breast milk manually or mechanically
Provide quiet
Encourage adequate rest
Ask the woman what makes her comfortable
Discuss possible pain-reducing measures
Provide a pain-relief measure of the person's choice
Give nonprescription drugs (analgesics)

Nursing Observations
Observe for complaints of pain duration
Evaluate pain for intensity and quality
Evaluate the effectiveness of the pain-relief measures

Health Teaching
Explain the causes of the pain (repeated breast stimulation, hormones)
Teach how to apply a breast binder
  OR
Recommend the use of a brassiere for breast support
Instruct not to massage the breast (massage stimulates more milk)
Teach how to apply cold therapy
Teach how to apply heat therapy
Recommend the use of a nipple shield or nipple padding (to protect clothing)
Explain the reason for and intended effect of the therapy (to promote comfort)

Medical Treatments Performed by Nurses
Give the prescribed drugs (estrogen and/or androgens)

EVALUATION

Record actual outcome

BREAST TENDERNESS [55,123,286]

ASSESSMENT

Data Collection

Subjective Data
• Localized aching (soreness) in the breasts
• Touching or pressure on the breasts increases tenderness
  When it occurs before menstruation, it is most frequent in women who have borne children

Objective Data
• Tenderness on palpation of the breasts

Data Analysis

Nursing Diagnosis
BREAST TENDERNESS (BREAST PAIN): Cutaneous sensitivity of the breast

Common Etiology (Stressors)
DISEASES: Fibrocystic disease, mastitis

INJURIES: Bruising of the breast

HUMAN BODY: *Body state*: Menstruation, pregnancy

HEALTH CARE FACTORS: *Drug therapy*: Hormone drugs

MAJOR PATHOPHYSIOLOGIC FACTORS CAUSING THE PROBLEM: Breast tenderness results from increased hormone activity 7–10 days before menstruation, causing fluid accumulation in breast tissue and pressure against breast nerve fibers, or nursing an infant on one breast and not alternating breasts

PLANNING

Unmet Needs

Comfort, protection from physical harm, freedom from pain, increased learning

Expected Outcome

Woman verbalizes increased comfort

No tenderness on palpation of the breasts

NURSING INTERVENTIONS

Nursing Treatments

Approach unhurriedly

Reassure that the pain will subside

Communicate nurse sensitivity to the person's pain

Handle gently

Position comfortably (off the tender area)

Apply a brassiere

Apply an ice bag (to the breast)

Remove constrictive clothing

Encourage decreased sodium-food intake (7–10 days before menstruation onset)

Ask the person what makes her comfortable

Discuss possible pain-reducing measures

Provide a pain-relief measure of the person's choice

Give nonprescription drugs (analgesics)

Nursing Observations

Observe for complaints of pain duration

Evaluate the pain for intensity and quality

Evaluate the effectiveness of the pain-relief measures

Health Teaching

Explain the causes of pain (fluid retention)

Teach how to apply cold therapy

Explain that nursing the infant on alternate breasts reduces tension

Explain the reason for and intended effect of the therapy (to promote comfort)

Medical Treatments Performed by Nurses

Give the prescribed drugs (testosterone, 7–10 days before menstruation onset)

EVALUATION

Record actual outcome

CRACKED NIPPLE(S) [55,123,286,527]

ASSESSMENT

Data Collection

Subjective Data

• Burning (stinging, smarting) pain localized at the breast nipple

- Persistent maternal complaints of pain during infant nursing

Objective
- Minute blisters or petechiae on the nipples
- Small fissures (cracks) or abrasions of the nipples
  Bleeding may be present

Data Analysis

Nursing Diagnosis
CRACKED NIPPLE(S): A painful cracking or splitting of the breast nipple

Common Etiology (Stressors)
DISEASES: Mastitis
HUMAN BODY: *Natural body function*: Breast-feeding after childbirth
MAJOR PATHOPHYSIOLOGIC FACTORS CAUSING THE PROBLEM: Cracked nipples result from the irritation and pressure of the sucking infant

PLANNING

Unmet Needs
Comfort, protection from physical harm, freedom from pain, increased learning

Expected Outcome
Woman verbalizes increased comfort
Smooth, intact breast nipples

NURSING INTERVENTIONS

Nursing Treatments
Approach unhurriedly
Reassure that the pain will subside or be relieved
Communicate nurse sensitivity to the woman's pain
Handle gently
Position comfortably
Apply a warm, moist compress (to the nipples)
Remove constrictive clothing
Lubricate the skin with cocoa butter, glycerine, lanolin, mineral oil, or olive oil
Apply an antibiotic ointment
Place a shield over the breast nipple
Caution about breast-feeding (which may further crack the nipple)
Ask the person what makes her comfortable
Discuss the possible pain-reducing measures
Provide a pain-relief measure of the person's choice
Give nonprescription drugs (analgesics)

Nursing Observations
Observe for complaints of pain duration
Evaluate the pain for intensity and quality
Evaluate the effectiveness of the pain-relief measures
Inspect for bleeding (from the nipples)

Health Teaching
Explain the causes of the pain (pressure and irritation from infant sucking)
Describe those symptoms that should be reported (bleeding)
Explain the reason for and intended effect of the therapy (to promote comfort)

Medical Treatments Performed by Nurses
Give the prescribed drugs (analgesics)

EVALUATION

Record actual outcome

DYSMENORRHEA [42,243,278]

ASSESSMENT

Data Collection

Subjective Data
• Abdominal, suprapubic, or back pain that sometimes radiates into the thighs
• Usually occurs before or at the onset of menstruation
• Pain lasts from 1 to several days
• Cramping (twisting, spasmodic) pain associated primarily with flow
• Dull, heavy backache

Objective Data
• Abdominal distention
  Grimacing
  Holding the abdomen with the hand

Data Analysis

Nursing Diagnosis
DYSMENORRHEA: The presence of pain and discomfort during menstrual flow

Common Etiology (Stressors)
DISEASES: Anemia, endometriosis, syphilis, uterine fibroid tumor, uterine retroversion
PSYCHOSOCIAL FACTORS: The threat of severe or chronic stress
MAJOR PATHOPHYSIOLOGIC FACTORS CAUSING THE PROBLEM: Imbalanced estrogen–progesterone
  levels, incomplete disintegration of abnormally thick endometrium resulting from corpus luteum overactivity, an exceptionally long cervix, uterine underdevelopment, uterine malposition, nerve-ending sensitivity in the uterine isthmus resulting in
  uncoordinated and highly irritable uterine contractions, vasoconstriction causing myo-
  metrium ischemia, vagus-nerve hyperexcitability because of hypersensitive autonomic
  nerves supplying the uterus, blood leaving the uterus in spasmodic spurts as the uterus contracts irregularly every 1–15 minutes, failure of the liver to destroy excessive
  hormone production by an overactive ovarian follicle, a decreased serum-calcium level
  causing muscle spasms, and recent research studies have found that excessive production of one or more of the prostaglandins causes uterine muscle spasms

PLANNING

Unmet Needs

Rest and relaxation, exercise, comfort, protection from physical harm, freedom from
  pain, increased learning

Expected Outcome

Woman verbalizes increased comfort
Calm, contented, relaxed facial expression
Normal posture
Freedom of body movement

NURSING INTERVENTIONS

Nursing Treatments

Approach unhurriedly
Reassure that the pain will subside or be relieved
Communicate nurse sensitivity to the woman's pain
Position comfortably
Place in the knee-chest position
Apply a heating pad
  OR   } To the abdomen
Apply a hot water bottle
Administer a hot foot bath
Give warm liquids

Refrain from giving iced liquids
Massage (the lumbar area) gently
Encourage increased calcium-food intake (one week before menstruation onset)
Encourage increased protein-food intake (daily)
Encourage adequate rest
Encourage moderate physical exercise
Ask the person what makes her comfortable
Discuss possible pain-reducing measures
Provide a pain-relief measure of the person's choice
Give nonprescription drugs (analgesics, muscle relaxants)
Make a referral (to a physician if the condition persists)

Nursing Observations

Observe for complaints of pain duration
Evaluate the pain for intensity and quality
Evaluate the effectiveness of the pain-relief measures

Health Teaching

Explain the causes of the pain (uterine ischemia, spasms)
Advise not to stand for prolonged periods
Teach how to apply heat therapy
Explain the reason for and intended effect of the therapy (to promote comfort)

Medical Treatments Performed by Nurses

Give the prescribed drugs (analgesics, hormones, antispasmodics)

EVALUATION

Record actual outcome

FAILURE OF LACTATION[291,527]

ASSESSMENT

Data Collection

Subjective Data
• Breast pain radiating to the back
  Breasts may or may not feel full

Objective Data
• Failure of milk to flow on stimulation of the breasts

Data Analysis

Nursing Diagnosis
FAILURE OF LACTATION (ANALACTIA): Inadequate secretion of breast milk

Common Etiology (Stressors)
DISEASES: Malnutrition, Simmond's disease
PSYCHOSOCIAL FACTORS: Excessive emotional excitement, the threat of severe or chronic stress

MAJOR PATHOPHYSIOLOGIC FACTORS CAUSING THE PROBLEM: Mammary gland undersecretion is due to decreased estrogen and progesterone secretion, inadequate sucking stimulus

PLANNING

Unmet Needs

Fluid and electrolyte balance, food balance, activity and exercise, comfort, cleanliness, protection from physican harm, increased learning

Expected Outcome

Adequate milk flow when breasts are stimulated by infant sucking

NURSING INTERVENTIONS

Nursing Treatments

Apply hot packs to the breast before breast feeding
Massage (the breasts) gently
Encourage increased (maternal) carbohydrate intake
Increase (maternal) fluid intake to about 3,000 cc daily
Supplement inadequate breast-feeding with bottle-feeding
Provide quiet (for the mother and infant during breast-feeding)

Nursing Observations

Inspect the breasts for abnormalities
Observe for evidence of a favorable response to therapy

Health Teaching

Explain that mothers have a choice of single or double breast-feeding (but double
    breast-feeding increases milk flow)
Inform of the recommended length of infant nursing periods (shorter, more frequent
    feedings stimulate breast milk)
Advise that highly emotional situations should be avoided (before and during breast-
    feeding, and that emotional excitement reduces milk flow)
Teach the principles of good nutrition
Explain the cause of the health problem (inadequate infant sucking, poor maternal nu-
    trition)

Medical Treatments Performed by Nurses

Give the prescribed drugs

EVALUATION

Record actual outcome

FALSE LABOR [55,123,286]

ASSESSMENT

Data Collection

Subjective Data
• Diffuse cramping (spasmodic, colicky) abdominal pain that does not radiate from the
    back to the front
• Intermittent, short pains
• Pain frequency does not increase
• Intensity does not become progressively stronger
    Walking may cause the pain to cease

Objective Data
• No regular, palpable uterine contractions

Data Analysis

Nursing Diagnosis
FALSE LABOR: Pains that at first appear to be labor pains but are not

Common Etiology (Stressors)
SIGNS AND SYMPTOMS: Fetal movements, flatulence
HUMAN BODY: *Body state*: Pregnancy

MAJOR PATHOPHYSIOLOGIC FACTORS CAUSING THE PROBLEM: Fetal activity before labor onset can stimulate mild pain often misinterpreted as labor pain

PLANNING

Unmet Needs

Comfort, protection from physical harm, freedom from pain, increased learning

Expected Outcome

Woman verbalizes an understanding of the difference between false and true labor pains

Verbalizes increased comfort

NURSING INTERVENTIONS

Nursing Treatments

Approach unhurriedly

Reassure that the pain will subside or be relieved

Communicate nurse sensitivity to the woman's pain

Ambulate the person

Give warm liquids

Refrain from giving iced liquids

Massage (the lumbar area) gently

Remove constrictive clothing

Ask the person what makes her comfortable

Discuss possible pain-reducing measures

Provide a pain-relief measure of the person's choice

Give nonprescription drugs (analgesics)

Nursing Observations

Observe for complaints of pain duration and of pain radiation

Evaluate the pain for intensity and quality

Evaluate the effectiveness of the pain-relief measures

Health Teaching

Explain the causes of the pain (fetal activity)

Describe those symptoms that should be reported (true labor pains)

Explain the difference between true and false labor pains (*True*: Occur at regular and shorter intervals, increase in intensity. *False*: Occur at irregular and long intervals, with no increased intensity)

EVALUATION

Record actual outcome

LABOR PAIN[55,123,286]

ASSESSMENT

Data Collection

Subjective Data

- Pain localized primarily in the center of the back during the first stage of labor, generalized in the anterior abdomen during the second stage of labor
- Pains occur every 10–15 minutes apart during the first stage of labor; continuous, every 2–3 minutes, lasting 50–100 seconds during the second stage of labor, finally becoming constant
- Mild intensity during the first stage of labor, gradually becoming more severe; during the second stage of labor and full cervical dilatation, the pains are very severe and frequently excruciating

• Cramping (twisting, spasmodic, colicky) pains during the first stage of labor, constrictive (squeezing, binding, pressing) pain in the second stage

Objective Data
• Palpable uterine contractions
• Restlessness

Data Analysis

Nursing Diagnosis
LABOR PAIN: Maternal, distressful hurting that occurs during the process of delivery of a child

Common Etiology (Stressors)
SITUATIONAL FACTORS: Termination of pregnancy
MAJOR PATHOPHYSIOLOGIC FACTORS CAUSING THE PROBLEM: Labor pain results from uterine contractions and cervical dilatation that occur in an effort to expel the infant from the uterus

PLANNING

Unmet Needs
Rest and relaxation, comfort, protection from physical harm, freedom from pain, increased learning

Expected Outcome
Active participation of the mother in the labor process
Woman deep breathes and uses relaxation techniques for the optimum comfort achievable during labor

NURSING INTERVENTIONS

Nursing Treatments
Approach unhurriedly
Reassure that the pain will subside (after delivery but can be reduced during labor)
Communicate nurse sensitivity to the woman's pain
Attend the person constantly
Demonstrate calmness
Provide an atmosphere of acceptance
Handle gently
Position comfortably
Change the person's position gradually
Ambulate the person
Encourage deep breathing (for relaxation)
Massage (the lumbar area) gently (during the first stage of labor)
Remove constrictive clothing
Refrain from jarring the bed
Provide quiet
Encourage adequate rest (as labor pains increase)
Ask the person what makes her comfortable
Discuss possible pain-reducing measures
Provide a pain-relief measure of the person's choice
Give nonprescription drugs (analgesics)

Nursing Observations
Observe for complaints of pain duration
Estimate the degree of pain experienced
Evaluate the effectiveness of the pain-relief measures

Health Teaching
Teach how to control breathing to aid the labor process (panting in short, shallow, rapid breaths during contractions will decrease the pain)
Describe those symptoms that should be reported (increased pain)

Explain that it is acceptable to admit the existence of pain (through moaning, crying out, etc.)

Medical Treatments Performed by Nurses
Give the prescribed drugs (analgesics)

EVALUATION
Record actual outcome

OVULATION PAIN[88,278]

ASSESSMENT
Data Collection
Subjective Data
- Cramping (spasmodic, colicky) pain localized in the lower abdomen, on either or both sides, sometimes on alternating sides each month
- Lasts about 24 hours
- Onset about 14 days before menstruation onset
- Residual lower abdominal soreness for 24–48 hours

Objective Data
- Clear vaginal discharge
  May have a palpable enlarged, tender ovary

Data Analysis
Nursing Diagnosis
OVULATION PAIN (MITTELSCHMERZ): Pain associated with the rupture of the graafian follicle and the discharge of the ovum from the ovary

Common Etiology (Stressors)
HUMAN BODY: *Body state*: Menstrual cycle
MAJOR PATHOPHYSIOLOGIC FACTORS CAUSING THE PROBLEM: Ovulation pain occurs when the graafian follicle ruptures and blood oozes from the ovulation site into the peritoneal cavity; when the egg escapes from the ovary during ovulation, the fluid in the sack surrounding the egg is discharged and temporarily irritates the sensitive inside lining of the pelvic cavity, causing a mild peritonitis

PLANNING
Unmet Needs
Rest, comfort, protection from physical harm, freedom from pain, increased learning
Expected Outcome
Woman verbalizes increased comfort

NURSING INTERVENTIONS
Nursing Treatments
Approach unhurriedly
Reassure that the pain will subside or be relieved
Communicate nurse sensitivity to the woman's pain
Position comfortably
Apply a hot water bottle
  OR

Soak in a sitz bath
Give warm liquids
Refrain from giving iced liquids (if cramping)
Encourage adequate rest
Ask the person what makes her comfortable
Discuss possible pain-reducing measures
Provide a pain-relief measure of the person's choice
Give nonprescription drugs (analgesics)

Nursing Observations
Observe for complaints of pain duration
Evaluate the pain for intensity and quality
Evaluate the effectiveness of the pain-relief measures

Health Teaching
Explain the causes of the pain (rupture of the graafian follicle)
Teach how to apply heat therapy
Teach how to take a sitz bath
Explain the reason for and intended effect of the therapy (to promote comfort)

EVALUATION

Record actual outcome

PELVIC CONGESTION [197,252]

ASSESSMENT

Data Collection

Subjective Data
• Heavy, weighted, lower abdominal sensation
• Feeling that the person's insides are about to fall out
  Urinary incontinence with sneezing or coughing, sometimes

Objective Data
None

Related Data
Most frequent in women who have had large babies, numerous pregnancies, or difficult
  labor

Data Analysis

Nursing Diagnosis
PELVIC CONGESTION: A feeling of congestion or weighted discomfort in the lower abdomen

Common Etiology (Stressors)
DISEASES: Bladder prolapse, uterus prolapse, cystic ovary
HUMAN BODY: *Body state*: Menstruation
MAJOR PATHOPHYSIOLOGIC FACTORS CAUSING THE PROBLEM: Pelvic congestion results from weak-
  ened musculature of the bladder and/or uterus as a result of traumatic childbirth or
  pelvic fluid congestion before menstruation onset

PLANNING

Unmet Needs
Comfort, protection from physical harm, freedom from pain, increased learning

Expected Outcome
Woman verbalizes increased comfort

NURSING INTERVENTIONS

Nursing Treatments
Approach unhurriedly
Reassure that the pain will subside or be relieved
Communicate nurse sensitivity to the woman's pain
Apply an abdominal support garment
Place in the foot-elevated, head-lowered (Trendelenburg) position
   OR
Place in the knee-chest position
Apply a heating pad ⎤
   OR   ⎬ To the abdomen
Apply a hot water bottle ⎦
   OR
Soak in a sitz bath
Give warm liquids
Remove constrictive clothing
Ask the person what makes her comfortable
Discuss possible pain-reducing measures
Provide a pain-relief measure of the person's choice
Give nonprescription drugs (analgesics)

Nursing Observations
Observe for complaints of pain duration
Evaluate the effectiveness of the pain-relief measures

Health Teaching
Explain the causes of the pain (fluid retention, weakened musculature)
Advise not to stand for prolonged periods
Recommend the use of an abdominal-support garment
Recommend the use of low-heeled shoes (to support body alignment)
Teach how to apply heat therapy
Teach how to take a sitz bath

EVALUATION

Record actual outcome

POSTPARTAL PERINEUM PAIN[55,123,286]

ASSESSMENT
Data Collection

Subjective Data
- Burning (stinging, smarting) pain
- Itching sensation
- Increased discomfort when sitting

Objective Data
- Perineal edema
  Perineal bruising
  Sutured laceration

Data Analysis

Nursing Diagnosis

POSTPARTAL PERINEUM PAIN: A painful, discomforting sensation in the perineal area following childbirth

Common Etiology (Stressors)

HUMAN BODY: *Natural body function*: Childbirth

HEALTH CARE FACTORS: *Surgical procedures*: Episiotomy

MAJOR PATHOPHYSIOLOGIC FACTORS CAUSING THE PROBLEM: Postpartal perineal pain results from the stretching of the birth canal and perineal structures, swelling from an episiotomy, discomfort of sutures pulling

PLANNING

Unmet Needs

Comfort, protection from physical harm, freedom from pain, increased learning

Expected Outcome

Gradual reduction of perineal edema
Woman verbalizes increased comfort

NURSING INTERVENTIONS

Nursing Teatments

Approach unhurriedly
Reassure that the pain will subside or be relieved
Communicate nurse sensitivity to the woman's pain
Handle gently
Position comfortably
Apply a heat lamp
   OR
Apply a heating pad
   OR   } To the perineum
Apply a hot water bottle
   OR
Apply a warm, moist compress
Soak in a sitz bath
Apply an analgesic ointment
Arrange pillows comfortably (under the buttocks)
Avoid placing tension on the (episiotomy) wound
Refrain from jarring the bed
Ask the person what makes her comfortable
Discuss possible pain-reducing measures
Provide a pain-relief measure of the person's choice
Give nonprescription drugs (analgesics)

Nursing Observations

Observe for complaints of pain duration
Evaluate the pain for intensity and quality
Evaluate the effectiveness of the pain-relief measures
Inspect for inflammation (of the perineum)

Health Teaching

Explain the causes of the pain (pressure of childbirth)
Teach how to apply heat therapy
Teach how to take a sitz bath
Explain the reason for and intended effect of the therapy (to promote comfort)

Medical Treatments Performed by Nurses

Give the prescribed drugs (analgesics)

EVALUATION

Record actual outcome

Knowledge Deficits Associated with the Reproductive System and Reproduction

UNKNOWLEDGEABLE ABOUT ABNORMAL VAGINAL BLEEDING[252,451]

ASSESSMENT

Data Collection

Subjective Data
• Person's discussion or questions indicate a need for additional information, clarification, or validation of information
  OR
• Person's lack of questions or comments indicates not wanting information or not knowing enough to seek information
• When questioned directly, the person's response or lack of response indicates that she does not know:
  When menstrual bleeding is abnormal
  That vaginal bleeding during pregnancy requires immediate medical attention
  That any abnormal vaginal bleeding should be brought to the physician's attention
  The causes of abnormal vaginal bleeding

Objective Data
• May exhibit behavior such as not seeking health care during abnormal vaginal bleeding

Related Data

Commonly Related Conditions
Cervical or endocervical polyps

Commonly Related Diseases
Uterine carcinoma, endometriosis, ectopic pregnancy

Data Analysis

Nursing Diagnosis
UNKNOWLEDGEABLE ABOUT ABNORMAL VAGINAL BLEEDING: Being without sufficient information about vaginal bleeding occurring in unusual amounts or at unusual intervals

Common Etiology (Stressors)
HEALTH CARE FACTORS: Lack of health information

PLANNING

Unmet Needs
Protection from physical harm, independence, increased learning

Expected Outcome
Correct verbal feedback of the information taught

NURSING INTERVENTIONS

Nursing Treatments
Approach unhurriedly
Encourage the person to ask questions

Nursing Observations
Determine teaching effectiveness by verbal feedback

Health Teaching
Describe the characteristics of abnormal vaginal bleeding (menstrual flow that requires

more than 4 sanitary napkins in an 8-hour period or 12 in a 24-hour period, bleeding
at times other than menstruation or after the onset of menopause)
Instruct to report serious symptoms immediately (any unusual bleeding)
Explain the causes of the health problem

EVALUATION

Record actual outcome

UNKNOWLEDGEABLE ABOUT POSTSURGICAL VAGINAL BLEEDING[252,397]

ASSESSMENT
Data Collection
Subjective Data
• Person's discussion or questions indicate a need for additional information, clari-
    fication, or validation of information
    OR
• Person's lack of questions or comments indicates not wanting information or not
    knowing enough to seek information
• When questioned directly, the person's response or lack of response indicates that she
    does not know:
    The fact that following a dilatation and currettement procedure, a red-brown bloody
        discharge can be expected for several days
    The fact that following a hysterectomy, bright blood, a red-brown discharge, or
        spotting can occur for as long as 6 weeks
    The causes of the bleeding
    Recommended methods for minimizing the bleeding
Objective Data
None
Data Analysis
Nursing Diagnosis
UNKNOWLEDGEABLE ABOUT POSTSURGICAL VAGINAL BLEEDING: Being without sufficient information
    about bleeding that normally occurs following vaginal surgery
Common Etiology (Stressors)
HEALTH CARE FACTORS: Lack of health instruction

PLANNING
Unmet Needs
Comfort, protection from physical harm, independence, increased learning
Expected Outcome
Correct verbal feedback of the information taught

NURSING INTERVENTIONS
Nursing Treatments
Approach unhurriedly
Encourage the person to ask questions
Reassure verbally (that the bleeding is expected to occur)
Encourage adequate rest
Nursing Observations
Determine teaching effectiveness by verbal feedback

Health Teaching

Explain the causes of the health problem (post–D and C bleeding is caused by surgical scraping of the uterine lining, and posthysterectomy bleeding is caused by slow healing of the surgical incision made at the top of the vagina in order to free the cervix from the vagina)

Describe those symptoms that should be reported (profuse bleeding)

Advise not to stand for prolonged periods

Inform that heavy lifting should be avoided

Instruct to avoid pushing and pulling activities

Advise against using tampons (which can irritate tissue and increase the bleeding)

Advise not to take enemas and laxatives

Inform that elimination straining should be avoided

Instruct that douching should be avoided

Advise daily bathing (in the shower, not the tub)

EVALUATION

Record actual outcome

UNKNOWLEDGEABLE ABOUT CHILDBIRTH[73,527]

ASSESSMENT

Data Collection

Subjective Data

• Person's discussion or questions indicate a need for additional information, clarification, or validation of information

>   OR

• Person's lack of questions or comments indicates not wanting information or not knowing enough to seek information

• When questioned directly, the person's response or lack of response indicates that the person does not know:

>   How to recognize the onset of labor
>
>   The physical changes to expect as labor progresses
>
>   The procedures that will be carried out during labor and delivery
>
>   Methods the mother can use to ease childbirth
>
>   Common behavior associated with childbirth

Objective Data

None

Data Analysis

Nursing Diagnosis

UNKNOWLEDGEABLE ABOUT CHILDBIRTH: Being without sufficient information about the natural process of labor and delivery

Common Etiology (Stressors)

HEALTH CARE FACTORS: Lack of health instruction

PLANNING

Unmet Needs

Comfort, protection from physical harm, independence, increased learning

Expected Outcome

Correct verbal feedback of the information taught

NURSING INTERVENTIONS

Nursing Treatments

Approach unhurriedly

Encourage the person to ask questions

Discuss the anticipated procedure (such as perineal shave, cleansing enema, rectal and vaginal examinations, monitoring fetal heart sounds, IV therapy)

Nursing Observations

Determine teaching effectiveness by verbal feedback

Health Teaching

Describe the manifestations of labor onset (lightening, mucous plug discharge, membrane rupture, labor pains)

Explain the difference between true and false labor pains (*True labor*: Pains occur at consistently shorter intervals, becoming progressively more intense and are initially located in the back. *False labor*: Pains are irregular, do not increase in intensity, and are located in the abdomen)

Explain the significance of premature membrane rupture and that it does not indicate a difficult labor

Describe the process of labor and delivery (the first stage of gradual to complete cervical dilatation, the second stage of expulsion and birth, the third stage of placenta delivery)

Explain that childbirth is a normal process

Describe the normal behavior pattern common during labor (anxiety, frustration, joy)

Teach how to control breathing to aid the labor process (deep breathing at the beginning of a contraction, shallow breathing at the peak of a contraction, slow and deep breathing as the contraction subsides)

Teach the specific method (proposed by Read and/or Lamaze for natural childbirth)

Explain the reason for and intended effects of the methods used (to ease childbirth and support a rewarding experience)

EVALUATION

Record actual outcome

UNKNOWLEDGEABLE ABOUT LACTATION SUPPRESSION[291,527]

ASSESSMENT

Data Collection

Subjective Data

• Person's discussion or questions indicate a need for additional information, clarification, or validation of information

  OR

• Person's lack of questions or comments indicates not wanting information or not knowing enough to seek information

• When questioned directly, the person's response or lack of response indicates that she does not know:

  The methods used to suppress lactation

  The breast changes expected

  Symptoms that should be reported

Objective Data

None

Data Analysis

Nursing Diagnosis

UNKNOWLEDGEABLE ABOUT LACTATION SUPPRESSION: Being without sufficient information about the prevention of breast-milk formation by therapeutic means

Common Etiology (Stressors)

HEALTH CARE FACTORS: Lack of health instruction

PLANNING

Unmet Needs

Protection from physical harm, independence, increased learning

Expected Outcome

Correct verbal feedback of the information taught

NURSING INTERVENTIONS

Nursing Treatments

Approach unhurriedly

Encourage the person to ask questions

Nursing Observations

Determine teaching effectiveness by verbal feedback

Health Teaching

Recommend the use of a brassiere for breast support (during the suppression therapy)

Teach how to apply cold therapy (ice bag or cold pack to the breasts)

Instruct not to massage the breasts or use a breast pump (since this will further stimulate the production of milk)

Describe those symptoms that should be expected (initially there is a breast fullness from the milk, fullness gradually subsides as the milk dries up in a few days)

Describe those symptoms that should be reported (if lactation does not subside)

EVALUATION

Record actual outcome

UNKNOWLEDGEABLE ABOUT MALE CLIMACERTIC[426]

ASSESSMENT

Data Collection

Subjective Data

• Person's discussion or questions indicate a need for additional information, clarification, or validation of information

   OR

• Person's lack of questions or comments indicates not wanting information or not knowing enough to seek information

• When questioned directly, the person's response or lack of response indicates that he does not know:

   When the male climacteric onset normally occurs

   The signs and symptoms of male climacertic

   The cause of male climacteric

   Good health practices recommended during male climacteric

Objective Data

None

Data Analysis

Nursing Diagnosis
UNKNOWLEDGEABLE ABOUT MALE CLIMACTERIC: Being without sufficient information about the life stage during which there is gradual reduction of male sexual potency

Common Etiology (Stressors)
HEALTH CARE FACTORS: Lack of health instruction

PLANNING

Unmet Needs
Comfort, protection from physical harm, independence, increased learning

Expected Outcome
Correct verbal feedback of the information taught

NURSING INTERVENTIONS

Nursing Treatments
Approach unhurriedly
Encourage the person to ask questions
Encourage adequate rest
Encourage moderate physical exercise

Nursing Observations
Determine teaching effectiveness by verbal feedback

Health Teaching
Describe the factors associated with the occurrence of the male climacteric (onset occurs around age 50 with almost complete quieting by age 60)
Describe the normal changes associated with male climacteric (decreased sexual desire, fatigue, palpitations, hot or cold flushes, dizziness, numbness and tingling, irritability, poor concentration, etc.)
Teach the principles of good nutrition (needed to maintain health as the body changes)
Explain the causes of the health problem (the onset of decreased androgen excretion from the adrenal cortex)
Describe those symptoms that should be reported (any symptom causing severe discomfort)

EVALUATION
Record actual outcome

UNKNOWLEDGEABLE ABOUT MALE PUBERTY[426]

ASSESSMENT

Data Collection

Subjective Data
• Person's discussion or questions indicate a need for additional information, clarification, or validation of information
  OR
• Person's lack of questions or comments indicates not wanting information or not knowing enough to seek information
• When questioned directly, the person's response or lack of response indicates that he does not know:
  When male puberty onset normally occurs
  The signs and symptoms of male puberty onset
  The physiology of male puberty

Normal emotional changes associated with male puberty
Good health practices recommended during male puberty

Objective Data
None

Data Analysis

Nursing Diagnosis
UNKNOWLEDGEABLE ABOUT MALE PUBERTY: Being without sufficient information about the life stage during which male reproductive organs become functionally mature

Common Etiology (Stressors)
HEALTH CARE FACTORS: Lack of health instruction

PLANNING

Unmet Needs
Comfort, protection from physical harm, independence, increased learning

Expected Outcome
Correct verbal feedback of the information taught

NURSING INTERVENTIONS

Nursing Treatments
Approach unhurriedly
Encourage the person to ask questions
Encourage adequate rest
Encourage moderate physical exercise

Nursing Observations
Determine teaching effectiveness by verbal feedback

Health Teaching
Describe the factors associated with the occurrence of male puberty (onset of male puberty occurs about age 14–15)
Describe the normal changes associated with male puberty (appearance of pubic, axillary, and facial hair; rapid growth; ejaculation; voice huskiness; accentuated Adam's apple)
Describe the normal behavior pattern common during male puberty (interest in the opposite sex, desire for independence, inconsistent attitudes)
Teach the principles of good nutrition (needed to maintain health as the body changes)
Explain the causes of the health problem (increased androgen excretion from the adrenal cortex)
Describe those symptoms that should be reported (any symptom causing severe discomfort)

EVALUATION

Record actual outcome

UNKNOWLEDGEABLE ABOUT MANAGING A NORMAL PREGNANCY[291,405,496,527]

ASSESSMENT

Data Collection

Subjective Data
• Person's discussion or questions indicate a need for additional information, clarification, or validation of information

OR
- Person's lack of questions or comments indicates not wanting information or not knowing enough to seek information
- When questioned directly, the person's response or lack of response indicates that she does not know about:
Weight control
Adequate hygiene
Breast care
Proper rest and exercise
Nutritional balance
Skin care
Comfortable clothing
Observation for and prevention of pregnancy complications

Objective Data
- May exhibit behavior such as changing from an active to sedentary life once pregnancy is diagnosed, may wear constrictive garments to reduce abdominal size, etc.

Data Analysis

Nursing Diagnosis
UNKNOWLEDGEABLE ABOUT MANAGING A NORMAL PREGNANCY: Being without sufficient information about the maintenance of health during the period from conception to the onset of labor

Common Etiology (Stressors)
HEALTH CARE FACTORS: Lack of health instruction

PLANNING

Unmet Needs
Comfort, protection from physical harm, independence, increased learning

Expected Outcome
Correct verbal feedback of the information taught

NURSING INTERVENTIONS

Nursing Treatments
Encourage adequate rest
Encourage moderate physical exercise
Encourage increased calcium-food intake, increased protein-food intake, increased residue-food intake, increased high-vitamin–food intake
Discourage the intake of oral stimulants
Discourage smoking

Nursing Observations
Determine teaching effectiveness by verbal feedback

Health Teaching
Inform that cleanliness is basic to health
Explain when showering should be substituted for tub bathing during pregnancy (when bleeding occurs, after membrane rupture, or after the mucus plug is passed)
Describe the breast changes expected during pregnancy (breasts become enlarged, feel stretched, full, tender; pigment around the nipples widens and darkens, sticky white fluid may be expressed from the nipple)
Recommend the use of a brassiere for breast comfort
Explain the advantages and disadvantages of breast-feeding (breast-milk is nutritious, free of bacteria, causes no allergy; breast-feeding requires a rigid schedule)
Explain how to prepare the breasts during pregnancy for postdelivery breast-feedings (breast massage, applying lanolin, pulling the nipples)
Explain how to adjust clothing to meet health problems (loose garments, maternity clothes)

Recommend the use of an abdominal-support garment (if back discomfort is a major concern)

Advise against wearing constrictive clothing (which might impair circulation)

Recommend the use of low-heeled shoes (for better balance)

Explain how to apply elastic stockings or an elastic bandage (to support better leg circulation)

Instruct to increase fluid intake (especially water)

Instruct that douching be avoided (because of possible introduction of bacteria into the vagina)

Advise not to take enemas and laxatives (habitually)

Advise against using mineral oil laxatives (which interfere with vitamin absorption)

Advise not to take *any* drugs (unless prescribed by a physician)

Teach the principles of good nutrition (needed for a healthy mother and child)

Explain how to control weight gain during pregnancy (limit weight gain to one-half pound each week from the fourth through the sixth month and three-quarters of a pound per week thereafter)

Inform that heavy lifting should be avoided

Emphasize the danger of x-ray exposure during early pregnancy (x-rays may injure the fetus or impair fetal development)

Explain that sexual activity should be temporarily limited (if there is a history of abortion, membrane rupture, or mucous-plug passage)

Describe the normal behavior pattern common during pregnancy (such as fear of death, mood swings)

Explain how to calculate the delivery date (count back 3 calendar months from the first day of the last menstrual period, then add 7 days)

Explain that childbirth is a normal process

Describe the danger signs of pregnancy (nausea, vomiting, dizziness, visual disturbance, edema, bleeding, pain, absence of fetal movement after the fourth month)

Instruct to report serious symptoms immediately (mentioned above)

EVALUATION

Record actual outcome

UNKNOWLEDGEABLE ABOUT MANAGING A NORMAL PUERPERIUM[291,405,496,527]

ASSESSMENT

Data Collection

Subjective Data

• Person's discussion or questions indicate a need for additional information, clarification, or validation of information
  OR
• Person's lack of questions or comments indicates not wanting information or not knowing enough to seek information
• When questioned directly, the person's response or lack of response indicates that she does not know:
  The importance of good nutrition during the puerperium
  The characteristics of normal lochia when menstruation begins
  How to establish the prepregnancy body shape through exercise
  What to observe for and how to prevent complications

Objective Data

None

Data Analysis

Nursing Diagnosis

UNKNOWLEDGEABLE ABOUT MANAGING A NORMAL PUERPERIUM: Being without sufficient information about the maintenance of health during the period following childbirth

Common Etiology (Stressors)

HEALTH CARE FACTORS: Lack of health instruction

PLANNING

Unmet Needs

Comfort, protection from physical harm, independence, increased learning

Expected Outcome

Correct verbal feedback of the information taught

NURSING INTERVENTIONS

Nursing Treatments

Approach unhurriedly
Encourage the person to ask questions
Encourage adequate rest
Encourage adequate physical exercise

Nursing Observations

Determine teaching effectiveness by verbal feedback

Health Teaching

Describe the characteristics of normal lochia (initially bloody with mucus, after 3 days changes to pink fluid, after 8 or 9 days becomes brownish, disappears within 3 weeks)
Explain when the postpartum flow normally resumes (about 8 weeks after delivery)
Describe those symptoms that should be reported (abnormal bleeding)
Inform that cleanliness is basic to health
Inform that heavy lifting should be avoided
Teach how to do postpartum exercises (back and pelvis, gluteal and pelvic strengthening exercises, knee-chest and monkey-trot postpartum exercises)
Teach the principles of good nutrition (the four basic food groups)
Describe those symptoms that should be reported (abnormal bleeding, pain, fatigue)

EVALUATION

Record actual outcome

UNKNOWLEDGEABLE ABOUT MENOPAUSE[158,252,426]

ASSESSMENT

Data Collection

Subjective Data
• Person's discussion or questions indicate a need for additional information, clarification, or validation of information
    OR
• Person's lack of questions or comments indicates not wanting information or not knowing enough to seek information
• When questioned directly, the person's response or lack of response indicates that she does not know:
    The signs and symptoms of menopause
    The normal behavior patterns associated with menopause
    The effect of menopause on sexual desire or response
    The factors related to its occurrence
    General health practice recommended to minimize the discomfort

Objective Data
• May exhibit behavior such as staying in bed for prolonged periods, indicating the perception of self as ill

Data Analysis

Nursing Diagnosis
UNKNOWLEDGEABLE ABOUT MENOPAUSE: Being without sufficient information about the life stage in which the cessation of menstruation has occurred for 1 year

Common Etiology (Stressors)
HEALTH CARE FACTORS: Lack of health instruction

PLANNING

Unmet Needs
Comfort, protection from physical harm, independence, increased learning

Expected Outcome
Correct verbal feedback of the information taught

NURSING INTERVENTIONS

Nursing Treatments
Approach unhurriedly
Encourage the person to ask questions
Encourage adequate rest

Nursing Observations
Determine teaching effectiveness by verbal feedback

Health Teaching
Describe the factors associated with the occurrence of menopause (usually occurs between ages 44 and 55 but normally occurs earlier in women who have not been pregnant)
Describe the normal changes associated with menopause (facial flushing, sweating, chills, irritability, fatigue, joint pain, sparsity of hair)
Describe the normal psychic changes common during menopause (emotional instability, weeping, excitement, fatigue)
Inform that menopause does not interfere with sex life (the emotional aspects of sexual desire and response remain)
Teach the principles of good nutrition (needed to maintain health as the body changes)
Advise that highly emotional situations should be avoided
Explain the causes of the health problem (decreased ovarian activity and increased pituitary activity, resulting in estrogen deficiency, or menopause)
Describe those symptoms that should be reported (any symptom causing severe discomfort)

EVALUATION
Record actual outcome

UNKNOWLEDGEABLE ABOUT MENSTRUATION[158,243,252,426]

ASSESSMENT

Data Collection

Subjective Data
• Person's discussion or questions indicate a need for additional information, clarification, or validation of information
  OR

- Person's lack of questions or comments indicates not wanting information or not knowing enough to seek information
- When questioned directly, the person's response or lack of response indicates that she does not know:
  When menstruation onset normally occurs
  The physiology of menstruation
  The signs and symptoms of premenstrual tension
  That bleeding from the nose, mouth, bladder, eyes, ears, breast, skin, or gums can occur during or just before menstruation
  Abnormalities associated with menstruation
  Normal emotional changes associated with the menstrual cycle
  The principles of good menstrual hygiene
  General health practices recommended during menstruation

Objective Data
- May exhibit behavior such as staying in bed for prolonged periods indicating the perception of self as ill

Data Analysis

Nursing Diagnosis

UNKNOWLEDGEABLE ABOUT MENSTRUATION: Being without sufficient information about the bloody discharge from the uterus occurring at regular intervals from puberty to menopause

Common Etiology (Stressors)

HEALTH CARE FACTORS: Lack of health instruction

PLANNING

Unmet Needs

Comfort, protection from physical harm, independence, increased learning

Expected Outcome

Correct verbal feedback of the information taught

NURSING INTERVENTIONS

Nursing Treatments

Approach unhurriedly

Encourage the person to ask questions

Encourage adequate rest

Encourage moderate physical exercise

Encourage moderate activity

Encourage decreased sodium-food intake (such as potato chips, pork, etc., for at least 1 week before menstrual onset)

Discourage the intake of oral stimulants (such as coffee, soft drinks, to reduce irritability)

Reassure verbally (that menstruation is a normal occurrence)

Nursing Observations

Determine teaching effectiveness by verbal feedback

Health Teaching

Describe the factors associated with the occurrence of menstruation (onset usually occurs when the young woman reaches 105 pounds of body weight, between the ages of 9 and 15)

Describe the manifestations of premenstrual tension (irritability, depression, backache, headache, edema, abdominal bloating, increased thirst and appetite, fatigue, weeping; it usually occurs 4–10 days before menstrual onset and primarily between the ages of 24 and 40)

Explain the causes of the health problem (premenstrual tension is caused by an increase in the estrogen but especially the progesterone level, which causes water retention throughout the body, especially in the brain and nerve tissue)

Advise that highly emotional situations be avoided (during the premenstrual period)

Explain the causes of the health problem (of nose, mouth, skin, gum bleeding before or during menstruation; a decreased platelet count that occurs 14 days before menstruation results in extragenital bleeding)

Explain those menstrual variations that indicate abnormality (when menstruation occurs more frequently than every 21 days, less frequently than every 35 days, or for a duration of less than 3 days or more than 7 days; when more than 12 perineal pads are used in 24 hours)

Teach menstrual cycle physiology

Teach menstrual hygiene (bathing, shampooing)

Recommend that perfumed vaginal products be avoided

Advise against using tampons (during a vaginal infection)

Teach the principles of good nutrition (needed to maintain health as the body changes)

Describe the emotional changes that normally occur during the menstrual cycle (mood changes from depression to feeling exceptionally well)

Describe those symptoms that should be reported (any symptoms that cause severe discomfort or abnormal bleeding)

EVALUATION

Record actual outcome

UNKNOWLEDGEABLE ABOUT PREMENOPAUSE [158,252,426]

ASSESSMENT

Data Collection

Subjective Data

- Person's discussion or questions indicate a need for additional information, clarification, or validation of information
  OR
- Person's lack of questions or comments indicates not wanting information or not knowing enough to seek information
- When questioned directly, the person's response or lack of response indicates that she does not know:
  The signs and symptoms of premenopause
  The many alterations in the menstrual cycle that can occur
  The factors related to its occurrence
  General health practices recommended to minimize the discomfort

Objective Data
None

Data Analysis

Nursing Diagnosis
UNKNOWLEDGEABLE ABOUT PREMENOPAUSE: Being without sufficient information about the life stages before and leading up to menstruation cessation

Common Etiology (Stressors)
HEALTH CARE FACTORS: Lack of health instruction

PLANNING

Unmet Needs

Comfort, protection from physical harm, independence, increased learning

Expected Outcome

Correct verbal feedback of the information taught

NURSING INTERVENTIONS

Nursing Treatments

Approach unhurriedly

Encourage the person to ask questions

Encourage adequate rest

Encourage moderate physical exercise

Nursing Observations

Determine teaching effectiveness by verbal feedback

Health Teaching

Describe the factors associated with the occurrence of premenopause (onset usually occurs after age 40 but normally occurs earlier in women who have not been pregnant than in women who have; it usually indicates that menopause is 2–4 years in the future)

Describe the normal changes associated with premenopause (weight gain, nervousness, depression, palpitations, headache, numbness and tingling, gradually decreasing flow, irregular cycle, shortened or lengthened regular cycle, etc.)

Explain the causes of the health problem (the temporary progesterone–pituitary gonadotropic hormone imbalance that occurs as the body adapts to the new hormone balance of menopause)

Teach the principles of good nutrition (needed to maintain health as the body changes)

Advise that highly emotional situations be avoided

Describe those symptoms that should be reported (any menstrual abnormality, any symptom causing severe discomfort)

EVALUATION

Record actual outcome

UNKNOWLEDGEABLE ABOUT FAMILY PLANNING[98,243,488]

ASSESSMENT

Data Collection

Subjective Data

• Person's discussion or questions indicate a need for additional information, clarification, or validation of information

   OR

• Person's lack of questions or comments indicates not wanting information or not knowing enough to seek information

• When questioned directly, the person's response or lack of response indicates that he does not know:

The options available for family planning
The side effects of some family planning methods
The contraindications for specific methods

Objective Data
• May exhibit behavior based on insufficient knowledge such as wearing charms around the neck or eating certain foods to ensure or prevent pregnancy

Data Analysis
Nursing Diagnosis
UNKNOWLEDGEABLE ABOUT FAMILY PLANNING: Being without sufficient information regarding methods for achieving, spacing, or preventing pregnancy

Common Etiology (Stressors)
HEALTH CARE FACTORS: Lack of health instruction

PLANNING
Unmet Needs
Comfort, increased learning

Expected Outcome
Correct verbal feedback of the information taught

NURSING INTERVENTIONS
Nursing Treatments
Approach unhurriedly

Encourage the person to ask questions (many will ask questions regarding the cost of the birth-control method, if it is painful, if it will affect the person's sex life, if it will cause cancer in later years, etc.)

Listen attentively (to each partner's needs; give special consideration to spiritual and cultural beliefs and practices and their effect on the person's choice of family planning methods; for example, the Catholic church does not sanction artificial birth control but does sanction natural birth control, and the Orthodox Jewish faith does not permit a man to do anything to interfere with his procreative ability)

Nursing Observations
Determine teaching effectiveness by testing or verbal feedback

Health Teaching
Explain normal reproductive organ function (so the person fully understands the function of the reproductive organs)

Explain the reproductive process (how procreation occurs)

Explain the options available for family planning (enumerating the various methods available such as oral contraceptives, rhythmic method, intrauterine device, etc.)

Explain the side effects of the various family planning methods (*Oral contraceptives*: Breast tenderness, hypertension, fluid retention, elevated glucose, altered thyroid function, amenorrhea after the pill has been stopped. *Intrauterine devices*: Bleeding, pain, or infection, etc.)

Explain the contraindications for various family planning methods (contraceptive pills should not be used when the woman has cancer of the breast or uterus, has active liver disease, hypertension, coronary artery disease or diabetes; intrauterine devices are not to be used during vaginal or uterine infection; the rhythm method is not reliable following childbirth and during menopause, etc.)

Explain how to determine the optimum time for conception (7 to 10 days after menstrual bleeding stops, when the clear and mucoid vaginal discharge occurs with ovulation)

EVALUATION
Record actual outcome

UNKNOWLEDGEABLE ABOUT THE REPRODUCTIVE PROCESS[371,527]

ASSESSMENT

Data Collection

Subjective Data
- Person's discussion or questions indicate a need for additional information, clarification, or validation of information
  OR
- Person's lack of questions or comments indicates not wanting information or not knowing enough to seek information
- When questioned directly, the person's response or lack of response indicates that he does not know:
  How fertilization takes place
  How fetal development occurs

Objective Data
None

Data Analysis

Nursing Diagnosis
UNKNOWLEDGEABLE ABOUT THE REPRODUCTIVE PROCESS: Being without sufficient information about the natural process of fertilization and fetal development

Common Etiology (Stressors)
HEALTH CARE FACTORS: Lack of health instruction

PLANNING

Unmet Needs
Comfort, protection from physical harm, independence, increased learning

Expected Outcome
Correct verbal feedback of the information taught

NURSING INTERVENTIONS

Nursing Treatments
Approach unhurriedly
Encourage the person to ask questions

Nursing Observations
Determine teaching effectiveness by verbal feedback

Health Teaching
Explain the reproductive process (the union of an egg with a spermatozoon; one egg is discharged from the ovary each month; it then works its way into the fallopian tube; if intercourse occurs at the right time, the spermatozoon penetrates the egg in the fallopian tube and fertilization takes place; the fertilized egg then moves into the uterus and embeds itself in the uterine lining, where fetal development begins)
Explain how the infant grows in utero (*First month*: Head and backbone develop. *Second month*: Face, arms and legs develop. *Third month*: Nails and teeth appear, sex is determined. *Fourth month*: Downy hair and fetal movement. *Fifth month*: Fetal heart tones are heard. *Sixth month*: Weighs 1.5 pounds. *Seventh month*: Weighs 2.5 pounds. *Eighth month*: Weighs 4 pounds. *Ninth month*: Weighs 6 pounds)

EVALUATION

Record actual outcome

UNKNOWLEDGEABLE ABOUT BREAST CANCER[26,73,158,474]

ASSESSMENT

Data Collection

Subjective Data
- Person's discussion or questions indicate a need for additional information, clarification, or validation of information
  OR
- Person's lack of questions or comments indicates not wanting information or not knowing enough to seek information
- When questioned directly, the person's response or lack of response indicates that she does not know:
  The signs and symptoms of breast cancer
  The factors associated with the occurrence of breast cancer
  The type of therapy suggested (usually a mastectomy or radiation therapy) and its effect

Objective Data
- May exhibit behavior such as not seeking health care despite breast changes

Related Data

Commonly Related Diseases
Fibroadenoma, lymphosarcoma, fibrosarcoma

Data Analysis

Nursing Diagnosis
UNKNOWLEDGEABLE ABOUT BREAST CANCER: Being without sufficient information about the signs, symptoms, causes and treatment of breast cancer

Common Etiology (Stressors)
HEALTH CARE FACTORS: Lack of health instruction

PLANNING

Unmet Needs
Comfort, protection from physical harm, independence, increased learning

Expected Outcome
Correct verbal feedback of the information taught

NURSING INTERVENTIONS

Nursing Treatments
Approach unhurriedly
Encourage the person to ask questions
Discuss the anticipated procedure (x-rays, surgery, etc.)

Nursing Observations
Determine teaching effectiveness by verbal feedback
Describe the factors associated with the occurrence of breast cancer (occurs most frequently between the ages of 20 and menopause and after age 65, in women with a familial tendency for breast cancer, in childless women with late menopause, in obese women, and with the use of hormone therapy beyond menopause; occurs least frequently in women with multiple pregnancies and prolonged nursing)
Explain the importance of periodic breast examination (for early detection of cancer)
Describe those symptoms that should be reported (breast lumps, nipple discharge, breast asymmetry)
Instruct to report serious symptoms immediately (mentioned above)
Explain the causes of the health problem (a disorganized proliferation of cell growth

that spreads from the original site to surrounding tissues; the cause is questionable but is associated with familial tendency and taking estrogen after the menopause)

Explain the reasons for and intended effect of the therapy (to remove the cancer and prevent metastasis)

EVALUATION

Record actual outcome

UNKNOWLEDGEABLE ABOUT PROSTATE CANCER[26,73,158]

ASSESSMENT

Data Collection

Subjective Data
- Person's discussion or questions indicate a need for additional information, clarification, or validation of information
  OR
- Person's lack of questions or comments indicates not wanting information or not knowing enough to seek information
- When questioned directly, the person's response or lack of response indicates that he does not know:
  The signs and symptoms of prostate cancer
  The factors associated with the occurrence of prostate cancer
  The value of a prostatectomy

Objective Data
None

Related Data

Commonly Related Diseases
Metatastic or primary carcinoma

Data Analysis

Nursing Diagnosis
UNKNOWLEDGEABLE ABOUT PROSTATE CANCER: Being without sufficient information about the signs, symptoms, causes, and treatment of prostate cancer

Common Etiology (Stressors)
HEALTH CARE FACTORS: Lack of health instruction

PLANNING

Unmet Needs
Comfort, protection from physical harm, independence, increased learning

Expected Outcome
Correct verbal feedback of the information taught

NURSING INTERVENTIONS

Nursing Treatments
Approach unhurriedly
Encourage the person to ask questions
Discuss the anticipated procedure (diagnostic studies or surgery)

Nursing Observations
Determine teaching effectiveness by verbal feedback

Health Teaching

Describe the factors associated with the occurrence of prostate cancer (most frequent in men between the ages of 60–90)

Describe those symptoms that should be reported (urinary frequency, severe backache, pain down the back of the leg)

Instruct to report serious symptoms immediately (mentioned above)

Explain the causes of the health problem (a disorganized proliferation of cell growth that spreads from the original site to surrounding tissues)

Explain the reason for and intended effect of the therapy (to remove the cancer and prevent metastasis)

EVALUATION

Record actual outcome

UNKNOWLEDGEABLE ABOUT UTERINE CANCER[26,73,158,474]

ASSESSMENT

Data Collection

Subjective Data

• Person's discussion or questions indicate a need for additional information, clarification, or validation of information
OR

• Person's lack of questions or comments indicates not wanting information or not knowing enough to seek information

• When questioned directly, the person's response or lack of response indicates that she does not know:
  The signs and symptoms of uterine cancer
  The factors associated with the occurrence of uterine cancer
  The meaning of different classes of Pap smear results
  The value of having the uterus removed when cancer is suspected

Objective Data
None

Related Data

Commonly Related Diseases
Cervical cancer, uterine carcinoma, endometriosis

Data Analysis

Nursing Diagnosis
UNKNOWLEDGEABLE ABOUT UTERINE CANCER: Being without sufficient information about the signs, symptoms, causes, and treatment of uterine cancer

Common Etiology (Stressors)
HEALTH CARE FACTORS: Lack of health instruction

PLANNING

Unmet Needs

Comfort, protection from physical harm, independence, increased learning

Expected Outcome

Correct verbal feedback of the information taught

NURSING INTERVENTIONS

Nursing Treatments

Approach unhurriedly

Encourage the person to ask questions

Discuss the anticipated procedure (Pap smear, surgery)

Nursing Observations

Determine teaching effectiveness by verbal feedback

Health Teaching

Describe the factors associated with the occurrence of uterine cancer (occurs most frequently between the ages of 30 and 50 in women who have had multiple pregnancies and who have a family history of uterine cancer)

Describe those symptoms that should be reported (abnormal vaginal bleeding, brown vaginal discharge, foul vaginal odor)

Instruct to report serious symptoms immediately (mentioned above)

Advise an annual gynecologic examination

Explain the meaning of the diagnostic report (Pap smear results are classified by Papanicolau as:

Class 1	No abnormal cells
Class 2	Some abnormal cells, no malignancy
Class 3	Abnormal cells suggesting possible malignancy
Class 4	Abnormal cells strongly suggesting malignancy
Class 5	Definite malignant cells)

Explain the causes of the health problem (a disorganized proliferation of cell growth that spreads from the original site to surrounding tissue; the cause is uncertain)

Explain the reason for and intended effect of the therapy (to remove the cancer and prevent metastasis)

EVALUATION

Record actual outcome

UNKNOWLEDGEABLE ABOUT YEAST INFECTIONS[42,88,371]

ASSESSMENT

Data Collection

Subjective Data

• Person's discussion or questions indicate a need for additional information, clarification, or validation of information

OR

• Person's lack of questions or comments indicates not wanting information or not knowing enough to seek information

• When questioned directly, the person's response or lack of response indicates that she does not know:

The causes of yeast infection

Methods for preventing yeast infection

Symptoms to be reported

Objective Data
None

Data Analysis

Nursing Diagnosis
UNKNOWLEDGEABLE ABOUT YEAST INFECTIONS: Being without sufficient information about the growth of yeast organisms in the intestines, respiratory tract, or vagina

Common Etiology (Stressors)
HEALTH CARE FACTORS: Lack of health instruction, lack of health-skill experience

PLANNING

Unmet Needs
Protection from physical harm, independence, increased learning

Expected Outcome
Correct verbal feedback of the information taught

NURSING INTERVENTIONS

Nursing Treatments
Approach unhurriedly
Encourage the person to ask questions

Nursing Observations
Determine teaching effectiveness by verbal feedback

Health Teaching
Instruct to eat yogurt or drink buttermilk (while on antibiotic therapy or to take Lactinex or acidophyllis tablets to prevent growth of yeast)
Instruct that douching be avoided (unless prescribed)
Describe those symptoms that should be reported (fever, malaise, vaginal or anal itching, white patches on the oral mucous membranes, brownish discoloration of nails, prolonged cough)
Explain the causes of the problem (when antibiotics destroy the bacteria for which they are intended, they also destroy normal bacteria; this allows organisms unaffected by the drug, which are no longer held in check by normal bacteria, to flourish and infect other body sites; adverse effects of prolonged, high doses of antibiotics such as penicillin, chloramphenicol, Aureomycin, and Terramycin, chronic and excessive use of douches; susceptibility to yeast infections as a side effect of diabetes mellitus)

EVALUATION

Record actual outcome

UNSKILLED AT SELF-BREAST EXAMINATION[26,73,362]

ASSESSMENT

Data Collection

Subjective Data
• Person's discussion or questions indicate a need for additional information,

clarification, or validation of information about performing the task of examining her own breasts
OR
• Person's lack of questions or comments indicates not wanting information or not knowing enough to seek information about performing the task of examining her own breasts
Person may not know:
The importance of breast examination
When to do the breast examination

Objective data
• Person cannot correctly demonstrate how to:
Perform a self-breast examination

Data Analysis

Nursing Diagnosis
UNSKILLED AT SELF-BREAST EXAMINATION: Being nonproficient, with or without knowledge, in the performance of the specific task of examining one's breasts for abnormal masses

Common Etiology (Stressors)
HEALTH CARE FACTORS: Lack of health instruction, lack of health-skill experience

PLANNING

Unmet Needs
Comfort, protection from physical harm, mastery and competence in skills, independence, increased learning

Expected Outcome
Correct verbal feedback of the information taught
Correct return demonstration of how to do a self-breast examination

NURSING INTERVENTIONS

Nursing Treatments
Approach unhurriedly
Encourage the person to ask questions

Nursing Observations
Determine teaching effectiveness by verbal feedback and return demonstration

Health Teaching
Explain the importance of periodic breast inspection (early detection and treatment of breast tumors saves lives)
Inform of when to do the breast examination (once a month, 1–2 days after completion of menstruation; after menopause, once a month at the same time each month)
Demonstrate how to do the breast examination (in the supine position, with one hand behind the head, gently feel with the opposite hand for a lump beginning at the outer breast and moving toward the nipple; examine the entire breast; repeat the examination in the sitting position with the same hand behind the head; reverse sides and repeat the examination on the other breast)
Describe those symptoms that should be reported (any breast lump, tissue thickening, nipple discharge, or breast asymmetry)
Instruct to report symptoms immediately

EVALUATION

Record actual outcome

Minor Health Problems Associated with the Respiratory System

CARBON DIOXIDE RETENTION[371]

ASSESSMENT

Data Collection

Subjective Data
- Dyspnea
- Drowsiness
  Dizziness
  Headache (throbbing, occipital)
  Confusion

Objective Data
- Absent or decreased breath sounds
- Prolonged expiratory breath sounds
- Decreased voice sounds
- Increased blood CO_2 content
  Cyanosis sometimes
  Papilledema sometimes

Data Analysis

Nursing Diagnosis

CARBON DIOXIDE RETENTION: The inability to eliminate carbon dioxide adequately from the lungs, resulting in the accumulation of large amounts of carbon dioxide in the blood

Common Etiology (Stressors)

BIRTH DEFECTS: Cystic fibrosis

DISEASES: Amyotrophic lateral sclerosis, asthma, atelectosis, bronchopneumonia, cerebral lesions, emphysema, Guillain–Barré syndrome, kyphoscoliosis, myastenia gravis, poliomyelitis, chronic pulmonary edema

INJURIES: Cerebral concussion, flail chest

HEALTH CARE FACTORS: *Drug therapy*: Respiratory depressants such as narcotics, sedatives, tranquilizers

HUMAN ERROR: Overdose of respiratory depressants

MAJOR PATHOPHYSIOLOGIC FACTORS CAUSING THE PROBLEM: Carbon dioxide is retained when there is alevolar hypoventilation due to a depressed respiratory center, or a disruption of nerve transmission to respiratory muscles, deformity or instability of the chest cage, or obstructing secretions of tissues in the lungs

PLANNING

Unmet Needs

Acid–base balance, waste elimination of carbon dioxide, comfort, protection from physical harm, increased learning

Expected Outcome

Normal breath sounds over the lung field
Ease of respirations
Normal serum CO_2 content

NURSING INTERVENTIONS

Nursing Treatments

Encourage coughing
Encourage deep breathing
Increase fluid intake to about 2,000 cc   To remove obstruction secretions
Suction the airway

Place in the sitting position
Do not place in the flat position
Remove constrictive clothing
Obtain a blood sample and send for analysis (blood gases)
Withhold the oxygen therapy (in chronic hypercapnia if the blood CO_2 content is 70–75 vol/100 ml and Po_2 is over 60)

Nursing Observations
Inspect the chest for respiratory rate and rhythm
Inspect the chest for symmetrical expansion
Auscultate the chest for abnormal breath sounds
Auscultate the chest for lung aeration
Auscultate the chest for adventitious sounds
Monitor the blood studies for arterial blood gases

Health Teaching
Explain the causes of the health problem (bronchial obstruction, thick secretions)
Describe those symptoms that should be reported (severe respiratory distress)
Teach how to do abdominal breathing (on inspiration have abdomen rise, on expiration have abdominal muscles contract)
Teach how to do resistive breathing exercises (place a weight on the abdomen and breathe against it, blow out a candle at increased distances)
Teach how to do bronchopulmonary hygiene measures
Explain the reason for and intended effect of the therapy (to reduce CO_2 retention)

Medical Treatments Performed by Nurses
Administer heated humidified oxygen (at no more than 1–2 liters/minute)
Administer intermittent positive-pressure breathing
Give the prescribed drugs (sedatives, bronchodilators)

EVALUATION
Record actual outcome

COUGH [125,371,451]

ASSESSMENT
Data Collection

Subjective Data
• Relates persistent coughing
• Fatigue
  Constrictive (squeezing, pressing) pain in the throat or chest, sometimes
  Productive or unproductive of sputum

Objective Data
• Rales, rhonchi, or wheezes may or may not be heard on auscultation
  Fever, sometimes

Data Analysis

Nursing Diagnosis
COUGH: The forceful expulsion of air from the lungs

Common Etiology (Stressors)
DISEASES: Aortic aneurysm, asthma, bronchiectasis, bronchitis, carcinoma of the lung, congestive heart failure, diptheria, emphysema, influenza, laryngitis, laryngotracheitis, pleurisy, pneumoconiosis, pneumonia, mitral stenosis, tuberculosis

INJURIES: Foreign body in the pharynx
LIFESTYLE: Smoking
ENVIRONMENTAL FACTORS: *Chemical substances*: Inhalation of toxic gases or vapors such as ammonia, pollution. *Pollen*: Ragweed
MAJOR PATHOPHYSIOLOGIC FACTORS CAUSING THE PROBLEM: Coughing results from pulmonary irritation or obstruction and from laryngeal spasms

PLANNING

Unmet Needs
Waste elimination of bronchopulmonary secretions, rest, comfort, protection from physical harm, increased learning

Expected Outcome
Person verbalizes that the coughing has decreased
Normal breath sounds over the entire lung field

NURSING INTERVENTIONS

Nursing Treatments
Elevate the head
　OR
Place in the sitting position
Increase fluid intake to about 2,000 cc daily
Administer vaporized air
Give warm liquids
Refrain from giving iced liquids (which stimulate coughing)
Refrain from giving milk or milk products (if they stimulate coughing)
Give coughdrops
Give nonprescription drugs (antitussives, coughdrops)
Encourage adequate rest
Discourage smoking
Remove constrictive clothing (around the neck and chest)
Maintain adequate atmospheric humidity
Maintain a warm room temperature
Make a referral (to a physician if the cough persists)

Nursing Observations
Inspect the chest for respiratory rate and rhythm
Inspect the chest for symmetrical expansion
Auscultate the chest for abnormal breath sounds
Auscultate the chest for lung aeration
Auscultate the chest for adventitious sounds
Monitor the laboratory findings of sputum analysis
Observe the characteristics of the cough (frequency, sound, productiveness)
Observe for complaints of pain or fatigue

Health Teaching
Advise against exposure to airborne irritants
Explain how to prevent coughing (slow, deep breathing)
Emphasize the danger of breathing cold air (it stimulates coughing)
Instruct to increase fluid intake (and avoid cold liquids, which stimulate coughing)
Instruct to change position frequently
Explain the causes of the health problem (respiratory irritation)
Explain the reason for and intended effect of the therapy (to promote comfort, loosen secretions)

Medical Treatments Performed by Nurses
Give the prescribed drugs

EVALUATION

Record actual outcome

HOARSENESS[88,371]

ASSESSMENT

Data Collection

Subjective Data
• Person relates having "lost my voice"
  Usually has no throat soreness

Objective Data
• Voice is barely audible
• Husky-sounding voice

Data Analysis

Nursing Diagnosis
HOARSENESS: A change in the voice sound from normal to a harshness or whisper sound

Common Etiology (Stressors)
DISEASES: Anemia (severe), aortic aneurysm located near the laryngeal nerve, angioneurotic edema, carcinoma of the larynx, Hansen's disease, lupus erythematosus, myasthenia gravis, myxedema, syphilis ulcer, tetanus, thyrotoxicosis, tuberculosis ulcer
INJURIES: Burn injury by swallowing extremely hot liquid, insect bite (vocal cord edema),
  poisoning by swallowing caustic fluid
SIGNS AND SYMPTOMS: Tetany (vocal cord spasm), uremia (vocal cord edema)
HEALTH CARE FACTORS: *Diagnostic procedures*: Broncoscopy, gastroscopy, laryngoscopy. *Drug
  therapy*: Atropinelike drugs (causing dryness), potassium iodide (cord edema). *Medical
  therapy*: Nasogastric or endotracheal intubation. *Surgical therapy*: Thyroidectomy with
  accidental cutting of the laryngeal nerve
LIFESTYLE: Smoking
ENVIRONMENTAL FACTORS: *Chemical substances*: Inhalation of chemical agents such as toxic
  gases
HUMAN ERROR: Prolonged shouting and cheering or excessive use of the voice as in giving
  speeches or teaching
MAJOR PATHOPHYSIOLOGIC FACTORS CAUSING THE PROBLEM: Hoareness results from irritation
  and edema of the vocal cords

PLANNING

Unmet Needs

Comfort, protection from physical harm, increased learning

Expected Outcome

Normal voice tone

NURSING INTERVENTIONS

Nursing Treatments

Reassure verbally (that the hoarseness will subside)
Give warm liquids
Encourage the use of a warm, saline gargle
Discourage smoking
Make a referral (to a physician, if the hoarseness persists more than 3 weeks)

Nursing Observations

Observe for evidence of a favorable response to therapy

Health Teaching

Advise limited talking (to promote vocal cord rest)
Explain the causes of the health problem (vocal cord edema or irritation, pressure on
  the vocal cord)

EVALUATION

Record actual outcome

HYPOVENTILATION[32,339]

ASSESSMENT

Data Collection

Subjective Data
- Dyspnea
  Anxiety

Objective Data
- Decreased chest movement with a respiratory rate of less than eight breaths/minute
- Absent or decreased breath sounds
- Percussion dullness
  Cyanosis, sometimes

Data Analysis

Nursing Diagnosis
HYPOVENTILATION: A reduced rate and depth of breathing resulting in inadequate pulmonary ventilation

Common Etiology (Stressors)
DISEASES: Amyotrophic lateral sclerosis, cerebral lesions, Guillain–Barré syndrome, myasthenia gravis, pneumonia, poliomyelitis
SIGNS AND SYMPTOMS: Abdominal distention, pain
HEALTH CARE FACTORS: *Drug therapy*: Narcotics, sedatives, tranquilizers, or other respiratory depressants. *Surgical therapy*: Anesthesia
MAJOR PATHOPHYSIOLOGIC FACTORS CAUSING THE PROBLEM: Hypoventilation results from decreased respiratory muscle strength, pain that inhibits normal respiratory depth, severe abdominal pressure causing pressure on the diaphragm, drug-depressed respirations, the disruption of nerve transmission to respiratory muscles, fluid in the pleural space that compresses the lung

PLANNING

Unmet Needs

Acid–base balance, tissue oxygenation or perfusion, waste elimination of carbon dioxide, protection from physical harm, increased learning

Expected Outcome

Respiratory rate of 16–20 in adults, 15–24 in adolescents, 20–30 in children, 30–60 in infants
Respiratory depth sufficient to verify lung aeration by auscultation
Normal skin, lip, earlobe, and nail color

NURSING INTERVENTIONS

Nursing Treatments

Change the person's position frequently
Encourage coughing
    AND   Periodically and frequently
Encourage deep breathing
Place in the sitting position
Ambulate the person (as soon and as often as possible)
Withhold the drugs (sedatives)

Nursing Observations

Inspect the chest for respiratory rate and rhythm
Inspect the chest for symmetrical expansion
Auscultate the chest for abnormal breath sounds
Auscultate the chest for lung aeration
Auscultate the chest for adventitious sounds
Monitor blood studies for arterial blood gases
Observe for cyanosis

Health Teaching

Explain the causes of the health problem (drugs, muscle weakness, fluid compression of the lungs)

Explain the reason for and intended effect of the therapy (adequate ventilation)

Medical Treatments Performed by Nurses

Administer heated humidified oxygen

Administer intermittent positive-pressure breathing

EVALUATION

Record actual outcome

LARYNGITIS[42,88,278]

ASSESSMENT

Data Collection

Subjective Data

- Person relates having "lost my voice"
- Burning, tickling, dryness of the throat
- Unproductive cough
  Constant urge to clear the throat
  Malaise

Objective Data

- Voice is barely audible
- Husky-sounding voice
  Laryngeal edema and redness visible by mirror examination
  Fever, sometimes

Data Analysis

Nursing Diagnosis

LARYNGITIS: Inflammation of the laryngeal mucosa

Common Etiology (Stressors)

DISEASES: Bronchitis, diphtheria, influenza, measles, pertussis, pneumonia, sinusitis, streptococcal pharyngitis

INJURIES: Foreign body in the larynx

LIFESTYLE: Smoking

ENVIRONMENTAL FACTORS: *Chemical substances*: Inhalation of chemical agents such as toxic gases

MAJOR PATHOPHYSIOLOGIC FACTORS CAUSING THE PROBLEM: Laryngeal inflammation results from the presence of infectious agents such as bacteria or viruses or from chronic, chemical, tissue irritation

PLANNING

Unmet Needs

Comfort, protection from physical harm, increased learning

Expected Outcome

Person verbalizes cessation of throat soreness

Absence of laryngeal inflammation or edema

NURSING INTERVENTIONS

Nursing Treatments

Reassure verbally (that the hoarseness will subside)

Give warm liquids (not hot)

Encourage the use of a warm, saline gargle

Administer vaporized air

Discourage smoking

Give nonprescription drugs (analgesic lozenges for the sore throat, antihistamines to reduce drainage, cough syrup for the cough)

Nursing Observations

Observe for evidence of a favorable response to therapy

Health Teaching

Advise limited talking (to promote vocal cord rest and healing)

Describe those symptoms that should be reported (dyspnea)

Explain the causes of the health problem (viral or bacterial infection, vocal cord irritation)

Medical Treatments Performed by Nurses

Give the prescribed drugs (antibiotics)

EVALUATION

Record actual outcome

PAINFUL RESPIRATIONS[72,88,451]

ASSESSMENT

Data Collection

Subjective Data
- Dyspnea
- Pain experienced on inspiration
  Stabbing (piercing, sharp) pain, sometimes
  Increased pain when coughing or laughing

Objective Data
- Shallow respirations
- Restricted chest movements
  May splint breathing by leaning to the painful side

Data Analysis

Nursing Diagnosis
PAINFUL RESPIRATIONS (POPOPNEA): Distressful hurting accompanying breathing

Common Etiology (Stressors)
DISEASES: Carcinoma of the lung, emphysema, pericarditis, pleural effusion, pleurisy,
pneumonia, pulmonary embolus, tuberculosis
INJURIES: Bone (rib) fracture, flail chest
HEALTH CARE FACTORS: *Surgical procedures*: Arterial bypass, cholecystectomy, mastectomy,
thoracentesis, thoracotomy
MAJOR PATHOPHYSIOLOGIC FACTORS CAUSING THE PROBLEM: Painful respirations result from
pleural inflammation or the rubbing of pleural spaces or from tension on an incisional
area

PLANNING

Unmet Needs

Rest, comfort, protection from physical harm, freedom from pain, increased learning

Expected Outcome

A respiration rate of 16–20 in adults, 15–24 in adolescents, 20–30 in children, 30–60 in
infants

Person verbalizes ease in breathing

Assumes a normal posture

Exhibits freedom of body movement

NURSING INTERVENTIONS

Nursing Treatments

Approach unhurriedly
Reassure that the pain will subside
Communicate nurse sensitivity to the person's pain
Handle gently
Position comfortably
Change the person's position gradually
Apply an elastic bandage (to the chest)
  OR
Place on the affected side
Splint the incisional area ⎤
Apply a heating pad   ⎥
  OR   ⎬ For pleuritic pain
Apply a hot water bottle ⎦
Massage gently (the posterior thorax area)
Maintain a warm room temperature
Refrain from performing nonessential procedures
Ask the person what makes him comfortable
Discuss possible pain-reducing measures
Encourage adequate rest
Provide a pain-relief measure of the person's choice
Give nonprescription drugs (analgesics)

Nursing Observations

Observe for complaints of pain duration or radiation
Evaluate the pain for intensity and quality
Inspect the chest for respiratory rate and rhythm
Inspect the chest for symmetrical expansion
Auscultate the chest for abnormal breath sounds
Auscultate the chest for lung aeration
Auscultate the chest for adventitious sounds
Evaluate the effectiveness of the pain-relief measures

Health Teaching

Explain the causes of the pain (pleural irritation or inflammation)
Describe those symptoms that should be reported (increased pain or air hunger)
Explain how to splint an incision (hold a pillow to the chest during deep breathing or coughing)
Teach how to apply heat therapy

Medical Treatments Performed by Nurses

Give the prescribed drugs (analgesics)

EVALUATION

Record actual outcome

RESPIRATORY DISTRESS [35,339,371]

ASSESSMENT

Data Collection

Subjective Data
• Air hunger
• Anxiety
  Fatigue
  Weakness

Objective Data
- Irregular or difficult chest movements
- Abnormal respiratory rate, rhythm, or depth
- Restlessness

Data Analysis

Nursing Diagnosis

RESPIRATORY DISTRESS: An uncomfortable, increased effort during respiratory inspiration and expiration

Common Etiology (Stressors)

DISEASES: Asthma, bronchiectasis, bronchitis, carcinoma of the lung, congestive heart failure, cystic fibrosis, emphysema, Guillian–Barré syndrome, laryngotracheobronchitis, pericarditis, pleural effusion, pleurisy, pneumoconiosis, pneumonia, poliomyelitis, pulmonary embolus, myasthenia gravis, tuberculosis

INJURIES: Bone (rib) fracture, flail chest, foreign body in the nose or pharynx

SITUATIONAL FACTORS: Impending death

MAJOR PATHOPHYSIOLOGIC FACTORS CAUSING THE PROBLEM: Respiratory distress results from airway obstruction, paralysis or impairment of respiratory musculature, or cyclic respiratory understimulation or overstimulation

PLANNING

Unmet Needs

Tissue oxygenation or perfusion, waste elimination of carbon dioxide, rest, comfort, protection from physical harm, increased learning

Expected Outcome

Respiratory rate of 16–20 in adults, 15–24 in adolescents, 20–30 in children, 30–60 in infants

Person verbalizes ease in breathing

Assumes a normal posture

Exhibits freedom of body movement

NURSING INTERVENTIONS

Nursing Treatments

Position comfortably

Elevate the head

   OR

Place in the sitting position

Encourage deep breathing

Suction the airway (as needed)

Administer vaporized air

Encourage adequate rest

Remove constrictive clothing

Maintain a cool room temperature

Maintain adequate atmospheric humidity

Maintain adequate room ventilation

Refrain from performing nonessential procedures

Discourage smoking

Nursing Observations

Inspect the chest for respiratory rate and rhythm

Inspect the chest for symmetrical expansion

Auscultate the chest for abnormal breath sounds

Auscultate the chest for lung aeration

Auscultate the chest for adventitious sounds

Monitor blood studies for arterial blood gases

Observe for complaints of pain, or fatigue

Observe for cyanosis

Observe for dyspnea

Health Teaching

Explain the causes of the health problem (poor oxygenation, respiratory muscle weakness, infection)

Explain the reason for and intended effect of the therapy (adequate ventilation)

Medical Treatments Performed by Nurses

Administer heated humidified oxygen

Administer intermittent positive-pressure breathing

Give the prescribed drugs

EVALUATION

Record actual outcome

PULMONARY CONGESTION[125,522]

ASSESSMENT

Data Collection

Subjective Data
- Chest tightness
- Breathing discomfort
  Cough
  Malaise
  Fatigue

Objective Data
- Rales, rhonchi, or wheezes are heard on chest auscultation
  Fever sometimes

Data Analysis

Nursing Diagnosis
PULMONARY CONGESTION: The presence of fluid or thick exudate in the lungs

Common Etiology (Stressors)
DISEASES: Asthma, bronchiectasis, bronchitis, congestive heart failure, emphysema, influenza, myocardial infarction, pneumonia, pulmonary edema, pulmonary embolus, tuberculosis
INJURIES: Drowning
HEALTH CARE FACTORS: *Medical therapy*: Prolonged bed rest
ENVIRONMENTAL FACTORS: *Chemical substances*: Inhalation of toxic gases or vapors
MAJOR PATHOPHYSIOLOGIC FACTORS CAUSING THE PROBLEM: Failure of the respiratory and cough reflexes to clear secretions from the respiratory system, pulmonary vasodilatation, excess fluid in pulmonary tissues (interstitial spaces)

PLANNING

Unmet Needs

Tissue oxygenation or perfusion, waste elimination of pulmonary secretions, sleep and rest, comfort, protection from physical harm, increased learning

Expected Outcome

Clear breath sounds over the entire lung field

Person verbalizes that breathing is more comfortable

NURSING INTERVENTIONS

Nursing Treatments

Administer vaporized air

Give warm liquids
Place in postural drainage
Change the person's position frequently
Encourage coughing, and
Encourage deep breathing
Give nonprescription drugs (decongestants)
Encourage adequate rest
Discourage smoking
Maintain adequate atmospheric humidity
Make a referral (to a physician for severe or persistant congestant)

Nursing Observations
Inspect the chest for respiratory rate and rhythm
Inspect the chest for symmetrical expansion
Auscultate the chest for abnormal breath sounds
Auscultate the chest for lung aeration
Auscultate the chest for adventitious sounds
Inspect the sputum for characteristics (yellow or green indicates bacterial infection)
Monitor the oral temperature (for fever)
Observe for complaints of pain, fatigue, weakness
Observe for dyspnea

Health Teaching
Advise against exposure to airborne irritants
Advise against exposure to inclement weather
Teach how to give vaporized-solution inhalation
Describe those symptoms that should be reported (dyspnea, pain)
Explain the causes of the health problem (accumulated secretions)
Explain the reason for and intended effect of the therapy (comfort and removal of secretions)

Medical Treatments Performed by Nurses
Administer heated humidified oxygen
Administer intermittent positive-pressure breathing

EVALUATION

Record actual outcome

SINUS CONGESTION [151,522]

ASSESSMENT

Data Collection

Subjective Data
- Malaise
- Headache
- Aching (soreness, tenderness)
- Pain in the forehead or above the eye (frontal sinus)
- Pain in the upper teeth, cheek, or side of the nasal bridge (maxillary sinus)
- Pain behind the eye (sphenoid or ethmoid sinus)
  Dizziness

Sensitivity to light
Nasal drainage

Objective Data
Sinus tenderness on palpation
Periorbital or forehead edema
Swollen nasal turbinates

Data Analysis

Nursing Diagnosis
SINUS CONGESTION: Increased fluid or swollen mucosa of the sinus cavity

Common Etiology (Stressors)
DISEASES: Allergic disorder, sinusitis
LIFESTYLE: Smoking
ENVIRONMENTAL FACTORS: *Biologic agents*: Viruses, bacteria (usually streptococci, pneumococci, or staphylococci). *Chemical substances*: Inhalation of toxic gases or vapors. *Pollen*: Ragweed, grass
MAJOR PATHOPHYSIOLOGIC FACTORS CAUSING THE PROBLEM: Thickened sinus mucosa results in inadequate drainage of the cavity

PLANNING

Unmet Needs
Fluid and electrolyte balance, waste elimination of sinus secretions, rest, comfort, cleanliness, protection from physical harm, increased learning

Expected Outcome
Person verbalizes increased comfort
Nontenderness on palpation of the sinus areas

NURSING INTERVENTIONS

Nursing Treatments
Apply a warm, moist compress (to the sinus area)
Administer vaporized air
Give warm liquids
Increase fluid intake to about 2,000 cc daily
Elevate the head (especially during sleep)
Position comfortably (on the unaffected side)
Give nonprescription drugs (decongestants and vasoconstricting nasal spray)
Discourage the intake of oral stimulants
Discourage smoking
Maintain adequate atmospheric humidity
Make a referral (to a physician if the drainage is yellow or green)

Nursing Observations
Observe for complaints of pain duration
Observe for complaints of pain radiation
Evaluate the pain for intensity and quality
Evaluate the effectiveness of the pain-relief measures

Health Teaching
Advise against exposure to airborne irritants
Advise against exposure to inclement weather
Advise gentle nose blowing
Explain the causes of the health problem (allergy, viral or bacterial infection)
Explain the reason for and intended effect of the therapy (to promote sinus drainage and removal of secretions)

Medical Treatments Performed by Nurses
Give the prescribed drugs (analgesics)

EVALUATION
Record actual outcome

Knowledge Deficits Associated with the Respiratory System

UNKNOWLEDGABLE ABOUT PULMONARY DISEASE[42,324,474]

ASSESSMENT

Data Collection

Subjective Data
- Person's discussion or questions indicate a need for additional information, clarification, or validation of information

  OR
- Person's lack of questions or comments indicates not wanting information or not knowing enough to seek information
- When questioned directly, the person's response or lack of response indicates that he does not know:

  The early signs and symptoms of lung disease

  That smoking is a primary cause of lung disease

  The fact that despite prolonged smoking, cessation of smoking greatly reduces the possibility of lung disease

  The need for periodic chest x-ray examinations

  How lung disease is treated

Objective Data
None

Related Data
Commonly Related Diseases
Pulmonary carcinoma, emphysema, tuberculosis, bronchitis, pneumonia

Data Analysis

Nursing Diagnosis
UNKNOWLEDGEABLE ABOUT PULMONARY DISEASE: Being without sufficient information about the signs, symptoms, cause, and treatment of lung disease

Common Etiology (Stressors)
HEALTH CARE FACTORS: Lack of health instruction

PLANNING

Unmet Needs
Comfort, protection from physical harm, independence, increased learning

Expected Outcome
Correct verbal feedback of the information taught

NURSING INTERVENTIONS

Nursing Treatments
Approach unhurriedly
Encourage the person to ask questions
Discuss the anticipated procedure (associated with the treatment of lung disease)
Make a referral (to programs for curing tobacco habituation, if appropriate)

Nursing Observations
Determine teaching effectiveness by verbal feedback

Health Teaching
Describe the early manifestations of lung disease (coughing, purulent or bloody sputum, dyspnea, weight loss, chest or shoulder pain)

Instruct to report serious symptoms immediately (mentioned above)

Explain the causes of the health problem (smoking, inhalation of irritants, familial tendency)

Recommend methods used to stop smoking (gradual or abrupt withdrawal, change of daily routine, substituting gum for cigarettes)

Describe those symptoms that should be reported (chronic cough, weight loss, dyspnea)

EVALUATION

Record actual outcome

UNSKILLED AT USING A RESPIRATORY DEVICE[72,451]

ASSESSMENT
Data Collection

Subjective Data
• Person's discussion or questions indicate a need for additional information, clarification, or validation of information about performing the task of using an assistive respiratory device
  OR
• Person's lack of questions or comments indicates not wanting information or not knowing enough to seek information about performing the task of using an assistive respiratory device
  Person may not know:
    The purpose of humidifiers, oxygenators, inhalators, positive-pressure machines, etc.
    When and for how long to take treatments
    The importance of machine cleanliness

Note: There may be no subjective data in unconscious, immature, or infirmed mental states

Objective Data
• Person cannot correctly demonstrate how to:
    Operate respiratory devices and machines
    Mix solutions put into the machine
    Dismantle and clean the equipment

Related Data
Commonly Related Diseases
Asthma, emphysema, pneumonia

Data Analysis
Nursing Diagnosis
UNSKILLED AT USING A RESPIRATORY DEVICE: Being nonproficient, with or without knowledge, in the performance of the specific task of using and maintaining devices that support improved respirations or respiratory hygiene

Common Etiology (Stressors)
HEALTH CARE FACTORS: Lack of health instruction, lack of health-skill experience

PLANNING
Unmet Needs
Tissue oxygenation or perfusion, comfort, protection from physical harm, mastery and competence in skills, independence, increased learning

Expected Outcome
Correct, on-time, therapeutic use of the respiratory device
Correct verbal feedback of the information taught

Correct return demonstration of how to operate and clean the respiratory device and mix the inhalation solution

NURSING INTERVENTIONS

Nursing Treatments

Provide temporary assistance until the skill is learned
Place in the sitting position
  OR
Place on the unaffected side (to aerate the involved lobes)
Encourage the patient and family to ask questions
Encourage self-performance
Make a referral (to a respiratory therapist if necessary)

Nursing Observations

Observe for readiness to assume self-care
Determine teaching effectiveness by testing, verbal feedback, and return demonstration

Health Teaching

Familiarize the person with the component parts of the respiratory equipment (how it is disassembled for cleaning, etc.)
Explain how the equipment works
Teach how to give vaporized-solution inhalation (with a vaporizer, tea kettle, etc.)
Teach how to give oxygen therapy (how to adjust the flow rate, apply a mask or cannula, fill the humidifier bottle)
Teach how to give positive-pressure breathing (how to adjust the flow rate, apply a mask or mouthpiece, breathe appropriately)
Explain the potential dangers of incorrect use of equipment/therapy (excessive oxygen intake can depress respirations, excessive IPPB pressure can damage tissues)
Explain the reason for and intended effect of the therapy (to promote the removal of secretions, increase lung ventilation and oxygen intake)
Describe those symptoms that should be reported (a rapid pulse, increased respiratory difficulty, chest pain)

EVALUATION

Record actual outcome

Minor Health Problems Associated with Sensory Responses

EYESTRAIN [42,139,732,733]

ASSESSMENT

Data Collection

Subjective Data
• Gradual onset during prolonged, close eye work
• Aching (soreness, tenderness) headache
• Pain localized in the eye orbit, above the eye, or in the forehead
• Does not subside immediately with eye rest
  Visual blurring sometimes

Objective Data
Person may or may not have impaired visual acuity, by Snellen test

Sclera may be reddened
Person may rub the eyes

Data Analysis

Nursing Diagnosis
EYESTRAIN: Eye pain associated with intense use of the eyes

Common Etiology (Stressors)
ENVIRONMENTAL FACTORS: *Light*: Inadequate environmental light
HUMAN ERROR: Engaging in prolonged, close eye work (reading, sewing, etc.)
MAJOR PATHOPHYSIOLOGIC FACTORS CAUSING THE PROBLEM: Prolonged contraction of the temporal, occipital, frontal, and/or extraocular muscles

PLANNING

Unmet Needs

Rest and relaxation, comfort, protection from physical harm, freedom from pain, increased learning

Expected Outcome

Person verbalizes increased comfort and vision

NURSING INTERVENTIONS

Nursing Treatments

Approach unhurriedly
Reassure that the pain will subside
Massage gently (the neck and shoulders, periorbital tissues)
Provide quiet
Ask the person what makes him comfortable
Discuss possible pain-reducing measures
Provide a pain-relief measure of the person's choice
Give nonprescription drugs (analgesics)
Encourage adequate rest
Make a referral (to an opthalmologist, if the condition persists)

Nursing Observations

Observe for complaints of pain duration
Evaluate the effectiveness of the pain-relief measures

Health Teaching

Instruct to avoid rubbing the eyes
Advise against letting light shine directly into the eyes
Explain how to illuminate a room correctly (close and distant illumination, placing the light over the left shoulder for righthanded persons)
Advise against wearing unprescribed eyeglasses

EVALUATION

Record actual outcome

SENSORY DEPRIVATION[13,14,529]

ASSESSMENT

Data Collection

Subjective Data
• Depression
• Heightened anxiety
• Fatigue

- Apathy or passiveness
- Little or no display of affection or feeling
  Brooding about imagined injustices
  Expressions of boredom
  Complaints of physical discomforts

Objective Data
Restlessness

Data Analysis

Nursing Diagnosis
SENSORY DEPRIVATION: A dulling of sensory responses following prolonged exposure to a nonstimulating environment

Common Etiology (Stressors)
DISEASES: Blindness, deafness
SIGNS AND SYMPTOMS: Anesthesia (loss of the touch sensation), anosmia (loss of the sense of smell), paralysis
HEALTH CARE FACTORS: *Health care environment*: Absence of *natural* light and dark in the health care environment. *Hospitalization*: Prolonged hospitalization. *Visitors*: Absence of visitors, restriction of visitors
DEVELOPMENTAL PHASES: Old age
ENVIRONMENTAL FACTORS: *Color*: Dull environmental colors. *Food substances*: Plain, poorly seasoned food. *Light*: Inadequate environmental light. *Noise*: Absence of noise. *Odors*: Absence of a variety of odors. *Windows*: Absence of windows
MAJOR PATHOPHYSIOLOGIC FACTORS CAUSING THE PROBLEM: In the absence of adequate external stimuli, the senses function at a minimal level

PLANNING

Unmet Needs
Activity, comfort, stimulation, protection from psychologic threat, warm and communicating relationships, sense of value and usefulness, increased learning, less of the familiar and more of the novel, increased pleasantness

Expected Outcome
Person expresses interest in the external world
Exhibits a normal display of emotions
Relates a positive approach to life

NURSING INTERVENTIONS

Nursing Treatments
Allow unlimited visiting
Assist the person to restructure his lifestyle (with more stimulating activity)
Dress the person in colorful clothing
Illuminate the room adequately
Keep the person's door open (for greater exposure to people)
Place by a window
Place (an infant) in an infant seat
Provide an attractive meal tray
Provide radio and television for diversion
Provide reading material for diversion
Encourage active diversional activities
Sit with the person
Talk with the person
Provide frequent contact with the person
Touch the person frequently

Nursing Observations
Observe for an excessive stress level (from the sensory deprivation)
Observe for evidence of a favorable response to therapy

Health Teaching

Recommend methods for increasing sensory stimulation (bright colors, thrilling TV, competitive activities, travel)

Explain the causes of the health problem (nonstimulating environment)

EVALUATION

Record actual outcome

SENSORY OVERLOAD[13,14,105]

ASSESSMENT

Data Collection

Subjective Data
- Verbal expressions of anxiety
- Desire to escape the situation
- Fatigue
- Nervousness

Objective Data
- Startle response to stimuli

Data Analysis

Nursing Diagnosis

SENSORY OVERLOAD: Excessive excitement of the sensory responses following excessive environmental stimulation

Common Etiology (Stressors)

PSYCHOSOCIAL FACTORS: The threat of severe, chronic stress

HEALTH CARE FACTORS: *Health care environment*: A crisis-oriented health care environment, exposure to intense human suffering of persons in the health care environment. *Diagnostic procedures*: Frequent, or frequent painful diagnostic procedures. *Medical therapy*: Frequent, or frequent painful medical procedures. *Surgical therapy*: Frequent, or frequent painful surgical procedures

LIFESTYLE: Excessive time and effort at employment, involvement in too many activities above the person's comfort level, nonallocation of leisure time

ENVIRONMENTAL FACTORS: *Housing*: Overcrowding. *Light*: Prolonged exposure to bright light. *Noise*: Prolonged exposure to loud noise

MAJOR PATHOPHYSIOLOGIC FACTORS CAUSING THE PROBLEM: Sensory overload results from the occurrence of multiple stress situations that require exhaustive coping or adaptation and sensory intake at maximum capacity

PLANNING

Unmet Needs

Rest, comfort, protection from physical harm, protection from psychologic threat, increased learning

Expected Outcome

Person has a calm, contented, relaxed facial expression

Person is not startled by minimal stimuli

NURSING INTERVENTIONS

Nursing Treatments

Arrange orderly surroundings

Arrange pleasant surroundings

Arrange a structured environment

Avoid causing intense emotional situations
Encourage adequate rest
Encourage quiet diversional activities
Handle gently
Keep the person's door closed
Plan undisturbed periods for the person
Provide frequent contact with the person
Provide quiet
Reduce the demands placed on the person
Refrain from performing nonessential procedures
Restrict unwanted visitors

Nursing Observations
Observe for an excessive stress level
Observe for evidence of a favorable response to therapy

Health Teaching
Recommend methods for reducing sensory stimulation (reduce the noise levels, minimize travel, keep the same job, live in a small community)
Describe the behavior pattern indicating overstimulation (fatigue, irritability, insomnia, panicky feeling)
Explain the reason for and intended effect of the therapy (to promote relaxation and reduce stress)

EVALUATION

Record actual outcome

Knowledge Deficits Associated with Sensory Responses

UNSKILLED AT ARTIFICIAL EYE CARE[362,451]

ASSESSMENT

Data Collection

Subjective Data
• Person's discussion or questions indicate a need for additional information, clarification, or validation of information about performing the task of caring for an artificial eye
  OR
• Person's lack of questions or comments indicates not wanting information or not knowing enough to seek information about performing the task of caring for an artificial eye
  Person may not know:
    Possible complications with the use of or failure to use the eye

Objective Data
• Person cannot correctly demonstrate how to:
    Insert and remove an artificial eye
    Clean and store the prosthesis

Data Analysis

Nursing Diagnosis

UNSKILLED AT ARTIFICIAL EYE CARE: Being nonproficient, with or without knowledge, in the performance of the specific task of using and caring for an artificial eye

Common Etiology (Stressors)

HEALTH CARE FACTORS: Lack of health instruction, lack of health-skill experience

PLANNING

Unmet Needs

Comfort, protection from physical harm, mastery and competence in skills, independence, increased learning

Expected Outcome

Correct verbal feedback of the information taught
Correct return demonstration of how to insert, remove, clean, and store an artificial eye
The artificial eye is correctly placed in the eye orbit
No inflammation or injury of the eye orbit
The artificial eye is clean and safely stored

NURSING INTERVENTIONS

Nursing Treatments

Provide temporary assistance until the skill is learned
Clean the artificial eye (with saline or tap water)
Insert and remove the artificial eye
Safeguard the person's artificial eye (in a case or container)
Encourage the person to ask questions
Encourage self-performance

Nursing Observations

Observe for signs of (orbit) irritation (redness, drainage)
Inspect the artificial eye for scratches, chipping, or other damage
Determine teaching effectiveness by testing, verbal feedback, and return demonstration

Health Teaching

Describe those symptoms that should be reported (orbit irritation from the artificial eye)
Teach how to care for an artificial eye (soak in normal saline or tap water)
Teach how to insert and remove an artificial eye (pull down the lower lid, gently slip the eye into position; to remove, place gentle pressure below the eye with an index finger until the prosthesis slips out)
Recommend the use of safety lens in eyeglasses (to protect the natural eye)
Explain the reason for and intended effect of the methods used (prevention of eye orbit irritation)

EVALUATION

Record actual outcome

UNSKILLED AT USING CONTACT LENSES[311,451]

ASSESSMENT

Data Collection

Subjective Data
• Person's discussion or questions indicate a need for additional information, clarification, or validation of information about performing the task of using contact lenses
  OR

- Person's lack of questions or comments indicates not wanting information or not knowing enough to seek information about performing the task of using contact lenses

  Person may not know:

  The methods of insertion, removal, and cleansing of the contact lenses

  The fact that contact lenses are affected by extreme cold or heat

  The dangers associated with wearing contact lenses

Objective Data

- Person cannot correctly demonstrate how to:

  Insert or remove contact lenses

  Clean the lenses in the proper fluid or container

  Safely store the lenses

Related Data

Commonly Related Conditions

Hyperopia, myopia

Commonly Related Diseases

Astigmatism

Data Analysis

Nursing Diagnosis

UNSKILLED AT USING CONTACT LENSES: Being nonproficient, with or without knowledge, in the performance of the specific task of caring for and using corrective, curved lenses placed directly over the cornea

Common Etiology (Stressors)

HEALTH CARE FACTORS: Lack of health instruction, lack of health-skill experience

PLANNING

Unmet Needs

Comfort, protection from physical harm, mastery and competence in skills, independence, increased learning

Expected Outcome

Correct verbal feedback of the information taught

Correct return demonstration of how to insert, remove, clean, and store contact lenses

NURSING INTERVENTIONS

Nursing Treatments

Provide temporary assistance until the skill is learned

Clean the contact lenses

Insert and remove the contact lenses

Safeguard the person's contact lenses

Encourage the person to ask questions

Encourage self-performance

Nursing Observations

Test the eyes for visual acuity (uncorrected and corrected vision with contact lens)

Inspect (the eyes) for signs of irritation (redness, tearing, blinking)

Observe for readiness to assume self-care

Determine teaching effectiveness by testing, verbal feedback, and return demonstration

Health Teaching

Advise that contact lenses not be used for eye-color change (any foreign object in the eye is a potential danger)

Describe the discomforts of adjusting to contact lens (tearing, burning, and light sensitivity are common)

Describe those symptoms that should be reported (eye inflammation, visual difficulty)

Explain that care should be taken to prevent scratching of the contact lenses (lens scratches irritate eye tissue)

Explain that extreme cold cracks and heat warps contact lenses

Instruct that contact lenses should not be worn beyond the prescribed time, during an eye disorder, or while sleeping

Instruct to avoid rubbing the eyes (when wearing contact lenses, since this irritates the eye)

Teach how to clean contact lenses (soak in sterile solution)

Teach how to insert and remove contact lenses (gently pull the upper and lower lid open, wet the inner side of the lens with a special solution, place the lens over the cornea; to remove, pull the outer canthus and pull the lids together, and the lens should pop out)

Explain the reasons for and intended effect of the methods used (to prevent eye irritation or infection)

EVALUATION

Record actual outcome

UNSKILLED AT USING EYEGLASSES[72,451]

ASSESSMENT

Data Collection

Subjective Data

• Person's discussion or questions indicate a need for additional information, clarification, or validation of information about performing the task of using eyeglasses
  OR
• Person's lack of questions or comments indicates not wanting information or not knowing enough to seek information about performing the task of using eyeglasses
  Person may not know:
    That broken or scratched glasses should not be worn
    The dangers of wearing someone else's glasses
    How to protect eyeglasses from damage
    That eyeglass lenses must be intermittently changed to support vision changes

Objective Data

• Person cannot correctly demonstrate how to:
    Correctly apply and remove eyeglasses
    Properly clean eyeglasses
    Protect the lens from scratching

Related Data

Commonly Related Conditions
Hyperopia, myopia

Commonly Related Diseases
Astigmatism, strabismus

Data Analysis

Nursing Diagnosis:
UNSKILLED AT USING EYEGLASSES: Being nonproficient, with or without knowledge, in the performance of the specific task of caring for and using eyeglasses

Common Etiology (Stressors)
HEALTH CARE FACTORS: Lack of health instruction, lack of health-skill experience

PLANNING

Unmet Needs

Comfort, protection from physical harm, mastery and competence in skills, independence, increased learning

Expected Outcome
Correct verbal feedback of the information taught
Correct return demonstration of how to apply, remove, and clean eyeglasses and how to
   safeguard the lens

NURSING INTERVENTIONS
Nursing Treatments
Provide temporary assistance until the skill is learned
Clean the eyeglasses
Safeguard the person's eyeglasses (in a case or drawer)
Encourage the person to ask questions
Encourage self-performance

Nursing Observations
Test the eyes for visual acuity (uncorrected and corrected vision with eyeglasses)
Observe for readiness to assume self-care
Determine teaching effectiveness by testing, verbal feedback, and return demonstration

Health Teaching
Advise against wearing unprescribed eyeglasses
Inform that eyeglasses should be kept clean, rested on their rims to prevent lens
   scratching, and placed in a case when unused
Advise against bending the ear frames when applying or removing eyeglasses
Explain that corrective eye lenses require periodic adjustment (usually yearly)
Recommend the use of safety lens in eyeglasses
Describe those symptoms that should be reported (vision change, dizziness, impaired
   coordination)

EVALUATION

Record actual outcome

UNSKILLED AT USING A HEARING AID[73,451]

ASSESSMENT
Data Collection
Subjective Data
• Person's discussion or questions indicate a need for additional information, clari-
   fication, or validation of information about performing the task of using a hearing
   aid
   OR
• Person's lack of questions or comments indicates not wanting information or not
   knowing enough to seek information about performing the task of using a hearing
   aid
   Person may not know:
      About different types of hearing aids
      How hearing aids are used

Objective Data
• Person cannot correctly demonstrate how to:
      Apply the hearing aid to the ear
      Adjust the amplification
      Intermittently change the batteries
      Store the hearing aid

Related Data
Commonly Related Diseases
Acoustic neuroma, labyrinthitis, otosclerosis, presbycusis

Data Analysis

Nursing Diagnosis

UNSKILLED AT USING A HEARING AID: Being nonproficient, with or without knowledge, in the performance of the specific task of caring for and using a hearing aid

Common Etiology (Stressors)

HEALTH CARE FACTORS: Lack of health instruction, lack of health-skill experience

PLANNING

Unmet Needs

Comfort, protection from physical harm, mastery and competence in skills, independence, increased learning

Expected Outcome

Correct verbal feedback of the information taught

Correct return demonstration of how to apply and adjust the hearing aid, change the batteries, care for the hearing aid parts

NURSING INTERVENTIONS

Nursing Treatments

Provide temporary assistance until the skill is learned

Provide hearing-aid care (clean the ear inserts, remove the batteries when the hearing aid is not in use)

Safeguard the person's hearing aid (in a case or drawer)

Encourage the person to ask questions

Encourage self-performance

Nursing Observations

Test the ears for hearing acuity (with and without the hearing aid)

Observe for readiness to assume self-care

Determine teaching effectiveness by testing, verbal feedback, and return demonstration

Health Teaching

Teach how to care for a hearing aid (how to clean the ear tips, remove the batteries, place the device in a safe place)

Teach how to apply and remove the hearing aid (by inserting and removing the ear piece, cord, and transmitter)

Teach how to adjust the hearing aid for optimum sensory intake (by changing the volume)

Explain the reason for and intended effect of the methods used (to improve hearing)

EVALUATION

Record actual outcome

Minor Health Problems Associated with Sleep

INSOMNIA [19,42,88,302,303]

ASSESSMENT

Data Collection

Subjective Data

• Person complains of not being able to sleep

- Chronic fatigue
  May fall asleep and suddenly awaken
  May lie awake for hours before falling asleep

Objective Data
Frequent yawning
Drawn facial expression
Slumped body posture
Dark circles under the eyes

Data Analysis

Nursing Diagnosis
INSOMNIA: Difficulty falling asleep

Common Etiology (Stressors)
DISEASES: Manic-depressive psychosis, psychoneurosis
SIGNS AND SYMPTOMS: Coughing, dyspnea, itching sensation, pain, palpitations
PSYCHOSOCIAL FACTORS: Excessive emotional excitement, the threat of real or imagined danger, the threat of severe or chronic stress
HUMAN BODY: *Natural body function*: Impending childbirth. *Body state*: Pregnancy
HEALTH CARE FACTORS: *Health care environment*: An unfamiliar health care environment. *Hospitalization*: Separation from a significant other during hospitalization. *Diagnostic procedures*: An impending diagnostic procedure. *Medical diagnosis*: An impending or unfavorable medical diagnosis. *Drug therapy*: Corticosteroids, epinephrine. *Medical therapy*: Impending medical therapy. *Surgical therapy*: Impending surgery
DEVELOPMENTAL PHASES: Middle age, old age
LIFESTYLE: Involvement in too many activities above the person's comfort level, overeating, high-caffeine and nicotine intake, overvigorous exercise, overwork
SITUATIONAL FACTORS: Impending death or death of a significant other, divorce, an impending marriage
ENVIRONMENTAL FACTORS: *Cataclysm*: Exposure to a cataclysm. *Environmental cold*: Low external temperature. *Environmental heat*: High external temperature. *Humidity*: High environmental humidity. *Light*: Bright light. *Noise*: Loud noise
MAJOR PATHOPHYSIOLOGIC FACTORS CAUSING THE PROBLEM: Any form of stress will disturb the normal sleep process

PLANNING

Unmet Needs
Sleep, rest, relaxation, comfort, protection from physical harm, increased learning

Expected Outcome
Adequate average sleep in 24 hours, 18–20 hours for infants, 10–14 hours for children, 7–9 hours for adults, 5–7 hours for the aged
No yawning or dark circles under the eyes
Clear conjunctiva
Good concentration and coordination

NURSING INTERVENTIONS

Nursing Treatments
Anticipate needs
Arrange pleasant surroundings
Administer a warm bath (before sleep)
Change the person's clothing at bedtime
Refresh the person before sleep (by washing the hands and face, combing the hair, etc.)
Cover with warm blankets
Give warm liquids (preferably milk)
Discourage the intake of oral stimulants (tea, cola, cocoa, and chocolate drinks)
Encourage bladder emptying before rest
Encourage an indifferent attitude toward sleep (not caring about falling asleep promotes relaxation and sleep)

Encourage light reading before sleep
Maintain the person's usual bedtime rituals
Massage gently (before sleep)
Position comfortably
Position on the left side (to slow the heart rate and reduce the circulation)
Darken the room (before sleep)
Provide quiet
Place in a private room
Plan undisturbed periods for the person

Nursing Observations
Observe the pattern of sleep
Observe for an excessive stress level
Observe for restlessness
Observe for the quantity and inquire about the quality of sleep
Observe for a favorable response to therapy (restful sleep)

Health Teaching
Recommend a regular sleeping schedule (going to bed at the same time each night)
Advise that highly emotional situations be avoided (before sleep)
Recommend methods for achieving total relaxation (controlled breathing, quiet time, listening to music)
Recommend the use of eye shields for sleeping (if light is a problem)
Instruct to eat only at mealtime (and not before going to bed, as eating stimulates metabolic activity)

EVALUATION

Record actual outcome

NIGHTMARES [19,42,105,302]

ASSESSMENT
Data Collection

Subjective Data
• Awakened suddenly in the middle or last third of the night
• Experiences anxiety or fear
• Does not scream on awakening
• Can remember the dream sequence in detail and that the threat factor, in the dream, awakened him

Objective Data
Person can be observed awakening from a nightmare
Pulse rate may be increased
Skin may be moist with perspiration

Data Analysis

Nursing Diagnosis
NIGHTMARES: Experiencing a frightening dream

Common Etiology (Stressors)
PSYCHOSOCIAL FACTORS: The threat of chronic or severe stress, the threat of deprivation of essential needs, the threat of real or imagined danger
HEALTH CARE FACTORS: *Health care environment*: An unfamiliar health care environment. *Hos-*

pitalization: Separation from a significant other during hospitalization. *Drug therapy*: Adverse effects of drugs. *Medical diagnosis*: An unfavorable medical diagnosis

DEVELOPMENTAL PHASES: Preschooler (age 3–6)

SITUATIONAL FACTORS: The death of a significant other, surviving a natural disaster, being victimized by combative or sexual assault

ENVIRONMENTAL FACTORS: *Cataclysm*: Such as an earthquake, flood, tornado, etc. *Television*: Scary or violent movies on television

MAJOR BEHAVIORAL FACTORS CAUSING THE PROBLEM: Small children may have nightmares because of their inability to distinguish between fantasy and reality

PLANNING

Unmet Needs

Sleep, rest, relaxation, comfort, protection from psychologic threat, increased reality perception

Expected Outcome

Person verbalizes that his sleep is peaceful
No sudden, fearful awakening from sleep

NURSING INTERVENTIONS

Nursing Treatments

Reassure verbally (that it was a dream and not reality)
Anticipate needs (following a nightmare the person has a need to be held close)
Demonstrate calmness
Encourage the expression of feelings (about the nightmare)
Sit with the person (or have a family member sit nearby until he falls asleep)
Provide a night light (to increase the feeling of safety while falling asleep or when suddenly awakening)
Refrain from teasing
Refrain from negatively cirticizing
Make a referral (to a physician for chronic episodes, especially in an older child or adult, or if the nightmares are drug-related)

Nursing Observations

Observe for a favorable response to therapy

Health Teaching

Advise that highly emotional situations be avoided (before sleep, such as family discord, violent or frightening television)
Explain that fatigue should be recognized as a stress factor (that children should not become overfatigued)
Explain the causes of the health problem (stress, hospitalization, drugs)

EVALUATION

Record actual outcome

SLEEP RHYTHM INVERSION[19,302,303]

ASSESSMENT

Data Collection

Subjective Data
• Person falls asleep when he would normally be awake
• Is awake and active when he would normally be asleep

Becomes annoyed if disturbed while sleeping at odd hours

Objective Data
• An unusual sleep pattern may be observed

Data Analysis

Nursing Diagnosis
SLEEP RHYTHM INVERSION: A change of sleep pattern so that sleep hours are reversed from one's normal pattern

Common Etiology (Stressors)
SIGNS AND SYMPTOMS: Impending hepatic coma, pain
HEALTH CARE FACTORS: *Health therapy*: Sleep interruption for therapy. *Adverse effects of medical or surgical therapy*: Daytime anesthesia followed by a wakeful night
SITUATIONAL FACTORS: Travel to time zone changes, the unregulated sleep schedule of an infant
MAJOR PATHOPHYSIOLOGIC FACTORS CAUSING THE PROBLEM: Patterns of sleep can be interrupted by many factors, but the person's normal circadian rhythm can be reestablished by enforcing the same sleep schudule as was the previous pattern

PLANNING

Unmet Needs
Sleep and rest, protection from physical harm, increased learning

Expected Outcome
A reestablished sleep cycle, normal for the individual

NURSING INTERVENTIONS

Nursing Treatments
Keep the person awake during the day (until the normal sleep pattern is reestablished)
Make a referral (to a physician if the condition persists)

Nursing Observations
Observe the pattern of sleep

Health Teaching
Recommend a regular sleeping schedule (at the usual hours)
Explain the causes of the health problem (infant adjustment, anesthesia, etc.)

EVALUATION

Record actual outcome

SLEEP TERROR DISORDER[19,302]

ASSESSMENT

Data Collection

Subjective Data
• Sudden awakening from sleep, 30 minutes to 3 hours after falling asleep
• Panicky scream
• Expresses a feeling of terror related to dreams
• Unable to remember the episode in the morning

Objective Data
• Dilated pupils

- Tachycardia
- Rapid breathing

Data Analysis

Nursing Diagnosis

SLEEP TERROR DISORDER (NIGHT TERRORS): Episodes of awakening from sleep with a panicky scream

Common Etiology (Stressors)

SIGNS AND SYMPTOMS: Fatigue

PSYCHOSOCIAL FACTORS: The threat of chronic or severe stress, the threat of deprivation of essential needs, the threat of real or imagined danger

HEALTH CARE FACTORS: *Health care environment*: An unfamiliar health care environment. *Hospitalization*: Separation from a significant other during hospitalization. *Drug therapy*: Adverse effects of drugs, especially tricyclic antidepressants and neuroleptic drugs

DEVELOPMENTAL PHASES: Preschooler (age 2–6) or school-aged (6–10) child, early adulthood (age 18–40 years)

SITUATIONAL FACTORS: The death of a significant other, surviving a natural disaster, being victimized by combative or sexual assault

ENVIRONMENTAL FACTORS: *Cataclysm*: Such as earthquake, flood, tornado, etc. *Television*: Scary or violent movies on television

MAJOR BEHAVIORAL FACTORS CAUSING THE PROBLEM: Small children may experience sleep terrors because of their inability to distinguish between fantasy and reality

PLANNING

Unmet Needs

Comfort, protection from psychologic threat, increased reality perception

Expected Outcome

Person verbalizes that his sleep is peaceful
No sudden, panicky awakening from sleep

NURSING INTERVENTIONS

Nursing Treatments

Reassure verbally (that it was a dream and not reality)
Anticipate needs (following night terrors the person has a need to be held close)
Demonstrate calmness
Encourage the expression of feelings (about the sleep terror)
Sit with the person (or have a family member sit nearby until he falls asleep)
Provide a night light (to increase the feeling of safety while falling asleep or when suddenly awakening)
Refrain from teasing
Refrain from negatively criticizing
Make a referral (to a physician for chronic episodes, especially in an older child or adult or if the night terrors are drug related)

Nursing Observations

Observe for a favorable response to therapy

Health Teaching

Advise that highly emotional situations be avoided (before sleep, such as family discord, violent or frightening television)
Explain that fatigue should be recognized as a stress factor (that children should not become overfatigued)
Explain the causes of the health problem (stress, hospitalization, drugs)

EVALUATION

Record actual outcome

SLEEPWALKING

ASSESSMENT

Data Collection

Subjective Data
- Person falls into a deep sleep
- Arises from the bed, while asleep, and walks about
- Onset 30 minutes to 3 hours after falling asleep
- Unresponsive to external awakening attempts
- Returns to bed
- Confusion or disorientation for a short time after awakening
- Unable to remember the sleepwalking episode

Objective Data
Episode can be observed

Data Analysis

Nursing Diagnosis
SLEEPWALKING: Episodes of walking about while asleep

Common Etiology (Stressors)
DISEASES: Central nervous system infections
INHERITED FACTORS: Familial tendencies
INJURIES: Trauma of any kind
SIGNS AND SYMPTOMS: Fatigue, fever, seizures
PSYCHOSOCIAL FACTORS: The threat of chronic or severe stress
HEALTH CARE FACTORS: *Drug therapy*: Adverse effects of sedatives or hypnotics
DEVELOPMENTAL PHASES: School-aged child (6–10) or early adulthood (age 18–40)
MAJOR PATHOPHYSIOLOGIC FACTORS CAUSING THE PROBLEM: Uncertain, but disturbances in the central nervous system probably alter mental processes during the sleep cycle

PLANNING

Unmet Needs
Protection from physical harm

Expected Outcome
Safe return to bed, unharmed

NURSING INTERVENTIONS

Nursing Treatments
Demonstrate calmness
Guide the sleepwalker back to bed
Sit with the person (if he awakens)
Talk with the person (about the episode)
Relate the time, day, place, and events occurring (since disorientation sometimes occurs after awakening)
Use a chest restraint (only in case of danger or self-injury during sleepwalking)
Keep the person's windows closed (if sleepwalking is chronic; use child-proof locks on windows and outside doors)

Nursing Observations
Observe for an excessive stress level (which could cause sleepwalking)

Health Teaching
Explain the causes of the health problem (fatigue, seizures, drugs)

EVALUATION

Record actual outcome

Knowledge Deficits Associated with Sleep

UNKNOWLEDGEABLE ABOUT JET LAG[564,649,657]

ASSESSMENT
Data Collection
Subjective Data
- Person's discussion or questions indicate a need for additional information, clarification, or validation of information
  OR
- Person's lack of questions or comments indicates not wanting information or not knowing enough to seek information
- When questioned directly, the person's response or lack of response indicates that he does not know:
  Which time zones cause jet lag
  The symptoms of jet lag
  The precautions to be taken

Objective Data
None

Data Analysis
Nursing Diagnosis
UNKNOWLEDGEABLE ABOUT JET LAG: Being without sufficient information about rapid adjustment to time changes in distant places while traveling by high-speed aircraft

Common Etiology (Stressors)
HEALTH CARE FACTORS: Lack of health instruction

PLANNING
Unmet Needs
Rest, comfort, protection from physical harm, independence, increased learning

Expected Outcome
Correct verbal feedback of the information taught

NURSING INTERVENTIONS
Nursing Treatments
Approach unhurriedly
Encourage the person to ask questions

Nursing Observations
Determine teaching effectiveness by verbal feedback

Health Teaching
Inform of the time-zone changes that cause jet lag (jet lag does not occur when flying north or south because the time zones are unchanged; jet lag does occur when flying east or west because of multiple time zones; adjustment is more difficult on flights away from home than on flights homeward bound)
Describe those symptoms that should be expected (jet lag causes fatigue, sleeplessness, body temperature and blood pressure changes, an irregular eating schedule, dehydration sometimes, and altered biophysiologic activity; physiologic changes are more persistent than psychologic changes)
Advise that positions that impair circulation should be avoided (while in flight, especially prolonged leg crossing; recommend that the person move about the plane at least every 2 hours)
Advise against wearing constrictive clothing (for comfort and good circulation)

Instruct to increase fluid (water) intake (while in flight, this helps maintain normal body functions)

Recommend eating and drinking in moderation (high-food intake increases the metabolic rate which stimulates the body and prevents sleep)

Recommend limiting jet-flying time to five consecutive hours when possible (A 4- to 5-hour time difference requires minimal adjustment, while a gain or loss of more than 6 hours or a day requires considerable adjustment)

Recommend that jet travelers reduce stress by arriving 24 hours before scheduled activity (this allows time for rest and adjustment to the time zone)

Recommend the use of eye shields for sleeping (while in flight, darkness promotes sleep)

Explain the causes of the health problem (rapid time changes temporarily disrupt the body's physiologic cycles that are dependent on a well-ordered internal clock or daily rhythm)

EVALUATION

Record actual outcome

UNKNOWLEDGEABLE ABOUT SLEEP/REST[99,302,371,465]

ASSESSMENT

Data Collection

Subjective Data
- Person's discussion or questions indicate a need for additional information, clarification, or validation of information
  OR
- Person's lack of questions or comments indicates not wanting information or not knowing enough to seek information
- When questioned directly, the person's response or lack of response indicates that he does not know:
  How many daily hours of sleep are needed for the health of their children, aging or sick relatives, or themselves
  How to promote rest for the body
  Why adequate rest is important to health

Objective Data
None

Data Analysis

Nursing Diagnosis
UNKNOWLEDGEABLE ABOUT SLEEP/REST: Being without sufficient information about healthy sleep patterns and methods of sleep promotion

Common Etiology (Stressors)
HEALTH CARE FACTORS: Lack of health instruction, lack of health-skill experience

PLANNING

Unmet Needs

Sleep, rest, relaxation, protection from physical harm, independence, increased learning

Expected Outcome

Correct verbal feedback of the information taught

Adequate sleep in 24 hours as recommended and individually appropriate, (*Infants*: 18–20 hours. *Children*: 10–14 hours. *Adults*: 7–9 hours. *Aged*: 5–7 hours)

Absence of complaints of fatigue

NURSING INTERVENTIONS

Nursing Treatments

Approach unhurriedly

Encourage the person to ask questions

Nursing Observations

Determine teaching effectiveness by verbal feedback

Health Teaching

Recommend a regular sleeping schedule (going to bed at the same time each night)

Recommend adherence to a pace of living with which the person is comfortable (taking on only what can realistically be accomplished, avoiding hurrying)

Explain that fatigue should be recognized as a stress factor (fatigue diminishes the energy level available for coping)

Explain that parental attitudes (toward sleep and rest) affect child development (insufficient sleep interferes with optimum child development)

Describe the characteristics of fatigue (yawning, irritability, poor concentration, feeling unable to go on)

Describe the specific dangerous effects of poor health practices (chronic, insufficient rest causes system breakdown with resulting illness)

Inform of the recommended minimum hours of sleep (*Infants*: 18–20 hours. *Children*: 10 –14 hours. *Adults*: 7–9 hours. *Aged*: 5–7 hours)

Recommend methods for achieving total relaxation (slow rhythmic breathing, quiet time, listening to soothing music, doing nothing for a while)

EVALUATION

Record actual outcome

UNSKILLED AT RELAXATION METHODS[263,475]

ASSESSMENT

Data Collection

Subjective Data

• Person's discussion or questions indicate a need for additional information, clarification, or validation of information about performing the task of relaxation techniques

  OR

• Person's lack of questions or comments indicates not wanting information or not knowing enough to seek information about performing the task of relaxation techniques

  Person may not know:

  Ways of promoting relaxation

Objective Data

• Person cannot correctly demonstrate how to:

  Perform relaxation technique

Data Analysis

Nursing Diagnosis

UNSKILLED AT RELAXATION METHODS: Being nonproficient, with or without knowledge, in the performance of the specific task of methods used for relief of inner tension

Common Etiology (Stressors)

HEALTH CARE FACTORS: Lack of health instruction, lack of health-skill experience

PLANNING

Unmet Needs

Relaxation, comfort, protection from physical harm, mastery and competence in skills, independence, increased learning

Expected Outcome

Correct verbal feedback of the information taught

Correct return demonstration of relaxation methods

Calm, serene facial expression, no startle response to normal stimuli, nonrigid body movements or posture following the relaxation therapy

NURSING INTERVENTIONS

Nursing Treatments

Approach unhurriedly

Administer a warm bath

Give warm liquids (especially milk)

Cover with warm blankets

Massage gently

Position comfortably

Encourage deep breathing

Darken the room

Provide quiet

Discourage the intake of oral stimulants (coffee, soft drinks, alcohol, tobacco, drugs)

Nursing Observations

Determine teaching effectiveness by verbal feedback and return demonstration

Health Teaching

Recommend methods for achieving total relaxation (*Controlled breathing*: Have the person consciously and gradually decrease respirations below 10 times a minute. *Soft music*: Have the person lay back, close his eyes, and relax all muscles while listening)

Explain the causes of the problem (pain, emotional distress, stimulation from overwork, oxygen insufficiency, steroid-therapy side effects)

Explain the reason for and intended effect of the therapy (to relax the neuromuscular system)

EVALUATION

Record actual outcome

Knowledge Deficits Associated with Procedures for Diagnosing and Treating Health Problems

UNKNOWLEDGEABLE ABOUT THE DIAGNOSTIC STUDY[86]

ASSESSMENT

Data Collection

Subjective Data

• Person's discussion or questions indicate a need for additional information, clarification, or validation of information

OR
- Person's lack of questions or comments indicates not wanting information or not knowing enough to seek information
- When questioned directly, the person's response or lack of response indicates that he does not know:
  Why the study is being done
  How to prepare for the study
  The procedure involved in the study
  What the results of the study mean

Objective Data
None

Related Data
Involves such studies as blood work, urinalysis, gastric analysis, pulmonary function studies, electrocardiogram, electroencephalogram, x-ray procedures such as cholecystogram, upper GI series, barium enema, pyleogram, cystogram, arteriogram, pulmonary angiography, chest film, bone films, and liver, brain, thyroid, or renal scan

Data Analysis
Nursing Diagnosis
UNKNOWLEDGEABLE ABOUT THE DIAGNOSTIC STUDY: Being without sufficient information about tests performed for the purpose of diagnosis

Common Etiology (Stressors)
HEALTH CARE FACTORS: Lack of health instruction, lack of health-skill experience

PLANNING

Unmet Needs
Comfort, independence, increased learning

Expected Outcome
Correct verbal feedback of the information taught
Person verbalizes increased comfort at knowing about and understanding the diagnostic study

NURSING INTERVENTIONS

Nursing Treatments
Approach unhurriedly
Discuss the anticipated procedure
Encourage the person to ask questions
Reassure verbally (that any discomforts of the diagnostic study will be treated and controlled)

Nursing Observations
Determine teaching effectiveness by verbal feedback

Health Teaching
Explain the reason for and intended effect of the study (why it should be done and if there are other options)
Explain how to prepare for the diagnostic study (give verbal and written details when possible)
Describe those symptoms that should be expected (during the study, such as a burning sensation during an angiogram, pain during the insertion of a needle, nausea during the insertion of a nasogastric tube, etc.)
Explain the meaning of the diagnostic report (in understandable terms)

EVALUATION
Record actual outcome

UNKNOWLEDGEABLE ABOUT THE MEDICAL/SURGICAL PROCEDURE[86]

ASSESSMENT

Data Collection

Subjective Data
- Person's discussion or questions indicate a need for additional information, clarification, or validation of information
    OR
- Person's lack of questions or comments indicates
    Not wanting information or not knowing enough to seek information
- When questioned directly, the person's response or lack of response indicates that he does not know:
    Why the medical or surgical procedure is to be done or was done
    How the medical or surgical procedure will be done
    What the effects of the procedure are
    If it is painless or painful
    How long recovery will take
    What the degree of expected recovery will be

Objective Data
None

Data Analysis

Nursing Diagnosis
UNKNOWLEDGEABLE ABOUT THE MEDICAL/SURGICAL PROCEDURE: Being without sufficient information about the performance of a medical or surgical procedure and the effects of the procedure

Common Etiology (Stressors)
HEALTH CARE FACTORS: Lack of health instruction

PLANNING

Unmet Needs
Comfort, protection from physical harm, independence, increased learning

Expected Outcome
Correct verbal feedback of the information taught
Person verbalizes increased comfort at knowing about and understanding the medical or surgical procedure

NURSING INTERVENTIONS

Nursing Treatments
Approach unhurriedly
Discuss the anticipated procedure (include details of what will be done, how it will be done, how long it will take, and how rapid the recovery will be)
Encourage the person to ask questions
Introduce to persons who have successfully undergone the same experience
Reassure verbally (that any discomforts from the procedure will be treated and controlled)

Nursing Observations
Determine teaching effectiveness by verbal feedback

Health Teaching
Explain the reason for and intended effect of the therapy (why it should be done and if there are other options)
Explain how to prepare for the procedure (give verbal and written details when possible)

Describe those symptoms that should be expected (during and following the procedure, such as pain from the incision, sleepiness after the anesthesia, no sensation during IV therapy or blood transfusion)

Describe those symptoms that should be reported (during and following the procedure, such as severe pain, nausea, vomiting, dyspnea)

EVALUATION

Record actual outcome

UNKNOWLEDGEABLE ABOUT THE PHYSICAL EXAMINATION[86]

ASSESSMENT

Data Collection

Subjective Data

- Person's discussion or questions indicate a need for additional information, clarification, or validation of information

    OR

- Person's lack of questions or comments indicates not wanting information or not knowing enough to seek information

- When questioned directly, the person's response or lack of response indicates that he does not know:

    The necessity for the physical examination

    How to prepare for the examination

    What the examination involves

    How often certain examinations are recommended

Objective Data

None

Data Analysis

Nursing Diagnosis

UNKNOWLEDGEABLE ABOUT THE PHYSICAL EXAMINATION: Being without sufficient information about a general or specific physical examination of the body

Common Etiology (Stressors)

HEALTH CARE FACTORS: Lack of health instruction

PLANNING

Unmet Needs

Comfort, protection from physical harm, independence, increased learning

Expected Outcome

Correct verbal feedback of the information taught

Person verbalizes increased comfort at knowing about and understanding the examination procedure

NURSING INTERVENTIONS

Nursing Treatments

Approach unhurriedly

Encourage the person to ask questions

Discuss the anticipated examination (in detail)

Nursing Observations

Determine teaching effectiveness by verbal feedback

Health Teaching

Describe those symptoms that should be expected (during the examination, such as pressure applied for palpation, the discomforts of palpating or inspecting body orifices)

Inform that elimination is advisable before abdominal examinations (this makes the palpation of organs easier)

Advise periodic examinations for known hereditary predispositions (such as diabetes, hypertension)

Advise an annual gynecologic examination

Instruct that douching be avoided (before a Pap smear for women)

Advise early correction of problems (discovered on examination)

Explain the reason for and intended effect of the examination

EVALUATION

Record actual outcome

Knowledge Deficits Associated with Diseases or Conditions

UNKNOWLEDGEABLE ABOUT THE DISEASE/CONDITION[86]

ASSESSMENT

Data Collection

Subjective Data

• Person's discussion or questions indicate a need for additional information, clarification, or validation of information
   OR
• Person's lack of questions or comments indicates not wanting information or not knowing enough to seek information
• When questioned directly, the person's response or lack of response indicates that he does not know:
   What the disease or condition is
   All of its signs and symptoms
   Its physiologic or pathologic effect on the body or mind
   How long recovery will take
   What the degree of recovery will be
   The significance of the disease or condition in terms of its effect on the length of life, ability to function or be productive, and current or future lifestyle

Objective Data
None

Data Analysis

Nursing Diagnosis
UNKNOWLEDGEABLE ABOUT THE DISEASE/CONDITION: Being without sufficient information about a particular disease or nonhealth condition and its effect on the person

Common Etiology (Stressors)
HEALTH CARE FACTORS: Lack of health instruction

PLANNING

Unmet Needs

Comfort, protection from physical harm, independence, increased learning

Expected Outcome

Correct verbal feedback of the information taught

Person verbalizes increased comfort at knowing about and understanding the disease or condition

NURSING INTERVENTIONS

Nursing Treatments

Approach unhurriedly

Encourage the person to ask questions

Reassure verbally

Provide reliable information (about the disease or condition in terms the person can fully understand)

Nursing Observations

Determine teaching effectiveness by verbal feedback

Health Teaching

Describe those symptoms that should be expected (and are indicative of the disease or condition)

Describe those symptoms that should be reported

Instruct to report serious signs and symptoms immediately

Advise early correction of (health) problems

EVALUATION

Record actual outcome

17 Nursing Diagnoses of PAIN PROBLEMS

Dual Domain of Nursing Expertise: Pain Problems

This chapter covers that sphere of nursing knowledge and skill related to the perception of distressful hurting experienced separately by each individual. These problems are solved by many health care providers, such as nurses, physicians, dentists, and pharmacists.

Views of Nursing Leaders That Support This Domain of Nursing Expertise

The physician checks on the complaint of pain by attempting to ascertain a cause for it. In much the same way as a physician determines whether or not a patient is sick, he also determines whether or not a patient should have pain. . . . The nurse's primary and unique responsibility seems to be more in the realm of assisting the patient to cope with pain regardless of the cause of the pain or whether the cause is known.

Margo McCaffery[310:6 & 7]

Whenever pain exists for a patient, nursing care must be directed toward reducing the pain or eliminating it and preventing other discomforts from aggravating the existing pain.

Valentia Fischer & Arlene Connolly[156:84]

Types of Pain

ACHING PAIN [42,88,125,244,310,358]

ASSESSMENT

Data Collection

Subjective Data

Skeletal
- Person complains of pain in the joints, skeletal muscles, tendons, or bones
- Relates experiencing the sensation of aching (soreness, tenderness, heaviness)
- Can accurately localize the pain

Visceral
- Person complains of pain in the internal organs or structures
- Relates experiencing the sensation of aching (soreness, tenderness)
- Has accompanying symptoms such as nausea, vomiting, headache, dizziness, dyspnea
- Cannot sharply localize the pain, describes it as being spread over an area

Skeletal and Visceral
- Anxiety (if the pain is acute)
- Depression and fatigue (if the pain is chronic)

Objective Data

Skeletal
- Tenderness on palpation of the skeletal muscle, tendon, bone, or joint
- Pain on movement, decreased by cessation of movement
- Normal or stable vital signs
  Edema
  Redness
  Heat
  Changes in skin color such as pallor, bruising
  Dilated pupils
  Grimacing
  Drawn facial expression
  Sweating
  Clenched jaws or hands
  Restlessness

Visceral
- Pain may occur or become worse without movement
- Decreased blood pressure
- Decreased pulse rate
  Dilated pupils
  Grimacing
  Drawn facial expression
  Sweating
  Clenched jaws or hands
  Restlessness
  Rubing the painful part
  Tensing the skeletal muscles

Data Analysis

Nursing Diagnosis
ACHING PAIN: A warning sign of irritation or damage to the tissue cells of joints, skeletal muscles, tendons, bones, or internal organs or structures manifested as a hurting soreness or tenderness

Common Etiology (Stressors)

DISEASES: Abscess, aplastic anemia, appendicitis, Buerger's disease, bursitis, cancer, cellulitis, Dengue fever, dysmenorrhea, fibromyositis, gastritis, hepatitis, influenza, leukemia, malaria, multiple myeloma, osteoma, osteomyelitis, otitis media, Paget's disease, paratitis, plague, Raynaud's disease, rheumatic fever, rheumatoid arthritis, rickets, Rocky Mountain spotted fever, spondylitis, thrombophlebitis, varicose veins

INJURIES: Contussion, bone fracture, bruising or hematoma, foreign body in the skin, sprains, strains

SIGNS AND SYMPTOMS: Inflammation, toothache

HEALTH CARE FACTORS: *Diagnostic procedures*: Pap smear, bone marrow. *Surgical therapy*: Positioning during surgery, lying on a hard surgical table during surgery

DEVELOPMENTAL PHASES: Old age

ENVIRONMENTAL FACTORS: *Environmental cold*: Low external temperature

MAJOR PATHOPHYSIOLOGIC FACTORS CAUSING THE PROBLEM: Cell and tissue receptors carry pain stimuli by way of the nerves and spinal cord to the thalamus; sensation is conducted along nerve fibers and pain perception occurs in the cerebral cortex; infection, inflammation also cause aching pain

PLANNING

Unmet Needs

Rest and relaxation, comfort, protection from physical harm, freedom from pain, increased learning

Expected Outcome

Person verbalizes increased comfort
Exhibits a calm, contented, relaxed facial expression
Assumes a normal posture
Exhibits freedom of body movement

NURSING INTERVENTIONS

Nursing Treatments

Approach unhurriedly
Reassure that the pain will subside or be relieved
Communicate nurse sensitivity to the person's pain
Handle gently
Position comfortably
Apply a heating pad
   OR
Apply a hot water bottle
   OR
Apply a warm, moist compress
   OR
Bathe in warm water
   OR
Apply a cold, moist compress
Apply mentholated ointment (for skeletal pain)
Massage gently
Ask the person what makes him comfortable
Discuss possible pain-reducing measures (medication, heat, positioning)
Provide a pain-relief measure of the person's choice
Offer assurance of other measures if the pain-relief method fails
Provide an atmosphere of acceptance (if the person cannot tolerate much pain)
Give nonprescription drugs (give aspirin or acetaminophen every 4–6 hours for mild or moderate pain)
Give the drug (narcotic) having the fewest side effects for the person, when drug choices are available
Give pain-relief drugs on a regular, preventive schedule, not PRN

Give one-half the narcotic dose PO and one-half IM before converting to a full PO dosage

Ask the person to relate the onset of returning pain, before the pain becomes severe

Refrain from equating sleep with the absence of pain (fatigue may have exhausted the person who is still feeling pain)

Nursing Observations

Before Giving Medication

Determine the person's physiologic factors that increase or decrease drug absorption (absorption is decreased with impaired circulation, tissue damage, and obesity; absorption is increased with rapid metabolism, in adolescents and young adults, underweight persons, and smokers)

Observe the level of arousal and the respiratory rate before giving an analgesic

Evaluate the pain for intensity and quality

Determine the urgency for pain relief (and administer accordingly)

After Giving Medication

Observe for complaints of pain duration (duration varies individually)

Observe for oversedation (difficult arousal, respiratory depression)

Observe for inadequate analgesic pain relief (pain that still exists 1 hour after the drug dose, pain that becomes severe before the next scheduled dose)

Evaluate the effectiveness of the pain-relief measures (the person verbalizes that the pain has been relieved, exhibits freedom of movement, has a relaxed facial expression)

Health Teaching

Explain that it is acceptable to admit the existence of pain (if the person denies or minimizes the pain)

Explain how to use nondrug methods for pain relief (heat, positioning, relaxation)

Recommend methods for distraction from pain (television, listening to music, counting, praying)

Explain the reason for the delay in giving a pain-relief drug (if the delay is due to the prescribed hours of drug administration)

Explain that immobility related to pain causes increased pain (in joint pain, in severe muscle pain)

Explain how to describe pain (aching, burning, constrictive, cramping, stabbing, throbbing)

Explain the causes of the pain (infection, inflammation)

Teach how to apply heat or cold therapy (for aching)

Medical Treatments Performed by Nurses

Give the prescribed drugs (ask the physician to order aspirin or acetaminophen with analgesics, or narcotics; combined, they affect both the peripheral nervous system and central nervous system for greater pain relief)

EVALUATION

Record actual outcome

BURNING PAIN [42,88,125,244,310,358]

ASSESSMENT

Data Collection

Subjective Data

• Person complains of pain near the skin surface or mucosal lining

• Relates experiencing the sensation of burning (stinging, smarting, hot, scalding, searing)

- Anxiety (if the pain is acute)
- Depression and fatigue (if the pain is chronic)
- Can accurately or sharply localize the pain

Objective Data
- Stroking the skin lightly produces pain
- Person guards against moving the affected area
  Elevated or decreased blood pressure
  Tachycardia or bradycardia
  Dilated pupils
  Grimacing
  Drawn facial expression
  Sweating
  Clenched jaws or hands
  Restlessness

Data Analysis

Nursing Diagnosis
BURNING PAIN: A warning sign of irritation or damage to tissue cells in the skin or mucosal surface, manifested in a localized, stinging hurting

Common Etiology (Stressors)
DISEASES: Beriberi, cystitis, dermatitis, duodenal ulcer, erythema multiforme, esophageal hernia, gastritis, gastric ulcer, herpes simplex, herpes zoster, hemorrhoids, indigestion, miliaria, peripheral neuritis, poison ivy, poison oak, tinea
INJURIES: Abrasion wound, burn wound, foreign body in skin, insect bites, venomous marine-life sting
SIGNS AND SYMPTOMS: Dysuria, heartburn, paresthesia, phantom pain
HEALTH CARE FACTORS: *Diagnostic procedures*: Angiography, bronchoscopy, cystoscopy, gastroscopy. *Medical therapy*: Urinary catheterization, nasogastric tube
ENVIRONMENTAL FACTORS: *Chemical substances*: Contact with chemical agents such as acids. *Environmental heat*: Fire and flames. *Friction*: Exposure to friction. *Objects*: Hot objects such as heaters, hot liquids, steam, stoves, torches. *Environmental radiation*: Ultraviolet light from the sun. *Wind*: Prolonged exposure to high wind
MAJOR PATHOPHYSIOLOGIC FACTORS CAUSING THE PAIN: Burning pain can be caused by inadequate circulation to peripheral nerves, injury to the peripheral nerve trunk, or increased temperature or movement; impaired kidney function elevates the serum phosphate, which decreases the calcium level, causing neuritis pain

PLANNING

Unmet Needs
Rest and relaxation, comfort, protection from physical harm, freedom from pain, increased learning

Expected Outcome
Person verbalizes increased comfort
Exhibits a calm, contented, relaxed facial expression
Assumes a normal posture
Exhibits freedom of body movement

NURSING INTERVENTIONS

Nursing Treatments
Approach unhurriedly
Reassure that the pain will subside or be relieved
Communicate nurse sensitivity to the person's pain
Handle gently
Position comfortably
Apply a cold, moist compress
   OR
Apply an ice bag

OR

Bathe in cool water

OR

Soak in cold water

Apply sodium bicarbonate to the skin

OR

Apply cornstarch to the skin

Apply an analgesic ointment (to burns or lesions)

Remove constrictive clothing

Remove tight bandaging

Apply a bed cradle

OR

Cover with lightweight blankets (for burning skin lesions)

Decrease drafts

Ask the person what makes him comfortable

Discuss possible pain-reducing measures (medication, heat, positioning)

Provide a pain-relief measure of the person's choice

Offer assurance of other measures if the pain-relief method fails

Provide an atmosphere of acceptance (if the person cannot tolerate much pain)

Give nonprescription drugs (give aspirin or acetaminophen every 4–6 hours for mild or moderate pain)

Give the drug (narcotic) with the fewest side effects for the person, if drug choices are available

Give pain relief drugs on a regular, preventive schedule, not PRN

Give one-half the narcotic dose PO and one-half IM before converting to a full PO dosage

Ask the person to relate the onset of the returning pain, before the pain becomes severe

Refrain from equating sleep with the absence of pain (fatigue may have exhausted the person feeling the pain)

Nursing Observations

Before Giving Medication

Determine the person's physiologic factors that increase or decrease drug absorption (decreased absorption occurs with impaired circulation, tissue damage, or obesity; increased absorption occurs with rapid metabolism, in adolescents and young adults, underweight persons, and smokers)

Observe the level of arousal and the respiratory rate before giving the analgesic

Determine the urgency for pain relief (and administer accordingly)

After Giving Medication

Observe for complaints of pain duration (duration varies individually)

Observe for oversedation (difficult arousal, respiratory depression)

Observe for inadequate analgesic pain relief (pain that still exists 1 hour after the drug dose; pain that becomes severe before the next scheduled dose)

Evaluate the effectiveness of the pain-relief measures (person verbalizes that the pain has been relieved, exhibits freedom of movement, has a relaxed facial expression)

Health Teaching

Explain that it is acceptable to admit the existence of pain (if the person denies or minimizes pain)

Explain how to use nondrug methods for pain relief (cold, positioning, relaxation)

Recommend methods for distraction from pain (television, listening to music, counting, praying)

Explain the reason for the delay in giving a pain-relief drug (if delay is due to the prescribed hours of drug administration)

Explain how to describe pain (aching, burning, constrictive, cramping, stabbing, throbbing)

Explain the causes of the pain (tissue irritation or damage)

Teach how to apply cold therapy

Medical Treatments Performed by Nurses

Give the prescribed drugs (ask the physician to order aspirin or acetaminophen with analgesics or narcotics; combined, they affect both the peripheral nervous system and central nervous system for greater pain relief)

EVALUATION

Record actual outcome

CONSTRICTIVE PAIN [42,88,125,244,310,358]

ASSESSMENT

Data Collection

Subjective Data

- Person complains of pain in the deep, internal organs or structures
- Relates experiencing the sensation of constriction (squeezing, crushing, binding, pressing, suffocating)
- Has accompanying symptoms such as nausea, vomiting, headache, dizziness, dyspnea
- Anxiety (if the pain is acute)
- Depression and fatigue (if the pain is chronic)
- Cannot sharply localize the pain, describes it as being spread over an area

Objective Data

- Pain may occur or become worse without movement
- Decreased blood pressure
- Decreased pulse rate
  Dilated pupils
  Grimacing
  Drawn facial expression
  Sweating
  Clenched jaws or hands
  Restlessness

Data Analysis

Nursing Diagnosis

CONSTRICTIVE PAIN: A warning sign of irritation or damage to tissue cells in internal organs or structures, manifested as a diffuse, squeezing hurt

Common Etiology (Stressors)

DISEASES: Angina pectoris, arteriosclerotic heart disease, esophageal stricture, myocardial infarction, syphilis

INJURIES: Burn wound scars

SIGNS AND SYMPTOMS: Abdominal distention (gastric dilatation), coughing

MAJOR PATHOPHYSIOLOGIC FACTORS CAUSING THE PROBLEM: Constrictive pain results from sensory nerve-fiber irritation by cardiac hypoxia, overdistention of some viscera, and infection of some nerve tissue

PLANNING

Unmet Needs

Rest and relaxation, comfort, protection from physical harm, freedom from pain, increased learning

Expected Outcome

Person verbalizes increased comfort
Exhibits a calm, contented, relaxed facial expression
Assumes a normal posture
Exhibits freedom of body movement

NURSING INTERVENTIONS

Nursing Treatments
Approach unhurriedly
Reassure that the pain will subside or be relieved
Communicate nurse sensitivity to the person's pain
Handle gently
Position comfortably
Apply a heating pad
　　OR
Apply a hot water bottle
　　OR
Apply a warm, moist compress
Give warm liquids
Refrain from giving iced liquids
Remove constrictive clothing
Insert a gastric tube and attach to suction (ET) (to decompress gastric dilatation)
Administer humidified oxygen (ET) (for cardiac ischemia)
Ask the person what makes him comfortable
Discuss possible pain-reducing measures (medication, positioning)
Provide a pain-relief measure of the person's choice
Encourage adequate rest
Offer assurance of other measures if the pain-relief method fails
Provide an atmosphere of acceptance (if the person cannot tolerate much pain)
Give nonprescription drugs (give aspirin or acetaminophen every 4–6 hours for mild or moderate pain)
Give the drug (narcotic) having the fewest side effects for the person, if drug choices are available
Give pain relief drugs on a regular, preventive schedule, not prn
Give one-half the narcotic dose PO and one-half IM before converting to a full PO dosage
Ask the person to relate the onset of the returning pain, before the pain becomes severe
Refrain from equating sleep with the absence of pain (fatigue may have exhausted the person feeling pain)

Nursing Observations
Before Giving Medication
Determine the person's physiologic factors that increase or decrease drug absorption (decreased absorption occurs with impaired circulation, tissue damage, or obesity; increased absorption occurs with rapid metabolism, in adolescents and young adults, underweight persons, and smokers)
Observe the level of arousal and the respiratory rate before giving the analgesic
Determine the urgency for pain relief (and give accordingly)

After Giving Medication
Observe for complaints of pain duration (duration varies individually)
Observe for oversedation (difficult arousal, respiratory depression)
Observe for inadequate analgesic pain relief (pain that still exists 1 hour after the drug dose, pain that becomes severe before the next scheduled dose)
Evaluate the effectiveness of the pain relief measures (Person verbalizes that the pain has been relieved, exhibits freedom of movement, has a relaxed facial expression)

Health Teaching
Explain that it is acceptable to admit the existence of pain (if the person denies or minimizes pain)
Explain how to use nondrug methods for pain relief (heat, positioning, relaxation)
Recommend methods for distraction from pain (television, listening to music, counting, praying)

Explain the reason for the delay in giving a pain-relief drug (if the delay is due to the prescribed hours of drug administration)

Explain how to describe pain (aching, burning, constrictive, cramping, stabbing, throbbing)

Explain the causes of the pain (ischemia, obstruction)

Teach how to apply heat therapy

Medical Treatments Performed by Nurses

Give the prescribed drugs (ask the physician to order aspirin or acetaminiphen with analgesics, or narcotics; combined, they affect both the peripheral nervous system and central nervous system for greater pain relief; give nitroglycerine for cardiac ischemia)

EVALUATION

Record actual outcome

CRAMPING PAIN [42,88,125,244,310,358]

ASSESSMENT

Data Collection

Subjective Data
• Person complains of pain in deep, internal organs or structures
• Experiences the sensation of cramping (twisting, spasm, colicky)
• Has accompanying symptoms such as nausea, vomiting, headache, dizziness, dyspnea
• Anxiety (if the pain is acute)
• Depression and fatigue (if the pain is chronic)
• Cannot sharply localize the pain, describes it as being spread over an area

Objective Data
• Pain may occur or become worse without movement
• Decreased blood pressure
• Decreased pulse rate
  Dilated pupils
  Grimacing
  Drawn facial expression
  Sweating
  Clenched jaws or hands
  Restlessness

Data Analysis

Nursing Diagnosis
CRAMPING PAIN: A warning sign of irritation or damage to tissue cells of internal organs or structures, manifested as a diffuse, colicky hurting

Common Etiology (Stressors)
DISEASES: Arteriosclerosis obliterans, bladder calculi, cholecystitis, cholelithiasis, Crohn's disease, diverticulitis, dysentery, dysmenorrhea, ectopic pregnancy, endometriosis, hypocalcemia, intermittent claudication, intussusception, pancreatitis, rabies, regional enteritis, renal calculi, salpingitis, sprue, strongyloidiosis, tabes dorsalis, ulcerative colitis, ureteral calculi, varicose veins
INJURIES: Poisoning (food, arsenic, lead)
SIGNS AND SYMPTOMS: Bladder spasms, constipation, diarrhea, flatulence, muscle spasm, pain (labor pain, afterbirth pain, ovulation pain)
HEALTH CARE FACTORS: *Diagnostic procedures*: Barium enema. *Drug therapy*: Adverse effects of antibiotics, cathartics. *Medical therapy*: Enemas, gastrostomy feeding, jejunostomy feeding, nasogastric feeding, hemodialysis, bladder or colonic irrigation, peritoneal dialy-

sis, traction. *Adverse effects of medical or surgical therapy*: Circulatory constriction from a cast or tight dressings

LIFESTYLE: Overvigorous exercise

ENVIRONMENTAL FACTORS: *Altitude*: High altitude. *Environmental cold*: Low external temperature. *Pressure*: Underwater pressure

MAJOR PATHOPHYSIOLOGIC FACTORS CAUSING THE PROBLEM: Cramping pain results from reduced blood supply to tissues or alternating forceful contraction and relaxation of muscle tissue

PLANNING

Unmet Needs

Rest and relaxation, comfort, protection from physical harm, freedom from pain, increased learning

Expected Outcome

Person verbalizes increased comfort
Exhibits a calm, contented, relaxed facial expression
Assumes a normal posture
Exhibits freedom of body movement

NURSING INTERVENTIONS

Nursing Treatments

Approach unhurriedly
Reassure that the pain will subside or be relieved
Communicate nurse sensitivity to the person's pain
Handle gently
Position comfortably
Apply a heating pad
    OR
Apply a hot water bottle
    OR
Apply a saline compress
    OR
Bathe in warm water
Massage gently
Remove constrictive clothing
Give warm liquids
Refrain from giving iced liquids
Introduce irrigating solutions slowly (if cramping pain is due to enema administration or the like)
Ask the person what makes him comfortable
Discuss possible pain-reducing measures
Provide a pain-relief measure of the person's choice
Offer assurance of other measures if the pain-relief method fails
Provide an atmosphere of acceptance (if the person cannot tolerate much pain)
Give nonprescription drugs (give aspirin or acetaminophen every 4–6 hours for mild or moderate pain)
Give the drug (narcotic) having the fewest side effects for the person, if drug choices are available
Give pain-relief drugs on a regular, preventive schedule, not PRN
Give one-half the narcotic dose PO and one-half IV before converting to a full PO dosage
Ask the person to relate the onset of the returning pain, before the pain becomes severe
Refrain from equating sleep with the absence of pain (fatigue may have exhausted the person feeling the pain)

Nursing Observations

Before Giving Medication

Determine the person's physiologic factors that increase or decrease drug absorption (decreased absorption occurs with impaired circulation, tissue damage, or obesity; increased absorption occurs with rapid metabolism, in adolescents and young adults, underweight persons, and smokers)

Observe the level of arousal and the respiratory rate before giving the analgesic

Determine the urgency for pain relief (and administer accordingly)

After Giving Medication

Observe for complaints of pain duration (duration varies individually)

Observe for oversedation (difficult arousal, respiratory depression)

Observe for inadequate analgesic pain relief (pain that still exists 1 hour after the drug dose, pain that becomes severe before the next scheduled dose)

Evaluate the effectiveness of the pain-relief measures (person verbalizes that the pain has been relieved, exhibits freedom of movement, has a relaxed facial expression)

Health Teaching

Explain that it is acceptable to admit the existence of pain (if the person denies or minimizes pain)

Explain how to use nondrug methods for pain relief (heat, positioning, relaxation)

Recommend methods for distraction from pain (television, listening to music, counting, praying)

Explain the reason for the delay in giving a pain-relief drug (if the delay is due to prescribed hours of drug administration)

Explain how to describe pain (aching, burning, constrictive, cramping, stabbing, throbbing)

Explain the causes of the pain (ischemia, obstruction)

Teach how to apply heat therapy

Medical Treatments Performed by Nurses

Give the prescribed drugs (ask the physician to order aspirin or acetaminophen with analgesics, or narcotics; combined, they affect both the peripheral nervous system and central nervous system for greater pain relief)

EVALUATION

Record actual outcome

GNAWING PAIN [42,88,125,165,244,310,358]

ASSESSMENT

Data Collection

Subjective Data

- Person complains of pain in deep, internal organs or structures
- Relates experiencing the sensation of gnawing (emptiness, hollowness, gnarling)
- Has accompanying symptoms such as nausea, vomiting, headache, dizziness, dyspnea
- Anxiety (if the pain is acute)
- Depression and fatigue (if the pain is chronic)
- Cannot sharply localize the pain, describes it as being spread over an area

Objective Data

- Pain may occur or become worse without movement
- Decreased blood pressure

• Decreased pulse rate
Dilated pupils
Grimacing
Drawn facial expression
Sweating
Clenched jaws or hands
Restlessness

Data Analysis

Nursing Diagnosis

GNAWING PAIN: A warning sign of irritation or damage to tissue cells of internal organs or structures, manifested as a diffuse, hurting emptiness

Common Etiology (Stressors)

DISEASES: Duodenal ulcer, gastric ulcer, hypoglycemia, peptic ulcer

SIGNS AND SYMPTOMS: Diarrhea, hunger

PSYCHOSOCIAL FACTORS: Excessive emotional excitement, the threat of real or imagined danger

ENVIRONMENTAL FACTORS: *Food substances*: Insufficient amounts of food available

MAJOR PATHOPHYSIOLOGIC FACTORS CAUSING THE PROBLEM: Gnawing pain results when gastric acid stimulates nerve endings in the ulcerated or gastric area

PLANNING

Unmet Needs

Acid–base balance, nutritional balance, rest and relaxation, comfort, protection from physical harm, freedom from pain, increased learning

Expected Outcome

Person verbalizes increased comfort
Exhibits a calm, contented, relaxed facial expression
Assumes a normal posture
Exhibits freedom of body movement

NURSING INTERVENTIONS

Nursing Treatments

Approach unhurriedly
Reassure that the pain will subside or be relieved
Communicate nurse sensitivity to the person's pain
Give milk
Give warm liquids
Refrain from giving iced liquids
Encourage decreased acid-food intake
Ask the person what makes him comfortable
Provide a pain-relief measure of the person's choice
Offer reassurance of other measures if the pain-relief method fails
Provide an atmosphere of acceptance (if the person cannot tolerate much pain)
Give nonprescription drugs (antacids)
Give pain relief drugs on a regular, preventive schedule, not PRN
Ask the person to relate the onset of the returning pain, before the pain becomes severe
Refrain from equating sleep with the absence of pain (fatigue may have exhausted the person feeling the pain)

Nursing Observations

Before Giving Medication

Determine the person's physiologic factors that increase or decrease drug absorption (decreased absorption occurs with impaired circulation, tissue damage, or obesity; increased absorption occurs with rapid metabolism, in adolescents and young adults, underweight persons, and smokers)

Observe the level of arousal and the respiratory rate before giving the analgesic

Determine the urgency for pain relief (and give accordingly)

After Giving Medication

Observe for complaints of pain duration (duration varies individually)

Observe for oversedation (difficult arousal, respiratory depression)

Observe for inadequate analgesic pain relief (pain that still exists 1 hour after the drug dose, pain that becomes severe before the next scheduled dose)

Evaluate the effectiveness of the pain-relief measures (person verbalizes that the pain has been relieved, exhibits freedom of movement, has a relaxed facial expression)

Health Teaching

Explain that it is acceptable to admit the existence of pain (if the person denies or minimizes pain)

Explain how to use nondrug methods for pain relief (food, positioning, relaxation)

Recommend methods for distraction from pain (television, listening to music, counting, praying)

Explain the reason for the delay in giving a pain-relief drug (if there is a delay)

Explain how to describe pain (aching, burning, constrictive, cramping, stabbing, throbbing)

Explain the causes of the pain (high gastric acidity, vigorous gastric movement)

Medical Treatments Performed by Nurses

Give the prescribed drugs (belladonna, phenobarbitol, Tagamet)

EVALUATION

Record actual outcome

STABBING PAIN[42,88,125,244,310,358]

ASSESSMENT

Data Collection

Subjective Data

- Person complains of pain near the skin surface
- Relates experiencing the sensation of stabbing (cutting, knifelike, piercing, sharp, lancinating, lightninglike, pricking)
- Anxiety (if the pain is acute)
- Depression and fatigue (if the pain is chronic)
- Can accurately or sharply localize the pain

Objective Data

- Stroking the skin lightly produces pain
- Person guards against moving the affected area
  Elevated or decreased blood pressure
  Tachycardia or bradycardia
  Dilated pupils
  Grimacing
  Drawn facial expression
  Sweating
  Clenched jaws or hands
  Restlessness

Data Analysis

Nursing Diagnosis

STABBING PAIN: A warning sign of irritation or damage to tissue cells in the skin or mucosal surface, manifested in a localized cutting, piercing, hurting sensation

Common Etiology (Stressors)

DISEASES: Bronchitis, glaucoma, neuralgia, otitis media, pericarditis, peripheral neuritis, peritonitis, pleurisy, pneumonia, pneumothorax, pulmonary embolus

INJURIES: Animal bite, bone fracture, foreign body in the skin, incision wound, insect bite, nonvenomous or venomous snake or spider bite

SIGNS AND SYMPTOMS: Photophobia

HUMAN BODY: *Natural body function*: Childbirth

HEALTH CARE FACTORS: *Diagnostic procedures*: Angiography, biopsy (kidney, liver, lung, muscle, skin, bone marrow), blood-analysis sampling, cisternal puncture, electromyogram. *Medical therapy*: Cardioversion (defibrillation), venipuncture for hemodialysis, intravenous infusion, needle injection, nerve-block injection, paracentesis, thoracentesis, blood transfusion. *Surgical incision*: Any

ENVIRONMENTAL FACTORS: *Biologic agents*: Bites of animals, insects, snakes. *Electricity*: Exposure to ungrounded electrical currents. *Environmental cold*: Freezing external temperature. *Objects*: Pointed or sharp objects. *Tools*: Powered or nonpowered. *Weapons*: Knives

MAJOR PATHOPHYSIOLOGIC FACTORS CAUSING THE PROBLEM: Stabbing pain results from short intervals of stimuli to sensory pain fibers, nerve injury and impaired peripheral circulation contribute to such pain

PLANNING

Unmet Needs

Rest and relaxation, comfort, protection from physical harm, freedom from pain, increased learning

Expected Outcome

Person verbalizes increased comfort
Exhibits a calm, contented, relaxed facial expression
Assumes a normal posture
Exhibits freedom of body movement

NURSING INTERVENTIONS

Nursing Treatments

Approach unhurriedly
Reassure that the pain will subside or be relieved
Communicate nurse sensitivity to the person's pain
Handle gently
Position comfortably
Place a pillow on the affected side
Remove constrictive clothing
Subdue the room lighting (for photophobia)
Ask the person what makes him comfortable
Provide a pain-relief measure of the person's choice
Offer assurance of other measures if the pain-relief method fails
Provide an atmosphere of acceptance (if the person cannot tolerate much pain)
Give nonprescription drugs (give aspirin or acetaminophen every 4–6 hours for mild or moderate pain)
Give the drug (narcotic) having the fewest side effects for the person, if drug choices are available
Give pain-relief drugs on a regular, preventive schedule, not PRN
Give one-half the narcotic dose PO and one-half IM before converting to a full PO dosage
Ask the person to relate the onset of the returning pain, before the pain becomes severe
Refrain from equating sleep with the absence of pain (fatigue may have exhausted the person feeling the pain)

Nursing Observations

Before Giving Medication

Determine the person's physiologic factors that increase or decrease drug absorption (decreased absorption occurs with impaired circulation, tissue damage, or obesity; increased absorption occurs with rapid metabolism, in adolescents and young adults, underweight persons, and smokers)

Observe the level of arousal and the respiratory rate before giving the analgesic

Determine the urgency for pain relief (and administer accordingly)

After Giving Medication

Observe for complaints of pain duration (duration varies individually)

Observe for oversedation (difficult arousal, respiratory depression)

Observe for inadequate analgesic pain relief (pain that still exists 1 hour after the drug dose, pain that becomes severe before the next scheduled dose)

Evaluate the effectiveness of the pain-relief measures (person verbalizes that the pain has been relieved, exhibits freedom of movement, has a relaxed facial expression)

Health Teaching

Explain that it is acceptable to admit the existence of pain (if the person denies or minimizes pain)

Explain how to use nondrug methods for pain relief (heat, cold, positioning, relaxation, splinting support)

Recommend methods for distraction from pain (television, listening to music, counting, praying)

Explain the reason for the delay in giving a pain-relief drug (if the delay is due to prescribed hours of drug administration)

Explain how to describe pain (aching, burning, constrictive, cramping, stabbing, throbbing)

Explain the causes of the pain (ischemia, edema, inflammation)

Medical Treatments Performed by Nurses

Give the prescribed drugs (ask the physician to order aspirin or acetaminophen with analgesics, or narcotics; combined, they affect both the peripheral nervous system and central nervous system for greater pain relief)

EVALUATION

Record actual outcome

THROBBING PAIN [42,88,125,244,310,358]

ASSESSMENT

Data Collection

Subjective Data

- Person complains of pain in the internal organs or structures
- Relates experiencing the sensation of throbbing (pounding, pulsating)
- Has accompanying symptoms such as nausea, vomiting, headache, dizziness, dyspnea
- Anxiety (if the pain is acute)
- Depression and fatigue (if the pain is chronic)
- Cannot sharply localize the pain, describes it as being spread over an area

Objective Data

- Pain may occur or become worse without movement
- Decreased blood pressure

- Decreased pulse rate
  Dilated pupils
  Grimacing
  Drawn facial expression
  Sweating
  Clenched jaws or hands
  Restlessness
  Pain often worsens with the lowering of the involved part

Data Analysis

Nursing Diagnosis

THROBBING PAIN: A warning sign of irritation or damage to tissue cells in the internal organs or structures, or to the extremities, manifested as a diffuse, hurting pulsation

Common Etiology (Stressors)

DISEASES: Abscess, arteritis (temporal), cellulitis, dental caries, headaches (cluster, or histamine; hypertensive, or vascular; menstrual migraine, migraine; postspinal; tension), phlebothrombosis, Raynaud's disease, thrombophlebitis

INJURIES: Contusion, subungual hemorrhage

SIGNS AND SYMPTOMS: Ischemia (venous congestion)

HEALTH CARE FACTORS: *Drug therapy*: Adverse effects of epinephrine causes headaches. *Medical therapy*: Circulatory constriction from a cast

ENVIRONMENTAL FACTORS: *Tools*: Powered or nonpowered

MAJOR PATHOPHYSIOLOGIC FACTORS CAUSING THE PROBLEM: Throbbing pain results from irritation stimuli to sensory pain fibers and the presence of vasodilation in a constricted area

PLANNING

Unmet Needs

Rest and relaxation, comfort, protection from physical harm, freedom from pain, increased learning

Expected Outcome

Person verbalizes increased comfort
Exhibits a calm, contented, relaxed facial expression
Assumes a normal posture
Exhibits freedom of body movement

NURSING INTERVENTIONS

Nursing Treatments

Approach unhurriedly
Reassure that the pain will subside or be relieved
Communicate nurse sensitivity to the person's pain
Handle gently
Position comfortably
Change the person's position gradually
Support the affected body part
Apply a cold, moist compress
   OR
Apply an ice bag
   OR
Apply a warm, moist compress
Refrain from tight bandaging
Remove constrictive clothing
Ask the person what makes him comfortable
Elevate the affected body part
Encourage adequate rest

Provide a pain-relief measure of the person's choice

Offer assurance of other measures if the pain-relief method fails

Provide an atmosphere of acceptance (if the person cannot tolerate much pain)

Give nonprescription drugs (give aspirin or acetaminophen every 4–6 hours for mild or moderate pain)

Give the drug (narcotic) having the fewest side effects for the person, if drug choices are available)

Give pain-relief drugs on a regular, preventive schedule, not PRN

Give one-half the narcotic dose PO and one-half IM before converting to a full PO dosage

Ask the person to relate the onset of the returning pain, before the pain becomes severe

Refrain from equating sleep with the absence of pain (fatigue may have exhausted the person feeling the pain)

Nursing Observations

Before Giving Medication

Determine the person's physiologic factors that increase or decrease drug absorption (decreased absorption occurs with impaired circulation, tissue damage, or obesity; increased absorption occurs with rapid metabolism, in adolescents and young adults, underweight persons, and smokers)

Observe the level of arousal and the respiratory rate before giving the analgesic

Determine the urgency for pain relief (and give accordingly)

After Giving Medication

Observe for complaints of pain duration (duration varies individually)

Observe for oversedation (difficult arousal, respiratory depression)

Observe for inadequate analgesic pain relief (pain that still exists 1 hour after the drug dose, pain that becomes severe before the next scheduled dose)

Evaluate the effectiveness of the pain-relief measures (person verbalizes that the pain has been relieved, exhibits freedom of movement, has a relaxed facial expression)

Health Teaching

Explain that it is acceptable to admit the existence of pain (if the person denies or minimizes pain)

Explain how to use nondrug methods for pain relief (heat, cold, positioning, relaxation)

Recommend methods for distraction from pain (television, listening to music, counting, praying)

Advise not to take hot baths (vasodilatation increases the pain of arteritis, caries, subungual hemorrhage, etc.)

Instruct to avoid coughing

Instruct to avoid elimination straining (pressure increases pain)

Explain the reason for the delay in giving a pain-relief drug (if the delay is due to prescribed hours of drug administration)

Explain that immobility related to pain causes increased pain

Explain how to describe pain (aching, burning, constrictive, cramping, stabbing, throbbing)

Explain the causes of the pain (vasodilatation)

Teach how to apply cold therapy

Teach how to apply heat therapy

Medical Treatments Performed by Nurses

Give the prescribed drugs (ask the physician to order aspirin or acetaminophen with analgesics, or narcotics; combined they affect both the peripheral nervous system and central nervous system for greater pain relief)

EVALUATION

Record actual outcome

Knowledge Deficits Associated with Pain

UNKNOWLEDGEABLE ABOUT PAIN-RELIEF METHODS [42,88,125,244,310,358]

ASSESSMENT

Data Collection
Subjective Data
- Person's discussion or questions indicate a need for additional information, clarification, or validation of information
  OR
- Person's lack of questions or comments indicates not wanting information or not knowing enough to seek information
- When questioned directly, the person's response or lack of response indicates that he does not know:
  Which drugs are appropriate for pain relief
  The fact that there are nondrug methods of pain relief
  Which pain-relief methods are most suitable to specific types of pain
  Person is concerned about relieving his own or the pain of another

Objective Data
None

Data Analysis
Nursing Diagnosis
UNKNOWLEDGEABLE ABOUT PAIN-RELIEF METHODS: Being without sufficient information about the many ways in which pain can be relieved

Common Etiology (Stressors)
HEALTH CARE FACTORS: Lack of health instruction

PLANNING

Unmet Needs
Comfort, protection from physical harm, freedom from pain, independence, increased learning

Expected Outcome
Correct verbal feedback of the information taught

NURSING INTERVENTIONS

Nursing Treatments
Approach unhurriedly
Encourage the person to ask questions

Nursing Observations
Determine teaching effectiveness by verbal feedback

Health Teaching
Explain how to use nondrug methods for pain relief (heat, cold, positioning, tension reduction, body alignment, supportive bandages and garments)
Explain that immobility related to pain causes increased pain (so the person should move about when possible)
Recommend methods for distraction from pain (television, listening to music, counting, praying)
Teach how or when to administer or take medications (for pain relief)

EVALUATION

Record actual outcome

18 Nursing Diagnoses of HEALTH MAINTENANCE AND PREVENTIVE HEALTH PROBLEMS

Dual Domain of Nursing Expertise: Health Maintenance and Preventive Health Problems

This chapter covers that sphere of nursing knowledge and skill related to identified sets of habits and characteristics that increase a person's chance of developing a specific disease or injury and that make the person's risk greater than that of the population as a whole. These problems are identified and preventive interventions are initiated by such health care providers as nurses, physicians, physicians' assistants, and nonprofessional private or government agencies.

Views of Nursing Leaders That Support This Domain of Nursing Expertise

The nurse may intervene at the primary prevention level which deals with the system before an encounter with a stressor occurs. The goal of primary prevention is to prevent the stressor from penetrating the normal line of defense or to lessen the degree of reaction by reducing the possibility of encounter with the stressor, reducing its strength, and/or strengthening the flexible line of defense.

Betty Neuman[410:136]

Preventive health is identified as an explicit function of nursing.

Florence Nightingale[379:65]

Self-care related to hazards includes (1) action to prevent events which may lead to hazardous conditions, (2) removal or protection of oneself from hazardous situations when they cannot be controlled, and (3) modification of hazardous situations to decrease danger to life and well-being when they are amenable to control. Specialized assistance may also be needed for individuals to understand the nature of hazardous conditions in particular environments as related to age, activity, or mere presence. It may also be necessary to learn preventive and protective practices.

Dorothea Orem[380:26]

Nursing as a service, involves helping the individual to become more self-directing in attaining or maintaining a healthy state of body.

Faye Abdellah[5:26]

Maintenance and promotion of health, prevention of disease . . . encompass the scope of nursing's goals.

Nursing is concerned with human beings, only some of whom are ill. The first approach toward building a healthy person lies in maintenance and promotion of health.

Martha Rogers[419:86–87 & 664:32]

At-Risk Factors for Accidental Injury

POTENTIAL FOR BURN INJURY[81,134,135,728,729,730]

ASSESSMENT

Data Collection

Subjective Data
• There are no actual symptoms of burn injury

Objective Data
• There are no actual signs of burn injury

Related Data
• There are one or more stressors present that increase the possibility that burn injury
  will occur:

HEALTH CARE FACTORS: *Medical therapy*: Cardioversion, diathermy, electroconvulsive therapy,
  application of heat (hot packs, heating pad, etc.), heated mist inhalation therapy, radiation therapy. *Drug therapy*: Infiltration of drugs into tissue. *Surgical procedures*: Cauterization by electrocautery. *Therapeutic equipment*: Safety restraints

DEVELOPMENTAL PHASES: Toddler or babyhood, old age

LIFESTYLE: Cigarette or tobacco smoking

ENVIRONMENTAL FACTORS: *Chemical substances*: Availability of chemicals. *Environmental heat*:
  High external temperature, fire and flames. *Environmental radiation*: Exposure to infrared rays, radiation, ultraviolet light

HUMAN ERROR: *Potential scald burn (hot fluid or steam)*: Person faces pot handles toward the
  front of the stove, bathes in very hot water, trips and falls while carrying hot liquids,
  allows self to be splattered by hot metals being poured. *Potential dry heat flash burn*:
  Holds matches near gas leaks, experiments with chemicals or gasoline. *Potential dry
  heat flame burn*: Fails to screen the fireplace and heaters (which can ignite clothing),
  wears plastic aprons or long sleeves around an open flame, plays with matches, stores
  matches in paper or wood containers, smokes in bed or around oxygen, leaves unused electrical equipment plugged in, allows frying pans to catch fire from cooking
  fat, allows grease to collect on stoves, uses thin worn pot holders or mits, gives children toys made from flammable materials. *Potential dry heat friction burn*: Takes little or
  no precaution when near rapid moving machinery, industrial pulleys, or belts, falls or
  slides on concrete or other hard surfaces when motorcycling or playing sports. *Potential electrical burn*: Uses faulty plugs and frayed wiring. *Potential chemical burn*: Takes little or no precaution when near or using acids or alkalis. *Potential flash burn*: Plays with
  fireworks or gunpowder. *Potential ice burn*: Fails to wear gloves when handling ice. *Potential radiation burn*: Overexposes self to sun, heat, or ultraviolet lamps

Data Analysis

Nursing Diagnosis
POTENTIAL FOR BURN INJURY: The presence of stressors that increase the possibility of the actual occurrence of tissue damage from heat, fire, chemical reaction, electricity, radiation, or friction

PLANNING

Unmet Needs
Protection from physical harm, increased learning

Expected Outcome
No signs or symptoms of a burn injury will occur
  OR

If signs and symptoms occur, they will be promptly recognized as an actual problem and will be treated appropriately

Person verbalizes an understanding of and practices preventive methods

NURSING INTERVENTIONS

Nursing Treatments
Minimize environmental dangers

Use a chest restraint (instead of limb restraints, which can cause burns)

Nursing Observations
Evaluate the safety of the environment

Observe for behavior modification (use of preventive measures)

Health Teaching
Advise against exposure to intense heat

Advise against prolonged skin exposure to the sun

Inform that the skin should be protected from windburn

Recommend safety measures to prevent a burn injury (such as keeping fireplaces and open heaters screened, storing matches in a metal container, keeping stoves grease free, not wearing long sleeves or plastic aprons around open flames, using well-padded pot holders, turning pot handles toward the back of the stove, not smoking around oxygen or in bed, avoiding the danger of fireworks and chemicals, washing chemically contaminated skin immediately)

Recommend safety measures to prevent electrical (burn) injury (such as immediately repairing worn electrical cords)

Emphasize that small children should always be attended

Advise not to use an electric blanket (on children, the aged, or persons with impaired touch perception)

Recommend the installation of a smoke alarm

Explain how to extinguish fires (if clothing is on fire, drop to the floor and roll over; cover pan fires with a lid; do not use water on flammable liquids or electrical fires; use dry chemical, carbon dioxide, or foam fire extinguishers on flammable liquids; use carbon dioxide on electrical fires)

Explain how to escape a fire (prepare escape routes and meeting places, leave the fire immediately, crawl along the floor of a smoke-filled room, do not use elevators, do not go back into the fire once outside)

Recommend strict adherence to safety rules

Explain why the potential problem could become actual (skin exposure to intense heat will result in burns)

Explain the reason for and intended effect of the preventive methods

EVALUATION

Record actual outcome

POTENTIAL FOR ELECTRICAL INJURY[20,22,399]

ASSESSMENT

Data Collection

Subjective Data

• There are no actual symptoms of electrical injury

Objective Data
• There are no actual signs of electrical injury

Related Data
• There are one or more stressors present that increase the possibility that electrical injury will occur:
ENVIRONMENTAL FACTORS: *Electricity*: Electrical currents. *Lightning*: Exposure to lightning
HUMAN ERROR: Person uses cut, frayed, or exposed electrical cord; disregards warm or hot equipment switches or switch plates; allows electrical equipment to become wet or places wet objects on such equipment; uses loose or broken wall outlets; overloads extension cords or outlets; does not use safety guards on electrical outlets to protect small children; uses two-pronged adaptors to plug into three-pronged plugs; leaves hot, sparking, or smoking electrical equipment plugged in; uses electrical appliances when showering or otherwise wet; touches faucets or metal pipes while simultaneously touching electrical appliances; does not avoid arcing machinery or power lines

Data Analysis
Nursing Diagnosis
POTENTIAL FOR ELECTRICAL INJURY: The presence of stressors that increase the possibility of the actual occurrence of being injured by electrical current

PLANNING
Unmet Needs
Protection from physical harm, increased learning
Expected Outcome
No signs or symptoms of electrical injury will occur
> OR

If signs and symptoms occur, they will be promptly recognized as an actual problem and will be treated appropriately
Person verbalizes an understanding of and practices preventive methods

NURSING INTERVENTIONS
Nursing Treatments
Minimize environmental dangers (unplug the electrical monitors during a bath, use only three-pronged electrical plugs, etc.)
Nursing Observations
Evaluate the safety of the environment
Observe for behavior modification (use of preventive measures)
Health Teaching
Recommend safety measures to prevent electrical injury (such as disconnecting unused electrical equipment; immediately repairing worn electrical cords, hot equipment switches, or plugs and hot or broken wall outlets; placing safety guards over electrical outlets; standing on dry surfaces and wearing insulated rubber gloves and rubber-soled shoes when working with electricity; never using electrical appliances near or in water; using only grounded electrical equipment and appliances; never plugging a two-pronged adaptor into a three-pronged plug; not overloading extension cords or wall outlets; never standing in an open field during an electrical storm)
Emphasize that small children should always be attended
Recommend strict adherence to safety rules
Explain why the potential problem could become actual (unless electricity is properly handled, the electrical current could pass through the body, causing severe or fatal injury)
Explain the reason for and intended effect of the preventive methods

EVALUATION
Record actual outcome

POTENTIAL FOR FALL INJURY[81,134,135,138]

ASSESSMENT

Data Collection

Subjective Data
• There are no actual symptoms of a fall injury

Objective Data
• There are no actual signs of a fall injury

Related Data
• There are one or more stressors present that increase the possibility that a fall injury will occur:

BIRTH DEFECTS: Blindness, brain tumor, cerebral palsy, clubfoot, deafness, Duchenne's muscular dystrophy, myasthenia gravis, Parkinson's disease

DISEASES: Cerebrovascular accident, epilepsy, multiple sclerosis, obesity, organic brain syndrome

INJURIES: Bone fracture

SIGNS AND SYMPTOMS: Coma, confusion, dizziness, unsteady gait, poor coordination, unconsciousness, weakness

HUMAN BODY: *Body states*: Pregnancy

HEALTH CARE FACTORS: *Health care environment*: Unfamiliar, hospital bed. *Medical therapy*: Prolonged bed rest, electroconvulsive shock, body casting, traction. *Drug therapy*: Barbiturates, narcotics, sedatives, tranquilizers. *Surgical therapy*: Anesthesia, recovery from anesthesia. *Therapeutic equipment*: Use of an artificial limb, brace, cane, crutches, walker, wheelchair, placement on a CircOlectric bed or Stryker frame

DEVELOPMENTAL PHASES: Infant (rolling over), toddler (learning to walk), preschooler (age 3–6 years), old age (age 60 and older)

LIFESTYLE: High alcohol intake, drug abuse, insufficient sleep and rest

SITUATIONAL FACTORS: Situational crisis, stress

ENVIRONMENTAL FACTORS: Darkness

HUMAN ERROR: Person polishes floors with slippery wax, allows snow to collect on stairs and walkways, uses slippery throw rugs or tub mats, uses unsteady ladders, does not maintain nonsturdy stair rails, leaves extension cords unanchored and loose, does not clean up litter or liquid spills on floors and stairways, allows children to play at the top of the stairs without a stair gate, walks into an unlighted room

Data Analysis

Nursing Diagnosis
POTENTIAL FOR FALL INJURY: The presence of stressors that increase the possibility of the actual occurrence of an injury by falling

PLANNING

Unmet Needs

Protection from physical harm, increased learning

Expected Outcome

No signs or symptoms of a fall injury will occur
   OR
If signs and symptoms occur, they will be promptly recognized as an actual problem and will be treated appropriately
Person verbalizes an understanding of and practices preventive methods

NURSING INTERVENTIONS

Nursing Treatments

Arrange orderly surroundings

Minimize environmental barriers
Minimize environmental dangers
Illuminate the room adequately
Assist with mobility
Provide safe play equipment for children
Restrain the patient (for safety purposes)
Safeguard with a crib dome
Safeguard with side rails and side rail padding
Provide a low-height bed
Cover the bed with netting
Place in a playpen (if the child is a toddler)
Apply a safety helmet to the head (of persons likely to fall)
Place in an uncrowded area
Discourage the intake of oral stimulants (specifically alcohol)

Nursing Observations
Evaluate the safety of the environment
Observe for behavior modification (use of preventive measures)

Health Teaching
Recommend safety measures to prevent falling (such as suction mats in tubs, securing
    extension cords in place, keeping the floors and stairways litter free and wax free, re-
    moving snow and ice from stairways, maintaining sturdy stair rails, using only sturdy
    ladders, using stairgates to prevent tumbles down stairs, using safety straps for poorly
    coordinated persons and in hazardous occupations, using hand rails, using nonskid
    throw rugs)
Emphasize that small children should always be attended
Explain that objects (furniture, etc.) should be consistently placed in the same location
    for the visually impaired
Explain how to illuminate a room correctly (so persons with decreased vision can see
    where they are going)
Recommend the use of a night-light
Recommend the use of low-heeled shoes (if the person is unsteady)
Explain why the potential problem could become actual (fall injuries result from dimin-
    ished perception of or becoming accustomed to environmental hazards, lack of expe-
    rience or misjudgment in interpreting dangerous stimuli as harmful, the absence of a
    sense of danger in young children, slowed reaction time to dangerous stimuli)
Explain the reason for and intended effect of the preventive methods

EVALUATION
Record actual outcome

POTENTIAL FOR MOTOR VEHICLE INJURY[81,134,135,295]

ASSESSMENT

Data Collection

Subjective Data
• There are no actual symptoms of an injury from a motor vehicle

Objective Data
• There are no actual signs of an injury from a motor vehicle

Related Data
• There are one or more stressors that increase the possibility that a motor vehicle injury will occur:

DISEASES: Alcoholism, cardiovascular disease, cataracts, diabetes mellitus, epilepsy, glaucoma, mental illness (persons with these diseases average twice as many motor vehicle injuries)

PSYCHOSOCIAL FACTORS: Lack of impulse control, the threat of chronic or severe stress

DEVELOPMENTAL FACTORS: Adolescence, old age

LIFESTYLE: High alcohol intake, drug abuse

SITUATIONAL FACTORS: Situational crisis or stress

HUMAN ERROR: Driving a mechanically unsafe vehicle, driving at a speed greater than 55 miles per hour (or above the city speed limit), failure to use seatbelts or child restraints, driving a car more than 8 years old (doubles the accident potential)

Data Analysis
Nursing Diagnosis
POTENTIAL FOR MOTOR VEHICLE INJURY: The presence of stressors that increase the possibility of the actual occurrence of body injury from an automobile accident

PLANNING
Unmet Needs
Protection from physical harm, increased learning

Expected Outcome
No signs or symptoms of motor vehicle injury will occur
OR
If signs and symptoms occur, they will be promptly recognized as an actual problem and will be treated appropriately
Person verbalizes an understanding of and practices preventive methods

NURSING INTERVENTIONS
Nursing Treatments
Discourage the intake of oral stimulants (alcohol use when driving)

Nursing Observations
Observe for behavior modification (use of preventive measures)

Health Teaching
Recommend safety measures to prevent motor vehicle injury (such as always fastening seatbelts, placing small children in safety seats, keeping the vehicle in good repair, driving no faster than the speed limit, respecting stop and yield signs, driving defensively)
Recommend strict adherence to safety rules
Advise not to take any drugs (such as antihistamines, tranquilizers, sedatives immediately before or while driving)
Explain why the potential problem could become actual (any moving object has the potential for causing injury, the faster the object moves, the greater the injury potential)
Advise not to drive for 3 hours after two alcoholic drinks
Explain that corrective eye lenses require periodic adjustment (for safe driving)
Instruct to restrict children to a fenced play area
Emphasize that small children should always be attended (when playing outside in an unfenced area)
Explain the reason for and intended effect of the preventive methods

EVALUATION
Record actual outcome

POTENTIAL FOR POISONING [81,134,135,490]

ASSESSMENT

Data Collection

Subjective Data
• There are no actual symptoms of poisoning

Objective Data
• There are no actual signs of poisoning

Related Data
• There are one or more stressors present that increase the possibility that poisoning will occur:

HEALTH CARE FACTORS: *Drug therapy*: Large supplies of drugs are made available

DEVELOPMENTAL PHASES: Toddler, preschooler

ENVIRONMENTAL FACTORS: *Chemical substances*: Availability of chemicals. *Housing*: Peeling paint or housing (lead poisoning)

HUMAN ERROR: Medicines stored in unlocked cabinets are accessible to children and confused persons, containers are poorly labeled, products have been placed in containers that are marked and intended for other products, dangerous products have been placed within the reach of children or confused persons, medicinal products or drugs prescribed for another person are being used for self-medication, outdated drugs are used

Data Analysis

Nursing Diagnosis
POTENTIAL FOR POISONING: The presence of stressors that increase the possibility of the actual occurrence of drugs or dangerous products being accidentally taken in doses sufficient to cause poisoning

PLANNING

Unmet Needs

Protection from physical harm, increased learning

Expected Outcome

No signs or symptoms of poisoning will occur
    OR
If signs and symptoms occur, they will be promptly recognized as an actual problem and will be treated appropriately
Person verbalizes an understanding of and practices preventive methods

NURSING INTERVENTIONS

Nursing Treatments

Minimize environmental dangers

Nursing Observations

Evaluate the safety of the environment
Observe for behavior modification (use of preventive measures)

Health Teaching

Recommend safety measures to prevent poisoning (such as storing dangerous products out of reach, locking medicine cabinets, clearly and correctly labeling all containers)
Emphasize the danger of mixing drugs and alcohol, the danger of sharing drugs between persons
Emphasize that outdated drugs should be discarded (destroyed)
Recommend that self-medication be avoided
Emphasize that small children should always be attended
Recommend strict adherence to safety rules

Explain why the potential problem could become actual (poisoning can result from lack of experience in interpreting dangerous stimuli as harmful, from lack of knowledge that a product is harmful)

Explain the reason for and intended effects of the preventive methods

EVALUATION

Record actual outcome

POTENTIAL FOR RADIATION INJURY[72,73]

ASSESSMENT

Data Collection

Subjective Data
• There are no actual symptoms of radiation injury

Objective Data
• There are no actual signs of radiation injury

Related Data
• There are one or more stressors present that increase the possibility that radiation injury will occur:

HEALTH CARE FACTORS: *Diagnostic procedures*: X-ray films. *Medical therapy*: Radiation and radioisotope therapy

Data Analysis

Nursing Diagnosis
POTENTIAL FOR RADIATION INJURY: The presence of stressors that increase the possibility of the actual occurrence of tissue damage from the rays of radioactive substances

PLANNING

Unmet Needs

Protection from physical harm, increased learning

Expected Outcome

No signs or symptoms of radiation injury will occur
Person verbalizes an understanding of and practices preventive methods

NURSING INTERVENTIONS

Nursing Treatments

Reassure verbally (that precautions are being taken)
Collect radiation-contaminated linen in a special laundry bag
Collect radiation-contaminated urine in a lead-lined container
Limit the amount of time visitors are exposed to radiation (no more than 30 minutes a day)
Limit the distance from which visitors approach the radiated patient (at least 3 feet from the patient)
Shield visitors from exposure to radiation (if for some reason a visitor must stay longer than 30 minutes, have him wear a lead-lined apron and sit behind lead-lined drapes)
Consult with the physician (if the radiation implants become dislodged from the insertion site)

Nursing Observations

Evaluate the safety of the environment (for family members and staff)

Health Teaching

Describe those symptoms that should be reported (if a person is overly exposed to radiation; nausea, vomiting, anorexia, malaise, hair loss, petechiae, nosebleed, mouth or throat inflammation, skin irritations)

Emphasize the danger of exposure to x-ray during the first three months of pregnancy (this could cause fetal injury)

Explain the reason for and intended effect of the preventive therapy

EVALUATION

Record actual outcome

POTENTIAL FOR SUFFOCATION[81,134,135]

ASSESSMENT

Data Collection

Subjective Data
• There are no actual symptoms of suffocation

Objective Data
• There are no actual signs of suffocation

Related Data
• There are one or more stressors present that increase the possibility that suffocation will occur:

HUMAN ERROR: Pillows are placed in an infant's crib, infant is placed in bed with an adult, an automobile is warmed in a closed garage, small children are allowed to play with plastic bags, children are allowed to play near discarded refrigerators or freezers, children are left unattended in bathtubs or pools, paint or lacquer are used in closed areas, heaters have not been vented to the outside, clotheslines are placed at a low level, a pacifier is hung around an infant's neck

Data Analysis

Nursing Diagnosis
POTENTIAL FOR SUFFOCATION: The presence of stressors that increase the possibility of the actual occurrence of inadequate air being available for inhalation

PLANNING

Unmet Needs

Protection from physical harm, increased learning

Expected Outcome

No signs or symptoms of suffocation will occur
 OR
If signs and symptoms occur, they will be promptly recognized as an actual problem and will be treated appropriately

Person verbalizes an understanding of and practices preventive methods

NURSING INTERVENTIONS

Nursing Treatments

Minimize environmental dangers

Nursing Observations

Evaluate the safety of the environment
Observe for behavior modification (use of preventive measures)

Health Teaching

Recommend safety measures to prevent suffocation (such as never starting a car in a closed garage, using fume-producing substances only in the open air, venting heaters to the outside, shredding or discarding plastic bags, locking unused refrigerators or removing the doors, placing infants in a pillow-free crib, never sleeping in the same bed with an infant, never smoking, not hanging a pacifier around an infant's neck, keeping clotheslines high enough to prevent stangulation, using protective measures against unattended entry into pools, checking for gas leakage)

Inform that airway noise indicates obstruction

Emphasize that small children should always be attended

Recommend strict adherence to safety rules

Explain why the potential problem could become actual (whenever there is decreased air space for breathing, suffocation can occur)

Explain the reason for and intended effect of the preventive measures

EVALUATION

Record actual outcome

POTENTIAL FOR WOUND INJURY[81,134,135]

ASSESSMENT

Data Collection

Subjective Data
• There are no actual symptoms of a wound injury

Objective Data
• There are no actual signs of a wound injury

Related Data
• There are one or more stressors present that increase the possibility that a wound injury will occur:

DEVELOPMENTAL PHASE: Toddler (up to age 3), preschooler (age 3–6)

HUMAN ERROR: Cracked dishware or glasses are used, knives are placed uncovered in drawers or in a dishpan of water, guns and ammunition are within easy reach, large icicles are left hanging from the roof, children are allowed to play in unfenced play areas, children are allowed to play with sharp-edged toys

Data Analysis

Nursing Diagnosis

POTENTIAL FOR WOUND INJURY: The presence of stressors that increase the possibility of the actual occurrence of a disruption of skin intactness from an injury

PLANNING

Unmet Needs

Protection from physical harm, increased learning

Expected Outcome

No signs or symptoms of a wound injury will occur
  OR
If signs and symptoms occur, they will be promptly recognized as an actual problem and will be treated appropriately

Person verbalizes an understanding of and practices preventive methods

NURSING INTERVENTIONS

Nursing Treatments

Minimize environmental dangers

Nursing Observations

Evaluate the safety of the environment
Observe for behavior modification (use of preventive measures)

Health Teaching

Recommend safety measures to prevent wound injuries (such as discarding cracked or broken dishware, using only covered knife racks, storing unloaded guns or ammunition in a locked cabinet or drawer, removing large icicles before they melt and fall, wearing a hard hat for head protection, avoiding giving children toys with sharp edges or that are sharp when broken)

Instruct to restrict children to a fenced play area

Emphasize that small children should always be attended

Recommend strict adherence to safety rules (regarding home, work, and play safety)

Explain why the potential problems should become actual (any hard or sharp object has the potential for causing injury)

Explain the reason for and intended effect of the preventive measures

EVALUATION

Record actual outcome

UNKNOWLEDGEABLE ABOUT WASTE SANITATION[134,135]

ASSESSMENT

Data Collection

Subjective Data

- Person's discussion or questions indicate a need for additional information, clarification, or validation of information
  OR
- Person's lack of questions or comments indicates not wanting information or not knowing enough to seek information
- When questioned directly, the person's respnse or lack of response indicates that he does not know the following:

  Exposed garbage allows flies and rats to carry infection

  Human wastes should be buried out of reach of flies

  Private sewage systems should never be closer than one acre apart

  Cesspools should never be near limestone, where the sewage can travel through the limestone crevices and contaminate underground wells and springs

  Solids from septic tanks must be periodically removed and buried

  Privies should be deep, have a floor above the ground, have an adequate seat cover, have screens over ventilation openings to prevent flies from entering, and have a tight door that prevents chickens, pigs, etc., from roaming inside

Objective Data

- May exhibit behavior such as acting inappropriately on the basis of insufficient knowledge, not taking precautions

Data Analysis

Nursing Diagnosis

UNKNOWLEDGEABLE ABOUT WASTE SANITATION: Being without sufficient information about satisfactory health measures for the disposal of human wastes

Common Etiology (Stressors)

HEALTH CARE FACTORS: Lack of health instruction

PLANNING

Unmet Needs

Protection from physical harm, independence, increased learning

Expected Outcome

Correct verbal feedback of the information taught

NURSING INTERVENTIONS
Nursing Treatments
Approach unhurriedly
Encourage the person to ask questions
Make a referral (to the city sanitation department, if needed)
Nursing Observations
Determine teaching effectiveness by verbal feedback
Health Teaching
Emphasize that food wastes should be burned in animal-inhabited outdoor areas
Emphasize that garbage should be covered
Emphasize that, in outdoor living, human wastes should be buried
Emphasize the need to use only an approved sewage facility
Inform that cleanliness is basic to health
Recommend strict adherence to safety rules

EVALUATION
Record actual outcome

UNKNOWLEDGEABLE ABOUT WATER SANITATION[134,135]

ASSESSMENT
Data Collection
Subjective Data
• Person's discussion or questions indicate a need for additional information, clarification, or validation of information
  OR
• Person's lack of questions or comments indicates not wanting information or not knowing enough to seek information
• When questioned directly, the person's response or lack of response indicates that he does not know the following:
  River water should not be used for bathing
  Unapproved water supplies should not be used
  Unpurified water from lakes and streams is unsafe
  It is dangerous to use wells and springs located in limestone where pollution from nearby cesspools, privies, or flooded lakes and streams can occur
  Safe wells and springs must be more than 50 feet from any source of contamination
  Wells must have properly constructed casings, a drainage system away from the well, and not be connected to a sewer system
  Ice cubes made from polluted water are as unsafe as the water itself

Objective Data
• May exhibit behavior such as acting inappropriately on the basis of insufficient knowledge, not taking precautions

Data Analysis
Nursing Diagnosis
UNKNOWLEDGEABLE ABOUT WATER SANITATION: Being without sufficient information about satisfactory health measures involving the consumption of drinking water

Common Etiology (Stressors)
HEALTH CARE FACTORS: Lack of health instruction

PLANNING

Unmet Needs
Protection from physical harm, independence, increased learning

Expected Outcome
Correct verbal feedback of the information taught

NURSING INTERVENTIONS

Nursing Treatments
Approach unhurriedly
Encourage patient questions
Make a referral (to the city sanitation department)

Nursing Observations
Determine teaching effectiveness by verbal feedback

Health Teaching
Emphasize that potentially unsafe water should be boiled for 10 minutes
Emphasize the need to use only an approved water supply
Inform that cleanliness is basic to health
Inform that halazone tablets should be added to potentially unsafe water
Inform that the color and taste of outdoor water do not indicate its safety
Recommend strict adherence to safety rules

EVALUATION

Record actual outcome

At-Risk Factors for Cardiovascular Disease

POTENTIAL FOR CARDIOVASCULAR DISEASE [146,295,346]

ASSESSMENT

Data Collection

Subjective Data
• There are no actual symptoms of cardiovascular disease

Objective Data
• There are no actual signs of cardiovascular disease

Related Data
• There are one or more stressors present that increase the possibility that cardiovascular disease will occur:
INHERITED FACTORS: *Familial tendency*: For coronary heart disease. *Sex*: More prevalent in men
DISEASES: Diabetes mellitus, hypertension, obesity
PSYCHOSOCIAL FACTORS: Type A personality (high achiever, competitive, hostile, rarely vacations, narrowed interests)

LIFESTYLE: High-cholesterol (lipid) diet (hyperlipidemia), high-triglyceride diet (hypertriglyceridemia), lack of exercise, cigarette or tobacco smoking

Data Analysis

Nursing Diagnosis

POTENTIAL FOR CARDIOVASCULAR DISEASE: The presence of stressors that increase the possibility of the actual occurrence of disease of the heart and coronary arteries

PLANNING

Unmet Needs

Protection from physical harm, increased learning

Expected Outcome

No signs or symptoms of cardiovascular disease will occur
    OR
If signs and symptoms occur, they will be promptly recognized as an actual problem and will be treated appropriately
Person verbalizes an understanding of and practices preventive methods

NURSING INTERVENTIONS

Nursing Treatments

Encourage moderate physical exercise
Encourage adequate rest
Discourage the intake of oral stimulants (coffee, tea, alcohol)
Discourage smoking
Encourage decreased carbohydrate intake (to maintain normal weight)
Encourage decreased fatty-food intake (to keep cholesterol and triglyceride blood levels low)
Encourage decreased sodium-food intake (to prevent blood pressure elevation)

Nursing Observations

Make a follow-up evaluation (periodically)
Auscultate the apical heartbeat for rate and rhythm (periodically)
Palpate the pulse for rate, rhythm, and volume
Monitor the blood pressure
Monitor blood studies for abnormal cardiac enzymes, abnormal chemistry, abnormal hematology
Monitor the ECG (periodically)
Observe for complaints of pain, weakness, fatigue
Observe for dyspnea
Observe for behavior modification (use of health-directed activities or methods)

Health Teaching

Emphasize the need to recognize fatigue as a stress factor
Emphasize the danger of crash dieting
Emphasize the danger of excessive body weight
Recommend adherence to a pace of living with which one is comfortable
Recommend methods for achieving total relaxation (controlled breathing, doing nothing, etc.)
Inform that a predisposition to the illness exists
Describe those symptoms that should be reported (chest pain, dyspnea, weakness)
Advise periodic examinations for known hereditary predispositions
Explain the importance of learning and practicing health principles
Explain why the potential problem could become actual (research verifies that certain stressors predispose to cardiovascular disease)
Explain the reason for and intended effect of the prevention methods

EVALUATION

Record actual outcome

POTENTIAL FOR CEREBROVASCULAR DISEASE[382]

ASSESSMENT

Data Collection

Subjective Data
• There are no actual symptoms of cerebrovascular disease

Objective Data
• There are no actual signs of cerebrovascular disease

Related Data
• There are one or more stressors present that increase the possibility that cerebrovascular disease will occur:
INHERITED FACTORS: *Familial tendency*: For stroke. *Sex*: Greater in females
DISEASES: Cardiovascular disease, hypertension (with a systolic above 160 mm/Hg and diastolic above 95 mm Hg)
HEALTH CARE FACTORS: *Drug therapy*: Adverse effects of contraceptive drugs
DEVELOPMENTAL FACTORS: Old age (over age 60)
LIFESTYLE: High-cholesterol diet, high saturated-fat diet, cigarette or tobacco smoking
HUMAN ERROR: Smoking

Data Analysis

Nursing Diagnosis
POTENTIAL FOR CEREBROVASCULAR ACCIDENT (POTENTIAL FOR STROKE): The presence of stressors that increase the possibility of the actual occurrence of a diminished blood supply to the brain as a result of the rupture, clotting, or sclerosis of a cerebral vessel

PLANNING

Unmet Needs
Protection from physical harm, increased learning

Expected Outcome
No signs or symptoms of cerebrovascular disease will occur
OR
If signs and symptoms occur, they will be promptly recognized as an actual problem and will be treated appropriately
Person verbalizes an understanding of and practices preventive methods

NURSING INTERVENTIONS

Nursing Treatments
Encourage adequate rest
Encourage moderate physical exercise
Discourage the intake of oral stimulants (coffee, tea, alcohol)
Discourage smoking
Encourage decreased fatty-food intake (to keep cholesterol and triglyceride blood levels low)
Encourage decreased sodium-food intake (to prevent blood pressure elevation)

Nursing Observations
Make a follow-up evaluation (periodically)
Monitor the blood pressure (for elevation)
Observe for complaints of dizziness, headaches, (facial) numbness and tingling, weakness, speech loss
Observe for behavior modification (use of health-directed activities or methods)

Health Teaching
Recommend adherence to a pace of living with which one is comfortable
Recommend methods for achieving total relaxation (controlled breathing, listening to soft music, etc.)

Inform that a predisposition to the illness exists

Describe those symptoms that should be reported (dizziness, recurring headaches, facial numbness, tingling or transient paralysis, intermittent confusion or memory lapses)

Advise periodic examinations for known hereditary predispositions

Explain the importance of learning and practicing health principles

Explain why the potential problem could become actual (research verifies that certain stressors predispose to cerebrovascular disease)

Explain the reason for and intended effect of the preventive methods

EVALUATION

Record actual outcome

POTENTIAL FOR HYPERTENSIVE DISEASE [61,181,225,278,295,491]

ASSESSMENT

Data Collection

Subjective Data
• There are no actual symptoms of hypertension

Objective Data
• There are no actual signs of hypertension

Related Data
• There are one or more stressors present that increase the possibility that hypertension will occur:

INHERITED FACTORS: *Familial tendency*: For hypertension. *Sex*: Greater in males than in females. *Race*: Black or white

DISEASES: Obesity, renal disease

DEVELOPMENTAL FACTORS: *Age*: Increases with age

LIFESTYLE: High alcohol intake, high-salt high-fat intake, cigarette or tobacco smoking, lack of exercise

Data Analysis

Nursing Diagnosis
POTENTIAL FOR HYPERTENSIVE DISEASE: The presence of stressors that increases the possibility of the actual occurrence of an abnormally high blood pressure level

PLANNING

Unmet Needs

Protection from physical harm, increased learning

Expected Outcome

No signs or symptoms of hypertensive disease will occur
    OR
If signs and symptoms occur, they will be promptly recognized as an actual problem and will be treated appropriately

Person verbalizes an understanding of and practices preventive methods

NURSING INTERVENTIONS

Nursing Treatments

Encourage physical exercise

Encourage adequate rest

Discourage the intake of oral stimulants (coffee, tea, alcohol)

Discourage smoking

Encourage decreased carbohydrate intake (to maintain normal weight)

Encourage decreased fatty-food intake (to keep cholesterol and triglyceride blood levels low)

Encourage decreased sodium-food intake (to prevent blood pressure elevation)

Nursing Observations

Monitor the blood pressure (for diastolic above 90 mm Hg)

Inspect the eyes for papilledema

Measure the body weight (for gain)

Observe for complaints of dizziness, headache, tinnitus, fatigue

Observe for behavior modification (use of health-directed activities or methods)

Health Teaching

Recommend a regular sleeping schedule

Advise that highly emotional situations be avoided

Explain that fatigue should be recognized as a stress factor

Emphasize the danger of excessive body weight

Advise that highly emotional situations be avoided

Recommend adherence to a pace of living with which one is comfortable

Recommend methods for achieving total relaxation (controlled breathing, doing nothing, etc.)

Inform that a predisposition to the illness exists

Describe those symptoms that should be reported (persistent headaches, dizziness, pounding heartbeat)

Advise periodic examinations for known hereditary predispositions

Explain the importance of learning and practicing health principles

Explain why the potential problem could become actual (research verifies that certain stressors predispose to hypertensive disease)

Explain the reason for and intended effects of the preventive methods

EVALUATION

Record actual outcome

At-Risk Factors for Dental Disease

POTENTIAL FOR DENTAL DISEASE[43,106]

ASSESSMENT

Data Collection

Subjective Data

• There are no actual symptoms of dental disease

Objective Data
• There are no actual signs of dental disease

Related Data
• There are one or more stressors present that increase the possibility that dental disease will occur:
SIGNS AND SYMPTOMS: Plaque accumulations
HUMAN BODY: *Anatomical abnormalities*: Abnormal formation of the mouth or teeth
HEALTH CARE FACTORS: *Medical therapy*: Radiation therapy. *Drug therapy*: Hydantoin (Dilantin) therapy
DEVELOPMENTAL PHASES: Infancy, toddler, preschooler, old age
LIFESTYLE: An insufficient or unbalanced diet, high-sugar diet, lack of dental hygiene, infrequent brushing, flossing, or use of a water jet
HUMAN ERROR: Disregarding dental prophylaxis, bottle-feeding an infant with milk or juice at the infant's bedtime

Data Analysis

Nursing Diagnosis
POTENTIAL FOR DENTAL DISEASE: The presence of stressors that increase the possibility of the actual occurrence of disease of the teeth or gums

PLANNING

Unmet Needs
Protection from physical harm, increased learning

Expected Outcome
No signs or symptoms of dental disease will occur
    OR
If signs and symptoms occur, they will be promptly recognized as an actual problem and will be treated appropriately
Person verbalizes an understanding of and practices preventive methods

NURSING INTERVENTIONS

Nursing Treatments
Encourage decreased carbohydrate intake (especially sucrose-containing products)

Nursing Observations
Inspect the teeth for abnormalities
Observe for complaints of (tooth) pain
Observe for behavior modification (use of health-directed activities or methods)

Health Teaching
Advise frequent and early dental attention
Advise against eating sweets
Advise that between-meal snacks be avoided
Recommend the use of a fluoride toothpaste
Advise early and consistent use of the toothbrush
Teach how to brush and floss the teeth correctly (including gum massage)
Instruct that only water, not milk or juice, be given in the infant's bottle at bedtime
Describe those symptoms that should be reported (tooth sensitivity or pain, bleeding gums, persistent bad breath)
Explain the importance of learning and practicing health principles
Explain why the potential problem could become actual (research verifies that certain stressors predispose to dental disease)
Explain the reason for and intended effects of the preventive methods

EVALUATION

Record actual outcome

At-Risk Factors for Endocrine Disease

POTENTIAL FOR DIABETES MELLITUS[73,137,202,399,458]

ASSESSMENT

Data Collection

Subjective Data
• There are no actual symptoms of diabetes mellitus

Objective Data
• There are no actual signs of diabetes mellitus

Related Data
• There are one or more stressors present that increase the possibility that diabetes mellitus will occur:

INHERITED FACTORS: *Familial tendency*: For diabetes. *Sex*: Both males and females
DISEASES: Acromegaly, Cushing's syndrome, obesity
PSYCHOSOCIAL FACTORS: The threat of severe or chronic stress (raises the blood glucose)
HUMAN BODY: *Body states*: Pregnancy
HEALTH CARE FACTORS: *Drug therapy*: Adverse effects of corticosteroids, phenytoin, thiazide diuretics, oral contraceptives. *History of*: A woman who has had multiple pregnancies, has delivered children weighing 10 lb or more, or who has had a myocardial infarction before the menopause; a man who has had a myocardial infarction before age 40
DEVELOPMENTAL PHASES: *Age*: Increased incidence with age, especially ages 45–70
LIFESTYLE: Chronic high-carbohydrate intake

Data Analysis

Nursing Diagnosis
POTENTIAL FOR DIABETES MELLITUS: The presence of stressors that increase the possibility of the actual occurrence of a disturbance in carbohydrate, protein, and fat metabolism resulting from a deficiency of or nonutilization of insulin

PLANNING

Unmet Needs
Protection from physical harm, increased learning

Expected Outcome
No signs or symptoms of diabetes mellitus will occur
    OR
If signs and symptoms occur, they will be promptly recognized as an actual problem and will be treated appropriately
Person verbalizes an understanding of and practices preventive methods

NURSING INTERVENTIONS

Nursing Treatments
Encourage decreased calorie intake
Encourage decreased carbohydrate intake (to maintain normal weight)
Encourage moderate physical exercise (as a regularly scheduled program)

Nursing Observations
Measure the body weight (for excessive gain or loss)
Monitor the blood pressure
Monitor blood studies for abnormal carbohydrate metabolism (elevated glucose, glucose tolerance, fatty acids, acetone)
Test the urine for sugar and acetone

Observe the breath for abnormal odor (sweet breath)
Observe for complaints of thirst, weakness, malaise, nocturia
Observe for behavior modification (use of health-directed activities or methods)
Make a follow-up evaluation

Health Teaching
Inform that a predisposition to the illness exists
Advise periodic examinations for known hereditary predispositions
Describe those symptoms that should be reported (slow healing wounds, increased appetite with weight loss, increased urine output)
Emphasize the danger of excessive body weight
Teach how to test the urine for sugar acetone
Explain the importance of learning and practicing health principles
Explain why the potential problem could become actual (research verifies that certain stressors predispose to diabetes mellitus)
Explain the reason for and intended effects of the preventive methods

EVALUATION
Record actual outcome

POTENTIAL FOR NONTOXIC GOITER[42,399]

ASSESSMENT
Data Collection

Subjective Data
• There are no actual symptoms of nontoxic goiter

Objective Data
• There are no actual signs of nontoxic goiter

Related Data
• There are one or more stressors present that increase the possibility that nontoxic goiter will occur:
INHERITED FACTORS: *Sex*: Greater in females than in males
HUMAN BODY: *Body states*: Pregnancy, menopause
DEVELOPMENTAL FACTORS: Puberty (age 10–14 years)
LIFESTYLE: Insufficient iodine intake
ENVIRONMENTAL FACTORS: *Geographic location*: Midwest, northwest, Great Lakes region.

Data Analysis

Nursing Diagnosis
POTENTIAL FOR NONTOXIC GOITER (POTENTIAL FOR SIMPLE GOITER): The presence of stressors that increase the possibility of the actual occurrence of an enlarged thyroid gland resulting from insufficient production of thyroid hormone

PLANNING
Unmet Needs
Protection from physical harm, increased learning

Expected Outcome
No signs or symptoms of nontoxic goiter will occur
    OR

If signs and symptoms occur, they will be promptly recognized as an actual problem and will be treated appropriately

Person verbalizes an understanding of and practices preventive methods

NURSING INTERVENTIONS

Nursing Treatments
Encourage increased high-iodine food intake
Give iodized salt (at mealtimes)

Nursing Observations
Make a follow-up evaluation
Monitor blood studies for abnormal thyroid function (decreased)
Palpate the thyroid gland for enlargement
Inspect the chest for respiratory rate and rhythm (wheezing)
Inspect the throat for an impaired swallowing reflex
Observe for behavior modification (use of health-directed activities or methods)

Health Teaching
Teach how to adjust the diet (to include high-iodine foods)
Recommend the use of iodized salt
Inform that a predisposition to the illness exists
Describe those symptoms that should be reported (wheezing, difficulty swallowing)
Explain the importance of learning and practicing health principles
Explain why the potential problem could become actual (research verifies that certain stressors predispose to nontoxic goiter)
Explain the reason for and intended effects of the preventive methods

EVALUATION
Record actual outcome

At-Risk Factors for Gastrointestinal Disease

POTENTIAL FOR COLORECTAL CANCER[295,474]

ASSESSMENT

Data Collection

Subjective Data
• There are no actual symptoms of colorectal cancer

Objective Data
• There are no actual signs of colorectal cancer

Related Data
• There are one or more stressors present that increase the possibility that colorectal cancer will occur:

INHERITED FACTORS: *Familial tendency*: For adenomatous polyposis
DISEASES: Ulcerative colitis
DEVELOPMENTAL PHASE: Middle age (over age 40)
LIFESTYLE: High-fat (animal) diet, low-fiber diet

Data Analysis

Nursing Diagnosis

POTENTIAL FOR COLORECTAL CANCER: The presence of stressors that increase the possibility of the actual occurrence of carcinogenic lesions of the colon and rectal areas

PLANNING

Unmet Needs

Protection from physical harm, increased learning

Expected Outcome

No signs or symptoms of colorectal cancer will occur
  OR
If signs and symptoms occur, they will be promptly recognized as an acutal problem and will be treated appropriately
Person verbalizes an understanding of and practices preventive methods

NURSING INTERVENTIONS

Nursing Treatments

Encourage increased residue-food intake (high-fiber diet)
Encourage decreased carbohydrate- and fatty-food intake

Nursing Observations

Make a follow-up evaluation
Observe for complaints of constipation, abdominal or rectal pain
Observe for diarrhea
Test the stool for occult blood by Hemoccult
Observe for behavior modification (use of health-directed activities and methods)

Health Teaching

Inform that a predisposition to the illness exists
Describe those symptoms which should be reported (persistent elimination irregularity, abdominal or rectal pain, bloody stools or rectal bleeding)
Explain the importance of learning and practicing health principles
Explain why the potential problem could become actual (research verifies that certain stressors predispose to colorectal cancer)
Explain the reason for and intended effects of the preventive methods

EVALUATION

Record actual outcome

POTENTIAL FOR GASTRIC OR DUODENAL ULCER[42,165]

ASSESSMENT

Data Collection

Subjective Data

• There are no actual symptoms of gastric or duodenal ulcer

Objective Data
• There are no actual signs of gastric or duodenal ulcer

Related Data
• There are one or more stressors present that increase the possibility that gastric or duodenal ulcer will occur:

INHERITED FACTORS: *Familial tendency*: For ulcers. *Sex*: More common in men; blood type A is especially susceptible to gastric ulcers

HEALTH CARE FACTORS: *Drug therapy*: Adverse effects of aspirin and drugs containing aspirin

DEVELOPMENTAL PHASE: *Age*: 45–55-year-old group

PSYCHOSOCIAL FACTORS: The threat of severe or chronic stress is especially predisposing to duodenal ulcers

LIFESTYLE: Cigarette smoking, high alcohol intake, spicy food intake

Data Analysis

Nursing Diagnosis
POTENTIAL FOR GASTRIC OR DUODENAL ULCER: The presence of stressors that increase the possibility of the actual occurrence of mucosal ulceration of the stomach or duodenum

PLANNING

Unmet Needs
Protection from physical harm, increased learning

Expected Outcome
No signs or symptoms of gastric or duodenal ulcer will occur
OR
If signs and symptoms occur, they will be promptly recognized as an actual problem and will be treated appropriately
Person verbalizes an understanding of and practices preventive methods

NURSING INTERVENTIONS

Nursing Treatments
Provide a balanced nutritional diet (but avoid hot spicy food)
Discourage the intake of oral stimulants (caffeine, alcohol, cigarette smoking)
Withhold all drugs (containing aspirin)
OR
Give enteric-coated aspirin

Nursing Observations
Observe for complaints of (epigastric or abdominal) pain, nausea, anorexia
Palpate the abdomen for tenderness
Observe for behavior modification (use of health-directed activities or methods)

Health Teaching
Make a follow-up evaluation
Teach how to adjust the diet (by reducing irritating foods and fluids)
Advise that between-meal snacks be avoided (to limit gastric acid stimulation to three times daily, at mealtimes)
Inform that a predisposition to the illness exists
Describe those symptoms that should be reported (abdominal or epigastric pain, nausea, vomiting, tarry stools)
Explain the importance of learning and practicing health principles
Explain why the potential problem could become actual (research verifies that certain stressors predispose to gastric and duodenal ulcers)
Explain the reason for and intended effects of the preventive methods

EVALUATION
Record actual outcome

At-Risk Factors for Genitourinary Disease

POTENTIAL FOR RENAL CALCULI[73,451,522,637]

ASSESSMENT

Data Collection

Subjective Data
• There are no actual symptoms of renal calculi

Objective Data
• There are no actual signs of renal calculi

Related Data
• There are one or more stressors present that increase the possibility that renal calculi will occur:

INHERITED FACTORS: *Familial tendency*: For renal calculi
DISEASES: Gout, hyperparathyroidism, urinary tract infection
SIGNS AND SYMPTOMS: Dehydration, prolonged immobility as with paralysis, urine retention
LIFESTYLE: High-calcium intake
HUMAN ERROR: Insufficient fluid intake, insufficient acid-ash food intake

Data Analysis

Nursing Diagnosis
POTENTIAL FOR RENAL CALCULI: The presence of stressors that increase the possibility of the actual occurrence of the formation of kidney or bladder stones

PLANNING

Unmet Needs
Protection from physical harm, increased learning

Expected Outcome
No signs or symptoms of renal calculi will occur
   OR
If signs and symptoms occur, they will be promptly recognized as an actual problem and will be treated appropriately
Person verbalizes an understanding of and practices preventive methods

NURSING INTERVENTIONS

Nursing Treatments
Ambulate the person (as much as possible)
Change the person's position frequently
Increase fluid intake to about 3,000 cc daily

For Potential Calcium Calculi
Encourage decreased calcium-food and fluid intake (no milk or milk products, dark leafy green vegetables, clams, oysters, yogurt)
Give urine-acidifying juices orally (apple, cranberry, plum, prune juice)
Refrain from giving bicarbonates, from giving milk or milk products, from giving carbonated beverages

For Potential Cystine or Uric Acid Calculi
Encourage decreased purine-food intake (no liver, kidney, poultry, fish, fried foods,

spinach, mushrooms, asparagus, peas, lentils, pastries, alcohol)
Encourage decreased calorie intake, decreased fatty-food intake
Give carbonated beverages
Give urine-alkalinizing juices orally (orange juice)

Nursing Observations
Test the urine for pH (high urine alkalinity favors calcium calculi formation, while acidity favors cystine and uric acid calculi formation)
Observe for complaints of dysuria, of flank pain
Test the urine by Dipstik (for hematuria)
Observe for behavior modification (use of health-directed activities or methods)

Health Teaching
Instruct to increase fluid intake (to at least eight 8-ounce glasses of fluid daily)
Explain how to keep urine within the desired pH range (with urine-acidifying and urine-alkalinizing juices and foods)
Recommend that alkalis be used conservatively (for potential calcium calculi)
Emphasize the need to avoid certain drugs (probenecid, which increases uric acid in the urine)
Describe those symptoms that should be reported (dysuria, flank pain, hematuria)
Explain the importance of learning and practicing health principles
Explain why the potential problem could become actual (an increase in parathyroid activity predisposes to increased excretion of calcium and phosphorous particles into the urine, immobility or reduced fluid intake prevents small particles from being flushed out of the kidney, where they continue to enlarge)
Explain the reason for and intended effects of the preventive methods

EVALUATION
Record actual outcome

At-Risk Factors For Hematologic Disease

POTENTIAL FOR IRON-DEFICIENCY ANEMIA[42,399]

ASSESSMENT

Data Collection

Subjective Data
• There are no actual symptoms of iron-deficiency anemia

Objective Data
• There are no actual signs of iron-deficiency anemia

Related Data
• There are one or more stressors present that increase the possibility that iron-deficiency anemia will occur:

BIRTH DEFECTS: Congenital heart disease
BIRTH STATUS: Low-birth-weight infants, multiple-birth infants, premature infant
INHERITED FACTORS: *Sex*: Females
DISEASES: Celiac disease (Sprue), chronic infection, hemorrhage, parasitic infestation
SIGNS AND SYMPTOMS: Bleeding, chronic diarrhea
HUMAN BODY: *Body states*: Pregnancy. *Natural body function*: Prolonged breast-feeding of infant, lactation
HEALTH CARE FACTORS: *Drug therapy*: Anticoagulant therapy, aspirin (high doses), corticosteroids
DEVELOPMENTAL PHASE: *Age*: More prevelant in children 6–24 months of age and in adolescents
LIFESTYLE: Insufficient or unbalanced diet, prolonged bottle-feeding of an infant with homogenized milk instead of milk and food

Data Analysis

Nursing Diagnosis
POTENTIAL FOR IRON-DEFICIENCY ANEMIA: The presence of stressors that increase the possibility of the actual occurrence of insufficient stores of body iron and decreased hemoglobin concentration

PLANNING

Unmet Needs
Protection from physical harm, increased learning

Expected Outcome
No signs or symptoms of iron-deficiency anemia will occur
> OR

If signs and symptoms occur, they will be promptly recognized as an actual problem and will be treated appropriately

NURSING INTERVENTIONS

Nursing Treatments
Provide a balanced nutritional diet
Encourage increased iron-food intake (lean meat, leafy green vegetables, enriched breads and cereals, dark molasses)

Nursing Observations
Make a follow-up evaluation
Monitor blood studies for abnormal hematology
Inspect the skin (and the inner, lower eyelids) for pallor
Observe for complaints of fatigue, weakness
Observe for behavior modification (use of health-directed activities and methods)

Health Teaching
Teach how to adjust the diet (to use iron-enriched products such as infant formula, cereals, breads, etc., to avoid drinking tea and calcium products that decrease the absorption of iron, to eat an orange or drink orange juice with iron-rich foods, since iron absorption is increased in an acid medium)
Inform that a predisposition to the illness exists
Describe those symptoms which should be reported (fatigue, pallor, listlessness)
Explain the importance of learning and practicing health principles
Explain why the potential problem could become actual (research verifies that certain stressors predispose to iron-deficiency anemia)
Explain the reason for and intended effects of the preventive methods

EVALUATION

Record actual outcome

At-Risk Factors for Immunologic Disease

POTENTIAL FOR ALLERGIC REACTION[386,401,475,487,639]

ASSESSMENT

Data Collection

Subjective Data
• There are no actual symptoms of an allergic reaction

Objective Data
• There are no actual signs of an allergic reaction

Related Data
• There are one or more stressors present that increase the possibility that an allergic reaction will occur:

INHERITED FACTORS: *Familial tendency*: For allergies

HEALTH CARE FACTORS: *History*: Person has a history of having had a skin rash as an infant before age 6 months, followed by colic episodes, then eczema from food, then nasal allergy

LIFESTYLE: High-protein intake (during pregnancy increases an infant's allergy potential)

ENVIRONMENTAL FACTORS: Dust, wind. *Pollen*: Ragweed, grass. *Chemical substances*: Pollution. *Biologic agents*: Dander from animals

HUMAN ERROR: The introduction of protein (eggs and meat) into a baby's diet before the age of 6–8 months

Data Analysis

Nursing Diagnosis
POTENTIAL FOR ALLERGIC REACTION: The presence of stressors that increase the possibility of the actual occurrence of an antigen–antibody reaction

PLANNING

Unmet Needs
Protection from physical harm, increased learning

Expected Outcome
No signs or symptoms of an allergic disorder will occur
   OR
If signs and symptoms occur, they will be promptly recognized as an actual problem and will be treated appropriately
Person verbalizes an understanding of and practices preventive methods

NURSING INTERVENTIONS

Nursing Treatments
Obtain a complete present and past history

Nursing Observations
Make a follow-up evaluation
Observe for a hypersensitivity response (for at least 30 minutes after exposure to an allergy-provoking substance)

Health Teaching
Inform that a predisposition to the illness exists
Describe those symptoms that should be reported (*Drug allergy*: Rash or hives, fever, respiratory difficulty, generalized weakness, joint pain. *Food allergy*: Rash, dyspnea, nasal stuffiness, mouth and lip swelling, diarrhea, vomiting, malaise. *Respiratory allergy*: Itching nose or eyes, headache, malaise. *Skin allergy*: Edema, redness, scaling, peeling, burning, stinging, itching)

Instruct to report early symptoms immediately

Explain how to take allergy precautions (avoid perfumes, scented products, swimming under water, dust, long-haired animals, plants, metals, plastics, dyes, wind; include instructions for allergy-proofing the home)

Inform that foods causing allergies fall into specific categories (dairy products, shellfish, fowl, etc.)

Instruct to introduce infants to only one new food each week and note allergic responses

Advise to delay introducing hyperallergenic foods until the child is 1 year old (cow's milk, eggs, wheat, fish, shellfish, chocolate, nuts, strawberries, citrus fruits, pork, chicken)

Explain the importance of learning and practicing health principles

Explain why the potential problem could become actual (research verifies that certain stressors predispose to an allergic reaction)

Explain the reason for and intended effects of the preventive methods

EVALUATION

Record actual outcome

At-Risk Factors For Neurologic Disease

POTENTIAL FOR TETANUS[73,278,522]

ASSESSMENT

Data Collection

Subjective Data
• There are no actual symptoms of tetanus

Objective Data
• There are no actual signs of tetanus

Related Data
• There are one or more stressors present that increase the possibility that tetanus will occur:

INJURY: animal bite, burn wound, contusion, compound bone fracture, incision, laceration, penetrating or puncture wound, any injury that breaks the skin

ENVIRONMENTAL FACTORS: *Dirt*: From roads, streets, or earth or from animal or human feces. *Objects*: A rusty or soiled wound-causing object

HUMAN ERROR: No initial tetanus immunizations or no tetanus booster within the past 5 years

Data Analysis

Nursing Diagnosis
POTENTIAL FOR TETANUS: The presence of stressors that increase the possibility of the actual occurrence of the introduction of clostridium tetani into the body through a wound, burn, or fracture

PLANNING

Unmet Needs

Protection from physical harm, increased learning

Expected Outcome

No signs or symptoms of tetanus will occur

OR

If signs and symptoms occur, they will be promptly recognized as an actual problem and will be treated appropriately

Person verbalizes an understanding of and practices preventive methods

NURSING INTERVENTIONS

Nursing Treatments

Clean with antiseptic solution (Betadine solution)

OR

Clean with hydrogen peroxide

OR

Clean with surgical soap

Give tetanus toxoid (ET) (0.5 ml IM within 24 hours after injury, if the patient has been previously immunized and if no previous immunizations have been given, give the initial dose and a second dose 4–6 weeks later)

Nursing Observations

Observe for a hypersensitivity response

Health Teaching

Advise adherence to the immunization schedule

Explain why the potential problem could become actual (research verifies that certain stressors predispose to tetanus)

Explain the reason for and intended effects of the preventive methods

Medical Treatments Performed by Nurses

Give the prescribed drugs

EVALUATION

Record actual outcome

At-Risk Factors for Nutritional Disease

POTENTIAL FOR MALNUTRITION[72,423,451,522]

ASSESSMENT

Data Collection

Subjective Data

• There are no actual symptoms of nutritional deficiency

Objective Data

• There are no actual signs of nutritional deficiency

Related Data

• There are one or more stressors present that increase the possibility that nutritional deficiency will occur:

BIRTH DEFECTS: Cystic fibrosis (pancreatic)

DISEASES: Alcoholism, carcinoma, celiac disease (sprue), gastritis, malabsorption syndrome, peptic ulcer, ulcerative colitis

SIGNS AND SYMPTOMS: Anorexia, difficulty sucking or swallowing, pain, nausea, vomiting

HEALTH CARE FACTORS: *Medical therapy*: Gastrostomy, jejunostomy, nasogastric feedings. *Surgical procedures*: Gastrectomy, small bowel resection, wiring of a mandible fracture

DEVELOPMENTAL FACTORS: Adolescence, old age (when there is diminished smell and taste sensation)

LIFESTYLE: Insufficient or unbalanced diet
SITUATIONAL FACTORS: Poverty, living alone

Data Analysis

Nursing Diagnosis

POTENTIAL FOR MALNUTRITION: The presence of stressors that increase the possibility of the actual occurrence of a state of nutritional deficiency

PLANNING

Unmet Needs

Protection from physical harm, increased learning

Expected Outcome

No signs or symptoms of malnutrition will occur
   OR
If signs and symptoms occur, they will be promptly recognized as an actual problem and will be treated appropriately
Person verbalizes an understanding of and practices preventive methods

NURSING INTERVENTIONS

Nursing Treatments

Provide a balanced nutritional diet
Encourage increased protein-food intake
Estimate the required daily calories
Give small frequent feedings
Give snacks
Grant special requests (for food)
Provide food selection

Nursing Observations

Make a follow-up evaluation
Measure the body weight (periodically)
Observe and record the food intake
Observe for diet intolerance
Observe for conditions indicating a need for increased nutritional requirements

Health Teaching

Teach the principles of good nutrition
Recommend a regular meal schedule
Explain the importance of learning and practicing health principles
Explain why the potential problem could become actual (research verifies that certain stressors predispose to malnutrition)
Explain the reason for and intended effects of the preventive methods

EVALUATION

Record actual outcome

POTENTIAL FOR OBESITY[42,72,423,451,522]

ASSESSMENT

Data Collection

Subjective Data
• There are no actual symptoms of obesity

Objective Data
• There are no actual signs of obesity

Related Data

• There are one or more stressors present that increase the possibility that obesity will occur:

INHERITED FACTORS: *Familial tendency*: For obesity

DISEASES: Cushing's syndrome, diabetes mellitus, hypothyroidism, major depression

PSYCHOSOCIAL FACTORS: Lack of impulse control, an attempt to attain pleasure, an attempt to relieve stress through eating

DEVELOPMENTAL PHASES: Middle age

LIFESTYLE: Overeating, lack of exercise

ENVIRONMENTAL FACTORS: Availability or abundance of food

HUMAN ERROR: Overfeeding an infant, insisting that a child always eat everything on his plate

Data Analysis

Nursing Diagnosis

POTENTIAL FOR OBESITY: The presence of stressors that increase the possibility of the actual occurrence of a condition of 20–30% or more excess body weight

PLANNING

Unmet Needs

Protection from physical harm, increased learning

Expected Outcome

No signs or symptoms of obesity will occur

OR

If signs and symptoms occur, they will be promptly recognized as an actual problem and will be treated appropriately

Person verbalizes an understanding of and practices preventive methods

NURSING INTERVENTIONS

Nursing Treatments

Provide a balanced nutritional diet

Estimate the required daily calories

Encourage decreased calories and decreased carbohydrate intake

Refrain from giving between-meal feedings

Encourage active diversional activities (as a substitute for eating during periods of stress and boredom)

Encourage moderate physical exercise

Nursing Observations

Make a follow-up evaluation

Measure the body weight (weekly)

Observe and record the food intake

Observe for behavior modification (use of health-directed activities or methods)

Health Teaching

Emphasize the danger of excessive body weight (can cause cardiovascular disease)

Advise against eating sweets

Advise that between-meal snacks be avoided

Recommend eating and drinking in moderation

Teach the principles of good nutrition

Recommend behavior modification for changing one's eating habits (purchase only foods that must be prepared, eat only when sitting down at a set table, keep food out of sight, etc.)

Explain the importance of learning and practicing health principles

Explain why the potential problem could become actual (research verifies that certain stressors predispose to obesity)

Explain the reason for and intended effects of the preventive methods

EVALUATION

Record actual outcome

At-Risk Factors for Psychologic Disorders

POTENTIAL FOR CHILD ABUSE[259,438,471]

ASSESSMENT

Data Collection

Subjective Data
• There are no actual symptoms of child abuse

Objective Data
• There are no actual signs of child abuse

Related Data
• There are one or more stressors present that increase the possibility that child abuse
   will occur:
PSYCHOSOCIAL FACTORS: The highly dependent personality of a parent, exposure as a child
   to an abusive or violent role model, use of ineffective defense mechanisms such as
   projecting anger onto the child
SITUATIONAL FACTORS: Situational crisis or stress

Data Analysis

Nursing Diagnosis
POTENTIAL FOR CHILD ABUSE: The presence of stressors that increase the possibility of the actual occurrence of an adult physically or emotionally injuring a child

PLANNING

Unmet Needs
Protection from physical harm, increased learning

Expected Outcome
No signs or symptoms of child abuse will occur
   OR
If signs and symptoms occur, they will be promptly recognized as an actual problem and
   will be treated appropriately
Person verbalizes an understanding of and practices positive parenting

NURSING INTERVENTIONS

Nursing Treatments
Approach unhurriedly
Provide an atmosphere of acceptance
Reassure verbally (that the nurse will be available whenever needed)
Encourage the expression of feelings (about having been abused when a child)
Listen attentively
   AND
Talk with the person
Offer feedback to the person's expressed feelings
Support a realistic assessment of the situation (that a child cannot meet all an adult's
   emotional needs, that a child cannot behave as an adult)
Explore with the person his strengths and resources (to control abusive impulses)
Provide meetings with supportive persons or groups
Set an example by role modeling (when nursing children)
Make a referral (to a psychiatric nurse specialist if needed)

Nursing Observations
Determine the degree of insight that the person has (into the potential for abuse)
Identify disturbing conversation topics (which reveal negative attitudes toward children
   or unreal expectations of children)

Observe for an excessive stress level (when the parent is with the child)
Observe for impaired self-attitudes (of the potential abuser)

Health Teaching

Explain the causes of the problem (poor role modeling by one's own parents)
Teach positive parenting behavior (how to rear a child with love and discipline)
Describe those symptoms that should be reported (uncontrollable anger directed at a child, feeling that a child does not meet one's expectations)
Explain the importance of persons offering emotional support to one another (when rearing children)
Explain the importance of maintaining a positive self-attitude (about one's parenting ability)
Explain how to channel emotional energy and obtain release from stress (running, bicycling, creative activities, crying, laughing, talking things over instead of using abusive behavior)
Explain the importance of learning and practicing (mental) health principles
Explain why the potential problem could become actual (research verifies that certain stressors predispose to child abuse)
Explain the reason for and intended effects of the preventive methods

EVALUATION

Record actual outcome

POTENTIAL FOR DEPRESSION[85,130,225,471]

ASSESSMENT

Data Collection

Subjective Data
• There are no actual symptoms of depression

Objective Data
• There are no actual signs of depression

Related Data
• There are one or more stressors present that increase the possibility that depression will occur:
BIRTH DEFECTS: Giving birth to an imperfect infant
DISEASES: Any
INJURIES: Any
SIGNS AND SYMPTOMS: Pain, paralysis, weakness
PSYCHOSOCIAL FACTORS: Any loss, lack of emotional support (positive reinforcement) from others, the exhaustion of adaptive reserves
PSYCHOSOCIAL FACTORS: The threat of change
HUMAN BODY: *Body appearance*: Change in body appearance, disfigured body. *Body function*: Loss of body function. *Natural body function*: Maternal energy depletion after childbirth. *Body states*: Menopause, male climacteric
HEALTH CARE FACTORS: *Hospitalization*: Of self or a significant other. *Medical diagnosis*: An unfavorable diagnosis. *Health therapy*: Unsuccessful or ineffective medical, drug, or surgical therapy. *Drug therapy*: Adverse effects of antihypertensive drugs, barbiturates, narcotics, sedatives, tranquilizers
DEVELOPMENTAL PHASES: Adolescence, old age
LIFESTYLE: An insufficient or unbalanced diet, alcohol or drug abuse, lack of exercise
SITUATIONAL FACTORS: Confinement in prison, death or impending death of a significant other, divorce, loss of employment, chronic illness, poverty, retirement, marital separation

Data Analysis

Nursing Diagnosis

POTENTIAL FOR DEPRESSION: The presence of stressors that increase the possibility of the actual occurrence of a mental state of gloom, sadness, and hopelessness

PLANNING

Unmet Needs

Protection from physical harm, increased learning

Expected Outcome

No signs or symptoms of depression will occur
  OR
If signs and symptoms occur, they will be promptly recognized as an actual problem and will be treated appropriately
Person verbalizes an understanding of and practices preventive methods, practices mental health principles

NURSING INTERVENTIONS

Nursing Treatments

Approach unhurriedly
Provide an atmosphere of acceptance
Encourage the expression of feelings
Listen attentively
  AND
Talk with the person
Offer feedback to the person's expressed feelings
Encourage gradual mastery of a situation
Encourage planned one-day-at-a-time living (especially during severe stress)
Reduce the demands placed on the patient
Refrain from performing nonessential procedures
Introduce one anxiety producing situation at a time
Introduce to persons who have successfully undergone the same experience
Encourage the identification of specific life values
Encourage the practical application of the accepted value system
Support a realistic assessment of the situation
Encourage laughter
Encourage meaningful activity
Encourage new goals at past goal achievement
Support the use of appropriate defense mechanisms
Avoid forcing the person into rapid adaptation to change by accepting the person's pattern of adjustment
Encourage the acceptance of self-limitations
Encourage adequate rest (needed for coping)
Make a referral (to a psychiatric nurse specialist if needed)

Nursing Observations

Determine the degree of insight that the person has (into potential depression)
Evaluate the significance of emotional distress mannerisms, of nonverbal communication
Identify disturbing conversation topics
Identify the appropriate use of defense mechanisms, the inappropriate use of defense mechanisms
Observe for an excessive stress level
Observe for impaired self-attitudes
Observe for evidence that the person is reaching out for emotional support
Observe for evidence of a favorable response to therapy

Health Teaching

Advise early correction of problems

Advise occasional respite from responsibility

Advise that negative responses from others be regarded with minimum significance (even though there are feelings about such responses)

Advise that significant persons express acceptance of one another, that significant persons express caring for one another

Explain the importance of persons offering emotional support to one another

Emphasize the need for realistic expectation of others

Explain the importance of recognizing tension within oneself

Explain that fatigue should be recognized as a stress factor

Explain the need to recognize highly stressful situations

Explain that some tension is normal

Explain how to channel emotional energy and obtain release from stress (running, swimming, bicycling, creative activities, crying, laughing, talking things over)

Teach how to use the problem-solving method (to reduce situational tension)

Explain the importance of maintaining a positive self-attitude

Explain the importance of learning and practicing health principles

Explain why the potential problem could become actual (research verifies that certain stressors predispose to depression)

Explain the reason for and intended effects of the preventive methods

EVALUATION

Record actual outcome

POTENTIAL FOR SUBSTANCE (ALCOHOL OR DRUG) ABUSE[17,19,35,93,445,471]

ASSESSMENT

Data Collection

Subjective Data
• There are no actual symptoms of substance abuse

Objective Data
• There are no actual signs of substance abuse

Related Data
• There are one or more stressors present that increase the possibility that substance abuse will occur:

DISEASES: Major depression, obesity

SIGNS AND SYMPTOMS: Chronic pain, constipation, headaches

PSYCHOSOCIAL FACTORS: Lack of competency in coping with everyday problems, the threat of repeated failure to achieve, an attempt to obtain pleasure, the threat of chronic or severe stress, the threat of peer pressure, a highly dependent personality, exposure to a substance-abuser role model

HEALTH CARE FACTORS: *Drug therapy*: Prolonged drug therapy (narcotics, sedatives, tranquilizers)

LIFESTYLE: High alcohol intake

SITUATIONAL FACTORS: Chronic illness

ENVIRONMENTAL FACTORS: *Chemical substances*: The availability of alcohol and drugs

HUMAN ERROR: Self-treatment with over-the-counter (OTC) drugs

Data Analysis

Nursing Diagnosis

POTENTIAL FOR SUBSTANCE (ALCOHOL OR DRUG) ABUSE: The presence of stressors that increase the possibility of the actual occurrence of the misuse of drugs or alcohol

PLANNING

Unmet Needs

Protection from physical harm, increased learning

Expected Outcome

No signs or symptoms of alcohol or drug abuse
  OR
If signs and symptoms occur, they will be promptly recognized as an actual problem and will be treated appropriately
Person verbalizes an understanding of and practices preventive methods, practices mental health principles

NURSING INTERVENTIONS

Nursing Treatments

Approach unhurriedly
Provide an atmosphere of acceptance
Reassure verbally (that the nurse will be available whenever needed)
Encourage the expression of feelings
Listen attentively
  AND
Talk with the person
Offer feedback to the person's expressed feelings
Give drugs judiciously for emotional repression
Explore with the person his strengths and resources (to overcome problems in constructive ways)
Provide meetings with supportive persons or groups
Make a referral (to a psychiatric nurse specialist if needed)

Nursing Observations

Determine the degree of insight that the person has (into potential substance abuse)
Observe for an excessive stress level (which could lead to substance abuse)
Observe for impaired self-attitudes

Health Teaching

Explain that drug abuse is an illness
Explain that drug use is not socially essential (for acceptance by peers)
Explain that it is essential to foster healthy drinking attitudes (moderation and positive attitudes toward alcohol consumption)
Explain that the use of drugs to solve problems is dangerous (it fails to solve problems and creates new ones)
Explain to families the importance of role modeling through abstinence from drug use
Explain the importance of staying well informed about drug abuse (well-informed parents can answer childrens' questions more accurately, being informed effects positive decision making)
Explain why persons resort to drug abuse (to obtain group acceptance, to cope with emotional problems, to hurt significant others, for experimental purposes)
Recommend that self-medication be avoided
Recommend new options for effective methods of coping (such as the problem-solving approach)
Describe those symptoms that should be reported (the use of alcohol or drugs for anxiety, pain, or problem relief)
Explain the importance of persons offering emotional support to one another (when resisting peer pressure or impulses to abuse substances)

Explain the importance of maintaining a positive self-attitude (which offsets the need for substance abuse)

Explain how to channel emotional energy and obtain release from stress (running, engaging in creative activities, laughing, talking things over) as opposed to substance-abuse behavior

Explain the importance of learning and practicing (mental) health principles

Explain why the potential problem could become actual (research verifies that certain stressors predispose to substance abuse)

Explain the reason for and intended effects of the preventive methods

EVALUATION

Record actual outcome

POTENTIAL FOR SUBSTANCE (ALCOHOL OR DRUG) DEPENDENCE[17,19,445,471]

ASSESSMENT
Data Collection

Subjective Data
• There are no actual symptoms of substance dependence

Objective Data
• There are no actual signs of substance dependence

Related Data
• There are one or more stressors present that increase the possibility that substance dependence will occur:

BIRTH DEFECTS: *Child*: The effects of maternal drug addiction on a child

DISEASES: Major depression

SIGNS AND SYMPTOMS: Chronic pain

PSYCHOSOCIAL FACTORS: Lack of competency in coping with everyday problems, the threat of repeated failure to achieve, an attempt to obtain pleasure, the threat of chronic or severe stress, the threat of peer pressure, a highly dependent personality, exposure to a substance-abuser role model

HEALTH CARE FACTORS: *Drug therapy*: Prolonged drug therapy (narcotics, sedatives, tranquilizers, etc.)

LIFESTYLE: Alcohol or drug abuse

SITUATIONAL FACTORS: Chronic illness

ENVIRONMENTAL FACTORS: *Chemical substances*: The availability of alcohol and drugs

Data Analysis

Nursing Diagnosis
POTENTIAL FOR SUBSTANCE (ALCOHOL OR DRUG) DEPENDENCE: The presence of stressors that increase the possibility of the actual occurrence of an inability to function without the use of alcohol or drugs

PLANNING
Unmet Needs
Protection from physical harm, increased learning

Expected Outcome
No signs or symptoms of substance dependence will occur
    OR
If signs and symptoms occur, they will be promptly recognized as an actual problem and will be treated appropriately

Person verbalizes an understanding of and practices preventive methods and practices mental health principles

NURSING INTERVENTIONS

Nursing Treatments

Approach unhurriedly

Provide an atmosphere of acceptance

Encourage the expression of feelings (about dependency needs)

Listen attentively

    AND

Talk with the person

Offer feedback to the person's expressed feelings

Accept and attempt to relieve unexplainable body complaints (with methods other than drugs)

Give drugs judiciously for emotional repression

Give nonprescription drugs (that do not support dependence)

Explore with the person his strengths and resources (to overcome problems in constructive ways)

Provide meetings with supportive persons or groups

Make a referral (to a psychiatric nurse specialist, if needed)

Nursing Observations

Determine the degree of insight that the person has (into potential substance dependence)

Observe for requests for increased drug dosage

Observe the newborn for signs of drug withdrawal (which could result in a lifetime of dependence)

Observe for an excessive stress level (which could lead to substance dependence)

Observe for impaired self-attitudes

Health Teaching

Explain that drug dependence is an illness

Explain that drug use is not socially essential (for acceptance by peers)

Explain that it is essential to foster healthy drinking attitudes (moderation and positive attitudes toward alcohol consumption)

Explain that long-term drug abuse reduces the pleasures derived from drug abuse

Explain that the use of drugs to solve problems is dangerous (it fails to solve problems and creates new ones)

Explain to families the importance of role modeling through abstinence from drug use

Explain why persons resort to drug abuse (to obtain group acceptance, to cope with emotional problems, to hurt significant others, for experimental purposes)

Recommend that self-medication be avoided

Recommend new options for effective methods of coping (such as the problem-solving approach)

Describe those symptoms that should be reported (gradually increasing the amount and/or frequency of drug or alcohol intake; complaints of illness-related pain long after pain normally should have subsided)

Explain the importance of persons offering emotional support to one another (when resisting peer pressure or impulses toward substance dependence)

Explain the importance of maintaining a positive self-attitude (which offsets the need for substance dependence)

Explain how to channel emotional energy and obtain release from stress (running, creative activities, laughing, talking things over)

Explain the importance of learning and practicing (mental) health principles

Explain why the potential problem could become actual (drugs or alcohol use is known to result in gradual dependence)

Explain the reason for and intended effect of the preventive methods

EVALUATION

Record actual outcome

POTENTIAL FOR SUICIDE[42,471]

ASSESSMENT

Data Collection

Subjective Data
• There are no actual symptoms of suicidal thoughts

Objective Data
• There are no actual signs of suicidal behavior

Related Data
• There are one or more stressors present that increase the possibility that a suicide attempt will occur:

DISEASES: Alcoholism, cancer, major depression, manic–depressive psychosis, schizophrenia

SIGNS OR SYMPTOMS: Chronic pain

PSYCHOSOCIAL FACTORS: Lack of emotional support from others, lack of impulse control, threat of chronic or severe stress, exposure to a role model who practiced poor coping skills, lack of hope for the present or future

HEALTH CARE FACTORS: *Previous history*: Suicide in the family. *Drug therapy*: Prescribed or over-the-counter (OTC) drugs. *Medical therapy*: Chronic hemodialysis

SITUATIONAL FACTORS: History of attempted suicides, intolerable situation(s), marital separation, divorce

ENVIRONMENTAL FACTORS: *Chemical substances*: The availability of chemicals. *Objects*: The availability of sharp or soft objects such as glass, ropes, sheets, plastic bags, extension cords. *Weapons*: Guns, knives, razors. *Windows*: High, unscreened windows

Data Analysis

Nursing Diagnosis
POTENTIAL FOR SUICIDE: The presence of stressors that increase the possibility of the actual occurrence of a person ending or attempting to end his life

PLANNING

Unmet Needs

Protection from physical harm, increased learning

Expected Outcome

No suicide attempts will occur

Person verbalizes an understanding of and practices preventive methods and practices mental health principles

NURSING INTERVENTIONS

Nursing Treatments

Approach unhurriedly

Provide an atmosphere of acceptance

Reassure verbally that the nurse will not allow the person to harm himself and will help him control impulses

Encourage the expression of feelings (such as anger, grief)

Listen attentively
    AND
Talk with the person

Offer feedback to the person's expressed feelings

Support a realistic assessment of the situation

Encourage both long-term and short-term goals (that convey a sense of hope)

Explore with the person his strengths and resources (to overcome problems)

Provide meetings with supportive persons or groups

Arrange geographic placement (so the person can be seen by the nurses)

Remove harmful objects from the environment (sharp objects, matches)

Consult with the physician (about giving drugs in blister packages, which are difficult to open, and about limiting the number of pills prescribed)

Make a referral (to a psychiatric nurse specialist if needed)

Nursing Observations

Determine the degree of insight that the person has (into the problem)

Identify disturbing conversation topics (that indicate thoughts of suicide)

Evaluate the significance of nonverbal communication (giving things away, making a will or funeral arrangements, withdrawing from social activities)

Evaluate the safety of the environment

Health Teaching

Explain the importance of maintaining a positive self-attitude

Recommend new options for effective methods of coping

Describe those symptoms that should be reported (depression, planning suicide, hopelessness)

Explain the long-term effects of suicide on children (poor role modeling, being a one-parent child, the child will feel abandoned and helpless)

Explain the importance of learning and practicing mental health principles

Explain the reason for and intended effects of the preventive methods

EVALUATION

Record actual outcome

At-Risk Factors for Reproductive Disease

POTENTIAL FOR BREAST CANCER[42,73,451,474]

ASSESSMENT

Data Collection

Subjective Data

• There are no actual symptoms of breast cancer

Objective Data

• There are no actual signs of breast cancer

Related Data

• There are one or more stressors present that increase the possibility that breast cancer will occur:

INHERITED FACTORS: *Familial tendency*: For breast cancer. *Sex*: Greater incidence in females

DISEASES: Chronic cystic mastitis

HEALTH CARE FACTORS: *History*: Previous unilateral breast cancer or endometrial or ovarian cancer, was not pregnant before the age of 30, menstruated for more than 35 years as a result of early onset of menses (before age 12) and late menopause (occurring at or after age 55), did not breast-feed her children. *Medical therapy*: Adverse effects of hormone therapy

ENVIRONMENTAL FACTORS: Exposure to radiation

Data Analysis

Nursing Diagnosis

POTENTIAL FOR BREAST CANCER: The presence of stressors that increase the possibility of the actual occurrence of carcinogenic lesions of the breast

PLANNING

Unmet Needs

Protection from physical harm, increased learning

Expected Outcome

If signs and symptoms of breast cancer occur, they will be detected during the early stages and treated

Woman verbalizes an understanding of and practices monthly screening for breast cancer

NURSING INTERVENTIONS

Nursing Treatments

Obtain a complete present and past history

Nursing Observations

Make a follow-up evaluation (periodically)

Palpate the breasts for nodules (or masses)

Inspect the breasts for abnormalities (dimpling, breast asymmetry, nipple discharge)

Health Teaching

Inform that a predisposition to the illness exists

Describe those symptoms that should be reported (breast lumps, nipple discharge, breast asymmetry)

Explain the importance of periodic breast examination

Inform of when to do the breast examination (same day each month)

Demonstrate how to do the breast examination

Explain the importance of learning and practicing health principles

Explain why the potential problem could become actual (research verifies that certain stressors predispose to breast cancer)

Explain the reason for and intended effects of the preventive methods

Advise early correction of problems

EVALUATION

Record actual outcome

POTENTIAL FOR CERVICAL CANCER[42,295,451,474]

ASSESSMENT

Data Collection

Subjective Data

• There are no actual symptoms of cervical cancer

Objective Data

• There are no actual signs of cervical cancer

Related Data

• There are one or more stressors present that increase the possibility that cervical cancer will occur:

INHERITED FACTORS: *Familial tendency*: For cervical cancer. *Race*: Lowest incidence among Jewish women, with a higher incidence among non-Jewish women

HEALTH CARE FACTORS: *History*: Early coitus during adolescence and before age 17, having more than one male sexual partner, in women having had multiple pregnancies

DEVELOPMENTAL PHASE: Middle age (peak incidence occurs during age 40–50).

Data Analysis

Nursing Diagnosis

POTENTIAL FOR CERVICAL CANCER: The presence of stressors that increase the possibility of the actual occurrence of carcinogenic lesions of the cervix

PLANNING

Unmet Needs

Protection from physical harm, increased learning

Expected Outcome

If signs of cervical cancer occur, they will be detected during the early stages and treated

Woman verbalizes an understanding of and seeks an annual Papanicoulaou (Pap) test for cancer screening

NURSING INTERVENTIONS

Nursing Treatments

Obtain a complete present and past history

Do a Pap test

Nursing Observations

Make a follow-up evaluation (periodically)

Monitor the Pap smear results for positive findings

Health Teaching

Inform that a predisposition to the illness exists

Advise an annual gynecologic examination

Describe those symptoms that should be reported (abnormal vaginal bleeding, brown vaginal discharge, foul vaginal odor)

Explain the meaning of the diagnostic report (the meaning of Pap smear classifications)

Explain the importance of learning and practicing health principles

Explain why the potential problem could become actual (research verifies that certain stressors predispose to cervical cancer)

Explain the reason for and intended effects of the preventive methods

Advise early correction of problems

EVALUATION

Record actual outcome

At-Risk Factors for Respiratory Disease

POTENTIAL FOR LUNG CANCER[295,451,474]

ASSESSMENT

Data Collection

Subjective Data

• There are no actual symptoms of lung cancer

Objective Data
• There are no actual signs of lung cancer

Related Data
• There are one or more stressors present that increase the possibility that lung cancer will occur:

INHERITED FACTORS: *Familial tendency*: For cancer. *Sex*: Greater in men than women

DEVELOPMENTAL PHASES: Middle age (increased incidence after age 50), old age (greatly increased risk after age 70)

LIFESTYLE: Cigarette or tobacco smoking

ENVIRONMENTAL FACTORS: *Chemical substances*: Inhalation of asbestos, arsenic, chromate nickel, or uranium, exposure to urban air pollution

Data Analysis

Nursing Diagnosis

POTENTIAL FOR LUNG CANCER: The presence of stressors that increase the possibility of the actual occurrence of carcinogenic lesions of the lung(s)

PLANNING

Unmet Needs
Protection from physical harm, increased learning

Expected Outcome
No signs or symptoms of lung cancer will occur
    OR
If signs and symptoms occur, they will be promptly recognized as an actual problem and will be treated appropriately
Person verbalizes an understanding of and practices preventive methods

NURSING INTERVENTIONS

Nursing Treatments
Discourage the intake of oral stimulants (cigarette, cigar smoking)

Nursing Observations
Make a follow-up evaluation (periodically)
Auscultate the chest for abnormal breath sounds (especially localized wheezing unrelated to an allergy)
Observe for coughing
Monitor the laboratory findings of sputum analysis
Observe for complaints of (chest) pain, fatigue

Health Teaching
Inform that a predisposition to the illness exists
Describe those symptoms that should be reported (coughing, brown or bloody sputum, dyspnea)
Explain the importance of learning and practicing health principles (such as air-cleaning techniques with respiratory filters and masks, the importance of an x-ray examination during the high-risk years and the need to avoid smoking)
Explain why the potential problem could become actual (research verifies that certain stressors predispose to lung cancer)
Explain the reason for and intended effects of the preventive methods
Advise early correction of problems

EVALUATION

Record actual outcome

At-Risk Factors for Sensory Disorders

POTENTIAL FOR HEARING LOSS[72,125,451]

ASSESSMENT

Data Collection

Subjective Data
• There are no actual symptoms of hearing loss

Objective Data
• There are no actual signs of hearing loss

Related Data
• There are one or more stressors present that increase the possibility that hearing loss will occur:

BIRTH STATUS: Premature infant (birth weight below 1,500 g or serum bilirubin greater than 20 mg/100 ml)

INHERITED FACTORS: Familial tendency toward deafness

DISEASES: Measles, Meniere's disease, mumps, otitis media, otosclerosis, impacted cerumen, meningitis (maternal disease), cytomegalovirus infection, herpes, rubella

INJURIES: Contusion of the ear, foreign object in the ear (beads, hairpins, etc.)

HUMAN BODY: *Anatomic abnormalities*: Deformed ear, nose, or throat

HEALTH CARE FACTORS: *Drugs*: Adverse effects, such as streptomycin, gentamicin

DEVELOPMENTAL PHASES: Old age

ENVIRONMENTAL FACTORS: *Altitude*: Altitude changes in an aircraft when the person has a cold. *Blast or explosion*: Exposure to a blast or explosion. *Noise*: Prolonged exposure to loud noise

HUMAN ERROR: Swimming and diving while having an ear infection

Data Analysis

Nursing Diagnosis
POTENTIAL FOR HEARING LOSS: The presence of stressors that increase the possibility of the actual occurrence of diminished hearing acuity

PLANNING

Unmet Needs

Protection from physical harm, increased learning

Expected Outcome

No signs or symptoms of hearing loss will occur
    OR
If signs and symptoms occur, they will be promptly recognized as an actual problem and will be treated appropriately
Person verbalizes an understanding of and practices preventive methods

NURSING INTERVENTIONS

Nursing Treatments

Minimize environmental dangers (to prevent traumatic hearing loss)
Consult with the physician (regarding drugs and dosages)
Withhold the drug

Nursing Observations

Inspect the ears with an otoscope (for abnormalities)
Test the hearing by a Weber test (place a vibrating tuning fork at the skull midline; normally, sound is heard equally in each ear; in conductive hearing loss the sound is heard in the impaired ear; in sensorineural loss, the sound is heard in the normal ear)

Test the hearing by a Rhinne test (with the patient covering one ear, place the vibrating tuning fork on the mastoid process of the other ear until the vibration is no longer heard (bone conduction); then place the tuning fork in front of the ear meatus where the person should continue to hear the fork vibrations (air conduction); normally, air conduction is twice as long as bone conduction)

Test the hearing by audiometry (determine the hearing level by tones of calibrated loudness)

Observe for evidence of diminished hearing (requests for repeating comments or questions; complaints that people do not speak loud enough to be heard; unresponsive or inappropriate responses to comments or questions)

Observe for complaints of tinnitus (ringing or roaring noises in the ears)

Health Teaching

Inform that a predisposition to the illness exists

Explain that yawning and swallowing will equalize ear pressure (when in high altitudes)

Emphasize the need to fly in pressurized airplanes (and to avoid flying when one has a cold, rhinitis, etc.)

Emphasize the danger of excessive exposure to noise

Recommend methods for noise reduction (using earplugs and ear mufflers, heavy drapes, carpeting, closed doors, and windows, etc.)

Inform that water should be kept out of infected ears

Explain how to remove earwax

Instruct not to insert foreign objects into body orifices

Recommend strict adherence to safety rules for hearing protection

Describe those symptoms that should be reported (ear pain, a sudden change in hearing ability, ear noises)

Instruct to report early symptoms immediately

Explain the importance of learning and practicing health principles

Explain why the potential problem could become actual (research verifies that certain stressors predispose to hearing loss)

Explain the reason for and intended effects of the preventive methods

EVALUATION

Record actual outcome

POTENTIAL FOR VISION LOSS/EYE INJURY[11,139,311,392,732,733]

ASSESSMENT

Data Collection

Subjective Data
• There are no actual symptoms of vision loss

Objective Data
• There are no actual signs of vision loss

Related Data
• There are one or more stressors present that increase the possibility that vision loss will occur:

DISEASES: Corneal ulcers, diabetes mellitus, keratitis, multiple sclerosis, gonorrhea (if transferred by the birth process or by hand contact with the eyes)

INJURIES: Contusion of eye, head, or face

SIGNS AND SYMPTOMS: Exophthalmia, lid lag, nonclosure of the eyelids when a person is in a coma

HEALTH CARE FACTORS: *Medical therapy*: Administration of a high concentration of oxygen above 40% to premature infants and above 50% to children and adults, phototherapy

DEVELOPMENTAL PHASES: Middle age, old age

ENVIRONMENTAL FACTORS: *Chemical substances*: Splashing of chemicals. *Objects*: Pointed, sharp, or hard objects such as bows and arrows, darts, javelins, hardballs, slingshots. *Weapons*: Guns, BB guns

HUMAN ERROR: Nonuse of safety eyeglasses; looking directly at the sun or sun eclipse; wearing contact lens while sleeping, during eye infections and disorders, or for prolonged periods; engaging in prolonged close eyework; person does not have regular eye examinations or seek treatment for eye disorders

Data Analysis

Nursing Diagnosis

POTENTIAL FOR VISION LOSS/EYE INJURY: The presence of stressors that increase the possibility of the actual occurrence of a decrease in visual acuity

PLANNING

Unmet Needs

Protection from physical harm, increased learning

Expected Outcome

No signs or symptoms of vision loss will occur
OR
If signs and symptoms occur, they will be promptly recognized as an actual problem and will be treated appropriately
Person verbalizes an understanding of and practices preventive methods

NURSING INTERVENTIONS

Nursing Treatments

Encourage adequate rest
Illuminate the room adequately
Limit the therapeutic oxygen concentrations to below 40%
Lubricate the eye and patch the eye (with a protective eye shield when the eye cannot be closed)
Minimize environmental dangers (to prevent eye injury)
Remove contact lenses (during sleep, eye infection, and coma)

Nursing Observations

Observe for complaints of visual disturbance
Test the eyes for visual acuity (by Snellen chart, or E chart for children)

Health Teaching

Recommend safety measures to prevent eye injury (such as wearing safety goggles; never sun gazing, even when wearing sunglasses; never wiping the eyes with soiled towels or hands; properly adjusting the television picture; viewing television from the front, not side angles; leaving a light on while viewing television; viewing television from a moderate distance; preventing children from playing with toys that could injure the eye)
Advise precaution when using chemicals
Instruct that contact lenses should not be worn beyond the prescribed time, during an eye disorder, or while sleeping (unless they are designed to be worn during sleep)
Instruct to avoid rubbing the eyes
Recommend the use of eyeglass safety lenses
Recommend strict adherence to safety rules
Advise against letting light shine directly into the eyes
Advise against wearing unprescribed eyeglasses

Explain how to illuminate a room correctly

Inform that large-print reading material is available

Describe those symptoms that should be reported (eye irritation, visual disturbance)

Instruct to report any early symptoms immediately

Explain the importance of learning and practicing health principles

Explain why the potential problem could become actual (research verifies that certain stressors predispose to vision loss)

Explain the reason for and intended effects of the preventive methods

EVALUATION

Record actual outcome

19 Nursing Diagnoses of SUSPECTED DISEASE PROBLEMS

Dual Domain of Nursing Expertise: Suspected Disease Problems

This chapter covers that sphere of nursing knowledge and skill related to the detection of clinical findings that suggest a specific disease or disorder. The detection of such clinical findings supports early recognition of health disorders. Screening for suspected disease problems is done by such health care providers as nurses, physicians, physicians' assistants, and nonprofessional private or government agencies.

Views of Nursing Leaders That Support This Domain of Nursing Expertise

The nurse may intervene at the secondary prevention level which deals with the system after an encounter with a stressor has occurred and is concerned mainly with early case finding.

Betty Neuman[410:136]

Primary care functions for which nurses are now generally responsible are case finding and medical referral. These activities usually are carried out by nurses who function in patient's homes, in community clinics, in schools, and in industrial settings, although identification of ills, actual and impending, is expected of all nurses.

Faye Abdellah[3:125]

Screening for Cardiovascular Disorders

POSITIVE SCREENING CUES FOR ABNORMAL NEWBORN APGAR[94,258]

ASSESSMENT

Data Collection

Subjective Data
• Infant is unable to relate significant symptoms

Objective Data
• Infant exhibits, during screening, clinical findings that are not within the normal standard range; at 1 minute and/or at 5 minutes after birth, the infant manifests an abnormal Apgar score based on heart rate, respiratory effort, muscle tone, color, and response to suctioning by catheter (*Apgar score 4–6*: Moderate depression or distress; examples of findings are heartbeat below 100 or above 160 beats per minute, slow and irregular respirations, muscle tone normal or diminished, cyanosis, and grimace in response to suctioning. *Apgar score 0–3*: Severe depression or distress; examples of findings are heartbeat below 100 beats per minute or absent, apnea or irregular respirations, limp body, pallor or cyanosis, nonresponsive to suctioning)

Data Analysis

Nursing Diagnosis
POSITIVE SCREENING CUES FOR ABNORMAL NEWBORN APGAR: Infant has presented significant, abnormal clinical findings during brief testing for the general condition of a newborn, based on Apgar standards

Common Etiology (Stressors)
BIRTH DEFECTS: Congenital heart disease (major defects of the heart or great vessels)
DISEASES: Hypoglycemia, respiratory distress syndrome
SIGNS AND SYMPTOMS: Hyponatremia
MAJOR PATHOPHYSIOLOGIC FACTORS: Asphyxia during or after delivery, intrauterine infection, neurologic problems such as cerebral deficit, brain damage, or intracranial bleeding

PLANNING

Unmet Needs
Protection from physical harm, increased learning

Expected Outcome
Infant will undergo further testing if recommended by the physician
Parents will accept and participate in the infant's treatment if testing verifies a physical abnormality

NURSING INTERVENTIONS

Nursing Treatments
Consult with a physician (about the results of the screening test)

Nursing Observations
Make a follow-up evaluation (to determine whether the infant's condition has improved or remained unchanged)

Health Teaching
Explain the causes of the problem (after the physician has evaluated the infant and the mother has rested)

EVALUATION

Record actual outcome

POSITIVE SCREENING CUES FOR
CARDIOVASCULAR DISEASE[167,501]

ASSESSMENT

Data Collection

Subjective Data

• Person may or may not relate the following significant symptoms:

 Dyspnea
 Chest pain
 Syncope
 Palpitations
 Edema
 Orthopnea
 Persistent hacking cough
 Fatigue

Objective Data

• Person exhibits, during screening, clinical findings that are not within the standard normal range:

Pulses

Absent, bounding, or unequal carotid, radial, bracheal, femoral, popliteal, dorsalis pedia, or posterior tibial pulses

Severe distention of the internal or external jugular veins or carotid arteries

Bradycardia or tachycardia

An irregular pulse

Pulse deficit (difference between apical and radial pulses)

Arterial bruits

Heart Sounds

Abnormal rate or rhythm such as gallops, friction rubs, ejection sounds

Systolic, diastolic, or continuous murmur of recent onset that has not been present since childhood

Skin Color

Cyanosis
 OR
Pallor

ECG Recordings

Abnormal ECG findings such as premature contraction, flutter, tachycardia, bradycardia, heart block

Data Analysis

Nursing Diagnosis

POSITIVE SCREENING CUES FOR CARDIOVASCULAR DISEASE: Person has presented significant abnormal clinical findings during brief testing for a disorder of the heart and circulation

Common Etiology (Stressors)

DISEASES: Aortic coarctation, insufficiency, regurgitation, or stenosis; angina pectoris; dissecting aneurysm; arteriosclerotic heart disease; bacterial endocarditis; congestive heart failure; coronary occlusion; mitral insufficiency, regurgitation, or stenosis; mitral valve prolapse; myocardial infarction; myocarditis; paroxysmal atrial tachycardia; pericarditis; tricuspid insufficiency, regurgitation, or stenosis; left or right ventricular failure

PLANNING

Unmet Needs

Protection from physical harm, increased learning

Expected Outcome

Person will accept and act upon referral to a physician

Person will undergo further testing if recommended by the physician

Person will accept and participate in treatment if testing verifies the suspected diagnosis

NURSING INTERVENTIONS

Nursing Treatments

Consult with a physician (about the results of the screening test)

OR

Make a referral to a physician (for immediate care if serious cardiac disease is suspected; in such conditions, instruct the person to avoid all effort or stress while enroute to the doctor)

Arrange safe transport (to the doctor, if needed)

Nursing Observations

Determine the degree of insight that the person has (into his symptoms and the significant of the screening outcome)

Make a follow-up evaluation (to determine whether further testing verified the suspected diagnosis)

Health Teaching

Explain the meaning of the diagnostic report (in terms of suspected disease requiring further medical investigation)

Advise early correction of problems

Inform of the resources available for health care (so the person has several options)

Following a Confirmed Medical Diagnosis

Explain the causes of the problem (tissue damage to the myocardium, poorly functioning valves, arterial obstruction, etc.)

Explain the reason for and intended effect of the therapy

EVALUATION

Record actual outcome

POSITIVE SCREENING CUES FOR CONGENITAL HEART DISEASE[739]

ASSESSMENT

Data Collection

Subjective Data

• Person may or may not relate the following significant symptoms:

Dyspnea

Recurrent respiratory infections

Difficulty with feeding or appetite

Specific to Children

Fatigue from mild exercise

Objective Data

• Exhibits, during screening, clinical findings that are not within the standard normal range:

Cyanosis

Heart murmur

Marked difference in the right and left blood pressure readings
Weak or absent femoral pulse

Specific to Infants
Cyanosis after feeding or when crying
Failure to gain weight
Stridor or choking spells
Tachycardia (more than 200 beats/minute)

Specific to Children
Poor physical development
Clubbing of fingers or toes
Elevated blood pressure
Squatting

Data Analysis

Nursing Diagnosis
POSITIVE SCREENING CUES FOR CONGENITAL HEART DISEASE: Person has presented significant abnormal clinical findings during brief testing for heart disease present at birth

Common Etiology (Stressors)
BIRTH DEFECTS: Atrial septal defect, coarctation of the aorta, patent ductus arteriosus, subaortic stenosis, tetralogy of Fallot, tricuspid atresia, truncus arteriosus, ventricular septal defect

PLANNING

Unmet Needs
Protection from physical harm, increased learning

Expected Outcome
Person (or parent) will accept and act upon the referral to a physician
Adult or child will undergo further testing if recommended by the physician
Person (or parent) will accept and participate in treatment, if testing verifies the suspected diagnosis

NURSING INTERVENTIONS

Nursing Treatments
Consult with a physician (about the results of the screening test)
    OR
Make a referral to a physician

Nursing Observations
Determine the degree of insight that the person or parent has (into the significance of the screening outcome)
Make a follow-up evaluation (to determine whether further testing verified the suspected diagnosis)

Health Teaching
Explain the meaning of the diagnostic report (in terms of suspected disease requiring further medical investigation)
Advise early correction of problems
Inform of the resources available for health care (so the patient has several options)

Following a Confirmed Medical Diagnosis
Explain the causes of the problem (heredity, prenatal factors, maternal infection or disease, alcohol or chemical ingestion, unknown causes)
Explain the reason for and intended effect of the therapy

EVALUATION

Record actual outcome

POSITIVE SCREENING CUES FOR HYPERTENSIVE DISEASE[255,282,491,748]

ASSESSMENT
Data Collection
Subjective Data
• Person may or may not relate the following significant symptoms:
Headaches
Dizziness
Changes in vision

Infants/Small Children
Irritability
Head-banging or rubbing
Awakes screaming (usually at night)

Objective Data
• Person exhibits, during screening, clinical findings that are not within the standard normal range:
Prepubertal children with consistent recordings of 140/90
Postpubertal children with consistent recordings of 150/100
Adults under age 50 with blood pressure above 140/90
Adults over age 50 with blood pressure above 160/95

Data Analysis
Nursing Diagnosis
POSITIVE SCREENING CUES FOR HYPERTENSIVE DISEASE: Person has presented significant abnormal clinical findings during brief testing for diseases associated with an elevated blood pressure

Common Etiology (Stressors)
BIRTH DEFECTS: Secondary to congenital adrenal hyperplasia
DISEASES: Essential hypertension, malignant hypertension, hypertension secondary to renal disease, primary aldosteronism, pheochromocytoma, coarctation of the aorta, Cushing's syndrome, hypothyroidism, hyperparathyroidism, acromegaly
INJURIES: Lead poisoning
HUMAN BODY: *Body states*: Secondary to pregnancy
HEALTH CARE FACTORS: *Drug therapy*: Adverse effects of contraceptives
HUMAN ERROR: Excessive ingestion of licorice

PLANNING
Unmet Needs
Protection from physical harm, increased learning
Expected Outcome
Person will accept and act upon referral to a physician
Person will undergo further testing if recommended by the physician
Person will accept and participate in treatment if testing verifies the suspected diagnosis

NURSING INTERVENTIONS
Nursing Treatments
Consult with a physician (about the results of the screening test)
OR
Make a referral to a physician
Nursing Observations
Determine the degree of insight that the person has (into the significance of the screening outcome)

Make a follow-up evaluation (to determine whether further testing verified the suspected diagnosis)

Health Teaching

Explain the meaning of the diagnostic report (in terms of suspected disease requiring further medical investigation)

Advise early correction of problems

Inform of the resources available for health care (so the person has several options)

Following a Confirmed Medical Diagnosis

Explain the causes of the problem (heredity, vascular or renal disease, the effect of renin secretion or of prostaglandins, etc.)

Explain the reason for and intended effect of the therapy

EVALUATION

Record actual outcome

POSITIVE SCREENING CUES FOR PERIPHERAL VASCULAR DISEASE[73,125]

ASSESSMENT

Data Collection

Subjective Data

• Person may or may not relate the following significant symptoms:
    Complaints of extremity pain
    Feelings of extremity cold or warmth
    Paresthesia

Objective Data

• Person exhibits, during screening, clinical findings that are not within the normal standard range:
    Abnormal color changes of the skin or nails (cyanosis, pallor, redness)
    Decreased nail growth
    Thickened ridged nails
    Shiny taut skin indicating edema
    Skin is unusually cold or warm on palpation
    Veins are enlarged or have abnormal pulsations
    Necrotic, gangrenous, or ulcerative lesions are present
    Extremity atrophy

Data Analysis

Nursing Diagnosis

POSITIVE SCREENING CUES FOR PERIPHERAL VASCULAR DISEASE: Person has presented significant abnormal clinical findings during brief testing for impaired circulation in the extremities

Common Etiology (Stressors)

DISEASES: Arteriosclerosis, atherosclerosis, Buerger's disease, diabetes mellitus, phlebitis, phlebothrombosis, polyarteritis nodosa, Raynaud's disease, thrombophlebitis, varicose veins

PLANNING

Unmet Needs

Protection from physical harm, increased learning

Expected Outcome

Person will accept and act upon referral to a physician

Person will undergo further testing if recommended by the physician
Person will accept and participate in treatment if testing verifies the suspected diagnosis

NURSING INTERVENTIONS

Nursing Treatments
Consult with a physician (about the results of the screening test)
   OR
Make a referral to a physician

Nursing Observations
Determine the degree of insight that the person has (into his symptoms and the significance of the screening outcome)
Make a follow-up evaluation (to determine whether the suspected diagnosis was verified)

Health Teaching
Explain the meaning of the diagnostic report (in terms of suspected disease requiring further medical investigation)
Advise early correction of problems
Inform of the resources available for health care (so the person has several options)

Following a Confirmed Medical Diagnosis
Explain the causes of the problem (insufficient peripheral circulation, a blood clot in a vessel, etc.)

EVALUATION
Record actual outcome

Screening for Dental Disorders

POSITIVE SCREENING CUES FOR DENTAL DISEASE[33,125]

ASSESSMENT

Data Collection

Subjective Data
• Person may or may not relate the following significant symptoms:
   Toothache
   Halatosis
   Bleeding gums
   Painful swelling of the gums

Infant/Small Child
Goes to sleep sucking on a bottle

Objective Data
• Person exhibits, during screening, clinical findings that are not within the standard normal range:
   Decay, malformation, discoloration, or absence of teeth
   Heavy accumulation of plaque
   Gum inflammation, bleeding or infection

Data Analysis

Nursing Diagnosis

POSITIVE SCREENING CUES FOR DENTAL DISEASE: Person has presented significant abnormal clinical findings during brief testing for disease of the teeth or gums

Common Etiology (Stressors)

INJURIES: Contusion of the mouth

DISEASES: Dental caries (bottle-mouth syndrome in toddlers), gingivitis, peridontitis

PLANNING

Unmet Needs

Protection from physical harm, increased learning

Expected Outcome

Adult (or parent) will accept and act upon referral to a dentist

Adult (or child) will undergo further testing if recommended by the dentist

Adult (or child) will accept and participate in treatment, if testing verifies the suspected diagnosis

NURSING INTERVENTIONS

Nursing Treatments

Consult with a dentist (about the results of the screening test)

   OR

Make a referral to a dentist

Nursing Observations

Determine the degree of insight that the person has (into the significance of the screening outcome)

Make a follow-up evaluation (to determine whether further testing verified the suspected diagnosis)

Health Teaching

Advise early correction of problems

Inform of the resources available for health care (so the person has several options)

Teach how to brush and floss the teeth correctly

EVALUATION

Record actual outcome

Screening for Gallbladder or Hepatic Disorders

POSITIVE SCREENING CUES FOR GALLBLADDER DISEASE[278,282,399,500]

ASSESSMENT

Data Collection

Subjective Data

• Person may or may not relate the following significant symptoms:

Anorexia

Nausea

Vomiting

Clay-colored stools

Acute, colicky, with upper quadrant abdominal pain radiating to the back, to the front of the chest, or between the shoulders

Objective Data

• Person exhibits, during screening, clinical findings that are not within the standard normal range:

Elevated serum bilirubin and alkaline phosphatase

Normal SGOT and LDH

Bilirubin in the urine (by Multistix test or by foam test; in the foam test, when a fresh urine sample of mahogany-colored urine is shaken, a yellow foam forms on top, indicating bilirubin in the uterine, which is normally absent)

Data Analysis

Nursing Diagnosis

POSITIVE SCREENING CUES FOR GALLBLADDER DISEASE: Person has presented significant abnormal clinical findings during brief testing for gallbladder disease

Common Etiology (Stressors)

DISEASES: Cholangitis, cholecystitis, choledocholithiasis, cholelithiasis, cholesterolesis, gallstone ileus

PLANNING

Unmet Needs

Protection from physical harm, increased learning

Expected Outcome

Person will accept and act upon referral to a physician

Person will undergo further testing if recommended by the physician

Person will accept and participate in testing, if testing verifies the suspected diagnosis

NURSING INTERVENTIONS

Nursing Treatments

Consult with a physician (about the results of the screening test)

   OR

Make a referral to a physician

Nursing Observations

Determine the degree of insight that the person has (into his symptoms and the significance of the screening outcome)

Make a follow-up evaluation (to determine whether further testing has verified the suspected diagnosis)

Health Teaching

Explain the meaning of the diagnostic report (in terms of suspected disease requiring further medical investigation)

Advise early correction of problems

Inform of the resources available for health care (so the person has several options)

Following a Confirmed Medical Diagnosis

Explain the causes of the problem (biliary obstruction, infection)

Explain the reason for and intended effect of the therapy (to improve gallbladder function or remove a diseased gallbladder)

EVALUATION

Record actual outcome

POSITIVE SCREENING CUES FOR HEPATIC DISEASE[278,283,399,500]

ASSESSMENT
Data Collection
Subjective Data
- Person may or may not relate the following significant symptoms:
  Anorexia
  Nausea
  Vomiting
  Lethargy
  Upper abdominal pain, sometimes
  Clay-colored stools, sometimes

Objective Data
- Person exhibits, during screening, clinical findings that are not within the standard normal range:
  Jaundice of the slcera or skin, sometimes
  Fever, sometimes
  Dark urine color
  Positive urine bilirubin
  Elevated serum bilirubin, alkaline phosphatase, SGOT, SGPT
  HAA (hepatitis-associated antigen) detection in serum is specific to hepatitis
  Palpable liver tenderness
  Liver enlargement on percussion

Data Analysis
Nursing Diagnosis
POSITIVE SCREENING CUES FOR HEPATIC DISEASE: Person has presented significant abnormal clinical findings during brief testing for liver disease

Common Etiology (Stressors)
DISEASES: Budd-Chiari syndrome, hepatic granulomata, hepatitis (viral or toxic), Laennec's cirrhosis, liver abscess, liver carcinoma, Wilson's disease

PLANNING
Unmet Needs
Protection from physical harm, increased learning

Expected Outcome
Person will accept and act upon referral to a physician
Person will undergo further testing if recommended by the physician
Person will accept and participate in treatment if testing verifies the suspected diagnosis

NURSING INTERVENTIONS
Nursing Treatments
Consult with a physician (about the results of the screening test)
  OR
Make a referral to a physician

Nursing Observations
Determine the degree of insight that the person has (into his symptoms and the significance of the screening outcome)
Make a follow-up evaluation (to determine whether further testing has verified the suspected diagnosis)

Health Teaching
Explain the meaning of the diagnostic report (in terms of suspected disease requiring

further medical investigation)
Advise early correction of problems
Inform of the resources available for health care (so the person has several options)

Following a Confirmed Medical Diagnosis
Explain the causes of the problem (liver damage, viral infection)
Explain the reason for and intended effect of the therapy (to heal the damaged liver cells and restore hepatic function)

EVALUATION
Record actual outcome

POSITIVE SCREENING CUES FOR HYPERBILIRUBINEMIA[73,313,500]

ASSESSMENT
Data Collection
Subjective Data
• Parent may or may not relate the following significant infant symptoms:
 Infant lethargy, sometimes
 Feeds poorly, sometimes

Objective Data
• Infant exhibits, during screening, clinical findings that are not within the normal standard range:
 Serum bilirubin level above 10 mg/100 ml in premature infants or above 15 mg/100 ml in full-term infants, over 5–8 mg/100 ml during the first 24 hours after birth or above 9 mg/100 ml after the first 24 hours
 Yellow skin or sclera
 Dark yellow urine
 Pale stools

Data Analysis
Nursing Diagnosis
POSITIVE SCREENING CUES FOR HYPERBILIRUBINEMIA: Infant has presented significant abnormal clinical findings during brief testing for ineffective and immature metabolism and excretion of bilirubin

Common Etiology (Stressors)
BIRTH STATUS: Premature infant, newborn
DISEASES: Diabetes mellitus (if the infant's mother has diabetes), hyaline membrane disease, hypothyroidism, hemolytic disease, septicemia
HUMAN BODY: *Natural body function*: Breast-feeding
HEALTH CARE FACTORS: *Drug therapy*: Adverse effects of drugs such as aspirin, chloramphenicol, morphine, novobiocin, pregnanediol, vitamin K

PLANNING
Unmet Needs
Protection from physical harm

Expected Outcome

Infant will receive therapy for hyperbilirubinemia

NURSING INTERVENTIONS

Nursing Treatments

Consult with a physician (about the results of the screening test)
 OR
Make a referral to a physician

Nursing Observations

Determine the degree of insight that the parent has (into the child's symptoms and the
 significance of the screening outcome)
Make a follow-up evaluation (to determine whether further testing has verified the suspected diagnosis)

Health Teaching

Explain the meaning of the diagnostic reports

Following a Confirmed Medical Diagnosis
Explain the causes of the problem (to the parents)

EVALUATION

Record actual outcome

Screening for Gastrointestinal Disorders

POSITIVE SCREENING CUES FOR GASTROINTESTINAL DISEASE[164,282,363,399,500]

ASSESSMENT

Data Collection

Subjective Data
• Person may or may not relate the following significant symptoms:
    Nausea
    Vomiting
    Diarrhea or constipation
    Anorexia
    Heartburn
    Eructation (frequent)
    Dysphagia (difficulty swallowing)
    Regurgitation
    Weight loss or gain
    Abdominal pain
    Pancreas (boring, bandlike pain generalized over the upper abdominal quadrants of-
        ten radiating to the back, pain less severe when sitting up or flexing at the waist)
    Peptic ulceration (burning, gnawing, hunger pain located in the epigastric area, re-
        lieved or caused by eating)

Objective Data
• Person exhibits, during screening, clinical findings that are not within the standard
  normal range:
  Auscultation (absent, rumbling, high- or low-pitched bowel sounds)
  Palpation (abdominal tenderness, rigidity, muscle guarding, or masses)
  Percussion (tympany)
  Inspection (abdominal distention)

Specific for Abdominal Bleeding
Positive Hemoccult test for occult blood (smear turns blue within 30–60 seconds after
  the application of 2 drops of developer)

Specific for Pancreatic Disease
Elevated serum amylase and serum lipase

Data Analysis

Nursing Diagnosis
POSITIVE SCREENING CUES FOR GASTROINTESTINAL DISEASE: Person has presented significant abnormal clinical findings during brief testing for disease of the stomach, intestines,
  and/or pancreas

Common Etiology (Stressors)
DISEASES: Appendicitis, celiac disease (sprue), Crohn's disease, diverticulitis, esophageal
  stricture, gastritis, gastroenteritis, hiatal hernia, ileitis, gastrointestinal cancer, intestinal obstruction, intussusception, pancreatitis, peptic ulcer, peritonitis, pilonidal disease, rectal prolapse, ulcerative colitis, viral enteritis, volvulus

PLANNING

Unmet Needs
Protection from physical harm, increased learning

Expected Outcome
Person will accept and act upon referral to a physician
Person will undergo further testing if recommended by the physician
Person will accept and participate in treatment if testing verifies the suspected diagnosis

NURSING INTERVENTIONS

Nursing Treatments
Consult with a physician (about the results of the screening test)
  OR
Make a referral to a physician

Nursing Observations
Determine the degree of insight that the person has (into his symptoms and the significance of the screening outcome)
Make a follow-up evaluation (to determine whether further testing has verified the suspected diagnosis)

Health Teaching
Explain the meaning of the diagnostic report (in terms of suspected disease requiring
  further medical investigation)
Advise early correction of problems
Inform of the resources available for health care (so the person has several options)

Following a Confirmed Medical Diagnosis
Explain the causes of the problem (bacterial infection, obstruction, mucosal irritation,
  etc.)
Explain the reason for and intended effect of the therapy (to restore maximum stomach
  and intestinal function for improved body nutrition)

EVALUATION

Record actual outcome

POSITIVE SCREENING CUES FOR ORAL CANCER[73,451,474]

ASSESSMENT

Data Collection

Subjective Data
- Person may or may not relate the following significant symptoms:
  May complain of a chronic lesion on the oral mucosa, lips, or tongue lasting over 2–3 weeks' duration
  Relates no pain (usually)

Objective Data
- Person exhibits, during screening, clinical findings that are not within the normal standard range:
  Oral lesions appear discolored, ulcerated, or bleeding
  Positive exfoliative cytology test (Papanicolaou smear) of a buccal mucosa scraping (*Positive results*: Class III, doubtful, requires a repeat Pap smear; class IV, probably malignant, requires a biopsy; class V, malignant, requires cancer therapy)

Data Analysis

Nursing Diagnosis
POSITIVE SCREENING CUES FOR ORAL CANCER: Person has presented significant abnormal clinical findings during brief testing for malignant lesions of the oral cavity

Common Etiology (Stressors)
DISEASES: Basal cell carcinoma, malignant melanoma, squamous cell carcinoma
LIFESTYLE: High alcohol intake, cigarette smoking, tobacco chewing, snuff dipping

PLANNING

Unmet Needs
Protection from physical harm, increased learning

Expected Outcome
Person will accept and act upon referral to a physician
Person will undergo further testing if recommended by the physician
Person will accept and participate in treatment if testing verifies the suspected diagnosis

NURSING INTERVENTIONS

Nursing Treatments
Consult with a physician (about the results of the screening test)
    OR
Make a referral to a physician

Nursing Observations
Determine the degree of insight that the person has (into his symptoms and the significance of the screening outcome)
Make a follow-up evaluation (to determine whether the suspected diagnosis was verified)

Health Teaching
Explain the meaning of the diagnostic report (in terms of suspected disease requiring further medical investigation)
Advise early correction of problems
Inform of the resources available for health care (so the person has several options)

Following a Confirmed Medical Diagnosis
Explain the causes of the problem (cell disorganization, tissue irritation from smoking, etc.)

EVALUATION

Record actual outcome

POSITIVE SCREENING CUES FOR PINWORM DISEASE[399,522]

ASSESSMENT

Data Collection

Subjective Data
- Person may or may not relate the following significant symptoms:
    Anal itching, especially at night
    Anal irritation
    Weight loss

Objective Data
- Person exhibits, during screening, clinical findings that are not within the normal standard range:
    Ova are found on a Graham scotch tape test

Data Analysis

Nursing Diagnosis
POSITIVE SCREENING CUES FOR PINWORM DISEASE (ENTEROBIASIS): Person has presented significant abnormal clinical findings during brief testing for pinworms

Common Etiology (Stressors)
LIFESTYLE: Lack of hygiene
ENVIRONMENTAL FACTORS: *Soil*: Contaminated soil
HUMAN ERROR: Walking barefooted

PLANNING

Unmet Needs

Protection from physical harm, increased learning

Expected Outcome

Person will accept and act upon referral to a physician
Person will undergo further testing if recommended by the physician
Person will accept and participate in treatment if testing verifies the suspected diagnosis

NURSING INTERVENTIONS

Nursing Treatments

Consult with a physician (about the results of the screening test)
    OR
Make a referral to a physician (for pyrantel, piperazine, or mebendazole)

Nursing Observations

Determine the degree of insight that the person has (into his symptoms and the significance of the screening outcome)
Make a follow-up evaluation (to determine whether further testing verified the suspected diagnosis)

Health Teaching

Explain the meaning of the diagnostic report (in terms of suspected disease requiring further medical investigation)
Advise early correction of problems
Inform of the resources available for health care (so the person has several options)

Following a Confimred Medical Diagnosis
Explain the causes of the problem (contact with soil contaminated with larvae and eggs, transmission by the person's hands and bare feet)

Explain the reason for and intended effect of the therapy
Advise against walking barefooted
Advise handwashing after elimination
Advise handwashing before meals
Inform that cleanliness is basic to health (that linens and clothes should be changed daily, that one should shower daily)

EVALUATION
Record actual outcome

Screening for Genitourinary Disorders

POSITIVE SCREENING CUES FOR RENAL DISEASE[71,84,282,399,500]

ASSESSMENT
Data Collection
Subjective Data
• Person may or may not relate the following significant symptoms:

Changes in Urination
Frequency
Dysuria
Nocturia
Hesitancy
Urgency or retention

Change in Urine Volume
Polyuria
Oliguria or anuria

Other
Flank, groin, or costovertebral angle pain
Edema
Anorexia, nausea, or vomiting

Objective Data
• Person exhibits, during screening, clinical findings that are not within the standard normal range:
  Elevated serum creatinine and blood urea nitrogen (BUN)
  Proteinuria, abnormal red blood cells (hematuria), abnormal white blood cells (pyuria), casts, bacteriuria (urine culture count of 100,000 or above), or glucose in the urine
  Urine specific gravity at or below 1.017
  Percussion may cause tenderness over the costovertebral angle
  Elevated blood pressure, sometimes
  Small stones in the urine
  Fever
  Painless abdominal mass (Wilms' tumor)

Data Analysis

Nursing Diagnosis

POSITIVE SCREENING CUES FOR RENAL DISEASE: Person has presented significant abnormal clinical findings during brief testing for detection of a disturbance in kidney function

Common Etiology (Stressors)

BIRTH DEFECTS: Polycystic kidney disease

DISEASES: Glomerulonephritis, glomerulosclerosis, nephritis, nephrosclerosis, nephrosis, nephrotic syndrome, pyleonephritis, renal calculi, renal failure, renal glucosuria, renal insufficiency, Wilms' tumor

PLANNING

Unmet Needs

Protection from physical harm, increased learning

Expected Outcome

Person will accept and act upon referral to a physician

Person will undergo further testing if recommended by the physician

Person will accept and participate in treatment if testing verifies the suspected diagnosis

NURSING INTERVENTIONS

Nursing Treatments

Consult with a physician (about the results of the screeing test)

   OR

Make a referral to a physician

Nursing Observations

Determine the degree of insight that the person has (into his symptoms and the significance of the screening outcome)

Make a follow-up evaluation (to determine whether further testing has verified the suspected diagnosis)

Health Teaching

Explain the meaning of the diagnostic report (in terms of suspected disease requiring further medical investigation)

Advise early correction of problems

Inform of the resources available for health care (so the person has several options)

Following a Confirmed Medical Diagnosis

Explain the causes of the problem (heredity, bacterial infection, renal tumors, etc.)

Explain the reason for and intended effect of the therapy (to restore renal function or prevent further damage to renal tissue)

EVALUATION

Record actual outcome

POSITIVE SCREENING CUES FOR URINARY TRACT INFECTION[71,282,399,500,652]

ASSESSMENT

Data Collection

Subjective Data

• Person may or may not relate the following significant symptoms:

   Frequency

Dysuria
Suprapubic pain
OR
Flank pain
Failure to thrive (infant)

Objective Data

* Person exhibits, during screening, clinical findings that are not within the standard normal range:
Fever
Hematuria (microscopic red blood cells in the urine or positive blood by Multistik)
Bacteriuria (urine culture count over 100,000 or positive nitrite by Multistik)
Unpleasant urinary odor (fishy)
Cloudy urine (pyuria)

Data Analysis

Nursing Diagnosis

POSITIVE SCREENING CUES FOR URINARY TRACT INFECTION: Person has presented significant abnormal clinical findings during brief testing for bacteria in the kidneys, ureters, bladder, or urethra

Common Etiology (Stressors)

DISEASES: Cystitis, pyelonephritis, urethritis

PLANNING

Unmet Needs

Protection from physical harm, increased learning

Expected Outcome

Person will accept and act upon referral to a physician
Person will undergo further testing if recommended by the physician
Person will accept and participate in treatment if testing verifies the suspected diagnosis

NURSING INTERVENTIONS

Nursing Treatments

Consult with a physician (about the results of the screening test)
OR
Make a referral to a physician

Nursing Observations

Determine the degree of insight that the person has (into his symptoms and the significance of the screening outcome)
Make a follow-up evaluation (to determine whether further testing verified the suspected diagnosis)

Health Teaching

Explain the meaning of the diagnostic report (in terms of suspected disease requiring further medical investigation)
Advise early correction of problems
Inform of the resources available for health care (so the person has several options)

Following a Confirmed Medical Diagnosis

Explain the causes of the problem (bacteria in the urinary system)
Explain the reason for and intended effect of the therapy (to reduce the bacterial count in the urinary tract, to prevent damage to bladder and kidney tissue)

EVALUATION

Record actual outcome

Screening for Hematologic Disorders

POSITIVE SCREENING CUES FOR ANEMIA[42,282,399,500]

ASSESSMENT

Data Collection

Subjective Data

• Person may or may not relate the following significant symptoms:
Fatigue
Lightheadedness
Dyspnea on exertion
Headache
Decreased tolerance to cold (easy chilling)
Glossitis
AND
Paresthesias of the extremities (specific for pernicious anemia)

Objective Data

• Person exhibits, during screening, clinical findings that are not within the standard normal range:
Pallor (especially of the conjunctiva)
A drop in the blood pressure and an increase in the pulse when the person stands
Hemoglobin below normal (*Females*: 12–14 g/dl Hgb. *Males*: 14–16 g/dl Hgb)
Hematocrit below normal (*Females*: 37–47% Hct. *Males*: 42–52% Hct)
Red blood cells (RBC) below normal (*Females*: 4.2–5 ml/mm³. *Males*: 4.7–6.1 ml/mm³)

Data Analysis

Nursing Diagnosis

POSITIVE SCREENING CUES FOR ANEMIA: Person has presented significant abnormal clinical findings during brief testing for impaired production, destruction, or excessive loss of red blood cells

Common Etilogy (Stressors)

BIRTH DEFECTS: Thalassemia
DISEASES: Aplastic anemia, folic acid deficiency, infection, iron deficiency anemia, hemolytic anemia, pernicious anemia, chronic renal failure
INJURIES: Hydrocarbon poisoning, lead poisoning
SIGNS AND SYMPTOMS: Bleeding and hemorrhage
HEALTH CARE FACTORS: Adverse effects of drugs such as chloramphenicol, phenylbutazone, mephenytoin
LIFESTYLE: An insufficient or unbalanced diet

PLANNING

Unmet Needs

Protection from physical harm, increased learning

Expected Outcome

Person will accept and act upon referral to a physician
Person will undergo further testing if recommended by the physician
Person will accept and participate in treatment if testing verifies the suspected diagnosis

NURSING INTERVENTIONS

Nursing Treatments

Consult with a physician (about the results of the screening test)
OR
Make a referral to a physician

Nursing Observations

Determine the degree of insight that the person has (into his symptoms and the significance of the screening outcome)

Make a follow-up evaluation (to determine whether further testing has verified the suspected diagnosis)

Health Teaching

Explain the meaning of the diagnostic report (in terms of suspected disease requiring further medical investigation)

Advise early correction of problems

Inform of the resources available for health care (so the person has several options)

Following a Confirmed Medical Diagnosis

Explain the causes of the problem (bleeding, malnutrition, food malabsorption, etc.)

Explain the reason for and intended effect of the therapy (to increase red blood cells and/or hemoglobin)

EVALUATION

Record actual outcome

POSITIVE SCREENING CUES FOR SICKLE CELL DISEASE[42,399,500]

ASSESSMENT

Data Collection

Subjective Data

• Person may or may not relate the following significant symptoms:

Relates irritability

Chronic colds or infection

Complains of pain in limbs, joints, abdomen, or chest

Parent may relate a child has delayed growth or onset of puberty

Weakness

Anorexia

Objective Data

• Person exhibits, during screening, clinical findings that are not within the standard normal range:

Sickle hemoglobin test (HbS) shows a positive sickle cell preparation

OR

Sickle-turbidity test (Sickledex) is positive for sickle cell trait and anemia (this test can give a false-negative result if the Hgb is below 10 g/100 ml; or if done on babies less than 4–6 months of age with a high level of fetal hemoglobin)

Data Analysis

Nursing Diagnosis

POSITIVE SCREENING CUES FOR SICKLE CELL DISEASE: Person has presented significant abnormal clinical findings during brief testing for sickle cell disease

Common Etiology (Stressors)

BIRTH DEFECTS: Sickle cell anemia, sickle cell trait

PLANNING

Unmet Needs

Protection from physical harm, increased learning

Expected Outcome

Person will accept and act upon referral to a physician

Person will undergo further testing if recommended by the physician

Person will accept and participate in treatment if testing verifies the suspected diagnosis

NURSING INTERVENTIONS

Nursing Treatments

Consult with a physician (about the results of the screening test)

OR

Make a referral to a physician

Nursing Observations

Determine the degree of insight that the person has (into his symptoms and the significance of the screening outcome)

Make a follow-up evaluation (to determine whether further testing has verified the suspected diagnosis)

Health Teaching

Explain the meaning of the diagnostic report (in terms of suspected disease requiring further medical investigation)

Advise early correction of problems

Inform of the resources available for health care (so the person has several options)

Following a Confirmed Medical Diagnosis

Explain the causes of the problem (heredity, sickling of cells)

Explain the reason for and intended effect of the therapy (to promote circulation and comfort, to prevent sickle cell crisis)

EVALUATION

Record actual outcome

Screening for Infectious Disorders

POSITIVE SCREENING CUES FOR GONORRHEA [42,88,500]

ASSESSMENT

Data Collection

Subjective Data

• Person may or may not relate the following significant symptoms:

History of sexual contacts

Reports purulent urethral (male) or vaginal (female) discharge

Dysuria

Inflammation at the site of infection

Some women may complain of peritonitis-like symptoms (abdominal pain, fever, constipation) if fallopian tubes are infected

Some persons are symptom free

Objective Data
- Person exhibits, during screening, clinical findings that are not within the standard normal range:
    Positive Gram stain of urethral (male) or vaginal (female) discharge

Data Analysis

Nursing Diagnosis

POSITIVE SCREENING CUES FOR GONORRHEA: Person has presented significant abnormal clinical findings during brief testing for the sexually transmitted disease, gonorrhea

Common Etiology (Stressors)
DISEASES: Gonorrhea

PLANNING

Unmet Needs
Protection from physical harm, increased learning

Expected Outcome
Person will accept and act upon referral to a physician
Person will undergo further testing if recommended by the physician
Person will accept and participate in treatment if testing verifies the suspected diagnosis

NURSING INTERVENTIONS

Nursing Treatments
Consult with a physician (about the results of the screening test)
    OR
Make a referral to a physician

Nursing Observations
Determine the degree of insight that the person has (into the significance of the screening outcome)
Make a follow-up evaluation (to determine whether the suspected diagnosis was verified)

Health Teaching
Explain the meaning of the diagnostic report (in terms of suspected disease requiring further medical investigation)
Advise early correction of problems
Inform of the resources available for health care (so the person has several options)

Following a Confirmed Medical Diagnosis
Explain the causes of the problem (sexual contact, bacterial infection)
Explain how to prevent cross-infection (the infected person should avoid direct contact with others)
Explain the reason for and intended effect of the therapy (to cure the infection)

EVALUATION
Record actual outcome

POSITIVE SCREENING CUES FOR HERPES GENITALIA [42,73]

ASSESSMENT

Data Collection

Subjective Data
- Person may or may not relate the following significant symptoms:

History of sexual contacts
Reports genital lesions
Dysuria
Itching
Genital pain
Neurologic pain several days before the appearance of lesions

Objective Data
• Person exhibits, during screening, clinical findings that are not within the standard normal range:
Small, vesicular, genital lesions
Painful lesions on palpation
Bilateral lymphadenopathy in the groin or abdomen
Female vaginal or male urethral discharge

Data Analysis

Nursing Diagnosis
POSITIVE SCREENING CUES FOR HERPES GENITALIA: Person has presented significant abnormal clinical findings during brief testing for the sexually transmitted disease, herpes genitalia

Common Etiology (Stressors)
DISEASES: Herpes genitalia

PLANNING

Unmet Needs
Protection from physical harm, increased learning

Expected Outcome
Person will accept and act upon referral to a physician
Person will undergo further testing if recommended by the physician
Person will accept and participate in treatment if testing verifies the suspected diagnosis

NURSING INTERVENTIONS

Nursing Treatments
Consult with a physician (about the results of the screening test)
    OR
Make a referral to a physician

Nursing Observations
Determine the degree of insight that the person has (into the significance of the screening outcome)
Make a follow-up evaluation (to determine whether the suspected diagnosis was verified)

Health Teaching
Explain the meaning of the diagnostic report (in terms of suspected disease requiring further medical investigation)
Advise early correction of problems
Inform of the resources available for health care (so the person has several options)

Following a Confirmed Medical Diagnosis
Explain the causes of the problem (sexual contact, herpes virus type II)
Explain how to prevent cross-infection (the infected person should avoid direct contact with others)
Explain the reason for and intended effect of the therapy (to heal the lesion, control the infection, relieve the discomfort)

EVALUATION
Record actual outcome

POSITIVE SCREENING CUES FOR INFECTIOUS MONONUCLEOSIS[42,88,500]

ASSESSMENT

Data Collection

Subjective Data
- Person may or may not relate the following significant symptoms:
  Sore throat for longer than 10 days
  Malaise
  Headache

Objective Data
- Person exhibits, during screening, clinical findings that are not within the standard normal range:
  Fever 100°–102° F
  Enlarged, tender lymph nodes
  Positive heterophil antibody test (Mono Spot)

Data Analysis

Nursing Diagnosis
POSITIVE SCREENING CUES FOR INFECTIOUS MONONUCLEOSIS: Person has presented significant abnormal clinical findings during brief testing for the viral disease, infectious mononucleosis

Common Etiology (Stressors)
DISEASES: Infectious mononucleosis

PLANNING

Unmet Needs
Protection from physical harm, increased learning

Expected Outcome
Person will accept and act upon referral to a physician
Person will undergo further testing if recommended by the physician
Person will accept and participate in treatment if testing verifies the suspected diagnosis

NURSING INTERVENTIONS

Nursing Treatments
Consult with a physician (about the results of the screening test)
  OR
Make a referral to a physician

Nursing Observations
Determine the degree of insight that the person has (into the significance of the screening outcome)
Make a follow-up evaluation (to determine whether the suspected diagnosis was verified)

Health Teaching
Explain the meaning of the diagnostic report (in terms of suspected disease requiring further medical investigation)
Advise early correction of problems
Inform of the resources available for health care (so the person has several options)

Following a Confirmed Medical Diagnosis
Explain the causes of the problem (the herpes, or Epstein-Barr, virus)
Explain how to prevent cross-infection (avoid close contact with the infected person, especially oral or airborne droplet contact)
Explain the reason for and intended effect of the therapy (to cure the infection)

EVALUATION
Record actual outcome

POSITIVE SCREENING CUES FOR OTITIS MEDIA[42,88,278]

ASSESSMENT

Data Collection

Subjective Data
• Person may or may not relate the following significant symptoms:
  Persistent, severe earache
  Nausea, vomiting, diarrhea (in small children)
  May complain of hearing loss
  Anorexia

Objective Data
• Person exhibits, during screening, clinical findings that are not within the standard normal range:
  Fever up to 105° F
  Otoscopic examination reveals erythematous and bulging tympanic membrane, indistinct landmarks, displaced light reflex, and possibly bloody or purulent drainage in the ear canal

Data Analysis

Nursing Diagnosis
POSITIVE SCREENING CUES FOR OTITIS MEDIA: Person has presented significant abnormal clinical findings during brief testing for middle-ear infection

Common Etiology (Stressors)
DISEASES: Adenoiditis, allergic rhinitis, hypertrophic adenoids, otitis media

PLANNING

Unmet Needs
Protection from physical harm, increased learning

Expected Outcome
Person will accept and act upon referral to a physician
Person will undergo further testing if recommended by the physician
Person will accept and participate in treatment if testing verifies the suspected diagnosis

NURSING INTERVENTIONS

Nursing Treatments
Consult with a physician (about the results of the screening test)
  OR
Make a referral to a physician

Nursing Observations
Determine the degree of insight that the person has (into the significance of the screening outcome)
Make a follow-up evaluation (to determine whether the suspected diagnosis was verified)

Health Teaching
Explain the meaning of the diagnostic report (in terms of suspected disease requiring further medical investigation)
Advise early correction of problems
Inform of the resources available for health care (so the person has several options)
Following a Confirmed Medical Diagnosis
Explain the causes of the problem (bacterial infection from *Hemophilus* or *Pneumococcus*)
Explain the reason for and intended effect of the therapy (to cure the infection)

EVALUATION

Record actual outcome

POSITIVE SCREENING CUES FOR STREPTOCOCCAL INFECTION[42,88]

ASSESSMENT

Data Collection

Subjective Data

• Person may or may not relate the following significant symptoms:
  Malaise
  Fatigue

Objective Data

• Person exhibits, during screening, clinical findings that are not within the standard normal range:
  Fever of 102–104° F
  Positive culture for streptococci
  Cellulitis (bright red, spreading area of inflammation on the skin)
  Impetigo (erythematous vesicular lesions, usually on the face)
  Pharyngitis/tonsillitis (white plaques of exudate on bright erythematous mucosa)
  Scarlet fever (a red, pinhead-size rash, more intense in the folds of the joints, absent on the face, a flushed face, a strawberry tongue)

Data Analysis

Nursing Diagnosis

POSITIVE SCREENING CUES FOR STREPTOCOCCAL INFECTION: Person has presented significant abnormal clinical findings during brief testing for the presence of streptococci in organ tissues

Common Etiology (Stressors)

DISEASES: Cellulitis, impetigo, pharyngitis, scarlet fever, tonsillitis

PLANNING

Unmet Needs

Protection from physical harm, increased learning

Expected Outcome

Person will accept and act upon referral to a physician
Person will undergo further testing if recommended by the physician
Person will accept and participate in treatment if testing verifies the suspected diagnosis

NURSING INTERVENTIONS

Nursing Treatments

Consult with a physician (about the results of the screening test)
  OR
Make a referral to a physician

Nursing Observations

Determine the degree of insight that the person has (into his symptoms and the significance of the screening outcome)
Make a follow-up evaluation (to determine whether the suspected diagnosis was verified)

Health Teaching

Explain the meaning of the diagnostic report (in terms of suspected disease requiring further medical investigation)
Advise early correction of problems
Inform of the resources available for health care (so the person has several options)
Following a Confirmed Medical Diagnosis
Explain the causes of the problem (a bacterial infection)
Explain how to prevent cross-infection (through hand washing, and avoiding direct contact with the infected person)

Explain the reason for and intended effect of the therapy (to cure the infection)

EVALUATION

Record actual outcome

POSITIVE SCREENING CUES FOR SYPHILIS[42,88,278,500]

ASSESSMENT

Data Collection

Subjective Data
• Person may or may not relate the following significant symptoms:
  History of sexual contacts
  Reports of genital, mouth, or skin lesions
  Variable rash (during the secondary stage)

Objective Data
• Person exhibits, during screening, clinical findings that are not within the standard normal range:
  Reactive VDRL (Venereal Disease Research Laboratory slide test) and RPR (rapid plasma reagin)
  OR
  Reactive FTA-ABS (Fluorescent Treponemal Antibody-Absorption test)

Data Analysis

Nursing Diagnosis
POSITIVE SCREENING CUES FOR SYPHILIS: Person has presented significant abnormal clinical findings during brief testing for the sexually transmitted disease, syphilis

Common Etiology (Stressors)
DISEASES: Syphilis

PLANNING

Unmet Needs
Protection from physical harm, increased learning

Expected Outcome
Person will accept and act upon referral to a physician
Person will undergo further testing if recommended by the physician
Person will accept and participate in treatment if testing verifies the suspected diagnosis

NURSING INTERVENTIONS

Nursing Treatments
Consult with a physician (about the results of the screening test)
  OR
Make a referral to a physician

Nursing Observations
Determine the degree of insight that the person has (into his symptoms and the significance of the screening outcome)
Make a follow-up evaluation (to determine whether the suspected diagnosis was verified)

Health Teaching
Explain the meaning of the diagnostic report (in terms of suspected disease requiring further medical investigation)
Advise early correction of problems
Inform of the resources available for health care (so the person has several options)

Following a Confirmed Medical Diagnosis
Explain the causes of the problem (sexual contact, bacterial infection)
Explain how to prevent cross-infection (the infected person should avoid direct contact
   with others)
Explain the reason for and intended effect of the therapy (to cure the infection)

EVALUATION

Record actual outcome

POSITIVE SCREENING CUES FOR TUBERCULOSIS[42,152,399]

ASSESSMENT
Data Collection
Subjective Data
• Person may or may not relate the following significant symptoms:
   Fatigue
   Anorexia
   Weight loss
   Night sweats
   Cough

Objective Data
• Person exhibits, during screening, clinical findings that are not within the standard
   normal range:
   Positive reaction to Mantoux (PPD) test (10 mm or more induration 48–72 hours af-
      ter intradermal injection of 0.1 ml serum)
   Positive reaction to tine or Mono Vacc test (5 mm or more induration 48–72 hours
      after intradermal injection)

Data Analysis
Nursing Diagnosis
POSITIVE SCREENING CUES FOR TUBERCULOSIS: Person has presented significant abnormal clini-
   cal findings during brief testing for tuberculosis

Common Etiology (Stressors)
DISEASES: Osteotuberculosis, pulmonary tuberculosis, spinal tuberculosis, tuberculosis
   meningitis, tuberculosis pericarditis, tuberculosis pyelonephritis

PLANNING
Unmet Needs
Protection from physical harm, increased learning

Expected Outcome
Person will accept and act upon referral to a physician
Person will undergo further testing if recommended by the physician
Person will accept and participate in treatment if testing verifies the suspected diagnosis

NURSING INTERVENTIONS
Nursing Treatments
Consult with a physician (about the results of the screening test)
   OR
Make a referral to a physician

Nursing Observations

Determine the degree of insight that the person has (into his symptoms and the significance of the screening outcome)

Make a follow-up evaluation (to determine whether the suspected diagnosis was verified)

Health Teaching

Explain the meaning of the diagnostic report (in terms of suspected disease requiring further medical investigation)

Advise early correction of problems

Inform of the resources available for health care (so the person has several options)

Following a Confirmed Medical Diagnosis

Explain the causes of the problem (a bacterial infection)

Explain how to prevent cross-infection (avoid contact with the infected person's sputum or airborne droplets)

Explain the reason for and intended effect of the therapy (to cure the infection, to prevent further infection)

EVALUATION

Record actual outcome

Screening for Integument Disorders

POSITIVE SCREENING CUES FOR SKIN CANCER[42,88,433,675]

ASSESSMENT

Data Collection

Subjective Data

• Person may or may not relate the following significant symptoms:
  Relates new sensations of pain, itching, or tenderness in a lesion

Objective Data

• Person exhibits during screening, clinical findings that are not within the standard normal range:

Changes in Skin, Including Warts, Moles, Birthmarks, Scars, Etc.

Color (a darkening, lightening, or spreading of color)

Size (a sudden increase in size)

Shape (the sudden elevation of a flat surface, smooth, regular borders becoming notched or irregular)

Surface (a scaling, flaking, ulceration, bleeding, bulging, mushrooming mass, a nonhealing wound)

Surrounding skin (redness or swelling of the surrounding skin, development of satellite lesions)

Data Analysis

Nursing Diagnosis

POSITIVE SCREENING CUES FOR SKIN CANCER: Person has presented significant abnormal clinical findings during brief testing for malignant lesions of the skin

Common Etiology (Stressors)

DISEASES: Basal cell carcinoma, malignant melanoma, squamous cell carcinoma

PLANNING

Unmet Needs

Protection from physical harm, increased learning

Expected Outcome

Person will accept and act upon referral to a physician

Person will undergo further testing if recommended by the physician

Person will accept and participate in treatment if testing verifies the suspected diagnosis

NURSING INTERVENTIONS

Nursing Treatments

Consult with a physician (about the results of the screening test)

    OR

Make a referral to a physician

Nursing Observations

Determine the degree of insight that the person has (into the significance of the screening outcome)

Make a follow-up evaluation (to determine whether the suspected diagnosis was verified)

Health Teaching

Explain the meaning of the diagnostic report (in terms of suspected disease requiring further medical investigation)

Advise early correction of problems

Inform of the resources available for health care (so the person has several options)

Following a Confirmed Medical Diagnosis

Explain the causes of the problem (exposure to the sun, changes in tissue cell structure)

Explain the reason for and intended effect of the therapy (to remove or arrest the cancer)

EVALUATION

Record actual outcome

Screening for Metabolic Disorders

POSITIVE SCREENING CUES FOR CYSTIC FIBROSIS[94,258]

ASSESSMENT

Data Collection

Subjective Data

• Parent may or may not relate the following significant symptoms:

    Recurrent pulmonary infections

    Diarrhea with greasy, floating stools

    Insatiable appetite

    History of meconium ileus

Objective Data

• Child exhibits, during screening, clinical findings that are not within the normal standard range:

    Retarded weight gain and growth measurements

    Infant's perspiration tastes salty

Elevated sodium and chloride in sweat (60 mEq/liter of sweat chloride is a positive sweat test)
Noisy, wheezing respirations
Cough with thick, tenacious secretions
Distended abdomen

Data Analysis

Nursing Diagnosis
POSITIVE SCREENING CUES FOR CYSTIC FIBROSIS (MUCOVISCIDOSIS): Child has presented significant abnormal clinical findings during brief testing for a disease of dysfunction of the pancreatic exocrine glands

Common Etiology (Stressors)
INHERITED FACTORS: Familial tendency
DISEASES: Cystic fibrosis

PLANNING

Unmet Needs
Protection from physical harm, increased learning

Expected Outcome
Parent will accept and act upon referral to a physician
Child will undergo further testing if recommended by the physician
Parent will accept and participate in treatment if testing verifies the suspected diagnosis

NURSING INTERVENTIONS

Nursing Treatments
Consult with a physician (about the results of the screening test)
  OR
Make a referral to a physician

Nursing Observations
Determine the degree of insight that the parents have (into the child's symptoms and the significance of the screening outcome)
Make a follow-up evaluation (to determine whether the suspected diagnosis was verified)

Health Teaching
Explain the meaning of the diagnostic report (in terms of suspected disease requiring further medical investigation)
Advise early correction of problems
Inform of the resources available for health care (so the parents have several options)

Following a Confirmed Medical Diagnosis
Explain the causes of the problem (hereditary dysfunction of the pancreas)

EVALUATION
Record actual outcome

POSITIVE SCREENING CUES FOR DIABETES MELLITUS[42,88,202]

ASSESSMENT

Data Collection

Subjective Data
• Person may or may not relate the following significant symptoms:
  Frequency of urination
  Thirst

Extreme hunger
Fatigue
Weakness
Blurred or changed vision
Weight loss

Objective Data
• Person exhibits, during screening, clinical findings that are not within the standard normal range:
Obesity (preceding the onset of symptoms)
Positive urine glucose test
Fasting blood glucose (FBS) above 120 mg/dl
Two-hour postprandial blood glucose (2-hour PPG) above 180 mg/dl

Data Analysis

Nursing Diagnosis
POSITIVE SCREENING CUES FOR DIABETES MELLITUS: Person has presented significant abnormal clinical findings during brief testing for an increased or decreased disturbance in the production of insulin or for impaired utilization of insulin

Common Etiology (Stressors)
INHERITED FACTORS: Infant of a diabetic mother, familial tendency for diabetes
DISEASES: Juvenile diabetes mellitus, adult diabetes mellitus, diabetes secondary to pancreatic cancer or chronic pancreatitis
HUMAN BODY: *Body state*: Secondary to pregnancy
HEALTH CARE FACTORS: *Drug therapy*: Adverse effects of contraceptives. *Surgical procedures*: Surgical removal of the pancreas

PLANNING

Unmet Needs
Protection from physical harm, increased learning

Expected Outcome
Person will accept and act upon referral to a physician
Person will undergo further testing if recommended by the physician
Person will accept and participate in treatment if testing verifies the suspected diagnosis

NURSING INTERVENTIONS

Nursing Treatments
Consult with a physician (about the results of the screening test)
    OR
Make a referral to a physician

Nursing Observations
Determine the degree of insight that the person has (into his symptoms and the significance of the screening outcome)
Make a follow-up evaluation (to determine whether further testing has verified the suspected diagnosis

Health Teaching
Explain the meaning of the diagnostic report (in terms of suspected disease requiring further medical investigation)
Advise early correction of problems
Inform of the resources available for health care (so the person has several options)

Following a Confirmed Medical Diagnosis
Explain the causes of the problem (impaired insulin secretion, excess production of glycogen, catecholamines, cortisol)
Explain the reason for and intended effect of the therapy (to reestablish adequate carbohydrate metabolism)

EVALUATION
Record actual outcome

POSITIVE SCREENING CUES FOR THYROID DISEASE[276,282,500]

ASSESSMENT

Data Collection

Subjective Data
• Person may or may not relate the following significant symptoms:

Hyperthyroidism
Tumor
Anxiety
Excessive appetite
Intolerance for heat
Weakness

Hypothryoidism
Lethargy
Intolerance for cold
Anorexia

Objective Data
• Person exhibits, during screening, clinical findings that are not within the standard normal range:

Hyperthyroidism
Elevated serum thyroxine (T7)
Visible swelling in the neck, sometimes
Palpable thyroid gland, sometimes
Bruit or thrill audible on auscultation of the thyroid gland
Tachycardia

Hypothyroidism
Decreased serum thyroxine (T7)
Bradycardia
Decreased tendon reflexes

Data Analysis

Nursing Diagnosis
POSITIVE SCREENING CUES FOR THYROID DISEASE: Person has presented significant abnormal clinical findings during brief testing for the thyroid gland's production and release of the hormone, thyroxine

Common Etiology (Stressors)
DISEASES: *Hyperthyroidism*: Thyrotoxicosis, thyroditis, thyroid carcinoma. *Hypothyroidism*: Myxedema (in adults), cretinism (in children)
HEALTH CARE FACTORS: *Surgical procedures*: Hypothyroidism from thyroidectomy or from radioactive iodine therapy

PLANNING

Unmet Needs
Protection from physical harm, increased learning

Expected Outcome
Person will accept and act upon referral to a physician
Person will undergo further testing if recommended by the physician
Person will accept and participate in treatment if testing verifies the suspected diagnosis

NURSING INTERVENTIONS

Nursing Treatments
Consult with a physician (about the results of the screening test)

OR

Make a referral to a physician

Nursing Observations

Determine the degree of insight that the person has (into his symptoms and the significance of the screening outcome)

Make a follow-up evaluation (to determine whether further testing has verified the suspected diagnosis)

Health Teaching

Explain the meaning of the diagnostic report (in terms of suspected disease requiring further medical investigation)

Advise early correction of problems

Inform of the resources available for health care (so the person has several options)

Following a Confirmed Medical Diagnosis

Explain the causes of the problem (excessive or decreased thyroxin production)

Explain the reason for and intended effect of the therapy (to reestablish normal thyroid function or maintain optimal replacement therapy)

EVALUATION

Record actual outcome

Screening for Musculoskeletal Disorders

POSITIVE SCREENING CUES FOR ARTHRITIC DISEASE[88,278,399,500]

ASSESSMENT

Data Collection

Subjective Data
- Person may or may not relate the following significant symptoms:
  Joint stiffness and aching
  Weakness
  Malaise

Objective Data
- Person exhibits, during screening, clinical findings that are not within the standard normal range:
  Joint swelling, tenderness, inflammation
  Weight loss
  Elevated sedimentation rate and/or positive C-reactive protein
  Decreased hemoglobin, hematocrit, and white blood cell count
  Positive rheumatoid factor
  Decreased range of motion of the affected joints

Data Analysis

Nursing Diagnosis

POSITIVE SCREENING CUES FOR ARTHRITIC DISEASE: Person has presented significant abnormal clinical findings during brief testing for conditions of joint inflammation or change in joint structure

Common Etiology (Stressors)

DISEASES: Bursitis, gout, myasitis, osteoarthritis, Raynaud's disease, rheumatic fever, rheumatoid arthritis, ulcerative colitis

PLANNING

Unmet Needs

Protection from physical harm, increased learning

Expected Outcome

Person will accept and act upon referral to a physician

Person will undergo further testing if recommended by the physician

Person will accept and participate in treatment if testing verifies the suspected diagnosis

NURSING INTERVENTIONS

Nursing Treatments

Consult with a physician (about the results of the screening test)

   OR

Make a referral to a physician

Nursing Observations

Determine the degree of insight that the person has (into his symptoms and the significance of the screening outcome)

Make a follow-up evaluation (to determine whether the suspected diagnosis was verified)

Health Teaching

Explain the meaning of the diagnostic report (in terms of suspected disease requiring further medical investigation)

Advise early correction of problems

Inform of the resources available for health care (so the person has several options)

Following a Confirmed Medical Diagnosis

Explain the causes of the problem (an inflammation reaction or degenerative changes in the joints)

EVALUATION

Record actual outcome

POSITIVE SCREENING CUES FOR GROWTH DISTURBANCE[234,462]

ASSESSMENT

Data Collection

Subjective Data

• Child may or may not relate the following significant symptoms:
   Growth problems

Objective Data

• Child exhibits, during screening, clinical findings that are not within the standard normal range:

Before Age 2

Variations of the head measurements, recumbent length, and standing height measurements, with a deviation above or below the two percentile lines on a growth chart

Variations in the child's weight for his height or length, a rate less than the 5th percentile indicating impaired growth, a rate greater than the 95th percentile indicating obesity

After Age 2

Only height and weight are evaluated

Data Analysis

Nursing Diagnosis

POSITIVE SCREENING CUES FOR GROWTH DISTURBANCE: A child has presented significant abnormal clinical findings during brief testing for variations from normal percentiles of growth in height, weight, and infant head circumference

Common Etiology (Stressors)

BIRTH DEFECTS: Cardiac anomalies, cleft lip and/or palate, craniostenosis, creatinism, cystic fibrosis, Down's syndrome, dwarfism, gastrointestinal tract atresia, giantism, hydrocephalus, microcephaly, Turner's syndrome

DISEASES: Celiac disease (sprue), malnutrition, other malabsorption syndromes, chronic renal insufficiency or failure

PSYCHOSOCIAL FACTORS: Lack of emotional stimuli from others

HEALTH CARE FACTORS: *Medical therapy:* Radiation therapy

PLANNING

Unmet Needs

Protection from physical harm, increased learning

Expected Outcome

Parent will accept and act upon referral of the child to a physician

Child will undergo further testing if recommended by the physician

Parent will accept and the child will participate in treatment if testing verifies the suspected diagnosis

NURSING INTERVENTIONS

Nursing Treatments

Consult with a physician (about the results of the screening test)
   OR
Make a referral to a physician

Nursing Observations

Determine the degree of insight that the parent has (into the significance of the screening outcome)

Make a follow-up evaluation (to determine whether the suspected diagnosis was verified)

Health Teaching

Explain the meaning of the diagnostic report (in terms of suspected disease requiring further medical investigation)

Advise early correction of problems

Inform of the resources available for health care (so the person has several options)

Following a Confirmed Medical Diagnosis

Explain the causes of the problem (if known, such as insufficient secretion of growth hormones, excessive food intake, etc.)

Explain the reason for and intended effect of the therapy (to support the maximum potential for growth)

EVALUATION

Record actual outcome

POSITIVE SCREENING CUES FOR LUMBAR DISC DISORDER[33,88,399]

ASSESSMENT

Data Collection

Subjective Data

• Person may or may not relate the following significant symptoms:
   Severe, sudden, unilateral low back pain

Unilateral pain radiation to the buttocks, legs, and feet
Numbness or tingling in the extremity
Burning pain in the foot

Objective Data

• Person exhibits, during screening, clinical findings that are not within the standard normal range:
Guarding position
Increased pain after coughing, sneezing, straining, or during the Valsalva maneuver
Posterior leg pain on straight-leg raising
Back pain on dorsiflexion of the foot
Limited range of motion of the back
Palpable tenderness over the intervertebral space
Depressed deep tendon reflexes (knee and ankle jerks)
Diminished sensory responses on pinprick examination

Data Analysis

Nursing Diagnosis

POSITIVE SCREENING CUES FOR LUMBAR DISC DISORDER: Person has presented significant abnormal clinical findings during brief testing for a disorder of the intervertebral discs

Common Etiology (Stressors)

INJURIES: Trauma to the back
DISEASES: Degenerative disc disease, degenerative joint disease of the spine

PLANNING

Unmet Needs

Protection from physical harm, increased learning

Expected Outcome

Person will accept and act upon referral to a physician
Person will undergo further testing if recommended by the physician
Person will accept and participate in treatment if testing verifies the suspected diagnosis

NURSING INTERVENTIONS

Nursing Treatments

Consult with a physician (about the results of the screening test)
OR
Make a referral to a physician

Nursing Observations

Determine the degree of insight that the person has (into his symptoms and the significance of the screening outcome)
Make a follow-up evaluation (to determine whether the suspected diagnosis was verified)

Health Teaching

Explain the meaning of the diagnostic report (in terms of suspected disease requiring further medical examination)
Advise early correction of problems
Inform of the resources available for health care (so the person has several options)

Following a Confirmed Medical Diagnosis

Explain the causes of the problem (heavy lifting, contusion injury, etc.)
Explain the reason for and intended effect of the therapy (to promote healing and reduce the pain)

EVALUATION

Record actual outcome

POSITIVE SCREENING CUES FOR MUSCULOSKELETAL DISEASE[33,399]

ASSESSMENT

Data Collection

Subjective Data

• Person may or may not relate the following significant symptoms:
Pain aggravated by joint movement or muscle use
Stiffness
Weakness
Fatigue

Objective Data

• Person exhibits, during screening, clinical findings that are not within the standard normal range:

Limitations in Range of Motion

Joints (swelling, deformity, redness, heat, tenderness)
Bones (crepitation, or a grating sensation on joint movement)
Muscle strength (decreased ability to grasp or squeeze a hand, difficulty pushing with the hand or foot against the examiner's palm, an abnormal gait)
Muscle tone (muscles are flaccid, spastic, rigid, or atrophied)

Data Analysis

Nursing Diagnosis

POSITIVE SCREENING CUES FOR MUSCULOSKELETAL DISEASE: Person has presented significant abnormal clinical findings during brief testing for the tone, strength, and functioning ability of muscles or for the alignment and integrity of skeletal bones

Common Etiology (Stressors)

BIRTH DEFECTS: Duchenne's muscular dystrophy
DISEASES: Acute tenosynovitis, bursitis, dermatomyositis, epicondylitis, ganglion, gout, Legg-Calve-Perthes disease, multiple sclerosis, osteoarthritis, polymyositis, rheumatoid arthritis, tendonitis

PLANNING

Unmet Needs

Protection from physical harm, increased learning

Expected Outcome

Person will accept and act upon referral to a physician
Person will undergo further testing if recommended by the physician
Person will accept and participate in treatment if testing verifies the suspected diagnosis

NURSING INTERVENTIONS

Nursing Treatments

Consult with a physician (about the results of the screening test)
    OR
Make a referral to a physician

Nursing Observations

Determine the degree of insight that the person has (into his symptoms and the significance of the screening outcome)
Make a follow-up evaluation (to determine whether the suspected diagnosis was verified)

Health Teaching

Explain the meaning of the diagnostic report (in terms of suspected disease requiring further medical investigation)
Advise early correction of problems
Inform of the resources available for health care (so the person has several options)

Following a Confirmed Medical Diagnosis
Explain the causes of the problem (heredity, immunologic changes, tissue injury, etc.)
Explain the reason for and intended effect of the therapy (to cure the disease and support maximum musculoskeletal function)

EVALUATION
Record actual outcome

POSITIVE SCREENING CUES FOR SCOLIOSIS[26,399]

ASSESSMENT
Data Collection

Subjective Data
• Child may or may not relate the following significant symptoms:
  Backache
  Fatigue
  Dyspnea
  Complains that clothing does not fit properly

Objective Data
• Child exhibits, during screening, clinical findings that are not within the standard normal range:

Examiner Seated, Examining Child from Rear
Child age 10–13 standing erect with feet together and arms hanging straight down exhibits:
  Unequal shoulder level
  Unequal hip level
  Uneven waistline
  Curved spine
  One usually prominent shoulder blade
  Unequal distances between the arms and body

Examiner Seated, Examining Child From Front and Rear
Child age 10–13 standing bent forward at the waist with feet together, knees unbent, arms hanging free, and palms together exhibits:
  Difference in the level between the two sides of the back
  Hump on one side of the upper back
  Hump on the other side of the lower back

Data Analysis

Nursing Diagnosis
POSITIVE SCREENING CUES FOR SCOLIOSIS: Child has presented significant abnormal clinical findings during brief testing for lateral curvature of the spine

Common Etiology (Stressors)
BIRTH DEFECTS: Cerebral palsy; dwarfism; Muscular dystrophy; myelomeningocele; wedged, fused, or hemivertebrae
DISEASES: Poliomyelitis, spinal cord tumor, nerve root irritation/inflammation, rheumatoid arthritis, rickets
INJURIES: Trauma to the back
HEALTH CARE FACTORS: *Medical therapy*: Radiation therapy (to the spine)

PLANNING
Unmet Needs
Protection from physical harm, increased learning

Expected Outcome
Person will accept and act upon referral to a physician
Person will undergo further testing if recommended by the physician
Person will accept and participate in treatment if testing verifies the suspected diagnosis

NURSING INTERVENTIONS

Nursing Treatments
Consult with a physician (about the results of the screening test)
  OR
Make a referral to a physician

Nursing Observations
Determine the degree of insight that the parent has (into the significance of the screening outcome)
Make a follow-up evaluation (to determine whether the suspected diagnosis was verified)

Health Teaching
Explain the meaning of the diagnostic report (in terms of suspected disease requiring further medical investigation)
Advise early correction of problems
Inform of the resources available for health care (so the person has several options)

Following a Confirmed Medical Diagnosis
Explain the causes of the problem (heredity, injury, infection, posture, etc.)
Explain the reason for and intended effect of the therapy (to reduce the deformity as much as possible)

EVALUATION
Record actual outcome

Screening for Neurologic Disorders

POSITIVE SCREENING CUES FOR DEVELOPMENTAL DELAY[234,239]

ASSESSMENT

Data Collection

Subjective Data
• Parent may or may not relate the following significant symptoms:
  Child's slowness
  Uncooperativeness
  Irritability
  Hypoactivity

Objective Data
• Child exhibits, during screening, clinical findings that are not within the standard normal range:

Denver Developmental Screening Test
Child fails to perform items performed by 90% of other children; this test includes the testing of gross motor and fine motor skills, language, and personal-social skills

Data Analysis
Nursing Diagnosis
POSITIVE SCREENING CUES FOR DEVELOPMENTAL DELAY: Child has presented significant abnormal

clinical findings during brief testing for a delay in the child's functioning ability at a specific age from infancy through the preschool years

Common Etiology (Stressors)
INHERITED FACTORS: Familial tendency of slow development
DISEASES: Anemia, autism, Down's syndrome, neurologic deficit, phenylketonuria (PKU)
SIGNS AND SYMPTOMS: Hearing loss, vision loss
PSYCHOSOCIAL FACTORS: Lack of emotional stimuli, lack of opportunity for play

PLANNING

Unmet Needs
Protection from physical harm, increased learning

Expected Outcome
Parent will accept and act upon referral of the child to a physician
Child will undergo further testing if recommended by the physician
Child will participate in treatment, if testing verifies the suspected diagnosis

NURSING INTERVENTIONS

Nursing Treatments
Consult with a physician (about the results of the screening test)
  OR
Make a referral to a physician

Nursing Observations
Determine the degree of insight that the parent has (into the significance of the screening outcome)
Make a follow-up evaluation (to determine whether the suspected diagnosis was verified)

Health Teaching
Explain the meaning of the diagnostic report (in terms of suspected disease requiring further medical investigation)
Advise early correction of problems
Inform of the resources available for health care (so the person has several options)

Following a Confirmed Medical Diagnosis
Explain the causes of the problem (heredity factors, malnutrition, poor nurturing)
Explain the reason for and intended effects of the therapy (to maximize the child's developmental potential)

EVALUATION
Record actual outcome

POSITIVE SCREENING CUES FOR NEUROLOGIC DISORDER [42,88,125,129]

ASSESSMENT

Data Collection

Subjective Data
• Person may or may not relate the following significant symptoms:
  Weakness
  Numbness
  Unsteadiness

Pain
Paresthesias
Double vision

Objective Data
• Person exhibits, during screening, clinical findings that are not within the standard normal range:
Mental status and speech
Impaired awareness, orientation, memory, intellectual performance, judgment, speech, mood, or affect

Sensory Changes
Impaired perception of:
Pain (pinprick test)
Vibration in the hands and feet (tuning-fork test)
Touch sensation (by cotton whisp or coin in the palm)
Temperature (hot or cold objects)

Abnormal Reflexes
Unilateral or bilateral increased or decreased deep tendon reflexes

Balance
Abnormal gait
Difficulty walking heel to toe in a straight line
Positive Rhomberg test (loss of balance when standing upright with feet together, and the eyes open and then closed)

Coordination (Position Sense)
Difficulty with point-to-point testing (inaccuracy in finger-to-nose and heel-down shin testing)
Difficulty with rapid, rhythmic alternating movements (touching each finger with the thumb in rapid sequence)

Muscle Tone and Strength
Decreased or increased muscle tone or rigidity when extremities are passively moved through range of motion
Diminished muscle strength, particularly with repetitive use of the muscle(s)

Cranial Nerves
Abnormal responses to cranial nerve testing, if such is done

Data Analysis

Nursing Diagnosis
POSITIVE SCREENING CUES FOR NEUROLOGIC DISORDER: Person has presented significant abnormal clinical findings during brief testing for disorders of the nervous system

Common Etiology (Stressors)
DISEASES: Amyotrophic lateral sclerosis, cerebrovascular accident, chronic alcoholism, diabetes mellitus, encephalitis, Guillain-Barré syndrome, Hansen's disease, intracranial hemorrhage, multiple sclerosis, myasthenia gravis, meningitis, neoplasms, neurosyphilis, Parkinson's disease, pernicious anemia
INJURIES: Cranial trauma, spinal trauma, peripheral nerve trauma, lead or mercury poisoning
HUMAN ERROR: Sniffing dangerous substances such as glue, benzene, gasoline

PLANNING

Unmet Needs
Protection from physical harm, increased learning

Expected Outcome
Person will accept and act upon referral to a physician
Person will undergo further testing if recommended by the physician
Person will accept and participate in treatment if testing verifies the suspected diagnosis

NURSING INTERVENTIONS

Nursing Treatments

Consult with a physician (about the results of the screening test)
> OR

Make a referral to a physician

Nursing Observations

Determine the degree of insight that the person has (into his symptoms and the significance of the screening outcome)

Make a follow-up evaluation (to determine whether the suspected diagnosis was verified)

Health Teaching

Explain the meaning of the diagnostic report (in terms of suspected disease requiring further medical investigation)

Advise early corrections of problems

Inform of the resources available for health care (so the person has several options)

Following a Confirmed Medical Diagnosis

Explain the causes of the problem (nerve degeneration, exposure to chemicals or radiation, tumors, etc.)

Explain the reason for and intended effect of the therapy (to reestablish maximum neurologic function)

EVALUATION

Record actual outcome

POSITIVE SCREENING CUES FOR NEWBORN NEUROMUSCULAR DEFICIT[133,239]

ASSESSMENT

Data Collection

Subjective Data

• Parent may or may not relate the following significant symptoms:
> Lethargy
> Somnolence
> Hypotonia (floppy baby)
> Periodic apnea

Objective Data

• Newborn exhibits, during screening, clinical findings that are not within the standard normal range:

Grasp Reflex

When the examiner's finger is placed across the newborn's palm, the infant does not grasp the finger as a normal infant would

Plantar Reflex

When the lateral sole of the foot is firmly but gently stroked from the heel upward to the toes the normal response of the newborn is the Babinski sign (dorsiflexion of the big toe and fanning of the other toes); curling of the toes downward or no toe movement is abnormal in the newborn

Rooting Reflex

When a finger is rubbed gently over the baby's cheek, lips, or corner of the mouth, the infant does not try to keep in contact with the finger as a normal infant would; instead he will only purse his lips

Sucking and Swallowing Reflex

When the infant's lips are touched, he does not suck and swallow as a normal infant would; instead he may not suck, suck only slightly, and have difficulty handling secretions

Absence of the Moro Reflex

During the first 3 months of life, when the infant is startled, he does not stiffen his body, bilaterally throw his arms up and out and draw up his legs as a normal infant would

Data Analysis

Nursing Diagnosis

POSITIVE SCREENING CUES FOR NEWBORN NEUROMUSCULAR DEFICIT: Newborn infant has presented significant abnormal clinical findings during brief testing for neuromuscular abnormalities

Common Etiology (Stressors)

BIRTH STATUS: Premature infant

BIRTH DEFECTS: Erythroblastosis fetalis, galactosemia

DISEASES: Hypoglycemia, kernicterus, septicemia

INJURIES: Birth injury (of the brain or spinal cord, intracranial bleeding)

SIGNS AND SYMPTOMS: Hypoxia, hypo-hyperkalemia

HEALTH CARE FACTORS: *Drug therapy*: Adverse drug effects (central nervous system depression from maternal sedation)

PLANNING

Unmet Needs

Protection from physical harm, increased learning

Expected Outcome

Parent will accept and act upon referral of the child to a physician

Child will undergo further testing if recommended by the physician

Parent will accept and will participate in the infant's treatment if testing verifies the suspected diagnosis

NURSING INTERVENTIONS

Nursing Treatments

Consult with a physician (about the results of the screening test)
> OR

Make a referral to a physician

Nursing Observations

Determine the degree of insight that the parent has (into the significance of the screening outcome)

Make a follow-up evaluation (to determine whether the suspected diagnosis was verified)

Health Teaching

Explain the meaning of the diagnostic reports (to the parents after the physician has consulted with the parents)

Advise early correction of problems

Inform of the resources available for health care (so the person has several options)

Following a Confirmed Medical Diagnosis

Explain the causes of the problem (prematurity, heredity, injury, etc.)

Explain the reason for and intended effect of the therapy (to prevent neurologic deterioration and support maximum function)

EVALUATION

Record actual outcome

POSITIVE SCREENING CUES FOR NEWBORN NEUROMUSCULAR OVERSTIMULATION[313]

ASSESSMENT

Data Collection

Subjective Data
• Parent may or may not relate the following significant symptoms:
  Irritability
  Crying, high-pitched screaming

Objective Data
• Newborn exhibits, during screening, clinical findings that are not within the normal standard range:
  Increased muscle tone (spasticity, rigidity)
  Jitteriness (jumps when touched)
  Abnormal posture
  Hyperactive deep-tendon reflexes

Data Analysis

Nursing Diagnosis
POSITIVE SCREENING CUES FOR NEWBORN NEUROMUSCULAR OVERSTIMULATION: Child has presented significant abnormal clinical findings during brief testing for excessive stimulation of the neurologic system

Common Etiology (Stressors)
BIRTH DEFECTS: Cerebral palsy (spastic)
DISEASES: Hypocalcemia, hypoglycemia, kernicterus, subarachnoid hemorrhage
HEALTH CARE FACTORS: *History*: A diabetic mother *Medical therapy*: Narcotic withdrawal

PLANNING

Unmet Needs
Protection from physical harm, increased learning

Expected Outcome
Parent will accept and act upon referral of the infant to a physician
Infant will undergo further testing if recommended by the physician
Parent will accept and will participate in the infant's treatment if testing verifies the suspected diagnosis

NURSING INTERVENTIONS

Nursing Treatments
Reduce infant handling to a minimum (except for the necessary examination)
Handle gently (but use firm, full-handed pressure when handling the infant)
Place only warm hands and objects on the infant
Consult with a physician (about the results of the screening test)
  OR
Make a referral to a physician

Nursing Observations
Determine the degree of insight that the parent has (into the infant's symptoms and the significance of the screening outcome)
Make a follow-up evaluation (to determine whether the suspected diagnosis was verified)

Health Teaching
Explain the meaning of the diagnostic report (in terms of suspected disease requiring further medical investigation)
Advise early correction of problems
Inform of the resources available for health care (so the parent has several options)
Advise minimal infant handling

Following a Confirmed Medical Diagnosis
Explain the causes of the problem (after the diagnosis is definite)
Explain the reason for and intended effect of the therapy (to reduce the excessive neurologic stimulation)

EVALUATION
Record actual outcome

POSITIVE SCREENING CUES FOR PHENYLKETONURIA [42,133,239,500]

ASSESSMENT
Data Collection
Subjective Data
• Parent may or may not relate the following significant symptoms:
  Failure to thrive
  Vomiting
  Irritability
  Screaming episodes
  Musty odor to the urine and perspiration

Objective Data
• Infant exhibits, during screening, clinical findings that are not within the standard normal range:
  Positive Phenistix for phenylketonuria
    OR
  Positive ferric chloride test for phenylketonuria
  Blonde, blue-eyed, very fair-skinned infant
  Eczematous lesions, frequently

Data Analysis
Nursing Diagnosis
POSITIVE SCREENING CUES FOR PHENYLKETONURIA: Infant has presented significant abnormal clinical findings during brief testing for evidence of a missing or inadequate liver enzyme phenylalanine hydroxylase, which may lead to mental retardation

Common Etiology (Stressors)
DISEASES: Phenylketonuria

PLANNING
Unmet Needs
Protection from physical harm, increased learning

Expected Outcome
Parent will accept and act upon referral of the child to a physician
Child will undergo further testing if recommended by the physician
Parent will accept and will participate in the child's treatment if testing verifies the suspected diagnosis

NURSING INTERVENTIONS
Nursing Treatments
Consult with a physician about the results of the screening test
  OR
Make a referral to a physician

Nursing Observations

Determine the degree of insight that the parent has (into the significance of the screening outcome)

Make a follow-up evaluation (to determine whether the suspected diagnosis was verified)

Health Teaching

Explain the meaning of the diagnostic report (in terms of suspected disease requiring further medical investigation)

Advise early correction of problems

Inform of the resources available for health care (so the person has several options)

Following a Confirmed Medical Diagnosis

Explain the causes of the problem (the absence of the enzyme phenylalanine hydroxylase causes an accumulation of phenylalanine in the blood; it is a hereditary factor)

Explain the reason for and intended effect of the therapy (to prevent developmental deficit)

EVALUATION

Record actual outcome

Screening for Pregnancy and Pregnancy Disorders

POSITIVE SCREENING CUES FOR PREGNANCY[214,527]

ASSESSMENT

Data Collection

Subjective Data

• Woman may or may not relate the following significant symptoms:
  Cessation of menstruation
  Increased breast size and fullness, pigmentation changes
  Frequent urination
  Nausea and vomiting (morning sickness)

Objective Data

• Woman exhibits, during screening, clinical findings that are not within the standard normal range for nonpregnancy:
  Positive serum pregnancy test (reliable as soon as the menstrual period is missed)
  Positive urine pregnancy test (95% reliable about 15 days after the first missed menstrual period)

Data Analysis

Nursing Diagnosis

POSITIVE SCREENING CUES FOR PREGNANCY: Woman has presented significant clinical findings during brief testing for verification that a woman has conceived a fetus

Common Etiology (Stressors)

HUMAN BODY: *Body state*: Pregnancy

PLANNING

Unmet Needs

Protection from physical harm, increased learning

Expected Outcome

Woman will accept and act upon referral to a physician

Woman will undergo further testing if recommended by the physician
Woman will accept and participate in prenatal care if testing verifies the suspected diagnosis

NURSING INTERVENTIONS

Nursing Treatments

Consult with a physician (about the results of the screening test)
   OR
Make a referral to a physician

Nursing Observations

Make a follow-up evaluation (to determine whether the suspected diagnosis was verified)

Health Teaching

Explain the meaning of the diagnostic reports
Inform of the resources available for health care (so the woman has several options)

Following a Confirmed Medical Diagnosis
Explain the reason for and intended effect of the prenatal care (to protect both mother and child and deliver a healthy infant)

EVALUATION

Record actual outcome

POSITIVE SCREENING CUES FOR A COMPLICATED PREGNANCY[214,527]

ASSESSMENT

Data Collection

Subjective Data
• Woman may or may not relate the following significant symptoms:
   Persistent vomiting beyond the 14th week of gestation
   Reports of vaginal bleeding
   Severe headaches
   Reports an absence of fetal movement later in the pregnancy
   Reports exposure to or contraction of an infection (measles, gonorrhea, syphilis, strep throat, etc.)

Objective Data
• Woman exhibits, during screening, clinical findings that are not within the standard normal range:
   Evidence of vaginal bleeding
   Hypertensive blood pressure (at or above 140/90; or a systolic rise of 30 mmHg or a diastolic rise of 15 mmHg above the baseline reading)
   Evidence of toxemia (hypertension, edema, proteinuria)
   Evidence of multiple fetuses (more than one fetal heart tone)
   Absence of fetal heart tones after 20 weeks' gestation
   Rh incompatibility revealed by an antibody screen (the paternal partner is Rh positive and the maternal partner Rh negative)
   Pregnancy extending beyond 42 weeks' gestation
   Premature labor (uterine contractions before 37 weeks' gestation)

Data Analysis

Nursing Diagnosis
POSITIVE SCREENING CUES FOR A COMPLICATED PREGNANCY: Woman has presented significant abnormal clinical findings during brief testing for evidence of an abnormal pregnancy

Common Etiology (Stressors)
BIRTH DEFECTS: Erythroblastosis fetalis, hydatidiform mole
INHERITED FACTORS: Maternal genetic Rh-negative factor
DISEASES: Abortion (spontaneous), abruptio placentae, cardiovascular disease, diabetes, hyperemesis gravidarum, placenta previa, sickle cell anemia

PLANNING
Unmet Needs
Protection from physical harm, increased learning

Expected Outcome
Woman will accept and act upon referral to a physician
Woman will undergo further testing if recommended by the physician
Woman will accept and participate in prenatal care if testing verifies the suspected diagnosis

NURSING INTERVENTIONS
Nursing Treatments
Consult with a physician (about the results of the screening test)
   OR
Make a referral to a physician

Nursing Observations
Determine the degree of insight that the woman has (into her symptoms and the significance of the screening outcome)
Make a follow-up evaluation (to determine whether the suspected diagnosis was verified)

Health Teaching
Explain the meaning of the diagnostic report (in terms of a suspected complication requiring medical investigation)
Advise early correction of problems (to prevent maternal or fetal injury)
Inform of the resources available for health care (so the woman has several options)

Following a Confirmed Medical Diagnosis
Explain the causes of the problem (a preexisting maternal disorder, malposition of the placenta, maternal nutritional/smoking/drinking habits, blood vessel spasm leading to hypertension, kidney damage, etc.)
Explain the reason for and intended effect of the therapy (to prevent injury to both mother and father)

EVALUATION
Record actual outcome

POSITIVE SCREENING CUES FOR A COMPLICATED LABOR AND DELIVERY[214,527]

ASSESSMENT
Data Collection
Subjective Data
• Woman may or may not relate the following significant symptoms:
   Excessively intense pain
   Fear or anxiety

Objective Data
• Woman exhibits, during screening, clinical findings that are not within the normal standard range:

Prolonged, or cessation of, uterine contractions

Prolonged, or cessation of, cervical dilatation (*Latent phase of labor*: Takes longer than 20 hours in a primigravida or 14 hours in a multigravida. *Active phase of labor*: Progresses less than or more than 1.25 cm/hour in a primigravida or 1.5 cm in a multigravida. *Deceleration phase*: Exceeds 3 hours in a primigravida or 1 hour in a multigravida, or no progress for 2 or more hours.)

Prolonged or arrested descent (progresses less than 1 cm/hour in primigravidas and 2 cm/hour in multigravidas or shows no descent in the second stage for at least 1 hour)

Hypotonic contractions (contractions of less than 40 seconds' duration or occurring more than 3 minutes apart)

Hypertonic contractions (ineffective contractions with a varied duration of 10–70 seconds, occurring 2–5 minutes apart)

Abnormal fetal presentation (breech, facial, or transverse presentation)

Umbilical cord prolapse

Slowed fetal heart tones

Data Analysis

Nursing Diagnosis

POSITIVE SCREENING CUES FOR A COMPLICATED LABOR AND DELIVERY: Woman has presented significant abnormal clinical findings indicating a complication during labor and delivery

PLANNING

Unmet Needs
Protection from physical harm, increased learning

Expected Outcome
Woman will immediately receive medical care

NURSING INTERVENTIONS

Nursing Treatments
Consult with a physician (immediately)

Attend the patient constantly (until a physician arrives)

Nursing Observations
Make a follow-up evaluation

Health Teaching
Explain the causes of the problem (whenever appropriate)

EVALUATION
Record actual outcome

POSITIVE SCREENING CUES FOR A COMPLICATED PUERPERIUM[214,527]

ASSESSMENT

Data Collection

Subjective Data

• Woman may or may not relate the following significant symptoms:

Reports of vaginal bleeding

Weakness, headache, pelvic pain, chills

Leg pain

Painful breasts, chills

Dysuria, frequency

Feeling depressed or "blue" for longer than 2 weeks

Objective Data
- Woman exhibits, during screening, clinical findings that are not within the standard normal range:

    Evidence of vaginal bleeding (normally, there is some blood flow for several hours postpartum, but it gradually decreases)

    Puerperal infection (fever above 38° C, 100.4° F, which occurs between the 2nd and 10th postpartum day and remains elevated for at least 24 hours, abdominal tenderness, profuse lochia or a foul odor from the lochia)

    Thrombophlebitis (unilateral leg edema and heat, Homan's sign, i.e., pain on dorsiflexion of the foot)

    Breast infection (fever of 39.4° C, 103° F, to 40° C, 104° F between the first and fourth weeks after delivery, breast redness, palpable breast hardness)

    Bladder or kidney infection (bacteriuria of 100,000 bacteria or more)

    Uterine subinvolution (palpation indicates a uterus that is larger and softer than is normal for the postpartum day, profuse and bright red lochia)

Data Analysis

Nursing Diagnosis
POSITIVE SCREENING CUES FOR A COMPLICATED PUERPERIUM: Woman has presented significant abnormal clinical findings during brief testing for abnormal findings during the 6-week period after maternal delivery

Common Etiology (Stressors)
DISEASES: Cystitis, diabetes, endometritis, mastitis, pyelitis, thrombophlebitis, thrombophlebosis

PLANNING

Unmet Needs
Protection from physical harm, increased learning

Expected Outcome
Woman will accept and act upon referral to a physician
Woman will undergo further testing if recommended by the physician
Woman will accept and participate in treatment if testing verifies the suspected diagnosis

NURSING INTERVENTIONS

Nursing Treatments
Consult with a physician (about the results of the screening test)
    OR
Make a referral to a physician

Nursing Observations
Determine the degree of insight that the woman has (into her symptoms and the significance of the screening outcome)
Make a follow-up evaluation (to determine whether the suspected diagnosis was verified)

Health Teaching
Explain the meaning of the diagnostic report (in terms of a suspected complication requiring further medical investigation)
Advise early correction of problems
Inform of the resources available for health care (so the person has several options)
Following a Confirmed Medical Diagnosis
Explain the causes of the problem (bacterial infection, birth trauma, retention of placental fragments)
Explain the reason for and intended effect of the therapy (to restore health)

EVALUATION
Record actual outcome

Screening for Psychosocial Behavioral Disorders

POSITIVE SCREENING CUES FOR CHILD ABUSE[259,438]

ASSESSMENT

Data Collection

Subjective Data

- Person (child or concerned adult) may or may not relate the following significant symptoms:

  Child relates distrust of adults

  Constantly fears doing something wrong or getting into trouble

  Wants desperately to please the abusing adult

  Child is aware that the parents' needs must be met first

  Parent has a history of being a victim of abuse

Objective Data

- Child exhibits, during screening, clinical findings that are not within the standard normal range:

Behavioral Findings

Child behaves positively toward the abusive adult, is hypervigilant on the watch to avoid trouble, is stoic, lacks spontaneity, displays little eye contact, is obedient and compliant

OR

Child is negative, aggressive, hyperactive, cannot play harmoniously with other children (hits other children, prescribes punishment for them), is inattentive to directions

Physical Findings

Physical injury such as bruises, welts, scratches, cuts, scars, burns, fractures, abdominal or central nervous system injury

OR

Child is underweight, yet when hospitalized and properly nourished will gain more than 2 ounces per day for at least 1 week

OR

Child is purposely drugged

OR

Child, under age 18, is sexually exploited

Other Findings

Child is not brought in for recommended medical care for chronic illness

OR

Child is abandoned

OR

Child, under age 12, is frequently left alone, day or night, without adult or baby sitter attendance

OR

Child is deprived of an education as guaranteed by law

Data Analysis

Nursing Diagnosis

POSITIVE SCREENING CUES FOR CHILD ABUSE: Child has presented significant clinical findings during brief testing for the characteristics of a child who has been a victim of violence or criminal negligence

Common Etiology (Stressors)

PSYCHOSOCIAL FACTORS: The highly dependent personality of a parent, exposure as a child to an abusive or violent role model, use of ineffective defense mechanisms such as projecting anger onto the child

SITUATIONAL FACTORS: Situational crisis or stress

PLANNING

Unmet Needs

Protection from physical harm and psychologic threat, increased learning

Expected Outcome

Person will accept and act upon referral of the child to a physician

Person will accept and participate in the child's treatment if testing verifies the suspected diagnosis

NURSING INTERVENTIONS

Nursing Treatments

Consult with a physician (about the results of the screening test)
   OR
Make a referral to a physician (who will report the child abuse to the appropriate agency as stipulated by law)

Nursing Observations

Determine the degree of insight that the person has (into the significance of the screening outcome)

Make a follow-up evaluation (to determine whether further investigation verified the suspected diagnosis)

Health Teaching

Explain the meaning of the diagnostic report (in terms of suspected abuse requiring further medical investigation)

Advise early correction of problems

Inform of the resources available for health care (so the child and abuser have several options)

Following a Confirmed Medical Diagnosis

Explain the causes of the problem (adult use of ineffective coping mechanisms)

Explain the reason for and intended effect of the therapy (to restore the child's health and prevent further abuse)

EVALUATION

Record actual outcome

POSITIVE SCREENING CUES FOR CHILD ABUSER[259,438]

ASSESSMENT

Data Collection

Subjective Data

• Person may or may not relate the following significant symptoms:
   Person has a history of having been abused as a child
   Did not receive positive nurturing from parental figures

Relates a continuous search for security and love that is never found

The abuser relates fantasizing that the child will meet his emotional needs and enable him to feel wanted and loved

Verbalizes strong dependency needs

Expresses intolerance for the child's dependency

Expects the child to perform as an adult

Objective Data

• Person exhibits, during screening, clinical findings that are not within the standard normal range:

Dependent Parental Behavior

Parent has the child waiting on him, has the child performing tasks inappropriate for the child's developmental level

Aggressive Parental Behavior

Continually shames or demeans the child

Becomes angry when the child cries, whines, or is unpleasant

Severely punishes the child when the child does not act as an adult

Data Analysis

Nursing Diagnosis

POSITIVE SCREENING CUES FOR CHILD ABUSER: Person has presented significant abnormal clinical findings during brief testing for the characteristics of a parental figure who uses violence against children

Common Etiology (Stressors)

PSYCHOSOCIAL FACTORS: The highly dependent personality of a parent, exposure as a child to an abusive or violent role model, use of ineffective defense mechanisms such as projecting anger onto a child

SITUATIONAL FACTORS: Situational crisis or stress

PLANNING

Unmet Needs

Child: Protection from physical harm and psychologic threat. *Abuser*: Increased learning

Expected Outcome

Abuser will accept and act upon referral to a physician, psychologist, etc.

Abuser will undergo further testing if recommended by the health professional

Abuser will accept and participate in treatment if testing verifies the suspected diagnosis

NURSING INTERVENTIONS

Nursing Treatments

Consult with a physician/psychologist (about the results of the screening test)

    OR

Make a referral to a physician/psychologist (and report child abuse to the appropriate agency as stipulated by law)

Nursing Observations

Determine the degree of insight that the abuser has (into the significance of the screening outcome)

Make a follow-up evaluation (to determine whether the suspected diagnosis was verified)

Health Teaching

Advise early correction of problems

Inform of the resources available for health care (so the person has several options)

Following a Confirmed Medical Diagnosis

Explain the causes of the problem (poor role modeling, ineffective coping, etc.)

Explain the reason for and intended effect of the therapy (to prevent further child abuse and support effective coping by the involved adult)

EVALUATION

Record actual outcome

POSITIVE SCREENING CUES FOR MALADAPTIVE BEHAVIOR[105,471]

ASSESSMENT
Data Collection
Subjective Data
• Person may or may not relate the following significant symptoms:
Person consistently fails to function in social roles
Does not live up to the expectations of his culture
Person does not know of more effective methods for meeting his needs

Objective Data
• Person exhibits, during screening, clinical findings that are not within the standard normal range:
Exhibits patterns of behavior that are a problem for himself or others

Data Analysis
Nursing Diagnosis
POSITIVE SCREENING CUES FOR MALADAPTIVE BEHAVIOR: Person has presented significant abnormal clinical findings during brief testing for severe difficulty in coping with daily living problems

Common Etiology (Stressors)
PSYCHOSOCIAL FACTORS: Lack of competency in coping with everyday problems, lack of early learning of effective coping mechanisms, the presence of reinforcing stimuli which maintain maladaptive behavior

PLANNING
Unmet Needs
Protection from physical harm and psychologic threat, increased learning
Expected Outcome
Person will accept and act upon referral to a psychiatrist or psychologist
Person will undergo further testing if recommended by the psychiatrist or psychologist
Person will accept and participate in treatment if testing verifies the suspected diagnosis

NURSING INTERVENTIONS
Nursing Treatments
Consult with a physician (about the results of the screening test)
  OR
Make a referral (to a psychiatric nurse specialist or psychiatrist so that the maladaptive behavior and the reinforcing stimuli for maladaptive behavior can be specifically identified)
Nursing Observations
Determine the degree of insight that the person has (into the significance of the screening outcome)
Make a follow-up evaluation (to determine what the specific diagnosis is)
Health Teaching
Advise early correction of problems
Inform of the resources available for health care (so the person has several options)

Following a Confirmed Medical Diagnosis
Explain the reason for and intended effect of the therapy (to promote effective coping)

EVALUATION
Record actual outcome

POSITIVE SCREENING CUES FOR SUBSTANCE (ALCOHOL OR DRUG) ABUSE[17,19,35,93,445,471]

ASSESSMENT

Data Collection

Subjective Data
- Person may or may not relate the following significant symptoms:
    Use of alcohol or drugs for a consistent period of time
    Need for daily use of the substance
    Repeated, unsuccessful attempts to withdraw from the use of the substance
    Use interferes with the functions of daily living and with interactions with others
    Amnesic periods during substance use

Objective Data
- Person exhibits, during screening, clinical findings that are not within the standard normal range:
    Elevated blood alcohol level
        OR
    Needle marks over veins
        OR
    Tissue damage in the nostrils
    Behavior indicating impaired function (slurred speech, confusion, staggering gait, illogical thinking)

Data Analysis

Nursing Diagnosis
POSITIVE SCREENING CUES FOR SUBSTANCE (ALCOHOL OR DRUG) ABUSE: Person has presented significant abnormal clinical findings during brief testing for the excessive use of alcohol or drugs

Common Etiology (Stressors)
LIFESTYLE: Alcohol abuse, drug abuse (barbiturates, sedatives, hypnotics, opioids, amphetamines, sympathomimetics, cannabis, cocaine, phencyclidine, arylcyclohexylamines, hallucinogens)

PLANNING

Unmet Needs
Protection from physical harm and psychologic threat, increased learning

Expected Outcome
Person will accept and act upon referral to a physician
Person will undergo further testing if recommended by the physician
Person will accept and participate in treatment if testing verifies the suspected diagnosis

NURSING INTERVENTIONS
Consult with a physician (about the results of the screening test)
    OR
Make a referral to a physician

Nursing Observations
Determine the degree of insight that the person has (into the significance of the screening outcome)
Make a follow-up evaluation (to determine whether the suspected diagnosis was verified)

Health Teaching
Explain the meaning of the diagnostic report (in terms of suspected abuse requiring further medical investigation)

Advise early correction of problems

Inform of the resources available for health care (so the person has several options)

Following a Confirmed Medical Diagnosis

Explain the causes of the problem (the use of ineffective coping methods)

Explain the reason for and intended effect of the therapy (to substitute substance abuse with more effective coping)

EVALUATION

Record actual outcome

POSITIVE SCREENING CUES FOR SUBSTANCE (ALCOHOL OR DRUG) DEPENDENCE[17,19,445,471]

ASSESSMENT

Data Collection

Subjective Data

• Person may or may not relate the following significant symptoms:

Use of alcohol or drugs for a consistent period of time

Need for daily use of the substance

Repeated unsuccessful attempts to withdraw from the substance

Compelling desire for the substance

Diminished effect felt with the regular use of the same dose of the drug or alcohol

Gradually increasing amount of the substance used to achieve the desired effect

Physiologic discomforts such as the "shakes" relieved by the substance or occur after the reduction or cessation of the use of the substance

Problems with the family, on the job, or with legal authorities

Amnesic periods during substance use

Objective Data

• Person exhibits, during screening, clinical findings that are not within the standard normal range:

Elevated blood alcohol level

OR

Needle marks over veins

Behavior indicating impaired function (slurred speech, confusion, staggering gait, illogical thinking)

Data Analysis

Nursing Diagnosis

POSITIVE SCREENING CUES FOR SUBSTANCE (ALCOHOL OR DRUG) DEPENDENCE: Person has presented significant abnormal clinical findings during brief testing for an inability to function without certain amounts of a drug or alcohol

Common Etiology (Stressors)

DISEASES: Alcoholism

LIFESTYLES: Alcohol dependence, drug dependence (barbiturates, sedatives, hypnotics, opioids, amphetamines, sympathomimetics, cannabis), high nicotine intake

PLANNING

Unmet Needs

Protection from physical harm and psychologic threat, increased learning

Expected Outcome

Person will accept and act upon referral to a physician

Person will undergo further testing if recommended by the physician

Person will accept and participate in treatment if testing verifies the suspected diagnosis

NURSING INTERVENTIONS

Nursing Treatments

Consult with a physician (about the results of the screening test)

OR

Make a referral to a physician

Nursing Observations

Determine the degree of insight that the person has (into the significance of the screening outcome)

Make a follow-up evaluation (to determine whether the suspected diagnosis was verified)

Health Teaching

Explain the meaning of the diagnostic report (in terms of suspected disease requiring further medical investigation)

Advise early correction of problems

Inform of the resources available for health care (so the person has several options)

Following a Confirmed Medical Diagnosis

Explain the causes of the problem (the use of ineffective coping mechanisms)

Describe the specific dangerous effects of poor health practices (the effects of alcohol and the specific drug on the body, such as liver cell damage, brain cell damage with impaired thinking ability)

Explain the reason for and intended effect of the therapy (to cure the substance dependency)

EVALUATION

Record actual outcome

Screening for Reproductive System Disorders

POSITIVE SCREENING CUES FOR A BREAST MASS [33,125,214]

ASSESSMENT

Data Collection

Subjective Data

• Person may or may not relate the following significant symptoms:

Awareness of a lump in the breast

Pain or tenderness in the breast

Objective Data
• Person exhibits, during screening, clinical findings that are not within the standard normal range:

Probable Benign Mass
Palpable round, rubbery, freely moving breast mass
One or more nodular masses
May have nipple discharge or retraction

Probable Malignant Mass
Palpable firm, dense, irregularly shaped mass
Found in the upper, outer breast quadrant
Palpable axillary lymph nodes
May have a nipple discharge or retraction
Usually a single mass
May have skin changes such as dimpling, orange-peel appearance, or ulceration

Data Analysis

Nursing Diagnosis
POSITIVE SCREENING CUES FOR A BREAST MASS: Person has presented significant abnormal clinical findings during brief testing for lumps in the breast

Common Etiology (Stressors)
DISEASES: *Benign masses*: Cystic hyperplasia, fibroadenoma, fibrocystic disease, intraductal papilloma, mammary duct ectasia. *Malignant masses*: Ductal carcinomas, adenocarcinomas

PLANNING

Unmet Needs
Protection from physical harm, increased learning

Expected Outcome
Person will accept and act upon referral to a physician
Person will undergo further testing if recommended by the physician
Person will accept and participate in treatment if testing verifies the suspected diagnosis

NURSING INTERVENTIONS

Nursing Treatments
Consult with a physician (about the results of the screening test)
　OR
Make a referral to a physician

Nursing Observations
Determine the degree of insight that the person has (into his symptoms and the significance of the screening outcome)
Make a follow-up evaluation (to determine whether the suspected diagnosis was verified)

Health Teaching
Explain the meaning of the diagnostic report (in terms of suspected disease requiring further medical investigation)
Advise early correction of problems
Inform of the resources available for health care (so the person has several options)

Following a Confirmed Medical Diagnosis
Explain the causes of the problem (a hormonal imbalance, adverse effects of drugs, changes in the tissue cell structure)
Explain the reason for and intended effect of the therapy (to reduce or remove the mass)

EVALUATION

Record actual outcome

POSITIVE SCREENING CUES FOR CERVICAL CANCER[214,474]

ASSESSMENT

Data Collection

Subjective Data

• Woman may or may not relate the following significant symptoms:
  Watery vaginal discharge
  Abnormal menstrual bleeding
  Intermenstrual bleeding
  Postmenopausal bleeding

Objective Data

• Woman exhibits, during screening, clinical findings that are not within the standard normal range:
  Papanicolaou test shows atypical cells shed from the cervix, listed as a class (III, doubtful; IV, suspicious for malignancy; V, malignancy present)

Data Analysis

Nursing Diagnosis

POSITIVE SCREENING CUES FOR CERVICAL CANCER: Woman has presented significant abnormal clinical findings during brief testing for evidence of abnormal cervical cells

Common Etiology (Stressors)

DISEASES: Adenocarcinoma, squamous cell carcinoma

PLANNING

Unmet Needs

Protection from physical harm, increased learning

Expected Outcome

Woman will accept and act upon referral to a physician
Woman will undergo further testing if recommended by the physician
Woman will accept and participate in treatment if testing verifies the suspected diagnosis

NURSING INTERVENTIONS

Nursing Treatments

Consult with a physician (about the results of the screening test)
  OR
Make a referral to a physician

Nursing Observations

Determine the degree of insight that the woman has (into the significance of the screening outcome)
Make a follow-up evaluation (to determine whether the suspected diagnosis was verified)

Health Teaching

Explain the meaning of the diagnostic report (in terms of suspected disease requiring further medical investigation)
Advise early correction of problem
Inform of the resources available for health care (so the woman has several options)

Following a Confirmed Medical Diagnosis

Explain the causes of the problem (hormonal changes, changes in the tissue cell structure)
Explain the reason for and intended effect of the therapy (to prevent metastasis of the cancer, to remove the cancer when possible)

EVALUATION

Record actual outcome

POSITIVE SCREENING CUES FOR A VAGINAL INFECTION[88,214]

ASSESSMENT
Data Collection
Subjective Data
- Woman may or may not relate the following significant symptoms:
    Vaginal itching
    Burning sensation
    Dysuria
    Dyspareunia

Objective Data
- Woman exhibits, during screening, clinical findings that are not within the standard normal range:

Vaginal discharge
    White, cheesy discharge (*Candida*)
    Yellowish-green, frothy, foul-smelling discharge (*Trichomonas*)
    Grayish-white foul-smelling discharge (*Hemophilus*)
    Thick, purulent discharge (bacteria or gonorrhea)

Data Analysis
Nursing Diagnosis
POSITIVE SCREENING CUES FOR A VAGINAL INFECTION: Woman has presented significant, abnormal clinical findings during brief testing for an infection of the vagina

Common Etiology (Stressors)
DISEASES: *Candida albicans*, cervicitis, diabetes mellitus, gonorrhea, *Hemophilus vaginalis*, *trichomonas vaginalis*
HEALTH CARE FACTORS: *Drugs*: Adverse antibiotics, oral contraceptives, vaginal suppositories
HUMAN ERROR: Chronic and excessive use of douches

PLANNING
Unmet Needs
Protection from physical harm, increased learning

Expected Outcome
Woman will accept and act upon referral to a physician
Woman will undergo further testing if recommended by the physician
Woman will accept and participate in treatment if testing verifies the suspected diagnosis

NURSING INTERVENTIONS
Nursing Treatments
Consult with a physician (about the results of the screening test)
    OR
Make a referral to a physician

Nursing Observations
Determine the degree of insight that the woman has (into her symptoms and the significance of the screening outcome)
Make a follow-up evaluation (to determine whether the suspected diagnosis was verified)

Health Teaching
Explain the meaning of the diagnostic report (in terms of suspected disease requiring further medical investigation)
Advise early correction of problems
Inform of the resources available for health care (so the woman has several options)

Following a Confirmed Medical Diagnosis
Explain the causes of the problem (yeast or bacterial infection, sexual contact, faulty hygiene)
Explain the reason for and intended effect of the therapy (to cure the infection)

EVALUATION
Record actual outcome

Screening for Respiratory Disorders

POSITIVE SCREENING CUES FOR RESPIRATORY DISORDER [33,125,150,399]

ASSESSMENT
Data Collection
Subjective Data
• Person may or may not relate the following significant symptoms:
Dyspnea
Cough
Sputum
Hemoptysis
Pain with chest movement
Anxiety
Night sweats
Objective Data
• Person exhibits, during screening, clinical findings that are not within the standard normal range:
Cyanosis
Abnormal chest configuration (barrel, tunnel, or region chest)
Abnormal respiratory rate (rapid or slow breathing)
Abnormal breathing pattern/rhythm (retraction or bulging of the interspaces, cessation of or periodic breathing, prolonged expiration, increased respiratory depth)
Increased effort to breathe
Percussion dullness (fluid or solid tissue instead of air in the lungs)
Abnormal breath sounds
Adventitious sounds (rales, rhonchi, wheezes, pleural friction rubs)
Absence of breath sounds (when an area is not ventilated, as in atelectasis or pneumothorax)
Stertorous (a snoring sound due to upper airway obstruction)
Stridor (a crowing sound on inspiration due to laryngeal obstruction)
Changes in vocal resonance
Egophony ("E" is heard through chest wall as "A")
Pectoriloquy (a whisper sound heard distinctly over consolidated lung tissue)
Abnormal blood gases (if available)
Abnormal spirometry (when available)

Data Analysis
Nursing Diagnosis
POSITIVE SCREENING CUES FOR RESPIRATORY DISORDER: Person has presented significant abnormal clinical findings during brief testing for a disorder of the respiratory or ventilating system

Common Etiology (Stressors)
DISEASES: Asthma, atelectasis, bronchitis, bronchogenic carcinoma, chronic obstructive pulmonary disease, emphysema, laryngitis, pleural effusion, pleurisy, pneumonia, pneumothorax, pulmonary embolus, pulmonary edema
INJURIES: Foreign body in larynx, nose, pharynx

PLANNING

Unmet Needs
Protection from physical harm, increased learning

Expected Outcome
Person will accept and act upon referral to a physician
Person will undergo further testing if recommended by the physician
Person will accept and participate in treatment if testing verifies the suspected diagnosis

NURSING INTERVENTIONS

Nursing Treatments
Consult with a physician (about the results of the screening test)
 OR
Make a referral to a physician

Nursing Observations
Determine the degree of insight that the person has (into his symptoms and the significance of the screening outcome)
Make a follow-up evaluation (to determine whether the suspected diagnosis was verified)

Health Teaching
Explain the meaning of the diagnostic report (in terms of suspected disease requiring further medical investigation)
Advise early correction of problems
Inform of the resources available for health care (so the person has several options)

Following a Confirmed Medical Diagnosis
Explain the causes of the problem (viral or bacterial infection, tumors, traumatic injury, bronchospasm)
Explain the reason for and intended effect of the therapy (to restore the maximum respiratory function)

EVALUATION

Record actual outcome

Screening for Sensory Disorders

POSITIVE SCREENING CUES FOR CATARACTS[33,124,278,731]

ASSESSMENT

Data Collection

Subjective Data
• Person may or may not relate the following significant symptoms:
 Blurred (or dimmed) vision for a prolonged period

No eye pain

Objective Data

• Person exhibits, during screening, clinical findings that are not within the normal standard range:

Flashlight Examination

The opacity (milky-white) of the lens may be seen through the pupil when a mature cataract ("ripe" or "overripe") is present, immature cataracts may not be seen with a flashlight

Ophthalmoscopic Examination

The opacity of the lens (immature cataracts) makes it difficult to see the retina and gives the appearance of black defects in the red retinal reflex, mature cataracts are centrally located and may completely block the red reflex

Data Analysis

Nursing Diagnosis

POSITIVE SCREENING CUES FOR CATARACTS: Person has presented significant abnormal clinical findings during brief testing for milky-white opacities of the lenses that adversely affect vision

Common Etiology (Stressors)

BIRTH DEFECTS: Congenital rubella, mongolism

DISEASES: Diabetes mellitus

INJURIES: Trauma to the lens, poisoning (with toxic chemicals or drugs)

DEVELOPMENTAL PHASES: Old age (over age 60)

ENVIRONMENTAL FACTORS: *Radiation*: Exposure to radiation

PLANNING

Unmet Needs

Protection from physical harm, increased learning

Expected Outcome

Person will accept and act upon referral to a physician

Person will undergo further testing if recommended by the physician

Person will accept and participate in treatment if testing verifies the suspected diagnosis

NURSING INTERVENTIONS

Nursing Treatments

Consult with a physician (about the results of the screening test)

   OR

Make a referral to a physician

Nursing Observations

Determine the degree of insight that the person has (into his symptoms and the significance of the screening outcome)

Make a follow-up evaluation (to determine whether the suspected diagnosis was verified)

Health Teaching

Explain the meaning of the diagnostic report (in terms of suspected disease requiring further medical investigation)

Advise early correction of problems

Inform of the resources available for health care (so the person has several options)

Explain the causes of the problem (after the diagnosis is definite)

EVALUATION

Record actual outcome

POSITIVE SCREENING CUES FOR GLAUCOMA [33,124,278,399]

ASSESSMENT

Data Collection

Subjective Data
• Person may or may not relate the following significant symptoms:
  Loss of peripheral vision
  Decreased visual acuity, especially at night
  Sees halos around lights
  Persistent dull eye pain, headache

Objective Data
• Person exhibits, during screening, clinical findings that are not within the standard normal range:
  Visual field test indicating narrowed peripheral vision
  Tonometry readings indicating increased intraoccular pressure (normal is 13 to 22)

Data Analysis

Nursing Diagnosis
POSITIVE SCREENING CUES FOR GLAUCOMA: Person has presented significant abnormal clinical findings during brief testing for the eye disease, glaucoma

Common Etiology (Stressors)
DISEASES: Chronic open-angle glaucoma

PLANNING

Unmet Needs
Protection from physical harm, increased learning

Expected Outcome
Person will accept and act upon referral to a physician
Person will undergo further testing if recommended by the physician
Person will accept and participate in treatment if testing verifies the suspected diagnosis

NURSING INTERVENTIONS

Nursing Treatments
Consult with a physician (about the results of the screening test)
  OR
Make a referral to a physician

Nursing Observations
Determine the degree of insight that the person has (into his symptoms and the significance of the screening outcome)
Make a follow-up evaluation (to determine whether the suspected diagnosis was verified)

Health Teaching
Explain the meaning of the diagnostic report (in terms of suspected disease requiring further medical investigation)
Advise early correction of problems
Inform of the resources available for health care (so the person has several options)

Following a Confirmed Medical Diagnosis
Explain the causes of the problem (hereditary predisposition, increased intraoccular pressure causing optic atrophy with vision loss)
Explain the reason for and intended effect of the therapy (to maximize vision, retard progression of the disease)

EVALUATION

Record actual outcome

POSITIVE SCREENING CUES FOR HEARING LOSS[33,282,399]

ASSESSMENT

Data Collection

Subjective Data
* Person may or may not relate the following significant symptoms:
  Decreased hearing acuity
  Does not pay attention
  Makes poor grades in school
  Responds inappropriately to questions/comments
  Tinnitus

Objective Data
* Person exhibits, during screening, clinical findings that are not within the standard normal range:
  Rinne test indicating longer bone conduction (BC) than air conduction (AC); normally AC is twice as long as BC
  Schwabach test indicating perceptive (sensorineural) hearing loss or conductive hearing loss as compared with the examiner's hearing; in conductive hearing loss, the person hears the tone (by tuning fork) longer than the examiner hears it; in perceptive hearing loss, the person hears the tone a shorter time than the examiner hears it
  Weber test indicating perceptive (sensorineural) hearing loss or conductive hearing loss; normally the tuning fork sound is heard equally in both ears; in perceptive hearing loss, the sound lateralizes to the normal ear; in conductive hearing loss, the sound lateralizes to the hearing-impaired ear
  Abnormal tone audiometry; audiometric readings are not within normal standards for the specific audiometer, which screens hearing responses to tones of calibrated loudness

Data Analysis

Nursing Diagnosis
POSITIVE SCREENING CUES FOR HEARING LOSS: Person has presented significant abnormal clinical findings during brief testing for the loss of hearing acuity

Common Etiology (Stressors)
DISEASES: Deafness, ear tumor, labyrinthitis, mastoiditis, Meniere's disease, multiple sclerosis, otitis media, otosclerosis, viral infection (measles, mumps)
INJURIES: Contusion of the ear, foreign object in the ear, rupture of the tympanic membrane
SIGNS AND SYMPTOMS: Excess cerumen
HEALTH CARE FACTORS: *Drug therapy:* Adverse effects of furosamide, gentamycin, quinine, streptomycin, tobramycin
ENVIRONMENTAL FACTORS: Noise (loud)

PLANNING

Unmet Needs
Protection from physical harm, increased learning

Expected Outcome
Person will accept and act upon referral to a physician
Person will undergo further testing if recommended by the physician
Person will accept and participate in treatment if testing verifies the suspected diagnosis

NURSING INTERVENTIONS

Nursing Treatments
Consult with a physician (about the results of the screening test)

OR

Make a referral to a physician

Nursing Observations

Determine the degree of insight that the person has (into his symptoms and the significance of the screening outcome)

Make a follow-up evaluation (to determine whether the suspected diagnosis was verified)

Health Teaching

Explain the meaning of the diagnostic report (in terms of suspected disease requiring further medical investigation)

Advise early correction of problems

Inform of the resources available for health care (so the person has several options)

Following a Confirmed Medical Diagnosis

Explain the causes of the problem (viral or bacterial infection, noise, nerve damage, tumor)

Explain the reason for and intended effect of the therapy (to prevent further tissue damage and restore hearing)

EVALUATION

Record actual outcome

POSITIVE SCREENING CUES FOR VISION LOSS[33,399,476]

ASSESSMENT

Data Collection

Subjective Data

• Person may or may not relate the following significant symptoms:

Decreased visual acuity

Frowning, squinting

Headaches, eye pain

Double vision, blurred vision

Photophobia

Objective Data

• Person exhibits, during screening, clinical findings that are not within the standard normal range:

Snellen eye test for adults reveals abnormality (normal is 20/20)

Snellen E chart or picture test for children over age 3 indicates abnormality (*Normal*: age 3, ±20/40; age 4–5, ±20/30; age 6–7, 20/20)

Ishihara's test indicates colorblindness

Data Analysis

Nursing Diagnosis

POSITIVE SCREENING CUES FOR VISION LOSS: Person has presented significant abnormal clinical findings during brief testing for loss of visual acuity

Common Etiology (Stressors)

DISEASES: Astigmatism, cataract, glaucoma, iritis, keratitis, multiple sclerosis, myasthenia gravis, myopia (nearsightedness), optic atrophy, presbyopia (farsightedness), retinal detachment

INJURIES: Burn wound of the eye (chemical or thermal), contusion of the eye, foreign body in eye

PLANNING

Unmet Needs

Protection from physical harm, increased learning

Expected Outcome

Person will accept and act upon referral to a physician

Person will undergo further testing if recommended by the physician

Person will accept and participate in treatment if testing verifies the suspected diagnosis

NURSING INTERVENTIONS

Nursing Treatments

Consult with a physician (about the results of the screening test)

   OR

Make a referral to a physician

Nursing Observations

Determine the degree of insight that the person has (into his symptoms and the significance of the screening outcome)

Make a follow-up evaluation (to determine whether the suspected diagnosis was verified)

Health Teaching

Explain the meaning of the diagnostic report (in terms of suspected disease requiring further medical investigation)

Advise early correction of problems

Inform of the resources available for health care (so the person has several options)

Following a Confirmed Medical Diagnosis

Explain the causes of the problem (eye tissue degeneration, infection, optic nerve damage, etc.)

Explain the reason for and intended effect of the therapy (to prevent further tissue damage and restore vision)

EVALUATION

Record actual outcome

20 Nursing Diagnoses of DRUG PROBLEMS

Dual Domain of Nursing Expertise: Drug Problems

This chapter covers that sphere of nursing knowledge and skill related to health problems involving the intake of chemical substances. These problems are solved by such health care providers as nurses, physicians, dentists, pharmacists, paramedics, and physicians' assistants.

Views of Nursing Leaders That Support This Domain of Nursing Expertise

In order to administer drugs intelligently, the nurse must be constantly vigilant. . . . Giving the patient information about the drugs he is receiving or will receive is a responsibility shared by nurse and physician.

Alice Rines and Mildred Montag[411:410]

Untoward Reactions to Drugs

ADVERSE DRUG EFFECT[30,277,299]

ASSESSMENT

Data Collection

Subjective Data
• Person may or may not relate any of the following:

Skin Abnormalities
Itching
Malaise
Sweating
Feeling excessively hot or cold

Cardiovascular Abnormalities
Palpitations
Feeling of faintness
Dizziness

Respiratory Abnormalities
Shortness of breath
Tightness of the chest or throat (larynx)

Gastrointestinal Abnormalities
Nausea
Diarrhea
Vomiting
Constipation
Indigestion

Central Nervous System Abnormalities
Dizziness
Drowsiness
Lightheadedness
Impaired memory

Kidney Abnormalities
Decreased urination

Blood Abnormalities
Fatigue
Malaise

Liver Abnormalities
Nausea
Vomiting
Abdominal pain

Ear Abnormalities
Vertigo
Tinnitus
Hearing loss

Eye Abnormalities
Blurring or dimming of vision

Objective Data
• Person exhibits any of the following:

Skin Abnormalities
Erythema

Urticaria
Scaling of the skin
Loss of hair or nails
Angioedema
Maculopapular rash
Pustules
Photosensitivity reaction
Blisters
Lymphadenopathy
Inflammation at an injection site or of a joint

Cardiovascular Abnormalities
Bradycardia
Tachycardia
Dysrhythmias
Increased or decreased blood pressure
Postural hypotension

Respiratory Abnormalities
Reduced or increased respirations
Respiratory wheezing
Laryngeal stridor

Gastrointestinal Abnormalities
Loud and excessive bowel sounds
Frequent stools, flatus
Liquid stools
Hematemesis
Melana

Central Nervous System Abnormalities
Impaired coordination
Depressed level of consciousness
Delirium
Overstimulation or excitement
Convulsions
Muscle weakness
Reduced ankle and knee reflexes
Impaired speech
Dyskinesia
Fever

Kidney Abnormalities
Hematuria
Casts in the urine
Proteinuria
Anuria
Oliguria
Edema
Uremia (elevated BUN and creatinine)
Hyperuricemia

Blood Abnormalities
Absence of granulocytes
Reduced number or leukocytes (WBCs) or red blood cells (RBCs)
Platelet deficiency
Hypokalemia
Hyperglycemia
Purpura
Petechiae
Hemolysis
Methemoglobinemia

Liver Abnormalities
Jaundice
Elevated liver studies (SGOT, SGPT, bilirubin)

Ear Abnormalities
Hearing tests indicating hearing loss (Weber, Rhinne, audiogram)

Eye Abnormalities
Nystagmus (rapid movement of the eyeballs)
Cataract growth

Data Analysis

Nursing Diagnosis
ADVERSE DRUG EFFECT: An unexpected or exaggerated reaction after the intake of a chemical substance for therapeutic reasons

Common Etiology (Stressors)
BIRTH DEFECTS: Glucose 6-phosphate dehydrogenase deficiency
BIRTH STATUS: Premature infant, low-birth-weight infant, newborn
DISEASES: Addison's disease, asthma, cerebral edema, congestive heart failure, hepatic insufficiency or failure, hypertension, infection (severe systemic), renal insufficiency or failure, septicemia, systemic lupus erythematosus, thyrotoxicosis, myocardial infarction
SIGNS AND SYMPTOMS: Dehydration, low body weight
HUMAN BODY: Natural body function, breast-feeding an infant
HEALTH CARE FACTORS: *Drug therapy*: Prolonged drug therapy; drug interactions; adverse effects of any drugs; Common drugs that cause specific reactions include the following. *Skin abnormalities*: Penicillin, sulfonamides, bromides, barbiturates, iodides, arsenic, gold, quinine, codeine, hydantoin, thiazides, antimalarial drugs. *Cardiac abnormalities*: Digitoxin, digitalis, antihistamines (Benadryl, Phenergan, etc.), meperidine, quinidine, rauwulfia. *Respiratory abnormalities*: Sedatives, narcotics, tranquilizers, barbiturates, alcohol, salicylates, mucomyst, neostigmine. *Gastrointestinal abnormalities*: Antibiotics, salicylates, iron, coumarin, digitalis, morphine, quinine, quinidine. *Central nervous system abnormalities*: Barbiturates, hypnotics, antianxiety and antidepressant agents, alcohol, ephedrine, atropine, belladonna, bromides, digitalis, isoniazid, morphine. *Kidney abnormalities*: Acetazolamide (Diamox), bromides, chloral hydrate, gold, hydantoin, kanamycin, neomycin, mercurials, quinine, quinidine, sulfonamides, vancomycin, tobramycin. *Blood abnormalities*: Sulfonamides, antibiotics such as chloramphenicol and streptomycin, acetazolamide, salicylates, antihistamines, gold, heparin, hydantoin, iodides, isoniazid, meprobamate, prophylthiouracil, quinine, quinadine. *Liver abnormalities*: Chloradiazepoxide (Librium), erythromycin, hydantoin, isoniazid, tetracyclines, cephradine, phenylbutazone (Butazolidin), acetaminophen, phenothiazines, steroids. *Ear abnormalities*: Antibiotics such as streptomycin, gentamicin, kanamycin, neomycin, vancomycin, and tobramycin, salicylates, diuretics such as ethacrynic acid, and furosemide, quinine, quinidine. *Eye abnormalities*: Corticosteroids, chloroquine, primaquine, phenathiazines
DEVELOPMENTAL PHASES: Infancy, old age
HUMAN ERROR: Self-treatment with over-the-counter drugs, duplication of drugs, taking incorrect drug dosages
MAJOR PATHOPHYSIOLOGIC FACTORS CAUSING THE PROBLEM: The different types of adverse drug effects include side effects, idiosyncratic responses, allergic (hypersensitive) reactions, and toxic effects. *Side effects*: Pharmacologic actions additional to those for which the drug is prescribed, such as drowsiness from antihistamines and orthostatic hypotension from meperidine. Adverse side effects occur from most drug administrations regardless of the person's physiologic status, and decreased dosage or discontinuation of the drug controls the adverse effects. *Idiosyncratic responses*: Occur when a person has an unusual physiologic susceptibility to the pharmacologic actions of a drug, such as when a normal dose of a hypnotic drug induces very deep sleep for 10–12 hours or a sedative drug causes hyperactivity instead of sedation; genetic defects in metabolism are frequently the basis for idiosyncratic responses. *Allergic reactions to drugs*: Occur most commonly in persons who demonstrate other forms of allergy (asthma, hay fe-

ver, food allergy) in persons with allergy-related diseases (systemic lupus erythematosus), with severe infections (septicemia, pneumonia), and in immunologically immune infants (under 1 year of age); in addition to the common skin manifestations (rashes, itching) of drug allergy, more serious responses may occur, such as anaphylaxis, serum sickness, bone marrow depression, and organ damage; the kidneys, liver, lungs, and blood vessel linings are especially likely to be damaged as a result of drug hypersensitivity; for example, when the metabolized products of methicillin combine with cellular protein in the kidneys, an immune response, an allergic reaction, results in interstitial nephritis; after local application or inhalation of the aerosols Mucomyst or neostigmine, allergic bronchospasm may result, with wheezing and chest tightness; a hypersensitivity response in the liver to isoniazid results in hepatocellular damage and necrosis, which are hepatitis manifestations; chlorpromazine causes bile stasis in the liver, resulting in jaundice; some adverse drug effects are not clearly classifiable as either allergic or toxic effects. *Toxic effects*: May be local, causing gastrointestinal irritation (oral dosages) and subcutaneous, muscular, or vascular irritation and damage (parenteral dosages); local toxicity is usually controlled by dose concentration and speed of administration rather than by dosage size; general toxicity is usually the result of an excessive dosage for the person's individual tolerance level or an accumulation of the drug due to ineffective metabolism and/or excretion of the drug by the kidneys and/or liver; the type of damage from toxic levels of a drug depend on the drug's propensity for specific tissues; for example, the glycosides (digitalis products) affect the cardiac pacemaker and impair circulation; the aminoglycosides (streptomycin, gentamicin, kanamycin, etc.) damage the VIII nerve (hearing loss) and renal structures (proteinuria, cylindruria, hematuria, oliguria); several drugs including alkylating agents (Cytoxan, Leukeran), chloramphenicol, mephenytoin, propylithiouracil and methimazole, cause bone marrow depression (agranulocytosis, aplastic anemia) while other drugs, including sulfonamides, nitrofurans, phenacetin, and salicylates cause hemolysis of red cells (hemolytic anemia); many drugs, including sedatives, atropine, digitalis, isoniazid, chlorpromazine, adversely affect the central nervous system (delirium, convulsions, somnolence, coma)

PLANNING

Unmet Needs
Waste elimination of toxic substances, protection from physical harm, increased learning

Expected Outcome
Person verbalizes that the adverse drug effects have either subsided or are minimized
Person no longer exhibits objective evidence of an adverse drug effect

NURSING INTERVENTIONS

Nursing Treatments
Withhold the drugs
   OR
Reduce the drug dosage
   OR
Increase the time interval between the drug doses
Give water orally (as much as the patient can comfortably tolerate, provided there are no fluid restrictions or acute renal failure)
Consult with the physician (about the drug dosage or drug changes)

Specific to Antihypertensive Drugs
Encourage decreased sodium-food/fluid intake
Encourage increased potassium-food/fluid intake
Restrict the fluid intake according to the weight gain
Reassure verbally that symptoms will subside in a few weeks

Specific to Adrenal-Steroid Drugs
Encourage decreased sodium-food/fluid intake
Encourage increased protein-food intake
Encourage increased potassium-food/fluid intake

Refrain from giving enemas
> AND

Refrain from giving laxatives (both of which will further deplete the potassium)
Restrict the fluid intake according to the weight gain

Specific to Alcohol Intake

Give hot coffee
> OR

Give hot tea
Give nonprescription drugs (aluminum hydroxide gel for the gastritis associated with alcohol intake)

Specific to Epinephrine

Discourage the intake of oral stimulants
Discourage smoking
Maintain a cool room temperature

Specific to Respiratory Depressants

Administer humidified oxygen (ET)
Ambulate the person (if possible)
Give hot coffee
> OR

Give hot tea
Stimulate by movement, touch, sternal pressure, or speech

Nursing Observations

Monitor the blood pressure
Palpate the pulse for rate, rhythm, and volume
Inspect the chest for respiratory rate and rhythm (and depth)
Observe for shock
Observe the level of consciousness
Inspect the eyes for pupil size, equality, and response to light
Measure the (urinary) output
Observe the urine for abnormal color, content, and odor
Inspect the skin for lesions (rash, purpura, etc.)

Health Teaching

Advise that the precipitating factor be avoided
Explain the causes of the problem
Explain the importance of wearing a Medic-Alert tag (for known adverse drug reactions)
Explain the reason for and intended effect of the therapy

Specific to Antihypertensive Drugs

Advise against exposure to intense heat
Advise not to stand for prolonged periods
Explain the need to avoid overexertion (especially strenuous exercise)
Explain how to apply elastic stockings or an elastic bandage (to the legs for dizziness, faintness, postural hypotension)
Instruct to change position gradually
Instruct to take medications immediately after meals (for nausea)

Medical Treatments Performed by Nurses

Give the prescribed drugs (drug or dosage changes)

EVALUATION

Record actual outcome

UNKNOWLEDGEABLE ABOUT ALCOHOL ABUSE [51,223,445,454]

ASSESSMENT

Data Collection

Subjective Data
- Person's discussion or questions indicate a need for additional information, clarification, or validation of information
  OR
- Person's lack of questions or comments indicates not wanting information or not knowing enough to seek information
- When questioned directly, the person's response or lack of response indicates that he does not know:
  Signs and symptoms of alcohol abuse
  Physiologic effects of alcohol consumption
  Reasons why people drink alcohol
  Where to obtain help for alcoholism

Objective Data
- Person may exhibit behavior based on insufficient knowledge, such as consuming excessive amounts of alcohol, drinking despite having liver or gastric disease, pressuring peers to drink heavily

Data Analysis

Nursing Diagnosis
UNKNOWLEDGEABLE ABOUT ALCOHOL ABUSE: Being without sufficient information regarding the frequent use of alcoholic beverages

Common Etiology (Stressors)
HEALTH CARE FACTORS: Lack of health instruction

PLANNING

Unmet Needs
Protection from physical harm, protection from psychologic threat, increased learning

Expected Outcome
Correct verbal feedback of the information taught

NURSING INTERVENTIONS

Nursing Treatments
Approach unhurriedly
Encourage the person to ask questions
Relate to the person on an adult–adult level, not on a parent–child level
Encourage the use of effective coping mechanisms (which may have to be taught to the person)
Make a referral (to supportive agencies such as Alcoholics Anonymous)

Nursing Observations
Determine teaching effectiveness by verbal feedback

Health Teaching
Advise early correction of problems
Describe the behavior pattern indicating early-, intermediate-, and late-stage alcohol abuse (*Early stage*: Drinking at the same time each day, eating irregularly, lying about or making excuses for drinking, drinking before a party begins. *Intermediate stage*: Carrying a supply of alcohol, weekend intoxication, impaired function at work or home, lost work time due to alcohol. *Late stage*: Drinking in the morning, drinking alone, frequent intoxication, family discord, loss of job, physical disease)

Describe the specific dangerous effects of poor health practices (liver damage, esophageal varices, increased potential for motor vehicle injury to himself or to another)

Explain that alcohol dependence is an illness

Explain that alcohol use is not socially essential

Explain that long-term alcohol abuse reduces the pleasures derived from alcohol abuse (that there is gradual deterioration of the quality of the experience)

Advise that the responsibility for alcohol abuse be placed on the abuser, not on other persons (the family must make it clear that the alcohol abuser is responsible for his obligations and behavior)

Explain that change must come from within the person

Explain that the use of alcohol to solve problems is dangerous (that it only creates one more problem)

Explain why persons resort to alcohol abuse (peer pressure, the inability to solve problems with effective coping methods)

Explain why persons should maintain self-control (out of respect for others and to reduce the potential for personal guilt or embarrassment later)

Relate the accepted criteria for commitment of alcohol abusers (if a person is a minor, is unable to function normally, or is not in touch with reality)

EVALUATION

Record actual outcome

UNKNOWLEDGEABLE ABOUT COPING WITH THE ALCOHOL ABUSER [51,223,445,454]

ASSESSMENT

Data Collection

Subjective Data
- Person's discussion or questions indicate a need for additional information, clarification, or validation of information
  OR
- Person's lack of questions or comments indicates not wanting information or not knowing enough to seek information
- When questioned directly, the person's response or lack of response indicates that he does not know:
  How to appropriately respond to the alcoholic
  How to help an alcoholic loved one
  How to pervent a loved one from becoming an alcoholic
  Where to seek help

Objective Data
- May exhibit behavior based on insufficient knowledge, such as nagging the alcoholic, confiscating the alcoholic's liquor supply, covering up for the alcoholic, etc.

Data Analysis

Nursing Diagnosis
UNKNOWLEDGEABLE ABOUT COPING WITH THE ALCOHOL ABUSER: Being without sufficient information about how one should respond to and attempt to help an alcoholic

Common Etiology (Stressors)
HEALTH CARE FACTORS: Lack of health instruction

PLANNING

Unmet Needs

Protection from physical harm, protection from psychologic threat, caring and communicating relationships, increased learning

Expected Outcome

Correct verbal feedback of the information taught

NURSING INTERVENTIONS

Nursing Treatments

Approach unhurriedly

Reassure verbally

Encourage the family to ask questions

Make a referral (to Al-Anon)

Nursing Observations

Determine teaching effectiveness by verbal feedback

Health Teaching

Advise early correction of problems

Describe the behavior pattern indicating early-, intermediate-, and late-stage alcohol abuse (*Early stage*: Drinking at the same time each day, eating irregularly, lying about or making excuses for drinking, drinking before a party starts. *Intermediate stage*: Carrying a supply of alcohol, weekend intoxication, impaired function at work or at home, lost work time due to alcohol. *Late stage*: Drinking in the morning, drinking alone, frequent intoxication, family discord, loss of job, physical disease)

Explain that alcohol dependence is an illness

Explain why persons resort to alcohol abuse (peer pressure, the inability to solve problems with effective coping methods)

Explain the importance of persons offering emotional support to one another

Advise against committing alcoholics to promises of sobriety (when the alcoholic breaks the promise not to drink, he feels guilty and loses self-respect, which further promotes drinking)

Advise against making emotional appeals to the alcoholic (such as "stop drinking if you really love me")

Advise against emphasizing past problems caused by another (this only reinforces past failures and decreases the alcoholic's sense of worth)

Advise against making excuses for the alcoholic (covering up for the alcoholic supports the maladaptive behavior)

Advise against questioning the alcoholic about drinking (when the person has been drinking it is evident, questioning him only increases his anxiety)

Advise against removing the alcoholic's liquor supply (this only increases deceptive practices the alcoholic must use in order to assure an adequate supply)

Advise against threatening the alcoholic (when feeling threatened, the alcoholic may become violent)

Advise that others should not assume the alcoholic's responsibilities (the family must clearly state that the alcoholic is responsible for his obligations and his behavior)

Recommend that behavioral limits be set (the alcoholic needs to know the behavior expected of him)

Explain that change must come from within the person

Advise that the alcoholic's illness be discussed only during sobriety (only then can the person fully comprehend and make objective decisions about his illness)

Explain the importance of setting an example through abstinence from alcohol use (alcoholics resent those who drink, when they are struggling to stop drinking)

Relate the accepted criteria for the commitment of alcohol users (if the person is a minor, is unable to function normally, or is not in touch with reality)

Explain the importance of meeting one's own needs as well as those of a significant other (family members must meet their needs as well as those of the alcoholic)

Advise that significant persons express caring for one another

Advise that significant persons express acceptance of one another

EVALUATION

Record actual outcome

UNKNOWLEDGEABLE ABOUT DRUG ABUSE [17,93,103,131,395,587]

ASSESSMENT

Data Collection

Subjective Data
- Person's discussion or questions indicate a need for additional information, clarification, or validation of information
  OR
- Person's lack of questions or comments indicates not wanting information or not knowing enough to seek information
- When questioned directly, the person's response or lack of response indicates that he does not know:
  Signs and symptoms of drug abuse
  Physiologic effects of drug abuse
  Reasons why people turn to drug abuse
  Where to obtain help

Objective Data
- Person may exhibit behavior based on insufficient knowledge, such as taking excessive amounts of drugs, consuming controlled drugs, pressuring others to use drugs

Data Analysis

Nursing Diagnosis
UNKNOWLEDGEABLE ABOUT DRUG ABUSE: Being without sufficient information regarding the excessive use of chemical, drug substances

Common Etiology (Stressors)
HEALTH CARE FACTORS: Lack of health instruction

PLANNING

Unmet Needs
Protection from physical harm, protection from psychologic threat, increased learning

Expected Outcome
Correct verbal feedback of the information taught

NURSING INTERVENTIONS

Nursing Treatments
Approach unhurriedly
Reassure verbally
Encourage the person to ask questions
Relate to the person on an adult–adult level, not on a parent–child level
Encourage the use of effective coping mechanisms (which may have to be taught to the person)
Make a referral (to a drug clinic, rehabilitation center, or agencies that provide supportive groups, etc.)

Nursing Observations
Determine teaching effectiveness by verbal feedback

Health Teaching
Advise early correction of problems
Describe the behavior pattern indicating drug abuse (behavioral changes, unusual activity or inactivity, unusual temper outbursts, indifference toward personal appearance, guarding one's possessions, frequent borrowing or stealing of money, wearing sunglasses or long-sleeved clothing at inappropriate times, deteriorating productivity such as poor school grades or decreased job effectiveness)
Describe the specific dangerous effects of poor health practices (systemic infection from needle punctures, impaired cerebral function from drug effects, increased potential

for motor vehicle injury to himself or another)

Explain that drug dependence is an illness

Explain that drug use is not socially essential

Explain that long-term drug abuse reduces the pleasures derived from drug abuse (that there is gradual deterioration of the quality of the experience)

Explain that the use of drugs to solve problems is dangerous (that it only creates one more problem)

Explain why persons resort to drug abuse (peer pressure, the inability to solve problems with effective coping methods)

Relate the accepted criteria for commitment of drug abusers (if a person is a minor, is unable to function normally, or is not in touch with reality)

EVALUATION

Record actual outcome

UNKNOWLEDGEABLE ABOUT COPING WITH THE DRUG ABUSER[17,93,103,131,395,587]

ASSESSMENT

Data Collection

Subjective Data

• Person's discussion or questions indicate a need for additional information, clarification, or validation of information
  OR
• Person's lack of questions or comments indicates not wanting information or not knowing enough to seek information
• When questioned directly, the person's response or lack of response indicates that he does not know:
  How to help the drug abuser
  How to prevent a loved one from becoming a drug abuser
  Where to seek help

Objective Data

• May exhibit behavior based on insufficient knowledge, such as searching the drug abuser's room for drugs, excluding the drug abuser from the family, covering up for the drug abuser

Data Analysis

Nursing Diagnosis

UNKNOWLEDGEABLE ABOUT COPING WITH THE DRUG ABUSER: Being without sufficient information regarding how one should respond to and attempt to help the drug abuser

Common Etiology (Stressors)

HEALTH CARE FACTORS: Lack of health instruction

PLANNING

Unmet Needs

Protection from physical harm, protection from psychologic threat, caring and communicating relationship, increased learning

Expected Outcome

Correct verbal feedback of the information taught

NURSING INTERVENTIONS

Nursing Treatments

Approach unhurriedly

Reassure verbally

Encourage the family to ask questions

Make a referral (to a drug clinic, rehabilitation center, or supportive group)

Nursing Observations

Determine teaching effectiveness by verbal feedback

Health Teaching

Advise early correction of problems

Describe the behavioral pattern indicating drug abuse (behavioral changes, unusual activity or inactivity, unusual temper outbursts, indifference toward personal appearance, guarding possessions, frequent borrowing or stealing of money, wearing sunglasses or long-sleeved clothing at inappropriate times)

Explain that drug dependence is an illness

Explain why persons resort to drug abuse (peer pressure, inability to solve problems with effective coping methods)

Explain the importance of persons offering emotional support to one another

Advise against emphasizing past problems caused by another (this only reinforces past failures and decreases the drug abuser's sense of worth)

Advise that the responsibility for drug abuse be placed on the abuser, not on other persons (the family must make it clear that the drug abuser is responsible for his obligations and behavior)

Recommend that behavioral limits be set (that the drug abuser needs to know the behavior expected of him)

Explain that change must come from within the person

Advise against intense surveillance of the drug user (this heightens his anxiety and sense of distrust)

Explain how to counteract the theories of drug users (drug use may be justified with the theory of free choice, but this defense can be counteracted by stating that certain behavior is unacceptable and that human dignity must not be diminished)

Explain the importance of setting an example through abstinence from drug use (drug abusers resent those who are using drugs, when they are struggling with drug withdrawal)

Advise acceptance of the drug user's return home (it often indicates a desire to return to normal living)

Explain the importance of staying well informed about drug abuse (parents need drug information to keep their children informed and to recognize the signs of drug abuse)

Recommend that the family not support the drug user's habit (financial support perpetuates the use of drugs)

Relate the accepted criteria for commitment of drug abusers (if the person is a minor, is unable to function normally, or is not in touch with reality)

Relate the accepted criteria for notifying authorities of drug abuse (when drugs are being sold to others)

Explain the importance of meeting one's own needs as well as those of a significant other (family members must meet their own needs as well as those of the drug abuser)

Advise that significant persons express caring for one another

Advise that significant persons express acceptance of one another

EVALUATION

Record actual outcome

21 Nursing Diagnoses of NUTRITION AND FOOD PROBLEMS

Dual Domain of Nursing Expertise: Nutrition and Food Problems

This chapter covers that sphere of nursing knowledge and skill related to health problems involving the intake and utilization of food substances. These problems are solved by such health care providers as nurses, physicians, dieticians, and dentists.

Views of Nursing Leaders That Support This Domain of Nursing Expertise

Adaptation level theory says that the patient's behavior will be more positive when there is less discrepancy between the level of the stimulus to which the patient must respond and all the other influencing factors. The nurse asks herself whether or not the focal stimulus can be changed to bring it closer to the level which the patient can handle. In this case, the nurse may decide to meet with the dietician to determine whether or not the diet can be modified to bring it closer to the patient's tastes and to the restrictions she can tolerate.

Sister Callista Roy[669:256]

The role of the nurse is primarily that of providing individuals and families with nutritional information. . . . Her first responsibility in this respect is getting expert information to the patient.

Alice Rines and Mildred Montag[411:298–299]

Nutrition-Related Disorders/Problems

MALNUTRITION [72,323,351,522]

ASSESSMENT

Data Collection

Subjective Data
- Dietary history of inadequate nutritional intake
- Weakness
  Fatigue
  Hunger or anorexia
  Paresthesia

Objective Data
- Underweight
- Little or no subcutaneous fat
  Pallor
  Sunken or swollen abdomen

Data Analysis

Nursing Diagnosis
MALNUTRITION: A state of nutritional deficiency

Common Etiology (Stressors)
DISEASES: Alcoholism, anorexia nervosa, cancer, cardiovascular disease, celiac disease (sprue), cholera, cholecystitis, cirrhosis, cystic fibrosis, diabetes, esophageal stricture, food allergy, hiatal hernia, kwashiorkor, major depression syndrome, pancreatitis, peptic ulcer, renal insufficiency or failure, schizophrenia (catatonic), thyrotoxicosis, ulcerative colitis

INJURIES: Starvation, burn injury, including caustic damage to the esophagus (from lye, etc.)

SIGNS AND SYMPTOMS: Anorexia, chronic diarrhea or vomiting

PSYCHOSOCIAL FACTORS: Threat of chronic and severe stress

HUMAN BODY: *Body states:* Pregnancy

LIFESTYLE: Fad dieting, an insufficient or unbalanced diet

HEALTH CARE FACTORS: *Surgical procedures:* Gastrectomy, small bowel resection. *Health therapy:* Radiation to the face, neck, or abdomen

HUMAN ERROR: Excessive intake of laxatives (cathartics)

MAJOR PATHOPHYSIOLOGIC FACTORS: Malnutrition results from the intake of fewer calories and nutrient components expended and needed for energy, activity, and tissue growth; it can also result from malabsorption in which inflammation or fibrosis of the intestinal mucosa or absence of essential factors disturbs the mechanisms of nutritional transport, diffusion, and absorption by gastrointestinal cells; decreased absorptive surface (from excision of the small bowel) and excessively rapid movement of nutrients through the intestines (from diarrhea) may also result in malabsorption and malnutrition

PLANNING

Unmet Needs
Fluid and electrolyte balance, nutritional balance, sleep and rest, protection from physical harm, increased learning

Expected Outcome
Person demonstrates an adequate and balanced food intake
Person's weight is within the normal range for his size and height

NURSING INTERVENTIONS
Nursing Treatments
Provide a balanced nutritional diet (one that includes the four basic food groups)

Estimate the required daily calories (by determining the desired body weight and multiplying that by 9 calories/lb)

Give small, frequent feedings

Grant special requests (for food)

Give buttermilk or yogurt (to improve absorption)

Encourage increased protein-food intake, increased carbohydrate intake, increased calorie intake

Encourage the substitution of undesirable (eating) habits with favorable habits (eating three times a day, eating quality foods rather than snack foods, relaxing instead of rushing at the mealtime)

Encourage adequate rest (to reduce the amount of energy expended)

Discourage smoking (which suppresses the appetite)

Nursing Observations
Measure the body weight (daily for fluid gain or loss, weekly for tissue gain or loss, or daily until the gain becomes established, and then weekly)

Observe and record the food intake

Review the dietary intake with the person to determine adherence to the prescribed diet

Health Teaching
Explain the causes of the health problem (an insufficient or unbalanced diet, malabsorption of nutrients)

Inform that underweight persons require additional sleep

Teach the principles of good nutrition (based on the four basic food groups)

Advise against the use of mineral oil laxatives (which deplete vitamins from the intestines)

Explain how to budget (for maximum food buying power, if insufficient food is the problem)

Medical Treatments Performed by Nurses
Give the prescribed diet

EVALUATION
Record actual outcome

OBESITY[32,110,351,371,522]

ASSESSMENT
Data Collection
Subjective Data
- Dietary history of excessive nutritional intake
- Fatigue on exertion or exercise

Objective Data
- A 20% or more excess of body weight
- Single skin fold thickness of more than 1 inch
- Excessive deposits of fat

Data Analysis
Nursing Diagnosis
OBESITY: An excessive amount of body weight with an accumulation of fatty or adipose tissue

Common Etiology (Stressors)

DISEASES: Diabetes mellitus, anterior hypopituitarism, hypothalamus lesion, hypothyroidism

PSYCHOSOCIAL FACTORS: The threat of chronic and severe stress, the pleasure of the sedative, relaxing effect and satisfaction gained from food, the substitution of food for the absence of love

LIFESTYLE: High calorie intake, lack of exercise, cultural and family habits of overeating

MAJOR PATHOPHYSIOLOGIC FACTORS: Obesity results from a calorie intake that exceeds the caloric requirements, resulting in the excessive storage of carbohydrates and fats, from damage to the satiation center in the hypothalamus, which regulates eating, and from endocrine disturbances in which the metabolic system is severely depressed

PLANNING

Unmet Needs

Fluid and electrolyte balance, nutritional balance, activity, exercise, protection from physical harm, increased learning

Expected Outcome

Person demonstrates a decreased and balanced food intake

Person is modifying eating habits

Person's weight is becoming within the normal range for his size and height

NURSING INTERVENTIONS

Nursing Treatments

Encourage decreased calorie intake, decreased carbohydrate intake

Estimate the required daily calories (by estimating the desired body weight and multiplying that by 9 calories/lb)

Encourage moderate physical exercise (dieting reduces the lean muscle mass and not the body's fat content, exercise is needed to reduce fat deposits)

Provide a balanced nutritional diet (including the four basic food groups)

Provide a nontempting environment (by keeping food and snacks out of sight)

Nursing Observations

Measure the body weight (weekly)

Observe and record the food intake

Review the dietary intake with the person to determine adherence to the prescribed diet

Health Teaching

Emphasize the danger of excessive body weight (excessive weight increases the cardiac workload, places a strain on the musculoskeletal system)

Teach the principles of good nutrition

Advise against eating sweets

Advise that between-meal snacks be avoided

Recommend eating and drinking in moderation

Recommend behavior modification for changing eating habits (behavior modification such as not eating while performing other activities, eating only when sitting down at a set table, eating only at mealtimes, purchasing only foods that must be prepared, eating slowly and chewing the food thoroughly, using a smaller than standard size plate)

Instruct to eat 25% of the daily calories at breakfast, 50% at lunch, and 25% at supper to achieve weight loss

Instruct to limit weight loss to 3 lb/week

Explain the causes of health problem (excessive caloric intake, a depressed metabolic system)

Medical Treatments Performed by Nurses

Give the prescribed diet

EVALUATION

Record actual outcome

Knowledge Deficits About Nutrition

UNKNOWLEDGEABLE ABOUT BALANCED NUTRITION[275,349]

ASSESSMENT

Data Collection

Subjective Data
- Person's discussion or questions indicate a need for additional information, clarification, or validation of information
  OR
- Person's lack of questions or comments indicates not wanting information or not knowing enough to seek information
- When questioned directly, the person's response or lack of response indicates that he does not know:
  Essential daily nutritional requirements
  Which foods contain specific nutrients
  How to prepare food so as to preserve maximum nutrients
  How to plan well-balanced meals from day to day
  How to balance nutrition when there are minimal financial resources

Objective Data
- May exhibit behavior based on sufficient knowledge, such as not eating a balanced diet, not eating three meals a day, consuming large amounts of snack food, preparing and serving inadequate meals to the family

Data Analysis

Nursing Diagnosis
UNKNOWLEDGEABLE ABOUT BALANCED NUTRITION: Being without sufficient information regarding the planning and preparation of a well-balanced food intake

Common Etiology (Stressors)
HEALTH CARE FACTORS: Lack of health instruction

PLANNING

Unmet Needs
Nutritional balance, protection from physical harm, increased learning

Expected Outcome
Correct verbal feedback of the information taught
Person exhibits recommended nutritional practices

NURSING INTERVENTIONS

Nursing Treatments
Approach unhurriedly
Encourage the person to ask questions

Nursing Observations
Determine teaching effectiveness by verbal feedback

Health Teaching
Teach the principles of good nutrition (based on the four basic food groups)
Teach how to prepare balanced meals (have the person write out menus)
Explain how to maintain maximum nutrients in food (by steaming instead of boiling food, by eating food raw instead of cooked)
Recommend a regular meal schedule
Explain how to budget (for maximum food-buying power)

Describe the specific dangerous effects of poor health practices (nutritional deficiencies, increasing the risk for diseases, decreased daily functioning ability)

Explain the need for increased nutrition during specific conditions (during blood loss or anemia, there is an increased need for high iron and protein foods, and during tissue healing, the protein intake should be increased, etc.)

EVALUATION

Record actual outcome

UNKNOWLEDGEABLE ABOUT DIETING[110,349]

ASSESSMENT

Data Collection

Subjective Data

• Person's discussion or questions indicate a need for additional information, clarification, or validation of information
  OR
• Person's lack of questions or comments indicates not wanting information or not knowing enough to seek information
• When questioned directly, the person's response or lack of response indicates that he does not know the following:
  It is not healthy to alternate from one diet to another
  Weight loss should be gradual and not rapid
  Weight loss by diet should be professionally supervised
  Excessive vitamin and mineral intake can have serious side effects
  Consistent, balanced nutrition is essential to health

Objective Data

• May exhibit behavior based on insufficient knowledge, such as losing weight and quickly regaining it, preparing diets that reflect poor nutrition, skipping meals and then eating a large meal at night

Data Analysis

Nursing Diagnosis

UNKNOWLEDGEABLE ABOUT DIETING: Being without sufficient information about the use of diets for weight loss

Common Etiology (Stressors)

HEALTH CARE FACTORS: Lack of health instruction

PLANNING

Unmet Needs

Nutritional balance, protection from physical harm, increased learning

Expected Outcome

Correct verbal feedback of the information taught
Cessation of improper dieting
Behavior modification involving a change to the recommended nutritional standards

NURSING INTERVENTIONS

Nursing Treatments

Approach unhurriedly
Encourage the person to ask questions
Encourage moderate physical exercise (dieting reduces the lean muscle mass and not the body's fat content, exercise is needed to reduce fat deposits, if dieting is to be permanently effective)

Nursing Observations

Determine teaching effectiveness by verbal feedback

Health Teaching

Teach the principles of good nutrition (by using the four basic food groups, and suggest that liquid protein and one-food diets be avoided)

Teach how to prepare balanced meals

Recommend a regular meal schedule

Emphasize the danger of the specific health practice of fad dieting (the occurrence of nutritional deficiencies, increasing the risk for diseases)

Instruct to avoid taking diet pills (they cause nervousness and difficulty sleeping and can accelerate certain disease processes such as adrenal, thyroid, or hypertensive conditions)

Recommend behavior modification for changing one's eating habits (such as not eating while performing other activities, eating only when sitting down at a set table, eating only at mealtimes, purchasing only foods which must be prepared, eating slowly and chewing the food thoroughly, using a smaller than standard size plate)

Instruct to eat 25% of the daily calories at breakfast, 50% at lunch, and 25% at supper to achieve weight loss

Instruct to limit weight loss to 3 lb/week

Suggest participation in group plans for weight reduction (so that the person has support from persons with the same goal)

Explain the reason for and intended effect of the methods used (to maintain good nutrition and reduce the potential for disease)

EVALUATION

Record actual outcome

UNSKILLED AT MANAGING A PRESCRIBED DIET[275,349,506]

ASSESSMENT

Data Collection

Subjective Data

• Person's discussion or questions indicate a need for additional information, clarification, or validation of information about performing the task
  OR

• Person's lack of questions or comments indicates not wanting information or not knowing enough to seek information about performing the task

  Person may not know:

  Why a special diet was prescribed

  Physiologic effect of the diet

  Specific foods that are and are not recommended

  Symptoms that indicate poor diet regulation

  How to determine which commercially prepared foods conform to the diet

Objective Data

• Person cannot demonstrate how to:

  Calculate the diet

  Plan menus and meals within the diet limitations

  Identify undesirable nutrients listed on product labels

Data Analysis

Nursing Diagnosis

UNSKILLED AT MANAGING A PRESCRIBED DIET: Being nonproficient, with or without knowledge, in the performance of the specific task of planning and preparing a prescribed diet

Common Etiology (Stressors)
HEALTH CARE FACTORS: Lack of health instruction, lack of health-skill experience

PLANNING
Unmet Needs
Nutritional balance, protection from physical harm, mastery and competence in skills, independence, increased learning

Expected Outcome
Correct verbal feedback of the information taught
Correct return demonstration of how to plan menus and prepare the prescribed foods
Person relates eating the prescribed foods, at the recommended times, in the required amounts

NURSING INTERVENTIONS
Nursing Treatments
Provide temporary assistance (with diet management) until the skill is learned
Provide a balanced nutritional diet
Provide food selection
Encourage patient questions
Encourage self-performance
Adjust the diet to the person's lifestyle (according to his likes and dislikes, allowable budget, needs for energy to work)

Nursing Observations
Determine teaching effectiveness by testing, verbal feedback, and return demonstration
Observe for readiness to assume self-care
Observe for diet intolerance (nausea, vomiting, abdominal distention, poor food intake)
Review the dietary intake with the patient to determine adherence to the prescribed diet (periodically, after the person has achieved skill in managing the diet)

Health Teaching
General Teaching
Teach the principles of good nutrition (using the four basic food groups)
Teach how to calculate a diet (using exchange lists when appropriate)
Teach how to prepare balanced meals
Instruct to eat only prescribed foods and amounts of food
Explain how to maintain maximum nutrients in food (by steaming instead of boiling the food, by eating fresh food instead of canned food)
Instruct to measure foods after cooking (to ensure accurate measurements)
Explain how to budget (for maximum food-buying power)
Emphasize what the person can, rather than cannot, eat

Specific to the Diabetic Diet
Explain which foods are or are not recommended for the diet (*Recommended*: Vegetables, meats, bread, and fruits according to the number of calories in the diabetic exchange lists, coffee, tea, salt, sugar substitutes, spices. *Not recommended*: Sugar, candy, honey, jam, jelly, marmalade, syrups, pie, cake, cookies, pastries, condensed milk, soft drinks, fried or creamed foods, alcoholic beverages)
Instruct to eat only at mealtime
Explain the importance of eating on time (in order to maintain carbohydrate metabolism in relation to the prescribed insulin dosage)
Instruct that diabetics should not fry foods (since the fats used for cooking have to be counted as part of the calorie intake)
Explain how to maintain a diabetic diet when away from home (by eating clear soups, unglazed, unbuttered, uncreamed foods, leafy salads, fresh fruits, avoid casseroles, use lemon and vinegar for dressings)

Explain the reason for and intended effect of the therapy (diabetics have low insulin secretion and cannot metabolize normal carbohydrate intake; by lowering the carbohydrate intake and regulating the insulin dosage, normal carbohydrate metabolism is achieved)

Specific to the Low-Potassium Diet

Explain which foods are or are not recommended for the diet (*Recommended*: Foods with minimal potassium content such as butter, margarine, salad oil, sugar, honey, cranberry juice and sauce, ginger ale, root beer, jelly beans, lollypops, popsicles, water ices, most spices, limited amounts of moderate potassium content in refined breads and cereals, eggs, milk, cheese, seafood, poultry, lamb, apples, applesauce, peaches, pears, green beans, beets, carrots, corn, peas, turnips, cucumber, onion; potassium content can be decreased by discarding the liquid from canned and cooked foods. *Not recommended*: Chocolate, coffee, cocoa, tea, dried fruit, peas or beans, milk desserts, ice cream, molasses, whole-grain breads and cereals, bananas, oranges, watermelon, apricots, spinach, nuts)

Explain the reason for and intended effect of the therapy (decreased potassium intake slows the development of hyperkalemia in renal insufficiency states and may delay the need for dialysis)

Specific to the Low-Sodium Diet

Explain which foods are or are not recommended for the diet (*Recommended*: Fresh or frozen vegetables and fruit, meat, or poultry, low-sodium bread, crackers, tuna, salmon, soups, butter, margarine, cheese, fresh or frozen fruit juices. *Not recommended*: Barbecued, smoked, or cured meats or fish, ham, bacon, sausage, salt pork, corned beef, processed lunch meats, and cheese, meat tenderizer, regular, canned vegetables and soups, bouillon, pizza, TV dinners, salted nuts and crackers, potato chips, pretzels, olives, pickles, ketchup, mustard, Gatorade)

Explain the difference between salt and sodium diet restriction (salt refers to table salt, sodium to various forms of sodium such as sodium bromide, sodium citrate)

Explain the reason for and intended effect of the therapy (in cardiac and renal disorders, there is reduced kidney excretion of sodium resulting in increased sodium retention; by decreasing the sodium intake, the osmotic pressure pulls sodium and water from the interstitial spaces into the bloodstream reducing tissue edema and lowering the blood pressure)

Specific to the Low-Triglyceride/Low-Fat or Low-Cholesterol Diet

Explain which foods are or are not recommended for the diet (*Recommended*: Fresh, frozen, or canned fruits, fruit juices and/or vegetables, cereals, rice, macaroni, noodles, clear broths and cream soups, lean, broiled, or roasted meats, fresh fish, chicken, or turkey without the skin, low-fat cottage cheese, skim milk, coffee, tea, carbonated beverages, baked goods made without whole milk, fat, or egg yolk. *Not recommended*: Fried or fatty meats such as bacon, cold cuts, hot dogs, fish canned in oil, buttered, creamed, or fried vegetables, butter, margarine, shortening, gravy, cream sauce, salad dressing, bakery goods made with whole milk, fat, or egg yolk, whole milk, cream, yogurt, avocado, ice cream, nuts, chocolate, peanut butter, and coconut)

Explain the reason for and intended effect of the therapy (decreased fatty food intake reduces bile secretion in the liver and bile volume stored in the gallbladder, the reduced organ activity promotes tissue healing of a diseased gallbladder, low fat and cholesterol intake decreases fat deposits in the arterial vessels, reducing the potential for arterial disorders)

Specific to the Low-Calorie Diet

Explain which foods are or are not recommended for the diet (*Recommended*: A good low-calorie diet uses the seven food exchanges; the size of the portions are determined by the calorie content of each food class; *vegetables, group A,* in amounts as desired (green vegetables such as asparagus, broccoli, cabbage, cauliflower, celery, squash, mushrooms); *vegetables, group B,* in limited amounts (beets, carrots, onions, peas, pumpkin, winter squash, turnips); *fruit, bread/cereal* (pasta, potatoes, dried beans), *milk/cheese/egg*, lean *meat*, fish, poultry and *fat* in limited amounts. *Not recommended*: Pure carbohydrates (sugar, jelly, candy, honey, etc.), alcoholic beverages, fatty meats (bacon, ham, etc.), saturated fats (cream, butter, etc.), snack foods, sauces, gravy, adding fats for flavor)

Explain the reason for and intended effect of the therapy (lowered calorie intake decreases body weight by using stored energy resources)

Specific to the High-Calorie Diet

Explain which foods are or are not recommended for the diet (*Recommended*: A balanced menu from the basic four food groups, supplemented by high-calorie, high-protein/high-fat milkshakes, ice cream, cheese, peanut butter and jelly sandwiches as between-meal and bedtime snacks. *Not recommended*: Snacks closer than 2 hours before mealtime, junk foods, and empty calories (chips, sugar candies, carbonated beverages, etc.) that promote poor dietary habits)

Explain the reason for and intended effect of the therapy (increased calorie intake supplies additional energy and fuel resources when needed to offset an increased metabolic rate, and illness)

Specific to the Low-Residue Diet

Explain which foods are or are not recommended for the diet (*Recommended*: Cottage, cream, and cheddar cheese; milk; eggs not fried or scrambled in fat; tender chicken, fish, ground beef, and lamb; broth, strained meat-base soups; cooked vegetables; beets, green beans, peas, carrots, squash, asparagus, spinach, potatoes (not fried); fruit juices, cooked and canned fruits (no skins, seeds or fiber); fresh bananas; refined bread and cereals, macaroni, spaghetti, noodles, rice, crackers; ices, ice creams, gelatin, custard, puddings, plain cake and cookies; tea, coffee, carbonated beverages, vegetable juice. *Not recommended*: Fried foods, meats not listed above, raw vegetables and fruits (except bananas), cooked vegetables and fruits that contain acid (strawberries, tomatoes, okra, etc.), nuts, whole-grain products)

Explain the reason for and intended effect of the therapy (foods containing low fiber decrease intestinal irritation, lessen gastrointestinal spasm, and reduce the volume of fecal elimination)

Specific to the High-Residue Diet

Explain which foods are or are not recommended for the diet (*Recommended*: Long-fibered vegetables such as greens, cabbage, and celery, raw vegetables and fruits, cooked fruits, whole-grain breads, nuts, and cereals)

Explain the reason for and intended effect of the therapy (increased food fiber increases bulk, improving the intestinal muscle tone and promoting comfortable fecal elimination)

Specific to the Low-Protein Diet

Explain which foods are or are not recommended for the diet (*Recommended*: Pure carbohydrates such as sugar, honey, jelly, hard candy; pure fats such as butter and margarine; protein foods of high biologic value, such as milk, eggs, and calves' liver, each in limited quantities. *Not recommended*: Cheese, meat, fish, poultry, bread, cereals, legumes, nuts, gelatin)

Explain the reason for and intended effect of the therapy (decreased protein intake reduces ammonia and/or urea blood levels in liver or kidney disorders)

Specific to the High-Protein Diet

Explain which foods are or are not recommended for the diet (*Recommended*: Milk, cheese, eggs, lean meats, fish, poultry, wheat bread and cereals, wheat germ, yeast, legumes, nuts, gelatin)

Explain the reason for and intended effect of the therapy (high protein intake promotes tissue growth and repair and increases resistance to infection and body heat production)

EVALUATION

Record actual outcome

Knowledge Deficits About Food

UNSKILLED AT SAFE FOOD HANDLING[349]

ASSESSMENT

Data Collection

Subjective Data
- Person's discussion or questions indicate a need for additional information, clarification, or validation of information about performing the task
  OR
- Person's lack of questions or comments indicates not wanting information or not knowing enough to seek information about performing the task
  Person may not know:
  It is necessary to wash one's hands prior to food handling
  Which foods require refrigeration
  Importance of using clean cooking utensils
  How to recognize unsafe cans/jars of food

Objective Data
- Person cannot correctly demonstrate how to:
  Clean raw fruits and vegetables properly
  How to package and store food

Data Analysis

Nursing Diagnosis
UNSKILLED AT SAFE FOOD HANDLING: Being nonproficient, with or without knowledge, in the performance of the specific task of using satisfactory methods in the preparation and storage of food

Common Etiology (Stressors)
HEALTH CARE FACTORS: Lack of health instruction, lack of health-skill experience

PLANNING

Unmet Needs
Cleanliness, protection from physical harm, mastery and competence in skills, increased learning

Expected Outcome
Correct verbal feedback of the information taught
Correct return demonstration of how to clean, prepare, and store food

NURSING INTERVENTIONS

Nursing Treatments
Provide temporary assistance until the skill is learned
Encourage the person to ask questions

Nursing Observations
Determine teaching effectiveness by testing, verbal feedback, and return demonstration

Health Teaching
Advise hand washing before meal preparation
Recommend adequate food refrigeration (for perishable foods, especially dairy products, eggs, meats, seafood, and foods labeled "to refrigerate")
Inform that clean cooking (and storage of) utensils are essential (to prevent bacteria growth and disease)
Emphasize that food in bulging cans and jars with bulging lids should be discarded
Emphasize that outdated foods should be discarded

Advise that fresh foods should be thoroughly washed (soaked and scrubbed)
Explain the reason for and intended effect of the methods used (to promote the cleanliness and nutrient value of the food)

EVALUATION
Record actual outcome

UNKNOWLEDGEABLE ABOUT FOREIGN FOOD HAZARDS[657]

ASSESSMENT
Data Collection

Subjective Data
• Person's discussion or questions indicate a need for additional information, clarification, or validation of information
  OR
• Person's lack of questions or comments indicates not wanting information or not knowing enough to seek information
• When questioned directly, the person's response or lack of response indicates that he does not know:
  Specific foods and fluids to avoid eating in foreign countries
  Foods and beverages that are safe
  How to protect oneself against the dangers of foreign foods

Objective Data
• May exhibit behavior based on insufficient knowledge, such as not taking precautions to prevent such disorders as amebic and bacillary dysentery

Data Analysis

Nursing Diagnosis
UNKNOWLEDGEABLE ABOUT FOREIGN FOOD HAZARDS: Being without sufficient information regarding the health dangers of eating certain foreign foods

Common Etiology (Stressors)
HEALTH CARE FACTORS: Lack of health instruction

PLANNING
Unmet Needs
Protection from physical harm, increased learning

Expected Outcome
Correct verbal feedback of the information taught
Person verbalizes having practiced preventive measures while traveling to foreign countries

NURSING INTERVENTIONS
Nursing Treatments
Approach unhurriedly
Encourage the person to ask questions
Nursing Observations
Determine teaching effectiveness by verbal feedback

Health Teaching

Specific to Food

Recommend eating only well-cooked meat and vegetables in foreign countries (since bacteria are killed by the extra cooking time)

Advise against eating raw fruits and vegetables in foreign countries (in some countries, human excreta is used for fertilizer, increasing the consumer's potential for dysentery)

Advise against eating dairy products (milk is not pasteurized in some countries, and intestinal distress can result from any product made from milk)

Advise against eating in unlicensed restaurants

Specific to Fluids

Emphasize that potentially unsafe water should be boiled for 10 minutes (to kill any bacteria, or only sealed, bottled, water should be used)

Advise against using ice cubes made from potentially unsafe water (freezing unsafe water does not kill the bacteria)

Inform that halazone tablets should be added to potentially unsafe water (chlorination of the water destroys bacteria)

Explain that teeth should not be brushed with potentially unsafe water (because one might swallow the water)

Inform that carbonated beverages are safe to drink in foreign countries (the carbonation process eliminates contamination)

Explain the causes of the problem (the food-processing techniques in South or Central America, Asia, Africa, eastern Europe, the Orient, and Mexico are not the same as those to which persons from other countries are accustomed)

EVALUATION

Record actual outcome

22 Nursing Diagnoses of PSYCHOSOCIAL NONADAPTATION

Dual Domain of Nursing Expertise: Psychosocial Nonadaptation

This chapter covers that sphere of nursing knowledge and skill related to emotional, mental, and social nonadjustment behavior during illness, developmental phases, and life crises. Such responses include those that are not considered normal and that deter personal growth and effective functioning. These problems are solved by such health care providers as nurses, psychiatric nurse specialists, physicians, psychiatrists, psychologists, psychiatric social workers, and psychiatric chaplins.

Views of Nursing Leaders That Support This Domain of Nursing Expertise

Long-term functions for which nurses and physicians share responsibility include providing continuous guidance for mentally ill patients and their families until all practical rehabilitation of the patient and family has been achieved, with a joint decision of therapists involved.

Faye Abdellah[3:128]

With a strong base of scientific knowledge, the nurse makes judgments of client adaptation or maladaptation. The nurse makes these judgments mutually with the client. Often . . . the client is the first to be aware of a coping failure. Maladaptive behavior, as well as adaptive behavior requiring support, becomes the focus of the nurse.

Sister Callistra Roy[187:207]

In Behavioral System theory, instability is described as behaviors that are not efficient and effective enough to meet the goals of the subsystems. . . . Nurses identify actual changes in overt behavior indicative of instability. These changes comprise categories that will be called behavioral discrepancies—disorderly, unpredictable, and purposeless.

Dorothy Johnson[410:225]

Nursing problems arise because there are disturbances in the structure or function of the subsystem or the system, or because the level of behavioral functioning is at less than a desired or optimal level. . . . The goal of nursing action in each case is to restore, maintain, or attain behavioral system balance and stability at the highest possible level for the individual.

Dorothy Johnson[410:214]

Nonadaptive Responses of Emotion (Affect): Anger

ACTING-OUT BEHAVIOR[471]

ASSESSMENT

Data Collection

Subjective Data
- Relates feelings of anger
- Does not understand the reason for his/her behavior

Objective Data
- A variety of behaviors that draw attention to the person:
  Dressing peculiarly
  Defying rules
  Engaging in overt sexual or seductive behavior
  Speaking very loudly
  Making hostile outbursts

Data Analysis

Nursing Diagnosis
ACTING-OUT BEHAVIOR: An attempt to gain the attention of others through impulsive actions

Common Etiology (Stressors)
PSYCHOSOCIAL FACTORS: An attempt to express an emotion indirectly or to control a life situation, the indirect expression of conflict, an attempt to avoid intimacy, lack of external limits or control, the threat of real or imagined danger, lack of competency in using effective coping mechanisms, an attempt to gain attention, the threat of chronic or severe stress, unlearned alternative behavior, the presence of reinforcing stimuli that maintain the maladaptive behavior

PLANNING

Unmet Needs
Psychologic stability, direct and communicating relationships, self-control, personal growth and maturity, increased learning, increased problem-solving ability

Expected Outcome
Person exhibits less impulsive behavior
Acknowledges that he thinks more about the outcome or results of his behavior
Verbalizes about recognizing and dealing with his own feelings in nondetrimental ways
Exhibits use of more appropriate coping mechanisms

NURSING INTERVENTIONS

Nursing Treatments
Approach unhurriedly
Demonstrate calmness
Provide an atmosphere of acceptance (of the person, not of the behavior)
Encourage the expression of feelings
Relate to the person on an adult–adult level, not on a parent–child level

Listen attentively

Talk with the person

Offer feedback to the person's expressed feelings

Explore with the person reasons for recurring problems (Why is acting out being repetitively exhibited?)

Explore with the person the effects of his behavior on others (it angers and embarrasses others, it causes conflict)

Encourage respect for the rights of others

Encourage participation in therapeutic group interaction (to gain insight into one's behavior and improve interpersonal relationships)

Suggest more appropriate means of emotional expression (such as talking things over)

Set an example by role modeling

Ignore undesirable behavior

   OR

Set limits on unacceptable behavior

Clearly communicate what is expected of the person

Hold the person responsible for his behavior (do not allow the person to blame others)

Provide seclusion (if needed)

Arrange a structured daily routine

Refrain from arguing, from negatively criticizing

Verbalize daily the person's successful progress (in changing behavior)

Provide emotional support for persons significant to the patient

Nursing Observations

Determine the degree of insight that the person has (into the acting-out behavior)

Determine the precipitating factors (that stimulate the acting out)

Identify disturbing conversation topics

Identify emotion-stimulating events

Identify potentially destructive behavior (such as high levels of irritability)

Observe for evidence that the person is reaching out for emotional support

Observe for behavior modification (resulting from the therapy)

Health Teaching

Explain how emotional responses occur (a situation is perceived in terms of its significance to the individual, an emotional response is experienced, physiologic changes accompany the response)

Emphasize the importance of recognizing tension within oneself (and reducing it before it becomes overwhelming)

Explain how to channel emotional energy and obtain release from stress (hammering, beating a pillow, bicycling, laughing, talking things over)

Recommend things to do when one begins to feel out of control (such as washing one's hands and face in cold water and taking deep breaths to give the person something to do besides feel)

Explain the importance of remaining calm (to conserve energy, and reduce internal tension, for a more realistic problem-solving approach)

Explain why persons should maintain self-control (out of respect for oneself and others, for role modeling, and to gain social approval)

Explain the importance of maintaining a positive self-attitude (positive attitudes promote positive behavior)

Explain that change must come from within the person (not from without)

Recommend that behavioral limits be set (by the family)

Explain how to set behavioral limits (the family should clearly state what constitutes acceptable and unacceptable behavior)

EVALUATION

Record actual outcome

AGGRESSIVE BEHAVIOR[19,455,471]

ASSESSMENT

Data Collection

Subjective Data
- Relates participation in physical violence against persons or property
- Repetitive, persistent behavior
- Relates feelings of anger

Objective Data
- Physical violence may be observed
  May speak loudly with emphasis or be quiet and withdrawn
  Uses prolonged, intrusive eye contact with others
  Uses threatening gestures (shaking the fist, stamping the feet)
  Stands in an erect, dominating posture with slight movement toward the other person

Data Analysis

Nursing Diagnosis
AGGRESSIVE BEHAVIOR (AGGRESSIVE DISORDER): Repetitive and persistent violation of the basic rights of others or of society's norms evidence by assaultive, violent, or destructive behavior

Common Etiology (Stressors)
DISEASES: Organic brain sydnrome
INJURIES: Cerebral concussion
PSYCHOSOCIAL FACTORS: Lack of emotional contact, lack of external limits or control, unlearned alternative behavior, the threat of real or imagined danger, lack of competency in using effective coping mechanisms, exposure to a violent role model, an attempt to control others or a life situation, the threat of chronic or severe stress, an attempt to enhance one's own self-esteem, the threat of rejection, the presence of reinforcing stimuli that maintain the maladaptive behavior

LIFESTYLE: Alcohol abuse, drug abuse, cultural norms
ENVIRONMENTAL FACTORS: *Chemical substances*: Inhalation of chemical substances

PLANNING

Unmet Needs
Psychologic stability, caring and communicating relationships, high evaluation of self, self-control, personal growth and maturity, increased learning, increased reality perception and problem-solving ability

Expected Outcome
Person demonstrates respect for the rights of others
Uses nonviolent methods to express feelings and accomplish goals
Relates increased feelings of self-esteem
Demonstrates having learned how to display aggression appropriately by hitting a pillow, hammering a board, punching a bag, etc.

NURSING INTERVENTIONS

Nursing Treatments
Approach unhurriedly
Demonstrate calmness
Provide an atmosphere of acceptance (of the person, not of the behavior)
Encourage the expression of feelings
Relate to the person on an adult–adult level, not on a parent–child level
Listen attentively
    AND

Talk with the person
Offer feedback to the person's expressed feelings
Encourage the use of normal coping mechanisms
Explore with the person his strengths and resources (to overcome the violent behavior)
Ask the person to identify the problem
Explore with the person if there is a pattern leading up to the behavior
Explore with the person the reasons for recurring problems (of aggression or violence)
Explore with the person the need to control
Ask for specifics, not generalizations, about the problem
Explore with the person the effects of his behavior on others (it is emotionally upsetting and angers and embarrasses others)
Encourage respect for the rights of others
Encourage participation in therapeutic group interaction (to learn about behavior and interpersonal relationships)
Suggest more appropriate means of emotional expression (such as talking things over, redirecting energy into creative activities)
Set an example by role modeling
Ignore undesirable behavior
   OR
Set limits on unacceptable behavior
Clearly communicate what is expected of the person
Iold the person responsible for his behavior (do not allow the person to blame others)
Remove the stimulus for the emotion (stimulus such as a person, or a job situation that may precipitate the violence)
Provide seclusion (if needed)
   OR
Restrain the person (if combative)
Reduce the demands placed on the person (so there is more energy for coping)
Refrain from arguing, from negatively criticizing
Refrain from using punitive measures (when exercising authority)
Verbalize daily the person's successful progress (in changing behavior)
Touch the person judiciously
Keep the person's door open (in case the nurse needs to exit rapidly during acute, uncontrollable violence)
Consult with the physician (about appropriate medication)
Provide emotional support for persons significant to the patient
Provide the family with information about the patient's progress (daily)

Nursing Observations
Determine the degree of insight that the person has (into the violent behavior)
Determine the precipitating factors (for the violence)
Evaluate the person's relatedness with others
Evaluate the significance of emotional distress mannerisms
Evaluate the significance of nonverbal communication
Identify disturbing conversation topics
Identify emotion-stimulating events
Identify potentially destructive behavior (threats of violence or destruction)
Determine the extent of group pressure conformity (in relationship to the destructive behavior)
Identify life values significant to the person (Is value placed on human life and property?)
Observe for evidence that the person is reaching out for emotional support
Observe for behavior modification (resulting from the therapy)

Health Teaching
Explain the causes of the problem (lack of emotional control, exposure to a poor role model, use of ineffective coping methods)

Explain what is considered justifiable aggression (self-defense in response to a real threat)

Advise that highly emotional situations be avoided (which can precipitate violence)

Explain how emotional responses occur (a situation is perceived in terms of its significance to the person, an emotional response is experienced, and physiologic changes accompany the response)

Emphasize the importance of recognizing tension within oneself (and reducing it before it becomes overwhelming)

Explain that change must come from within the person (not from without)

Explain how to channel emotional energy and obtain release from stress (by hammering, beating on a pillow, bicycling, running, laughing, working out with exercise equipment and through hobbies, travel, work, etc.)

Recommend things to do when one begins to feel out of control (such as washing one's face and hands in cold water, taking deep breaths, and counting to 500, to give the person something to do besides feel)

Explain the importance of remaining calm (to conserve energy and reduce internal tension for a more realistic problem-solving approach)

Explain why persons should maintain self-control (out of respect for oneself and others, to provide role modeling, to gain social approval, for reasons of attaining positive behavior and its end results)

Explain the importance of maintaining a positive self-attitude (positive attitudes support positive behavior)

Explain the importance of learning and practicing health principles (good mental health supports a fulfilling life)

Recommend that behavioral limits be set (by the family)

Explain how to set behavioral limits (the family should clearly state what is acceptable and unacceptable behavior)

Explain the reason for and intended effect of the methods used (to prevent the person from harming himself or others, and include an explanation of nursing's legal responsibility to prevent a person from harming himself or others)

EVALUATION

Record actual outcome

EXPLOSIVE BEHAVIOR[19,471]

ASSESSMENT

Data Collection

Subjective Data
• Acute, aggressive onset with quick remission
• History of explosive behavior
  Relates regret or self-reproach after the episode

Objective Data
• Sudden violent outbursts
• Behavior is out of proportion to the stressor
• Absence of aggressive or impulsive behavior between explosive episodes

Data Analysis

Nursing Diagnosis
EXPLOSIVE BEHAVIOR (EXPLOSIVE DISORDER): Loss of control of aggressive impulses resulting in an assault on persons or destruction of property

Common Etiology (Stressors)
BIRTH DEFECTS: Developmental deficit
DISEASES: Encephalitis, epilepsy

INJURIES: Cerebral concussion or contusion, perinatal trauma
PSYCHOSOCIAL FACTORS: An attempt to control others
LIFESTYLE: Alcohol or drug abuse, cultural norms

PLANNING

Unmet Needs

Psychologic stability, caring and communicating relationships, self-control, personal
growth and maturity, increased learning, increased reality perception and problem-
solving ability

Expected Outcome

Person verbalizes how to anticipate cues that indicate an impending explosive outburst
Makes plans to use control measures such as self-isolation
Demonstrates how to display aggression appropriately by hitting a pillow, hammering a
board, punching a bag, etc.
Uses nonviolent methods to express feelings and accomplish goals
Demonstrates respect for the rights of others

NURSING INTERVENTIONS

Nursing Treatments

Approach unhurriedly
Demonstrate calmness
Provide an atmosphere of acceptance (of the person, not of the behavior)
Relate to the person on an adult–adult level, not on a parent–child level
Encourage the expression of feelings
Listen attentively
Talk with the person
Explore with the person whether there is a pattern leading up to the behavior (the pre-
cise sequence of events or situations leading up to the behavior)
Explore with the person his strengths and resources (to overcome the explosive behav-
ior)
Ask the person to identify the problem
Ask for specifics, not generalizations, about the problem (such as cues that indicate an
impending outburst of explosive behavior)
Set limits on unacceptable behavior (even though the basis for the behavior may be
physiologic)
Clearly communicate what is expected of the person
Hold the person responsible for his behavior (do not allow the person to blame others)
Provide seclusion (if needed)
Explore with the person the effects of his behavior on others (it is emotionally upsetting
and it angers and embarrasses others)
Encourage respect for the rights of others
Suggest more appropriate means of emotional expression (such as talking things over)
Refrain from arguing and from negatively criticizing
Refrain from using punitive measures (when exercising authority)
Verbalize daily the person's successful progress (in changing behavior)
Touch the person judiciously
Keep the person's door open (in case the nurse needs to rapidly exit during an acute,
explosive episode)
Consult with the physician (about appropriate medication)
Provide emotional support for persons significant to the patient
Provide the family with information about the person's progress (daily)

Nursing Observations

Determine the degree of insight that the person has (into the cues that indicate an
impending episode and the causes of the explosive behavior itself)
Identify emotion-stimulating events (such as alcohol or drug abuse, exposure to loud
music)

Observe for evidence that the person is reaching out for emotional support
Observe for behavior modification (resulting from the therapy)

Health Teaching

Explain the causes of the problem (brain cell abnormalities or alcohol or drug effects that result in decreased impulse control)

Explain what is considered justifiable aggression (self-defense in response to a real threat)

Advise that highly emotional situations be avoided

Recommend methods for reducing sensory stimulation (such as eliminating loud noises, flashing or bright lights, rapidly moving objects)

Emphasize the importance of recognizing tension within oneself (as a cue to impending explosive behavior, and recommend that the person use the technique of self-imposed isolation if the explosive episodes are uncontrollable)

Explain how to channel emotional energy and obtain release from stress (by hammering, beating on a pillow, running, laughing and through work, hobbies, etc.)

Recommend methods for achieving total relaxation (deep breathing, listening to soft music, doing nothing)

Explain why persons should maintain self-control (out of respect for oneself and others)

Explain the importance of maintaining a positive self-attitude (positive attitudes support positive behavior)

Recommend that behavioral limits be set (by the family)

Explain how to set behavioral limits (the family should clearly state what constitutes acceptable and unacceptable behavior)

Explain the reason for and intended effect of the methods used (to prevent the person from harming himself or others, and include an explanation of nursing's responsibility to prevent a person from harming oneself or others)

EVALUATION

Record actual outcome

PASSIVE–AGGRESSIVE BEHAVIOR[19,471]

ASSESSMENT

Data Collection

Subjective Data
- Relates that the behavior is long-term
- Relates ineffective performance and nonachievement of goals
- Verbalizes the intention to do one thing but does something else
  May use sarcasm
  Uses derogatory humor

Objective Data
- Demonstrates resistance behavior such as procrastination, stubbornness, forgetfulness, dawdling
- Continues to use passive–aggressive behavior even when self-assertion is possible
  Little eye contact
  Assumes slouched posture with arms close to the body
  May fidget considerably

Data Analysis

Nursing Diagnosis
PASSIVE–AGGRESSIVE BEHAVIOR (PASSIVE–AGGRESSIVE DISORDER): The indirect expression of anger

Common Etiology (Stressors)
PSYCHOSOCIAL FACTORS: The threat of being overly controlled, the threat of real or imagined danger, lack of competency in using effective coping mechanisms, unlearned al-

ternative behavior, an attempt to express anger indirectly, lack of control of a life situation, the presence of reinforcing stimuli that maintain the maladaptive behavior

PLANNING

Unmet Needs

Psychologic stability, direct and communicating relationships, personal growth and maturity, increased learning, increased problem-solving ability

Expected Outcome

Person directly verbalizes his feelings and needs

Demonstrates how to display aggression appropriately by hitting a pillow, hammering a board, punching a bag, etc.

NURSING INTERVENTIONS

Nursing Treatments

Approach unhurriedly

Demonstrate calmness

Provide an atmosphere of acceptance (of the person, not of the behavior)

Relate to the person on an adult–adult level, not on a parent–child level

Encourage the expression of feelings (directly instead of indirectly)

Listen attentively

Talk with the person

Offer feedback to the person's expressed feelings

Explore with the person his strengths and resources (to overcome the passive–aggressive behavior)

Ask the person to identify the problem

Explore with the person reasons for recurring problems (of passive–aggressive behavior)

Ask for specifics, not generalizations, about the problem

Explore with the person the effects of his behavior on others (it irritates and angers others)

Encourage participation in therapeutic group interaction (to learn about behavior and interpersonal relationships)

Suggest more appropriate means of emotional expression (by calmly and directly relating one's feelings of anger)

Set an example by role modeling

Ignore undesirable behavior

    OR

Set limits on unacceptable behavior

Clearly communicate what is expected of the person

Hold the person responsible for his behavior (do not allow the person to blame others)

Refrain from arguing, from negatively criticizing

Refrain from using punitive measures (when exercising authority)

Verbalize daily the person's successful progress (in changing the behavior)

Provide the family with information about the patient's progress (and work with the family, helping them change how they relate to the person)

Nursing Observations

Determine the degree of insight that the person has (into the passive–aggressive behavior)

Determine the precipitating factors (dominating significant other, conflicting goals of different persons)

Evaluate the person's relatedness with others

Evaluate the significance of emotional distress mannerisms

Evaluate the significance of nonverbal communication

Identify disturbing conversation topics (which reveal what the person is really angry about)

Identify life values significant to the person (such as a distaste for open aggression)

Observe for evidence that the person is reaching out for emotional support

Observe for behavior modification (resulting from the therapy)

Health Teaching

Explain the causes of the problem (being overly controlled, unlearned alternative behavior, the indirect expression of anger, the unfavorable consequences of being direct)

Emphasize the importance of recognizing tension within oneself (and coping effectively with it)

Explain that change must come from within the person (not from without)

Explain how to channel emotional energy and obtain release from stress (by hammering, beating on a pillow, running, laughing and through work, sports, travel, etc.)

Recommend methods for achieving total relaxation (deep breathing, biofeedback)

Explain the importance of maintaining a positive self-attitude (positive attitudes support positive behavior)

Explain the importance of learning and practicing health principles (as a means to a more positive life)

Recommend that behavioral limits be set (by the family)

Explain how to set behavioral limits (the family should state clearly what constitutes acceptable and unacceptable behavior)

EVALUATION

Record actual outcome

Nonadaptive Responses of Emotion (Affect): Anxiety

COMPULSIVE BEHAVIOR[19,471]

ASSESSMENT

Data Collection

Subjective Data
• Relates being compelled to perform certain behaviors despite a desire to resist the compulsion
• Performance is excessive
• Derives tension release from the activity
• Relates impaired social or role functioning
• May perceive the behavior to be senseless

Objective Data
• Repetitive behaviors can be observed

Data Analysis

Nursing Diagnosis
COMPULSIVE BEHAVIOR (COMPULSIVE DISORDER): A recurring, irresistible impulse to perform the same act over and over as an expression of anxiety

Common Etiology (Stressors)
DISEASES: Major depression, organic brain syndrome, schizophrenia, Tourette's syndrome
PSYCHOSOCIAL FACTORS: An attempt to express overwhelming anxiety or guilt indirectly, the threat of real or imagined danger, lack of competency in using effective coping mechanisms, an excessively rigid conscience

PLANNING

Unmet Needs

Comfort, protection from physical or psychologic threat, psychologic stability, self-control, personal growth and maturity, increased learning, increased reality perception and problem-solving ability

Expected Outcome

Person no longer performs compelling acts
Demonstrates the use of more appropriate coping mechanisms
Verbalizes feelings of relaxation and comfort

NURSING INTERVENTIONS

Nursing Treatments

Approach unhurriedly
Provide an atmosphere of acceptance
Encourage the expression of feelings (about the anxiety causing the compulsive behavior)
Listen attentively
Talk with the person
Offer feedback to the person's expressed feelings
Communicate nurse sensitivity to the person's problem
Relate to the person on an adult–adult level, not on a parent–child level (which causes increased anxiety)
Ask for specifics, not generalizations, about the problem
Support a realistic assessment of the situation (which may not be as threatening as perceived)
Assist the person to convert the anxiety into a specifically identified fear (so the problem can be recognized and dealt with)
Explore with the person whether there is a pattern leading up to the behavior (Is there a sequence of events leading up to the behavior? Can that sequence be changed?)
Support the use of appropriate defense mechanisms
Refrain from negatively criticizing
Set limits on unacceptable behavior (for example, the person may only wash his hands five times daily)
Verbalize daily the person's successful progress (in overcoming the compulsive behavior)
Make a referral (to a physician for possible medication therapy)

Nursing Observations

Determine the degree of insight that the person has (into the compulsive behavior)
Identify disturbing conversation topics (which reveal the underlying anxiety)
Observe for evidence of a favorable response to therapy (decreased compulsive and more appropriate behavior)

Health Teaching

Explain the causes of the problem (it is an indirect expression of anxiety)
Explain that anxiety often disguises itself (and the expressed anxiety may be a substitute for a less socially acceptable anxiety)
Explain how to use the stop-and-think technique (have the person shout "stop" to himself, an act that interrupts the compulsive behavior and gives the person time to substitute another behavior)
Explain the importance of learning and practicing mental health principles
Emphasize the importance of recognizing tension within oneself (before the tension becomes overwhelming)
Explain that some tension is normal
Explain how to channel emotional energy and obtain release from stress (running, creative activities, laughing, etc.)

EVALUATION

Record actual outcome

OBSESSIVE THOUGHTS[19,471]

ASSESSMENT

Data Collection

Subjective Data
- Person relates recurring ideas, images, thoughts, or impulses
- Relates that they are unwanted and cannot be dismissed
- Perceives them to be senseless or repugnant
- Relates impaired social or role functioning
  Conversation focuses on obsessive thoughts
  Experiences anxiety

Objective Data
None

Data Analysis

Nursing Diagnosis
OBSESSIVE THOUGHTS (OBSESSIVE DISORDER, RUMINATION): The persistent recurrence of involuntary unwanted thoughts

Common Etiology (Stressors)
DISEASES: Major depression, schizophrenia
PSYCHOSOCIAL FACTORS: An attempt to express overwhelming anxiety or guilt indirectly, the threat of real or imagined danger, lack of competency in using effective coping mechanisms, an excessively rigid conscience

PLANNING

Unmet Needs

Comfort, protection from psychologic threat, psychologic stability, personal growth and maturity, increased learning, increased reality perception and problem-solving ability

Expected Outcome

Person verbalizes that the unwanted thoughts are no longer persistent or, if persistent, are no longer disturbing
Demonstrates the use of more appropriate coping mechanisms

NURSING INTERVENTIONS

Nursing Treatments

Approach unhurriedly
Provide an atmosphere of acceptance
Encourage the expression of feelings (about the anxiety causing the obsessive thoughts)
Listen attentively
Talk with the person
Offer feedback to the person's expressed feelings
Communicate nurse sensitivity to the person's problem
Relate to the person on an adult–adult level, not on a parent–child level (which could increase the anxiety)
Ask for specifics, not generalizations, about the problem
Support a realistic assessment of the situation (which may not be as threatening as perceived)
Assist the person to convert the anxiety into a specifically identified fear (so the problem can be recognized and dealt with)
Explore with the person the reasons for recurring problems (of obsessive thoughts)
Support the use of appropriate defense mechanisms
Refrain from negatively criticizing
Encourage active diversional activities (such as whistling, humming a tune, gardening, or reading, to divert one's attention from the unwanted thoughts)

Make a referral (to a physician for possible medication therapy)

Nursing Observations

Determine the degree of insight that the person has (into the obsessive thoughts)

Identify disturbing conversation topics (that reflect underlying anxiety)

Observe for evidence of a favorable response to therapy (decreased obsessive thoughts)

Health Teaching

Explain the causes of the problem (it is an indirect expression of anxiety)

Explain that anxiety often disguises itself (and the expressed anxiety may be a substitute for a less socially acceptable anxiety)

Explain how to use the stop-and-think technique (have the person shout "stop" to himself, an act that interrupts the obsessive thought and gives the person time to substitute another thought)

Explain the importance of learning and practicing mental health principles

Emphasize the importance of recognizing tension within oneself (before the tension becomes overwhelming)

Explain that some tension is normal

Explain how to channel emotional energy and obtain release from stress (through creative activities, sports, laughing, etc.)

EVALUATION

Record actual outcome

OBSESSIVE–COMPULSIVE BEHAVIOR[19,471]

ASSESSMENT

Data Collection

Subjective Data

- Relates recurring ideas, images, thoughts, or impulses that are unwanted and that cannot be dismissed
- Relates being compelled to perform certain behaviors despite the desire to resist the compulsion

Objective Data

- Repetitive compulsive behavior can be observed, such as persistent hand washing, following ritualistic patterns

Data Analysis

Nursing Diagnosis

OBSESSIVE–COMPULSIVE BEHAVIOR (OBSESSIVE-COMPULSIVE DISORDER): A combined persistent recurrence of unwanted thoughts and the performance of compelling activity

Common Etiology (Stressors)

DISEASES: Major depression, organic brain syndrome, schizophrenia, Tourette's syndrome

PSYCHOSOCIAL FACTORS: An attempt to express overwhelming anxiety or guilt indirectly, the threat of real or imagined danger, lack of competency in using effective coping mechanisms, an excessively rigid conscience

PLANNING

Unmet Needs

Comfort, protection from psychologic threat, psychologic stability, self-control, personal growth and maturity, increased learning, increased reality perception and problem-solving ability

Expected Outcome

Person no longer performs compelling acts

Verbalizes that unwanted thoughts are no longer persistent or, if persistent, are no longer disturbing

Uses more appropriate coping mechanisms

NURSING INTERVENTIONS

Nursing Treatments

Approach unhurriedly

Provide an atmosphere of acceptance

Encourage the expression of feelings (about the anxiety causing the compulsive behavior)

Listen attentively

Talk with the person

Offer feedback to the person's expressed feelings

Communicate nurse sensitivity to the person's problem

Relate to the person on an adult–adult level, not on a parent–child level (which could increase anxiety)

Ask for specifics, not generalizations, about the problem

Support a realistic assessment of the situation (which may not be as threatening as perceived)

Assist the person to convert the anxiety into a specifically identified fear (so the problem can be recognized and dealt with)

Explore with the person whether there is a pattern leading to the behavior

Explore with the person the reasons for recurring problems (of obsessive–compulsive behavior)

Support the use of appropriate defense mechanisms

Refrain from negatively criticizing

Encourage active diversional activities (such as whistling or humming a tune to divert one's attention from the unwanted thoughts)

Set limits on unacceptable behavior (such as the number of times per day the person exhibits compulsive behavior)

Verbalize daily the person's successful progress (in overcoming compulsive behavior)

Make a referral (to a physician for possible medication therapy)

Nursing Observations

Determine the degree of insight that the person has (into the obsessive–compulsive behavior)

Identify disturbing conversation topics (that reflect the underlying anxiety)

Observe for evidence of a favorable response to therapy (reduced compulsive behavior and expressed relief that obsessive thoughts have decreased)

Health Teaching

Explain the causes of the problem (it is an indirect expression of anxiety)

Explain that anxiety often disguises itself (and the expressed anxiety may be a substitute for a less socially acceptable anxiety)

Explain how to use the stop-and-think technique (have the person shout "stop" to himself, an act that interrupts the obsessive thought and gives the person the time to substitute another thought)

Explain the importance of learning and practicing mental health principles

Emphasize the importance of recognizing tension within oneself (before tension becomes overwhelming)

Explain that some tension is normal

Explain how to channel emotional energy and obtain release from stress (through sports, creative activities, etc.)

EVALUATION

Record actual outcome

OVERANXIOUS BEHAVIOR[19,105]

ASSESSMENT

Data Collection

Subjective Data
- Unrealistic worry of the child about future events
- Preoccupation with appropriateness of past behavior
- Overconcern about personal competence in school and socially
  May refuse to participate in school or in social activities

Objective Data
- No physical findings despite complaints of headache, stomachache, etc.
  Nail biting
  Pulling at one's own hair
  Poor school performance
  Inattentiveness

Data Analysis

Nursing Diagnosis
OVERANXIOUS BEHAVIOR (OVERANXIOUS DISORDER): A child's excessive concern with the future or past events

Common Etiology (Stressors)
PSYCHOSOCIAL FACTORS: The threat of real or imagined danger, the absence or loss of a significant other (usually a parent), the gain of a significant other (a new baby in the family), the threat of change (a new home or school)

PLANNING

Unmet Needs

Comfort, protection from psychologic threat, psychologic stability, personal growth and maturity, increased learning, increased reality perception and problem-solving ability

Expected Outcome

Child no longer exhibits worry or somatic complaints
Becomes attentive and finds school a rewarding experience
Interacts satisfactorily with peers

NURSING INTERVENTIONS

Nursing Treatments

Approach unhurriedly
Provide an atmosphere of acceptance
Provide frequent contact with the person
Demonstrate calmness
Reassure verbally (that the nurse and significant others will help the child through the situation)
Encourage the expression of feelings (about future and past events)
Listen attentively
Talk with the child
Offer feedback to the child's expressed feelings
Support a realistic assessment of the situation (which may not be as threatening as perceived)
Explore with the child his strengths and resources (to meet and enjoy the changes such as going to a new school or having a new sibling)
Provide reliable information (which will ease the anxiety)
Provide emotionally safe experiences
Reduce the demands placed upon the patient
Refrain from performing nonessential procedures (during the overanxious period)

Refrain from negatively criticizing

Involve the family (and help them provide the child with a consistent family support system)

Make a referral (to a psychiatric nurse specialist if needed)

Nursing Observations

Determine the degree of insight that the child has (into the overanxious behavior)

Evaluate the child's relatedness with others (such as parents, siblings, peers)

Evaluate the significance of emotional distress mannerisms

Evaluate the significance of nonverbal communication

Identify disturbing conversation topics

Identify emotion-stimulating events

Observe for evidence of a favorable response to therapy (decreased anxiety)

Health Teaching

Describe those factors that intensify anxiety (such as being alone, being in the dark)

Emphasize the importance of recognizing tension within oneself (before it becomes overwhelming)

Explain how to channel emotional energy and obtain release from stress (through sports, creative activities, schoolwork)

Explain that the situation is temporary (that the child will feel more comfortable in time)

Explain that persons must make adjustments at their own pace

Advise that significant persons express caring for one another (which reduces the anxiety)

EVALUATION

Record actual outcome

PANIC DISORDER [19,455,471]

ASSESSMENT

Data Collection

Subjective Data
* Sudden onset of intense dread and terror
* Feeling of impending doom
* Relates that it has occurred at least three times a week for a 3-week period
* Not associated with either severe physical exertion or a life-threatening situation
* Complaints such as palpitations, chest pain, choking, dyspnea, dizziness, unsteadiness, extremity tingling, hot or cold flashes, trembling
  Rapid speech
  Crying episodes

Objective Data
  Increased motor activity
  Unable to maintain normal function, even with direction

Data Analysis

Nursing Diagnosis
PANIC DISORDER (ANXIETY ATTACK): The sudden onset of very severe, intense anxiety

Common Etiology (Stressors)
DISEASES: Asthma, hyperthyroidism, hypoglycemia, mitral valve prolapse, pheochromocytoma
SIGNS AND SYMPTOMS: Confusion, delusions, severe pain, hallucinations

PSYCHOSOCIAL FACTORS: The threat of painful unconscious thoughts emerging into the consciousness, the threat of or deprivation of essential needs, the threat of intimacy, the threat of physical closeness, loss of or separation from a significant other, the threat of real or imagined danger, lack of competency in using effective coping mechanisms

HEALTH CARE FACTORS: *Hospitalization*: Separation from a significant other during hospitalization. *Diagnostic procedure*: Unfamiliar diagnostic procedures. *Medical diagnosis*: An unfavorable medical diagnosis. *Medical diagnosis of a significant other*: Unfavorable medical diagnosis of a significant other. *Drug therapy*: Adverse effects of amphetamines, corticosteroids, epinephrine. *Medical therapy*: Unfamiliar medical therapy, withdrawal from alcohol or drugs. *Surgical therapy*: Impending surgery. *Therapeutic devices*: Enforced confinement with safety restraints

LIFESTYLE: Drug abuse with lysergic acid diethylamide (LSD), marijuana, phencyclidine (PCP)

SITUATIONAL FACTORS: Confinement in a prison, death of a significant other, divorce, acute illness or injury, acute illness or injury of a significant other, impending marriage, loss of employment, birth of a first child

ENVIRONMENTAL FACTORS: *Cataclysm*: Exposure to an earthquake, flood, etc.

PLANNING

Unmet Needs
Comfort, protection from psychologic threat, psychologic stability, caring and communicating relationships, sense of adequacy, self-control, personal growth and maturity, increased learning, increased reality perception and problem-solving ability

Expected Outcome
Person verbalizes feeling calm and in control
Maintains self-initiated daily activities
No longer exhibits somatic complaints

NURSING INTERVENTIONS

Nursing Treatments
General Interventions
Approach unhurriedly
Demonstrate calmness
Express empathy
Provide an atmosphere of acceptance
Touch the person judiciously
Reassure verbally (that the intense anxiety can be controlled)
Attend the person constantly (until he feels sufficiently comfortable to be alone)
Provide frequent contact with the person (thereafter)
Encourage the expression of feelings
Listen attentively
Talk with the person
Offer feedback to the person's expressed feelings
Communicate nurse sensitivity to the person's problem
Relate to the person on an adult–adult level, not on a parent–child level (which could increase anxiety)
Ask for specifics, not generalizations, about the problem
Support a realistic assessment of the situation (which may not be as threatening as perceived)
Provide reliable information (which may ease the anxiety, and explain the physiologic reason for body sensations that mimic anxiety)
Assist the person to convert the anxiety into a specifically identified fear (so the problem can be recognized and dealt with)
Encourage the person to face the anxiety (avoidance increases anxiety)
Explore with the person if there is a pattern leading up to the behavior (if a specific se-

quence of events leads up to the behavior, that sequence can be changed)
Encourage the use of normal coping mechanisms
Reduce the demands placed on the person (so that more energy is available for coping)
Do not allow unpleasant surprise situations (which increase anxiety)
Avoid placing the person on enforced inactivity (which heightens anxiety)
Massage gently
    OR
Bathe in warm water (for the relaxation effect)
Call the person's family (to the bedside if the person desires such)
Encourage telephone calls with significant persons
Arrange a structured daily routine (suitable to the person)
Arrange orderly surroundings
Provide quiet
Acknowledge dependency (if the panic condition severely reduces the person's ability to function)
Restrict unwanted visitors
Explore with the person the reasons for recurring problems (related to the anxiety)
Encourage active diversional activities (to promote periods of rest from the anxiety)
Encourage gradual mastery of the situation (causing the anxiety)
Encourage planned one-day-at-a-time living
Make a referral (to a psychiatric nurse specialist if needed)
Consult with a physician (about medication to reduce the panic)

Nursing Observations
Determine the degree of insight that the person has
Determine the precipitating factors, the relieving factors
Evaluate the significance of emotional distress mannerisms
Evaluate the significance of nonverbal communication
Identify disturbing conversation topics
Identify abnormal perceptions (hallucinations, illusions)
Identify abnormal thought content (delusions)
Identify attention span abnormalities
Observe for impaired judgment (which could cause the person to harm himself, taking appropriate precautionary action)
Observe for side effects of drug
    (to caffeine or epinephrine)
Monitor blood studies for
    abnormal (decreased) glucose
Monitor blood studies for
    abnormal (increased) thyroid
    function   } Indicating that the panic is of a
Monitor blood studies for   physical origin
    arterial blood gases (decreased O_2 level)
Monitor blood studies for
    abnormal (increased) adrenal function
Monitor blood studies for
    increased lactic acid
Observe for evidence of a favorable response to therapy (reduced anxiety, identified fear, increased functioning ability)

Health Teaching
Advise against fighting anxiety (which reinforces the anxiety)
Explain and offer hope that the emotional pain will decrease with time
Describe those factors that intensify anxiety (being alone, or in the dark)
Emphasize the importance of recognizing tension within oneself (before it becomes overwhelming)

Explain the need to recognize highly stressful situations (and to be prepared to cope with them)

Explain how to channel emotional energy and obtain release from stress (talking things over, laughing, participating in sports, creative activities)

Explain how to use the stop-and-think technique (have the person shout "stop" to himself, an act that interrupts the panic-provoking thoughts and gives the person time to substitute calm thoughts)

Explain the difference between freedom from anxiety and freedom from problems (people will always have problems, but approaching them with positive solutions reduces anxiety)

Recommend methods for achieving total relaxation (controlled breathing, listening to quiet music, doing nothing)

Explain that the situation is temporary (if it is, and that the anxiety will decrease as he feels more comfortable with the anxiety-provoking situation)

Explain that persons must make adjustments at their own pace

Advise that significant persons express caring for one another (which reduces anxiety)

Explain the causes of the problem (both physical and psychologic)

EVALUATION

Record actual outcome

SEPARATION ANXIETY[19,471]

ASSESSMENT

Data Collection

Subjective Data
- Child expresses concern that his major attachment figure will be harmed, will leave, or will never return
- Child is concerned that he will be harmed and separated from his major attachment figure
- Expresses reluctance to go to school, with preference for staying home
- Physical complaints of headache, stomachache, etc.

Objective Data
- Temper tantrums, crying, or pleading either before or when the attachment figure leaves

Data Analysis

Nursing Diagnosis
SEPARATION ANXIETY: A child's excessive concern with separation from a major attachment figure

Common Etiology (Stressors)
PSYCHOSOCIAL FACTORS: The absence of, loss of, or separation from a significant other
HEALTH CARE FACTORS: *Hospitalization of a significant other*: Separation during the hospitalization of a significant other
DEVELOPMENTAL PHASES: Childhood, preschooler aged 3–6
SITUATIONAL FACTORS: Being a foster child, death of a significant other, divorce, extensive travel by a significant other, loss or relocation of a home

PLANNING

Unmet Needs

Comfort, protection from psychologic threat, psychologic stability, independence, self-control, personal growth and maturity, increased learning

Expected Outcome

Child no longer has somatic complaints
Goes to school willingly
Functions at his or her developmental level

NURSING INTERVENTIONS

Nursing Treatments

Approach unhurriedly
Provide an atmosphere of acceptance
Provide frequent patient contact
Demonstrate calmness
Reassure verbally (that the nurse is available, that the significant other is safe and will return)
Encourage the expression of feelings (about the anxiety)
Listen attentively
Talk with the child
Offer feedback to the child's expressed feelings
Support a realistic assessment of the situation (that separation is a normal part of life)
Provide reliable information (which will reduce the anxiety)
Explore with the person his strengths and resources (to overcome the problem)
Encourage telephone calls with significant persons
Encourage active diversional activities
Provide emotionally safe experiences (until the anxiety decreases)
Arrange orderly surroundings
Arrange a structured daily routine
Do not allow unpleasant surprise situations (which increase anxiety)
Reduce the demands placed on the person
Refrain from performing nonessential procedures
Refrain from negatively criticizing
Set limits on unacceptable behavior (such as temper tantrums, crying)
Involve the family (and help them provide the child with a consistent family support system)
Make a referral (to a psychiatric nurse specialist if needed)

Nursing Observations

Determine the degree of insight that the person has (into the anxiety)
Evaluate the person's relatedness with others (especially the attachment figure)
Evaluate the significance of emotional distress mannerisms, the significance of nonverbal communication
Identify disturbing conversation topics
Identify emotion-stimulating events
Observe for evidence of a favorable response to therapy (reduced anxiety, increased comfort with the separation)

Health Teaching

Explain that the situation is temporary (if the separation is temporary, and relate when a reunion will occur)
Explain that persons must make adjustments (to separations) at their own pace
Advise that significant persons express caring for one another (to reduce the trauma of separation)

EVALUATION

Record actual outcome

Nonadaptive Responses of Emotion (Affect): Attachment

MATERNAL-CHILD NONBONDING[105,207,251,471,776]

ASSESSMENT
Data Collection

Subjective Data

Maternal Responses
- Mother verbalizes negative comments about and finds fault with the infant
- Enjoys leaving the infant with someone else
- Relates that she seldom thinks about the infant while away
- Little or no verbal interaction with the child

Objective Data

Maternal Responses
- No *en face* positioning, with little or no eye contact
- Does not affectionately touch or gently explore the infant and neither caresses nor cuddles the child

  Will allow the child to "cry it out"

  Pays little attention to the feeding infant

  Rarely takes the infant out

  Rejects the child's efforts for physical contact with the mother

  Punishes the child inappropriately

  Interferes with the child's activities

  Mother has a fixed facial expression and tense body movements

Child's Responses
- Child makes little effort to approach or contact the mother after a separation
- May ignore or turn away from the mother
- Child tends to turn away from persons in favor of objects in the environment

Data Analysis

Nursing Diagnosis

MATERNAL–CHILD NONBONDING: The absence of emotional closeness and caring that bind a mother to a child

Common Etiology (Stressors)

BIRTH DEFECTS: Giving birth to an imperfect infant

DISEASES: Schizophrenia

PSYCHOSOCIAL FACTORS: The threat of inadequacy as a mother, differences between maternal prebirth fantasies and postbirth realities about the infant, the threat of responsibility beyond the mother's developmental phase, lack of emotional support (positive reinforcement) from others, the threat of intimacy, loss of a significant other (recent loss makes the mother unable to attach to another), loss of the expected normal child, lack of the expected, positive infant response to mothering, the threat of possibly harming the infant

HEALTH CARE FACTORS: *Complications*: A complicated pregnancy or delivery

SITUATIONAL FACTORS: Chronic maternal or infant illness

DEVELOPMENTAL PHASES: Adolescence

SITUATIONAL FACTORS: Placing a child up for adoption, an unwanted and unplanned pregnancy, unwed parents, multiple births, having been abused as a child

PLANNING

Unmet Needs

Acceptance, caring and communicating relationships, a sense of adequacy, personal growth and maturity, increased learning, increased reality perception

Expected Outcome

Parent will verbalize an understanding of the nonbonding behavior
Will verbalize feelings about the relationship
Will modify current behavior and exhibit a bonding relationship to the child

NURSING INTERVENTIONS

Nursing Treatments

Approach unhurriedly
Demonstrate calmness
Provide an atmosphere of acceptance (that bonding has not occurred)
Encourage the expression of feelings (about the lack of bonding between parent and infant)
Listen attentively
Talk with the person
Offer feedback to the person's expressed feelings
Communicate nurse sensitivity to the person's problem
Clearly communicate what is expected of the person (in her culture when she becomes a mother)
Hold the person responsible for her behavior (do not allow the woman to blame others for her nonbonding behavior)
Set an example by role modeling (show how to care for and relate to the infant by your example)
Encourage the mother/father to explore the newborn (to unwrap and undress the infant and to look at and feel the infant's body)
Ask the mother what makes her comfortable (and provide such when her infant visits, especially if the mother feels ill)
Encourage patience in developing relationships (point out that bonding takes time)
Offer praise (when the mother successfully completes caring activities, both physical and emotional)
Encourage the acceptance of responsibility (for the child)
Encourage an awareness of positive responses from the child (infant smiling, responses to rocking and feeding, etc.)
Encourage participation in therapeutic group interaction
Encourage recognition of one's various roles in life
Encourage role-playing to develop sensitivity
Encourage the use of normal coping mechanisms
Explore superficial topics and reasons for avoiding in-depth feelings
Explore with the person her strengths and resources (to be a successful mother)
Make a referral (if efforts to establish bonding fail consider referral to a psychiatric nurse specialist or if the mother wishes to give away the infant refer to the appropriate social agency and consider referral to visiting nurses who can observe for possible abuse)

Nursing Observations

Determine the degree of insight that the mother has (into her attitude toward the infant)
Evaluate the significance of nonverbal communication
Identify disturbing conversation topics
Identify life values significant to the person
Observe for an excessive stress level
Observe for evidence that the person is reaching out for emotional support
Observe performance level and problems involved in completing the task (as the mother cares for the infant)

Observe for readiness to assume infant care (if bonding occurs)

Observe for evidence of a favorable response to therapy (successful bonding between parent and child)

Make a follow-up evaluation (to assess whether the nonbonding is detrimental to the infant's physical or emotional health)

Health Teaching

Explain about the unique personality of each child (that the newborn is often not what one expects, that one needs to look at and accept what the child is)

Advise that significant persons express acceptance of one another, that significant persons express caring and love for one another

Explain the importance of maintaining a positive self-attitude

Explain that parental attitudes affect child development

EVALUATION

Record actual outcome

SIGNIFICANT-OTHER NONBONDING [105,207,471,776]

ASSESSMENT

Data Collection

Subjective Data
- Person relates little or no interest in the other person
- Admits to seldom thinking about the other person
- May verbalize negative comments about and find fault with the other person
  May enjoy being away from the other person

Objective Data
- No overt expressions of caring such as touching, sitting close to another, offering comfort
- Quick to relinquish responsibility for the other person to whomever will assume it

Data Analysis

Nursing Diagnosis

SIGNIFICANT-OTHER NONBONDING: The absence of emotional closeness and caring between persons usually considered significant in one's life such as parents and older children, siblings, spouses, husband or wife, grandparents, and other extended family members

Common Etiology (Stressors)

PSYCHOSOCIAL FACTORS: The threat of inadequacy or of intimacy, lack of communications with others, an attempt to resist control by others, lack of emotional support from a significant other, lack of early training in socialization, differences in person's values

SITUATIONAL FACTORS: Stepparenting, being a stepchild, confinement (of the parent) in a prison, runaway parent

PLANNING

Unmet Needs

Comfort, protection from psychologic threat, acceptance, caring and communicating relationships, personal growth and maturity, increased learning, increased reality perception and problem-solving ability

Expected Outcome

Person verbalizes feelings about the nonbonding

Acknowledges that bonding may not occur, if such is true

Will modify current behavior and exhibit a bonding relationship if such is possible

Accepts and plans for other relationships in which bonding is likely

NURSING INTERVENTIONS

Nursing Treatments

Approach unhurriedly

Demonstrate calmness

Provide an atmosphere of acceptance (that bonding has not occurred)

Encourage the expression of feelings (about the absence of bonding)

Listen attentively

Talk with the person

Offer feedback to the person's expressed feelings

Communicate nurse sensitivity to the person's problem

Encourage patience in developing relationships (point out that bonding takes time)

Encourage honesty in presenting oneself to others (if both persons are free to be themselves, bonding is more likely to occur)

Encourage the sharing of common interests with others

Encourage the identification of specific life values (common to both persons)

Encourage the use of normal coping mechanisms (such as temporary withdrawal until persons are more comfortable with each other)

Encourage awareness of positive responses from others (which may indicate possible future bonding)

Support a realistic assessment of the situation (bonding may never occur, and persons involved may only live in peaceful coexistence)

Make a referral (if efforts to establish bonding fail and if bonding is essential to personal growth, consider referral to a psychiatric nurse specialist, psychologist, etc.)

Nursing Observations

Observe for an excessive stress level

Determine the degree of insight that both persons have

Observe for disturbing conversation topics (between the involved persons)

Observe for evidence of a favorable response to therapy (if it occurs)

Health Teaching

Advise that significant persons express acceptance of one another, that significant persons express caring and love for one another

Advise against causing defensive responses in others

Explain that the person's response is both appropriate and commonly experienced (especially where relationships were not sought by the person, but resulted from circumstances)

Recommend new options for effective methods of coping (living in peaceful coexistence, terminating a relationship)

EVALUATION

Record actual outcome

Nonadaptive Responses of Emotion (Affect): Depression

DEPRESSIVE REACTION [19,85,105,455,471]

ASSESSMENT

Data Collection

Subjective Data

• Relates a poor appetite

- Insomnia or hypersomnia
- Fatigue
- Feelings of worthlessness, guilt, failure, self-reproach, hopelessness
- Complaints of poor concentration, slowed thinking, emotional flatness or emptiness, unable to find pleasure in things
  Considers suicide
  Somatic complaints of backache, chest pain, dizziness, loss of sexual desire

Objective Data
- Slow activity in speech and movements
- Unable to maintain usual functions
  Sad facial expression
  Tearfulness
  Little or no eye contact
  Stooped posture
  Self-neglect

Data Analysis

Nursing Diagnosis
DEPRESSIVE REACTION: A change in mood reflecting loss of interest or pleasure in one's usual activities

Common Etiology (Stressors)
INHERITED FACTORS: Familial tendency to depression
PSYCHOSOCIAL FACTORS: The threat of or deprivation of essential needs, the threat of repeated failure to achieve, loss (of a relationship, role, significant other, or valued object), lack of emotional support from others, lack of competency in using effective coping mechanisms, an attempt to express anger indirectly
HUMAN BODY: *Body appearance*: Disfigured body. *Body function*: Loss of body function. *Body part*: Loss of a body part
HEALTH CARE FACTORS: *History*: Family history of depression
DEVELOPMENTAL PHASES: Aging
LIFESTYLE: Alcohol or drug abuse
SITUATIONAL FACTORS: Chronic or terminal illness, launching grown children, loss of employment, dying self, death of a significant other, divorce from a spouse, divorce of parents, marital separation, loss of or relocation of a home, lack of finances, retirement
ENVIRONMENTAL FACTORS: *Cataclysm*: Earthquake, flood, tornado, tidal wave, etc.

PLANNING

Unmet Needs
Protection from psychologic threat, psychologic stability, high evaluation of self, personal growth and maturity, increased learning, increased reality perception and problem-solving ability

Expected Outcome
Person verbalizes positive feelings about himself
Maintains self-initiated daily activities
Relates experiencing the usual pleasures of life
No longer exhibits somatic complaints

NURSING INTERVENTIONS

Nursing Treatments
Approach unhurriedly
Reassure verbally (that you will help the person overcome his depression)
Demonstrate calmness
Provide an atmosphere of acceptance
Encourage the expression of feelings (of moodiness, sadness, helplessness)
Listen attentively

Talk with the person
Offer feedback to the person's expressed feelings
Communicate nurse sensitivity to the person's problem
Relate to the person on an adult–adult level, not on a parent–child level (which could increase the depression)
Ask the person to identify the problem
Ask for specifics, not generalizations, about the problem
Support a realistic assessment of the situation (Is it really as he perceives it to be?)
Provide reliable information (which often reduces depression)
Reveal the person's depression feelings (if he is unaware that depression is what he is feeling)
Encourage mutual problem solving
Encourage the sharing of common problems with others
Encourage the acceptance of self-limitations (if nonacceptance of limitations is causing the depression)
Encourage an awareness of positive responses from others
Explore with the person whether there is a pattern leading up to the behavior (if a specific sequence of events is leading up to the behavior, the sequence can be changed)
Explore with the person the reasons for self-criticism (since self-criticism reinforces depression)
Explore with the person his strengths and resources (to overcome the depression)
Acknowledge dependency
    BUT
Encourage self-performance
Encourage meaningful activity, a full day of activities, active diversional activities (all of which divert attention from the depression and focus attention on the external)
Encourage planned one-day-at-a-time living
Encourage pride in appearance (in spite of the depression)
Offer hope
Introduce to persons who have successfully undergone the same experience
Reduce the demands placed upon the person (so that more energy is available for coping)
Refrain from criticizing negatively
Stimulate by touch or speech
Provide frequent contact with the person (share as much time with the person as possible)
Arrange a structured daily routine (suitable and familiar to the person)
Arrange pleasant surroundings
Do not allow unpleasant surprise situations (which require additional coping energy)
Avoid attempting to cheer up the depressed person (the inability to respond cheerfully makes the depressed person more depressed)
Encourage the patient to make a verbal no-suicide contract (there is always a suicide risk in depression)
Call the person's family (to the bedside)
    OR
Encourage telephone calls with significant persons

    If the patient prefers or strongly needs significant others and if the significant others are available as a support system

Make a referral (to a psychiatric nurse specialist, if needed)
Consult with a physician (about antidepressant medication)

Nursing Observations
Determine the degree of insight that the person has (into the depression)
Determine the precipitating factors and the relieving factors
Evaluate the person's relatedness with others (and its effect on the depression)
Observe for an excessive stress level

Monitor blood studies for abnormal (decreased) adrenal function
Monitor blood studies for abnormal (decreased) glucose   } Indicating that the depression is of a physical origin
Monitor blood studies for (increased) dexamethasone suppression level

Observe for a favorable response to therapy (decreased moodiness, sadness)

Health Teaching

Describe the factors associated with the occurrence of the problem (explain that complaints such as insomnia, tiredness, wanting to sleep excessively, etc., are normal parts of depression)

Explain and offer hope that the emotional pain will decrease with time (that the depression will eventually end despite the present discomfort)

Advise that significant persons express acceptance of one another

Advise that significant persons express caring for one another

Explain the importance of offering emotional support to one another

Explain the importance of maintaining a positive self-attitude

Advise that negative responses from others be regarded with minimum significance (even though they may cause intense feelings)

Emphasize the importance of recognizing tension within oneself (so that tension can be dealt with in the early stages)

Explain the need to recognize highly stressful situations

Describe those symptoms that should be reported (severe depression in which one cannot function or in which one considers suicide)

Teach how to use the problem-solving method

EVALUATION

Record actual outcome

Nonadaptive Responses of Emotion (Affect): Fear

SIMPLE PHOBIA[19,455]

ASSESSMENT

Data Collection

Subjective Data
• Relates experiencing a persistent fear
• Has a compelling desire to avoid the object or fearful situation
• Aware of and disturbed about others recognizing that the fear is irrational
  Usually seeks information about situations in which hy may encounter the phobic object

Objective Data
Profuse sweating
Poor motor control
Tachycardia
Increased blood pressure

Impairment of function may be minimal

Angry outbursts against persons who cause or arrange encounters with the phobic object

Data Analysis

Nursing Diagnosis

SIMPLE PHOBIA: A persistent excessive fear that is out of proportion to actual threat is directed toward a specific person or situation

Common Etiology (Stressors)

PSYCHOSOCIAL FACTORS: An attempt to express anger, anxiety, or dependency indirectly, lack of competency in using effective coping mechanisms, the threat of chronic or severe stress

HEALTH CARE FACTORS: *Medical therapy*: Withdrawal from drugs (amphetamines)

LIFESTYLE: *Drug abuse*: Marijuana

PLANNING

Unmet Needs

Relaxation, comfort, protection from psychologic threat, psychologic instability, a predictable and orderly world, caring and communicating relationships, adequacy, self-control, personal growth and maturity, increased learning, increased reality perception and problem-solving ability

Expected Outcome

Person verbalizes that the fear no longer occurs when the person is exposed to the phobic object or situation

Relates the use of more appropriate coping mechanisms

NURSING INTERVENTIONS

Nursing Treatments

Approach unhurriedly

Reassure verbally (that the nurse will help the person overcome his fear)

Demonstrate calmness

Provide an atmosphere of acceptance

Encourage the expression of feelings (about the phobia)

Listen attentively

Talk with the person

Offer feedback to the person's expressed feelings (about the phobia)

Communicate nurse sensitivity to the person's problem

Relate to the person on an adult–adult level, not on a parent–child level (which could increase the fear)

Attend the person constantly (until he feels sufficiently comfortable to be alone)

Provide frequent contact with the person (thereafter)

Ask the person to identify the problem

Ask for specifics, not generalizations, about the problem

Support a realistic assessment of the situation (reality reduces fear)

Provide reliable information (about the feared object)

Ask how the person normally copes with fear (What does he usually do when fearful that reduces the fear?)

Provide whatever the person needs to use his usual coping mechanisms (if he wants to talk out the problem the nurse listens, if he wants to cry the nurse provides privacy, etc.)

Encourage the person to face the fear (when able, to reduce the fear)

Explore with the person his strengths and resources (to overcome the phobia)

Provide emotionally safe experiences (whenever possible)

Provide objects that symbolize safeness

Do not allow unpleasant surprise situations (which increase fear)

Avoid placing the person on enforced inactivity (which heighten fear)
Reduce the demands placed on the person (so that more energy is available for coping)
Involve the family (as an appropriate support system)
Make a referral (to a psychiatric nurse specialist)

Nursing Observations
Observe for an excessive stress level (resulting from the fear)
Determine the degree of insight that the person has (into the phobia)
Observe for evidence that the person is reaching out for emotional support
Observe for evidence of a favorable response to therapy (reduced fear and increased comfort)

Health Teaching
Advise against fighting fear (which reinforces the emotion)
Explain that fear often disguises itself (that the expressed phobia is often a substitute for an underlying fear that the person is unable to cope with)
Teach how to use a systematic desensitization technique (teach deep breathing and exhaling to promote relaxation; then introduce the anxiety-producing object or situation at levels of closer proximity until it can be tolerated without anxiety at each level and finally at outright confrontation)
Explain the importance of recognizing tension within oneself (so that the tension can be dealt with during the early stages)
Explain that fatigue should be recognized as a stress factor (which heightens fear)
Explain the need to recognize highly stressful situations (which could precipitate the phobic episode)
Explain how to channel emotional energy and obtain release from stress (running, swimming, creative activities, laughing, talking things over)
Recommend methods for achieving total relaxation (controlled breathing, quietly listening to music, doing nothing)
Recommend a habitual, positive mental attitude
Teach how to use the problem-solving method

EVALUATION
Record actual outcome

Nonadaptive Responses of Emotion (Affect): Grief

DELAYED GRIEF REACTION [297,471,568,575]

ASSESSMENT
Data Collection

Subjective Data
• Sense of emotional numbness
• Absence of feeling

Objective Data
• Person remains emotionally composed
• Does not weep
  Continues to perform routine functions

Does not discuss or seldom discusses the loss

Behavior changes begin to occur sometime after the loss, especially around anniversaries

Data Analysis

Nursing Diagnosis

DELAYED GRIEF REACTION: Failure to express sorrow and inner distress at the time of a significant loss

Common Etiology (Stressors)

PSYCHOSOCIAL FACTORS: The threat of unpleasant reality, the absence of a significant other (with whom one can grieve), lack of emotional expression due to inhibiting social norms, the threat of having to deal with strong emotions, the use of exaggerated defense mechanisms

HEALTH CARE FACTORS: *Drug therapy*: Tranquilizers (which prevent the person from feeling grief and result in a delayed response when the tranquilizers are no longer taken)

PLANNING

Unmet Needs

Comfort, protection from psychologic threat, psychologic stability, caring and communicating relationships, personal growth and maturity, increased learning

Expected Outcome

Person acknowledges the loss

Person outwardly exhibits grief behavior

States that he feels comfortable with his ability to work through the normal grief process

NURSING INTERVENTIONS

Nursing Treatments

Approach unhurriedly

Provide an atmosphere of acceptance

Express empathy

Reassure verbally (that it is acceptable to show grief and that the emotional pain will diminish with the passage of time)

Communicate that the nurse feels comfortable with the person's discussions of death (in relationship to a departed loved one)

Encourage the expression of feelings (about the loss)

Listen attentively

Talk with the person

Offer feedback to the person's expressed feelings

Encourage the use of normal coping mechanisms (such as crying)

Explore superficial topics and reasons for avoiding in-depth feelings

Explore with the person his strengths and resources (to endure overt grieving)

Support a realistic assessment of the situation (that the loss has actually occurred)

Nursing Observations

Determine the degree of insight that the person has (into his delayed grieving and the grief process)

Evaluate the person's relatedness with others (especially with the lost person)

Evaluate the significance of emotional distress mannerisms

Evaluate the significance of nonverbal communication

Identify disturbing conversation topics

Observe for evidence that the person is reaching out for emotional support

Observe for evidence of a favorable response to therapy (the ability to grieve)

Health Teaching

Advise that significant persons express caring for one another (especially after a loss)

Explain the importance of persons offering emotional support to one another

Describe the normal stages of grief (denial, anger, bargaining, depression, acceptance)

Emphasize the importance of recognizing tension within oneself

Explain how to channel emotional energy and obtain release from stress (talking things over, crying, laughing)

Advise that children participate in grief-related activities

EVALUATION

Record actual outcome

PROLONGED GRIEF REACTION[297,471,568,575]

ASSESSMENT

Data Collection

Subjective Data

- Preoccupation with thoughts of the deceased
- Intense feelings of anxiety, fear, guilt, helplessness, anger, self-devaluation
- Prolonged mourning for longer than 1 year from the time of loss

Objective Data

- Overt sadness and slowness or agitation and elation

Data Analysis

Nursing Diagnosis

PROLONGED GRIEF REACTION: An exaggerated grief reaction out of proportion to normal grief responses

Common Etiology (Stressors)

PSYCHOSOCIAL FACTORS: An indirect expression of conflict with the lost person, an indirect expression of guilt feelings

PLANNING

Unmet Needs

Comfort, protection from psychologic threat, psychologic stability, caring and communicating relationships, high evaluation of self, personal growth and maturity, increased learning, increased reality perception and problem-solving ability

Expected Outcome

Person verbalizes the reason for the prolonged grieving

States he is resolving the conflict about the lost person

Moves forward to a nongrieving fulfilled life

NURSING INTERVENTIONS

Nursing Treatments

Approach unhurriedly

Provide an atmosphere of acceptance

Reassure verbally (that the nurse will help the person work through the grief process)

Express empathy

Encourage the expression of feelings (about the loss and what the loss means in terms of one's self identity)

Listen attentively

Talk with the person

Offer feedback to the person's expressed feelings

Use direct eye contact to terminate excessive crying (have the person look directly into your eyes for several minutes)

Explore with the person his strengths and resources (to overcome the grief)

Explore with the person the effects of his behavior on others (when he grieves excessively)

Support a realistic assessment of the situation (that the loved one is gone and that those left behind must continue to live)

Assist the person in restructuring his lifestyle (without the loved one, especially if he lived his life through the other person)

Avoid attempting to cheer up the grieving person (the inability to respond cheerfully causes the grieving person to feel less about himself)

Encourage the acceptance of the right to pleasure (in spite of the loss)

Encourage a full day of activities

Encourage enhanced involvement in already established relationships

Encourage meaningful activity

Encourage planned one-day-at-a-time living

Encourage the use of normal coping mechanisms

Introduce to persons who have successfully undergone the same experience

Refrain from negatively criticizing

Encourage involvement in helping others

Make a referral (for possible medication therapy, for evaluation of the need for psychotherapy)

Nursing Observations

Determine the degree of insight that the person has (into the prolonged grieving)

Estimate the degree of stress experienced

Evaluate the person's relatedness with others (especially with the deceased: Is guilt involved in the relationship and prolonging the grief? Has the grieving person lived through the other person and no longer feels alive to himself?)

Evaluate the significance of emotional distress mannerisms

Evaluate the significance of nonverbal communication

Identify disturbing conversation topics

Observe for evidence of a favorable response to therapy (control of the grief, acceptance of the loss)

Health Teaching

Explain and offer hope that the emotional pain will decrease with time

Advise that significant persons express caring for one another

Explain the importance of persons offering emotional support to one another

Describe the normal stages of grief (denial, anger, bargaining, depression, acceptance)

Explain how to channel emotional energy and obtain release from stress (talking things over, laughing, participating in sports, creative activities, etc.)

EVALUATION

Record actual outcome

Nonadaptive Responses of Emotion (Affect): Guilt

NONADAPTIVE GUILT[105,471]

ASSESSMENT

Data Collection

Subjective Data

• Condemnation of self and self-devaluation

- Dwells on the past
- Unable to forgive oneself
  Convinced that he can never be fully forgiven
  Feels no satisfaction in anything he does
  Fears punishment for actions

Objective Data
Person may project blame on others for his misdeeds

Data Analysis

Nursing Diagnosis
NONADAPTIVE GUILT (PATHOLOGIC GUILT): A pathologic response of feelings of blame for a particular action

Common Etiology (Stressors)
PSYCHOSOCIAL FACTORS: Lack of competency in using effective coping mechanisms, an excessively rigid conscience, failure to achieve unrealistic expectations of oneself

PLANNING

Unmet Needs
Comfort, protection from psychologic threat, psychologic stability, acceptance, caring and communicating relationships, high evaluation of self, personal growth and maturity, increased learning

Expected Outcome
Person verbalizes the inappropriateness of the guilt behavior
Relates the use of more appropriate coping mechanisms
Verbalizes he is willing to forget the past, accept forgiveness, and move toward a fulfilling future

NURSING INTERVENTIONS

Nursing Treatments
Approach unhurriedly
Reassure verbally (that the nurse will help the person solve his problem)
Demonstrate calmness
Provide an atmosphere of acceptance
Encourage the expression of feelings (about the guilt)
Listen attentively
Talk with the person
Offer feedback to the person's expressed feelings
Communicate nurse sensitivity to the person's problem
Relate to the person on an adult–adult level, not on a parent–child level (which could increase the guilt feelings)
Ask the person to identify the problem (that is causing the guilt)
Ask for specifics, not generalizations, about the problem
Support a realistic assessment of the situation (that the pathologic guilt prevents the person from growing and getting the most out of life)
Provide reliable information (which may clarify facts and reduce guilt)
Encourage the admission of wrongdoing
Explore with the person the reasons for self-criticism
Explore with the person the effects of his behavior on others (when guilt affects his ability to function)
Suggest that reparation will diminish guilt (if the person feels he can offer reparation)
Encourage the acceptance of forgiveness offered by others
Explore with the person the difference between his child and adult conscience (the child conscience is based on fear of punishment, while the adult conscience is based on mature judgment)
Encourage the use of normal coping mechanisms
Encourage active diversional activities (to divert attention from preoccupation with guilt)
Refrain from negatively criticizing

Nursing Observations

Evaluate the significance of emotional distress mannerisms

Evaluate the significance of nonverbal communication

Identify disturbing conversation topics (reflecting guilt)

Identify life values significant to the person (which may reinforce the guilt)

Observe for evidence that the person is reaching out for emotional support

Observe for evidence of a favorable response to therapy (the acceptance of forgiveness)

Health Teaching

Explain and offer hope that the emotional pain will decrease with time

Recommend new options for effective methods of coping (making reparation when possible)

Advise that negative responses from others be regarded with minimum significance (even though there are intense feelings about such responses)

Advise that significant persons express acceptance of one another

Advise that significant persons express caring for one another (especially when one person feels guilty)

Explain the importance of persons offering emotional support to one another

Explain the importance of maintaining a positive self-attitude

Explain how to channel emotional energy and obtain release from stress (through running, swimming, creative activities, laughing, talking things over)

EVALUATION

Record actual outcome

Nonadaptive Responses of Emotional (Affect): Fluctuation

IMPULSE CONTROL DISORDER[19,455]

ASSESSMENT

Data Collection

Subjective Data

• Feelings of tension before an action

• A strong desire to perform a particular act that is harmful to oneself or others

• Experiences pleasure or gratification after committing the act

• May or may not feel regret or guilt after the act

Objective Data

Chronically gambles

OR

May practice kleptomania, or pyromania

Data Analysis

Nursing Diagnosis

IMPULSE CONTROL DISORDER: The inability to restrain inner tensions to perform specific harmful acts suddenly and without thought

Common Etiology (Stressors)

DISEASES: Alcoholism, schizophrenia, organic brain syndrome

PSYCHOSOCIAL FACTORS: The threat of chronic or severe stress, exposure to an impulse-directed role model, an attempt to express anger or anxiety indirectly, lack of competency in using effective coping mechanisms, lack of impulse control

PLANNING
Unmet Needs
Protection from physical harm, psychologic stability, acceptance, direct and communicating relationships, high evaluation of self, self-control, personal growth and maturity, increased learning, increased reality perception and problem-solving ability

Expected Outcome
Person demonstrates control of inner tensions that direct impulsive actions
Verbalizes that he has learned to think before acting
Verbalizes that he feels satisfied with increased control over his behavior

NURSING INTERVENTIONS
Nursing Treatments
Approach unhurriedly
Reassure verbally (that the nurse will help the person)
Demonstrate calmness
Provide an atmosphere of acceptance (of the person, not of the behavior)
Encourage the expression of feelings
Relate to the person on an adult–adult level, not on a parent–child level
Listen attentively
Talk with the person
Offer feedback to the person's expressed feelings
Explore with the person whether there is a pattern leading up to the behavior (Is there a sequence of events preceding the behavior? Can that sequence be interrupted?)
Explore with the person the reasons for recurring problems (why the person repeatedly fails to control impulses)
Explore with the person the effects of his behavior on others (others cannot rely on what behavior to expect from the person and may respond with defensive behavior toward the person)
Encourage participation in therapeutic group interaction (to gain insight into the impulse control disorder)
Set an example by role modeling
Ignore undesirable behavior
    OR
Set limits on unacceptable behavior
Clearly communicate what is expected of the person
Hold the person responsible for his behavior (do not allow the person to blame others)
Provide seclusion (if needed)
Minimize environmental dangers (by removing all harmful objects from the environment)
Refrain from arguing, from negatively criticizing
Verbalize daily the person's successful progress (in changing behavior)
Provide emotional support for persons significant to the patient
Make a referral (for possible medication therapy and for evaluation of the need for psychotherapy)

Nursing Observations
Determine the degree of insight that the person has (into the impulse control disorder)
Determine the precipitating factors (for impulsive behavior)
Observe for behavior modification (resulting from therapy)

Health Teaching
Emphasize the importance of recognizing tension within oneself (as an early sign of impending impulsive behavior)
Recommend things to do when one begins to feel out of control (such as washing one's hands and face in cold water, slowly counting to 500, and withdrawing from the situation, which give the person something to do besides feel)
Explain the importance of remaining calm (for energy conservation, to reduce internal

tension, for a more realistic problem-solving approach)

Explain why persons should maintain self-control (out of respect for oneself and for others)

Recommend that behavioral limits be set (by the family)

Explain how to set behavioral limits (the family should clearly state what constitutes acceptable and unacceptable behavior)

EVALUATION

Record actual outcome

LABILE AFFECT[471]

ASSESSMENT

Data Collection

Subjective Data
• Verbalizes rapid change of feelings from joy to sadness and from sadness to joy

Objective Data
• Abrupt emotional swing from laughter to tearfulness or from tearfulness to laughter
• Response is unrelated to the current situation

Data Analysis

Nursing Diagnosis
LABILE AFFECT (LABILE PERSONALITY): A sudden fluctation of emotional responses, usually in direct contrast to one another

Common Etiology (Stressors)
DISEASES: Central nervous system disorder, cerebrovascular accident, major depression, manic–depressive psychosis, organic brain syndrome, schizophrenia
DEVELOPMENTAL PHASES: Adolescence, old age.

PLANNING

Unmet Needs

Psychologic stability, acceptance, caring and communicating relationships, dignity

Expected Outcome

Person verbalizes an awareness of the labile affect

Gains control of his emotions if possible

Demonstrates minimal anxiety about the fluctuating emotions, when control is not possible

If the labile affect is unresolvable, significant others verbalize an understanding of the cause and exhibit acceptance

NURSING INTERVENTIONS

Nursing Treatments

Approach unhurriedly

Provide an atmosphere of acceptance

Encourage the expression of feelings (in spite of their fluctuation)

Relate to the person on an adult–adult level, not on a parent–child level (which could increase tension and the frequency of emotional fluctuations)

Listen attentively

Talk with the person (disregarding the fluctuating emotions as much as possible during the conversation)

Reassure verbally (that the labile emotions do not decrease the person's self-worth or prevent meaningful communication with others)

Make a referral (for evaluation of a need for psychotherapy)

Nursing Observations

Determine the degree of insight that the person has (into the labile emotions)

Determine the precipitating factors and the relieving factors

Observe for evidence of a favorable response to therapy (decreased frequency of emotional fluctuation, calm acceptance of the uncontrollable fluctuations)

Health Teaching

Explain the causes of the problem (to the patient and family so they understand that the problem results from organic brain syndrome, cerebrovascular accident, central nervous system disorder)

Advise that significant persons express caring for one another

Advise that significant persons express acceptance of one another

Emphasize the importance of recognizing tension within oneself (increased tension predisposes the person to exhibit fluctuating emotions)

Explain the importance of remaining calm (reduced tension helps control labile emotions, calmness helps others accept the emotional changes with less anxiety and concern)

Explain the importance of maintaining a positive self-attitude

EVALUATION

Record actual outcome

MANIC BEHAVIOR[19,105,471]

ASSESSMENT

Data Collection

Subjective Data

- Relates little need for sleep
- Relates grandiose ideas about self
- Relates involvement in foolish activities
  Expresses feelings of well-being, optimism, good health
  Too busy to eat or attend to hygiene
  May alternate with depressed feelings

Objective Data

- Increased physical activity
- Persistent talking
- Flight of ideas
- Easily distracted
  Monopolizes the conversation
  Does not follow through on plans

Data Analysis

Nursing Diagnosis

MANIC BEHAVIOR (MANIC REACTION): The occurrence of an expansive or euphoric mood

Common Etiology (Stressors)

DISEASES: Manic–depressive psychosis, schizophrenia

PSYCHOSOCIAL FACTORS: An attempt to express anger, anxiety, hopelessness, rejection indirectly, an attempt to redirect feelings into activity

PLANNING

Unmet Needs

Sleep, rest and relaxation, protection from physical harm, protection from psychologic threat, psychologic stability, caring and communicating relationships, self-control, personal growth and maturity, increased learning

Expected Outcome

Person verbalizes an awareness of the causes and effects of the manic behavior
Relates the use of more appropriate coping mechanisms
Verbalizes that he feels calm and in control of himself and of his behavior
Exhibits controlled behavior

NURSING INTERVENTIONS

Nursing Treatments

Approach unhurriedly
Demonstrate calmness
Provide an atmosphere of acceptance (of the person, not of the behavior)
Encourage the expression of feelings (in a calm, rather than expansive mood)
Relate to the person on an adult–adult level, not on a parent–child level
Listen attentively
Talk with the person (keep comments and explanations short and concise)
Explore with the person whether there is a pattern leading up to the behavior (Is there a sequence of events preceding the behavior? Can that sequence be changed?)
Explore with the person the reasons for recurring problems (of manic behavior)
Explore with the person the effects of his behavior on others (others are unable to predict his behavior, which makes the person an unstable force in others' lives)
Encourage participation in therapeutic group interaction (to gain insight into the behavior)
Set an example by role modeling
Minimize environmental dangers (by removing all harmful objects)
Ignore undesirable behavior
   OR
Set limits on unacceptable behavior
Clearly communicate what is expected of the person
Hold the person responsible for his behavior
Provide seclusion (if needed)
Refrain from arguing, from negatively criticizing
Verbalize daily the person's successful progress (in changing behavior)
Provide emotional support for persons significant to the patient
Make a referral (if medication is needed)

Nursing Observations

Determine the degree of insight that the person has (into the manic behavior)
Determine the precipitating factors
Identify disturbing conversation topics
Identify emotion-stimulating events
Identify potentially destructive behavior (during manic states)
Observe for impaired judgment (which could cause the person to harm himself)
Observe for behavior modification (resulting from therapy)

Health Teaching

Emphasize the importance of recognizing tension within oneself
Recommend things to do when one begins to feel out of control (such as taking a long walk, washing one's hands and face in cold water, and scrubbing the sink, which give the person something to do besides feel)
Recommend new options for effective methods of coping
Explain the importance of remaining calm (it conserves energy and reduces internal tension)
Recommend that behavioral limits be set (by the family)
Explain how to set behavioral limits (the family should clearly state what constitutes acceptable and unacceptable behavior)

EVALUATION
Record actual outcome

Nonadaptive Responses of Self-Esteem (Self-Worth)

SELF-DESTRUCTIVE BEHAVIOR[105,471]

ASSESSMENT

Data Collection

Subjective Data
- Person experiences anxiety
- Relates overeating, use of tobacco, reckless driving, involvement in dangerous sports or other activities, the use of drugs, the excessive use of alcohol, persisting in underachievement
- Relates feelings of worthlessness, loneliness

Objective Data
- Overweight
- Smoking

Data Analysis

Nursing Diagnosis
SELF-DESTRUCTIVE BEHAVIOR: Exhibiting behaviors in which one takes risks with his own life or behaves in a manner that will ultimately hurt him

Common Etiology (Stressors)
PSYCHOSOCIAL FACTORS: Lack of competency in using effective coping mechanisms, the threat of chronic or severe stress, an attempt to express anger, anxiety, or guilt indirectly, lack of impulse control, an attempt to control others or to test one's own omnipotence, lack of self-esteem

PLANNING

Unmet Needs

Protection from psychologic threat, psychologic stability, love and affection, acceptance, caring and communicating relationships, high evaluation of self, sense of adequacy, self-control, personal growth and maturity, increased learning, increased reality perception and problem-solving ability

Expected Outcome

Person verbalizes an awareness that the current behavior is self-destructive
Ceases to use the specific self-destructive behavior
Relates the use of more appropriate coping mechanisms
Exhibits behavior that leads to personal growth

NURSING INTERVENTIONS

Nursing Treatments

Approach unhurriedly
Reassure verbally (that the nurse will help the person)
Demonstrate calmness
Provide an atmosphere of acceptance (of the person, not of the behavior)
Encourage the expression of feelings (about oneself and about destructive behavior)

Listen attentively

Talk with the person

Offer feedback to the person's expressed feelings

Communicate nurse sensitivity to the person's problem

Relate to the person on an adult–adult level, not on a parent–child level (which could reduce self-esteem)

Hold the person responsible for his behavior (do not allow the person to blame others)

Clearly communicate what is expected of the person

Explore with the person his value as an individual

Explore with the person his positive characteristics (his use of nondestructive behavior)

Explore with the person his strengths and resources (to overcome the self-destructive behavior)

Explore with the person the reasons for criticism by others (concern for his well-being)

Support a realistic assessment of the situation (that continuing such behavior leads to self-destruction)

Encourage the use of normal coping mechanisms

Nursing Observations

Determine the degree of insight that the person has (into the self-destructive behavior)

Observe for impaired self-attitudes (that lead to self-destructive behavior)

Observe for evidence that the person is reaching out for emotional support

Observe for evidence of a favorable response to therapy

Health Teaching

Explain the cause of the problem (it is an expression of anger and can result from the use of ineffective coping mechanisms)

Advise that negative responses from others be regarded with minimum significance (even though there are feelings about such responses)

Explain that change must come from within the person (not from without)

Advise that significant persons express acceptance of one another

Explain the importance of person's offering support to one another

Explain the importance of maintaining a positive self-attitude

Recommend new options for effective methods of coping (nondestructive behavior)

EVALUATION

Record actual outcome

SUICIDE THREATS[105,471]

ASSESSMENT

Data Collection

Subjective Data
- Person experiences severe anxiety
- Relates feelings of worthlessness, loneliness
- May verbally indicate suicide intentions such as "I'll soon be gone"

Objective Data
- Nonverbal indications such as giving away possessions, making funeral arrangements, drawing up a will

Data Analysis

Nursing Diagnosis

SUICIDE THREATS: Verbal statements or nonverbal actions indicating an intention to commit suicide

Common Etiology (Stressors)
DISEASES: Major depression
PSYCHOSOCIAL FACTORS: Lack of competency in using effective coping mechanisms, an attempt to express anger or ambivalence about suicide indirectly, an attempt to gain attention, the threat of having needs for help unfulfilled through constructive behavior, which results in negative or destructive behavior, an attempt to test the love of a significant other or to punish a significant other, overwhelming stress

PLANNING

Unmet Needs
Protection from psychologic threat, psychologic stability, love and affection, acceptance, caring and communicating relationships, high evaluation of self, sense of adequacy, personal growth and maturity, increased learning, increased reality perception and problem-solving ability

Expected Outcome
Person no longer uses suicide threats
Verbalizes that he has learned and uses more appropriate coping mechanisms
Verbalizes that he feels satisfied with his personal growth and looks forward to a fulfilling future

NURSING INTERVENTIONS

Nursing Treatments
Approach unhurriedly
Demonstrate calmness
Provide an atmosphere of acceptance (of the person but not of the behavior)
Encourage the expression of feelings (the person has about himself and his attitude toward suicide)
Listen attentively
Talk with the person (in an effort to improve communication patterns)
Offer feedback to the person's expressed feelings
Communicate nurse sensitivity to the person's problem
Relate to the person on an adult–adult level, not on a parent–child level (which could reduce self-esteem)
Help the suicidal person set goals to preserve his life (goals such as wanting to survive, informing the staff of impulses to hurt himself, verbalizing reasons for not hurting himself)
Explore with the person his value as an individual
Explore with the person his positive characteristics
Encourage an awareness of positive responses from others
Explore with the person his strengths and resources (to overcome problems)
Explore with the person the reasons for self-criticism (and for self-destructive behavior)
Support a realistic assessment of the situation
Encourage the use of normal coping mechanisms (by helping the person set up a strong support system)
Encourage the person to make a verbal no-suicide contract (agreeing not to kill himself or get himself killed until the next time he sees you)
Clearly communicate what is expected of the person
Hold the person responsible for his behavior (do not allow him to blame others)
Arrange geographic placement (so the person can be seen by the nurse)
Provide frequent contact with the person
Remove harmful objects from the environment (which could be used for suicide)
Consult with the physician (about limiting the number of prescribed pills with each prescription)
Consult with the pharmacist (about providing pills, each of which is separately blister packed, because if each pill has to be opened separately, the person is less likely to consume large quantities at one time)

Make a referral (for evaluation of the need for psychotherapy, to support groups, to a suicide crisis line)

Involve the family (have them express their feelings about the suicide threats, and plan responses to future threats)

Nursing Observations

Determine the degree of insight that the person has (into the suicide threats)

Evaluate the person's relatedness with others

Identify disturbing topics of conversation

Identify life values significant to the person

Observe for an excessive stress level

Observe for impaired self-attitudes (which lead to self-destructive behavior)

Observe for evidence that the person is reaching out for emotional support (through suicide threats)

Evaluate the safety of the environment

Observe for evidence of a favorable response to therapy

Health Teaching

Explain the causes of the problem (it is a means of expressing anger, of testing significant others, of gaining attention, etc.)

Advise that negative responses from others be regarded with minimum significance (even though there are feelings about such responses)

Advise that significant persons express acceptance of one another

Explain the importance of persons offering support to one another

Explain the importance of maintaining a positive self-attitude

EVALUATION

Record actual outcome

SUICIDE ATTEMPT[105,471]

ASSESSMENT

Data Collection

Subjective Data
• Person experiences severe anxiety
• Relates feelings of intensely low self-worth
• Feelings of helplessness, hopelessness, dependency, severe loneliness
  May have a specific plan for self-inflicted death

Objective Data
• Uses lethal methods to terminate life such as drugs, gases, guns, knives, hanging oneself, jumping from high places
  May use methods that allow time to be discovered before death occurs

Data Analysis

Nursing Diagnosis
SUICIDE ATTEMPT (SUICIDE GESTURE): Self-initiated destructive behaviors that, if uninterrupted, could lead to the person's death

Common Etiology (Stressors)
DISEASES: Major depression, organic brain syndrome, schizophrenia
PSYCHOSOCIAL FACTORS: Lack of competency in using effective coping mechanisms, an attempt to express anger, anxiety, hopelessness indirectly, an attempt to gain attention, the threat of having needs for help unfulfilled through constructive behavior resulting in negative or destructive behavior, an attempt to test the love of a significant other or punish a significant other, overwhelming stress, lack of impulse control

PLANNING

Unmet Needs

Protection from psychologic threat, psychologic stability, love and affection, acceptance, caring and communicating relationships, high evaluation of self, sense of adequacy, personal growth and maturity, increased learning, increased reality perception and problem-solving ability

Expected Outcome

Person verbalizes an awareness of the reasons for attempting suicide

Ceases to attempt suicide

Verbalizes he has learned and uses more appropriate coping mechanisms

Verbalizes that he feels satisfied with his personal growth and looks forward to a fulfill-ing future

NURSING INTERVENTIONS

Nursing Treatments

Approach unhurriedly

Demonstrate calmness

Provide an atmosphere of acceptance (of the person, but not of the behavior)

Encourage the expression of feelings (about oneself and about the suicide attempt)

Listen attentively

Talk with the person (in an effort to improve communication patterns)

Offer feedback to the person's expressed feelings

Communicate nurse sensitivity to the person's problem

Relate to the person on an adult–adult level, not on a parent–child level (which could reduce self-esteem)

Help the suicidal person set goals to preserve his life (goals such as wanting to survive, informing the staff of impulses to hurt himself, stating reasons for not hurting him-self)

Explore with the person his value as an individual

Explore with the person his positive characteristics

Encourage an awareness of positive responses from others

Explore with the person whether there is a pattern leading up to the behavior (if there is a sequence of events preceding the suicide attempts, the sequence can be changed)

Explore with the person his strengths and resources (to overcome his problems)

Explore with the person the reasons for self-criticism (and self-destructive behavior)

Support a realistic assessment of the situation

Encourage the use of normal coping mechanisms (by helping the person set up a strong support system)

Encourage the person to make a verbal no-suicide contract (agreeing not to kill himself or get himself killed until the next time you see him)

Clearly communicate what is expected of the person

Hold the person responsible for his behavior (do not allow him to blame others)

Arrange geographic placement (so the person can be seen by the nurses)

Provide frequent contact with the person

Remove harmful objects from the environment (which could be used for suicide)

Consult with the physician (about limiting the number of prescribed pills with each pre-scription)

Consult with the pharmacist (about providing pills each of which is separately blister packed, because if each pill has to be opened separately, the person is less likely to consume large quantities at one time)

Make a referral (for psychotherapy, to support groups, to a suicide crisis line)

Involve the family (have them express their feelings about the suicide attempt and plan responses to further attempts)

Nursing Observations

Determine the degree of insight that the person has (into the suicide attempt)

Evaluate the person's relatedness with others

Identify disturbing conversation topics
Identify life values significant to the person
Observe for an excessive stress level
Observe for impaired self-attitudes (which lead to self-destructive behavior)
Observe for evidence that the person is reaching out for emotional support (through suicide attempts)
Evaluate the safety of the environment
Observe for evidence of a favorable response to therapy

Health Teaching

Explain the causes of the problem (it is a means of expressing anger, of testing significant others, of gaining attention, etc.)
Advise that negative responses from others be regarded with minimum significance (even though there are feelings about such responses)
Advise that significant persons express acceptance of one another
Explain the importance of persons offering support to one another
Explain the importance of maintaining a positive self-attitude
Recommend new options for effective methods of coping

EVALUATION

Record actual outcome

Nonadaptive Responses of Self-Identity (Self-Image)

DISTURBED BODY IMAGE[471]

ASSESSMENT
Data Collection
Subjective Data
- Person does not like his body
- Verbalizes displeasure, low worth to his body
  Relates anxiety feelings
  May have a sense of unreality about body parts such as limbs being detached, stepping outside the body and observing it
Objective Data
- Bizarre clothing may be worn

Data Analysis
Nursing Diagnosis
DISTURBED BODY IMAGE: Severely distorted conscious or unconscious attitudes of the person toward his body
Common Etiology (Stressors)
PSYCHOSOCIAL FACTORS: The threat of change or forced adaptation to change, the threat of loss of self-esteem or identity, lack of competency in using effective coping mechanisms, the use of exaggerated defense mechanisms, the use of exaggerated defense mechanisms and indirect expression of conflict, overwhelming stress, loss of a valued concept of self

PLANNING
Unmet Needs
Protection from psychologic threat, psychologic stability, acceptance, caring and commu-

nicating relationships, high evaluation of self, dignity, personal growth and maturity, increased learning, increased reality perception and problem-solving ability

Expected Outcome

Person verbalizes his feelings about his unacceptable body
Verbalizes that he recognizes the dignity of the self, despite an abnormal body
Verbalizes the acceptance of and contentment with his body
Exhibits caring for the body through cleanliness and appropriate dress

NURSING INTERVENTIONS

Nursing Treatments

Approach unhurriedly
Demonstrate calmness
Provide an atmosphere of acceptance (of the person, but not of the behavior)
Encourage the expression of feelings (about the displeasure with the body)
Listen attentively
Talk with the person
Offer feedback to the person's expressed feelings
Communicate nurse sensitivity to the person's problem
Explore with the person his value as an individual (that because he is a human being, he is a person of worth despite changes in his body)
Ask questions that encourage answers reflecting reality perceptions (questions about his worth, his positive characteristics, his value to others)
Encourage the identification of specific life values, of success standards, of values acquired from one's own culture, of values in common with the values of others
Encourage the differentiation between self-ideal and actual self
Encourage an awareness of positive responses from others (about the body changes)
Offer praise (for positive attitudes toward the body image)

Nursing Observations

Determine the degree of insight that the person has (into his body image)
Observe for an excessive stress level
Observe for evidence that the person is reaching out for emotional support
Observe for evidence of a favorable response to therapy (verbalized satisfaction with the changed body)

Health Teaching

Recommend new options for effective methods of coping (new ways to perceive one's changed body as acceptable to oneself)
Explain the importance of maintaining a positive self-attitude
Advise that negative responses from others be regarded with minimum significance (even though there are feelings about such responses)
Explain (to the family) that persons must make adjustments at their own pace
Explain that ill persons are often hypersensitive (about their bodies)

EVALUATION

Record actual outcome

GENDER-IDENTITY DISORDER[13,19,432,540]

ASSESSMENT

Data Collection

Subjective Data

• Person cannot accept himself as a man or herself as a woman
• Desires to be a person of the opposite sex

• Persistently denies the existence of own male or female anatomy

Objective Data

Female
• Displays generally accepted male behavior and dress
  Prefers to work in male-identified occupations
  Is competitive
  Is aggressive
  Has coarse body movements

Male
• Displays generally accepted female behavior and dress
  Is preoccupied with domestic affairs
  Prefers female-identified occupations and working with women rather than with men
  Prefers sentimental and romantic movies and literature
  Has feminine body movements

Data Analysis

Nursing Diagnosis
GENDER-IDENTITY DISORDER: Feeling dissatisfied with one's own sex and wanting to be of the opposite sex

Common Etiology (Stressors)
PSYCHOSOCIAL FACTORS: A direct expression of conflict over gender identity, lack of an affectionate rewarding relationship with the parent of the same sex, lack of a role model of the same sex, an attempt to express indirectly fear or hate of the parent of the opposite sex, the absence of a significant other (usually a parent whose absence forced the child into the absent parent's role)

PLANNING

Unmet Needs
Comfort, sexuality, protection from psychologic threat, psychologic stability, acceptance, caring and communicating relationships, high evaluation of self, personal growth and maturity, increased learning, increased reality perception and problem-solving ability

Expected Outcome
Person verbalizes an awareness of the causes of the problem
Demonstrates a clear identity of his or her own sex
Relates the acceptance of oneself

NURSING INTERVENTIONS

Nursing Treatments
Approach unhurriedly
Provide an atmosphere of acceptance (of the person, but not of the behavior)
Encourage the expression of feelings (about the gender-identity disorder)
Listen attentively
Talk with the person
Offer feedback to the person's expressed feelings
Communicate nurse sensitivity to the person's problem
Explore with the person his value as an individual (that because he is a human being, he is a person of worth)
Ask questions that encourage answers reflecting reality perception (questions about one's worth, individual characteristics, group status)
Encourage the identification of specific life values, of success standards, of values acquired from one's own culture, of values in common with the values of others
Encourage the differentiation between self-ideal and actual self
Encourage an awareness of positive responses from others
Explore with the person his strengths and resources
Encourage the use of normal coping mechanisms

Refrain from negatively criticizing
Involve the family (have them express their feelings about the gender-identity disorder)

Nursing Observations

Determine the degree of insight that the person has (into the gender-identity disorder)
Observe for impaired self-attitudes
Observe for evidence that the person is reaching out for emotional support
Observe for evidence of a favorable response to therapy (verbalized satisfaction with oneself)

Health Teaching

Recommend new options for effective methods of coping
Explain the importance of maintaining a positive self-attitude
Advise that negative responses from others be regarded with minimum significance (even though there are feelings about such responses)
Advise that significant persons express acceptance of one another
Explain the importance of persons offering emotional support to one another
Explain the need for realistic expectations of others

EVALUATION

Record actual outcome

IDENTITY DISORDER [19,105,432]

ASSESSMENT

Data Collection

Subjective Data
• Person verbalizes "Who am I?"
• Relates being unable to decide on a career choice, on a set of moral values for himself, on group loyalties, on religious affiliation, on sexual behavior patterns for himself, or on friendship choices

Objective Data
• Overt evidence of poor social or occupational functioning

Data Analysis

Nursing Diagnosis
IDENTITY DISORDER: The inability of an adolescent to choose or adopt a life pattern

Common Etiology (Stressors)
PSYCHOSOCIAL FACTORS: The threat of inadequacy, differences in parental and children's values, differences in personal, peer, and community values, changes in cultural practices and values, lack of clearly defined values, the threat of multiple options available

PLANNING

Unmet Needs

Protection from psychologic threat; psychologic stability; acceptance; caring, direct, and communicating relationships; high evaluation of self; sense of adequacy; personal growth and maturity; increased learning; identification of values; increased reality perception and problem-solving ability

Expected Outcome

Person verbalizes his feelings about his self-identity
Demonstrates having made a decision regarding his life choices
Exhibits productive social and occupational functioning

NURSING INTERVENTIONS

Nursing Treatments

Approach unhurriedly

Reassure verbally (that a clear identity will evolve)

Demonstrate calmness

Provide an atmosphere of acceptance (of the person, but not of the behavior)

Encourage the expression of feelings (about oneself and one's life choices)

Listen attentively

Talk with the person

Offer feedback to the person's expressed feelings

Communicate nurse sensitivity to the person's problem

Explore with the person his value as an individual (that because he is a human being, he is a person of worth)

Ask questions that encourage answers that reflect reality perception (questions about one's worth, positive characteristics, group status, life philosophy)

Encourage the identification of specific life values, of success standards, of values acquired from one's own culture, of values in common with the values of others

Encourage the differentiation between self-ideal and actual self

Encourage an awareness of positive responses from others

Make a referral (to groups with similar problems)

Nursing Observations

Determine the degree of insight that the person has (into his identity disorder)

Observe for an excessive stress level

Observe for impaired self-attitudes (that delay identity clarification)

Observe for evidence that the person is reaching out for emotional support

Observe for evidence of a favorable response to therapy (the choice of a life pattern)

Health Teaching

Recommend new options for effective methods of coping (new ways to perceive one's characteristics, status among others, and philosophy of life)

Explain the importance of maintaining a positive self-attitude

Advise that negative responses from others be regarded with minimum significance (even though there are feelings about such responses)

Explain (to the family) that persons must make adjustments at their own pace

EVALUATION

Record actual outcome

Nonadaptive Responses of Psychosexual Function

FUNCTIONAL DYSPAREUNIA[19,278,471]

ASSESSMENT

Data Collection

Subjective Data

- Woman complains of persistent genital pain during intercourse
- Complaints of discomfort externally (at the introitus) or internally (within and beyond the genital canal)
- Relates marital difficulties

Objective Data
None

Data Analysis

Nursing Diagnosis
FUNCTIONAL DYSPAREUNIA: Psychologically induced pain during intercourse

Common Etiology (Stressors)
PSYCHOSOCIAL FACTORS: The threat of a deteriorating relationship, an attempt to control the sexual partner, an attempt to express anxiety, anger, or rejection indirectly, the threat of intimacy and/or physical closeness, the threat of inadequacy, lack of enjoyment of a particular role (as a sexual partner) with another person, the threat of pregnancy, unresolved feelings about having been a victim of rape

PLANNING

Unmet Needs

Comfort, protection from psychologic threat, acceptance, caring and communicating relationships, high evaluation of self, control over others or situations, personal growth and maturity, increased learning, increased reality perception and problem-solving ability

Expected Outcome

Person verbalizes an awareness of the causes of the problem
No longer verbalizes somatic complaints
Relates having satisfying and fulfilling relationships with the sexual partner

NURSING INTERVENTIONS

Nursing Treatments

Approach unhurriedly
Reassure verbally
Demonstrate calmness
Provide an atmosphere of acceptance (of the person but not of the behavior)
Obtain a complete present and past history (including a sexual history)
Make a referral (to a physician if needed)
Encourage the expression of feelings (about sexual concerns, about anxiety, anger, or conflict)
Listen attentively
Talk with the person
Offer feedback to the person's expressed feelings
Communicate nurse sensitivity to the person's problem (regarding sexual matters)
Relate to the person on an adult–adult level, not on a parent–child level
Ask the person to identify the problem (which is usually an interpersonal or marriage problem)
Ask for specifics, not generalizations, about the problem
Explore superficial topics and reasons for avoiding in-depth feelings (about sexual concerns)
Explore with the person the need to control
Support a realistic assessment of the situation
Explore with the person her strengths and resources (to overcome the problem)
Encourage the use of normal coping mechanisms

Nursing Observations

Perform a physical examination and evaluate if the findings are normal (or if there is any suspicion of nonfunctional dyspareunia from endometriosis, vaginal infection, or estrogen depletion with menopause)
Determine the degree of insight that the person has
Evaluate the person's relatedness with others (especially the sexual partner)
Identify disturbing conversation topics
Observe for impaired self-attitudes (affecting sexual function)

Identify life values significant to the person (and related to her sexuality)

Observe for evidence of a favorable response to therapy (woman verbalizes nonpainful sexual intercourse)

Health Teaching

Explain the cause of the problem (it is an indirect expression of anxiety, anger, or rejection of another, or it is a response to the threat of pregnancy, etc.)

Recommend the use of a water-soluble lubricant (before coitus)

Explain that relaxation is essential for a successful sexual response

Recommend alternative approaches to sexual activity (such as changing the coital position to reduce the pain)

EVALUATION

Record actual outcome

FUNCTIONAL VAGINISMUS[19,471]

ASSESSMENT

Data Collection

Subjective Data
- Woman complains of vaginal spasms during intercourse
- Dreads sexual relations
- Relates marital difficulties
  Woman feels she is being used by her partner and is not getting any satisfaction from the relationship

Objective Data
None

Data Analysis

Nursing Diagnosis
FUNCTIONAL VAGINISMUS: Psychologically induced vaginal spasms during intercourse

Common Etiology (Stressors)
PSYCHOSOCIAL FACTORS: The threat of a deteriorating relationship, an attempt to control the sexual partner, an attempt to express anxiety, anger, or rejection indirectly, the threat of intimacy and/or physical closeness, the threat of inadequacy, lack of enjoyment of a particular role (as a sexual partner) with another person, the threat of pregnancy, unresolved feelings about having been a victim of rape

PLANNING

Unmet Needs

Comfort, protection from psychologic threat, acceptance, caring and communicating relationships, high evaluation of self, control over others or situations, personal growth and maturity, increased learning, increased reality perception and problem-solving ability

Expected Outcome

Person verbalizes an awareness of the causes of the problem

No longer verbalizes somatic complaints

Relates having satisfying and fulfilling relationships with the sexual partner

NURSING INTERVENTIONS

Nursing Treatments

Approach unhurriedly

Reassure verbally
Demonstrate calmness
Provide an atmosphere of acceptance (of the person, but not of the behavior)
Obtain a complete present and past history (including a sexual history)
Encourage the expression of feelings (about her low self-esteem)
Listen attentively
Talk with the person
Offer feedback to the person's expressed feelings
Communicate nurse sensitivity to the person's problem (regarding sexual matters)
Relate to the person on an adult–adult level, not on a parent–child level
Ask the person to identify the problem (which is usually an interpersonal or marriage
problem)
Ask for specifics, not generalizations, about the problem
Explore superficial topics and reasons for avoiding in-depth feelings (about sexual concerns)
Explore with the person the need to control (others and situations)
Support a realistic assessment of the situation
Explore with the person her strengths and resources (to overcome the problem)
Encourage the use of normal coping mechanisms

Nursing Observations

Perform a physical examination and evaluate whether the findings are normal (determine whether there is any suspicion of nonfunctional vaginismus)
Determine the degree of insight that the person has (into the problem)
Evaluate the person's relatedness with others (especially the sexual partner)
Identify disturbing conversation topics
Observe for impaired self-attitudes (affecting sexual function)
Identify life values significant to the person (and related to her sexuality)
Observe for evidence of a favorable response to therapy (woman verbalizes having
nonpainful sexual intercourse)

Health Teaching

Explain the cause of the problem (it is an indirect expression of anxiety, anger, or rejection of another, or it is a response to the threat of pregnancy, etc.)
Recommend the use of a water-soluble lubricant (before coitus)
Explain that relaxation is essential for a successful sexual response

EVALUATION

Record actual outcome

INHIBITED SEXUAL DESIRE[19,67,262]

ASSESSMENT

Data Collection

Subjective Data
• Person relates a decreased sexual desire and responsiveness
• Perceives sexual activities as undesirable
• Woman perceives herself as merely an instrument of male gratification, not a love
object
Feelings of guilt
Blames the reduced response on a natural or surgical menopause or on a hormonal
deficiency
Complains of changed attitudes in the partner
Partner may relate anxiety and frustration

Objective Data
The person's previously aggressive personality becomes passive

Data Analysis

Nursing Diagnosis
INHIBITED SEXUAL DESIRE: A decrease in the frequency and desire for sexual activity

Common Etiology (Stressors)
DISEASES: Diabetes mellitus, hypopituitarism, renal failure
PSYCHOSOCIAL FACTORS: Severe stress, the threat of a deteriorating relationship, an attempt to control the sexual partner, an attempt to express anger, anxiety, or rejection indirectly, the threat of intimacy and/or physical closeness, lack of enjoyment of a particular role (as a sexual partner) with another person, the threat of pregnancy
HEALTH CARE FACTORS: *Medical therapy:* Hemodialysis. *Drug therapy:* Adverse effects of Tagamet and antihypertensive drugs (Inderal)
LIFESTYLE: Marijuana drug abuse, religious beliefs
SITUATIONAL FACTORS: Child rearing, divorce, a new job, the illness or injury of oneself or a significant other

PLANNING

Unmet Needs
Comfort, sexuality, protection from psychologic threat, acceptance, caring and communicating relationships, high evaluation of self, personal growth and maturity, increased learning, increased reality perception and problem-solving ability

Expected Outcome
Person verbalizes an awareness of the causes of the problem
Relates the acceptance of self-limitations in sexual matters
Relates contentment with achievable sexual experiences

NURSING INTERVENTIONS

Nursing Treatments
Approach unhurriedly
Provide an atmosphere of acceptance (of the person, but not of the behavior)
Express empathy
Reassure verbally
Encourage the expression of feelings (about sexual concerns)
Listen attentively
    AND
Talk with the person
Offer feedback to the person's expressed feelings
Ask the person to identify the problem
Ask for specifics, not generalizations, about the problem
Explore superficial topics and reasons for avoiding in-depth feelings
Explore with the person the reasons for recurring problems
Explore with the person the effects of his behavior on others (the partner)
Encourage an awareness of positive responses from others (the partner)
Make a referral (to a psychiatric or sexuality nurse specialist if needed)
Consult with the physician (if therapy or drugs are the cause)

Nursing Observations
Determine the degree of insight that the person has (into the sexual problem)
Evaluate the person's relatedness with others (especially the partner)
Evaluate the significance of emotional distress mannerisms
Evaluate the significance of nonverbal communication
Identify disturbing conversation topics
Identify life values significant to the person (and related to sexuality)
Observe for evidence that the person is reaching out for emotional support
Observe for evidence of a favorable response to therapy

Health Teaching

Explain the emotional causes of reduced sexual response (it is an indirect expression of anger, anxiety, or rejection of another, it is a response to the threat of intimacy or pregnancy, etc.)

Explain the physical causes of reduced sexual response (diabetes, drug therapy, hemodialysis, etc.)

Explain that sexual response normally varies (according to the person's mood, level of fatigue, life situation, or activities and emphasize that sexual response cannot always be at a high level)

Recommend alternative approaches to sexual activity (such as different precoital activities)

Explain the need for realistic expectations of others (including one's sexual partner)

Explain that relaxation is essential for a successful sexual response

Explain the importance of maintaining a positive self-attitude

Relate the criteria for a successful sexual response (if the person experiences satisfaction, completeness, euphoria, or contentment, the experience is considered successful)

EVALUATION

Record actual outcome

INHIBITED SEXUAL EXCITEMENT[19,67,262]

ASSESSMENT

Data Collection

Subjective Data
• Person relates being partially or totally unable to perform the sexual act
• Focuses more on preintercourse sexual activity
• Expresses diminished sexual satisfaction
  Worries about the mate's reaction
  Male perceives himself as less of a man

Objective Data
None

Data Analysis

Nursing Diagnosis
INHIBITED SEXUAL EXCITEMENT (FRIGIDITY, IMPOTENCE): The limited ability or inability to perform the sexual act

Common Etiology (Stressors)
DISEASES: Cerebrovascular accident, multiple sclerosis, renal failure, syphilis
INJURIES: Fracture and compression of the spinal cord
PSYCHOSOCIAL FACTORS: Severe stress, the threat of a deteriorating relationship, the threat of intimacy and/or physical closeness, lack of enjoyment of a particular role (as a sexual partner) with another person, the threat of pregnancy
HEALTH CARE FACTORS: *Medical therapy*: Hemodialysis. *Drug therapy*: Adverse effects of Tagamet and antihypertensive drugs (Inderal)
DEVELOPMENTAL PHASES: Old age
LIFESTYLE: Marijuana drug abuse, religious beliefs

PLANNING

Unmet Needs

Relaxation, comfort, sexuality, protection from psychologic threat, love and affection, acceptance, caring and communicating relationships, high evaluation of self, sense of adequacy, personal growth and maturity, increased learning, increased reality perception and problem-solving ability, increased pleasantness

Expected Outcome

Person verbalizes an awareness of the causes of the problem
Relates the acceptance of self-limitations in sexual matters
Relates contentment with his achievable sexual experiences

NURSING INTERVENTIONS

Nursing Treatments

Approach unhurriedly
Provide an atmosphere of acceptance (of the person but not of the behavior)
Express empathy
Reassure verbally
Encourage the expression of feelings (about sexual concerns)
Listen attentively
Talk with the person
Offer feedback to the person's expressed feelings
Ask the person to identify the problem
Ask for specifics, not generalizations, about the problem
Explore superficial topics and reasons for avoiding in-depth feelings
Explore with the person the reasons for recurring problems
Explore with the person the effects of his behavior on others (the partner)
Encourage an awareness of positive responses from others (the partner)
Make a referral (to a psychiatric or sexuality nurse specialist if needed)
Consult with the physician (if the disease, therapy, or drugs are the cause)

Nursing Observations

Determine the degree of insight that the person has (into the sexual problem and into motivations of sexual activity)
Evaluate the person's relatedness with others (especially the partner)
Evaluate the significance of emotional distress mannerisms
Evaluate the significance of nonverbal communication
Identify disturbing conversation topics
Identify life values significant to the person (and related to sexuality)
Observe for evidence that the person is reaching out for emotional support
Observe for evidence of a favorable response to therapy

Health Teaching

Explain the emotional causes of reduced sexual response (fracture and compression of the spinal cord, cerebrovascular accident, multiple sclerosis, syphilis, drug therapy or drug abuse, aging)
Explain that sexual response normally varies (according to the person's mood, level of fatigue, life situation, or activities and emphasize that sexual response cannot always be at a high level)
Recommend alternative approaches to sexual activity (such as different coital positions)
Explain the need for realistic expectations of others (including one's sexual partner)
Explain that relaxation is essential for a successful sexual response
Explain the importance of maintaining a positive self-attitude
Relate the criteria for a successful sexual response (if the person experiences satisfaction, completeness, euphoria, or contentment, the experience is considered successful)

EVALUATION

Record actual outcome

SEXUAL ACTING OUT[262,348]

ASSESSMENT

Data Collection

Subjective Data

- Person relates an increased interest in sex
- Perceives sexual exploits as self-glorifying, as a validation of maleness or femaleness
  Enjoys having many sexual conquests
  Expects immediate gratification of needs
  Feels no guilt or anxiety about sexual exploits

Objective Data

- Person presents a charming facade
  Exhibits flirtations or intimate behavior (such as verbalizing about sex, making direct body contact with others)

Data Analysis

Nursing Diagnosis

SEXUAL ACTING OUT (EXCESSIVE LIBIDO): Experiencing and outwardly expressing feelings of an exaggerated sexual drive

Common Etiology (Stressors)

DISEASES: Manic–depressive psychosis, organic brain syndrome, personality disorder, schizophrenia

PSYCHOSOCIAL FACTORS: The threat of inadequacy, lack of self-esteem, an attempt to control mortality by becoming pregnant, an attempt to test sexual functioning and desirability, lack of impulse control, an indirect expression of anxiety, anger, or guilt

PLANNING

Unmet Needs

Psychologic stability, acceptance, caring and communicating relationships, sense of adequacy, self-control, personal growth and maturity, increased learning, increased reality perception and problem-solving ability

Expected Outcome

Person verbalizes an awareness of the causes of the problem
Relates the acceptance of having to place limitations on sexual behavior
Exhibits control over sexual behavior

NURSING INTERVENTIONS

Nursing Treatments

Approach unhurriedly
Reassure verbally
Demonstrate calmness
Provide an atmosphere of acceptance (of the person but not of the behavior)
Encourage the expression of feelings (about the person's sexual drive)
Explore superficial topics and reasons for avoiding in-depth feelings (about sexual concerns)
Listen attentively
Talk with the person
Offer feedback to the person's expressed feelings
Communicate nurse sensitivity to the person's problem
Relate to the person on an adult–adult level, not on a parent–child level
Explore with the person the effects of his behavior on others (that the behavior angers and embarrasses others)
Encourage respect for the rights of others
Encourage participation in therapeutic group interaction (to gain insight into the behavior and improve interpersonal relationships)

Set limits on unacceptable behavior (at the same time being careful not to reject the person)

Clearly communicate what is expected of the person

Hold the person responsible for his behavior (do not allow the person to blame others)

Refrain from arguing, from negatively criticizing

Verbalize daily the person's successful progress (in changing the behavior)

Make a referral (to a psychiatric or sexuality nurse specialist as needed)

Consult with a physician (about medications, if appropriate) .

Nursing Observations

Determine the degree of insight that the person has (into his sexuality and his acting-out behavior)

Determine the precipitating factors (for sexual acting out)

Identify disturbing conversation topics

Evaluate the significance of emotional distress mannerisms

Evaluate the significance of nonverbal communication

Observe for evidence that the person is reaching out for emotional support

Observe for behavior modification (resulting from the therapy)

Health Teaching

Explain the causes of the problem (inadequacy feelings, attention seeking, an indirect expression of anxiety, anger, or guilt)

Emphasize the importance of recognizing tension within oneself (prior to the impulse of acting-out; and of recognizing the origin of tension as sexual or nonsexual)

Explain how to channel sexual energy and obtain release from stress (through sports, work, travel, creative activity)

Recommend things to do when one begins to feel out of control (wash hands and face with cold water, take a long walk, etc.)

Explain why the person should maintain self-control (out of respect for oneself and others, for role modeling, etc.)

Explain the importance of maintaining a positive self-attitude (which supports positive behavior)

Recommend that behavioral limits be set (by significant others)

Explain how to set behavioral limits (by clearly stating acceptable and unacceptable behavior)

EVALUATION

Record actual outcome

Nonadaptive Responses to Stress

ADJUSTMENT REACTION[19,471]

Note: This category is used only when specific disorders are not listed elsewhere

ASSESSMENT

Data Collection

Subjective Data

• Person relates an encounter with a stressor that took place within the past 3 months

• Person verbalizes about experiencing many emotions

- Relates concern about impaired social or occupational functioning

Objective Data
- Person exhibits overt emotional responses that are exaggerated
- The exaggerated emotional response occurs more than once

Data Analysis

Nursing Diagnosis

ADJUSTMENT REACTION: A maladaptive reaction that occurs within 3 months after an encounter with a stressor, the reaction will remit after the stressor ceases or when the person reaches a new level of adaptation

Common Etiology (Stressors)

PSYCHOSOCIAL FACTORS: An attempt to adjust to change, the threat of change, the threat of lack of control over a life situation, the use of exaggerated defense mechanisms, the threat of real or imagined danger, lack of emotional support from others, the threat of inadequacy, a change in a vital life role, the threat of having needs unfulfilled through constructive behavior, which results in negative behavior

SITUATIONAL FACTORS: Adoption of a child, confinement in a prison, death of a significant other, disaster, divorce, loss of employment, loss or relocation of a home, illness or injury of a significant other, marriage, retirement, entry into or change of school, marital separation, situational crisis

PLANNING

Unmet Needs

Comfort, protection from psychologic threat, psychologic stability, acceptance, caring and communicating relationships, sense of adequacy, control over others or over situations, personal growth and maturity, increased learning, increased reality perception and problem-solving ability

Expected Outcome

Person verbalizes his feelings about the life change that requires adjustment
Demonstrates the use of coping mechanisms appropriate to the situation
Verbalizes acceptance of the life change
Exhibits competent social and occupational functioning

NURSING INTERVENTIONS

Nursing Treatments

Approach unhurriedly
Reassure verbally
Demonstrate calmness
Provide an atmosphere of acceptance (of the person, but not of the behavior)
Encourage the expression of feelings (about the problem)
Listen attentively
Talk with the person
Offer feedback to the person's expressed feelings
Communicate nurse sensitivity to the person's problem
Relate to the person on an adult–adult level, not on a parent–child level
Ask the person to identify the problem
Ask for specifics, not generalizations, about the problem
Encourage the use of normal coping mechanisms
Hold the person responsible for his behavior (do not allow him to blame others)
Clearly communicate what is expected of the person
Arrange situations that encourage the person's autonomy (to increase the sense of control over the situation)
Encourage a positive life approach (to maintain positive attitudes)
Explore with the person his positive characteristics
Explore with the person previous achievements of success (in adjusting)

Explore with the person the effects of his behavior on others (effects such as worry, anger, embarrassment)

Reduce the demands placed on the person (so that more energy is available for coping)

Refrain from performing nonessential procedures (that add stress and slow adaptation)

Encourage gradual mastery of the situation

Encourage participation in therapeutic group interaction (to gain insight into the problem)

Encourage both long- and short-term goals

Introduce to persons who have successfully undergone the same experience (if appropriate)

Support a realistic assessment of the situation

Nursing Observations

Determine the degree of insight that the person has (into the problem)

Identify disturbing conversation topics

Evaluate the significance of emotional distress mannerisms

Identify the inappropriate use of defense mechanisms

Observe for a favorable response to therapy (behavior modification)

Health Teaching

Explain the causes of the problem (the threat of change, lack of control of a situation, the use of exaggerated defense mechanisms)

Recommend new options for effective methods of coping (appropriate to the situation)

Explain the importance of remaining calm (calmness decreases internal tension, which results in higher levels of functioning)

Explain that the situation is temporary

Explain that persons must make adjustments at their own pace

Explain the importance of maintaining a positive self-attitude (positive attitudes yield positive behavior)

Advise that significant persons express caring for one another (especially during adjustment periods)

Explain the importance of persons offering emotional support to one another

Teach how to use the problem-solving method

EVALUATION

Record actual outcome

Nonadaptive Ego Defense Responses

DEPENDENCY REACTION[19,105,471]

ASSESSMENT

Data Collection

Subjective Data

• Person relates that another person (spouse, parent) makes his decisions for him
• He does not make demands of persons on whom he is dependent
• Verbally belittles himself
• Relates perceiving himself as helpless
  May express anxiety, depression
  Feels an intense discomfort when left alone
  Has social and occupational limitations
  Does not question that which affects him, but blindly accepts everything

Objective Data
• Little or no overt evidence of self-initiated activity

Data Analysis

Nursing Diagnosis
DEPENDENCY REACTION (DEPENDENT PERSONALITY DISORDER): Allowing others to assume responsibility for the significant decisions and events in one's life

Common Etiology (Stressors)
PSYCHOSOCIAL FACTORS: The threat of inadequacy, the absence of, separation from, or loss of a significant other, an attempt to control others, to express anger indirectly, an attempt to gain attention or to reduce present life responsibilities and assume a less demanding personal status
DEVELOPMENTAL PHASES: Old age
SITUATIONAL FACTORS: Chronic illness

PLANNING

Unmet Needs
Protection from psychologic threat, psychologic stability, acceptance, sense of adequacy, independence, personal growth and maturity, increased learning, increased reality perception and problem-solving ability

Expected Outcome
Person arrives at his own decisions
Independently initiates and completes any attempted activity
Relates satisfaction with self-growth

NURSING INTERVENTIONS

Nursing Treatments
Approach unhurriedly
Reassure verbally (that the person is mature and capable of managing his own life)
Demonstrate calmness
Provide an atmosphere of acceptance (of the person, but not of the behavior)
Encourage the expression of feelings (discuss with him what it means to be independent and explore some of his feelings about independence such as whether it makes him fearful, etc.)
Listen attentively
Talk with the person
Offer feedback to the person's expressed feelings
Communicate nurse sensitivity to the person's problem
Relate to the person on an adult–adult level, not on a parent–child level (which could reinforce the dependent reaction)
Encourage decision making (by the dependent person)
Encourage self-performance
Encourage the acceptance of responsibility
Arrange situations that encourage the person's autonomy
Explore with the person his strengths and resources (to be independent)
Support a realistic assessment of the situation (that independence characterizes maturity)
Set limits on unacceptable (dependent) behavior
 OR
Ignore undesirable (dependent) behavior
Clearly communicate what is expected of the person
Offer praise (for decision making and independent action)

Nursing Observations
Determine the degree of insight that the person has (into the dependency)
Evaluate the person's relatedness with others (in regard to dependence–independence)
Observe for impaired self-attitudes (that support dependency)

Observe for evidence that the person is reaching out for emotional support

Observe for evidence of a favorable response to therapy (the achievement of maximum independence attainable, increased comfort feelings)

Health Teaching

Recommend a habitual, positive mental attitude (to overcome dependency feelings)

Explain the causes of the problem (a sense of inadequacy, attempts to gain attention or control others)

EVALUATION

Record actual outcome

HYPOCHONDRIASIS [13,14,19,105,432]

ASSESSMENT

Data Collection

Subjective Data
• Person relates a preoccupation with body function
• Feels certain he has a serious disease
• Person perceives his body as vulnerable and sickly
  Has strange inner sensations directed toward different organs
  Worries excessively about his health
  May develop an illness after exposure to conversation about the illness
  Relates an endless verbal description of ailments
  Warns others about germs and infection
  Presents his physical history in great detail
  May relate having been to many physicians without finding satisfactory health care

Objective Data
• Absence of physical findings to explain the disorder

Data Analysis

Nursing Diagnosis
HYPOCHONDRIASIS: An unrealistic preoccupation with or fear of having a serious disease

Common Etiology (Stressors)
DISEASES: Dependent personality disorder
PSYCHOSOCIAL FACTORS: An attempt to gain attention, lack of competency in using effective coping mechanisms, an attempt to express an emotion such as anger, anxiety, or dependency indirectly, an attempt to control others or a life situation, the threat of having needs unfulfilled through constructive behavior resulting in negative behavior, lack of emotional support from others, an attempt to reduce present life responsibilities and assume a less demanding personal status

PLANNING

Unmet Needs

Comfort, protection from psychologic threat, psychologic stability, acceptance, caring and communicating relationships, sense of adequacy, attention, personal growth and maturity, increased learning, increased reality perception and problem-solving ability, increased pleasantness

Expected Outcome

Person relates an awareness of the causes of the problem
Verbally expresses his underlying emotions
Demonstrates the use of more appropriate coping mechanisms
No longer relates somatic complaints

NURSING INTERVENTIONS

Nursing Treatments

Approach unhurriedly

Provide an atmosphere of acceptance (of the person, but not of the behavior)

Encourage the expression of feelings (about the underlying problem)

Listen attentively

Talk with the person

Offer feedback to the person's expressed feelings

Communicate nurse sensitivity to the person's problem

Relate to the person on an adult–adult level, not on a parent–child level (which could reinforce the reaction)

Ask the person to identify the problem

Ask for specifics, not generalizations, about the problem

Encourage the use of normal coping mechanisms

Provide reliable information (about the health status)

Explore with the person the reasons for recurring problems

Explore with the person the effects of his behavior on others (effects such as worry, anger, frustration)

Explore with the person the need for attention, the need to control

Explore with the person his positive characteristics

Support a realistic assessment of the situation (that the person is physically well)

Refrain from negatively criticizing

Nursing Observations

Determine the degree of the insight that the person has (into the problem)

Determine the precipitating factors, the relieving factors

Evaluate the person's relatedness with others (and its effect on behavior)

Evaluate the significance of emotional distress mannerisms, the significance of nonverbal communication

Identify disturbing conversation topics

Observe for evidence that the person is reaching out for emotional support

Observe for evidence of a favorable response to therapy (behavior modification)

Health Teaching

Explain the causes of the problem (an attempt at attention seeking, control of persons or situations, ineffective coping mechanisms)

Advise that significant persons express caring for one another

Explain the importance of persons offering emotional support to one another

EVALUATION

Record actual outcome

HYSTERIA [19,471]

ASSESSMENT

Data Collection

Subjective Data

• Person relates physical symptoms inconsistent with the symptoms of the physical disorder

• Expresses some psychologic conflict

• Relates some undesirable situation that the person would prefer to avoid

May express a need for emotional support

Objective Data
• Absence of physical findings to explain the disorder

Data Analysis

Nursing Diagnosis
HYSTERIA (CONVERSION DISORDER): A loss of physical functioning as an expression of psychologic need

Common Etiology (Stressors)
DISEASES: Personality disorder
PSYCHOSOCIAL FACTORS: Overwhelming stress, an attempt to express anxiety or guilt indirectly, lack of competency in using effective coping mechanisms, an attempt to gain attention and to control others, lack of emotional support from others, an attempt to reduce the present life responsibilities and assume a less demanding personal status, the threat of having needs unfulfilled through constructive behavior resulting in negative behavior

PLANNING

Unmet Needs
Comfort, protection from psychologic threat, psychologic stability, acceptance, caring and communicating relationships, sense of adequacy, attention, personal growth and maturity, increased learning, increased reality perception and problem-solving ability, increased pleasantness

Expected Outcome
Person relates an awareness of the causes of the problem
Verbally expresses psychologic conflicts
Demonstrates the use of more appropriate coping mechanisms
Regains and maintains normal physical functioning

NURSING INTERVENTIONS

Nursing Treatments
Approach unhurriedly
Provide an atmosphere of acceptance (of the person but not of the behavior)
Encourage the expression of feelings (his own feelings such as fear, anger)
Listen attentively
Talk with the person
Offer feedback to the person's expressed feelings
Communicate nurse sensitivity to the person's problem
Relate to the person on an adult–adult level, not on a parent–child level
Ask the person to identify the problem
Ask for specifics, not generalizations, about the problem
Encourage the use of normal coping mechanisms
Provide reliable information (about the health status)
Explore with the person the reasons for recurring problems
Explore with the person the effects of his behavior on others (effects such as worry, anger, frustration)
Explore with the person the need for attention, the need to control
Explore with the person his positive characteristics
Support a realistic assessment of the situation (that the person is physically well)
Refrain from negatively criticizing

Nursing Observations
Determine the degree of insight that the person has (into the problem)
Determine the precipitating factors, the relieving factors
Evaluate the person's relatedness with others (and its effect on his behavior)
Evaluate the significance of emotional distress mannerisms, the significance of nonverbal communication
Identify disturbing conversation topics

Observe for evidence that the person is reaching out for emotional support
Observe for evidence of a favorable response to therapy (behavior modification)

Health Teaching

Explain the causes of the problem (an attempt at attention seeking, to control persons or situations, the use of ineffective coping mechanisms)
Advise that significant persons express caring for one another
Explain the importance of persons offering emotional support to one another

EVALUATION

Record actual outcome

MANIPULATIVE BEHAVIOR[471,661]

ASSESSMENT

Data Collection

Subjective Data
- Person perceives all interpersonal relationships as an opportunity for self-gain
- May appear to be emotionally involved with others, but involvement is only self-oriented
- Believes he must maintain control or others will take advantage of him
- Feels he is deserving of special consideration

Objective Data
- Person uses charming overt behavior
  May bargain, demand, intimidate, flatter, play one person against another, act helpless
  Violates rules or disrupts routines

Data Analysis

Nursing Diagnosis
MANIPULATIVE BEHAVIOR (MANIPULATION): Relating to others as if they were objects for self-gain

Common Etiology (Stressors)
DISEASES: Personality disorder
PSYCHOSOCIAL FACTORS: An attempt to control others or a life situation, lack of competency in using effective coping mechanisms, an attempt to achieve one's own goals by using others, lack of training in social skills, the threat of a deteriorating relationship

PLANNING

Unmet Needs

Protection from psychologic threat, psychologic stability, sense of adequacy, self-control, personal growth and maturity, increased learning, increased reality perception and problem-solving ability

Expected Outcome

Person relates an awareness of using manipulative behavior
Demonstrates the use of effective and acceptable coping mechanisms
Demonstrates increasing skill in establishing and maintaining rewarding and trusting relationships

NURSING INTERVENTIONS

Nursing Treatments

Approach unhurriedly
Demonstrate calmness

Provide an atmosphere of acceptance (of the person, but not of the behavior)
Encourage the expression of feelings
Listen attentively
Talk with the person (but do not allow the person to evade the subject, and do refocus on the topic of discussion)
Set limits on unacceptable behavior (clarify exactly what the person can or cannot do)
OR
Ignore the unacceptable behavior (giving attention to the person reinforces the manipulative behavior)
Clearly communicate what is expected of the person (in positive terms)
Hold the person responsible for his own behavior (do not allow the person to blame others)
Encourage respect for the rights of others
Encourage role-playing to develop sensitivity
Explore with the person the effects of his behavior on others
Explore with the person the need to control
Maintain consistent staff behavior (both in behavioral expectations and in responses to behavior)
Recommend new options for effective methods of coping (direct help seeking, talking things over)
Encourage decision making (which gives the person some control, but it may be necessary to limit the choices)
Arrange a structured daily routine (to reduce anxiety, which decreases the need for manipulative behavior)
Avoid assuming that all behavior is manipulative (some complaints or requests will be valid)
Offer praise (for behavior modification)
Involve the family (work with the family if possible, and help them learn how not to be manipulated)

Nursing Observations

Determine the degree of insight that the person has (into the manipulative behavior)
Evaluate the patient's relatedness with others (does the patient play one person against another)
Observe for evidence of a favorable response to therapy (behavior modification)

Health Teaching

Explain the causes of the problem (high anxiety levels, poor training in social skills, an attempt to control)
Recommend (to the family) that behavioral limits be set (on manipulative methods)
Explain (to the family) how to set behavioral limits (by clearly stating what constitutes acceptable and unacceptable behavior)
Teach the problem-solving method (offer the person multiple nonmanipulative options for solving the problem)

EVALUATION

Record actual outcome

NONADAPTIVE DENIAL[105,525]

ASSESSMENT

Data Collection

Subjective Data
• Person exhibits verbal rejection of the occurring reality

- Prolongs denial for an extended period beyond the normal adjustment time
Person disregards clear evidence of a threatening situation

Objective Data
- Exhibits behavior as though the threatening situation did not exist

Data Analysis

Nursing Diagnosis
NONADAPTIVE DENIAL: The use of denial as a defense mechanism beyond the point at which denial is usually effective

Common Etiology (Stressors)
PSYCHOSOCIAL FACTORS: Overwhelming stress, the threat of unpleasant reality, lack of competency in using effective coping mechanisms, an attempt to control a life situation, lack of emotional support from others, the threat of inadequacy or of having to deal with strong emotions

PLANNING

Unmet Needs
Protection from psychologic threat, psychologic stability, acceptance, caring and communicating relationships, sense of adequacy, control over others or situations, personal growth and maturity, increased learning, increased reality perception or problem-solving ability

Expected Outcome
Person verbalizes an awareness of the cause of the denial
Demonstrates the use of more appropriate coping mechanisms
Relates feeling comfortable with the perceived threat and confident about meeting the demands of the problem

NURSING INTERVENTIONS

Nursing Treatments
Approach unhurriedly
Reassure verbally
Demonstrate calmness
Provide an atmosphere of acceptance (of the person but not of the behavior)
Encourage the expression of feelings (exploring with him the feelings he might have if he viewed the situation as a reality)
Listen attentively
Talk with the person
Offer feedback to the person's expressed feelings
Communicate nurse sensitivity to the person's problem
Ask the person to identify the problem (to the degree that he is psychologically able)
Ask for specifics, not generalizations, about the problem (specifics may penetrate the denial)
Ask questions that encourage answers that reflect reality perception (such as "Do you think you are sick?" "Do you think your wife will die?" to support a sense of reality; then if the person asks why he hurts, direct him to answer the question, noting that he will respond with the level of truth acceptable to him at the time)
Periodically verbalize the denied reality ("You'll be going for radiation therapy this afternoon," "Your divorce is final the end of the month")
Act out the reality the person cannot accept (visibly and openly care for an amputation stump, verbalize about the special needs of paralyzed limbs while providing care, demonstrate teaching methods used for children with developmental deficits in specialized classes or schools)
Share with the person objective data that verify the health status (show him laboratory reports, let him listen to his own lung sounds, etc.)
Ensure the person's feeling of safety before introducing unpleasantness (which might increase the denial)

Support the use of appropriate defense mechanisms (by allowing the denial if it is the person's most effective defense mechanism)

Explore with the person his strengths and resources (awareness of one's strength may reduce the need for denial)

Encourage gradual mastery of the situation (face the reality one step at a time)

Nursing Observations

Determine the degree of insight that the person has (into the denial)

Identify disturbing conversation topics

Evaluate the significance of emotional distress mannerisms

Identify cues indicating some acceptance of reality (statements such as "I'm half dead. Everyone in my family has had cancer—why should I be different?")

Observe for an excessive stress level (talkativeness, pacing, nervousness, heavy smoking)

Observe for evidence that the person is reaching out for emotional support

Observe for evidence of a favorable response to therapy (the acceptance of reality)

Health Teaching

Explain the causes of the problem (overwhelming stress, the threat of an unpleasant reality, an attempt to control)

Recommend new options for effective methods of coping (talking about the problem, developing new skills to compensate for lost functions, planning for a positive future)

Explain that persons must make adjustments at their own pace

Teach how to use the problem-solving method

EVALUATION

Record actual outcome

PARANOIA [19,105]

ASSESSMENT

Data Collection

Subjective Data
- Person verbalizes extreme suspiciousness
- Relates having feelings of powerlessness
- Blames others for his own unacceptable impulses
- Relates delusional thinking but otherwise acts normally
- States he is being taken advantage of or plotted against

Objective Data
None

Data Analysis

Nursing Diagnosis
PARANOIA (PARANOID DISORDER): Person believes himself to be persecuted or mistreated by others

Common Etiology (Stressors)
PSYCHOSOCIAL FACTORS: Lack of competency in using effective coping mechanisms, the threat of a deteriorating relationship, the threat of inadequacy, an attempt to conceal unacceptable impulses, the threat of real or imagined danger, the threat of lack of control of a life situation, lack of early training in socialization

PLANNING

Unmet Needs
Comfort, protection from psychologic threat, psychologic stability, acceptance, caring

and communicating relationships, sense of adequacy, personal growth and maturity, increased learning, increased reality perception and problem-solving ability

Expected Outcome
Person verbalizes the causes of the problem
Demonstrates the use of more appropriate coping mechanisms
Verbalizes about satisfying and trusting interrelatedness

NURSING INTERVENTIONS
Nursing Treatments
Approach unhurriedly
Provide an atmosphere of acceptance (of the person, but not of the behavior)
Demonstrate calmness (and matter-of-fact behavior)
Arrange situations that encourage the person's autonomy
Encourage the expression of feelings (about distrusting others)
Offer feedback to the person's expressed feelings
Listen attentively
Talk with the person
> BUT
Terminate emotionally threatening conversation immediately
Support a realistic assessment of the situation
Ask for specifics, not generalizations, about the problem (regarding who or what is distrusted)
Explore with the person the reasons for recurring problems
Explore with the person the effects of his behavior on others
Ensure the person's feeling of safety before introducing unpleasantness
Introduce one anxiety-producing situation at a time
Provide emotionally safe experiences
Provide objects that symbolize safeness
Limit the touching of suspicious persons
Maintain consistent staff behavior
Maintain social formality or informality (whichever is most acceptable to the person)
Refrain from making promises
> BUT
Follow through on promises (which are made)
Provide reliable information
Refrain from arguing, from teasing, from negatively criticizing
Refrain from performing nonessential procedures (that deplete energy needed for coping)
Set limits on unacceptable behavior

Nursing Observations
Determine the degree of insight that the person has (into the paranoia)
Determine the precipitating factors, the relieving factors
Evaluate the person's relatedness with others
Evaluate the significance of emotional distress mannerisms, the significance of nonverbal communications
Identify disturbing conversation topics
Identify potentially destructive behavior
Observe for evidence of a favorable response to therapy (increased trust)

Health Teaching
Advise that negative responses from others be regarded with minimum significance (even though there are feelings about such responses)
Advise that significant persons express acceptance of one another
Advise that significant persons express caring for one another
Explain the importance of offering emotional support to one another
Explain the need for realistic expectations of others (that one cannot expect perfection from others)

Explain the causes of the health problem
Recommend that behavioral limits be set (for excessive distrust)
Explain how to set behavioral limits (by clearly stating what constitutes acceptable and unacceptable behavior)

EVALUATION

Record actual outcome

PSYCHOGENIC PAIN DISORDER[19,530,663]

ASSESSMENT

Data Collection

Subjective Data
• Person complains of severe, prolonged pain
• Expresses some psychologic conflict
  Focuses on and is preoccupied with the pain

Objective Data
• Physical findings are inconsistent with the complaint of pain

Data Analysis

Nursing Diagnosis
PSYCHOGENIC PAIN DISORDER: A complaint of pain in the absence of validating physical findings and in the presence of psychologic conflict

Common Etiology (Stressors)
PSYCHOSOCIAL FACTORS: An indirect expression of conflict, the threat of severe or chronic stress, lack of emotional support from others, lack of competency in using effective coping mechanisms

PLANNING

Unmet Needs
Relaxation, comfort, protection from physical harm, protection from psychologic threat, freedom from pain, personal growth and maturity, increased learning, increased reality perception and problem-solving ability

Expected Outcome
Person relates an awareness of the cause of the problem
Verbally expresses the psychologic conflict
Demonstrates the use of more appropriate coping mechanisms
Relates feeling satisfied with his personal growth

NURSING INTERVENTIONS

Nursing Treatments
Approach unhurriedly
Reassure that the pain will subside or be relieved
Communicate nurse sensitivity to the person's pain
Demonstrate calmness
Listen attentively
Provide an atmosphere of acceptance (of the person but not of the behavior)
Provide frequent contact with the person
Massage gently (for the relaxation effect)

Encourage adequate rest
Reduce the demands placed on the person
Refrain from performing nonessential procedures (that increase stress)
Encourage the expression of feelings (about inner conflicts)
Reveal the person's ambivalent feelings (if the person cannot do so)
Support a realistic assessment of the situation
Encourage mutual problem solving
Accept and attempt to relieve unexplainable body complaints
Ask the person that makes him (or her) comfortable
Discuss possible pain-reducing measures
Provide a pain-relief measure of the person's choice
Make a referral (to a psychiatric nurse specialist if needed)

Nursing Observations

Determine the precipitating factors, the relieving factors
Determine the degree of insight that the person has (into the cause of the pain)
Observe for complaints of pain duration
Evaluate the pain for intensity and quality
Evaluate the effectiveness of the pain-relief measures
Observe for evidence of a favorable response to therapy (behavior modification)

Health Teaching

Explain the causes of the problem (the indirect expression of conflict)
Explain the relationship between conflict and psychologic pain (psychogenic pain symbolizes subconscious emotional conflict)
Explain how to channel emotional energy and obtain release from stress (through sports, creative activities, talking things over, laughing, etc.)
Emphasize the importance of recognizing tension within oneself (in its early phase before it becomes overwhelming, and of dealing with conflicts as soon as they occur).

EVALUATION

Record actual outcome

SOMATIC REACTION [471,530,663]

ASSESSMENT

Data Collection

Subjective Data
• Person relates a recent emotional trauma, often a loss, and intense feelings of tension
• Expresses feelings of helplessness, of being overwhelmed
• Complains of pain

Objective Data
• Physical findings are appropriate to the complaint
  Tense facial expression
  Restlessness

Related Data

Commonly Related Conditions and Diseases
Colitis, constipation, diarrhea, duodenal ulcer, gastritis, headache, muscle cramps, sinusitis, vaginismus

Data Analysis

Nursing Diagnosis
SOMATIC REACTION (SOMATIZATION REACTION, PSYCHOSOMATIC PAIN): A distressful hurting that occurs in the presence of a physical disorder brought on by intense stress

Common Etiology (Stressors)
PSYCHOSOCIAL FACTORS: An indirect expression of conflict, the threat of severe or chronic stress, lack of emotional support from others, lack of competency in using effective coping mechanisms

MAJOR PATHOPHYSIOLOGIC FACTORS: Organic pain results from muscle tension and nerve stimulation in response to stressful situations, psychologic stress has been subconsciously channeled to visceral organs, constitutional physical weakness is accentuated by intense stress and causes physical disorders, the pain itself results from nerve excitation and is considered an autonomic nervous system disorder

PLANNING

Unmet Needs
Sleep, rest and relaxation, comfort, protection from physical harm, protection from psychologic threat, freedom from pain, personal growth and maturity, increased learning, increased reality perception and problem-solving ability

Expected Outcome
Person relates an awareness of the cause of the problem
Verbally expresses his feelings about the threatening emotion
Demonstrates the use of more appropriate coping mechanisms
Relates feeling satisfied with personal growth

NURSING INTERVENTIONS

Nursing Treatments
Approach unhurriedly
Reassure that the pain will subside or be relieved
Communicate nurse sensitivity to the person's pain
Demonstrate calmness
Listen attentively
Provide an atmosphere of acceptance (of the person but not of the behavior)
Provide frequent patient contact
Massage gently (for the relaxation effect)
Encourage adequate rest
Reduce the demands placed upon the person
Refrain from performing nonessential procedures (that increase stress)
Encourage the expression of feelings (about inner conflicts)
Support a realistic assessment of the situation
Ask the person what makes him (or her) comfortable
Discuss possible pain-reducing measures
Provide a pain-relief measure of the person's choice

Nursing Observations
Observe for complaints of pain duration
Evaluate the pain for intensity and quality
Determine the degree of insight the person has (into the causes of the pain)
Evaluate the effectiveness of the pain-relief measures
Observe for evidence of a favorable response to therapy (behavior modification)

Health Teaching
Explain the psychologic causes of organic pain (muscle tension and nerve stimulation resulting from stress)
Explain how to channel emotional energy and obtain release from stress (through sports, creative activities, talking things over, laughing, etc.)

Emphasize the importance of recognizing tension within oneself (in its early phase before it becomes overwhelming)

Explain how to reduce muscular tension (stretching and suddenly letting the muscles go limp)

Recommend methods for achieving total relaxation (controlled breathing, listening to soft music, doing nothing for a while)

EVALUATION

Record actual outcome

SUSPICIOUSNESS [105,130,225,471]

ASSESSMENT

Data Collection

Subjective Data
- Person doubts the integrity of the other person's motivation
- Questions the competency of others in detail
- Checks and rechecks all interactions with others to be sure he has not been taken advantage of

Fears that the effects of the actions of others may prove harmful to him

May accuse persons of causing him injury when such was neither intended nor inflicted

Objective Data
- May display uncooperative behavior

Susceptible to displays of jealousy

Data Analysis

Nursing Diagnosis

SUSPICIOUSNESS: The inability to feel confident regarding the competency and reliability of other persons

Common Etiology (Stressors)

DISEASES: Organic brain syndrome

PSYCHOSOCIAL FACTORS: The threat of inadequacy, the threat of loss of self-esteem, exposure to a suspicious role model, lack of control of others or of a life situation, the threat of having needs unfulfilled through constructive behavior resulting in negative behavior, lack of early training in socialization, nonachievement of developmental trust

DEVELOPMENTAL PHASES: Old age

ENVIRONMENTAL FACTORS: Violence on television, being a victim of violence

PLANNING

Unmet Needs

Comfort, protection from psychologic threat, psychologic stability, a predictable and orderly world, acceptance, caring and communicating relationships, high evaluation of self, personal growth and maturity, increased learning, increased reality perception and problem-solving ability

Expected Outcome

Person relates an awareness of the causes of the problem

Demonstrates the use of more appropriate coping mechanisms

Verbalizes about satisfying and trusting interrelatedness

NURSING INTERVENTIONS

Nursing Treatments
Approach unhurriedly
Provide an atmosphere of acceptance (of the person, but not of the behavior)
Demonstrate calmness
Arrange situations that encourage the person's autonomy
Encourage the expression of feelings (about distrusting others)
Offer feedback to the person's expressed feelings
Listen attentively
Talk with the person
    BUT
Terminate emotionally threatening conversation immediately
Support a realistic assessment of the situation
Ask for specifics, not generalizations, about the problem (regarding who or what is distrusted)
Explore with the person the reasons for recurring problems
Explore with the person the effects of his behavior on others
Ensure the person's feeling of safety before introducing unpleasantness
Introduce one anxiety-producing situation at a time
Provide emotionally safe experiences
Provide objects which symbolize safeness
Limit the touching of suspicious persons
Maintain consistent staff behavior
Maintain social formality or informality (whichever is most acceptable to the person)
Refrain from making promises
    BUT
Follow through on promises (when they are made)
Provide reliable information
Refrain from arguing, from teasing, from negatively criticizing
Refrain from performing nonessential procedures
Set limits on unacceptable behavior

Nursing Observations
Determine the degree of insight that the person has (into the suspiciousness)
Determine the precipitating factors, the relieving factors
Evaluate the person's relatedness with others
Evaluate the significance of emotional distress mannerisms, the significance of nonverbal communications
Identify disturbing conversation topics
Identify potentially destructive behavior
Observe for evidence of a favorable response to therapy (increased trust)

Health Teaching
Advise that negative responses from others be regarded with minimum significance (even though there are feelings about such responses)
Advise that significant persons express acceptance of one another
Advise that significant persons express caring for one another
Explain the importance of persons offering emotional support to one another
Explain the need for realistic expectations of others (that one cannot expect perfection from others)
Explain the causes of the health problem
Recommend that behavioral limits be set (for excessive distrust)
Explain how to set behavioral limits (by clearly stating what constitutes acceptable and unacceptable behavior)

EVALUATION
Record actual outcome

Nonadaptive Responses of Families

FALTERING FAMILY[293,408,471,682,775]

ASSESSMENT

Data Collection

Subjective Data

• Family members relate attitudes and behavior such as the following:

Power

The spouses share an unequal relationship; each tries to achieve an advantage over the other

Each spouse perceives the other as hostile

Intimacy

One spouse (usually the wife) relates wanting closeness and affection, but the other spouse (usually the husband) relates feeling emotionally isolated and does not openly share his thoughts or feelings; he relates perceiving his wife as demanding, difficult, and depressed; she relates that her husband is a loner, keeps all his feelings inside and is not affectionate

Each partner seeks an intimate relationship with another family member such as a child, parent, etc.

Emotional Aspects

One spouse does not openly express feelings

One spouse relates that his/her emotional needs are not met by the other spouse, both relate being unhappy

Family members do not openly express emotions, but instead avoid and mask feelings; they are not emotionally spontaneous

The children usually do not develop emotional illness

Basic Family Mood

Family members are polite to each other, but cautious about arousing conflict between the spouses

Personal Growth of Family Members

Parents focus on the growth and development of the children

Despite the parental problems, the children do move toward independence and self-direction

Each family member is definitely an individual

Family members relate having a strong sense of responsibility

Socialization

Family members relate that they participate in recreational, leisure, and other activities together

Problem Solving

The family solves both simple and difficult problems efficiently

The spouses are unable to solve the problem of their unhappy relationship, because each blames the other as being the source of the problem

Sexual Relations

Spouses relate that sexual relations do not provide deep satisfaction; the desire for intimacy may lead to extramarital relations

Stress Management

Family members are usually free of physical complaints; the wife is the most likely one to complain, as an expression of her unhappiness

Objective Data
• Family members are involved in activities and practices such as the following:

Roles and Tasks
Each family member functions effectively in his/her specific role
The husband provides economic security and gives mostly money, not affection, to his family; he gains satisfaction from the achievement of projects, not from working with people

Child Rearing
The family relates few difficulties in child rearing
Children are expected to assume responsibility and be independent

Family Value System
The family relates that there are consistent values among family members

Communications
Family members openly and clearly communicate thoughts and ideas

Physical Needs
The physical needs of all family members are met
Preventive health measures are practiced

Environment
The family environment is clean, orderly, in good repair, and free of hazards, provides the basic resources of heat, light, water, etc., and each person has adequate privacy

Community Involvement
Family members are involved in community activities

Data Analysis

Nursing Diagnosis
FALTERING FAMILY: A family that is essentially well except that the relationship of the spouses does not meet the emotional needs of either person

Common Etiology (Stressors)
PSYCHOSOCIAL FACTORS: Unlearned alternative behavior, lack of competency in using effective coping mechanisms, the presence of reinforcing stimuli that maintain maladaptive behavior, exposure to a role model who practiced poor coping skills

PLANNING

Unmet Needs
Protection from psychologic threat, psychologic stability, love and affection, caring and communicating relationships, family growth and maturity, increased learning, increased reality perception and problem-solving ability

Expected Outcome
Family members will learn and practice the principles of a well family
Family members will exhibit the behaviors of a well family

NURSING INTERVENTIONS

Nursing Treatments
Approach unhurriedly
Demonstrate calmness
Provide an atmosphere of acceptance (of each person, but not of the dysfunctional behavior)
Relate to the spouses on an adult–adult level, not on a parent–child level
Listen attentively (to all sides of the issue)
Talk with the spouses (either separately, or together, depending on the situation)
Encourage the expression of feelings (of all family members, and support verbal interaction between members without participating in the interaction)
Ask for specifics, not generalizations, about the problem (obtain descriptions of behavior rather than feelings)

Offer feedback to the person's expressed feelings

Explore with the spouses the reasons for recurring problems

Explore with the spouses the effects of one's behavior on the other (demanding behavior causes emotional distancing, distancing results in increased demands)

Encourage respect for the rights of others

Encourage participation in therapeutic group interaction (in which the spouses can share their problems and gain solutions)

Encourage role playing to develop sensitivity (to each other)

Ignore undesirable behavior
> OR

Set limits on unacceptable behavior (behavioral boundaries between spouses must be clearly defined)

Clearly communicate what is expected of each spouse

Hold the person (each spouse) responsible for his behavior (to not allow one to blame the other)

Explore with the family its strengths and resources

Make a referral (to a psychiatric nurse specialist, psychologist, etc.)

Nursing Observations

Identify the appropriate use of defense mechanisms (such as open communications, freedom to alternate emotional closeness and distancing to support the separateness of the self, allowing each spouse to achieve personal growth)

Identify the inappropriate use of defense mechanisms (point out dysfunctional coping methods such as emotional isolation, the use of fixed triangles, reacting emotionally rather than intellectually)

Determine the degree of insight each spouse has (into the problem)

Determine the precipitating factors (and assist the spouses to identify what triggers their behavior)

Identify potentially destructive behavior (between the spouses)

Identify life values significant to the spouses (have the spouses identify their values and the sources of their values, including an exploration of the values of past generations in a family and their effect on the current generation)

Observe for behavior modification (between spouses)

Health Teaching

Explain how emotional responses occur (the person perceives a situation in terms of its significance to him, an emotional response is experienced accompanied by physiologic changes)

Explain how thinking occurs (information is perceived and is then interpreted on the basis of language skills, sensory-motor development, remembering, reasoning, imaging, and evaluation, then compare the emotional and thought processes and encourage the spouses to separate feeling and thinking)

Advise against causing defensive responses in others

Advise against emphasizing past problems caused by another

Explain the need for realistic expectations of others

Explain that undesirable thoughts and feelings are normal (even when about one's spouse)

Emphasize the importance of recognizing tension within oneself (and dealing with it in the early stages)

Advise against communicating double-meaning messages (messages that convey two conflicting feelings and that confuse the person receiving the message)

Explain the dysfunctional family system of fixed triangles (which consists of using three people, two people and a group, or two people and an issue as a triangle in which the third party or issue is used as a fixed scapegoat for reducing the tensions of the other two people; persons can then avoid the uncomfortable emotion that is really troubling them as long as they focus on the third part of the triangle, for example, two parents focus on the misbehavior of a child in order to avoid their own personal conflict)

Teach how to detriangle dysfunctional fixed triangles (at least one person in the triangle needs to identify his emotional responses to the second party and the behavior of the second party causing the emotional response, since by changing their emotional responses the triangle system will be interrupted)

Inform the spouses of the need for both emotional closeness and separateness (each person needs to feel close to others, yet remain a separate individual)

Explain that change must come from within the person (change does not occur by attempting to change others)

Recommend that behavioral limits be set (on such issues as authority, expectations of significant others)

Explain that one's rank and sex among siblings affects how one interrelates (a person often relates to a spouse as one related to siblings during childhood)

Advise that significant persons express acceptance of one another, that significant persons express caring for one another

Explain the importance of persons offering emotional support to one another (at all times, but especially during crisis)

Advise early correction of problems

Teach how to use the problem-solving method (for making decisions with a minimum of conflict)

Explain the importance of learning and practicing health principles (in personal interaction)

EVALUATION

Record actual outcome

TROUBLED, DOMINATED FAMILY[293,408,471,682,775]

ASSESSMENT

Data Collection

Subjective Data
• Family members relate attitudes and behavior such as the following:

Power
The family is controlled and dominated by one powerful spouse who is the final authority on all matters

One spouse is dominant, the other is submissive

Power is the primary focus of the relationship

Intimacy
In this relationship, the spouses share little intimacy because the dominant spouse cannot tolerate the vulnerability associated with intimacy; the submissive spouse often seeks an intimate relationship with another family member, such as a child, parent, etc.

Emotional Aspects
Family members relate that it is dangerous to express one's feelings around the dominant spouse

Family members are either withdrawn and shy, impulsive and rebellious, or depressed and fearful

When there is open emotional conflict, there is much emotional pain and strife

The dominant spouse often lacks emotional control

There is often at least one mentally ill person in the family

Basic Family Mood
Family members are cautious not to arouse the anger of the dominant spouse; they feel controlled and insecure

Personal Growth of Family Members
The effect of the dominant spouse causes individual family members to avoid assuming responsibility
Autonomy is difficult for other family members to achieve
Differences in family members are discouraged

Socialization
The dominant spouse controls the amount and kinds of family socialization

Problem Solving
Problem solving is solely the prerogative of the dominant spouse, who portrays himself as an expert in all areas of life

Sexual Relations
The dominant spouse controls the sexual relatedness of the couple; if the other spouse enjoys the submissive role, there may be satisfaction in the relationship

Stress Management
The family does not deal well with change, and especially loss
The family is under daily stress and tension
Family members lack confidence in their ability to deal with stress because of being controlled

Objective Data
• Family members are involved in activities and practices such as the following:

Roles and Tasks
The dominant spouse delegates all roles and tasks

Child Rearing
Child rearing is rigid, frequently with unrealistic expectations of the children for their age and developmental phase

Family Value System
The family rules are rigid and enforced by the dominant person who has set up an authoritarian value system; the dominant person makes the rules and punishes those who deviate from them

Communications
The dominant spouse communicates clearly
There is little negotiation with other family members
Differences of opinion are perceived by the dominant spouse to be a cue for arguing
Fear of the anger of the dominant spouse causes other family members to project blame or find a scapegoat
Spontaneous communication is lacking

Physical Needs
The physical needs of the family may or may not be met

Environment
The family environment may or may not be in accordance with accepted health standards

Community Involvement
The family may or may not be involved in community activities

Data Analysis

Nursing Diagnosis
TROUBLED, DOMINATED FAMILY: A family that is controlled by one very powerful spouse

Common Etiology (Stressors)
PSYCHOSOCIAL FACTORS: Unlearned alternative behavior, lack of competency in using effec-

tive coping mechanisms, the presence of reinforcing stimuli that maintain maladaptive behavior, exposure to a role model who practiced poor coping skills

PLANNING
Unmet Needs
Protection from psychologic threat, psychologic stability, love and affection, caring and communicating relationships, family growth and maturity, increased learning, increased reality perception and problem-solving ability

Expected Outcome
Family members will learn and practice the principles of a well family
Family members will exhibit the behaviors of a well family

NURSING INTERVENTIONS
Nursing Treatments
Approach unhurriedly

Demonstrate calmness

Provide an atmosphere of acceptance (of each person, but not of the dysfunctional behavior)

Relate to the family on an adult–adult level, not on a parent–child level

Listen attentively (to all sides of the issue)

Talk with the family members (either separately, in twos, or as a group, depending on the situation)

Explore with the person (the spouse) the need to control (Why does the dominating person feel he has to rigidly control others? What are his insecurities, his fears? Is he mimicking a role model? etc.)

Encourage the expression of feelings (of all family members, and support verbal interaction between members without participating in the interaction)

Ask for specifics, not generalizations, about the problem (obtain descriptions of behavior rather than feelings)

Offer feedback to the family's expressed feelings

Explore with the family members the reasons for recurring problems

Explore with the family members the effects of one's behavior on others (dominating behavior prevents the autonomy of others, whereas submissive behavior encourages dominant behavior)

Encourage respect for the rights of others

Encourage participation in therapeutic group interaction (family therapy with just the involved family members or multiple family therapy in which several families share their problems and solutions)

Encourage role playing to develop sensitivity (among family members, but especially of the dominant spouse)

Ignore undesirable behavior
OR

Set limits on unacceptable behavior (behavioral boundaries among family members must be clearly defined)

Clearly communicate what is expected of each family member

Hold the person (each family member) responsible for his behavior (do not allow one person to blame another)

Encourage family-shared responsibility (for specific family tasks, and do not allow the dominant person to keep others dependent)

Refrain from arguing, from negatively criticizing

Explore with the family its strengths and resources

Make a referral (to a psychiatric nurse specialist, psychologist, etc.)

Nursing Observations
Identify the appropriate use of defense mechanisms (such as open communications, freedom to alternate emotional closeness and distancing to support the separateness of the self, individual autonomy in a family, allowing each member to achieve personal growth)

Identify the inappropriate use of defense mechanisms (point out dysfunctional coping methods such as overcontrolling family members, reacting emotionally rather than intellectually)

Determine the degree of insight that the family members have (into their disturbed interaction)

Determine the precipitating factors (and assist family members to identify that which triggers the dominating behavior)

Identify potentially destructive behavior (between family members)

Identify life values significant to family members (have the individuals, especially spouses, identify their values and the source of their values, including an exploration of the values of past generations in a family and their effect on the current generation)

Observe for behavior modification (between family members)

Health Teaching

Explain how emotional responses occur (the person perceives a situation in terms of its significance to him, an emotional response is experienced and physiologic changes accompany the response)

Explain how thinking occurs (information is perceived, which is then interpreted on the basis of language skills, sensory-motor development, remembering, reasoning, imaging, and evaluation, then compare the emotional and thought processes, encourage family members to separate feeling and thinking, explain that family members should be able to discuss issues of conflict with intelligent rather than controlling responses)

Advise against causing defensive responses in others

Advise against emphasizing past problems caused by another

Explain the need for realistic expectations of others

Advise against verbally comparing significant others

Explain that undesirable thoughts and feelings are normal (even when about family members)

Emphasize the importance of recognizing tension within family members (and effectively dealing with it in the early stages)

Advise against communicating double-meaning messages (messages that convey two conflicting feelings and confuse the person receiving the message)

Explain about the unique personality of each individual (in the family, and explain that difference should be encouraged, not discouraged, in a family)

Inform family members of the need for both emotional closeness and separateness (each person needs to feel close to others, yet remain a separate individual)

Explain that change must come from within the person or family (in order to change the dominant situation, each family member must change his behavioral response so as not to reinforce the dominant behavior)

Recommend that behavioral limits be set (for the dominant spouse)

Explain that one's rank and sex among siblings affects how one interrelates (a person often relates to a spouse as one related to siblings during childhood)

Advise that significant persons express acceptance of one another, that significant persons express caring for one another

Explain the importance of persons offering emotional support to one another (at all times, but especially during crisis)

Explain the need for family restructuring during developmental stages (families restructure as the composition of family members change, and behavior aimed at preventing or controlling change can result in severe family strife)

Advise early correction of (family) problems

Teach how to use the problem-solving method (for making family decisions with a minimum of conflict)

Explain the importance of learning and practicing health principles (in family interaction)

EVALUATION

Record actual outcome

TROUBLED, CONFLICTED FAMILY[293,408,471,682,775]

ASSESSMENT

Data Collection

Subjective Data

• Family members relate attitudes and behavior such as the following:

Power

The spouses relate being in a constant struggle to control each other

They relate that their relationship is intensely competitive

Intimacy

The spouses do not share or disclose their most private thoughts and feelings with one
another

Emotional Aspects

The spouses openly express their anger with each other; feelings of love and caring are
not expressed

Each spouse seeks allies such as friends or family members, especially their children

The family has difficulty coping with loss, since loss forces them to deal with guilt feelings

May relate having children with childhood behavior disorders or adulthood depression

Basic Family Mood

The basic mood in the family is one of high tension and constant warfare; there is emotional caution and distance

Personal Growth of Family Members

Family members are not encouraged to accept responsibility for their behavior

Despite the conflict, the children are often self-directed

The children become involved in parental conflicts that inhibit the child's achievement
of developmental tasks

Socialization

A child may relate involvement in drug or alcohol abuse, antisocial behavior, etc., as an
expression of anger at the conflicting parents

Problem Solving

The spouses have poor problem-solving skills because of their inability to negotiate

They are unable to decide which of the two will make the necessary decisions

Family members often use distancing to solve problems

Sexual Relations

Since there is little intimacy, sexual satisfaction may be sought in extramarital affairs

Stress Management

The family is in a constant state of stress

During times of crisis, one spouse may use the crisis as a weapon against the other

Objective Data

• Family members are involved in activities and practices such as the following:

Roles and Tasks

The parents are unable to provide a role model of intimate relatedness for their children

Child Rearing

Children become caught up in their parents' attacking behavior; the children often take
sides

OR

Alternately take sides with a different parent

There may be little or no disciplinary control of the children because of the parents'
preoccupation with their own conflict

Family Value System

The primary family value is to win, and this end may justify the means

The spouses are unable to set consistent rules for the family because of their inability to agree

Communications

The spouses communicate clearly and spontaneously but do so in an attacking manner

Communications are used to acquire weapons for further verbal attacks

There is frequent projection of blame on others

Physical Needs

The family's physical needs may or may not be met

Environment

The family environment may or may not be in accordance with accepted health standards

Community Involvement

The family may or may not be involved in community activities

Data Analysis

Nursing Diagnosis

TROUBLED, CONFLICTED FAMILY: A family in which both spouses are engaged in a competitive struggle to control each other

Common Etiology (Stressors)

PSYCHOSOCIAL FACTORS: Unlearned alternative behavior, lack of competency in using effective coping mechanisms, the presence of reinforcing stimuli that maintain maladaptive behavior, exposure to a role model who practiced poor coping skills

PLANNING

Unmet Needs

Protection from psychologic threat, psychologic stability, love and affection, caring and communicating relationships, family growth and maturity, increased learning, increased reality perception and problem-solving ability

Expected Outcome

Family members will learn and practice the principles of a well family

Family members will exhibit the behaviors of a well family

NURSING INTERVENTIONS

Nursing Treatments

Approach unhurriedly

Demonstrate calmness

Provide an atmosphere of acceptance (of each person, but not of the dysfunctional behavior)

Relate to the spouses on an adult–adult level, not on a parent–child level

Listen attentively (to all sides of the issue)

Talk with the family members (either separately, in twos or a group, depending on the situation)

Encourage the expression of feelings (of all family members, and support verbal interaction between members without participating in the interaction)

Ask for specifics, not generalizations, about the problem (obtain descriptions of behavior rather than feelings)

Offer feedback to the person's expressed feelings

Explore with the spouses the reasons for recurring problems

Explore with the spouses the effects of their behavior on others (attacking behavior causes high tension levels in the family, serves as a poor role model, fails to resolve problems)

Encourage respect for the rights of others

Encourage participation in therapeutic group interaction (family therapy with just the involved family members, or multiple family therapy in which several families share their problems and solutions)

Encourage role playing to develop sensitivity of the spouses to each other

Ignore undesirable behavior

OR

Set limits on unacceptable behavior (behavioral boundaries between the spouses must be clearly defined)

Clearly communicate what is expected of each family member

Hold the person (each family member) responsible for his behavior (do not allow one person to blame another)

Refrain from arguing, from negatively criticizing

Explore with the family its strengths and resources

Make a referral (to a psychiatric nurse specialist, psychologist, etc.)

Nursing Observations

Identify the appropriate use of defense mechanisms (such as open communications, freedom to alternate emotional closeness and distancing to support the separateness of the self, individual autonomy in the family, allowing each member to achieve personal growth, gaining family emotional support from the extended family)

Identify the inappropriate use of defense mechanisms (point out dysfunctional coping methods such as aggressive behavior, the use of fixed triangles, reacting emotionally rather than intellectually)

Determine the degree of insight the family members have (into the disturbed interaction)

Determine the precipitating factors (and assist the spouses to identify what triggers their attacking behavior)

Identify life values significant to the spouses (have the spouses identify their values and the sources of their values, including an exploration of the values of past generations in a family and their effect on the current generation)

Observe for behavior modification (between family members)

Health Teaching

Explain how emotional responses occur (the person perceives a situation in terms of its significance to him, an emotional response is experienced and physiologic changes accompany the response)

Explain how thinking occurs (information is perceived and is then interpreted on the basis of language skills, sensory-motor development, remembering, reasoning, imagining, and evaluation; then compare the emotional and thought processes, encourage family members to separate feeling and thinking, explain that family members should be able to discuss issues of conflict with intelligent rather than assaultive responses)

Advise against causing defensive responses in others

Advise against emphasizing past problems caused by another

Explain the need for realistic expectations of others

Advise against verbally comparing significant others

Explain that undesirable thoughts and feelings are normal (even when about family members)

Emphasize the importance of recognizing tension within family members (and dealing with it in the early stages)

Advise against communicating double-meaning messages (messages that convey two conflicting feelings and confuse the person receiving the message)

Explain the dysfunctional family system of fixed triangles (which consists of using three people, two people and a group, or two people and an issue as a triangle in which the third party or issue is used as a fixed scapegoat for reducing the tensions of the other two people; persons can then avoid the uncomfortable emotion that is really troubling them as long as they focus on the third part of the triangle, for example, two spouses focus on the issue of family finances in order to avoid feelings that are the basis of their conflict)

Teach how to detriangle dysfunctional fixed triangles (at least one person in the triangle needs to identify his emotional responses to the second party and the behavior of the second party causing the emotional response, since by changing their emotional responses the triangle system will be interrupted)

Explain about the unique personality of each individual (in the family and that difference should be encouraged, not discouraged, in a family)

Inform family members of the need for both emotional closeness and separateness (each person needs to feel close to others, yet remain a separate individual)

Explain that change must come from within the person or family (change does not occur by attempting to change one's spouse)

Recommend that behavioral limits be set (for each spouse on such issues as authority, expectations of significant others, interference from parents or extended family, specific individual tasks)

Explain that one's rank and sex among siblings affects how one interrelates (a person often relates to a spouse as one related to siblings during childhood)

Explain how to keep a positive, emotional family relationship (remembrances of special occasions, maintaining emotional control, avoiding emotional triangles)

Advise that significant persons express acceptance of one another, that significant persons express caring for one another

Explain the importance of persons offering emotional support to one another (at all times, but especially during crisis)

Advise early correction of (family) problems

Teach how to use the problem-solving method (for making family decisions with a minimum of conflict)

Explain the importance of learning and practicing health principles (in family interaction)

EVALUATION

Record actual outcome

TROUBLED, CHAOTIC FAMILY[293,408,471,682,775]

ASSESSMENT

Data Collection

Subjective Data
• Family members relate attitudes and behavior such as the following:

Power
No one in the family has adequate power to lead an organized, structured family group

Intimacy
The spouses are excessively fused together
  OR
The spouses cling to each other but experience a deep sense of emptiness
Excessively strong ties may exist with the spouses' parents

Emotional Aspects
Emotions are often denied
Everyone in the family is expected to have the same emotional responses to a situation
Family members do not provide emotional support during a crisis
Family members have difficulty coping with change because they refuse to recognize that change has occurred
May have one or more family member who is emotionally disturbed (severely)

Basic Family Mood
The basic family mood is one of despair and hopelessness

Personal Growth of Family Members
The family discourages efforts toward individuality, independence, or self-direction
Family members refuse to accept change that could lead to personal growth

Socialization
Family members seldom, if ever, socialize outside the family

Problem Solving
Family problems are not dealt with; they are either denied or ignored
Family members do not face reality and reinforce distortions of reality
The family fails to plan ahead for foreseeable difficulties

Sexual Relations
Sexual relations may enhance the feeling of fusion between the spouses

Stress Management
Family members do not effectively cope with stress because they refuse to recognize the existence of the stressful situation

Objective Data
• Family members are involved in activities and practices such as the following.

Roles and Tasks
Children are exposed to emotionally unhealthy parental role models
Family members do not use constructive, task-oriented behavior

Child Rearing
Children are not encouraged to demonstrate growing-up behavior because this would require a change within the family

Family Value System
The family primarily values the excessive fusion of its members
All family members must adhere to the family value system

Communications
Family members often disregard each other during communications
A family may develop its own language and nonfamily members may find it difficult to understand them
Family members are expected to have the same opinions

Physical Needs
Family members often have severe, chronic illnessess

Environment
The environment may or may not be in accordance with accepted health standards

Community Involvement
The family is not involved in community affairs

Data Analysis

Nursing Diagnosis
TROUBLED, CHAOTIC FAMILY: A family that is severely disorganized and isolated

Common Etiology (Stressors)
PSYCHOSOCIAL FACTORS: Unlearned alternative behavior, lack of competency in using effective coping mechanisms, the presence of reinforcing stimuli that maintain maladaptive behavior, exposure to a role model who practiced poor coping skills

PLANNING

Unmet Needs
Protection from psychologic threat, psychologic stability, love and affection, caring and communicating relationships, family growth and maturity, increased learning, increased reality perception and problem-solving ability

Expected Outcome

Family members will learn and practice the principles of a well family
Family members will exhibit the behaviors of a well family

NURSING INTERVENTIONS

Nursing Treatments

Approach unhurriedly
Demonstrate calmness
Provide an atmosphere of acceptance (of each person but not of the dysfunctional behavior)
Relate to the family on an adult–adult level, not on a parent–child level
Talk with the family members (either separately, in twos, or in a group, depending on the situation)
Encourage the expression of feelings (of all family members, and support verbal interaction between members without participating in the interaction)
Ask for specifics, not generalizations, about the problem (obtain descriptions of behavior rather than feelings)
Offer feedback to the person's expressed feelings
Explore with the family members the reasons for recurring problems
Explore with the family members the effects of the spouses' behavior on others (excessive fusing prevents normal growth and development of all family members, isolation from the outside world limits family's resources)
Encourage participation in therapeutic group interaction (family therapy with just the involved family members, or multiple family therapy in which several families share their problems and solutions)
Ignore undesirable behavior
OR
Set limits on unacceptable behavior (behavioral boundaries among family members must be clearly defined)
Clearly communicate what is expected of each family member
Hold each family member responsible for his behavior (do not allow one person to blame another)
Encourage family-shared responsibility (for specific family tasks)
Explore with the family its strengths and resources
Make a referral (to a psychiatric nurse specialist or psychologist, etc.)

Nursing Observations

Identify the appropriate use of defense mechanisms (such as open communications, freedom to alternate emotional closeness and distancing to support the separateness of the self, individual autonomy in the family, allowing each member to achieve personal growth)
Identify the inappropriate use of defense mechanisms (point out isolation from others, excessive family fusion, etc.)
Determine the degree of insight that the spouses have (into the disturbed family interaction)
Determine the precipitating factors (and assist family members to identify what triggers abnormal behavior)
Identify life values significant to family members (have the individuals, especially spouses, identify their values and the sources of their values; this includes exploring the values of past generations in a family and their effect on the current generation)
Observe for behavior modification (between family members)

Health Teaching

Explain how emotional responses occur (the person perceives a situation in terms of its significance to him, an emotional response is experienced and physiologic changes accompany the response)
Explain how thinking occurs (information is perceived and is then interpreted on the

basis of language skills, sensory-motor development, remembering, reasoning, imaging, and evaluation, then compare the emotional and thought processes, encourage family members to separate feeling and thinking, explain that family members should be able to discuss issues of conflict with intelligent, rather than assaultive, responses)

Emphasize the importance of recognizing tension within family members (and dealing with it in the early stages)

Advise against communicating double-meaning messages (messages that convey two conflicting feelings and confuse the person receiving the message)

Explain about the unique personality of each individual (in the family and that differences should be encouraged, not discouraged, in a family)

Inform family members of the need for both emotional closeness and separateness (each person needs to feel close to others, yet remain a separate individual)

Explain that change must come from within the person or family (change does not occur by attempting to change others)

Recommend that behavioral limits be set (on such family issues as authority, expectations of significant others, interference from parents or extended family, specific individual tasks, etc.)

Explain that one's rank and sex among siblings affects how one interrelates (a person often relates to a spouse as he related to siblings during childhood)

Advise that significant persons express acceptance of one another, express caring for one another

Explain the importance of persons offering emotional support to one another (at all times, but especially during crisis)

Explain the need for family restructuring during developmental stages (families restructure as the composition of family members change, as tasks change, etc.)

Advise early correction of (family) problems

Teach how to use the problem-solving method (for making family decisions with a minimum of conflict)

Explain the importance of learning and practicing health principles (in family interaction)

EVALUATION

Record actual outcome

Knowledge Deficits Associated with Psychosocial Problems

UNKNOWLEDGEABLE ABOUT COPING WITH THE MENTALLY ILL[46,118,199,586,591]

ASSESSMENT

Data Collection

Subjective Data
- Person's discussion or questions indicate a need for additional information, clarification, or validation of information
  OR
- Person's lack of questions or comments indicates not wanting information or not knowing enough to seek information
- When questioned directly, the person's response or lack of response indicates that he does not know:

How to help the mentally ill person
Where to obtain health assistance for the mentally ill

Objective Data
• May exhibit behavior such as acting inappropriately toward the mentally ill based on insufficient knowledge and not taking precautions against combative or suicidal behavior
May treat the person as a child, placing him in an excessively dependent role
May argue with the person and/or make disparaging remarks about his behavior
May verbally reject the person rather than the undesirable behavior

Data Analysis

Nursing Diagnosis
UNKNOWLEDGEABLE ABOUT COPING WITH THE MENTALLY ILL: Being without sufficient information about how to approach and help persons who are mentally ill

Common Etiology (Stressors)
HEALTH CARE FACTORS: Lack of health instruction

PLANNING

Unmet Needs
Comfort, protection from psychologic threat, independence, increased learning

Expected Outcome
Correct verbal feedback of the information taught
Person relates having successfully coped with the mentally ill person

NURSING INTERVENTIONS

Nursing Treatments
Approach unhurriedly
Reassure verbally
Encourage the person to ask questions
Provide reliable information
Make a referral (to agencies that specialize in specific mental health problems, to a psychiatric nurse specialist, psychiatrist, psychologist)

Nursing Observations
Determine teaching effectiveness by testing or verbal feedback

Health Teaching
Advise early correction of (behavior) problems
Advise against causing defensive responses (in the mentally ill)
Advise against communicating double-meaning messages (messages that are unclear or that relate opposing emotions such as "You're a good driver, but you can't take the car while it's raining")
Advise against emphasizing past problems caused by another (being reminded of past mistakes causes defensive behavior)
Advise against verbally comparing significant others (comparing one person to another promotes feelings of inadequacy)
Advise that highly emotional suituations be avoided (until the mental illness is stabilized)
Advise that significant persons express acceptance of one another
Advise that significant persons express caring for one another
Explain the importance of persons offering emotional support (positive reinforcement) to one another
Explain that ill persons are often hypersensitive (especially mentally ill persons)
Explain that the behavior of one family member is not a reflection on other family members
Explain that undesirable thoughts and feelings are normal (and not necessarily a sign of mental illness)

Explain the importance of remaining calm (since it reduces inner tension and supports maximum functioning ability)

Explain that persons must make adjustments at their own pace

Explain the need for realistic expectations of others

Recommend that behavioral limits be set

Explain how to set behavioral limits (by clearly stating what constitutes acceptable and unacceptable behavior)

Describe those symptoms that should be reported (combative behavior, loss of emotional control, inability to maintain daily function)

Relate the criteria for determining mental illness (behavioral changes such as severe depression, confusion, hearing voices, seeing visions, complaints of unverifiable pain, abuse of others or self)

Relate the accepted criteria for commitment of the mentally ill (when the person is in danger of harming himself or others; or when unable to maintain daily functions)

EVALUATION

Record actual outcome

UNKNOWLEDGEABLE ABOUT MENTAL HEALTH PRINCIPLES[52,118,372,405,587,727]

ASSESSMENT

Data Collection

Subjective Data

• Person's discussion or questions indicate a need for additional information, clarification, or validation of information

  OR

• Person's lack of questions or comments indicates not wanting information or not knowing enough to seek information

• When questioned directly, the person's response or lack of response indicates that he does not know:

  Signs of good mental health

  How to improve a basically healthy mental status

  How to foster mental health in others

Objective Data

• May exhibit behavior such as not channeling emotional energy into constructive activities but using destructive methods, seldom including recreation in his lifestyle or placing excessive value on winning in recreational games, inconsistent or inappropriate behavioral approaches in meeting the other person's (especially a child's) needs

Data Analysis

Nursing Diagnosis

UNKNOWLEDGEABLE ABOUT MENTAL HEALTH PRINCIPLES: Being without sufficient information about sound principles and their appropriate use in maintaining mental health

Common Etiology (Stressors)

HEALTH CARE FACTORS: Lack of health instruction

PLANNING

Unmet Needs

Comfort, protection from psychologic threat, independence, increased learning

Expected Outcome

Correct verbal feedback of the information taught

Person relates the practice of mental health principles

NURSING INTERVENTIONS

Nursing Treatments
Approach unhurriedly
Reassure verbally
Encourage the person to ask questions
Provide reliable information

Nursing Observations
Determine teaching effectiveness by testing or verbal feedback

Health Teaching
Describe the behavior patterns indicating mental health (explain that emotional maturity is reflected by many factors as suggested by the Mental Health Association. *The person feels comfortable and good about himself*: The person is not overcome by his emotions, is able to accept disappointments and personal shortcomings, is able to laugh at himself, neither under- or overestimates his abilities, feels comfortable when alone, has respect for himself, enjoys everyday pleasures, is able to commit himself to philosophical views and consistent values that give life purpose and direction. *The person feels good about other people*: The person is able to give to others without expecting gain, feels entitled to and able to accept love from others, is able to establish close emotional ties and still remain independent, expects to like and trust others and have others like and trust him, is able to respect the differences in people, does not attempt to control others or allow oneself to be controlled, the person feels he is part of a group, feels a sense of responsibility to others, is able to work harmoniously with others. *The person feels able to meet life's demands*: The person feels capable of dealing with most situations, is able to make undelayed independent decisions, is sufficiently objective about life to find humor in difficult situations, welcomes new ideas and experiences, sets realistic goals, uses his natural abilities, does his best in all efforts and gains satisfaction from doing and accomplishing)
Advise that significant persons express acceptance of one another (feeling accepted promotes positive self-attitudes)
Advise that significant persons express caring for one another
Explain the importance of persons offering emotional support to one another (positive reinforcement from others supports positive behavior)
Explain the need for realistic expectations of others (realistic expectations support positive achievement and personal growth, and when expectations are unachievable feelings of failure result)
Explain the importance of maintaining a positive self-attitude (positive attitudes foster positive behavior)
Explain that parental attitudes affect child development
Explain that recreation aids total health, supports personal growth, and is not an escape mechanism (recreation provides a change from the stress of work and responsibility, enriches and develops the personality)
Explain that undesirable thoughts and feelings are normal (in mentally well persons)
Emphasize the importance of planning and anticipating future activities (looking forward to an event provides a positive approach to the future and the predictable world needed for mental health)
Explain the need to predict and plan for change (which gives the person a healthy control of his life)
Explain how to channel emotional energy and obtain release from stress (through sports, creative activities, and work, all of which can bring satisfaction)
Teach how to use the problem-solving method (for effective coping with resulting mental health)

EVALUATION
Record actual outcome

UNKNOWLEDGEABLE ABOUT CHILD SOCIALIZATION/DISCIPLINE[94,313,762]

ASSESSMENT

Data Collection

Subjective Data
• Person's discussion or questions indicate a need for additional information, clarification, or validation of information
  OR
• Person's lack of questions or comments indicates not wanting information or not knowing enough to seek information
• When questioned directly, the person's response or lack of response indicates that he does not know:
  How to guide a child
  How to correctly provide discipline
  How to cope with a child who responds differently than most children

Objective Data
• May exhibit behavior such as acting inappropriately based on insufficient knowledge, using disciplined action or allowing liberties inappropriate to the child's age
  May be inconsistent in disciplining and/or reward action
  May use fear-creating or humiliating approaches to control the child's behavior

Data Analysis

Nursing Diagnosis
UNKNOWLEDGEABLE ABOUT CHILD SOCIALIZATION/DISCIPLINE: Being without sufficient information about the correct methods to use in providing for the social development of a young person

Common Etiology (Stressors)
HEALTH CARE FACTORS: Lack of health instruction

PLANNING

Unmet Needs
Comfort, protection from psychologic threat, independence, increased learning

Expected Outcome
Correct verbal feedback of the information taught
Person relates success with child socialization

NURSING INTERVENTIONS

Nursing Treatments
Approach unhurriedly
Reassure verbally
Encourage the person to ask questions
Provide reliable information

Nursing Observations
Determine teaching effectiveness by testing or verbal feedback

Health Teaching
Advise early correction of problems (with child socialization)
Advise against verbally comparing significant others (comparing a child with siblings or peers promotes feelings of inadequacy)
Emphasize that children need guidance (children need and want guidance because of their lack of experience and poorly developed judgment)
Explain that parental attitudes affect child development (parental attitudes affect the child's perception of himself and his world)
Advise that discipline be consistent (predictable discipline promotes consistent behavior)

Inform that bribing and threatening are ineffective child discipline methods (bribing causes the child to expect rewards for normal behavior, threatening arouses child hostility)

Inform that isolation, loss of treat, and restriction are effective child discipline methods (the loss of pleasure and the need to compensate for misbehavior cause the child to realize the value of acceptable behavior)

Recommend that independence be encouraged (since it increases the child's sense of adequacy)

Relate the criteria for successful child rearing (frequent physical contact with the child; constant exposure of the child to some form of positive reinforcement; discipline based on informing the child of what is and is not acceptable and pleasing; punishment that is dealt at the time of the unacceptable behavior, that is appropriate to the child's age, that does not inflict physical harm, and that is consistent; there should be a gradual lessening of adult restraint with greater assumption of behavior control and responsibility by the child)

EVALUATION

Record actual outcome

UNKNOWLEDGEABLE ABOUT SEXUALITY[262,348]

ASSESSMENT
Data Collection
Subjective Data
- Person's discussion or questions indicate a need for additional information, clarification, or validation of information
  OR
- Person's lack of questions or comments indicates not wanting information or not knowing enough to seek information

When questioned directly, the person's response or lack of response indicates that he does not know:

About the anatomy and physiology involved in sexuality

About normal sexual tensions and responses

Of the methods for engaging in sexual activity

That sexuality is but one part of human development

About stereotyped sexual roles

Whether myths about sex are factual

Whether sexual thoughts and fantasies are normal or abnormal

Objective Data
- May exhibit behavior such as:
  Excessive modesty during examination or treatment procedures requiring exposure of breasts or genitalia
  Nervousness, restlessness, or irritability when sexual discussions are brought up
  Possessing pornographic or erotic materials to gain information

Data Analysis
Nursing Diagnosis
UNKNOWLEDGEABLE ABOUT SEXUALITY: Being without sufficient information about the factors associated with being male or female

Common Etiology (Stressors)
HEALTH CARE FACTORS: Lack of health instruction

PLANNING

Unmet Needs

Comfort, protection from physical harm and psychologic threat, independence, increased reality perception, increased learning

Expected Outcome

Correct verbal feedback of the information taught

Person relates increased comfort with and growth in sexuality

NURSING INTERVENTIONS

Nursing Treatments

Approach unhurriedly

Reassure verbally

Encourage the person to ask questions

Provide reliable information (about sexual myths and stereotyped roles)

Nursing Observations

Determine teaching effectiveness by testing or verbal feedback

Health Teaching

Explain the physical changes that occur during periods of growth and development (and their effect on our sexuality)

Explain about normal sexual tensions (onset in adolescence, an inner stirring and attraction to the opposite sex, sexual tensions prevail throughout life, and that sexual satisfaction is as essential as eating, sleeping, etc., and that sexual fantasies are normal in adolescence)

Relate that sexual response normally varies (according to one's mood, level of fatigue, life situations, or activities, and emphasize that sexual response cannot always be at a high level)

Explain that relaxation is essential for a successful sexual response

Recommend alternative approaches to sexual activity (such as different precoital activities, coital positioning)

Explain that pregnancy can result from sexual activity

Explain that sexual activity is not always an expression of intimacy (but can be an expression of anger, anxiety, or conflict)

Explain that sexuality is but one part of human development (that while the media may portray sexuality as the primary life focus, human development involves the tasks of daily living, intellectual pursuits, goal seeking, nonsexual pleasures, etc.)

Relate the criteria for a successful sexual response (if the person experiences satisfaction, completeness, euphoria or contentment the experience is considered successful)

EVALUATION

Record actual outcome

UNKNOWLEDGEABLE ABOUT STRESS MANAGEMENT[141,380,487]

ASSESSMENT

Data Collection

Subjective Data

• Person's discussion or questions indicate a need for additional information, clarification, or validation of information

OR

- Person's lack of questions or comments indicates not wanting information or not knowing enough to seek information
- When questioned directly, the person's response or lack of response indicates that he does not know:
  How to recognize stress
  How to control or avoid excessively stressful situations
  How to cope effectively with stress

Objective Data
- May exhibit behavior based on insufficient knowledge, such as not taking precautions against excessive stress, not planning for change, being involved in too many stressful activities at one time
  May exhibit signs that indicate excessive stress or poor coping with stress such as nervousness, irritability, cries easily, easily startled by sound, adamant resistance to change

Data Analysis

Nursing Diagnosis
UNKNOWLEDGEABLE ABOUT STRESS MANAGEMENT: Being without sufficient information about methods used for reducing and coping with stress

Common Etiology (Stressors)
HEALTH CARE FACTORS: Lack of health instruction

PLANNING

Unmet Needs
Comfort, protection from physical harm and psychologic threat, independence, increased learning

Expected Outcome
Correct verbal feedback of the information taught
Person relates reduced feelings of tension and increased comfort in dealing with stress

NURSING INTERVENTIONS

Nursing Treatments
Approach unhurriedly
Reassure verbally
Encourage the person to ask questions
Provide reliable information
Encourage the expression of feelings (talking about one's problems reduces stress)

Nursing Observations
Determine teaching effectiveness by testing or verbal feedback

Health Teaching
Teach the specific methods (for stress management)
Recommend that the person adhere to the basic principles of stress management:
  Obtain adequate sleep each night since sufficient rest is essential to reduce stress and to provide energy for coping with stress
  Maintain a balanced nutritional diet since a poorly nourished body is under stress and good nutrition provides energy for coping
  Participate consistently in moderate physical exercise at least three times a week since exercise relieves tension
  Restructure lifestyle so that the stress of the daily routine is reduced or minimized and, if boredom is the source of stress, engage in a more active lifestyle to reduce the stress
  Accept own limitations since trying to be perfect predisposes a person to the stress of failure as perfection is impossible to achieve
  Accept the limitations of others since expecting perfection from others increases tension through frustration

Avoid setting time limits whenever possible since time limits result in hurrying, hence tension

Set both short- and long-term goals since short-term goals bring immediate satisfaction and reduce the stress of frustration encountered in long-term goals

Engage primarily in noncompetitive activities since exposure to constant competition increases tension

Recognize that some tension is normal and is needed to motivate us to activity

Be aware of highly stressful situations and do whatever possible to alter the situation's potential for tension

Recognize when tension is beginning to build up and cope with the tension in the early stages before it becomes overwhelming by removing yourself from the scene for a few moments or counting slowly to 20 or washing your face with cool water to regain equilibrium

Avoid staying constantly "stirred up" over routine things and save your energy for coping with real crises

Remain calm since calmness reduces inner stress and diminishes the stress we place on other persons and approach each task in a calm organized manner

Adhere to a pace of living with which you are comfortable and do not allow others to set your pace of living; avoid accepting tasks that increase stress to an uncomfortable level

Pursue only one activity at a time since stress levels can be controlled by performing one task at a time and attempting multiple tasks increases the demand for human energy

Predict and plan for change since having control over a situation reduces stress, and whenever possible prevent multiple simultaneous changes such as having a baby and moving to a new city

Plan and anticipate future pleasurable activities since looking forward to pleasurable events reduces stress through an awareness that a current stress will soon end

Gradually master difficult situations by setting priorities and doing one thing each day and recognize that "everything" does not have to be done today since gradual accomplishment reduces tension

Avoid making decisions when under severe stress since decision making is an added stress and wise decisions are best made in a calm objective climate

Take occasional respite from responsibility as a temporary tension-reducing measure

Avoid unpleasant stress-inducing conversations by focusing on subjects that require adaptive energy, and do not allow others to draw you into unpleasant conversation or arguments that deplete your energy reserves

Include recreation in the daily routine not as a form of escape but because recreation aids total health while supporting personal growth and reestablishing psychological balance

Use methods for achieving total relaxation such as listening to soft music, doing nothing, and engaging in deep-breathing exercises, biofeedback, and meditation

Use methods for reducing sensory stimulation such as subduing the room lighting, turning off radios and televisions, staying away from crowds, being employed in a small office, living in a small community, traveling to familiar places, taking traffic routes that are less traveled, shopping during the quiet hours, visiting quiet places such as churches, art museums, the oceanside

Recognize that fatigue is a primary stress factor, and remember to take intermittent breaks from stressful endeavors and not to work harder and longer when fatigued in order to complete a task as this only increases the level of stress

Take a mental health day when tension begins to build up or just to engage in sound health practices and spend one day doing what pleases you

Channel emotional energy constructively and release anger, disappointment and anxiety by running, swimming, cleaning out closets, hitting a pillow, ball, or punching bag, laughing, talking things over, writing a letter of complaint but not mailing it, verbalizing one's anger into a tape recorder and then erasing the tape,

becoming involved in hobbies such as sewing, painting, wood chopping, and doing something pleasant such as seeing a comic movie or strolling through a garden

When problems seem insurmountable become involved in helping others since this
activity serves to distract from worrying about yourself and helps you feel good
about yourself

Avoid self-defeating thoughts such as belittling oneself for nonaccomplishments, failing to forgive oneself for being human or making human errors, thinking negatively about one's worth, thinking of oneself as "poor me," and worrying about
trifling matters since negative attitudes intensify stress

Practice a habitual, positive mental attitude since thinking well of oneself or confi-
dently about a situation reduces stress and leads to constructive living

Do not blame others or situations for the stress one feels, and look objectively at
how one has contributed to one's own stress level, as the choices one has or has
not made are almost always the cause of one's stress, and recognize that everyone
is responsible for his own stress level

Explain the importance of persons offering support to one another (as a deterrent to
stress and as a relief from stress)

Explain the importance of meeting one's own needs as well as those of a significant other (to keep family stress at a minimum, all members must have their needs met)

Describe those persons who have a decreased tolerance for stress (premature infants, ill
or injured persons, the aged)

Explain the causes of the problem (tension can result from such factors as change, difficult relationships, unfinished tasks, illness, injury, money problems, changes in family
structure)

EVALUATION

Record actual outcome

Altered Responses in Thought Process

ATTENTION-DEFICIT DISORDER [19,105]

ASSESSMENT
Data Collection

Subjective Data
• Person does not follow through on requests from others
• Does not seem to listen to others

Objective Data
• Person does not finish what he starts
• Interrupts others by restless activity or unrelated comments when they are speaking to
him
• Is easily distracted
Impulsive behavior, sometimes
Excess motor activity involves running about and being unable to sit still or stay seated
for a time

Data Analysis

Nursing Diagnosis
ATTENTION-DEFICIT DISORDER: Persistent difficulty maintaining attention to subjects or tasks

Common Etiology (Stressors)

BIRTH DEFECTS: Developmental deficit, cerebral palsy

DISEASES: Epilepsy, manic–depressive psychosis, schizophrenia

PSYCHOSOCIAL FACTORS: The threat of real or imagined danger, lack of competency in using effective coping mechanisms, lack of consistent discipline, the threat of rejection

DEVELOPMENTAL PHASES: Preschooler (aged 3–6)

LIFESTYLE: High sugar intake, drug abuse

SITUATIONAL FACTORS: Frequent change of parents as when one is a foster child or the child of a separated couple

ENVIRONMENTAL FACTORS: *Environmental disorder*: Clutter, noise, moving persons, etc.

PLANNING

Unmet Needs

Protection from psychologic threat, a predictable and orderly world, acceptance, caring and communicating relationships, high evaluation of self, dignity, increased learning, increased reality perception and problem-solving ability

Expected Outcome

Person verbalizes an awareness of the problem

Learns and uses methods for increasing his attention span

Exhibits increased attention to the subjects or tasks

NURSING INTERVENTIONS

Nursing Treatments

Approach unhurriedly

Demonstrate calmness

Provide an atmosphere of acceptance (of the person but not of the behavior)

Clearly communicate what is expected of the person

Encourage the expression of feelings (if anxiety is the cause)

Listen attentively

Offer feedback to the person's expressed feelings

Arrange orderly surroundings

Arrange a structured daily routine

Provide quiet

Provide seclusion (if needed to prevent distraction while the person attempts tasks)

Remove the stimuli that support the attention deficit (reduce the stimuli to a single stimulus)

Touch the person (to get his attention before attempting to communicate)

Encourage the person to listen attentively (have the person look at you when you are speaking)

Give explicit directions (that are clear, concise, and simple)

Ask simple, direct questions (while speaking slowly and distinctly)

Limit the conversation to short discussions

Allow time for thought comprehension (after communicating with the person, and do not expect an immediate response)

Divide tasks into multiple, simple steps (to make it easier to achieve tasks)

Encourage decision making (by the person whenever possible)

Reduce the demand for cognitive functioning when the person is ill or fatigued (limit the demands for thinking to simple processes)

Avoid demands for abstract thinking if the person can only think in concrete terms (such demands cause feelings of inadequacy and failure)

Reduce physical discomforts that could interfere with cognitive function (be certain the person is not in pain, feeling hungry, wet, chilled, too warm, etc., since such discomforts distract his attention)

Provide finger foods (that can be held in the hand if the person cannot sit long enough to eat a meal)

Encourage decreased carbohydrate intake (avoiding high sugar intake and chemical additives in the diet when a hypersensitivity to these substances contributes to the disorder)

Provide frequent contact with the person

Verbalize daily the person's successful progress (in changing his behavior if behavioral change is possible)

Provide emotional support for persons significant to the patient

Consult with a physician (if medications are needed)

Involve the family (in methods for coping with the attention-deficit disorder)

Nursing Observations

Determine the degree of insight that the person has (into the attention-deficit disorder)

Evaluate the safety of the environment (in relationship to the attention deficit)

Observe for a favorable response to therapy (an increased attention span)

Health Teaching

Explain the causes of the problem (neurologic deficit, high anxiety level)

Explain that persons with limited attention span require message repetition

Advise that highly emotional situations be avoided (before attempting tasks; emotional states will distract the person from task performance)

Explain how thinking occurs (incoming information is perceived and is interpreted on the basis of language skills, sensory-motor development, remembering, reasoning, imagining, and evaluation)

EVALUATION

Record actual outcome

CONFUSION [53,422,471,497,305]

ASSESSMENT

Data Collection

Subjective Data
• Person relates difficulty comprehending what is being said
 Verbalizes an awareness of the confusion during lucid moments
 Relates feeling frightened by the confusion

Objective Data
• Rambling, incoherent speech
• Unable to deal with abstract thinking
 Restlessness
 Fluctuating mental clarity

Data Analysis

Nursing Diagnosis
CONFUSION: Diminished mental clarity

Common Etiology (Stressors)
DISEASES: Alcoholism, anemia (severe), arrhythmias, arteriosclerosis, brain abscess or tumor, cardiovascular disease, cerebrovascular accident, major depression, eclampsia, encephalitis, epilepsy, hemorrhage, hepatic failure, hyper- or hypoglycemia, hyper- or hypothyroidism, meningitis, myocardial infarction, organic brain syndrome, psychosis, renal failure, schizophrenia, senility, subarachnoid hemorrhage, subdural hematoma, syphilis of the central nervous system

INJURIES: Burn wound, cerebral concussion or contusion, electric shock, fracture and compression of the spinal cord, heat exhaustion or stroke, poisoning

SIGNS AND SYMPTOMS: Convulsions, dehydration, fever, hypothermia, hypoxia, pain, shock

PSYCHOSOCIAL FACTORS: The threat of chronic, severe, or overwhelming stress, decreased sensory input, loss of a significant other

HEALTH CARE FACTORS: *Health care environment*: An unfamiliar environment. *Institutional routine*: An unflexible institutional routine. *Health therapy*: Unfamiliar therapy. *Medical therapy*: Cardioversion, electroconvulsive therapy, hemodialysis, inhalation therapy, oxygen therapy, alcohol or drug withdrawal. *Drug therapy*: Adverse effects of drugs. *Surgical therapy*: Anesthesia. *Surgical procedures*: Burr holes, craniotomy, etc.

DEVELOPMENTAL PHASES: Old age

LIFESTYLE: Alcohol or drug abuse, insufficient rest and sleep

SITUATIONAL FACTORS: A disaster, the relocation of a home (if elderly)

ENVIRONMENTAL FACTORS: Darkness. *Chemical substances*: Inhalation or ingestion of chemicals. *Noise*: Loud noise

PLANNING

Unmet Needs

Protection from psychologic threat, a predictable and orderly world, acceptance, caring and communicating relationships, high evaluation of self, dignity, increased learning, increased reality perception and problem-solving ability

Expected Outcome

Person and/or family verbalizes an awareness of the problem
Verbalizes an understanding of the causes of the confusion
Learns and uses methods to reduce the confusion
Person exhibits decreased confusion if such is physiologically possible

NURSING INTERVENTIONS

Nursing Treatments

Approach unhurriedly
Demonstrate calmness
Provide an atmosphere of acceptance
Provide quiet (noise increases confusion)
Arrange orderly surroundings
Arrange a structured daily routine
Illuminate the room adequately (so there are no disturbing shadows)
Provide a night light
Provide desired personal articles (which are items significant and familiar to the person)
Touch the person (to get his attention before attempting to communicate)
Encourage the person to listen attentively (have the person look at you when you speak)
Give explicit directions (that are clear and simple)
Ask simple, direct questions (while speaking slowly and distinctly)
Limit the conversation to short discussions
Allow time for thought comprehension (after communicating with the person, and do not expect an immediate response, as confused persons need time to comprehend)
Divide tasks into multiple, simple steps (to make it easier to achieve tasks)
Encourage decision making (by the person whenever possible)
Reduce the demand for cognitive functioning when the person is ill or fatigued (limit the demand for thinking to simple processes)
Avoid demands for abstract thinking if the person can only think in concrete terms (confused persons can deal better with concrete/specific ideas)
Reduce physical discomforts that could interfere with cognitive function (be certain the person is not in pain, does not feel hungry, is not wet, etc; such discomforts interfere with thinking)
Refrain from performing nonessential procedures (that could increase confusion)
Discuss the anticipated procedure (so the person is prepared for what will occur)

Plan undisturbed periods (of sleep) for the person (being awakened during sleep often increases confusion)

Correct misinterpreted messages immediately

Provide frequent contact with the person

Escort the person during off-ward activities

Limit visitors (if numerous visitors increase the person's confusion)

Consult with the physician (if drugs, therapy, or physiologic imbalance are causing the confusion)

Involve the family (in methods of coping with the confusion, and encourage the family to provide the person with meaningful tasks and responsibilities which often diminish confusion)

Nursing Observations

Determine the degree of insight that the person has (into the confusion)

Compare the preoperative and postoperative response level

Observe for an excessive stress level (resulting from the confusion)

Evaluate the safety of the environment (in relationship to the degree of confusion)

Observe for evidence of a favorable response to therapy (decreased confusion)

Health Teaching

Explain the causes of the problem (organic disease, pain, severe stress)

Explain how thinking occurs (incoming information is perceived and is interpreted on the basis of language skills, sensory-motor development, remembering, reasoning, imagining, and evaluation)

Advise that highly emotional situations be avoided (before attempting tasks, as emotional states can increase confusion, making tasks more difficult)

Explain that persons with impaired cerebral function require close observation

EVALUATION

Record actual outcome

DISORIENTATION[53,422,471,497]

ASSESSMENT

Data Collection

Subjective Data
• Person cannot identify time, place and/or persons
• Cannot recognize the surroundings
  Aware of the disorientation during lucid moments
  Feels frightened by the disorientation

Objective Data
• Fluctuating mental clarity

Data Analysis

Nursing Diagnosis
DISORIENTATION: An inability to recognize the time period (hour, day, or year), place, or persons

Common Etiology (Stressors)
DISEASES: Alcoholism, anemia (severe), arrhythmias, arteriosclerosis, brain abscess or tu-

mor, cardiovascular disease, cerebrovascular accident, major depression, eclampsia, encephalitis, epilepsy, hemorrhage, hepatic failure, hyper- or hypoglycemia, hyper- or hypothyroidism, meningitis, myocardial infarction, organic brain syndrome, psychosis, renal failure, schizophrenia, senility, subarachnoid hemorrhage, subdural hematoma, syphilis of the central nervous system

INJURIES: Burn wound, cerebral concussion or contusion, electric shock, fracture and compression of the spinal cord, heat exhaustion or stroke, poisoning

SIGNS AND SYMPTOMS: Convulsions, dehydration, fever, hypothermia, hypoxia, pain, shock

PSYCHOSOCIAL FACTORS: The threat of chronic, severe, or overwhelming stress, decreased sensory input

HEALTH CARE FACTORS: *Health care environment*: An unfamiliar environment. *Institutional routine*: An inflexible routine. *Health therapy*: Unfamiliar health therapy. *Medical therapy*: Cardioversion, electroconvulsive therapy, hemodialysis, inhalation therapy, oxygen therapy, alcohol or drug withdrawal. *Drug therapy*: Adverse effects of drugs. *Surgical therapy*: Anesthesia. *Surgical procedures*: Burr holes, craniotomy, etc.

DEVELOPMENTAL PHASES: Old age

LIFESTYLE: Alcohol or drug abuse, insufficient rest and sleep

SITUATIONAL FACTORS: A disaster

ENVIRONMENTAL FACTORS: Darkness. *Chemical substances*: Inhalation or ingestion of chemicals. *Noise*: Loud noise

PLANNING

Unmet Needs

Protection from psychologic threat, a predictable and orderly world, acceptance, caring and communicating relationships, high evaluation of self, dignity, increased learning, increased reality perception

Expected Outcome

Person and/or family verbalizes an awareness of the problem
Verbalizes an understanding of the causes of the disorientation
Learns and uses methods to reduce the disorientation
Person exhibits decreased disorientation if such is physiologically possible

NURSING INTERVENTIONS

Nursing Treatments

Approach unhurriedly
Demonstrate calmness
Provide an atmosphere of acceptance (of the person but not of the behavior)
Provide quiet
Arrange orderly surroundings
Arrange a structured environment and daily routine
Illuminate the room adequately (so the person can see where he is)
Provide a night light
Use the person's name frequently (so he knows who he is, a large sign on which his name is written often helps)
Relate the time, day, place, and events occurring
Provide a clock, a calendar
Provide desired personal articles (items significant to the person and on which the person can concentrate his attention)
Communicate recent nonthreatening news events to the disoriented person (so he feels in touch with the outside world)
Touch the person (to get his attention before attempting to communicate)
Encourage the person to listen attentively (have the person look at you when you speak)
Ask simple, direct questions (while speaking slowly and distinctly)
Allow time for thought comprehension (after communicating with the person, as disoriented persons need time to comprehend)
Correct misinterpreted messages immediately
Involve the family (in methods of coping with the disorientation)

Nursing Observations

Compare the preoperative and postoperative response level

Observe for an excessive stress level (resulting from the disorientation)

Evaluate the safety of the environment (in relationship to the degree of disorientation)

Observe for evidence of a favorable response to therapy (full orientation of the person)

Health Teaching

Explain the causes of the problem (a change in the environment, drug side effects, surgery, organic disease)

EVALUATION

Record actual outcome

ILLOGICAL THOUGHT PROCESSES[471]

ASSESSMENT

Data Collection

Subjective Data

- Person's ideas are poorly organized and vague with an uncertain meaning
- Idea associations are illogical
- Is unable to relate abstractions and understand symbols
- Cannot move from one topic to another with ease
- Has little thought continuity, ideas do not reach a goal

  There is little connection between one thought and the next

  New words may be made up to express an idea

Objective Data

- Unable to interpret proverbs used for testing thought process correctly (for example, explain the proverb "a stitch in time saves nine")

Data Analysis

Nursing Diagnosis

ILLOGICAL THOUGHT PROCESSES: Unclear, unreasonable, or faulty thinking

Common Etiology (Stressors)

DISEASES: Major depression, manic–depressive psychosis, organic brain syndrome, schizophrenia

PSYCHOSOCIAL FACTORS: Unlearned alternative behavior, lack of problem-solving skills

PLANNING

Unmet Needs

Protection from psychologic threat, a predictable and orderly world, acceptance, caring and communicating relationships, high evaluation of self, dignity, increased learning, increased reality perception and problem-solving ability

Expected Outcome

Person and/or family verbalizes an awareness of the problem

Verbalizes an understanding of the causes of the illogical thought process

Learns and uses methods of logical thought

Person exhibits a greater degree of logical thought

NURSING INTERVENTIONS

Nursing Treatments

Approach unhurriedly

Demonstrate calmness

Provide an atmosphere of acceptance

Arrange orderly surroundings

Arrange a structured environment and daily routine

Relate to the person on an adult–adult level, not on a parent–child level

Touch the person (to get his attention before attempting to communicate, and touch him and interrupt him when thought processes become disorganized)

Encourage the person to listen attentively (have the person look at you when you speak)

Give explicit directions (which are clear and simple)

Ask simple, direct questions (while speaking slowly and distinctly)

Limit the conversation to short discussions (short, simple messages)

Allow time for thought comprehension (after communicating with the person as persons exhibiting illogical thought need time to comprehend)

Divide tasks into multiple simple steps

Encourage decision making (by the person whenever possible)

Reduce the demand for cognitive functioning when the person is ill or fatigued (limit the demand for thinking to simple processes)

Avoid demands for abstract thinking if the person can only think in concrete terms (illogically thinking persons can deal better with concrete/specific ideas)

Reduce physical discomforts that could interfere with cognitive function (be certain the person is not in pain, does not feel hungry, is not wet, etc., as such discomforts interfere with thinking)

Discuss the anticipated procedure (so the person is prepared for what will occur)

Correct misinterpreted messages immediately

Refrain from arguing (perceived threat impairs logical thinking)

Involve the family (in methods of coping with the illogical thought)

Nursing Observations

Determine the degree of insight that the person has (into the illogical thinking)

Observe for an excessive stress level

Observe for evidence of a favorable response to therapy (increased logical thinking)

Health Teaching

Explain the causes of the problem (organic disease, excessive stress)

Explain how thinking occurs (incoming information is perceived and is interpreted on the basis of language skills, sensory-motor development, remembering, reasoning, imagining, and evaluation)

Teach how to use the problem-solving method (as a process of logical thinking)

EVALUATION

Record actual outcome

IMPULSIVENESS[19,105,471]

ASSESSMENT

Data Collection

Subjective Data
- Person relates that he acts before thinking
- Frequently shifts from one activity to another
- Difficulty organizing work

Objective Data
- May vocally interrupt others
- Difficulty waiting his turn when in a group

Data Analysis

Nursing Diagnosis
IMPULSIVENESS: A sudden drive to act without previous thought about doing so

Common Etiology (Stressors)
BIRTH DEFECTS: Developmental deficit
DISEASES: Cerebral disease (involving the posterior orbital areas of the frontal lobes), neurosis, senility (agitated)
SIGNS AND SYMPTOMS: Confusion, hyperactivity
PSYCHOSOCIAL FACTORS: Lack of impulse control, chronic or severe stress, an attempt to redirect feelings into activity, lack of the perception of danger or threat, exposure to an impulse-directed role model
HEALTH CARE FACTORS: *Surgical procedures*: Prefrontal lobotomy

PLANNING

Unmet Needs

Protection from physical harm, psychologic stability, acceptance, caring and communicating relationships, high evaluation of self, personal growth and maturity, self-control, increased learning, increased reality perception and problem-solving ability

Expected Outcome

Person gains control of inner tensions that direct impulsive actions
Exhibits behavior that indicates he is thinking before acting
Verbalizes satisfaction with increased control over his behavior

NURSING INTERVENTIONS

Nursing Treatments

Approach unhurriedly
Reassure verbally (that the nurse will help the person)
Demonstrate calmness
Provide an atmosphere of acceptance (of the person, not of the behavior)
Encourage the expression of feelings
Relate to the person on an adult–adult level, not on a parent–child level
Listen attentively
Talk with the person
Explore with the person the reasons for recurring problems (why the person repeatedly does not think before acting)
Explore with the person the effects of his behavior on others (others cannot rely on what behavior to expect from the person and may respond with defensive behavior toward the person)
Set an example by role modeling (calm decision making followed by action)
Clearly communicate what is expected of the person (responsible thought and activity)
Hold the person responsible for his behavior (do not allow the person to blame others)
Minimize environmental dangers (if the person could harm himself during impulsive behavior)
Refrain from negatively criticizing
Verbalize daily the person's successful progress (in changing his behavior)
Provide emotional support for persons significant to the patient
Involve the family (in methods of coping with impulsiveness)

Nursing Observations

Determine the degree of insight that the person has (into the impulsive behavior)
Determine the precipitating factors (for the impulsive behavior)
Evaluate the safety of the environment (in relation to the impulsiveness)
Observe for behavior modification (resulting from therapy)

Health Teaching

Emphasize the importance of recognizing tension within oneself (as an early sign of impending impulsive behavior)

Explain how thinking occurs (incoming information is perceived and is interpreted on the basis of language skills, sensory-motor development, remembering, reasoning, imagining, and evaluation)

Teach how to use the problem-solving method (to prevent impulsive actions)

EVALUATION

Record actual outcome

Altered Responses in Thought Content

DELUSIONAL THINKING [105,471]

ASSESSMENT

Data Collection

Subjective Data
- Person persists in beliefs that are illogical
- Disregards evidence which proves the beliefs to be false
  May believe others are against him
  May believe himself to be someone of greatness

Objective Data
- Exhibits behavior consistent with the delusional thinking

Data Analysis

Nursing Diagnosis
DELUSIONAL THINKING (DELUSION): The holding of false beliefs despite evidence that the belief is not true

Common Etiology (Stressors)
DISEASES: Organic brain syndrome, paranoia, schizophrenia

PLANNING

Unmet Needs

Comfort, protection from psychologic threat, a predictable and orderly world, acceptance, caring and communicating relationships, increased learning, increased reality perception and problem-solving ability

Expected Outcome

Person and/or family verbalizes an awareness of the problem
Verbalizes an understanding of the cause of the delusional thinking
Learns and uses methods to reduce the delusional thinking
Person relates decreased delusional thinking if such is physiologically possible

NURSING INTERVENTIONS

Nursing Treatments

Approach unhurriedly
Demonstrate calmness
Provide an atmosphere of acceptance (of the person but not of the delusion)
Encourage the expression of feelings (about the false beliefs)
Encourage the person to listen attentively (have the person look at you when you speak)
Give explicit directions (that are clear and simple)

Encourage active diversional activities (that will divert the person from the delusional ideas and support reality orientation)

Refrain from supporting the person's delusions (do not agree with or participate in the delusional thinking)

Avoid situations that would cause conflict with the delusional thinking (if the person believes he is a composer, do not remove his musical instrument)

Cast doubt about the reality of the delusional thinking (by comments such as "You believe you are a king, but I wonder if you are")

Refrain from arguing, from teasing (which heightens the person's anxiety and reduces his self-esteem)

Encourage the use of normal coping mechanisms

Correct misinterpreted messages immediately (so they are not incorporated into the existing delusions)

Involve the family (in methods of coping with the delusional thinking)

Nursing Observations

Determine the degree of insight that the person has (into the delusional thinking)

Evaluate the safety of the environment (in relationship to the character of the delusional thinking, for instance, the person may believe he is an indestructable bionic man)

Observe for a favorable response to therapy (orientation to reality)

Health Teaching

Explain the causes of the problem (paranoia, schizophrenia, organic disease)

EVALUATION

Record actual outcome

MEMORY LOSS[471,774]

ASSESSMENT

Data Collection

Subjective Data
• Person is unable to recall recent events or information
• Usually able to recall past events
  Listens for clues from others that might restore the memory
  Feels frightened
  Hopes others will not notice the memory loss

Objective Data
Confabulates when unable to remember in an attempt to maintain self-esteem

Data Analysis

Nursing Diagnosis
MEMORY LOSS: Decreased ability to recall recent events or information

Common Etiology (Stressor)
DISEASES: Alcoholism, arteriosclerosis, cerebrovascular accident, epilepsy, Korsakoff's syndrome, organic brain syndrome, senility, subarachnoid hemorrhage, subdural hematoma, syphilis of the central nervous system

INJURIES: Cerebral concussion or contusion

SIGNS AND SYMPTOMS: Hypoxia (cerebral), severe pain

PSYCHOSOCIAL FACTORS: Severe or overwhelming stress

HEALTH CARE FACTORS: *Medical therapy*: Cardioversion, electroconvulsive therapy. *Drug therapy*: Adverse effects of drugs. *Surgical therapy*: Anesthesia

DEVELOPMENTAL PHASES: Old age
LIFESTYLE: Alcohol or drug abuse, a chronically unbalanced diet

PLANNING

Unmet Needs

Comfort, protection from psychologic threat, a predictable and orderly world, acceptance, caring and communicating relationships, high evaluation of self, sense of adequacy, dignity, increased learning, increased reality perception

Expected Outcome

Person and/or family verbalizes an awareness of the problem
Verbalizes an understanding of the cause of the memory loss
Learns and uses methods to reduce the memory loss
Person exhibits decreased memory loss if such is physiologically possible

NURSING INTERVENTIONS

Nursing Treatments

Approach unhurriedly
Demonstrate calmness
Reassure verbally (that the memory loss is not complete, that the memory will return, or that adaptation to the memory loss is possible)
Provide an atmosphere of acceptance (of the person, not of the behavior)
Arrange a structured environment (consistent placement of objects, etc.) and a structured daily routine
Encourage the person to listen attentively (for cues that could stimulate the memory)
Ask simple, direct questions (if the person cannot remember the answer, restate the question in another way, such as offering a leading question)
Allow time for thought comprehension (persons with memory loss need time to comprehend)
Divide tasks into multiple, simple steps (if there is memory loss about a task performance)
Stimulate the memory by repeating the person's last expressed thought
Encourage the person to write down what he wants to remember (this will increase his confidence in his ability to remember)
Refrain from teasing (which decreases self-esteem)
Refrain from arguing (when the person confabulates, and recognize that it is being done to maintain self-esteem)
Consult with the physician (if the memory loss is a side effect of drugs or therapy)
Involve the family (in the methods of coping with the memory loss)

Nursing Observations

Determine the degree of insight that the person has (into the memory loss)
Observe for an excessive stress level (about the memory loss)
Evaluate the safety of the environment (if there is severe memory loss, for example, the person may have forgotten that knives are sharp)
Observe for evidence of a favorable response to therapy (satisfaction with methods for coping with the memory loss)

Health Teaching

Explain the essential factors that affect memory (we must understand that we are trying to remember, we remember only what is important to us, what we learn must be reinforced, the unique and outstanding are best remembered, a relaxed uncluttered mind receives information best)
Teach methods for improving the memory (such as linking ideas together, paying strict attention when receiving information, reinforcing the memory with the five senses, such as touching, smelling, and visualizing a flower, reviewing the information within 10 minutes, again within 24 hours, and when going to sleep, making lists, exercising to improve cerebral circulation, using memory games, rereading, retelling, rehearing,

reviewing, and reinforce the information, thinking positively about remembering)
Explain the causes of the problem (excessive stress, organic disease, etc.)

EVALUATION
Record actual outcome

Altered Responses in Perception

HALLUCINATIONS [53,105,278,399,471]

ASSESSMENT
Data Collection
Subjective Data
• Person perceives objects that are not based on reality
• May smell, taste, or hear that which is nonexistent

Objective Data
• Responds as though the hallucinatory object is real
  Withdrawal behavior (decreases interaction with real people)
  Decreased ability to function

Data Analysis
Nursing Diagnosis
HALLUCINATIONS: The perception of sensory phenomena without appropriate external
  stimuli

Common Etiology (Stressors)
DISEASES: Alcoholism, arteriosclerosis, bacterial infection (toxic), brain tumor, encephalitis, hepatic failure, malaria, organic brain syndrome, paranoia, renal failure, schizophrenia
INJURIES: Concussion
SIGNS AND SYMPTOMS: Delirium, high fever
PSYCHOSOCIAL FACTORS: The threat of danger not clearly identified or perceived redirected
  into an object outside of oneself, the threat of acute sensory deprivation, decreased
  sensory input
MAJOR PATHOPHYSIOLOGIC FACTORS: Brain cell damage or specific stimulation causing the
  person to project perceptions, sensations, and thoughts into the environment as
  though they were independent of the individual
HEALTH CARE FACTORS: Adverse effects of drugs such as atropine, scopolamine. *Medical therapy*: Alcohol or drug withdrawal
LIFESTYLE: Drug abuse, the use of drugs such as lysergic acid diethylamide (LSD), mesca-
  line, or phencyclidine (PCP), prolonged lack of sleep (exhaustion)

PLANNING
Unmet Needs
Comfort, protection from psychologic threat, a predictable and orderly world, acceptance, caring and communicating relationships, increased learning, increased reality
  perception

Expected Outcome
Person and/or family relates an awareness of the problem
Verbalizes an understanding of the causes of the hallucinations
Learns and uses methods to reduce the hallucinatory perceptions

Person verbally expresses the anxiety causing the hallucinations
Person relates decreased hallucinations if such is possible

NURSING INTERVENTIONS

Nursing Treatments
Approach unhurriedly
Demonstrate calmness
Provide an atmosphere of acceptance (of the person, but not of the hallucinations)
Encourage the expression of feelings (about the hallucinations and the anxiety causing or resulting from them)
Arrange a structured environment and daily routine (to reduce the anxiety)
Provide frequent contact with the person (as evidence of caring and for reality orientation)
Encourage active diversional activities (that will divert the person from the hallucinations and have him interact with others to support reality orientation)
Refrain from supporting the person's hallucinations (do not agree with or participate in the hallucinations)
Cast doubt about the reality of the hallucinations (state that "You may believe the voices you hear are real, but I wonder if they are")
Refrain from arguing, from teasing (which heightens anxiety)
Encourage the use of normal coping mechanisms
Explore with the person his strenghts and resources (to overcome the problem)
Involve the family (in methods of coping with the hallucinations)

Nursing Observations
Determine the degree of insight that the person has (into the hallucinations)
Identify disturbing conversation topics
Determine the precipitating factors, the relieving factors
Evaluate the safety of the environment (in relationship to the character of the hallucinations, for example, the voices may say such degrading and destructive things that the person will attempt suicide to escape them)
Observe for evidence of a favorable response to therapy (reality orientation)

Health Teaching
Explain the causes of the problem (the projection of high levels of anxiety into the external world, organic disease)
Advise (the family) against denouncing erroneous perceptions (this tendency increases the patient's anxiety)

EVALUATION
Record actual outcome

ILLUSIONAL THINKING [105,471]

ASSESSMENT

Data Collection

Subjective Data
• Person relates perceiving an external object as different than it really is
  May perceive a lace curtain to be a spider, a bed rail as a jail bar

Objective Data
• Responds to the object as he perceives it to be

Data Analysis
Nursing Diagnosis
ILLUSIONAL THINKING: The incorrect perception of existing objects in the environment

Common Etiology (Stressors)
DISEASES: Alcoholism, brain tumor, organic brain syndrome, paranoia, schizophrenia
PSYCHOSOCIAL FACTORS: An attempt to express anxiety, fear, or guilt indirectly
MAJOR PATHOPHYSIOLOGIC FACTORS: Brain cell damage causes a misinterpretation of the environment

PLANNING

Unmet Needs
Comfort, protection from psychologic threat, a predictable and orderly world, acceptance, caring and communicating relationships, increased learning, increased reality perception

Expected Outcome
Person and/or family relates awareness of the problem
Verbalizes understanding of the causes of the illusions
Learns and uses methods to reduce illusional perceptions
Person verbally expresses emotions causing the illusions
Person relates decreased illusions if such is possible

NURSING INTERVENTIONS

Nursing Treatments
Approach unhurriedly
Demonstrate calmness
Provide an atmosphere of acceptance (of the person, not of the delusional thinking)
Encourage the expression of feelings (about the illusions and the anxiety causing them)
Arrange a structured environment and daily routine (to reduce anxiety)
Illuminate the room adequately (to reduce the potential for incorrect perception)
Provide frequent contact with the person (as evidence of caring and to promote reality orientation)
Encourage active diversional activities (that will divert the person from the illusions and support reality perception)
Refrain from supporting the person's illusions (do not agree with the illusion)
Cast doubt about the reality of the illusions (make statements such as "You may believe that you see a spider on the wall, but all I can find is a place where the paint is chipped off")
Remove the stimuli that support the misperception
Refrain from arguing, from teasing (which heightens anxiety)
Encourage the use of normal coping mechanisms
Involve the family (in methods of coping with the illusions)

Nursing Observations
Determine the degree of insight that the person has (into the illusions)
Identify disturbing topics of conversation
Determine the precipitating factors, the relieving factors
Observe for evidence of a favorable response to therapy (reality orientation)

Health Teaching
Explain the causes of the problem (the projection of high levels of anxiety into the external world, organic disease)
Advise (the family) against denouncing erroneous perceptions (this tendency increases the anxiety)

EVALUATION

Record actual outcome

Knowledge Deficits Associated with Cognitive Function

UNKNOWLEDGEABLE ABOUT PROBLEM-SOLVING METHODS[653]

ASSESSMENT

Data Collection

Subjective Data
- Person's discussion or questions indicate a need for additional information, clarification, or validation of information
  OR
- Person's lack of questions or comments indicates not wanting information or not knowing enough to seek information
- When questioned directly, the person's response or lack of response indicates that he does not know:
  How to identify the problem
  Methods for determining a solution to the problem
  How to make choices effectively, even though he may know of multiple solutions
  May relate being preoccupied with the problem rather than the solution

Objective Data
- May exhibit behavior based on insufficient knowledge, such as not taking precautions, making the problem worse

Data Analysis

Nursing Diagnosis
UNKNOWLEDGEABLE ABOUT PROBLEM-SOLVING METHODS: Being without sufficient information about methods used to solve problems effectively

Common Etiology (Stressors)
HEALTH CARE FACTORS: Lack of health instruction

PLANNING

Unmet Needs
Independence, increased learning and problem-solving ability

Expected Outcome
Correct verbal feedback of the information taught

NURSING INTERVENTIONS

Nursing Treatments
Approach unhurriedly
Provide an atmosphere of acceptance (of the person but not of the behavior)
Encourage the person to ask questions
Provide reliable information
Encourage mutual problem solving
Support a realistic assessment of the situation
Encourage gradual mastery of a situation
Encourage both long- and short-term goals
Discourage decision making when one is under severe stress

Nursing Observations
Observe for evidence of a favorable response to therapy (improved problem-solving ability)

Health Teaching

Teach how to use the problem-solving method

Inform of the resources available (for solving the specific problem)

EVALUATION

Record actual outcome

23 Nursing Diagnoses of PHYSICAL AND SPEECH REHABILITATION

Dual Domain of Nursing Expertise: Physical and Speech Rehabilitation

This chapter covers that sphere of nursing knowledge and skill related to restoring or maximizing a person's ability to function with a disability. Physical rehabilitation focuses on restoring neuromuscular and orthopedic function. Speech rehabilitation focuses on the restoration of impaired verbal communication. These problems are solved by such health care providers as nurses, physicians, and physical and speech therapists.

Views of Nursing Leaders That Support This Domain of Nursing Expertise

Nursing as a service involves . . . helping the individual to adjust to his limitations.

Faye Abdellah[4:25]

Modern nursing is by no means limited to the giving of expert physical care to the sick, important as this is. It is more far reaching, including as it does helping the patient to adjust to unalterable situations.

Hester Frederick and Ethel Northam[379:68]

Nursing is a humanistic science dedicated to compassionate concern for maintaining and promoting health, preventing illness, and caring for and rehabilitating the sick and disabled.

Martha Rogers[419:vii]

Although the nurse seeks to help the patient meet his needs during a period of dependency, she also tries to shorten this period. Before she carries out any act for him, she asks herself what part of it could he himself perform. . . . In other words, the rehabilitation of all patients in the hands of a nurse begins with her first service to him.

Virginia Henderson[221:27]

Knowledge Deficits Associated with Physical Rehabilitation

UNKNOWLEDGEABLE ABOUT COPING WITH ARCHITECTURAL BARRIERS[356,477]

ASSESSMENT

Data Collection

Subjective Data
• Person's discussion or questions indicate a need for additional information, clarification, or validation of information
    OR
• Person's lack of questions or comments indicates not wanting information or not knowing enough to seek information
• When questioned directly, the person's response or lack of response indicates that he does not know:
    About methods of home adaptations that facilitate ease of mobility

Objective Data
• May exhibit behavior such as mobilizing with difficulty based on insufficient knowledge of alternative methods

Data Analysis

Nursing Diagnosis
UNKNOWLEDGEABLE ABOUT COPING WITH ARCHITECTURAL BARRIERS: Being without sufficient information about methods for promoting independent, normal activity of disabled persons in spite of obstructive structural designs of a dwelling or building

Common Etiology (Stressors)
HEALTH CARE FACTORS: Lack of health instruction

PLANNING

Unmet Needs
Comfort, independence, increased learning, increased problem-solving ability

Expected Outcome
Correct verbal feedback of the information taught
Person verbalizes about and demonstrates an increased ease in mobility

NURSING INTERVENTIONS

Nursing Treatments
Encourage the person to ask questions
Make a referral (to the National Self-Help Clearinghouse for a complete list of home adaptations)

Nursing Observations
Determine teaching effectiveness by verbal feedback

Health Teaching
Recommend home adaptations appropriate for persons in a wheelchair (such as living in a single-level ground-floor dwelling, using outdoor carpeting instead of deep carpeting or tile floor coverings, removing unnecessary doors when possible, having hallways at least 48 inches wide, using a narrow wheelchair, having windowsills, door knobs, and light switches no higher than 36 inches from the floor, placing electrical outlets 18 inches from the floor, using polyethylene instead of wood or metal doorsills, using front-loading washers and dryers and front stove controls, having low storage cabinets and revolving cabinet shelves and low clothing racks)

Recommend home adaptations appropriate for persons unable to stoop (such as using hand rails, high electrical outlets, top-loading washers and dryers, top stove controls, high storage closets and clothing racks, use of foot pedals on appliance doors)

Explain that objects should be placed consistently in the same location for the visually impaired

Explain the reason for and intended effect of the methods used

EVALUATION

Record actual outcome

UNSKILLED AT USING A BRACE[356,477]

ASSESSMENT

Data Collection

Subjective Data

• Person's discussion or questions indicate a need for additional information, clarification, or validation of information about performing the task
  OR
• Person's lack of questions or comments indicates not wanting information or not knowing enough to seek information about performing the task

Person may not know:

How to apply and remove a brace

The proper clothing to be worn with a brace

The safety precautions related to wearing a brace

How to attain maximum mobility with a brace

How to care for and protect a brace

Objective Data

• Person cannot correctly demonstrate how to:

Apply and remove the brace

Oil and clean the appliance

Walk with the brace

Data Analysis

Nursing Diagnosis

UNSKILLED AT USING A BRACE: Being nonproficient, with or without knowledge, in the performance of the specific task of manipulating and caring for a brace

Common Etiology (Stressors)

HEALTH CARE FACTORS: Lack of health instruction, lack of health-skill experience

PLANNING

Unmet Needs

Comfort, exercise, protection from physical harm, dependence, mastery and competence in skills, independence, increased learning

Expected Outcome

Correct verbal feedback of the information taught

Correct return demonstration of how to apply, remove, oil, clean, and walk with a brace

Person verbalizes that he has a clean, fitted, fully functional brace

NURSING INTERVENTIONS

Nursing Treatments

Provide temporary assistance (with the brace) until the skill is learned

Dress in nonrestrictive clothing

Limit the patient's mobility distance (until he becomes skilled at using the brace)

Encourage the person to ask questions

Encourage self-performance

Nursing Observations

Inspect the skin for breakdown (around the brace)

Observe for mobility capabilities (with the brace)

Determine teaching effectiveness by testing, verbal feedback, and return demonstration

Health Teaching

Explain how to adjust clothing to meet health problems (the person should wear culottes, wide pants, shifts, and A-line dresses and should avoid wearing loose-knit underwear and pants with unfinished inside seams)

Instruct to use a wide supportive stance for good body balance (the feet should be placed at equal distances from the body midline)

Teach how to apply and remove a leg brace (cross the affected leg over the unaffected leg, turn the brace shoe slightly inward and insert the toes at a right angle, pull the shoe upward and lace, etc.)

Teach how to elevate from a sitting to a standing position with leg braces (using his locked brace and a chair to support the body)

Teach mobility down stairs and curbs with leg braces (using the stair rail and crutches to support the body)

Teach mobility from a standing to a sitting position with leg braces (by unlocking the braces and using the arms of the chair for support)

Teach mobility up a curb with leg braces (swinging one leg back and up onto the curb while leaning on both crutches)

Teach mobility up stairs with leg braces (using the stair rail and crutches for support as he lifts his legs up each step)

Explain how to recognize when a brace has been outgrown (evident when the brace joints do not coincide with the body joints)

Explain how to care for a leg brace (such as storing the unused brace in an aligned position, oiling the brace locks and joints once a week with one drop of machine oil, washing the brace straps with soap and water and replacing them when frayed, removing lint from the locks and joints, and keeping the shoe heels in good repair to maintain a balanced walking surface)

Explain that persons wearing leg braces should avoid contact sports

Explain the reason for and intended effect of the methods used (to assure effective use of the brace)

Medical Treatments Performed by Nurses

Mobilize with the prescribed brace

EVALUATION

Record actual outcome

UNSKILLED AT USING A CANE[356,477]

ASSESSMENT

Data Collection

Subjective Data

• Person's discussion or questions indicate a need for additional information, clarification, or validation of information about performing the task

OR
- Person's lack of questions or comments indicates not wanting information or not knowing enough to seek information about performing the task
  Person may not know:
  - When to use a cane
  - How to properly use a cane
  - The safety precautions related to using a cane
  - How to recognize an incorrect cane length

Objective Data
- Person cannot correctly demonstrate:
  How to walk with a cane

Data Analysis

Nursing Diagnosis
UNSKILLED AT USING A CANE: Being nonproficient, with or without knowledge, in the performance of the specific task of using a cane to promote balance and/or to decrease weight-bearing on one leg

Common Etiology (Stressors)
HEALTH CARE FACTORS: Lack of health instruction, lack of health-skill experience

PLANNING

Unmet Needs
Comfort, protection from physical harm, mastery and competence in skills, independence, increased learning

Expected Outcome
Correct verbal feedback of the information taught
Correct return demonstration of how to walk with a cane

NURSING INTERVENTIONS

Nursing Treatments
Provide temporary assistance until the skill is learned
Assist with mobility
Limit the patient's mobility distance (until he becomes skilled with the cane)
Encourage the person to ask questions
Encourage self-performance

Nursing Observations
Check the cane for correct length (if the cane is the correct length, the person's arm will be at a 30-degree angle)
Observe for mobility capabilities (with a cane)
Determine teaching effectiveness by testing, verbal feedback, and return demonstration

Health Teaching
Explain how to determine the proper cane length (the arm should be at a 30-degree angle)
Instruct to check the cane safety-tip regularly for needed replacement
Teach how to use a cane for balancing and weight-bearing (*For balancing*: Hold the cane on the side of the strong leg, move the cane forward at the same time one moves the weak leg forward. *For weight-bearing*: Hold the cane on the side of the weak leg and bear weight on the cane when stepping forward with the good leg)
Explain the reason for and intended effect of the methods used (to assure safe mobility)

EVALUATION

Record actual outcome

UNSKILLED AT USING CRUTCHES[356,477]

ASSESSMENT

Data Collection

Subjective Data

• Person's discussion or questions indicate a need for additional information, clarification, or validation of information about performing the task
  OR
• Person's lack of questions or comments indicates not wanting information or not knowing enough to seek information about performing the task
  Person may not know the following:
  Type of crutches to use
  How to prepare for crutch walking
  When crutches are too long or too short
  How to attain maximum mobility with crutches
  Precautions to take with crutches

Objective Data

• Person cannot correctly demonstrate how to:
  Walk, climb stairs and curbs or manipulate the body into and out of cars, chairs, etc., with crutches

Data Analysis

Nursing Diagnosis

UNSKILLED AT USING CRUTCHES: Being nonproficient, with or without knowledge, in the performance of the specific task of using crutches for mobility

Common Etiology (Stressors)

HEALTH CARE FACTORS: Lack of health instruction, lack of health-skill experience

PLANNING

Unmet Needs

Comfort, protection from physical harm, mastery and competence in skills, independence, increased learning

Expected Outcome

Correct verbal feedback of the information taught
Correct return demonstration of how to walk, climb stairs and curbs, manipulate self into and out of cars, chairs, etc., proper crutch-walking gait and stance

NURSING INTERVENTIONS

Nursing Treatments

Provide temporary assistance (with mobility) until the skill is learned
Limit the patient's mobility distance (until he is skilled at crutch walking)
Encourage the person to ask questions
Encourage self-performance

Nursing Observations

Check the crutches for correct length (the crutches should extend 6 inches out from the heel and fit comfortably under the arm)
Check the crutches for intact rubber tips (and replace if worn)
Check the crutch hand bar for position (when the hand is relaxed on the hand bar the elbow flexion should be at about 30 degrees)
Check to ensure that the top of the crutch does not press into the axilla
Observe for mobility capabilities (with the crutches)
Determine teaching effectiveness by testing, verbal feedback, and return demonstration

Health Teaching

Explain how to determine the proper crutch length (the crutches should measure the same as the length from the axilla to a point 6 inches out from the side of the foot when the person is standing)

Inform that the use of nonadjustable crutches for heavy persons is preferable (a solid piece of wood provides greater support than does wood held together with nuts and bolts)

Instruct to check the crutch safety tip regularly for needed replacement

Instruct to use wide crutch tips

Instruct to use a wide supportive stance for good body balance (the feet should be placed at equal distances from the body midline)

Recommend the use of low-heeled shoes (for balanced mobility)

Teach the proper gait to use with crutches (two-point crutch walking, three-point crutch walking, etc.)

Teach correct weight-bearing on the crutch handbar (and not on the top of the crutches)

Teach good crutch-walking posture (full extension of the hips and knees, looking forward and not downward during mobility)

Teach how to elevate from a sitting to a standing position with crutches (using the crutches and the chair arm rest to stand up)

Teach mobility from a standing to a sitting position with crutches (using the crutches and arm of the chair to support the body when sliding into the chair)

Teach mobility down a curb with crutches (placing the crutches down and off the curb, then moving the weak leg forward, followed by the strong leg)

Teach mobility up a curb with crutches (by stepping onto the curb with the strong leg, then lifting the weak leg and the crutches up onto the curb)

Teach mobility down stairs with crutches (using the stair rail and crutches to support the body)

Teach mobility up stairs with crutches (using the stair rail and crutches for weight-bearing as he moves the strong leg, followed by the weak leg and the crutches)

Teach how to do pre-crutch-walking exercises (by doing pushups or lifting weights and sandbags)

Explain the reason for and intended effect of the methods used (to provide safe crutch-walking)

Medical Treatments Performed by Nurses

Mobilize with the prescribed crutches

EVALUATION

Record actual outcome

UNSKILLED AT USING A LIMB PROSTHESIS[356,477]

ASSESSMENT

Data Collection

Subjective Data

• Person's discussion or questions indicate a need for additional information, clarification, or validation of information about performing the task
  OR

• Person's lack of questions or comments indicates not wanting information or not knowing enough to seek information about performing the task

  Person may not know:

  How to prepare for the use of a prosthesis

Precautions to be taken when wearing a prosthesis

Objective Data
• Person cannot correctly demonstrate how to:
Apply and remove a limb prosthesis
Walk with the prosthesis

Data Analysis

Nursing Diagnosis
UNSKILLED AT USING A LIMB PROSTHESIS: Being nonproficient, with or without knowledge, in the performance of the specific task of caring for and using an artificial limb

Common Etiology (Stressors)
HEALTH CARE FACTORS: Lack of health instruction, lack of health-skill experience

PLANNING

Unmet Needs
Comfort, protection from physical harm, mastery and competence in skills, independence, increased learning

Expected Outcome
Correct verbal feedback of the information taught
Correct return demonstration of how to apply and remove the prosthesis and how to walk with the prosthesis

NURSING INTERVENTIONS

Nursing Treatments
Provide temporary assistance until the skill is learned
Limit the patient's mobility distance (until he is skilled with the prosthesis)
Encourage the person to ask questions
Encourage self-performance

Nursing Observations
Observe for mobility capabilities (with the prosthesis)
Inspect the skin (on the limb stump) for breakdown
Observe for readiness to assume self-care
Determine teaching effectiveness by testing, verbal feedback, and return demonstration

Health Teaching
Advise not to stand for prolonged periods (when first starting to use the prosthesis)
Instruct to increase the wearing time of the prosthesis gradually (a little longer each day)
Instruct to avoid artificial leg abduction (that is, moving the leg to the side and outward when walking)
Instruct to avoid hiking the shoulder when walking with a leg prosthesis (one shoulder should not be raised higher than the other when walking)
Instruct to use a wide supportive stance for good body balance (the feet should be placed at equal distances from the body midline)
Teach good posture when walking with a leg prosthesis (the person should take steps of equal length with both feet and should avoid hiking the hip)
Recommend the use of low-heeled shoes (for balanced walking)
Teach how to apply a stump sock (smoothly over the stump)
Instruct that several stump socks should not be worn simultaneously
Instruct to wash the stump sock frequently
Teach how to percuss the amputation stump (by gently taping the stump against a soft pillow, one's hand, and finally against a firm surface)
Teach how to use a temporary prosthesis (only 10% of the body weight should be applied to the prosthesis, and a stump wrap should be applied at night)
Explain the reason for delaying the prosthesis application (to allow time for the stump tissue to heal)

Medical Treatments Performed by Nurses
Apply the prescribed prosthesis

EVALUATION
Record actual outcome

UNSKILLED AT USING A WALKER[356,477]

ASSESSMENT
Data Collection
Subjective Data
- Person's discussion or questions indicate a need for additional information, clarification, or validation of information about performing the task
  OR
- Person's lack of questions or comments indicates not wanting information or not knowing enough to seek information about performing a task
  Person may not know:
    The kind of walker to use
    How to determine if the walker height is correct
    How to manipulate the walker
    The precautions to take with a walker

Objective Data
- Person cannot correctly demonstrate how to:
    Ambulate with a walker
Data Analysis
Nursing Diagnosis
UNSKILLED AT USING A WALKER: Being nonproficient, with or without knowledge, in the performance of the specific task of ambulating with a walker for improved balance and/or decreased weight-bearing on the leg(s)

Common Etiology (Stressors)
HEALTH CARE FACTORS: Lack of health instruction, lack of health-skill experience

PLANNING
Unmet Needs
Comfort, exercise, protection from physical harm, mastery and competence in skills, independence, increased learning

Expected Outcome
Correct verbal feedback of the information taught
Correct return demonstration of how to ambulate with a walker

NURSING INTERVENTIONS
Nursing Treatments
Provide temporary assistance until the skill is learned
Limit the patient's mobility distance (until skilled at using the walker)
Encourage the person to ask questions
Encourage self-performance

Nursing Observations
Check the walker for proper height (if the walker height is correct, the person's elbow will be bent at a 30° angle)
Observe for mobility capabilities (with the walker)

Observe for readiness to assume self-care

Determine teaching effectiveness by testing, verbal feedback, and return demonstration

Health Teaching

Advise not to stand for prolonged periods (which tires and weakens the person)

Explain how to determine the proper walker height (the person's elbows should be bent at a 30° angle)

Inform that the use of a walker without wheels is preferable (the absence of wheels increases the stability of the walker)

Recommend the use of low-heeled shoes (for balanced walking)

Teach the proper gait to use with a walker (by moving the walker forward, then moving the right foot forward, followed by the left)

Explain the reason for and intended effect of the methods used (to support safe ambulation

EVALUATION

Record actual outcome

UNSKILLED AT USING A WHEELCHAIR[356,477]

ASSESSMENT

Data Collection

Subjective Data

• Person's discussion or questions indicate a need for additional information, clarification, or validation of information about performing the task

    OR

• Person's lack of questions or comments indicates not wanting information or not knowing enough to seek information about performing the task

  Person may not know:

    Kind of wheelchair to use

    Dangers to be avoided when using a wheelchair

Objective Data

• Person cannot correctly demonstrate how to:

    Move into and out of a wheelchair effectively

    Propel the chair

    Manipulate in doorways, halls, and tight places

Data Analysis

Nursing Diagnosis

UNSKILLED AT USING A WHEELCHAIR: Being nonproficient, with or without knowledge, in the performance of the specific task of using a wheelchair for mobility

Common Etiology (Stressors)

HEALTH CARE FACTORS: Lack of health instruction, lack of health-skill experience

PLANNING

Unmet Needs

Comfort, protection from physical harm, mastery and competence in skills, independence, increased learning

Expected Outcome

Correct verbal feedback of the information taught

Correct return demonstration of how to move into and out of a wheelchair, propel the chair, negotiate in doorways and halls, etc.

NURSING INTERVENTIONS

Nursing Treatments
Provide temporary assistance until the skill is learned
Limit the person's mobility distance (until skilled at using the wheelchair)
Encourage the person to ask questions
Encourage self-performance
Make a referral (to a supplier of wheelchairs who can show the patient the wheelchairs that are available and help evaluate and select the type that best meets the patient's personal needs)

Nursing Observations
Observe for mobility capabilities (with the wheelchair)
Observe for readiness to assume self-care
Determine teaching effectiveness by testing, verbal feedback, and return demonstration

Health Teaching
Teach how to transfer from a bed to a wheelchair (with the front of the wheelchair facing the side of the bed, the person can slide his body backward off the bed, into the chair)
Teach how to transfer from a wheelchair to a bed (with the front of the wheelchair facing the bed, the person can stand and then pivot his body onto the bed)
Teach how to transfer from a bathtub to a wheelchair (with the front of the wheelchair facing the bathtub, the person can move his body backward into the wheelchair)
Teach how to transfer from a wheelchair to a bathtub (with the front of the wheelchair facing the side of the bathtub, the person can lift himself and then lower himself into the bathtub)
Teach how to transfer from a chair to a wheelchair (with the chair and wheelchair facing each other, the person can pivot his body from the chair to the wheelchair)
Teach how to transfer from a wheelchair to a chair (with the wheelchair and chair facing each other, the person can pivot his body from the wheelchair to the chair)
Teach how to transfer from a wheelchair to an automobile (with the front of the wheelchair facing the side of the car, the person can use the car's window ledge and the wheelchair arm to lift his body onto the car seat)
Teach how to transfer from an automobile to a wheelchair (with the front of the wheelchair facing the side of the car, the person can swing his legs out of the car and lift his body into the wheelchair)
Instruct to lock the wheelchair before transferring
Teach how to propel the wheelchair (by using long, even strokes)
Instruct to do wheelchair pushups (to reduce pressure on the skin)
Inform about various assistive devices for the wheelchair (hand grips on the wheel rims, apparatus for narrowing the chair to permit passage through doorways)
Inform that the use of a lightweight wheelchair is preferable
Recommend home adaptations appropriate for persons in a wheelchair (using a tile floor or firm carpeting, removing unnecessary doors, widening narrow doors, using safety rails for toilet and bathtub transfer, living in a single-level ground-floor dwelling, using polyethylene instead of metal door sills, having low window sills, using front-loading washers and dryers and front stove controls, having low clothing racks and low storage cabinets)
Explain the reasons for and intended effects of the methods used

EVALUATION
Record actual outcome

UNSKILLED AT EXERCISE METHODS[110,746]

ASSESSMENT

Data Collection

Subjective Data
• Person's discussion or questions indicate a need for additional information, clarification, or validation of information about performing the task
  OR
• Person's lack of questions or comments indicates not wanting information or not knowing enough to seek information about performing a task
  Person may not know:
     How often to exercise
     The length of time to exercise during each session
     The most effective types of exercise
     The warning signs that indicate that exercise should be stopped
     The contraindications for exercise

Objective Data
• Person cannot correctly demonstrate how to:
     Perform exercise

Data Analysis

Nursing Diagnosis
UNSKILLED AT EXERCISE METHODS: Being nonproficient, with or without knowledge, in the performance of the specific task of repeated physical exertion designed to maintain body strength and function

Common Etiology (Stressors)
HEALTH CARE FACTORS: Lack of or incorrect health instruction

PLANNING

Unmet Needs

Exercise, protection from physical harm, mastery and competence in skills, increased learning

Expected Outcome

Correct verbal feedback of the information taught
Correct return demonstration of how to exercise
Person participates in an exercise program

NURSING INTERVENTIONS

Nursing Treatments

Provide temporary assistance until the skill is learned
Encourage the person to ask questions

Nursing Observations

Observe for fatigue, for complaints of pain
Observe for readiness to assume self-care
Determine teaching effectiveness by testing, verbal feedback, and return demonstration

Health Teaching

Instruct to exercise at least three times a week on nonconsecutive days
Instruct to exercise 20–30 minutes each session (warm-up 3–5 minutes, conditioning 10–20 minutes, cooling 3–5 minutes)
Explain that rhythmic and repetitive exercises are most effective (arm and leg movements should be performed over and over again)
Instruct to increase exercise tolerance gradually (over several months)
Inform of the warning signs to stop exercising (abnormal heart rate or rhythm, pain or pressure in the arm, throat, or chest, dizziness, impaired coordination, confusion, cold sweats, pallor or cyanosis, fainting)

Inform of the warning signs to exercise less vigorously (nausea and vomiting, severe breathlessness, prolonged fatigue, front or side leg pain and muscle cramps, pain beneath the ribs, acute insomnia, an elevated heart rate persisting 5–10 minutes after ceasing to exercise)

Inform of the contraindications to exercise (fever, acute illness, elevated blood pressure, cardiac condition, chest pain, emphysema, gout, hyperthyroidism, dyspnea, intermittent claudication, or any chronic illness)

Inform of the American Heart Association's recommended exercise schedule (see specifics in Part Four)

Explain how to evaluate the pulse after exercise (count for 10 seconds and multiply by 6 immediately after stopping the exercise, and check for a normal pulse range)

Teach how to locate and count the pulse (if needed)

Explain the reason for and intended effect of the methods used (exercise strengthens muscles, increases circulation, lowers blood pressure, uses up excess calories)

EVALUATION
Record actual outcome

Knowledge Deficits Associated with Speech Impairment

UNSKILLED AT ESOPHAGEAL SPEECH [705,706,707]

ASSESSMENT
Data Collection
Subjective Data
- Person's discussion or questions indicate a need for additional information, clarification, or validation of information about performing the task
  OR
- Person's lack of questions or comments indicates not wanting information or not knowing enough to seek information about performing the task
  Person may not know:
    About esophageal speech
    Whom to contact to learn esophageal speech

Objective Data
- Person cannot correctly demonstrate how to:
    Perform esophageal speech

Data Analysis
Nursing Diagnosis
UNSKILLED AT ESOPHAGEAL SPEECH: Being nonproficient, with or without knowledge, in the performance of the specific task of speaking through control of the esophagus rather than the larynx

Common Etiology (Stressors)
HEALTH CARE FACTORS: Lack of health instruction, lack of health-skill experience

PLANNING
Unmet Needs
Communication, mastery and competence in skills, increased learning

Expected Outcome
Correct verbal feedback of the information taught
Correct return demonstration of how to use esophageal speech

NURSING INTERVENTIONS
Nursing Treatments
Provide temporary assistance until the skill is learned
Encourage the person to ask questions
Limit the conversation to short discussions (when esophageal speech is being learned)
Make a referral (to a speech therapist)
Encourage the use of esophageal speech as directed by the speech therapist

Nursing Observations
Determine teaching effectiveness by testing, verbal feedback, and return demonstration

Health Teaching
Explain that communication should be encouraged despite impairment
Explain that ill persons are often hypersensitive (about their speech impairment)
Explain the reason for and intended effect of the therapy

EVALUATION
Record actual outcome

UNKNOWLEDGEABLE ABOUT COPING WITH A SPEECH-IMPAIRED PERSON [47,381,448,490,679]

ASSESSMENT
Data Collection
Subjective Data
- Person's discussion or questions indicate a need for additional information, clarification, or validation of information
  OR
- Person's lack of questions or comments indicates not wanting information or not knowing enough to seek information
- When questioned directly, the person's response or lack of response indicates that he does not know:
  The best methods to use when communicating with a person having impaired communication
  About assistive communication devices
  The most effective psychologic approach to use with persons having impaired communication
  The resources available, such as speech therapists

Objective Data
- May exhibit behavior such as acting inappropriately based on insufficient knowledge by shouting at the speech-impaired person or criticizing the speech-impaired person when his attempts to communicate fail

Data Analysis
Nursing Diagnosis
UNKNOWLEDGEABLE ABOUT COPING WITH A SPEECH-IMPAIRED PERSON: Being without sufficient information regarding the most effective approach for communicating with a person having an impaired ability to exchange thoughts and ideas with others

Common Etiology (Stressors)
HEALTH CARE FACTORS: Lack of health instruction

PLANNING

Unmet Needs
Comfort, caring and communicating relationships, increased learning

Expected Outcome
Correct verbal feedback of the information taught
Person exhibits behavior modification in communicating with the speech-impaired person

NURSING INTERVENTIONS

Nursing Treatments
Encourage the person or family to ask questions
Encourage simple signal language during impaired communication (signals for yes or no, such as blinking the eyes and moving the fingertip up and down)
Make a referral (to a speech therapist if needed)

Nursing Observations
Determine teaching effectiveness by verbal feedback

Health Teaching
Advise against whispering around ill persons
Advise that communications be delayed during fatigue (and that messages be given only when the person is receptive)
Describe those behaviors that usually occur in communication impairment (frustration, embarrassment, irritation, agitation)
Explain that communication should be encouraged despite impairment (since it reduces the sense of isolation from others)
Explain that questions need to be phrased for yes and no answers when there is impaired speech delivery
Explain the importance of correct message interpretation
Instruct to use simple words when speaking with persons having impaired communication reception
Recommend the use of slow, distinct speech with persons having impaired communication reception
Relate specific methods for improving communications with speech-impaired persons (such as allowing time for thought comprehension, immediately correcting misinterpreted messages, using nonverbal communication, limiting communication to one person at a time, keeping discussions short, using assistive devices such as alphabet letters, word and phrase cards, and a writing pad and pencil, not asking a person to repeat a message too often, not shouting at the person, waiting for a response to one message before delivering another)
Advise that normal, not accentuated, lip movements be used when speaking to hearing-impaired persons
Recommend communication by gesture (if needed)
Advise against responding to gesture speech (of a child aged 1–3, who prefers gesturing to verbalizing)
Explain the reason for and intended effects of the methods used

EVALUATION

Record actual outcome

24 Nursing Diagnoses of SPIRITUAL CARE

Dual Domain of Nursing Expertise: Spiritual Care

This chapter covers that sphere of nursing knowledge and skill related to problems of human spiritual or religious relationships as they are affected by illness and suffering. These problems are solved by nurses, physicians, ministers, and chaplains.

Views of Nursing Leaders That Support This Domain of Nursing Expertise

Nursing practice focuses on human beings—on man in his entirety and wholeness.

Martha Rogers[419:127]

By basic nursing care I mean helping the patient to worship according to one's faith.

The nurse will be alert to what gives the patient physical and spiritual comfort and will seek out for him the person's needs to attain this comfort.

Virginia Henderson[221:16 & 27]

As a part of the nursing process nurses must be aware of the existence of spiritual needs and must provide for them in the plan of care when the occasion arises.

Alice Rine and Mildred Montag[111:71]

Spiritual Problems Associated with Illness and Suffering

SPIRITUAL AWARENESS RELATED TO A LIFE SITUATION[157,266,456,599,771]

ASSESSMENT

Data Collection

Subjective Data
- Person verbalizes that he alone is not sufficient
- Relates a need for a more meaningful spiritual relationship
- May request spiritual assistance
  May relate searching for a spiritual source of strength
  May verbalize about a broken or neglected spiritual relationship
  Relates an increased interest in spiritual matters

Objective Data
- May exhibit behavior such as reading spiritual books, viewing or listening to spiritual programs, attending religious services, engaging in quiet contemplation

Data Analysis

Nursing Diagnosis
SPIRITUAL AWARENESS RELATED TO A LIFE SITUATION: An ongoing consciousness of a need for a more positive spiritual force in one's life during a difficult life situation

Common Etiology (Stressors)
BIRTH DEFECTS: Giving birth to an imperfect infant
DISEASES: Any serious disease
INJURIES: Severe trauma of any kind
SIGNS AND SYMPTOMS: Pain, weakness
PSYCHOSOCIAL FACTORS: An attempt to change the direction of one's life, the threat of loss of control of a life situation, lack of emotional support from others, the threat of inadequacy, lack of meaning and purpose in one's life, the threat of chronic or severe stress
HEALTH CARE FACTORS: *Medical diagnosis*: An unfavorable diagnosis. *Health therapy*: Painful medical, drug, or surgical health therapy, long-term therapy. *Prognosis*: An unfavorable prognosis
SITUATIONAL FACTORS: Surviving an accident or disaster, death of a significant other, divorce from a spouse or of parents, loss of employment, lack of finances, loss of a home, terminal illness, living alone, childrearing, pregnancy

PLANNING

Unmet Needs
Comfort, acceptance, personal growth and maturity, spiritual satisfaction

Expected Outcome
Person verbalizes feelings about spiritial matters
Relates satisfaction with personal spiritual growth

NURSING INTERVENTIONS

Nursing Treatments
Provide an atmosphere of acceptance
Encourage the expression of feelings
Encourage discussion of the person's spiritual values

Listen attentively
Provide desired spiritual articles
Provide spiritual reading material
Encourage the chaplain's visit
Provide information (about spiritual programs on the radio and television or in the chapel and as to how the person can reach the chaplain)

Nursing Observations
Evaluate the significance of spirituality in the person's life
Observe for a favorable response to spiritual care

Health Teaching
Explain that the person's response is both appropriate and commonly experienced

EVALUATION
Record actual outcome

SPIRITUAL DISTRESS RELATED TO DISRUPTED SPIRITUAL PRACTICES [157,266,456,599,771]

ASSESSMENT
Data Collection
Subjective Data
• Person verbalizes definite spiritual/religious values
• Expresses concern that the values are being threatened
• May request assistance with spiritual matters
  May relate that it is difficult to take part in usual spiritual practices such as attendance at spiritual services and obtaining and conforming to specific food requirements for the particular religious belief
  May relate that suggested therapy is contrary to one's basic spiritual beliefs

Objective Data
• May exhibit behavior such as demanding and controlling behavior, unusual quietness, crying, sleeplessness, restlessness

Data Analysis
Nursing Diagnosis
SPIRITUAL DISTRESS RELATED TO DISRUPTED SPIRITUAL PRACTICES: Troubled concern about threats to one's belief system when one is unable to practice familiar spiritual rituals

Common Etiology (Stressors)
DISEASES: Any severe disease
INJURIES: Any severe injury
SIGNS AND SYMPTOMS: Pain, weakness
HEALTH CARE FACTORS: *Health care system*: Rigid health care system. *Hospitalization/Institutionalization:* Any
DEVELOPMENTAL PHASES: Old age

PLANNING
Unmet Needs
Comfort, protection from psychologic threat, caring and communicating relationships, spiritual satisfaction

Expected Outcome
Person will have the required foods, spiritual articles, etc., needed to maintain spiritual practices

Will relate feeling satisfied with his spiritual practices even if ability to participate is limited

NURSING INTERVENTIONS

Nursing Treatments

Provide an atmosphere of acceptance

Honor religious dietary regulations

Encourage the bringing in of outside food (if the institution cannot supply special foods)

Assist with bedside spiritual observances

Guide the person in simple prayer (if such is desired)

Pray with the person (if he requests that someone pray with him)

Provide desired spiritual articles (such as a bible)

Provide information (about substitute spiritual programs on the radio or television or in the chapel)

Provide spiritual reading material (if requested)

Listen attentively (to the person's spiritual concerns)

Encourage the expression of feelings

Encourage chapel service attendance

Encourage the chaplain's visit (or that of other spiritual advisors)

Prepare the patient for the clergy's visit

Nursing Observations

Observe for evidence of a favorable response to spiritual care (expressions of satisfaction with special foods, spiritual articles, prayers)

Health Teaching

Explain the reason for and intended effect of the spiritual care (to meet the needs of the whole person)

EVALUATION

Record actual outcome

SPIRITUAL DISTRESS RELATED TO A LIFE SITUATION [156,266,456,599,771]

ASSESSMENT

Data Collection

Subjective Data

• Person verbalizes definite spiritual/religious values

• Expresses concern that the values are being threatened

• May request assistance with spiritual matters

Person is unable to perceive the situation as having meaning to himself or others

Cannot determine why the situation has occurred or what good will come from it

May question the purpose of his own existence

May openly discuss a loss of confidence in the spiritual forces in his life

Objective Data

• May exhibit behavior such as changes in spiritual rituals, displaced anger toward religious representatives such as a chaplain, priest, or minister, as well as unusual quietness, crying, restlessness, sleeplessness

Data Analysis

Nursing Diagnosis

SPIRITUAL DISTRESS RELATED TO A LIFE SITUATION: Troubled concern about threats to one's belief system during a difficult life situation

Common Etiology (Stressors)

BIRTH DEFECTS: Giving birth to an imperfect infant

DISEASES: Any serious disease

INJURIES: Severe trauma of any kind

SIGNS AND SYMPTOMS: Pain, weakness

PSYCHOSOCIAL FACTORS: The threat of loss of control of a life situation, lack of emotional support from others, lack of meaning and purpose in one's life

HEALTH CARE FACTORS: *Medical diagnosis*: An unfavorable diagnosis. *Prognosis*: An unfavorable prognosis

SITUATIONAL FACTORS: The death of a significant other, divorce from a spouse or of parents, loss of employment, lack of finances, loss of a home, terminal illness

PLANNING

Unmet Needs

Comfort, acceptance, caring and communicating relationships, personal growth and maturity, spiritual satisfaction

Expected Outcome

Person verbalizes feelings about spiritual matters

Relates comfort and satisfaction from spiritual resources during a difficult life situation

NURSING INTERVENTIONS

Nursing Treatments

Provide an atmosphere of acceptance

Encourage the expression of feelings

Encourage discussion of the person's spiritual values

Assist the person in setting standards of a meaningful existence

Explore with the person his (spiritual) strengths and resources

Support a realistic assessment of the situation

Encourage the chaplain's visit

Nursing Observations

Evaluate the significance of spirituality in the person's life

Observe for a favorable response to spiritual care

Health Teaching

Explain that the person's response is both appropriate and commonly experienced

EVALUATION

Record actual outcome

25 Nursing Diagnoses of WELLNESS

Dual Domain of Nursing Expertise: Wellness

This chapter covers that sphere of nursing knowledge and skill related to patterns of healthy behavior and lifestyle that promote a high level of health in an asymptomatic person. This domain involves supporting health behavior that makes healthy persons healthier, and it includes normal body changes during developmental phases and reproduction. These diagnoses are identified and supported by nurses and physicians.

Views of Nursing Leaders That Support This Domain of Nursing Expertise

The concept of wellness as the maximum level of well-being that an individual can achieve is a relatively recent development in the health field. Precise determination of an individual's level of wellness is largely in the realm of untested theory. But nurses have a clear responsibility to make an estimate of the level of wellness of each patient and to attempt to help him raise that level to its maximum potential.

Alice Rine & Mildred Montag[411:183]

Professional practice in nursing seeks to promote symphonic interaction between man and environment, to strengthen the coherence and integrity of the human field, and to direct and redirect patterning of the human and environmental fields for realization of maximum health potential.

Martha Rogers[419:122]

If the patient is adapting, the nursing goal is to maintain that response.

Sister Callista Roy[410:140]

Nurses have a primary role . . . in promoting wellness—living to one's fullest capacity.

Pamela Mitchell[379:79]

Wellness Responses of Children

WELL BABY/INFANT[94,313,323]

ASSESSMENT

Data Collection

Subjective Data
• Parent may relate data about the baby
Objective Data
• Age from birth through 12 months
• Developmental and physical findings include:

Emotional Development
Exhibits trust by behavior such as cooing, smiling, sleeping after being fed, waiting for
    short periods without protest to be fed or diapered

Cognitive (Mental) Development
Loud noises stimulate the Moro reflex, a touch on the face elicits the rooting reflex, a
    stroke on the sole of the foot elicits the Babinski reflex
Age 1–4 months:
    Focuses attention on objects
    Reaches for and grasps object
    Sucks on grasped objects
    Discriminates by sucking on one object and discarding another
Age 4–7 months:
    Shakes a rattle, to hear the noise
    Repeats the same action with other objects
    Recognizes his bottle, stops fussing when he sees it
Age 7–10 months:
    Searches for objects out of view
    Can move objects
    Becomes investigative
    Touches, shakes, bites, and tastes objects

Language Development
Babbles at about 6 months
Uses double syllables such as "dada" and "mama" at about 8 months
Speaks two or three words at about 12 months

Growth and Physical Changes
Length:
    Birth length is 47.5–53.7 cm (19–21.5 inches); in relationship to total body length the
        head is 25%, trunk 50%, legs 25%
    Up to age 6 months length is increased by approximately 1 inch/month
    At age 7–12 months length is increased by approximately 0.5 inch/month
Weight:
    Birth weight is from 2.500–4.300 g (4.5–9.5 lb)
    At age 5 months birth weight is doubled
    At age 12 months birth weight is tripled
Head:
    34–35 cm (13.5–14 inches in circumference)
    At age 3–4 months posterior fontanelle is closed
    At age 12–18 months anterior fontanelle is closed
Chest:
    At birth the chest circumference is about 1 inch less than the head circumference
    By 1–2 years the chest and head circumference are about equal

Teeth:
  Newborn has no teeth
  At age 6–9 months the central incisors erupt
  At age 12 months has eight teeth, and the lower and upper central and lateral incisors
    erupt
Hearing:
  Responds appropriately to sound
Vision:
  Visually follows a bright object from side to side
  Newborn responds visually only to near objects
  At age 12 months the child responds visually to distant objects
Heart and pulse rate:
  Newborn: 120–140 beats/minute
  Age 12 months: 120–140 beats/minute
Blood pressure:
  Newborn: 80/46 mm Hg
  Age 12 months: 96/66 mm Hg
Respirations:
  Newborn: 30–80 breaths/minute
  Age 12 months: 20–40 breaths/minute
Temperature:
  Slightly higher than an adult's
Hemoglobin:
  Newborn: 19 g/100 ml of blood
  Age 12 months: 12 g/100 ml of blood
Hematocrit:
  Newborn: 55%–68%
  Age 12 months: 29%–41%

Motor Development
Birth through 3 months:
  Infant sucks, roots, jerks, and spreads his limbs in response to external stimuli
  Can lift the head when prone and crawl forward
  Opens and closes his hands
  Moves his fists to his mouth and moves his arms about freely
Age 4–6 months:
  Infant uses his arms, shoulders and legs to turn over
  When pulled to a sitting position, he holds his head in line with his back
  May sit momentarily without support
  Kicks his legs
  Can grasp objects and move them to his mouth
Age 7–9 months:
  Infant assumes the sitting position alone
  Can pull himself up
  Will walk around his crib holding onto the sides
  Crawls and creeps
  Can transfer objects from one hand to another
  Bangs two objects together
  Holds his own bottle
Age 10–12 months:
  Infant can easily change from a lying to a sitting to a standing position
  Walks when holding someone's hand
  Stands alone for a moment or so
  Takes a step or two alone before falling
  Climbs onto furniture, boxes, and up stairs on all four limbs
  Grasps small objects
  Uses a cup and possibly a spoon

Nutrition
Infant breast- or bottle-feeds
Around age 6 months, he eats puréed or strained foods, as one at a time are introduced
into the diet

Sleeping
Newborn sleeps 16–20 hours/day
At age 6 months, the infant sleeps 10 hours at night, taking three naps a day
At age 12 months, he sleeps 10–12 hours at night and takes one long nap or two short
naps during the day

Eating
Newborn consumes breast or bottle milk every 2 hours
At age 6–8 months, the infant consumes breast or bottle milk three or four times a day,
eats three meals a day, has hand-to-mouth motions, and can feed himself a cracker
At age 9–12 months, he holds his bottle and drinks from a cup with help, feeds himself
finger foods, and begins to hold a spoon

Play
Moves about to entertain himself
Responds to stimulating objects such as mobiles

Data Analysis

Nursing Diagnosis
WELL BABY/INFANT: An infant, from birth to age 12 months, who shows evidence of conforming to standards of normalcy for that developmental level

Common Etiology
INHERITED FACTORS: The inheritance of normal genes/chromosomes *Note*: A baby may have
an inherited deformity resulting from abnormal chromosomes and still be considered
a well baby, for instance, a child with a cleft lip may essentially be a well child.
HUMAN BODY: A state of physiologic homeostasis
HEALTH CARE FACTORS: High-quality health care delivery
LIFESTYLE (MATERNAL LIFESTYLE): The consistent practice of sound health principles by the
newborn's mother during pregnancy
SITUATIONAL FACTORS: The presence of adequate resources for the gratification of basic
physiologic and psychologic needs

PLANNING

Unmet Needs
Continued development of potential, continued learning

Expected Outcome
The toddler's parent or care provider relates feelings of personal satisfaction for having
achieved wellness for the child
The toddler's parent or care provider continues to practice wellness behavior

NURSING INTERVENTIONS

Nursing Treatments
Encourage new goals at past goal achievement (new goals for higher levels of wellness)
Encourage the parent to ask questions (about wellness behavior)
Encourage the expression of feelings (about the satisfaction of practicing wellness be-
havior)
Offer praise (for the parents' practice of wellness behavior)

Nursing Observations
Make a follow-up evaluation (at a later date to determine whether the state of wellness
still exists and if wellness behavior is still being practiced)

Health Teaching
Recommend the continued practice of wellness behavior

EVALUATION

Record actual outcome

WELL TODDLER[94,313,323]

ASSESSMENT

Data Collection

Subjective Data
• Parent may relate data about the toddler

Objective Data
• Age 12–30 months
• Developmental and physical findings include the following:

Emotional Development

Exhibits autonomy by independent behaviors such as negativism in which he separates himself from his parents by stating "no," having temper tantrums, going limp when he does not want to be picked up, exploring his limited world, and moving toward some degree of self-control over impulses

He exhibits self-awareness by behaviors such as exploring his body and naming body parts

Cognitive (Mental) Development

Toddler uses his memory to imitate his parents

Solves problems by imitating others, at about age 12 months

Exhibits new ways to solve problems by use of his intelligence, at about 24 months of age

Uses words to symbolize objects such as "dooe" for dog

Uses objects as symbols such as a block for a train

Does not understand logic because he can only understand from his point of view and not from the viewpoint of others

Language Development

At age 12–18 months uses only a few words meaningfully

At age 18 months and after demonstrates having learned new words each day, learns nouns first such as "kitty," "ball," etc.

Growth and Physical Changes

Height:

   By age 24 months the birth height is doubled and the toddler reaches approximately half his adult height

   Head and trunk growth slows considerably

   Arms and legs begin to lengthen

Weight:

   By age 24 months the birth weight has quadrupled

   After 24 months normal weight gain is considered to be 4 ½–6 lb/year

Head:

   At age 1–2 years, the head and chest are about equal in circumference

   Age 18 to 19 months the anterior fontanelles are closed

Chest:

   After 2 years of age, the chest becomes larger than the head

Teeth:

   At age 24 months, toddler has 20 primary teeth

Hearing:
  Responds to sound with acute hearing
Vision:
  After age 24 months the toddler can identify the pictures of a tree, house, or car on
    the Allen cards
  After age 30 months the child can correctly identify the direction the Es are facing on
    the Denver Eye Screening Test (DEST, E test)
Heart and pulse rate
  90–100 beats/minute
Blood pressure:
  About 95/65
Respirations:
  About 25 breaths/minute
Hemoglobin:
  At age 24 months 11–12 g/100 ml of blood
Hematocrit:
  At age 12 months 40%
  At age 24 months 43%

Motor Development
Age 13–15 months:
  Progresses from a few unsteady steps to a "waddling" walk and even running, can
    walk forward and backward
  Can stack two blocks
  Uses a spoon for soft foods
  Scribbles with a pencil or crayon
At age 18 months:
  Toddler walks well
  Runs while pulling toys
  Walks up stairs but not down stairs
  Can push stools, chairs, small tables
  Can climb to get things
  Puts small objects through an opening
  Stacks two or three blocks and knocks them down
  Uses a spoon and cup, but often spills food and drink
  Scribbles with a pencil or crayon
At age 24 months:
  Walks up and down stairs
  Jumps and runs
    Pedals a riding toy
  Climbs on furniture
  Stacks blocks and delights in smashing them down
  Draws with a pencil and crayon, but prefers finger painting
  Feeds self with only an occasional spill
  Puts on some of his clothes by himself
At age 30 months:
  Can put puzzles together
  Fits objects into the right slot

Nutrition
At age 24 months the toddler:
  Wants to decide what he eats
  Needs and eats less food
  Enjoys using a spoon
  No longer drinks from a bottle, so he decreases his fluid intake

Sleeping
At age 13 to 15 months he sleeps 16–20 hours/day
Beyond 15 months of age he sleeps about 12 hours a night
Sleeps 2 hours during the afternoon

Eating
Eats three meals a day
Requires a mid-morning and mid-afternoon snack to prevent irritability
Likes to eat finger foods

Toilet Training
Learns anal and bladder sphincter control

Play
Learns to socialize with peers while playing
Does not share things with others yet

Data Analysis

Nursing Diagnosis
WELL TODDLER: A young child, from age 12–30 months, who shows evidence of conforming to standards of normalcy for that developmental level

Common Etiology
INHERITED FACTORS: The inheritance of normal genes/chromosomes
HUMAN BODY: A state of physiologic homeostasis
HEALTH CARE FACTORS: High-quality health care delivery
LIFESTYLE (OF TODDLER'S SIGNIFICANT OTHERS): The consistent practice of sound health principles by the toddler's parents or care providers

SITUATIONAL FACTORS: The presence of adequate resources for the gratification of basic physiologic and psychologic needs

PLANNING

Unmet Needs
Continued development of potential, continued learning

Expected Outcome
The infant's parent or care provider relates feelings of personal satisfaction for having achieved wellness for the infant
The infant's parent or care provider continues to practice wellness behavior

NURSING INTERVENTIONS

Nursing Treatments
Encourage new goals at past goal achievement (new goals for higher levels of wellness)
Encourage the parent to ask questions (about wellness behavior)
Encourage the expression of feelings (about the satisfaction of practicing wellness behavior)
Offer praise (for the parents' practice of wellness behavior)

Nursing Observations
Make a follow-up evaluation (at a later date to determine whether the state of wellness still exists and whether wellness behavior is still being practiced)

Health Teaching
Recommend the continued practice of wellness behavior

EVALUATION
Record actual outcome

WELL PRESCHOOL CHILD[94,313,323]

ASSESSMENT

Data Collection

Subjective Data
• Parent or child may relate any data

Emotional Development
Believes that his wishes cause things to happen
Achieves sexual identity by usually identifying with the parent of the same sex

Objective Data
• Age 3–6 years
• Developmental and physical findings include:

Emotional Development
Exhibits initiative by assuming some responsibility
Takes risks by attempting and accomplishing new tasks and endeavors
Explores his world and questions the "why" of things
Actions are based on a developing sense of conscience
Exhibits behavior relating creative thinking
May talk to or about an imaginary friend who helps him cope with the normal fears and anxieties of his age
Begins to investigate his body
Exhibits interest in where babies come from by asking questions

Cognitive (Mental) Development
Exhibits the behavior of focusing on only one thing at a time
Begins to learn and understand the concepts of time, space, number, class, and causality

Language Development
By age 6 years:
  Uses about 2,500 words
  Understands and speaks in sentences
  Participates in noncomplex family discussions
  Repeatedly uses his favorite words "why," "what," "when," and "how"
  May stutter, since he thinks faster than he can speak
  May use "bad" words for shock effect or as a way of breaking rules

Growth and Physical Changes
Height:
  Gains approximately 7 cm, or 2.75 inches, each year
  Arms and legs are longer in proportion to the trunk
  Has a slimmer, taller appearance
Weight:
  Gains approximately 2 kg (4.5 lb) each year
Head and chest:
  Chest grows more rapidly than the head
Teeth:
  No loss or gain of teeth
Hearing:
  Responds to sound with acute hearing
Vision:
  Early preschool age: 20/40 visual acuity
  Later preschool age: 20/20 or 20/30 visual acuity
Heart and pulse rate:
  90–100 beats/minute
Blood pressure:
  About 100/65

Respirations:
   About 20–30 breaths/minute
Hemoglobin:
   Early preschool age: 11.5 to 12.5 g/100 ml
      Later preschool age: 12 to 13 g/100 ml
Hematocrit:
   Age 3–6 years: 43%

Motor Development
Age 3 years:
   Walks up and down stairs
   Runs at full speed
   Climbs on climbing equipment
   Jumps from place to place
   Draws, colors, and paints
   Uses scissors with difficulty
Age 4 years:
   Runs, jumps, climbs with confidence
   Rides a bicycle
   Draws pictures in recognizable shapes
   Skillfully cuts large objects with a scissor
Age 5 years:
   Plays marching or dancing games
   Sits and listens to brief stories
   Practices fine and gross motor skills

Nutrition
Likes to choose and plan what he will eat
Prefers finger foods

Sleeping
May no longer nap during the day
Sleeps longer at night

Eating
Demonstrates an interest in and begins to learn table manners

Play
Age 3 years:
   Begins to share willingly
Age 4 years:
   Enjoys groups and group games

Data Analysis

Nursing Diagnosis
WELL PRESCHOOL CHILD: A child, age 3–6 years, who shows evidence of conformity to standards of normalcy for that developmental level

Common Etiology
INHERITED FACTORS: The inheritance of normal genes/chromosomes
PSYCHOSOCIAL FACTORS: Exposure to a role model who practices wellness behavior, positive self-attitudes, positive health attitudes
HUMAN BODY: A state of physiologic and psychosocial homeostasis
HEALTH CARE FACTORS: High-quality health care delivery
LIFESTYLE: The consistent practice of sound health principles by the preschool child and his parents or care providers.
SITUATIONAL FACTORS: The presence of adequate resources for the gratification of basic physiologic and psychologic needs

PLANNING

Unmet Needs
Continued development of potential, continued learning

Expected Outcome
The preschool child relates feelings of personal satisfaction for having achieved wellness
The child continues to practice wellness behavior

NURSING INTERVENTIONS

Nursing Treatments
Encourage new goals at past goal achievement (new goals for higher levels of wellness)
Encourage the parents and child to ask questions (about wellness behavior)
Encourage the expression of feelings (about the satisfaction of practicing wellness behavior)
Offer praise (for the child's practice of wellness behavior)

Nursing Observations
Make a follow-up evaluation (at a later date to determine whether the state of wellness still exists and whether wellness behavior is still being practiced)

Health Teaching
Recommend the continued practice of wellness behavior

EVALUATION
Record actual outcome

WELL SCHOOL-AGE CHILD[94,313,323]

ASSESSMENT

Data Collection

Subjective Data
• Parent or child may relate any data

Emotional Development
Feels the pressure of persons outside the family such as peers and teachers
By age 12 years, can assess his strengths and weaknesses without severe inferiority feelings
Questions parental values
Understands the concept of death and feels anxious about it

Objective Data
• Age 6–12 years
• Developmental and physical findings include the following:

Emotional Development
Person exhibits industry by attempting to accomplish a task and completing it to the satisfaction of the standards he has set
Interacts with and learns to relate to peers and adults outside the family
Yields to peer pressure in play, dress, hobbies, and language
Joins a group of schoolchildren of the same sex and rigidly adheres to the group's rules

Cognitive (Mental) Development
Person exhibits conceptual and logical thinking in concrete situations, but not in abstract situations
Understands and can complete several related steps in achieving task or problem solving
Is capable of thinking in reverse, from finish to start
Is able to categorize objects according to characteristics

Language Development
Person uses complex sentence structure
Participates in enjoyable rhymes, riddles, and chants
Uses language for problem solving

Growth and Physical Changes
Height:
   Gains about 5 cm (2 inches) each year
   At age 9 girls begin a growth spurt
   At age 11 boys begin a growth spurt
   Arms and legs lengthen faster than the trunk
   General body appearance is thin
Weight:
   Gain of 3 kg (6.6 lb) each year, mostly during the later school years
   Average weight is 37–41 kg (81–90 lb)
Head:
   Little head growth
Chest:
   No significant change
Teeth:
   At about age 6 years primary teeth begin to loosen
   At about age 12 years all primary teeth are gone
   Permanent teeth erupt
Hearing:
   Responds to sound with acute hearing
Vision:
   Visual acuity of 20/20, with 20/30 being acceptable
Heart and pulse rate:
   67–90 beats/minute
Blood pressure:
   About 110/60 in late school age
Respirations:
   About 19 breaths/minute
Hemoglobin:
   14 g/100 ml
Hematocrit:
   Age 6 years: 43%
   Age 7 to 12 years: 46%

Motor Development
Person shows a preference for either right or left hand dominance
Competes in sports activities
Writes well, draws, paints
Exhibits interest in hobbies, electronic games

Nutrition
Has a daily intake of 2,200–2,400 calories
During prepubescent growth, child takes in an additional 400 calories/day

Sleeping
Early school age: about 10–12 hours of sleep nightly
Older school age: about 8–10 hours of sleep nightly

Eating
Person eats and requires three meals a day and an afterschool snack

Play
Person is involved in games, hobbies, and organized sports
Collects things

Data Analysis

Nursing Diagnosis
WELL SCHOOL-AGE CHILD: A child, age 6–12 years, who shows evidence of conforming to the standards of normalcy for that developmental level

Common Etiology
INHERITED FACTORS: The inheritance of normal genes/chromosomes

PSYCHOSOCIAL FACTORS. Positive self-attitudes, positive health attitudes, exposure to a role model who practices or practiced wellness behavior

HUMAN BODY: A state of physiologic and psychosocial homeostasis

HEALTH CARE FACTORS: High-quality health care delivery, correct and sufficient health instruction

LIFESTYLE: The consistent practice of sound health principles by the school-age child and his parents or care providers

SITUATIONAL FACTORS: The presence of adequate resources for gratification of basic physiologic and psychologic needs

PLANNING

Unmet Needs

Continued development of potential, continued learning

Expected Outcome

School-age child relates feelings of personal satisfaction for having achieved wellness
Continues to practice wellness behavior

NURSING INTERVENTIONS

Nursing Treatments

Encourage new goals at past goal achievement (new goals for higher levels of wellness)
Encourage the child and parents to ask questions (about wellness behavior)
Encourage the expression of feelings (about the satisfaction of practicing wellness behavior)
Offer praise (for the child's practice of wellness behavior)

Nursing Observations

Make a follow-up evaluation (at a later date to determine whether the state of wellness still exists and whatever wellness behavior is still being practiced)

Health Teaching

Recommend the continued practice of wellness behavior

EVALUATION

Record actual outcome

WELL ADOLESCENT[26,233,463]

ASSESSMENT

Data Collection

Subjective Data
• Parent or adolescent may relate any data

Emotional Development
Person may relate the onset of sexual feelings
Achieves self-acceptance

Objective Data
• Age 12–20 years
• Developmental and physical findings include:

Emotional Development
Person exhibits independence by behavior that makes him emotionally independent of parents and adults
Assumes appropriate masculine or feminine roles
Assumes increased social responsibility
Attempts different methods of coping with life situations

Tests different value systems as a basis for self-behavior
Experiments with dating and sexual relatedness

Cognitive (Mental) Development
Person develops intellectual skills
Displays increasing use of ability to reason, assess, and evaluate
Capable of abstract thinking and complex relationships such as the relationship of
    speed, distance, and time in traveling
Begins to think beyond the present into the future
Selects a future occupation

Language Development
Person makes full use of the cultural language
Has a set of special words for group communications

Growth and Physical Changes
Height:
    Girls gain 5–25 cm (2–10 inches)
    Boys gain 10–30 cm (4–12 inches)
    Evidence of a growth spurt, representing the final 20–25% of growth
    Gangly, awkward appearance
Weight:
    Girls gain of 6.8–24.8 kg (15 to 55 lbs) increased subcutaneous fat
    Boys gain of 6.8–29 kg (15–65 lb), increased muscle mass and strength
Head:
    Brain and skull reach near adult size by age 15
    Facial structures change and enlarge during adolescence, forehead becomes higher
        and wider, nose lengthens, and jaw enlarges to adult size
Chest:
    The chest size increases first in breadth, then in depth
    Breast tissue develops in adolescent girls
Teeth:
    The second permanent molars are present by age 12 years
    Braces for straightening malpositioned teeth may be applied
Third permanent molars, the wisdom teeth, usually erupt in late adolescence (18–25
    years)
Hearing:
    Acute
Vision:
    Visual acuity of 20/20
Heart and pulse rate:
    Approximately 70–75 beats/minute
Blood pressure:
    About 120/60
Respirations:
    About 16–18 breaths/minute
Temperature:
    About 98.6°F
Hemoglobin:
    Adult level (*Male*: 14–18 g/100 ml. *Female*: 12–16 g/100 ml)
Hematocrit:
    Adult level (*Male*: 40–54%. *Female*: 37–47%)

Secondary Sex Characteristics
Girls:
    Breast development
    Growth of pubic hair
    Growth of axillary hair about 1 year after appearance of pubic hair
    Menstruation
    Ovulation about 1 year after menstruation onset

Boys:
  Growth of testes and scrotum which appear to be red, wrinkled, and coarse
  Growth of pubic hair
  Growth of penis about 1 year later
  Maturation of the prostate and seminal vesicles
  Ejaculation
  Some increase in breast size
  Facial, axillary, and body hair growth about 2 years after pubic hair growth
  Deepening of the voice tone

Motor Development
Rapid skeletal growth occurs, but is accompanied by a significant lag in muscular growth (especially in girls)
Sports, weight lifting, and gymnastics develop muscles and promote good posture and graceful movement, overcoming the awkwardness
Motor skills development becomes more intricate and involved (dancing, sports, driving motor vehicles, needlework)

Nutrition
In girls, caloric intake of 2,300–2,500 per day
In boys, caloric intake of 2,800–3,000 per day
Increased protein intake (needs 50–60 g/day)
Learns to regulate nutritional needs

Sleeping
Person learns to regulate sleep needs
Increased rest and sleep are needed to balance the increased activity and high stress levels

Eating
Person learns to regulate food and fluid intake
Has an increased appetite

Play and Exercise
Person participates in sports and physical fitness programs
Learns to regulate exercise needs
Prefers group and team activities, especially paired couples activities (dancing, movies, etc.)

Data Analysis

Nursing Diagnosis
WELL ADOLESCENT: A young person, aged 12–20 years, who shows evidence of conforming to the standards of normalcy for that developmental level

Common Etiology
INHERITED FACTORS: The inheritance of normal genes/chromosomes
PSYCHOSOCIAL FACTORS: Positive self-attitudes, positive health attitudes, exposure to a role model who practices wellness behavior
HUMAN BODY: State of physiologic and psychosocial homeostasis
HEALTH CARE FACTORS: High-quality health care delivery, correct and sufficient health instruction
LIFESTYLE: The consistent practice of sound health principles by the adolescent
SITUATIONAL FACTORS: The presence of adequate resources for the gratification of basic physiologic and psychologic needs

PLANNING

Unmet Needs
Continued development of potential, continued learning

Expected Outcome
Adolescent relates feelings of personal satisfaction for having achieved wellness
Continues to practice wellness behavior

NURSING INTERVENTIONS

Nursing Treatments

Reassure verbally (that the body changes are normal and to be expected)

Encourage new goals at past goal achievement (new goals for higher levels of wellness)

Encourage the person to ask questions (about wellness behavior)

Encourage the expression of feelings (about the satisfaction of practicing wellness behavior)

Offer praise (for the adolescent's practice of wellness behavior)

Nursing Observations

Make a follow-up evaluation (at a later date to determine whether the state of wellness still exists and whether wellness behavior is still being practiced)

Health Teaching

Recommend the continued practice of wellness behavior

EVALUATION

Record actual outcome

Wellness Responses of Young Adults

HIGH-LEVEL WELL, YOUNG ADULT[24,26,110,136,140,162,463,485]

ASSESSMENT

Data Collection

Subjective Data
• Person relates using energy to move in a forward direction of expanding personal growth
• Verbalizes that the future is perceived as an opportunity to develop unique potential
• Relates an interest in all aspects of life involving the total person, including a history of the following:

Self-Responsibility
Relates feeling responsible for his own wellness
States that he feels in control of personal choices

Emotional Development
Young adult relates changes in his psychologic view of himself
Relates he is learning to cope with the gain or loss of significant others
Verbalizes about adapting to environmental changes, such as moving to a new city or home, buying a new car or clothes
Relates being able to adjust to changes in his body image or physical self

Developmental Achievements or Tasks
Person has achieved or is in the process of achieving all the developmental tasks expected at this life phase
Relates being involved in the following:
  Achieving emotional, physical, and economic independence from parents
  Defining and practicing his own sense of values by altering, retaining, or modifying the moral, ethical, political, or religious values of his parents or society
  Forming intimate relationships with persons outside the family
  Choosing a mate, starting a family, rearing children, managing a home
  Establishing a lifestyle

Assuming social responsibility
Identifying his unique personal identity
Selecting and pursuing a career in which he can develop his unique self

Sexuality
Person exhibits peak interest in sexual activity before age 20
Expresses satisfaction with own sexuality and with sexual relatedness with another

Communications
Person openly expresses feelings, ideas, and thoughts while maintaining sensitivity to
the feelings of others
Relates feeling comfortable when expressing love and concern for others

Creativity or Productivity
Person is constantly involved in self-motivated creative activity
Relates feeling good about his life work and life plan
States that specific efforts are made to continue the growth of the mind even if the body
grows weak

Spirituality
Person has or is in the process of identifying values satisfactory to himself
Consistently applies the same values to multiple life roles

Safety Awareness
Person practices most all recommendations for personal and environmental safety

Environmental Awareness
Person relates a sensitivity to nature's beauty
Concerned with saving and restoring environmental resources

Community Involvement
Person is well informed about local, national, and international events
Consistently participates in community events (such as voting) and community organiza-
tions (social, church, or political groups)

Stress Management
Person uses effective methods for tension relief
Avoids destructive coping mechanisms (alcohol, drugs, violence)
Spaces major life changes so that he feels comfortable with the changes
Relates being aware of personal behavior that indicates he is under excessive stress (irri-
tability, foot tapping, etc.)
Enjoys leisure time and recreation
Takes an annual vacation
Relates feeling confident and emotionally calm
Relates feeling good about important relationships
Expresses a sense of confidence about obtaining support from close persons

Preventive Health
Person maintains periodic health appraisals
Uses preventive health measures (immunizations, dental prophylaxis)

Physical Status
Maintains the highest level of physical health attainable by the person
Relates no significant physical complaints
Relates being able to complete all tasks of daily living without fatigue
Has an energy reserve sufficient for leisure or evening activities

Sleep Status
Person relates that the amount of sleep obtained is adequate to restore energy, usually
8 hours daily

Exercise Status
Person maintains a consistent exercise schedule (such as running, walking, or bicycling
for at least 30 minutes three times a week)

Nutritional Status
Person eats a balanced diet based on the essential food groups
Avoids or limits the intake of harmful foods such as sweets, salt, fats, or preservatives
Modifies the dietary intake as needed, such as increasing protein intake when under stress

Objective Data
Person is 20–39 years of age

Cognitive (Mental) Functioning
Person exhibits intellectual maturity by carrying out problem-solving skills, refines intellectual capacities with education or job skills

Physical Findings and Characteristics
Person has a fully matured body
All body systems are within normal limits on examination

Data Analysis

Nursing Diagnosis
HIGH-LEVEL WELL, YOUNG ADULT: The use of human energy toward the pursuit of one's highest potential for personal growth by a person 20–39 years of age

Common Etiology
INHERITED FACTORS: The inheritance of normal genes/chromosomes
PSYCHOSOCIAL FACTORS: Positive self-attitudes, positive health attitudes, exposure to a role model who practices or practiced young-adult wellness behavior
HUMAN BODY: A state of physiologic and psychosocial homeostasis
HEALTH CARE FACTORS: High-quality health care delivery, correct and sufficient health instructions
LIFESTYLE: The consistent practice of sound health principles by the young adult
SITUATIONAL FACTORS: The presence of adequate resources for gratification of basic physiologic and psychologic needs

PLANNING

Unmet Needs
Continued development of potential, continued learning

Expected Outcome
The young adult relates feelings of personal satisfaction for having achieved wellness
Continues to practice wellness behavior

NURSING INTERVENTIONS

Nursing Treatments
Reassure verbally (that the body changes are normal and to be expected)
Encourage new goals at past goal achievement (new goals for higher levels of wellness)
Encourage the person to ask questions (about wellness behavior)
Encourage the expression of feelings (about the satisfaction of practicing wellness behavior)
Offer praise (for the person's practice of wellness behavior)

Nursing Observations
Make a follow-up evaluation (at a later date to determine whether the state of wellness still exists and whether wellness behavior is still being practiced)

Health Teaching
Recommend the continued practice of wellness behavior

EVALUATION
Record actual outcome

MODERATE-LEVEL WELL, YOUNG ADULT[24,26,110,136,140,162,463,486]

ASSESSMENT

Data Collection

Subjective Data

• Person relates using energy to maintain the status quo and for occasional efforts at personal growth
• Expresses a primary concern with today, occasionally perceiving that the future offers opportunity for growth
• Relates an interest in only some aspects of life involving the total person, including a history of the following:

Self-Responsibility

Person relates some responsibility for his own wellness, but also relies on others to keep him well (needs reminding to take medications, to keep appointments, etc.)

Emotional Development

Person relates having the capacity, most of the time, to maintain emotional control and to cope effectively with life stressors and situations

Developmental Achievements or Tasks

Person has achieved most of the developmental tasks, but not all the tasks, at this life stage and may compensate for or attempt to achieve tasks that are unrealized
The tasks expected to be achieved are:
  Achieving emotional, physical, and economic independence from his parents
  Defining and practicing his own sense of values by altering, retaining, or modifying the moral, ethical, political, or religious values of his parents or society
  Forming intimate relationships with persons outside the family
  Choosing a mate, starting a family, rearing children, managing a home
  Establishing a lifestyle
  Assuming social responsibility
  Identifying his unique personal identity
  Selecting and pursuing a career in which he can develop his unique self

Sexuality

Person may or may not exhibit peak interest in sexuality before age 20
May or may not express satisfaction with his own sexuality and with sexual relatedness with another

Communications

Person relates having difficulty expressing feelings, ideas, and thoughts and can usually do so with selected persons
Relates being occasionally uncomfortable when expressing love and concern for others

Creativity or Productivity

Person occasionally becomes involved in self-motivated creative activity
Accepts but is not enthusiastic about his life work or life plan

Spirituality

Person has some well-defined spiritual values and some that are vague
May or may not consistently apply the same values to multiple life roles

Safety Awareness

Person practices some recommendations for personal and environmental safety and considers others of no value

Environmental Awareness

Person relates sometimes feeling sensitive to nature's beauty
Has some but not much concern for saving and restoring environmental resources

Community Involvement
Person is fairly well informed about local, national, and international events
Person sometimes participates in community events (such as voting) and community organizations (social, church, or political groups)

Stress Management
Person uses some methods for tension relief, but some are unsatisfactory
May occasionally use destructive coping mechanisms (alcohol, drugs, violence)
Sometimes spaces major life changes so close together that he feels uncomfortable with the change
Relates being aware, only sometimes, of personal behavior that indicates he is under excessive stress (rushing about, yelling at others)
Relates only limited enjoyment of leisure time and recreation
Does not always take an annual vacation
Relates fluctuating feelings of self-confidence
Relates being emotionally calm much of the time with occasional lack of emotional control

Preventive Health
Person sporadically obtains health appraisals
Person uses selected preventive health measures (takes only certain immunizations)

Physical Status
Person maintains a satisfactory level of physical health, but not as high a level as is attainable by the person

Sleep Status
Person relates that the amount of sleep obtained only partially restores energy

Exercise Status
Person exercises sporadically

Nutritional Status
Person eats a partially balanced diet based on the essential food groups
Eats some harmful foods such as sweets, salt, fats, or preservatives
Intermittently modifies the dietary intake but does not persist with the modification, such as increasing protein intake the first day or two of a stressful situation, but then forgetting it

Objective Data
Person is 20–39 years of age

Cognitive (Mental) Functioning
Person carries out reasonable problem-solving abilities and may delay coping with a problem

Physical Findings and Characteristics
Person has a fully matured body
All body systems are within normal limits on examination

Data Analysis

Nursing Diagnosis
MODERATE-LEVEL WELL, YOUNG ADULT: The use of human energy to maintain life's essentials and to move occasionally toward personal growth by a person 20–39 years of age

Common Etiology (Stressors)
PSYCHOSOCIAL FACTORS: Lack of emotional support from others (to achieve high-level wellness), lack of exposure to a role model who practices or practiced young-adult wellness behavior
LIFESTYLE: Cultural norms or traditions

PLANNING

Unmet Needs
Continued development of potential, continued learning

Expected Outcomes

Person verbalizes a desire to achieve a higher level of wellness
Relates a knowledge of the standards of high-level wellness
Demonstrates wellness behavior at his highest achievable level

NURSING INTERVENTIONS

Nursing Treatments

Reassure verbally (that the body changes are normal and to be expected)
Encourage the person to ask questions (about wellness behavior)
Offer praise (for the degree of wellness the person practices)

Nursing Observations

Make a follow-up evaluation (at a later date to determine whether wellness behavior is
    being practiced and to provide positive reinforcement for continued wellness prac-
    tices)

Health Teaching

Explain that change must come from within the person
Teach the specific procedure or method (for achieving a higher level of wellness, such
    as nutrition, exercise, stress management)
Explain the reason for and intended effect of the wellness behavior

EVALUATION

Record actual outcome

LOW-LEVEL WELL, YOUNG ADULT[24,26,110,136,140,162,463,485]

ASSESSMENT

Data Collection

Subjective Data
• Person relates using energy to maintain the status quo
• Verbalizes that the concept of personal growth has little meaning
• Relates primary interest in those aspects of life that involve essential needs, while
    other aspects of life are as follows:

Self-Responsibility
Person relates feeling little or no responsibility for his own wellness
States that the health professionals are responsible for wellness

Emotional Development
Person relates having some difficulty maintaining emotional control and coping effec-
    tively with life stresses and situations

Developmental Achievements or Tasks
Person has achieved few of the developmental tasks expected during this or previous
    life phases
Rarely attempts to achieve those developmental tasks that are unrealized
The tasks expected to be achieved are the following:
    Achieving emotional, physical, and economic independence from his parents

Defining and practicing his own sense of values by altering, retaining, or modifying the moral, ethical, political, or religious values of his parents or society
Forming intimate relationships with persons outside the family
Choosing a mate, starting a family, rearing children, managing a home
Establishing a lifestyle
Assuming social responsibility
Identifying his unique personal identity
Selects and pursues a career in which he can develop his unique self

Sexuality
Person may or may not exhibit peak interest in sexuality before age 20 and may or may not express satisfaction with his own sexuality and with sexual relatedness with another

Communications
Person cannot openly express feelings, ideas, or thoughts or does so with little or no sensitivity to the feelings of others
Relates feeling uncomfortable when expressing love and concern for others

Creativity or Productivity
Person rarely becomes involved in self-motivated creative activity
Relates little enthusiasm for his life work or life plan

Spirituality
Person has poorly defined values for himself
Values change as the person assumes different life roles

Safety Awareness
Person practices very few recommendations for personal and environmental safety

Environmental Awareness
Person relates little sensitivity to nature's beauty
Unconcerned with saving and restoring environmental resources

Community Involvement
Person is uninformed about local, national, and international events
Rarely participates in community events (such as voting) and community organizations (social, church, or political groups)

Stress Management
Person uses few effective methods for tension relief
Often uses destructive coping mechanisms (alcohol, drugs, child abuse, wife battering)
Relates being seldom aware of personal behavior that indicates he is under excessive stress (irritability, shouting)
Seldom takes or enjoys leisure time
May never take a vacation
Relates a persistent feeling of lack of self-confidence
Relates feeling easily threatened and having little emotional control

Preventive Health
Person rarely obtains a health appraisal
Rarely uses preventive health measures (does not make use of immunizations or dental prophylaxis)

Physical Status
Person maintains a level of health far below that which is attainable by the person

Sleep Status
Person relates that the amount of sleep obtained is not adequate to restore energy and is chronically tired

Exercise Status
Person seldom exercises

Nutritional Status
Person eats an unbalanced diet not based on the essential food groups
Eats harmful foods such as sweets, salt, fats, preservatives
Does not modify the dietary intake for special needs

Objective Data
Person is 20–39 years of age

Cognitive (Mental) Functioning
Person demonstrates limited problem-solving abilities
Relies on others to solve the problems

Physical Findings and Characteristics
Person has a fully matured body
All body systems are within normal limits on examination

Data Analysis

Nursing Diagnosis
LOW-LEVEL WELL, YOUNG ADULT: The use of human energy to maintain life's essentials with little or no movement toward personal growth by a person 20–39 years of age

Common Etiology (Stressors)
PSYCHOSOCIAL FACTORS: Unlearned alternative behavior, lack of competency in using effec-
tive coping mechanisms, lack of emotional support from others (to achieve a higher
level of wellness), lack of a defined goal; lack of exposure to a role model who prac-
tices or practiced young-adult wellness behavior
HEALTH CARE FACTORS: Lack of health instruction
LIFESTYLE: Cultural norms or traditions
SITUATIONAL FACTORS: Lack of finances, poverty

PLANNING

Unmet Needs
Continued development of potential, continued learning

Expected Outcome
Person verbalizes a desire to achieve a higher level of wellness
Relates a knowledge of the standards of high-level wellness
Demonstrates wellness behavior at his highest achievable level

NURSING INTERVENTIONS

Nursing Treatments
Reassure verbally (that the body changes are normal and to be expected)
Encourage the person to ask questions (about wellness behavior)
Offer praise (for the degree of wellness the person practices)

Nursing Observations
Make a follow-up evaluation (at a later date to determine whether wellness behavior is
being practiced and to provide positive reinforcement for continued wellness practices)

Health Teaching
Explain that change must come from within the person
Teach the specific procedure or method (for achieving a higher level of wellness, such
as nutrition, exercise, stress management)
Explain the reason for and intended effect of the wellness behavior

EVALUATION
Record actual outcome

Wellness Responses of Middle-Aged Adults

HIGH-LEVEL WELL, MIDDLE-AGED ADULT[24,26,110,136,140,162,463,485]

ASSESSMENT

Data Collection

Subjective Data
- Person relates using energy to move in a forward direction of expanding personal growth
- Verbalizes that the future is perceived as an opportunity to develop his unique potential
- Relates an interest in all aspects of life involving the total person, including a history of the following:

Self-Responsibility
Person relates feeling responsible for his own wellness
States that he feels in control of personal choices

Emotional Development
Person relates having the capacity to maintain emotional control and to cope effectively with life's stresses and situations

Developmental Achievements or Tasks
Person has achieved or is in the process of achieving all the developmental tasks of his life phase
Relates involvement in the following:
  Accepting and adjusting to physiologic changes
  Adjusting to children leaving home and to the loss of the parent role
  Fostering a relationship with his children's spouses
  Adjusting to the grandparent role
  Adjusting to his parents growing old
  Increasing his self-esteem through self-awareness that involves experimenting with what he can and cannot do
  Reviewing and modifying his value system
  Fostering a more clearly defined relationship with his spouse
  Redefining vocational and occupational goals (may change jobs or acquire additional education to achieve these goals)
  Assuming adult social and civic responsibility
  Preparing financially for a future of retirement and old age
  Expanding areas of enjoyment so that he will have many interests when retirement comes

Sexuality
Person relates that he is adjusting to changes in sexual patterns
Expresses satisfaction with his own sexuality and with sexual relatedness with another

Communications
Person openly expresses feelings, ideas, and thoughts while maintaining sensitivity to the feelings of others
Relates feeling comfortable when expressing love and concern for others

Creativity or Productivity
Person is consistently involved in self-motivated creative activity
Relates feeling good about his life work and life plan

States that specific efforts are made to continue the growth of the mind, even if the body grows weak

Spirituality
Person has identified spiritual values satisfactory to himself
Consistently applies the same values to multiple life roles

Safety Awareness
Person practices most all recommendations for personal and environmental safety

Environmental Awareness
Person relates a sensitivity to nature's beauty
Concerned with saving and restoring environmental resources

Community Involvement
Person is well informed about local, national, and international events
Consistently participates in community events (such as voting) and community organizations (social, church, or political groups)

Stress Management
Person uses effective methods for tension relief
Avoids destructive coping mechanisms (alcohol, drugs, violence)
Spaces major life changes so that he feels comfortable with the changes
Relates being aware of personal behavior that indicates he is under excessive stress (irritability, foot tapping, etc.)
Enjoys leisure time and recreation
Takes an annual vacation
Relates feeling confident and emotionally calm
Relates feeling good about important relationships
Expresses a sense of confidence about obtaining support from close persons

Preventive Health
Person maintains periodic health appraisals
Uses preventive health measures (immunizations, dental prophylaxis)

Physical Status
Person maintains the highest level of physical health attainable by the person
Relates some physical complaints such as the following:
    Difficulty reading small print (presbyopia)
    Decreased visual adaptation to the dark
    Hearing difficulties
    Decreased taste sensitivity
    Joint aching
    Chronic backache
    Gastric complaints such as acidity and belching
    Decrease in energy and the capacity for physical work, resulting in less social involvement and the spreading out of social events to accommodate the decreased energy level

Sleep Status
Person relates that the amount of sleep obtained is adequate to restore energy, usually 8 hours daily

Exercise Status
Person maintains a consistent exercise schedule (such as running, walking, bicycling for at least 30 minutes three times a week)

Nutritional Status
Person eats a balanced diet based on the essential food groups
Avoids or limits the intake of harmful foods such as sweets, salts, fats, or preservatives
Modifies the dietary intake as needed, such as increasing protein intake when under stress

Objective Data
Person is 40–60 years of age

Cognitive (Mental) Functioning
Person exhibits intellectual maturity by carrying out problem-solving skills
Refines intellectual capacities with education or job skills

Physical Findings and Characteristics
Person has a fully matured body
All body systems are within normal limits on examination with the following normal changes:
  Weight gain
  Graying hair
  Thinning hair in women
  Baldness in men
  Muscle flabbiness
  Sagging, wrinkled, and dry, scaly skin
  More bony facial appearance with a more dominant nose
  Eye examination reveals farsightedness and decreased peripheral vision
  Audiometry may reveal hearing changes

Data Analysis

Nursing Diagnosis
HIGH-LEVEL WELL, MIDDLE-AGED ADULT: The use of human energy toward the pursuit of one's highest potential for personal growth by a person 40–60 years of age

Common Etiology
INHERITED FACTORS: The inheritance of normal genes/chromosomes
PSYCHOSOCIAL FACTORS: Positive self-attitudes, positive health attitudes, exposure to a role model who practices or practiced middle-age adult wellness behavior
HUMAN BODY: A state of physiologic and psychosocial homeostasis
HEALTH CARE FACTORS: High-quality health care delivery, correct and sufficient health instructions
LIFESTYLE: The consistent practice of sound health principles by the middle-age adult
SITUATIONAL FACTORS: The presence of adequate resources for gratification of basic physiologic and psychologic needs

PLANNING

Unmet Needs
Full development of potential, continued learning

Expected Outcome
Middle-aged adult relates feelings of personal satisfaction for having achieved wellness
Continues to practice wellness behavior

NURSING INTERVENTIONS

Nursing Treatments
Reassure verbally (that the body changes are normal and to be expected)
Encourage new goals at past goal achievement (new goals for higher levels of wellness)
Encourage the person to ask questions (about wellness behavior)
Encourage the expression of feelings (about the satisfaction of practicing wellness behavior)
Offer praise (for the person's practice of wellness behavior)

Nursing Observations
Make a follow-up evaluation (at a later date to determine whether the state of wellness still exists and whether wellness behavior is still being practiced)

Health Teaching
Recommend the continued practice of wellness behavior

EVALUATION

Record actual outcome

MODERATE-LEVEL WELL, MIDDLE-AGED ADULT[24,26,110,136,140,162,463,485]

ASSESSMENT

Data Collection

Subjective Data
- Person relates using energy to maintain the status quo and for occasional efforts at personal growth
- Expresses a primary concern with today, occasionally perceiving that the future offers opportunity for growth
- Relates an interest in only some aspects of life involving the total person, including a history of the following:

Self-Responsibility
Person relates feeling some responsibility for his own wellness, but also relies on others to keep him well (needs reminding to take medications, keep appointments, etc.)

Emotional Development
Person relates having the capacity, most of the time, to maintain emotional control and to cope effectively with life stresses and situations

Developmental Achievement and Tasks
Person has achieved most of the developmental tasks at this and other life stages and may compensate for or attempt to achieve those that are unrealized
Person relates involvement in the tasks expected to be achieved at this developmental stage:
  Accepting and adjusting to the physiologic changes
  Adjusting to children leaving home and to the loss of the parent role
  Fostering a relationship with his children's spouse
  Adjusting to the grandparent role
  Adjusting to his parents growing old
  Increasing his self-esteem through self-awareness, which involves experimenting with what he can and cannot do
  Reviewing and modifying his value system
  Fostering a more clearly defined relationship with his spouse
  Redefining vocational and occupational goals (may change jobs or acquire additional education to achieve these goals)
  Assuming adult social and civic responsibility
  Preparing financially for a future of retirement and old age
  Expanding one's area of enjoyment so that he will have many interests when retirement comes

Sexuality
Person may or may not relate that he is adjusting to changes in sexual patterns and may or may not express satisfaction with his own sexuality and with sexual relatedness with another

Communications
Person relates having difficulty expressing feelings, ideas, and thoughts but can usually do so with selected persons
Relates being occasionally uncomfortable when expressing love and concern for others

Creativity or Productivity
Person occasionally becomes involved in self-motivated creative activity
Accepts but is not enthusiastic about his life work or life plan

Spirituality
Person has some well-defined spiritual values and some that are vague
May or may not consistently apply the same values to multiple life roles

Safety Awareness
Person practices some recommendations for personal and environmental safety
Considers others of no value

Environmental Awareness
Person relates sometimes feeling sensitive to nature's beauty
Has some but not much concern for saving and restoring environmental resources

Community Involvement
Person is fairly well informed about local, national, and international events
Sometimes participates in community events (such as voting) and community organizations (social, church, or political groups)

Stress Management
Person uses some methods for tension relief, but some are unsatisfactory
May occasionally use destructive coping mechanisms (alcohol, drugs, violence)
Sometimes spaces major life changes so close together that he feels uncomfortable with the change
Relates being aware, only sometimes, of personal behavior that indicates he is under excessive stress (rushing about, yelling at others)
Relates only limited enjoyment of leisure time and recreation
Does not always take an annual vacation
Relates fluctuating feelings of self-confidence
Relates being emotionally calm much of the time, with occasional lack of emotional control

Preventive Health
Person sporadically obtains health appraisals
Uses selected preventive health measures (takes only certain immunizations and occasionally uses dental prophylaxis)

Physical Status
Person maintains a satisfactory level of physical health, but not as high a level as is attainable by the person
Relates some physical complaints such as:
    Difficulty reading small print (presbyopia)
    Decreased visual adaptation to the dark
    Hearing difficulties
    Decreased taste sensitivity
    Joint aching
    Chronic backache
    Gastric complaints such as acidity and belching
    Decrease in energy and the capacity for physical work, resulting in less social involvement and the spreading out of social events to accommodate the decreased energy level

Sleep Status
Person relates that the amount of sleep obtained only partially restores energy

Exercise Status
Person exercises sporadically

Nutritional Status
Person eats a partially balanced diet based on the essential food groups
Eats some harmful foods such as sweets, salt, fats, or preservatives
Intermittently modifies the dietary intake but does not persist with the modification, such as increasing protein intake the first day or two of a stressful situation, but then forgetting it

Objective Data
Person is 40–60 years of age

Cognitive (Mental) Functioning
Person carries out reasonable problem-solving abilities
May delay coping with a problem

Physical Findings and Characteristics
Person has a fully matured body
All body systems are within normal limits on examination with the following normal changes:
Weight gain
Graying hair
Thinning hair in women
Baldness in men
Muscle flabbiness
Sagging, wrinkled, and dry, scaly skin
More bony facial appearance with a more dominant nose
Eye examination reveals farsightedness and decreased peripheral vision
Audiometry may reveal hearing changes

Data Analysis

Nursing Diagnosis
MODERATE-LEVEL WELL, MIDDLE-AGED ADULT: The use of human energy to maintain life's essentials and to move occasionally toward personal growth between 40 and 60 years of age

Common Etiology (Stressors)
PSYCHOSOCIAL FACTORS: Lack of emotional support from others (to achieve high-level wellness), lack of exposure to a role model who practices or practiced middle-aged adult wellness behavior.
LIFESTYLE: Cultural norms or traditions

PLANNING

Unmet Needs
Continued development of potential, continued learning

Expected Outcome
Person verbalizes a desire to achieve a higher level of wellness
Relates a knowledge of the standards of high-level wellness
Demonstrates wellness behavior at his highest achievable level

NURSING INTERVENTIONS

Nursing Treatments
Reassure verbally (that the body changes are normal and to be expected)
Encourage the person to ask questions (about wellness behavior)
Offer praise (for the degree of wellness the person practices)

Nursing Observations
Make a follow-up evaluation (at a later date to determine whether wellness behavior is being practiced, and to provide positive reinforcement for continued wellness practices)

Health Teaching
Explain that change must come from within the person
Teach the specific procedure or method (for achieving a higher level of wellness, such as nutrition, exercise, stress management)
Explain the reason for and intended effect of the wellness behavior

EVALUATION

Record actual outcome

LOW-LEVEL WELL, MIDDLE-AGED ADULT [24,26,110,136,140,162,463,485]

ASSESSMENT

Data Collection

Subjective Data
- Person relates using energy to maintain the status quo
- Verbalizes that the concept of personal growth has little meaning
- Relates primary interest in those aspects of life that involve essential needs, and other aspects of life are as follows:

Self-Responsibility
Person relates feeling little or no responsibility for his own wellness
States that the health professionals are responsible for wellness

Emotional Development
Person relates having some difficulty maintaining emotional control and coping effectively with life stresses and situations

Developmental Achievements and Tasks
Person has achieved few of the developmental tasks during this and other life phases
Rarely attempts to achieve those developmental tasks that are unrealized
The tasks expected to be achieved at this developmental stage are:
  Adjusting to children leaving home and to the loss of the parent role
  Fostering a relationship with his children's spouses
  Adjusting to the grandparent role
  Adjusting to his parents growing old
  Increasing his self-esteem through self-awareness that involves experimenting with what he can and cannot do
  Reviewing and modifying his value system
  Fostering a more clearly defined relationship with his spouse
  Redefining vocational and occupational goals
  Assuming adult social and civic responsibility
  Preparing financially for a future of retirement and old age
  Expanding areas of enjoyment so that he will have many interests when retirement comes

Sexuality
Person may or may not relate that he is adjusting to changes in sexual patterns and may or may not express satisfaction with his own sexuality and with sexual relatedness with another

Communications
Person cannot openly express feelings, ideas, or thoughts or does so with little or no sensitivity to the feelings of others
Relates feeling uncomfortable when expressing love and concern for others

Creativity or Productivity
Person rarely becomes involved in self-motivated creative activity
Relates little enthusiasm for his life work or life plan

Spirituality
Person has poorly defined values for himself
Values change as the person assumes different life roles

Safety Awareness
Person practices very few recommendations for personal and environmental safety

Environmental Awareness
Person relates little sensitivity to nature's beauty
Unconcerned with saving and restoring environmental resources

Community Involvement
Person is uninformed about local, national, and international events
Rarely participates in community events (such as voting) and community organizations
(social, church, or political groups)

Stress Management
Person uses few effective methods for tension relief
Often uses destructive coping mechanisms (alcohol, drugs, child abuse, wife battering)
Relates being seldom aware of personal behavior that indicates he is under excessive
stress (irritability, shouting)
Seldom takes or enjoys leisure time
May never take a vacation
Relates a persistent feeling of lack of self-confidence
Relates feeling easily threatened and having little emotional control

Preventive Health
Person rarely obtains a health appraisal
Rarely uses preventive health measures (does not make use of immunizations or dental
prophylaxis)

Physical Status
Person maintains a level of health far below that attainable by the person
Relates some physical complaints such as the following:
    Difficulty reading small print (presbyopia)
    Decreased visual adaptation to the dark
    Hearing difficulties
    Decreased taste sensitivity
    Joint aching
    Chronic backache
    Gastric complaints such as acidity and belching
    Decrease in energy and the capacity for physical work, resulting in less social involve-
    ment and the spreading out of social events to accommodate the decreased energy
    level

Sleep Status
Person relates that the amount of sleep obtained is not adequate to restore energy and
is chronically tired

Exercise Status
Person seldom exercises

Nutritional Status
Person eats an unbalanced diet not based on the essential food groups
Eats harmful foods such as sweets, salts, fats, and preservatives
Does not modify the dietary intake for special needs

Objective Data
Person is 40–60 years of age

Cognitive (Mental) Functioning
Demonstrates limited problem-solving abilities
Relies on others to solve the problems

Physical Findings and Characteristics
Person has a fully matured body

All body systems are within normal limits on examination with the following normal changes:
Weight gain
Graying hair
Thinning hair in women
Baldness in men
Muscle flabbiness
Sagging, wrinkled, and dry, scaly skin
More bony facial appearance with a more dominant nose
Eye examination reveals farsightedness and decreased peripheral vision
Audiometry may reveal hearing changes

Data Analysis

Nursing Diagnosis
LOW-LEVEL WELL, MIDDLE-AGED ADULT: The use of human energy to maintain life's essentials with little or no movement toward personal growth, during 40–60 years of age

Common Etiology (Stressors)
PSYCHOSOCIAL FACTORS: Unlearned alternative behavior, lack of competency in using effective coping mechanisms, lack of emotional support from others (to achieve a higher level of wellness), lack of a defined goal, lack of resources to achieve a goal, lack of exposure to a role model who practices or practiced middle-aged adult wellness behavior
HEALTH CARE FACTORS: Lack of health instruction
LIFESTYLE: Cultural norms or traditions
SITUATIONAL FACTORS: Lack of finances, poverty

PLANNING

Unmet Needs
Continued development of potential, continued learning

Expected Outcome
Person verbalizes a desire to achieve a higher level of wellness
Relates a knowledge of the standards of high-level wellness
Demonstrates wellness behavior at his highest achievable level

NURSING INTERVENTIONS

Nursing Treatments
Reassure verbally (that the body changes are normal and to be expected)
Encourage the person to ask questions (about wellness behavior)
Offer praise (for the degree of wellness the person practices)

Nursing Observations
Make a follow-up evaluation (at a later date to determine whether wellness behavior is being practiced and to provide positive reinforcement for continued wellness practices)

Health Teaching
Explain that change must come from within the person
Teach the specific procedure or method (for achieving a higher level of wellness, such as nutrition, exercise, stress management)
Explain the reason for and intended effect of the wellness behavior

EVALUATION
Record actual outcome

Wellness Responses of Aged Adults

HIGH-LEVEL WELL, AGED ADULT[24,26,110,136,140,162,463,485]

ASSESSMENT

Data Collection

Subjective Data

- Person relates using energy to move in a forward direction of expanding personal growth
- Verbalizes that the future is perceived as an opportunity to develop his unique potential
- Relates an interest in all apsects of life involving the total person, including a history of the following:

Self-Responsibility
Person relates feeling responsible for his own wellness
States that he feels in control of personal choices

Emotional Development
Person relates having the capacity to maintain emotional control and to cope effectively with life stresses and situations

Developmental Achievements or Tasks
Person has achieved or is in the process of achieving all the developmental tasks expected at this life phase
Person relates being involved in:
  Thinking of aging as a positive experience, focusing on what he learned from life instead of on what he did wrong, and using introspection to resolve his concerns with the past
  Making adjustments to physical limitations through changes in living accommodations, role, and so forth
  Gaining greater control of his daily schedule than he had in the past and structuring his day to fit his own pleasure
  Adjusting to driving at mid-morning and early afternoon for safety reasons
  Maintaining self-esteem by being of service to someone else and enriching the lives of others, and working through church, senior citizens, and volunteer groups
  Making preparations for death by completing unfinished business and discussing death with his family and how he wishes to die or be buried
  Deciding when he will retire, and where he will live when retired, and determining how to supplement retirement income if such is needed

Sexuality
Person may relate a continued interest in sex and participation in the normal sexual activity of an aged person and expresses satisfaction with his own sexuality and with sexual relatedness with another

Communications
Person openly expresses feelings, ideas, and thoughts while maintaining sensitivity to the feelings of others
Relates feeling comfortable when expressing love and concern for others

Creativity or Productivity
Person is consistently involved in self-motivated creative activity
Relates feeling good about his life work and life plan
States that specific efforts are made to continue the growth of the mind, even if the body grows weak

Spirituality
Person has identified spiritual values satisfactory to himself
Consistently applies the same values to multiple life rules

Safety Awareness
Person practices most all recommendations for personal and environmental safety

Environmental Awareness
Person relates a sensitivity to nature's beauty
Concerned with saving and restoring environmental resources

Community Involvement
Person is well informed about local, national, and international events
Consistently participates in community events (such as voting) and community organizations (social, church, or political groups)

Stress Management
Person uses effective methods for tension relief
Avoids destructive coping mechanisms (alcohol, drugs, violence)
Spaces major life changes so that he feels comfortable with the changes
Relates being aware of personal behavior that indicates he is under excessive stress (irritability, foot tapping)
Enjoys leisure time and recreation
Takes an annual vacation
Relates feeling confident and emotionally calm
Relates feeling good about important relationships
Expresses a sense of confidence about obtaining support from close persons

Preventive Health
Person maintains periodic health appraisals
Uses preventive health measures (immunizations, dental prophylaxis)

Physical Status
Maintains the highest level of physical health attainable by the person
Relates some physical complaints such as the following:
  Decreased visual acuity (caused by loss of lens elasticity, reduced pupil size)
  Chilliness (due to loss of fatty tissue and impaired temperature regulation)
  Dry, itchy skin
  Skin easily bruises (due to fragile blood vessels)
  Dizziness (due to decreased cerebral circulation)
  Joint aching and stiffness
  Loss of teeth
  Decreased sense of taste and smell
  Constipation
  Poor appetite
  Urinary retention, incontinence, and dribbling (in men due to the enlarged prostate)
  Decreased energy level (in men due to a sharp decrease in testosterone levels, which causes a decline in muscle strength and aggressiveness)
  Hot flashes, sweating, depression, and nightmares (in men during their 70s)
  Vaginal dryness and painful intercourse (in women due to a decreased estrogen level)

Sleep Status
Person relates that he sleeps shorter hours at night and may nap during the day

Exercise Status
Person consistently participates in moderate exercise such as brisk walking

Nutritional Status
Person eats a balanced diet based on the essential food groups
Has appropriate calorie intake (women eat approximately 1,800 calories daily, men eat approximately 2,000 calories daily)

Avoids or limits the intake of harmful foods such as sweets, salt, fats, or preservatives

Modifies the dietary intake as needed, such as increasing protein intake when under stress

Objective Data

Person is over 60 years of age

Cognitive (Mental) Functioning

Person may not readily learn new concepts because of loyalty to old values

Needs more time when integrating changes

Takes longer to reach conclusions

Exhibits poor memory for recent events and good memory for remote events

Shows reduced interest in creative thinking

Physical Findings and Characteristics

Nose becomes elongated

Skin wrinkles

Shoulders stoop

Abdomen bulges and droops

Chin doubles

Nails become thick, tough, and brittle

Breasts shrink and droop in women

Enlargement of the prostate gland in men (due to decreased hormone secretion)

Audiometer may reveal decreased hearing (due to increased rigidity of the middle ear bones)

Slower reaction time (due to a decreased rate of conduction of nerve impulses)

Decreased muscle strength

Increased systolic blood pressure

Data Analysis

Nursing Diagnosis

HIGH-LEVEL WELL, AGED ADULT: The use of human energy, toward the pursuit of one's highest potential for personal growth by an individual older than 60 years of age

Common Etiology

INHERITED FACTORS: The inheritance of normal genes

PSYCHOSOCIAL FACTORS: Positive self-attitudes, positive health attitudes, exposure to a role model who practices or practiced aged-adult wellness behavior

HUMAN BODY: A state of physiologic and psychosocial homeostasis

HEALTH CARE FACTORS: High-quality health care delivery, correct and sufficient health instructions

LIFESTYLE: The consistent practice of sound health principles by the aged adult

SITUATIONAL FACTORS: The presence of adequate resources for gratification of basic physiologic and psychologic needs

PLANNING

Unmet Needs

Continued development of potential, continued learning

Expected Outcome

Aged person relates feelings of personal satisfaction for having achieved wellness

Continues to practice wellness behavior

NURSING INTERVENTIONS

Nursing Treatments

Reassure verbally (that the body changes are normal and to be expected)

Encourage new goals at past goal achievement (new goals for higher levels of wellness)

Encourage the person to ask questions (about wellness behavior)

Encourage the expression of feelings (about the satisfaction of practicing wellness behavior)

Offer praise (for the person's practice of wellness behavior)

Nursing Observations

Make a follow-up evaluation (at a later date to determine whether the state of wellness still exists and whether wellness behavior is still being practiced)

Health Teaching

Recommend the continued practice of wellness behavior

EVALUATION

Record actual outcome

MODERATE-LEVEL WELL, AGED ADULT[24,26,110,136,140,162,463,485]

ASSESSMENT

Data Collection

Subjective Data

- Person relates using energy to maintain the status quo and for occasional efforts at personal growth
- Expresses a primary concern with today, occasionally perceiving that the future offers opportunity for growth
- Relates an interest in only some aspects of life involving the total person, including a history of the following:

Self-Responsibility

Person relates feeling some responsibility for his own wellness, but also relies on others to keep him well (needs reminding to take medications, to keep appointments, etc.)

Emotional Development

Person relates having the capacity, most of the time, to maintain emotional control and to cope effectively with life stresses and situations

Developmental Achievements

Person has achieved most of the developmental tasks expected at different life stages and may compensate for or attempt to achieve those that are unrealized

Person relates being involved in the tasks expected to be achieved at this life stage:

Thinking of aging as a positive experience, focusing on what he learned from life instead of on what he did wrong, and using introspection to resolve his concerns with the past

Making adjustments to his physical limitations through changes in living accommodations, role, etc.

Gaining greater control of his daily schedule than he had in the past and structuring his day to fit his own pleasure

Adjusting to driving at mid-morning and early afternoon for safety reasons

Maintaining self-esteem by being of service to someone else and enriching the lives of others and working through church, senior citizen, and volunteer groups

Making preparations for death by completing unfinished business and discussing death with his family and how he wishes to die or be buried

Deciding when he will retire, where he will live when retired, and how to supplement retirement income if such is needed

Communications

Person relates having difficulty expressing feelings, ideas, and thoughts and can usually do so with selected persons

Relates being occasionally uncomfortable when expressing love and concern for others

Creativity or Productivity

Person occasionally becomes involved in self-motivated creative activity

Accepts but is not enthusiastic about his life work or life plan

Spirituality
Person has some well-defined spiritual values and some that are vague
May or may not consistently apply the same values to multiple life roles

Safety Awareness
Person practices some recommendations for personal and environmental safety
Considers others of no value

Sexuality
Person may or may not relate a continued interest in sex and participation in the normal sexual activity of an aged person and may or may not express satisfaction with his own sexuality and with sexual relatedness with another

Environmental Awareness
Person relates sometimes feeling sensitive to nature's beauty
Has some but not much concern for saving and restoring environmental resources

Community Involvement
Person is fairly well informed about local, national, and international events
Sometimes participates in community events (such as voting) and community organizations (social, church, or political groups)

Stress Management
Person uses some methods for tension relief, but some are unsatisfactory
May occasionally use destructive coping mechanisms (alcohol, drugs, violence)
Sometimes spaces major life changes so close together that he feels uncomfortable with the change
Relates being aware, only sometimes, of personal behavior that indicates he is under excessive stress (rushing about, yelling at others)
Relates only limited enjoyment of leisure time and recreation
Does not always take an annual vacation
Relates fluctuating feelings of self-confidence
Relates being emotionally calm much of the time with occasional lack of emotional control

Preventive Health
Person sporadically obtains health appraisals
Uses selected preventive health measures (takes only certain immunizations)

Physical Status
Person maintains a satisfactory level of physical health, but not as high a level as is attainable by the person
Relates some physical complaints such as the following:
    Decreased visual acuity (due to loss of lens elasticity, reduced pupil size)
    Chilliness (due to loss of fatty tissue and impaired temperature regulation)
    Dry, itchy skin
    Skin easily bruises (due to fragile blood vessels)
    Dizziness (due to decreased cerebral circulation)
    Joint aching and stiffness
    Loss of teeth
    Decreased sense of taste and smell
    Constipation
    Poor appetite
    Urinary retention, incontinence, and dribbling (in men due to the enlarged prostate)
    Decreased energy level (in men due to a sharp decrease in testosterone levels, which causes a decline in muscle strength and aggressiveness)
    Hot flashes, sweating, depression, and nightmares (in men during their 70s)
    Vaginal dryness and painful intercourse (in women due to a decreased estrogen level)

Sleep Status
Person relates that the amount of sleep obtained only partially restores energy

Exercise Status
Person exercises sporadically

Nutritional Status
Person eats a partially balanced diet based on the essential food groups
Eats some harmful foods such as sweets, salt, fats, or preservatives
Intermittently modifies the dietary intake, but does not persist with the modification, such as increasing protein intake the first day or two of a stressful situation, but then forgetting it

Objective Data
Person is over age 60 years

Cognitive (Mental) Functioning
Person may not readily learn new concepts due to loyalty to old values
Needs more time when integrating changes
Takes longer to reach conclusions
Exhibits poor memory for recent events and good memory for remote events
Shows reduced interest in creative thinking

Physical Findings and Characteristics
Nose becomes elongated
Skin wrinkles
Shoulders stoop
Abdomen bulges and droops
Chin doubles
Nails become thick, tough, and brittle
Breasts shrink and droop in women
Enlargement of the prostate gland in men (due to decreased hormone secretion)
Audiometer may show decreased hearing (due to increased rigidity of the middle ear bones)
Slower reaction time (due to a decreased rate of conduction of nerve impulses)
Decreased muscle strength
Increased systolic blood pressure

Data Analysis

Nursing Diagnosis
MODERATE-LEVEL WELL, AGED ADULT: The use of human energy to maintain life's essentials and to move occasionally toward personal growth by an individual older than 60 years of age

Common Etiology (Stressors)
PSYCHOSOCIAL FACTORS: Lack of emotional support from others (to achieve high-level wellness), lack of exposure to a role model who practices or practiced aged-adult wellness behavior
LIFESTYLE: Cultural norms or traditions

PLANNING

Unmet Needs
Continued development of potential, continued learning

Expected Outcome
Person verbalizes a desire to achieve a higher level of wellness
Relates a knowledge of the standards of high-level wellness
Demonstrates wellness behavior at his highest achievable level

NURSING INTERVENTIONS

Nursing Treatments
Reassure verbally (that the body changes are normal and to be expected)
Encourage the person to ask questions (about wellness behavior)
Offer praise (for the degree of wellness the person practices)

Nursing Observations

Make a follow-up evaluation (at a later date to determine whether wellness behavior is being practiced and to provide positive reinforcement for continued wellness practices)

Health Teaching

Explain that change must come from within the person

Teach the specific procedure or method (for achieving a higher level of wellness, such as nutrition, exercise, stress management)

Explain the reason for and intended effect of the wellness behavior

EVALUATION

Record actual outcome

LOW-LEVEL WELL, AGED ADULT[24,26,110,136,140,162,463,485]

ASSESSMENT

Data Collection

Subjective Data

• Person relates using energy to maintain the status quo
• Verbalizes that the concept of personal growth has little meaning
• Relates primary interest in those aspects of life that involve essential needs, while other aspects of life are as follows:

Self-Responsibility

Person relates feeling little or no responsibility for his own wellness

States that the health professionals are responsible for wellness

Emotional Development

Person relates having some difficulty maintaining emotional control, and coping effectively with life stresses and situations

Developmental Achievements

Person has achieved few of the developmental tasks expected during the life phases

Rarely attempts to achieve those developmental tasks unrealized

The tasks that are to be expected to be achieved are:

   Thinking of aging as a positive experience, focusing on what he learned from life instead of on what he did wrong, and using introspection to resolve his concerns with the past

   Making adjustments to physical limitations through changes in living accommodations, role, etc.

   Gaining greater control of his daily schedule than he had in the past and structuring his day to fit his own pleasure

Adjusting to driving at mid-morning and early afternoon for safety reasons

Maintaining self-esteem by being of service to someone else and enriching the lives of others and working through church, senior citizen, and volunteer groups

   Making preparations for death by completing unfinished business and discussing death with his family and how he wishes to die or be buried

   Deciding when he will retire, where he will live when retired, and how to supplement retirement income if such is needed

Sexuality

Person may or may not relate a continued interest in sex and participation in the normal sexual activity of an aged person and may or may not express satisfaction with his own sexuality and with sexual relatedness with another

Communications
Person cannot openly express feelings, ideas, or thoughts or does so with little or no sensitivity to the feelings of others
Relates feeling uncomfortable when expressing love and concern for others

Creativity or Productivity
Person rarely becomes involved in self-motivated creative activity
Relates little enthusiasm for his life work or life plan

Spirituality
Person has poorly defined values for himself
Values change as the person assumes different life roles

Safety Awareness
Person practices very few recommendations for personal and environmental safety

Environmental Awareness
Person relates little sensitivity to nature's beauty
Unconcerned with saving and restoring environmental resources

Community Involvement
Person is poorly informed about local, national, and international events
Rarely participates in community events (such as voting) and community organizations (social, church, or political groups)

Stress Management
Person uses few effective methods for tension relief
Often uses destructive coping mechanisms (alcohol, drugs, child abuse, wife battering)
Relates being seldom aware of personal behavior that indicates he is under excessive stress (irritability, shouting)
Seldom takes or enjoys leisure time
May never take a vacation
Relates a persistent feeling of lack of self-confidence
Relates feeling easily threatened and having little emotional control

Preventive Health
Person rarely obtains a health appraisal
Rarely uses preventive health measures (does not make use of immunizations or dental prophylaxis)

Physical Status
Person maintains a level of health far below that which is attainable by the person
Relates some physical complaints such as the following:
    Decreased visual acuity (due to loss of lens elasticity, reduced pupil size)
    Chilliness (due to loss of fatty tissue and impaired temperature regulation)
    Dry, itchy skin
    Easily bruised skin (due to fragile blood vessels)
    Dizziness (due to decreased cerebral circulation)
    Joint aching and stiffness
    Loss of teeth
    Decreased sense of taste and smell
    Constipation
    Poor appetite
    Urinary retention, incontinence, and dribbling (in men due to the enlarged prostate)
    Decreased energy level (in men due to a sharp decrease in testosterone levels, which causes a decline in muscle strength and aggressiveness)
    Hot flashes, sweating, depression, and nightmares (in men during their 70s)
    Vaginal dryness and painful intercourse (in women due to a decreased estrogen level)

Sleep Status
Person relates that the amount of sleep obtained is not adequate to restore energy, is chronically tired

Exercise Status
Person seldom exercises

Nutritional Status
Person eats an unbalanced diet not based on the essential food groups
Eats harmful foods such as sweets, salt, fats, and preservatives
Does not modify dietary intake for special needs

Objective Data
Person is over 60 years of age

Cognitive (Mental) Functioning
Person may not readily learn new concepts due to loyalty to old values
Needs more time when integrating changes
Takes longer to reach conclusions
Exhibits poor memory for recent events and good memory for remote events
Shows reduced interest in creative thinking

Physical Findings and Characteristics
Nose becomes elongated
Skin wrinkles
Shoulders droop
Abdomen bulges and droops
Chin doubles
Nails become thick, tough, and brittle
Breasts shrink and droop in women
Enlargement of the prostate gland in men (due to decreased hormone secretion)
Audiometer may reveal decreased hearing (due to increased rigidity of the middle ear bones)
Slower reaction time (due to a decreased rate of conduction of nerve impulses)
Decreased muscle strength
Increased systolic blood pressure

Data Analysis

Nursing Diagnosis
LOW-LEVEL WELL, AGED ADULT: The use of human energy to maintain life's essentials with little or no movement toward personal growth by an individual older than 60 years of age

Common Etiology (Stressors)
PSYCHOSOCIAL FACTORS: Lack of emotional support from others (to achieve high-level wellness), lack of exposure to a role model who practices or practiced old-age wellness behavior
LIFESTYLE: Cultural norms or traditions
SITUATIONAL FACTORS: Lack of finances, poverty

PLANNING

Unmet Needs
Continued development of potential, continued learning

Expected Outcome
Person verbalizes a desire to achieve a higher level of wellness
Relates a knowledge of the standards of high-level wellness
Demonstrates wellness behavior at his highest achievable level

NURSING INTERVENTIONS

Nursing Treatments
Reassure verbally (that the body changes are normal and to be expected)
Encourage the person to ask questions (about wellness behavior)
Offer praise (for the degree of wellness the person practices)

Nursing Observations

Make a follow-up evaluation (at a later date to determine whether wellness behavior is being practiced and to provide positive reinforcement for continued wellness practices)

Health Teaching

Explain that change must come from within the person

Teach the specific procedure or method (for achieving a higher level of wellness, such as nutrition, exercise, stress management)

Explain the reason for and intended effect of the wellness behavior

EVALUATION

Record actual outcome

Wellness Responses of Women in Pregnancy

NORMAL PREGNANCY[50,239,388,527]

ASSESSMENT

Data Collection

Subjective Data

Early Pregnancy
Woman relates the cessation of menstruation
Relates a feeling of breast fullness
Complains of fatigue
No history of complicating diseases or injuries

Sixth Week of Pregnancy
Woman may relate morning or afternoon nausea

First 3–4 Months of Pregnancy
Woman relates increased urinary frequency

Fourth Month of Pregnancy
Woman relates feeling a quickening sensation or fetal movement

Throughout the Pregnancy
Woman may complain of the following:
  Nausea
  Vomiting
  Heartburn
  Flatulence
  Constipation
  Varicose veins
  Hemorrhoids
  Leg cramps
  Shortness of breath
  Dizziness during position change
  Abdominal pain from stretching of the round ligaments
  Backache
  Fatigue

Insomnia
Yellow or white vaginal discharge
Itching

Objective Data
Early Pregnancy
Increased breast size and firmness
Enlargement and darkening of the breast nipples and areolae
Prominence of the breast veins
Pale yellow discharge from the breast nipples
Chadwich's sign (a dark blue or purple appearance of the vaginal lining)
Appearance of abdominal striae

Second Month of Pregnancy
Goodell's sign (softening of the uterus)

Sixth Week of Pregnancy
Hegar's sign (the isthmus of the uterus feels soft and compressible)

First 3–4 Months of Pregnancy
On palpation, the uterus feels round, soft, and doughy
Enlargement of the abdomen
Normal weight gain of about 2–4 lb during the first 3 months

Fourth and Fifth Months of Pregnancy
Ballottement (rebounding of the fetus to its original position when the examiner pushes against the abdomen)
Fetal heart tones can be heard at a rate of 120–160 beats/minute
Normal weight gain of about 1 lb/week, until the pregnancy terminates, with a total gain of about 24–28 lb

Fifth Month of Pregnancy
Active fetal movement can be felt on palpation of the abdomen

Throughout the Pregnancy
Braxton-Hicks contractions (alternately hard and soft, palpable, uterine contractions)
Measurement in centimeters, from the symphysis pubis to the top of the fundus, is approximately the same as the number of weeks of gestation (for example, if the fundus height is 32 cm, gestation is 32 weeks)

Laboratory Findings
Hematocrit (34% or above)
White blood count (increased white blood cells up to 12,000/mm^3)
Rh-positive blood type
Urinalysis and urine culture (within normal limits)
Serology (negative)
Cervical smear (negative for gonorrhea and Papanicolaou screening)
Rubella screen (positive antibody titer for rubella)
Blood sugar (within normal limits)

Data Analysis
Nursing Diagnosis
NORMAL PREGNANCY (NORMAL ANTEPARTUM PERIOD) (UNCOMPLICATED PREGNANCY): A condition of being with child in which the woman and fetus show evidence of conformity to standards of normalcy during pregnancy

Common Etiology
HUMAN BODY: A state of physiologic and psychologic homeostasis
HEALTH CARE FACTORS: High-quality health care delivery, correct and sufficient health information or instruction
LIFESTYLE: The consistent practice of sound health principles

PLANNING

Unmet Needs

Protection from physical harm, increased learning

Expected Outcome

Woman will practice sound health principles in order to maintain normal pregnancy

NURSING INTERVENTIONS

Nursing Treatments

Provide a balanced nutritional diet
Encourage moderate physical exercise
Encourage adequate rest
Discourage the intake of oral stimulants
Discourage smoking
Withhold all drugs (unless prescribed by a physician)

Nursing Observations

Specific to the Initial Visit
Measure the pelvic size
Monitor blood studies for blood type
Monitor blood studies for Rh factor
Monitor blood studies for positive VDRL
Monitor the Papanicolaou smear results for positive findings
Obtain a bacterial culture (for evidence of gonorrhea)

Initial and Follow-up Visits
Monitor the fetal heart sounds
Palpate the uterus for fundus height
Inspect the breasts for abnormalities
Inspect for edema and for bleeding
Inspect the vagina for discharge (especially bleeding)
Measure the body weight
Monitor the blood pressure
Monitor blood studies for abnormal hematology (especially for anemia or infection)
Observe for complaints of constipation, of backache, of (vaginal) itching
Test the urine for protein
Test the urine for sugar and acetone

Health Teaching
Recommend that self-medication be avoided
Teach the principles of good nutrition
Explain how to control weight gain during pregnancy
Inform that heavy lifting should be avoided
Emphasize the danger of x-ray exposure during early pregnancy
Describe the danger signs of pregnancy (persistent headache, nausea or vomiting, dizziness, edema, vaginal bleeding or fluid, abdominal pain, absence of fetal movement after the fourth month, acute illness, high fever)
Instruct to report any serious symptoms immediately
Explain why the potential problem could become actual (existing disease or conditions can dangerously affect both mother and fetus)
Explain the reason for and intended effect of the therapy

EVALUATION

Record actual outcome

NORMAL LABOR AND DELIVERY[50,239,388,527]

ASSESSMENT

Data Collection

Subjective Data

Impending Labor

Lightening, that is, she may relate that she felt the infant drop in the abdomen and finds it easier to breathe because of decreased pressure against the diaphragm but now feels increased pelvic pressure

Complains of increased urinary frequency

May complain of leg cramps

First Stage of Labor

Woman complains of a dull, low backache and abdominal tightness

Woman first relates weak, infrequent (10–20 minutes apart) contractions with pain in the back and later in the lower abdomen, lasting 15–30 seconds and gradually increasing in intensity until they are 3–4 minutes apart and last 50–75 seconds

Second Stage of Labor

Woman experiences very forceful contractions

Has an urge to bear down

Third Stage of Labor

Woman experiences minimal or no discomfort during contractions

Relates a feeling of exhilaration at the birth of her child, followed by a feeling of exhaustion

Objective Data

Impending Labor

Lightening, that is, the top of the fundus drops to about midway between the umbilicus and xyphoid process

Bloody show (a pinkish, mucoid vaginal discharge)

First Stage of Labor

Examiner can feel the firmness of the uterus during a contraction by palpating the abdomen

Gradual cervical dilatation to approximately 10 cm that takes no longer than 24 hours

Audible fetal heart sounds

Membranes may rupture during this period

Second Stage of Labor

Rupture of the membranes if they have not already ruptured

Forceful contractions occurring every 2–3 minutes and lasting 50–90 seconds

Increasing perineal bulging

Appearance of the infant head at the perineal opening

Gradual descent of the infant through the birth canal

Amniotic fluid gushes out of the vagina

Third Stage of Labor

Palpation of the uterus reveals a firm mass

Top of the fundus lies slightly below the umbilicus

Before placenta separation, the uterus has a round shape during contractions and a flat shape during relaxation

After placenta separation, the uterus has a round shape during both contractions and relaxation

Placenta descends to the lower uterine segment

Expulsion of the placenta and fetal membranes

Bleeding from the vagina

Data Analysis

Nursing Diagnosis

NORMAL LABOR AND DELIVERY (NORMAL INTRAPARTUM PERIOD, UNCOMPLICATED PREGNANCY): Period leading up to and including childbirth in which there is evidence of conformity to standards of normalcy during labor and delivery

Common Etiology

HUMAN BODY: A state of physiologic and psychologic homeostasis

HEALTH CARE FACTORS: High-quality health care delivery, correct and sufficient health information or instruction

LIFESTYLE: The consistent practice of sound health principles

PLANNING

Unmet Needs

Protection from physical harm, increased learning

Expected Outcome

Woman received the support of her partner and the health staff during all phases of the labor and delivery

A healthy infant is delivered

Parents relate feelings of personal satisfaction with their achievement

NURSING INTERVENTIONS

Nursing Treatments

First Stage of Labor

Attend the patient constantly

Reassure verbally

Provide quiet

Do a perineal prep

Administer an enema (cleansing enema given slowly and as comfortably as possible)

Ambulate the patient (as much as possible during the early first stage)

Give small, frequent drinks (during the early first stage)

Restrict the intake to nothing by mouth (food is restricted during the entire first stage and fluid is restricted during the advanced first stage)

Position comfortably (as the first stage advances)

Massage gently (the lumbosacral area and effeurage the abdomen)

Toilet frequently

Touch the patient judiciously

Refrain from performing nonessential procedures

Provide radio and television for diversion (if the patient desires)

Encourage visiting by significant others

Second Stage of Labor

Place in the lithotomy (dorsosacral) position (on the delivery table)

Place on sterile linens

Drape modestly

Position comfortably (as much as possible)

Restrain the patient (for safety)

Do a perineal prep (cleansing only)

Facilitate the delivery by gently guiding the infant through the vulva

Third Stage of Labor

Tie off and cut the umbilical cord

Await delivery of the placenta

Refrain from pulling the umbilical cord during expulsion of the placenta

Refrain from removing the placenta except during a uterine contraction

Massage the uterine fundus (if it fails to contract)

Nursing Observations

First Stage of Labor
Monitor the fetal heart sounds
Palpate the cervix for dilatation
Palpate the uterus for contraction quality
Time the uterine contractions
Monitor the blood pressure (every hour)
Monitor the oral temperature
Palpate the pulse for rate, rhythm, and volume
Inspect the chest for respiratory rate and rhythm
Observe for uterine membrane rupture
Inspect the amnoitic fluid for meconium
Inspect the vagina for a prolapsed umbilical cord
Observe for complaints of pain, of fatigue
Observe for an excessive stress level
Test the urine for protein
Test the urine for sugar and acetone

Second Stage of Labor
Monitor the fetal heart sounds (until birth occurs)

Third Stage of Labor
Inspect for bleeding
Inspect the placenta for abnormalities
Inspect the umbilical cord for abnormalities
Palpate the uterus for firmness
Monitor the blood pressure
Palpate the pulse for rate, rhythm, and volume

Health Teaching

Teach how to control breathing to aid the labor process (panting in short, shallow, rapid breaths during contractions will decrease the pain)
Describe those symptoms that should be reported (contractions, membrane rupture, pink "show," bleeding)

Medical Treatments Performed by Nurses

Give the prescribed drugs

EVALUATION

Record actual outcome

NORMAL PUERPERIUM[50,239,388,527]

ASSESSMENT

Data Collection

Subjective Data
Woman may relate experiencing fatigue
May have mood swings

Objective Data
Breasts are full with milk
Top of the fundus can be palpated as a firm, round mass, and the fundus height decreases each day
Bladder may be full
Presence of bright red lochia that gradually fades to pink and has no odor
Temperature may rise slightly after labor, but is normal within 24 hours
Pulse rate may be normal or slow
Blood pressure is stable

No evidence of thrombophlebitis

Gradual return to normal of the white blood count, hemoglobin, hematocrit, and red blood count

No infection or inflammation of the episeotomy

Data Analysis

Nursing Diagnosis

NORMAL PUERPERIUM (NORMAL POSTPARTUM PERIOD): A 6-week period after labor and delivery in which there is evidence of conformity to standards of normalcy after pregnancy termination

Common Etiology

HUMAN BODY: A state of physiologic and psychologic homeostasis

HEALTH CARE FACTORS: High-quality health care delivery, correct and sufficient health information or instruction

LIFESTYLE: The consistent practice of sound health principles

PLANNING

Unmet Needs

Protection from physical harm, increased learning

Expected Outcome

Woman practices sound health principles in order to maintain a normal puerperium

NURSING INTERVENTIONS

Nursing Treatments

Encourage adequate rest

Cover with warm blankets

Give warm liquids

Provide quiet

Massage the uterine fundus (if it becomes relaxed)

Ambulate the patient (as soon as possible, if there are no contraindications)

Encourage moderate physical exercise

Nursing Observations

Inspect for (vaginal) bleeding

Inspect the skin for perspiration abnormality (profuse perspiration)

Measure the intake and output

Monitor the blood pressure

Monitor the oral temperature (for fever)

Inspect for edema, inflammation, and bleeding (of the incision site if an episiotomy was done)

Inspect the vagina for discharge

Observe for complaints of thirst

Palpate the uterus for firmness (every 15 minutes)

Palpate the uterus for fundus height

Palpate the bladder for distension

Palpate the pulse for rate, rhythm, and volume

Monitor blood studies for evidence of infection

Monitor blood studies for abnormal hematology

Monitor urine studies for evidence of urinary tract infection

Health Teaching

Describe those symptoms that should be reported (bleeding, pain, etc.)

Teach how to do postpartum exercises (when the woman feels ready for such)

Explain the reason for and intended effect of the therapy

EVALUATION

Record actual outcome

Wellness Responses of the Family

WELL FAMILY[293,408,471,682,775]

ASSESSMENT

Data Collection

Subjective Data
- Family relates that together they are moving in a forward direction of expanding personal growth
- Family perceives the future as offering an opportunity to develop unique potential
- Family members relate attitudes and behaviors of wellness such as the following:

Power
Spouses share equal or nearly equal power in their relationship
As parents, they are not authoritarian, and their children do not resent their authority

Intimacy
Spouses share deep levels of intimacy without feeling vulnerable, yet still maintain individuality
They relate being able to disclose their most private thoughts and feelings to one another

Emotional Aspects
Family relates little difficulty adapting to change
Family relates feeling strongly connected, and contact is maintained between family members and across generations
Members relate feeling safe and secure within the family
Family members openly express both positive and negative feelings, and love and concern are expressed for one another
All members maintain emotional control and calm
Members trust each other and have an attitude that people are generally good
Each spouse relates feeling comfortable when focusing on the relationship with the other spouse
Family members are present during a crisis
Family members deal openly with loss and share their grief
A positive emotional climate is maintained, through positive family interaction

Basic Family Mood
Family relates that most of the time the family mood is one of warmth, humor, and concern for one another

Personal Growth of Family Members
Personal growth and creativity are encouraged by the recognition and support of individual differences
Each person is accepted as human and likely to make mistakes
Family members focus on their stages of growth and on the achievement of developmental tasks
Members are given the support they need to expand their world outside the family

Socialization
Family members relate that they participate in recreational, leisure, and other activities together

Problem Solving
Spouses relate being able to face reality and deal objectively with both simple and difficult problems as they arise and outside help is sought when needed
Family members identify problems early and solve their problems together

Each two persons who have a problem are expected to solve it and a third person or issue is not used to take the focus off the problem or solution

Family has set specific goals for the future

Needs of both individual members and the group as a whole are considered before decisions are made

Family does not worry about trivial matters

Members use the expertise within the group to the benefit of all

Use the material resources within the group to benefit all

Sexual Relations

Spouses relate that their sexual relations are important and gratifying and they see no need for sexual satisfaction outside the marriage

Stress Management

Family members are usually free of physical complaints and when symptoms are present, they are of short duration and are not severe (related to actual stress such as life events or significant decisions)

Objective Data

• Family members are involved in activities and practices that are wellness oriented, such as the following:

Roles and Tasks

Each family member effectively functions in his specific role

Family members equally share family tasks and provide each other with task-oriented assistance

Family relates that the roles and functions of family members are flexible

Parents express confidence in their roles as mates, parents, wage earners, and as members of society

Child Rearing

Family relates few difficulties in child-rearing practices

Children are expected to assume responsibility and enjoy the privileges associated with the child's age

Children are listened to

Children and parents verbalize respect for each other

Family Value System

Family relates that there are clearly defined, consistent values among family members

Family acknowledges that their value system is based on rational conclusions and feelings, not on authoritarian rule

Communications

Family members openly and spontaneously communicate feelings and needs

Members are directly in touch with one another

Exhibit sound family communication patterns by using a common language, pleasant gestures, and eye contact and letting each person know they are heard by a nod, wink, etc.

They do not project blame on others

Differences of opinion are openly accepted and are not considered to be grounds for arguing

Physical Needs

Physical needs of all family members are met

Preventive health measures are practices

Environment

Family environment is clean, orderly, in good repair, free of accident hazards and provides the basic resources (heat, light, water, etc.)

Each person has adequate privacy

Community Involvement

Family members are involved in community activities

Data Analysis

Nursing Diagnosis

WELL FAMILY: Use of human energy, by persons living together, toward the pursuit of the highest potential for personal growth of the group as a whole

Common Etiology

PSYCHOSOCIAL FACTORS: Positive self-attitudes of family members, positive health attitudes of family members, exposure to a family role model who practices or practiced family wellness behavior

HEALTH CARE FACTORS: Correct and sufficient health information or instruction

LIFESTYLE: The consistent practice of sound health principles by family members

SITUATIONAL FACTORS: The presence of adequate resources for gratification of basic physiologic and psychologic needs of the family members

PLANNING

Unmet Needs

Continued development of potential, continued learning

Expected Outcome

Family members relate feelings of personal satisfaction for having achieved wellness

Family continues to practice wellness behavior

NURSING INTERVENTIONS

Nursing Treatments

Encourage new goals at past goal achievement (new goals for the maintenance of and higher levels of wellness)

Encourage the person to ask questions (about wellness behavior)

Encourage the expression of feelings (about the satisfaction of practicing wellness behavior)

Offer praise (for the family's practice of wellness behavior)

Nursing Observations

Make a follow-up evaluation (at a later date to determine whether the state of wellness still exists and whether wellness behavior is still being practiced)

Health Teaching

Recommend the continued practice of wellness behavior

EVALUATION

Record actual outcome

Wellness Responses of Competency

COMPETENCE IN SELF-CARE[775]

ASSESSMENT

Data Collection

Subjective Data

• Person (or family) verbalizes the ability to and knowledge of how to handle self-care

Specific to an Individual Person

Person relates that he does all he can for himself that is adequate to meet his needs

Relates a sense of responsibility for his own care

Specific to a Family
Dependent person is encouraged to do all that he can for himself
Physical care of the dependent person is shared by all family members
Family members are cared for and none is neglected

Objective Data
• Person (or family) correctly demonstrates the ability to handle the problem or complete the task
  Person appears well cared for and is clean, well-nourished, and hydrated, comfortable, and rested

Data Analysis

Nursing Diagnosis
COMPETENCE IN SELF-CARE: Person (or family) gives evidence of adequate ability, knowledge, or proficiency in providing physical care for self or a dependent person

Common Etiology
PSYCHOSOCIAL FACTORS: Exposure to a role model who demonstrates competence
HEALTH CARE FACTORS: Correct and sufficient information and instruction
DEVELOPMENTAL FACTORS: The achievement of one's developmental tasks
SITUATIONAL FACTORS: Experience in handling the problem of self-care

PLANNING

Unmet Needs
Continued development of potential

Expected Outcome
Person relates feelings of personal satisfaction for having achieved competency
Person continues to practice competence in self-care

NURSING INTERVENTIONS

Nursing Treatments
Encourage new skill development (if and when appropriate)
Encourage the desire for satisfactory achievement (of the skill on a long-term basis)
Provide nursing availability (assure the person that the nurse is available by phone or in person if there is a question about self-care)
Encourage the expression of feelings (about the satisfaction of having achieved competency)

Nursing Observations
Make a follow-up evaluation (at a later date to determine whether the person has maintained competency)

Health Teaching
Explain the reason for and intended effect of the methods used (for self-care)

EVALUATION
Record actual outcome

COMPETENCE IN MANAGING HEALTH THERAPY[207,525,775]

ASSESSMENT

Data Collection

Subjective Data
• Person (or family) verbalizes the ability to and knowledge of how to handle health therapy

Specific to an Individual Person
Person does all he can for himself that is adequate to meet his needs
Feels a sense of responsibility for his own care

Specific to a Family
Verbalizes a willingness to manage health therapy for a dependent family member

Objective Data
• Person (or family) correctly demonstrates the ability to handle the problem or complete the task
Person (or family) carries out all prescribed treatments and procedures
Therapy is carried out safely
Methods are performed as prescribed and correctly demonstrated

Data Analysis

Nursing Diagnosis
COMPETENCE IN MANAGING HEALTH THERAPY: Person (or family) gives evidence of adequate ability, knowledge or proficiency in carring out prescribed treatments and procedures

Common Etiology
PSYCHOSOCIAL FACTORS: Exposure to a role model who demonstrates competence
HEALTH CARE FACTORS: Correct and sufficient health information and instruction
SITUATIONAL FACTORS: The presence of adequate resources to achieve a task, experience in handling the problem

PLANNING

Unmet Needs
Continued development of potential

Expected Outcome
Person relates feelings of personal satisfaction for having achieved competency
Continues to practice competence in health therapy management

NURSING INTERVENTIONS

Nursing Treatments
Encourage new skill development (if and when appropriate)
Encourage the desire for satisfactory achievement (of the skill on a long-term basis)
Provide nursing availability (assure the person that the nurse is available by phone or in person if there is a question about the health therapy)
Encourage the expression of feelings (about the satisfaction of having achieved competency)

Nursing Observations
Make a follow-up evaluation (at a later date to determine whether the person has maintained competency)

Health Teaching
Explain the reason for and intended effect of the methods used (in the health therapy)

EVALUATION

Record actual outcome

COMPETENCE IN HEALTH KNOWLEDGE/SKILLS[775]

ASSESSMENT

Data Collection

Subjective Data
• Person (or family) verbalizes the ability to and knowledge of how to handle a problem

Person or family members have sufficient information
Information is correct
Understands the underlying principles, causes, and effects
Knows where to obtain additional knowledge if needed

Objective Data
• Person (or family) correctly demonstrates the ability to handle the problem or to complete the task

Data Analysis

Nursing Diagnosis
COMPETENCE IN HEALTH KNOWLEDGE/SKILL: Person (or family) gives evidence of adequate ability, knowledge, or proficiency in acquiring and putting into action knowledge to maintain or promote health

Common Etiology
PSYCHOSOCIAL FACTORS: Positive health attitudes, exposure to a role model who demonstrates competence
HEALTH CARE FACTORS: Correct and sufficient (health) information or instruction
SITUATIONAL FACTORS: Experience in handling the problem, presence of adequate resources to achieve a health skill

PLANNING

Unmet Needs
Continued development of potential

Expected Outcome
Person relates feelings of personal satisfaction for having achieved competency
Practices sound health principles based on the acquired health knowledge or skills

NURSING INTERVENTIONS

Nursing Treatments
Encourage new skill development (if and when appropriate)
Encourage the desire for satisfactory achievement (of the skill on a long-term basis)
Provide nursing availability (assure the person that the nurse is available by phone or in person if there is a question about the health knowledge subject or skill)
Encourage the expression of feelings (about the satisfaction of having achieved competency)

Nursing Observations
Make a follow-up evaluation (to determine whether the person has maintained the competency)

Health Teaching
Explain the reason for and intended effect of the methods used (when acquiring health knowledge or skills)

EVALUATION
Record actual outcome

COMPETENCE IN PARENTING[94,133]

ASSESSMENT

Data Collection

Subjective Data
• Person (or family) verbalizes the ability to and knowledge of how to care for and socialize a child

Parent provides the child's economic needs of food, clothing, and shelter
Loves and cares for the child according to his developmental stage
Guides and disciplines the child using positive reinforcement and a system of reward
Teaches the child how to communicate and fosters continuous learning
Protects the child against physical and emotional harm
Encourages, praises, and supports the development of the child's potential

Objective Data
• Person (or family) correctly demonstrates the ability to handle the problem or complete the task
Parents exhibit a warm relationship between themselves and the child
Parents demonstrate a consistent, rational approach to directing the child's activities and behavior

Data Analysis

Nursing Diagnosis
COMPETENCE IN PARENTING: Person (or family) gives evidence of adequate ability, knowledge, or proficiency in the caring for and socializing of a child

Common Etiology
PSYCHOSOCIAL FACTORS: Exposure to a role model who demonstrated competence in parenting
HEALTH CARE FACTORS: Correct and sufficient information and instruction
LIFESTYLE: The consistent practice of sound health principles in child rearing
SITUATIONAL FACTORS: Experience in handling the problem, presence of adequate resources to achieve competence in parenting

PLANNING

Unmet Needs
Continued development of potential

Expected Outcome
Person relates feelings of personal satisfaction for having achieved competency
Continues to practice competence in parenting

NURSING INTERVENTIONS

Nursing Treatments
Encourage new skill development (if and when appropriate)
Encourage the desire for satisfactory achievement (of the skill on a long-term basis)
Provide nursing availability (assure the person that the nurse is available by phone or in person if there is a question about parenting)
Encourage the expression of feelings (about the satisfaction of having achieved competency)

Nursing Observations

Make a follow-up evaluation (at a later date to determine whether the person has maintained competency)

Health Teaching
Explain the reason for and intended effect of the methods used (in parenting)

EVALUATION
Record actual outcome

COMPETENCE IN MANAGING PSYCHOLOGIC ADAPTATION[105,775]

ASSESSMENT

Data Collection

Subjective Data
- Person (or family) verbalizes the ability to or knowledge of how to handle psychologic adaptation

  Person relates a conscious and realistic recognition that new requirements are being made of him

  Relates feeling competent to meet the requirements of the situation

  Relates a realistic appraisal of alternative action that can be taken to meet the new demands

  Relates satisfaction that his needs have been met

Objective Data
- Person (or family) correctly demonstrates the ability to handle psychologic adaptation

  Person has taken a coordinated and integrated sequence of steps in initiating appropriate action to meet the adjustive demands

  Has relied on or changed established behavior or changed the external environment in order to meet the new demands

  Overtly exhibits the ability to function well

Data Analysis

Nursing Diagnosis
COMPETENCE IN MANAGING HEALTH THERAPY: Person (or family) gives evidence of adequate ability, knowledge, or proficiency in using effective, task-oriented coping mechanisms to adjust to psychologic stress

Common Etiology
PSYCHOSOCIAL FACTORS: Exposure to a role model who practices or practiced psychologic wellness behavior
HEALTH CARE FACTORS: High-quality health care delivery, correct and sufficient health information or instruction
LIFESTYLE: The consistent practice of sound health principles
SITUATIONAL FACTORS: Experience in handling situations and problems, presence of adequate resources to achieve a task

PLANNING

Unmet Needs
Continued development of potential

Expected Outcome
Person relates feelings of personal satisfaction for having achieved competency
Continues to practice competence in psychologic adaptation

NURSING INTERVENTIONS

Nursing Treatments
Encourage new skill development (if and when appropriate)
Encourage the desire for satisfactory achievement (of the skill on a long-term basis)
Provide nursing availability (assure the person that the nurse is available by phone or in person if there is a question about psychologic adaptation)
Encourage the expression of feelings (about the satisfaction of having achieved competency)

Nursing Observations
Make a follow-up evaluation (at a later date to determine whether the person has maintained competency)

Health Teaching

Explain the reason for and intended effect of the methods used (in managing psychologic adaptation)

EVALUATION

Record actual outcome

COMPETENCE IN UTILIZING COMMUNITY RESOURCES[775]

ASSESSMENT

Data Collection

Subjective Data

- Person (or family) verbalizes the ability to and knowledge of how to use available community resources

  Knows when to seek help

  Knows what community resources are available

  Chooses the appropriate and suitable facilities

  Feels secure in relationship with professionals at the facility

Objective Data

- Person (or family) correctly demonstrates the ability to handle the problem or complete the task

  Person (or family) has made and kept an appointment with the agency representative

Data Analysis

Nursing Diagnosis

COMPETENCE IN UTILIZING COMMUNITY RESOURCES: Person (or family) gives evidence of adequate ability, knowledge, or proficiency in utilizing available community resources to meet unmet needs

Common Etiology

HEALTH CARE FACTORS: Correct and sufficient (health) information or instruction

SITUATIONAL FACTORS: Experience in handling situations or problems

PLANNING

Unmet Needs

Continued development of potential

Expected Outcome

Person relates feelings of personal satisfaction for having achieved competence

Continues to practice competence in utilizing community resources as long as the resources are needed

NURSING INTERVENTIONS

Nursing Treatments

Encourage new skill development (if and when appropriate)

Encourage the desire for satisfactory achievement (of the skill on a long-term basis)

Provide nursing availability (assure the person that the nurse is available by phone or in person if there is any question about community resources)

Encourage the expression of feelings (about the satisfaction of having achieved competency)

Nursing Observations

Make a follow-up evaluation at a later date (to determine whether the person has maintained the competency)

Health Teaching

Explain the reason for and intended effect of the methods used (when utilizing community resources)

EVALUATION

Record actual outcome

Knowledge Deficits Associated with Well Persons

UNKNOWLEDGEABLE ABOUT COPING WITH AGED PERSONS [121,124,222,497,531]

ASSESSMENT

Data Collection

Subjective Data

- Person's discussion or questions indicate a need for additional information, clarification or validation of information
  OR
- Person's lack of questions or comments indicates not wanting information or not knowing enough to seek information
- When questioned directly, the person's response or lack of response indicates that he does not know the following:
  What to expect of the older person
  How to respond to the older person's needs
  How it feels to be an aged person
  What losses occur with old age

Objective Data

- Person may exhibit behavior indicating insufficient knowledge, such as performing tasks for an older person who is capable of independence or moving an aged person into the household when it is not necessary

Data Analysis

Nursing Diagnosis

UNKNOWLEDGEABLE ABOUT COPING WITH AGED PERSONS: Being without sufficient information about successful methods for meeting older person's needs

Common Etiology (Stressors)

HEALTH CARE FACTORS: Lack of health instruction

PLANNING

Unmet Needs

Comfort, protection from physical harm and psychologic threat, increased reality perception and problem solving, increased learning

Expected Outcome

Correct verbal feedback of the information taught
Person relates increased satisfaction when coping with the aged person
Aged person relates greater satisfaction in having needs met

NURSING INTERVENTIONS

Nursing Treatments
Approach unhurriedly
Reassure verbally
Encourage the person to ask questions
Provide reliable information (about the aged)

Nursing Observations
Determine teaching effectiveness by testing or verbal feedback

Health Teaching
Teach the specific methods (for dealing with problems that result from the aging of significant others); teach the individual the following:

Independence vs. Dependence
Encourage aged persons to remain independent as long as possible
Give the aged the responsibility to make decisions about their own lives, and let them have the final word as to what happens to them
Encourage the aged to maintain their own self-care whenever possible

Energy Level
Help the aged determine priorities for using limited energy reserves, as the person may be able to modify rather than give up activities, such as playing golf for 4 hours instead of 6 hours
Take notice of nonverbal cues that the aged person is becoming fatigued (such as slumped shoulders, sitting down, snoozing, yawning) and of requests that he be taken home
Postpone activities until he is rested

Hygiene
Recognize that daily bathing is not necessary (aging skin is dry and perspires little)

Nutrition
Encourage the aged to partake of a balanced diet
Recognize that a decreased appetite is due to an impaired sense of taste and smell and that denial of these physiologic changes often results in complaints about present food and glorification of past foods eaten, so avoid confrontations over such complaints by recognizing their cause
Avoid fussing about the aged person's eating habits, and instead provide the foods he wants and enjoys
Utilize "Meals on Wheels" or a similar service when needed
Recognize that some aged persons prefer to eat five or six small meals a day
Encourage the aged to eat with others, since eating is a social event

Sleep
Encourage the aged to obtain adequate sleep
Emphasize that sleep patterns change in old age, and that it is not necessary to adhere to former sleep patterns. The sleep cycle can be adjusted to meet current needs

Communications
Recognize that aged persons usually have hearing or vision loss
Provide large-print books or taped books for the visually impaired
Communicate in a quiet, rather than a noisy, environment
Touch the person and face him before speaking to him if hearing is impaired
Expect that aged persons will take longer to respond to conversation
Wait for the aged to respond to the first communicated idea before relating a second idea
Limit communications to verbal exchanges if the aged person has difficulty writing
Place a telephone near the person's bed and in strategic places in the home and recommend a cordless telephone for moving about

Provide special telephone devices available for the hearing impaired
Call at prearranged times once or twice a day to communicate with aged persons
Suggest that two aged friends call daily to check on one another
Utilize a telephone service to check daily on the aged person
Allow the older person to tell the same story repeatedly or to go into minute details in conversations, as telling stories is a way to relate to other persons
Use large clocks and calendars to communicate time and date
Carefully explain anything new before it occurs

Exercise
Encourage the aged to exercise moderately in order to promote circulation, relaxation, and relief of stiff joints

Mental Abilities
Recognize that mental decline does not usually occur in aged persons unless there is a health problem

Emotional Factors
Stay in frequent contact with the aged person, reassuring him frequently that he is loved and wanted
Reassure the aged person that you will return whenever you leave him and, if known, mention when you will return
Recognize that anger expressed by the aging person is due to loss of identity with work, loss of companionship, loss of financial compensation, loss of health, and a feeling of helplessness about what is happening to him

Personal Growth
Encourage the aged person to seek new experiences, knowledge, and creativity
Help the aged recognize that aging represents the complete person who has experienced more of life than younger generations
Support the concept that aging is a time to enjoy simply for the experience of enjoyment and not for reasons of productivity and help the person learn to cope with free time, encouraging him to create pleasure through self-ingenuity by smelling the flowers, watching people, eating a picnic lunch at the lake
Recognize that reminiscence leads to self-growth (a means of maintaining self-esteem, of reaffirming self-identity, of working through losses, of finding meaning in life, and of permitting the person to see the connection between the end and beginning of his life and where he is now and what choices to make for the future) and encourage the aged to reminisce together to promote a common bond between them and about happy events, which can be a source of gratification

Sexual Activity
Recognize that it is normal for the aged to remain sexually active if a sexual partner is available

Activity
Keep the aged person mobile as long as possible in order to support health and independence
Keep the aged person busy doing something meaningful when underfoot and undirected or when idle and preoccupied with bodily processes

Socialization
Encourage the aged to maintain contact with old friends, as the continuity of sharing life experiences with persons of the same age is especially significant, and do not insist that the aged socialize with their childrens' friends
Encourage the aged to participate in senior-citizen group activities
Link the aged with the outside world through church or social agencies, reading, television, rides in cars, out-of-home lunches, excursions, etc.
Recognize that, socially, the aged person may prefer to observe rather than participate

Environment

Encourage the aged to live at home instead of in an institution

Keep him in familiar surroundings, where he functions best

Recognize that older persons may prefer outdated appliances because of their simplicity and do not insist that they have modern, new equipment

Check for safety precautions throughout the house (nail down rugs, use safety rails in bathrooms, use night lights, etc.)

Encourage the aged to keep and use old, significant belongings and let him be surrounded by his own possessions

If the aged person is concerned about drafts or chills, set aside a warm place for him, by the fire, etc.

Transportation

When there is a question about whether an aged person should continue to drive, let his physician make the decision

Utilize special transportation services for the aged whenever needed

Retirement

If the aged person perceives retirement as psychologically or financially unacceptable, encourage gradual retirement such as reducing work hours, or gradually moving from a highly responsible to a less responsible position

Encourage a positive attitude toward retirement and support the idea that, although it brings change, retirement presents a new opportunity for personal growth

Recognize that most retired persons must adjust to a reduced income that raises realistic concerns

Health Maintenance

Encourage health examinations once a year to reassure the aged person that he is healthy and despite chronic complaining to get early attention for significant physical complaints, since the elderly are more vulnerable to illness and critical physical changes can occur rapidly in old age

Recognize that older persons often prefer an older physician or nurse with whom he can relate

If the person becomes ill, remember that recovery is slower in aged persons so do not expect a rapid recovery

Care Providers for the Aged

Since people now live longer, caring for the aged should be expected to be a long-term commitment

Recognize the activity restrictions the care provider will have to endure, and take measures to reduce the restrictions as much as possible

If financially feasible, obtain outside help, such as home health aids, to assist in the care of the helpless aged, as old persons feel less dependent when cared for by nonfamily members, and recommend that the family be subtle when offering help, so as to reduce dependency feelings

Death and Dying

Openly discuss dying with the person if he wants to talk about it, understanding that since death is such an important event in life, the aged usually want to share and prepare for it with significant persons

On Being Aged

Help the person perceive aging as a successful phase of life, and do not let him live the stereotyped role of depression and dependence

If a person denies being old, do not remind him of his age, as reminding the person of an age unacceptable to him makes him feel older than he actually feels he is

Avoid fussing over the aged person or calling attention to his age unless he finds it gratifying

Recognize and emphasize that being old does not mean being sick
Physiologic changes that occur in aging are normal
Explain the reason for and intended effects of the methods used (to maintain self-esteem of the aged and to promote a meaningful and independent life)

EVALUATION

Record actual outcome

26 Nursing Diagnoses of HEALTH RESOURCE PROBLEMS

Dual Domain of Nursing Expertise: Health Resource Problems

This chapter covers that sphere of nursing knowledge and skill related to problems involving the use of professional assistive resources available to persons in a community. These problems are solved by nurses, physicians, and social workers.

Views of Nursing Leaders That Support This Domain of Nursing Expertise

Primary care functions for which nurses and physicians share responsibility include making referrals to appropriate agencies.

Faye Abdellah[3:125–127]

Providing a person with this type of support [material resources] is not the specialized work of nurses. Nonetheless, nurses often assist their patients in obtaining the resources available to them from institutions or agencies. . . . In assisting individuals in their development, it is not enough to supply resources. It may also be necessary to show them how to use these resources.

Dorothea Orem[380:65,66]

Modern nursing is by no means limited to the giving of expert physical care to the sick, important as this is. It is more far reaching, including . . . helping a person to use the available community resources.

Hester Frederick and Ethel Northam[379:68]

Deficits in Utilizing Health Care Resources

DIFFICULTY UTILIZING COMMUNITY RESOURCES[492,682,685]

ASSESSMENT

Data Collection

Subjective Data
- Person (or family) relates that it is difficult to attain his social needs
- Verbalizes unsuccessful methods attempted
  Person (or family) relates knowing when to seek outside help
  May relate choosing resources that were neither appropriate nor suitable
  May ask for clarification about the available resources
  Verbalizes feeling comfortable when relating to nurses, doctors, social workers, teachers, etc.

Objective Data
- Person (or family) has demonstrated repeated efforts to attain help through community resources
- Person (or family) may exhibit behavior indicating that methods attempted are partially but not completely effective, may go to the health department for free immunizations but not for a needed x-ray film of the chest, may go to a church for spiritual guidance but does not use the church-offered food and recreational assistance

Data Analysis

Nursing Diagnosis
DIFFICULTY UTILIZING COMMUNITY RESOURCES: Person (or family) is only partially effective in using those resources provided for the common good, when such resources are needed

Common Etiology (Stressors)
PSYCHOSOCIAL FACTORS: Lack of skill in self-direction, lack of or loss of control of a life situation, a highly dependent personality, lack of emotional support from others, lack of problem-solving skills
HEALTH CARE FACTORS: Lack of correct information
SITUATIONAL FACTORS: Loss of property by disaster, loss of employment, poverty

PLANNING

Unmet Needs
Comfort, protection from physical harm, dependence, independence, increased learning

Expected Outcome
Person relates successful use of community resources

NURSING INTERVENTIONS

Nursing Treatments
Approach unhurriedly
Anticipate needs
Talk with the person or family (about their problems)
Encourage the person to ask questions
Ask the person or family to identify the problem (with which they need help)
Encourage mutual problem solving (between the involved persons)
Make a referral (to the appropriate agency, institution, etc.)

Nursing Observations
Observe for evidence of a favorable response to assistance (through the use of community resources)

Health Teaching

Inform of the resources available

EVALUATION

Record actual outcome

INABILITY TO UTILIZE COMMUNITY RESOURCES[492,682,685]

ASSESSMENT

Data Collection

Subjective Data

• Person (or family) relates being unable to meet his social needs
• May or may not know of or have attempted solution methods
  Person or family may not recognize that they need outside help to meet their needs
  Relates not having sought outside help
  May relate feeling uncomfortable in their relationship with nurses, doctors, social workers, teachers, etc.

Objective Data

• Person (or family) may exhibit behavior indicating that the solution/goal has not been achieved, person or family may be borrowing money to pay medical bills when they could be using free medical services, a parent may be leaving children unattended while at work when free day-care services are available

Data Analysis

Nursing Diagnosis

INABILITY TO UTILIZE COMMUNITY RESOURCES: Person (or family) is ineffective in using those resources provided for the common good, when such resources are needed

Common Etiology (Stressors)

PSYCHOSOCIAL FACTORS: Lack of skill in self-direction, lack of or loss of control of a life situation, a highly dependent personality, lack of emotional support from others, lack of problem-solving skills

HEALTH CARE FACTORS: Lack of correct information

SITUATIONAL FACTORS: Loss of property by disaster, loss of employment, poverty

PLANNING

Unmet Needs

Comfort, protection from physical harm, dependence, independence, increased learning

Expected Outcome

Person relates successful use of community resources

NURSING INTERVENTIONS

Nursing Treatments

Approach unhurriedly

Anticipate needs

Talk with the person or family (about their problems)

Encourage the person to ask questions

Provide an atmosphere of acceptance (that it is acceptable to obtain outside help)

Ask the person or family to identify the problem (which could be resolved by outside help)

Encourage mutual problem solving (among family members so that there is mutual acceptance of outside help)

Make a referral (to the appropriate agency, institution, etc.)

Nursing Observations

Observe for evidence of a favorable response to assistance (through the use of community resources)

Health Teaching

Inform of the resources available

EVALUATION

Record actual outcome

Knowledge Deficits in Utilizing Health Care Sources

UNKNOWLEDGEABLE ABOUT COMMUNITY RESOURCES[492,682,685]

ASSESSMENT

Data Collection

Subjective Data
• Person's (or family's) discussion or questions indicate a need for additional information, clarification, or validation of information
 OR
• Person's (or family's) lack of questions or comments indicates not wanting information or not knowing enough to seek information
• When questioned directly, the person's (or family's) response or lack of response indicates that he does not know:
 What community resources are available
 Services offered by each
 Criteria for admittance to the agency
 Requirements the agency places upon the client

Objective Data
• May exhibit behavior such as acting inappropriately based on insufficient knowledge such as not taking a sick family member to the hospital, drinking polluted water instead of calling the health department, not obtaining aid for a disabled person, etc.

Data Analysis

Nursing Diagnosis
UNKNOWLEDGEABLE ABOUT COMMUNITY RESOURCES: Being without sufficient information about those resources that the community has made available for the well-being of persons in the community

Common Etiology (Stressors)
HEALTH CARE FACTORS: Lack of instruction

PLANNING

Unmet Needs

Comfort, protection from physical harm, dependence, independence, increased learning

Expected Outcome

Correct verbal feedback of the information taught

Person relates successful use of community resources

NURSING INTERVENTIONS

Nursing Treatments

Encourage the person to ask questions

Make a referral (to an appropriate agency)

Nursing Observations

Determine teaching effectiveness by verbal feedback

Health Teaching

Inform of the resources available (for health care, the criteria for admittance to agencies, the services provided, etc.)

Explain the reason for and intended effects of using the community resource

EVALUATION

Record actual outcome

PART FOUR
NURSING INTERVENTIONS

NURSING TREATMENTS

Accept and attempt to relieve unexplainable body complaints When the person persists in complaining of physical ailments that cannot be diagnosed medically, do not indicate that the ailment is imaginary or of psychic origin. Accept the complaint and take measures to relieve it.

Rationale: The attention and love derived as a result of functional complaints tend to alleviate the functional discomfort or pain. Comfort is promoted through effective communication with others. Nonacceptance of body complaints heightens anxiety or psychologic threat and increases the stress of adaptation, with resulting energy depletion. Complaints are the most reliable guide to nonhealth conditions.

Fulfilled Needs: Comfort, protection from physical harm, protection from psychologic threat, acceptance

Acknowledge dependency For a limited period of time, permit the person to rely on others to meet basic physiologic and psychologic needs.

Rationale: Any physiologic or psychologic disequilibrium is potentially threatening. Regressive behavior is a defensive reaction to threatening situations and a temporary adaptive mechanism toward future equilibrium.

Fulfilled Needs: Comfort, protection from physical harm, protection from psychologic threat, dependence

Act out the reality the person cannot accept If a person refuses to accept a reality, demonstrate the reality through deliberate action. Do for the person what he could be doing if he accepted the reality. If a person refuses to accept that a loved one is ill, care for the loved one in a visible, open manner. If the person denies an amputated limb, clean the stump and change the dressing in a manner visible to the person. If the person denies the reality of permanent blindness, count aloud the number of steps he takes from the bed to the bathroom, the chair, etc; move his hand to the clock-face areas of his dinner plate to locate each type of food; verbally identify sounds while in his presence ("That's the food cart coming," "I hear Dr. G's steps in the hall"). As he develops functional skills, he can face the reality of blindness. If the person denies the reality that socializing is possible when the person has a colostomy, clean the colostomy well, apply a clean appliance, insist the person put on make-up or shave, etc., and get dressed. Arrange for the least-stressful visitors such as family, chaplain, other health personnel to visit. Arrange for a visit by an attractive ostomate.

Rationale: When persons in the environment act out a denied reality, the denying person is forced to perceive the reality. In time, the reinforcement of reality brings about the acceptance of reality.

Fulfilled Needs: Increased reality perception

Add an emollient to the bath water To the bath water, add one-half to one ounce of a substance that soothes the skin, such as Alpha-Keri, Lubath, Nivea oil, mineral oil or olive oil.

Rationale: Use of an emollient in the bath water helps keep skin well moisturized.

Fulfilled Needs: Comfort, protection from physical harm

Adjust the diet to the person's lifestyle When attempting to change dietary patterns, obtain a history of the person's daily routine and available food resources. Adjust the diet so that the person can best fit the dietary change into his everyday life. If he

1417

goes to work at 4:30 AM, do not expect him to eat a large breakfast at that hour; instead, let him set his dietary schedule. If a diabetic child cannot obtain the needed food for lunch at school, show him how to pack an adequate sack lunch.

Rationale: The more a dietary change can be adjusted to the person's lifestyle, the higher the potential for compliance.

Fulfilled Needs: Comfort, nutritional balance

Administer a drug sensitivity test Before administering any highly antigenic drug, subcutaneously inject a few drops and note any reaction.

Rationale: Protection from physical harm.

Fulfilled Needs: Protection from physical harm

Administer a hot foot bath Place the feet in a tub or pan of plain or saline water at about 110° F and soak for 20–30 minutes.

Rationale: Hot foot soaks promote comfort by drawing excess fluid from congested body parts and by stimulating circulation

Fulfilled Needs: Hypotension, dizziness, impaired peripheral circulation of the lower extremity

Contraindications: Hypotension, dizziness, impaired peripheral circulation of the lower extremity

Administer a vaginal douche Gently insert an irrigating nozzle into the vagina after cleansing the external genitalia with surgical soap and water. Allow an irrigating solution at approximately 105° F to flow in and out of the vagina slowly by careful nozzle rotation.

Rationale: Vaginal irrigations cleanse, discourage bacterial growth, remove foul and irritating discharges, and provide heat or cold therapy.

Fulfilled Needs: Comfort, cleanliness, protection from physical harm

Contraindications: Pregnancy, vaginal bleeding, recent vaginal surgery

Administer an enema Dispense an enema into the colon. Select the amount, type, and temperature of the solution according to the desired result.

Rationale: One quart of fluid for an adult and less than 500 cc for a small child distends the colon sufficiently to stimulate peristalsis. The addition of heat (105° F) and a mild soap solution acts as an irritant and further increases peristalsis. A hot soap-solution enema will stimulate uterine contractions. A 0.85% sodium chloride solution is isotonic with the blood and does not irritate the colon; tap water is hypotonic and may disrupt water balance. A hypertonic saline solution of 100 cc sodium phosphate and biphosphate pulls fluid by osmotic attraction into the colon, causing colonic distention and stimulating peristalsis and the urinary (micturition) reflex. A small amount of oil (100–200 cc) given as a retention enema softens hard fecal masses and is especially effective when given 2–3 hours before a cleansing enema.

Fulfilled Needs: Waste elimination of food residue and intestinal gases, comfort, stimulation, cleanliness, protection from physical harm

Contraindications: *Any enema:* Hypokalemia, intestinal spasms, uterine or rectal bleeding, afterbirth pains, during peritoneal dialysis, nausea, vomiting, acute abdominal pain, premature onset of labor, the presence of a ureterosigmoidostomy

Soap-solution enema: Ulcerative or inflammatory intestinal conditions

Saline and sodium phosphate enema: Hypernatremia

Tap-water enema: Hyponatremia, edema, ascites, when there is a potential for water intoxication, as in small children or infants

Administer heated humidified oxygen (ET)* Dispense water-vaporized oxygen by bubbling oxygen down a stem immersed in electrically heated sterile water.

Rationale: Normally, 40% of body humidity is breathed in from external air. The internal respiratory tract supplies 60% of the nearly 100% humidity required. Heating

---

*(ET) means emergency treatment.

water to 100–105° F and diffusing oxygen gas out of the water increase the capacity of oxygen in external air to hold water (humidity) at 90% humidity. Therefore, the internal respiratory tract needs to supply only 10% humidity instead of the normal 60%. This decreases respiratory tissue dryness, prevents tissue friction during respirations, and loosens and thins mucus secretions. Normally, a person breathes in 97% of the 20.95% oxygen in ordinary air, or 20.32% oxygen. Oxygen therapy builds up a slightly higher oxygen intake by elevating the oxygen concentration of ordinary air from 20.32% to 22.31–33.95%. This increased oxygen intake eases breathing and promotes comfort.

Fulfilled Needs: Tissue oxygenation or perfusion, waste elimination of bronchopulmonary secretions, comfort, protection from physical harm

Contraindications: High fever, oxygen toxicity, increased metabolic rate

Administer humidified oxygen (ET) Dispense water-vaporized oxygen by bubbling oxygen down a stem immersed in sterile water at room temperature.

Rationale: When oxygen is humidified, the dry gas is converted to approximately the same moisture level as the humidity of room air. The vapor thus created decreases the drying effect of oxygen on the respiratory mucosa. Oxygen therapy builds up a higher oxygen intake than provided by ordinary air. This increased oxygen intake eases breathing and promotes comfort. When blood volume is low, administering oxygen saturates the hemoglobin of the remaining blood cells. In conditions of increased metabolic rate, administered oxygen helps ease excessive oxygen consumption. Cool vapor is preferable because heated mist further accelerates the metabolic rate.

Fulfilled Needs: Tissue oxygenation or perfusion, comfort, protection from physical harm

Contraindications: Oxygen toxicity, severe chronic obstructive pulmonary disease in which relief of hypoxia with oxygen therapy could precipitate apnea

Administer intermittent positive-pressure breathing (ET) Give pressurized air into the lungs during inhalation by mechanically induced intermittent positive pressure.

Rationale: Intermittent positive-pressure breathing provides inhalation of air having above-normal atmospheric pressure. This pressure, applied by mouthpiece or mask, inflates the lungs. It pushes pressurized air past mucus and stimulates coughing, which eliminates secretions. On exhalation, the pressure returns to normal atmospheric pressure. Intermittent positive-pressure breathing expands alveoli and promotes diffusion of oxygen, increasing the oxygen saturation level of the blood.

Fulfilled Needs: Tissue oxygenation or perfusion, waste elimination of bronchopulmonary secretions, protection from physical harm

Contraindications: Pulmonary embolus, pulmonary hemorrhage, impaired cardiac output as in myocardial infarction

Administer intravenous fluids (ET) Infuse physiologic saline solution, glucose, or other intravenous solutions into the vein.

Rationale: Intravenous infusions provide an immediate source of water, electrolytes, and nutrients for the purpose of maintenance, replacement, or as an avenue for drug administration. The basic composition of IV fluid is isotonic, but hypotonic fluid may be given (to correct hypertonic dehydration) and hypertonic fluid may be given (to reduce cerebral edema). IV fluids increase the vascular pressure, especially when administered rapidly, when, during shock, there is a disproportion between the blood volume and the vascular space. IV fluids stimulate urine production during decreased output associated with shock and, when there is fever, replaces fluid lost from dehydration so that the body can perspire and cool itself.

Fulfilled Needs: Fluid and electrolyte balance, normal temperature, stimulation, protection from physical harm

Contraindications: Circulatory overload as evidenced by venous distention or other signs, thrombophlebitis, suspected air embolism, dextrose solutions above 10% and solutions containing alcohol are given only if ordered by a physician

Administer isotonic saline intravenous fluid between the blood transfusion and glucose infusion   When a blood transfusion has been completed and a glucose solution is ordered to follow, flush the tubing with normal saline IV fluid first or use new tubing.

Rationale: Isotonic saline is compatible with blood and will not cause blood clotting within the tubing. Glucose solution causes hemolysis of the red blood cells in the tubing, resulting in microemboli.

Fulfilled Needs: Protection from physical harm

Administer mechanical ventilation (ET)   Administer some form of ventilation by machine or bag until the person is able to maintain respirations without assistance.

Rationale: Mechanical ventilation assists the person with respirations and gas exchange until such time as assistance is no longer needed

Fulfilled Needs: Tissue oxygenation or perfusion, comfort, protection from physical harm

Administer vaporized air   Dispense water vapor through a bubble or diffuse humidifier or vaporizer. Electrically heat the water to 100–105° F.

Rationale: The use of a vaporizer decreases respiratory tissue dryness, prevents friction during respirations, loosens and thins mucus, decongests sinuses, prevents mouth dryness, and promotes comfort.

Fulfilled Needs: Waste elimination of bronchopulmonary secretions, comfort, protection from physical harm

Contraindications: High fever

Allow a significant other (family member) to sit quietly at the bedside   When treatments are not in progress, provide a comfortable chair by the person's bedside. Encourage one significant other to sit quietly by the person, to offer reassurance, to meet certain needs.

Rationale: The presence of significant others during times of illness, reassures the patient that a caring loved one will see that his needs are met. It prevents a break in their normal bonding and supports mutual growth in their interrelatedness.

Fulfilled Needs: Comfort, protection from psychologic threat, psychologic stability, caring and communicating relationships, unity with loved ones, personal growth and maturity

Allow time for thought comprehension   After delivery of a verbal message, allow sufficient time for the person to receive and interpret the message.

Rationale: Rapidity of message reception and interpretation depends on the degree of physiologic and psychologic equilibrium. Psychologic comfort is promoted through effective communication with others.

Fulfilled Needs: Comfort, caring and communicating relationships

Allow unlimited visitors (unlimited visiting)   Permit visitors freedom to come and go as the patient desires and at their own discretion.

Rationale: Psychologic equilibrium is fostered by an awareness that the person is not threatened with aloneness. Human contact relieves fear and anxiety. The physical presence and involvement of loved ones reassures the person that he will be cared for.

Fulfilled Needs: Protection from psychologic threat, caring and communicating relationships, unity with loved ones

Ambulate the person   Walk the person as much as possible, especially after surgery or an immobilizing illness or disease.

Rationale: Ambulation promotes and helps restore normal physiologic function, stimulates circulation, increases pulmonary ventilation and the movement of secretions, stimulates peristalsis, empties the renal pelvis, promotes the passage of stones, and increases muscle strength and endurance. Improved physiologic function reduces the dependency of illness. During labor, ambulation promotes fetal head descent by placing pressure on the lower uterus and stimulating contractions.

Fulfilled Needs: Tissue oxygenation or perfusion; waste elimination of food residue, intestinal gases, and bronchopulmonary secretions; activity and exercise; energy; comfort; stimulation; protection from physical harm; dependence

Contraindications: Temperature elevation above 103° F, head or spinal cord injury, internal hemorrhage, coma or semicoma, severe energy depletion, life-threatening situations

Anchor the tubing securely   When the person has an intravenous infusion or a urinary, gastric, chest, or any other type of tube, anchor the tubing so that the person's movements will not displace the tubing. Loop a section of the tubing, then secure it in place with adhesive tape or a bandage.

Rationale: Anchoring tubing provides comfort by minimizing the replacement of dislodged tubes.

Fulfilled Needs: Comfort, protection from physical harm

Anticipate needs/anticipate and provide for needs   Supply the person's requirements before they are sought or asked for.

Rationale: Physical or psychologic needs unknown to or unmet by the person could be potentially threatening to health equilibrium. Meeting unsolicited needs offers security, attention, recognition, and acceptance, promotes comfort, restores physical strength, allows for necessary dependency, and nonverbally recognizes the person's value and dignity.

Fulfilled Needs: Energy, comfort, protection from physical harm, protection from psychologic threat, dependence, acceptance, sense of value, high evaluation of self, recognition, dignity, attention

Apply a bed cradle   Place a metal or plastic frame over the body, between the sheets and the person, and cover the cradle with bed linens.

Rationale: Bed cradles prevent bedding from touching the body, yet maintain warmth around the body. A cradle prevents skin irritation and promotes comfort. In paralysis, sheets touching the skin can stimulate the reflex arc or lower motor neurons and cause severe muscle spasm.

Fulfilled Needs: Comfort, protection from physical harm

Apply a brassiere   Apply or have the person apply a brassiere to the breasts, especially during pregnancy and lactation. The brassiere should have a sufficiently large cup, over all breast tissue in the underarm area, and have wide supportive straps.

Rationale: The application of a supportive brassiere during pregnancy or to an engorged or lactating breast aids in preventing fluid congestion, shields the breast for cleanliness, relieves discomfort from breast weight by offering support, and prevents backache by enhancing good posture.

Fulfilled Needs: Comfort, cleanliness, protection from physical harm

Apply a breast binder   Apply a wide binder and encircle it around the breasts. Hold the breasts in the normal position while the binder is being applied snugly but not too tightly. Pin the binder from the bottom up.

Rationale: The application of a breast binder to an engorged or lactating breast aids in preventing fluid congestion, shields the breast for cleanliness, relieves discomfort from breast weight by offering support, and prevents backache by enhancing good posture.

Fulfilled Needs: Comfort, cleanliness, protection from physical harm

Apply a butterfly bandage or closure strips   Place an adhesive strip on one side of an open wound. Pull the wound edges together. Bring the tape over and to the other side of the wound. When the wound edges appear aligned, anchor the tape to the skin. Several adhesive strips sometimes are required to hold one incisional line closed.

Rationale: Alignment of wound edges promotes healing, comfort, and cleanliness.

Fulfilled Needs: Comfort, cleanliness, protection from physical harm

Apply a cold/cool, moist compress Apply a cold/cool, wet, absorbent cloth by soaking a towel or wool cloth in cold water. Wring it out thoroughly and place it on the skin surface.

Rationale: Cold causes vasoconstriction, which decreases bleeding, pain, and pressure from tissue fluid and gas. Cold especially reduces pain due to burns.

Fulfilled Needs: Comfort, protection from physical harm, freedom from pain

Contraindications: Avoid cold applications to decubitus ulcers, gangrenous tissue, skin-graft areas, varicose veins, areas of paralysis or sensation loss, and aged or debilitated skin

Apply a cool, damp cloth to the face Gently touch the face with a cool damp cloth when the person experiences such discomforts as dizziness, nausea or vomiting, faintness, etc.

Rationale: Coolness constricts blood vessels, sending the blood supply away from the skin to vital organs. It refreshes the face, thus promoting comfort.

Fulfilled Needs: Comfort, stimulation

Apply a cortisone ointment Apply an ointment that contains a small amount of cortisone to the skin

Rationale: Cortisone is an anti-inflammatory drug that reduces inflammation and itching. Its properties promote comfort, decrease the inflammatory response and reduce the severity of allergic and other immune responses.

Fulfilled Needs: Comfort, protection from physical harm

Apply a greasy substance over the tick If a tick imbeds itself in the skin or hair, cover the tick with petrolatum, cold cream, lard, margarine, or another greasy substance. Nail polish also may be used.

Rationale: Grease or nail polish smothers the tick, facilitating easy removal.

Fulfilled Needs: Protection from physical harm

Apply a heat cradle/heat lamp Expose the body or body part to dry heat from an electric light bulb. Suspend the bulb from a frame over the body or from a gooseneck lamp and enclose with a sheet for concentrated warmth.

Rationale: Dry heat increases circulation through mild vasodilatation, relieves pain and congestion, promotes muscle relaxation, and draws pus to the skin surface. With skin burns, peripheral vessels cannot contract to retain body heat. External heat helps maintain normal body temperature.

Fulfilled Needs: Tissue oxygenation or perfusion, normal temperature, relaxation, comfort, protection from physical harm, freedom from pain

Contraindications: Avoid applying heat to areas of paralysis or sensation loss, edema, vasodilatation, or allergic responses, to any body part after heart surgery, to areas of hemorrhage or trauma, to febrile persons, and to persons who are unable to cooperate with safety instructions such as children or confused persons

Apply a heating pad Expose the body to dry heat by using an electric heating pad.

Rationale: Dry heat increases circulation through mild vasodilatation, relieves pain and congestion, promotes muscle relaxation, and draws pus to the skin surface. Heat on the bladder stimulates voiding and relieves bladder spasms.

Fulfilled Needs: Tissue oxygenation or perfusion, relaxation, comfort, protection from physical harm, freedom from pain

Contraindications: Avoid applying a heating pad on a child or a confused or comatose person; to areas of paralysis or sensation loss, edema, vasodilatation, or allergic responses; to any body part after heart surgery; to areas of hemorrhage or trauma; and to febrile persons

Apply a hot water bottle/hot pack On the affected body part, place a rubber or plastic bag filled with temperature-tested hot water or apply a hot pack. Encase them in linen or towel outer coverings.

Rationale: Heat increases circulation through vasodilatation, relieves pain and congestion, promotes muscle relaxation, and draws pus to the skin surface. Heat applied to the bladder stimulates voiding and relieves bladder spasms.

Fulfilled Needs: Tissue oxygenation or perfusion, relaxation, comfort, protection from physical harm, freedom from pain

Contraindications: Never use a hot-water bottle or hot pack on a child, or a confused or comatose person; avoid heat application to areas of paralysis or sensation loss, edema, vasodilatation, or allergic responses, to any body part after heart surgery, to areas of hemorrhage or trauma, and in conditions where fever exists

Apply a precordial thump (ET) In cases where the onset of cardiac arrest is witnessed by the nurse, administer a sharp blow to the midsternum from a height of 8–12 inches, using the soft side of the fist.

Rationale: The shock force from a sternal blow should stimulate heart muscle contractions if administered very soon after a cardiac arrest.

Fulfilled Needs: Tissue oxygenation or perfusion, stimulation, protection from physical harm

Contraindications: Do not use this therapy on children, do not administer if faint heartbeats can be detected or if the heartbeat has ceased for longer than one minute because the hypoxic heart will not respond to the blow, and there will be tissue damage

Apply a pressure dressing Apply a firmly anchored sterile bandage or binder. Apply the binder snugly but prevent tightness that may interrupt blood flow.

Rationale: Pressure application prevents bleeding and wound seepage and promotes comfort.

Fulfilled Needs: Comfort, protection from physical harm

Apply a safety helmet to the head Whenever there is danger of head trauma during ambulation, apply a football helmet to the head.

Rationale: Head trauma can damage the vital life centers of the brain.

Fulfilled Needs: Protection from physical harm

Apply a saline compress Apply a sterile dressing, dampened with warm or cool isotonic (0.85%) saline solution.

Rationale: A wet, saline compress is nonirritating to open wounds, promotes growth of granulation tissue, cleans wounds by debridement, softens wound discharges, promotes drainage, and localizes area infection.

Fulfilled Needs: Comfort, cleanliness, protection from physical harm

Apply a sterile dressing Apply a dry, sterile bandage over a wound

Rationale: Sterile wound coverings enhance cleanliness, prevent infection and trauma, restrict motion, and absorb secretions.

Fulfilled Needs: Comfort, cleanliness, protection from physical harm

Apply a stump sock Snugly apply a soft, absorbent, cone-shaped sock to the amputated stump.

Rationale: The stump sock's porous material allows good stump ventilation. Pressure application reduces edema. The sock protects the skin from prosthesis pressure and irritation.

Fulfilled Needs: Comfort, protection from physical harm

Apply a supportive splint When the body has been traumatized and is in danger of further injury if moved, immobilize the body part with a supporting splint.

Rationale: Immobilization and support prevents further injury and provides physiologic rest and comfort.

Fulfilled Needs: Rest, comfort, protection from physical harm

Apply a tenderizer paste to the lesion Mix a small amount of water with meat tenderizer until a paste is formed. Then apply this to insect bites and stings

Rationale: The enzyme in the tenderizer chemically changes the venom from bee and wasp stings (plus other insect bites and stings), thus decreasing discomfort and allergic reactions.

Fulfilled Needs: Comfort, protection from physical harm

Apply a tourniquet between the extremity wound and the body Apply a tourniquet 2–4 inches above the injury site on the extremity, between the wound and the body torso. The tourniquet should be loose enough so a finger will fit under it and the arterial pulses can still be felt. Some oozing of the wound will also occur. If there is swelling above the tourniquet, apply another tourniquet a few inches above the first one, leaving the first one in place. Maintain the tourniquet application until medical care is obtained.

Rationale: The application of a tourniquet minimizes the amount of snake venom absorbed into the circulatory system. In trauma, it reduces the degree of hemorrhage.

Fulfilled Needs: Protection from physical harm

Apply a warm, moist compress Apply warm, wet heat by soaking a towel or wool cloth in hot water, wringing it almost dry, and placing it on the skin surface. Unsterile compresses may be used on intact skin, but sterile normal saline compresses are essential over open lesions.

Rationale: Moist heat increases circulation through intense vasodilatation, relieves pain and congestion, promotes muscle relaxation, enhances drainage, localizes infection, and draws pus to the skin surface.

Fulfilled Needs: Tissue oxygenation or perfusion, comfort, cleanliness, protection from physical harm, freedom from pain

Contraindications: Avoid applying heat to areas of paralysis or sensation loss, edema, vasodilatation, or allergic responses, to any body part after heart surgery, to areas of hemorrhage or trauma, and to febrile persons

Apply after-bath powder Apply a thin layer of powder, usually talcum or zinc oxide, to the skin. Use it sparingly in the winter because of its drying effect. Do not powder the skin folds or between the toes, or apply only a thin film in these areas.

Rationale: Powder has a drying action, permits movement of skin against skin, allows for good air circulation over the skin, reduces friction, and promotes cooling and drying of inflamed skin.

Fulfilled Needs: Comfort, protection from physical harm

Contraindications: Dry skin, allergic reactions, do not apply powders containing zinc on the skin of patients receiving radiation therapy

Apply alcohol to the skin/lesion Rub the body with full-strength alcohol or sponge with alcohol mixed with tepid water.

Rationale: Rubbing the body surface with alochol stimulates circulation and inhibits bacterial growth on the skin. Alcohol evaporates at a relatively low temperature, rapidly removing heat and cooling the body surface.

Fulfilled Needs: Normal temperature, comfort, cleanliness

Contraindications: Dry skin, respiratory distress in which the alcohol fumes might irritate the respiratory mucosa, during oxygen administration in which alcohol fumes might precipitate an explosion

Apply aluminum paste to the skin Cover the skin surrounding the colostomy stoma or a ureterostomy with a thin layer of a mixture of half aluminum powder and half oil.

Rationale: Aluminum paste neutralizes the acidity of digestive enzymes found in bowel content. It minimizes skin irritation and excoriation by preventing exudates from coming in contact with the skin.

Fulfilled Needs: Comfort, protection from physical harm

Apply an abdominal support garment Apply to the abdomen, or suggest that the person wear, clothing articles that uphold the abdominal wall, its contents, and healing tissue. Such garments would include binders and girdles.

Rationale: Supportive pressure decreases stress on abdominal muscles and organs, promotes comfort, and reduces pain.

Fulfilled Needs: Comfort, protection from physical harm, freedom from pain

Apply an analgesic ointment Apply an anesthetizing ointment to the skin in order to reduce pain or itching.

Rationale: Decreased pain promotes comfort and rest.

Fulfilled Needs: Rest, comfort

Apply an antibiotic ointment (or spray) Locally apply a salve or spray containing an antibiotic drug. Use it on mildly inflamed areas and on nonbleeding or crusted eruptions. Use on open skin areas rather than in skin folds.

Rationale: Antibiotic ointments and sprays reduce or prevent bacterial growth and infection. Ointments retard water evaporation from the skin, soften scabs and scales, and promote comfort.

Fulfilled Needs: Comfort, protection from physical harm

Contraindications: Known drug allergy

Apply an antiperspirant to the axillary region After cleansing the skin of the axilla, apply a chemical product under the axilla to control skin odor and inhibit sweating.

Rationale: Body odor is controlled by oxidizing odoriferous material or by inhibiting bacterial growth and decaying putrefaction. Control of body odor promotes comfort. It offers aid in illness dependency.

Fulfilled Needs: Comfort, dependence

Contraindications: Axillary irritation or inflammation

Apply an arm sling Support the arm, elbow, hand, and shoulder by application of a triangular sling for temporary use or a commercial sling for long-term use.

Rationale: Support of a traumatized body part prevents further injury and promotes rest for that part.

Fulfilled Needs: Rest, comfort, protection from physical harm

Apply an elastic bandage Wrap a rubberized stretch bandage around the affected body area.

Rationale: The gentle, supportive pressure of an elastic bandage around a body part reduces venous stasis and fluid accumulation by increasing circulation.

Fulfilled Needs: Tissue oxygenation or perfusion, comfort, stimulation, protection from physical harm

Apply an external urinary catheter Apply an external collection device to the urinary orifice.

Rationale: A urinary collection apparatus promotes accurate output measurement, maintains dryness, cleanliness, and comfort, and improves sleep and rest by decreasing frequent bathroom visits.

Fulfilled Needs: Sleep and rest, comfort, cleanliness, protection from physical harm

Contraindications: Irritation or inflammation of the external genitalia

Apply an ice bag (cold pack, ice pack) On the affected body part, place a rubber or plastic bag filled with ice or a cold pack. Encase each in a linen or towel cover. Apply cold to the breast for about 48 hours after delivery while the breasts are engorged with milk. When the body temperature is severely elevated, place ice bags or cold packs along the torso and extremities. Stop the treatment when the temperature drops to 101° F, or shock may occur. Interrupt ice applications for a few minutes every hour to ensure adequate skin circulation.

Rationale: Dry cold decreases circulation through mild vasoconstriction, relieves pain and congestion, and reduces pus formation, swelling, and bleeding.

Fulfilled Needs: Normal temperature, comfort, protection from physical harm, freedom from pain

Contraindications: Avoid cold applications to decubitus ulcers, gangrenous tissue, skin-graft areas, varicose veins, areas of paralysis or sensation loss, and aged or debilitated skin

Apply an ice collar On the neck, place a collar-shaped rubber or plastic bag filled with ice and wrapped with a linen cover.

Rationale: Dry cold decreases circulation through mild vasoconstriction, relieves pain and congestion, and reduces pus formation, swelling, and bleeding. Coldness around the neck depresses nerve fiber activity and produces vasoconstriction in the carotid vessels, reducing tachycardia.

Fulfilled Needs: Normal temperature, comfort, protection from physical harm, freedom from pain

Contraindications: Avoid cold applications to areas of decubitus ulcer, gangrenous tissue, skin-graft areas, areas of paralysis or sensation loss, and aged or debilitated skin

Apply an occlusive dressing Apply a dressing in which the outer covering is a plastic wrap placed around the dressing.

Rationale: An occlusive dressing prevents the evaporation of the medication being applied by the dressing, assuring more effective use of the medication, which promotes the comfort of healing. It also offers the protection of cleanliness.

Fulfilled Needs: Comfort, cleanliness

Apply calamine lotion Apply a solution of zinc oxide and ferric oxide to the skin. Cover the skin surrounding an ileostomy stoma or a ureterileostomy with a thin layer of calamine. Since it has a drying effect, it is best used in skin folds and where two skin surfaces come together.

Rationale: Calamine lotion soothes the skin's surface. It hardens and contracts superficial skin cells by coagulating cell albumin and forming a thin coating over the cells. It protects against skin irritation and promotes healing. The lotion dries up weeping, oozing areas and reduces skin inflammation. Evaporation of the moisture in the lotion causes cooling and drying. The powder in the lotion absorbs oozing and weeping serum.

Fulfilled Needs: Comfort, protection from physical harm

Apply camphor to the lesion Apply a liquid or ointment containing camphor to fever blisters and cold sores. Campho-Phenique is commonly used.

Rationale: Camphor has a drying effect that dries up the lesion and reduces swelling.

Fulfilled Needs: Comfort, protection from physical harm

Apply cornstarch to the skin Using a powder puff for even skin distribution, apply cornstarch. Prevent starch from collecting in skin folds.

Rationale: The powdery consistency of cornstarch is absorbent, soothes irritated skin, relieves itching, and cleanses the skin. It should be used sparingly because as starch absorbs water, the starch granules swell and, when placed in skin folds, cakes and irritates the skin.

Fulfilled Needs: Comfort, cleanliness, protection from physical harm

Apply diapers loosely Diaper the child with a loose diaper that does not rub against the perineum.

Rationale: A loose diaper prevents friction against the circumcision site, irritated perineum, or buttocks and allows for better ventilation of the area.

Fulfilled Needs: Comfort, protection from physical harm

Apply elastic stockings Put properly measured, rubberized, stretch stockings (elastic hose) on the lower limbs.

Rationale: The application of supportive pressure to the lower limbs reduces blood stagnation and speeds the flow of deeper venous blood back to the heart.

Fulfilled Needs: Tissue oxygenation or perfusion, comfort, stimulation, protection from physical harm

Contraindications: Circulatory embolus or thrombus

Apply fine mesh gauze Place fine mesh gauze over wounds and between burned skin surfaces.

Rationale: Fine mesh gauze is an absorbent material. Its close weave prevents granulation tissue from growing between the threads, yet it allows air to reach the wound. Placing it between burned surfaces keeps the surfaces from growing together during the growth of granulation tissue and decreases the chance for infection by allowing for ventilation.

Fulfilled Needs: Comfort, protection from physical harm

Apply hot packs to the breast before breast-feeding Apply a hot water bottle or other heat to the breast 15–20 minutes before breast-feeding.

Rationale: Vasodilatation of blood vessels of the breast promotes lactating milk flow and comfort.

Fulfilled Needs: Comfort

Apply karaya powder to skin Karaya powder, also called Swun gum powder, should be applied to the skin surface around an ileostomy. It is for external use only.

Rationale: Karaya powder protects the skin from excoriation and erosion when exposed to ileostomy drainage.

Fulfilled Needs: Comfort, protection from physical harm

Apply manual pressure over the bleeding area (over the potential bleeding area Apply pressure with the hand over a specific bleeding structure, organ, or area.

Rationale: Pressure application prevents blood and body fluid from escaping outside the circulatory system or tissue structures. It promotes comfort when used to reduce pain.

Fulfilled Needs: Comfort, protection from physical harm

Apply mentholated ointment Lubricate the skin with cream containing oil of peppermint or mint oils (camphor). Rub deep into the skin.

Rationale: Mentholated ointment produces deep, penetrating warmth that relieves mild pain, muscle spasm, and irritation of deeper structures.

Fulfilled Needs: Comfort, freedom from pain

Contraindications: Skin irritation

Apply milk of magnesia to the skin Cover the skin surrounding an ileostomy stoma or a ureterileostomy with a thin layer of milk of magnesia.

Rationale: Milk of magnesia neutralizes the acidity of digestive enzymes found in ileostomy bowel content. It prevents skin irritation and excoriation.

Fulfilled Needs: Comfort, protection from physical harm

Apply ostomy adhesive and then an ostomy appliance Apply an external collection device for a colostomy, ileostomy, ileal conduit, ureterostomy, etc.

Rationale: An ostomy collection apparatus prevents skin irritation from fecal and digestive enzymes or urine. It promotes dryness, cleanliness, comfort, and accurate output measurement.

Fulfilled Needs: Comfort, cleanliness, protection from physical harm

Apply providone-iodine sponges around the tubing connections After changing the hyperalimentation tubing, tape sponges that have been soaked with providone-iodine around the tubing connections.

Rationale: The application of antiseptic-filled sponges around the hyperalimentation tubing connections prevents bacterial invasion into the tubing and eventually into the body.

Fulfilled Needs: Protection from physical harm

Apply rotating tourniquets (ET)[26,73] Place a tourniquet above the elbow or above the knee on three extremities. At 15-minute intervals, alternate the application and removal of the tourniquets. Remove one tourniquet every 15 minutes and place it on the extremity that has no tourniquet. Follow a clockwise or counterclockwise pattern.

7:00 AM	off right leg	on right arm, left arm, left leg
7:15	off right arm	on left arm, left leg, right leg
7:30	off left arm	on left leg, right leg, right arm
7:45	off left leg	on right leg, right arm, left leg

Place padding, such as 4″ × 4″ gauze squares, under each tourniquet to protect the underlying tissue. If tourniquets are not available, blood pressure cuffs may be used and inflated to a pressure between the systolic and diastolic blood pressure. To remove all tourniquets, remove them one at a time at 15-minute intervals.

Rationale: The application of tourniquets interferes with venous return by trapping blood in the extremities. This reduces the volume of blood reaching the lungs and prevents excessive fluid collection in the lungs.

Fulfilled Needs: Protection from physical harm

Apply sodium bicarbonate (baking soda) to an odiferous cast Sprinkle generous amounts of baking soda onto the cast. Leave on for 1 or 2 hours. Then dust off and repeat if needed.

Rationale: Baking soda absorbs unpleasant odors and will refresh an odiferous cast.

Fulfilled Needs: Comfort

Apply sodium bicarbonate (baking soda) to the skin Cover a local, moistened skin area with household baking soda.

Rationale: Sodium bicarbonate relieves the discomfort of stinging pain from insects.

Fulfilled Needs: Comfort, protection from physical harm, freedom from pain

Apply sterile petrolatum gauze Apply sterile gauze covered with transparent, sterile petrolatum.

Rationale: Petrolatum lubricates and smoothes skin, has a neutral (neither acid or alkaline) effect on the skin, prevents skin drying and cracking, promotes comfort, and maintains cleanliness by covering the skin.

Fulfilled Needs: Comfort, cleanliness, protection from physical harm

Apply the Heimlich maneuver   When a person is choking on a foreign object, make a fist with one hand. Place that hand with the thumb side against the abdomen slightly above the navel but below the sternum. Quickly press or thrust the fist into the abdomen above the umbilicus and below the sternum to move the diaphragm upward. Or press the patient's abdomen against the back of a chair, stair railing, table edge, or similar object.

Rationale: Thrusting movements in the diaphragmatic area force air from the lungs into the throat. The air pressure dislodges the foreign object.

Fulfilled Needs: Protection from physical harm

Apply tincture of benzoin   Apply tincture of benzoin (a balsic resin from various trees) over areas of potential or acute skin breakdown. To remove the stickiness associated with benzoin, apply a fine film of powder over the dried benzoin.

Rationale: Tincture of benzoin provides a tough protective coating for threatening or impending decubitus ulcers or other skin surfaces threatened by excess pressure. A sticky benzoin surface adheres to linen and clothing and pulls off skin, causing further tissue trauma, unless powder is applied over the benzoin.

Fulfilled Needs: Protection from physical harm

Contraindications: Do not use on deep, raw (granulating) wounds

Apply zinc oxide to the skin/lesions   Cover the skin surrounding a colostomy stoma or ureterostomy with a thin layer of zinc oxide paste ointment. This mixture is one-half zinc powder and one-half oil.

Rationale: Zinc oxide paste inhibits bacterial growth. It hardens and contracts superficial skin cells by coagulating cell albumin and forming a thin coating over the cells. It protects against skin irritation and promotes healing by preventing exudates from coming in contact with the skin.

Fulfilled Needs: Comfort, protection from physical harm

Approach unhurriedly   Communicate concern through an unrushed attitude.

Rationale: When there are physical or psychologic limitations to performance, an unhurried approach eliminates additional tension, especially if tension already exists. An unhurried approach communicates sufficient recognition and respect for the person to warrant the use of another's valuable time.

Fulfilled Needs: Comfort, protection from physical harm, protection from psychologic threat, caring and communicating relationships, high evaluation of self, recognition, dignity, attention

Arrange a predischarge planning conference   Bring health team members together to help the patient evaluate his health situation and contribute to problem solving.

Rationale: Comprehensive health planning reduces potential physical and psychologic problems and offers the patient the comfort of a predictable future.

Fulfilled Needs: Comfort, protection from physical harm, protection from psychologic threat, predictable and orderly world, increased learning, increased reality perception and problem-solving ability

Arrange a structured environment/daily routine   Offer a routine that is basically the same each day. Discover the person's previous routines and make every effort to reestablish the same daily habits in relation to time and detail.

Rationale: Feelings of threat result from the disruption of established behavior patterns by illness. Feelings of safety arise from familiar and predictable situations that have been handled successfully in the past.

Fulfilled Needs: Comfort, protection from psychologic threat, psychologic stability, predictable and orderly world

Arrange easy access to the bed-positioning switch Show the person the location of, and how to use, the switch that lowers and raises the foot, head and total bed. Arrange the bed linens so they do not cover or become entangled in the switch.

Rationale: Being able to change position without assistance supports independence and increased mobility.

Fulfilled Needs: Comfort, independence

Arrange geographic placement Locate the patient in a room accessible to maximum physical and emotional care, observation, socialization, etc. Assure him that he is close to available nursing care.

Rationale: Close supervision facilitates recognition of health disorders. Human contact relieves fear and anxiety. Psychologic comfort is promoted through a sense of nearness to others. Placement in an environment conducive to activity increases sensory stimulation.

Fulfilled Needs: Comfort, stimulation, protection from physical harm, protection from psychologic threat, caring and communicating relationships, attention

Arrange orderly surroundings Provide surroundings in which the furniture and accessories are so placed to give a neat, uniform appearance.

Rationale: An orderly environment establishes the whereabouts of objects, decreasing potential injury. It reduces misperceptions and promotes safety feelings in a familiar and predictable situation. Orderliness reduces the anxiety of environmental confusion.

Fulfilled Needs: Comfort, protection from physical harm, protection from psychologic threat, predictable and orderly world

Arrange pillows comfortably Place pillows under the head and body parts so they support but in no way impair circulation.

Rationale: Pressure prevention and support of a body area promote comfort and assist in illness dependency.

Fulfilled Needs: Comfort, dependence

Arrange pleasant surroundings Provide surroundings in which the decor lends a cheerful and attractive atmosphere.

Rationale: The perception of a pleasant environment promotes comfort which has a positive physiologic and psychologic effect.

Fulfilled Needs: Comfort, protection from physical harm, protection from psychologic threat, increased pleasantness

Arrange safe transport Make arrangements for the person to be safely transported to their destination. Transportation may be by ambulance, automobile, aircraft, etc.

Rationale: Persons undergoing the effects of illness often need special transportation to ensure their safety.

Fulfilled Needs: Comfort, protection from physical harm

Arrange situations that encourage the person's autonomy Offer the person a choice of experiences therapeutically selected to encourage him to control the situation. Suggest that he choose his own food, arrange his furniture, pick companions, decide which activities to attend, etc.

Rationale: Independence evolves from making choices. Comfort and safety evolve from an awareness that the person can cope successfully with life and can exert sufficient control to prevent harm to himself.

Fulfilled Needs: Comfort, protection from psychologic threat, adequacy, self-reliance, independence, control over others

Ask for specifics, not generalizations, about the problem Ask the person to give detailed information about the problem rather than to use indefinite terms or make general assumptions. If he states that he has pain, ask for a description of the pain, the time of day it occurs, what he is doing when it occurs, etc. If a woman states that her spouse is violent, ask for a detailed description of the violence.

Rationale: Detailed verbalization clarifies mental imagery and enhances growth toward total perception of the situation.

Fulfilled Needs: Protection from psychologic threat, personal growth and maturity, increased reality perception and problem-solving ability

Ask how the person normally copes with stress (fear, etc.) Have the person explain those activities or methods he uses to reduce the tension of stress. Request specifics such as jogging every morning, doing needle work, taking a brisk walk, playing tennis, going sailing, going to church, etc.

Rationale: Knowing how a person usually copes with stress helps the nurse provide similar circumstances so the person can use his normal coping methods in the present situation.

Fulfilled Needs: Comfort, increased reality perception and problem-solving ability

Ask questions that encourage answers that reflect reality perception Ask the dying person straightforward questions such as "Do you feel sick today? How much progress do you think you are making? Do you think your treatments are doing you any good?" Ask persons experiencing guilt, conflict, etc. questions appropriate to the situation.

Rationale: Straightforward questions offer an opportunity for greater reality perception while still providing the safety of denial answers if there is psychologic threat.

Fulfilled Needs: Protection from psychologic threat, increased reality perception and problem-solving ability

Ask simple, direct questions When speaking to persons having impaired message reception or delivery, ask only simple, direct questions that are easily understood and answered.

Rationale: Simple and direct communication enhances perception and reduces frustration and anxiety. Psychologic comfort is promoted through effective communication with others.

Fulfilled Needs: Comfort, caring and communicating relationships

Ask the person what makes him comfortable Discover the particular situations or conditions that make the person comfortable. Then, provide these comforts.

Rationale: Comfort evolves from an awareness that comfort needs will be met and that previously experienced comforts will be repeated.

Fulfilled Needs: Comfort, caring and communicating relationships

Ask the person to identify the problem Have the person state in clear, concise terms the nature of his problem. It may take nursing guidance for the person to accomplish this.

Rationale: Clearly identifying a problem is the first step to solving a problem.

Fulfilled Needs: Increased reality perception and problem-solving ability

Ask the person to relate the onset of returning pain before the pain becomes severe Ask the person to call the nurse as soon as pain begins to return. Advise that he should not wait until the pain is severe.

Rationale: An analgesic given at the onset of returning pain is more effective than when given after the pain is severe.

Fulfilled Needs: Comfort, protection from physical harm

Ask when the coping mechanisms failed Have the person relate when his usual coping methods were no longer effective, when tension was not reduced by such methods, and when he felt emotionally overwhelmed.

Rationale: Knowledge of when the coping mechanisms failed can help to pinpoint the problem.

Fulfilled Needs: Comfort, increased reality perception and problem-solving ability

Assist the dying person with detachment from life[279] When the dying person reaches total acceptance and indicates his readiness to detach himself from the world, help him do so. Clues that he is detaching himself from the world include turning the television off, especially at news time, wanting visitor limitations with gradual restriction to family members only, and lack of concern with environmental events.

Rationale: Detachment from the world eases the pain of losses anticipated by the dying person. Awareness that others support detachment brings comfort and rest.

Fulfilled Needs: Rest, comfort, protection from psychologic threat

Assist the dying person with unfinished business[279] When a person says that he cannot allow his death to occur because of commitments such as caring for a sick relative, paying debts, etc., offer assistance in the resolution of these problems whenever possible. It is preferable that these matters be attended to when the patient is still feeling reasonably well.

Rationale: The threatening responsibilities of unfinished business prevent the dying person from experiencing the peace of total acceptance.

Fulfilled Needs: Comfort, protection from psychologic threat, psychologic stability

Assist the family to prepare for life changes that will occur after the loved one's death[279] Discuss with family members their plans for daily living after their loved one has died. This includes housing, finances, changes in social life, etc.

Rationale: Preparation for the future reduces the adaptive stress through the recognition of predictable problems. Discussion of what life will be like without a loved one promotes adaptation to the reality that the time is approaching when the loved one will no longer be a part of the person's life.

Fulfilled Needs: Protection from psychologic threat, psychologic stability, increased reality perception and problem-solving ability

Assist the person or family to restructure his/their lifestyle Motivate and help the person to plan changes in his daily living habits. Have him set down on paper a revised daily schedule suitable to his needs.

Rationale: To restructure a lifestyle for the benefit of health requires mature reality perception. It includes behavior changes that specifically meet situational demands and individual needs. When the person is able to restructure a new pattern of daily living, he is providing himself with a reasonably predictable world.

Fulfilled Needs: Protection from physical harm, predictable and orderly world, personal growth and maturity, awareness of potential, full development of potential, increased reality perception and problem-solving ability

Assist the person to convert the anxiety into a specifically identified fear Ask questions and guide the person so that the vague anxiety feelings can be identified as a specific fear.

Rationale: Vague anxiety is difficult to cope with because the person has not identified the problem to be dealt with. When anxiety is recognized as a specific fear, the problem is subject to solution.

Fulfilled Needs: Comfort, protection from psychologic threat, personal growth and maturity, increased learning

Assist the person to define consistent life standards Assist the person in defining for himself a set of values that can be applied consistently to the broad scope of general living. Discourage different value systems for varying life situations.

Rationale: An accepted value system significantly influences behavioral responses.

Fulfilled Needs: Comfort, protection from psychologic threat, psychologic stability, improved values

Assist the person to set standards of a meaningful existence   Help the person set standards that give significant meaning to his life. In our affluent society, meaningfulness must be more than the basic needs of food, shelter, and clothing.

Rationale: In a society where basic needs have been met, working toward meeting survival needs offers little meaning. Therefore, activities must be developed that are time consuming and give people a sense of value, motivation, and satisfying ideals.

Fulfilled Needs: Comfort, protection from psychologic threat, psychologic stability

Assist with bedside spiritual observances   When bedside prayers or services are being held, assist in any way possible. Directions from the clergyman, patient, or family are excellent sources for knowing how to offer proper and needed assistance.

Rationale: Religious observances help people to express spiritually their relationship with God and to recognize outwardly the Supreme Being.

Fulfilled Needs: Comfort; dignity; dependence; spiritual, religious, or philosophic satisfaction

Assist with dressing and undressing   Help the person put his clothes on.

Rationale: Clothing maintains body warmth and promotes comfort. Assistance with dressing meets dependency needs.

Fulfilled Needs: Comfort, protection from physical harm, dependence

Assist with feeding   Help feed the person and help prepare food and utensils for feeding.

Rationale: Balanced nutritional intake is essential to body cell activity and energy production. Relief of visceral hunger promotes comfort. Assistance with feeding meets dependency needs.

Fulfilled Needs: Nutritional balance, energy, comfort, protection from physical harm, dependence

Assist with hygiene (hair, nails, oral, skin hygiene)   Help with hygiene and grooming activities of the hair, nails, teeth, and skin.

Rationale: Assistance with personal hygiene and cleanliness meets dependency needs and provides the comfort of being refreshed and of knowing that the personal appearance is pleasing.

Fulfilled Needs: Comfort, cleanliness, protection from physical harm, dependence

Assist with mobility   Help the person to walk, sit, stand, and move about.

Rationale: Mobility is necessary for meeting daily needs and for the maintenance of health. Assistance with mobility meets dependency needs.

Fulfilled Needs: Comfort, protection from physical harm, dependence

Attach the chest tube to a water-seal drainage   Attach the chest tube to the tubing that leads to chest bottles or a plastic (Pleur-Evac) water-seal drainage. The apparatus should be sterile and contain sufficient sterile water so the long tube within the closed system is about 1 inch below the surface of the sterile water. When using chest bottles, to prevent the tube from kinking, tape a tongue blade to the tubing located at the entry site to the bottle. Tape all connectors to prevent leakage.

Rationale: Water-seal drainage prevents additional air from entering the pleural space while fluid and blood drain from the pleural space. It facilitates reexpansion of a collapsed lung.

Fulfilled Needs: Protection from physical harm

Attach the collection appliance (or tube) to straight drainage and a collection container   Connect the collection appliance of an ileal conduit, a ureterostomy, an indwelling urinary catheter, etc., to a closed system of tubing and a collection container.

Rationale: A closed system of straight drainage and a collection container help control the hazards of infection, promote accurate output measurement, prevent skin irritation and promote dryness, cleanliness, and comfort.

Fulfilled Needs: Comfort, cleanliness, protection from physical harm

Attach the tube to a leg urinal Connect a plastic or waterproof bag to the urinary drainage tube and attach the bag to the person's leg.

Rationale: A urinary collection bag promotes accurate output measurement, maintains dryness, cleanliness, and comfort, allows for unlimited mobility, and reduces the threat of social embarrassment.

Fulfilled Needs: Waste elimination of urine, comfort, cleanliness, protection from physical harm, protection from psychologic threat

Attend the person constantly Remain with the person constantly.

Rationale: Constant attendance facilitates recognition of health disorders. Psychologic equilibrium is fostered by an awareness that the person is not threatened with aloneness. Human contact relieves fear and anxiety. Comfort is promoted through a sense of adequate communication with others.

Fulfilled Needs: Comfort, protection from physical harm, protection from psychologic threat, caring and communicating relationships

Avoid activities that increase intracranial pressure Refrain from performing any activity that could increase intracranial pressure such as placing the person in the prone position, hyperflexing the legs at the hips, positioning the head at or below the heart level, arousing the person suddenly, flexing the neck so veins are compressed.

Rationale: Avoiding activities that increase intracranial pressure keeps the intracranial pressure at a minimal level or prevents an excessively high plateau from occurring.

Fulfilled Needs: Protection from physical harm, physiologic stability

Avoid assuming that all behavior is manipulative Even though much of a person's behavior is manipulative, do not assume that all behavior is manipulative. Recognize complaints and requests that are valid. Investigate when there is doubt.

Rationale: The acceptance of nonmanipulative behavior communicates to the person that he is trusted. It also encourages him to trust the nursing staff. It indirectly expresses approval of nonmanipulative behavior.

Fulfilled Needs: Protection from psychologic threat, acceptance, approval from others

Avoid attempting to cheer up the depressed (grieving) person Do not try to make the depressed person happy by using cheering methods such as telling jokes, comic television programs, etc.

Rationale: Depressed or grieving persons cannot respond to external cheering up because of the nature of their emotion. Being aware that they are unable to respond to others trying to cheer them tends to make them feel worse.

Fulfilled Needs: Protection from psychologic threat, psychologic stability

Avoid causing embarrassing situations Do not create situations that will cause uncomfortable or shameful feelings in the person. If such situations exist take measures to alter them.

Rationale: Feelings of safety evolve from an awareness that a person can cope successfully with the life situation.

Fulfilled Needs: Comfort, protection from psychologic threat, dignity

Avoid causing intense emotional situations Do not create circumstances that arouse highly excitable or emotional responses in the person.

Rationale: Highly emotional responses deplete body energy and may stimulate irritating regulatory secretions. Emotional situations reduce sleep and rest and increase already existing fear and anxiety.

Fulfilled Needs: Sleep and rest, energy, comfort, protection from physical harm, protection from psychologic threat, psychologic stability

Avoid demands for abstract thinking if the person can only think in concrete terms If the person's highest level of thought process is limited to concrete terms (specifics), do not make an effort to have the person think in abstractions (generalizations).

Rationale: Efforts to have persons think in abstract terms, who are limited to concrete thinking, result in failure. Such failure is detrimental to self-esteem.

Fulfilled Needs: Comfort, protection from psychologic threat, sense of adequacy

Avoid forceful removal of the yellowish-white exudate at the circumcision site Do not remove the exudate that collects around the circumcision site. Instead, allow it to fall off by itself.

Rationale: Forceful removal of exudate can damage delicate tissues and cause pain and bleeding.

Fulfilled Needs: Comfort, protection from physical harm

Avoid forcing the person into rapid adaptation to change by accepting the person's unique pattern of adjustment Acknowledge that the person must adapt to changes in life situations according to his age, stage of development, past life experiences, and physical and psychologic health. Support adjustment at the person's own pace.

Rationale: When there are physical or psychologic limitations in performance, an unhurried approach eliminates additional tension to the already tension-filled threat of inadequacy. Reduced tension provides more energy for physical healing and psychologic coping.

Fulfilled Needs: Comfort, protection from physical harm, protection from psychologic threat

Avoid misshaping the wet cast When raising a wet cast off a flat surface, pull upward with the entire palm of the hand, not with the fingers.

Rationale: Finger indentations in soft plaster change the cast's shape and, through pressure, decrease circulation to tissues enclosed in the cast.

Fulfilled Needs: Protection from physical harm

Avoid overheating or chilling the person Perform such activities as maintaining a normal room temperature, dressing the person in moderate clothing, using blankets sparingly, keeping drafty windows closed, etc. Personal warmth or cold is a highly individual situation and requires interventions specific to the person.

Rationale: Overheating or chilling a person increases their oxygen consumption.

Fulfilled Needs: Protection from physical harm, physiologic stability

Avoid placing tension on the wound Do not allow pulling or stretching of tissue to occur around a wound site.

Rationale: Stress around a wound site heightens pain, increases the time needed for healing, and usually distorts tissue replacement.

Fulfilled Needs: Comfort, protection from physical harm

Avoid placing the person on enforced inactivity Do not allow the person to be totally restricted or to restrict himself from all activity.

Rationale: Enforced inactivity increases stress by requiring adaptation to the threat of frustration. Adaptation and adjustment require energy that, in illness, is needed for healing.

Fulfilled Needs: Energy, comfort, protection from physical harm, protection from psychologic threat

Avoid situations that could cause conflict with the delusional thinking
When a person is engaged in delusional thinking, avoid activities that conflict with that thinking. When a person believes he has contact with outer space (Mars, etc.) through his radio, do not take the radio from him. When an elderly widow believes the dead husband will come home "soon," do not dispose of the husband's clothing, etc.; do not remove the table-setting she has placed for him; do not insist she move to a smaller house or where he "cannot find her." If the person believes he is a composer, do not remove his musical instrument. If a person thinks his goodluck piece protects him from evil forces, illness, etc., permit him to retain the object even though some kind of adaptation for safety may be necessary.
Rationale: Activities that conflict with delusional thinking heighten an already high level of anxiety and support increased delusional thinking.
Fulfilled Needs: Protection from psychologic threat

Avoid the use of restraints   Do not apply restraints to the person's extremities or chest.
Rationale: Restraints, which limit body movements, cause increased anxiety and a sense of powerlessness. The application of restraints should be avoided whenever possible.
Fulfilled Needs: Comfort, protection from psychologic threat

Avoid using rough-textured bed linens   Do not allow use of bed linens made from coarse materials such as muslin or rough-textured cotton. Use only soft cotton (if possible, percale) sheets.
Rationale: Rough-textured linens cause friction irritation, and skin breakdown.
Fulfilled Needs: Comfort, protection from physical harm

Avoid verbal communications   When the person is hoarse or has difficulty speaking, temporarily avoid communications that necessitate a verbal response. When, in an emotional situation, the person prefers not to communicate verbally, delay the verbal exchange until later.
Rationale: Speech places stress and discomfort on irritated vocal cords. Avoiding verbal communication at inappropriate times reduces psychologic threat.
Fulfilled Needs: Comfort, protection from physical harm, protection from psychologic threat

Avoid written communications   Do not give the person printed or written material that requires his interpretation through reading.
Rationale: Ill persons are hypersensitive to their weaknesses. Awareness of severe health impairment increases feelings of threat.
Fulfilled Needs: Comfort, protection from psychologic threat

Await delivery of the placenta   Wait 10–20 minutes until the placenta delivers itself through the vulva. Do not under any circumstances force the delivery.
Rationale: Assisting with placenta expulsion promotes maternal safety.
Fulfilled Needs: Protection from physical harm

Balance fluid intake to equal output   Maintain a daily balanced fluid intake by offering the patient the same amount of fluid that is put out. Normally, older children and adults need a fluid intake of 1,500–3,600 cc/day due to 1,500 cc urine loss, 500–1,000 cc sweat loss, 400 cc loss through respirations, and 500 cc fecal loss. Normally, infants and small children need 125 cc of water for every 2.2 lb of body weight per day. In nonhealth states, the output may be above or below normal. The intake should be balanced accordingly so both are equal.

Rationale: Balanced fluid intake and output are essential to cell functioning. Fluid alterations damage and impair cell activity. Adequate intake is essential for glomerular filtration of nitrogen waste products. Balanced fluid intake reduces the number of foreign particles, such as fat, in the circulation.

Fulfilled Needs: Fluid and electrolyte balance, waste elimination of nitrogenous and other toxic substances, comfort, protection from physical harm

Bandage with a draining-wound dressing   Apply a fluffed and loosely packed sterile dressing to the draining wound.

Rationale: Loosely packed gauze draws drainage away from its source. It promotes air circulation, resulting in moisture evaporation and area heat reduction. It maintains cleanliness and comfort.

Fulfilled Needs: Comfort, cleanliness, protection from physical harm

Bathe daily   Cleanse the person's body daily by bed bath, sponge bath, shower, or tub.

Rationale: Cleanliness prevents bacterial growth and promotes comfort. It assists in illness dependency. Gently touching the person's skin during bathing can express concern and relatedness toward the person.

Fulfilled Needs: Comfort, cleanliness, protection from physical harm, dependence

Contraindications: Partial baths should be substituted several times a week for persons with very dry skin

Bathe in a shower   Wash the body with soap and rinse it with water in spray form.

Rationale: The gentle pressure of sprayed water cleanses the skin of infecting microorganisms, promotes comfort, and stimulates peripheral circulation. Steam from a shower helps moisten the lungs of persons with a laryngectomy. It assists in illness dependency.

Fulfilled Needs: Tissue oxygenation or perfusion, comfort, cleanliness, protection from physical harm, dependence

Bathe in a tub   Immerse the body in a tub of clean water. Wash with soap and rinse with water.

Rationale: Tub bathing cleanses the skin of infecting microorganisms, promotes comfort, facilitates musculoskeletal movement, and stimulates peripheral circulation. Tub bathing does not pose the threat of water entering the vagina and so is safe during early pregnancy. It assists in illness dependency.

Fulfilled Needs: Tissue oxygenation or perfusion, comfort, cleanliness, protection from physical harm, dependence

Contraindications: Avoid tub bathing once the membrane has ruptured, the mucous plug appears, or if there is vaginal bleeding during pregnancy

Bathe in cool water   Apply cool water to the skin either in a bath or by local sponge application.

Rationale: Liquid solutions in contact with heat change into vapor. When water comes in contact with excessively warm skin, the liquid vaporizes and reduces body temperature. Cooling the body surface promotes comfort.

Fulfilled Needs: Normal temperature, comfort

Bathe in vinegar water   Place the person in a tub or bathe with a washcloth, using a vinegar-water solution of 2 tablespoons vinegar to 1 pint water.

Rationale: Vinegar-water solution reduces uremic itching by dissolving and removing uremic urate salts from the skin.

Fulfilled Needs: Comfort, cleanliness, protection from physical harm

Bathe in warm water   Apply warm water (90–100°F) to the skin either by bath or local sponge application.

Rationale: Bathing in warm water increases body temperature, relaxes muscles, promotes comfort, increases extremity circulation through vessel dilatation, stimulates voiding, and relieves bladder spasms.

Fulfilled Needs: Tissue oxygenation or perfusion, waste elimination of urine, normal temperature, relaxation, comfort, protection from physical harm

Bathe locally Using soap and water, cleanse any body area that frequently becomes soiled. Include areas of drainage, incontinence, and prolonged bleeding.

Rationale: Irritating body discharges promote skin breakdown. Bathing removes skin irritating substances, cleanses infecting microorganisms, and promotes comfort. It assists in illness dependency.

Fulfilled Needs: Comfort, cleanliness, protection from physical harm, dependence

Bathe with oil Use mild oil to bathe a premature infant. Do not use soap and water.

Rationale: Soap and water may irritate the fragile skin of premature infants. Oil cleanses the skin.

Fulfilled Needs: Cleanliness, protection from physical harm

Bathe with water only Wash the skin with nothing but clear, clean water.

Rationale: Chemical substances on sensitive skin irritate cutaneous tissue and promote skin breakdown. Bathing in clean water cleanses the skin, refreshes, and promotes comfort.

Fulfilled Needs: Comfort, cleanliness, protection from physical harm

Bivalve and spread the cast to relieve pressure (ET) When evidence of severe tissue edema or circulatory impairment exists in a casted limb and medical assistance is not available, the cast should be split along both sides. The anterior and posterior cast is then adjusted to allow for the problem and taped or bandaged in place so it still fulfills its function of maintaining immobility.

Rationale: Pressure on edematous tissues could puncture the skin, and prolonged, impaired circulation could cause tissue necrosis and nerve damage.

Fulfilled Needs: Tissue oxygenation or perfusion, comfort, protection from physical harm

Boil the milk When an allergy or intolerance to milk exists, cook the milk to boiling, cool, and serve.

Rationale: In milk intolerance, boiling milk destroys enzymes and supports easier and more rapid digestion and absorption, and, in milk allergy, breaks down protein, reducing allergy responses.

Fulfilled Needs: Nutritional balance, comfort, protection from physical harm

Brush and comb the hair Stroke the hair with a brush and comb several times a day.

Rationale: Brushing the hair removes dirt particles and dead scalp cells, promotes comfort, and conserves energy in weak persons.

Fulfilled Needs: Energy, comfort, cleanliness, dependence

Brush and floss the teeth Using a toothbrush and abrasive agent, clean the person's teeth and surrounding tissues. Using dental floss, apply it between the teeth to remove debri.

Rationale: Since illness predisposes mouth tissue to infection, cleanliness reduces bacterial action and promotes comfort. Brushing and flossing the person's teeth for him conserves energy needed for healing and aids in illness dependency.

Fulfilled Needs: Energy, comfort, cleanliness, protection from physical harm, dependence

Brush the infant's hair with a soft hairbrush Stroke the infant's hair with a soft-bristled brush several times a day.

Rationale: A soft hairbrush prevents irritation to tender skin, removes dirt particles, and promotes comfort.

Fulfilled Needs: Comfort, cleanliness, protection from physical harm, dependence

Brush the teeth with a soft toothbrush   When brushing the teeth of a person with injured, degenerating, or bleeding gums, use a soft toothbrush.

Rationale: Using a soft toothbrush prevents trauma to gums and oral mucosa, while maintaining gum stimulation and clean teeth.

Fulfilled Needs: Comfort, protection from physical harm

Brush the tongue   Apply the stroking action of a toothbrush to the tongue surface.

Rationale: Friction from brushing removes coatings or food accumulations from mucous membrane surfaces, reduces irritation, and promotes comfort. Persons having a laryngectomy need an exceptionally clean mouth because of impaired taste and smell.

Fulfilled Needs: Comfort, cleanliness, protection from physical harm

Call the person's family, physician   Contact the person's loved ones by telephone, inform them of the person's condition, and ask that they come and stay with the person. Call the physician as needed.

Rationale: The presence of loved ones during illness promotes comfort and emotional support. Early notification of a relative's serious illness gives family members time to adapt to the stressful situation.

Fulfilled Needs: Comfort, unity with loved ones

Cast doubt about the reality of the hallucinations (illusions, delusional thinking)   Let the person know that the nurse questions if the person's thinking or perceptions are correct. Make a statement such as "You may think you are a king, but I wonder if you are"; or "You may see a tiger, but I don't see it." Avoid direct verbal attacks on the perception or thinking.

Rationale: Casting doubts on the reality of perceptions or thinking promotes reality orientation.

Fulfilled Needs: Increased reality perception and problem-solving ability

Catheterize with an indwelling urinary catheter   Introduce a sterile catheter through the urethra into the bladder. Inflate the catheter and leave it in place.

Rationale: An indwelling catheter facilitates urine flow from the bladder, maintains normal elimination of nitrogenous and other toxic wastes, promotes comfort by relieving bladder pressure, and prevents skin irritation from incontinence.

Fulfilled Needs: Waste elimination of urine, comfort, cleanliness, protection from physical harm

Contraindications: Susceptibility to or existing genitourinary infection, hematuria, urethral obstruction

Caution about breast-feeding   When there is breast inflammation or possible nipple cracking, allow the mother to breast-feed, but caution her against allowing extreme sucking pressure or prolonged feeding.

Rationale: Infant sucking irritates breast tissue.

Fulfilled Needs: Comfort, protection from physical harm

Contraindications: During severe breast-tissue irritation or infection, breast-feeding is to be avoided

Change the catheter each time the airway is suctioned   Dispose of the airway suctioning catheter immediately after use and obtain a new, sterile catheter, especially when suctioning tracheostomy and endotracheal tubes. Wear sterile gloves.

Rationale: Airway suctioning with sterile catheters minimizes the introduction of microorganisms into the respiratory system.

Fulfilled Needs: Cleanliness, protection from physical harm

Change the dressing frequently Check the wound dressing for drainage at least every 4 hours and apply a clean, dry, sterile dressing immediately when soiled.

Rationale: Dry, sterile wound coverings minimize bacterial growth and promote cleanliness and comfort.

Fulfilled Needs: Comfort, cleanliness, protection from physical harm

Change the hyperalimentation tubing with each dressing change Remove all the used hyperalimentation tubing, except the subclavian Intracath, and replace with new sterile tubing at each dressing change. Maintain absolute sterile technique, especially at the tubing tips.

Rationale: Clean therapeutic equipment minimizes infection.

Fulfilled Needs: Cleanliness, protection from physical harm

Change the ostomy appliance as needed If the person has a colostomy, an ileostomy, a ureterostomy, or a ureteroileostomy, etc., change the drainage receptacle as often as needed to maintain cleanliness and comfort. Appliances attached with adhesive are changed less frequently but require intermittent emptying.

Rationale: Frequently changing the ostomy appliance promotes comfort. It maintains cleanliness, reducing the possibility of infection and skin irritation.

Fulfilled Needs: Comfort, cleanliness, protection from physical harm

Change the person's clothing at bedtime Before bedtime, change the clothes that the person has been wearing all day. Provide a clean gown.

Rationale: Clean clothes are refreshing, promote comfort, and assist in illness dependency.

Fulfilled Needs: Comfort, cleanliness, dependence

Change the person's position frequently At least every 2 hours both day and night, move the person's body from one position to another, from side to side and back to abdomen. Turn frequenty.

Rationale: Body-position changes prevent respiratory congestion, prolonged pressure on body areas, and contractures. They promote circulation and expectoration, reduce fatigue, and stimulate voiding. Position change assists in illness dependency.

Fulfilled Needs: Tissue oxygenation or perfusion, waste elimination of urine and bronchopulmonary secretions, comfort, protection from physical harm, dependence

Contraindications: Spinal cord injuries or bone fractures requiring complete body immobilization

Change the person's position gradually Slowly raise the person from a lying or sitting position to a step-by-step elevated position.

Rationale: Gradual position change reduces severe arterial and venous blood pressure adaptations, promotes uniform circulation, prevents sudden eye pressure changes, decreases pressure on bones, and in hyperalimentation decreases possible catheter clogging.

Fulfilled Needs: Tissue oxygenation or perfusion, comfort, protection from physical harm, freedom from pain

Change the sanitary pads/tampons frequently Replace the saturated sanitary pad with a clean one as often as needed, preferably every 4 hours.

Rationale: Cleanliness prevents infection and promotes comfort. Changing pads assists in illness dependency.

Fulfilled Needs: Comfort, cleanliness, protection from physical harm, dependence

Change the tracheostomy tube When the inserted tracheostomy tube becomes encrusted with secretions and cannot be cleaned properly while in place, gently remove the tube, use forceps to hold the stoma open, and insert a new tube.

Rationale: A patient airway is essential to normal oxygen and carbon dioxide exchange. Cleanliness prevents respiratory tract infection and promotes comfort.

Fulfilled Needs: Tissue oxygenation or perfusion, comfort, cleanliness, protection from physical harm

Change the urinary catheter Replace the indwelling urinary catheter when the present catheter is no longer aseptically clean or patent.

Rationale: A sterile catheter minimizes bacterial spread from catheter to urinary tract. A patent catheter facilitates urine flow, maintaining normal elimination of nitrogenous and other toxic wastes, and promotes comfort.

Fulfilled Needs: Waste elimination of urine, comfort, cleanliness, protection from physical harm

Change the urinary drainage apparatus Replace the urinary drainage bag every 24 hours if urinary infection exists. Change it at least every 3 days if no infection exists and if it serves as a receptacle for urine from an indwelling catheter.

Rationale: Urinary drainage bag cleanliness prevents infection.

Fulfilled Needs: Cleanliness, protection from physical harm

Change the wet diaper immediately Check often to determine when diapers are wet and replace them with dry diapers immediately.

Rationale: Urine ammonia causes skin irritation. Skin dryness promotes cleanliness and comfort.

Fulfulled Needs: Comfort, cleanliness, protection from physical harm

Clamp the chest tube but for only a short time[686] If the closed-chest-drainage system breaks, clamp off the chest tube as quickly as possible with a rubberized hemostat. Limit the clamping of the tube to the least possible time, preferably no more than several minutes. Immediately release the clamp if signs of tension pneumothorax (tracheal deviation, severe cyanosis and dyspnea, shock) occur.

Rationale: When a person has had lung surgery or has a large pneumothorax, if there is leakage of air from the lung, clamping the chest tube will cause air to build up in the chest, increasing the pleural pressure resulting in lung collapse (tension pneumothorax). A clamped chest tube prevents air from being sucked into the thoracic cavity when the closed-chest-drainage system has been interrupted.

Fulfilled Needs: Comfort, protection from physical harm

Clamp the indwelling urinary catheter intermittently When retraining is essential to maintain bladder control, intermittently clamp the catheter to prevent urinary flow. At first the catheter should be clamped for periods of 1–2 hours, gradually working up to 4-hour periods.

Rationale: Catheter clamping increases urine volume in the bladder. The increased pressure on bladder tissues and nerves improves bladder muscle tone and stimulates the voiding reflex. Bladder control is essential to the removal of body wastes, the maintenance of dryness to prevent skin irritation, and comfort.

Fulfilled Needs: Waste elimination of urine, comfort, protection from physical harm

Clean the artificial eye Use normal saline or tap water to remove unclean particles from an artificial eye.

Rationale: Cleansing the artificial eye prevents infection and promotes comfort. It offers assistance during illness dependency.

Fulfilled Needs: Comfort, cleanliness, protection from physical harm, dependence

Clean the contact lenses Using the appropriate cleaning fluid, remove all dirt and smudge from the contact lenses.

Rationale: Clean contact lenses reduce the potential for eye infection and aid good vision.

Fulfilled Needs: Comfort, cleanliness, protection from physical harm, dependence

Clean the dentures Place the person's artificial teeth in cleansing solution. Brush the teeth with a toothbrush, rinse them with cool water, and then soak them in mouthwash for a short period. Table salt or sodium bicarbonate may be used as a cleansing agent.

Rationale: Since illness predisposes mouth tissue to infection, cleanliness reduces bacterial action and promotes comfort. Cleansing the person's dentures helps conserve energy and offers assistance during illness dependency.

Fulfilled Needs: Energy, comfort, cleanliness, protection from physical harm

Clean the eye(s)/ears Use sterile gauze to remove accumulated secretions from the eye. Use a soft or flexible cotton swab to gently clean the ears.

Rationale: Eye cleansing prevents tissue irritation and infection. It promotes comfort and visual acuity. Cleaning the ears promotes hygiene and auditory acuity.

Fulfilled Needs: Comfort, cleanliness, protection from physical harm

Clean the eyeglasses Remove soil, dirt, lint, or cloudiness from the eyeglasses before the person wears them. To prevent scratching, be sure the lens is wet before cleaning, and always use a soft cloth rather than paper tissue.

Rationale: Cleaning eyeglasses promotes visual acuity essential to physical safety and comfort and offers assistance during illness dependency.

Fulfilled Needs: Comfort, cleanliness, protection from physical harm, dependence

Clean the nails Soak the finger- and toenails, then use an orange stick to remove dirt from under and around the nails.

Rationale: Cleanliness minimizes microorganism transfer into and onto body areas that have finger contact. It promotes comfort and offers assistance during illness dependency.

Fulfilled Needs: Comfort, cleanliness, protection from physical harm, dependence

Clean the skin with a drying soap Wash the skin with an oil-removing soap that causes skin dryness. Such soaps include Fels Naptha and Kirkman's soap.

Rationale: Drying soaps remove oils that obstruct sebaceous glands, causing inflammation.

Fulfilled Needs: Cleanliness, protection from physical harm

Contraindications: Avoid using on dry skin

Clean the skin with a nondrying soap Clean the skin with soap which does not dry out the skin such as Dove, Neutrogena, Alpha-Keri, Shepard's soap.

Rationale: Use of a nondrying soap helps keep the skin well moisturized.

Fulfilled Needs: Comfort, protection from physical harm

Clean the skin with an astringent Wash the skin with an astringent, metallic salt solution such as zinc oxide or aluminum acetate.

Rationale: Astringent chemicals cause vasoconstriction in superficial tissues, and their drying effect on the skin reduces skin oiliness. Cleanliness promotes comfort.

Fulfilled Needs: Comfort, cleanliness, protection from physical harm

Contraindications: Avoid using on dry skin

Clean the tracheostomy (or laryngectomy) tube inner cannula Remove and wash the tracheostomy (or laryngectomy) tube inner cannula with hydrogen peroxide and clean it with pipe cleaners or sterile gauze. After cleaning the cannula, soak it for a few moments in sterile water to remove any cleansing agents that might irritate tracheal tissue.

Rationale: Oxygen and carbon dioxide exchange through respirations is essential to life. Cleanliness inhibits the growth of infecting microorganisms into the respiratory tract.

Fulfilled Needs: Tissue oxygenation or perfusion, cleanliness, protection from physical harm

Clean the urinary catheter externally at the meatus Using benzalkonium (Zephiran) chloride, hydrogen peroxide, or surgical soap, clean the outside of the urinary catheter, especially in the area surrounding the meatus.

Rationale: Cleanliness minimizes the number of infecting microorganisms entering the urinary meatus and promotes comfort.

Fulfilled Needs: Comfort, cleanliness, protection from physical harm

Clean with alcohol Remove skin dirt and bacteria through a friction application of alcohol.

Rationale: Alcohol in 70% solution stops bacterial growth. Cleanliness promotes comfort.

Fulfilled Needs: Comfort, cleanliness, protection from physical harm

Contraindications: Avoid using alcohol on an open wound since it causes severe pain; do not use if it causes chilling of the skin

Clean with antiseptic solution Clean the skin or wound with a chemical agent that prevents microorganism growth, such as the skin antiseptic ethyl alcohol or wound antiseptic potassium permanganate.

Rationale: Antiseptics inhibit bacterial growth, preventing infection and promoting cleanliness and comfort.

Fulfilled Needs: Comfort, cleanliness, protection from physical harm

Clean with castile or lanolin soap Wash dirt and bacteria from the skin using castile soap (made from olive oil and caustic soda) or lanolin soap (made from wool fat or grease).

Rationale: Castile and lanolin soap oils soothe the skin and prevent epidermal irritation. Soap friction promotes the comfort of cleanliness.

Fulfilled Needs: Comfort, cleanliness, protection from physical harm

Clean with hydrogen peroxide Wash the wound or skin with a 3% hydrogen peroxide solution.

Rationale: Hydrogen peroxide destroys bacteria through oxidation and removes adhered exudates and debris from areas where microorganisms might grow. Cleanliness promotes comfort.

Fulfilled Needs: Comfort, cleanliness, protection from physical harm

Contraindications: Avoid using in closed body cavities (bladder, chest tubes, open wounds into cavities) because excess pressure will result when the gas produced by the hydrogen peroxide becomes trapped in the cavity

Clean with surgical soap (antibacterial soap, an antibacterial agent) Remove skin dirt and bacteria through the use of antibacterial or surgical soap or agents and sterile water.

Rationale: Surgical or antibacterial soap or agents remove skin bacteria, preventing infection. Soap friction promotes the comfort of cleanliness.

Fulfilled Needs: Comfort, cleanliness, protection from physical harm

Clear nasal secretions Free the internal nares of dirt and secretions by gently inserting a moistened cotton-tipped applicator or folded tissue into the nares and removing undesirable substances.

Rationale: Cleaning the internal nares allows for free passage of respiratory gases. It promotes comfort and offers assistance during illness dependency.

Fulfilled Needs: Tissue oxygenation or perfusion, comfort, cleanliness, protection from physical harm, dependence

Clearly communicate what is expected of the person Specifically communicate to the person the behavior that you expect. Make it clear that deviations from such behavior are unacceptable.

Rationale: Clearly communicated behavioral expectations encourage the person toward positive behavioral responses. The fulfillment of such expectations provides the satisfaction of positive responses from others.

Fulfilled Needs: Predictable and orderly world, approval from others, high evaluation of self, personal growth and maturity, increased reality perception

Clothe in disposable incontinent briefs Apply disposable, protective briefs that absorb moisture during incontinence. Change immediately when soiled.

Rationale: Collecting urine or fecal wastes in absorbent material reduces skin wetness, decreasing potential skin irritation from waste products. Cleanliness promotes comfort.

Fulfilled Needs: Cleanliness, comfort, protection from physical harm

Clothe in flannel pajamas at night Cover the body with soft woolen clothing during nighttime sleeping hours.

Rationale: Flannel fabric absorbs excessive moisture on the skin from sweating and prevents the discomfort of chilling.

Fulfilled Needs: Normal temperature, comfort

Collect radiation-contaminated linen in a special laundry bag Place in a special laundry bag, linens used by a person receiving radium implants or other radioactive substances producing gamma rays. Label the bag for special handling.

Rationale: Radiation causes physical harm to exposed persons.

Fulfilled Needs: Protection from physical harm

Collect radiation-contaminated urine in a lead-lined container Place in jugs inside lead-lined boxes, urine excreted by a person receiving radium implants or other radioactive substances producing gamma rays. Do not remove the urine until radioactivity has decreased to 30 millicuries.

Rationale: Radiation causes physical harm to exposed persons.

Fulfilled Needs: Protection from physical harm

Comb the dandruff up from the scalp Press the teeth of the comb against the scalp and comb the dandruff away from the scalp.

Rationale: Removal of dead scalp tissue promotes cleanliness and reduces the discomfort of itching. When sebaceous gland inflammation exists, dandruff accumulation promotes hair loss or thinning.

Fulfilled Needs: Comfort, cleanliness, protection from physical harm

Communicate by gesture Send messages by expressing ideas through the use of hand motions and facial changes.

Rationale: Nonverbal gesturing clarifies the meaning of words. Psychologic comfort is promoted through a sense of adequate communication with others. Increased external stimuli enhance perception and response to stimuli.

Fulfilled Needs: Comfort, stimulation, caring and communicating relationships

Communicate nurse sensitivity to the person's pain/problem Verbally and nonverbally communicate that the nurse experiences feelings for the person's suffering or situation and will make every effort to perceive the pain or problem as the person sees it.

Rationale: Feelings of control evolve from an awareness that the person is not threatened with aloneness. Relief measures, in terms of the person's perception of pain or a problem, result from the nurse's sensitivity to the situation.

Fulfilled Needs: Comfort, protection from psychologic threat

Communicate recent nonthreatening news events to the disoriented person   Acquaint the person with the environment by telling him important current happenings going on in the world and in the local community. Be cautious about sharing disturbing information.

Rationale: The ability to comprehend the environment in regard to time, place, persons, and events prevents confusion and anxiety.

Fulfilled Needs: Protection from psychologic threat, increased reality perception

Communicate that the nurse feels comfortable with the person's discussion of death (of sex, of sexuality)   Express to the person that the nurse is comfortable with and not threatened by discussions of death, sex, or sexuality. Let the person know that when he wants to talk, he need only call for the nurse to listen. Do not run off, change the subject, or deal in trivial conversation when death, sex, or sexuality are mentioned.

Rationale: The person who senses that health personnel are threatened by discussions of death, sex, or sexuality, feels isolated and unable to resolve conflicts. Dying persons sometimes pretend denial in order to maintain the comfort of health personnel. A discussion of death, sex, or sexuality at the person's pace promotes comfort and reduces threat.

Fulfilled Needs: Comfort, protection from physiologic threat, caring and communicating relationships

Confine the animal suspected of being infected   If an animal has inflicted injury on a person, lock the animal in a specific area where it can be observed.

Rationale: Confining an animal offers opportunity to observe it for the presence of disease and prevents the animal from inflicting further injury on others.

Fulfilled Needs: Protection from physical harm

Connect the mother to the fetal/maternal ultrasound monitor   Turn the monitor on. Place the transducers against the abdomen and attach with an elastic belt around the mother's abdomen and back for uterine contraction readings and fetal heart tones.

Rationale: Monitoring fetal activity promotes early detection and correction of fetal distress.

Fulfilled Needs: Protection from physical harm

Connect the person to a respiratory monitor   Place leads on the person's chest and attach them to a respiratory monitor; or place the infant's chest and abdomen on the apnea pad, which is connected to a respiratory monitor.

Rationale: The respiratory monitor visually records the person's rate of respirations. It signals when respirations go below the safe limit.

Fulfilled Needs: Protection from physical harm

Connect the person to an ECG monitor   Attach the person to the electrocardiogram monitor by placing ECG leads on the person's chest, arms, and legs. Position the person comfortably. Adjust the ECG monitor to the correct setting and turn on the alarms.

Rationale: The electrocardiogram displays and records the electrical activity of the heart. Use of an ECG monitor provides instant recognition of cardiac activity, abnormal cardiac rhythm and myocardial damage.

Fulfilled Needs: Protection from physical harm

Consult with the/a physician On behalf of the person, discuss with the physician the person's problem and the alternatives available for solving the problem.
Rationale: Nursing consultation with the person's physician provides safety and comfort for the person
Fulfilled Needs: Comfort, protection from physical harm

Control ileostomy/colostomy odor by deodorization Disagreeable odors from an ileostomy or colostomy can be controlled by keeping the patient, his clothes, and the appliance clean; by inserting deodorant tablets such as charcoal, chlorophyll, and aspirin into the bag following each emptying; by placing an alcohol-saturated cloth or tissue in the bag; by using spray deodorant; or by applying an extra plastic covering such as kitchen wrap over the bag.
Rationale: Freedom from body odors promotes comfort.
Fulfilled Needs: Comfort

Control offensive odors by removing the source When odors are disagreeable, remove the source from which the odors come, such as urinals, bedpans, soiled sheets, genitorurinary collection bags, soiled dressings, or soiled ostomy bags.
Rationale: Offensive odors irritate olfactory senses, causing severe discomfort. Illness produces hypersensitive olfactory sensory perception, which heightens the irritation.
Fulfilled Needs: Comfort

Correct misinterpreted messages immediately If there is evidence that a message has been interpreted incorrectly, immediately correct this misinterpretation.
Rationale: Message reception and interpretation is influenced by physiologic and psychologic disequilibrium. Psychologic comfort is promoted through a sense of adequate communication with others.
Fulfilled Needs: Protection from physical harm, protection from psychologic threat, caring, and communicating relationships

Cover the bed with netting Put fine netting over the bed when there are flying insects in the environment or when there is potential for a child to fall out of bed.
Rationale. Insects transmit viral and bacterial disease, and their bites reduce human comfort. Netting prevents children from climbing over the sides of beds.
Fulfilled Needs: Comfort, protection from physical harm

Cover the hands with mittens Place the person's hand in a mitten or mitten substitute to restrict finger movements of a small child or an incoherent adult.
Rationale: Limiting finger movements decreases the ability to cause skin irritation and infection through scratching.
Fulfilled Needs: Protection from physical harm

Cover the sucking wound immediately Cover a sudden, open-chest wound immediately so that air cannot be sucked into the pleural cavity. Use available dressings, clothes, or even the palm of the hand.
Rationale: Air entering the pleural space increases intrapleural pressure and causes lung collapse.
Fulfilled Needs: Protection from physical harm

Cover with lightweight blankets Place lightweight sheets and blankets over the person.
Rationale: Lightweight blankets maintain body heat with a minimum of pressure and weight. They prevent excessive warming of the body, thereby supporting a normal metabolic rate and lessening the burden on an ailing cardiac or respiratory system. In shock, lightweight covers maintain peripheral coolness so the circulating blood can meet

the needs of vital internal organs.

Fulfilled Needs: Normal temperature, comfort, protection from physical harm

Contraindications: Very low body temperature

Cover with warm blankets   Place warm sheets and blankets over the person.

Rationale: Warm bed covering promotes comfort by increasing environmental heat surrounding the body and maintaining normal temperature. It decreases body heat loss to the environment.

Fulfilled Needs: Normal temperature, comfort, protection from physical harm

Contraindications: Avoid warm blankets during shock and increased metabolic rate

Create giving situations   Create circumstances in which the person has the opportunity to give emotionally to others without receiving a reward. Usually, this situation occurs between loved ones and friends. However, if a person lacks affection from significant persons, nursing personnel can offer warmth and friendship as a temporary substitute.

Rationale: Love given unconditionally requires a high degree of maturity. Self-esteem is nourished by the development of interpersonal skills and from positive responses from others.

Fulfilled Needs: Comfort, caring and communicating relationships, approval from others, sense of usefulness, high evaluation of self, personal growth and maturity, increased pleasantness or pleasure

Cut off the electrical power source causing the injury   Stop the flow of electricity into a person by curtailing the source of power. Use insulated wire cutters or gloves if it is necessary to come in direct contact with the electrical source.

Rationale: The disruption of the electrical power source terminates the injuring force.

Fulfilled Needs: Protection from physical harm

Cut the food into bite-size pieces   Slice the food into small pieces so it can be handled easily when placed in the mouth.

Rationale: The intake of food determines the nutritional state. With involuntary or absent tongue movements, food cannot be properly masticated. Cutting food into small bites aids the digestive process and meets dependency needs. It promotes the comfort of ease in chewing or swallowing, and it prevents choking and aspiration.

Fulfilled Needs: Nutritional balance, comfort, protection from physical harm, dependence

Dangle the legs   Gradually bring the person to a sitting position and slowly move his feet and legs off the side of the bed. Provide foot support with a chair.

Rationale: Dangling, the first step in reestablishing activity, supports strength renewal. The downward gravitational force improves the vascular tone of the muscles, which, in turn, improves circulation. Assistance with activity meets illness dependency needs.

Fulfilled Needs: Tissue oxygenation or perfusion, activity, protection from physical harm, dependence

Contraindications: Avoid dangling when there is leg edema or impaired peripheral circulation

Darken the room   Turn off or remove all light sources within the immediate environment.

Rationale: Light stimuli promote wakefulness. Adequate sleep is essential in that the decreased metabolic rate occurring during sleep restores depleted cell energy reserves that result from body adaptation requirements.

Fulfilled Needs: Sleep, rest, relaxation, energy, comfort, protection from physical harm

Decrease drafts   Reduce the volume of air currents in the environment.

Rationale: Decreasing drafts allows low body temperature to return to normal by reducing the evaporation of perspiration. It prevents itching of irritated skin and reduces body chilling. Drafts over a wet cast cause coldness, which may result in the discomfort of a chill. Drafts stimulate open nerve endings of an open stump and cause pain or phantom sensation. Drafts stimulate the reflex arc or lower motor neurons in paralyzed muscles, causing severe muscle spasm.

Fulfilled Needs: Normal temperature, comfort, protection from physical harm

Decrease environmental stimuli   Decrease the amount of stimulus the person receives from the environment. This includes minimal light and sound, limited visitors.

Rationale: Decreased environmental stimulation promotes rest and healing.

Fulfilled Needs: Comfort, protection from physical harm

Decrease the time interval between infant feedings   Feed the infant more often than the present schedule. If he has been eating every 4 hours, feed him every 3 hours. This applies to both bottle- and breast-feeding.

Rationale: More frequent feedings satisfy the infant's desire for prolonged sucking, provide a greater quantity of food, and promote comfort.

Fulfilled Needs: Nutritional balance, comfort

Defer speech communications for 72 hours after a partial laryngectomy
Following a partial laryngectomy, suggest that the person not attempt to make any sound for at least 72 hours.

Rationale: Vibrations made when attempting to speak can traumatize healing tissue.

Fulfilled Needs: Protection from physical harm

Defibrillate the heart muscle (ET)   Discharge an electrical current into the heart muscle just after the R-wave of the QRS complex, if cardiac arrythmia exists. If ventricular fibrillation occurs, no QRS complex will exist, so timing the electrical shock is not dependent on the R-wave, and the procedure should be performed immediately.

Rationale: The discharge of an electrical current into the heart muscle promotes simultaneous contraction and relaxation of all cardiac muscles at appropriate intervals, thus facilitating the flow of oxygen-saturated blood to body tissues. Inadequate oxygenation causes damage or death to body tissue.

Fulfilled Needs: Tissue oxygenation or perfusion, protection from physical harm

Deflate the airway-tube cuff periodically   Release air from the endotracheal or tracheostomy tube cuff. Suction during cuff deflation. Usually the cuff is deflated for 5–15 minutes every 1 to 4 hours. The cuff often is deflated immediately after intermittent positive-pressure breathing and meals and is not inflated again until the next treatment or meal.

Rationale: Deflation of an airway-tube cuff relieves pressure on the tracheal and laryngeal mucosa. It decreases potential tissue necrosis from inflation pressure.

Fulfilled Needs: Protection from physical harm

Delay bathing   Temporarily put off bathing.

Rationale: Water, on evaporation, tends to cool the body. A chilled body may already be too cool and uncomfortable for bathing. In severe illness, the activity of bathing may further deplete energy reserves.

Fulfilled Needs: Energy, comfort, protection from physical harm

Delay communications   Put off communicating until the person is ready to express his thoughts and feelings.

Rationale: Thoughts and feelings are the person's internal world, the privacy of which should be respected until there is a desire for external expression. Information is poorly communicated when a person is emotionally disturbed, distracted, or preoccupied.

Fulfilled Needs: Protection from psychologic threat, dignity

Delay teaching Do not offer health care teaching while a person is preoccupied with survival or crisis. Plan the teaching for a future date when the person is more receptive.

Rationale: During periods of threats to survival and crisis, human energy is directed toward self-preservation and homeostasis. At such times, there is no energy for learning. Teaching must, therefore, be put off until the crisis subsides and energy can again be directed outward.

Fulfilled Needs: Comfort, protection from physical harm, protection from psychologic threat

Demonstrate attitudes consistent with the child's parents' attitudes Maintain the same behavioral approach as parents display toward their child provided the parental attitude is healthy.

Rationale: Feelings of safety arise from familiar and predictable situations that have been handled successfully in the past.

Fulfilled Needs: Comfort, protection from psychologic threat, predictable and orderly world

Demonstrate calmness Assume a calm, although concerned, attitude about the person's problem. Display confidence, knowledge, and decisive judgment in helping the person.

Rationale: Identification with the positive attitudes of other people reduces fear and anxiety and promotes positive self-attitudes.

Fulfilled Needs: Comfort, protection from psychologic threat

Detect communicable disease cases Find persons who have been exposed to or have contracted a communicable disease. Report such findings to the health department.

Rationale: Persons who have contracted or have been exposed to a communicable disease can potentially transmit that disease to others.

Fulfilled Needs: Protection from physical harm

Dilute the medication Thin the medication consistency with water or syrup, giving the same dosage but in a larger volume.

Rationale: Dilution of medications reduces gastric irritation, damage to teeth, and unpleasant taste.

Fulfilled Needs: Comfort, protection from physical harm

Dilute the milk Mix milk with water to decrease the concentration of the milk.

Rationale: The gastrointestinal system tolerates diluted milk more easily. The kidneys of infants under 4 months of age have difficulty handling cow's milk since it contains four times the solute content of breast milk. Therefore, infants can handle diluted milk more easily.

Fulfilled Needs: Comfort, protection from physical harm

Discontinue the blood transfusion/intravenous infusion Stop the infusion of typed and crossmatched blood by clamping off the blood flow or removing the injection needle. When intravenous fluids have infiltrated tissues, have become contaminated, or have been completed, remove the needle immediately.

Rationale: Circulatory overload, infusion-transmitted infection, severe allergic reactions, or hemolytic reactions to incompatible blood pose a serious threat to life. Edema pressure within the tissues from an infiltrated IV causes tissue trauma. Certain drugs intended for intravascular use may cause severe damage when they come in contact with extravascular tissue. Contaminated fluids can cause serious infection. Removal of a needle on fluid completion supports comfort.

Fulfilled Needs: Comfort, protection from physical harm

Discourage decision making when the person is under severe stress
Point out that it is not wise to make important decisions while under severe stress. Such decisions should be withheld until there has been time for adjustment to the crisis and reality perception has been reestablished. A widow should not sell her home immediately after the death of her husband. A divorced daughter should not move back home until she has had time to adjust and consider the situation realistically.

Rationale: Decisions made during times of severe stress often reflect distorted thinking or the opinions of others and often are regretted at a later date. Important decisions require full attention to problem solving and are best made when stress is not an influencing factor.

Fulfilled Needs: Protection from psychologic threat, increased reality perception and problem-solving ability

Discourage smoking Suggest restraint from smoking tobacco products.
Rationale: Tobacco fumes irritate nasal and pulmonary tissue, causing increased secretions. The fumes paralyze tracheobronchial cilia with the resulting danger of secretion retention. The constriction of circulatory blood vessels by tobacco's chemical irritants results in decreased tissue oxygenation, in impaired extremity circulation, and in a decrease of 1–2°F in skin temperature. Tobacco smoke moves from the throat to the eustachian canal and irritates the inner ear. Smoking discolors teeth and irritates gums. During pregnancy, smoking causes a high carbon monoxide blood level in the fetus. This, and the nicotine vasoconstrictive effect, is suspected of causing cardiac anomalies in infants. Breast milk from heavy smoking mothers contains nicotine, which can be harmful to the child. Smoking inhibits peristaltic activity, which contributes to constipation. It delays gastric emptying, which inhibits normal digestion. It decreases the hunger sensation by deadening the taste receptors. Smoking stimulates the heart rate 8–10 beats faster per minute and, by doing so, often makes sleeping difficult. Its stimulative effect can alter cardiac patterns being recorded by a monitor.

Fulfilled Needs: Tissue oxygenation or perfusion, comfort, cleanliness, protection from physical harm

Discourage strenuous activities Suggest that the person not participate in activities that greatly increase the metabolic rate and body energy requirements.
Rationale: Fatigue results from activity or energy-depleting responses to physiologic stress stimuli.
Fulfilled Needs: Energy, comfort, protection from physical harm

Discourage talking while eating and/or drinking Suggest that the person refrain from talking while eating or drinking.
Rationale: Avoiding talking while eating or drinking reduces the possibility of aspiration or swallowing air into the stomach. Since all activity requires energy, refraining from talking provides the extremely fatigued person with a little more energy to direct toward food and fluid consumption.
Fulfilled Needs: Protection from physical harm

Discourage the intake of oral stimulants Suggest restraint from using coffee, tea, amphetamines, alcohol, chocolate, or cola drinks.
Rationale: Oral stimulants can alter cardiac patterns being recorded by a monitor. Alcohol and coffee increase peristaltic activity, increase bladder irritability, and stimulate voiding. Alcohol causes skin vasodilatation with decreased vasoconstriction. Alcohol depresses the central nervous system even though initially it appears to stimulate it. Caffeine causes vasodilatation and has a temporary stimulative effect. Caffeine, in both cof-

fee and tea, heightens fever. Caffeine stimulates the adrenal cortex to produce adrenalin, causing the liver to change glycogen into glucose and raising the blood glucose. Stimulants produce a temporary increase in metabolic rate, cause excitement of nerve and muscle tissue, and increase the general level of body activity, ultimately decreasing energy reserves and threatening the healing process.

Fulfilled Needs: Sleep, rest, relaxation, comfort, protection from physical harm

Discourage the setting of time limits   Suggest that the person not set a specific date or a specific time for reaching a goal.

Rationale: Failure to meet self-expectations results in the threat of frustration. The stimulus of needing to hurry causes muscular tension requiring the use of energy, which, in illness, is vital to healing.

Fulfilled Needs: Energy, comfort, protection from physical harm, protection from psychologic threat, sense of adequacy

Discuss possible pain-reducing measures   Mention all possible measures available for pain relief. Emphasize measures other than drugs. Let the person make his own choice of pain relief. Offer such measures as heat and cold applications, respositioning, relief of pressure or constriction, relaxation measures, attention diversion, and subdued lighting.

Rationale: Awareness that pain-relief measures other than drugs are available reduces the anxiety of potential drug addiction. Comfort feelings are enhanced by awareness that the person has choices and has sufficient independent control to prevent harm and bring comfort to self.

Fulfilled Needs: Comfort, protection from psychologic threat, freedom from pain, caring and communicating relationships

Discuss priority setting   Speak with the person about the need for giving health care a high rank among those life activities that the person considers important.

Rationale: Health care requires a reasonably high priority among life's important activities. Without health, limited function results, which reduces the pleasure and productivity of life.

Fulfilled Needs: Protection from physical harm, independence, identification of priorities, increased reality perception and problem-solving ability

Discuss the anticipated procedure/examination   Provide a clear description of the procedure confronting the person and verbally illustrate what can be expected to occur. In addition, use drawings, pictures, models of organs, toys, and sensory information for clarification.

Rationale: Positive preparation before an occurrence promotes psychologic safety by reducing fear and anxiety of the unknown. Safety feelings arise from familiar and predictable situations.

Fulfilled Needs: Comfort, protection from psychologic threat, predictable and orderly world, increased learning

Disguise drugs with fruit-flavored syrup   Mix a distasteful drug with syrup that is the flavor of a favorite fruit.

Rationale: Enhancing the favorable taste of drugs increases the probability of the drug being taken.

Fulfilled Needs: Comfort

Disinfect contaminated articles   Cleanse objects or materials that have been exposed to infecting microorganisms with disinfectant solution. Whenever possible, expose the objects or materials to open air and sunlight for 12–24 hours.

Rationale: Removal of infectious microorganisms from surfaces decreases the potential for transfer of disease from one person to another.

Fulfilled Needs: Cleanliness, protection from physical harm

Distribute the fluid intake over 24 hours   When fluids are restricted, divide the intake of allowable fluids so they are available over the entire 24 hours. Give three-fourths during waking hours and save one-fourth for thirst during sleeping hours. If possible, have the patient divide the intake as it most pleases him.

Rationale: Awareness that fluids are available to quench thirst 24 hours a day provides comfort.

Fulfilled Needs: Comfort

Distribute the intravenous fluid infusion over 12 to 24 hours   When administering intravenous fluids, distribute the total volume over a 12- to 24-hour period instead of administering fluids over a few short hours.

Rationale: Fluids infused over a long period provide a more balanced fluid and electrolyte level than those given over a short time.

Fulfilled Needs: Fluid and electrolyte balance, protection from physical harm

Divide tasks into multiple, simple steps   Take a complete task and separate it into as many simple steps as possible. If a person is brushing his teeth, break the task into steps such as gathering equipment, putting paste on the toothbrush, brushing the teeth, rinsing the mouth, replacing the equipment.

Rationale: Persons functioning at a level below normal can often maintain independent activities if they do so one step at a time.

Fulfilled Needs: Independence, increased problem-solving ability

Do a papanicolaou (Pap) test   Perform a Pap smear. First, insert a speculum lubricated with warm water or saline. Then scrape secretions from the woman's cervix with a saline moistened Pap stick. Spread the secretions on a slide. Immerse the slide into or spray with a fixative. Remove the speculum.

Rationale: The Papanicolaou test is used for detecting early evidence of malignant cells in the cervix.

Fulfilled Needs: Protection from physical harm

Do a pregnancy test   Obtain the first morning urine sample and do a pregnancy test according to directions or send a blood sample to the laboratory for pregnancy determination.

Rationale: Pregnancy tests of urine or blood samples can verify whether or not a woman is pregnant.

Fulfilled Needs: Comfort, protection from physical harm

Do a surgical/perineal prep   Before surgery or delivery, prepare the skin by thoroughly cleansing and removing all hair from the appropriate skin area.

Rationale: Cleansing and removing bacteria and hair from the skin decreases the potential for infection.

Fulfilled Needs: Cleanliness, protection from physical harm

Do not allow air into the dialysis instillation tubing   Do not allow air to enter the tubing through which the dialysis fluid flows into the peritoneum. Clamp the tubing when the fluid level reaches the neck of the bottle.

Rationale: Air flowing into the peritoneal cavity increases pressure and causes pain.

Fulfilled Needs: Comfort, protection from physical harm

Do not allow skin surfaces (overlapping skin surfaces or burned skin surfaces) to touch   Do not allow body surfaces to touch one another. Separate fingers, toes, legs, skin folds, and the area under the breasts. Place gauze between burned fingers to keep them separated during healing. Under the breasts and between the buttocks, apply a gauze padding to keep the skin apart, absorb moisture, and allow air to pass over the skin.

Rationale: Body surfaces that touch produce friction irritation.

Fulfilled Needs: Protection from physical harm

Do not allow unpleasant surprise situations Reduce fear by preventing elements of surprise and confusion in stressful or fearful situations.

Rationale: The threat of fear is reduced when there is time to prepare for the threat and adapt with appropriate defenses.

Fulfilled Needs: Comfort, protection from psychologic threat

Do not disguise drugs in food   Do not attempt to hide bad-tasting drugs by mixing the drug in food.

Rationale: Drugs mixed in food frequently make food distasteful, causing dislike or rejection of that food. When drugs are disguised in food, unless all the food is eaten, an undetermined portion of the drug is not taken.

Fulfilled Needs: Protection from physical harm

Do not encourage or reinforce hope (the denial) Avoid reinforcing a person's hope or denial. Do not give false information or reassurance that things are better than they are. Do not divert the person's attention from the reality.

Rationale: Reinforcing hope or denial postpones the person's acceptance of the truth and his appropriate coping with the threatening situation.

Fulfilled Needs: Personal growth and maturity, increased reality perception

Do not give a blood transfusion or medications via the hyperalimentation catheter Do not give a blood transfusion or allow medications to be given through the subclavian Intracath being used for hyperalimentation.

Rationale: Blood cells or drug chemicals will coat the internal catheter surface and obstruct the catheter, altering the flow rate of the hyperalimentation solution.

Fulfilled Needs: Protection from physical harm

Do not give blood that is more than 3 weeks old   Do not administer blood by transfusion if it is more than 3 weeks old.

Rationale: The oxygen-carrying capacity of blood decreases with age.

Fulfilled Needs: Protection from physical harm

Do not give blood unrefrigerated for more than 1 hour   If blood for transfusion has been left unrefrigerated for 1 hour or more, it should not be administered. Blood should never be allowed to warm, be recooled, and then be administered.

Rationale: Blood that has been kept under proper refrigeration, when left unrefrigerated, will increase in temperature $10°$ F in 1 hour. This $10°$ F temperature increase allows for bacterial growth.

Fulfilled Needs: Protection from physical harm

Do not induce vomiting   Do not perform any procedure that would cause vomiting.

Rationale: Vomiting ingested caustic poisons further traumatizes intestinal mucosa as the highly irritating chemicals pass over the tissue a second time.

Fulfilled Needs: Protection from physical harm

Do not inject drugs into a blood transfusion Drugs should never be injected into blood being transfused intravenously.

Rationale: Many drugs, especially calcium, are incompatible with blood and cause blood clotting.

Fulfilled Needs: Protection from physical harm

Do not massage   Do not rub any body area where circulatory impairment, thrombus, or frostbite exists.

Rationale: Massage may dislodge a thrombus, sending it into the bloodstream where it might occlude the blood supply to a vital organ. Massaging an area of impaired circulation or frostbite may cause gangrene because massage increases the tissue's need for blood that cannot be provided when blood vessels are severely damaged or diseased.

Fulfilled Needs: Protection from physical harm

Do not neutralize the chemical injuring the eye   Do not attempt to counteract chemical reactions in the eye by using an alkali on an acid or an acid on an alkali. Instead, flush the eye with clean water from the nasal corner to the outer corner of the eye.

Rationale: Neutralization of chemicals brings about a chemical heat reaction that can further damage the eye.

Fulfilled Needs: Protection from physical harm

Do not place in the flat position   Do not allow the person to lie flat who is in respiratory distress, who has potential for increased intracranial pressure, who has severe hypertension or any other condition in which the flat position would contribute to discomfort.

Rationale: The flat position inhibits air flow during respiratory distress, increases intracranial pressure when there is potential for pressure elevation, and increases the blood pressure within the brain to an abnormally high degree if the blood pressure is already elevated.

Fulfilled Needs: Comfort, protection from physical harm

Do not place the amputation stump in the flexion position   Do not allow the person with a below-knee amputation stump to bend (flex) the stump backward. Instead, the stump should be kept straight (extended) and in alignment with the rest of the body. Do not place a pillow under the thigh or knee.

Rationale: Extension alignment of an amputated stump prevents flexion contractures and promotes positioning conducive to successful prosthesis walking.

Fulfilled Needs: Protection from physical harm

Do not start IVs or draw blood in the affected extremity   When the extremity is severely swollen or tissue has been traumatized, do not start intravenous fluids or draw blood from the veins in the affected extremity.

Rationale: Needle punctures in edematous or traumatized tissue further injure the tissue.

Fulfilled Needs: Protection from physical harm

Do not withdraw by catheter more than 1,000 cc of urine at one time
When voiding is not possible and a catheter is inserted to promote urinary flow, do not allow more than 1,000 cc of urine to be drained at one time. If it appears that the bladder contains more than 1,000 cc of fluid, clamp the catheter after the first 1,000 cc of urine have been withdrawn. Wait 30–40 minutes and then allow up to another 1,000 cc of urine to be withdrawn.

Rationale: The sudden pressure changes created by emptying an overdistended bladder can cause hypotension and will retard the return of the bladder's muscle tone.

Fulfilled Needs: Protection from physical harm

Drain the condensation from the nebulizer tubing periodically   When giving aerosol nebulization, drain the accumulated water or liquid from the aerosol tubing into a waste container every 1 or 2 hours. The accumulation is evident by a bubbling sound.

Rationale: Heated condensation in an aerosol tubing may splash and burn the skin

or be sucked into the airway, causing death from drowning.
Fulfilled Needs: Comfort, protection from physical harm

Drape for warmth   When covering the person for bathing or examinations, make certain that the drape is sufficient and properly placed to ensure comfortable body warmth.
Rationale: Normal body warmth promotes comfort and prevents chilling, which often stimulates muscle spasms.
Fulfilled Needs: Comfort, protection from physical harm

Drape modestly   Keep the person's body covered at all times and prevent the unnecessary display of the uncovered body, especially during examinations and procedures.
Rationale: Comfort and safety feelings are increased when normal sociocultural values are upheld, despite dependency on others. Awareness of esteem from others results from satisfactory and respectful relationships with others.
Fulfilled Needs: Comfort, protection from psychologic threat, dignity

Dress and undress the person   Clothe the person completely without his assistance.
Rationale: When the person is unable to clothe himself, meeting such needs offers comfort and meets dependency needs.
Fulfilled Needs: Comfort, dependence, dignity

Dress in easily removable clothing   Dress the person in clothes that can be removed quickly and without difficulty. Clothes that open in front, have medium-sized buttons, or loose snaps are best for children and persons with impaired finger motion.
Rationale: Easily removable clothes allow the person to be independent during such activities as toileting.
Fulfilled Needs: Comfort, independence

Dress in lightweight clothing   Clothe the person in garments made of light material.
Rationale: Lightweight clothing increases heat lost to the environment, causing a reduction in body temperature and increased comfort. Such clothing reduces pressure on skin lesions and decreases fatigue by preventing strain or pull on shoulder muscles. Lightweight socks lessen foot perspiration.
Fulfilled Needs: Normal temperature, energy, comfort, protection from physical harm
Contraindications: Subnormal temperature, tendency to chill

Dress in minimum clothing   Dress the person in the least amount of clothing essential to modesty.
Rationale: Minimum clothing, by increasing the amount of heat lost to the environment, helps to decrease an elevated body temperature to within normal limits. Minimum clothing gives persons bothered by incontinence the comfort of being able to easily remove garments. In peritoneal dialysis and ascites, a minimum of clothing reduces the sensation of pressure within the peritoneum and promotes comfort.
Fulfilled Needs: Normal temperature, energy, comfort, protection from physical harm
Contraindications: Subnormal temperature, reduced metabolic rate, low environmental temperature

Dress in nonconstrictive/nonrestrictive clothing   Remove clothing that causes tightness around the person's body or that limits free, normal body movements.
Rationale: Constriction that prevents venous return will impair circulation and result

in tissue damage. Limitations placed on body movements prevent normal mobility.

Fulfilled Needs: Tissue oxygenation or perfusion, comfort, protection from physical harm, freedeom from pain

Dress in personal clothing   Have the person wear his own clothing each day.

Rationale: Safety feelings are promoted by objects that represent past pleasure and security. Certain material objects provide symbolic identification of the self.

Fulfilled Needs: Comfort, protection from psychologic threat

Dress in warm clothing   Clothe the person in layered clothing and garments made of wool, fur, etc., which protect the body against exposure to severe temperature changes.

Rationale: Warm clothing increases environmental heat surrounding the body, decreases heat lost to the environment, promotes comfort of normal body temperature.

Fulfilled Needs: Normal temperature, comfort, protection from physical harm

Contraindications: Fever, increased metabolic rate, allergic reactions

Dress the person in colorful clothing   When there is evidence that the person's spirit or mood is low, suggest that brightly colored clothing be worn.

Rationale: Bright colors often promote comforting sensory stimulation.

Fulfilled Needs: Comfort, stimulation

Dust the skin with an antiperspirant powder   Apply powder to the feet or under the arms to reduce sweat gland secretion. Do not powder skin folds or between the toes, or apply only a thin film in these areas.

Rationale: Inhibiting sweat gland secretion reduces skin odor and promotes comfort. Powder has a drying action, permits movement of the skin against skin, allows good air circulation over the skin, reduces friction, and promotes cooling and drying of inflamed skin.

Fulfilled Needs: Comfort, protection from physical harm

Dust the skin with medicated powder   Apply a medicated powder to the skin. Do not powder skin folds or between the toes, or apply only a thin film to these areas. Apply fairly heavy amounts to open, inflamed skin.

Rationale: Medicated powder soothes the skin surface and absorbs moisture. Powder has a drying action, permits movement of skin against skin, allows good air circulation over the skin, reduces friction, and promotes cooling and drying of inflamed skin. An antibacterial powder minimizes bacterial growth on the skin and inhibits skin odor.

Fulfilled Needs: Comfort, protection from physical harm

Contraindications: Known medication allergy

Elevate the affected body part   Raise the body part by placing a pillow comfortably beneath it.

Rationale: Body-part elevation promotes circulation and decreases edema by reducing pressure in veins and capillaries, thus facilitating fluid reabsorption.

Fulfilled Needs: Tissue oxygenation or perfusion, comfort, protection from physical harm

Elevate the extremity   Lift or raise the limb above the normal flat level to either a 20- or 30-degree angle. When elevating the arm, be sure the hand is higher than the elbow, and the elbow is higher than the shoulder. Extremity elevation can be done by using a pillow or by using a sling made from a stockinette slipped over the extremity and attached to an IV pole.

Rationale: Decreasing the pulling effect of gravity reduces or prevents fluid accumulation in interstitial spaces. Excessive fluid accumulation in body tissues results in discomfort.

Fulfilled Needs: Tissue oxygenation or perfusion, rest, comfort, protection from physical harm, freedom from pain

Elevate the foot of the bed Raise the foot of the bed and then raise the knee gatch until the knees are no longer in hyperextension (stretched out).

Rationale: Foot elevation enhances circulation, reduces pressure on the injured limb, and prevents the person from slipping down in bed.

Fulfilled Needs: Tissue oxygenation or perfusion, comfort, protection from physical harm

Contraindications: Hypertension, increased intracranial or intraocular pressure, respiratory distress, ascites, congestive heart failure, severe peripheral arterial disease

Elevate the head Lift or raise the head above the level of the heart.

Rationale: Head elevation decreases intracranial pressure, promotes venous blood flow from the brain to the heart, reduces potential damage to brain centers controlling the vital signs, increases peripheral blood flow, and clears the airway for improved respiratory ventilation. Raising the head decreases pain from intracranial pressure when the pain results from the inability of the skull to expand. During peritoneal dialysis, pressure placed on the diaphragm from the dialysis fluid in the peritoneal cavity can cause respiratory difficulty. Elevating the head reduces the pressure on the diaphragm, facilitating ease of respirations. Elevation of the body after death prevents discoloration of the exposed body and gives an appearance of sleep.

Fulfilled Needs: Tissue oxygenation or perfusion, comfort, protection from physical harm, freedom from pain

Contraindications: Shock, labrynthitis vomiting, potential fainting, meningitis and cerebral conditions (especially tumors) in which gravity pulls the brain further downward into the cranium (tentorium), causing increased pressure on the medulla breathing center, resulting in respiratory failure

Eliminate undesirable light and noise Take measures to do away with light and noise that disturb the person. Change the lighting so that the person feels comfortable with the arrangement. Turn off the radio, television, and nonessential equipment to reduce the noise. Keep doors and windows closed if necessary.

Rationale: Illness increases sensitivity to noxious stimuli. The elimination of undesirable light and noise promotes comfort and rest.

Fulfilled Needs: Rest, comfort, protection from physical harm

Empty the collection appliance (or container) Remove from the collection appliance or container the fluid or substance that has drained into the container. Measure the amount emptied.

Rationale: Emptying collection appliances or containers removes disagreeable sights and odors, promotes cleanliness, and provides for observation of new drainage that may have changed character from previous drainage.

Fulfilled Needs: Comfort, cleanliness, protection from physical harm

Encourage a full day of activities Involve the person in external activity for the entire day, beginning at the time of arising and ending at bedtime.

Rationale: Focusing attention on external stimuli temporarily relieves the tension of internal stress, enhances involvement with reality, and promotes comfort.

Fulfilled Needs: Comfort, stimulation, protection from psychologic threat, increased reality perception

Encourage active (passive or quiet) diversional activities *Active diversional activities:* Suggest that the person participate in an activity in which something is produced; for example, fishing, doing crossword puzzles, woodburning, making jewelry, making crepe paper flowers, lettering, crayoning, clay modeling, weather forecasting, box gardening, photography, creative writing, stamp collecting, coin collecting, stuffing toys, painting pictures, knitting, potting, basket weaving.

Passive diversional activities: Suggest that the person participate in nonphysical activities in which there is sensory intake but little or no productivity. These include watching television or movies; listening to records, tapes, and radio; reading newspapers, magazines, or books; bird-watching; star-gazing; riding in a car or wheelchair.

Quiet diversional activities: Offer activities that can be performed noiselessly and in a relatively noise-free environment.

Rationale: Focusing attention on external stimuli temporarily relieves the tension of internal stress. It promotes temporary escape from conscious perception of threats of fear, anxiety, and pain and decreases energy consumption. Quiet supports easier adaptation to stress.

Fulfilled Needs: Comfort, stimulation, protection from physical harm, protection from psychologic threat, freedom from pain

Encourage adequate rest Encourage a minimum of 6–8 hours rest a day for persons who are well. Encourage about 9–12 hours of partial rest a day for persons who have a localized infection, who only a few days previously had an elevated temperature that is now normal, who feel weak and are gradually attempting to restore energy, who are gradually increasing mobility activities, who are convalescing, or who have a slight illness. Encourage about 13–17 hours of moderate rest a day for persons with a slight temperature elevation of 99–101° F, who have conditions in which energy is depleted fairly quickly, who are moderately ill, or who are slowly restoring mobility activites. Encourage about 18–23 hours of intensive rest a day for persons who have a moderate temperature of 101–103° F, who have a moderate blood pressure elevation, who have conditions in which there is severe energy depletion, or who have a serious illness. Since travel is stressful, encourage persons going on trips to rest adequately during the days before the trip to minimize the degree of stress placed on the body.

Rationale: Rest is essential to the maintenance of body function. Rest replenishes cell energy, which the body uses for the maintenance of life and physical and emotional activity, and promotes healing and comfort.

Fulfilled Needs: Sleep and rest, energy, comfort, protection from physical harm, protection from psychologic threat

Encourage alternate rest and activity For each hour of activity, have the person rest for 10 minutes. As fatigue is reduced, increase the length of activity with less frequent rest periods.

Rationale: Fatigue, feelings of tiredness, and weariness result from activity or energy requiring responses to physiologic and psychologic stress stimuli. Fatigue conditions are decreased by reducing stress stimuli or by restoring energy by means of reducing metabolic requirements during rest. The accomplishment of activity without fatigue promotes comfort.

Fulfilled Needs: Rest, energy, comfort, protection from physical harm, protection from psychologic threat

Encourage an awareness of positive responses from others Suggest that the person consciously make mental notes each time someone responds favorably to him. At the end of the day, have the person enumerate those responses.

Rationale: Positive feelings regarding self result from positive responses from others.

Fulfilled Needs: Comfort, protection from psychologic threat, acceptance, approval from others, high evaluation of self

Encourage an indifferent attitude toward sleep Suggest that the person assume an "I don't care" attitude about whether or not he falls asleep.

Rationale: When a person does not consciously try to go to sleep, the body relaxes and sleep occurs. Adequate sleep is essential in that the decreased metabolic rate occurring during sleep restores the depleted cell energy reserves.

Fulfilled Needs: Sleep, rest, relaxation, energy, comfort, protection from physical harm

Encourage bladder emptying before rest Suggest to the person that he empty his bladder just before resting.

Rationale: A full bladder produces a certain degree of bladder tension as the muscles stretch to contain urine. The relief of this muscular tension through bladder emptying promotes relaxation.

Fulfilled Needs: Relaxation, comfort

Encourage both long- and short-term goals While long-term goals are being attempted, suggest short-term objectives that can be accomplished intermittently along with the extended goal.

Rationale: The accomplishment of short-term goals reduces the adaptation to frustration that accompanies long-term goals. Adaptation and adjustment require energy that, in illness, is needed for healing. Successful achievement in overcoming barriers to a goal enhances the ability to cope, with a resulting increased sense of adequacy.

Fulfilled Needs: Energy, comfort, protection from physical harm, protection from psychologic threat, adequacy, goal achievement

Encourage chapel-service attendance While the patient is hospitalized, inform him of available chapel services and provide transportation to the chapel.

Rationale: Religious observances help people to express spiritually their relationship with God and outwardly to recognize the Supreme Being.

Fulfilled Needs: Comfort, spiritual, religious, or philosophic satisfaction

Encourage coughing Place the person in a sitting position. Have him inhale deeply, then forcefully exhale with a cough.

Rationale: The forceful movement of air from the lower to the upper respiratory tract propels thick mucus from the tracheobronchial tree, improving respirations and removing infectious material.

Fulfilled Needs: Tissue oxygenation or perfusion, waste elimination of bronchopulmonary secretions, protection from physical harm

Contraindications: Increased intrathoracic, intraocular, intraabdominal, or intracranial pressure; pulmonary hemorrhage

Encourage decision making Assist the person in making decisions by himself regarding situations, problems, or matters affecting him and his future.

Rationale: The ability to maintain self-direction and be free from control of others requires clear self-identity, knowledge, competence, and adult values. The ability to overcome the ambivalence of dependency–independency needs is essential to growth and maturity. Feelings of safety evolve from an awareness that the person can cope successfully with life. Vulnerability to the outcome of decisions made by others produces anxiety.

Fulfilled Needs: Comfort, protection from psychologic threat, adequacy, self-reliance, independence, personal growth and maturity

Contraindications: Confusion states

Encourage decreased acid-ash-food intake Suggest that the person decrease the intake of highly acid-ash food. Foods to avoid include meat, fish, poultry, eggs, cheese, plums, cranberries, prunes, all breads, cakes, cookies, cereals, crackers, macaroni, spaghetti, noodles, brazil nuts, peanuts, walnuts, corn, and lentils.

Rationale: A reduced acid-ash diet will cause a more alkaline urine, resulting in less uric acid and cystine stone formation.

Fulfilled Needs: Protection from physical harm

Contraindications: Potential calcium or phosphate calculi

Encourage decreased acid-food intake   Suggest that the person decrease the intake of highly acidic foods. Foods to avoid include citrus fruits and juices, pickles, vinegar, sauerkraut.

Rationale: Decreased intake of highly acidic foods reduces saliva stimulation, irritation of the intestinal tract, and promotes a neutral acid–base balance.

Fulfilled Needs: Acid–base balance, comfort, protection from physical harm, freedom from pain

Contraindications: Reduced saliva secretion, alkalosis

Encourage decreased calcium-food/fluid intake   Suggest that the person decrease the intake of high-calcium food and fluids. Foods and fluids to avoid include milk and milk products; meat and poultry; dark green leafy vegetables such as mustard greens, turnip greens, and broccoli; sardines, clams, oysters; and yogurt.

Rationale: Decreased calcium intake reduces the potential for the formation of calcium urinary stones, especially in existing kidney disease and illness-enforced immobility. It helps maintain normal acid–base balance.

Fulfilled Needs: Fluid and electrolyte balance, acid–base balance, protection from physical harm

Contraindications: Blood-clotting abnormalities, poor lactation, impaired bone growth, persons receiving large volumes of citrated blood by transfusion

Encourage decreased calorie intake   Suggest that the person reduce the intake of foods having high fuel and energy value. Foods to avoid include potatoes, bread, butter, cream, sugar, sweets, greasy foods, and alcoholic beverages. Low-calorie foods are recognized by their thin, watery dilutions, high fiber content, and crispness due to excess water.

Rationale: Lowered calorie intake decreases body weight by forcing the body to use stored energy resources. Since the calorie intake available for fuel and energy does not meet daily requirements, decreased body weight reduces the cardiac work load and improves tissue oxygenation.

Fulfilled Needs: Nutritional balance, protection from physical harm

Contraindications: Increased metabolic rate, excessive weight loss, underweight persons

Encourage decreased carbohydrate intake   Suggest that the person decrease the intake of foods having high sugar and starch value. Foods to avoid include breads, cereals, sugar, candy, cakes with icing, pies, pastry, milk, ice cream, sauces, gravies, chocolate, syrups, honey, puddings, and cocktails. Foods to eat include meat, poultry, fish, eggs, butter, margarine, limited vegetables and fruits.

Rationale: Lowered carbohydrate intake decreases body weight by forcing the body to use stored energy resources since the carbohydrates available for fuel and energy do not meet daily requirements. The decreased body weight reduces the cardiac workload and improves tissue oxygenation. Low-carbohydrate intake is compatible with steroid (cortisone) therapy since steroids cause increased blood and urine sugar with diminished carbohydrate tolerance. The physician orders a low-carbohydrate diet for diabetics in whom insulin secretion is inadequate to metabolize normal carbohydrate intake.

Fulfilled Needs: Nutritional balance, protection from physical harm

Contraindications: Increased metabolic rate, renal failure, excessive weight loss, underweight persons

Encourage decreased cholesterol-food intake   Suggest that the person decrease the intake of foods more highly composed of unsaturated than saturated fats. Foods to avoid include egg yolks; butter; cream cheese; shellfish such as lobster, crab, and shrimp; organ meats such as liver, brains, heart, kidney, and sweet breads.

Rationale: Lowered cholesterol intake decreases fat deposits in arterial tissue, reducing the threat of arterial degeneration.

Fulfilled Needs: Protection from physical harm

Encourage decreased fatty-food intake   Suggest that the person decrease the intake of foods high in triglyceride or lipid content. Foods to avoid include fatty meat; gravy; salad dressings; rich and heavy desserts; fried foods; highly flavored vegetables such as legumes and melons; packaged, canned, or frozen foods and dinners; and poultry skin. Foods to eat include meat, gravy from meat drippings that have been chilled and the fat removed, vegetable oils, whole or skim milk, eggs, cottage cheese, bread and vegetables, fruits, and cereals.

Rationale: Fatty foods increase abnormal bile secretion in the liver and bile volume stored in the gallbladder. They stimulate pancreatic secretions. Decreased fat intake reduces organ activity, allowing for tissue healing and reduced tissue trauma. The physician orders a low-fat diet in gallbladder and pancreatic disease.

Fulfilled Needs: Comfort, protection from physical harm, freedom from pain

Contraindications: Gastric hyperacidity, hypoglycemia

Encourage decreased gas-forming-food intake   Suggest that the person decrease the intake of foods causing stomach or intestinal gas. Foods to avoid include kidney, lima, and navy beans, broccoli, brussels sprouts, cabbage, cauliflower, corn, cucumbers, kohlrabi, leeks, lentils, onions, black-eyed and split peas, green peppers, pimento, radishes, rutabagas, sauerkraut, scallions, shallots, turnips, soybeans, cantaloupe, honeydew melon, raw apples, avocados, and watermelon.

Rationale: Flatulence results from fermentation (oxidative decomposition by microorganisms) or putrefaction (decomposition by bacteria or fungi). The ingestion of foods causing decreased fermentation and putrefaction reduces flatulence. Flatulence causes pressure within the intestinal walls, resulting in severe, sharp pain and discomfort.

Fulfilled Needs: Comfort, protection from physical harm, freedom from pain

Encourage decreased potassium-food intake   Suggest that the person decrease the intake of foods high in potassium. Foods to avoid include cereals, dried peas and beans, nuts, molasses, fresh fish and poultry, cocoa, fresh vegetables such as spinach, unstrained orange juice, prunes, tangerines, grapefruit and tomatoes, coffee, milk, cream, eggs, bananas, raisins, dried apricots.

Rationale: Normal blood-potassium level is essential to intracellular fluid balance, osmotic pressure regulation, acid–base balance, and the conduction of nerve impulses in muscle tissue. The physician orders a low-potassium diet in kidney failure because kidney failure inhibits the normal elimination of potassium.

Fulfilled Needs: Fluid and electrolyte balance, acid–base balance, protection from physical harm

Contraindications: Diarrhea; vomiting; diuresis; impaired muscle function; profuse colostomy, ileostomy, ileal conduit or T-tube drainage; when persons are on steroid therapy or receiving large volumes of IV dextrose or saline

Encourage decreased protein-food intake   Suggest that the person decrease the intake of foods high in nitrogenous compounds. Foods to avoid include cheese, meat, fish, poultry, bread, cereals, legumes, nuts, and gelatin. Use protein-foods of high biologic value (milk and eggs or commercial formulas of essential amino acids) to provide the limited amount of protein allowed. Protein-free foods include pure carbohydrates (sugar, honey, jelly, hard candy) and pure fats (butter and margarine).

Rationale: The liver breaks down amino acids into keto acid and ammonia and coverts the ammonia into urea which is excreted by the kidneys. In severe liver disease, ammonia is formed more rapidly than it can be converted to urea, and high ammonia-blood levels result, contributing to hepatic coma. In kidney failure, urea is not eliminated as rapidly as it is formed, and high blood-urea levels result, contributing to uremia. Decreasing the intake of protein, and limiting the protein to essential amino acids, results in a decreased amount of ammonia and/or urea accumulation and provides the essential amino acids needed for maintenance and repair of tissue. In liver and renal failure, the physician orders specific amounts of dietary protein.

Fulfilled Needs: Protection from physical harm

Contraindications: Edema not associated with liver or renal failure, during the growth years, when persons are burned

Encourage decreased purine-food intake Encourage the person to avoid foods high in purine such as liver, kidneys, poultry, fish, fried foods, spinach, mushrooms, asparagus, peas, lentils, pastries, and alcohol.

Rationale: Foods of a high purine content break down during metabolism, to form uric acid. High uric-acid content in the urine increases the potential for renal calculi.

Fulfilled Needs: Protection from physical harm

Encourage decreased residue-food intake Suggest that the person decrease the intake of foods containing considerable bulk and fat. Increase foods that are almost completely absorbed, leaving little or no intestinal waste. Foods to avoid include milk, cheese, vegetables, fruits, coarse breads and cereals, relishes, sweets, fried foods, tough meats, and condiments. Foods to eat include tender meat, fish, poultry, refined bread and cereals, fat-free clear soup, plain gelatin, coffee, tea, sugar, butter, and margarine.

Rationale: Reduced residual waste matter decreases intestinal irritation, lessens gastrointestinal spasms, prevents contamination of a ureterosigmoidostomy site, and promotes the comfort of reduced bowel elimination.

Fulfilled Needs: Comfort, protection from physical harm

Contraindications: Constipation

Encourage decreased sodium-food/fluid intake Suggest that the person decrease the intake of foods and fluids containing sodium. Suggested low-sodium fluids include orange juice, pineapple juice, cranberry juice, cola drinks, gingerale, tea. Low-sodium foods include fresh or frozen meat or poultry, low-sodium canned tuna and salmon, asparagus, green beans, lima beans, navy beans, broccoli, brussel sprouts, cabbage, cauliflower, chicory, corn, cucumbers, eggplant, lentils, mushrooms, lettuce, okra, onions, yellow and green peas, red and green peppers, sweet and white potatoes, pumpkin, radishes, yellow turnips, tomatoes, squash, turnip greens, fresh fruits, low-sodium bread, salt-free cakes and cookies, rice, hominy grits, oatmeal, noodles, spaghetti, flour, and unsalted butter and oils.

Rationale: A normal level of sodium salts is essential for electrolyte balance, regulation of osmotic pressure in cells and fluid, and acid–base balance. In severe cardiac damage, venous stasis and increased pressure prevent sodium and water from returning from interstitial tissues to the bloodstream to be excreted by the kidneys. When kidney excretion of sodium is reduced, restricted sodium intake decreases the blood-sodium level. Osmotic pressure then pulls sodium and water from the interstitial spaces into the bloodstream, relieving tissue edema. In cardiac and renal disorders, the physician orders specific amounts of dietary sodium.

Fulfilled Needs: Fluid and electrolyte balance, acid–base balance, protection from physical harm

Contraindications: Diarrhea; vomiting; excessive sweating; diuresis; second- or third-degree burns; repetitive paracentesis; fever; profuse colostomy, ileostomy, ileal conduit, fistula, or T-tube drainage; persons receiving large volumes of IV dextrose.

Encourage decreased yellow fruit and vegetable intake Suggest that the person lower the intake of yellow fruits and vegetables. Suggest a balanced intake of yellow, green, white, and other vegetables.

Rationale: Excessive ingestion of yellow fruits and vegetables discolors the skin.

Fulfilled Needs: Nutritional balance, protection from physical harm

Encourage deep breathing   Have the person slowly inhale air to maximum chest expansion and then slowly exhale. Have him deep breathe for a 10–15-minute period three to four times a day.

Rationale: Lung expansion increases arterial oxygen concentrations, facilitates gas exchange within the lungs, increases negative pressure in the thorax, promotes emptying of large veins, stimulates the cough reflex by placing pressure on mucous secretions, and promotes muscle relaxation. Forceful inhalation and exhalation when covering a chest wound helps to reexpand the collapsed lung.

Fulfilled Needs: Tissue oxygenation or perfusion, waste elimination of carbon dioxide and bronchopulmonary secretions, relaxation, protection from physical harm

Contraindications: Pulmonary hemorrhage, respiratory alkalosis

Encourage discussion of the person's spiritual values   Initiate conversation about the person's spiritual life and its value. Help him clarify his values and renew his spiritual goals.

Rationale: Spiritual goals assist in developing an understanding of the essential meaning of life.

Fulfilled Needs: Personal growth and maturity; identification of spiritual, religious, or philosophic satisfaction.

Encourage early replacement of dwindling therapeutic/drug supplies
Suggest that the person procure additional supplies approximately 1 week before they are needed.

Rationale: Anticipating the need for and acquiring therapeutic supplies in advance supports uninterrupted therapeutic treatment.

Fulfilled Needs: Protection from physical harm

Encourage enhanced involvement in already established relationships
Attempt involving one person in the feelings of another. Direct activities that will increase feeling intensity between persons with established relationships.

Rationale: Sensitivity responses are more frequent in established friendships and group situations than in newly developed relationships. Awareness of feelings in another arouses a corresponding emotional effect and promotes a more realistic perception of another's emotional world.

Fulfilled Needs: Caring and communicating relationships, personal growth and maturity

Encourage exploration of the dark when fearful of the dark   Suggest that fear of the dark can be prevented or reduced by accompanying the person into the darkened area and allowing him to search the area with a flashlight.

Rationale: Since fear stems from a sense of helplessness in the face of danger, a sense of adequacy in confronting the danger reduces fear. Adequacy evolves from an awareness of a person's ability to cope with life. Sound health approaches to behavioral problems bring about safety, comfort, growth, and maturity.

Fulfilled Needs: Comfort, protection from psychologic threat, sense of adequacy, personal growth and maturity, increased reality perception

Encourage family-shared responsibility   Suggest that all family members be included in the person's direct or indirect care and that relatives divide the responsibility so no one family member is burdened.

Rationale: Mutually shared responsibility promotes feelings of safety, adequacy, and comfort. Involvement in meeting the needs of others promotes self-esteem.

Fulfilled Needs: Comfort, protection from psychologic threat, unity with loved ones, sense of usefulness, sense of adequacy, endurance, personal growth and maturity, increased reality perception and problem-solving ability

Encourage family support of the person's acceptance of death   Offer the family of a dying person, who has reached the acceptance stage, an understanding of the feelings of the person. Show them how they can comfort their loved one by sharing in his acceptance of the approaching death.

Rationale: When a dying person reaches the acceptance stage but perceives that loved ones cannot accept the inevitable, he experiences intense inner conflict until his family also reaches the point of acceptance.

Fulfilled Needs: Comfort, protection from psychologic threat, acceptance, unity with loved ones, personal growth and maturity

Encourage frequent vacationing   Suggest that the person change his surroundings by taking a pleasant trip or doing things that change his usual daily routine. To vacation three or four times a year is ideal.

Rationale: A change of scene and carefree distraction promotes temporary escape from threatening situations and supports emotional healing. Involvement in new interests interrupts habitual patterns of thought.

Fulfilled Needs: Comfort, protection from psychologic threat, psychologic stability, less of the familiar and more of the novel

Encourage gradual mastery of a/the situation   Assist the person to move gradually into an emotional disturbing situation. Encourage him to overcome the problem slowly, gaining increased confidence with each success. For instance, if he is afraid of heights, have him go one story higher in a building each day.

Rationale: Unpleasant situations can be less threatening when experienced in small doses. Feelings of adequacy arise from an awareness of a person's ability to cope with life. Gradual success supports gradual recognition of strengths.

Fulfilled Needs: Comfort, protection from psychologic threat, sense of adequacy, endurance

Encourage honesty in presenting oneself to others   Suggest that when a person presents himself to others as he really is, he has greater assurance of being loved for what he is.

Rationale: Honesty relieves the anxiety of anticipated detection of dishonesty. Self-esteem is maintained as long as a person sees himself as living up to cultural expectations. Sound health approaches to behavioral problems promote safety, comfort, growth, and maturity.

Fulfilled Needs: Comfort, protection from psychologic threat, acceptance, high evaluation of self, personal growth and maturity, increased reality perception

Encourage increased acid-ash-food intake   Suggest that the person raise the intake of foods that promote an acid state. Foods to increase include meat, fish, poultry, eggs, cheese, plums, cranberries, prunes, all breads, cakes, cookies, cereals, crackers, macaroni, spaghetti, noodles, brazil nuts, peanuts, walnuts, corn, and lentils.

Rationale: An increased acid-ash diet will cause a more acid urine, resulting in a diminished potential for infection and calcium and phosphate stone formation.

Fulfilled Needs: Protection from physical harm

Contraindications: Potential uric acid or cystine stones

Encourage increased acidic-food intake   Suggest that the person increase the intake of highly acidic foods. Foods to increase include citrus fruits and juices, pickles, vinegar, sauerkraut.

Rationale: Increased intake of acidic foods will stimulate salivation

Fulfilled Needs: Acid–base balance, protection from physical harm

Contraindications: Excessive salivary flow, gastric hyperacidity

Encourage increased calcium-food/fluid intake   Suggest that the person raise the intake of high-calcium foods such as milk; milk products; meat and poultry; dark green leafy vegetables like mustard greens, turnip greens, and broccoli; sardines, clams, oysters; and yogurt.

Rationale: A high-calcium diet provides calcium for normal bone growth and function, assists in blood clotting, promotes lactation, enhances nerve and muscle functioning, and activates enzymes.

Fulfilled Needs: Fluid and electrolyte balance, protection from physical harm

Contraindications: Potential calcium urinary calculi, illness-enforced immobility, potential cardiac arrhythmia, persons having a high-alkali intake

Encourage increased calorie intake
Suggest that the person raise the intake of foods having a high fuel and energy value. Include all regular foods plus additional amounts of cereals, potatoes, bread, butter, cream, sugars, and sweets.

Rationale: Increased metabolic rate and illness causing weight loss require added energy and fuel resources to promote oxidation and provide nutrition to body tissue.

Fulfilled Needs: Nutritional balance, energy, protection from physical harm

Contraindications: Obesity, severe cardiac damage with impaired circulation, diabetes mellitus ˙

Encourage increased carbohydrate intake
Suggest that the person raise the intake of foods having high- sugar and starch value. Include syrups and jellies; fine cereals and breads; starch puddings; high-carbohydrate vegetables like potatoes, beets, carrots, peas, beans, lentils, turnips, and parsnips; high-carbohydrate fruits such as bananas, raisins, prunes, dried dates, and figs; ice cream, fruit pies, and cakes.

Rationale: Increased metabolic rate and illness causing weight loss require high-carbohydrate intake that will yield sufficient calories to produce adequate energy and fuel resources to promote oxidation and provide nutrition to body tissue. In renal failure, the physician orders a high-carbohydrate diet to reduce the conversion of tissue protein into urea, since the failing kidneys cannot excrete the urea.

Fulfilled Needs: Nutritional balance, energy, protection from physical harm

Contraindications: Obesity, severe cardiac damage with impaired circulation, diabetic states, person's receiving steroid therapy

Encourage increased fatty-food intake
Suggest that the person increase the intake of foods with triglyceride or lipid content. Include cream, butter, bacon, salad oils and dressings, meat, eggs, and cheese.

Rationale: Fats combine with oxygen and release energy for tissue cell oxidation and nutrition. Fatty foods are digested slowly and remain in the stomach longer than other foods. The prolonged digestion reduces and neutralizes acidity, decreases pain, and defers hunger. The physician orders a high-fat diet in hypoglycemia because fatty foods depress Isle of Langerhans activity, causing reduced insulin production.

Fulfilled Needs: Nutritional balance, comfort

Contraindications: Cholecystitis, cholelithiasis, cholangitis, pancreatitis

Encourage increased high-iodine food intake
Explain that foods containing high amounts of iodine should be eaten. Such foods include seafood, especially halibut and cod, and seaweed, a common food in Japan.

Rationale: Iodine affects the production of thyroid hormone, which regulates thyroid metabolism.

Fulfilled Needs: Protection from physical harm, increased learning

Encourage increased high-pectin food intake
Explain that foods containing high levels of pectin should be eaten. Such foods include the pulp of fruits such as the apple, pear, or ripe banana.

Rationale: Pectin is a carbohydrate found in fruits and vegetables that forms a gelatinous mass when digested. It slows peristalsis by its soothing, nonirritating, emolient effect.

Fulfilled Needs: Comfort, protection from physical harm, increased learning

Encourage increased high-vitamin food intake Suggest that the person increase the intake of foods having high vitamin content.

Vitamin A: Milk, cod liver oil, egg yolks, leafy green and yellow vegetables, limes, oranges, liver, pineapples, cantalopes, and prunes.

Vitamin B: Egg yolks, fruits and vegetables, whole grain breads and cereals, nuts, legumes, and yeast, poultry and meat, rice, and bran.

Vitamin C: Oranges, strawberries, pears, apricots, plums, peaches, pineapples, tomatoes, raw cabbages, carrots, lettuce, celery, onions, green peppers, radishes, and rutabagas.

Vitamin D: Egg yolks, butter, fat, cod liver oil, and milk.

Vitamin K: Oats, wheat, rye, alfalfa, and fats.

Rationale: Vitamins increase the conversion of food into energy although they are not an energy source in themselves. Vitamins prevent deficiency diseases that occur from poor nutritional intake.

Fulfilled Needs: Nutritional balance, energy, protection from physical harm

Contraindications: Avoid an excessively high intake of any high-vitamin food

Encourage increased iron-food intake Suggest that the person increase the intake of foods having a high-iron content. Include sardines, lobster, clams, liver, oysters, shellfish, kidney, heart, lean meat, tongue, leafy vegetables, egg yolks, dried peas and beans, dried fruits, dark molasses, enriched breads and cereals.

Rationale: The liver must store sufficient iron for the manufacture of hemoglobin in new red blood cells. Hemoglobin is necessary to form oxyhemoglobin, which provides tissue oxidation and nutrition.

Fulfilled Needs: Nutritional balance, energy, protection from physical harm

Encourage increased potassium-food/fluid intake Suggest that potassium be replaced following episodes of diarrhea, vomiting, or diuresis by eating foods and drinking fluids high in potassium, such as tea, coffee, chocolate or cocoa drinks; meat, poultry, or fish; fresh or dried nuts; spinach; whole-grain cereals; milk solids such as ice cream; dried peas and beans; fresh fruits, especially grapefruit, tangerines, oranges, bananas, prunes, and tomatoes.

Rationale: In diarrhea, potassium is lost in the feces. In vomiting, potassium is lost in the gastric juices. In diuresis, fluid reabsorption from the renal tubules is prevented with a resulting loss of potassium in the urine. A normal potassium level is essential to salt balance, acid–base balance, normal osmotic pressure, and nerve-impulse conduction, especially to muscle and cardiac tissue.

Fulfilled Needs: Fluid and electrolyte balance, acid–base balance, protection from physical harm

Contraindications: Hyperkalemia, renal failure with oliguria or anuria, during the shock state of severe second- or third-degree burns or crushing injuries, adrenal insufficiency, ventricular fibrillation, patients receiving IV infusions containing potassium

Encourage increased protein-food intake Suggest that the person increase the intake of foods high in protein content. Include milk, cheese, eggs, lean meats, fish, poultry, wheat bread and cereals, wheat germ, yeast, legumes, nuts gelatin, chicken breasts, tuna fish, leg of lamb, beef, and loin pork.

Rationale: Proteins are essential for tissue growth and repair. Proteins increase immunity, resistance to infection, and body heat production. They provide cell oxidation and nutrition and decrease negative nitrogen balance caused by steroid therapy. Normally, the protein level is higher in the blood than it is in interstitial fluid. When the blood-protein level is low, the return of fluid from the interstitial tissues to the blood is decreased, contributing to edema and ascites. If the protein intake increases, the elevated blood-protein level reestablishes the normal return of the fluid from the interstitial tissues to the blood, supporting fluid balance. In cirrhosis, hypertension exists within the portal vein, forcing fluid and albumin from the blood into the tissues with resulting ascites. With increased protein intake, a balanced colloid osmotic pressure is established between the blood and the tissues allowing the blood to retain fluid at its normal level and decrease fluid (ascites) in the tissues. Increased protein intake is especially important after prolonged starvation and in burns and proteinuria. The physician orders a high-protein diet when there is liver damage without liver failure, after the shock stage of burns, and for hypoproteinemia when there is no kidney failure.

Fulfilled Needs: Fluid and electrolyte balance, nutritional balance, normal temperature, energy, protection from physical harm

Contraindications: Impending hepatic coma, renal insufficiency or failure

Encourage increased residue-food intake   Suggest that the person raise the intake of foods containing considerable bulk. Include long-fibered vegetables such as greens, cabbage and celery, raw vegetables and fruits, cooked fruits, and whole-grain bread and cereals.

Rationale: An increased quantity of residue waste matter after food is digested and absorbed improves intestinal muscle tone, promoting comfortable intestinal elimination.

Fulfilled Needs: Waste elimination of food residue, comfort, protection from physical harm

Contraindications: Intestinal irritation, gastrointestinal spasm, ureterosigmoidostomy; rectal bleeding, irritation, or inflammation

Encourage increased sodium-food/fluid intake   Suggest that sodium be replaced after episodes of diarrhea, vomiting, diuresis, profuse drainage or excessive sweating from high environmental temperatures, fever, or heavy exercising. Sodium can be replaced by eating foods such as ham, bacon, salted nuts, salted or frozen fish, potato chips, salted crackers, pretzels, peanut butter, ketchup, mustard, bread, butter, milk, frozen peas, lima beans, cake, cookies, artichokes, sauerkraut, beets, carrots, celery, hominy, mustard greens, spinach, white turnips, cheese, or table salt. Fluids high in sodium include milk, root beer, instant and dry coffee, and dutch chocolate.

Rationale: Sodium and chloride are essential to fluid and acid–base balance. Sodium is the principal electrolyte of the plasma and other body fluids and is essential to fluid balance, electrolyte balance, normal osmotic pressure, and acid–base balance. Normal sodium loss occurs in the urine, but abnormal amounts are lost when there is profuse perspiration and when reabsorption of intestinal secretions is hindered, as in vomiting, diarrhea, or drainage from a tube, sinus, or wound. Profuse losses of sodium and water result in circulatory failure unless replacement is maintained. Replacement of water and sodium losses with low-sodium fluids (water, Coca Cola, 7-Up, apple juice, orange juice, etc.) may result in water intoxication.

Fulfilled Needs: Fluid and electrolyte balance, acid–base balance, protection from physical harm

Contraindications: Impaired renal function, edema, ascites, hypernatremia, cardiac damage with impaired circulation, dehydration, patients on steroid therapy who are receiving large volumes of IV saline or are on a low-sodium diet

Encourage involvement in totally new interests   Help the person to participate in interesting and stimulating activities in which he has had no previous involvement. Promote interests from which satisfaction and pleasure can be experienced.

Rationale: Involvement in totally new interests fosters growth and development of potential. Novel interests prevent boredom.

Fulfilled Needs: Comfort, stimulation, personal growth and maturity, awareness of potential, full development of potential, less of the familiar and more of the novel

Encourage laughter   Help the person view the problem with a sense of humor.
Rationale: Laughter brings problems into realistic perspective and assists in reducing tension.
Fulfilled Needs: Comfort, protection from psychologic threat, psychologic stability, increased reality perception

Encourage light reading before sleep   Suggest that the person read unemotional and preferably boring material while in bed, just before sleep.
Rationale: Lack of stimulation from boredom promotes sleep. Adequate sleep is essential in that the decreased metabolic rate occurring during sleep restores depleted cell energy reserves.
Fulfilled Needs: Sleep, rest, relaxation, energy, comfort, protection from physical harm

Encourage meaningful activity   Involve the person in some activity that he sees as having value and importance.
Rationale: The perception of an activity as being important supports motivation toward accomplishing the activity, which in turn supports a positive self-image since the achievement has a positive value.
Fulfilled Needs: Comfort, sense of usefulness, high evaluation of self

Encourage moderate activity   Suggest that the person set for himself a schedule of reasonable, nonstrenuous activity.
Rationale: Moderate activity supports normal functioning of body systems and reduces internal tension. During impaired health, it is preferable to excessive activity, in that it provides a reduction in the amount of energy expended for adaptation, making available more energy for healing.
Fulfilled Needs: Activity, energy, comfort, protection from physical harm, protection from psychologic threat

Encourage moderate physical exercise   Promote muscular and joint activity through the performance of daily chores.
Rationale: Muscular exertion through exercise enhances free-joint mobility, strengthens muscle tone, develops coordination, prevents nonfunctional contractures, and promotes increased blood circulation. Exercise uses up excessive body calories. Exercise improves pelvic circulation and stretches pelvic ligaments, reducing menstrual pain.
Fulfilled Needs: Tissue oxygenation or perfusion, activity and exercise, protection from physical harm
Contraindications: Fever, states of severe energy depletion, any nonhealth condition in which the performance of daily chores is incompatible with health maintenance

Encourage modes of travel other than flying   Recommend to persons for whom air travel is unsuitable that they travel by bus, car, train, or boat.
Rationale: Human safety and comfort are promoted when there is exposure to lesser atmospheric pressure changes in a bus, car, train, or boat, as compared to greater pressure changes in an airplane.
Fulfilled Needs: Comfort, protection from physical harm

Encourage mutual problem solving   Interact with and help the person to identify problems and discover methods for solving them. Assist the patient in dealing objectively with the difficulty.
Rationale: Knowledge of oneself and problem situations, plus the pursuit of realistic goals, promotes growth, maturity, increased adequacy, and reduced anxiety. Comfort arises from a sense of effective communication with others.
Fulfilled Needs: Comfort, protection from physical harm, protection from psychologic threat, caring and communicating relationships, sense of adequacy, goal achievement,

mastery and competence in skills, personal growth and maturity, increased learning, increased reality perception and problem-solving ability

Encourage new goals at past goal achievement
As the person achieves one goal successfully, immediately present a new goal to be accomplished.

Rationale: A positive self-image is supported when new and important goals are anticipated in the near future.

Fulfilled Needs: Comfort, protection from psychologic threat, sense of usefulness, high evaluation of self

Encourage new skill development
Suggest new skills that the person might enjoy performing. Assist, if possible, with the learning of these previously unknown abilities.

Rationale: The ability to maintain self-direction through personal competencies supports feelings of adequacy and self-esteem. The ability to maintain independence is essential to growth and maturity.

Fulfilled Needs: High evaluation of self, sense of adequacy, self-reliance, mastery and competence in skills, independence, personal growth and maturity, full development of potential

Encourage noncompetitive activities
Involve the person in activities and relationships in which there is minimum or no competition.

Rationale: Competition is a stimulus for aggressive behavior and can result in regrettable conduct when there is difficulty maintaining emotional control. Suspicious people strive to prove their superiority through competition but are highly threatened on losing, which often results in heightened distrust.

Fulfilled Needs: Comfort, protection from psychologic threat, caring and communicating relationships

Encourage normal use of the involved limb
Have the person use the remaining strength in a limb as frequently as possible in everyday activities even if at first the use is limited.

Rationale: The exertion of muscular activity through exercise promotes circulation and free-joint mobility, strengthens muscle tone, develops coordination, and prevents nonfunctional contractures.

Fulfilled Needs: Tissue oxygenation or perfusion, exercise, comfort, protection from physical harm

Encourage participation in therapeutic group interaction
Suggest that the person become involved in interaction between a number of group members for a period of several weeks or months.

Rationale: Group interaction protects against threatening individual involvement and promotes interpersonal satisfaction when the relationships prove to be nonthreatening. Behavioral insight gained through group interaction promotes emotional growth.

Fulfilled Needs: Comfort, protection from psychologic threat, caring and communicating relationships, personal growth and maturity

Encourage part-time employment
Suggest that part-time employment is possible and profitable. Some part-time endeavors include typing, babysitting, running a mail-order business, and creating artistic works or crafts.

Rationale: Part-time employment provides socialization and a sense of meaningfulness, maintains status, and offers financial security.

Fulfilled Needs: Comfort, protection from psychologic threat, sense of usefulness, high evaluation of self

Encourage patience in developing relationships
Point out that it takes time for persons to know each other and to develop a significant relationship. For instance, a

stepparent may not feel close to a stepchild for a year or two; a new in-law may not be significant for some time.

Rationale: Significance in relationships is based on knowing the person, developing trust, and having common interests, all of which take time.

Fulfilled Needs: Comfort, protection from psychologic threat

Encourage patience in illness adjustment Reassure both the person and his family that adjustment to illness can be very slow and painstaking and that these adaptations require endurance on the part of all concerned and are vital to regaining health.

Rationale: In severe physiologic or psychologic disequillibrium, the healing process requires considerable time. Knowing what to expect supports endurance, promotes comfort, and increases reality perception.

Fulfilled Needs: Comfort, protection from physical harm, protection from psychologic threat, endurance, increased reality perception

Encourage planned one-day-at-a-time living In the morning, help the person to look no further than that day. In the evening, if the person desires, help him to look no further than the next day.

Rationale: Stress is reduced by limiting the demands to a single day's responsibilities. This reduction in stress enhances clear perception and allows concentrated use of powers to meet demands adequately. When the threat of death appears relatively imminent, concentration on the immediate future promotes realistic goals and gives a feeling of the extension of a meaningful life. Planning for the next day promotes the safety of a predictable future.

Fulfilled Needs: Comfort, protection from psychologic threat, predictable and orderly world, sense of adequacy, endurance

Encourage pride in appearance Direct the person toward good grooming and appropriate dress so his appearance will be satisfying to himself and to others.

Rationale: Self-esteem requires that a person experience positive feelings about himself and positive response from others.

Fulfilled Needs: Comfort, approval from others, high evaluation of self

Encourage recognition of the person's various roles in life Help the person to identify clearly how he sees himself in the role most important to him.

Rationale: A positive self-image is fostered by behavior compatible with a person's perception of his significant roles.

Fulfilled Needs: Comfort, sense of usefulness, high evaluation of self

Encourage relationships between persons with common interests and goals Foster a pleasant relationship between persons who have similar interests and goals.

Rationale: Psychologic comfort is promoted through a sense of effective communication with others. When group goals are clearly perceived, group unity tends to increase because of participation in reaching those goals.

Fulfilled Needs: Comfort, caring and communicating relationships, group companionship

Encourage respect for the rights of others Help the person to fulfill his own needs. At the same time, help him recognize that his needs can be met only as long as they do not infringe on the rights of others.

Rationale: Properly managed aggression contributes to strength of character by control of self-assertion, which in turn reduces the threat of social disapproval. Self-esteem is maintained when a person perceives himself as living up to cultural expectations and receiving the approval of others. Maturity and growth involve reality perception and behavioral changes that appropriately meet situational demands and individual needs.

Fulfilled Needs: Protection from psychologic threat, approval from others, high evaluation of self, personal growth and maturity, increased reality perception and problem-solving ability

Encourage role playing to develop sensitivity
Suggest that the person act out the situation of another as if he were that person.

Rationale: The ability to assume the role of another person promotes sensitivity feelings for the behavior of others.

Fulfilled Needs: Personal growth and maturity, increased reality perception

Encourage self-performance
Suggest that the person do as much as possible for himself and that he rely on his own capabilities.

Rationale: The ability to maintain self-direction and be free from control of others requires clear self-identity, knowledge, and competencies. The ability to overcome the ambivalence of dependency–interdependency needs is essential to growth and maturity. Independence is built on successful past experience.

Fulfilled Needs: High evaluation of self, sense of adequacy, self-reliance, mastery and competence in skills, independence, dignity, personal growth and maturity, full development of potential

Encourage simple signal language during impaired communication
When attempting to communicate with a person who cannot relay messages verbally, encourage the use of simple signals for yes and no, such as blinking the eyes or moving the fingertips up and down. Avoid using complex symbols or signals that the person may find difficult to understand.

Rationale: Simple signal language supports improved communication when there is communication impairment.

Fulfilled Needs: Comfort, caring and communicating relationships

Encourage social and community activities
Promote activities in which there is contact with other people and in which the person can relate to others. Such activities include sewing together, dancing, playing music and games, choral groups, talent shows, and discussion groups, volunteering in hospitals and other agencies.

Rationale: Comfort and safety feelings evolve from an awareness that the person is not threatened with aloneness.

Fulfilled Needs: Comfort, protection from psychologic threat, caring and communicating relationships, group companionship

Encourage striving toward realistic goals
Assist the person in choosing and striving toward realistic objectives. Initially support attempts at small-goal achievements that most likely will be accomplished with success. Gradually support more difficult goals as the minor aims are overcome.

Rationale: Safety feelings and adequacy evolve from an awareness that a person can cope successfully with life. Self-esteem is enhanced by the development of new competencies and the achievement of important goals. Honest evaluation of self and situation plus the pursuit of realistic goals promotes growth and maturity.

Fulfilled Needs: Comfort, protection from psychologic threat, high evaluation of self, sense of adequacy, self-reliance, goal achievement, personal growth and maturity, increased reality perception and problem-solving ability

Encourage telephone calls with significant persons
Suggest that the person and his distant family speak to each other by telephone as frequently as possible.

Rationale: Comfort is promoted through a sense of effective communication with others. Unity with loved ones reduces stress and strengthens the capacity to cope with it.

Fulfilled Needs: Comfort, protection from physical harm, caring and communicating relationships, unity with loved ones

Encourage the acceptance of forgiveness offered by others
Assist the per-

son in reappraising his relationship with other people and with a supreme being, if he believes in one. Help him recognize that forgiveness is available if he will accept it.

Rationale: The healing of guilt comes not in erasing it, but in the ability to see oneself as worthy of accepting the forgiveness offered. Safety feelings require that a person experience awareness of acceptance by others.

Fulfilled Needs: Comfort, protection from psychologic threat, acceptance, high evaluation of self

Encourage the acceptance of interdependency
Verbally reinforce the truth that people must be interdependent if they are to enjoy a rich, full life. Stress the fact that at times people must be willing to help one another and at other times be able to accept help from others without shame.

Rationale: When a person is forced into dependency, he needs care that is physically and emotionally reminiscent of the safe mother–child relationship. Psychologic comfort is promoted through a sense of relatedness to others and the ability to communicate needs. Self-esteem requires that a person experience positive responses from others.

Fulfilled Needs: Comfort, protection from psychologic threat, dependence, caring and communicating relationships, high evaluation of self

Encourage the acceptance of limitations in others
Teach that all human beings have weaknesses of one sort or another. Suggest that it is best to look on other human beings favorably despite human frailties and not to expect perfection from others.

Rationale: Safety and comfort are promoted through a sense of adequate communication with others. Sound health approaches to behavioral problems promote safety and comfort, enhance the natural tendency to organize perceptual data into relationships and selections, and promote growth and maturity.

Fulfilled Needs: Protection from psychologic threat, caring and communicating relationships, personal growth and maturity, increased reality perception and problem-solving ability

Encourage the acceptance of partial goal satisfaction
When the person attempts to withdraw totally from goals that he cannot accomplish, suggest ways he can gain satisfaction through partial accomplishment of those same goals.

Rationale: Withdrawal removes the person from perceived threat. Negative perception can be altered through identification with the positive perceptions of another and result in reduced threat. Comfort and safety feelings evolve from an awareness that the person can cope successfully with life. The anticipation of satisfying achievement leads to activity.

Fulfilled Needs: Comfort, protection from psychologic threat, sense of adequacy, goal achievement, increased reality perception and problem-solving ability

Encourage the acceptance of responsibility
Assist the person in accepting tasks or duties and in fulfilling the obligation assumed.

Rationale: The acceptance of responsibility results from a sense of clear self-identity, competencies, and adult values. The ability to overcome the ambivalence of dependency–interdependency needs is essential to growth and maturity.

Fulfilled Needs: High evaluation of self, sense of adequacy, self-reliance, mastery and competence in skills, independence, personal growth and maturity, full development of potential, identification of values

Encourage the acceptance of self-limitations
Assist the person in recognizing that all human beings have weaknesses and that limitations are not unique. Suggest that the person look on himself favorably despite human frailties.

Rationale: A positive self-image can be developed only when self-expectations are in harmony with the realistic self. Comfort and adequacy are fostered by an awareness that personal weaknesses are not unique.

Fulfilled Needs: Comfort, protection from psychologic threat, high evaluation of self, personal growth and maturity, increased reality perception

Encourage the acceptance of the right to pleasure Assist the person in realizing that he has a right to enjoy pleasure.

Rationale: A positive self-image results from positive responses from others. Persons receiving reasonable amounts of pleasure experience a more positive approach to life and more successfully tolerate unpleasant experiences.

Fulfilled Needs: Protection from psychologic threat, high evaluation of self, increased pleasantness

Encourage the admission of wrongdoing Assist the person to express verbally the details of the wrongdoing to whomever is appropriate.

Rationale: Confession relieves the anxiety of anticipated detection and punishment, reestablishes an inner sense of love-worthiness, and can divert punishment and gain approval. Self-esteem requires that a person experience positive responses from others.

Fulfilled Needs: Comfort, protection from psychologic threat, acceptance, approval from others

Encourage the bringing in of outside food Suggest to families and friends that they bring the person food prepared outside the hospital.

Rationale: Balanced nutritional intake and comfort are enhanced by the availability of familiar and desired foods.

Fulfilled Needs: Nutritional balance, comfort

Contraindications: Special diet restrictions

Encourage the chaplain's visit Call the chaplain or a clergyman to bring spiritual aid to the ill person.

Rationale: Clergy provide spiritual guidance designed to bring spiritual peace and understanding.

Fulfilled Needs: Comfort; spiritual, religious, or philosophic satisfaction

Encourage the desire for satisfactory achievement Suggest that specific goals be sought for the purpose of realizing a sense of satisfaction and reward that accompanies achievement.

Rationale: Anticipation of satisfying achievement leads to activity

Fulfilled Needs: Goal achievement, increased pleasantness

Encourage the differentiation between self-ideal and actual self Help the person evaluate the difference between the self he sees as ideal and the actual functioning self. Help him incorporate into his frame of reference realism and harmony between the two.

Rationale: A poorly organized self-concept leads to disorganized behavior because behavior is consistent with the self-concept. Increased and accurate information about self leads to mature reality perception, awareness of potential, value clarification, and enhanced adequacy in solving problems and making decisions.

Fulfilled Needs: Sense of adequacy, personal growth and maturity, awareness of potential, identification of values, increased reality perception and problem-solving ability

Encourage the expression of feelings Foster communication with the nurse or between significant persons in which emotional feelings are revealed. Communicate to the person that the verbal expression of feelings, ideas, hopes, and doubts will be received favorably and that there need be no fear of humiliation, embarrassment, or punishment.

Rationale: Feeling ventilation supports honesty and objectivity of the situation in which the people are involved. Awareness of another's feelings arouses a corresponding emotional effect and promotes a more realistic perception of another's emotional world.

When differences can be accepted, people feel free to look at themselves fearlessly and no longer feel restricted in growth.

Fulfilled Needs: Comfort, protection from psychologic threat, caring and communicating relationships, acceptance, high evaluation of self, personal growth and maturity, increased reality perception and problem-solving ability

Encourage the identification of specific life values

Help the person to define for himself specific values for successful living and to avoid situations in which intense value conflict exists.

Rationale: The threat of anxiety results when there is a value conflict, when the person does not trust his own valuing process or when there is a breakdown of cultural values. Feelings of adequacy and comfort evolve from an awareness that the person can cope successfully with life within a framework of well-defined values.

Fulfilled Needs: Comfort, protection from psychologic threat, sense of adequacy, identification of values

Encourage the identification of success standards

Assist the person in clearly identifying those qualities that he sees as associated with success.

Rationale: A positive self-image can be enhanced by identifying and behaving in accordance with qualities compatible to the person's perception of success.

Fulfilled Needs: High evaluation of self

Encourage the identification of values acquired from the person's own culture

Help the person identify, in detail, those values imposed by his own culture. Promote an awareness of why those values exist and, if possible, their origin.

Rationale: Culture is a principal element in human development. Each society teaches concepts, values, and desired behavior in an effort to meet needs and perpetuate the society. The realization of how cultural values affect the person leads to greater self-insight, acceptance, and problem solving. It provides the basis for improved values when current cultural values are unacceptable.

Fulfilled Needs: Comfort, acceptance, personal growth and maturity, identification of values, increased reality perception and problem-solving ability

Encourage the identification of values in common with the values of others

Help the person to exchange verbally and to define those standards that he has in common with others.

Rationale: Psychologic comfort is promoted through a sense of commonality among persons. An accepted value system significantly influences behavioral responses.

Fulfilled Needs: Comfort, protection from psychologic threat, acceptance, approval from others, increased reality perception and problem-solving ability

Encourage the mother/father to explore the newborn

Suggest that the mother and father unwrap and undress their newborn. Have them look at and feel the face, hands, toes, and other body parts.

Rationale: Since the newborn is a person unknown to the parents, exploring the infant helps the parents to familiarize themselves with the child. It also helps the infant to know what the parents are like. Exploratory touching is an important part of the infant–parent bonding process.

Fulfilled Needs: Comfort, unity with loved ones, increased learning

Encourage the mother/father to see and touch the newborn immediately after birth

As soon as the infant is born, place the child on the mother's abdomen or in her arms. Permit the father to hold the infant at the earliest possible time.

Rationale: Immediate contact between infant and mother (father) at birth supports attachment for each other. It is the beginning of a lifetime of bonding.

Fulfilled Needs: Comfort, caring and communicating relationships

Encourage the person, parent, or family to ask questions Offer the person every opportunity to ask questions and emphasize the importance of his inquiring to better understand the health problem.

Rationale: Adequate health knowledge increases a person's ability to protect his health and prevent harm to himself.

Fulfilled Needs: Comfort, protection from physical harm, protection from psychologic threat, increased learning, increased reality perception and problem-solving ability

Encourage the person to face the fear (anxiety or grief) Suggest that the person face the unknown that is causing his fear or anxiety and to face painful emotions such as grief.

Rationale: Fear is reduced when the safe reality of a situation is confronted. Facing fear promotes comfort, growth, and maturity. Painful emotions tend to diminish when dealt with realistically.

Fulfilled Needs: Comfort, protection from psychologic threat, personal growth and maturity, increased reality perception and problem-solving ability

Encourage the person to listen attentively Call to the person's attention the need to listen carefully to what others are saying before drawing conclusions about the meaning of the message being sent. Also, suggest he listen carefully to his own spoken messages.

Rationale: Message reception is influenced by the person's current needs and interests and can result in pleasurable or threatening interpretation. Preoccupation and emotionally charged thinking interfere with correct delivery, reception, and interpretation of messages.

Fulfilled Needs: Protection from psychologic threat, caring and communicating relationships

Encourage the person to make a verbal no-suicide contract Encourage the person to make a verbal commitment in which he states that he will not take his life accidentally or intentionally without calling the nurse first. Set a time limit of 1 day, 1 week, 1 month, or whatever is suitable to the person. When the time limit expires, have the person renew the contract for another length of time. Give the person your phone number and be available to him 24 hours a day. When the therapeutic relationship is terminated, encourage the person to give you a long-term commitment.

Rationale: Encouraging the person to make a no-suicide contract makes him feel that he is important to someone; therefore, he feels important to himself.

Fulfilled Needs: Protection from physical harm, protection from psychologic threat, caring and communicating relationships, high evaluation of self, dignity

Encourage the person to seek one goal at a time Suggest that only one objective be attempted at a time. After one goal has been accomplished, then another can be sought.

Rationale: Multiple goal seeking requires intense diversion of thought, which often results in mental confusion and nonachievement of any goal. Successfully overcoming barriers to a goal enhances the ability to cope and results in increased adequacy feelings.

Fulfilled Needs: Comfort, protection from psychologic threat, adequacy, goal achievement

Encourage the person to write down what he wants to remember Suggest that the person with poor memory, write down whatever is important. Have him carry messages with him to facilitate recall.

Rationale: Written messages are easily retrieved and increase confidence in the person's ability to remember.

Fulfilled Needs: Comfort, protection from psychologic threat, sense of adequacy

Encourage the practical application of the accepted value system Help the person objectively assess his situation in light of his value system. Help him to state in detail how his values can be applied to successful living.

Rationale: Maturity and growth involve the ability to perceive and cope with the demands and limitations of the real world and to organize perceptions into a meaningful whole.

Fulfilled Needs: Personal growth and maturity, increased reality perception and problem-solving ability

Encourage the sharing of common interests with others Support the sharing of common interests among persons. Encourage people to explore their common interests and to pursue them together.

Rationale: The sharing of common interests fosters emotional ties between persons.

Fulfilled Needs: Comfort, caring and communicating relationships, unity with loved ones

Encourage the sharing of common problems with others Suggest that persons having similar difficulties verbally share their problems and methods for solving the problems.

Rationale: Psychologic comfort is promoted through a sense of effective communications. The exchange of common problems enhances realistic perception, the solution of the person's own problems, and growth and maturity.

Fulfilled Needs: Comfort, personal growth and maturity, increased reality perception and problem-solving ability

Encourage the substitution of undesirable habits with favorable habits Suggest that injurious habits can be changed by substituting a pleasant habit in its place. Nail biting can be replaced with gum chewing. Smoking can be substituted with sucking on hard candy.

Rationale: Sound health approaches promote safety, growth, maturity, and increased problem-solving ability.

Fulfilled Needs: Protection from physical harm, protection from psychologic threat, personal growth and maturity, increased reality perception and problem-solving ability

Encourage the use of a warm, saline gargle Suggest that a warm, salt solution gargle be used two to four times a day.

Rationale: A warm saline gargle promotes soothing comfort to irritated mucosa and minimizes infection through cleansing

Fulfilled Needs: Cleanliness, comfort

Contraindications: Hypernatremia, when on a low-sodium diet

Encourage the use of an artificial larynx (or esophageal speech) as directed by the speech therapist Encourage the person to follow the directions of the speech therapist in using either an artificial larynx or esophageal speech. In using an artificial larynx, the vibrator is placed either externally against the side of the neck or internally toward the side and back of the mouth. In using esophageal speech, air it taken into the mouth, the lips are brought together tightly, and air is forced into the esophagus. As pressure increases in the upper esophagus, a tonal vibration is produced.

Rationale: An artificial larynx and/or esophageal speech offer methods for verbal communication when such communication has been interrupted by a laryngectomy.

Fulfilled Needs: Comfort, caring and communicating relationships

Encourage the use of normal/effective coping mechanisms Encourage the use of normal adaptive methods for dealing with emotions.

Rationale: The development and use of adaptive psychologic mechanisms fosters safety, comfort, and psychologic equilibrium. External attempts to remove psychologic defenses increase anxiety.

Fulfilled Needs: Comfort, protection from psychologic threat, psychologic stability

Encourage the use of spiritual resources   Suggest that spiritual assistance can give direction and purpose to a floundering life and that feelings of helplessness or fear can be reduced through the development of internal strength drawn from the unlimited strength of a spiritual source.

Rationale: Awareness of the value of spirituality leads to closer God–human relationships, which bring about the satisfaction of strength, comfort, and maturity.

Fulfilled Needs: Comfort; protection from psychologic threat; endurance; personal growth and maturity; spiritual, religious, or philosophic satisfaction; increased pleasantness

Encourage the use of the bathroom   If at all possible, encourage the person to get out of bed and use the bathroom facilities.

Rationale: Use of the bathroom promotes relaxation, comfort, and normal body function.

Fulfilled Needs: Waste elimination of food residue and urine, comfort, cleanliness

Contraindications: Prescribed 24-hour bed rest

Encourage visiting by significant others   Suggest that persons significant to the person visit as frequently as possible.

Rationale: The presence of significant persons promotes comfort and assurance that the person will be cared for properly.

Fulfilled Needs: Comfort, protection from psychologic threat, unity with loved ones

Encourage volunteers to visit the sick/lonely   Encourage volunteers from churches or social organizations to visit sick or lonely persons routinely.

Rationale: Positive feelings about self result from positive responses from others and an awareness that the person is not threatened with aloneness.

Fulfilled Needs: Comfort, caring and communicating relationships

Encourage youths toward goal achievements that please significant others   Arouse positive behavior by suggesting that goals be achieved for loved ones or for persons with whom there is close identification.

Rationale: When youths earn awards, etc., their self-esteem is enhanced as a result of the esteem they receive from significant others.

Fulfilled Needs: Unity with loved ones, high evaluation of self, goal achievement, sense of adequacy

Ensure the person's feelings of safety before introducing any unpleasantness   Choose a time when the person is under little or no tension or threat to convey to him any unpleasantness or bad news.

Rationale: When a person feels secure, threatening situations are less frightening than at times when he feels less secure. When a person feels well, he has greater strength for adaptation to bad news. When a state of psychologic safety exists, perception tends to identify associated objects and situations as nonthreatening.

Fulfilled Needs: Comfort, protection from psychologic threat

Escort the person during off-ward activities   When the person goes off the nursing unit for therapeutic or other reasons, provide constant accompaniment by a responsible staff member.

Rationale: Aloneness offers a person with self-destructive tendencies an opportunity to harm himself physically. Recognition of potentially harmful physical threats promotes safety. Respect for the basic worth of human beings promotes the support of life whenever possible.

Fulfilled Needs: Protection from physical harm

Estimate the required daily calories   Determine the approximate number of daily calories required by an adult involved in normal daily activity. Base this estimate on average daily requirements of 9 calories per pound of body weight. To maintain a constant weight base, the calorie estimate is determined by the present weight. To bring about weight loss or gain, determine the desired weight and multiply that by 9 calories per pound.

Rationale: Normal body weight enhances normal body function. Calorie intake should approximate caloric output.

Fulfilled Needs: Nutritional balance, protection from physical harm

Evert the eyelid   Lay a cotton-tipped applicator across the eyelid edge. Gently grasp the eyelashes with the fingers of the other hand. Pull the lid outward from the eye and turn it upward.

Rationale: Eyelid eversion facilitates visualization of foreign bodies in the eye and prevents eye-tissue irritation caused by eyelid inversion.

Fulfilled Needs: Comfort, protection from physical harm

Exercise in range of motion   Promote muscular and joint activity by carrying out the total exercising of muscles and joints. This may be done solely by the person or with nursing assistance.

Rationale: Muscular exertion through exercise promotes circulation and free-joint mobility, strengthens muscle tone, develops coordination, and prevents nonfunctional contractures.

Fulfilled Needs: Tissue oxygenation or perfusion, exercise, protection from physical harm

Contraindications: Circulatory embolus-thrombus, severe inflammation or pain, fracture, recent surgery on or near the joint

Explore superficial topics and reasons for avoiding in-depth feelings
Help the person to examine why he avoids discussing his feelings. Let him know that feelings are natural and should be experienced. Discuss happy, sad, and angry feelings and explain that feelings are good in themselves.

Rationale: Exploring provides an opportunity to perceive and express the person's own deep feelings regarding an emotional topic. Increased knowledge of self leads to maturity.

Fulfilled Needs: Personal growth and maturity, increased reality perception and problem-solving ability

Explore with the person his normal (individual, positive) characteristics
Frequently point out to the person those personal qualities that he shares with others. Include those characteristics that make him an individual and those that are positive rather than negative.

Rationale: An awareness of a person's normal and positive characteristics fosters a sense of adequacy and comfort. Individual characteristics that set us apart from others can be a source of pride.

Fulfilled Needs: Comfort, high evaluation of self, sense of adequacy, personal growth and maturity, increased reality perception

Explore with the person/family his/their strengths and resources   Help the person to give a verbal, detailed account of his resources and capabilities. Include such areas as physical, intellectual, emotional, financial, social, and specific ability resources. Help the person become aware that he has great physical and emotional reserves that will support him during times of stress.

Rationale: A positive attitude toward self promotes positive behavior. Increased and accurate information about self leads to mature reality perception, awareness of potential, value clarification, increased meaningfulness, and enhanced adequacy in solving problems and making decisions. An awareness of man's enduring strength builds confidence in self that reduces fear and promotes comfort, growth, and maturity.

Fulfilled Needs: Comfort, protection from psychologic threat, sense of adequacy, personal growth and maturity, awareness of potential, increased reality perception and problem-solving ability

Explore with the person his value (worth) as an individual Make the person aware that he is contributing something worthwhile and that his ideas and feelings are valuable. Emphasize that he has something to give to others, that because he is a human being, he is a person of worth.

Rationale: A positive response from others indicates acceptance and promotes self-esteem.

Fulfilled Needs: Comfort, acceptance, approval from others, high evaluation of self, sense of adequacy

Explore with the person whether there is a pattern leading up to the behavior Help the person determine if his behavior results from a specific sequence of events or situations that precede the behavior.

Rationale: Being aware of the sequence of events or situations that result in a particular behavior gives the person an opportunity to alter preexisting patterns leading to the behavior.

Fulfilled Needs: Protection from psychologic threat, personal growth and maturity, increased reality perception and problem solving ability

Explore with the person previous achievements of success Help the person to enumerate verbally past life experiences in detail that in his perception have been unsuccessful.

Rationale: Memories of past success promote positive self-attitudes toward present tasks.

Fulfilled Needs: Comfort, protection from psychologic threat, high evaluation of self, sense of adequacy

Explore with the person previous displays of courage Help the person to recall those life experiences in which he displayed courage and to enumerate the details of that courage.

Rationale: A positive, detailed image of qualities, capabilities, and strengths promotes a positive self-image.

Fulfilled Needs: Comfort, protection from psychologic threat, high evaluation of self, sense of adequacy

Explore with the person the difference between his child and adult conscience Help the person to distinguish between the childhood conscience based on fear of punishment and the adult conscience based on self-ideal. Indicate the need to use self-judgments rather than parentally imposed judgments of what is right or wrong. Help the person develop an adult conscience based on an evaluation of what he ought to do as related to his feelings of individual obligation and not based on blind rigidity to society's standards and values.

Rationale: The rigid conscience results from painful human relations with early authorities and, when maintained in adulthood, perpetuates similar relationships. Modifying the rigid conscience allows for internal self-direction based on realistic values. The capacity to make moral judgements and justify actions enhances self-esteem.

Fulfilled Needs: Comfort, protection from psychologic threat, psychologic stability, high evaluation of self, increased reality perception and problem-solving ability

Explore with the person the effects of his behavior on others Help the person to recognize that his behavior is a stimulus that causes responses in other persons. These responses may be favorable or unfavorable in the life of the person responding.

Rationale: Awareness that a person's behavior has an effect on others promotes greater consideration for others with resulting increased harmony in interpersonal relationships.

Fulfilled Needs: Personal growth and maturity, increased reality perception and problem-solving ability

Explore with the person the need for approval Help the person to determine the extent of his need for positive regard from others and if that need is so great as to thwart personal growth and freedom.

Rationale: The need for approval stems from people's interdependency and from the realization that assistance from others is acquired through socially approved behavior. Increased self-insight leads to mature reality perception.

Fulfilled Needs: Personal growth and maturity, increased reality perception and problem-solving ability

Explore with the person the need for attention Help the person to determine motives behind his attempts to bring attention to himself.

Rationale: Attention-seeking results from underlying feelings of inadequacy or from having basic needs unmet. An awareness of such causes can result in personal growth.

Fulfilled Needs: Personal growth and maturity, increased reality perception and problem-solving ability

Explore with the person the need to control Help the person to determine the extent of his need to control others, the reasons for it, and responses that dominating behavior elicits from others.

Rationale: The need to exert control stems from a perceived threat. An awareness of the effects of controlling behavior on others can result in behavior modification with improved interrelatedness.

Fulfilled Needs: Personal growth and maturity, increased reality perception and problem-solving ability

Explore with the person the reasons for criticism by others Help the person to identify, in detail, reasons why other persons criticize him.

Rationale: Exploring how others react to a person leads to mature reality perception. Such information helps the person to solve problems of relatedness with others.

Fulfilled Needs: Personal growth and maturity, increased reality perception and problem-solving ability

Explore with the person the reasons for criticism of others Help the person to identify, in detail, his motives for criticizing other persons.

Rationale: An awareness that chronic criticism of others is an effort to enhance a person's own self-esteem leads to mature reality perception. It assists the person to relate more positively to others and to correct his low self-esteem.

Fulfilled Needs: Personal growth and maturity, increased reality perception and problem-solving ability

Explore with the person the reasons for recurring problems Help the person to identify, in detail, motives, reasons, and circumstances that evolve around a frequently recurring emotional reaction.

Rationale: An awareness of those factors that affect a recurring problem often leads to behavioral changes that solve or diminish the problem.

Fulfilled Needs: Personal growth and maturity, increased reality perception and problem-solving ability

Explore with the person the reasons for self-criticism Help the person to identify, in detail, his motives for looking negatively at himself.

Rationale: Self-criticism is the result of a poorly developed self-image and/or lack of positive feedback from others. Awareness of these causes can result in positive self-attitudes.

Fulfilled Needs: Personal growth and maturity, increased reality perception and problem-solving ability

Expose the drying cast to air   When an orthopedic cast has been applied, expose it to the circulating air and protect it from dampness for at least 24 hours. A wet cast will be gray, dull, feel damp, and have a musty odor. When dry, it will be shiny white and firm. Normally, it takes 24–48 hours for complete drying.

Rationale: A therapeutic cast provides immobility and support to injured limbs, preventing further injury and enhancing healing.

Fulfilled Needs: Protection from physical harm

Expose the skin to sunlight   Place the person in the outdoor sun for short periods several times a day or by an open window or door through which the sun rays can come.

Rationale: Ultraviolet sun rays reduce the yellowness in jaundiced skin.

Fulfilled Needs: Comfort, protection from physical harm

Expose the wound (burn, decubitus, umbilical cord, lesions) to air   Expose an injured, burned, infected, degenerating, or ulcerated body area to the air without a protective dressing.

Rationale: Wound exposure to air promotes exudate drying and crusting, which supports skin regeneration beneath the crust and protects the wound from bacterial invasion.

Fulfilled Needs: Protection from physical harm

Express breast milk manually/mechanically   Breast milk may be expressed by either a hand or electric pump. When a hand pump is used, apply the suction cup to the nipple and alternately squeeze and release the suction bulb; or gently massage the breast for a few moments. Place one hand on top of the other above the breast. Bring the hands down over the breast, turn the fingers downward as the hands are drawn apart and encircle the breast. Use three fingers to cup and support under the breast as well as bring the breast forward and upward. Place the forefinger below and the thumb above the alveoli and apply gentle pressure until the milk flows in a stream. Gently rotate the fingers around the alveoli until all milk is expressed. The opposite hand should be used for holding a sterile container. When an electric pump is used, apply the suction cup to the nipple with a low degree of vacuum. Breast suctioning should be gradual, intermittent, continued for no more than 15 minutes, and stopped earlier if the breast is empty. The milk is measured and saved in a sterile container for later infant feeding. Handwashing is essential before expressing breast milk.

Rationale: When breast-feeding is temporarily curtailed, breast milk must be removed artificially or lactation will be inhibited permanently. The expression of milk from the lactating breast promotes comfort.

Fulfilled Needs: Comfort, protection from physical harm

Contraindications: Intentional lactation suppression

Facilitate the delivery by gently guiding the infant through the vulva   As the infant presents himself at the vulva opening, gently lift his chin up through the vulva. To assist in delivering the anterior (upper) shoulder, gently guide the infant's head downward. Gently turn the head upward to deliver the lower shoulder.

Rationale: Assisting with childbirth promotes maternal and infant safety.

Fulfilled Needs: Protection from physical harm

Feed by bottle   Nourish an infant with liquids by means of a bottle and artificial nipple.

Rationale: Balanced nutritional intake is essential to body cell activity and energy production from food. Relief of the visceral hunger sensation promotes comfort. Feeding meets dependency needs.

Fulfilled Needs: Fluid and electrolyte balance, nutritional balance, energy, comfort, protection from physical harm, dependence

Feed by cup Offer the child a drink with a cup.

Rationale: Eating, being a social event, requires learning socially acceptable conduct. A child's use of a cup supports independence.

Fulfilled Needs: Comfort, independence

Feed by rubber-tipped medicine dropper Provide liquid food for the premature infant by using a medicine dropper.

Rationale: A medicine dropper provides sufficiently small amounts of food so premature infants may swallow safely without choking. Feeding meets dependency needs.

Fulfilled Needs: Fluid and electrolyte balance, nutritional balance, protection from physical harm, dependence

Feed by syringe Administer oral fluids or pureed foods with a syringe.

Rationale: Balanced nutritional intake is essential to body cell activity and energy production from food. Relief of the visceral hunger sensation promotes comfort. Feeding meets dependency needs.

Fulfilled Needs: Fluid and electrolyte balance, nutritional balance, comfort, protection from physical harm, dependence

Feed the patient (person) Place food and drink into the person's mouth when he cannot do so himself.

Rationale: Food is essential to life maintenance. Feeding meets dependency needs.

Fulfilled Needs: Fluid and electrolyte balance, nutritional balance, protection from physical harm, dependence

Feed unhurriedly/slowly Unhurriedly nourish the person with food and fluids. Allow adequate time for chewing, swallowing, and pauses between food bites.

Rationale: The stress of hurrying causes intestinal spasms with reduced digestive functioning. Relaxed eating promotes comfort.

Fulfilled Needs: Relaxation, comfort, protection from physical harm

File the nails in one direction and only on the underside File the nails in one direction, not back and forth. File on the under surface of the nail and not on the upper or side surface. Use a metal file for shaping long, hard nails. Use the coarse side of an emery board for shaping normal nails and the fine side to finish the shaping.

Rationale: Filing the nails in one direction and only on the underside prevents nail splitting. Ragged or excessively long fingernails are prone to catch on objects with which they come in contact, causing nail injury.

Fulfilled Needs: Protection from physical harm

Fill the drinking cup (glass) only one-half full When a person has difficulty holding or manipulating a cup or glass, fill the cup or glass only one-half full even if it requires several fillings.

Rationale: The contents of a half-full cup or glass are less likely to spill. Persons unable to maintain good control of cups or glasses feel a greater sense of success when there is no spilling.

Fulfilled Needs: Comfort, mastery and competence in skills

Follow distasteful drugs with fruit juices When drugs taste bad and the taste cannot be disguised, give a favorite fruit juice immediately after the drug is taken.

Rationale: Fruit juice following distasteful drug ingestion provides the comfort of a desirable flavor in the mouth.
Fulfilled Needs: Comfort
Contraindications: Avoid giving fruit juices with drugs that have decreased absorption when combined with juices

Follow feedings with water   After food- or bottle-feeding is completed, give a glass or bottle of water.
Rationale: Following food or liquid intake with water flushes particles from the mouth that might support bacterial growth.
Fulfilled Needs: Protection from physical harm

Follow quick-acting glucose with long-acting carbohydrates and proteins
After the person with hypoglycemia has received a quick-acting glucose source (orange juice or candy), follow this with long-acting carbohydrates such as bread or crackers.
Rationale: A quick-acting glucose source immediately raises the blood sugar, but only for a short period. When a long-acting carbohydrate is given to follow the quick-acting glucose source, the blood sugar will be maintained at a normal level for a longer period.
Fulfilled Needs: Nutritional balance, protection from physical harm, physiologic stability

Follow through on promises   When the nurse gives her word that she will do something for a person, she should be absolutely certain that the commitment is fulfilled in the allotted time. If, for some reason, the promise cannot be carried out, she should give a thorough explanation as to why and offer a substitute commitment.
Rationale: Trust is enhanced when important matters pertaining to the person are considered matters of concern by others.
Fulfilled Needs: Comfort, protection from psychologic threat, caring and communicating relationships

Fully support the drying cast on pillows   While the cast is wet, do not lay it on a hard bed surface. Instead, place soft, fluffy pillows under the wet cast.
Rationale: A wet cast placed on a hard surface will become flattened over bony prominences with the resulting pressure causing decreased circulation to tissues enclosed in the cast.
Fulfilled Needs: Comfort, protection from physical harm

Give a charcoal solution orally   Give between 100 and 200 cc of activated charcoal orally.
Rationale: Charcoal absorbs poisons, reducing tissue damage.
Fulfilled Needs: Protection from physical harm, physiologic stability

Give a pacifier to the infant   Place a plastic or rubber nipple or teething ring in the baby's mouth.
Rationale: Use of a pacifier during tube-feeding promotes digestion and speeds the development of the infant's sucking ability. It promotes sucking contentment when contentment from human contact is limited or when adequate sucking is not sufficient during feeding.
Fulfilled Needs: Comfort, stimulation
Contraindications: Avoid using a pacifier to keep the child quiet

Give a salt–soda solution orally   Give a salt–soda solution made up of 1 teaspoon of salt and $\frac{1}{2}$ teaspoon of baking soda added to 1 quart of water. Adults should be given 4 ounces every 15 minutes; children (ages 1–12 years), 2 ounces; and infants (less than 1 year), 1 ounce. If not contraindicated, lemon or lime may be added for flavor.

Rationale: A salt–soda solution provides adequate fluid and electrolyte replacement to assist in reversing shock.

Fulfilled Needs: Fluid and electrolyte balance, protection from physical harm, physiologic stability

Give a salt solution orally   Give a mixture of 1 teaspoon of salt in a glass of water. Give one-half glass every 15 minutes for 1 hour.

Rationale: Salt solution provides adequate electrolyte replacement to assist in reversing acidosis.

Fulfilled Needs: Fluid and electrolyte balance, protection from physical harm, physiologic stability

Give a starch solution orally   Give a drinkable, pastelike mixture of cornstarch and water.

Rationale: A starch antidote neutralizes ingested tincture of benzoin and reduces the harmful effects.

Fulfilled Needs: Protection from physical harm, physiologic stability

Give a whole-milk substitute   When an allergy or intolerance to milk exists, milk substitutes such as skim milk, soybean formula, evaporated milk, or protein hydrolysate formulas can be given. Milk also can be diluted with water.

Rationale: A milk substitute provides an alternate to milk, maintains the nutrition of whole milk, and minimizes undesirable physical responses.

Fulfilled Needs: Nutritional balance, comfort, protection from physical harm

Give an antidote as recommended on the poison container label   Read the container label of the ingested product and use the suggested antidote for that particular product as stated on the label.

Rationale: A proper antidote will neutralize the harmful effects of a poison.

Fulfilled Needs: Protection from physical harm, physiologic stability

Give bland foods   Give foods low in residue, acid, and spice content. These include milk, eggs, cream, butter, mild cheese, tender meat, poultry and fish, low-residue and low-acid fruits and vegetables, white bread, refined cereals, plain desserts, and starches like potatoes, rice, and macaroni. Avoid giving foods containing seeds, coarse fibers and skins, heavy seasoning, caffeine, and alcohol.

Rationale: Bland foods neutralize acids, reduce gastric juice secretion and peristalsis, and will not stimulate salivation to the degree that seasoned foods will.

Fulfilled Needs: Nutritional balance, energy, comfort, protection from physical harm

Give buttermilk or yogurt   Give a glass of buttermilk or a serving of yogurt.

Rationale: Buttermilk and yogurt contain lactobacilli that increase the absorption of nutritional substances such as vitamins. During and following antibiotic therapy or diarrhea, buttermilk or yogurt restore normal intestinal bacteria, which improves digestion and promotes comfort. Yogurt is a good source of calcium, riboflavin, and protein.

Fulfilled Needs: Comfort, protection from physical harm

Give carbonated beverages   Dispense an effervescent drink.

Rationale: Vomiting removes hydrochloric acid from the stomach, causing alkalosis. The carbon dioxide (effervescence) in carbonated beverages is acid. When alkalosis exists, it helps restore normal pH and increases fluid intake. Carbonated beverages cause air in the stomach to bubble and move up the esophagus relieving the discomfort of trapped air. Carbonated beverages produce alkaline urine. The ginger root, a basic ingredient in ginger ale, soothes the intestinal mucosa.

Fulfilled Needs: Fluid and electrolyte balance, acid–base balance, comfort

Contraindications: Acidosis, high susceptibility to tooth decay, gastric hyperacidity, potential or existing calcium renal calculi, abdominal distention from intestinal disorders, respiratory disorders in which there is carbon dioxide retention

Give citrus fruit juice   Give citrus-fruit juice to the person who has swallowed a corrosive alkali poison. If a child is 1–5 years old, give 1–2 cups of juice. If he is over 5 years of age, give up to 1 quart (1,000 cc) of juice. Citrus-fruit juices include orange and grapefruit juice. If a person is in shock, give citrus-fruit juice only if he is able to swallow.

Rationale: The high-acid content of citrus-fruit juices neutralizes the alkali in alkali poisons and in alkalosis. The high-glucose content of citrus-fruit juices tends to offset shock.

Fulfilled Needs: Fluid and electrolyte balance, acid–base balance, protection from physical harm

Give clear-liquid foods   Give water and nutritional liquids including tea with lemon and sugar, coffee, carbonated beverages, fat-free broth, flavored gelatin, fruit ices, and strained or clear fruit juices.

Rationale: Clear-liquid foods replace lost fluids. Their nonirritating effect reduces flatulence and excessive peristaltic stimulation. Relief of visceral hunger promotes comfort.

Fulfilled Needs: Fluid and electrolyte balance, nutritional balance, comfort, protection from physical harm

Give drugs judiciously for emotional repression   Recognize that drugs can be given appropriately for the repression of emotions during times of crisis, but that the drugs should no longer be given when the crisis is over.

Rationale: Drugs during a time of crisis help to repress intense emotions and assist the person in coping with the situation. Once the crisis is over, drugs should no longer be given since the person needs to face his emotions in the now less stressful situation. If emotions are repressed constantly, they will surface at a later time, causing a painful, inappropriate experience. Honest confrontation with emotions promotes growth, maturity, and reality perception.

Fulfilled Needs: Comfort, protection from psychologic threat, personal growth and maturity, increased reality perception and problem-solving ability

Give dry crackers   Give the person experiencing nausea or vomiting dry, preferably salted, crackers to eat.

Rationale: Dry crackers absorb and neutralize intestinal acids and promote comfort.

Fulfilled Needs: Acid–base balance, comfort, protection from physical harm

Contraindications: Avoid salted crackers in salt- or sodium-restricted diets

Give enteric-coated medications   Give medications coated with a substance that prevents their destruction until after they pass through the stomach.

Rationale: Enteric-coated medications do not disintegrate and are not absorbed until they reach the small intestine. They protect the stomach against irritation from the drug and protect the drug from exposure to gastric acid.

Fulfilled Needs: Comfort, protection from physical harm

Contraindications: Restricted sugar intake

Give explicit directions   Give firm, simple directions that can be understood and acted on easily.

Rationale: Simple, direct communications enhance perception and reduce threats of frustration and anxiety. Lengthy directions reduce available time for thinking and deciphering messages and result in confusion and discomfort. When a person cannot make decisions because of overtaxed adaptation needs, direction from a person uninvolved in the crisis reduces threat and promotes comfort.

Fulfilled Needs: Comfort, protection from physical harm, protection from psychologic threat, dependence

Give flavor-intensified food Give foods whose flavor has been accentuated by adding monosodium glutamate.

Rationale: Monosodium glutamate intensifies food flavor without adding new flavor. When taste is physiologically impaired, improved flavor promotes comfort and the desire to eat.

Fulfilled Needs: Nutritional balance, comfort

Contraindications: Sodium-restricted diet, intolerance to monosodium glutamate

Give fresh fruits/fruit juices Dispense nonprocessed fruits or fruit juices that are in the natural state, such as apples, oranges, plums, grapes, pineapple.

Rationale: Fresh fruits and fruit juices contain indigestible cellulose that supplies bulk for normal comfortable elimination. Fresh fruits and juices supply nutritional vitamins.

Fulfilled Needs: Nutritional balance, waste elimination of food residue, comfort

Contraindications: Diarrhea, hyperperistalsis, gastric ulceration

Give full-liquid foods Give liquid or semiliquid foods that are free of cellulose and spices. Include carbonated beverages, milk, coffee, tea, cocoa, strained or fine whole-grain cereals, custards, plain gelatin, ice cream, sherbert, junket, cornstarch puddings, raw or softly cooked eggs, strained juices, strained or creamed meat and vegetable soups, butter, sugar, salt, and eggnog.

Rationale: When food is tolerated poorly, a full-liquid diet supplies nourishment and facilitates easy digestion. Relief of visceral hunger promotes comfort. Salivation is increased by mechanical stimulation of taste buds with full-liquid foods.

Fulfilled Needs: Fluid and electrolyte balance, nutritional balance, comfort, protection from physical harm

Give hard candy Dispense hard candy for sucking.

Rationale: Sucking on hard candy (especially lemon and peppermint) promotes comfort and hygiene by refreshing the mouth and sour breath. It prevents mouth dryness and is a quick source of glucose. Candy is a substitute for less desirable oral satisfactions such as smoking, chewing tobacco, etc. Lemon candy increases salivation.

Fulfilled Needs: Energy, comfort, protection from physical harm

Contraindications: Do not give when sugar intake is restricted, except in emergency insulin shock; susceptibility to tooth decay

Give high-calcium fluids orally Give milk or liquids such as milk shakes, malts, milk sodas, melted ice cream, cocoa, milk punch.

Rationale: High-calcium fluids increase a low-calcium blood level and help maintain acid–base and fluid balance.

Fulfilled Needs: Fluid and electrolyte balance, acid–base balance, protection from physical harm

Contraindications: Potential or existing calcium urinary calculi, high-alkali intake, prolonged illness-enforced mobility or bed rest, nausea, vomiting, diarrhea, respiratory infection, high fever

Give high-glucose fluids orally Give liquids such as lemonade, orange juice, or tea or coffee with sugar, honey, or corn syrup.

Rationale: Glucose ingestion raises a low blood-sugar level to normal, produces energy from food, and balances fluid intake and body acid–base.

Fulfilled Needs: Fluid and electrolyte balance, acid–base balance, energy, protection from physical harm

Contraindications: Do not give when sugar intake is restricted, except in emergency insulin shock; susceptibility to tooth decay

Give high-magnesium fluids orally Raise the intake of high-magnesium liquids. Include milk, cocoa, chocolate, prune juice.

Rationale: A normal magnesium level is essential to osmotic pressure balance, enzyme activation, nerve and muscular activity, normal bone development, and acid–base balance.

Fulfilled Needs: Fluid and electrolyte balance, protection from physical harm

Contraindications: Hypermagnesemia, diabetic acidosis, dehydration, profuse sweating

Give high-magnesium snacks Give snacks that have a high-magnesium content such as nuts, bananas, oranges, chocolate, peanut butter, ice cream.

Rationale: A normal magnesium level is essential to osmotic pressure balance, enzyme activation, nerve and muscular activity, normal bone development, and acid-base balance.

Fulfilled Needs: Fluid and electrolyte balance, protection from physical harm

Give high-potassium fluids orally Dispense fluids containing high levels of potassium. Include grape, grapefruit, orange, prune, tangerine, or tomato juice, and tea, coffee, chocolate, and meat broth.

Rationale: Normal blood-potassium level is essential to intracellular fluid balance, osmotic pressure regulation, acid–base balance, and the conduction of nerve impulses in muscle tissue. High-potassium intake offsets the tendency of steroid drugs to cause negative nitrogen balance and replaces potassium loss from diuresis, diarrhea and vomiting.

Fulfilled Needs: Fluid and electrolyte balance, acid–base balance, protection from physical harm

Contraindications: Hyperkalemia, renal failure with oliguria or anuria, adrenal insufficiency, ventricular fibrillation, during the shock stage of severe second- or third-degree burns or crushing injuries, persons receiving IV infusions containing potassium

Give high-sodium fluids orally Dispense liquids having a high sodium content, such as milk, root beer, instant or dry coffee, Dutch chocolate, tomato juice.

Rationale: A normal sodium level is essential to fluid and electroyte balance, normal osmotic pressure, and acid–base balance. It replaces sodium lost through diarrhea and vomiting.

Fulfilled Needs: Fluid and electrolyte balance, acid–base balance, protection from physical harm

Contraindications: Impaired renal function, edema, ascites, cardiac damage with impaired circulation, persons receiving steroid therapy, large volumes of intravenous saline, or on a low-sodium diet

Give hot coffee Offer a cup of hot coffee, preferably without sugar or cream.

Rationale: Hot coffee reduces fatigue through its stimulative effect. It increases circulation, counteracts overdoses of barbiturates and sleeping pills, increases fluid intake, and promotes bowel and bladder elimination.

Fulfilled Needs: Tissue oxygenation or perfusion, fluid and electrolyte balance, waste elimination of food residue and urine, comfort, stimulation, protection from physical harm

Contraindications: Impaired blood supply to the cardiac muscle, poisonous snakebites, electrical shock, excessive peristalsis, urinary frequency, vasodilatation, nervousness or irritability, hypoglycemia, increased metabolic rate, cracked or sensitive teeth, sensitive gums or oral mucous membranes

Give hot tea Offer a cup of hot tea, preferably without sugar and cream.

Rationale: Vomiting removes hydrochloric acid from the stomach, causing alkalosis. The tannic acid in tea helps reestablish normal pH, and the fluid increases liquid intake. Theine in tea makes it mildly stimulating, causing temporarily improved circulation, fatigue reduction, and ease of fatigue headaches. It counteracts overdoses of barbiturates and sleeping pills.

Fulfilled Needs: Circulation (tissue oxygenation or perfusion), fluid and electrolyte balance, acid-base balance, comfort, stimulation, protection from physical harm

Contraindications: Impaired blood supply to the cardiac muscle, poisonous snakebites, electrical shock, excessive peristalsis, urinary frequency, vasodilatation, nervousness or irritability, hypoglycemia, increased metabolic rate, cracked or sensitive teeth, sensitive gums or oral mucous membranes

Give iced (or cool) liquids Give fluids that are chilled or iced, such as ice water or fruit juices.

Rationale: Cold liquids in the stomach and duodenum stimulate the gastrocolic reflex, causing colon contractions and peristalsis. Iced liquids reduce elevated body temperature and stimulate the vagus nerve to slow the heart. Cool liquids cause vasoconstriction, which prevents mouth bleeding.

Fulfilled Needs: Fluid and electrolyte balance, normal temperature, comfort, protection from physical harm

Contraindications: Low body temperature, impaired blood circulation, bladder or intestinal spasms, diarrhea or hyperperistalsis, cracked or sensitive teeth, sensitive or receding gums

Give important messages only when the person is receptive Convey thoughts and ideas of importance only in a nondistracting environment when the person's attention can be focused on the message.

Rationale: The quality of message reception and interpretation is reduced by distracting environmental influences and events. Comfort is promoted through a sense of effective communication with others.

Fulfilled Needs: Comfort, protection from psychologic threat, caring and communicating relationships

Give iodized salt Dispense salt fortified with either sodium or potassium iodide.

Rationale: The use of iodized salt before or during the early stages of iodine deficiency usually will correct the problem. Iodine is essential to thyroxin production necessary for normal thyroid function.

Fulfilled Needs: Protection from physical harm

Contraindications: Hypernatremia, hyperkalemia

Give isotonic drinks orally Dispense liquid drinks containing a 0.9% water solution of sodium chloride. These drinks can be individually prepared or obtained from commercial manufacturers.

Rationale: Sodium and chloride are essential to fluid and acid–base balance. When large amounts of sodium chloride are lost through urine, sweating, vomiting, and diarrhea, body cells become overhydrated because of failure to maintain equal concentrations of water and solute (osmosis) within the cells. Isotonic drinks reestablish normal osmotic pressure so water can pass to and from the cells equalizing the solute and water concentration. Isotonic drinks maintain fluid, salt, and acid–base balance.

Fulfilled Needs: Water–salt balance, acid–base balance, protection from physical harm

Contraindications: Hypernatremia, hyperchloremia

Give light foods Give a light snack of easily digestible foods.

Rationale: Light foods alleviate the discomfort of hunger while providing nutrition when persons have difficulty eating. The metabolic rate is stimulated less with light foods than with a heavy meal.

Fulfilled Needs: Energy, comfort, protection from physical harm

Give low-calcium fluids orally   Dispense fluids containing little or no milk.

Rationale: Decreased calcium intake reduces the potential formation of calcium urinary stones especially in existing kidney disease and illness-enforced immobility. It increases fluid intake and helps restore electrolyte balance when the blood-calcium level is elevated.

Fulfilled Needs: Fluid and electrolyte balance, protection from physical harm

Contraindications: Blood-clotting abnormalities, poor lactation, impaired bone growth, persons receiving large volumes of citrated blood by transfusion

Give low-magnesium fluids orally   Decrease the intake of high-magnesium liquids, such as milk, fruit juice, cocoa, and chocolate.

Rationale: A normal magnesium level is essential for osmotic pressure balance, enzyme activation, nerve and muscular activity, normal bone development, and acid–base balance.

Fulfilled Needs: Fluid and electrolyte balance, protection from physical harm

Contraindications: Hypomagnesemia, impaired bone development

Give low-potassium fluids orally   Dispense liquids having little potassium content such as cranberry juice, ginger ale, root beer, 7-Up, Pepsi Cola.

Rationale: In kidney failure, potassium cannot be eliminated, causing an elevated blood-potassium level. A normal blood-potassium level is essential to intracellular fluid balance, osmotic pressure regulation, acid–base balance, and the conduction of nerve impulses in muscle tissue.

Fulfilled Needs: Fluid and electrolyte balance, acid–base balance, protection from physical harm

Contraindications: Diarrhea, vomiting, diuresis, impaired muscle function, profuse colostomy, ileostomy, ileal conduit, or T-tube drainage, persons on steroid therapy or receiving large volumes of IV dextrose or saline.

Give low-sodium fluids orally   Dispense liquids having little sodium content. Salt-free tomato juice, dry roasted coffee, orange juice, pineapple juice, apple juice, cranberry juice, prune juice, tangerine juice, cola drinks, Kool-Aid, lemonade, tea, and ginger ale are recommended.

Rationale: A normal blood-sodium level is essential for electrolyte balance, osmotic pressure regulation in cells, and fluid and acid–base balance. In severe cardiac damage, venous stasis and increased venous pressure prevent the return of sodium and water from interstitial tissues into the bloodstream for excretion by the kidneys. When kidney excretion of sodium is reduced, restricted sodium intake decreases the blood-sodium level. Osmotic pressure then pulls sodium and water from the interstitial spaces into the bloodstream relieving tissue edema.

Fulfilled Needs: Fluid and electrolyte balance, acid–base balance, protection from physical harm

Contraindications: Diarrhea, vomiting, excessive sweating, diuresis, second- or third-degree burns, repetitive paracentesis, fever, profuse colostomy, ileostomy, ileal conduit, fistula, or T-tube drainage; persons receiving large volumes of IV dextrose

Give magnesium sulfate solution orally   Give 2 tablespoons of magnesium sulfate in two glasses of water. In bichloride of mercury poisoning, give 1 ounce of magnesium sulfate in a pint of water.

Rationale: Magnesium sulfate has a neutralizing effect on specific poisons, including overdoses of codeine, paregoric, bromides, sleeping pills, and barbiturates. It also neutralizes poisoning by the ingestion of food, bichloride of mercury, DDT, and mushrooms.

Fulfilled Needs: Protection from physical harm, physiologic stability

Give mechanically soft foods   Give mechanically soft foods that can be chewed easily. Such foods include ground or minced meats, soft breads, chopped or diced cooked vegetables, soft raw vegetables such as tomatoes and lettuce, soft fruits such as apricots, peaches, bananas, oranges, grapefruit, berries, pears, and finely chopped dried fruits and nuts, mashed potatoes, ice cream, custards and gelatin.

Rationale: The normal digestive process includes the reduction of food to small particles by the teeth. The edentulous diet allows for the omission of mastication in the digestive process when teeth are missing. Balanced nutritional intake is essential to body cell activity and energy production from food. Relief of the visceral hunger sensation promotes comfort.

Fulfilled Needs: Nutritional balance, energy, comfort, protection from physical harm

Give milk   Give homogenized milk.

Rationale: Milk neutralizes the harmful effects of acids and promotes comfort. It dilutes the effects of overdoses of pep pills, iron compounds, alcohol, aspirin, headache and cold drugs, paregoric, codeine, and belladonna. It offsets the corrosive effects of poisons such as sodium fluoride, arsenic, strychnine, iodine, bichloride of mercury, chlorine bleach and disinfectant, oil of Wintergreen, rubbing alcohol, carbolic acid disinfectant, furniture polish, gasoline, kerosene, pine oil, and turpentine.

Fulfilled Needs: Comfort, protection from physical harm

Contraindications: Milk intolerance, infants younger than 4–6 months of age.

Give milk with medications   Dispense milk when administering oral medications that irritate the stomach lining.

Rationale: The soothing effect of milk on the stomach lining promotes comfort and reduces irritation.

Fulfilled Needs: Comfort, protection from physical harm

Contraindications: Milk intolerance, when giving medications that have adverse reactions with milk, conditions of decreased gastric absorption

Give (apply) nonprescription drugs   Give medical substances readily available to the public that do not require a prescription to be obtained.

Rationale: Drugs consist of chemicals that combine with body processes to either alter or improve body function, to promote comfort or elimination, to regulate body temperature, and to protect from inflammatory or infectious conditions.

Fulfilled Needs: Comfort, protection from physical harm, freedom from pain

Contraindications: Hypersensitivity to the drug; presence of diseased conditions that may be affected adversely, persons taking prescription drugs that are incompatible with the nonprescription drug

Give one direction at a time   Direct the person toward accomplishing one activity at a time. Avoid giving further direction until that activity has been completed.

Rationale: Impaired cerebral function limits the accomplishment of more than one activity at a time.

Fulfilled Needs: Comfort, protection from psychologic threat

Give one-half the narcotic dose PO and one-half IM before converting to full PO dosage[627,628]   When attempting to wean a person from narcotic injections to oral dosage, give half the medication dosage IM and half orally. Increase the oral dose so that its strength equals half the IM dose. Convert the person to a full oral dosage as is appropriate and after consulting with a physician.

Rationale: Giving half IM and half PO drug dosages helps persons reluctant to convert to full PO dosage by supporting a gradual change in medications.

Fulfilled Needs: Comfort

Give pain-relief drugs on a regular, preventive schedule, not PRN[627,628]

Give pain-relief drugs on a regular schedule. Do not wait until the person is in pain and requests relief. Anticipate that oral narcotics have an onset time of 1 hour and a peak effect at 2 hours, while injections have an onset time of 30 minutes and a peak effect at 1 hour.

Rationale: Giving pain-relief drugs on a preventative basis prevents the person from having to needlessly endure 30 minutes or an hour of pain before the drug takes effect. Pain that is not allowed to become severe is more easily controlled.

Fulfilled Needs: Comfort, protection from physical harm

Give perineal care Give perineal care by cleansing the vulva and perineum and pouring water over the external female genitalia.

Rationale: Cleanliness minimizes bacterial growth leading to infection and reduces tissue irritation from diseased conditions.

Fulfilled Needs: Comfort, cleanliness, protection from physical harm

Give prune juice Dispense a glass of prune juice at least once a day.

Rationale: Prune juice promotes intestinal mobility through the byproduct of the prune called dihydroxyphenylisatin. Normal elimination promotes comfort.

Fulfilled Needs: Waste elimination of food residue, comfort

Contraindications: Diarrhea, hyperperistalsis, hypercalcemia

Give pureed foods Give foods boiled to a pulp consistency and strained through a sieve.

Rationale: Pureed foods are swallowed and digested easily because of their pulp consistency and minimal cellulose. Salivation is increased by mechanical stimulation of the taste buds with pureed foods. Balanced nutritional intake is essential to body cell activity and energy production from food. Relief of visceral hunger promotes comfort.

Fulfilled Needs: Nutritional balance, energy, comfort, protection from physical harm

Give raw egg white orally Give two raw egg whites beaten up or mixed with water.

Rationale: Raw egg whites have a neutralizing effect on specific poisons such as household ammonia, washing soda, and carbolic acid disinfectant.

Fulfilled Needs: Protection from physical harm, physiologic stability

Give raw vegetables When small children reject soft, mushy food such as cooked vegetables, give raw, firm vegetables.

Rationale: The ability to grasp food firmly makes eating easier and more pleasurable for the child whose small muscle coordination is not developed fully.

Fulfilled Needs: Comfort

Give regular diet (foods) Give the person a general diet including any foods he desires.

Rationale: A general diet of varied foods provides good nutrition.

Fulfilled Needs: Nutritional balance, protection from physical harm, increased learning

Give rice cereal or rice water When diarrhea occurs, give the person cereal made from rice; or cook the rice, drain off the water, and cool, and offer the rice water as a drink or place it in a bottle for an infant.

Rationale: Rice and rice water have a constipating effect and will stop the diarrhea. It is especially appropriate for infants who should not be taking drugs.

Fulfilled Needs: Fluid and electrolyte balance, protection from physical harm, increased learning

Give small, frequent drinks Give small amounts of fluid, but give it at frequent intervals such as every 1–2 hours.

Rationale: Small amounts of fluids given at frequent intervals can provide adequate fluid intake, promote comfort, and meet dependency needs.

Fulfilled Needs: Fluid and electrolyte balance, comfort, protection from physical harm, dependence

Contraindications: Restricted oral intake

Give small, frequent feedings Give nourishing food in small amounts at least six times a day.

Rationale: Small food amounts at frequent intervals are easily digested, prevent fatigue and abdominal distention, and maintain balanced nutritional intake. Relief of visceral hunger promotes comfort. The intake of small, frequent feedings requires less physical exertion, which reduces oxygen consumption in severe cardiac and pulmonary disorders.

Fulfilled Needs: Nutritional balance, energy, comfort, protection from physical harm

Give snacks Between meals, give foods that add to the nutrients of the day. Include foods like milk products, fruits, and sandwiches instead of nonnutritious foods such as concentrated sweets and carbonated beverages.

Rationale: Balanced nutritional intake is essential to body cell activity and energy production from food. Relief of visceral hunger promotes comfort.

Fulfilled Needs: Nutritional balance, energy, comfort

Contraindications: Obesity

Give sodium bicarbonate solution orally Orally, give a solution of 1 tablespoon sodium bicarbonate in 1 quart water. For an overdose of iron compounds, mix 2 teaspoons of sodium bicarbonate in a glass of warm water.

Rationale: Sodium bicarbonate has a neutralizing effect on overdoses of iron compounds, alcohol, aspirin, headache and cold drugs. It counteracts poisoning from phosphorous, oil of Wintergreen, and rubbing alcohol. It assists in reversing acidosis.

Fulfilled Needs: Acid–base balance, protection from physical harm, physiologic stability

Give soft foods Give foods that are soft, easily digested, not highly seasoned, and contain no harsh fibers. Such foods include bread, dry or cooked cereals, mild cheese, angel food and sponge cakes, custards, gelatin salads with fruit, sherbert, ice creams and pudding, creamed soups, cookies, tender meats, vegetables without skins, all beverages, eggs except when fried, canned or cooked fruit.

Rationale: Soft foods decrease intestinal irritation and bowel spasm and promote comfort. Balanced nutritional intake is essential to body cell activity and energy production from food.

Fulfilled Needs: Nutritional balance, energy, comfort, protection from physical harm

Give strongly seasoned foods Give foods highly seasoned with herbs, spices, and salts that enhance food tastes.

Rationale: Strong seasoning increases taste when taste has been physiologically impaired and promotes a greater desire to eat.

Fulfilled Needs: Nurtitional balance, comfort

Contraindications: Avoid in oral-tissue injury, gastric or intestinal irritation

Give sugar During persistent hiccoughs, give several teaspoons of table sugar orally.

Rationale: Swallowing sugar crystals stops hiccoughs by stimulating the vagus and phrenic nerves.

Fulfilled Needs: Comfort

Contraindications: Restricted sugar intake

Give tetanus toxoid (ET) If the person has received a severe wound, especially a burn, puncture, or deep wound, he should receive tetanus immunization. If he has been immunized fully with tetanus toxoid and has received a booster within the last 5 years, no additional tetanus toxoid is needed. If the last booster is older than 5 years, he should receive a booster dose of toxoid. If the person has never received tetanus toxoid, he should receive tetanus immune globulin (human) for immediate protection and begin tetanus toxoid immunization as soon as his condition permits. Use tetanus antitoxin (animal serum) only if human globulin is not available because of the dangerous sensitivity reactions possible.

Rationale: The injection of antigens into the body produces antibodies that react against the infectious organisms that attack the body.

Fulfilled Needs: Protection from physical harm

Contraindications: Known hypersensitivity reactions to tetanus immunization

Give the drug (narcotic) having the fewest side effects for the person, when drug choices are available[627,628]   When administering narcotics, give the drug that has the fewest undesirable side effects for the person. Avoid drugs that oversedate or cause nausea and vomiting. Persons often know which drugs have adverse effects on them. Short-acting drugs are best for persons with organ damage such as hepatic or renal disorders.

Rationale: The fewer the side effects of a drug, the less harmful it is, and the more effective its intended results.

Fulfilled Needs: Comfort, protection from physical harm

Give the infant a chilled teething ring to chew on   Give the teething infant a soft, gel-like teething ring that has been cooled in the refrigerator. Let him chew on it.

Rationale: Cold causes vasoconstriction, which relieves pain and swelling.

Fulfilled Needs: Comfort, protection from physical harm, freedom from pain

Give the medication by injection or in liquid form instead of pills   When medication in pill form causes gastric irritation, give the same medication either by injection or as a liquid.

Rationale: Liquid medications are absorbed more easily by the gastric mucosa, and medication by injection has no contact with the gastric mucosa.

Fulfilled Needs: Comfort, protection from physical harm

Contraindications: Drugs that require a different dosage when given parenterally instead of orally must be reordered by the physician

Give urine-acidifying juices orally   Give acid–ash juices of apple, cranberry, plum, or prune juice.

Rationale: Increased urine acidity decreases the formation of calcium urinary stones. Effective urinary tract hydration prevents the separation of potential calculi particles from solution and decreases stone formation. Following digestion and oxidation, acid–ash juices alter the bladder pH toward an acid level that deters bacterial growth.

Fulfilled Needs: Fluid and electrolyte balance, protection from physical harm

Contraindications: Hyperuricemia, cystine renal stones

Give urine-alkalinizing juices orally   Give carbonated beverages, orange juice, and other fruit juices except cranberry, apple, prune, and plum juice.

Rationale: Increased alkaline in the urine decreases uric acid and cystine urinary stone formation. Effective urinary tract hydration prevents the separation of potential calculi particles from solution and decreases stone formation.

Fulfilled Needs: Fluid and electrolyte balance, protection from physical harm

Contraindications: Calcium renal stones, urinary tract infection

Give warm liquids/fluids   Offer heated liquids.

Rationale: Warm liquids increase body temperature, promote relaxation, enhance circulation, which decreases pain, reduce bladder spasms, promote comfort, increase fluid intake, and promote elimination.

Fulfilled Needs: Tissue oxygenation or perfusion, fluid and electrolyte balance, waste elimination of food residue, normal temperature, sleep, rest, relaxation, comfort, protection from physical harm, freedom from pain

Give warm liquids after meals Suggest that fluids not be taken with meals and then offer a warm drink at the end of the meal.

Rationale: Warm fluids after a meal reduce flatulence.

Fulfilled Needs: Comfort

Give water orally Give water orally to the person who has swallowed a poison or is in impending or early shock. If a child is 1–5 years of age, give 1–2 cups. If he is over 5-years old, give up to 1 quart (1,000 cc).

Rationale: Water dilutes poisons, reducing their irritating effect on mucous membranes. Water increases the circulating blood volume and thereby assists in reversing shock.

Fulfilled Needs: Fluid and electrolyte balance, protection from physical harm

Contraindications: Do not give oral fluids if the person is well into shock because the existing hypoxia generally stops peristalsis and oral fluids would result in abdominal distention and vomiting

Give wine, whiskey, brandy Offer a small glass of wine or liquor 30 minutes before meals.

Rationale: The alcohol content of wine causes vasodilatation, which enhances peripheral circulation, relieves internal congestion, and increases appetite.

Fulfilled Needs: Tissue oxygenation or perfusion, comfort, protection from physical harm

Contraindications: Do not give alcoholic beverages to persons with an alcohol dependency

Gradually increase the amount of feedings Initially, offer small amounts of food and liquids. As the small amounts are tolerated, add a little more with each feeding until normal nutritional quantity is established.

Rationale: Small food amounts in the stomach prevent pressure against the cardiac sphincter and reduces possible regurgitation. Gradually increasing nutritional intake promotes slow stomach filling and thorough digestion by gastric juices. Infants require a gradual increase in feedings as the child makes the transition from liquids to solids.

Fulfilled Needs: Comfort, protection from physical harm

Gradually increase the amount of ventilator pressure When artificial ventilation disturbs the person, use a very low-pressure setting at first. After the person is comfortable with that pressure, gradually increase it, keeping in mind individual pressure tolerances.

Rationale: Low-pressure ventilation offers comfort and slow adjustment to greater pressure settings.

Fulfilled Needs: Comfort

Grant special requests If the person wishes to have a particular favor granted, willingly offer to do it.

Rationale: Positive self-attitudes are reinforced by positive responses from others. Granting requests meets dependency needs.

Fulfilled Needs: Comfort, dependency, high evaluation of self, recognition, diginity, attention

Guide the person in simple prayer If the person is unable to pray, guide him in short meaningful prayer, such as; "My God, I offer You all my suffering," or "Thank you, Lord, for all your blessings," or "My God, I love you."

Rationale: Communication with God promotes comfort and understanding and fosters closer God-human relationships.

Fulfilled Needs: Comfort; spiritual, religious, or philosophic satisfaction

Guide the sleepwalker back to bed   If a person is sleepwalking, slowly guide him toward and into the bed.

Rationale: Returning the sleepwalker back to bed prevents injury during the episode.

Fulfilled Needs: Protection from physical harm

Handle gently   Move the person's body slowly and carefully. Avoid jarring or sudden movements.

Rationale: Nerve fibers throughout skin layers convey pain impulses. The greater the external stimuli on nerve fibers, the greater the pain potential. Respect for the human body promotes dignity.

Fulfilled Needs: Comfort, protection from physical harm, freedom from pain, dignity

Help the suicidal person set goals to preserve his life   Assist the person to set long- and short-term goals that will result in positive self-preservation. Such goals include instilling in the person a desire to survive, having the person voluntarily inform the staff of impulses to harm himself, and verbalizing reasons why he does not want to hurt himself.

Rationale: By setting goals for the preservation of life, the person is counteracting intents of self-destruction.

Fulfilled Needs: Protection from physical harm, high evaluation of self, control over self, personal growth and maturity

Hold the infant while feeding   While feeding, elevate the infant's head above his stomach and hold the infant in your arms and close to your body.

Rationale: Head elevation above the stomach during feeding prevents food aspiration into the lungs. Human contact during infant feeding supports an association of love with food and promotes comfort.

Fulfilled Needs: Comfort, protection from physical harm, caring and communicating relationships

Hold the person responsible for his behavior   Make it clear that the person, and no one else, is responsible for his or her behavior. Do not allow the person to blame others for his behavior.

Rationale: When a person is held responsible for his behavior and is not allowed to blame others, that person is forced to recognize and deal with the reality of his behavior.

Fulfilled Needs: Personal growth and maturity, increased reality perception

Honor religious dietary regulations   Be certain that the person's religious dietary regulations are met. Seek guidance in this matter from the person and his family.

Rationale: Religious observances assist people in spiritually expressing and outwardly recognizing their relationship with God.

Fulfilled Needs: Comfort; dignity; spiritual, religious, or philosophic satisfaction

Ignore undesirable behavior   Refuse to take notice of undesirable behavior by acting as if it never occurred. Instead, satisfy the need for attention by noticing favorable behaviors.

Rationale: Self-esteem is acquired through acceptable sociocultural behavior. Ignoring undesirable behavior prevents diminished self-esteem, which would result from social disapproval. It supports increased perception that attention cannot be acquired by socially unacceptable behavior.

Fulfilled Needs: Protection from psychologic threat, increased reality perception

Illuminate the room adequately   Provide suitable room lighting according to individual needs.

Rationale: Adequate lighting supports maximum visual acuity, decreases sensory misinterpretation, and promotes comfort. It meets dependency needs.

Fulfilled Needs: Comfort, protection from physical harm, protection from psychologic threat, dependence

Immobilize the affected body part (the fractured body part, the graft site)
Stabilize the injured or surgical body area and the joints above and below the injury or surgery. Place the person in the injury-assumed position or in a comfortable position. When there is an existing or suspected spinal cord injury, place the person on a firm board before transporting to medical services.

Rationale: Immobilization and support of a traumaticed body area prevents further injury and possible circulation loss through vascular damage and decreases fluid loss in burns. It promotes rest and comfort and supports healing.

Fulfilled Needs: Rest, comfort, protection from physical harm

Increase drafts   Increase the volume of air currents in the environment.

Rationale: Increased drafts decrease elevated body temperature by perspiration vaporization and promote comfort.

Fulfilled Needs: Normal temperature, comfort

Increase environmental stimuli   Increase the amount of stimulation the person receives from the environment. This includes more visitors, radio and television, mobiles above the bed, and a wide mirror for enlarging the field of vision.

Rationale: Increased environmental stimulation supports the perception of reality, diverts attention from preoccupation with self, and acts as a motivating force for action.

Fulfilled Needs: Comfort, stimulation, increased reality perception

Increase fluid intake according to weight loss   Weigh the person and increase his fluid intake 500 cc for each pound of weight lost on the previous day.

Rationale: A 1-pound weight loss in 24 hours is considered a 500 cc fluid loss.

Fulfilled Needs: Fluid and electrolyte balance, protection from physical harm

Increase fluid intake to about 2,000 cc daily   Increase the daily fluid intake to 2,000 cc (eight 8-ounce glasses) or 500 cc above the normal daily requirement of 1,500 cc. Fluids include water, fruit juice, Jello, Kool-Aid, tea, ginger ale, etc.

Rationale: Conditions of fever, excessive perspiration, dehydration due to vomiting or diarrhea require large fluid intake to replace fluid loss. Increased fluid intake moistens mucous membranes, dilutes chemical materials within the body that cause itching, distends a prolapsed bladder by helping to reestablish muscle tone, dilutes alcohol in the blood, reducing its effect, and promotes comfort.

Fulfilled Needs: Fluid and electrolyte balance; waste elimination of food residue, urine, toxic substances, bronchopulmonary secretions; normal temperature; comfort; protection from physical harm

Contraindications: Edema, ascites, renal insufficiency or failure, congestive heart failure

Increase fluid intake to about 3,000 cc daily   Increase the daily fluid intake to 3,000 cc (twelve 8-ounce glasses of liquid). Fluids can include water, fruit juice, Jello, Kool-Aid, tea, ginger ale, etc.

Rationale: Effective urinary tract hydration prevents separation of calculi particles from solution, decreasing stone formation. Increased fluid intake assists in moving urinary calculi through and out of the urinary tract. It prevents burning on urination, dilutes ingested poisons, and reduces their effects. Fluid balance promotes comfort.

Fulfilled Needs: Fluid and electrolyte balance; waste elimination of food residue, urine, toxic substances, bronchopulmonary secretions; comfort; protection from physical harm

Contraindications: Edema, ascites, renal insufficiency or failure, congestive heart failure

Increase fluids at mealtime   Give an increased quantity of liquids with each meal.

Rationale: Saliva moistens food and aids swallowing. When saliva production is low, liquids can be substituted to moisten foods.

Fulfilled Needs: Comfort, protection from physical harm

Contraindications: Excessive flatulence, postmeal diarrhea resulting from the dumping syndrome

Increase the intravenous infusion flow rate   Raise the intravenous flow rate above the maintenance rate until the blood pressure reaches normal. Then return the flow rate to 60 drops/minute.

Rationale: When the blood volume is less than the volume of vascular space available for blood, circulation becomes inadequate, causing arteries to lose normal tone with resulting blood-pressure drop and cardiac failure. Rapid replacement of fluid volume increases arterial tone, and the blood pressure returns to normal, supplying the heart with an adequate blood volume for tissue oxygenation. An output of less than 15–20 cc of urine per hour indicates more rapid fluid loss than replacement and that normal fluid requirements are not being met.

Fulfilled Needs: Fluid and electrolyte balance, protection from physical harm

Contraindications: Circulatory overload, when the output is more than 80 cc of urine per hour because of overhydration; neurogenic or vasogenic shock; renal failure

Increase the time interval between the drug doses   Lengthen the amount of time between each dose of the drug; determine the increased interval on the basis of the amount of adverse drug effect, its intended effect, and consultation with the physician when appropriate.

Rationale: Increasing the interval between drug doses will often eliminate or reduce adverse drug effects.

Fulfilled Needs: Comfort, protection from physical harm, physiologic stability

Increase the weaning time off the therapeutic device(s) gradually   Gradually increase the time during which a person is free of life-supporting measures or machines.

Rationale: Awareness that a person can sustain his own life without supportive measures promotes comfort. Professional recognition of potential danger resulting from sudden, complete withdrawal of life-supporting measures promotes safety. Gradually increased self-dependency enhances self-reliance and adequacy, while reducing stress and anxiety.

Fulfilled Needs: Comfort, protection from physical harm, protection from psychologic threat, sense of adequacy, self-reliance

Induce vomiting immediately   Give an oral solution that causes vomiting, such as warm tap water, warm salt water (1 teaspoon salt to one-half glass water), mustard water (1 teaspoon mustard to one-half glass water), syrup of ipecac (15–20 cc given once and then repeated once 15 minutes later), or induce vomiting by inserting the finger down the throat. *Note*: If syrup of ipecac does not produce vomiting within 30 minutes, wash it out of the stomach.

Rationale: Vomiting removes poisons from the stomach.

Fulfilled Needs: Protection from physical harm, physiologic stability

Contradications: Avoid inducing vomiting when caustic poisons have been ingested such as household ammonia, lye, washing soda, or when oily preparations such as pine oil, kerosene, or gasoline are taken

Inflate the airway tube cuff   Inject air into the endotracheal or tracheostomy tube cuff until no breath escapes around the cuff. Then release the air slowly until a small leak occurs. Leave the cuff at this pressure or put enough air back into the cuff to stop the leak.

Rationale: Airway-cuff inflation prevents air leakage during ventilation procedures and food aspiration during meals.

Fulfilled Needs: Protection from physical harm

Initiate endotracheal intubation (ET)   Pass an endotracheal tube through the mouth or nose into the trachea. Use a laryngoscope to guide the tube in place. This treatment is performed only in emergencies by nurses specifically trained in this skill.

Rationale: Endotracheal intubation provides an open airway when other methods have failed.

Fulfilled Needs: Tissue oxygenation or perfusion, protection from physical harm

Initiate external cardiac massage (ET)   Rhythmically compress the heart between the lower sternum and thoracic vertebrae.

Rationale: Rhythmic pressure over the sternum compresses the heart and reestablishes arterial circulation bringing oxygen to tissue cells.

Fulfilled Needs: Tissue oxygenation or perfusion, protection from physical harm

Insert a colon tube   Place a short rectal tube into the colon through the anus about 4–5 inches.

Rationale: Colon tubes promote removal of irritating flatulence and prevent abdominal distention. When a ureterosigmoidostomy tube is in place, a colon tube keeps the rectosigmoid area empty, decreasing urinary leakage that may occur through anastomosis.

Fulfilled Needs: Waste elimination of intestinal gases, comfort, protection from physical harm

Contraindications: Rectal bleeding, severe rectal irritation or pain, do not insert a colon tube earlier than 1 week after perineal surgery, fecal impaction, diarrhea, rectal stricture, bradycardia, cardiac arrhythmias

Insert a gastric (nasogastric) tube and attach to suction (ET)   Pass a gastric tube through the nose, down the esophagus, and into the stomach. Anchor the tube at the nasal orifice to prevent tube movement or displacement. Attach to a suction machine.

Rationale: The insertion of a patent tube into the stomach permits withdrawal and analysis of stomach contents and relieves distention discomfort.

Fulfilled Needs: Waste elimination of food residue and intestinal gases, comfort, protection from physical harm

Insert a padded tongue blade   Place a wooden tongue blade, padded to a thickness equal to or greater than the tongue, between the upper and lower teeth on one side of the mouth. If a tongue blade is unavailable, use a substitute.

Rationale: Tongue-blade insertion between the teeth prevents tongue tissue trauma when the teeth are involuntarily brought together.

Fulfilled Needs: Protection from physical harm

Contraindications: When teeth are diseased and very fragile, when missing teeth reduce the stability of the remaining teeth so that tongue blade pressure might loosen the existing teeth, during a convulsive seizure while the jaw muscles already are contracted

Insert an oiled cotton pledget into the ear   When an insect ventures into an ear, soak a cotton ball with a drop of oil and place it in the ear for a few seconds. Then, remove both the cotton and the immobilized insect. Chloroform may be used instead of oil.

Rationale: Oil prevents insect movement.

Fulfilled Needs: Comfort, protection from physical harm

Insert an oral airway   Place an artificial airway device in the mouth, above the tongue, to maintain a clear air passage for respiratory gas exchange. If the person has fragile teeth, use a rubber airway instead of the standard plastic type.

Rationale: Oxygen and carbon dioxide exchange through respirations is essential to tissue-cell life. Oral airways frequently prevent biting on an endotracheal tube. A rubber airway prevents damage to fragile teeth.

Fulfilled Needs: Tissue oxygenation or perfusion, waste elimination of carbon dioxide, protection from physical harm

Insert and remove the artificial eye   To insert an artificial eye, pull down on the lower eyelid or use a suction cup and gently slip the eye into position. To remove an artificial eye, place gentle pressure below the eye, with the finger or suction cup, until the prosthesis slips out of its socket.

Rationale: Artificial-eye insertion promotes comfort, prevents eye-socket shrinkage, supports positive body image, and aids in dependency. Removal of the artifical eye permits prosthesis cleansing, offers protection against infection, and reduces eye orbit irritation.

Fulfilled Needs: Comfort, cleanliness, protection from physical harm, dependence

Contraindications (for Insertion):   Eye socket irritation, inflammation, or infection

Insert and remove the contact lens   To insert a contact lens, pull the upper lid up and the lower lid down with the index finger and thumb of one hand. Moisten the contact lens with wetting solution. Place the outer surface of the lens on the tip of the index finger of the other hand and gently put the left lens on the left cornea and the right lens on the right cornea. Most right contact lens are identified by a black dot. In order to remove a contact lens from the cornea, open the person's eye. Pull the side of the eye (near the ear) outward with one hand. With the other hand, gently pull the lids together and the lens should pop out. Before attempting to remove a lens, be sure it is over the cornea. If it is not, gently close the eyelid and with very gentle pressure, move the lens toward the cornea. After removing the lens, be careful to place them in the lens case or in a safe container. Do not mix the right and left lens.

Rationale: Contact lens insertion promotes visual acuity essential to safety and comfort and aids in illness dependency. Prolonged wearing of contact lens may cause corneal injury.

Fulfilled Needs: Comfort, cleanliness, protection from physical harm, dependence

Contraindications (for Insertion):   Eye irritation, inflammation, or infection; do not insert if the person is confused, sedated, or likely to have his eyes closed for a prolonged period

Insert and remove the dentures   Place the person's artificial teeth in his mouth if he is unable to do so. Take the person's artificial teeth out of his mouth at appropriate times.

Rationale: Artificial teeth aid in chewing and digestion, maintain natural jaw contour, promote comfort and dignity through a pleasant appearance, and aid in illness dependency. Removal of artificial teeth allows for denture cleansing and oral hygiene.

Fulfilled Needs: Nutritional balance, comfort, cleanliness, protection from physical harm, dependence, dignity

Contraindications (for Insertion):   Oral mucosa irritation; gum inflammation and infection; when persons are comatose, confused, or helpless; when there is the possibility of vomiting

Instill warm oil into the ear   Drop a small amount of warm olive oil or mineral oil into the ear.

Rationale: Warm oil relieves ear dryness, soothes ear pain, softens hardened earwax, and smothers insects that enter the ear.

Fulfilled Needs: Comfort, protection from physical harm

Contraindications: Perforated eardrum, evidence of ear infection

Introduce irrigating solutions slowly When introducing solution into a body opening, minimize the pressure of solution flow by maintaining a slow-flow rate.

Rationale: Pressure prevention promotes comfort and reduces the potential for tissue injury from rapid organ distention.

Fulfilled Needs: Comfort, protection from physical harm

Introduce one anxiety-provoking situation at a time When the person is facing several stressful situations, assist in scheduling them one at a time. If x-ray studies are scheduled for one day, delay instructions on colostomy care until the next day. If the person is in pain, withhold unfavorable news until the pain subsides.

Rationale: Meeting one stressful situation at a time reduces the degree of physical and emotional adaptation and promotes comfort.

Fulfilled Needs: Comfort, protection from physical harm, protection from psychologic threat

Introduce the person to replacement personnel before an impending separation Gradually bring the therapeutic relationship to a close by notifying the person of the impending separation and by introducing him to the new person.

Rationale: Gradual changes decrease adaptation stress, physiologic comfort is promoted from predictable situations

Fulfilled Needs: Comfort, protection from psychologic threat, predictable and orderly world.

Introduce to persons (or groups) who have successfully undergone the same experience Acquaint the person who is threatened with an unsafe situation with someone who successfully encountered the same experience.

Rationale: Feelings of safety increase through identification with persons who have successfully met the same situation.

Fulfilled Needs: Comfort, protection from psychologic threat

Involve the family Include the person's family or other significant persons in as much planning and care as possible. Keep them continuously informed of all happenings. Verbalize to the person their participation in his care.

Rationale: Family members experience fear and anxiety from lack of factual information and noninvolvement in the care of their loved ones. The involvement of loved ones reassures the patient that he will be cared for. Encouraging families to care for their own provides the opportunity for expressions of love. When guilt exists, it helps the family member make amends for past misdeeds or omissions.

Fulfilled Needs: Comfort, protection from physical harm, protection from psychologic threat, unity with loved ones

Irrigate the ear with alcohol (water or saline) Instill an alcohol solution, warmed to body temperature, into the ear containing a foreign object. Irrigate the ear with water or normal saline for removal of cerumen.

Rationale: Objects that absorb water swell and, when located in a small body orifice, obstruct the opening. Alcohol prevents swelling.

Fulfilled Needs: Comfort, protection from physical harm

Contraindications: Perforated eardrum

Irrigate the eye Instill isotonic sterile saline at body temperature into the eye and allow it to flow gently over the eye tissue, escaping from the outer canthus.

Rationale: Irrigations have cleansing and antiseptic effects that minimize infection. They promote comfort by reducing pain through solution warmth.

Fulfilled Needs: Comfort, cleanliness, protection from physical harm

Irrigate the gastric tube with saline   Introduce 10–30 cc of normal saline into the gastric tube after releasing it from the suction apparatus. Gently inject the solution and aspirate the same amount.

Rationale: Gastric-tube irrigation ensures patency, facilitates removal of gastric contents by suction, and prevents abdominal distention. Irrigation of a gastric tube with saline prevents chloride loss that would occur from the use of hypotonic fluid (water).

Fulfilled Needs: Fluid and electrolyte balance, protection from physical harm

Irrigate the nose   Gently introduce small amounts of warm sodium bicarbonate, normal saline, or other solution into one nostril. Have the person tilt his head backward, allowing the fluid to flow out.

Rationale: Nasal irrigation cleanses infected tissue while the warm solution promotes comfort.

Fulfilled Needs: Comfort, cleanliness, protection from physical harm

Irrigate the urinary catheter   Introduce 50 cc of sterile saline or other solution into an indwelling urinary catheter at periodic intervals. Allow the solution to return by gravity flow.

Rationale: A patent catheter facilitates urine flow from the bladder and promotes comfort.

Fulfilled Needs: Waste elimination of urine, comfort, protection from physical harm

Contraindications: It is not necessary to irrigate a Silastic catheter, since it is designed to prevent residue from attaching itself to the catheter

Irrigate the wound   Flush a wound with a sterile saline or other solution until the tissue appears clean and free from harmful debris.

Rationale: Wound irrigations promote comfort and healing by cleansing tissue and removing foreign particles.

Fulfilled Needs: Comfort, cleanliness, protection from physical harm

Isolate infected persons   When a person is infected with a contagious disease, restrict him to the confines of his home, or, if traveling, detain him from entering the country.

Rationale: Pathogen transfer from person to person is decreased through limited human contact.

Fulfilled Needs: Protection from physical harm

Isolate persons exposed to communicable disease   When a person has been exposed to a communicable disease, but has not contracted the disease, restrict him to the confines of his home, or, if traveling, detain him from entering the country.

Rationale: Pathogen transfer from person to person is decreased through limited human contact.

Fulfilled Needs: Protection from physical harm

Keep the drainage container below bladder (chest, stomach, nephrostomy, or t-tube) level   Keep the drainage container below the level of the tube-insertion site. If the container must be moved to a level higher than the tube-insertion site, the drainage tubing should be clamped off securely so fluid cannot flow backward.

Rationale: The backflow of drainage into an internal organ site would cause pressure on the organ resulting in tissue drainage or organ collapse. The backflow of drainage contaminated with bacteria poses the threat of infection.

Fulfilled Needs: Protection from physical harm

Keep the hyperalimentation tube patent with 5% dextrose in water   If the hyperalimentation infusion runs dry, add 5% dextrose in water to keep the subclavian catheter patent. Remove all air bubbles and run the D5W until another bottle of hyperalimentation solution is available.

Rationale: A clotted subclavian catheter has to be replaced, causing the person unnecessary pain. Air embolus allowed to flow into the subclavian vein can prove fatal.

Fulfilled Needs: Comfort, protection from physical harm

Keep the person's door closed   Protect the person from environmental stimuli and exposure to other persons by keeping the door to his room closed.

Rationale: Comfort and safety feelings are increased when privacy is respected. Doors act as barriers to noise and reduce noise level.

Fulfilled Needs: Comfort, protection from physical harm, protection from psychologic threat, dignity

Keep the person's door open   Keep the door to the person's room open to increase exposure to external stimuli and to afford the person an opportunity to investigate the world outside his room.

Rationale: External stimuli increases sensory perception.

Fulfilled Needs: Stimulation, increased reality perception

Keep the person's windows closed   Protect the person from environmental discomforts and stimuli by keeping the windows in his area closed.

Rationale: Closed windows keep out pollen that causes hypersensitivity reactions or weather elements that cause discomfort. Windows act as a barrier to noise and reduce the noise level.

Fulfilled Needs: Rest, comfort, protection from physical harm

Keep the treatment equipment (collection equipment) out of sight   Keep treatment equipment out of sight of the person on whom it has been or will be used. Also keep it out of sight of visitors if the presence of the equipment causes embarrassment for the person. Genitourinary bags can be covered with a sheet, etc.

Rationale: Equipment previously associated with pain or discomfort can serve as emotional stimuli for anxiety. Keeping equipment out of sight of visitors protects the person from the embarrassment of being exposed when in a position of social disadvantage.

Fulfilled Needs: Comfort, protection from psychologic threat

Lavage the stomach (ET)   Insert a nasogastric tube into the stomach and wash out the stomach contents with water or normal saline. Instill no more than 300 cc of the solution in an adult stomach at one time.

Rationale: Gastric lavage removes substances harmful to the gastric mucosa or general body systems.

Fulfilled Needs: Protection from physical harm

Lift with a hydraulic hoist   Raise the person off a flat surface using a hydraulic hoist

Rationale: The use of a hydraulic hoist for lifting provides even body distribution, limited pressure on cutaneous nerves, and aids in illness dependency.

Fulfilled Needs: Comfort, protection from physical harm, dependence

Limit blood-pressure–cuff inflation to a few moments   As soon as the blood-pressure cuff is inflated, immediately read the monometer and release the cuff pressure. If the reading needs rechecking, wait until the cuff is completely depressurized and wait for a period of 2 minutes before repeating the procedure.

Rationale: Pressure prevention in any body area promotes comfort. Keeping the blood pressure cuff inflated or reinflating the cuff before completely emptying it causes vasomotor changes that give a false blood-pressure reading.

Fulfilled Needs: Comfort, protection from physical harm

Limit communication to one person at a time   When a person has impaired message reception or delivery, allow only one person at a time to communicate verbally with the person.

Rationale: The reception and interpretation of messages is enhanced by nondistracting environmental influences. Psychologic comfort is promoted through a sense of effective communications with others.

Fulfilled Needs: Comfort, caring and communicating relationships

Limit infant crying by feeding on schedule and immediately changing soiled diapers   Reduce the infant's crying to an absolute minimum by providing food on or before the schedule and by changing the diaper just as soon as it is soiled.

Rationale: Infant crying increases intracranial pressure, depletes energy needed for healing, and places a strain on already painful areas.

Fulfilled Needs: Energy, comfort, protection from physical harm

Limit IPPB treatments to short periods   If artificial ventilation disturbs the person, refrain from lengthy treatments. Administer the first few treatments only so long as the person is comfortable and remove the ventilator when the person is uncomfortable.

Rationale: Short-treatment periods promote comfort and support adjustment to longer treatments.

Fulfilled Needs: Comfort

Contraindications: Acute or life-threatening respiratory distress

Limit patient use of the telephone   Do not allow persons who have difficulty with message reception or delivery to use the telephone.

Rationale: Persons experiencing asphasic conditions can only understand tone over the telephone and receive little of the message being delivered. The inability to see the other person also impairs message reception and heightens anxiety. Fear that others will hang up if silence occurs on the telephone causes excitement and confusion in the asphasic person.

Fulfilled Needs: Comfort, protection from psychologic threat

Limit the amount of time visitors are exposed to radiation   When a person receives radium implants or other radioactive substances emitting gamma rays, limit the time that relatives and friends stay with the person. Exposure to radiation over a year should not exceed 5 rads or 5,000 millirads. In 1 hour of contact, the exposed person will receive 20 millirads. It is recommended that a person receive no more than 10 millirads a day. This means that radiation exposure should not exceed 30 minutes a day.

Rationale: Body exposure to radioactive substances results in blood cell disturbances, sterility, internal burns, genetic changes, gastrointestinal upsets, and altered tissue cell structure.

Fulfilled Needs: Protection from physical harm

Limit the conversation to short discussions   When speaking to a person who has impaired message reception or delivery, limit the conversation to short uninvolved discussions.

Rationale: Simple and direct communications enhance perception and reduce the threat of frustration and anxiety. Comfort is promoted through effective communications with others.

Fulfilled Needs: Comfort, caring and communicating relationships

Limit the distance from which visitors approach the radiated patient (person)   When a person receives radium implants or other radioactive substances emitting gamma rays, limit relative and friends to a distance of at least 3 feet from the person, but as far away as possible. Each time the distance is doubled (from 2 to 4 feet, 4 to 8 feet, 8 to 16 feet), the radiation intensity is cut by one-quarter.

Rationale: The rate of radiation exposure decreases as the square of the distance from the radiated person increases. Body exposure to radioactive substances results in blood-cell disturbances, sterility, internal burns, genetic changes, gastrointestinal upsets, and altered tissue cell structure.

Fulfilled Needs: Protection from physical harm

Limit the person's mobility distance Limit the area in which the person moves about to one in which nursing supervision is possible.

Rationale: Supervision of health disorders promotes safety.

Fulfilled Needs: Protection from physical harm

Limit the therapeutic oxygen concentration to below 40% Do not allow persons, especially premature infants, to receive oxygen concentrations above 40% over prolonged periods.

Rationale: High-oxygen concentrations cause spasms of the retinal vessels. This leads to blood and serum filtration through the vessel walls into the retinal tissue with resulting blindness.

Fulfilled Needs: Protection from physical harm

Limit the touching of suspicious persons Avoid close physical contact with the person, especially skin contact.

Rationale: Suspicious persons frequently feel threatened by touch because of misinterpretations of the social meaning of personal contact. They may feel that touch is an invasion of privacy, or that it has evil connotations.

Fulfilled Needs: Protection from psychologic threat

Limit visitors Control the persons and number of persons who visit, especially during acute illness.

Rationale: Visitor limitations provide rest and comfort, reduce stress, and conserve energy for healing which would be used for socialization. Infected visitors should stay away from other ill persons.

Fulfilled Needs: Rest, energy, comfort, protection from physical harm, protection from psychologic threat

Listen attentively Listen with full attention to the message being communicated and observe for the full meaning of the message.

Rationale: Attentive listening conveys sufficient recognition and respect for a person to warrant the use of another's valuable time. It also supports feeling ventilation.

Fulfilled Needs: Comfort, caring and communicating relationships, recognition, dignity, attention, increased reality perception and problem-solving ability

Lubricate the eye/eye globes Instill one drop of sterile mineral oil into each eye.

Rationale: Mineral-oil instillation into the eye prevents loss of visual acuity due to eye tissue dryness.

Fulfilled Needs: Comfort, protection from physical harm

Lubricate the skin with a protective ointment or cream Apply an ointment or cream which will protect against moisture and skin irritation. Use Desitin or A&D ointment or cream.

Rationale: Protective ointments and creams prevent skin irritation.

Fulfilled Needs: Comfort, protection from physical harm

Lubricate the skin with baby oil, bath oil, or body lotion Apply a thin coating of baby oil, bath oil, or body lotion to the skin. Use only on intact skin.

Rationale: The lubricating effect of baby oil, bath oil, or body lotion promotes comfort by soothing the skin and preventing cracking and drying.

Fulfilled Needs: Comfort, protection from physical harm

Contraindications: Do not use on skin that remains wet from perspiration, such as when the person is lying on a bed covered with a plastic mattress cover. Do not use in skin folds, such as under the breast. Avoid using when there is a known allergic response.

Lubricate the skin with cocoa butter, glycerine, lanolin, mineral oil, or olive oil Apply a thin coating of cocoa butter, glycerine, lanolin, mineral oil, or olive oil to the skin. Use moderately on inflamed eruptions or in areas of poor circulation such as the skin over varicose veins. Glycerine is most effective when diluted with water or applied after the skin has been moistened with water.

Rationale: Emollients promote comfort by softening and soothing the skin. They are less drying than lotions because they retard water evaporation from the skin, while preventing cracking and drying. When applied following removal of a cast, they loosen crusting and dead skin residue.

Fulfilled Needs: Comfort, protection from physical harm

Contraindications: Avoid using on oozing or weeping eruptions, do not use in skin folds or when there is a known allergic response

Lubricate the skin (lesions, lips, external nares) with petrolatum Apply to the skin, lesions, lips, or external nares a transparent, fatlike substance obtained from petroleum (petrolatum). Use on areas of long-term, mild inflammation or eruption and on scaling skin. It is more effective on open skin than on skin folds.

Rationale: Petrolatum produces a soothing, comforting effect. It has a neutral (neither acid or alkaline) effect and prevents skin drying or cracking. It softens scales by retarding moisture evaporation from the skin.

Fulfilled Needs: Comfort, protection from physical harm

Maintain a clean environment Remove all dust and dirt particles from the immediate surroundings.

Rationale: Dust and dirt particles irritate mucous membranes and carry microorganisms. The reduction of irritating environmental factors promotes comfort and assists in illness dependency.

Fulfilled Needs: Comfort, cleanliness, protection from physical harm, dependence

Maintain a cool room temperature Keep the room temperature at about 65° F.

Rationale: A cool room temperature decreases environmental heat surrounding the body and increases heat loss to the environment, promoting decreased or normal body temperature. It assists in maintaining fluid and electrolyte balance because of the reduced need for perspiration cooling. It decreases oxygen and energy consumption since the body's metabolic requirements are lower than in warm surroundings. In states of shock, a cool environment helps maintain peripheral vasoconstriction, which supports adequate blood supply to vital organs.

Fulfilled Needs: Fluid and electrolyte balance, normal temperature, energy, comfort, protection from physical harm

Maintain a normal room temperature Keep the room temperature between 68–72°F.

Rationale: Normal environmental temperature promotes comfort by reducing the body's stress and adaptation requirements to temperature extremes. It prevents burn crusts from softening and separating as would occur in an excessively warm room.

Fulfilled Needs: Normal temperature, comfort, protection from physical harm

Maintain a steady intravenous infusion flow rate Keep the intravenous infusion at a consistent rate of flow. Prevent the fluids from running excessively slow or fast.

Rationale: A consistent rate of intravenous flow prevents a fluid deficit and prevents the circulatory volume from expanding with resulting increased circulatory pressure.

Fulfilled Needs: Fluid and electrolyte balance, protection from physical harm

Maintain a warm body temperature for the newborn Carry out procedures that will ensure the newborn of a warm body temperature. Wrap the infant in a dry, warm towel or blanket. Place on a dry, warm surface, in an open bed with radiant overhead heat, or next to the mother's skin.

Rationale: At birth, the infant's body temperature is unstable for 8–36 hours. Keeping the infant's body warm assists him to establish stability of body temperature.

Fulfilled Needs: Normal temperature, comfort, protection from physical harm

Maintain a warm room temperature Keep the room temperature between 75–78° F. In premature nurseries, maintain the temperature at 80° F.

Rationale: A warm room temperature increases environmental heat surrounding the body, decreases heat lost to the environment and raises the body temperature. Premature infants require warmth because they cannot maintain body heat due to lack of insulating skin fat, poor reflex control of skin capillaries, and small muscle inactivity. A warm room reduces chilling, often responsible for urinary frequency, bedwetting or muscle spasm.

Fulfilled Needs: Normal temperature, comfort, protection from physical harm

Contraindications: Fever, oxygen deficiency, shock, increased metabolic rate

Maintain adequate atmospheric humidity Keep the air moisture between 40–50% by regulating the room humidifier. In premature nurseries, maintain the humidity at between 55–65%.

Rationale: Normal air humidity supports normal lung production of moisture. A higher than normal humidity for premature infants decreases their tendency toward dehydration which is often responsible for weight loss and body temperature instability. Atmospheric humidity at 40–50% prevents burn crusts from cracking. Adequate atmospheric humidity reduces crusting of nasal mucosa, especially in perforated nasal septum.

Fulfilled Needs: Fluid and electrolyte balance, normal temperature, comfort, protection from physical harm

Maintain adequate room ventilation Inquire as to the amount of fresh air preferred by the person and maintain the desired ventilation, provide sufficient air movement to remove stagnant air.

Rationale: Pleasant environmental factors promote comfort. Cool room ventilation helps maintain normal body temperature and refreshes the air. Adequate air currents ventilating a room remove discomforting odors and infectious agents. Attending to room ventilation offers assistance in illness dependency.

Fulfilled Needs: Normal temperature, comfort, protection from physical harm, dependence

Maintain body alignment Position and support the extremities, head, and other body parts in a normal line of function or in a therapeutic position. For example: When a person is lying on his back (supine), support his knees in a slightly flexed position to prevent hyperextension of the knees. When he is lying on his abdomen (prone), support his ankles and shins to prevent plantar flexion of his feet. When he is lying on his side, support the upper leg and arm with pillows to prevent internal rotation of the hip and shoulder joints. When a fracture of the neck is known or suspected, maintain the neck in a straight line (neither flexed nor extended) while transporting to the hospital. When an extremity is in traction, maintain the same alignment that was established when the traction was applied (or adjusted).

Rationale: Functional body alignment promotes circulation and comfort, helps prevent joint deformities, painful stretching or shortening of tendons, and further damage to vital tissues by fractured bones. Nonfunctional or therapeutic alignment of extremities in traction may be necessary to hold the fractured bone pieces in position for healing.

Fulfilled Needs: Tissue oxygenation or perfusion, comfort, protection from physical harm

Maintain consistent staff behavior Demonstrate staff behavior that remains constant in attitude and performance. Avoid discrepancy between the spoken word and actions.

Rationale: Safety feelings and confidence in others increase when consistent and predictable attitudes and behaviors are demonstrated by others.

Fulfilled Needs: Comfort, protection from psychologic threat, predictable and orderly world

Maintain countertraction force Maintain a constant equal pull in two opposing directions while the patient is in traction. When there is an upper extremity fracture, the countertraction force is maintained by the patient's body weight and friction against the bed. When there is a lower extremity fracture, the countertraction is maintained by the person's body weight and may be increased by elevating the foot of the bed.

Rationale: Countertraction helps maintain proper direction and force of the applied traction.

Fulfilled Needs: Protection from physical harm

Maintain dry, clean linen Immediately change wet linen and replace with clean, dry linen. Frequently check for wet linens where there is incontinence or profuse drainage.

Rationale: Any wet substance in prolonged contact with the skin may damage or irritate the skin. Maintaining clean, dry linens promotes comfort and aids in illness dependency.

Fulfilled Needs: Comfort, cleanliness, protection from physical harm, dependence

Maintain dry (clean) skin When the skin becomes wet from perspiration, discharges, or excretions, remove such substances with mild soap and water, and dry the skin thoroughly. Frequently check for wet skin where there is incontinence or profuse drainage. Immediately after hot pack or ice bag applications, dry the wet or damp skin.

Rationale: Any wet substance in prolonged contact with the skin may damage or irritate the skin. Maintaining a dry skin surface promotes cleanliness and comfort and aids in illness dependency.

Fulfilled Needs: Comfort, cleanliness, protection from physical harm, dependence

Maintain isolation technique Carry out precautionary measures to prevent the spread of infectious conditions. These include wearing a gown and mask, maintaining room cleanliness, disinfecting clothing, linens, dishes, etc.

Rationale: Isolation technique minimizes the contact of noninfected persons with the bacteria present in infected persons, reducing infection transmission.

Fulfilled Needs: Protection from physical harm

Maintain patient wakefulness during the day During the day, periodically awaken the person despite a possible annoyance response from him. Keep him awake until his normal bedtime hour.

Rationale: Reestablishing normal sleeping hours promotes the comfort of sound nighttime sleep. Maintaining wakefulness throughout the day maintains stimulation and reduces withdrawal.

Fulfilled Needs: Sleep, rest, comfort, stimulation

Maintain reverse isolation Approach persons highly susceptible to infection only when wearing a mask and gown and after thorough handwashing.

Rationale: Pathogen transfer from person to person decreases through the protective shield of a gown, mask, and hand-washing. During periods of high-infection susceptibility, resistance is very low and could result in severe or fatal infectious conditions.

Reverse isolation protects the ill person from exposure to bacteria carried by the health staff, family, and visitors.

Fulfilled Needs: Protection from physical harm

Maintain silence Maintain a state of silence when the person indicates the need or when attempting to promote conversation in another.

Rationale: When the person indicates a need for silence as an adaptive mechanism, maintaining such fosters feelings of safety. When attempting to promote therapeutic conversation, remaining silent often makes the person so uncomfortable that he will initiate conversation to relieve the discomfort.

Fulfilled Needs: Comfort, protection from psychologic threat, caring and communicating relationships

Maintain social formality or informality Contribute attitudes toward a formal interpersonal relationship that indicates respectful, psychologic distance and restraint. Contribute attitudes toward an informal interpersonal relationship that indicates freedom and ease in communication.

Rationale: Social formality protects the person's psychologic defenses against closeness. Social informality provides relief from rigid social standards that decreases fear and anxiety by reducing tension.

Fulfilled Needs: Comfort, protection from psychologic threat, caring and communicating relationships, less rigid conventionality

Maintain the person's usual bedtime rituals Ask the person about the rituals he performs before going to sleep and see that these rituals are carried out. Presleep rituals include such activities as drinking a glass of milk, tucking sheets a certain way, using special blankets or pillows, saying nighttime prayers.

Rationale: Customary rituals before sleep promote relaxation. Adequate sleep is essential to restore depleted cell energy.

Fulfilled Needs: Sleep, rest, relaxation, energy, comfort, predictable and orderly world

Maintain wrinkle-free sheets Keep the bed sheets smooth, flat, and without wrinkles.

Rationale: Wrinkled sheets cause pressure on and irritation of skin surfaces with resulting tissue trauma and discomfort. Providing wrinkle-free sheets offers assistance in illness dependency.

Fulfilled Needs: Comfort, protection from physical harm, dependence

Make a referral When certain needs can be met by an allied health agency or individual, write or call the agency or individual and make arrangements for the person to benefit from the services offered.

Rationale: Community resources often provide health care not available in other health agencies. They often support sound approaches to problem-solving and may be a resource for developing potential, independence, and self-reliance.

Fulfilled Needs: Comfort, protection from physical harm; protection from psychologic threat, independence, increased reality perception and problem-solving ability, full development of potential

Contraindications: Medical referrals are usually the prerogative of the physician

Make an appointment for the person's health care Call the appropriate office, agency or institution and set up a date and time for the person to receive the desired health care. Verify with the person that the appointment time is satisfactory.

Rationale: People are often reluctant or unable to obtain health care appointments. If the nurse makes the appointment, stress is often reduced, there is reaffirmation of the necessity for care, and nurses can often gain quick entry into the health care system when others cannot.

Fulfilled Needs: Comfort, protection from physical harm, dependence

Massage bony prominences   Rhythmically stimulate and manipulate body areas having prominent bony structures. Such areas include the heels, ankles, knees, iliac crest, scapula and clavicle, wrists, elbows, chin, nose, ear pinna, and sacrum.

Rationale: Prolonged pressure of bone against skin results in decreased area circulation with increased susceptibility to irritation, necrosis, and discomfort. Stimulation of these areas promotes circulation, which prevents tissue damage.

Fulfilled Needs: Tissue oxygenation or perfusion, comfort, stimulation, protection from physical harm

Contraindications: Circulatory thrombus, severe circulatory impairment

Massage gently   With rhythmic gentle stroking, manipulate the body muscles in appropriate areas, producing a soothing effect. Use either alcohol or an emollient preparation.

Rationale: Gentle massage promotes muscle relaxation, stimulates circulation, conditions the skin, relieves muscle tension, and produces relaxation of nerve fibers, which relieves pain. Gentle massage stimulates flow of breast milk. During labor, gentle circular strokes over the abdomen are used as a diversional method to ease labor pain.

Fulfilled Needs: Tissue oxygenation or perfusion, sleep, rest, relaxation, comfort, protection from physical harm, freedom from pain

Contraindications: Do not massage extremities (especially calves) in the presence of thrombi and any tissue with seriously impaired circulation; avoid massaging where there is spinal cord injury with the potential for nerve damage

Massage the gums   With one finger, gently rub the infant's gum surface.

Rationale: Gum massage promotes circulation and reduces pain.

Fulfilled Needs: Tissue oxygenation or perfusion, comfort

Massage the uterine fundus   Place one hand on the person's abdomen, grasp the body of the uterus and externally massage by applying moderate pressure.

Rationale: Uterine fundus massage reduces hemorrhage.

Fulfilled Needs: Protection from physical harm

Contraindications: Avoid uterine massage if the fundus is firm

Massage vigorously   Using rhythmic, strong strokes, manipulate muscular tissue to produce an invigorating effect.

Rationale: Vigorous muscular stroking greatly increases circulation and promotes comfort and stimulation.

Fulfilled Needs: Tissue oxygenation or perfusion, comfort, stimulation, protection from physical harm

Contraindications: Circulatory thrombus, severe circulatory impairment, emotional overstimulation

Minimize environmental barriers   Decrease to a minimum objects in the way of the person attempting mobility. This entails moving furniture to its most efficient and nonobstructive position.

Rationale: The removal of mobility barriers enhances freedom of movement, reduces injury potential, aids in illness dependency, and promotes the comfort of successful coping. Short or tall persons frequently are confronted with environmental barriers unknown to average height persons.

Fulfilled Needs: Energy, comfort, protection from physical harm, dependence

Minimize environmental dangers   Keep harmful objects out of the person's reach. These include objects such as knives, cleaning fluids, matches, glass objects.

Rationale: The removal of potential danger prevents illness, injury, and disease. It aids in safeguarding dependent persons.

Fulfilled Needs: Protection from physical harm, dependence

Mobilize with a cane   Help the person to move about by providing a cane while walking.

Rationale: Moving about reduces pulmonary fluid congestion, stimulates circulation, restores normal physiologic function, promotes comfort and independence, and aids in illness dependency.

Fulfilled Needs: Tissue oxygenation or perfusion, activity and exercise, comfort, protection from physical harm, dependence, independence

Contraindications: Severe energy depletion, impaired body balance

Mobilize with a walker   Help the person to move about by providing a supportive frame within which he can walk.

Rationale: Moving about reduces pulmonary fluid congestion, stimulates circulation, restores normal physiologic function, promotes comfort and independence, and aids in illness dependency.

Fulfilled Needs: Tissue oxygenation or perfusion, activity and exercise, comfort, protection from physical harm, dependence, independence

Contraindications: Severe energy depletion

Mobilize with a wheelchair   Help the person to move about by placing him in a wheelchair. When able, encourage him to propel himself about.

Rationale: Moving about reduces pulmonary fluid congestion, stimulates circulation, restores normal physiologic function, promotes comfort and independence, and aids in illness dependency.

Fulfilled Needs: Tissue oxygenation or perfusion, activity and exercise, comfort, protection from physical harm, dependence, independence

Contraindications: Unstabilized head or spinal cord injury, internal hemorrhage, coma or semicoma, temperature above 103°F, any life-threatening situation

Moisten the dressing before removal   When a dressing becomes dried onto or encrusted around a wound, soak the dressing with sterile normal saline before removing.

Rationale: Moistening a dressing before removal minimizes tissue trauma and bleeding and reduces pain and discomfort.

Fulfilled Needs: Comfort, protection from physical harm, freedom from pain

Moisten the hair with conditioning formula   Use conditioner on the hair shafts following shampoo.

Rationale: Conditioning solutions replace hair oils for maintenance of healthy, untraumatized hair shafts.

Fulfilled Needs: Comfort, protection from physical harm, dependence

Moisten the mouth with cracked ice   Moisten the lips and mouth with ice chips. Do so according to fluid intake allowance and restrictions. Include ice chips on the fluid intake record.

Rationale: The coolness and wetness of ice refreshes, soothes, and comforts the lips and mouth without significantly increasing fluid intake.

Fulfilled Needs: Comfort

Move the entire body as a single unit   When turning or moving the person's body, use four persons to move the body as a whole unit. Maintain complete support of the total body area.

Rationale: Moving the body as a single unit prevents pressure on any particular body area and reduces the potential for injury.

Fulfilled Needs: Protection from physical harm

Obtain a blood/urine sample and send for analysis   Secure a sample of blood and urine. Send the specimens for laboratory analysis appropriate to the health situation.

Rationale: Blood and urine analysis reveals pathologic changes in physiologic function and offers clues for the diagnosis of diseases and conditions.

Fulfilled Needs: Protection from physical harm, goal achievement

Obtain a complete present and past history   Ask the person or family members for pertinent, precise, and complete information in the following categories:

> The present illness and/or health problem and the person's understanding of the problem and expectations from health care
> Past illnesses and health problems, including family history of disease
> Social and cultural factors that influence the person's behavior, including information about significant others
> Usual patterns of living and ways of coping with health problems in the past

Rationale: A precise history provides clues for diagnosing existing health problems and information for developing an organized plan of care, including prevention of disease. Giving a history allows the person to express concerns about health problems and helps establish the beginning nurse–patient relationship.

Fulfilled Needs: Protection from physical harm, goal achievement

Obtain feedback to the communicated message   Have the listener repeat the message he received.

Rationale: Feedback of messages clarifies the extent to which the original idea was correctly received. Comfort is promoted through effective communications with others.

Fulfilled Needs: Protection from physical harm, protection from psychologic threat, caring and communicating relationships

Obtain permission for procedures   Before performing a therapeutic procedure or nursing care, ask the person or family if such activities are favorable with them.

Rationale: Comfort and independence are enhanced by having sufficient control to prevent harm to self and through respectful relationships with others.

Fulfilled Needs: Comfort, protection from psychologic threat, independence, dignity

Offer assurance of other measures if the pain-relief method fails   After administering pain relief, assure the patient that if the present measure fails, other measures are available.

Rationale: An awareness that pain can be terminated decreases pain intensity by relieving tension produced by the anxiety of pain anticipation.

Fulfilled Needs: Comfort, protection from psychologic threat

Offer assurance that decisions are revokable   Point out that a decision is not necessarily a final, unchangeable determination. Decisions can be altered by the person, and at times, external forces alter decisions.

Rationale: Awareness that decisions are revokable reduces anxiety and promotes comfort.

Fulfilled Needs: Comfort, protection from psychologic threat

Offer assurance that return visits are acceptable despite termination of the therapeutic relationship   Gradually bring the therapeutic relationship to a close by notifying the person of the impending separation and favorably suggest that he come back to visit whenever he so desires.

Rationale: Gradual changes decrease adaptation stress. Comfort is promoted through relatedness to others, predictable situations, and having sufficient control of a situation.

Fulfilled Needs: Comfort, protection from psychologic threat, predictable and orderly world, caring and communicating relationships

Offer environmental stimulation through contact with varied personnel, environmental change, and variety in the daily routine When a person is confined to the hospital for a prolonged period, offer environmental stimulation by frequently changing familiar personnel who care for him, moving the person to a new room, rearranging the room, taking him outside for short periods, and adding variety to his daily routine.

Rationale: Perception of the external environment is enhanced by the degree of external stimuli.

Fulfilled Needs: Stimulation

Offer feedback to the person's expressed feelings Restate what the person has said in such a way as to emphasize those words that carry emotional significance.

Rationale: Reflected feelings promote insight into emotional responses, which, in turn, supports growth and maturity.

Fulfilled Needs: Personal growth and maturity, increased reality perception and problem-solving ability

Offer hope Offer the dying, or permanently ill, person the anticipated trust that new drugs, treatments, techniques, and research will extend or improve life. Offer this hope with a genuine belief that all things are possible.

Rationale: Hopelessness brings feelings of isolation that result in depression. Hope reestablishes confidence in the future.

Fulfilled Needs: Comfort, protection from psychologic threat

Contraindications: Once predeath acceptance has occurred, avoid reinforcing hope

Offer praise Verbally express praise for the efforts that the person puts forth regardless of success or failure.

Rationale: A high self-esteem results from positive responses from others. Rewards transform the threat of frustration into motivation by giving ego satisfaction.

Fulfilled Needs: Comfort, approval from others, high evaluation of self, sense of adequacy, appreciation from others

Offer reading material with familiar content When a person has impaired message reception, give him only reading material with contents that are familiar to him.

Rationale: Safety and comfort feelings arise from familiar situations that have been handled successfully in the past.

Fulfilled Needs: Comfort, caring and communicating relationships

Open packaged foods Open cereal boxes, milk cartons, salt and pepper shakers, packaged utensils, and peel fresh fruit.

Rationale: Assistance in making food easily available promotes comfort and aids in illness dependency.

Fulfilled Needs: Comfort, dependence

Pack sterile cotton between the ingrown nail and the skin Gently pack sterile cotton under the ingrown nail so it no longer touches the skin.

Rationale: Packing cotton between an ingrown nail and the skin takes the pressure off the skin area and promotes normal nail growth.

Fulfilled Needs: Comfort, protection from physical harm

Pack the draining wound with fine mesh gauze Gently insert sterile, fine mesh gauze into a wound cavity until that cavity is filled.

Rationale: Fine mesh gauze inserted into a wound promotes cleanliness, soaks up drainage, protects the wound from injury, and prevents the wound from sealing off at the skin surface before granulation tissue fills the wound.

Fulfilled Needs: Comfort, cleanliness, protection from physical harm

Pad the bedpan Before offering a bedpan to a person with potential or existing skin breakdown, pad the top surface of the bedpan with a folded towel or foam rubber.

Rationale: Soft padding reduces pressure and irritation on the skin surface and promotes comfort.

Fulfilled Needs: Comfort, protection from physical harm

Pad the bony prominences Apply gauze, elastic bandages, polystyrene foam blocks, fitted sheepskin, or similar substances to prominent bony structures. Include the heels, ankles, knees, iliac crest, scapula and clavicle, wrists, elbows, chin, nose, and ears.

Rationale: Prolonged pressure of bone against skin results in decreased area circulation with increased susceptibility to irritation and potential necrosis. Soft padding reduces pressure and irritation of the skin surface and promotes comfort.

Fulfilled Needs: Comfort, protection from physical harm

Pad the rough cast edges/the traction connections Cover hard cast edges with stockinette. If, however, the cast edges are rough or sharp, add felt padding, soft gauze, or other protective material.

Rationale: Pressure from cast edges causes irritation and discomfort and could puncture the skin.

Fulfilled Needs: Comfort, protection from physical harm

Patch the eye(s) Place a protective sterile covering over the eye.

Rationale: Protective eye coverings reduce injury or strain and maintain cleanliness, which prevents infection. Eye tissue exposed to air for prolonged periods will become traumatized from the drying of tissue, dust, and dirt.

Fulfilled Needs: Rest, comfort, cleanliness, protection from physical harm

Percuss the amputation stump to increase firmness Begin by gently tapping the stump of an amputated limb against a soft pillow or the hand. Gradually increase the pressure by tapping on firmer surfaces until a hard surface can be used. Percussion must be done in relation to gradual decrease in stump pain sensitivity.

Rationale: Percussion of an amputated stump toughens the skin by gradually decreasing nerve sensitivity, it prepares the stump for the pressure of a prosthesis

Fulfilled Needs: Protection from physical harm

Contraindications: Stump bleeding or nonhealing

Perform a tracheostomy Make a vertical incision through the tracheal cartilage. Insert a tracheostomy tube if it is available or any clean tubing as a temporary measure.

Rationale: An emergency tracheostomy provides an airway through which gas exchange is possible and life is sustained.

Fulfilled Needs: Tissue oxygenation or perfusion, waste elimination of carbon dioxide, protection from physical harm

Perform the specific procedure of (name the procedure) Carry out the therapeutic procedure that is specific to the health problem. Such procedures may be nursing or medical in nature.

Rationale: Therapeutic procedures are designed to support cure or improved function of the body or person as a whole.

Fulfilled Needs: Protection from physical harm, dependence

Periodically verbalize the denied reality Remind the person of the reality of a situation by comments such as "You'll be going for your chemotherapy in the morning." "Your colostomy drainage is irritating your skin." "You have to be in the divorce court on the fifteenth of the month."

Rationale: Verbalizing realities increases the perception of reality, which brings about the acceptance of reality.

Fulfilled Needs: Increased reality perception

Pierce the nail with a nail drill and express the blood   Using a nail drill, place a hole in the nail. Then apply pressure to the nail and express accumulated blood.

Rationale: The release of blood from under the injured nail reduces pressure and decreases pain.

Fulfilled Needs: Comfort, protection from physical harm, freedom from pain

Place a bed board under the mattress   Put a plywood board between the mattress and bedsprings. Have the board cover as many of the springs as possible.

Rationale: A firm mattress prevents body sagging, maintains body alignment, and promotes comfort. A sagging mattress causes flexion contractures of an amputated stump.

Fulfilled Needs: Comfort, protection from physical harm, freedom from pain

Place a blanket directly against the skin   Place a blanket beneath the sheet directly next to the person's body.

Rationale: Warmth promotes vasodilatation which results in relaxation, sleep, and relief of fatigue and pain.

Fulfilled Needs: Sleep, rest, relaxation, energy, comfort, protection from physical harm

Contraindications: Increased metabolic rate, sensitivity to wool

Place a footboard at the feet   Put a board at the foot of the bed and position the soles of the feet against the board.

Rationale: Foot placement against a board maintains dorsal flexion, keeps pressure from bed covers off the feet, and promotes foot circulation through pressing exercises against the board.

Fulfilled Needs: Protection from physical harm

Place a footstool at the bedside   Put a footstool at the bedside if the bed is too high for the person to reach the floor easily.

Rationale: A stepping stool diminishes potential injury from falling and allows for comfortable movement into and out of bed.

Fulfilled Needs: Comfort, protection from physical harm

Place a hand roll under the fingers   In the palm of the hand and under the fingers, place a hand roll.

Rationale: A hand roll helps maintain proper hand positioning, which prevents contractures and assures further functional hand use.

Fulfilled Needs: Protection from physical harm

Place a knee rest under the knees   Roll a blanket or pillow and place it under the knees.

Rationale: Knee rests promote comfort by relieving strain on abdominal muscles and on tendons beneath the knees.

Fulfilled Needs: Comfort, protection from physical harm

Contraindications: Circulatory thrombus, under a below-knee amputation stump

Place a pillow between the knees   Place a soft pillow lengthwise between the person's knees when he is lying flat or turned with knees flexed.

Rationale: A pillow between the knees prevents friction irritation, discomfort, and pressure. It aligns the knees, reducing internal rotation.

Fulfilled Needs: Comfort, protection from physical harm

Place a pillow on the affected side   If a person complains of pain, place a pillow adjacent to the body part affected with pain.
Rationale: Pillow placement gives support to the injured body area and relieves strain and tension that cause pain.
Fulfilled Needs: Comfort, protection from physical harm, freedom from pain

Place a smoldering match on the imbedded tick   Light a match and blow out the flame. While the match is still smoking and hot, apply it to the tick imbedded in the skin. Be extremely careful not to touch the person's skin with the match.
Rationale: When an embedded tick is touched with a smoldering match, the tick will back out of his entrenched position and then can be removed easily.
Fulfilled Needs: Protection from physical harm

Place a trochanter roll for positioning   Fold a sheet or blanket to one-fourth its size lengthwise. Place the narrow dimension tight against the outer thigh and slightly under the hip line.
Rationale: Trochanter roll support holds the legs in good alignment, prevents outward leg rotation, and reduces contractures.
Fulfilled Needs: Protection from physical harm

Place a urinal at the perineum   Keep the urinal placed at the perineum so that the container will catch involuntary urine flow. An emesis basin also may be used.
Rationale: Urine collection in a container reduces the area of skin wetness, decreasing potential skin irritation. Cleanliness promotes comfort.
Fulfilled Needs: Comfort, cleanliness, protection from physical harm

Place absorbent pad(s) under the person   Place pads that will absorb moisture under the person. When the person is lying on a plastic covered or foam mattress that reflects body heat back to the person, absorbent padding is needed to provide some insulation and to absorb perspiration.
Rationale: Absorbent padding insulates the skin against some of the heat reflected back by plastic or foam materials, thus aerating the skin and decreasing the chances for heat rash, maceration, and other heat-related lesions.
Fulfilled Needs: Comfort, protection from physical harm

Place air freshener in the room   Place a commercial preparation in the room that absorbs odors and/or adds pleasant odors.
Rationale: The absorption of unpleasant odors supports personal comfort and enhances social comfort.
Fulfilled Needs: Comfort
Contraindications: Avoid air freshners if the scent of flowers causes allergic symptoms

Place by a window   Locate the person next to a window with a pleasurable view. In case of depression, be certain the window is tightly secured.
Rationale: Outside activities perceived through a window divert attention from internal stress, promoting comfort. Light from a window stimulates persons in mild coma.
Fulfilled Needs: Comfort, stimulation, protection from physical harm, increased pleasantness
Contraindications: Avoid placing suicidal or confused ambulatory persons by a window if they are likely to harm themselves

Place drug tablets in a gelatin capsule   If a drug has an unfavorable taste or is irritating to the stomach, place the tablet inside a gelatin capsule. Crush or break the tablet, if necessary.
Rationale: Gelatin capsules are tasteless and prevent unfavorable tastes of drugs in-

side the capsule from reaching the taste buds. Gelatin capsules prevent digestion of the medication in the stomach and, therefore, reduce stomach irritation.
Fulfilled Needs: Comfort

Place in a heavily draped, carpeted room to reduce noise Decrease the person's exposure to noise by placing him in a heavily draped, thickly carpeted room.
Rationale: Heavy drapes and carpeting absorb noise, reducing the noise level. Certain levels of quiet are essential to normal physical and emotional function.
Fulfilled Needs: Comfort, protection from physical harm, protection from psychologic threat

Place in a playpen Put a child who is learning to walk in a playpen.
Rationale: Playpens allow children to experiment with walking while maintaining safety through restricted wandering.
Fulfilled Needs: Protection from physical harm

Place in a private room Arrange for the person to be in a room by himself.
Rationale: A private room provides quiet, reduces the stress of environmental stimuli, allows for individual regulation of room temperature, and provides the comfort of privacy.
Fulfilled Needs: Sleep, rest, relaxation, comfort

Place in a whirlpool bath Put the person in a bath of swirling water.
Rationale: Swirling warm water dilates blood vessels, stimulates circulation, promotes muscle relaxation, which relieves spasticity, and promotes comfort and cleanliness.
Fulfilled Needs: Tissue oxygenation or perfusion, relaxation, comfort, cleanliness, protection from physical harm

Place in an infant seat Place the infant in a vertical position in an infant seat.
Rationale: The vertical position prevents aspiration after eating and promotes comfort through greater awareness and visualization of the surroundings.
Fulfilled Needs: Comfort, stimulation, protection from physical harm

Place in an uncrowded area Arrange for the person to be in an area where there is considerable space between persons and where there are few persons.
Rationale: Decreased sensory input reduces stress and promotes comfort. Stress reduction decreases energy consumption for the diseased body. Uncrowded areas allow for maximum mobility when motor function is impaired. An uncrowded area is cooler and offers comfort to persons with heat intolerance.
Fulfilled Needs: Rest, comfort, protection from physical harm, protection from psychologic threat

Place in postural drainage Determine the lobe of the lung that needs drainage and position the patient accordingly for 5–15 minutes.
Right or left upper lobes: Place in a sitting position.
Right or left anterior upper lobes: Lean backward 30 degrees.
Right or left posterior upper lobes: Lean forward 30 degrees.
Right or left anterior lower lobes: Place the person on his back with two pillows under the hips so his head is 30–45 degrees downward.
Right or left posterior lower lobes: Place the person on his abdomen with two pillows under his hips so his head is 30–45 degrees downward.
Right upper lateral (side) lobe: Place on the right side.
Left lower lateral (side) lobe: Place on the left side.
Rationale: Postural drainage facilitates secretion removal from the lung through the pull of gravity.

Fulfilled Needs: Waste elimination of bronchopulmonary secretions, protection from physical harm

Contraindications: Hypertension, increased intracranial or intraocular pressure, ascites, esophageal bleeding, if dyspnea is increased or if traction is disrupted by the position

Place in the face-down (prone) position   Lay the person flat on his abdomen with face turned to the side, palms turned downward, and feet extended.

Rationale: The prone position relieves sacral area pressure. It promotes hip-joint hyperextension, which preserves the normal gait, provides secretion drainage, and promotes comfort.

Fulfilled Needs: Comfort, protection from physical harm

Contraindications: Respiratory distress

Place in the face-upward (supine) position   Place the head, face up, in a neutral, straight position so it is in perfect alignment with the rest of the body.

Rationale: The neutral position is less likely to cause further spinal cord injury when cervical vertebrae are fractured.

Fulfilled Needs: Protection from physical harm

Place in the flat position   Lay the person horizontally on his back (supine or dorsal position) so the body is level.

Rationale: General blood circulation is most adequate and the heart's workload is least when the body is flat. The flat position reduces enlarged hemorrhoids, increases blood flow to the brain during shock, and when the head is turned to the side, prevents aspiration of emesis into the lungs. The flat position is preferred during peritoneal dialysis; otherwise, intraperitoneal pressure may become too great, causing pain and injury.

Fulfilled Needs: Tissue oxygenation or perfusion, rest, comfort, protection from physical harm, freedom from pain

Contraindications: Hypertension, increased intracranial pressure, ascites, severe respiratory distress

Place in the foot-elevated, head-lowered (Trendelenburg) position   Raise the foot of the bed, elevating the legs and feet at a 45 degree angle, with the head lower than the hips.

Rationale: The Trendelenburg position facilitates drainage by gravity, pushes abdominal contents into the upper abdomen near the diaphragm, increases cerebral blood flow, holds back the presenting infant from the birth canal, and prevents pressure from cutting off an infant's oxygen supply in case of a prolapsed cord.

Fulfilled Needs: Tissue oxygenation or perfusion, comfort, protection from physical harm

Contraindications: Hypertension, increased intracranial or intraocular pressure, ascites, respiratory distress

Place in the functional position   Place the hands, feet, and knees in the natural position of function. Position the hand so that the wrist is slightly hyperextended (slight upward position), the fingers slightly flexed (bent), the thumb flexed and adducted (rotated inwardly) toward the first finger. Position the feet in the neutral position at a right angle with the leg, and avoid outward rotation. Position the knee in a slightly flexed (bent) position.

Rationale: Placing the hands or feet in the functional position increases the potential for normal use after the current injury is healed.

Fulfilled Needs: Protection from physical injury

Place in the knee-chest position   Have the person rest her chest and knees on the bed, keeping the thighs erect and the abdomen off the bed. Place her arms above and on either side of her head. Encourage the person to empty her bladder before assuming this position.

Rationale: The knee-chest position corrects uterus or ovary displacement, causes the fetal head to move away from the pelvis, reducing pressure on a prolapsed cord, and relieves lower pelvic pain.

Fulfilled Needs: Comfort, protection from physical harm

Contraindications: Do not place a mother in the knee-chest position until 3 weeks after delivery

Place in the lithotomy (dorsosacral) position   Have the patient lie on her back with legs and thighs flexed and knees held widely apart.

Rationale: The lithotomy position facilitates exposure of the perineal, rectal and vaginal areas for examination and for the administration of therapeutic procedures.

Fulfilled Needs: Protection from physical harm

Place in the side-lying (Sims', lateral, semiprone) position   Place the patient on his left side with the upper arm forward, the under leg slightly flexed, and the upper leg flexed at the thigh and knee. Support the knee and head with a pillow.

Rationale: The side-lying position aids drainage of body cavities, helps prevent postoperative pulmonary and circulatory complications, minimizes aspiration of regurgitated food, prevents the tongue from falling backward, causing airway obstruction, is favorable for examination of the female pelvis and the administration of enemas.

Fulfilled Needs: Comfort, protection from physical harm

Contraindications: Pulmonary hemorrhage, atelectasis, pneumonitis (pneumonia), pleural effusion

Place in the sitting position   Put in a sitting position with the back resting comfortably against a firm surface. Place a pillow under each arm for comfortable support.

Rationale: The sitting position facilitates abdominal drainage, supports improved respirations, reduces tracheal edema and abdominal pressure on the diaphragm during ascites, provides room for pulmonary expansion by lowering the diaphragm, and promotes comfort.

Fulfilled Needs: Tissue oxygenation or perfusion, comfort, protection from physical harm

Contraindications: Shock, potential fainting, labrinythitis vomiting

Place in the slight foot-elevated head-lowered (semi-Trendelenburg) position   Raise the foot of the bed, elevating the legs and feet at a 20 degree angle. Place the head lower than the hips.

Rationale: The semi-Trendelenburg position facilitates drainage by gravity, displaces intestines into the upper abdomen, and increases cerebral blood flow. It holds back the presenting infant from the birth canal by exerting mild pressure against the presenting part and prevents pressure from cutting off an infant's oxygen supply in the case of prolapsed cord. In shock resulting from blood loss, this position increases arterial blood flow to the brain and promotes venous blood flow from the lower extremities to the right atrium.

Fulfilled Needs: Tissue oxygenation or perfusion, comfort, protection from physical harm

Contraindications: Hypertension, increased intracranial or intraocular pressure, ascites, respiratory distress

Place in the slight-sitting (semi-Fowler's semirecumbent) position   Raise the head of the bed approximately 12 inches above normal bed level and elevate the knees.

Rationale: The slight-sitting position improves respiratory ventilation, lessens fluid accumulation in the lungs, relieves painful tension on surgical incisions, minimizes the liver's pressure on the diaphragm, and promotes pelvic drainage.

Fulfilled Needs: Tissue oxygenation or perfusion, comfort, protection from physical harm

Contraindications: Shock, potential fainting

Place objects out of reach   Place objects so the person cannot reach them or so they cannot be reached by persons who should not have access to them. This is especially true of harmful objects such as alcohol, drugs, cleaning fluid, etc.

Rationale: The elimination of potentially harmful threats promotes safety.

Fulfilled Needs: Protection from physical harm

Place objects within reach   Place objects to facilitate their easiest possible use in meeting the needs of the particular person.

Rationale: Easy access to needed objects promotes independence, prevents unnecessary use of energy, and aids in illness dependency.

Fulfilled Needs: Energy, comfort, protection from physical harm, dependence, independence

Place on a bedpan at the first sign of full-bladder clues   Response to signs of a full bladder when normal bladder sensations are absent promotes control. Such signs include perspiration, headache, goose pimples, feelings of abdominal fullness, and restlessness. When these signs occur during bladder retraining, the person should be given the urinal immediately or placed on the bedpan.

Rationale: Bladder control is essential to the maintenance of skin dryness, cleanliness, comfort, and socialization.

Fulfilled Needs: Comfort, cleanliness, protection from physical harm

Place on a CircOlectric bed   Put the person on a frame and canvas bed in which position change can be electrically controlled.

Rationale: The CircOlectric bed allows for position change while maintaining immobility, for gradual head elevation, gradually increased standing tolerance, and aids in maintaining circulation.

Fulfilled Needs: Protection from physical harm

Place on a flotation mattress   Place the person on a water bed. Periodically, observe the mattress for holes that might allow leakage, for proper positioning of the mattress on the bed, and appropriate water temperature.

Rationale: A flotation mattress relieves pressure against the skin and improves tissue oxygenation. It reduces surface tension and decreases body weight through partial submergence in water.

Fulfilled Needs: Protection from physical harm

Place on a polyurethane foam pad   Put a pad made of porous, resilient, easily compressible polyurethane between the person and the mattress.

Rationale: Polyurethane foam prevents friction irritation against cutaneous tissue, reducing pressure on tissue and promoting comfort.

Fulfilled Needs: Comfort, protection from physical harm

Place on a rocking bed   Lay the person on a motorized bed that alternately raises and lowers the head and feet in a seesaw motion.

Rationale: Alternately elevating and lowering the body improves circulation and assists respiration through diaphragmatic movement.

Fulfilled Needs: Tissue oxygenation or perfusion, protection from physical harm

Contraindications: Increased intracranial or intraocular pressure, hypertension, ascites

Place on a sheepskin   Lay sheep's wool under the person who must lie or sit for prolonged periods.

Rationale: Air spaces in the sheepskin keep the skin area dry. Skeepskin softness eases pressure on the skin, preventing decubitus formation, while the oil from the lamb's wool lubricates the skin.

Fulfilled Needs: Comfort, protection from physical harm

Place on a silicone pad Place a gel foam pad, which has the consistency of human fat, under the person who must lie or sit for prolonged periods.

Rationale: Gel foam pads support body weight and, by preventing friction between the pad and the person, reduce the potential for decubitus formation. Its softness promotes comfort.

Fulfilled Needs: Comfort, protection from physical harm

Place on a split-foam mattress Place a thick foam mattress, split so that the buttocks are suspended in mid-air, under the patient who must lie in bed for prolonged periods.

Rationale: The suspension of bony prominences in air reduces pressure and maintains normal skin circulation.

Fulfilled Needs: Protection from physical harm

Place on a Stryker frame Put the person on a frame and canvas bed that can be turned anteriorly and posteriorly.

Rationale: A Stryker frame allows for position change while maintaining immobility.

Fulfilled Needs: Protection from physical harm

Place on an alternating pressure mattress Place the person on a mattress that alternately fills and empties with air.

Rationale: The reduction of constant pressure on any body area by alternately changing the pressure point increases blood circulation to tissues, preventing tissue degeneration.

Fulfilled Needs: Protection from physical harm

Place on an orthopedic bed Put the person on a fracture bed with an overhead frame to which can be added traction and assistive moving devices. These beds are usually 3–6 inches longer than ordinary beds.

Rationale: The orthopedic bed provides a flat, firm surface for fractured limbs and facilitates the use of devices such as traction and overhead bars. It provides comfort for very tall persons.

Fulfilled Needs: Comfort, protection from physical harm

Place on complete bed rest Place the person on 24-hour bed rest. This applies to instances such as sudden cardiac episodes, during high or severe temperature elevations of 103–108°F, in head or spinal cord injuries, hemorrhage, coma or semicoma, during severe energy depletion, very high blood pressure elevations, or in any life-threatening situation.

Rationale: Complete bed rest prevents further tissue injury and reduces the probability of complications associated with activity. It replenishes cell energy that the body uses for the maintenance of life and activity and promotes healing and comfort.

Fulfilled Needs: Sleep and rest, energy, comfort, protection from physical harm

Place on nonadherent sheeting For burns use a special sheeting that will not stick to the open wound.

Rationale: Nonadherent sheeting reduces pain and trauma by preventing sheeting from sticking to and pulling against injured tissue.

Fulfilled Needs Comfort, protection from physical harm

Place on sterile linens When there are severe burns or open wounds or when the person is highly susceptible to infection, cover the bed and the person with linens that have been sterilized.

Rationale: Reduced exposure to microrrganisms minimizes infection.

Fulfilled Needs: Cleanliness, protection from physical harm

Place on the affected side   When there is evidence of pulmonary hemorrhage, pleural fluid or inflammation, or when one lung is not ventilating adequately, position the person on the affected side.

Rationale: Pressure applied to a bleeding area reduces and localizes blood flow. When applied to the chest in pleura inflammation, it stabilizes the chest wall and reduces pain. Placement on the affected side localizes fluid accumulation and prevents compression of the other lung. When one lung has diminished ventilation, it supports maximum ventilation of the other lung.

Fulfilled Needs: Tissue oxygenation or perfusion, comfort, protection from physical harm, freedom from pain

Contraindications: Atelectasis

Place on the unaffected side   Place the person on the body side that is free of the troublesome symptom. If there is pain, position on the painfree side. If there is tinnitis, position on the side of the quiet ear. If the heart is pounding, place the person on the right side so the pounding is less perceptible.

Rationale: Positioning on the unaffected side decreases the amount of pressure in the body area of a troublesome symptom, resulting in a reduction of the intensity of the symptom.

Fulfilled Needs: Comfort

Place only warm hands and objects on the person   Do not touch the person with anything that is cold. Run warm water over the surface of the bedpan before it is used. Before touching the person, rub hands together so they will be warm. Rub the stethoscope between hands to warm it.

Rationale: Sudden coldness disturbs skin receptors while warmth promotes comfort. Warmth prevents chilling, which often stimulates muscle spasms.

Fulfilled Needs: Comfort, protection from physical harm

Place the amputation stump in the extension position   Have the person with a below-knee amputation turn from side to side or lie on his abdomen so that the amputated stump is extended and maintained in alignment with the rest of the body.

Rationale: Extension alignment of an amputated stump prevents contractures and promotes positioning conducive to successful prosthesis walking.

Fulfilled Needs: Protection from physical harm

Place the call light within reach   Arrange the call light so it is easily accessible and can be reached without difficulty.

Rationale: Awareness that help can be easily obtained reduces anxiety and meets dependency needs.

Fulfilled Needs: Comfort, protection from physical harm, protection from psychologic threat, dependence

Place the equipment (or object) within sight   Keep within visual range, objects or equipment that the person uses to meet hygienic and other basic needs. Also keep within sight pictures of loved ones, as well as flowers and cards from family and friends.

Rationale: Seeing familiar objects or equipment that represents safety promotes comfort.

Fulfilled Needs: Comfort

Place the feet in hard-soled ankle-top shoes   Place the feet in bootlike high-ankle shoes. Pad the inside of the shoe to prevent skin breakdown. Place the shoe soles against a footboard.

Rationale: Ankle-top shoes prevent plantar flexion by maintaining ankle alignment.

Fulfilled Needs: Protection from physical harm

Place the foot in the dorsiflexion position Bend the foot and toes up toward the knee.

Rationale: Dorsiflexion position inhibits the transmission of motor nerve impulses to a spastic muscle. This decreases muscle tension and relieves the pain and discomfort of foot and leg spasms.

Fulfilled Needs: Comfort, freedom from pain

Place the infant on an apnea pad Place the infant so its chest and abdomen are on the apnea pad that is covered with one thickness of linen. Connect the pad to the monitor, which is set to sound an alarm when respirations cease for 10–15 seconds or the time specified by the physician. Turn the alarm switch to the "on" position.

Rationale: Use of an apnea monitor provides early warning of infant respiratory distress. Early detection supports immediate, effective treatment.

Fulfilled Needs: Protection from physical harm

Place the newborn/infant in an incubator Place the newborn or premature infant in a temperature-regulated incubator.

Rationale: Newborn infants cannot regulate their own temperature for 8–36 hours following birth. Premature infants cannot regulate their body temperature until they reach considerable maturity. The incubator maintains a stable environmental temperature.

Fulfilled Needs: Normal temperature, protection from physical harm

Place the person in a room with someone having a favorable prognosis When a person is aware that death is approaching, do not place him in a room with someone who is likely to die before he does or who is dying a painful death. Put him in a room with someone who probably will get well.

Rationale: The presence of death heightens anxiety even in well persons. Awareness that an experience can be very painful decreases the potential for a satisfactory experience.

Fulfilled Needs: Comfort, protection from psychologic threat

Plan undisturbed periods for the person Adjust nursing activities and visiting schedules so there will be a period during the day when the person will be undisturbed.

Rationale: Undisturbed periods support rest, relaxation, and renewal of energy resources needed for healing.

Fulfilled Needs: Rest and relaxation, energy, comfort

Position comfortably Place the body in a position suitable and comforting to the person. Be sure the position supports body areas without applying pressure. When restfully positioning an infant for breast-feeding, place the child in the mother's arms so he can grasp the whole nipple and not just the end. Avoid pressing the infant's nose against the breast. When bottle feeding, restfully position the infant's head slightly to one side.

Rationale: Restful positioning, with lack of pressure on any body surface, promotes comfort. Comfort arises through association with positions previously experienced as comforting. Proper positioning meets illness dependency needs.

Fulfilled Needs: Sleep, rest, relaxation, comfort, freedom from pain, dependence

Contraindications: Avoid any positioning that will cause or increase body injury

Position on the left side Suggest that the person lie on his left side when ready to go to sleep.

Rationale: Lying on the left side causes slowed heart action and reduces circulation which promotes sleep.

Fulfilled Needs: Sleep, rest, relaxation, comfort, protection from physical harm

Contraindications: Right-sided pulmonary hemorrhage or inflammation. Pleural fluid, left-sided atelectasis

Position the affected limb lower than the rest of the body   Place the limb wounded by a poisonous snake or spider at a level lower than the rest of the body.

Rationale: Lowering the limb wounded by a snake or spider decreases the rapidity with which the venom circulates through the blood.

Fulfilled Needs: Protection from physical harm

Position the infant with the head elevated for burping   Bubble the infant by raising his head and gently rubbing or patting the posterior chest midway and after bottle-feeding.

Rationale: External stimulation brings stomach air up the esophagus with resulting pressure and pain relief.

Fulfilled Needs: Comfort, protection from physical harm, freedom from pain

Contraindications: Meningitis

Position the pacemaker generator box comfortably   While the person is in bed, place the generator box so there is neither strain on the wires nor any discomfort.

Rationale: Proper positioning of the pacemaker generator box safeguards against the wires being accidentally pulled out and provides comfort.

Fulfilled Needs: Comfort, protection from physical harm

Position to promote drainage of the infected area   If a draining infection exists, position that body area so the pull of gravity will exert pressure and increase drainage flow. For instance, if the left ear is draining, raise the right side of the head with a pillow so the left ear is the lowest part of the head.

Rationale: Drainage of infected material promotes healing, prevents infection spread to adjacent body parts, reduces pressure, and decreases pain.

Fulfilled Needs: Comfort, protection from physical harm, freedom from pain

Position with pillows   Assist with the maintenance of a desired body position by propping the body with pillows.

Rationale: Pillows will support the body in alignment without placing undue pressure against body tissue.

Fulfilled Needs: Comfort, protection from physical harm

Positon with sandbags   Place canvas bags filled with sand around the body part after proper positioning.

Rationale: Sandbag weight promotes immobilization and protects against poor alignment and contractures.

Fulfilled Needs: Protection from physical harm

Postpone feeding when the person/child is fatigued   If the person is fatigued, withhold food until he is well rested, usually after having slept.

Rationale: Fatigue reduces appetite.

Fulfilled Needs: Comfort

Pray with the person   If the person wishes to pray, stand beside him and offer to pray with him.

Rationale: The turning of heart and mind toward God promotes spiritual growth.

Fulfilled Needs: Comfort, spiritual, religious, or philosophic satisfaction

Prepare the person for a/the painful experience   When a person is to be faced with a painful experience, calmly tell him what can be expected and that every effort will be made to minimize the pain as much as possible.

Rationale: Anxious anticipation of pain increases tension, which enhances the painfulness of the actual experience. Preparation before a painful experience decreases tension, which reduces pain.

Fulfilled Needs: Comfort, protection from psychologic threat

Prepare the person for the clergy's visit   In anticipation of a clergy member's visit, refresh the person and dress him in clothing respectful of the clergyman. Provide a clean, neat environment and privacy so the person may feel free to discuss religious or other problems.

Rationale: Preparation for a clergyman's visit promotes comfort.

Fulfilled Needs: Comfort

Present change gradually   Slowly present for acceptance alterations and substitutions for that which currently exists.

Rationale: Gradual change decreases adaptation stress. Safety feelings arise from predictable situations.

Fulfilled Needs: Comfort, protection from psychologic threat, predictable and orderly world, sense of adequacy

Prop with a back rest   Provide a supportive back rest for comfortable sitting.

Rationale: Back support promotes relaxation and comfort.

Fulfilled Needs: Relaxation, comfort

Protect the person wearing a pacemaker by practicing safety measures
Take special precautions to protect the person wearing a pacemaker such as: avoid simultaneously touching electrical equipment and the patient; do not use multiple electrical machines around a pacemaker; do not use extension cords, worn electrical cords, plugs or outlets; disconnect unused electrical equipment, insulate exposed pacemaker electrodes, place the person on a nonelectric bed.

Rationale: Persons wearing pacemakers need to be protected against leaking electrical currents that could result in electrocution.

Fulfilled Needs: Protection from physical harm

Protect the water-seal drainage apparatus from damage   If chest bottles are used for water-seal drainage, place them in a wooden cradle or holder so the bottles will not be broken accidentally. If a plastic apparatus is used, position it so it is not subject to puncture or tearing.

Rationale: Water-seal drainage systems must be protected from damage because if the system is interrupted, the atmospheric pressure will cause air to enter the chest cavity and collapse the lung.

Fulfilled Needs: Protection from physical harm

Protect with absorbent padding   Lay padding that will soak up liquid excretions and drainage under the patient and around draining wounds.

Rationale: Absorbent materials draw wetness that otherwise would lay in contact with the skin. This lessens skin irritation and promotes cleanliness and comfort.

Fulfilled Needs: Comfort, cleanliness, protection from physical harm

Protect with a plastic bib   Place a water-repellent bib over the neck and chest.

Rationale: Cleanliness promotes comfort.

Fulfilled Needs: Comfort, cleanliness

Protect with plastic pants   When the person is incontinent, but up and about, have him wear plastic pants.

Rationale: Plastic pants prevent skin irritation by limiting the skin area exposed to wetness, preventing soiled clothes, promoting comfort, and reducing the potential for embarrassment.

Fulfilled Needs: Comfort, cleanliness, protection from physical harm, protection from psychologic threat
Contraindications: Diaper rash or severe skin irritation

Provide a balanced nutritional diet Maintain a balanced diet by providing the four basic food groups daily. They include meat, milk and milk products, bread and cereal, and fruits and vegetables.
Rationale: A balanced nutritional diet is essential to body cell activity and energy production from foods. Relief of visceral hunger promotes comfort.
Fulfilled Needs: Nutritional balance, energy, comfort, protection from physical harm

Provide a bedpan/a urinal Provide a bedpan or urinal for elimination purposes for persons confined to bed.
Rationale: Less energy is required to use a bedpan or urinal than to walk to the bathroom for elimination purposes. Limited mobility often requires the use of a bedpan or urinal. Adequate elimination facilities promote comfort and cleanliness.
Fulfilled Needs: Energy, comfort, cleanliness, protection from physical harm

Provide a bedside commode Place a portable commode at the person's bedside for elimination purposes.
Rationale: Less energy is required to use a bedside commode than to use a bedpan or to walk to the bathroom for elimination purposes. Adequate elimination facilities promote comfort and cleanliness.
Fulfilled Needs: Energy, comfort, protection from physical harm
Contraindications: Maximum 24–hour bed rest

Provide a calendar Acquaint the person with the environment by providing a large, single-day calendar and placing it on the wall where it is easily seen.
Rationale: The ability to comprehend the environment with regard to time, place, and person identity prevents confusion and anxiety.
Fulfilled Needs: Protection from psychologic threat, increased reality perception

Provide a clean, comfortable bed Provide freshly washed bed linen on a bed with a firm mattress.
Rationale: Clean bed linen refreshes the skin, promotes comfort and rest, protects against bacterial infection, and assists in illness dependency.
Fulfilled Needs: Sleep and rest, comfort, cleanliness, protection from physical harm, dependence

Provide a clock Acquaint the person with the environment by providing a large clock and placing it where it can be seen easily.
Rationale: The ability to comprehend the environment with regard to time, place, and person identity prevents confusion and anxiety.
Fulfilled Needs: Protection from psychologic threat, increased reality perception

Provide a compatible room companion Place the person in a room with someone having a compatible personality and whose length of stay approximates that of the person.
Rationale: Persons with compatible personalities associate comfortably and support positive feelings between each other.
Fulfilled Needs: Comfort, caring and communicating relationships

Provide a convenient bed (or meal) tray Furnish an over-the-bed or meal tray within easy reach and adjust to proper height.
Rationale: Accessibility to needed objects promotes comfort and supports independence when there is illness dependency.

Fulfilled Needs: Comfort, dependence, independence

Provide a drinking straw Furnish a straw through which liquids may be sucked into the mouth.

Rationale: A straw facilitates easy ingestion of liquids, especially during limited range of motion or muscular weakness. It prevents staining or injury by allowing liquids to by-pass the teeth and keeps glass pressure from traumatizing lip blisters and pustules.

Fulfilled Needs: Comfort, protection from physical harm

Contraindications: Traumatized, bleeding, or sutured oral mucosa; excessive flatulence

Provide a firm mattress Furnish a mattress that has a solid compact surface and does not sag under body weight.

Rationale: A firm mattress offers a smooth, level lying surface that results in good back support and body alignment. It provides comfort, distributes body weight, and promotes even distribution of circulation.

Fulfilled Needs: Tissue oxygenation or perfusion, comfort, protection from physical harm, freedom from pain

Provide a fracture bedpan For persons confined to bed, provide an extremely shallow, almost flat vessel for elimination purposes. Have them use the fracture pan instead of the standard size bedpan.

Rationale: Less energy is required to raise the body over a nearly flat surface than over an elevated surface for elimination purposes. A flat surface under the body provides minimal disturbance of body alignment and minimizes movement pain and discomfort.

Fulfilled Needs: Energy, comfort, protection from physical harm

Provide a home visit Go to the person's home, observe the total situation, identify needs, and provide nursing care.

Rationale: The home situation indicates the person's overall lifestyle, physical and emotional needs, and resources. A home visit communicates caring.

Fulfilled Needs: Comfort, protection from physical harm, protection from psychologic threat, caring and communicating relationships

Provide a language interpreter When attempting to communicate with a person who does not speak the same language, furnish an interpreter.

Rationale: Comfort is promoted through a sense of effective communication with others.

Fulfilled Needs: Comfort, protection from psychologic threat, caring and communicating relationships

Provide a low-height bed Furnish a bed low enough for the person to place his feet on the floor while sitting on the side of the bed.

Rationale: A low-height bed diminishes the potential for injury from falling and allows for comfortable movement out of and into the bed.

Fulfilled Needs: Comfort, protection from physical harm, independence

Provide a magnifying glass Furnish a magnifying glass which enlarges objects many times.

Rationale: Enlarged objects promote visual acuity, reduce eyestrain, and promote comfort.

Fulfilled Needs: Comfort, protection from physical harm

Provide a mirror for reflection of the self (the room) Give the person a mirror so that he can see himself frequently or place the person's bed in a position facing a mirror.

Rationale: Frequent visualization of physical appearance helps establish self-image. The new mother viewing herself and her newborn child in the mirror receives reinforcement for the realization of her new role. When death is approaching, the reflection of self in the mirror may promote acceptance.

Fulfilled Needs: Increased reality perception

Contraindications: It is sometimes best not to let a person see himself in the mirror after severe trauma such as burns, contusions with swelling, and mutilations until the severity of the situation has lessened; jaundiced persons often do better not viewing themselves in the mirror

Provide a night light Furnish a night light so there is a sufficient amount of illumination for seeing in the dark.

Rationale: Illumination of the dark prevents accidents, allows minimal disturbance of sleep, and prevents distorted perception.

Fulfilled Needs: Comfort, protection from physical harm, protection from psychologic threat, increased reality perception

Provide a nontempting environment Remove objects from the environment that entice the person to perform unhealthy actions from which restraint is difficult. This includes keeping candy out of sight of a diabetic and cigarettes away from a heavy smoker.

Rationale: Decreased sensory perception of desired but harmful objects or situations reduces internal conflict or threat and the harm the object or situation can produce.

Fulfilled Needs: Comfort, protection from physical harm, protection from psychologic threat

Provide a pain-relief measure of the person's choice Give the person a choice as to the pain-relief measure preferred and administer the one indicated.

Rationale: Comfort is enhanced by the availability of choices and having sufficient control to bring comfort or prevent harm to oneself.

Fulfilled Needs: Comfort, protection from psychologic threat, freedom from pain

Provide a paper bag for breathing Furnish a paper bag into which the person may breathe and rebreathe his own exhaled air.

Rationale: Rebreathing accumulations of excessively exhaled carbon dioxide collected within a paper bag raises the blood level of carbon dioxide to normal and reestablishes respiratory acid–base balance.

Fulfilled Needs: Acid–base balance, protection from physical harm

Contraindications: Increased blood–carbon-dioxide level, emphysema

Provide a paper bag for tissue disposal Pin a paper bag on the side of the bed so used tissues may be discarded easily and will not be touched by persons other than the patient.

Rationale: Proper disposal of infectious material prevents the spread of infection from one person to another.

Fulfilled Needs: Comfort, cleanliness, protection from physical harm

Provide a pleasant buffer sound to mask uncontrollable noise When noise exists that cannot be turned off, buffer the sound with a pleasant sound such as soft music, a gentle blowing fan or air conditioner, etc.

Rationale: Pleasant sounds that buffer noxious sounds provide comfort.

Fulfilled Needs: Comfort, sleep and rest, protection from physical harm

Provide a short drinking straw Furnish a short, 4- or 5-inch, drinking straw.

Rationale: A short drinking straw reduces fatigue because less energy is required for sucking.

Fulfilled Needs: Energy, comfort

Provide a sputum container Make available a clean, covered container for sputum collection.

Rationale: Placing specimens in a container prevents infection spread from one person to another.

Fulfilled Needs: Comfort, cleanliness, protection from physical harm

Provide a sugar substitute When the dietary intake of sugar is restricted, furnish artificial sugar.

Rationale: Sugar substitutes prevent the metabolic imbalances caused by natural sugar in certain disorders, and their sweet taste promotes comfort.

Fulfilled Needs: Comfort, protection from physical harm

Provide a transfer board Provide a wide, flat, firm board to bridge the gap and support the person's weight as he moves from the bed to the wheelchair. Take extra care that the person does not slide across the board and produce friction against tender skin.

Rationale: A transfer board allows for independent transfer from bed to wheelchair and back to bed.

Fulfilled Needs: Activity and exercise, independence

Provide a trapeze bar and/or bed rope Furnish a swinging, overhead bar immediately above the person's head.

Rationale: Pulling exercises performed on a trapeze bar promote muscle strength. A trapeze bar allows for easier in-bed movement and increases in and out of bed mobility.

Fulfilled Needs: Activity and exercise, comfort, independence

Provide airtight drainage containers Use drainage containers that have an airtight, closed system.

Rationale: Airtight drainage containers lock odors within the closed system.

Fulfilled Needs: Comfort

Provide an alternate method of communication appropriate to the person's specific needs and abilities Make available alternate methods of communication such as paper and pencil, words and phrases cards, picture cards of objects, alphabet letters for word composition, typewriter, magic slate, hand and eye signals, computerized devices.

Rationale: The loss of speech, whether temporary or permanent, is accompanied by acute, severe anxiety. Having a substitute method for communicating needs and desires reduces the anxiety and increases the person's sense of security.

Fulfilled Needs: Comfort, caring and communicating relationships

Provide an atmosphere of acceptance Display accepting attitudes that create an environment in which the person feels that he is favorably received as a person. Acceptance involves communicating the worth of the person because he is a person. It does not indicate approval of unacceptable behavior.

Rationale: Psychologic safety requires that a person experience awareness of acceptance by others. Acceptance allows for testing reality and the reactions of others. Acceptance is acquired through cultural roles and the relationships with others and promotes mutual respect.

Fulfilled Needs: Comfort, protection from psychologic threat, acceptance, high evaluation of self, dignity, personal growth and maturity

Provide an attractive meal tray Furnish a colorful, nicely set meal tray.

Rationale: Attractive meal trays enhance the appearance of food which promotes appetite.

Fulfilled Needs: Comfort, protection from physical harm

Provide an over-the-bed table for the leaning-forward position   Make available an over-the-bed table with a soft pillow on top of it so that the orthopneic person may lean forward and ease difficult breathing.
Rationale: Proper positioning in respiratory difficulty promotes comfort and improves ventilation.
Fulfilled Needs: Tissue oxygenation or perfusion, comfort

Provide and manage the health therapy   Direct and carry out the therapy, specific for the person, according to the proper procedure, at recommended times and in correct amounts. Such therapy may be either nursing or medical in nature.
Rationale: Directing and carrying out therapy for persons increases the probability of reestablishing health and meets dependency needs.
Fulfilled Needs: Comfort, protection from physical harm, dependence

Provide assistance until the person is fully able to assume self-care   Help the person with those activities that he finds difficult to do, until such time as he is capable of doing the activities for himself. Allow him to do as much as he can for himself, but not to overdo.
Rationale: Assistance with activities helps the person conserve energy for the healing process and helps meet dependency needs.
Fulfilled Needs: Comfort, protection from physical harm, dependency

Provide braille reading material   Make available reading material that has been printed with raised dots representing language symbols.
Rationale: Braille allows those who cannot see the printed words to read by touch.
Fulfilled Needs: Comfort, mastery and competence in skills, independence

Provide clean clothing   Provide freshly washed or cleaned clothing.
Rationale: Clean clothing refreshes the skin, promotes comfort, reduces bacterial entrance into wounds, and assists in illness dependency.
Fulfilled Needs: Comfort, cleanliness, protection from physical harm, dependence

Provide cold water for mouth rinsing but not swallowing   Give the person a small amount of cold water with which he can rinse his mouth. Be sure that the water is not swallowed but discarded after the rinsing.
Rationale: Cold water moistens dry oral mucosa and refreshes the mouth, temporarily relieving thirst.
Fulfilled Needs: Comfort

Provide conditions that the person desires for peaceful dying   Provide whatever conditions the person requires for a peaceful death. These usually include dying at home, dying surrounded by family, visits from dear friends, the company of a faithful pet, the beauty of flowers in the room, having a chance to communicate with God, quiet surroundings, favorite drinks and food, or any other individual preferences.
Rationale: Recognition of a person's wishes indicates attitudes of value and dignity toward him.
Fulfilled Needs: Comfort, protection from psychologic threat, unity with loved ones, dignity

Provide desired personal articles   Furnish personal articles that the person may desire such as clothing, knick-knacks, a special blanket.
Rationale: Familiar articles promote safety and comfort feelings.
Fulfilled Needs: Comfort, protection from psychologic threat

Provide desired spiritual articles   Furnish spiritual articles that the person may desire such as a Bible, statues, crucifix, rosary, prayerbook, religious candles.
Rationale: Spiritual articles assist man to express his relationship with God.
Fulfilled Needs: Comfort; spiritual, religious, or philosophic satisfaction

Provide disposable tissue Provide paper handkerchiefs that can be discarded after use.
Rationale: Disposable handkerchiefs prevent the transfer of infectious respiratory conditions from one person to another.
Fulfilled Needs: Comfort, cleanliness

Provide emotional support for persons significant to the patient Sustain persons who are important to the patient by meeting their needs as they become evident.
Rationale: Awareness that there is concern for one's loved ones promotes comfort. Support from others promotes feelings of strength, reducing fear and anxiety.
Fulfilled Needs: Comfort, protection from psychologic threat, endurance

Provide emotionally safe experiences Set up situations in which the person feels free from all threat. These should be situations in which he previously experienced comfort and success.
Rationale: Safety feelings arise from familiar and predictable situations successfully handled in the past and from an awareness that one can cope successfully with life.
Fulfilled Needs: Comfort, protection from psychologic threat, predictable and orderly world, sense of adequacy

Provide finger foods Offer foods that can be eaten with the fingers, such as celery, carrot and bread sticks, crackers, apple slices, crisp bacon, raw vegetables, fruits.
Rationale: The consistency of finger foods gives pleasure when taste is undeveloped. Finger foods are helpful in chewing and swallowing problems, and are good for children who have difficulty holding up their head. They are a substitute for such behaviors as thumb sucking and nail biting. When persons are hyperactive and cannot sit still to eat, or are slow eaters, finger foods can be caried about.
Fulfilled Needs: Nutritional balance, comfort

Provide firm eating utensils Supply knives, forks, spoons, glasses, and dishes made of hard material that does not bend.
Rationale: During limited hand motion, muscular weakness, and developing coordination of the small child, manipulation of objects is often difficult. Utensils that do not bend against pressure are easiest to manipulate.
Fulfilled Needs: Comfort, mastery and competence in skills

Provide fluid selection Furnish a number of liquids and juices to choose from.
Rationale: Balanced fluid intake is enhanced by the availability of familiar and desired liquids. Fluid selection promotes comfort.
Fulfilled Needs: Fluid and electrolyte balance, comfort
Contraindications: Dietary restrictions such as salt and potassium

Provide foam-rubber pillows Make available pillows made of foam rubber. Avoid using cotton or down-filled pillows.
Rationale: Foam-rubber pillows are nonirritating to hypersensitive respiratory systems.
Fulfilled Needs: Comfort, protection from physical harm

Provide foods and toys for chewing When a small child needs to bite, supply the child with apples, crackers, cookies, or chewing toys.
Rationale: Biting and chewing meet the oral activity needs of a developing child. Providing appropriate objects for biting reduces the potential for inappropriate biting of humans and animals by children.
Fulfilled Needs: Comfort

Provide foods at their most appetizing temperature Give foods that are heated or cooled to their most desirable temperature. Be certain that the coffee is hot and the ice cream is cold when the patient receives it.

Rationale: Proper food temperature offers the comfort of improved taste and oral palatability and assets in illness dependency.
Fulfilled Needs: Comfort, dependence

Provide food selection   Furnish a choice of foods, particularly those especially liked and desired. When introducing a child to new foods, place the foods on a plate. Leave the child alone and let him select what he wants.
Rationale: Balanced nutritional intake is enhanced by the availability of familiar and desired foods. The privilege of being able to select foods promotes comfort.
Fulfilled Needs: Nutritional balance, comfort
Contraindications: Special diet restrictions reduce the amount of selection

Provide frequent contact with the person   Attend to the person for short periods at frequent intervals and be certain that the person is aware of your presence.
Rationale: Fear and anxiety are reduced by an awareness that the person is not threatened with aloneness. Frequent contact enhances the probability of detecting abnormal physical conditions.
Fulfilled Needs: Comfort, protection from physical harm, protection from psychologic threat, attention

Provide fresh drinking water   Furnish and frequently replace cool, fresh water at the bedside.
Rationale: Cool water relieves thirst, promotes comfort, and assists in illness dependency.
Fulfilled Needs: Comfort, dependence

Provide glucose ice chips   Make available ice cubes made from 20–50% glucose.
Rationale: When fluid intake is restricted but caloric intake needs to be maintained, glucose ice cubes can fill both needs.
Fulfilled Needs: Nutritional balance, protection from physical harm
Contraindications: Caloric dietary restrictions

Provide hearing-aid care   Properly care for the person's hearing aid by removing the batteries when the aid is not in use, cleaning the ear inserts, and safeguarding it against damage.
Rationale: A well-maintained hearing aid promotes improved auditory function.
Fulfilled Needs: Comfort, dependence

Provide heavyweight utensils   Make available eating utensils, pencils, etc., made of heavyweight material. Avoid lightweight plastic objects.
Rationale: In impaired proprioception, the position of heavily weighted objects is most easily determined.
Fulfilled Needs: Comfort
Contraindications: Muscle or motor impairment, severe weakness

Provide information (reliable information)   Communicate knowledge and facts about whatever subject is important to the person.
Rationale: Information provides the person with data needed for physical and emotional health and assists the person to adapt to nonhealth situations. Fear and anxiety result from misperceptions due to lack of factual information. Adequacy and comfort evolve from factually analyzing situations and coping with them.
Fulfilled Needs: Comfort, protection from psychologic threat, sense of adequacy

Provide large-print reading material   Furnish reading matter printed in very large type and found in most public libraries.
Rationale: As eye muscle tone decreases, large print is more easily read and its use

prevents eyestrain. Reading promotes focused attention on external stimuli which temporarily relieves internal stress.

Fulfilled Needs: Comfort, protection from physical harm

Provide lightweight utensils Supply knives, forks, spoons, glasses, and dishes made of lightweight plastic material.

Rationale: Lightweight utensils are easily held when there is muscle or motor impairment or fatigue.

Fulfilled Needs: Comfort, independence

Contraindications: Impaired proprioception

Provide loose bedding with toe pleats Avoid tightly tucked bed sheets over the toes by putting toe pleats in the top sheet at the bottom of the bed.

Rationale: Pressure from tight bedding holds the foot in plantar flexion. Such prolonged pressure could tighten the heel cord and eventually prevent the person from placing his heel flat on the floor when standing. Toe pleats prevent pressure, yet allow for neatly tucked linen.

Fulfilled Needs: Comfort, protection from physical harm

Provide meetings with supportive persons or groups Arrange for a meeting between the individual and another person or group of people who can offer support.

Rationale: Support from others reduces the sense of aloneness, enhances the awareness that others care, and renews psychologic strength.

Fulfilled Needs: Comfort, protection from psychologic threat, caring and communicating relationships, group unity, companionship, personal growth and maturity

Provide needed supplies Furnish equipment needed to perform a desired function.

Rationale: Providing task tools promotes the comfort of independent action.

Fulfilled Needs: Comfort, independence

Provide nursing availability Reassure the person that a professional nurse is easily attainable and readily accessible whenever the need arises.

Rationale: Illness often presents a situation where some needs cannot be met by independent action, causing the person to rely on others to meet those needs. Safety feelings arise from the assurance that help is available for need satisfaction.

Fulfilled Needs: Comfort, protection from physical harm, protection from psychologic threat, dependence, caring and communicating relationships, attention

Provide objects related to the message When speaking to a person who has impaired message reception, give the person the object about which you are speaking. For instance, if you want him to scrub his teeth, tell him so and give him a toothbrush.

Rationale: Visual perception enhances reception of verbal messages. Comfort is promoted through effective communications with others.

Fulfilled Needs: Comfort, caring and communicating relationships

Provide objects that symbolize safeness Furnish the person with material objects identified with past pleasure and safety, such as a child's blanket, an adult's favorite book.

Rationale: Feelings of safety arise from the presence of objects representing past pleasure and security. Stability evolves from the possession of objects perceived as permanent.

Fulfilled Needs: Comfort, protection from psychologic threat, psychologic stability

Provide objects that symbolize sex identity Provide the person with objects symbolically identified with his or her particular sex. Male objects would include a pipe, objects associated with male sports, pictures of rugged scenes, work tools, model ships, boats, cars. Women would enjoy feminine clothes, perfumes, beauty products, recipes, needlework, dainty wall decorations. In order to meet the person's needs, these objects must be highly individualized.

Rationale: Objects that are strongly identified with sexuality clarify the self-image and promote comfort

Fulfilled Needs: Comfort, sexuality, high evaluation of self

Provide oral hygiene   Provide measures that keep the mouth clean such as brushing the teeth and dentures; rinsing the mouth with salt solution, one-half solution of water and hydrogen peroxide, or a commercial mouthwash; lubricating the lips or oral tissue with glycerine.

Rationale: Oral hygiene refreshes the mouth with the comfort of cleanliness.

Fulfilled Needs: Comfort, cleanliness, protection from physical harm

Provide orthopedic pin care   Gently clean around the orthopedic pin with a sterile cotton-tipped applicator soaked with hydrogen peroxide. Remove the hydrogen peroxide with normal saline. Apply a nonocclusive antibacterial agent, Betadine Helafoam, and allow to air dry.

Rationale: A clean orthopedic pin reduces the potential for bacterial growth that could cause wound and bone infection.

Fulfilled Needs: Protection from physical harm

Contraindications: Do not use Betadine in instances of allergy to Betadine

Provide pleasant experiences with the feared object   Associate a pleasurable sensation or event with the feared object.

Rationale: The threat of fear is reduced when a pleasurable emotion can be associated with the fear.

Fulfilled Needs: Comfort, protection from psychologic threat

Provide prior notification of an impending separation   Gradually bring the therapeutic relationship to a close by notifying the person of the impending separation ahead of time.

Rationale: Gradual change decreases adaptation stress. Safety feelings arise from predictable situations.

Fulfilled Needs: Comfort, protection from physical harm, protection from psychologic threat, predictable and orderly world

Provide prism eyeglasses   When a person must continuously lie flat and is unable to hold a book for reading, furnish prism eyeglasses.

Rationale: The cut of glass into prisms allows for the upward reflection of objects. The ability to read promotes focused attention on external stimuli that temporarily relieves internal stress.

Fulfilled Needs: Comfort

Provide privacy   Protect the person from the observation of others by means of a curtain or screen, closing a door, or providing a private room. This is especially important during bathing, meals, periods of severe pain or illness, and during emotional episodes.

Rationale: Privacy allows the person to relax normal sociocultural values during times of stress or dependency without the risk of decreased esteem from others. It reduces stress in that there is no need to cope with external stimuli. Providing privacy conveys respect for the person's personal life.

Fulfilled Needs: Comfort, protection from psychologic threat, dignity

Provide quiet   Offer peaceful and tranquil surroundings.

Rationale: A quiet environment reduces the need for adaptation to stress.

Fulfilled Needs: Sleep, rest, relaxation, comfort, protection from physical harm

Provide radio, television, reading material, and conversation for diversion (for distraction)   Provide radio or television, furnish books and magazines, or provide verbal distraction about subjects that do not relate to the person's problem. Periodically check to be sure that the radio or television topic has not changed to one that could disturb the person.

Rationale: Focusing attention on external stimuli relieves internal stress by promoting temporary escape from conscious perception of threats such as fear, anxiety, and pain. It allows the body or emotions time for restoring balance.

Fulfilled Needs: Comfort, stimulation, protection from physical harm, protection from psychologic threat, freedom from pain

Provide rooming-in   Whenever possible, encourage the mother to accept having her newborn infant to stay with her in the hospital room. Provide adequate facilities for such.

Rationale: Physical closeness of mother and newborn promotes emotional closeness. It supports early knowledge of one to the other as well as increasing family involvement.

Fulfilled Needs: Comfort, caring and communicating relationships, unity with loved ones, increased learning

Provide safe banging objects   Offer such objects as pots, rag dolls, old boards, and punching bags that can be banged on without injury to the person or object.

Rationale: Release of emotion in nonharmful ways prevents injury. Since banging is a normal developmental activity of children, safe banging objects should be provided.

Fulfilled Needs: Comfort, protection from physical harm, protection from psychologic threat

Provide safe play equipment for children   Provide play equipment that is safe and suitable to the age of the child. Furnish the infant with such playthings as rattles, balls, rings to chew on, soft dolls and animals, noisemakers, bathtub toys, large blocks, pull toys, linen books. Furnish the preschool child with blocks, a sandbox with shovel and pail, a wagon, kiddy car, bicycle, rocking horse, boxes, balls, toys for playing house or store, dolls, trains, trucks, automobiles, airplanes, fire engines, stuffed animals, crayons and coloring books, chalk and blackboard, clay paints, mallets and hammers, picture books of all types, and large-piece puzzles. Furnish the school-age child with roller and ice skates, baseballs, footballs, jumping rope, croquet, tennis, complicated puzzles, nondangerous tools, games of all kinds, and books of adventure, suspense, and heros.

Rationale: Infant play should stimulate manipulation and investigation, gradually increase motor skills, lay the foundation for learning about size, shape, and texture, and promote development of large muscles. Preschool play should promote motor skills, sensory perception, physical development, creative imagination, and social relations with peers. School-age play should develop special interests and promote perfection of already learned skills, and skill competition between peers. All play should be safe.

Fulfilled Needs: Comfort, protection from physical harm

Provide seclusion   Place the emotionally disturbed person in an area or room totally away from contact with others.

Rationale: External control of behavior supports internal control when the latter cannot be maintained. Limitations protect against future shame resulting from presently uncontrolled behavior.

Fulfilled Needs: Comfort, protection from physical harm, protection from psychologic threat, high evaluation of self

Provide spiritual reading material   Provide reading material having a spiritual theme. Include books, magazines, tapes, etc.

Rationale: Spiritual reading elevates people's thoughts to higher resources.

Fulfilled Needs: Comfort; spiritual, religious, or philosophic satisfaction

Provide standby equipment (and/or drugs) Furnish equipment or drugs that may be needed in an emergency. Keep them close to the person as long as the possibility of an emergency exists. These include oxygen, airways, tongue blades, rubber-tipped hemostats, tracheostomy tubes and trays, tourniquets, wire cutters, endotracheal tubes, defibrillators, suction machines, etc.

Rationale: Readily available emergency equipment and drugs can save a life when time is of the utmost importance.

Fulfilled Needs: Protection from physical harm

Provide sufficiently long tubing to allow freedom of movement Whenever tubing is inserted into the body, make certain it is long enough for the patient to freely turn and move about.

Rationale: Freedom of movement is essential to good circulation, general comfort and care.

Fulfilled Needs: Comfort, protection from physical harm

Provide sunglasses Furnish eyeglasses containing colored lenses.

Rationale: Glare reduction prevents damage to optic tissue and nerves.

Fulfilled Needs: Comfort, protection from physical harm

Contraindications: Impaired vision where reduced illumination will raise the potential that the person might fall

Provide temporary assistance until the skill is learned Help the person with those treatments that, until learning is acquired, he cannot do for himself. While performing the skill for the person, teach that which is appropriate at the time.

Rationale: Until a health skill is accurately learned and is usable, it will not be effective for health. When nurses assist with health skills during the learning phase, there is greater assurance of effective health therapy and more accurate learning.

Fulfilled Needs: Comfort, protection from physical harm, dependency, increased learning

Provide the child with a play-practice doll or cloth that has a zipper, laces, buttons, and snaps Give the child a doll, wearing clothes that can be zippered, buttoned, snapped, or laced. Help the child to perform these activities during play.

Rationale: As the doll is being dressed and undressed, the child acquires skills that can be used to dress and undress himself. Introduced as a play activity, the child considers it pleasurable.

Fulfilled Needs: Mastery and competence in skills, increased learning

Provide the family with information about the person's progress Give the family as much information as possible about the condition of their loved one. Be specific about what has occurred, is occurring, and when possible, what is expected to occur. Do so at least once and preferably twice daily.

Rationale: Information about an ill loved one promotes family comfort and reassurance that their loved one is being cared for.

Fulfilled Needs: Comfort, protection from psychologic threat, unity with loved ones

Provide toilet hygiene Following the elimination of excreta, wipe or wash the buttocks, genitalia, or other body areas clean. If clothing or linens are soiled, replace them with fresh substitutes.

Rationale: Cleanliness after elimination provides comfort and reduces skin irritation and infection.

Fulfilled Needs: Cleanliness, comfort, protection from physical harm, dependence

Provide unbreakable objects Supply articles made of materials that will not break when dropped.

Rationale: Unbreakable objects, when dropped, will not result in physical injury.

Fulfilled Needs: Comfort, protection from physical harm

Provide whatever the person needs to use his usual coping mechanisms

Once the person explains how he usually copes with a situation, provide whatever will foster the use of those effective mechanisms. If he usually cries, provide privacy; if he talks out the problem, listen; if he goes for a walk, accompany him on a stroll. Such coping methods vary with each person.

Rationale: Supporting normal coping mechanisms helps the person maintain emotional stability. It reduces energy consumption by allowing the use of established, instead of new, mechanisms.

Fulfilled Needs: Comfort, protection from psychologic threat, psychologic stability

Read to the person When a person is unable to read due to visual impairment, brain damage, or position, offer to do it for him.

Rationale: Reading is a major source of comfort in communication of ideas and thoughts.

Fulfilled Needs: Comfort

Reassure that the pain will subside or be relieved While offering some measure for pain relief, verbally assure the person that the pain will soon be alleviated.

Rationale: Awareness that pain relief has been initiated promotes relaxation, which, in itself, decreases pain and promotes comfort.

Fulfilled Needs: Relaxation, comfort, protection from psychologic threat

Contraindications: In intractable pain, it is better to reassure the person that pain will be reduced rather than alleviated

Reassure verbally Place the person's mind at ease by verbal assurance that problems can be solved and that the nurse will help solve these problems.

Rationale: Identification with the positive attitudes of other persons reduces fear and anxiety and promotes comfort.

Fulfilled Needs: Comfort, protection from psychologic threat, caring and communicating relationships

Recognize the need for superstition Permit belief in superstition, but do not agree with such beliefs.

Rationale: Interference with deeply accepted superstitions causes feelings of threat and heightened anxiety.

Fulfilled Needs: Protection from psychologic threat

Record the battery-change date on the pacemaker generator box

Whenever the battery is changed in a pacemaker, place the date of change on the box where it is clearly visible.

Rationale: Since pacemaker batteries have a potential 3-year life, it is essential to know the replacement date to maintain a functional pacemaker.

Fulfilled Needs: Protection from physical harm

Reduce infant handling to a minimum Handle the infant (especially the irritable child) only when it is absolutely necessary. At all other times, leave him undisturbed.

Rationale: Decreased external stimuli reduces the need for adaptive responses, promotes sleep, and decreased energy depletion.

Fulfilled Needs: Sleep, rest, relaxation, energy, comfort, protection from physical harm

Reduce physical discomforts that could interfere with cognitive function

Before attempting to increase cognitive functioning, make certain that the person is comfortable. Take care of problems such as pain, hunger, thirst, wetness, chilliness, excess warmth, etc. before attempting activities involving thought processes.

Rationale: Physical discomforts distract the person, decreasing his ability to think in complex terms.

Fulfilled Needs: Comfort, protection from psychologic threat

Reduce the demand for cognitive functioning when the person is ill or fatigued
If a person is ill or fatigued, avoid situations that require the use of intense thought processes. Limit demands for thinking to the more simple processes. For example, give directions in short, clear sentences instead of complex, explanatory statements; offer simple choices (milk or coffee?) instead of major decisions such as (what would you like to drink?).

Rationale: Persons who are ill or fatigued lack sufficient energy to successfully think through complicated thought processes. If that person has a previous deficit in thought processes, the thinking task will be even more difficult.

Fulfilled Needs: Comfort, protection from psychologic threat

Reduce the demands placed on the person
Decrease the requirements placed on the person and include only those that are essential.

Rationale: Adaptation and adjustment to demands require energy that, in illness, is needed for healing. Safety feelings evolve from an awareness that the person can cope successfully with life.

Fulfilled Needs: Comfort, protection from physical harm, protection from psychologic threat, sense of adequacy

Reduce the drug dosage
Decrease the amount of the drug the person is taking; determine the amount to be decreased on the basis of the adverse effect of the drug, its intended effect, and consultation with the physician when appropriate.

Rationale: Reduction of a drug dosage will often eliminate adverse drug effects.

Fulfilled Needs: Comfort, protection from physical harm, physiologic stability

Refrain from administering gastric lavage
Do not insert a nasogastric tube into the stomach for the purpose of washing out stomach contents.

Rationale: A gastric lavage performed after the ingestion of strong caustic poisons could cause perforation of the injured tissue.

Fulfilled Needs: Protection from physical harm

Refrain from applying pressure to the body part
Do not apply pressure to the body part by palpating the part, applying pressure dressings, or positioning with pillows.

Rationale: Pressure on a body part could break or fracture a delicate or injured organ.

Fulfilled Needs: Protection from physical harm

Refrain from arguing
Avoid all verbal disputes despite the attempt of another to coax the nurse into an argument.

Rationale: Emotionally charged interaction interferes with effective communications and is perceived as threatening.

Fulfilled Needs: Protection from psychologic threat, caring and communicating relationships

Refrain from asking the person to repeat the message too often
When attempting to communicate with a person having an impaired ability to send messages, do not ask him to repeat the message over and over again. If the message is not understood on the first attempt, stop all other activity, ask the person to repeat the message, and concentrate fully on interpreting what is being said. If the message is still not un-

derstood, come to an agreement with the person on a more effective method of communication.

Rationale: Loss of the ability to communicate causes anxiety. Effective communication promotes comfort.

Fulfilled Needs: Comfort, protection from psychologic threat

Refrain from cleansing with alcohol Do not clean the wound or injured body area with alcohol.

Rationale: Alcohol causes pain on burned areas and severely irritates some wounds.

Fulfilled Needs: Comfort, protection from physical harm, freedom from pain

Refrain from dislodging blood clots Do not touch a blood clot formed to seal off hemorrhage. Do not force a blood clot lodged in a needle into the vein.

Rationale: The disruption of blood clots formed to prevent hemorrhage can cause renewed hemorrhage. Dislodging clots from a needle into a vein can result in circulatory obstruction with tissue damage or death.

Fulfilled Needs: Protection from physical harm

Refrain from distracting the person while he swallows Do not take the person's attention away from the task of swallowing. Avoid conversation and laughing.

Rationale: Pharyngeal or esophageal trauma, obstruction, impaired nerve or muscle function, inflammation, or congenital defects can make swallowing sufficiently difficult to require total concentration. Difficulty swallowing poses the potential threat of food aspiration into the lungs.

Fulfilled Needs: Protection from physical harm

Refrain from doing a rectal/vaginal examination Do not insert a finger into the rectum for examination purposes.

Rationale: A foreign object inserted into the rectum causes mechanical stimulation of the defecation reflex and increases tissue injury, infection potential, and discomfort. Rectal stimulation results in vagus nerve stimulation that decreases the heart rate.

Fulfilled Needs: Comfort, protection from physical harm

Refrain from drawing blood studies via the hyperalimentation catheter Do not draw blood or allow blood to be drawn for laboratory analysis through the subclavian catheter being used for hyperalimentation.

Rationale: Blood cells will coat the internal catheter surface and obstruct the catheter, altering the flow rate of the hyperalimentation solution.

Fulfilled Needs: Protection from physical harm

Refrain from elevating the bed at the knee gatch Do not raise the bed under the person's knee when there is venous stasis in the lower extremity.

Rationale: Elevating the bed at the knee gatch places pressure behind the knee, decreasing circulation.

Fulfilled Needs: Protection from physical harm

Refrain from equating sleep with the absence of pain Do not assume that pain has subsided because the person has fallen asleep.

Rationale: Pain can cause exhaustion that induces sleep during which pain is still felt.

Fulfilled Needs: Comfort, protection from physical harm

Refrain from forcing distasteful drugs Do not forcibly insist that bad-tasting medicine be taken. Instead, attempt to promote free choice regarding how the medication will be taken.

Rationale: Forcing bad-tasting drugs may cause aspiration and decreases the chance of future voluntary medication ingestion.

Fulfilled Needs: Comfort, protection from physical harm

Refrain from forcing the treatment Avoid insisting or physically forcing a person to accept unwanted health treatment.

Rationale: Forcing treatments causes intense anxiety and feelings of threat. The realization that the person has sufficient control to prevent harm to himself promotes comfort. Awareness that others respect the person's wishes reinforces human dignity.

Fulfilled Needs: Comfort, protection from psychologic threat, dignity

Contraindications: When persons are legally considered incapable of making appropriate decisions, some force may be required, but it should be kept at an absolute minimum

Refrain from giving an alcohol rub Do not apply friction to the skin by means of an alcohol rub.

Rationale: Alcohol has a drying effect on the skin. Alcohol fumes irritate respiratory mucosa. Since alcohol is highly volatile, it is never used on person's receiving oxygen.

Fulfilled Needs: Protection from physical harm

Refrain from giving animal or vegetable oil orally Do not give a poison antidote that contains animal or vegetable oil.

Rationale: Animal or vegetable oils are not soluble in insect or rat poisons that contain phosphorous and are therefore ineffective.

Fulfilled Needs: Protection from physical harm

Refrain from giving between-meal feedings Do not allow the person with gastric ulceration to eat between meals. Provide three well-balanced meals a day with antacids between meals. Do not give food between meals to obese persons.

Rationale: Each time food is placed in the stomach, gastric secretions are stimulated, causing further irritation of ulcerated mucosa. When gastric secretions are stimulated only three times a day, there is less irritation and more time for healing. Between-meal feedings increase the caloric intake, compounding the problem of obesity.

Fulfilled Needs: Protection from physical harm

Refrain from giving bicarbonates Do not give any foods or drugs that contain carbonic acid.

Rationale: Bicarbonate ingestion will increase the possibility that hypokalemia will result from metabolic alkalosis.

Fulfilled Needs: Fluid and electrolyte balance, acid–base balance, protection from physical harm

Contraindications: Severe acidosis

Refrain from giving carbonated beverages Do not give effervescent drinks. If they must be given, vigorously stir the drink and let it stand until the effervescence is gone.

Rationale: The carbon dioxide (effervescence) in carbonated beverages is acid and can irritate sensitive gastrointestinal tissue, damage tooth enamel, and enhance acidosis by increasing the blood's carbon dioxide content. Carbonated beverages cause an alkaline urine, which enhances the chance of calcium calculi formation and forms a carbon gas in the stomach, which increases abdominal distention.

Fulfilled Needs: Acid–base balance, comfort, protection from physical harm

Refrain from giving continuous positive-pressure breathing Do not allow continuous inhalation and exhalation of air into the lungs through mechanically induced positive pressure.

Rationale: Continuous inhalation and exhalation under positive pressure impairs normal cardiac output and increases intrathoracic pressure, which decreases venous return. It is especially threatening when the blood volume has been lowered due to excessive fluid or blood loss.

Fulfilled Needs: Protection from physical harm

Refrain from giving crumbling, flaking foods Do not give foods that crumble and flake, such as cookies, crackers, cakes, coconut, dry cereals, hard biscuits.

Rationale: Crumbling or flaking foods can enter a tracheostomy and cause airway irritation or obstruction.

Fulfilled Needs: Protection from physical harm

Refrain from giving enemas Do not administer fluid into the rectum and colon.

Rationale: Enemas deplete body potassium and will further decrease low-blood potassium levels. They increase peristalsis and intestinal spasm as a result of colon distention and, by stimulating peristalsis increase uterine contractions, causing severe afterbirth pains or uterine bleeding. When a ureterosigmoidostomy is performed, the pressure of an enema may force feces into the ureters. During peritoneal dialysis, the intraabdominal pressure from the simultaneous instillation of enema fluid and dialysis fluid could rupture a visceral organ. When there is an inflamed appendix, the increased pressure from an enema may rupture the organ and cause peritonitis. Any time nausea, vomiting, or abdominal pain are present, enemas should not be given.

Fulfilled Needs: Fluid and electrolyte balance, protection from physical harm

Refrain from giving hot liquids Do not give very hot liquids such as coffee, tea, or soup.

Rationale: Hot liquids increase body temperature, injure oral mucous membranes or gums, increase the metabolic rate, cause vasodilatation, which in severe cardiac impairment results in stagnation of the blood flow with reduced tissue oxygenation, increases peristalsis, which is undesirable in diarrhea, and may cause expansion of a cracked tooth or pain in a cracked or sensitive tooth.

Fulfilled Needs: Normal temperature, comfort, protection from physical harm

Refrain from giving iced (cold) liquids Do not give extremely cold liquids.

Rationale: Iced liquids decrease body temperature, promote muscular and bladder spasm, cause vasoconstriction with resulting decreased blood supply to tissues, stimulate peristalsis, which is undesirable during diarrhea, and cause retraction of a cracked tooth or pain in a cracked or sensitive tooth.

Fulfilled Needs: Normal temperature, comfort, protection from physical harm

Refrain from giving insulin Do not allow the person to receive insulin.

Rationale: Persons with Addison's disease have a chronically low blood-glucose level. The administration of insulin will further lower the blood-glucose level, causing death.

Fulfilled Needs: Protection from physical harm

Refrain from giving intravenous or intramuscular injections Do not give intravenous or intramuscular injections for at least 4–6 hours immediately after hemodialysis.

Rationale: Heparinization during hemodialysis enhances the bleeding tendency.

Fulfilled Needs: Protection from physical harm

Refrain from giving laxatives Do not give purgative and cathartic medications.

Rationale: Laxatives stimulate peristalsis, contractions, and cramping that can further damage irritated, traumatized, or poison-corroded intestinal mucosa. Harsh laxation causes dehydration. When laxatives are given during uterine bleeding, the heightened peristalsis increases uterine contractions causing more severe bleeding.

Fulfilled Needs: Comfort, protection from physical harm

Refrain from giving local cold applications Do not apply cold to decubitus ulcers, gangrenous tissue, varicose veins, areas of vascular grafts, paralysis or sensation loss, or to age-debilitated skin. Cold is usually not applied to skin grafts.

Rationale: Cold applications decrease body temperature, can stimulate chills, and can cause vasoconstriction, which reduces tissue circulation.

Fulfilled Needs: Comfort, protection from physical harm

Refrain from giving local heat applications   Do not apply heat to areas of paralysis or sensation loss, edema, hemorrhage or trauma, the right lower abdomen in suspected appendicitis, the head following injury, or any body part after heart surgery.

Rationale: Heat applied to areas of diminished or absent sensation may result in a burn. When applied to enclosed tissues where the vasodilating effect expands tissue fluids or gases, it may cause increased pain, swelling, or rupture of tissues. Applications of heat increase tissue metabolism, which in turn increases the cardiac workload. Warmth promotes the itching and discomfort of allergic reactions. Heat applied to the scrotum will destroy spermatozoa.

Fulfilled Needs: Protection from physical harm

Refrain from giving magnesium laxatives or antacids   Do not give laxatives or antacids that contain a magnesium compound.

Rationale: The ingestion of magnesium salts increases the blood-magnesium level.

Fulfilled Needs: Fluid and electrolyte balance, protection from physical harm

Refrain from giving milk or milk products   Do not give milk, milk shakes, malts, ice cream, cream soups, etc.

Rationale: After digestion, milk produces a large amount of solid wastes that must be eliminated through the kidneys. In any condition where there is an increased need for fluids (fever, upper respiratory infection, etc.) milk will further increase the need for fluid resulting in dehydration and thickening of secretions.

Fulfilled Needs: Comfort, protection from physical harm

Refrain from giving oral analgesics   Do not administer oral analgesics immediately after surgery.

Rationale: Disturbances in gastrointestinal function following surgery result in unpredictable drug absorption.

Fulfilled Needs: Protection from physical harm

Refrain from giving oral stimulants   Do not give coffee, tea, amphetamines, or alcohol.

Rationale: During electrical shock or when the myocardial blood supply is impaired, oral stimulants can cause ventricular fibrillation resulting in death. After a snake bite, oral stimulants increase circulation thereby hastening the flow of venom throughout the body.

Fulfilled Needs: Protection from physical harm

Refrain from giving positive-pressure breathing   Do not introduce air into the lungs during inhalation by mechanically induced intermittent positive pressure.

Rationale: When the person already has an inadequate cardiac output such as in myocardial infarction, IPPB reduces filling of the right side of the heart and thereby further reduces cardiac output. When the lung has been ruptured, the pressure from IPPB causes air to enter the pleural space building up pressure, which results in shock. IPPB spreads active tuberculosis and increases pulmonary hemorrhage.

Fulfilled Needs: Protection from physical harm

Refrain from giving potassium-containing drugs and solutions   Do not give drugs such as penicillin G potassium or whole blood containing potassium to persons with an elevated blood-potassium level.

Rationale: Potassium drugs and solutions further elevate an already increased blood-potassium level.

Fulfilled Needs: Fluid and electrolyte balance, protection from physical harm

Refrain from giving saline laxatives   Do not give purgative or cathartic medications containing sodium. Such laxatives include magnesium citrate, magnesium sulfate, sodium potassium tartrate, sodium sulfate, sodium phosphate.

Rationale: Saline laxatives, by the process of osmosis, cause fluid withdrawal from body tissues and circulation into the intestines. If saline laxatives are given frequently, fluid loss will result in dehydration.

Fulfilled Needs: Fluid and electrolyte balance, protection from physical harm

Refrain from giving table salt Do not give iodized sodium chloride traditionally used as table salt.

Rationale: Decreasing sodium intake reduces the blood-sodium level. Osmotic pressure then pulls sodium and water from the interstitial spaces into the blood, relieving tissue edema.

Fulfilled Needs: Fluid and electrolyte balance, protection from physical harm

Refrain from inserting a rectal tube Do not insert a rectal tube into the colon.

Rationale: A foreign object inserted into the rectum causes mechanical stimulation of the defecation reflex and increases tissue injury, infection potential, and discomfort. Rectal stimulation results in vagal nerve stimulation, which decreases the heart rate.

Fulfilled Needs: Comfort, protection from physical harm

Refrain from inserting objects into a bleeding orifice Tubes or other objects should not be inserted into any bleeding orifice until the exact cause of bleeding has been determined.

Rationale: Irritating objects placed into a bleeding orifice promote further bleeding or cause increased tissue damage.

Fulfilled Needs: Protection from physical harm

Refrain from irrigating Do not irrigate a wound or body orifice, especially when there is severe tissue damage.

Rationale: Irrigations increase pressure on tissues and further damage already traumatized tissue.

Fulfilled Needs: Protection from physical harm

Refrain from jarring the bed Do not allow the bed to be shaken or vibrated.

Rationale: Jarring can stimulate muscle spasms, severe pain, drainage of wounds and fistulas, and in hyperparathyroidism can cause bone breakage.

Fulfilled Needs: Comfort, protection from physical harm

Refrain from making a specific length-of-life estimate[279] When a person asks how long he will live, do not answer in months or days. Explain that there are many variables such as individual strength, disease progression, and treatments. An exception should be considered when the anticipated lifespan is short and the person has significant responsibilities. Even in these cases the time should be expressed as "not very long" or "a very short time."

Rationale: Setting specific anticipated death dates heightens anxiety and increases hopelessness.

Fulfilled Needs: Comfort, protection from psychologic threat

Refrain from making promises Avoid making promises and commitments that are difficult to keep.

Rationale: Refraining from making promises reduces the potential for distrust when promises cannot be met.

Fulfilled Needs: Protection from psychologic threat

Refrain from negatively criticizing Do not make destructive remarks regarding a person's personality or character.

Rationale: Negative responses from others usually are perceived as threatening, while positive responses enhance positive self-evaluation.

Fulfilled Needs: Comfort, protection from psychologic threat, acceptance, caring and communicating relationships, high evaluation of self

Refrain from performing nonessential procedures Avoid doing treatments and procedures that are not absolutely necessary.

Rationale: Therapeutic procedures often present irritating external stimuli frequently perceived as threatening. They require adaptations that drain energy needed for the healing process. Many procedures cause embarrassment or increase anxiety if the person feels his privacy is invaded.

Fulfilled Needs: Sleep, rest, relaxation, energy, comfort, protection from physical harm, protection from psychologic threat

Refrain from placing a pillow under the knee Do not put a pillow or rolled blanket under the knee when there is venous stasis.

Rationale: Pressure applied under the knee decreases circulation.

Fulfilled Needs: Protection from physical harm

Refrain from pulling the person across the sheets Do not pull the person's body across the sheet surface. Instead, lift the body from one position to another.

Rationale: Pulling the body across a sheet causes friction irritation of the skin.

Fulfilled Needs: Comfort, protection from physical harm

Refrain from pulling the umbilical cord during expulsion of the placenta Never attempt removal of the placenta by pulling the umbilical cord.

Rationale: Pulling the umbilical cord before the placenta is expelled can turn the uterus inside out.

Fulfilled Needs: Protection from physical harm

Refrain from rapidly replacing lagging hyperalimentation solution Do not rapidly increase the flow rate of hyperalimentation solution in an effort to make up for a slowed rate. Instead, reassess the desired fluid intake and readjust the flow rate at a moderate pace.

Rationale: The excessive metabolic stress caused by the rapid infusion of hyperalimentation solution can cause shock.

Fulfilled Needs: Protection from physical harm

Refrain from removing the placenta except during a uterine contraction Never attempt to remove the placenta when the uterus is not firmly contracted.

Rationale: Removing the placenta from a relaxed uterus will turn the uterus inside out.

Fulfilled Needs: Protection from physical harm

Refrain from restricting fluids Do not limit the intake of fluids.

Rationale: During pregnancy, it is the high-salt intake, not the fluid intake, that causes edema. Fluids are essential to the maintenance of normal body function during pregnancy. In diabetes insipidus, limiting fluids will not reduce the output of urine, since the cause is not the amount of fluid intake but failure of the body to produce adequate antidiuretic hormone.

Fulfilled Needs: Protection from physical harm

Refrain from saying anything not intended for the person to hear Avoid speaking in a whisper in the presence of the person or discussing any topic that would be distressing or disturbing to him.

Rationale: During illness, comments made by others often are misinterpreted. The illness may be such that clarification of the message is impossible. If the message reveals unpleasantness, the additional stress may increase anxiety and inhibit rest needed for healing.

Fulfilled Needs: Protection from physical harm, protection from psychologic threat

Refrain from sealing the feeding (nasogastric, urinary) tube with a heavy clamp Do not close off tubes with large heavy metal clamps. Use lightweight small clamps.

Rationale: Heavy clamps pull tubing out of place and add the discomfort of having the tube reinserted.

Fulfilled Needs: Protection from physical harm

Refrain from shouting at persons with communication disorders Do not use a loud voice when speaking to persons with aphasic disorders, partial deafness, a stroke, in a coma, or who speak a foreign language. Changing the voice to a higher or lower tone, rather than making it louder, often facilitates communications.

Rationale: Loud voice sounds frequently cause mental confusion and emotional stress. Voice tone changes are more readily perceptible.

Fulfilled Needs: Comfort, protection from psychologic threat

Refrain from simultaneously powdering and lubricating the skin Do not powder and oil the skin at the same time. It is preferable not to powder until all oils have soaked into the skin, to powder without applying oil, or to oil without applying powder.

Rationale: A mixture of oil and powder on the skin causes caking and irritation.

Fulfilled Needs: Comfort, cleanliness, protection from physical harm

Refrain from strapping the ventilator mask in place When artificial ventilation disturbs the person, refrain from strapping the mask onto his face. Instead, have him hold the mask tightly against the face with his hand or use a mouthpiece.

Rationale: The ability to control an undesirable or frightening object that affects respirations, promotes comfort.

Fulfilled Needs: Comfort

Refrain from supporting the person's delusions (illusions or hallucinations) Do not participate actively in the person's delusions, illusions, or hallucinations. If he says that he is a king and asks for a crown, do not pretend to give him one. If, when hallucinating, he sees snakes, do not agree with him. If he thinks a lace curtain is a spider web, do not support the illusion.

Rationale: Other person's noninvolvement in delusional, hallucinatory, or illusional behavior enhances reality perception.

Fulfilled Needs: Increased reality perception

Refrain from taking rectal temperatures Do not take the temperature rectally. Instead use the oral or axillary method.

Rationale: Thermometer insertion into the rectum may cause pain, bleeding, stimulation of the defecation reflex, or vagal nerve stimulation, which decreases the heart rate. It increases existing tissue injury and when worm lavae come in contact with the rectal thermometer, causes further contamination thereby increasing the potential for infection.

Fulfilled Needs: Protection from physical harm

Refrain from teasing Do not verbally jest or make satirical remarks.

Rationale: Persons with sensitive perception may interpret teasing as a negative and threatening response from others.

Fulfilled Needs: Comfort, protection from psychologic threat

Refrain from tight bandaging Do not apply bandages so tightly that they will constrict blood flow. Do not apply tape so it completely encircles an extremity.

Rationale: Injured tissues require unimpaired circulation for healing. Swelling following an injury may cause a snug bandage to impair circulation with resulting tissue damage.

Fulfilled Needs: Comfort, protection from physical harm

Refrain from using a cotton-filled gauze tracheostomy dressing Do not use cotton-filled gauze when changing a tracheostomy dressing. Nonwoven or premade molded gauze is preferable.

Rationale: Cotton gauze shreds. When pieces of cotton are sucked into the tracheostomy on inhalation, respiratory obstruction can occur.

Fulfilled Needs: Protection from physical harm

Refrain from using a cream-based soap Do not use soap having a base of cream such as cold cream.

Rationale: Cream-based soaps add oil to the skin and further obstruct overactive sebaceous glands.

Fulfilled Needs: Protection from physical harm

Contraindications: Very dry skin

Refrain from using a ventilator nose clip When artificial ventilation disturbs the person, refrain from placing a ventilator clip on the nose. Instead, have the person hold his nose with his fingers.

Rationale: The ability to control an undesirable or frightening object that affects respirations promotes comfort.

Fulfilled Needs: Comfort

Refrain from using an alkaline soap on the skin Use soaps that are combined with oils and do not have a high percentage of alkali.

Rationale: Excessive alkali in soap is a potential source of skin irritation.

Fulfilled Needs: Protection from physical harm

Refrain from using punitive measures Avoid the use of mannerisms or verbalization that could be interpreted as punishment. A quiet, unassuming, firm manner can be used to communicate a need for behavior change, without imposing the threat of punishment.

Rationale: Punishment is associated with dependency, which poses the threat of loss of control.

Fulfilled Needs: Comfort, protection from psychologic threat, caring and communicating relationships

Refresh the person before sleep Use hygienic measures to refresh the body before sleep.

Rationale: Cleanliness promotes comfort and relaxation, which supports rest and sleep.

Fulfilled Needs: Sleep, rest, relaxation, comfort

Refresh with a mouth freshener Spray a chemically refreshing solution into the mouth.

Rationale: Mouth freshner promotes the comfort of a clean, fresh mouth.

Fulfilled Needs: Comfort, cleanliness

Refresh with a mouthwash Offer a refreshing and cleansing solution to swirl in the mouth. If oral tissues are inflamed or irritated, dilute the mouthwash with water.

Rationale: The removal of decaying food by bubbling action and the reduction of bacteria controls bad breath and promotes cleanliness. Alkaline mouthwashes cause less saliva stimulation than acid mouthwashes. Alkaline mouthwashes contain calcium, magnesium, potassium, or sodium hydroxide.

Fulfilled Needs: Comfort, cleanliness, protection from physical harm, dependence

Contraindications: Avoid using alkaline mouthwashes in hypernatremia, hyperkalemia, hypercalcemia, and sodium-restricted diets

Reinforce concern throughout the entire illness Frequently assure the person that every possible thing will be done for him in the way of treatment and comforting measures. Throughout the entire illness, assure him that all health personnel are available and sincerely concerned for his welfare.

Rationale: Awareness that others are supportive prevents feelings of isolation, anxiety, and hopelessness.

Fulfilled Needs: Comfort, protection from psychologic threat, high evaluation of self, endurance, dignity

Relate the time, day, place, and events occurring Reinforce the person's awareness of where he is, what time of day it is, the day of the week, and the events occurring. Be very specific so he is well-oriented to the environment.

Rationale: Correct orientation to the environment is essential to normal human functioning. It also reduces anxiety and feelings of helplessness.

Fulfilled Needs: Protection from psychologic threat, increased reality perception

Relate to (interact with) the person on an adult–adult level, not on a parent–child level When communicating with the person, let the behavior reflect an adult role and an expected adult role from the other person. Avoid acting as a parent, which causes a child response from the other person.

Rationale: Adult–adult relationships are more successful than parent–child relationships, which put the person responding as a child at a disadvantage.

Fulfilled Needs: Comfort, protection from psychologic threat, increased learning

Release restraints and walk the person periodically Remove the person's restraints at least every 6 hours. If possible, ambulate or sit the person up. Maintain constant nursing supervision during this time.

Rationale: Long-term restraint impairs tissue circulation because of limited motion. Release from restraints reduces anxiety associated with forced immobility.

Fulfilled Needs: Comfort, protection from physical harm, protection from psychologic threat

Contraindications: Extreme agitation

Remove adhesive tape and adhesive debris Gently remove the adhesive tape from the skin. Remove the adhesive debris by applying baby oil, cold cream, acetone, or peanut butter to the area and then wiping it clean.

Rationale: Removing adhesive tape and the remaining adhesive debris promotes skin cleanliness and reduces irritation.

Fulfilled Needs: Comfort, cleanliness, protection from physical harm

Remove blisters from the burned area[49] If a large skin area is burned, use mild pressure with sterile gauze, a sterile scalpel, or sterile scissors to break the blisters. If the burned area is small, leave the blisters intact.

Rationale: When blisters cover a large burned area, they cannot be protected from breaking. Breaking the blisters under sterile conditions facilitates the maintenance of a clean skin area.

Fulfilled Needs: Cleanliness, protection from physical harm

Remove constrictive clothing   Remove clothing that is very tight around a body part; clothing such as garters, girdles, head bands, tight belts, socks or hose.
Rationale: Constrictive clothing impairs circulation to the body part.
Fulfilled Needs: Protection from physical harm

Remove food from the mouth   When a person is choking, manually remove unchewed food from his mouth or have him spit the food out.
Rationale: Foreign objects in the mouth can be aspirated into the lung during a choking episode, causing impaired pulmonary ventilation.
Fulfilled Needs: Tissue oxygenation or perfusion, cleanliness, protection from physical harm

Remove hair with a depilatory cream   Use a chemical cream compound that will remove hair.
Rationale: Hair removal with a depilatory cream minimizes the potential for being cut with a razor and promotes thorough cleansing of the body part.
Fulfilled Needs: Comfort, protection from physical harm
Contraindications: Any evidence of skin irritation before or after using the cream

Remove harmful objects from the environment   Watch for and remove all objects that could cause physical harm such as knives, razors, sheets, belts, cleaning fluids, electric sockets, utensils, glasses, dishes.
Rationale: Certain common objects, when possessed by persons with self-destructive tendencies, can be used to carry out physical self-harm. Recognition of potential physical threats promotes safety. Respect for the basic worth of people promotes the support of life whenever possible.
Fulfilled Needs: Protection form physical harm, dignity

Remove immediately to a safe area   When a person has been harmed by some environmental condition, move the person away from the area of danger.
Rationale: An unsafe environment increases the potential for health impairment.
Fulfilled Needs: Protection from physical harm

Remove the bedpan immediately following its use   Remove the bedpan immediately after it has been used and wash and dry it.
Rationale: Quickly removing the bedpan reduces pressure on the skin, decreases tissue irritation, and offers assistance in illness dependency.
Fulfilled Needs: Comfort, protection from physical harm, dependence

Remove the colon tube for bowel elimination and then reinsert about 4 inches   When the person has a ureterosigmoidostomy, a rectal tube is kept in place for the first 10 postoperative days. When the person needs to have a bowel elimination, gently remove the tube. Following elimination, reinsert it 4 inches into the rectum.
Rationale: With ureterosigmoidostomy, a colon tube is placed in the rectum for urine drainage. Since feces cannot pass through the tube, it is removed for bowel elimination.
Fulfilled Needs: Waste elimination of food residue and urine

Remove the contact lens   If the person has an eye infection or is going to sleep, remove his contact lenses if he is unable to do so. In order to remove a contact lens from the cornea, open the person's eye. Pull the side of the eye (near the ear) outward with one hand. With the other hand, gently pull the lids together and the lens should pop out. Before attempting to remove a lens, be sure it is over the cornea. If it is not, gently close the eyelid and, with very gentle pressure, move the lens toward the cornea. After removing the lenses, be careful to place them in a case or a safe container. Do not mixup the right and left lens.

Rationale: Wearing contact lenses during sleep or eye infection may cause corneal injury, unless the contact lens is designed for long-term use.

Fulfilled Needs: Comfort, cleanliness, protection from physical harm, dependence

Remove the dentures   Take the person's artificial teeth out of his mouth.

Rationale: The removal of artificial dentures prevents respiratory obstruction in unconscious or confused states. When the dentures are irritating the oral mucosa, their removal prevents tissue trauma.

Fulfilled Needs: Protection from physical harm

Remove the fecal impaction manually   With a slightly lubricated gloved finger, gently remove accumulated feces tightly wedged in the colon.

Rationale: Removal of hard fecal material promotes comfort and elimination. It prevents loss of rectal muscle tone from prolonged distention.

Fulfilled Needs: Waste elimination of food residue, comfort, protection from physical harm

Remove the/all foreign objects/debris   Remove any object from the skin or body orifice that does not normally belong there. This may require the use of forceps, irrigations, and so forth. When removing foreign objects from the eye, use moistened sterile gauze. Never use cotton in the eye. Remove foreign objects with great care so further injury does not occur.

Rationale: Foreign particles may cause mucosal irritation, infection, or obstruction of passages such as the airway.

Fulfilled Needs: Tissue oxygenation or perfusion, comfort, protection from physical harm

Remove the insect stinger   When a person is bitten by an insect with a stinger, remove the stinger by pulling it out of the skin.

Rationale: Removing an insect stinger eliminates the source of pain.

Fulfilled Needs: Comfort, freedom from pain

Remove the loose burned skin with a gauze pad and slight pressure[49]   In the early stage of burn, while the skin is still soft, gently rub the skin with a gauze pad and, with a slight pressure, gently remove the burned tissue from the living tissue.

Rationale: The removal of loose burned skin minimizes infection by eliminating areas under which bacteria collect.

Fulfilled Needs: Cleanliness, protection from physical harm

Remove the person from the electrocuting source with a nonconducting material   Use dry objects made of wood, rubber, or rope to remove the person from the source of electrical shock.

Rationale: Rubber, wood, and rope do not conduct electricity and will prevent the electrical current from harming the rescuer.

Fulfilled Needs: Protection from physical harm

Remove the stimuli that support the misperception (the attention deficit)   When the environment contains stimuli that the person perceives as disturbing, remove those stimuli whenever possible. Example: If a statue of a kitten is perceived to be a dangerous tiger, remove it from the room. Replace the object when the person's condition improves.

Rationale: The removal of objects misperceived as threatening promotes rest and comfort.

Fulfilled Needs: Sleep, rest, relaxation, comfort, protection from psychologic threat

Remove the stimulus for the emotion   Remove persons, objects, or situations that arouse severely unpleasant or disturbing feelings.

Rationale: An awareness that controls exist to prevent harm to self promote comfort and safety feelings.

Fulfilled Needs: Comfort, protection from physical harm, protection from psychologic threat

Remove the sutures When healing appears to have occurred, about the fifth or sixth day after suturing, remove the sutures. Using forceps to lift each suture, cut the suture near the skin with surgical scissors, and pull them out one by one.

Rationale: Once healing has occurred, sutures are no longer needed. Removing them reduces their potential for causing a wound infection.

Fulfilled Needs: Comfort, protection from physical harm

Remove the therapeutic tube when the treatment is terminated Gently remove such tubes as gastric, hyperalimentation, colon, or T-tubes, urinary or venous catheters, etc. when they are no longer needed for treatment.

Rationale: The removal of unneeded tubes increases comfort and reduces the injury and infection potential.

Fulfilled Needs: Comfort, cleanliness, protection from physical harm

Remove the tick with tweezers If a tick has imbedded itself in the skin or hair, use tweezers rather than your fingers to remove it.

Rationale: Removal of the tick with tweezers enhances the chance of complete removal and prevents the tick from striking the person attempting to remove it with his fingers.

Fulfilled Needs: Protection from physical harm

Repeat the message until it is understood Repeat messages not properly interpreted until they are correctly understood.

Rationale: Message repetition enhances communication by reinforcing perception of the intended ideas and thoughts.

Fulfilled Needs: Caring and communicating relationships

Replace the pacemaker batteries Between 30 and 36 months after batteries have been installed in a pacemaker, exchange them for new batteries.

Rationale: Proper pacemaker function is essential to life. Awareness that such a device is functioning properly supports comfort.

Fulfilled Needs: Comfort, protection from physical harm

Replace the prolapsed umbilical cord into the vagina When the umbilical cord is prolapsed, wash the protruding portion of the umbilical cord with a sterile soap solution and, using sterile gloves, replace the cord into the vagina.

Rationale: A sterile umbilical cord must be maintained to prevent infection of the birth canal.

Fulfilled Needs: Protection from physical harm

Respond immediately to the person's call When a person signals for help, provide immediate attention and effective measures to resolve the difficulty.

Rationale: Early recognition of abnormalities by health personnel promotes safety. Psychologic comfort is fostered by an awareness that the person is not alone when threatened with pain, fear, or anxiety.

Fulfilled Needs: Comfort, protection from physical harm, protection from psychologic threat, attention

Restrain the person Limit the person's freedom of movement with restraining devices only after due consideration of safety and the legal factors involved.

Rationale: Gentle restraint protects the person from accidental injury.

Fulfilled Needs: Protection from physical harm

Contraindications: When the use of physical force threatens the person's integrity, promotes distrust or aggressive behavior, or when restraint benefits institutional routine and not the safety of the person

Restrict fluids at the mealtime Do not give fluids with the meal, though warm fluids may be sipped after the meal.

Rationale: In the dumping syndrome, fluid ingestion during a meal causes the production of a hypertonic solution in the small intestine. This hypertonic solution pulls fluid from the blood into the intestine, causing intestinal distention and irritation, which results in diarrhea.

Fulfilled Needs: Protection from physical harm

Restrict head movements with a cervical collar, pillows, or sandbags Place a cervical collar around the neck or place sandbags or pillows snugly against the side of the face to prevent sudden turning or movement of the head.

Rationale: Sudden head movements may increase pressure within the eye, causing visual damage in eye disorders. In trauma, sudden head movements frequently cause further injury.

Fulfilled Needs: Protection from physical harm

Restrict the blood transfusion rate to 500 cc every 2 to 4 hours Regulate the rate of blood being transfused to no more than 500 cc over a 2- to 4-hour period. In cases of severe emergency and blood depletion, up to 100 cc/minute may be given.

Rationale: A rapid increase in circulating fluid volume can cause pulmonary edema or fluid and electrolyte imbalance.

Fulfilled Needs: Fluid and electrolyte balance, protection from physical harm

Restrict the fluid intake according to the weight gain Limit the amount of fluid taken in a 24-hour period to the amount of weight gained in the past 24 hours. For every pound of weight gained, limit fluid intake 500 cc.

Rationale: When water balance is maintained, the body weight remains unchanged if the person is in nutritional balance and not in negative-nitrogen balance. A loss or gain of solid tissue is accompanied by a loss or gain of water. A 1-pound weight gain in 24 hours is considered to be a 500 cc accumulation of excess fluid.

Fulfilled Needs: Fluid and electrolyte balance, protection from physical harm

Restrict the fluid intake to 600 cc plus the output Maintain the person's fluid intake at 600 cc plus the amount of output lost through urine, gastric secretions, profuse perspiration, wound drainage, etc.

Rationale: Fluid intake at 600 cc is essential for normal renal function under conditions of normal body and environmental temperature. The additional intake of other output losses prevents dehydration.

Fulfilled Needs: Fluid and electrolyte balance, protection from physical harm

Contraindications: Pregnancy, diabetes insipidus

Restrict the glucose intravenous solution rate according to the weight Intravenous solutions of glucose should be given at a calculated hourly rate of 0.5 g of glucose per kilogram of body weight.

Rationale: Rapid intravenous glucose infusions can cause glucosuria or potassium depletion.

Fulfilled Needs: Fluid and electrolyte balance, protection from physical harm

Restrict the hypertonic intravenous solution rate to 200 cc per hour Regulate the rate of a hypertonic intravenous solution containing more than 0.9% salt or over 5% sugar in water so it does not exceed 200 cc/hr. Check bottle labels indicating which fluids are hypertonic.

Rationale: When hypertonic solutions are introduced into the circulatory system, the fact that they contain more salt or sugar and less water (increased osmotic pressure) than the blood causes them to pull fluid from the blood cells to equalize the pressure differences between the fluid and the cell contents. This physiologic change results in shrinkage of the blood cells and should not be allowed to occur at a rapid rate.

Fulfilled Needs: Fluid and electrolyte balance, protection from physical harm

Restrict the hypotonic intravenous solution rate to 400 cc per hour Regulate the rate of a hypotonic intravenous solution containing less than 0.9% salt or less than 5% sugar in water so it does not exceed 400 cc/hr. Check bottle labels indicating which fluids are hypotonic.

Rationale: When hypotonic solutions are introduced into the circulatory system, the fact that they contain less salt or sugar and more water (decreased osmotic pressure) than the blood causes fluid to be pulled from the solution into the blood cells to equalize the pressure differences between the fluid and the cell contents. This physiologic change results in swelling of the blood cells and should not be allowed to occur at a rapid rate.

Fulfilled Needs: Fluid and electrolyte balance, protection from physical harm

Restrict the intake to nothing by mouth Do not allow the intake of any food or fluid.

Rationale: Withholding food and fluids decreases gastric juice secretion, irritation of intestinal mucosa, and stimulation of peristalsis. A clean intestinal tract is necessary for many diagnostic studies.

Fulfilled Needs: Comfort, protection from physical harm

Contraindications: In severe debilitation and in very young children, limit the NPO restriction to as short a time as possible

Restrict the intravenous potassium to 20 mEq per hour or 200 mEq per 24 hours When administering potassium containing intravenous infusions, regulate the potassium so that the adult receives no more than 20 mEq each hour.

Rationale: Potassium, given too rapidly, causes cardiac irritability with resulting arrhythmia and potential cardiac standstill.

Fulfilled Needs: Fluid and electrolyte balance, protection from physical harm

Restrict the isotonic intravenous solution rate to 600 cc per hour Regulate the rate of an isotonic intravenous solution containing 0.9% salt or 5% sugar in water so it does not exceed 600 cc/hr. Preferably it is given at a much slower rate. However, in cases of severe emergency and fluid depletion, as much as 2,000 cc may be given per hour. Check bottle labels indicating which fluids are isotonic.

Rationale: When isotonic solutions are introduced into the circulatory system, the fact that they contain a concentration of salt or sugar (osmotic pressure) equal to that of the blood makes them safe to give at a fairly rapid rate. Isotonic solutions maintain the blood cells in a relatively normal state and do not produce the shrinkage effect of hypertonic solutions or the swelling effect of hypotonic solutions on cells.

Fulfilled Needs: Fluid and electrolyte balance, protection from physical harm

Restrict unwanted visitors Prevent specifically named persons from visiting the patient when it is evident that these persons are a disturbing influence. Limits should be enforced when the patient expresses negative feelings toward persons but is himself unable to control the visiting without a breakdown in interpersonal relationships.

Rationale: Highly emotional conditions deplete body energy and stimulate irritating regulatory secretions. Safety feelings evolve from an awareness that sufficient control can be exerted to prevent harm to oneself.

Fulfilled Needs: Comfort, protection from physical harm, protection from psychologic threat

Retract and clean the foreskin Each time the male infant is bathed, gently pull back the penal foreskin and clean the head of the penis. Gently pull the skin back in place once cleansing is completed.

Rationale: Cleanliness prevents infection.

Fulfilled Needs: Cleanliness, protection from physical harm

Return the blood to the blood bank after a reaction When a blood transfusion reaction occurs, return the remaining blood and a reaction report to the blood bank.

Rationale: Checking for blood incompatibility or bacterial contamination reduces the potential for further harm to the person.

Fulfilled Needs: Protection from physical harm

Reveal the person's ambivalent (angry or depressed) feelings Bring to the person's attention feelings that his behavior indicates he is experiencing.

Rationale: Insight into the person's own feelings promotes growth, maturity, and problem solving.

Fulfilled Needs: Personal growth and maturity, increased reality perception and problem-solving ability

Rinse the mouth with dilute hydrogen peroxide Using a solution of one-half water and one-half hydrogen peroxide, have the person rinse his mouth several times a day.

Rationale: The oxidizing action of hydrogen peroxide acts as a cleansing agent and discourages the growth of certain microorganisms.

Fulfilled Needs: Cleanliness, protection from physical harm

Safeguard the person's dentures (eyeglasses, artificial eye, contact lenses, hearing aid, personal belongings) Protect the person's dentures, eyeglasses, artificial eye, or hearing aid by placing it in a case or container. Place contact lenses in a lens wetting solution or plain water and in their protective case. Keep articles belonging to the person in a secure place and properly labeled with adequate identification. Be certain to inform the person of their whereabouts.

Rationale: Artificial teeth aid in the chewing and digestion of food, maintain a natural jaw contour, and promote comfort. Protecting the artificial eye prevents scratches on it that could cause socket irritation, minimizes breakage, and maintains cleanliness, which prevents infection. Eyeglass and contact lens safety supports visual acuity and reduces the economic stress of having to replace them. Protection of the hearing aid ensures its availability to function properly.

Fulfilled Needs: Comfort, protection from physical harm

Safeguard with a crib dome Protect the child from falling or getting out of bed by applying a plastic crib dome over the bed.

Rationale: Adequate safety measures prevents severe injury.

Fulfilled Needs: Protection from physical harm

Safeguard with accurate indentification Protect the person with a correct identification band.

Rationale: Accurate identification promotes safety and exhibits dignity through concern for the person.

Fulfilled Needs: Protection from physical harm, dignity

Safeguard with siderails/siderail padding Place bedrails on either side of the bed. Cushion the bedrails when such is needed.

Rationale: Adequate safety measures prevent severe injury.

Fulfilled Needs: Protection from physical harm

Save the poison container for content analysis   If a poisonous substance has been ingested and the identification of the product is unknown, keep the container and send it with the person when he seeks medical care.

Rationale: Knowledge of the substance ingested allows for effective treatment with appropriate antidotes.

Fulfilled Needs: Protection from physical harm.

Schedule toileting   Take the person to the bathroom or place him on the bedpan or bedside commode at specific times, periodically throughout the day or night. Select a time compatible with the person's usual elimination schedule and his current daily activities.

Rationale: Offering the opportunity for elimination prevents accidents and promotes elimination. When bowel or bladder retraining is essential to maintain elimination control, the body systems adapt more readily to routine functioning than to unscheduled activity.

Fulfilled Needs: Waste elimination of food residue and urine, comfort, cleanliness, protection from physical harm, dependence

Season the food for individual taste   Add garlic, herbs, and spices to already prepared foods in amounts preferred by the person.

Rationale: Seasoning food enhances flavor and promotes greater desire to eat.

Fulfilled Needs: Comfort

Contraindications: Avoid salt in salt-restricted diets

Secure all tubing so there is no interference with mobility   Whenever the person has any type of therapeutic tubing, adjust or attach the tubing so that the person has complete freedom of movement. Be certain that the tubing cannot become entangled in an extremity or in clothing.

Rationale: Freedom of movement is essential to good circulation, general comfort, and care.

Fulfilled Needs: Comfort, protection from physical harm

Send a blood sample for type and crossmatch   Obtain a clotted-blood sample and send for analysis of the type (A, B, AB, O, Rh factor) of blood the person has. Request crossmatching with the recipient's and donor's blood.

Rationale: Blood-type analysis determines the various factors in the person's blood in order to prevent the highly dangerous antigen–antibody agglutination reaction that results from transferring the incorrect type of blood. Crossmatching establishes the compatibility of the recipient's and donor's blood. Having blood typed and crossmatched, and thus readily available, protects the ill person from delay of a needed transfusion.

Fulfilled Needs: Protection from physical harm

Set an example by role modeling   When exhibiting behavior expected to be performed by another, do so with preciseness and clarity. Be aware that what the person sees you doing, he will repeat in his own behavior.

Rationale: Role modeling sets an example of behavior for others to follow. It is a method of teaching.

Fulfilled Needs: Mastery and competence in skills, personal growth and maturity, increased learning

Set limits on unacceptable behavior   Request cooperation in curtailing unacceptable behavior by clearly defining roles, responsibilities, routines, and what the person can and cannot do. Limits may be set by verbal comments or judicious restraint.

Rationale: External control of behavior supports internal control when the latter cannot be maintained. Limitations protect against future shame resulting from presently uncontrolled behavior. Esteem needs from others promote acceptance of and conformity to expectations of others.

Fulfilled Needs: Comfort, protection from psychologic threat, personal growth and maturity, increased reality perception and problem-solving ability

Shampoo the hair/scalp   Clean the hair with soap and water or shampoo.

Rationale: Cleanliness prevents infection and promotes comfort.

Fulfilled Needs: Comfort, cleanliness, protection from physical harm

Contraindications: Skull fracture, potential or existing intracranial hemorrhage, extra caution should be taken when there are skull tongs for cervical traction

Share with the person objective data that verify the health status   Show the person reports such as ECGs, blood and urine analysis, radiology reports, and the like. Explain their meaning in relation to the person's condition.

Rationale: Tangible evidence of a person's state of health reinforces the reality of that state.

Fulfilled Needs: Protection from physical harm, increased learning, increased reality perception

Shave the hair surrounding the burned area[49]   Using shaving cream and a safety razor or Weck blade, remove the hair on the injured skin around a burned area. Heat from the burn usually removes the hair from the burned area. If some hair still remains, it too should be shaved gently.

Rationale: Hair around or on a burn collects bacteria, which heightens the potential for infection.

Fulfilled Needs: Cleanliness, protection from physical harm

Shield the tracheostomy (or laryngectomy stoma) from water   Cover a tracheostomy or laryngectomy stoma with a protective shield such as a folded washcloth or the hand whenever the person takes a shower. Never use a plastic bag as a covering.

Rationale: Water in a tracheostomy tube or laryngectomy stoma obstructs the airway.

Fulfilled Needs: Protection from physical harm

Shield visitors from exposure to radiation   When a visitor stays with a person receiving radiation therapy, protect that person through radiation shielding. Have him wear a lead-lined apron and sit behind lead-lined drapes or a thick concrete wall.

Rationale: Certain materials decrease the spread of radiation rays. Body exposure to radioactive substances results in blood cell disturbances, sterility, internal burns, genetic changes, gastrointestinal upsets, and altered tissue cell structure.

Fulfilled Needs: Protection from physical harm

Sit the person in an armchair   Assist the person into a well-supported sitting position in a comfortable armchair.

Rationale: Sitting up prevents fluid congestion in the lungs, stimulates circulation, restores normal physiologic function, and promotes comfort. An armchair provides the safety of a supportive structure against which the weakened person may lean.

Fulfilled Needs: Rest and relaxation, activity and exercise, comfort, stimulation, protection from physical harm

Contraindications: Temperature elevation above 103° F, head or spinal cord injury, internal hemorrhage, coma or semicoma, severe energy depletion, life-threatening situations

Sit with the person   Sit in a chair beside the person either silently or engaging in activity and conversation.

Rationale: Psychologic comfort results from an awareness that a person is not alone.

The presence of another person is stimulative, provides attention, and supports inter-personal communications.

Fulfilled Needs: Comfort, stimulation, protection from psychologic threat, caring and communicating relationships, attention

Slow the intravenous infusion (or blood transfusion) flow rate Decrease the intravenous flow rate to 20–40 drops/minute. If the blood pressure rises, further de-crease the drops per minute.

Rationale: Excessive fluid entering the circulation increases arterial pressure, which results in a loss of fluid into tissue spaces, causing edema. Slowing the intravenous infu-sion prevents edema and blood pressure elevation because it reduces circulatory over-load. The excretion of more than 80 cc of urine/hour indicates that fluid intake is far more rapid than fluid output and that fluid imbalance or circulatory overload exists.

Fulfilled Needs: Fluid and electrolyte balance, protection from physical harm

Contraindications: Circulatory failure, hypotension

Soak in a colloidal bath Immerse the body in an oatmeal or corn starch bath, taking care not to allow large amounts of starch to gather in skin folds.

Rationale: Starch or oatmeal have an emollient effect, relieving irritation and itching and cleansing the skin. As starch absorbs water, the starch granules swell in skin folds and cause irritation.

Fulfilled Needs: Comfort, cleanliness, protection from physical harm

Soak in a germicidal solution Wash the skin with a solution that will destroy germs. Such solutions include Betadine and iodine.

Rationale: The destruction of germs by germicidal solutions prevents or reduces in-fection.

Fulfilled Needs: Cleanliness, protection from physical harm

Soak in a sitz bath Apply hot (96–106° F) water to the pelvic area by having the person sit in a tub filled with water up to the navel.

Rationale: Moist heat promotes relaxation and healing by cleansing. It relieves pain through local vasodilatation of the pelvic area.

Fulfilled Needs: Comfort, cleanliness, freedom from pain

Contraindications: Persons subject to episodes of hypotension must be observed closely, especially when getting out of the tub

Soak in cold water Submerge the burned skin area in cold, clean water, not ice wa-ter.

Rationale: Cold water reduces the pain of burns.

Fulfilled Needs: Comfort, protection from physical harm, freedom from pain

Contraindications: Avoid on areas of decubitus ulcers, gangrenous tissue, skin graft, varicose veins, paralysis or sensation loss, or with aged, debilitated skin

Soak in providone-iodine (Betadine) solution Soak the skin area in the iodine preparation Betadine.

Rationale: Betadine has a prolonged antiseptic effect. It kills skin bacteria, fungus, viruses, yeasts, and protozoa. It is used to treat chronic skin infection (pyoderma), fresh lacerations, and beginning decubitus.

Fulfilled Needs: Cleanliness, protection from physical harm

Contraindications: Known Betadine allergy

Soak in saline solution Immerse the arm, hand, fingers, leg, foot, or toes in a warm hypertonic (2 teaspoons of salt to 500 cc of water) saline solution for approxi-mately 20–30 minutes, three to four times a day. Apply only to intact skin.

Rationale: The local application of a warm saline solution supports cleanliness and has an astringent effect that promotes the relief of pain and edema of inflamed tissues by improving circulation to the area.

Fulfilled Needs: Comfort, cleanliness, protection from physical harm

Contraindications: Open wounds should be soaked in isotonic solutions since plain water or a hypertonic saline solution causes a burning sensation

Soak the nails in warm oil When the nails are brittle or the cuticles are ragged, soak them in warm olive oil or liquid lanolin for 15–20 minutes.

Rationale: Soaking the nails in warm oil loosens dead cuticles and replaces the natural oils and moisture of the dried nails.

Fulfilled Needs: Comfort, protection from physical harm

Soften and remove the earwax Place a few drops of mineral oil into the ear for 30 minutes to 1 hour or put two drops of liquid stool softener (Colace) into the ear. Compress the ear opening several times to push the softening agent into the ear. Wait 2–5 minutes. Then wash the wax out with a bulb syringe or remove with a cerumen spoon.

Rationale: Removal of ear wax improves hearing when hearing loss is due to wax accumulations. It also promotes the comfort of cleanliness and offers assistance during illness dependency.

Fulfilled Needs: Comfort, cleanliness, protection from physical harm, dependence

Contraindications: Earache, ear infection

Soften the hair with a cream rinse After shampooing the hair, rinse with a mild, oily hair cream.

Rationale: Cream rinse softens the hair shafts, prevents tangling, and promotes comfort.

Fulfilled Needs: Comfort, protection from physical harm

Solicit the family's assistance in understanding the person's speech When attempting to communicate with a person having impaired communication ability, seek the assistance of family members to interpret the person's message.

Rationale: Familiarity with a person's nonverbal methods of communication facilitates clarity of message interpretation. Comfort is promoted through effective communication with others.

Fulfilled Needs: Comfort, caring and communicating relationships

Space necessary activities that increase intracranial pressure Space the times far apart for performing activities that increase intracranial pressure. Do not perform two activities at the same time if at all possible. Such activities include turning; suctioning; painful procedures such as injections, dressing changes, exercises, checking for fecal impactions, etc.

Rationale: By reducing the number of stressors at one time that increase intracranial pressure, the pressure is kept at a minimal level or prevents an excessively high plateau from occurring.

Fulfilled Needs: Protection from physical harm, physiologic stability

Splint the incisional area Hold a pillow firmly against the area of a fresh abdominal or chest incision while the patient coughs, turns in bed, or gets up to a sitting position.

Rationale: Supportive pressure decreases stress on incisional areas, promotes comfort, and reduces pain.

Fulfilled Needs: Comfort, freedom from pain

Sponge the wound clean Soak up wound drainage by gently inserting sterile, absorbent, gauze into the wound. Immediately remove after it has become saturated and replace it with clean gauze.

Rationale: Removal of wound drainage promotes cleanliness and rapid healing.

Fulfilled Needs: Comfort, cleanliness, protection from physical harm

Stand the man for urination   When a man has difficulty voiding while in bed, allow him to assume the standing position for a brief period.

Rationale: The standing position increases gravity pull within the bladder, promoting urine flow, and is the natural voiding position for men.

Fulfilled Needs: Waste elimination of urine, comfort

Contraindications: Temperature elevations above 103° F, head or spinal cord injury, internal hemorrhage, coma or semicoma, severe energy depletion, life-threatening situations

Start the infant on breast-feedings   Begin the infant on breast-feeding when both infant and mother are ready.

Rationale: Breast-milk provides the infant with the best nutritional composition known for infants and fulfills an essential psychologic need for both the infant and mother.

Fulfilled Needs: Food balance, comfort

Sterilize the bedpan after each use   Each time the bedpan is used, sterilize it thoroughly before it is used again.

Rationale: Cleanliness prevents the spread of infection.

Fulfilled Needs: Cleanliness, protection from physical harm

Stimulate by movement, touch, sternal pressure, or speech   Arouse a response by repeatedly speaking to the person, touching him, applying sternal pressure, or moving him about.

Rationale: Stimuli promote full orientation of the person with impaired cerebral activity, bring attention to current needs, and promote realistic perception of objects and situations.

Fulfilled Needs: Stimulation, protection from physical harm, protection from psychologic threat, increased reality perception and problem-solving ability

Contraindications: Avoid sternal pressure when there is a chest injury

Stimulate the infant with back stroking, foot thumping, or spanking   Arouse the infant by lightly rubbing his back with the hand or thumping the bottom of his feet with a finger.

Rationale: Infant stimulation brings about crying, which aerates the lungs. It enhances perception of available food and the surrounding environment.

Fulfilled Needs: Tissue oxygenation or perfusion, stimulation, protection from physical harm

Stimulate the infant with a mobile   Arouse the infant's perception by placing, above and in front of him, a structure whose parts move by air currents.

Rationale: A moving mobile enhances perception of shapes, sizes, motion, and color.

Fulfilled Needs: Stimulation

Stimulate the memory by repeating the person's last expressed thought   When there is difficulty in recall, repeat the last few words or sentences that the person spoke or mention the general trend of thought.

Rationale: Repetition of recent verbally expressed thoughts reinforces thought content and reduces the threat and anxiety of memory failure.

Fulfilled Needs: Stimulation, protection from psychologic threat

Stimulate the reflex bladder by applying cold to the abdomen, stroking the inner thigh, or running water When retraining for bladder control, the reflex bladder may be stimulated by applying a cold towel to the abdomen, stroking the inner thigh, turning on the water faucet, or pulling pubic hair.

Rationale: External stimulation triggers the bladder's spastic reflex. Bladder control is essential to the maintenance of dryness, comfort, cleanliness, and to the prevention of skin irritation.

Fulfilled Needs: Comfort, cleanliness, protection from physical harm

Contraindications: Do not apply cold to the abdomen if the person has bladder spasms

Stimulate the reflex bowel by abdominal stroking and anal stimulation When retraining for bowel control, the reflex bowel can be stimulated by stroking downward on the abdomen, applying pressure in front of, in back of, and to the side of the anus, inserting the finger into the anus and manually stimulating it.

Rationale: External stimulation triggers the bowel's spastic reflex. Bowel control is essential to the maintenance of dryness, comfort, cleanliness, and to the prevention of skin irritation.

Fulfilled Needs: Comfort, cleanliness, protection from physical harm

Contraindications: If there is any anal tissue injury

Stimulate the sucking reflex through jaw and lip pressure Promote the sucking reflex in an infant during feeding by gently stroking the cheeks or near the lips.

Rationale: The stimulation of infant sucking is essential to food and fluid intake.

Fulfilled Needs: Stimulation

Strip the chest tubing Hold the chest tube securely with the fingers of one hand. Lubricate the fingers of the other hand and clamp them below those of the first hand, pulling the clamped fingers down the tubing to empty it of fluid and air.

Rationale: Chest-tube stripping maintains chest-tube patency since the negative pressure created by the stripping dislodges clots and sediment in the tubing.

Fulfilled Needs: Protection from physical harm

Subdue the room lighting Prevent glare from windows or artificial lamps from reaching the person. Tilt or close blinds or shades. Use only soft room lighting.

Rationale: In conditions such as cerebral edema, measles, meningitis, or drug reactions, light glare irritates nerves and tissue, causing pain. Subdued lighting decreases external stimuli and promotes sleep and comfort.

Fulfilled Needs: Sleep, rest, relaxation, comfort, protection from physical harm

Contraindications: Impaired vision where poor lighting might cause injury

Substitute artificial salt When natural sodium chloride is restricted from the diet, offer an artificial salt substitute.

Rationale: Seasoning food enhances flavor and increases the desire to eat.

Fulfilled Needs: Comfort, protection from physical harm

Contraindications: Conditions in which increased potassium intake is not advisable, such as hyperkalemia

Substitute caffeine-free coffee or tea When regular coffee or tea is restricted from the diet, offer a noncaffeine substitute.

Rationale: Noncaffeine coffee or tea does not cause the gastric acidity, cardiac and respiratory stimulation, and diuretic effects of regular coffee or tea.

Fulfilled Needs: Comfort, protection from physical harm

Suction the airway Using a catheter or bulb syringe, suction the mouth, nose, pharynx, or trachea and remove obstructing secretions.

Rationale: Secretion removal maintains a patent airway, allowing for respiratory gas exchange.

Fulfilled Needs: Tissue oxygenation or perfusion, waste elimination of bronchopulmonary secretions, protection from physical harm

Suction the snake (or spider) venom   When a poisonous snake or spider bite has occurred, incise the site of the bite and, with a suction cup or by mouth, draw out the venom. Do not use the mouth for suctioning if there are mouth ulcers or lacerations, and take care not to swallow the venom.

Rationale: Removal of venom prevents its toxic effects from harming the body.

Fulfilled Needs: Protection from physical harm

Suggest more appropriate means of need gratification   When a person is gaining need satisfaction through demands or impositions on others, suggest less damaging and more fulfilling ways in which those needs can be met.

Rationale: Gratification of needs without imposition on others results in more favorable response from others, which in itself heightens need gratification.

Fulfilled Needs: Protection from psychologic threat, personal growth and maturity

Suggest nursing home care   Suggest that the person consider going to a nursing home where care can be given 24 hours a day.

Rationale: Nursing homes provide continuous custodial care, companionship, and activity for lonely persons.

Fulfilled Needs: Comfort, dependence, increased reality perception and problem-solving ability

Suggest possible child adoption   When a couple cannot have children of their own, suggest they consider adoption.

Rationale: Adopted children provide the same need gratification as biologic children.

Fulfilled Needs: Comfort, sexuality, sense of usefulness, high evaluation of self, sense of adequacy

Contraindications: Avoid suggesting adoption if there is a high potential for rejection by the adoption agency

Suggest private nurse care   Suggest that the person might consider employing a private nurse to come into the home and administer care.

Rationale: Private nursing care allows a person to remain in the security of his home despite illness.

Fulfilled Needs: Comfort, dependence, increased reality perception and problem-solving ability

Suggest substitute means of goal attainment   Suggest alternate means by which anticipated goals can be reached when the present approach seems ineffective.

Rationale: Successful achievement in overcoming barriers to a goal enhances the ability to cope and results in increased adequacy feelings.

Fulfilled Needs: Comfort, protection from physical harm, protection from psychologic threat, sense of adequacy, goal achievement, increased reality perception and problem-solving ability

Suggest that one relative remain with the dying person   When death is fast approaching and all family members cannot remain at the bedside because of other commitments, suggest that the family member who feels most comfortable in the stressful situation remain at the bedside.

Rationale: The presence of one relative with a dying family member assures the others who must leave that death was not met with loneliness. This reduces the potential for guilt feelings.

Fulfilled Needs: Comfort, caring and communicating relationships, unity with loved ones

Suggest that reparation will diminish guilt Suggest that guilt will diminish when a person makes amends for damage done to another.
Rationale: When a guilty person makes reparation, the injured party usually responds in a positive manner, offering acceptance and approval.
Fulfilled Needs: Comfort, protection from psychologic threat

Suggest that volunteers (friends) might offer assistance with home care Suggest that the sick person consider obtaining assistance from volunteers. This service sometimes is offered by church organizations or close friends.
Rationale: Assistance with daily care in illness dependency and allows the person to remain in his desired environment.
Fulfilled Needs: Comfort, dependence, increased problem-solving ability

Supplement inadequate breast-feeding with bottle-feeding Give the infant bottle-feedings in addition to breast-feedings if lactation deficiency exists.
Rationale: Adequate nutrition is essential to life and health.
Fulfilled Needs: Nutritional balance, protection from physical harm

Support a realistic assessment of the situation Help the person evaluate the situation not from assumption but from factual data. Have him explain the situation in detail and draw conclusions from his explanation. Assist in the reevaluation of the situation.
Rationale: Growth and maturity involve the ability to perceive and cope with the demands and limitations of the real world and to organize perceptions into a meaningful whole.
Fulfilled Needs: Protection from psychologic threat, personal growth and maturity, increased reality perception and problem-solving ability

Support the affected body part When moving the person, support the body part that is injured, infected, inflamed, or traumatized.
Rationale: Support of a traumatized body area prevents further injury and promotes comfort.
Fulfilled Needs: Comfort, protection from physical harm, freedom from pain

Support the use of appropriate defense mechanisms Encourage the person to use defense mechanisms that maintain psychologic equilibrium such as identification, sublimation, temporary denial, rationalization, etc.
Rationale: The use of appropriate defense mechanisms is essential for the maintenance of psychologic homeostasis.
Fulfilled Needs: Protection from physical harm, psychologic stability, personal growth and maturity

Support with a binder Offer support to the pelvic area by applying a single-tailed or T-binder, to the torso by applying a straight binder, and to any body area needing support by applying a many-tailed or Scultetus' binder.
Rationale: Binders provide a firm support against uncomfortable movement and the painful or tiring gravity pull on tissues.
Fulfilled Needs: Comfort, protection from physical harm

Suture the wound After thorough cleansing, stitch together the skin and tissue that have been separated by an injury.
Rationale: Suturing promotes the healing of separated skin and tissue and reduces the potential for infection of internal tissue.
Fulfilled Needs: Comfort, protection from physical harm
Contraindications: When a wound infection is highly probable, the wound should be left open for drainage

Swab the mouth with diluted glycerine   Soak a cotton-tipped applicator or a gauze-tipped tongue blade in a 50% water-glycerine solution and cleanse the oral mucous membranes. For flavor, add a little lemon.

Rationale: Diluted glycerine breaks down mucous collections in the mouth and removes it from teeth and gums. It cleanses and lubricates the mouth.

Fulfilled Needs: Comfort, cleanliness

Contraindications: Do not add the lemon flavor if there is excessive salivation or mucosal ulcerations

Take nasal and oral secretion precautions   Dispose of nasal and oral secretions in approved sanitation facilities. Be careful not to have hand contact with the secretions.

Rationale: Pathogen transfer from person to person is decreased by control and precaution when handling pathogens.

Fulfilled Needs: Cleanliness, protection from physical harm

Take needle-syringe precautions   Carefully dispose of all needles and plastic syringes so they cannot be reused accidentally. If glass syringes are being used instead of the disposable ones, soak the needles and syringes in strong disinfecting solution then autoclave them.

Rationale: Pathogens, especially for hepatitis and malaria, are readily transferred by contaminated needles and syringes.

Fulfilled Needs: Cleanliness, protection from physical harm

Take skin-contact precautions   Wear gloves to prevent direct contact with communicable skin lesions.

Rationale: Pathogen transfer from person to person can be decreased by avoiding contact with the pathogens.

Fulfilled Needs: Cleanliness, protection from physical harm

Take sputum precautions   Dispose of infective sputum in approved sanitation facilities. Avoid hand contact with secretions.

Rationale: Pathogen transfer from person to person is decreased by control and precaution in handling pathogens.

Fulfilled Needs: Cleanliness, protection from physical harm

Take stool precautions   Dispose of stools in approved sanitation facilities. Avoid hand contact with the stool.

Rationale: Pathogen transfer from person to person is decreased by control and precaution when handling the pathogens. In typhoid fever, flies and hands carry organisms from feces to food, and the food, when eaten, transmits the organisms.

Fulfilled Needs: Cleanliness, protection from physical harm

Take urine precautions   Dispose of urine contaminated with infectious organisms or radioactive isotopes in approved sanitation facilities. Avoid hand contact with the urine.

Rationale: Pathogen transfer from person to person is decreased by control and precaution when handling pathogens.

Fulfilled Needs: Cleanliness, protection from physical harm

Talk with the person (family, visitor, or significant others)   Converse with the person(s) for as long as necessary to meet his (their) needs.

Rationale: The exchange of verbal responses assures the person of concern, reduces loneliness, supports positive interpersonal relationships, and provides stimulation.

Fulfilled Needs: Comfort, protection from psychologic threat, stimulation, caring and communicating relationships

Tape the pacemaker wire to the person Position the pacemaker wire so that it does not fall under the person. Coil it to the proper length and tape it to the chest.

Rationale: Proper positioning of the pacemaker wire provides safety and comfort.

Fulfilled Needs: Comfort, protection from physical harm

Tape the urinary catheter onto the abdomen When a man has prolonged insertion of an indwelling catheter, tape the end of the catheter onto the abdomen.

Rationale: Taping the urinary catheter onto the abdomen prevents ulceration on the penal-scrotal junction by keeping pressure off the glans and urethra.

Fulfilled Needs: Protection from physical harm

Contraindications: Abdominal surgical incision

Terminate emotionally threatening conversation immediately Whenever the person indicates a desire to talk about the death or an incurable disease, support such discussions. However, the moment the person changes the subjects to a life-oriented topic, the previous discussion should no longer be pursued.

Rationale: When truth can no longer be tolerated, denial becomes essential to prevent intense physiologic threat. Respectful attitudes toward a person's limitations support dignity.

Fulfilled Needs: Protection from psychologic threat, dignity

Tie off and cut the umbilical cord Tie umbilical tape around the umbilical cord about 4–5 inches from the infant's umbilicus, making sure the cord is completely obstructed. Tie a second knot about 2 inches away from the original knot toward the mother. Then cut the cord between the two knots with sterile scissors.

Rationale: Tying off the umbilical cord prevents hemorrhage. Cutting the umbilical cord frees the infant from its mother so it may assume independent life.

Fulfilled Needs: Protection from physical harm

Toilet frequently Offer the bedpan or urinal or take the person to the bathroom at consistently close intervals.

Rationale: Frequently emptying the bladder promotes elimination, prevents the embarrassment of elimination accidents, promotes comfort and cleanliness, and helps relieve intraabdominal pressure during labor.

Fulfilled Needs: Comfort, cleanliness, protection from physical harm, protection from psychologic threat

Touch the person (frequently or judiciously) Express concern and human relatedness by touching the person's skin. This can be done in one of many ways: cuddling a child, playing touch games such as patti-cake and ring-around-the-rosey, holding the person's hand, rocking the child, placing a hand on the person's shoulder or an arm around the waist, patting or stroking, or squeezing the person's arm, or touching the person when dressing or bathing him. Use discretion when touching a person who is suspicious and might misinterpret the intent.

Rationale: The expression and perception of emotional feelings can be activated through stimulation of skin nerves. Touch meets people's most basic need for relatedness to others. The feel of the body is basic to self-perception.

Fulfilled Needs: Comfort, stimulation, caring and communicating relationships

Contraindications: Avoid touch communications in nearness tension or when working with suspicious persons

Tour the health care facility with the person When a person experiences anxiety associated with health care, escort him through the facility and introduce him to the personnel.

Rationale: Safety and comfort arise from familiar and predictable situations.

Fulfilled Needs: Comfort, protection from psychologic threat, predictable and orderly world
Contraindications: Delay if the tour heightens anxiety

Turn off audible monitor signals When loud monitor signals are disturbing the
person, turn the signals off. This will require the nurse to concentrate on the visual
monitor signals.
Rationale: Turning off audible monitor signals provides a quiet environment that
promotes comfort.
Fulfilled Needs: Comfort, sleep and rest, protection from physical harm

Turn the mattress frequently Turn the bed mattress end-over-end and side-over-
side alternately every day if possible and not less than once a week.
Rationale: Mattress rotation prevents the formation of weakened, sagging mattress
areas. It provides a smooth, level lying surface for good back support, body alignment,
comfort, and provides assistance in dependency needs.
Fulfilled Needs: Comfort, protection from physical harm, dependence

Use a chest restraint Use chest restraints so that free movement of the limbs is still
possible. Be sure that the restraint is tied to the bed, with the person close enough to
the head of the bed, so that he cannot slip down or off the side of the bed and strangle
himself.
Rationale: Limb restraints result in the discomfort of arm and leg immobility, increased pressure on skin tissue, and heightened anxiety when loss of mobility is realized. Chest restraints allow arm and leg mobility, and promote comfort in the
knowledge that one is not completely powerless.
Fulfilled Needs: Comfort, protection from physical harm, protection from psychologic threat

Use a large-holed nipple for feeding When an infant is struggling to obtain liquid through a nipple or when the infant is in a weakened condition and will have to ex-
pend large amounts of energy to obtain milk, use a nipple with a larger than usual hole.
Rationale: When the amount of energy expended to obtain nourishment approaches
the amount of energy produced by the nutrients, the infant will fail to thrive.
Fulfilled Needs: Fluid and electrolyte balance. Nutritional balance, comfort
Contraindications: Swallowing difficulty

Use a small-holed nipple for feeding When feeding the infant a bottle, use a
nipple with a small hole.
Rationale: A small-holed nipple increases the length of feeding time and satisfies the
infant's desire for prolonged sucking.
Fulfilled Needs: Comfort
Contraindications: Infant weakness, intense infant hunger

Use a waist safety strap during mobility When a person is relearning to walk or
is very weak when walking, place a safety strap around his waist. Hold the strap and
stand behind the person during his relearning efforts.
Rationale: Safety straps allow for mobility freedom, protect against potential falling,
and assist in illness dependency.
Fulfilled Needs: Protection from physical harm, dependence

Use direct eye contact to terminate excessive crying When a depressed
person cries excessively, sit directly in front of him, hold his hand, and ask him to look
into your eyes. This technique usually stops crying.
Rationale: The termination of exhaustive crying reduces energy consumption and
promotes comfort.

Fulfilled Needs: Comfort, protection from physical harm

Use either the head-tilt or jaw-thrust maneuver to maintain an airway[20]

When there is evidence that air is not moving through the person's airway, place the person flat on his back.

Head-tilt maneuver: With the fingers of one hand, lift the lower jaw forward. With the other hand on the person's forehead, tip the head backward.

Jaw-thrust maneuver: Place three fingers behind the angle of the lower jaw, apply pressure, and thrust the lower jaw into a jutting-out position.

Rationale: Upward jaw movement brings the tongue forward and maintains an open airway.

Fulfilled Needs: Tissue oxygenation or perfusion, protection from physical harm

Use methods for stimulating urination

If a person is having difficulty urinating, try several methods. Have a man stand or a woman assume the usual sitting position, provide the sound of nearby running water, pour water over the perineum, or sit the person in a tub of warm water, if such is not contraindicated.

Rationale: The standing or sitting position increases gravity pull within the bladder, promoting urine flow, and is a natural voiding position. Sitting in a tub of warm water stimulates the bladder by increasing its circulation and relaxes the meatal sphincter. Running water or pouring water over the perineum psychologically suggests voiding.

Fulfilled Needs: Waste elimination of urine

Use paper or transparent tape instead of adhesive on the skin

Instead of using adhesive tape on the skin, use paper or transparent tape.

Rationale: Paper or transparent tape is nonirritating, prevents tissue trauma, and promotes comfort.

Fulfilled Needs: Protection from physical harm

Use pleasant odors to mask unpleasant odors

When there are odors that cannot be removed as in cancer or infection, mask the unpleasant odor with a scented candle, wick deodorizer, spray deodorizer, or place bars of perfumed soap about or cotton balls with a drop of oil of wintergreen on them.

Rationale: When odors cannot be removed, masking the odors with pleasant scents will bring relief from the intense odor.

Fulfilled Needs: Comfort

Contraindications: An allergy to scented products.

Use separate hyperalimentation infusion sets for incompatible solutions

When administering hyperalimentation solutions of fat, carbohydrates, and amino acids, use different infusion sets.

Rationale: Incompatible solutions clump, cause tube clogging, and change the rate of infusion.

Fulfilled Needs: Protection from physical harm

Use simple words and short sentences

When persons have impaired communication ability, use short sentences composed of simple, common words.

Rationale: The use of simple words and sentences facilitates ease in understanding messages.

Fulfilled Needs: Comfort, caring and communicating relationships

Use small-gauge injection needles

When injecting a person who bleeds easily, use the smallest possible needle gauge.

Rationale: The smaller the needle puncture, the lower the probability of severe bleeding.

Fulfilled Needs: Protection from physical harm

Use sterile technique   Maintain sterile technique when doing procedures that involve sterile equipment, sterile body cavities (bladder, trachea), or wounds.

Rationale: Sterile technique minimizes microorganism entrance into the catheters, wounds, etc.

Fulfilled Needs: Cleanliness, protection from physical harm

Use the person's name frequently   Whenever the opportunity arises, call the person by name.

Rationale: The comprehension of identity minimizes disorientation. A person's name is his most basic core of identity.

Fulfilled Needs: Comfort, protection from psychologic threat, recognition

Ventilate the person (ET)   When respirations have ceased as a result of accident or a cardiopulmonary pathologic state, immediately administer artificial ventilation. Remove foreign matter from the mouth and pharynx. Bend the head backward. Push the jaw outward to move the tongue from the back of the throat. Pinch the nostrils closed. Open the person's mouth wide. Take a deep breath. Place your mouth on his and blow vigorously into his airway. Remove your mouth and watch for chest movement and returned air through the mouth and nose. Repeat the procedure approximately 12 times a minute until respirations are spontaneous or mechanical respirator assistance is available. If the person is a child, place your mouth over the child's nose and mouth and promote shallow breaths about 20 times a minute. Moderate intermittent pressure on the diaphragm also will stimulate respirations. The pressure should be applied only for inspiration and omitted momentarily for expiration.

Rationale: Oxygen and carbon dioxide exchange is essential to life and the prevention of brain tissue damage.

Fulfilled Needs: Tissue oxygenation or perfusion, waste elimination of carbon dioxide, protection from physical harm

Ventilate the person mouth-to-stoma or bag-to-stoma when the person has a laryngectomy/tracheostomy (ET)   When a person who has had a laryngectomy requires resuscitation, place the person on his back. Place your mouth around the stoma (or tracheostomy tube) and blow air into the trachea until the chest rises. Allow time for the chest to fall and repeat the procedure. If the chest fails to rise, place the palm of the hand over the lips and mouth. Hold the jaw upward and pinch the nose closed before resuscitation.

Rationale: When a person has a total laryngectomy, air cannot reach the lungs by way of the mouth or nose and must be administered through the stoma.

Fulfilled Needs: Tissue oxygenation or perfusion, waste elimination of carbon dioxide, protection from physical harm

Verbalize daily the person's successful progress   At the end of each day, assist the person to enumerate verbally the success and progress made since the previous day, no matter how small that progress may be.

Rationale: Focusing attention on success promotes positive self-attitudes.

Fulfilled Needs: Comfort, protection from psychologic threat, high evaluation of self, sense of adequacy

Wait for a response to one message before delivering another   When a person has communication difficulties, wait until there is clear evidence that the first message has been received and interpreted before going on to the second message.

Rationale: The reception and interpretation of messages is reduced by perceptual overload. Comfort is promoted through effective communication with others.

Fulfilled Needs: Comfort, caring and communicating relationships

Walk with the person   When a person indicates a need to move about to decrease internal stress, is in need of companionship, or requires close supervision, walk with the person.

Rationale: Comfort and safety are promoted through relatedness to others, the ability to communicate needs, and protection associated with physical limitations.

Fulfilled Needs: Comfort, protection form physical harm, protection and psychologic threat, caring and communicating relationships

Warm the dialysis fluid before instillation Warm the dialysis fluid to body temperature (98–99° F) before instilling it into the peritoneal cavity.

Rationale: Warming dialysis fluid prevents abdominal cramping and helps maintain normal body temperature.

Fulfilled Needs: Normal temperature, comfort

Wash the brush and comb with a parasiticide Make a water and parasiticide solution. Soak the comb and brush of a person with hair infestations in the solution.

Rationale: A parasiticide kills lice or nits transferred to the comb and brush from infected hair.

Fulfilled Needs: Cleanliness, protection from physical harm

Wash the person's hands Wash the person's hands before meals and after elimination.

Rationale: Cleanliness, through hand-washing, prevents infection and promotes comfort.

Fulfilled Needs: Comfort, cleanliness, protection from physical harm

Wash your hands between contacts Wash hands thoroughly with water, soap, friction rubbing, and rinsing. Repeat after each contact with a person or contaminated articles.

Rationale: Surface removal of infectious microorganisms decreases the potential for the transfer of disease from one person to another.

Fulfilled Needs: Cleanliness, protection from physical harm

Wear a clean gown and mask Wear a fresh gown and mask with each patient contact and discard them afterward.

Rationale: A clean gown and mask prevent the transfer of pathogen from person to person. Reuse of gowns and masks reduces the safety factor because of bacteria accumulation.

Fulfilled Needs: Cleanliness, protection from physical harm

Wear a mask when suctioning When suctioning a person with a tracheostomy, wear a mask.

Rationale: Since suctioning requires proximity with the person, wearing a mask prevents the spread of bacteria into the trachea by the person suctioning.

Fulfilled Needs: Cleanliness, protection from physical harm

Wear sterile gloves Wear sterile gloves when doing sterile procedures such as suctioning a tracheostomy, dressing changes, sterile soaks, packing a wound, and catheterizations.

Rationale: Sterile gloves prevent the transfer of bacteria from one person to another.

Fulfilled Needs: Cleanliness, protection from physical harm

Withhold food until the person requests it Inform the person that his food will not be served until he asks for it.

Rationale: The availibility of choice enhances the person's control over a situation. When there is gastric distress, food will be most comforting when the person feels hungry or desires food.

Fulfilled Needs: Comfort

Contraindications: Prolonged periods of no food intake

Withhold the/all drug(s) Refrain from giving drugs that cause toxic, allergic, or other harmful side effects in the person.

Rationale: Harmful effects from drugs may increase in severity with each dose taken, even causing death. Some drugs cause insidious effects such as electrolyte imbalance.

Fulfilled Needs: Protection from physical harm

Contraindications: When drugs are essential to the maintenance of life, consult with the physician before withholding them

Withhold the oxygen therapy Remove the oxygen equipment when the person who has received large and prolonged doses of oxygen therapy suddenly develops decreased respirations.

Rationale: Excessive oxygenation of the blood reduces the respiratory stimulating effect of carbon dioxide resulting in depressed respirations.

Fulfilled Needs: Protection from physical harm

Wrap the amputation stump Wrap an elastic bandage around the amputation stump. Begin at the mid-anterior thigh, bringing one length of bandage down to the stump, under the stump, and up over the anterior stump and thigh. A crisscross or figure-eight pattern is used, never a circular pattern. Apply the bandage with even pressure and change in the morning, afternoon, and before bedtime.

Rationale: Wrapping the stump shrinks and shapes it in preparation for a prosthesis, gives support to soft tissue, decreases edema, and promotes comfort.

Fulfilled Needs: Comfort, protection from physical harm

NURSING
OBSERVATIONS

Auscultate and palpate the arteriovenous shunt for patency   Place the stethoscope on the venous side of the shunt and listen for a bruit. Place your fingers over the shunt and feel for a thrill.

Rationale: Absence of a bruit or a palpable thrill indicates inadequate blood flow or pressure within the vein due to clotting within the arteriovenous shunt.

Fulfilled Needs: Protection from physical harm

Auscultate the abdomen for abnormal bowel sounds[125,253]   Place the stethoscope bell over each abdominal quadrant and listen for absent, diminished, gurgling, or rushing bowel sounds, succussion splash, bruit, and peritoneal friction rub.

Rationale: Absent or diminished bowel sounds indicate peritoneal irritation or intestinal obstruction. Gurgling bowel sounds, which sound like broken, noisy current, are associated with partial pyloric or intestinal obstruction and excessive intestinal contraction as in diarrhea or colic. Rushing bowel sounds, which sound like rushing water, indicate obstruction. Succussion splash, which sounds like fluid striking or dashing about, is associated with excessive abdominal fluid, gastric dilatation, and obstruction of the stomach. This sound is normal after the intake of large amounts of fluid. A bruit is heard as a whish-whish, blowing sound over the abdominal aorta. It indicates arterial occlusion or dilatation and is associated with an aneurysm. Peritoneal friction rub, which sounds like two pieces of leather being rubbed together, suggests peritoneal inflammation and is most commonly associated with splenic infarction.

Fulfilled Needs: Protection from physical harm

Auscultate the abdomen for renewed bowel sounds   When abdominal bowel sounds have been absent, listen periodically for the return of normal bowel sounds.

Rationale: Renewed bowel sounds indicate that an intestinal obstruction has been cleared or that bowel function has returned after gastrointestinal surgery.

Fulfilled Needs: Protection from physical harm

Auscultate the apical heartbeat and palpate the radial pulses for a pulse deficit   Count the radial pulse rate and listen to and count the heartbeat. If the rates differ, a pulse deficit exists.

Rationale: A pulse deficit indicates the presence of atrial fibrillation, during which some of the ventricular contractions do not produce enough blood to result in a radial pulse.

Fulfilled Needs: Protection from physical harm

Auscultate the apical heartbeat for rate and rhythm   Place the stethoscope diaphragm over the apex (the point of maximum impulse) and listen for a normal heart rate and rhythm.

Rationale: Auscultation of the apical heartbeat allows for accurate counting of the pulse of infants, young children, and critically ill persons. It also indicates the adequacy of cardiac function, since abnormalities are readily recognized.

Fulfilled Needs: Protection from physical harm

Auscultate the bone for crepitus[125]   Listen with the stethoscope for a grating sound heard when the body part is cautiously moved.

Rationale: Crepitus bone sounds indicate bone fracture.

Fulfilled Needs: Protection from physical harm

Auscultate the carotid arteries for bruit[125]   With the stethoscope, listen over the carotid artery for the whish-whish blowing sound of a bruit (murmur).

Rationale: A bruit over the carotid artery indicates arterial constriction or dilatation and is associated with aneurysm, arteriosclerosis, and thyroid artery dilatation in thyrotoxicosis.

Fulfilled Needs: Protection from physical harm

Auscultate the chest for abnormal breath sounds[125,253]   In a quiet place, have the person sit upright and breathe deeply through his mouth. With a stethoscope, proceed from the chest top downward and from right to left. Listen for and identify duration of breath sounds. Normally, there is a long inspiratory phase and a short expiratory phase with a "whishing" sound over the lung surface. Listen for the quality of sound such as absent, diminished, bronchial, bronchovesicular, asthmatic, and amphoric breath sounds.

Rationale: Absent and diminished breath sounds indicate airflow obstruction. They are associated with atelectasis, pleural effusion, emphysema, airway obstruction, pneumothorax, or consolidation. Bronchial (tubular) breath sounds are short inspiratory and prolonged expiratory breath sounds. On expiration, there is a harsh, high-pitched lung sound like wind going through a hollow tube or breathing through a clay pipe. They are associated with pulmonary consolidation or compression of pulmonary tissue. Bronchovesicular breathing is normal except when heard in areas other than the manubrium sterni and upper interscapular region. In such cases, it indicates pulmonary consolidation or compression of pulmonary tissue. Asthmatic (wheezing) breath sounds have a hissing, whistling sound. They indicate airflow obstruction and are associated with atelectasis, pulmonary edema, and airway obstruction. Amphoric (cavernous) breath sounds, which sound like air being blown over the mouth of a bottle, indicate a pulmonary cavity.

Fulfilled Needs: Protection from physical harm

Auscultate the chest for abnormal heart sounds[33,125,253,780]   Using the stethoscope diaphragm, listen over the entire anterior chest wall as follows:

1. Listen to and count the heartbeat.
2. Listen for a regular or irregular rhythm.
3. Identify the first and second heart sounds.
4. In the aortic area (right second intercostal space) the S_2 (diastolic sound) is normally louder than the S_1 (systolic sound).
5. In the pulmonic area (left second intercostal space), S_2 is also louder than S_1.
6. Physiologic (normal) splitting may be heard in the pulmonic area and normally varies with respirations. Listen for splitting of the second heart into two sounds, resulting in a duplication, or doubling sound. In an abnormally wide physiologic split, there is no variation with respiraions.
7. In the tricuspid area (fifth left interspace close to the sternum) and mitral area

(fifth left interspace medial to the midclavicular line), S_1 is normally louder than S_2.

8. Listen for extra sounds in systole and diastole, such as S_3 (Ken-tucky), S_4 (Tenn-e-ssee), systolic and diastolic murmurs, pericardial friction rubs, gallops, and venous hums.

9. Upon hearing a murmur, determine if it is innocent or organic. An innocent murmur is systolic, grade 1–3, and does not radiate; the heart sounds are normal, and there are no cardiac symptoms. An organic murmur is diastolic, grade 3–6, radiates to other areas, and has a harsh quality; the person presents with significant cardiac complaints.

10. After listening with the stethoscope diaphragm, which reveals high-pitched sounds, repeat the procedure with the stethoscope bell, which reveals low-pitched sounds.

Rationale: Abnormal heart sounds indicate specific pathology.

Loud first heart sound: Mitral stenosis, anemia, hyperthyroidism, exercise, hypertension, emotional excitement.

Diminished first heart sound: Obesity, emphysema, pericardial or pleural effusion, first-degree AV block, rheumatic heart disease, arteriosclerotic heart disease, myocardial infarction, cardiac failure.

Splitting of the first heart sound: Bundle branch block; sometimes this can be normal.

Loud aortic second heart sound: Arterial hypertension, aortic regurgitation, aortic coarctation, aortic aneurysm.

Diminished aortic second heart sound: Aortic stenosis.

Loud pulmonic second heart sound: Mitral stenosis, left ventricular failure, pulmonary hypertension, atrial septal defect, truncus arteriosus.

Diminished pulmonic second heart sound: Pulmonic stenosis, atrial septal defect.

Inspiratory splitting of the second heart sound: Right bundle branch block, atrial septal defect, pulmonary stenosis, mitral regurgitation.

Expiratory splitting of the second heart sound: Aortic stenosis, left bundle branch block.

Third heart sound: This is normal in children, young adults, and pregnant women. In older persons, when heard in the apical area, it indicates overfilling of a failing ventricle.

Fourth heart sound: AV block; it indicates unsynchronized ventricular beats or forceful atrial contractions from left ventricular hypertrophy.

Fulfilled Needs: Protection from physical harm

Auscultate the chest for abnormal voice sounds (pectoriloquy, bronchophony, or egophony)[125,253]   In a quiet place, have the patient sit upright. With a stethoscope, proceed from the chest top downward and from right to left, while the person repeatedly whispers "ninety-nine" or "one-two-three." Listen for pectoriloquy, in which these sounds are transmitted distinctly through the lung though they are whispered. Listen for bronchophony, in which spoken voice sounds are greatly increased. Then, have the patient say "e" out loud. Listen for egophony, in which the "e" sounds like an "a."

Rationale: Pectoriloquy indicates increased lung volume and is associated with pulmonary consolidation, embolus, or atelectasis. Bronchophony indicates a hollow lung space or increased lung volume and is associated with pulmonary consolidation. Egophony indicates increased lung volume or the presence of pleural fluid and is associated with pulmonary consolidation or pleural effusion.

Fulfilled Needs: Protection from physical harm

Auscultate the chest for crepitus[125,253]   In a quiet place, have the person sit upright and breathe deeply through his mouth. With a stethoscope, proceed from the chest top downward and from right to left. Listen for a grating sound.

Rationale: Crepitus rib sounds indicate rubbing fractured rib ends and are associated with rib fracture.

Fulfilled Needs: Protection from physical harm

Auscultate the chest for lung aeration[125,253]   Using the stethoscope diaphragm or bell, listen for the sound of air moving through the lungs on inspiration and expiration.

Rationale: Proper lung aeration is essential to normal body function and gas exchange.

Fulfilled Needs: Protection from physical harm

Auscultate the chest for pleural friction rub[125,253]   In a quiet place, have the patient sit upright and breathe deeply through his mouth. With a stethoscope, proceed from the chest top downward and from right to left. Listen with each inspiration and expiration for a sound like rubbing sandpaper or a leather creaking sound.

Rationale: Friction rub sounds indicate pulmonary inflammation or rubbing pulmonary membranes. They are associated with pulmonary embolus and pleurisy.

Fulfilled Needs: Protection from physical harm

Auscultate the chest for rales and/or rhonchi (adventitious sounds)[125,253] In a quiet place, have the patient sit upright and breathe deeply through his mouth. With a stethoscope, proceed from the chest top downward and from right to left. Listen for gurgling, bubbling and crackling rales, and musical or sonorous rhonchi.

Rationale: Gurgling rales are loud, low-pitched, intermittent noisy current sounds best heard at the beginning of inspiration. They indicate fluid in the large bronchi and are associated with pulmonary edema and airway obstruction. Bubbling rales sound like bubbles being blown underwater or fizzling carbonated beverages. They are best heard halfway through inspiration. Bubbling rales indicate thin fluid moving in small bronchi and are associated with pulmonary congestion, edema, consolidation, embolus, cavity, and infection. Crackling rales sound like crackling cellophane and are heard either at the end of inspiration or on both inspiration and expiration. They indicate thick exudate or inflamed edematous lung alveoli. They are associated with pulmonary consolidation, congestion, cavity, embolus, and infection. Musical rhonchi have a high-pitched, tinkling sound. Sonorous rhonchi have a snoring sound. They indicate pulmonary inflammation, bronchial or pulmonary fluid, or thick exudate. Both are associated with pulmonary congestion or edema.

Fulfilled Needs: Protection from physical harm

Auscultate the head for cranial bruit[125,253]   Place the stethoscope bell over the cranium and listen for a blowing sound over the mastoid process, the temples, or each closed eye.

Rationale: Cranial bruit sounds indicate dilatation or constriction of cranial vessels. They are associated with aneurysms.

Fulfilled Needs: Protection from physical harm

Auscultate the head for cranial crepitus[125,253]   Place the stethoscope bell over

the cranium and listen over the mastoid process, the temples, and each closed eye. Listen for a grating sound.
Rationale: Cranial crepitus sounds indicate cranial bone fracture.
Fulfilled Needs: Protection from physical harm

Auscultate the head for cranial friction sounds[125,253]   Place the stethoscope bell over the cranium and listen over the mastoid process, the temples, and each closed eye for sounds like sandpaper being rubbed or leather creaking during bone movement.
Rationale: Cranial friction sounds indicate bone fracture.
Fulfilled Needs: Protection from physical harm

Auscultate the thyroid for bruit[125,253]   Place the stethoscope over the thyroid gland and listen for a blowing sound. It is heard near the center of the thyroid gland.
Rationale: As the thyroid gland enlarges, accelerated blood flow through the thyroid arteries causes the hum. Thyroid bruits are associated with thyrotoxicosis.
Fulfilled Needs: Protection from physical harm

Check for fluctuation of the fluid level in the water-seal container   Periodically check to see that the level of the water in the long tubing inside the chest drainage container goes up and down simultaneously with respiratory inspiration and expiration.
Rationale: Proper fluctuation of fluid within the water-seal drainage system indicates that the system is functioning properly. When fluctuation stops, the tubing is either obstructed or the lung has reexpanded.
Fulfilled Needs: Protection from physical harm

Check for infiltration of the solution   Watch for signs that the solution may have leaked into the subcutaneous tissue, evident by swelling at the injection site.
Rationale: Solution infiltration into tissues could cause tissue damage.
Fulfilled Needs: Protection from physical harm

Check suction equipment for correct functioning   Determine if the suction equipment is functioning adequately. Note the amount of suction force. Check the quality of drainage, as well as the amount and any unusual characteristics.
Rationale: Well-functioning suction equipment is essential to the drainage of undesirable substances from body cavities. Removal of these substances often produces comfort.
Fulfilled Needs: Comfort, protection from physical harm

Check that the traction weights are hanging free   Periodically check that the traction weights are hanging free, have not fallen to the floor, and are not caught in the bed grooves or chairs.
Rationale: Free-hanging traction weights allow for constant pulling pressure against specific bones, maintaining the healing position.
Fulfilled Needs: Protection from physical harm

Check the cane/crutches for correct length   *Cane:*   Have the person stand erect and hold the cane head. Place the cane tip a few inches in front and to the side of the patient's foot. If the cane is at the proper height, the person's arm will be at a 30° angle. If the cane is too long, remove its rubber tip and saw it to the correct length.
   Crutches: Have the person lay supine. Measure from the anterior fold of the axilla to a point 6 inches out from the person's heel. This is the length that the crutch should

measure and be adjusted to if it is an inaccurate length.

Rationale: Proper cane and crutch length is essential for correct body alignment, weight bearing, comfort, and mobility.

Fulfilled Needs: Protection from physical harm

Check the chest bottle drainage for quantity and character Check the chest drainage system for bright bloody drainage. Determine the amount of drainage every hour and report an excess of 125 cc/hour.

Rationale: Bright red blood or copious chest drainage indicates blood loss, tissue damage, or imbalanced thoracic pressure.

Fulfilled Needs: Protection from physical harm

Check the crutches for intact rubber tips Periodically check the rubber tips on crutches for adequate width, for wearing on one side, and for secure attachment to the crutch.

Rationale: A firm, stable base is essential to safe ambulation and prevention of falling.

Fulfilled Needs: Protection from physical harm

Check the crutch handbar for position Check that the crutch handbar is positioned properly so when the patient places weight on the bar, his elbow is flexed at a 30-degree angle.

Rationale: A properly positioned crutch handbar is essential for correct body alignment, weight bearing, and mobility.

Fulfilled Needs: Protection from physical harm

Check the dialysis circuit for leakage Watch for a leak in either the peritoneal or hemodialysis setup.

Rationale: Leakage within the dialysis circuit causes fluid loss and heightens the infection potential.

Fulfilled Needs: Protection from physical harm

Check the drainage system for leakage Intermittently, look over the chest, genitourinary, gastrointestinal, etc., drainage system for any sign of leakage around connection sites.

Rationale: A closed drainage system minimizes the potential for bacterial invasion into the tubing insertion site. The water-seal drainage, which is closed to atmospheric pressure, prevents air from replacing drainage and permits return of the normal intrapleural negative pressure.

Fulfilled Needs: Protection from physical harm

Check the environmental controls on the incubator periodically Check that the premature infant's incubator is being controlled at an environmental temperature of 32–36° C, that oxygen concentrations are individualized according to blood gases, and that the humidity is around 40–60%.

Rationale: Warm environmental temperature is essential to the life of the premature infant because the child is unable to maintain body heat, due to lack of insulating skin fat, poor reflex control of skin capillaries, and inactive small muscles. High air humidity is essential because of the infant's tendency toward dehydration, which results in weight loss and temperature instability. Oxygen concentrations must meet his individualized needs.

Fulfilled Needs: Protection from physical harm

Check the general functioning of the hemodynamic monitoring system[249] Check the electronic devices that monitor arterial, venous, pulmonary artery, and intracranial pressure. Check for patency and placement of the catheter and for proper balance, calibration, and airtightness of the system. Check that electrical signals and alarms are working efficiently.

Rationale: Correct pressure measurements are essential for the maintenance of life in the critically ill. The recording of such measurements is dependent on an efficiently functioning hemodynamic monitoring system.

Fulfilled Needs: Protection from physical harm

Check the hemodialysis AV shunt for cleanliness and patency   Check the AV shunt for blood clotting, tube kinking, and for signs of infection.

Rationale: The arterial tube of the dialysis shunt carries toxic blood to be filtered into the dialysis machine and the venous tube carries the detoxified blood back to the person. Recognition and correction of nonfunctioning, inefficient therapeutic devices promote safety and assure their therapeutic effect.

Fulfilled Needs: Protection from physical harm

Check the hemodialysis equipment for mechanical breakdown   Watch for signs that the artificial kidney is not mechanically sound. Look for clotting in the shunt or coils, rupture of the cellophane membrane, or decreased blood flow through the machine.

Rationale: Proper artificial kidney functioning is essential to patient safety and successful removal of body wastes.

Fulfilled Needs: Protection from physical harm

Check the hyperalimentation solution for cloudiness and precipitation   Check that the hyperalimentation fluid is not cloudy and that no precipitation of particles exists.

Rationale: The administration of therapeutically safe hyperalimentation solution is essential to patient safety.

Fulfilled Needs: Protection from physical harm

Check the label on the blood container for correct patient identification   Check the person's hospital identification number and his name, blood type, and Rh factor against the same data on the blood container.

Rationale: The infusion of blood intended for another person could lead to a serious blood transfusion reaction and even death.

Fulfilled Needs: Protection from physical harm

Check the monitor electrodes for placement periodically   Periodically check the placement and attachment of monitor electrodes on the skin. Placement should be as follows: #1 and #2 negative beneath the right clavicle, lead #1 positive beneath the left clavicle, lead #2 positive on the left upper thigh, and ground electrode on the right chest side.

Rationale: Recognition and correction of nonfunctioning, inefficient therapeutic devices promote safety and assure the intended effect of the device.

Fulfilled Needs: Protection from physical harm

Check the oxygen flow rate   When administering oxygen with a nonrebreathing mask, watch the bag as the patient inspires. If the bag completely collapses on inspiration, the oxygen flow rate is too low. If the bag collapses only partially on inspiration, the oxygen flow rate is sufficient.

Rationale: An adequate volume of oxygen is essential for blood and tissue oxygenation and life maintenance.

Fulfilled Needs: Protection from physical harm

Check the pacemaker for pacing rate   Verify pacemaker effectiveness. Count the apical pulse. Determine whether the generator light flashes and the dial needle

moves immediately before the pulse beat. Run an EKG strip and determine if a long or short straight line exists before each QRS complex.

Rationale: In a well-functioning pacemaker, one electrical stimulus coincides with each single heartbeat. If pacing occurs intermittently or if the straight line "blip" does not appear before each QRS complex on the EKG strip, it indicates an altered catheter position, dislodged or broken catheter, or some failure of the monitor equipment. If the pacing occurs more often than one electrical stimulus to one heartbeat, it may indicate a tissue reaction to the catheter or possible infection.

Fulfilled Needs: Protection from physical harm

Check the peritoneal dialysis catheter for leakage or displacement Continuously check the peritoneal catheter for leakage around or displacement from the abdominal site of insertion.

Rationale: The normal flow of dialysate solution into and out of the peritoneal cavity removes diffusible toxins, urea, and electrolytes through the peritoneal membrane from the blood.

Fulfilled Needs: Protection from physical harm

Check the peritoneal dialysis fluid for bloody or cloudy return Watch for blood or milkiness in the dialysis fluid being withdrawn from the peritoneum.

Rationale: Heparin placed in the dialysis fluid could precipitate bleeding. Cloudy dialysis fluid return indicates protein loss.

Fulfilled Needs: Protection from physical harm

Check the peritoneal dialysis fluid for retention or drainage in excess of 500 cc Continuously check to determine if there is an excess of 500 cc of dialysate solution retained or drained from the peritoneal cavity.

Rationale: An excessive amount of fluid lost through peritoneal drainage will result in excessive electrolyte loss. When large amounts of dialysate fluid are not returned during peritoneal drainage, it indicates that an excess amount has been absorbed and could lead to circulatory overload.

Fulfilled Needs: Protection from physical harm

Check the respirator/mechanical ventilator for proper functioning Check how well the respirator or ventilator is functioning, especially if changes in the patient's respirations alter the respirator's cycling.

Rationale: The proper exchange of oxygen and carbon dioxide through respirations is essential to life.

Fulfilled Needs: Protection from physical harm

Check the solution for flow rate Check that fluids are not flowing at either excessively slow or rapid rates, including intravenous fluids, hypodermoclysis, tidal drainage, tube feeding, dialysis, and hyperalimentation.

Rationale: Excessively slow flow rates may contribute to inadequate hydration or nutrition and ineffective therapy. Excessively rapid flow rates can contribute to circulatory overload, shock, or gastric dilatation.

Fulfilled Needs: Protection from physical harm

Check the traction ropes and pulleys for alignment Periodically check if the traction ropes are secure in the pulley wheel grooves, the supporting apparatus is free of the pulleys, and good alignment exists. Watch for frayed cords and loosened knots.

Rationale: Properly aligned traction ropes and pulleys allow for constant pulling pressure against specific bones so the healing position is uninterrupted.

Fulfilled Needs: Protection from physical harm

Check the tube for patency and/or cleanliness Check that tubes are not obstructed by kinking, secretions, or other collected material. Watch for free-flowing

drainage of fluids (includes intravenous, genitourinary, gastric, airway, chest, local drainage tubes).
Rationale: Recognition and correction of nonfunctioning tubes associated with therapeutic procedures promote safety and assure the therapeutic effect of the treatment.
Fulfilled Needs: Protection from physical harm

Check the tube placement before giving the tube feeding Before giving tube feeding, check that the tube is located in the stomach by aspirating for gastric contents with a syringe. Place the open end of the tube in water. If bubbles appear on exhalation, the tube is in the respiratory tract and the feeding should not be given. If there are no bubbles, the tube is in the stomach and feeding may proceed.
Rationale: The introduction of liquids or food into a feeding tube accidentally located in or proximal to the lungs can cause death.
Fulfilled Needs: Protection from physical harm

Check the walker for proper height Have the person grasp the top of the walker frame. If the walker height is correct, the patient's elbow will be bent at a 30° angle. If the height is incorrect, a new walker should be provided.
Rationale: Proper walker height is essential for correct body alignment, weight bearing, and mobility.
Fulfilled Needs: Protection from physical harm

Check to ensure that the top of the crutch does not press into the axilla When the person is using the crutch or resting on it, check to be certain that the crutch top does not put pressure on the axilla.
Rationale: Pressure on the axilla from the top of a crutch can cause nerve damage that could paralyze the arm.
Fulfilled Needs: Protection from physical harm

Compare the preoperative and postoperative response level Determine whether the person's level of cerebral response is the same as before surgery, especially for patients whose surgery required artificial oxygenation or circulation maintenance by pump.
Rationale: Inadequate oxygenation of cerebral tissues will result in impaired cerebral function.
Fulfilled Needs: Protection from physical harm

Count the number of sanitary pads used Count the number of saturated sanitary pads used within an 8-hour period. Determine the amount of saturation by one-fourth, one-half, three-fourths, or totally saturated.
Rationale: If more than four sanitary pads are saturated in an 8-hour period, it indicates excessive vaginal bleeding.
Fulfilled Needs: Protection from physical harm

Determine teaching effectiveness by testing, verbal feedback, and return demonstration Determine if learning has occurred after the person has been taught. Note if there are adequate scores on written tests, if the person can verbalize the new information, and if he can correctly demonstrate the health material or skills taught. Observe for increased self-direction and for verbalization that the information is meaningful to the patient.
Rationale: By testing, feedback, and demonstration, we can determine if teaching has been achieved. Information and skills that have not been learned need to be retaught until learning occurs.
Fulfilled Needs: Protection from physical harm, protection from psychologic threat, mastery and competence in skills, increased learning

Determine the cerebral perfusion pressure[249] Determine the amount of blood being circulated to the brain. Normally, cerebral perfusion pressure (PP) is equal to the mean arterial pressure (MAP). The PP is determined by MAP minus the intracranial pressure (ICP).

Rationale: When the cerebral PP is decreased, it indicates that the ICP is increased. When the ICP equals the cerebral PP, cerebral blood flow ceases.

Fulfilled Needs: Protection from physical harm

Determine the degree of insight that the person has Watch for verbal and nonverbal clues as to the person's understanding of the problem. Observe if he recognizes its existence, knows why and how it occurred, and how it might be resolved.

Rationale: The degree of insight greatly affects the recognition and resolution of problems.

Fulfilled Needs: Protection from physical harm, protection from psychologic threat

Determine the extent of group pressure conformity Watch for the person's strength or weakness in conforming to group pressure.

Rationale: Self-confidence and well-defined values are compatible with strong resistance to group pressure. Persons lacking self-confidence and well-defined values perceive group pressure as threatening and submit to that pressure by conforming.

Fulfilled Needs: Protection from psychologic threat

Determine the extent of lack of information Determine the person's overall general level of knowledge.

Rationale: The person's general level of knowledge usually indicates interests, the extent of formal education, and the capacity to recognize and solve problems.

Fulfilled Needs: Protection from physical harm, protection from psychologic threat

Determine the extent of the child's comprehension of death Watch for verbal and nonverbal clues as to the child's concept of what death is and of how he copes with it.

Rationale: At different levels of growth and development, a child's perception of death and his adaptation responses to stress vary.

Fulfilled Needs: Protection from psychologic threat

Determine the infant's Apgar score Determine the status of the newborn during the first 10 minutes of life. Score the following conditions as 0, 1, or a high of 2: heart rate, respiratory effort, muscle tone, reflex irritability, and color. Total the score of all the conditions. An Apgar score of 7–10 indicates a good infant condition; 4–6 is fair; 0–3 is very poor.

Rationale: The infant's Apgar score serves as a baseline of information from which to plan patient care.

Fulfilled Needs: Protection from physical harm

Determine the influence of culture on the pain reaction After discovering the person's cultural background, watch for pain reactions frequently associated with that culture, such as the following: Italians react with fear of pain and need quick relief, Jewish persons become anxious over the source of pain and its meaning as it relates to family responsibility, and descendants of pioneer American families minimize pain and seldom complain.

Rationale: Awareness that persons react to pain according to cultural standards affects the nursing approach to the treatment of pain.

Fulfilled Needs: Protection from physical harm, protection from psychologic threat

Determine the need that the denial is serving Determine whether the denial is being used as a temporary mechanism to maintain emotional stability when the threat of crisis is emotionally overwhelming and the denial prevents complete disorganization or whether it is being used as an escape from problems, responsibility, and personal growth instead of more effective coping methods.

Rationale: By determining the reasons why the person is using denial, the nurse can more accurately initiate nursing interventions that will help and support the person.

Fulfilled Needs: Protection from psychologic threat

Determine the physiologic factors that increase or decrease drug absorption Determine which factors, specific to the person, increase or decrease his absorption of the drug. Drug absorption is decreased with impaired circulation, edema, tissue damage, old age, or obesity. Drug absorption is increased with rapid metabolic rate, in adolescents and young adults, underweight persons, and smokers.

Rationale: Awareness of increased or decreased drug absorption should result in the administration of correct drug dosages.

Fulfilled Needs: Comfort, protection from physical harm

Determine the precipitating factors Watch for and identify those factors that bring about pain, cyanosis, weakness, rapid pulse, etc.

Rationale: Awareness of those factors that contribute to distress supports prevention of their future occurrence.

Fulfilled Needs: Protection from physical harm

Determine the relieving factors Watch for and identify those situations and therapies that bring about cessation of the specific abnormality such as pain and dizziness.

Rationale: Awareness of factors that relieve impaired health is valuable in initiating therapy to relieve the condition.

Fulfilled Needs: Protection from physical harm

Determine the urgency for pain relief Determine how quickly pain relief needs to be given. If the cause of pain is life threatening, as in myocardial infarction, relief should be immediate. When a person has endured pain for a prolonged period, his tolerance for pain is decreased and he requires immediate relief. If moderate pain exists, then perhaps some delay may be tolerated. In all painful conditions, relief should be given as quickly as possible.

Rationale: Pain is a signal of threat or disruption of body integrity. Its degree reveals the severity of the threat and the rapidity with which relief must be given.

Fulfilled Needs: Protection from physical harm, protection from psychologic threat

Determine whether the denial is adaptive or nonadaptive Determine if the denial is an adaptive response to a crisis situation. Adaptive denial focuses on the threat, is temporary, and permits the person to function. When denial is nonadaptive, it persists for a long period, reduces functioning ability, and drains the person's psychic energy. It is nonadaptive when a person denies his own health needs or refuses to accept the implications of a health problem.

Rationale: Adaptive denial is a temporary stabilizing force. Nonadaptive denial can lead to severe psychologic disturbance. By determining the type of denial being used, the nurse can help the person by initiating therapeutic interventions.

Fulfilled Needs: Protection from psychologic threat

Determine whether the prosthesis is effective Determine if the patient is getting effective usefulness from the prosthesis or if it is causing any undesirable effects.

Rationale: A prosthesis assists the person in carrying out normal daily activities. Proper fit and quality are essential for safety.

Fulfilled Needs: Protection from physical harm

Estimate the amount of feeding the baby will need Determine the approximate amount of milk or similar feeding the child will need at different age levels.

1–2 months	3–4 oz feeding (24 oz total)
2–3 months	4–5 oz feeding (25 oz total)
3–4 months	6–8 oz feeding (24–28 oz total)
4–5 months	7–8 oz feeding (32 oz total)
5–6 months	1 quart of milk a day

Rationale: Adequate nutrition is essential to healthy growth and development.

Fulfilled Needs: Protection from physical harm

Estimate the blood volume loss Visually inspect for and estimate the amount of blood lost.

Rationale: A blood loss of 1,500 cc or more in an adult threatens life because a severely decreased circulating blood volume results in inadequate tissue oxygenation.

Fulfilled Needs: Protection from physical harm

Estimate the degree of pain experienced[769] Determine the approximate level of pain that the person is experiencing. Use the pain assessment tool developed by Kuempel, based on ratings from 1 to 10:

Childbirth	10
Passing kidney stones	10
Postsurgical coughing	10
Gallbladder attack	10
Spinal headache	10
Immediate postsurgical pain	10
Bone pain	8
Burn pain	7–8
Coronary thrombosis	4–6
Hand contractions	5
Migraine headache	5
Back pain	2–4
48-hour postsurgical pain	1–4
Stomach ulcer	2–3.5
Postsurgical walking	2
Toothache	2
Ordinary headache	0.5–1.5

Rationale: Although pain brings about highly individualized reactions in different persons and in the same person under different circumstances, the threshold for recognition of pain stimuli remains approximately equal from one person to another in whom the nervous system is functionally normal.

Fufilled Needs: Protection from physical harm

Estimate the degree of stress experienced Using the Social Readjustment Rating Scale* of Holmes and Rohe, estimate how much stress the person is experiencing in his present situation.

Life Event	Mean Value
1. Death of spouse	100
2. Divorce	73
3. Marital separation	65
4. Jail term	63
5. Death of close family member	63

---

*Reprinted with permission from T.H. Holmes and R.H. Rohe and from the Pergamon Press Ltd. The Social Readjustment Scale, *Journal of Psychosomatic Research* 11:213–218, 1967.

6.	Personal injury or illness	53
7.	Marriage	50
8.	Fired at work	47
9.	Marital reconciliation	45
10.	Retirement	45
11.	Change in health of family member	44
12.	Pregnancy	40
13.	Sex difficulties	39
14.	Gain of new family member	39
15.	Business readjustment	39
16.	Change in financial state	38
17.	Death of close friend	37
18.	Change to different line of work	36
19.	Change in number of arguments with spouse	35
20.	Mortgage over $10,000	31
21.	Foreclosure of mortgage or loan	30
22.	Change in responsibilities at work	29
23.	Son or daughter leaving home	29
24.	Trouble with in-laws	29
25.	Outstanding personal achievement	28
26.	Wife begins or stops work	26
27.	Begin or end school	26
28.	Change in living conditions	25
29.	Revision of personal habits	24
30.	Trouble with boss	23
31.	Change in work hours or conditions	20
32.	Change in residence	20
33.	Change in schools	20
34.	Change in recreation	19
35.	Change in church activities	19
36.	Change in social activities	18
37.	Mortgage or loan less than $10,000	17
38.	Change in sleeping habits	16
39.	Change in number of family get-togethers	15
40.	Change in eating habits	15
41.	Vacation	13
42.	Christmas	12
43.	Minor violations of the law	11

Rationale: Awareness of the amount of stress being experienced by the person supports a more realistic approach to therapeutic care.

Fulfilled Needs: Protection from psychologic threat

Evaluate the adequacy of the housing Determine if the facilities in which the person is housed have sufficient room, adequate sanitation, ventilation, lighting, heating, and furnishings and if they are safe and well kept.

Rationale: Adequate shelter is essential to protect us from the environment and for the maintenance of health.

Fulfilled Needs: Protection from physical harm

Evaluate the effectiveness of the pain-relief measures Look for clues that the pain-relief measures have been effective. Observe for verbalization of pain relief, relaxation of tense facial expressions, freedom of movement when movement was previously restricted, decreased restlessness, and a return of normal skin color.

Rationale: Evaluating the effectiveness of pain-relief measures determines if comfort has been provided or if another relief approach should be tried.

Fulfilled Needs: Protection from physical harm

Evaluate the pain for intensity and quality Watch for the severity and nature of the experienced pain. Pain intensity includes intractable, severe, moderate, or mild pain. Pain quality includes aching, burning, constrictive, cramping, gnawing, neuralgic, pleuritic, stabbing, stinging, throbbing, and tingling pain, as well as tenderness.

Rationale: Pain intensity and quality signal the degree of body threat and determines the relief approach.

Fulfilled Needs: Protection from physical harm, protection from psychologic threat

Evaluate the person's relatedness with others Determine the person's ability to interact with others. This includes communication abilities, acceptance of role and place in the life situation, and the ability to form meaningful relationships with skill and success.

Rationale: Psychologic comfort is promoted through the ability to relate to others.

Fulfilled Needs: Protection from psychologic threat

Evaluate the safety of the environment Watch for existing and potential safety hazards within the environment. These include high beds, spills on floors, belongings placed too far out of reach, fire hazards, poorly placed furniture, ineffective call buttons, inadequate lighting, and any other situation deemed unsafe for the person.

Rationale: A safe environment is essential to health.

Fulfilled Needs: Protection from physical harm

Evaluate the significance of emotional distress mannerisms Watch for nonverbal indications of emotional upset such as crying, hand wringing, floor pacing, chain smoking, lip and nail biting, fidgeting.

Rationale: When psychologic defenses are threatened, mannerisms give evidence of that threat.

Fulfilled Needs: Protection from psychologic threat

Evaluate the significance of nonverbal communication Watch for facial expressions, hand gestures, body postures and movements, clothing attire, associations with other persons, and preferences in life style peculiar to the person.

Rationale: Nonverbal communications reveal much about and promote understanding of the person.

Fulfilled Needs: Protection from psychologic threat

Evaluate the significance of spirituality in the person's life Determine how important the spiritual aspects of life are to the person by listening to his conversation and noticing his involvement in spiritual affairs.

Rationale: When spiritual involvement is important in health, it should be recognized as significant during illness.

Fulfilled Needs: Protection from psychologic threat

Identify abnormal perceptions Watch for indications that the person is receiving abnormal sensory input. Note any inability to discriminate between persons, distortion of one's self-image or the image of others, illusions in which one misperceives the identity of persons or objects, or hallucinations of an auditory, visual, olfactory, or tactile nature.

Rationale: Persons react to situations as they perceive them. Faulty perceptions are often the cause of abnormal behavior.

Fulfilled Needs: Protection from psychologic threat

Identify abnormal thought content Watch for indications that the person thinks about false beliefs, delusions regarding self or others, involuntary and unsuppressible obsessive thoughts, irrational phobias, autistic thinking, or prolonged fixed ideas.

Rationale: The thought process is impaired by physiologic or psychologic disequilibrium.

Fulfilled Needs: Protection from physical harm, protection from psychologic threat

Identify attention span abnormalities   Watch for inability to focus attention for any length of time or the concentration of attention on a single subject.
Rationale: The ability to function is impaired by attention span abnormalities.
Fulfilled Needs: Protection from physical harm, protection from psychologic threat

Identify cues that indicate some acceptance of reality   Listen for cues of the person's ability to accept the reality of the situation. In health situations, such cues would include statements such as, "I'm dying bit by bit," "I'm half dead," "I'm almost 6 feet under," and "I'm a peg-legged sailor." There are times when the person has not been told of a poor prognosis, yet he exhibits these cues because he has perceived the truth through nonverbal cues.
Rationale: Ill persons frequently come to accept the reality of situations through the nonverbal communications of others. They quickly perceive changes in the amount of attention they receive, new approaches by health personnel, and saddened family members who cannot hide their feelings. The ill person frequently returns the communication through indirect inferences. An awareness of the patient's level of perception and acceptance highly influences the course of treatment.
Fulfilled Needs: Protection from psychologic threat

Identify disturbing conversation topics   Listen for discussion of topics that cause tension or emotional upset.
Rationale: When psychologic defenses are threatened, emotional responses give evidence of that threat.

Fulfilled Needs: Protection from psychologic threat

Identify emotion-stimulating events/situations   Identify those environmental stimuli and situations that arouse undesirable feelings and cause stressful emotional reactions.
Rationale: Emotional comfort and safety are influenced by environmental stimuli.
Fulfilled Needs: Protection from psychologic threat

Identify inappropriate emotional responses   Determine if the person's emotional responses are appropriate to the situation. Does he laugh in a happy situation, or does he cry inappropriately when laughter is in order? Take into account cultural influences.
Rationale: When stress becomes so threatening that normal defenses become inadequate, response through inappropriate emotions becomes evident.
Fulfilled Needs: Protection from psychologic threat

Identify life values significant to the person   Identify those moral values that are important to the person.
Rationale: Value codes are essential to human safety and comfort.
Fulfilled Needs: Protection from psychologic threat

Identify potentially destructive behavior   Watch for potential suicide, assaultive, or threatening behavior.
Rationale: Potentially destructive behavior must be curtailed to preserve the safety of persons involved.
Fulfilled Needs: Protection from physical harm, protection from psychologic threat

Identify the appropriate use of defense mechanisms[416]   Recognize those unconscious mental mechanisms that the patient is using appropriately in an effort to maintain psychologic equilibrium. Appropriate defense mechanisms are as follows:

Identification that contributes to growth of conscience, gives the child a model for patterns of success, provides parental approval, reinforces the parent's positive attitudes toward the child, and develops the characteristic of empathy within the person.

Sublimation of sexual and aggressive impulses that is directed into socially acceptable behavior.

Repression that can involuntarily exclude from the consciousness unacceptable internal impulses and ideas, thus reducing anxiety and allowing the remaining tensions to be used constructively.

Denial that blocks out the occurrence of intolerable thoughts and situations only long enough to give the person time to adjust to that which is intolerable and move on to acceptance.

Reaction formation that denies the consciousness of unacceptable thoughts and feelings through the expression of directly opposite but acceptable thoughts and feelings.

Compensation that results in increasing self-esteem and feelings of security that occur from the person's strivings to overcome the sources of insecurity.

Rationalization that conceals the person's real motives with the result that self-esteem is maintained and guilt feeling resolved.

Substitution that provides an alternate but satisfactory goal in place of the original goal is always appropriate.

Displacement that allows the individual to avoid recognizing unacceptable feelings toward a person by displacing those same feelings toward another person or objects that represent that person.

Projection that provides comfort by recognizing in others those unfavorable characteristics in ourselves that we prefer not to admit exist.

Symbolism that results in merely transferring an emotional value to an object.

Regression that maintains some adult behavior along with the regressed behavior and that is used to support the process of adjustment.

Fixation and dissociation are not appropriate.

Rationale: Defense mechanisms are essential for the maintenance of psychologic equilibrium. Recognition of their appropriate use offers assurance that the person is coping adequately and making a satisfactory adjustment. It is a clue to the nurse to support such coping mechanisms.

Fulfilled Needs: Protection from psychologic threat, personal growth and maturity

Identify the current dominant emotion Identify the person's prevailing mood. Through verbal and nonverbal communications, discover present emotions such as depression, anger, anxiety, joy, hatred, ambivalence, and grief.

Rationale: Current emotional states affect experiences of perception, thinking, motivation, and internal safety feelings.

Fulfilled Needs: Protection from physical harm, protection from psychologic threat

Identify the inappropriate use of defense mechanisms[416] Recognize those unconscious mental mechanisms that the patient is using inappropriately in an effort to maintain psychologic equilibrium. Inappropriate defense mechanisms are as follows:

Identification that causes the child to assume undesirable characteristics of the parent or when one transfers the identification of one person to another similar person.

Repression that is insufficient to reduce anxiety, and that impairs the capacity for reality perception, often resulting in hallucinations or delusions.

Denial that permanently blocks out the occurrence of intolerable thoughts and situations and does not lead to later acceptance, or denial that results in malingering.

Reaction formation that becomes exaggerated or inappropriate or when it interferes with adjustment.

Compensation that results in unrealistic self-esteem such as delusions of grandeur that occur from the excessive strivings to overcome the insecurity.

Rationalization that conceals one's true motives and is based on such false causes as to prevent goal seeking, causes self-depreciation, or results in delusions.

Displacement that uses symbols to avoid recognizing unacceptable feelings, such as a phobia.

Projection that results in the unrealistic perception of oneself, disrupts favorable interpersonal relationships through excessive criticism, hostility, and prejudice, promotes the suspiciousness of paranoia, causes ideas of reference, illusions, hallucinations, and delusions.

Symbolism that results in forbidden impulses being expressed by acceptable physical symptoms, obsessive thoughts, compulsive acts, phobias, or undoing behavior.

Fixation that prevents mature and independent personality development by limiting personality growth to a past era of satisfaction.

Regression that brings about disorganization of the personality such as in schizophrenia.

Dissociation that results in loss of control over the integration of the personality and is expressed in automatic writing, sleep-walking, fugue states, dual or multiple personalities, and conversion reactions

Rationale: Defense mechanisms that are used inappropriately are failing to maintain psychologic equilibrium. Recognition of their inappropriateness can serve as a guide to direct the patient toward the appropriate use of defense mechanisms and the reestablishment of psychologic balance.

Fulfilled Needs: Protection from psychologic threat, personal growth and maturity

Inspect and palpate the painful site   Look for inflammation, edema, bruising, bone distortion, distention, etc., of the painful area. Palpate for rigidity, tenderness, subcutaneous swelling, skin warmth, etc. If the area itself is not painful, look for foreign objects in the bed linen or clothing (pins, splinters, etc.) that may be the source of pain.

Rationale: Inspection of the painful site offers clues as to the cause of pain and supports action to reduce pain.

Fulfilled Needs: Protection from physical harm

Inspect for abnormal body movements   Look for unusual body movements, such as irregular jerking, purposeless, spastic twitching, worm-like movements and tremors.

Rationale: Abnormal body movements occur with nervous system degeneration or organic brain disease.

Fulfilled Needs: Protection from physical harm

Inspect for an abnormal body discharge   With the aid of a light, look for abnormal excretions through body orifices, including the eyes, ears, nose, mouth, vagina, anus, and urethra.

Rationale: Purulent and odoriferous discharges indicate infection. Hardened discharges may cause obstruction. Bloody discharges indicate tissue injury.

Fulfilled Needs: Protection from physical harm

Inspect for bleeding: Remove the patient's clothing and look for small amounts of bloody discharge from wounds or body orifices. A light may facilitate visualization. Observe for the amount, color, flow rapidity, and source.

Rationale: Bleeding can lead to reduced circulating blood volume that, if prolonged, can threaten life.

Fulfilled Needs: Protection from physical harm

Inspect for body alignment   Inspect the body for straight alignment of all parts.

Rationale: Nonalignment of the body can indicate disease, deformity, or cause of illness.

Fulfilled Needs: Protection from physical harm

Inspect for deformity Look for abnormal structural formation in any or all body areas.
Rationale: Recognition and correction of deformities often improves body function.
Fulfilled Needs: Protection from physical harm

Inspect for dehydration Watch for signs of insufficient body fluid, including thinness, sunken eyes, parched or cracked lips, dry thick tongue coating, hollow cheeks, gray skin discoloration, poor skin turgor, sunken fontanels, lethargy, or irritability.
Rationale: Altered fluid balance damages and impairs cell activity.
Fulfilled Needs: Protection from physical harm

Inspect for drainage Look for oozing or flow of fluid or pus from a cavity, wound, or other area. Note the color, consistency, amount, and odor.
Rationale: Purulent drainage indicates the presence of infection. Excessive drainage indicates delayed healing. Inadequate drainage indicates obstruction.
Fulfilled Needs: Protection from physical harm

Inspect for edema Look for swollen body areas. Press those areas and watch for deep impressions resulting from finger pressure. Such swelling usually occurs in the feet, ankles, fingers, eyelids, or sacral area.
Rationale: Edema is an abnormal accumulation of fluid in the interstitial spaces and may be the result of many disorders including increased permeability of capillary walls, increased capillary pressure (venous obstruction, congestive heart failure), lymphatic obstruction, impaired kidney function, inadequate plasma protein, fluid and electrolyte imbalance, inflammatory reactions, and hormone imbalance.
Fulfilled Needs: Protection from physical harm

Inspect for foreign bodies Look for small objects in any body opening.
Rationale: Foreign objects cause irritation, inflammation, infection, and respiratory obstruction.
Fulfilled Needs: Protection from physical harm

Inspect for hemorrhage Remove the person's clothing and look for evidence of severe blood loss. Observe for the amount, color, rapidity of flow, and the source. After delivery, watch the mother for vaginal bleeding of 500 cc or more. Especially watch mothers with large babies, large amounts of amniotic fluid, premature placenta separation, or multiple births.
Rationale: Hemorrhage decreases the circulating blood volume, resulting in circulatory impairment or collapse. Even though approximately 5,000 cc of blood normally circulates through the adult body, the rapid loss of more than 500 cc of blood seriously threatens life.
Fulfilled Needs: Protection from physical harm

Inspect for impaired circulation Inspect the extremities for pallor or cyanosis. Touch the extremity skin, feeling for normal body warmth, and check for capillary refill.
Rationale: Diminished tissue oxygenation results from impaired circulation, which increases the potential for tissue necrosis.
Fulfilled Needs: Protection from physical harm

Inspect for inflammation Look for redness, heat, swelling, pain, and loss of function (especially if a joint is involved).
Rationale: An inflammatory response is a natural body defense indicating a tissue reaction to irritation from toxic, bacterial, chemical, or mechanical injury.
Fulfilled Needs: Protection from physical harm

Inspect for necrosis Check the area for signs of dead tissue. Necrotic tissue is a brownish or black color, and there is sloughing of the tissue. It is usually surrounded by healthy tissue.
Rationale: Tissue necrosis results in loss of tissue and a breach of the skin's resistance to infection. This process needs to be interrupted before it becomes a serious threat to the body.
Fulfilled Needs: Protection from physical harm

Inspect for renewed bleeding Once bleeding has stopped, check every 15 minutes to 1 hour for resumed bleeding.
Rationale: Renewed bleeding can cause decreased circulating blood volume or shock.
Fulfilled Needs: Protection from physical harm

Inspect for signs of infection Look for signs indicating an infection such as pain, redness, swelling, heat, and impaired function.
Rationale: The recognition of infection supports the initiation of treatment to reduce the infection.
Fulfilled Needs: Protection from physical harm

Inspect for signs of irritation Look over the skin for signs of redness.
Rationale: Signs of skin irritation when heeded can prevent skin breakdown.
Fulfilled Needs: Protection from physical harm

Inspect for stool abnormalities Look for watery or hard feces, abnormal shapes such as ribbon or cylinder stool, abnormal color such as clay or tarry stools, and obvious abnormal content such as undigested food, blood, or mucus. Note the time of occurrence, frequency, and accompanying discomforts.
Rationale: Abnormal stools indicate gastrointestinal disorders.
Fulfilled Needs: Protection from physical harm

Inspect for the percentage of burned area[768] Look over the burned adult body surface and estimate the percentage of injury. The entire head is considered 9%, each arm 9%, each leg 18%, front torso 18%, back torso 18%, and genital area 1%.
Rationale: Therapy and prognosis are determined by the percentage of burned body surface.
Fulfilled Needs: Protection from physical harm

Inspect the abdomen for ascites Watch for a single curved profile of the abdomen, an inverted umbilicus, and bulging flanks.
Rationale: Ascites indicates an excessive fluid accumulation in the peritoneal cavity.
Fulfilled Needs: Protection from physical harm

Inspect the abdomen for distention Inspect for taut, abdominal wall stretching with umbilical protrusion and thin, glossy abdominal skin.
Rationale: Gas or fluid accumulation in the intestines or peritoneal cavity results in abdominal distention and severe pain.
Fulfilled Needs: Protection from physical harm

Inspect the abdomen for vein engorgement[125,253] Look for abnormal, prominent veins (venation) over the abdominal walls. If present, inspect the direction of blood flow in the following manner. Place both the right and left index fingertips over the vein and compress it. Maintaining the same pressure, slide the fingers apart in opposite directions. Release the right finger and watch for venous filling from that side. Repeat the same test, releasing the left finger instead of the right.

Rationale: An upward, venous blood flow from the lower abdomen indicates inferior vena cava obstruction. An upward flow from the upper abdomen indicates portal obstruction. A downward flow from the upper abdomen indicates superior vena cava obstruction.

Fulfilled Needs: Protection from physical harm

Inspect the abdomen for visible peristalsis[125,253] Inspect the upper abdomen for waves of intestinal contractions that begin at the upper left quadrant and slant downward toward the right lower quadrant.

Rationale: Visible peristalsis indicates excessive intestinal contraction or obstruction.

Fulfilled Needs: Protection from physical harm

Inspect the adenoids for enlargement[125,253] With a small light, look into the open mouth. Inspect the tonsil area for oversized adenoids.

Rationale: Enlarged adenoids affect speech sounds, cause mouth breathing, respiratory obstruction, and permit infectious agents to pass from the throat to the auditory tube and infect the ear.

Fulfilled Needs: Protection from physical harm

Inspect the amniotic fluid for meconium During the labor process, watch for a greenish stool substance in the amniotic fluid, especially at the time of uterine membrane rupture.

Rationale: Meconium in amniotic fluid indicates fetal distress or breech presentation.

Fulfilled Needs: Protection from physical harm

Inspect the arms and hands for venous distention[125,253] Watch for arm and hand veins that appear swollen or are pulsating with a bounding thrust when the hands and arms are held at heart level.

Rationale: Distention of arm and hand veins indicates circulatory fluid overload or the presence of a trauma-related or congenital arteriovenous fistula.

Fulfilled Needs: Protection from physical harm

Inspect the artificial eye for scratches, chipping, or other damage Look over the artificial eye before insertion. Be sure its surface is smooth and undamaged.

Rationale: A scratched or chipped artificial eye will tear or damage orbital tissue. It may eventually cause inflammation and infection.

Fulfilled Needs: Comfort, protection from physical harm

Inspect the breasts for abnormalities Inspect the breasts for symmetry, vein distention, flat, depressed, or inverted nipples, excessive or diminished lactation, bloody nipple discharge, dimpling, engorgement, lumps, inflammation, or cracked nipples.

Rationale: Breast irregularities indicate abnormal conditions or diseases.

Fulfilled Needs: Protection from physical harm

Inspect the cast for tightness Watch for evidence that a cast is too tight on a limb. Such evidence includes swelling, toe or finger pallor or cyanosis, pain, numbness, and inadequate capillary filling. Check the skin at the edges of the cast for evidence of excessive pressure, including redness, pain, and abrasion.

Rationale: A tight cast can impair tissue circulation, cause tissue necrosis, and produce severe pain.

Fulfilled Needs: Protection from physical harm

Inspect the chest for precordial bulge[125,253] Inspect for a chest swelling or protrustion, especially in the right ventricle and upper sternal area.

Rationale: Precordial bulge indicates cardiac enlargement or aortic aneurysm.

Fulfilled Needs: Protection from physical harm

Inspect the chest for respiratory rate and rhythm Count the number of respirations that occur each minute. Watch for abnormal respiratory patterns such as abdominal, Cheyne-Stokes, dyspneic, orthopneic, rapid, shallow, slow, noisy, jerky, wheezing, mouth breathing, and sighing respirations. Watch for deviations from normal newborn respirations of 30–50 per minute and normal adult respirations of 16–20 per minute.

Rationale: Normal respirations are essential to blood and tissue oxygenation.

Fulfilled Needs: Protection from physical harm

Inspect the chest for symmetrical expansion Inspect for chest movements in which both sides of the chest move up and down at the same time.

Rationale: Asymmetrical chest expansion indicates that both lungs are not receiving the same amount of air at the same time.

Fulfilled Needs: Protection from physical harm

Inspect the ears and nose for cerebrospinal fluid leakage Watch for a yellowish fluid leaking from the nose, ear, or head wound. Spinal fluid feels slick or oily and will give a positive glucose reaction on Tes-Tape.

Rationale: Spinal fluid loss indicates a skull fracture.

Fulfilled Needs: Protection from physical harm

Inspect the ears with an otoscope[125,253] Use a lighted speculum to visualize the inner canal of the ear and the tympanic membrane. When examining adults, gently pull the ear upward and backward. With infants and children, gently pull the ear downward. Inspect for a normal, shiny, pearl-gray membrane.

Rationale: A blue internal ear membrane indicates blood in the middle ear. A chalky white membrane indicates pus. An amber or yellow membrane indicates serum. A dull membrane indicates fibrosis. An amber membrane with air bubbles indicates fluid accumulation.

Fulfilled Needs: Protection from physical harm

Inspect the eyelids for drooping/for incomplete closure Watch for an inability to keep the eyelid open voluntarily or for the lid to fall involuntarily lower than normal, when the eye is open. Watch for indications that the person is unable to close his eye(s) tightly.

Rationale: Poor control of the eyelid indicates an oculomotor nerve disorder. Eyelid closure protects the eye from damage caused by foreign particles.

Fulfilled Needs: Protection from physical harm

Inspect the eyes for discoloration With a light, look for yellow or red color changes in the normally white sclera.

Rationale: Scleral jaundice indicates that red blood cell pigments are not being normally excreted through the bile. Scleral redness indicates eye-strain or infection.

Fulfilled Needs: Protection from physical harm

Inspect the eyes for exophthalmia Examine the eyes for lid retraction, a widened opening between the eyelids, lid lag, a staring expression, forward displacement of a swollen eye, and a limited upward gaze.

Rationale: Exophthalmia most often indicates thyrotoxicosis.

Fulfilled Needs: Protection from physical harm

Inspect the eyes for papilledema[125,253] Examine the eye with an ophthalmoscope and look for blurring of the upper and lower nasal disk margins with extended blurring to diverging vessels. The eye veins appear distended and pulseless and may appear to bend sharply over the edge of the disk.

Rationale: Papilledema indicates increased intracranial pressure. The central retinal vein is compressed and the return of blood from the eye is obstructed, causing edema and potential blindness.

Fulfilled Needs: Protection from physical harm

Inspect the eyes for pupil size, equality, and response to light Examine the pupils for equal size. Shine a light into each eye and determine if the pupil constricts quickly and if both constrict with equal rapidity.

Rationale: The third cranial nerve controls pupillary response and, because of the nerve's location, it provides an accurate sign of increased intracranial pressure.

Fulfilled Needs: Protection from physical harm

Contraindications: Conditions that cause photophobia, such as meningitis and measles.

Inspect the fingers for clubbing[125,253] Determine if the fingernail sets at a 10-degree or 20-degree angle to the finger. Press the skin near the cuticle with your fingertip. In finger clubbing, you can feel the nail plate move toward the bone and then spring back when your finger pressure is released. The fingers may have a stub or stunted shape.

Rationale: Finger clubbing is associated with blood disorders, thyroid enlargement, cardiac inflammation, tuberculous, pulmonary infection, pulmonary tumor, and liver cirrhosis.

Fulfilled Needs: Protection from physical harm

Inspect the genitalia for abnormalities Look for edema, irritation, inflammation, loss of pubic hair, and abnormal organ development of the genitalia.

Rationale: Genitalia abnormalities may reveal disorders of the reproductive organs.

Fulfilled Needs: Protection from physical harm

Inspect the gums for abnormalities Inspect the fleshy tissue at the base of the teeth for bleeding, inflammation, ulceration, receding, tenderness, discoloration, paleness, swelling, and hyperplasia.

Rationale: Poor gum conditions reflect basic health disorders. Sore gums indicate niacin deficiency. Bleeding gums occur in leukemia, vitamin C deficiency, excessive tartar deposits, and gum infection. Gum inflammation occurs with vitamin C deficiency. Gum hyperplasia may occur during prolonged Dilantin therapy.

Fulfilled Needs: Protection from physical harm

Inspect the hair for abnormalities Watch for unusual hair conditions such as excessive dryness or oiliness, thinning, matting, hair loss, parasites, bleeding onto the hair, or abnormal hair distribution.

Rationale: Hair abnormalities indicate poor hygiene or physiologic disorders.

Fulfilled Needs: Protection from physical harm

Inspect the head for Battle's sign Inspect for a spongy area on the temple and behind the ear, which may appear bruised.

Rationale: A positive Battle's sign indicates skull fracture.

Fulfilled Needs: Protection from physical harm

Inspect the joints for abnormalities Look for joint disorders such as limited joint movement, muscle atrophy around a joint, swelling, tenderness, pain, increased joint size, and heat.

Rationale: Normal fibrous connective tissue and cartilage are essential for freely moveable joints.

Fulfilled Needs: Protection from physical harm

Inspect the joints for impending contractures Look for a drooping hand or foot, chronically bent knees or elbows, turning of the neck toward one side, flexed fingers, or decreased finger movement.

Rationale: Muscle shortening prevents normal functional use of the joints. Early treatment of contractures maintains normal joint movement.

Fulfilled Needs: Protection from physical harm

Inspect the mouth for abnormal salivation Look for excessive accumulation or production of saliva or decreased salivation.

Rationale: Excessive saliva can cause choking. Excessive production of saliva is evident in poisonous spider bites and epileptic seizures. Decreased saliva occurs with salivary gland obstruction.

Fulfilled Needs: Protection from physical harm

Inspect the mucous membranes for abnormalities Look for abnormalities of the mucous membranes of the mouth, nose, throat, and vagina. These include inflammation, edema, exudates, irritation, trauma, allergy responses, pallor, yellow discoloration of the hard palate, rashes, lesions, and dryness.

Rationale: Healthy mucous membranes are moist and well lubricated and protect the underlying tissue. Traumatized oral mucosa impairs eating and drinking and reduces comfort. Abnormal mucous membranes may indicate other underlying disorders.

Fulfilled Needs: Protection from physical harm

Inspect the nails for abnormalities Inspect the fingernails and toenails for cleanliness, excessive length, ragged edges, hangnails, abnormal nail formation, thickness, discoloration, splitting, or ulcers appearing around the nail.

Rationale: Nail changes occur in nutritional deficiencies, systemic illnesses, and local infection.

Fulfilled Needs: Protection from physical harm

Inspect the nasal turbinates for abnormalities Using a light, gently inspect the inner nasal tissue for redness, paleness, or swelling.

Rationale: Pale, swollen nasal turbinates occur with hay fever and allergies. Red, swollen nasal turbinates occur with the common cold.

Fulfilled Needs: Protection from physical harm

Inspect the neck veins for distention Determine if the neck veins appear swollen or if they pulsate with a bounding thrust.

Rationale: Distended neck veins of a person resting with the head elevated at a 45° angle indicate venous congestion that may be the result of left ventricular failure, severe pulmonary obstructive disease, or vascular overload.

Fulfilled Needs: Protection from physical harm

Inspect the nose for asymmetry With a light, examine the nasal septum, externally and internally, for marked deviation to one side of the face. If the nasal passages are not of equal size, then the septum is not straight.

Rationale: Asymmetric nasal passages can cause nasal obstruction or inadequate sinus drainage.

Fulfilled Needs: Protection from physical harm

Inspect the nose for epistaxis Look for nose bleeding, especially serious bleeding.

Rationale: Rapid loss of more than 1 pint (500 cc) of blood in an adult poses a threat to life.

Fulfilled Needs: Protection from physical harm

Inspect the nose for polyps   With a light, look for small growths protruding from the nasal lining.
Rationale: Nasal polyps obstruct normal air flow.
Fulfilled Needs: Protection from physical harm

Inspect the nose, mouth, and throat for evidence of burns   With a light, look for scorched hairs in the nose and abnormal coloration and drying of the mucous membrane.
Rationale: Nose, mouth, or throat burns may indicate burns extending into the lungs.
Fulfilled Needs: Protection from physical harm

Inspect the orthopedic pin site   Periodically check the entrance site of the orthopedic pin into the skin. Look for infection, crusting, and drainage.
Rationale: Exudate at a wound opening promotes bacterial growth causing wound and bone infection. If the pin slips out of position, it pulls the contaminated pin into the tissue.
Fulfilled Needs: Protection from physical harm

Inspect the palms for coloration   With the fingers stretched, look for white, pink, or red coloring in the lines of the hand or yellow pigment on the palm.
Rationale: White or no coloring in the lines of the hands indicates anemia. Bright red coloring indicates polycythemia vera. Yellow palm discoloration indicates liver disease or myxedema.
Fulfilled Needs: Protection from physical harm

Inspect the person's mouth for concealed medications   When giving oral medications, check the person's mouth carefully for medications that have not been swallowed.
Rationale: Small, therapeutic doses of drugs can be collected and, when taken in large doses, cause death.
Fulfilled Needs: Protection from physical harm

Inspect the placenta for abnormalities   Look for separation of the placenta into two parts, atrophy, incomplete placenta, and umbilical cord attachment at the margins.
Rationale: Placental abnormalities indicate potential uterine or hemorrhage disorders. When portions of the placenta are missing, it indicates that some of the placenta has been retained in the uterus.
Fulfilled Needs: Protection from physical harm

Inspect the skin for abnormal perspiration   Look for discolored perspiration, excessive sweating at night, absent perspiration, profuse sweating, frosty or snowlike perspiration, or excessively salty sweating.
Rationale: Excessive perspiration may lead to dehydration or may indicate the need for body temperature regulation. Frosty, snowlike perspiration indicates uremia. Discolored sweat indicates toxicity. Excessive salty sweating may lead to electrolyte imbalance. Absent perspiration indicates an inability of the body to cool itself.
Fulfilled Needs: Protection from physical harm

Inspect the skin for breakdown   Look for redness, irritation, duskiness, blistering, and broken skin.
Rationale: Skin breakdown supports infection and reduces circulation, which furthers tissue necrosis.
Fulfilled Needs: Protection from physical harm

Inspect the skin for color/discoloration   Look for changes in skin color, such as cherry redness, blanching, purple color, cyanosis (blueness), pallor (whiteness), erythema (redness), jaundice (yellowness), bronzing.

Rationale: Cherry redness indicates carbon monoxide poisoning. Blueness, purple color, or blanching suggest impaired oxygenation of tissue. Pallor is seen in decreased circulation and number of red blood cells, as in anemias and chronic disease. Redness indicates inflammation, vasomotor disturbances, or burns. Yellow skin suggests liver disorders and biliary obstruction. Bronzing is evident in adrenal disorders.

Fulfilled Needs: Protection from physical harm

Inspect the skin for lesions/for infectious lesions   Look for open sores, fever, swelling, redness, crusting, ulceration, warts, rashes, pain, chains or clusters of blisters, vesicles, discolored lumps, gummas, chancre, or thick, leathery, nodular skin lesions.

Rationale: Invasion of the skin by viruses, bacteria, and fungus causes infection and discomfort.

Fulfilled Needs: Protection from physical harm

Inspect the skin for pallor   Look for lack of color and whiteness of the skin.

Rationale: Localized pallor results from peripheral blood vessel constriction, localized edema, or obstructed arterial flow. Generalized pallor indicates shock.

Fulfilled Needs: Protection from physical harm

Inspect the skin for petechiae   Look for small, purplish, hemorrhagic spots on the skin.

Rationale: Petechiae indicate a blood clotting disorder, capillary fragility, or a severe systemic disorder such as meningococcal septicemia or bacterial endocarditis.

Fulfilled Needs: Protection from physical harm

Inspect the skin for skin spiders   Look over the face, neck, upper trunk, and arms for small, reddened spiderlike vascular abnormalities. They may pulsate enough for the pulsation to be seen and felt.

Rationale: Most vascular spiders are arterioles and, although they are associated with cirrhosis, their specific cause is not known.

Fulfilled Needs: Protection from physical harm

Inspect the sputum for characteristics   Look for the amount, consistency, and appearance of the sputum.

Rationale: Blood-tinged sputum indicates respiratory tract inflammation. Pink sputum is evident in pneumonia and pulmonary edema. Very bloody sputum occurs with tuberculosis, embolism, and carcinoma. Rusty sputum is seen in pneumococcal pneumonia. Stringy sputum is associated with asthma, and frothy sputum with pulmonary edema. Yellow, green, or dirty gray (purulent) sputum indicates lung infection. Gelatinous sputum suggests pneumonia. Soot in the sputum may indicate that burns have extended into the respiratory system.

Fulfilled Needs: Protection from physical harm

Inspect the teeth for abnormalities   Inspect the teeth for caries, chipping, cracking, discoloration, and alignment.

Rationale: Teeth are essential to chewing and digestion, maintenance of natural jaw contour, and comfort.

Fulfilled Needs: Protection from physical harm

Inspect the throat for an impaired swallowing reflex   Touch the posterior pharyngeal wall with an applicator stick and note if gagging occurs. If there is question as to the ability to swallow, have the patient suck a piece of ice or drink small sips of water and note how well he swallows.

Rationale: Swallowing is necessary for the passage of food and fluid into the digestive system. An impaired swallowing reflex indicates soft palate paralysis, stroke, head injury or trauma and may result in choking.

Fulfilled Needs: Protection from physical harm

Inspect the tongue for abnormalities Inspect the tongue for scars, tremors, sharp pointedness, protrustion, enlargement, atrophy, bleeding, inflammation, cracking, dryness, longitudinal furrows, tenderness, ulceration, rashes, discoloration, coatings, paleness, swelling, and deviations from the midline.

Rationale: A normal tongue is essential to food manipulation, chewing, taste perception, and speech. An abnormal tongue may indicate other underlying disorders.

Fulfilled Needs: Protection from physical harm

Inspect the umbilical cord for abnormalities At childbirth, inspect the umbilical cord for the presence of two arteries and one vein. During the infant's first few weeks of life, inspect the umbilical cord area for a weeping discharge, excessive bulging, or hemorrhage.

Rationale: The absence of umbilical cord arteries or vein indicates a congenital abnormality. Other abnormalities indicate poor healing, infection, or herniation.

Fulfilled Needs: Protection from physical harm

Inspect the vagina for a prolapsed umbilical cord After membrane rupture and the gush of amniotic fluid, look for protrusion of the umbilical cord through the vagina.

Rationale: An umbilical cord visible at the vagina indicates umbilical cord prolapse. A prolapsed umbilical cord, compressed between the fetal head and pelvis, can cause fetal strangulation or fatal circulatory impairment.

Fulfilled Needs: Protection from physical harm

Inspect the vagina for discharge Inspect for normal and abnormal vaginal discharges. Normal vaginal discharges include the following:

> A clear, mucoid discharge occurring with normal ovulation
> Lochia, which is a moderate, bloody, mucus flow during the first 3 days; decreases and becomes watery and pink from about the fourth to the ninth day; becomes thin, colorless, and scant after the tenth day; usually disappears or is just a slight brownish, mucoid discharge at 21 days post partum; lochia should never have an offensive odor
> Menstruation of moderate flow and duration
> A bright red or red-brown discharge or spotting lasting 3–6 weeks after a hysterectomy
> A red-brown discharge lasting for several days after a dilatation and curettage (D and C)
> Abnormal vaginal discharges include the following:
> A brown or chocolate-colored discharge associated with endometriosis or uterine carcinoma
> A cheesy discharge occurring with *Monilia* infection
> A creamy, white discharge occurring with streptococcal or staphyloccal infection or radiation therapy
> A frothy white discharge indication *Trichomonas* infection or radiation therapy
> A mucoid, yellow discharge associated with streptococcal or staphylococcal infection
> A thick, yellow discharge occurring with *Gonococcus* infection

Rationale: Early detection and treatment of reproductive disorders prevent progression to serious disease.

Fulfilled Needs: Protection from physical harm

Inspect the vocal cords for lesions With a small light, a tongue depressor, and a dental mirror, look through the open mouth into the lower pharynx for vocal cord tumors.

Rationale: Vocal cord tumors affect the ability to speak and to communicate. When large enough, such tumors cause respiratory obstruction or difficulty swallowing food.

Fulfilled Needs: Protection from physical harm

Inspect the wound dressing frequently Inspect the wound dressing at least every 4 hours, and more often if necessary. Look for wetness, cleanliness, adequate wound coverage, bleeding, and drainage. Inspect the bed and clothing underneath the wound, since drainage sometimes seeps out from under the dressing instead of being absorbed by it.

Rationale: Frequent observation of wound dressings supports detection of abnormalities and the need for dressing change.

Fulfilled Needs: Protection from physical harm

Inspect the wound for evisceration Determine if a surgically closed wound has broken open and area organs are exposed.

Rationale: Wound evisceration poses the threat of infection and shock.

Fulfilled Needs: Protection from physical harm

Interpret laboratory results and notify the physician of abnormalities Look at the laboratory results and determine their meaning and significance in each individual situation. Report significant changes to the physician.

Rationale: Early recognition and interpretation of laboratory results are essential for patient protection and support immediate therapy in life-threatening situations.

Fulfilled Needs: Protection from physical harm

Keep a dialysis flow sheet Record the time that each dialysis treatment is begun and when each drainage period is concluded. Also, include the amount of fluid instilled, the volume drained, and any medications given.

Rationale: An accurate record of the dialysis process assists the physician in evaluating the treatment being given and promotes patient safety.

Fulfilled Needs: Protection from physical harm

Make a follow-up evaluation Make contact with the person, after a given time, to determine the status of the person and of the problem being treated. Look for objective evidence to verify the evaluation.

Rationale: Follow-up evaluation verifies the outcome of health therapy. If the outcome is undesirable, new therapy can be initiated in an effort to solve the problems.

Fulfilled Needs: Comfort, protection from physical harm

Measure the body weight Determine the body weight by using a standard scale that gives body weight in pounds or kilograms or a metabolic scale that records weight in kilograms only (each kilogram equals 2.2 lbs).

Rationale: Body weight changes indicate loss or retention of fluids, food intake changes, food absorption abnormalities, or increased adaptation requirements on body processes. Kilograms are used to measure body weight when accuracy is essential for computing drug dosage, fluids, and nutrient intake.

Fulfilled Needs: Protection from physical harm

Measure the chest drainage after clamping the chest tube, and attaching a new drainage system Clamp the chest tube close to the insertion site. Remove the present water-seal drainage system and immediately replace it with a new, sterile system. Remove the clamp from the chest tube and check that it is patent. Then measure the amount of drainage in the old container by measuring the total volume and subtracting from it the amount of sterile water originally placed in the water-seal drainage system.

Rationale: Measuring the chest drainage gives an estimate of the amount of blood lost and facilitates equivalent blood or fluid replacement.

Fulfilled Needs: Protection from physical harm

Measure the girth/circumference of the (specific body part) Measure the circumference of a body area with a tape measure as often as necessary.

Rationale: The abdominal or extremity girth increases with fluid accumulation in tissues. A child's head circumference increases abnormally with increased intracranial pressure.

Fulfilled Needs: Protection from physical harm

Measure the height Measure in feet and inches (meters and cm) the distance between the person's feet and the top of his head.

Rationale: Measuring height allows for determination of normal and abnormal growth patterns and proportional body development between height and weight. Normal child growth is 3–5 inches a year.

Fulfilled Needs: Protection from physical harm

Measure the intake Measure the volume of fluids taken in over a 24-hour period. This includes all liquids, such as water, milk, soups, soft drinks, intravenous fluids, ice cream, Jell-O, juices, ice, ice chips, and irrigating fluids that have not been withdrawn.

Rationale: Accurate intake and output measurement is essential for correct fluid replacement therapy. Balanced fluid intake and output is essential to cell functioning. Severely altered fluid balance damages and impairs cell activity.

Fulfilled Needs: Protection from physical harm

Measure the output Measure and record the fluid volume and wastes excreted from the body within a 24-hour period. Include urine, liquid feces, approximate plasma loss from burns, gastrointestinal drainage, T-tube bile drainage, excessive wound drainage, chest drainage, etc.

Rationale: Accurate intake and output measurement is essential for correct fluid replacement therapy. Balanced fluid intake and output are essential to cell functioning. Severely altered fluid balance damages and impairs cell activity.

Fulfilled Needs: Protection from physical harm

Measure the pelvic size Using a pelvimeter, determine if the pelvic diameter size is large enough for normal delivery. Normal measurements should be: Externally, 26 cm between the iliac spines, 29 cm between the iliac crests, 31 cm between the great trochanters, 20 cm between the last lumbar spine and the pubic front surface. Internally, 12.5 cm from the pubic outer edge to the sacral promontory (diagonal conjugate), 11 cm from the inner symphysis pubis to the sacral promontory (true conjugate), 11.5 cm between the ischial spines, 11 cm between the ischial tuberosities, 11.5 cm between the sacrum and pubis.

Rationale: The birth canal must be sufficiently large for the infant to pass safely through without harm.

Fulfilled Needs: Protection from physical harm

Measure the residual urine Measure the urine volume that remains in the bladder after voiding. Have the patient void, then insert a catheter into the bladder to remove the remaining urine and measure the volume.

Rationale: Retained urine of 50 cc or more after voiding indicates decreased bladder efficiency.

Fulfilled Needs: Protection from physical harm

Measure the urine output hourly   Measure the urine volume excreted within 1 hour. Normal adult urine excretion is approximately 60 cc/hr with a minimum of 30 cc/hour.

Rationale: The excretion of less than 15–20 cc of urine per hour indicates failure of the kidneys to excrete, inadequate fluid intake, excessive salt intake, overproduction of antidiuretic hormones, shock, transfusion reaction, or excess fluid loss through burns or diarrhea. The excretion of more than 80 cc of urine per hour indicates failure of the kidneys to concentrate the urine, deficient production of antidiuretic hormones, or excessive intravenous or oral fluid intake.

Fulfilled Needs: Protection from physical harm

Monitor blood studies for abnormal acid-base[173,287]   Watch for laboratory analysis reports indicating abnormal acid–base levels. These studies include tests for alkali reserve, base excess, bicarbonate, pH, and carbon dioxide.

Rationale: *Alkali reserve:*   A normal blood alkali is essential to neutralize blood acids. Increased blood alkali reserve occurs with metabolic alkalosis or respiratory acidosis. Decreased blood alkali reserve occurs with metabolic acidosis or respiratory alkalosis.

Base excess: A normal blood base is essential for neutralizing acids. An abnormality indicates a change in the blood buffer base at a given level of hemoglobin concentration. It reveals the amount of nonvolatile acid or base accumulated in the blood. Elevated base excess occurs with metabolic alkalosis or respiratory acidosis.

Bicarbonate: This study reveals the amount of salt that results when carbonic acid is not completely neutralized or when carbon dioxide mixes in excessive amounts with a base. Increased blood bicarbonate occurs with metabolic alkalosis or respiratory acidosis. Decreased blood bicarbonate occurs with metabolic acidosis, renal acidosis, or respiratory alkalosis.

pH: This study reveals the blood's hydrogen ion concentration by indicating the ratio between bicarbonate and carbonic acid blood levels. It shows the blood's acid-alkaline concentration. Increased blood pH occurs with respiratory and metabolic alkalosis. Decreased blood pH occurs with metabolic, respiratory, and renal acidosis.

Carbon dioxide: This test reveals the amount of carbon dioxide present in the blood. Increased blood carbon dioxide occurs with respiratory acidosis and metabolic alkalosis. Decreased blood carbon dioxide occurs with respiratory alkalosis and metabolic acidosis.

Fulfilled Needs: Protection from physical harm

Monitor blood studies for abnormal adrenal function[173,287]   Watch for laboratory analysis reports indicating adrenal hyperactivity or insufficiency. These studies include tests for cortisol, sodium, and glucose.

Rationale: *Cortisol:*   Increased blood cortisol indicates adrenal hyperactivity (Cushing's syndrome). Decreased blood cortisol indicates adrenal insufficiency (Addison's disease).

Sodium: Increased blood sodium indicates adrenal hyperactivity. Decreased blood sodium reveals adrenal insufficiency and is the result of impaired sodium reabsorption by the kidneys.

Glucose: Increased blood glucose indicates adrenal hyperactivity. Decreased blood glucose indicates adrenal insufficiency.

Fulfilled Needs: Protection from physical harm

Monitor blood studies for abnormal carbohydrate metabolism[173,287]   Watch for laboratory analysis reports indicating the ability of the body to metabolize carbohydrates. These studies include tests for glucose tolerance, glucose, acetone, fatty acids.

Rationale: *Glucose tolerance:*   This test reveals the body's ability to metabolize glucose over a 4–5 hour period. Increased blood glucose tolerance can occur with diabetes mellitus.

Glucose: Increased blood levels can indicate diabetes mellitus and decreased levels are associated with hypoglycemia.

Acetone: When increased, this test indicates an elevation in the ketone end products of fat metabolism that occurs with impaired carbohydrate metabolism.

Fatty acids: Fatty acids are hydrocarbons resulting from fat digestion. They are increased with impaired carbohydrate metabolism.

Fulfilled Needs: Protection from physical harm

Monitor blood studies for abnormal cardiac enzymes[173,287]   Watch for laboratory analysis reports indicating cardiac tissue necrosis. These studies include tests for aldolase, creatine phosphokinase (CPK), lactate dehydrogenase (LDH), SGOT and SGPT (transaminase).

Rationale: *Aldolase:*   Aldolase is a muscle enzyme necessary for conversion of glycogen into lactic acid. Increased blood aldolase occurs with myocardial ischemia and necrosis.

CPK: Increased blood CPK occurs with myocardial ischemia and necrosis.

LDH: Lactate dehydrogenase is an enzyme causing lactic acid to lose hydrogen through oxidation. The numbers of hydrogens (H) lost help determine the organ in which the disorder exists. Elevated LDH occurs with tissue necrosis.

SGOT and SGPT: These enzymes are generally present in tissues. When tissue injury occurs, the enzymes are released into the bloodstream. Increased SGOT and SGPT occurs with myocardial ischemia and necrosis.

Fulfilled Needs: Protection from physical harm

Monitor blood studies for abnormal chemistry   Examine laboratory analysis reports promptly upon receipt for indications of abnormal changes in the body's chemical levels.

Rationale: Changes in blood chemistry levels indicate the presence of existing or potential pathologic processes or evidence of the recovery process.

Fulfilled Needs: Protection from physical harm

Monitor blood studies for abnormal cholesterol[287]   Watch for laboratory results indicating an increased blood cholesterol (lipids).

Rationale: Increased blood cholesterol is associated with familiar hypercholesterolemia, which is believed to predispose to arteriosclerotic disease.

Fulfilled Needs: Protection from physical harm

Monitor blood studies for abnormal clotting mechanism[173,287]   Watch for laboratory analysis reports indicating an abnormality in blood coagulation. These studies include tests for bleeding time, clotting time, prothrombin time, partial thromboplastin time (PTT), fibrinogen, and the antihemophilic factor.

Rationale: *Bleeding time:*   This test reveals how long it takes blood to cease flowing following a small wound puncture. An increased bleeding time occurs with prolonged small blood vessel nonconstriction, or anticoagulant therapy.

Clotting time: An increased blood clotting time occurs with a clotting factor deficiency or anticoagulant therapy.

Prothrombin time: This study reveals the level of the prothrombin protein essential to coagulation. Prothrombin is formed in the liver in the presence of vitamin K. When there is impaired liver function, the liver cannot adequately absorb vitamin K from the intestines and so prothrombin cannot be adequately formed. Prothrombin formation is also dependent on fibrinogen, calcium, and factors V, VIII, and X. If any of these essentials is missing, there will be a tendency toward bleeding. The number of seconds in which prothrombin forms and coagulation occurs is increased when there is liver cell damage or necrosis, a deficiency of a clotting factor, or during anticoagulant therapy.

PTT: This test reveals deficiencies of essential coagulation factors. Increased blood

PTT occurs when there are deficiencies in clotting factors VIII, IX, and X.

Antihemophilic factor: Decreased blood antihemophilic factor occurs with a deficiency of clotting factor VIII and indicates potential abnormal bleeding.

Fibrinogen: A normal fibrinogen level is essential for conversion of thrombin into fibrin for normal blood clotting. Increased blood fibrinogen occurs with noninflammatory kidney degeneration, acute infection, hemoconcentration, lung inflammation, and pregnancy.

Fulfilled Needs: Protection from physical harm

Monitor blood studies for abnormal electrolytes[173,287] Watch for laboratory analysis reports indicating an abnormality in blood sodium, potassium, chloride, calcium, and magnesium levels.

Rationale: *Sodium:* A normal blood sodium level is essential for fluid and electrolyte balance, normal osmotic pressure, and acid–base balance. Increased blood sodium levels occur with kidney inflammation, diuresis caused by insufficient antidiuretic hormone, dehydration, adrenal hyperactivity, hemoconcentration, aldosterone hypersecretion, obstructed intestines, excessive sodium intake, and as a side effect of steroid therapy. Decreased blood sodium levels occur with overhydration, renal acidosis, adrenal and pituitary insufficiency, diarrhea and vomiting, metabolic acidosis, and diminished cardiac output.

Potassium: This mineral is essential to fluid balance, acid–base balance, normal osmotic pressure, and nerve impulse conduction, especially to muscle and cardiac tissue. Potassium is found in large amounts in cells and in small amounts in serum. Increased blood potassium levels occur with kidney failure, adrenal insufficiency, excessive potassium intake, impaired carbohydrate metabolism, renal acidosis, and diminished myocardial excitability and conduction rate in diastole. Decreased blood potassium levels occur with kidney inflammation, upper and lower gastrointestinal fluid loss, diuretic fluid loss, adrenal hyperactivity, aldosterone hypersecretion, impaired carbohydrate metabolism, diminished cardiac output, overhydration, as a side effect of steroid therapy, and with diminished myocardial excitability and conduction rate in systole.

Chloride: This salt is essential to balanced osmotic pressure and electrolytes. Increased blood chloride levels occur with metabolic acidosis, respiratory alkalosis, insufficient antidiuretic hormone causing diuresis and dehydration, kidney inflammation, genitourinary obstruction, and dehydration. Decreased blood chloride levels occur with metabolic alkalosis, respiratory acidosis, loss of plasma, obstructed intestines, adrenal hyperactivity, lung inflammation, diminished cardiac output, vomiting, and diarrhea.

Calcium: Calcium is a metallic element essential to blood coagulation, normal bone and tooth development, lactation, muscle, nerve, and enzyme activity, and electrolyte balance. Increased blood calcium levels occur with metabolic alkalosis, parathyroid hypersecretion, kidney inflammation, and excessive cardiac muscle contraction. The intake of alkali impairs the renal excretion of calcium. Calcium is then excessively absorbed from cow's milk, elevating the blood level. Decreased blood calcium levels occur with diminished cardiac contraction, excessive neuromuscular irritability, renal acidosis, noninflammatory kidney degeneration, parathyroid hyposecretion, small intestine malabsorption, diarrhea, and as a steroid therapy side effect.

Magnesium: The mineral magnesium maintains osmotic pressure, electrolyte balance, muscle and nerve activity, and enzyme functioning. An increased blood magnesium level occurs with kidney failure. Decreased blood magnesium levels occur with pregnancy toxicity, vomiting, excessive neuromuscular irritability, aldosterone hypersecretion, and kidney failure.

Fulfilled Needs: Protection from physical harm

Monitor blood studies for abnormal/normal glucose[173,287] Watch for laboratory results indicating an elevated or decreased blood glucose.

Rationale: *Glucose:* Glucose results from carbohydrate metabolism. Glucose is essential to the maintenance of body energy, especially in muscles and nerves. Increased blood glucose levels occur with adrenal hyperactivity, impaired glucose metabolism, early stage pituitary hypersecretion, excessive thyroid production, kidney inflammation or failure, pregnancy, and as a side effect of steroid therapy. Decreased blood glucose levels occur with impaired carbohydrate metabolism, adrenal insufficiency, insulin excess, prolonged pituitary hypersecretion, thyroid insufficiency, and liver cell necrosis.

Fulfilled Needs: Protection from physical harm

Monitor blood studies for abnormal hematology[173,287]
Watch for laboratory analysis reports indicating an abnormality in blood gas exchange. These include erythrocyte count (RBC), hematocrit, hemoglobin, mean corpuscular hemoglobin (MCH), mean corpuscular volume (MCV), mean corpuscular hemoglobin concentration (MCHC), plasma total volume, platelet count, reticulocytes, and sedimentation rate.

Rationale: *Erythrocyte count:* Normal erythrocyte levels are essential for carrying oxygen to and carbon dioxide from tissues, acid–base balance, and the development of bile pigment. Increased erythrocyte count occurs with water deprivation, diminished cardiac output, impaired pulmonary gas exchange, fluid intolerance dehydration, lower gastrointestinal fluid loss, excessive red blood cell production, and as a steroid therapy side effect. Decreased erythrocyte count occurs with vitamin B_6 and B_{12} deficiencies, iron deficiency, chronic infections, chronic renal insufficiency, pathologic conditions, and bone marrow failure.

Hematocrit: This test indicates the percentage of red blood cells in the total blood volume. Increased blood hematocrit occurs with dehydration, impaired pulmonary gas exchange, increased red blood cell volume, diminished cardiac output, hemoconcentration and adrenal insufficiency. Decreased blood hematocrit occurs with blood loss, malnutrition, decreased red blood cell and plasma volume, anticoagulant therapy, and red blood cell destruction.

Hemoglobin: A normal hemoglobin is essential for carrying oxygen from the lungs to body tissues. Increased blood hemoglobin occurs with diminished cardiac output, increased red blood cell volume, impaired pulmonary gas exchange, and dehydration. A decreased blood hemoglobin occurs with decreased red blood cell and plasma volume, blood loss, malnutrition, decreased red blood cell oxygenation, and red blood cell destruction.

MCH: The MCH level indicates the amount of hemoglobin found in each red blood cell. Increased blood MCH occurs with excessive red blood cell hemoglobin.

MCV: The MCV indicates the volume of red blood cells. Increased blood MCV occurs with excessive red blood cell volume. Decreased blood MCV occurs with a low red blood cell volume.

MCHC: The MCHC indicates the percentage of hemoglobin concentration in each red blood cell. Decreased blood MCHC occurs with a low red blood cell hemoglobin and with overhydration.

Plasma total volume: This study reveals the proportion of blood in the body as related to total body weight. Increased blood plasma total volume occurs with a reduced secretion of antidiuretic hormone. Decreased blood plasma total volume occurs with upper and lower gastrointestinal fluid loss or dehydration.

Platelet count: This study reveals the number of thrombocytes (platelets) in the blood. A normal platelet count is essential, for these cells clump together and form clots to stop bleeding. An increased platelet count occurs with generalized infection and increased red blood cell volume, and after surgery, trauma, and delivery. A decreased platelet count occurs with impaired red blood cell production, acute infection, diminished blood coagulation, excessive white blood cell production, capillary fragility, and bone marrow failure.

Reticulocytes: Reticulocytes are immature red blood cells. Their quantity reveals how rapidly they are being released from bone marrow in relation to the norm. Increased blood reticulocytes occur with excessive bone marrow activity, infection, and hemorrhage. Decreased blood reticulocytes occur with impaired bone marrow activity and excessive white blood cell production.

Sedimentation rate: This test reveals the speed at which red blood cells settle in a test tube after an anticoagulant has been added to the blood. Increased sedimentation rate occurs with infection, tissue cell destruction, and pregnancy.

Fulfilled Needs: Protection from physical harm

Monitor blood studies for abnormal liver function[522]   Watch for laboratory analysis reports indicating impaired liver function. These include alkaline phosphatase, bilirubin, lactate dehydrogenase (LDH), prothrombin time, cephalin flocculation, thymol turbidity, total protein, SGOT and SGPT (transaminase), bromosulfthalein (BSP) test.

Rationale: *Alkaline phosphatase:*   In liver disease, increased levels of the alkaline phosphatase enzyme are released into the bloodstream.

Bilirubin: Increased serum bilirubin indicates hepatic jaundice.

LDH: This enzyme causes lactic acid to lose hydrogen through oxidation. The number of hydrogens (H) lost helps determine the organ in which the disorder exists. Elevated LDH occurs with tissue necrosis.

Prothrombin time: This study reveals the level of prothrombin, a protein essential to coagulation. Prothrombin is formed in the liver in the presence of vitamin K. When there is severely impaired liver function, the liver cannot adequately use vitamin K absorbed from the intestines, so prothrombin production is reduced.

Cephalin flocculation: This study reveals changes in globulin protein. These protein changes cause the fatty substance cephalin to collect into small clumps (flocculate). Since protein metabolism occurs in the liver, the clumping of cephalin indicates liver damage that may or may not affect other systems. Increased blood cephalin flocculation occurs with liver cell necrosis, diminished cardiac output, infection, and lung inflammation.

Thymol turbidity: Thymol is a gamma globulin protein. When in solution and serum is added to it, the solution becomes cloudy if the proteins are concentrated. Since protein metabolism occurs in the liver, this test reveals liver damage. Increased thymol turbidity occurs with liver cell necrosis.

Total protein: This study reveals the ratio of albumin, globulin, and fibrinogen to total protein. An increased globulin level in the protein occurs with liver disease.

SGOT and SGPT: These enzymes are generally present in tissues. When tissue injury occurs, the enzymes are released into the bloodstream. Increased blood SGOT and SGPT levels occur with liver cell damage, necrosis, or inflammation.

BSP: This test reveals the adequacy of liver cells to remove BSP dye from the blood. Elevated BSP occurs with liver cell damage.

Fulfilled Needs: Protection from physical harm

Monitor blood studies for abnormal pancreatic function[173,287]   Watch for laboratory analysis reports indicating impaired pancreatic function. These include amylase, lipase, and SGOT.

Rationale: *Amylase:*   Amylase is a digestive enzyme found in pancreatic secretions. An increased blood amylase level occurs with acute pancreatic inflammation or obstruction.

Lipase: Lipase is an enzyme that is secreted by the pancreas and aids in fat digestion. An increased lipase level indicates pancreatic inflammation.

SGOT: This enzyme is generally present in tissues. When tissue injury occurs, the enzyme is released into the bloodstream. An increased SGOT level occurs with pancreatic inflammation.

Fulfilled Needs: Protection from physical harm

Monitor blood studies for abnormal parathyroid function[173,287]   These studies include tests for calcium and phosphate.

Rationale: *Calcium:*   Calcium regulation is maintained by the parathyroid hormone. An elevated calcium can indicate hyperactivity of the parathyroid gland. A decreased calcium level may indicate impaired parathyroid function.

Phosphate: This study reveals the blood level of the salt phosphoric acid that maintains acid–base balance through its buffering action. Increased blood phosphate occurs with parathyroid hyposecretion.

Calcium and phosphate have a reciprocal relationship, when one goes up, the other goes down.

Fulfilled Needs: Protection from physical harm

Monitor blood studies for abnormal pituitary function[173,287] Watch for a laboratory analysis report of cortisol indicating impaired pituitary function.

Rationale: A decreased blood cortisol level indicates pituitary insufficiency.

Fulfilled Needs: Protection from physical harm

Monitor blood studies for abnormal renal function[173,287] Watch for laboratory analysis reports indicating impaired kidney function. These include urea, urea nitrogen, creatinine, and albumin.

Rationale: *Urea and urea nitrogen:* Normally, the kidney excretes urea and urea nitrogen after protein metabolism. When adequate amounts are not excreted, the blood level rises. Increased blood urea levels occur with kidney inflammation, degeneration, or failure.

Creatinine: Creatinine is an alkaline nonprotein blood component and results from creatinine metabolism. Normal blood levels are maintained by daily creatinine excretion through the kidneys. An increased blood creatinine level occurs with kidney inflammation or failure and during rejection of kidney transplant.

Albumin: A decreased blood albumin level occurs with the nephrotic syndrome.

Fulfilled Needs: Protection from physical harm

Monitor blood studies for abnormal thyroid function[368] Look for laboratory analysis reports revealing impaired thyroid function. These studies include radioimmunoassay (RIA) tests for thyroxine (T_4), triiodothyronine (T_3), and thyrotropin (TSH).

Rationale: *T_4 and T_3:* The serum levels of thyroid hormones are increased in hyperthyroidism (thyrotoxicosis and some tumors) and decreased in hypothyroidism (myxedema, cretinism). The T_4 level is normally higher during the first few weeks of life. These are the major tests for checking the amount of hormone being produced.

TSH (RIA): The serum level of thyrotropin measured by a RIA is a test for hypothyroidism. The normal level is below 10 μU/ml. Levels elevated over 20 μU/ml indicate hypothyroidism; levels between 10–20 μU/ml suggest a decreased thyroid reserve. Levels are low in hyperthyroidism.

Fulfilled Needs: Protection from physical harm

Monitor blood studies for arterial blood gases[173,287] Watch for laboratory study reports indicating an abnormality in blood gas exchange. These studies include tests for O_2 saturation, PaO_2, CO_2 combining power, CO_2 content, $PaCO_2$, and hemoglobin.

Rationale: *CO_2 combining power:* This study reveals the amount of carbon dioxide that is absorbed by or combines with the blood at a specific temperature and pressure. Increased blood CO_2 combining power occurs with respiratory acidosis, metabolic alkalosis, and upper gastrointestinal fluid loss. Decreased blood CO_2 combining power occurs with metabolic acidosis, obstructed intestines, traumatic shock, and diarrhea.

CO_2 content: This test reveals the amount of carbon dioxide present in the blood. Increased blood carbon dioxide content occurs with upper gastrointestinal fluid loss, impaired pulmonary gas exchange, and obstructed intestines. A decreased blood carbon dioxide content occurs with respiratory alkalosis, diarrhea, renal acidosis, kidney inflammation, and pregnancy toxicity.

O_2 saturation: This study indicates the ratio of oxygen in the blood in relation to the amount of oxygen the blood is capable of holding. Increased blood O_2 saturation occurs with excessive blood oxygenation caused by oxygen therapy. Decreased blood O_2

saturation occurs with decreased red blood cell oxygenation, diminished cardiac output, and impaired pulmonary gas exchange.

PaO₂: This study shows the partial pressure of oxygen in the arteries. It reveals the amount of pressure being exerted against the artery by oxygen. Decreased blood PaO_2 occurs with impaired pulmonary gas exchange or diminished cardiac output.

PaCO₂: This study indicates the partial pressure of carbon dioxide in the arteries. It reveals the amount of pressure being exerted against the artery by carbon and oxygen gases when chemically combined. The blood level is in proportion to the amount of carbon dioxide produced by the cells and the rate of gas exchange in alveolar ventilation. Increased blood $PaCO_2$ occurs with metabolic alkalosis, respiratory acidosis, and impaired pulmonary gas exchange. Decreased blood $PaCO_2$ occurs with metabolic acidosis or respiratory alkalosis.

Hemoglobin: A normal hemoglobin is essential for carrying oxygen from the lungs to body tissues. An increased blood hemoglobin occurs with impaired pulmonary gas exchange. A decreased hemoglobin predisposes red blood cells to carry less oxygen.

Fulfilled Needs: Protection from physical harm

Monitor blood studies for biliary obstruction[173,287]
Watch for laboratory analysis reports indicating obstruction of bile flow from either the liver, gallbladder, or biliary ducts. These studies include tests for direct bilirubin, icterus index, leucine aminopeptidase, cholesterol, lipase, alkaline phosphatase, SGOT, and SGPT.

Rationale: *Direct bilirubin:* Direct bilirubin is a measurement of how the liver manages the bilirubin and is increased when there is biliary obstruction.

Icterus index: Increased blood icterus index occurs with biliary obstruction and indicates an increased ratio of bilirubin to blood.

Leucine aminopeptidase, cholesterol, lipase, alkaline phosphatase, SGOT, and SGPT: All are elevated when there is biliary obstruction.

Fulfilled Needs: Protection from physical harm

Monitor blood studies for blood type
Note the type of blood that laboratory analysis indicates the person has. Types include A, B, AB, and O. The blood may be Rh positive or negative.

Rationale: During pregnancy, detecting that the mother has Rh-negative blood and could produce antibiotics against the antigens in the infant's red blood cells causing hemolysis of the infant's cells supports early treatment for infant safety. When plans are being made for a kidney transplant, both the donor and the recipient must have the same blood types. When a person is given a blood type incompatible with his type, the results could be fatal.

Fulfilled Needs: Protection from physical harm

Monitor blood studies for dexamethasone suppression level[596]
The dexamethasone suppression test (DST) is done as follows: The person is given dexamethasone 1 mg by mouth at bedtime. The following day serum cortisol levels are drawn at 4 o'clock PM and 11 o'clock PM, or a single level is drawn at 4 o'clock PM. If any of the cortisol levels is greater than 5 μg/dl, the test is considered positive. If both cortisol levels are less than 5 μg/dl, the test is negative.

Rationale: In 96% of cases, a positive DST verifies the diagnosis of physiologic (endogenous, biologic, vital, or melancholic) depression. A positive DST also identifies those persons who are likely to relapse into depression when antidepressant and ECT therapy are terminated. If the person is not likely to relapse into depression, the DST level will gradually become normal. The regulation of emotion occurs in the hypothalamus and limbic system. The hypothalamus stimulates the pituitary gland to produce corticotropin (ACTH), which in turn stimulates the adrenal gland to produce cortisol. In normal persons, high levels of cortisol inhibit the release of additional ACTH. Glucocorticoid drugs, including dexamethasone, will also suppress the release of ACTH. However, in most persons with depression, there is an excessive production of cortisol with failure of the normal mechanism of ACTH suppression, so that the administration of dexamethasone does not produce the normally expected ACTH suppression.

Fulfilled Needs: Protection from physical and psychologic threat

Monitor blood studies for evidence of gastric ulceration[173,287]
Watch for laboratory analysis reports revealing the presence of gastric ulceration. These studies include tests for amylase and lipase.

Rationale: *Amylase:* Amylase is a digestive enzyme found in intestinal secretions. An increased blood amylase level occurs with gastric ulceration.

Lipase: A normal lipase level maintains adequate fat digestion. An increased blood lipase level occurs with gastrointestinal ulceration.

Fulfilled Needs: Protection from physical harm

Monitor blood studies for evidence of infection[173,287,368]
Watch for laboratory analysis reports revealing infection. These studies include tests for the leukocyte count, sedimentation rate, and WBC differential.

Rationale: *Leukocyte Count:* A normal leukocyte count is essential for body defense and tissue repair. An increased leukocyte count occurs with bacterial infection and excessive white blood cell production. A decreased leukocyte count occurs with viral infection.

Sedimentation rate: An increased sedimentation rate occurs with infection.

WBC differential: This report gives the percentage of each type of white blood cell contained in the blood specimen examined and points to specific infections.

Neutrophils normally make up more than 60% of the white blood cells. Their primary function is to attack bacteria (phagocytosis) so an increased neutrophil level indicates infection. A decreased neutrophil level indicates either an overwhelming infection because of the excessive destruction of cells or a viral infection. Certain drugs and chemicals also cause a decreased level.

Monocytes make up 2–6% of the WBC count. An elevated number of monocytes indicates recovery from serious infection, subacute bacterial endocarditis, tuberculosis, Rocky Mountain spotted fever, and typhoid fever.

Lymphocytes make up 20–40% of the white blood cells. An increased number of lymphocytes occur in many viral infections such as influenza, mumps, German measles, and infectious mononucleosis. Children and young adolescents have a normally higher percentage of lymphocytes than adults. A decreased lymphocyte count occurs with severe stress, as in burns or trauma, and in patients taking drugs such as epinephrine, ACTH, and cortisone.

Eosinophils and basophils comprise only 1–4% of the white blood count. An increased eosinophil count occurs with allergic reactions, parasite infestations, and brucellosis. A decreased count occurs when epinephrine, ACTH, or large doses of insulin are given. Basophils are increased in chronic granulocytic leukemia and hemolytic anemia.

The presence of immature WBCs occurs in leukemia and severe, acute infection.

The WBC may normally vary as much as 2,000/cu mm from morning to evening because of such activities as exercise, eating, or emotional stress.

Fulfilled Needs: Protection from physical harm

Monitor blood studies for evidence of kidney rejection[72,451]
Look for blood analysis studies of creatinine, urea nitrogen, protein, and white blood cells indicating that the transplanted kidney is being rejected by the immunological system.

Rationale: Increased levels of these substances indicate kidney rejection.

Fulfilled Needs: Protection from physical harm

Monitor blood studies for increased drug (barbiturate, digitalis, quinidine, salicylate, etc.) level
Look for a laboratory report indicating an abnormally high level of a specific drug in the blood.

Rationale: An elevated serum drug level indicates excessive consumption of the drug or impaired excretion of the drug.

Fulfilled Needs: Protection from physical harm

Monitor blood studies for increased lactic acid[173,287] Look for laboratory reports indicating elevated lactic acid. Lactic acid results from glycogen breakdown after muscle activity. When in excess, the lactate ion binds the calcium ion. This interferes with the normal calcium function of transmitting nerve impulses and causes intense anxiety associated with the increased blood level.

Rationale: An elevated lactic acid level occurs with increased muscular activity, decreased tissue oxygenation, and metabolic acidosis.

Fulfilled Needs: Protection from physical harm

Monitor blood studies for increased triglycerides[173,287] Look for indications that the blood triglyceride level is elevated. Triglycerides are fatty acids and glycerol. Their concentration in the blood causes the degree of cloudiness seen in the serum when the blood is centrifuged.

Rationale: An elevated blood triglyceride level occurs in myocardial ischemia and necrosis.

Fulfilled Needs: Protection from physical harm

Monitor blood studies for increased uric acid[173,287] Look for indications that the blood uric acid level is abnormally elevated. Uric acid results from purine metabolism. Normally, sufficient amounts are excreted daily through the urine in order to maintain a balanced blood level.

Rationale: Increased blood uric acid levels occur with kidney inflammation, pregnancy toxicity, excessive white blood cell production, and excessive purine metabolism.

Fulfilled Needs: Protection from physical harm

Monitor blood studies for positive VDRL Look for a positive VDRL blood report.

Rationale: This study is a screening test for syphilis. It does not confirm the diagnosis but supports the need for further laboratory studies.

Fulfilled Needs: Protection from physical harm

Monitor blood studies for Rh factor[73,158] Look for laboratory reports indicating whether the mother has Rh-positive or Rh-negative blood. If she has Rh-negative blood, then the father's Rh factor must also be checked. If the mother has Rh-negative blood and the father has Rh-positive blood, then referral to a physician should be made.

Rationale: When the mother has Rh-negative blood and the father has Rh-positive blood, the mother will produce antibodies against the antigens in the baby's blood, causing destruction of red blood cells.

Fulfilled Needs: Protection from physical harm

Monitor cerebrospinal fluid studies for abnormalities[173,287] Look for laboratory reports indicating abnormalities in cerebrospinal fluid. These include chloride level, cell count, and protein level.

Rationale: *Chloride:* Decreased levels of spinal fluid chloride occur with infection.
  Cell count: Increased spinal fluid cell count occurs with infection.
  Protein: Increased levels of spinal fluid protein occur with meningeal irritation and spinal cord tumor.

Fulfilled Needs: Protection from physical harm

Monitor gastric analysis studies for abnormalities[173,287] Look for laboratory reports indicating abnormal gastric analysis studies. These studies include tests for combined acid and total acid studies.

Rationale: *Combined acid:* A study showing increased combined acid indicates excessive gastric hydrochloric acid. A study showing decreased combined acid indicates gastric inflammation.

Total acid: Increased gastric total acidity occurs with gastrointestinal ulceration. Decreased gastric total acidity occurs in the presence of malignant gastric cells.

Fulfilled Needs: Protection from physical harm

Monitor the axillary temperature Measure body heat by placing a thermometer into the axilla so that the thermometer bulb has good skin contact. Axillary temperatures are taken when oral and rectal temperatures are contraindicated; they are also indicated for premature infants. Normal axillary temperature is 98.1° F (36.7° C).

Rationale: Abnormal body temperatures are caused by the body's protective mechanisms and are indicative of excessive body heat production or loss or poor temperature regulating mechanisms. Axillary temperatures are perferable for patients with self-destructive tendencies, as they lessen the possibility of ingestion of glass.

Fulfilled Needs: Protection from physical harm

Monitor the blood pressure Determine the pressure exerted by the blood on arterial walls by use of a mercury manometer and aircuff. Note abnormalities in blood pressure readings. Normal adult blood pressure consists of a systolic reading of 100–140 mm Hg and a diastolic reading of 60–90 mm Hg. In the infant the normal systolic reading is 55–90 mm Hg and the diastolic is 40–60 mm Hg.

Rationale: Blood pressure is controlled by heartbeat force, vessel tone, and blood volume and viscosity. Systolic blood pressure indicates the circulatory pressure during ventricular contraction. Decreased systolic blood pressure is associated with reduced circulating blood volume and cardiac output. Increased systolic blood pressure is associated with excessive water and sodium in the blood, which causes increased blood volume. It may also involve increased tension in arterial walls, plugging of arterial walls with fat deposits, decreased arterial dimensions caused by scar tissue, or severe stress causing contraction of arterial wall muscles and resulting in increased arterial pressure. Diastolic blood pressure indicates the circulatory pressure during ventricular relaxation. Decreased diastolic blood pressure is associated with reduced peripheral resistance caused by vasodilatation. Increased diastolic blood pressure is associated with increased peripheral resistance caused by vasoconstriction.

Fulfilled Needs: Protection from physical harm

Contraindications: Do not monitor the blood pressure of persons in whom an extremity has a fractured bone or in whom there is a circulatory embolus, AV shunt or fistula, lymphatic obstruction, or IV infusion.

Monitor the body/oral temperature Measure body heat by inserting a thermometer into the mouth. Wait 30 minutes after intake of hot or cold foods. Oral temperatures are most frequently used to measure body heat and are most valuable when rectal temperatures are contraindicated. Normal oral temperature is 98.6° F (37° C).

Rationale: Abdominal body temperatures are caused by the body's protective mechanisms and are indicative of excessive body heat production or loss or poor temperature regulating mechanisms.

Fulfilled Needs: Protection from physical harm

Contraindications: Do not take oral temperatures of infants or unconscious or confused persons or when there is mouth breathing, respiratory congestion, a wired jaw, or a convulsive disorder.

Monitor the cardiac output[249] The cardiac output is determined by the use of a pulmonary artery flow-directed thermodilution catheter connected to a cardiac output computer measuring the stroke volume (amount of blood pumped to the body during each ventricular contraction) multiplied by the heart rate per minute. Normally, the cardiac output is 4–7 liters/minute in an adult.

Rationale: Cardiac output levels provide data about the cardiac function of the right and left ventricle. It supports early recognition and treatment of ventricular failure.

Fulfilled Needs: Protection from physical harm

Monitor the cardiogram/the ECG   Record and interpret signals indicating regular or irregular heart action by using a surveillance device that records electrical discharges from the heart.

Rationale: Electrocardiograph recordings indicate the heart's electrical activity as levels of excitation in the different cardiac chambers. Recognition of inadequate circulation and cardiac inadequacies prevents damage to body tissues and tissue death.

Fulfilled Needs: Protection from physical harm

Monitor the central venous pressure[73]   After the central venous pressure (CVP) catheter has been inserted through the arm or neck vein into the superior vena cava, attach the catheter to the water manometer and intermittently monitor and record the CVP reading. Normal CVP is 5–15 cm H_2O. Since CVP readings are influenced by blood pressure, respiratory rate, emotional state, urine output, and intravenous fluids, several readings are desirable; one should not rely on a single abnormal reading.

Rationale: CVP reflects the circulating blood volume, the efficiency of cardiac function, and the vascular tone. Increased CVP indicates increased circulating blood volume and impaired cardiac function. Decreased CVP occurs with blood or fluid loss.

Fulfilled Needs: Protection from physical harm

Monitor the external counterpulsation pressure suit apparatus[249]   Check the functioning of the external pressure suit, which encloses the legs and pelvis and provides external counterpulsation. Monitor the control console for timing and synchronization of the pump.

Rationale: The pressure suit assists the circulation of the failing heart by increasing the return of peripheral venous blood to the right heart during diastole. It improves the cardiac output and somewhat reduces the workload of the left ventricle. Counterpulsation limits the size of the infarction by increasing coronary blood flow.

Fulfilled Needs: Tissue oxygenation or perfusion, protection from physical harm

Monitor the fetal heart sounds   Place the stethoscope or headscope over the maternal anterior abdominal wall and listen to the heart sounds of the unborn infant. Listen between contractions or at contraction termination. Listen for irregular, rapid, or slow heartbeats and for fetal heart sounds immediately after the uterine membrane has ruptured and again 10 minutes later. If the fetal pulse is greatly accelerated or decreased, also watch for meconium in the amniotic fluid indicating fetal distress.

Rationale: Fetal heart sounds assist in determining if there is fetal life. Movement of fetal heart sounds can give clues to the progress of labor. If umbilical cord prolapse occurs, it will be evidenced by fetal distress immediately or shortly after membrane rupture. During maternal seizures, fetal circulation is impaired, and fetal heart sounds can warn of fetal distress. When the fetal head is exerting pressure on the umbilical cord, abnormally rapid or abnormally slow fetal heart sounds signal distress.

Fulfilled Needs: Protection from physical harm

Monitor the flow rate of the intravenous fluids   Watch the rate of flow of the intravenous fluids, counting the number of drops per minute being infused.

Rationale: The flow rate of intravenous fluids is monitored to ensure the correct administration of the fluids ordered for the day and to protect against fluid overload or fluid depletion.

Fulfilled Needs: Fluid and electrolyte balance, protection from physical harm

Monitor the infant for apnea   Place a monitor under the crib sheet and place the infant on it with his chest positioned directly over it.

Rationale: Monitoring infants for apnea can facilitate early recognition and treatment of respiratory distress.

Fulfilled Needs: Protection from physical harm

Monitor the internal counterpulsation intra-aortic balloon apparatus[249]

Check the functioning of the balloon catheter inserted into the femoral artery and threaded up into the artery, just below the left subclavian artery. Observe the timing of inflation with diastole and deflation with systole. Observe for obstruction of the arterial blood flow to the leg used for cannulation. Monitor for signs of shock and insufficient blood flow to the leg.

Rationale: The intra-aortic balloon pump assists the circulation of the failing heart. It reduces the workload of the left ventricle, which, in turn, reduces the body's oxygen requirements.

Fulfilled Needs: Tissue oxygenation or perfusion, protection from physical harm

Monitor the intracranial pressure recordings[249]

If the person has an intracranial monitoring line inserted, monitor the recordings. The normal intracranial pressure (ICP) level is 110–140 mm H_2O, or 0–10 mm Hg.

Rationale: Pressures elevated above 200 mg H_2O or 15 mm Hg indicate increased intracranial pressure.

Fulfilled Needs: Protection from physical harm

Monitor the laboratory findings of sputum analysis[173,287]

Look for laboratory reports of sputum analysis.

Rationale: Analysis of sputum specimens can indicate respiratory system disorders. Clear thin (mucoid) sputum occurs with early bronchitis. Thick, frothy, greenish (mucopurulent) sputum indicates late bronchitis, pneumonia, or tuberculosis. Thick yellow (purulent) sputum occurs with lung abscess, bronchiectasis, empyema, or late tuberculosis. Gelatinous rusty sputum indicates pneumonia. Offensive dark brown (prune juice) sputum occurs with pneumonia, pulmonary gangrene, or early lung growth. Jellylike blood-clotted (red currant jelly) sputum indicates early lung growth.

Fulfilled Needs: Protection from physical harm

Monitor the mean arterial pressure[73]

The mean arterial pressure is one-half the sum of the systolic and diastolic pressure. For example, for an arterial pressure of 120/80, MAP = 200 ÷ 2 = 100.

Rationale: The MAP represents the average amount of pressure pushing blood through the circulatory system. A minimum of 70 mm Hg MAP is necessary for kidney function.

Fulfilled Needs: Protection from physical harm

Monitor the oxygen saturation status by ear oximeter or transcutaneous monitor[249]

The ear oximeter is a noninvasive device that works by trans-illumination of the ear, giving a continuous reading of the oxygen saturation status. The transcutaneous monitor is also noninvasive. An electrode (skin sensor) is applied (it is usually put on the abdomen of premature infants) and a continuous reading of the partial arterial pressure of oxygen (PO_2) is given.

Rationale: These devices are used for persons on respirators to determine when adjustments of the fraction of inspired oxygen (FIO_2) is needed.

Fulfilled Needs: Protection from physical harm

Monitor the Papanicolaou smear results for positive findings[125]

Look for laboratory reports of a positive Papanicolaou (Pap) smear. Pap smears can be performed on uterine cells and on fluid expressed from the prostate. Pap smear results are classified by Papanicolau as:

Class 1	No abnormal cells
Class 2	Some abnormal cells, no malignancy
Class 3	Abnormal cells suggesting possible malignancy
Class 4	Abnormal cells strongly suggesting malignancy
Class 5	Definite malignant cells

Rationale: A positive Pap smear supports early detection and treatment of cancer.

Fulfilled Needs: Protection from physical harm

Monitor the pulmonary artery pressure (and/or the pulmonary capillary wedge pressure) by Swan-Ganz catheter[249]

Check the functioning of the Swan-Ganz catheter, a multilumen catheter inserted into the femoral vein. It is then threaded into the right side of the heart and passed into the pulmonary artery. Pulmonary artery (PA) pressure is monitored continuously, while the pulmonary capillary wedge pressure (PCWP) is read by intermittently inflating the catheter balloon. Observe carefully for complications such as inflammation, balloon rupture, pulmonary hemorrhage, infarction, right-sided premature ventricular contractions, or ventricular fibrillation from stray or leaky electrical current.

Rationale: The Swan-Ganz catheter provides for measurement of systolic, diastolic, and mean pulmonary artery pressures, and of mean PCWP. The PA diastolic and PCWP represent the pressure in the left ventricle just before contraction (end-diastolic). In general, an increase in these two pressure readings signifies an increased blood volume, and a decrease indicates a decreased volume, so impending circulatory overload, hypovolemia, and cardiac failure can be recognized early. A thermistor wire included in some of the catheters measures the blood temperature and is used to measure cardiac output by the thermodilution technique.

Fulfilled Needs: Protection from physical harm

Monitor the pulse pressure

Subtract the diastolic blood pressure reading from the systolic blood pressure reading to obtain pulse pressure. If the pulse pressure is more than 50 points or less than 30 points, it is abnormal.

Rationale: Pulse pressure indicates the tone of the arterial walls. A pulse pressure of more than 50 points indicates decreased arterial elasticity (increased arterial rigidity), which reduces arterial blood flow and impairs normal oxygen transport. A pulse pressure of less than 30 points indicates insufficient blood circulating volume, which results in decreased tissue oxygenation.

Fulfilled Needs: Protection from physical harm

Monitor the rectal temperature

Measure body heat by inserting the bulb of a thermometer into the rectum. Rectal temperatures are taken when oral temperatures are contraindicated. The normal range of rectal temperature is 99.1–99.6° F (32.2° C–37.5° C.)

Rationale: Abnormal body temperatures are caused by the body's protective mechanisms and are indicative of excessive body heat production or loss or poor temperature regulating mechanisms.

Fulfilled Needs: Protection from physical harm

Contraindications: Rectal surgery, fecal impaction, diarrhea, rectal stricture, rectal pain or bleeding, bradycardia, cardiac arrhythmias, intestinal worms.

Monitor tidal volume studies for decreased lung capacity

Look for laboratory reports indicating a decrease in the total volume of air inspired and expired with each normal breath.

Rationale: Decreased tidal volume indicates decreased pulmonary muscle strength or increased pulmonary tissue or airway resistance.

Fulfilled Needs: Protection from physical harm

Monitor urine studies for abnormal adrenal function[173,287]

Look for urinalysis reports that indicate impaired adrenal function. Levels of aldosterone, sodium, 17-hydroxycorticoids, and 17-ketosteroids are monitored.

Rationale: *Aldosterone:* Aldosterone is a mineralocorticoid that is essential for balanced sodium, potassium, and chloride metabolism. Increased urinary levels of aldosterone occur with adrenal cortex hypersecretion of aldosterone.

Sodium: Increased urinary levels of sodium occur with adrenal insufficiency.

Decreased urinary levels of sodium occur with diuresis resulting from insufficient antidiuretic hormone, adrenal hyperactivity, and aldosterone hypersecretion.

17-hydroxycorticoids: 17-Hydroxycorticoids are involved primarily in regulating carbohydrate and protein metabolism. Their secretion is dependent on ACTH production. Decreased urinary levels of 17-hydroxycorticoids occur with adrenal insufficiency (Addison's disease). Increased urinary levels of 17-hydroxycorticoids indicate adrenal hyperactivity (Cushing's syndrome).

17-ketosteroids: The 17α- and 17β-ketosteroids are produced in the adrenal cortex and gonads and are normally excreted in the urine. Decreased urinary levels of 17-ketosteroids occur with adrenal insufficiency. Increased urinary levels of 17-ketosteroids occur with adrenal hyperactivity.

Fulfilled Needs: Protection from physical harm

Monitor urine studies for abnormal carbohydrate metabolism[173,287] Look for urinalysis reports indicating impaired carbohydrate metabolism. Levels of acetone, glucose, and ammonia are monitored.

Rationale: *Acetone:* The presence of acetone in the urine indicates that the ketone and other products of fat metabolism have spilled into the urine. The presence of acetone in the urine indicates impaired carbohydrate metabolism that has caused excessive fat metabolism.

Glucose: The sugar level results from carbohydrate metabolism. Excesses are spilled into the urine. Increased urinary levels of glucose occur with impaired glucose metabolism.

Ammonia: Ammonia gas results from the metabolism of proteins and amino acids by the liver. Increased urinary levels of ammonia occur with impaired glucose metabolism.

Fulfilled Needs: Protection from physical harm

Monitor urine studies for abnormal liver function[173,287] Look for urinalysis findings indicating impaired liver function. Levels of ammonia, urobilinogen, copper, and porphobilinogen are monitored.

Rationale: *Ammonia:* Ammonia gas results from the metabolism of proteins and amino acids by the liver. The liver then converts the ammonia to urea for excretion by the kidneys. Increased urinary levels of ammonia occur with liver cell damage.

Urobilinogen: Normally, urobilinogen is absorbed by the circulatory system and returned to the liver. Increased urinary levels of urobilinogen indicate that the liver cannot adequately convert urobilinogen to urobilin because of impaired liver function.

Copper: Copper is normally found in the liver and is excreted by the kidneys. Increased urinary levels of copper occur with liver cell damage.

Porphobilinogen: Porphobilinogen is one of several porphyrin compounds that unite with the protein globin to form hemoglobin. A standard test will reveal excessive excretion of porphobilinogen, which occurs with chronic liver disease.

Fulfilled Needs: Protection from physical harm

Monitor urine studies for abnormal parathyroid function[173,287] Look for urinalysis findings indicating impaired thyroid function. Rate of phosphate clearance and level of calcium are monitored.

Rationale: *Phosphate clearance:* A standard test reveals the kidney's ability to excrete phosphate. Increased urinary levels of phosphate occur with parathyroid hypersecretion. Decreased urinary levels of phosphate occur with parathyroid hyposecretion.

Calcium: A standard test reveals the ratio of calcium to phosphorus. If the urinary level of calcium is excessive, the urinary level of phosphorus will be low. Increased urinary levels of calcium occur with parathyroid hypersecretion.

Fulfilled Needs: Protection from physical harm

Monitor urine studies for abnormal pituitary function[173,287] Look for urinaly-

sis studies indicating impaired pituitary function. Levels of 17-hydroxycorticoids, potassium, and pituitary gonadotropin are monitored.

Rationale: *17-hydroxycorticoids:* 17-Hydroxycorticoids are involved primarily in regulating carbohydrate and protein metabolism. Their secretion is dependent on ACTH production. Decreased urinary levels of 17-hydroxycorticoids occur with pituitary insufficiency.

Potassium: Decreased urinary levels of potassium occur with pituitary insufficiency.

Pituitary gonadotropin: The pituitary gonadotropin hormones are released by the anterior pituitary; they include follicle-stimulating hormone, interstitial-cell-stimulating hormone, luteinizing hormone, and luteotropic hormone. Decreased urinary levels of pituitary gonadotropin occur with pituitary insufficiency.

Fulfilled Needs: Protection from physical harm

Monitor urine studies for abnormal renal function[173,287]
Look for urinalysis findings indicating impaired renal function. Rates of creatinine clearance and urea clearance, levels of protein (albumin), phosphorus, urea, uric acid, and phenolsulfonaphthalein (PSP), and specific gravity are monitored.

Rationale: *Creatinine clearance:* The rate of creatinine clearance indicates the kidney's ability to excrete creatinine. A decreased rate of urinary creatinine clearance occurs with kidney glomerular dysfunction.

Protein: Proteins (albumin) appear in the urine when there is impaired renal function caused by inflammation of glomeruli, excessive pressure within renal arteries, or urinary tract infection. Increased urinary levels of protein occur with kidney inflammation.

Phosphorus: Decreased urinary levels of phosphorus occur with kidney inflammation.

Urea and urea clearance: Normally the kidneys excrete a specific amount of urea following protein metabolism. Decreased urinary levels of urea occur with kidney failure.

Uric acid: Uric acid results from purine metabolism and is excreted in normal amounts daily. Decreased urinary levels of uric acid occur with kidney inflammation.

PSP: The level of PSP indicates the quality of the kidney's excretory functioning and its ability to concentrate urine and maintain body fluid and electrolyte balance. Decreased urinary levels of PSP occur with kidney tubule dysfunction and genitourinary infection or obstruction.

Specific gravity: The test for specific gravity reveals the degree of urine concentration. Decreased urinary specific gravity indicates a decreased ability to concentrate urine. Increased specific gravity indicates a decreased ability to reabsorb sodium, etc.

Fulfilled Needs: Protection from physical harm

Monitor urine studies for abnormal thyroid function[368]
Look for urinalysis findings indicating impaired thyroid function. Studies include a test for radioactive iodine uptake.

Rationale: *Radioactive iodine uptake:* Following oral ingestion of radioactive iodine, the thyroid removes some of the iodide from the blood, and the remainder is excreted by the kidneys within a 24-hour period. In addition to a Geiger counter survey of the neck, the entire 24-hour urine output is checked for radioactivity. Excretion of 40% or less of the radioactive iodine during the 24-hour period indicates thyrotoxicosis.

Fulfilled Needs: Protection from physical harm

Monitor urine studies for biliary obstruction[173,287]
Look for urinalysis reports that indicate biliary obstruction. Levels of bilirubin and urobilinogen are monitored.

Rationale: *Bilirubin:* When an obstruction prevents bile from flowing into the intestines, it goes into the blood and is excreted by the kidneys. With increased urinary levels of bilirubin, the bile pigment colors the urine dark yellow, green yellow or brown.

Urobilinogen: When the liver excretes bile, it is broken down into bilirubin and goes into the intestines. The intestinal bacteria break it down further into urobilinogen. The intestinal circulation absorbs some of the urobilinogen and returns it to the liver to be converted into urobilin. Normally a specific amount leaves the circulation and is excreted in the urine. If the kidneys excrete large amounts, this may indicate that the liver is unable to convert urobilinogen to urobilin. Increased urinary levels of urobilinogen occur with incomplete biliary obstruction. Decreased urinary levels of urobilinogen occur with complete biliary obstruction.

Fulfilled Needs: Protection from physical harm

Monitor urine studies for decreased D-xylose absorption[173,287] Look for an abnormally low urinary D-xylose level.

Rationale: Decreased urinary levels of D-xylose occur with malabsorption in the small intestine.

Fulfilled Needs: Protection from physical harm

Monitor urine studies for evidence of kidney rejection[451] Look for urinalysis studies indicating that the transplanted kidney is being rejected by the immunologic system. The level of protein and the white blood cell (lymphocyte) count are monitored.

Rationale: Increased urinary levels of protein and increased white blood cell counts indicate kidney rejection.

Fulfilled Needs: Protection from physical harm

Monitor urine studies for evidence of urinary tract infection[173,287] Look for urinalysis studies indicating infection of the genitourinary system, as indicated by the presence of erythrocytes, hemoglobin, hyaline casts, leukocytes, and tubular casts.

Rationale: *Erythrocytes:* The presence of these red blood cells in the urine indicates urinary tract inflammation or irritation. Increased urinary levels of erythrocytes occur with genitourinary infection and kidney inflammation or failure.

Hemoglobin: The presence of hemoglobin in the urine indicates the abnormal presence of red blood cells. Increased urinary levels of hemoglobin occur with kidney inflammation.

Hyaline casts: The presence of pale, cylinder-shaped hyaline casts indicates kidney irritation. Increased urinary levels of hyaline casts occur with genitourinary infection and kidney inflammation, degeneration, or failure.

Leukocytes: White blood cells in the urine occur with genitourinary infection and kidney inflammation.

Tubular casts: The presence of tube-shaped waxy casts indicates separation of dead epithelial cells from the renal system. Increased urinary levels of tubular casts occur with noninflammatory kidney degeneration, kidney failure, genitourinary infection, and renal acidosis.

Fulfilled Needs: Protection from physical harm

Monitor urine studies for increased Bence Jones protein[173,287] Look for the presence of Bence Jones protein in the urine. This protein dissolves when urine is boiled and precipitates when the urine cools.

Rationale: Bence Jones protein occurs in the urine of patients with bone tumors, lymph tissue malignancy and hyperplasia, excessive white blood cell production, brittle bones, and parathyroid hypersecretion.

Fulfilled Needs: Protection from physical harm

Monitor urine studies for increased catecholamines[173,287] Look for urinalysis reports showing elevated urinary levels of catecholamines. The test reveals the levels of epinephrine and norepinephrine being excreted by the adrenal medulla.

Rationale: Increased urinary levels of catecholamines occur with tumor of the adrenal medulla and peripheral vasoconstriction.

Fulfilled Needs: Protection from physical harm

Monitor urine studies for increased drug (salicylate, barbiturate, etc.) level

Look for urinalysis reports showing an elevated drug level.

Rationale: Increased urinary drug levels occur with excessive drug doses.

Fulfilled Needs: Protection from physical harm

Monitor urine studies for increased gonadotropins[173,287] Look for urinalysis reports indicating elevated urinary levels of gonadotropins.

Rationale: Gonadotropins (hormones) stimulate the sex glands, which are responsible for cell formation in human reproduction. During pregnancy the gonadotropin level is elevated.

Fulfilled Needs: Protection from physical harm

Monitor urine studies for increased uric acid[173,287] Look for indications that the urinary level of uric acid is abnormally elevated. Uric acid is derived from purine metabolism and is excreted in normal amounts daily.

Rationale: Increased urinary levels of uric acid occur with excessive white blood cell production, with excessive purine metabolism, and as a side effect of steroid drugs.

Fulfilled Needs: Protection from physical harm

Monitor urine studies for increased VMA[173,287] Look for urinalysis reports showing elevated levels of vanillylmandelic acid (VMA). VMA is a product of catecholamine metabolism.

Rationale: Increased urinary levels of VMA occur with tumor of the adrenal medulla and peripheral vasoconstriction, which causes hypertension.

Fulfilled Needs: Protection from physical harm

Observe and record the food/fluid intake Record the amounts and kinds of solid and semisolid foods and liquids the patient eats or drinks within a 24-hour period. Sometimes this record is referred to a dietitian for a calorie count.

Rationale: A record of food and fluid intake provides a basis from which to initiate a balanced nutritional and fluid intake.

Fulfilled Needs: Protection from physical harm.

Observe for a blood transfusion reaction Observe the patient for sudden complaints of chest pain or tightness, fever, chills, facial burning, back pain, bloody urine, absent or decreased urine output, dyspnea, cyanosis, skin rash or hives, decrease in blood pressure, nausea, vomiting, laryngeal edema, wheezing, and distended neck veins.

Rationale: A blood transfusion reaction may result from an excessive increase in blood volume, which causes circulatory overload, or from the transmission of viruses, bacteria, or parasites from a donor to the recipient who usually forms antibodies to the allergens contained in the donor blood. When incompatible blood is administered, the red blood cells received from the donor clump together (agglutinate) in the plasma of the recipient. The red cells are rapidly broken down by enzymes, exceeding the liver's ability to detoxify the products, which results in damage of the kidney tubules when the excess is excreted.

Fulfilled Needs: Protection from physical harm

Observe for a halo sign When there is a possibility of spinal fluid leakage, notice if drainage from the nose or ears, onto linen leaves a blood-tinged center spot surrounded by a lighter-colored ring.

Rationale: The presence of a halo sign indicates spinal fluid leakage from the ears or nose.

Fulfilled Needs: Protection from physical harm

Observe for a hypersensitivity response Look for an unfavorable antigen-antibody reaction manifested by the symptoms of frequent sneezing, tearing, dyspnea, wheezing, skin rashes and inflammation, nausea, vomiting, diarrhea, local edema, itching, cyanosis, choking, weak and rapid pulse, hypotension, clammy skin, or convulsions.

Rationale: Foreign bodies introduced into the body act as antigens. The antigen reacts with antibodies that respond to the specific antigen. When the antigen-antibody reaction is unfavorable, adjacent cells and tissue are damaged.

Fulfilled Needs: Protection from physical harm

Observe for a positive skin test   After a small amount of toxin or antigen has been injected under the skin, watch for an area of redness. Depending on the drug, the redness will be evident 24–48 hours after injection. This applies to toxins for diphtheria, tuberculosis (Mantoux), and the systemic fungal disease (histoplasmosis, coccidioidomycosis, etc.)

Rationale: When the blood does not contain enough antitoxin to protect the patient against the toxin of a disease, a positive reaction of redness will occur at the point of injection. In such cases a prophylactic immunization should be given to protect against the disease.

Fulfilled Needs: Protection from physical harm

Observe for abnormal gait   Look for unsteadiness, shuffling, staggering, limping, stooped walking, high stepping, propulsion walking, weaving, waddling, spastic gait, scissor gait, chorea gait, or atactic gait.

Rationale: Abnormal gait indicates musculoskeletal, neurologic, or circulatory disorders.

Fulfilled Needs: Protection from physical harm

Observe for acute pain onset   Look for indications that pain has suddenly occurred.

Rationale: Acute pain is generally associated with inflammatory conditions, coronary artery disease, muscle spasms, and trauma.

Fulfilled Needs: Protection from physical harm

Observe for adequate hydration   Look for signs that the person is receiving sufficient fluid. Such signs include consistent weight, rapid capillary refill, pink moist skin, mucous membranes, and pinched skin that rapidly returns to normal position.

Rationale: Adequate hydration is essential to normal cardiopulmonary function.

Fulfilled Needs: Protection from physical harm

Observe for airway obstruction/choking   Observe whether the airway is clear for adequate gas exchange. Airway obstruction may be evidenced as respiratory distress, restlessness, airway noise, cyanosis, or anxious behavior.

Rationale: A patent airway is essential for the maintenance of life.

Fulfilled Needs: Protection from physical harm

Observe for an excessive stress level   Determine whether the person perceives an extreme threat and believes that it is imposed on him and is beyond his control, whether a great number of adjustive demands are being made within a short time, or whether extremely important needs are not being met. Signs of an excessive stress level include irritability, intense resistance to change, startle reflex to noise, and overactivity.

Rationale: Excessive stress causes severe disequilibrium because adaptive capacities are overtaxed.

Fulfilled Needs: Protection from physical harm. Protection from psychologic threat

Observe for apathy   Notice if the person's facial expression and body movements reveal a lack of feeling. He may make verbal comments about disinterest or unconcern.

Rationale: Apathy results when frustration and stress reach very high levels and the person feels unable to cope. The coping method then used is one of unconcern.

Fulfilled Needs: Protection from psychologic stress

Observe for behavior modification   Look for changes from unhealthy behavioral patterns to the healthy behavioral patterns that have been suggested.

Rationale: A change to healthy behavioral patterns will support the development of improved health in the future.

Fulfilled Needs: Protection from physical harm

Observe for chewing difficulty   Look for signs that the person cannot chew or is having difficulty chewing.

Rationale: Chewing is essential to food breakdown before digestion.

Fulfilled Needs: Protection from physical harm

Observe for clothing that constricts circulation or movement   Look for tight clothing that constricts circulation or freedom of movement, such as garters, girdles, hatbands, belts, or purse straps over the arm.

Rationale: Constricting clothing impairs circulation, reducing tissue oxygenation and preventing freedom of movement.

Fulfilled Needs: Protection from physical harm

Observe for cold, clammy skin   Touch the skin and feel for cold or moistness.

Rationale: Cold, clammy skin is caused by activation of sweat glands, with concomitant peripheral blood vessel constriction. It indicates circulatory impairment.

Fulfilled Needs: Protection from physical harm

Observe for complaints of anorexia   Listen for complaints of prolonged loss of appetite. The person relates having little or no interest in food.

Rationale: Anorexia may indicate chemical disturbances in the body, adverse drug effects, or excessive psychologic stress.

Fulfilled Needs: Protection from physical harm

Observe for complaints of anxiety/apprehension/fear   Watch for signs that the person is experiencing anxiety or fear. Such signs include sleeplessness, demanding behavior, avoiding persons or situations, and nervous gestures.

Rationale: Being aware of the person's anxiety or fear, the nurse can respond appropriately and meet the person's needs.

Fulfilled Needs: Comfort, protection from psychologic threat

Observe for complaints of chills   Listen for complaints of intermittent internal coldness. Chills may or may not be accompanied by shaking, pallor, teeth chattering, or external skin coldness. Note the length and severity of the chill.

Rationale: Chills indicate the body's need for increased temperature or the existence of a fever.

Fulfilled Needs: Protection from physical harm

Observe for complaints of constipation   Listen for complaints of difficult passage of hard, dry stools.

Rationale: Constipation may be associated with inactivity, pregnancy, gastrointestinal disorders, trauma to the intestinal tract during surgery, or inadequate intake of bulk food or fluid.

Fulfilled Needs: Protection from physical harm

Observe for complaints of difficulty concentrating   Listen for complaints that the person finds it hard to focus his thoughts on a particular subject or task.

Rationale: Impaired concentration may indicate adverse drug effects, excessive psychologic stress requiring large amounts of energy for coping with the stress, or neurologic problems.

Fulfilled Needs: Protection from physical harm

Observe for complaints of dizziness   Listen for complaints of a whirling sensation in the head, with or without giddiness or confusion. Watch for unstable walking.

Rationale: Dizziness may indicate a circulatory or neurologic disorder.

Fulfilled Needs: Protection from physical harm

Observe for complaints of dysuria Listen for complaints of painful or difficult urination.

Rationale: Dysuria may occur with bladder or urethral inflammation, urethral stricture, uterine prolapse, prostate enlargement or ulceration, painful menstruation, or cervical carcinoma.

Fulfilled Needs: Protection from physical harm

Observe for complaints of excessive flatulence Listen for complaints of stomach or intestinal gas.

Rationale: Excessive flatulence may occur with liver and gastrointestinal problems. It causes pressure within the stomach or intestines, resulting in severe sharp pain and discomfort.

Fulfilled Needs: Protection from physical harm

Observe for complaints of fatigue Look for signs of fatigue, such as yawning, irritability, dark shadows under the eyes, uncoordinated movements, inability to concentrate, shortness of breath, rapid pulse, and complaints of being tired.

Rationale: Fatigue results when the body cells, because of adaptation requirements, have depleted their energy reserves and require a period of restoration.

Fulfilled Needs: Protection from physical harm

Observe for complaints of headache Listen for complaints of pressure or pain within the cranium.

Rationale: Headache indicates a disorder within the head, scalp, sinuses, or other body area.

Fulfilled Needs: Protection from physical harm

Observe for complaints of itching Watch for scratching of any body part as indicative of the itching sensation.

Rationale: Itching may indicate internal or external skin irritation or a sensitivity reaction to a specific agent.

Fulfilled Needs: Protection from physical harm

Observe for complaints of lightheadedness Listen for complaints that the person feels as though his head is floating or unsteady.

Rationale: Lightheadedness may indicate adverse drug effects, lack of sleep or nutrition, or chemical imbalance.

Fulfilled Needs: Protection from physical harm

Observe for complaints of malaise Listen for complaints of a generalized feeling of being barely able to function.

Rationale: Malaise is common during infection and general body dysfunction.

Fulfilled Needs: Protection from physical harm

Observe for complaints of menstruation cycle abnormalities Observe for complaints that menstruation is occurring more frequently than every 21 days, occurring less frequently than every 35 days, or having a duration of less then 3 days or more than 7 days.

Rationale: Abnormal menstruation is frequently indicative of endocrine or reproductive system disorders.

Fulfilled Needs: Protection from physical harm

Observe for complaints of nasal congestion Look and listen for evidence of obstructing secretions or swollen tissues in the nose, such as inability to breathe in and out of one or both nostrils, frequent nasal drainage, and noisy breathing when the mouth is closed.

Rationale: Nasal congestion can result in airway obstruction and severe discomfort.

Fulfilled Needs: Protection from physical harm

Observe for complaints of nausea Listen for complaints of the sensation of stomach queasiness.

Rationale: Nausea can indicate gastric irritation, intestinal obstruction, motion sickness, increased intracranial pressure, severe pain, toxic and disease states, or psychogenic disturbances.

Fulfilled Needs: Protection from physical harm

Observe for complaints of nervousness Observe the person for signs of easy excitability and agitation.

Rationale: Nervousness may indicate that the body's regulatory mechanisms are in a state of disorder or that the nervous system has been overstimulated.

Fulfilled Needs: Protection from physical harm

Observe for complaints of nocturia Listen for the person's complaints of having to get up to void during the night time. Note the number of times the person voids at night.

Rationale: Being awakened at night to void indicates bladder or kidney disorders.

Fulfilled Needs: Protection from physical harm

Observe for complaints of noise sensitivity Note complaints that noise greatly disturbs the patient. Indications of sensitivity include irritability when in a noisy environment, closing oneself off from noise, startle reactions when noises occur, and asking others to turn off radios and televisions.

Rationale: Hypersensitivity causes heightened responses to environmental stimuli and requires increased adaptation to stress.

Fulfilled Needs: Protection from physical harm

Observe for complaints of numbness and tingling Listen for complaints of loss of sensation or complaints of pinprick sensations in some body area.

Rationale: Numbness and tingling occur when there is inadequate circulation to peripheral nerves or when there is nerve damage.

Fulfilled Needs: Protection from physical harm

Observe for complaints of orthopnea Look for difficulty in breathing during which the person elevates his head and thorax while resting.

Rationale: Orthopnea may indicate severe cardiac or respiratory disorder.

Fulfilled Needs: Protection from physical harm

Observe for complaints of pain/tenderness/backache Listen for complaints of distressful hurting anywhere in the body.

Rationale: Pain is the body's signal of impending or existing tissue damage.

Fulfilled Needs: Protection from physical harm, protection from psychologic threat

Observe for complaints of pain duration Listen for a description of the length of time a person's pain lasts. Determine its duration (minutes, hours, or days) and whether it is intermittent or continuous.

Rationale: Pain duration assists in determining the cause. Prolonged pain is usually perceived as threatening.

Fulfilled Needs: Protection from physical harm, protection from psychologic threat

Observe for complaints of pain radiation Listen for complaints of pain occurring in areas other than the area of its first appearance, including radiation to the back, shoulder, arm, hand, jaw, neck, head, or any body area.

Rationale: Pain radiation follows nerve pathways and signals body distress. During the instillation of peritoneal dialysis fluid, pain may occur in the left shoulder, indicating diaphragmatic irritation from fluid pressure within the peritoneum.

Fulfilled Needs: Protection from physical harm

Observe for complaints of respiratory muscle weakness   Listen for complaints of not having strength to breathe.

Rationale: Respiratory muscle weakness occurs in endocrine, metabolic, and nervous system disorders.

Fulfilled Needs: Protection from physical harm

Observe for complaints of thirst   Listen for complaints of a dry cottony feeling in the mouth.

Rationale: Thirst indicates physiologic body changes related to fluid or electrolyte imbalance. It occurs with dehydration, when it may be associated with fever, vomiting, diarrhea, hemorrhage, shock, or polyuria. Thirst results when there is decreased fluid volume, in which loss of water is disproportionately higher than loss of salt. It also occurs when there is increased fluid volume, in which salt losses are disproportionately higher than water losses. Potassium depletion and drug side effects also cause thirst.

Fulfilled Needs: Protection from physical harm

Observe for complaints of tinnitus   Listen for complaints that the patient is hearing ringing or buzzing sounds or the like. These sounds usually seem louder at night.

Rationale: Tinnitus may indicate a hearing disorder, a drug side effect, impacted earwax, tension, a foreign body in the ear, inflammation, or skull fracture.

Fulfilled Needs: Protection from physical harm

Observe for complaints of urinary frequency   Determine whether the adult voids more often than every 5 hours. Normal urine output is 30–60 cc/hour. Normal bladder capacity is approximately 450 cc before the elimination reflex is activated. Observe the patient for the intake of large amounts of liquids, especially tea and coffee. Determine whether the increased intra-abdominal pressure of pregnancy is the cause of frequency.

Rationale: Urinary frequency may result from kidney inflammation, pressure against the bladder, high urea or uric acid concentrations, reflex stimulation of calculi in the ureter, or loss of bladder tone.

Fulfilled Needs: Protection from physical harm

Observe for complaints of visual disturbance   Listen for complaints of changes in vision, such as blurring, double vision, and light flashes.

Rationale: Visual distrubances are often associated with physiologic disorders such as cerebral pressure, vascular disorders, acid–base balance, and respiratory gas-exchange disorders, as well as with digitalis and atropine overdosage.

Fulfilled Needs;   Protection from physical harm

Observe for complaints of warmth   Notice if the person complains of feeling unusually warm or flushed.

Rationale: Unusual warmth indicates peripheral dilatation, which can result from hormonal changes, drug side effects, fever, and excessive environmental temperature (as when in an oxygen tent).

Fulfilled Needs: Protection from physical harm

Observe for complaints of weakness   Listen for complaints of decreased strength, such as weakness on exertion, a desire to lie down, muscle tremors, irritability, nervousness, clumsy movements, rapid breathing, and inability to deal with complex problems. Note any increase or decrease in blood pressure or any increase in pulse pressure.

Rationale: Muscle weakness may result from impaired nerve supply, decreased circulation, muscle disuse, inadequate nutrition, muscle glycogen depletion, or lactic acid accumulation.

Fulfilled Needs: Protection from physical harm

Observe for conditions indicating a need for increased nutritional requirements   Watch for the onset of conditions in which the person will need additional nourishment, such as endocrine disorders, fever, severe tissue damage, pregnancy, lactation, rapid growth during childhood, or loss of body weight. Determine if the person needs more protein, carbohydrates, or other foods than is usually required of an individual.

Rationale: In certain conditions, such as tissue healing, weakness, malabsorption, physical growth, and pregnancy, additional food intake is needed to maintain and promote health.

Fulfilled Needs: Nutritional balance, protection from physical harm, increased learning

Observe for confusion   Determine if the person is bewildered or perplexed.

Rationale: Confusion may occur with inadequate brain oxygenation or with disorganization of thought or emotion resulting from excessive physiologic or emotional stress.

Fulfilled Needs: Protection from physical harm

Observe for contradictory verbal and nonverbal messages   Observe for overt behavior that seems contrary to what the person states verbally, such as staying in bed when he says he feels fine, crying when he says he's stopped grieving, and pacing when he says he's not fearful.

Rationale: Contradictory verbal and nonverbal messages reveal that the problem is unsolved.

Fulfilled Needs: Protection from psychologic threat

Observe for convulsions/seizures   Look for involuntary muscle contraction and relaxation, often accompanied by loss of consciousness. These convulsions/seizures include tonic contractions, which are often seen in infants, Jacksonian seizures of localized twitching or jerking, and petit mal seizures, in which there is momentary cessation of activity and thought.

Rationale: Convulsions may indicate brain, nerve, or chemical disorders. They increase the possibility of physical harm from environmental sources and can cause inadequate pulmonary ventilation during and after the episode.

Fulfilled Needs: Protection from physical harm

Observe for coughing and the cough's characteristics   Watch to see if the person is coughing. Observe characteristics such as frequency, sound, productiveness, and precipitating factors of the cough.

Rationale: Coughing indicates respiratory tract stimulation caused by irritation.

Fulfilled Needs: Protection from physical harm

Observe for cyanosis   Look for blue, gray, slate, or dark purple discoloration in the nail beds and skin, around the lips, and in the earlobe.

Rationale: Normal oxygen saturation of hemoglobin is 97%, or 14.5 g. Cyanosis indicates oxygen deficiency in the blood. Cyanosis occurs when there are 5 g or more of reduced hemoglobin in the blood.

Fulfilled Needs: Protection from physical harm

Observe for dehiscence   Look for signs that a wound has begun to open, such as serosanguineous fluid at the incision site, complaints of a sharp pulling sensation, and breaking of some but not all sutures.

Rationale: Early detection of dehiscence can prevent wound evisceration.

Fulfilled Needs: Protection from physical harm

Observe for delayed healing Observe wounds that fail to heal within the average 4–7 days or wounds that intermittently heal and reopen.

Rationale: Delayed wound healing may be related to inadequate blood supply, failure to keep wound edges together, serious nutritional deficits, or malignant cells.

Fulfilled Needs: Protection from physical harm

Observe for delirium Notice if the person exhibits a mental disturbance of confused excitement. His speech may be rambling and body movements poorly organized.

Rationale: Delirium results from such conditions as high fever, alcohol intake, and acute toxic states.

Fulfilled Needs: Protection from physical harm

Observe for depression Notice if there are signs of depression, such as slowed activity, inability to function in a normal capacity, weeping, decreased interest in usual activities, and focusing on a recent loss.

Rationale: Depression can result from physiochemical imbalances, drug side effects, and severe psychologic stress related to loss.

Fulfilled Needs: Protection from physical harm, protection from psychologic threat

Observe for developing Cushing's phenomenon[249] Watch for signs of Cushing's phenomenon, such as increased systolic blood pressure with a widened pulse pressure, decreased pulse rate, and change in respiration rate.

Rationale: Cushing's phenomenon indicates a decrease in cerebral perfusion pressure resulting from increased intracranial pressure.

Fulfilled Needs: Protection from physical harm

Observe for developmental deficits Observe the person for an inability to learn at a normal rate, poor physical development, or behavior difficulties. Estimate the degree of deficit by observing the patient's abilities in regard to self-care, responses to others, and command of language, as well as by comparing the patient to average children:

At *3–4 months* the normal child balances his head, smiles, laughs, reaches, squirms, and turns his head toward sound.

At *6–7 months* the normal child reaches, grasps, sits, rolls over, bounces up and down, laughs when laughed at, and makes increasing sounds.

At *9 months* the normal child sits without support, creeps, pulls up to stand, feeds himself crackers and a bottle, and copies sounds.

At *12 months* the normal child stands alone, takes a few steps, attempts to eat with a spoon, squeals, and imitates familiar words.

At *18 months* the normal child begins to run, pulls toys, hugs dolls, cooperates in dressing himself, claims possession of his own things, knows between 5 and 20 single words, and chatters.

The normal *2-year-old* child runs well, walks up and down stairs, assists in dressing himself, uses a spoon with some spilling, and combines two to three words to express ideas.

At *3 years of age* the normal child rides a tricycle, throws a ball, marks with crayon or pencil, participates in some cooperative play, uses long sentences, and refers to himself as "I."

At *4 years of age* the normal child runs, skips, climbs, does simple tricks, uses imaginative play, counts to 10, and is social and talkative.

At *5 years of age* the normal child can roller-skate, jump rope, sing and dance, and participate in competitive play. He uses connective words such as "but" and "and."

The normal *6-year-old* child plays simple table games, uses a telephone, counts to 30, writes or prints his name, and has become sensitive to others.

If the child's development seems to be between 50% and 75% that of the normal child, then the exceptional child is educable, and his IQ will range between 50 and 75. If his development seems to be between 25% and 50% of normal, the exceptional child is trainable, and his IQ will range between 25 and 50. If his development seems to be less than 25% of normal, the child is totally dependent, and his IQ will be below 25.

Rationale: Persons with developmental deficits need the supervision of more mature persons to ensure their safety and require special training in order to meet their own daily needs.

Fulfilled Needs: Protection from physical harm, protection from psychologic threat

Observe for diarrhea/for complaints of diarrhea   Watch to see if the person has frequent unformed and liquid stools.

Rationale: Diarrhea is associated with gastrointestinal disorders.

Fulfilled Needs: Protection from physical harm

Observe for diet intolerance   Observe the person for any inability to tolerate food, such as refusal to eat, nausea, vomiting, abdominal distention after eating, and complaints that the food is poorly tolerated.

Rationale: Foods incompatible with the person's physiologic state irritate the stomach and intestinal mucosa and disrupt the digestive process.

Fulfilled Needs: Protecton from physical harm

Observe for disorientation   Determine if the person is aware of time, of place, of environment, of who he is, of who others are, and of what is happening.

Rationale: Disorientation is associated with toxic states, brain trauma, psychic disturbances, and social isolation.

Fulfilled Needs: Protection from physical harm, protection from psychologic threat

Observe for dyspnea   Look for signs of difficult breathing, such as gasping, anxiety, rapid and shallow breathing, dilated nostrils, moist and cyanotic skin, and retraction respirations.

Rationale: Respiratory difficulty prevents adequate blood and tissue oxygenation and may threaten life.

Fulfilled Needs: Protection from physical harm

Observe for emotional instability   Look for verbal and nonverbal emotional responses that are inconsistent and indicative of instability. Determine whether these are habitual feeling responses or newly adopted responses.

Rationale: Behavioral patterns are influenced by physiologic and psychologic disorders.

Fulfilled Needs: Protection from physical harm, protection from psychologic threat

Observe for euphoria   Look for indications of sudden feelings of unusual well-being, such as sudden bursts of energy, unusual cheerfulness, and overactivity.

Rationale: Euphoria, when it appears in a previously depressed patient, may indicate unresolved conflict and a decision to commit suicide. While experiencing euphoria, a person tends to minimize danger and to indulge in unsafe activities. Persons who are potential drug abusers often become euphoric on drugs given for therapeutic effect. Euphoria should be a clue to prescribe as little drug therapy as possible.

Fulfilled Needs: Protection from physical harm, protection from physchologic threat

Observe for evidence of a favorable response to therapy   Observe whether the person's therapy is having the effect that was intended. Determine whether it is reducing the fever, blood pressure, or pain, promoting healing, or altering emotional responses.

Rationale: Therapy that does not produce the intended effect should be reevaluated and new therapy initiated.

Fulfilled Needs: Protection from physical harm

Observe for evidence of diminished hearing Observe for behavior that indicates that the person is having difficulty hearing, such as requests for repeating comments or questions, complaints that people do not speak loud enough to be heard, and unresponsive or inappropriate responses to comments or questions.

Rationale: Behavior indicating diminished hearing may be the first cue of auditory disease, for which early treatment may prevent further ear damage.

Fulfilled Needs: Protection from physical harm

Observe for evidence of pressure on the skin Look for areas of redness or indentation on the skin.

Rationale: Pressure on a body area impairs circulation to that area and could result in tissue necrosis.

Fulfilled Needs: Protection from physical harm

Observe for evidence that the patient/family is reaching out for emotional support Look for signs indicating that the person is seeking emotional support from others. Such signs include frequently turning on the call light, crying, unwarranted angry outbursts, withdrawal of various degrees, chronic complaining, holding out the arm or hands to reach for others, returning to thumb sucking, holding onto a blanket or toy while sleeping, excessive eating, and excessive talking.

Rationale: Emotional support from others reduces the intensity of suffering. When persons feel unable to directly ask for emotional support, they will reach out by using indirect behavioral methods.

Fulfilled Needs: Protection from psychologic threat

Observe for excessive talking Watch for the person who talks at an excessively rapid rate or who talks consistently without pause.

Rationale: Excessive talking may indicate rapid metabolic rate, intracranial pressure, neurologic or circulatory brain disorders, or anxiety.

Fulfilled Needs: Protection from physical harm, protection from psychologic threat

Observe for heart failure Look for signs that the heart is unable to deliver adequate oxygenated blood to meet the body's needs. Such signs include dyspnea on exertion, a nonproductive cough, a need to sleep on several pillows, jugular vein distention, nausea, chest pain, dependent edema, gallop heart rhythm, and crackling rales at the base of the lung.

Rationale: Heart failure reduces blood flow, resulting in circulatory impairment.

Fulfilled Needs: Protection from physical harm

Observe for hemoptysis Look for evidence that the person is coughing up blood.

Rationale: Hemoptysis indicates lung hemorrhage.

Fulfilled Needs: Protection from physical harm

Observe for hiccoughs Listen for the short, sharp sound of intermitent diaphragmatic spasms.

Rationale: Hiccoughs indicate diaphragmatic irritation, often due to peritoneal inflammation.

Fulfilled Needs: Protection from physical harm

Observe for hyperactivity Look for signs of overactivity in which the person is seldom or never quiet.

Rationale: Hyperactivity may indicate hormonal imbalance, emotional stress, drug or chemical side effects, or cerebral dysfunction.

Fulfilled Needs: Protection from physical harm, protection from psychologic threat

Observe for impaired conceptual thinking Observe the person's ability to think clearly and rationally and to comprehend the various factors involved in an idea.
Rationale: The thought process is influenced by the physiologic and psychologic states.
Fulfilled Needs: Protection from physical harm, protection from psychologic threat

Observe for impaired judgment Observe the person's ability to identify problems and arrive at adequate solutions.
Rationale: An ability to solve problems indicates integration of self, creativity, knowledge, and experience. It is affected by the physiologic and psychologic states.
Fulfilled Needs: Protection from physical harm. Protection from psychologic threat

Observe for impaired learning ability Observe the person for any impairment of ability to learn. Compare the person's responses with normal responses or with previous responses
Rationale: Impaired learning ability may indicate central nervous system disorder or psychologic disequilibrium.
Fulfilled Needs: Protection from physical harm, protection from psychologic threat

Observe for impaired self-attitudes Observe the person for expressions of self-doubt, distorted self-image, diminished feelings of usefulness, unrealistic levels of aspiration, and other poor attitudes toward the self.
Rationale: An integrated self-concept is essential to emotional maturity and safety feelings.
Fulfilled Needs: Protection from psychologic threat

Observe for inadequate analgesic pain relief Watch for signs that the analgesic is not adequate for the person. For example, the person still feels pain 1 hour after the injection, which should be the peak time of pain relief, or the pain becomes severe before the next scheduled dose.
Rationale: Awareness of inadequate analgesic pain relief should result in an altered drug dose or scheduling that does give relief.
Fulfilled Needs: Comfort, protection from physical harm

Observe for incoherent thinking Observe the person for disorganization and instability of thought processes, including conversations and expressions of ideas in which thoughts are loosely connected or totally disconnected.
Rationale: The thought process is influenced by physiologic and psychologic states.
Fulfilled Needs: Protection from physical harm, protection from psychologic threat

Observe for incontinence Observe the person for inability to control the urinary sphincter and to retain urine.
Rationale: Urinary incontinence may result from cerebral impairment, spinal cord injury or pressure, urinary tract irritation, or nerve or muscle degeneration.
Fulfilled Needs: Protection from physical harm

Observe for infant head rolling Watch for head movements in which the infant chronically turns his head from side to side, usually accompanied by profuse perspiration on the face and forehead.
Rationale: Infant head rolling may indicate rickets or an attempt to focus poorly coordinated eyes.
Fulfilled Needs: Protection from physical harm

Observe for intestinal obstruction Look for indications that the intestinal lumen is blocked. Such indications include wavelike abdominal pains, diarrhea or passage of blood or mucus without passage of fecal matter or flatus, fecal vomiting, drowsiness, malaise and aching, intense thirst, abdominal distention, weak and rapid pulse, lowered temperature and blood pressure, cold and clammy skin.

Rationale: Intestinal obstruction prevents the waste elimination essential to life.

Fulfilled Needs: Protection from physical harm

Observe for irritability Look for signs of a high level of susceptibility to stimuli, such as quick excitement responses, quickness to anger, impatience, and becoming easily annoyed or frustrated.

Rationale: Irritability may indicate body chemical imbalance or high physical or emotional stress levels.

Fulfilled Needs: Protection from physical harm, protection from psychologic threat

Observe for laryngeal edema Look for swelling in the laryngeal area, especially after intubation. Signs include hoarseness, difficulty in swallowing, and difficulty breathing.

Rationale: Laryngeal swelling obstructs the airway.

Fulfilled Needs: Protection from physical harm

Observe for lethargy Observe the person for severe drowsiness and sluggishness.

Rationale: Lethargy indicates interference with normal cerebral and sensory function. It is often evident before convulsions or with meningitis.

Fulfilled Needs: Protection from physical harm

Observe for memory impairment Observe the person for any inability to remember facts and events or difficulty with recall. Notice whether memory gaps begin and end abruptly, whether they are confined to one particular period or are scattered over a lengthy time, whether they are associated with only unpleasant events or with both pleasant and unpleasant events, whether they are related to lack of attention or to poor retention and recall, and whether the person is aware of the memory problem.

Rationale: Impaired recall is influenced by current physiologic and psychologic states and affects the capacity to function.

Fulfilled Needs: Protection from physical harm, protection from psychologic threat

Observe for mental blocking During conversations, watch for moments during which the patient is temporarily unable to think. Take into account the topic being discussed when the blocking or hesitancy occurs.

Rationale: Anxiety can give rise to hesitant speech patterns and thought disorganization.

Fulfilled Needs: Protection from psychologic threat

Observe for mobility capabilities Observe the person's ability to move about. Determine whether the child can crawl at the age of 9 months, walk with assistance at 12 months, walk alone at 15 months, run successfully at 18 months, and jump at 2 years. Determine whether the adult can walk or run without assistance and, if not, what his mobility capabilities are.

Rationale: Normal mobility is essential to uninhibited activity as well as safety.

Fulfilled Needs: Protection from physical harm

Observe for mouth breathing Note whether the person consistently breathes through his mouth.

Rationale: Mouth breathing indicates nasal obstruction.

Fulfilled Needs: Protection from physical harm

Observe for muscle twitching/jerking Look for sudden quick jerks of the muscles.

Rationale: Muscle twitching may indicate increased blood potassium, decreased blood calcium, hypoglycemia, or a neurologic or psychosomatic disorder.

Fulfilled Needs: Protection from physical harm

Observe for nasal flare Determine whether the lower nares are full and expanded outward during respirations. This occurs most frequently during sleep.

Rationale: Nasal flaring is characteristic of dyspnea in infants, especially with atelectasis and other obstructions.

Fulfilled Needs: Protection from physical harm

Observe for nonverbal communication of pain Look for nonverbal indications of pain, such as skin redness, pallor, restlessness, excessive perpiration, increased respirations, bedfastness, distorted facial expression (drawn expression, clenched teeth, wrinkled forehead), or fatigue. Note posture variations, such as lying perfectly straight and still, knee flexion, kneeling, and stooping.

Rationale: Swelling and redness occur with inflammatory pain. Pallor is associated with painful circulatory constriction. The severe intensity of colicky pain resulting from intestinal, kidney, or biliary tract disorders causes restlessness and sometimes vomiting. Pain increases perspiration secretion. Pain stimulates the autonomic nervous system, which controls respirations. Withdrawal from normal activity to bed rest reveals a disruption or threat of disruption in normal body function. Facial grimaces reveal pain. The stress of body adaptation while experiencing pain quickly produces fatigue. Deviations from normal posture indicate efforts at self-protection against pain and discomfort.

Fulfilled Needs: Protection from physical harm

Observe for oversedation Watch the person for signs of having received too much analgesic, such as difficulty being aroused and respiratory depression. Restlessness and dyspnea may occur when the respiratory depression causes pulmonary secretions to pool, with resulting hypoxia.

Rationale: Oversedation reduces the function of vital body parts. In addition, it makes the person unnecessarily dependent.

Fulfilled Needs: Protection from physical harm

Observe for poor communication skills Look for signs that the person has difficulty sending or receiving messages. These signs include stuttering, stammering, dysarthria, inappropriate emotional responses to messages, disorganization in the message sent, message misinterpretation, lack of interest in communicating, and making inferences not intended.

Rationale: Psychologic comfort and safety are promoted through effective communications with others.

Fulfilled Needs: Protection from psychologic threat

Observe for pulmonary edema[249] Watch for signs of pulmonary edema, such as restlessness, cough with frothy sputum, dyspnea, orthopnea, cyanosis, distended neck veins, tachycardia, wheezing, bubbling rales, severe anxiety.

Rationale: Pulmonary edema is the presence of fluid in the alveoli, which reduces the amount of lung tissue available for gas exchange. It is usually caused by left ventricular failure. Its life-threatening nature makes it imperative that it be recognized in the early stages.

Fulfilled Needs: Protection from physical harm

Observe for pulsus paradoxicus Notice if the pulse volume becomes weaker with respiratory inspiration and stronger with expiration.

Rationale: Pulsus paradoxicus is sometimes seen with constrictive pericarditis, pericardial effusion, or hemopericordium.

Fulfilled Needs: Protection from physical harm

Observe for readiness to assume self-care/infant care Determine those activities of daily living that the person can perform and is ready to perform. Such activities may include moving about in bed, obtaining objects from a bedside table, grooming and personal hygiene, dressing and undressing, feeding himself, walking or pushing a wheelchair, and activity involving use of the hands and fingers, such as writing, turning on lights, turning book pages, smoking, and winding a watch. Notice when a mother is ready to care for her newborn infant. The exhaustion that follows labor delays the mother's interest in caring for her infant. After adequate rest, the interest is renewed.

Rationale: When a person cannot carry on the activities of daily living, his needs must be met by others.

Fulfilled Needs: Protection from physical harm

Observe for readiness to learn Look for signs that the person is able and wants to learn. Such signs include observing curiously, asking questions, and reading about the subject on his own.

Rationale: Learning cannot occur until the person is physically and mentally well enough to understand and acquire new knowledge and skill.

Fulfilled Needs: Protection from physical harm, protection from psychologic threat

Observe for requests for increased drug dosage Note any requests for drugs at more frequent intervals or at increased dosages.

Rationale: As the body builds up tolerance to a habit-forming drug, the amount and frequency of the drug must be increased in order to obtain the desired effect. This is a clue that the patient may be inclined toward drug habituation.

Fulfilled Needs: Protection from physical harm

Observe for restless-leg phenomenon Notice if the person moves his legs in a compelling manner. Also, note complaints of a painful tension or jumping leg sensation, usually worse at the end of the day in persons with the idiopathic form of the disorder, and particularly if the legs are restrained in persons with the uremic form.

Rationale: The restless leg syndrome is an idiopathic disorder. In uremia, the cause is believed to be nerve irritation of toxic substances, but other causes are yet to be discovered. Restless leg syndrome is observed so that it can be distinguished from restlessness. The legs are often restrained in restlessness. However, leg restraints applied during restless leg syndrome intensify the pain and may cause damage to ankle tissue. Leg movement helps decrease the pain in restless leg syndrome.

Fulfilled Needs: Comfort, protection from physical harm

Observe for restlessness Watch for frequent movements when the person is attempting to rest or sleep.

Rationale: Poor tissue oxygenation, pain, discomfort, internal stress, or tension may cause restlessness.

Fulfilled Needs: Protection from physical harm

Observe for shock Look for signs and symptoms of circulatory collapse, such as rapid pulse, pallor, cool and clammy skin, increased respirations, restlessness, hypotension, lethargy or anxiety, thirst, decreased urine output by the kidneys, coma or stupor, and dilated pupils.

Rationale: Shock results from decreased cardiac output, severe blood or fluid loss, severe pain, septicemia, or nervous system disorder.

Fulfilled Needs: Protection from physical harm

Observe for side effects of drugs/therapy Look for drug reactions, such as allergic responses (rash, itching, etc.), anaphylactic responses (difficulty in breathing, circulatory failure), and toxic or overdose effects specific to the drug. Certain types of therapy can also produce side effects, such as vomiting associated with radiation.

Rationale: Early recognition and treatment of drug or therapy reactions can reduce their harmful effects on the body.

Fulfilled Needs: Protection from physical harm

Observe for signs or healing Look for evidence that the wound is being restored to health by healing. Evidence of healing includes no inflammation or drainage, closure of the wound edges, and the formation of granulation tissue to fill the area between the wound edges.

Rationale: Healing is essential to good functional use of body areas.

Fulfilled Needs: Protection from physical harm

Observe for signs of physiologic stability Watch for signs that the body system is functioning in a stable, effective manner. Stability exists when clinical findings indicate that body function falls within the standards of normalcy.

Rationale: Recognition of signs of physiologic stability are essential for the termination of illness therapy and for the initiation of supportive measures leading to physiologic function independent of therapeutic care.

Fulfilled Needs: Physiologic stability

Observe for sneezing Be alert to the onset of sneezing episodes.

Rationale: Sneezing may be an early sign of impending upper respiratory infection. Awareness of its significance can prevent the transmission of infection to other persons. Sneezing may also indicate a hypersensitivity response.

Fulfilled Needs: Protection from physical harm

Observe for speech loss Notice if the person has lost his ability to speak, if speech is severely impaired, or if the speech cannot be interpreted.

Rationale: Loss of speech indicates a neurologic disorder.

Fulfilled Needs: Protection from physical harm

Observe for suicidal threats Look for signs of a sense of unusual well-being and serenity in a person who has previously displayed self-destructive behavior.

Rationale: Once the decision of self-destruction has been made, the person may perceive his troubles as being resolved and may exhibit a sense of well-being. Recognition of potentially harmful physical threats can promote safety. A sense of the basic worth of the individual supports the continuance of life.

Fulfilled Needs: Protection from physical harm

Observe for tetany Observe the person for tonic, muscular spasms.

Rationale: Tetany is most often seen with hyperventilation or alkalosis or in the early postoperative period after thyroidectomy.

Fulfilled Needs: Protection from physical harm.

Observe for the quantity and inquire about the quality of sleep Determine the characteristics and the kind of sleep the person experiences, including light, normal, deep, or interrupted sleep.

Rationale: During sleep, body energy is used for healing. Loss of sleep can delay restoration to health and threaten good health.

Fulfilled Needs: Protection from physical harm

Observe for the stages of grief[279] As the person moves from one stage to another, determine where they are on the grief continuum. Stages of grief are *denial*, a feeling of disbelief; *anger*, feeling hostile and aggressive; *bargaining*, negotiating in an attempt to control the situation; *depression*, a feeling of intense sadness; *acceptance*, a time of peaceful and quiet expectation of death or peaceful acceptance of the situation.

Rationale: Determining the stage of grief being experienced provides a guideline for nursing intervention, which assists the person toward growth through the experience.

Fulfilled Needs: Protection from psychologic threat

Observe for the sudden absence of severe pain   Take note when the person who has been experiencing severe pain states that the pain is suddenly gone.

Rationale: Sudden disappearance of severe pain often indicates rupture of the affected organ or passage of a kidney stone. It also occurs at the onset of shock in peritonitis.

Fulfilled Needs: Protection from physical harm

Observe for tremors   Watch for shaking of the hands, extremities, or head. Tremors can be minimal or severe.

Rationale: Tremors indicate the presence of a primary or secondary neurologic problem.

Fulfilled Needs: Protection from physical harm

Observe for uterine membrane rupture   Be alert for the release of the amniotic and chorionic fluid that surrounds the unborn infant in a membranous sack.

Rationale: Uterine membrane rupture at the normal stage of labor indicates normal progress toward delivery. Delayed or early uterine membrane rupture may require therapeutic intervention. Once the uterine membrane ruptures, the potential for uterine infection exists.

Fulfilled Needs: Protection from physical harm

Observe for voice changes   Listen for voice changes, such as hoarseness, loss of voice, whispering, and changes in tone.

Rationale: Marked voice changes indicate pressure on or inflammation of the vocal cord or pharynx. A husky voice during puberty is evidence of the maturing youth.

Fulfilled Needs: Protection from physical harm

Observe for vomiting   Determine the quantity of emesis, force of projection, color, consistency, and those factors that precipitate its occurrence.

Rationale: Vomiting may indicate gastric irritation, intestinal obstruction, motion sickness, increased intracranial pressure, severe pain, toxic or disease states, or a psychogenic disturbance.

Fulfilled Needs: Protection from physical harm

Observe for water intoxication   Observe the person for indications of overhydration, such as anxiety, disorientation, confusion, shouting, inattention, convulsions, anorexia, nausea, vomiting, hyperventilation, sudden weight gain and edema, headache, gurgling respirations, pulse irregularity, and tremors.

Rationale: When the person has received excess fluid and the circulatory system is overloaded with more water than the kidneys can excrete, the potential for shock and pulmonary edema exists.

Fulfilled Needs: Protection from physical harm

Observe infant for adequate sucking reflex   Notice if the infant's sucking ability is sufficiently strong to provide a fluid intake to satisfy his hunger.

Rationale: Adequate infant sucking is essential to balanced food and fluid intake.

Fulfilled Needs: Protection from physical harm

Observe performance level and problems involved in completing the task/activities of daily living   Look for the level of independent performance that the person is displaying. Determine if the person is completely independent, requires the use of equipment or devices, requires assistance from other persons and/or equipment, or is a dependent nonparticipant. Look for specific problems that hinder the individual from completing the desired task.

Rationale: Observation of levels of performance serves as a baseline for determining needs for assistance and protection and for supporting self-care.

Fulfilled Needs: Protection from physical harm, dependence, mastery and competence in skills, independence

Observe personal hygiene habits   Observe the person's practice of hygiene, including bath, hair care, nail care, mouth care, and general cleanliness.

Rationale: Cleanliness can have an effect on the growth and transmission of microorganisms that cause illness and disease. Attitudes toward personal hygiene reflect internal self-attitudes.

Fulfilled Needs: Protection from physical harm, protection from psychologic threat

Observe spontaneous body movements   Observe how the person moves his body without deliberation. Do both sides move the same? Is one side weaker than the other? Does either side function more normally than the other?

Rationale: When both sides do not function equally, there may be increased intracranial pressure or neurologic damage.

Fulfilled Needs: Protection from physical harm

Observe the amputation stump for odor   Note any unpleasant odor coming from an amputated stump.

Rationale: Infection or tissue necrosis may be manifested by an unpleasant odor.

Fulfilled Needs: Protection from physical harm

Observe the breath for abnormal odors   Determine whether the patient has abnormal breath odors, such as mousy, acid-fruit (acetone), fermented, ammonia, fecal, or foul odor. Note any sour or disagreeable breath or the smell of blood.

Rationale: A mousy odor is associated with liver disease; and acid-fruit (acetone) odor is associated with diabetes; a fermented odor is associated with alcohol consumption; an ammonia odor is associated with uremia. Disagreeable breath may be caused by spicy foods, smoking, or a dirty or infected mouth. A fecal odor is associated with lower intestinal obstruction; sour breath is associated with digestive disorders; a foul odor is associated with potential renal acidosis. The smell of blood occurs with gastrointestinal bleeding and esophageal varices.

Fulfilled Needs: Protection from physical harm

Observe the cast for an expanding bleeding area   When bleeding appears on a cast, outline the area with pencil or pen and mark the time and date of each outline. Periodically check for bleeding that spreads beyond the marked area.

Rationale: Bleeding reduces circulating blood volume, and a wet cast provides an opening for the entry of infectious organisms.

Fulfilled Needs: Protection from physical harm

Observe the cast for odor   Note any unpleasant odor coming from a cast.

Rationale: Unseen tissue necrosis beneath the cast covering can be detected because of an unpleasant odor.

Fulfilled Needs: Protection from physical harm

Observe the characteristics of the child's cry   Listen for variations in the crying of the infant that may indicate abnormalities or unmet needs.

Rationale: Different qualities of the infant's cry may indicate various types of distress. Pain may be indicated by a shrill, loud cry interrupted by whimpering and groaning, as well as by a short, sharp, piercing cry. Discomfort is evidenced by a low whimpering cry. Hunger is communicated by a loud cry with interrupted sucking motions. Fatigue is indicated by crying accompanied by eye rubbing, yawning, and eyelid drooping. Fear or apprehension may be evidenced by crying, clinging to the mother, and turning away from the frightening situation. Brain damage may be indicated by a weak, infrequent cry. Neurologic infection should be suspected when there is a shrill, weak cry. Nervous tension is indicated by excessive crying when there is no physical problem but when an apprehensive atmosphere exists within the family. Colic may be evidenced by a piercing scream and abdominal distention, with the infant pulling his legs up and stiffening his legs. A spoiled child may cry angrily until someone appears, then suddenly stop crying.

Fulfilled Needs: Protection from physical harm, protection from psychologic threat

Observe the ECG monitor Watch the computerized ECG monitor for recording of an irregular heart rhythm.

Rationale: The ECG monitor computerizes and records the electrical activity of the heart in different cardiac chambers. The rapid recognition of electrical cardiac instability supports immediate treatment of cardiac abnormalities, thereby preventing myocardial tissue damage or death.

Fulfilled Needs: Protection from physical harm

Observe the fetal/maternal ultrasound monitor[388] Observe the monitor strip chart for the following abnormalities: severe variable, late or prolonged decelerations, bradycardia, the absence of variablity, or an unstable heart rate.

Rationale: Early recognition of fetal distress promotes early and successful intervention.

Fulfilled Needs: Protection from physical harm

Observe the level of arousal and respiratory rate before giving analgesics Before giving an analgesic with sedative or depressant actions, observe how quickly the person responds to external stimuli as well as his respiratory rate per minute.

Rationale: A baseline level of arousal, and respiratory rate, before giving analgesics can be used to detect oversedation from analgesics.

Fulfilled Needs: Protection from physical harm

Observe the level of consciousness Determine the person's level of response. Check for alertness or lethargy, ability to cooperate or inability to cooperate, orientation or disorientation as to time, place, other people, oneself (does not respond to own name), response to painful stimuli (purposeful, in which he tries to pull away from stimulus or push the stimulus away, versus purposeless, in which he moves about irrelevantly or hyperventilates, versus no response at all), and corneal and gag reflexes (when these are absent, the patient is comatose).

Rationale: Levels of consciousness are altered by pathologic conditions involving the cerebral cortex and brain stem. Levels of consciousness affect behavior patterns and the capacity of function.

Fulfilled Needs: Protection from physical harm

Observe the newborn for signs of drug withdrawal Observe the newborn for signs of drug withdrawal; these may appear immediately after birth, several hours later, or within 4 days, depending on the quantity of drug taken by the mother and the time of last ingestion. Signs of drug withdrawal include hyperirritability, tremors, shrill and high-pitched crying, sneezing, sweating, vomiting, diarrhea, ravenous appetite, and abrasions caused by the rubbing of skin on sheets. Without treatment, the child will develop convulsions, apnea, fever, and dehydration progressing to circulatory collapse and death.

Rationale: The newborn drug withdrawal syndrome, when untreated, is potentially fatal.

Fulfilled Needs: Protection from physical harm

Observe the onset time of infant jaundice Note the number of hours or days between birth and the appearance of the first signs of infant jaundice.

Rationale: Jaundice beginning within 36 hours of birth indicates erythroblastosis fetalis, which is the excessive formation of erythroblasts in the blood caused by production of maternal antibodies in an Rh-negative mother against an Rh-positive fetus. Jaundice beginning within 48–72 hours of birth indicates physiologic jaundice, in which there is a sudden increase in the destruction rate of red blood cells shortly after birth.

Jaundice beginning 3–4 days after birth is usually caused by septicemia. Jaundice beginning about the second week of life indicates bile duct obstruction.

Fulfilled Needs: Protection from physical harm

Observe the pattern of sleep Note the times of day that the person sleeps and how consistently the sleep schedule is followed. Note whether he sleeps at night or during the day, whether he goes to bed at the same time every day, and whether the pattern suddenly changes.

Rationale: A consistent sleep pattern is essential to good health and to normal functioning of the internal clock. Altered sleep patterns should be returned to the normal pattern as soon as possible.

Fulfilled Needs: Protection from physical harm

Observe the seizure characteristics Monitor the occurrence of any seizure, and determine the circumstances surrounding the seizure. This includes the factors involved in its onset, the areas of body involvement, the severity of muscle twitching, the length of the episode, the level of consciousness, the sequence of movement, and any preseizure and postseizure signs and symptoms.

Rationale: Seizures indicate neurologic disorder.

Fulfilled Needs: Protection from physical harm

Observe the time of the first meconium stool Determine when meconium is passed from the infant's rectum and is replaced by normal yellow stool. This usually occurs within the first 10 hours of life.

Rationale: Anal malformation or bowel obstruction may prevent passage of meconium.

Fulfilled Needs: Protection from physical harm

Observe the time of the newborn's first voiding Determine whether the newborn infant voids within the first 24–36 hours of life.

Rationale: Newborn infants normally void within the first 36 hours of life.

Fulfilled Needs: Protection from physical harm

Observe the urine by implementing the three-bottle procedure In the three-bottle procedure, three urine specimen bottles are used for serial urine specimen collections. The first voiding is put into bottle #1, and so forth through the third voiding. At the fourth voiding, bottle #1 is emptied, cleaned, and used, as bottle #3. This rotating method continues with the oldest specimen discarded to provide a bottle for each new specimen. For a patient with an indwelling catheter, a regular schedule of collection from the catheter is made.

Rationale: The three-bottle procedure is used to determine the amount and characteristics of the urine. Each bottle is evaluated in relationship to the others for evidence of changing renal function.

Fulfilled Needs: Protection from physical harm

Observe the urine for abnormal color, content, and odor Inspect the urine for pigment (color) other than the normal yellow, orange, or brownish yellow. Inspect the urine for mucus, fat globules, blood, or other visible solids and determine whether there is any unusual urine odor.

Rationale: Bile-colored urine may be associated with jaundice. Black urine may indicate malignant tumors, hemorrhage, or mercury, lead, or phenol poisoning. Blue urine indicates prior use of methylene blue or indigo. Milky white urine is associated with fat globules. Red urine indicates bleeding. Cloudiness is associated with pus and urinary tract infection.

Mucus in the urine is associated with inflammation. Albumin is associated with fever, excessive physical exercise or exertion, Bright's disease, and scoliosis. Fat in the urine indicates kidney degeneration. Sugar indicates faulty carbohydrate metabolism. White precipitate suggests excessive phosphates, while pink precipitate suggests excessive uric acid. Blood in the urine indicates hemorrhage, urinary tract trauma, blood dyscrasias, or renal disease. Foam suggests protein loss and the nephrotic syndrome.

Acetone urine odor is associated with the excessive fat metabolism of diabetes. Ammonia odor indicates uremia. Fecal odor indicates intestinal or urinary fistulas. Fishy odor suggests kidney inflammation.

Fulfilled Needs: Protection from physical harm

Observe the vagina for abnormal odor   Determine if the patient has an abnormal vaginal odor. Usually such odor will be foul smelling and accompanied by discharge.

Rationale: The presence of vaginal odor indicates vaginal infection. In addition to the common infections, bacterial growth can be due to failure to remove a tampon.

Fulfilled Needs: Protection from physical harm

Obtain a bacterial culture   Using sterile technique, collect a specimen of body fluid, drainage, or secretion and have it incubated for bacterial growth.

Rationale: A culture of body secretions may reveal potentially harmful infection.

Fulfilled Needs: Protection from physical harm

Obtain standard laboratory studies and evaluate for normal levels   Have blood and urine studies done according to the standard procedure of the institution or organization in which practice is being conducted.

Rationale: Laboratory studies help determine normal and abnormal health status.

Fulfilled Needs: Protection from physical harm

Palpate for arterial pulsations/peripheral pulses[169]   Count the expansions of the arterial wall occurring in 1 minute by placing the fingertips over the artery. Determine whether there is soreness, distention, or bounding pulsation and whether right and left pulses are of equal strength. Examine the temporal artery at the temple above and outside the eye, the external maxillary artery (facial), the carotid artery on the side of the neck, the brachial artery on the inner arm above the elbow joint, the radial artery on the thumb side of the wrist, the femoral artery in the groin, the popliteal artery behind the knee, and the arteria dorsalis pedis on the top of the foot near the ankle.

Rationale: Pulsation and expansion of the arterial walls occur with each ventricular contraction. Abnormalities indicate cardiac or circulatory pathology.

Fulfilled Needs: Protection from physical harm

Palpate for fetal position   Palpate the maternal abdomen, feeling for the fetal head, buttocks, and extremities. Determine whether the fetus is facing left or right.

Rationale: Palpation for fetal position helps locate the back of the fetus, where fetal heart sounds are most easily heard. Fetal position indicates whether the infant will be delivered in cephalic or breech presentation.

Fulfilled Needs: Protection from physical harm

Palpate for tenderness   Feel body areas for soreness or sensitivity to pain when palpation is attempted.

Rationale: Abdominal tenderness may indicate organ distention or inflammation of the abdominal viscera, wall, or peritoneum. Calf tenderness may result from a localized blood clot. Cranial tenderness may occur with trauma, fracture, or abrasions. Thoracic tenderness may indicate injury.

Fulfilled Needs: Protection from physical harm

Palpate the abdomen for tenderness, rigidity, and masses[125,253]   Gently press the hand into each of the four abdominal quadrants. The person may feel rebound tenderness, in which the sudden release of pressure causes pain. Palpate for rigidity, in which there is a feeling of resistance. Feel for masses.

Rationale: Rebound tenderness occurs with inflammation. Abdominal rigidity may indicate inflammation, peritoneal irritation, or abdominal tissue growth.

Fulfilled Needs: Protection from physical harm

Palpate the abdominal aorta for increased pulsation[125,253]   Feel for an increased or bounding epigastric pulsation and for a pulsating mass. Normally there is only slight epigastric pulsation.

Rationale: Very strong pulsation in the abdominal aorta indicates arterial dilatation and may be associated with aneurysm or aortic insufficiency.

Fulfilled Needs: Protection from physical harm

Palpate the bladder for distention[125,253]   Feel for an enlarged bladder by placing the fingers over the lower middle abdomen. Feel for distention and masses. An empty bladder cannot be palpated.

Rationale: Bladder distention indicates urine retention. Abnormal bladder masses can be detected by palpation.

Fulfilled Needs: Protection from physical harm

Palpate the breasts for nodules/masses[125,253]   Examine the person for breast nodules or masses in the following manner: Ask the person to raise both her arms. Carefully observe breast tissue for bulging, edema, and dimpling. Compare the sizes and shapes of the breasts. Carefully palpate the tissue in all four quadrants of the breasts for increased heat, tenderness, and masses. Beginning at the breastbone, gently palpate the inner half of the breast. With the flat part of the fingers, palpate the nipple. Ask the patient to place her arm at her side. Then feel the tissues that extend to the axilla. Examine the upper and lower outside quadrants of the breast.

Rationale: Breast palpation reveals abnormalities that can be resolved if detected and treated early.

Fulfilled Needs: Protection from physical harm

Palpate the cervix for dilatation   With the person flat on her back with knees flexed, slowly insert a lubricated index finger into the rectum. Feel for a depression surrounded by a circular ridge, and determine the extent of cervical expansion by the size of the circular ridge. Dilatation begins with 1 cm and ends with 10 cm. The progression is as follows: 1 cm (½-inch circular ridge), 2 cm (¾-inch circular ridge), 3 cm (1¼-inch circular ridge), 4 cm (1½-inch circular ridge), 5 cm (2-inch circular ridge), 6 cm (2¼-inch circular ridge), 8 cm (3-inch circular ridge), 10 cm (3¾-inch circular ridge).

Rationale: Cervical dilatation measures the progress of labor and allows for recognition of abnormalities.

Fulfilled Needs: Protection from physical harm

Palpate the chest for a precordial heave[125,253]   On the anterior chest, look for and then palpate for any pulsation at the left 5th interspace, the right 3rd, 4th, and 5th interspaces, and the lower sternum.

Rationale: A precordial heave may indicate increased myocardial tone (from increased metabolic rate) and right ventricular hypertrophy (from a failing cardiac valve). It may be associated with pulmonary or tricuspid insufficiency, with mitral, pulmonary, or tricuspid stenosis, or with thyrotoxicosis.

Fulfilled Needs: Protection from physical harm

Palpate the chest for a thrill[125,253]   Feel for vibrations over the chest precordium. The feeling is similar to that felt when placing a hand on the chest of a purring cat.

Rationale: A thrill indicates that blood is flowing through an abnormal heart or arteries. It is associated with aortic or mitral stenosis.

Fulfilled Needs: Protection from physical harm

Palpate the chest for abnormal vocal fremitus[125,253]   Moving the hand over the anterior thorax from left to right, feel the costal cartilages, ribs, and rib interspaces.

Apply the fingers of one hand to the interspaces and ask the person to say "ninety-nine." Feel for a strong tremor, a diminished tremor, or the absence of a tremor within the chest wall.

Rationale: Increased tremor within the chest wall indicates increased lung volume and is associated with pulmonary consolidation. Decreased tremor within the chest wall occurs with airflow obstruction and is associated with pleural effusion and pneumothorax.

Fulfilled Needs: Protection from physical harm

Palpate the chest for an abnormal precordial thrust[125,253]
Feel for the normal cardiac pulsation at the point of maximum impulse (PMI). Determine whether the pulsation is weak or excessively forceful and whether it covers a wider area than normal.

Rationale: An excessively forceful precordial thrust may indicate increased myocardial tone (from increased metabolic rate) or left ventricular hypertrophy (from a failing cardiac valve). It may be associated with hypertension, with aortic or mitral insufficiency, aortic stenosis, or with thyrotoxicosis.

Fulfilled Needs: Protection from physical harm

Palpate the cranial suture line for separation
Feel for nonclosure of the arrow-shaped (sagittal) and long (longitudinal) skull bones that connect the two fontanels. Run a hand over the baby's head and feel the skull bone with the fingertips.

Rationale: A separated infant suture line indicates increased intracranial pressure.

Fulfilled Needs: Protection from physical harm

Palpate the eyeballs for tension
Place the tip of the forefinger on the closed eyelid. Gently press the eyeball with the finger. Determine whether the eyeball firmness is approximately the same as that of a normal eye.

Rationale: Increased eyeball tension indicates glaucoma. Decreased eyeball tension indicates severe dehydration.

Fulfilled Needs: Protection from physical harm

Palpate the fontanelles for abnormality/bulging/tightness
Feel for variations in the soft space between the cranial skull bones of the baby. Such variations may include delayed closure of the posterior fontanel beyond 2 months, delayed closure of the anterior fontanel beyond 18 months, premature fontanel closure before 10 months, or bulging or depression of the anterior fontanel. Palpate by running a hand over the baby's head and feeling the fontanel with the fingertips.

Rationale: Delayed fontanel closure may indicate insufficient intake or absorption of calcium or vitamin D. Premature fontanel closure prevents normal brain growth. Fontanel bulging indicates increased intracranial pressure. Fontanel depression indicates dehydration.

Fulfilled Needs: Protection from physical harm

Palpate the head for a cranial bulge
Grasp the infant's head in the fingertips and firmly press over the entire cranial and facial bone surface. Examine for areas of cranial projection or protuberance and for unusually hard or soft areas.

Rationale: Cranial bulge may be indicative of trauma, tumor, or congenital defect.

Fulfilled Needs: Protection from physical harm

Palpate the liver for enlargement[125,253]
Examine the liver by placing the palm of the left hand over the lower anterior ribs of the right thorax. Strike the back of the left hand lightly with a right-handed fist and determine whether pain or tenderness is experienced. Feel the liver for enlargement and determine whether it moves with each arterial pulsation.

Rationale: Liver enlargement indicates congestion caused by cardiac failure, poor nutrition, or impaired liver function. It may be associated with an intraabdominal mass, cardiac failure, liver damage, liver failure, or malnutrition.

Fulfilled Needs: Protection from physical harm

Palpate the lymph nodes for enlargement[125,253]   Stand behind the patient and gently palpate the entire neck, under the jaw, and behind and in front of the ears. Determine whether there is tenderness, and feel for heat or swelling in the nodes. Then palpate the axillary area for the same symptoms.

Rationale: Lymph node swelling may indicate infection of lymph node or lymph vessel disease or obstruction.

Fulfilled Needs: Protection from physical harm

Palpate the parotid gland for swelling[125,253]   Feel for enlargement of the parotid glands located near each ear.

Rationale: Parotid gland swelling may indicate viral or bacterial infection.

Fulfilled Needs: Protection from physical harm

Palpate the pulse(s) for rate, rhythm, and volume   Count the expansions of the arterial wall occurring in 1 minute by placing the fingertips over the wrist artery. Normal pulse rate is 70–80 pulses/minute in adults, 85–110 in children, and 130–140 in infants. Rhythm should be consistent, and volume should be moderate.

Rationale: Pulsation of the arterial walls occurs with each left ventricular contraction. Abnormalities indicate cardiac or circulatory pathology.

Fulfilled Needs: Protection from physical harm

Palpate the sinuses for tenderness   Place slight pressure over the maxillary, submaxillary, and sphenoid sinuses. Ask if pressure causes tenderness or pain.

Rationale: Tenderness or pain in the sinus area indicates sinus infection.

Fulfilled Needs: Protection from physical harm

Palpate the skin for crepitation   Feel the skin areas over the chest, neck, extremities, and face for a bubbling, crackling sensation.

Rationale: Skin crepitation indicates air in subcutaneous tissues. It may occur in the neck when there is tracheal or esophageal injury, in the extremities with gas gangrene, and in the face when there is major trauma.

Fulfilled Needs: Protection from physical harm

Palpate the skin for temperature   Feel the skin for levels of heat and cold. Determine if the skin is warm or hot, cool or cold. Use the backs of the fingers (rather than the palmar surface) to feel for temperature changes.

Rationale: Very warm or hot skin indicates fever, exposure to high temperatures, marked vasodilatation, or inflammation. Cold skin suggests shock, lowered blood pressure, fear, poor or obstructed circulation, or vasomotor spasms.

Fulfilled Needs: Protection from physical harm

Palpate the spleen for enlargement[125,253]   Have the person lie on his back and place his left fist under his 11th rib, near his waist. Curl the fingers of both your hands around the left costal margin so that they fit up under the ribs. Ask the person to breathe in deeply. The margin of the spleen can be felt with the fingertips. If it is enlarged, it will be displaced downward from behind the thoracic cage toward the right iliac fossa, or it may extend to the midline.

Rationale: A moderately enlarged, soft spleen with blunt edges may indicate infection or increased red blood cell destruction. A firm, hard spleen with sharp edges may indicate chronic disease. An enlarged spleen also may indicate congestion caused by cardiac failure or circulatory disturbance.

Fulfilled Needs: Protection from physical harm

Palpate the thyroid gland for enlargement[125,253]   Examine the thyroid gland by standing behind the person. Place the tips of two or three fingers of each hand on each side of the trachea. Ask the patient to swallow. Feel for nodule fullness, which will glide upward if there is an abnormality.

Rationale: Thyroid nodules and thyroid enlargement may occur with tumorous growth, tissue hyperplasia, or thyroid hyperactivity.

Fulfilled Needs: Protection from physical harm

Palpate the trachea for deviation[125,253] Feel the trachea and determine whether it is in the normal midline position with the sternal notch.

Rationale: If there is pressure on the trachea, it may shift its location to the right or left side of the sternal notch. Tracheal deviation may be associated with pulmonary atelectasis, pulmonary cavity, or pleural effusion.

Fulfilled Needs: Protection from physical harm

Palpate the uterus for contraction quality Place one finger on the abdomen above the uterine area and attempt to indent the finger into the uterine wall when a contraction and pain occur.

Rationale: When an excellent uterine contraction occurs, finger indentation cannot occur. When a moderately good contraction occurs, slight finger indentation is possible. When a poor contraction occurs, finger indentation occurs easily. Contractions cease completely in uterine rupture.

Fulfilled Needs: Protection from physical harm

Palpate the uterus for firmness Feel the uterus and determine whether it is hard or soft.

Rationale: Normally the uterus is hard. A soft or boggy quality indicates internal uterine bleeding.

Fulfilled Needs: Protection from physical harm

Palpate the uterus for fundus height[527] Feel the uterus during different stages of pregnancy to determine whether it is enlarging appropriately. At the end of the third month, the uterus should have enlarged sufficiently that it can be felt at the level of the symphysis pubis. At the end of the fifth month, it should be at the level of the umbilicus. At the middle of the eighth month, it should be palpable at the xiphoid cartilage located near the lower sternum. After childbirth, feel the uterine fundus through the abdominal wall. Immediately after birth, the fundus is felt halfway between the umbilicus and the bony prominence under the pubic hair. It gradually rises until about 12 hours after birth, when it lies slightly above the umbilicus. Each day the fundus height should be palpated. It should normally decrease about ½ inch/day until the 10th day, when it is no longer detectable.

Rationale: Gradual enlargement of the uterus during pregnancy permits estimation of the size of the fetus and determination of whether growth is adequate. A uterine fundus that does not descend approximately ½ inch/day may indicate poor uterine muscle tone, retained placental tissue, or endometrium inflammation.

Fulfilled Needs: Protection from physical harm

Percuss the abdomen for abnormal resonance[125,253] Percuss each abdominal quadrant. Normally a resonant, vibrating sound should be heard. Listen for decreased resonance (dullness) or for a hollow drumlike (tympany) sound.

Rationale: A dull abdominal percussion sound may indicate peritoneal cavity fluid or a full bladder. Tympanic abdominal sounds may indicate air or gas within the stomach, intestines, or peritoneal cavity.

Fulfilled Needs: Protection from physical harm

Percuss the chest for abnormal resonance[125,253] Begin under the clavicle and work downward from right to left, percussing each symmetric rib interspace. Normally a resonant, vibrating sound should be heard, except in areas of cardiac dullness. Listen for decreased resonance. Have the person pull his shoulders forward. Working down the posterior chest from right to left, percuss each rib interspace. Normally the resonant sounds end about the ninth rib. Listen for dullness (decreased resonance), flatness (absence of resonance), hyperresonance, and tympany (hollow, drumlike sound)

Rationale: Dull thoracic sounds may indicate pulmonary fluid, increased lung volume, or a deflated lung. They are associated with pulmonary atelectasis, pulmonary consolidation, and pulmonary congestion. Flat thoracic sounds may indicate chest fluid and increased lung volume and are associated with pulmonary consolidation, pleural effusion, and pulmonary congestion. Increased resonance sounds may indicate increased lung volume and pleural fluid. When heard over the upper lung, they are associated with emphysema or pleural effusion. Tympanic thoracic sounds indicate a hollow lung space and are associated with a pulmonary cavity.

Fulfilled Needs: Protection from physical harm

Percuss the posterior chest for decreased diaphragmatic descent[125,253]
With the person in a forward-bent position, percuss the posterior thorax from the scapula downward. Note the point at which dullness is heard. Then ask the person to take a deep breath and hold it. Continue percussion to a point where a new level of dullness is heard. Measure the distance between the two points; normally it should be 4–6 cm (1½–2½ inches). Compare the two sides of the chest to determine whether the measurements are equal.

Rationale: On inspiration, the diaphragm descends as the lungs fill with air. When one side of the diaphragm does not descend as far as the other, one should suspect atelectasis in that lung.

Fulfilled Needs: Protection from physical harm

Perform a physical examination and evaluate whether the findings are normal
Examine the person according to the standard procedure followed by the institution or organization in which the practice is being conducted. Include all body systems.

Rationale: By means of a physical examination, it can be determined whether the patient's health status is normal or abnormal.

Fulfilled Needs: Protection from physical harm

Review the dietary intake with the person to determine adherence to the prescribed diet
Have the person describe his complete dietary intake over a particular period. Determine whether this intake is correct in relationship to the diet prescribed for his condition.

Rationale: Adherence to a prescribed diet is essential for maintenance of health.

Fulfilled Needs: Protection from physical harm

Strain the urine
Filter all urine output through gauze or a strainer in order to catch renal stones.

Rationale: Filtering out renal stones confirms passage of the stones. Analysis of renal stones provides information that supports the use of preventive measures against future stone formation.

Fulfilled Needs: Protection from physical harm

Test and observe for nystagmus
Test for involuntary movement of the eyeballs. First, have the person fix his gaze on the nurse's finger for about 30 seconds. Then, have the person look upward, downward, and to each side, permitting the gaze to remain fixed in each position for about 5–10 seconds. Observe for involuntary eye movements in each of the test positions.

Rationale: Nystagmus may indicate neurologic disorders, particularly of cerebellar and brain stem lesions.

Fulfilled Needs: Protection from physical harm

Test for a positive Babinski sign[125]
Using a hard object, stroke the sole of the

foot from the heel up along the outer edge and across the ball of the foot. Note any abnormal upward movement (dorsal extension) of the big toe or spreading of the other toes. Normally the great toe should flex downward when the sole of the foot is stroked. A positive Babinski sign is normally found in the newborn infant, but it should disappear after approximately 1 year.

Rationale: A positive Babinski sign may indicate an immature nervous system or upper motor neuron lesion.

Fulfilled Needs: Protection from physical harm

Test for a positive Homans' sign[125,253]

When the person complains of calf tenderness, bend the foot up toward the knee (dorsiflexion) and observe for complaints of pain in the calf.

Rationale: A positive Homans' sign indicates thrombosis.

Fulfilled Needs: Protection from physical harm

Test for a positive Trousseau's sign[125]

Apply pressure to the brachial artery on the inside of the upper arm by inflating a blood pressure cuff above that area. Between the systolic and diastolic readings, determine if the hand bends downward (Palmar flexion). If spasmodic contractions of the muscles occur, this is a positive Trousseau's sign.

Rationale: A positive Trousseau's sign indicates tetany caused by decreased blood calcium levels.

Fulfilled Needs: Protection from physical harm

Test for abnormal deep-reflex responses[125,253]

Strike a sudden blow with a rubber hammer over the tendon (pectoralis, biceps, brachioradial, pronator, triceps, quadriceps, adductor, Achilles) of a muscle. Look for a highly sensitive response or a weak response of a nerve impulse occurring on external stimulation.

Rationale: An increased deep-reflex response is caused by loss of normal reflex control of the reflex arc as a result of an injury in the spinal cord at a level higher than the reflex arc. A decreased deep-reflex response indicates an interrupted reflex arc.

Fulfilled Needs: Protection from physical harm

Test for Chvostek's sign[125]

Lightly tap the face just below the temple and watch for twitching. This sign is normal in infants up to 6 months of age, but otherwise it is abnormal.

Rationale: A positive Chvostek's sign indictes calcium deficit.

Fulfilled Needs: Protection from physical harm

Test for decreased vibratory sensation

Place the vibrating tuning fork over a bony prominence and have the person indicate when the vibration ceases. Then place the tuning fork over the examiner's bony prominence to determine whether the vibration has stopped.

Rationale: When the examiner feels vibratory sensation longer than the person does, the test indicates that the person has decreased perception of vibration sensation. This problem is found in aging, peripheral neuropathy, and posterior column disease.

Fulfilled Needs: Protection from physical harm

Test for fluid deficit

Fluid deficit exists when pinched skin takes 30 seconds or more to flatten, when mucous membranes are dry, or when the skin is scaly. Babies have diminished or absent tears and a sunken fontanel, when in fluid deficit.

Rationale: The recognition of fluid deficit supports immediate treatment and resolution of the problem.

Fulfilled Needs: Protection from physical harm

Test for heat and cold perception

Test for the degree of heat and cold sensation the person can perceive. Have the person close his eyes. Place a cold object and then a warm object against the skin. Ask the person to identify the difference.

Rationale: Decreased heat or cold perception indicates neurologic impairment. It also raises the potential for injury.

Fulfilled Needs: Protection from physical harm

Test for hyperesthesia[125,253] Using a pin, lightly stroke the abdomen from the umbilicus downward, or stroke the extremities. Have the person indicate whether the pin feels sharper in any area.

Rationale: Hyperesthesia may indicate visceral, peritoneal, or extremity nerve irritation or inflammation.

Fulfilled Needs: Protection from physical harm

Test for impaired balance[33] Do a Romberg test. Have the person close his eyes and stand with his feet together. Normally, he should sway very little. If abnormal, he will lean to either the right or left.

Rationale: Impaired balance indicates a neurologic disorder.

Fulfilled Needs: Protection from physical harm

Test for impaired coordination[125] Look for signs that the normally smooth integration of body movements is impaired. This may be done in several ways. Have the person walk a straight line, placing each foot directly in front of the other. Have the person bring the tip of his index finger to the tip of his nose, once with his eyes open and once with his eyes closed. With the person lying flat, have him extend one leg and then run the heel of the other foot from the knee to the foot of the extended leg. Observe the person's ability to write, to button and unbutton clothing, to tie shoelaces, and to pick up small objects such as pins and needles.

Rationale: Impaired coordination may indicate a cerebellar lesion or extrapyramidal disorder.

Fulfilled Needs: Protection from physical harm

Test for impaired smell perception Listen for complaints of decreased ability to smell. Watch for lack of response to odor-producing objects such as flowers, food, etc.

Rationale: Impaired smell perception may result from nasal masses, nasal packing, dry nasal mucous membranes, or nerve injury. Smell perception affects taste perception, which in turn affects nutritional intake.

Fulfilled Needs: Protection from physical harm

Test for impaired taste perception Listen for complaints of decreased ability to taste. Watch for lack of response to foods such as pickles and lemons.

Rationale: Impaired taste perception may result from brain or nerve damage, tongue or oral mucosa inflammation, or decreased smell perception. Taste perception affects nutritional intake.

Fullfilled Needs: Protection from physical harm

Test for range of motion Test to determine if there is full or limited range of motion of the joints. Have the person flex, extend, and rotate each joint as appropriate to that joint. Observe the person's ability to move both arms and legs normally.

Rationale: Abnormal range of motion indicates a joint or muscle disorder.

Fulfilled Needs: Protection from physical harm

Test for sensory abilities of location and position Have the person close his eyes. Touch parts of the body with a piece of cotton and have him identify the location of the cotton on his body. Then, grasp the person's large toe and randomly move the toe up and down. Ask the person to identify the position of the toe.

Rationale: Abnormalities in sensory location and position indicate neurological disorders.

Fulfilled Needs: Protection from physical harm

Test for the degree of muscle/motor strength[125]   Have the person actively move the muscles being tested. Pull against the person's tensed muscles and have him attempt resistance. The degrees of muscle strength are as follows:

Minimum muscle weakness: Complete joint movement with almost complete muscle contraction when resistance is applied against the joint.

Mild muscle weakness: Complete joint movement with some muscle contraction when resistance is applied against the joint.

Moderate muscle weakness: Complete joint movement with some muscle contraction as long as there is no application of resistance against the joint.

Severe muscle weakness: No joint movement, some muscle contraction.

Complete muscle weakness: No joint movement, no muscle contraction.

Rationale: Testing the person's muscle strength gives an indication of his activity capabilities.

Fulfilled Needs: Protection from physical harm

Test for urine phenylalanine with ferric chloride   Apply a ferric chloride solution to a freshly saturated diaper. Interpret the chemical reaction.

Rationale: A reaction producing a green color indicates phenylketonuria, which indicates the possibility of developmental deficit.

Fulfilled Needs: Protection from physical harm

Test motor function   Test the functional ability of the muscles by the use of counterpressure in the flexion, extension, and lateral positions. Have the person press or push his finger against your finger or his extremity against your hand.

Rationale: Abnormal motor function in the extremities indicates a nerve or muscle disorder.

Fulfilled Needs: Protection from physical harm

Test the amniotic fluid pH   Using Nitrazine paper, determine the pH level of the amniotic fluid once the membrane has ruptured or if it is suspected that the membrane has ruptured. Normal vaginal secretions have a pH of 4.5–5.5 while amniotic fluid pH is 7.0–7.5.

Rationale: When fluid is escaping from the vagina, but there is doubt about whether the membrane has ruptured, this test will determine whether the fluid is amniotic or is from another source.

Fulfilled Needs: Protection from physical harm

Test the blood for glucose level   Do a finger stick. Place a drop of blood on the Dextrostix and determine the person's glucose level. Use a glucometer if available.

Rationale: Abnormal blood glucose level, whether increased or decreased, occurs with impaired carbohydrate metabolism. Results of the test reveal the effectiveness of diabetic therapy.

Fulfilled Needs: Protection from physical harm

Test the cranial nerves[33]   Determine whether lesions are associated with any of the 12 cranial nerves. *Olfactory nerve,* test smell. *Optic nerve,* test visual acuity, color vision, visual fields. For *oculomotor, trochlear, Abduces nerves,* test for extraocular movement, nystagmus, upper lip elevation, and pupil constriction. *Trigeminal nerve,* test facial sensation and jaw closure. *Facial nerve,* test facial muscle movement and eye closure. *Acoustic nerve,* test hearing. *Glossopharyngeal* and *vagus nerve,* test uvula position, swallowing, gag reflex. *Accessory nerve,* test head movement, shoulder shrugging. *Hypoglossal nerve,* test for protrusion of tongue and tremor of tongue.

Rationale: Testing the cranial nerves reveals neurologic deficits.

Fulfilled Needs: Protection from physical harm

Test the ears for hearing acuity[125,253]   To do the whisper test, begin whispering 20 feet from the patient and decrease the distance 5 feet at a time until the person can hear the whisper. To do the Weber test, hold a tuning fork at the skull midline and have the person compare the sound intensities in his two ears. To do the Rhinne test, place a tuning fork against the patient's mastoid process (bone conduction) and count the number of seconds until he no longer hears the sound. Then hold the tuning fork 1 inch from his ear (air conduction) and time his hearing again.

Rationale: Impaired hearing is said to exist when a person cannot hear a whisper at 10 feet, when there is a higher intensity of sound in one ear with the Weber test, or when the Rhinne test indicates that bone-conducted sound is heard as long as or longer than air-conducted sound.

Fulfilled Needs: Protection from physical harm

Test the eyes for decreased corneal reflex[253]   Test each eye separately and have the person look to one side while being tested. Gently place a whisp of sterile cotton on the cornea. Normally the eyelids will blink when the cornea is touched. If the corneal reflex is decreased, there will be little or no blinking.

Rationale: A decreased corneal reflex may indicate a lesion of the fifth or seventh cranial nerve.

Fulfilled Needs: Protection from physical harm

Test the eyes for impaired coordination[125,253]   Hold a light at the level of the person's eyes, then move the light in a U pattern, from top to bottom, across, and bottom to top. Ask the patient to follow the light with his eyes.

Rationale: Jerky eye movements indicate impaired eye muscle coordination. If, after the age of 6 months, an infant cannot coordinate his eyes, there may be impaired neuromuscular development.

Fulfilled Needs: Protection from physical harm

Test the eyes for light sensitivity   Watch for unusual light intolerance such as squinting, frowning, wearing sunglasses when others do not need them, and complaints of headache.

Rationale: Light sensitivity may occur with inflammatory conditions, vitamin deficiency, or increased intracranial pressure.

Fulfilled Needs: Protection from physical harm

Test the eyes for visual acuity[253]   Place a Snellen chart 20 feet in front of the person. In the visual acuity formula (e.g., 20/20) the first number is the distance the patient is standing from the chart. The first line on the chart is normally read at 200 feet, the second line at 50 feet, the third line at 40 feet, the fourth line at 30 feet, the fifth line at 20 feet, the sixth line at 15 feet, and the seventh line at 10 feet. Ask the person to read as far down the chart as he can. Indentify the number of the line to which he can read (e.g., line 7). Then insert as the second number in the visual acuity formula the normal number of feet for that line (e.g., 10 feet for line 7). Thus the patient has 20/10 vision.

If no chart is available, hold up any number of fingers and ask the person to identify the number.

Also notice whether the person bumps into things, refuses to read, requests brighter lights, squints when reading, cannot locate nearby objects, or misidentifies other people.

Rationale: As measured by the Snellen chart, vision of 20/30 or below ((20/20 or 20/10 is normal) is considered normal. Any higher rating (20/40, 20/50, etc.) indicates impaired vision.

Fulfilled Needs: Protection from physical harm

Test the hearing by a Rhinne test[33]   Place a vibrating tuning fork on the mastoid process until the vibration is no longer heard (bone conduction). Then place the still vibrating tuning fork in front of the ear meatus where the patient should continue to hear vibrations (air conduction).

Rationale: In normal hearing air conduction is twice as long as bone conduction. If bone conduction is longer than air conduction the Rhinne test is negative, indicating hearing loss.

Fulfilled Needs: Protection from physical harm

Test the hearing by a Weber test[33] Place a vibrating tuning fork at the skull midline on the forehead. Ask the person if he hears the vibration in one or both ears.

Rationale: In normal hearing the vibration sound is heard equally in both ears. Lateralization of the sound to one ear indicates bone conduction loss in that ear or perceptive loss in the other ear.

Fulfilled Needs: Protection from physical loss

Test the hearing by audiometry Using an audiometry machine, test the level of tones the person can hear.

Rationale: Audiometers determine the degree of hearing loss through the use of tones in calibrated loudness.

Fulfilled Needs: Protection from physical harm

Test the infant for the Moro reflex[253] Suddenly change the infant's position, and provide jarring or loud noise stimuli. Notice whether the infant appears startled, tenses his muscles, makes a wide embracing motion with his arms, and extends his legs.

Rationale: The Moro reflex is normal in children younger than 8 weeks of age. If it lasts beyond 4 months, it may indicate an inability to walk.

Fulfilled Needs: Protection from physical harm

Test the infant for the neck-righting reflex Place the child on his back and turn his head to one side. Normally he will turn his whole body in an effort to maintain alignment with his head. This reflex is normal up to the age of 5 months, but it should disappear between 6 and 8 months of age.

Rationale: When the neck-righting reflex lasts beyond 8 months of age, it may indicate an inability to walk.

Fulfilled Needs: Protection from physical harm

Test the infant for the rooting reflex[253] Touch the infant on the cheek. Normally he will turn his head in the direction of the touch in an effort to find or root for food. When something is placed in his mouth, normally he will suck on it in an effort to obtain food.

Rationale: If the infant does not respond normally with the rooting reflex, this may indicate central nervous system or intracranial injury.

Fulfilled Needs: Protection from physical harm

Test the skin for impaired feeling perception Have the person close his eyes. With a pin, touch the skin and watch for a decreased pain response. Touch the person with heat or cold and determine if the response is normal.

Rationale: Impaired feeling perception indicates nerve or circulatory damage and increases the potential for tissue trauma.

Fulfilled Needs: Protection from physical harm

Test the stool for occult blood by Hemoccult Ask the person to collect a stool specimen and put a small amount on the Hemoccult guaiac paper. Drop some Hemoccult developing solution onto the back of the guaiac paper (over the fecal smear), and look for a blue color, which indicates the presence of fecal blood.

Rationale: The presence of occult blood in the stool may occur in several disease states and during certain drug therapies. It is particularly important as a screening test for cancer of the colon.

Fulfilled Needs: Protection from physical harm

Test the strength and equality of the hand grasps Have the person squeeze your hand and determine if the strength of the squeeze is normal. Determine the person's grasping ability. Notice if he is able to close safety pins, button clothing, pick up coins, and perform other activities requiring precise finger movements.

Rationale: The inability to firmly grasp objects is indicative of brain or nerve cell damage. Skilled voluntary movements are dependent on an intact corticospinal tract. The inability to perform daily living skills is usually perceived as threatening.

Fulfilled Needs: Protection from physical harm

Test the urine by Dipstick (Multistix) Use a Dipstick or Multistix to test for urobilinogen, nitrite, blood, glucose, acetone, protein, and pH.

Rationale: Testing the urine by Dipstick can reveal physiologic abnormalities, such as may occur in liver disease, urinary tract infection, and diabetes.

Fulfilled Needs: Protection from physical harm

Test the urine for pH Determine the urine acidity or alkalinity with litmus or Nitrazine paper or other chemical agents. The first morning urine specimen is usually more acidic than any other sample during the day.

Rationale: The urine pH (acidity or alkalinity) has an influence on the tendency to form renal stones.

Fulfilled Needs: Protection from physical harm

Test the urine for protein Use a commercial product such as Combistix or Urostix to determine the presence of protein in the urine.

Rationale: Protein in the urine may indicate impaired kidney function, impending pregnancy toxemia, impending kidney transplant rejection, prostatitis, or epididymitis.

Fulfilled Needs: Protection from physical harm

Test the urine for sugar and/or acetone/ketone Use a commercial product such as Clinitest, Diastix, or Tes-Tape to determine the presence of sugar in the urine. Use Acetest or Ketostix to determine the presence of acetone in the urine.

Rationale: Sugar in the urine indicates that insulin secretion is insufficient to break down glucose carbohydrates for storage in the liver as energy. This causes sugars to appear in the urine and brings about an acid state. Acetone in the urine indicates that body fat is being used for energy in place of sugar.

Fulfilled Needs: Protection from physical harm

Time the uterine contractions Place a warm hand just above the umbilicus and feel the uterus rise in the abdominal cavity, contract, become very hard, and then relax. Count the number of seconds that the uterus remains very hard, the duration of a contraction. Determine the interval between contractions by counting the minutes between the beginning of one contraction and the beginning of the next. The relaxation time is the time between the end of one contraction and the beginning of the next.

Rationale: Timing uterine contractions determines whether the uterus is progressing toward cervical dilatation. Uterine contractions will cease completely if there is uterine rupture.

Fulfilled Needs: Protection from physical harm

HEALTH
TEACHING

Advise a gradual return to activity   Suggest that the person gradually take on more activities. When one activity has been accomplished successfully several times without fatigue, have him take on another.

Rationale: Feelings of comfort and safety arise from an awareness that one can successfully and independently cope with and master the skills of everyday living. The accomplishment of activities without fatigue promotes comfort.

Fulfilled Needs: Protection from physical harm, protection from psychologic threat, sense of adequacy, independence, increased learning

Advise acceptance of the drug user's return home[445]   When a family member has temporarily left the family to join other drug users, but then suddenly wants to return home, suggest that his return be accepted without bitterness and reproach.

Rationale: On realizing his mistake, the young drug user may wish to return to normal life. Acceptance by loved ones allows for a new beginning.

Fulfilled Needs: Comfort, protection from psychologic threat, unity with loved ones, increased learning

Advise adherence to the immunization schedule   Suggest that periodic immunizations be maintained according to the recommended schedule of health officials. The generally accepted immunization routine as recommended by the American Academy of Pediatrics [313:312]:

Age	Immunization
2 months	First dose of diphtheria/tetanus/pertussis vaccine, first dose of polio vaccine
4 months	Second dose of diphtheria/tetanus/pertussis vaccine and polio vaccine
6 months	Third dose of diphtheria/tetanus/pertussis vaccine, third dose of polio vaccine
15 months	Measles, mumps, rubella
18 months	Boosters for diphtheria/tetanus/pertussis and polio
4–6 years	Boosters for diphtheria/tetanus/pertussis and polio
14–16 years	Tetanus/diphtheria toxoid
Following years	Tetanus/diphtheria toxoid every 10 years

Rationale: Immunizations protect against potentially threatening disease.

Fulfilled Needs: Protection from physical harm, increased learning

Advise against bending the ear frames when applying or removing eyeglasses   Suggest that when applying or removing eyeglasses, the person use both hands, one on each ear frame, to keep the frames in straight alignment with the face. Eyeglasses should not be pulled off or put on at an angle using only one hand on one ear frame.

Rationale: Removing or applying eyeglasses at an angle to the face bends the ear frame, changing the lens alignment with the eye and distorting vision.

Fulfilled Needs: Comfort, protection from physical harm, increased learning

Advise against causing defensive responses in others   Suggest that the person never place another person in such a position that the person feels compelled to protect his sense of pride. This can only result in defensive behavior.

Rationale: Behavior based on defensive attitudes is often socially unacceptable; it can result in shame or guilt at a later time.

Fulfilled Needs: Protection from psychologic threat. Personal growth and maturity. Increased learning. Increased reality perception and problem-solving ability.

Advise against chewing gum Suggest that gum chewing be avoided when the person suffers from excessive flatulence.

Rationale: As gum is chewed, air is swallowed and added to intestinal gases, further increasing flatulence and the associated pressure discomfort.

Fulfilled Needs: Comfort, protection from physical harm, increased learning

Advise against committing alcoholics to promises of sobriety[445] Suggest that the family not ask the alcoholic to promise that he will stop drinking.

Rationale: If an alcholic promises not to drink and then breaks the promise, he suffers guilt feelings and loss of self-respect, which further promote drinking.

Fulfilled Needs: Comfort, increased learning

Advise against communicating double-meaning messages Suggest that messages that convey conflicts of feeling be avoided. Point out that it is unwise to make such statements as these: "I know you're capable, but I doubt you can meet the challenge." "Your friend is a fine person, but you're not to associate with him."

Rationale: Double-meaning messages cause confusion and doubt. They do not convey a single clear meaning, and they render the receiver unable to determine the real intent of the message and unable to determine an appropriate response.

Fulfilled Needs: Protection from psychologic threat, personal growth and maturity, increased learning, increased reality perception and problem-solving ability

Advise against correlating God's love and death to children Suggest that a child not be told that a family member was taken to heaven because God loved him.

Rationale: Loss of a loved one causes anger. If the loss is associated with God, it can result in anger toward God, with the potential for depression and anxiety over moral conflict.

Fulfilled Needs: Protection from psychologic threat, increased learning

Advise against denouncing erroneous perceptions When delusional, illusional, or hallucinational ideas are expressed, suggest that they not be laughed at and that the person expressing them not be told he is "crazy" or is mistaken. Instead, it should be made known to him that he has a right to his feelings, but that others may not agree with him.

Rationale: When persons are told that they are mistaken about their perceptions, they are threatened with confusion, anxiety, and fear. Acceptance associated with disagreement supports a return to realistic perception.

Fulfilled Needs: Protection from psychologic threat, increased reality perception, increased learning·

Advise against drawing secretions to the back of the throat Suggest that nasal secretions not be drawn to the back of the throat, but be removed by blowing the nose.

Rationale: Drawing secretions to the back of the throat causes pressure changes on sinus tissue and pulls fluid into the sinuses. If the secretions are infectious and the material is swallowed into the digestive tract, this increases the potential for generalized infection.

Fulfilled Needs: Protection from physical harm, increased learning

Advise against drinking alcohol for warmth Explain that drinking alcoholic beverages may produce temporary body warmth but that the end result is decreased circulation with lowered body temperature.

Rationale: Alcohol causes an immediate vasodilatation that gives an immediate feeling of internal body warmth. Later, vasoconstriction occurs, impairing systemic circulation and reducing the body temperature.

Fulfilled Needs: Protection from physical harm, increased learning

Advise against eating dairy products in foreign countries   Suggest that persons traveling to foreign countries avoid milk, ice cream, cream sauces, or soft cheeses.

Rationale: In some foreign countries milk is not pasteurized, and it can cause intestinal distress to persons unaccustomed to raw milk.

Fulfilled Needs: Protection from physical harm, increased learning

Advise against eating in unlicensed restaurants   Suggest that one look for a license from the local health authority on the wall of a restaurant before eating there.

Rationale: To receive a license to operate, a restaurant must meet sanitation standards.

Fulfilled Needs: Protection from physical harm, increased learning

Advise against eating raw fruits and vegetables in foreign countries   Suggest to persons traveling to foreign countries that raw fruits and vegetables not be eaten. Only those that are well cooked are safe.

Rationale: Many foreign countries use human excreta for fertilizing fruits and vegetables; this practice increases food contamination with dysentery organisms. Hygienic standards for food handling in many foreign countries are low.

Fulfilled Needs: Protection from physical harm, increased learning

Advise against eating sweets   Suggest that sweets be avoided. This includes sugar, candy, honey, jam, jelly, marmalade, syrups, pies, cakes, cookies, pastries, condensed milk, soft drinks, and candy-coated gum.

Rationale: Since a diabetic's pancreas fails to produce sufficient insulin to metabolize glucose adequately, foods high in glucose are not converted into energy, but instead disrupt metabolic equilibrium. Sugar on the teeth promotes bacterial growth, which leads to decay.

Fulfilled Needs: Protection from physical harm, increased learning

Advise against emphasizing past problems caused by another   Suggest that it is inadvisable to remind another person that he was the cause of past failures or unpleasant experiences.

Rationale: Being reminded of past failures reinforces feelings of guilt and shame and supports defensive behavior.

Fulfilled Needs: Comfort, protection from psychologic threat, sense of adequacy, personal growth and maturity, increased learning, increased reality perception and problem-solving ability

Advise against exposure to airborne irritants   Suggest that persons with allergies or artificial airways avoid environments in which dust levels or pollen counts are high. If airborne irritants are unavoidable, suggest that a mask of filtering material be worn over the nose or artificial airway.

Rationale: Respiratory irritation may stimulate coughing, cause bronchial spasm, or injure tissue.

Fulfilled Needs: Comfort, protection from physical harm, increased learning

Advise against exposure to inclement weather/extreme cold   Suggest that cold, windy, or damp weather be avoided in nonhealth conditions.

Rationale: Cold weather causes vasoconstriction and increases cardiac workload as the heart pumps blood through constricted vessels. Cold decreases the metabolic rate.

Cold causes bronchoconstriction causing dyspnea.

Fulfilled Needs: Normal temperature, comfort, protection from physical harm, increased learning

Advise against exposure to intense heat Suggest that an effort be made to avoid high environmental temperatures and hot objects.

Rationale: Intense environmental heat causes vasodilatation and sluggish blood flow which, in impaired cardiac function, overtaxes the heart; increases the metabolic rate causing energy consumption and malaise; and alters fluid and electrolyte balance by increasing perspiration. Sunrays and contact with hot objects can cause severe skin burns.

Fulfilled Needs: Normal temperature, comfort, protection from physical harm, increased learning

Advise against fighting fear/anxiety Explain that a mental effort to fight fear or anxiety reinforces the emotion and maintains focus on it. Fear is best conquered by facing the cause of the fear, using logic, constructive thinking and action.

Rationale: Since fear and anxiety stem from a sense of helplessness in the face of danger, fighting fear and anxiety merely reinforces that sense of helplessness, while logical thinking supports adequacy through realistic perception of the danger.

Fulfilled Needs: Comfort, protection from psychologic threat, personal growth and maturity, increased learning, increased reality perception and problem-solving ability

Advise against gulping food and drink Suggest that food and drink not be swallowed rapidly in large amounts at one time.

Rationale: While gulping food and drink, large amounts of air are carried into the stomach and added to intestinal gases. This further increases flatulence and the associated pressure discomfort. Gulping food and drink heightens the potential for aspiration.

Fulfilled Needs: Comfort, protection from physical harm, increased learning

Advise against intense surveillance of the drug user[25] Suggest that parents who suspect their child of using drugs avoid searching through personal possessions, listening in on telephone conversations, and monitoring mail.

Rationale: When persons are aware that they are being watched, they begin to distrust those who are watching them, and communication may be seriously threatened.

Fulfilled Needs: Protection from psychologic threat, caring and communicating relationships, increased learning

Advise against letting light shine directly into the eyes Suggest that light never be allowed to shine directly into the eyes and that light bulbs always be shaded.

Rationale: Reduced glare can prevent damage to optic tissue and nerves.

Fulfilled Needs: Comfort, protection from physical harm, increased learning

Advise against making emotional appeals to the alcoholic Suggest that the family avoid appeals such as these: "Will you stop drinking out of love for me?" "If you cared for your family, you'd stop drinking."

Rationale: Emotional appeals to the alcoholic who cannot stop drinking increase his sense of guilt, which in turn supports further drinking.

Fulfilled Needs: Comfort, increased learning

Advise against making excuses for the alcoholic[445] Suggest that the family not try to cover up the real reason why the alcoholic hasn't gone to work or met other commitments.

Rationale: Encouraging the alcoholic to employ readily available excuses fosters behavioral disorders.

Fulfilled Needs: Increased learning, increased reality perception and problem-solving ability

Advise against mingling in crowds Suggest that the person stay away from crowds and from persons with infections.

Rationale: Exposure to crowds enhances the potential for infection.

Fulfilled Needs: Protection from physical harm, increased learning

Advise against piercing or squeezing the skin/lesions Suggest that skin lesions not be opened with objects such as pins, needles, and the like. If a lesion has come to a head, it should be incised and drained by qualified persons using sterile technique. Suggest that skin pustules not be squeezed. To hasten their removal, the skin should be thoroughly washed and heat should be applied, permitting pustules to dry naturally.

Rationale: Piercing or squeezing the skin bruises and traumatizes tissue and may force pathogenic microorganisms into the bloodstream.

Fulfilled Needs: Protection from physical harm, increased learning

Advise against prolonged skin/scalp exposure to the sun and/or the water Suggest that prolonged body exposure to the sunrays be avoided. Suggest that the skin not be exposed to water, especially salty or chemically treated water, for prolonged periods.

Rationale: Prolonged exposure to sunrays activates melanin pigment and discolors and burns the skin. Prolonged exposure to water removes natural skin oils and causes skin irritation.

Fulfilled Needs: Comfort, protection from physical harm, increased learning

Advise against pulling off dead skin/scabs When underlying skin has not adequately healed, or when scabs have formed over a wound, suggest that dead skin or scabs not be pulled off. Skin should be removed only if healing is adequate, and no discomfort or bleeding should result. Scabs should be allowed to fall off.

Rationale: Pulling off dead skin or scabs before they are ready to fall off may traumatize the underlying skin, cause pain and bleeding, and permit the entrance of bacteria into the open wound.

Fulfilled Needs: Comfort, protection from physical harm, increased learning

Advise against questioning the alcoholic about drinking Suggest that it is inadvisable to question the alcoholic about whether he has been drinking.

Rationale: If an alcoholic has been drinking, it will soon become evident; the distrust aroused by questioning him will increase his anxiety, thus precipitating further drinking.

Fulfilled Needs: Protection from psychologic threat, increased learning, increased reality perception and problem-solving ability

Advise against reading or looking out the window while in a moving vehicle Suggest that reading or looking out the window while riding in a car, airplane, boat, or train be avoided if one is susceptible to motion sickness.

Rationale: The eye movement that occurs when reading or when watching passing scenery increases motion stimuli to the medulla, thus raising the potential for motion sickness.

Fulfilled Needs: Protection from physical harm, increased learning

Advise against removing the alcoholic's liquor supply Suggest that the family not throw away or hide liquor from the alcoholic.

Rationale: Once the alcoholic realizes that his liquor supply is threatened, he will resort to deceptive practices to assure an available supply.

Fulfilled Needs: Protection from psychologic threat, increased learning, increased reality perception and problem-solving ability

Advise against responding to gesture speech Suggest that parents who have children with delayed or impaired speech patterns respond only to verbal communications, not to gesturing or jargon.

Rationale: When children become aware that adults respond only to verbal communications, they will find it essential to develop appropriate speech skills.

Fulfilled Needs: Caring and communicating relationships, mastery and competence in skills, increased learning

Advise against scratching Suggest that an effort be made to avoid scratching skin that itches; substitute methods such as dabbing the itching area with an alcohol sponge or applying a cool cloth or ice cubes.

Rationale: Scratching further irritates already inflamed oversensitive skin. Reduced scratching can diminish skin irritation and promote comfort.

Fulfilled Needs: Comfort, protection from physical harm, increased learning

Advise against threatening the alcoholic Suggest that the family not threaten, argue with, or put intense pressure on the alcoholic in an effort to stop his drinking.

Rationale: When severely threatened, the alcoholic may respond with violence.

Fulfilled Needs: Increased learning, increased reality perception and problem-solving ability

Advise against using ice cubes made from potentially unsafe water Suggest that ice cubes never be used in drinks if they are made with water that might be contaminated. For cooling, set the glass or container in a bucket of ice with the ice around it, not in it.

Rationale: Freezing contaminated water does not destroy bacteria.

Fulfilled Needs: Protection from physical harm, increased learning

Advise against using mineral oil laxatives Suggest that the chronic use of mineral oil laxatives be avoided.

Rationale: Mineral oil in the intestinal tract interferes with absorption of fat-soluble vitamins, especially vitamins A and K.

Fulfilled Needs: Protection from physical harm, increased learning

Advise against using tampons Suggest that tampons not be used whenever there is an infectious vaginal discharge, when the person has undergone a hysterectomy, or when there is nonmenstrual vaginal bleeding.

Rationale: Tampons obstruct the flow of an infectious vaginal discharge and prevent proper drainage. After a hysterectomy, tampons irritate the incised vagina.

Fulfilled Needs: Protection from physical harm, increased learning

Advise against verbally comparing significant others Suggest that verbal comparisons of the qualities of significant persons be avoided. If evaluation is necessary, it should be confined to one person.

Rationale: Comparisons with others may promote feelings of inadequacy. Comfort feelings require that a person experience acceptance from others and relatedness to others.

Fulfilled Needs: Comfort, protection from psychologic threat, sense of adequacy, increased learning, increased reality perception and problem-solving ability

Advise against walking barefoot Explain that bare feet are subject to injury and infection.

Rationale Walking barefoot subjects the feet to injury from sharp objects, to the larvae of fecal worms present in the soil, to insect and snakebites, and to poisonous plants and fungus growth.

Fulfilled Needs Protection from physical harm, increased learning

Advise against wearing constrictive/restrictive clothing Suggest that tight clothing such as girdles, hatbands, belts, ties, and garters either not be worn or be fastened loosely. Suggest that clothing that restricts body movement be avoided, such as tight skirts and jackets.

Rationale: Constriction prevents adequate venous return, and this impairs blood circulation and results in tissue damage. Restrictive clothing reduces freedom of body movement.

Fulfilled Needs: Protection from physical harm, increased learning

Advise against wearing unprescribed eyeglasses   Suggest that eyeglasses manufactured for general use or those prescribed for another person not be worn.

Rationale: Unprescribed eyeglasses may cause eye damage because the correction in the glass may be inappropriate to the visual problem.

Fulfilled Needs: Protection from physical harm, increased learning

Advise against weight bearing   Recommend that the person not put his body weight on the injured or diseased body part. Show him how to shift the weight to a stronger body area or to a crutch or walker, if the leg is involved.

Rationale: Keeping an injured or diseased body part free from the pressure of body weight gives that body part the rest needed to promote healing.

Fulfilled Needs: Protection from physical harm, increased learning

Advise against whispering around ill persons   Suggest that persons visiting a sick person refrain from speaking in whispers.

Rationale: Whispering between two visitors can contribute to tension in the patient and lead to misinterpretation. The patient knows that something is being said, but can only guess what it is.

Fulfilled Needs: Comfort, increased learning

Advise an annual gynecologic examination   Suggest that a yearly examination of the female reproductive organs and a vaginal smear be done. This is especially important for women who have had children.

Rationale: Annual physical examinations are a means of early disease detection.

Fulfilled Needs: Protection from physical harm, increased learning

Advise daily bathing   Suggest that a bath be taken daily to maintain cleanliness.

Rationale: Cleanliness prevents bacterial growth and promotes comfort.

Fulfilled Needs: Comfort, cleanliness, protection from physical harm, increased learning

Contraindications: When a person has excessively dry skin, a complete bath and a partial bath should be taken on alternate days.

Advise early and consistent use of the toothbrush   Suggest that a child be taught to use a toothbrush as soon as he is able to manipulate the brush.

Rationale: Brushing the teeth removes food particles, reduces the potential for decay, and provides the comfort of a refreshed mouth.

Fulfilled Needs: Cleanliness, protection from physical harm, increased learning

Advise early correction of problems   Suggest that small health problems be corrected as soon as they are noticed.

Rationale: If corrected in the early stages, most problems cause minimal distress and never have cumulative effects.

Fulfilled Needs: Protection from physical harm, protection from psychologic threat, increased learning

Advise frequent and early dental attention   As soon as a child has fully developed teeth, suggest that he receive dental attention at least once a year and preferably every 6 months.

Rationale: Early recognition and treatment of caries can prevent the spread of caries.
Fulfilled Needs: Protection from physical harm, increased learning

Advise frequent hair brushing   Suggest that the hair be brushed well at least daily.
Rationale: Hair brushing stimulates circulation and normal secretion of sebaceous glands, removes dirt particles and dead scalp cells, and promotes comfort.
Fulfilled Needs: Comfort, cleanliness, protection from physical harm, increased learning

Advise frequent sanitary pad/tampon change   Suggest that clean perineal pads be applied every few hours when there is vaginal discharge.
Rationale: Cleanliness prevents infection and promotes comfort.
Fulfilled Needs: Comfort, cleanliness, protection from physical harm, increased learning

Advise gentle nose blowing   Suggest that the nose be blown with minimum force or pressure.
Rationale: Harsh nose blowing irritates the nasal mucous membrane and forces infected material into the ears and sinuses.
Fulfilled Needs: Protection from physical harm, increased learning

Advise hand washing after elimination   Suggest that the hands be washed thoroughly with soap and water after each bowel or urinary elimination.
Rationale: Cleanliness through hand washing prevents the spread of infection from one body part to another and from person to person.
Fulfilled Needs: Cleanliness, protection from physical harm, increased learning

Advise hand washing before meals/before meal preparation   Suggest that the hands be washed thoroughly with soap and water before each meal.
Rationale: Cleanliness through hand washing prevents the introduction of bacteria into the mouth.
Fulfilled Needs: Cleanliness, protection from physical harm, increased learning

Advise how to integrate the therapeutic procedure (dialysis, chemotherapy, physical therapy, etc.) into the daily routine   Make suggestions that will assist the person to fit therapeutic procedures into his daily routine. Whenever possible, adjust appointments for the convenience of the person.
Rationale: Therapeutic procedures that cause the least disruption of the person's usual lifestyle are the most likely to be accepted and completed.
Fulfilled Needs: Comfort, increased learning

Advise limited talking   When the patient's throat is irritated, suggest that he avoid speaking except for essentials. When the patient talks excessively, suggest that he limit his speaking to brief conversation.
Rationale: Excessive talking irritates the vocal cords and, when associated with vocal cord disease, can permanently damage speech. Excessive talking can irritate other people and reduce favorable social responses.
Fulfilled Needs: Protection from physical harm, protection from psychologic threat, increased learning

Advise limited use of hair spray   Suggest that hair spray be used in small quantities or not at all when scalp and hair problems exist.
Rationale: Hair sprays may irritate scalp tissue, damage hair follicles, and contribute to uncleanliness.
Fulfilled Needs: Cleanliness, protection from physical harm, increased learning

Advise limited use of powder on the skin   When dusting powder is being applied to the skin, suggest that the powder be sprinkled onto the hands; the hands should then be rubbed together lightly, removing excess powder, and rubbed over the skin, leaving only a light film.

Rationale: Heavy layers of dusting powder on the skin tend to cake in skin folds and irritate the skin surface. Sprinkling powder directly on the baby causes inhalation of powder particles, which results in respiratory irritation.

Fulfilled Needs: Comfort, protection from physical harm, increased learning

Advise minimal infant handling Suggest that irritable infants be handled only when it is absolutely necessary and at other times be left undisturbed.

Rationale: Decreasing the external stimuli reduces the need for adaptive responses, promotes sleep, and decreases energy depletion.

Fulfilled Needs: Protection from physical harm, protection from psychologic threat, increased learning

Advise moderation in douching Explain that it is not necessary to douche daily, after menstruation, or after sexual intercourse. Douching should be used only for cleanliness and therapeutic purposes.

Rationale: Consistent douching may lead to vaginal irritation. Since douching removes the natural vaginal flora, it increases the potential for vaginal infection from other organisms.

Fulfilled Needs: Protection from physical harm, increased learning

Advise mouth rinsing when brushing is inconvenient When the person is unable to brush his teeth after each meal, suggest that the mouth be rinsed with water.

Rationale: Removing food particles from the teeth reduces the potential for decay and provides the comfort of a refreshed mouth.

Fulfilled Needs: Comfort, cleanliness, protection from physical harm, increased learning

Advise not to drive for 3 hours after two alcoholic drinks Suggest that one not drive any sooner than 3 hours after ingesting two alcoholic drinks.

Rationale: Oxidation of alcohol in the blood takes 3 hours to occur. Before this oxidation is accomplished, the nervous system experiences impaired perception and motor skills.

Fulfilled Needs: Protection from physical harm, increased learning

Advise not to move or use joints immediately distal and proximal to the fracture Suggest that the joints immediately distal and proximal to a fracture not be used or moved until the fracture is sufficiently immobilized or healed to resist disalignment.

Rationale: When the joints approximating a fracture are immobilized, healing can occur more rapidly and completely.

Fulfilled Needs: Protection from physical harm, increased learning

Advise not to partake of very hot or cold foods and drinks Suggest that very hot or cold foods and drinks be avoided and that warm foods and drinks be chosen instead.

Rationale: Extreme temperatures in food and drink can cause injury to oral and gastric tissue. Very hot food or drink can cause vasodilatation, and coldness can cause vasoconstriction.

Fulfilled Needs: Normal temperature, comfort, protection from physical harm, increased learning

Advise not to stand for prolonged periods Suggest that standing be limited to short periods or alternated with walking or sitting.

Rationale: Prolonged standing causes blood pooling in the lower extremities, reducing circulation throughout the body. Prolonged standing puts pressure on the venous system, predisposing to varicosities. Standing puts pressure on hemorrhoids, and if they are severe, standing can precipitate bleeding.

Fulfilled Needs: Tissue oxygenation or perfusion, comfort, protection from physical harm, increased learning

Advise not to take any drugs   Advise the person that drugs are not to be taken unless prescribed by a physician. This includes all over-the-counter drugs. It is especially important during pregnancy.

Rationale: Taking drugs during pregnancy can adversely affect normal fetal development. Taking unprescribed drugs can complicate existing disease states.

Fulfilled Needs: Protection from physical harm, increased learning

Advise not to take enemas and/or laxatives   Suggest that it is inadvisable to take enemas and laxatives habitually for bowel elimination and that they should not be taken when there is abdominal pain or vaginal bleeding.

Rationale: Frequent use of enemas and laxatives gradually makes the intestinal mucosa insensitive to normal elimination stimulation and decreases the normal muscle tone required for elimination. When there is abdominal pain, the pressure caused by enemas and laxatives may precipitate organ rupture, when there is vaginal bleeding, the pressure may precipitate hemorrhage.

Fulfilled Needs: Protection from physical harm, increased learning

Advise not to take hot baths   Suggest that lukewarm baths, not hot baths, be taken. A bath is too hot when it reddens the skin.

Rationale: Hot baths cause vasodilatation, which can reduce blood pressure in persons subject to hypotension and can cause engorgement of scalp vessels, resulting in increased headache pain.

Fulfilled Needs: Normal temperature, protection from physical harm, increased learning

Advise not to use a harsh dentifrice   Point out that toothpastes and tooth powders should never cause excessive friction and should bear the mark of approval of the American Dental Association.

Rationale: Harsh dentifrices traumatize the gums.

Fulfilled Needs: Protection from physical harm, increased learning

Advise not to use adhesive tape on the skin   Suggest that adhesive tape not be used for prolonged periods and that it not be used at all on tender skin. Transparent or paper tape is more appropriate.

Rationale: The sticky surface of adhesive tape irritates skin tissue; when it must be removed frequently from tender skin, it pulls off the surface layer of skin.

Fulfilled Needs: Protection from physical harm, increased learning

Advise not to use an electric blanket   Explain that electric blankets should not be used by small children or by anyone who has experienced loss of touch sensation.

Rationale: When the skin cannot perceive heat correctly, serious burns can result from electric blankets.

Fulfilled Needs: Protection from physical harm, increased learning

Advise occasional respite from responsibility   Explain that the stress of responsibility can be reduced if a person is relieved of responsibility by others at reasonable intervals.

Rationale: Occasional relief from intense stress is essential to physical and emotional health.

Fulfilled Needs: Comfort, protection from physical harm, protection from psychologic threat, increased learning

Advise periodic examinations for known hereditary predispositions Suggest that persons whose blood relatives have diabetes, hypertension, and other genetically transmitted diseases have frequent examinations to determine early evidence of disease.

Rationale: Early treatment tends to be more successful than treatment administered after the disease has become serious.

Fulfilled Needs: Protection from physical harm, increased learning

Advise precaution when using chemicals Whenever and for whatever purpose chemicals are used, suggest that they be used with extreme care. Such agents include strong household cleaning agents containing poison, lye, lime, or ammonia.

Rationale: Exercising caution when using chemicals can prevent physical injury.

Fulfilled Needs: Protection from physical harm, increased learning

Advise that a poor prognosis be shared with significant others Suggest that it is best not to keep a poor prognosis a secret from family members and other significant persons.

Rationale: Sharing the information that there is a poor prognosis gives family members the satisfaction and consolation of reaching acceptance together and supporting one another.

Fulfilled Needs: Protection from psychologic threat. Unity with loved ones, endurance, increased learning

Contraindications: Sometimes it is best to delay telling a severely ill family member of a poor prognosis of another family member

Advise that between-meal snacks be avoided Explain to overweight persons that between-meal snacks add carbohydrates and calories to their daily food intake, thus increasing body weight.

Rationale: Intake of calories should equal energy expenditure if weight gain is to be avoided.

Fulfilled Needs: Protection from physical harm, increased learning

Contraindications: Increased metabolic rate, as with fever, burns, or hyperthyroidism

Advise that children participate in grief-related activities Suggest that children be included in activities that occur during and following the death of a family member.

Rationale: Participation by children in the family's expression of grief reassures them that they are not alone with their feelings; it provides comfort and enhances their perception of death as a part of life.

Fulfilled Needs: Comfort, protection from psychologic threat, unity with loved ones, personal growth and maturity, increased learning

Advise that communication be delayed during fatigue Suggest that important messages be delayed whenever an ill person becomes temporarily fatigued.

Rationale: Messages received during a state of fatigue are poorly perceived. If the message is unpleasant, the potential for stress is increased by the fatigue.

Fulfilled Needs: Protection from physical harm, protection from psychologic threat, increased learning

Advise that contact lenses not be used for eye color change Explain that contact lenses should be worn only for therapeutic correction of visual disorders and never for esthetic eye coloring.

Rationale: Whenever an object is placed in the eye, there is risk of corneal injury.

Fulfilled Needs: Protection from physical harm, increased learning

Advise that discipline be consistent Suggest that discipline be consistently firm and that it be such that the child can easily relate it to unacceptable behavior. The use of discipline on one occasion, while letting the same behavior go undisciplined on other occasions, is to be discouraged.

Rationale: Familiar and predictable situations support learning, comfort, and safety feelings.

Fulfilled Needs: Comfort, protection from psychologic threat, predictable and orderly world, personal growth and maturity, increased learning, increased reality perception and problem-solving ability

Advise that fresh foods should be thoroughly washed   Explain that raw fruits and vegetables should be soaked in clear water and scrubbed clean.

Rationale: Washing raw fruits and vegetables removes dirt particles and bacteria, thus reducing the potential for intestinal disturbances.

Fulfilled Needs: Protection from physical harm, increased learning

Advise that highly emotional situations be avoided   Suggest that situations that tend to arouse intense emotions be avoided, whenever possible, by those with certain health disorders.

Rationale: Intense emotions stimulate adrenal secretions, which affect cardiovascular, respiratory, and gastric activity.

Fulfilled Needs: Protection from physical harm, protection from psychologic threat, increased learning

Advise that infants be started on solid foods no later than 6 months of age   Explain that infants should be on solid foods no later than 6 months of age and that the foods should be rich in iron and protein. Such foods include fruits, vegetables, meats, and eggs.

Rationale: At the age of 6 months an infant's iron reserves are depleted and need to be supplemented. Protein foods are essential for rapid growth.

Fulfilled Needs: Nutritional balance, protection from physical harm, increased learning

Advise that lanolin be applied to brittle nails   Suggest that lanolin be applied under the cuticles and around the nail area.

Rationale: Lanolin softens the nail and surrounding area, decreases skin cracking, and facilitates healing.

Fulfilled Needs: Protection from physical harm, increased learning

Advise that negative responses from others be regarded with minimum significance   Suggest that negative responses from others are relatively unimportant if the person's behavior has satisfied his inner self and has met personal value commitments. Suggest that such negative responses might sometimes serve as clues to self-improvement but that they should not be dwelled on at length.

Rationale: A positive self-image is nourished by the achievement of goals that the person perceives as important.

Fulfilled Needs: Comfort, protection from psychologic threat, high evaluation of self, sense of adequacy, increased learning

Advise that normal, not accentuated, lip movements be used when speaking to hearing impaired persons   Suggest that normal lip movements be used when speaking to a deaf person and that accentuated pronunciations be avoided.

Rationale: Deaf persons are taught to read normal lip movements. Accentuated pronunciations confuse the lip reader and impair message reception.

Fulfilled Needs: Comfort, caring and communicating relationships, increased learning

Advise that others should not assume the alcoholic's responsibilities   Suggest that, whenever possible, families refrain from performing those duties and obligations that are the responsibility of the alcoholic.

Rationale: When the family assumes the alcoholic's responsibilities, his sense of value and usefulness is diminished.

Fulfilled Needs: Comfort, personal growth and maturity, increased learning

Advise that persons attending the sick economize their energies Suggest that it is better for several persons to stay for short periods with a sick person than for one person to remain continuously at the bedside.

Rationale: The capacity to function is most effective when there is a balance between serving others and meeting our own needs. A person cannot function well under the stress of constant awareness of illness.

Fulfilled Needs: Rest and relaxation, protection from physical harm, protection from psychologic threat, increased learning

Advise that positions that impair circulation be avoided Suggest that prolonged knee bending, leg crossing, standing, and pressure behind the knee be avoided.

Rationale: Positions that compress the veins or that decrease muscle activity impair venous flow and promote thrombosis.

Fulfilled Needs: Tissue oxygenation or perfusion, comfort, protection from physical harm, freedom from pain, increased learning

Advise that significant persons express acceptance of one another Suggest that persons who care for each other openly communicate to one another that each perceives the other as a person of worth simply because he is a unique person.

Rationale: Psychologic safety requires that a person be aware that he has worth simply because he is himself and that his worth will continue even when his behavior is unacceptable.

Fulfilled Needs: Comfort, protection from psychologic threat, high evaluation of self, increased learning

Advise that significant persons express caring/love for one another Suggest that persons who care for each other communicate their love and affection through words, loving gestures of touch, gift giving, and general respect for one another.

Rationale: Psychologic comfort is promoted through communicated love and affection. Unity with significant others increases a person's self-esteem and sense of value.

Fulfilled Needs: Comfort, protection from psychologic threat, caring and communicating relationships, love and affection, unity with loved ones, high evaluation of self, personal growth and maturity, increased learning, increased reality perception and problem-solving ability

Advise that the alcoholic's illness be discussed only during sobriety Suggest that the family of the alcoholic not discuss the problem while the alcoholic is intoxicated. They should discuss it with him only when he is sober.

Rationale: During intoxication, the alcoholic cannot respond favorably or decisively to attempts at correcting the situation.

Fulfilled Needs: Comfort, increased learning, increased reality perception and problem-solving ability

Advise that the precipitating factor(s) be avoided Suggest that the person stay away from food, drugs, situations, environments, etc., that can disrupt health.

Rationale: By avoiding factors that can cause poor health states, the chance for good health is increased.

Fulfilled Needs: Protection from physical harm, increased learning

Advise that the responsibility for drug/alcohol abuse be placed on the abuser, not on other persons Suggest that it be made clear to the drug user that his abuse involves a rational decision that he alone has made, one that can affect the course of his life. Do not allow him to excuse his abuse as an uncontrollable result of life's traumas.

Rationale: Being held responsible for decisions usually precipitates careful consideration or reevaluation of those decisions.

Fulfilled Needs: Protection from psychologic threat, personal growth and maturity, increased learning, increased reality perception and problem-solving ability

Advise that toilet training failures be ignored Suggest that failure to control elimination during the period of toilet training be overlooked and that punishment and disapproving communications be avoided.

Rationale: Learning is more easily acquired in a positive environment.

Fulfilled Needs: Comfort, increased learning

Advise the child about the front and back of clothes, right and left shoe, and armholes versus pants legs Explain to the child the different parts of a garment and where the body parts fit. Be specific so that he clearly understands the use of clothing. The use of color coding (a red tag for the right armhole, a red mark inside right shoe, etc.) will help the child learn to distinguish right from left.

Rationale: Specific knowledge about clothing helps a small child to grasp the skill of dressing himself more readily.

Fulfilled Needs: Independence, increased learning

Advise to delay introducing hyperallergenic foods until the child is 1 year old Advise that certain foods, if introduced to an at-risk (allergy-susceptible) infant before the age of 1 year, can cause allergies. Such foods, which should not be given until after 1 year, include cow's milk, eggs, wheat, fish, shellfish, chocolate, nuts, strawberries, citrus fruits, pork, and chicken.

Rationale: Restricting the intake of hyperallergenic foods until after the child's immune system becomes more mature reduces the potential for development of allergic reactions.

Fulfilled Needs: Protection from physical harm, increased learning

Advise to observe for signs of infection Teach the person to look for signs of infection in himself, such as fever, inflammation, drainage, pus, heat in tissues, pain, and swelling.

Rationale: Early awareness and treatment of infection prevents severe illness and stress to the body associated with infection.

Fulfilled Needs: Protection from physical harm, increased learning

Advise to warm numbed tissues by immersing the body part in warm water Explain that tissues numbed by severe cold should be immersed in warm water (100°–105° F), not hot water. Maintain the water temperature until the numbness is relieved.

Rationale: Tissues numbed from environmental cold have severely impaired circulation, which should be rapidly improved by warmth. Immersion in warm rather than hot water provides gradual warming without damaging the tissues.

Fulfilled Needs: Protection from physical harm, increased learning

Advise voiding every 4 hours during waking hours Suggest that the person urinate every 4 hours during the waking hours. Discourage prolonged periods of nonvoiding.

Rationale: Frequent voiding removes urine from the bladder and prevents bacterial growth in retained urine. Voiding before the bladder is full decreases the chances for urine backflow into the ureters (which causes renal infection).

Fulfilled Needs: Waste elimination of urine, protection from physical harm, increased learning

Correct misinformation regarding breast-feeding Many untruths about breast-feeding have been passed down from generation to generation. Whenever possible, correct such misinformation. Explain that breast size does not affect the amount of lactation, that properly supported breasts will maintain good shape, that neither cesarean section nor Rh factor has any effect on breast-feeding, that drugs should be avoided during breast-feeding, and that balanced nutrition is essential during lactation.

Rationale: Misinformation about breast-feeding may deprive the mother and child of the advantages it offers.

Fulfilled Needs: Comfort, protection from physical harm, increased learning

Demonstrate how to do the breast examination[73] Assist the person to develop skill in performing the breast examination. Provide her with appropriate literature after demonstrating the examination method. Have the woman lie down and place her left hand behind her head. With her right fingers flat, have her gently palpate her left breast. Begin at the outer breast and move toward the nipple. Palpate the entire breast. Repeat the examination in the sitting position with the left hand behind the head. Repeat the entire procedure on the right breast, putting the right hand behind the head and palpating with the left hand.

Rationale: Early detection of breast abnormalities reduces the potential for severe and advanced breast disease.

Fulfilled Needs: Protection from physical harm, increased learning

Demonstrate how to feed an infant/a dependent person Inform the person of the correct technique for feeding another person, including how to hold or sit the infant or adult and how to put the spoon well back into the mouth, giving moderate, not large, food portions with each spoonful. Describe the differences and similarities in feeding oneself and a dependent person.

Rationale: Proper feeding methods promote comfort, adequate nutritional intake, and protection from aspiration.

Fulfilled Needs: Comfort, protection from physical harm, mastery and competence in skills, independence, increased learning

Contraindications: Delay spoon feeding if the person is susceptible to vomiting.

Describe the behavioral pattern indicating affection deprivation Explain that the signs indicating that a person is, or feels he is, lacking love include verbal expressions of being unloved, withdrawal, seeking affection from insignificant persons, and frequent weeping.

Rationale: Feeling loved is essential to psychologic safety and comfort.

Fulfilled Needs: Protection from psychologic threat, increased learning, increased reality perception and problem-solving ability

Describe the behavioral pattern indicating drug abuse[25] Explain the clues that can alert one to drug dependence in another.

General clues: Sudden changes of behavior to patterns that are out of character with previous conduct, sudden changes in job performance, unusual activity or inactivity, sudden displays of emotion or temper, indifference toward personal appearance, guarding personal possessions, wearing sunglasses and long-sleeved clothes at inappropriate times and places, frequent borrowing of money or stealing when unable to borrow.

More specific clues: Glue sniffing: odor of glue on the breath and clothes, excessive secretion from nasal and oral mucous membranes, red watering eyes, carrying of plastic or paper bags or handkerchiefs containing plastic cement, an intoxicated appearance, poor motor control, double vision, tinnitus, drowsiness, stupor, or unconsciousness following use of glue

Use of depressants (barbiturates or tranquilizers): staggering or stumbling, falling into a deep sleep, lack of interest, disorientation

Use of stimulants (amphetamines and related drugs): excessive activity, irritability, argumentativeness, nervousness, inability to sit still, dilated pupils, frequent licking of lips to overcome mouth dryness, long periods without sleeping or eating

Use of narcotics (paregoric, heroin, etc.): red, raw nostrils when inhaling powdered narcotics, injection marks along veins in the feet and ankles as well as arms, availability of injection equipment, lethargy or drowsiness, pupil constriction

Use of marijuana (pot): loud, rapid talking with excessive bursts of laughter, followed by stupor or sleep, as well as dilated pupils and odor of burned rope on breath and clothing

Use of hallucinogens (LSD): sitting in a dreamlike or trancelike state, possibly extreme fearfulness

Rationale: Early recognition of behavior patterns indicating drug abuse can lead to early treatment.

Fulfilled Needs: Protection from physical harm, protection from psychologic threat, increased learning

Describe the behavioral pattern indicating early-, intermediate-, and late-stage alcohol abuse[445] Explain that the early symptoms of alcohol dependence include drinking at regular times each day, eating irregularly, breaking promises, lying about drinking, gulping drinks, drinking before a party starts, and making excuses for drinking. The intermediate symptoms include carrying a secret supply of alcohol, eating irregularly, frequent intoxication, (especially on weekends), nervousness, missing work because of drinking, minimizing drinking, and unusual behavior. The late symptoms include drinking alone, drinking in the morning, irritability, frequent and severe episodes of intoxication, loss of job, substituting alcohol for food, severe family discord, delirium tremens, and deficiency diseases.

Rationale: Recognition of harmful behavior promotes safety and increases reality perception.

Fulfilled Needs: Protection from physical harm, protection from psychologic threat, increased learning, increased reality perception and problem-solving ability

Describe the behavioral pattern indicating mental health[727] Explain that emotional maturity is reflected by many factors, as suggested by the Mental Health Association:

The person feels comfortable and good about himself: Is not overcome by his emotions, is able to accept disappointments and personal shortcomings, is able to laugh at himself, neither under- nor overestimates his abilities, feels comfortable when alone, has respect for himself, enjoys everyday pleasure, is able to commit himself to philosophical views and consistent values that give his life purpose and direction.

The person feels good about other people: Is able to give to others without expecting gain, feels entitled to and able to accept love from others, is able to establish close emotional ties and still remain independent, expects to like and trust others and have others like and trust him, is able to respect the differences among people, does not attempt to control others or allow himself to be controlled, feels he is part of a group, feels a sense of responsibility to others, is able to work harmoniously with others.

The person feels able to meet life's demands: Feels capable of dealing with most situations, is able to make undelayed and independent decisions, is sufficiently objective about life to find humor in difficult situations, welcomes new ideas and experiences, sets realistic goals, uses his natural abilities, does his best in all efforts and gains satisfaction from doing and accomplishing.

Rationale: Awareness of normal patterns of behavior promotes comfort and provides motivation toward such behavior.

Fulfilled Needs: Comfort, protection from psychologic threat, personal growth and maturity, increased learning, increased reality perception and problem-solving ability

Describe the behavioral pattern indicating overstimulation   Explain that when the nervous system is overstimulated, palpitations, tremors, fatigue, insomnia, confusion, irritability, and panicky feelings occur.

Rationale: Awareness of harmful behavioral patterns promotes safety and increased reality perception.

Fulfilled Needs: Protection from physical harm, protection from psychologic threat, increased learning, increased reality perception and problem-solving ability

Describe the breast changes expected during pregnancy   Explain that during pregnancy the breasts become enlarged; they feel stretched, full, firm, and tender. There may be tingling and throbbing. The pigmented area around the nipples widens and becomes darker and swollen. As early as the fourth month a sticky white fluid may be expressed from the nipple, and breast blood vesels become enlarged.

Rationale: An awareness of what to expect promotes comfort and safety.

Fulfilled Needs: Comfort, protection from physical harm, increased learning

Describe the cardiac signs of physical overactivity   Explain that the signs of an overworked, weakened heart include chest pain, labored breathing, palpitations, limited endurance, rapid pulse, pallor, and extreme weakness.

Rationale: Overexertion creates an increased demand for circulation to the muscles, which the weakened heart struggles to provide. As cardiac effort is increased, the heart's own blood supply must be increased; if it is not, as in many diseased states, such signs as chest pain will develop.

Fulfilled Needs: Protection from physical harm, increased learning

Describe the characteristics of abnormal vaginal bleeding   Explain that the use of more than four saturated sanitary napkins in an 8-hour period, or more than 12 napkins in a 24-hour period, indicates excessive vaginal bleeding. Any bleeding that occurs at times other than at menstruation or any bleeding after the onset of menopause is abnormal.

Rationale: Knowledge that supports early detection of physiologic abnormalities promotes comfort.

Fulfilled Needs: Protection from physical harm, increased learning

Describe the characteristics of controlled diabetes   Explain that a feeling of well-being, maintenance of normal body weight on a well-balanced diet, negative urine tests, and normal levels of blood sugar and acetone indicate well-controlled diabetes.

Rationale: Control of diabetes is essential to the relative health and comfort of the diabetic.

Fulfilled Needs: Comfort, protection from physical harm, increased learning

Describe the characteristics of edema   Explain that the characteristics of edema include swelling of subcutaneous tissue, weight gain, and shiny, tight skin.

Rationale: Edema results when fluid moves from the circulating blood into interstitial tissues. Knowledge of potentially harmful physical threats promotes safety.

Fulfilled Needs: Protection from physical harm, increased learning

Describe the characteristics of fatigue   Explain that yawning, irritability, inability to concentrate, shortness of breath, rapid pulse, and a feeling of being unable to go on are characteristics of fatigue.

Rationale: Awareness that fatigue results from depleted energy reserves and that it requires a period of restoration supports human safety.

Fulfilled Needs: Protection from physical harm, increased learning

Describe the characteristics of normal lochia   Explain that immediately after delivery the vaginal discharge should appear bloody, with small amounts of mucus. After 3 days the lochia gradually changes to a pink serous fluid. After 8 or 9 days the discharge becomes brownish. Within 3 weeks the discharge usually disappears.

Rationale: Awareness of normal physiologic processes promotes comfort and safety.

Fulfilled Needs: Comfort, protection from physical harm, increased learning

Describe the danger signs of pregnancy Explain that during pregnancy the following signs should be reported immediately: persistent headache, nausea and vomiting, dizziness, visual disturbances, epigastric pain, edema (of hands, face, or legs), decreased urinary output, constipation, vaginal bleeding, severe lower abdominal pain, shortness of breath, lumbar pain in the early months, absence of fetal movements during the fourth to ninth months, any acute illness, sudden discharge of vaginal fluid

Rationale: Awareness of physiologic abnormalities promotes safety.

Fulfilled Needs: Protection from physical harm, increased learning

Describe the discomforts of adjusting to contact lens Explain that during the period of adjustment to contact lenses, tearing, itching, burning, and light sensitivity are common.

Rationale: Awareness of what to expect promotes comfort and safety.

Fulfilled Needs: Comfort, protection from physical harm, increased learning

Describe the early manifestations of lung disease Explain that early signs and symptoms of lung disease include coughing of purulent or bloody sputum, a cough that persists longer than 3 weeks, breathlessness, weight loss, wheezing, and chest or shoulder pain.

Rationale: Knowledge that supports early disease detection promotes safety.

Fulfilled Needs: Protection from physical harm, increased learning

Describe the emotional changes that normally occur during the menstrual cycle Explain that varying hormone levels during the menstrual cycle cause women to experience different emotions at different times of the month. From the first day to the fourth day, when hormone levels are low, a woman feels tired, blue, and depressed. From the fifth day to the 14th day, when the estrogen level is high, the woman feels quite well. This feeling gradually increases, reaching a peak on the day of ovulation. From the 14th day to the 20th day, when both estrogen and progesterone levels are high, she feels her best. After the 20th day, as both hormones reach low levels, she again feels tired, blue, and depressed.

Rationale: Awareness of normal physiologic processes promotes comfort and safety.

Fulfilled Needs: Comfort, protection from psychologic threat, increased learning

Describe the factors associated with the occurrence of (name the problem) Describe those factors commonly linked with a particular problem, such as the life stage, during which the problem usually occurs, its probability in certain races, its limitations to geographic areas, and its frequency in the population.

Rationale: Knowledge of the factors associated with a problem can help overcome the problem.

Fulfilled Needs: Protection from physical harm, increased learning

Describe the manifestations of a drug reaction Explain that undesirable reactions to the drug being taken will cause specific signs and symptoms. Teach the person exactly what to watch for and what to do if these signs and symptoms occur.

Rationale: Hypersensitivity to drugs as well as cumulative toxic responses and other undesirable effects from drug therapy are always possibilities. An informed person can recognize early evidence of such reactions and obtain medical assistance before the condition becomes critical.

Fulfilled Needs: Protection from physical harm, increased learning

Describe the manifestations of an impending seizure Explain that seeing bright flashes of light, hearing unusual noises, smelling strange odors, and experiencing confusion and lightheadedness signal an impending seizure.

Rationale: Some patients have an aura that warns of impending seizure. Early identification of such warnings and prompt action can prevent many seizure-related injuries.

Fulfilled Needs: Protection from physical harm, increased learning

Describe the manifestations of circulatory impairment Explain that the signs indicating diminished blood flow to a body part include skin coldness, cyanosis, nonpalpable pulse, numbness and tingling, and slowed capillary filling.

Rationale: A diminished supply of oxygen to tissues resulting from impaired circulation causes tissue death.

Fulfilled Needs: Protection from physical harm. Increased learning

Describe the manifestations of impending cataracts Explain that blurred vision, inability to find light bright enough to read by, double vision, spots before the eyes, and frequent need for new glasses are warning signs of impending cataract.

Rationale: Awareness of impending cataract can prevent serious visual impairment.

Fulfilled Needs: Protection from physical harm, increased learning

Describe the manifestations of impending diabetic coma Explain that frequent copious urination, constant thirst, persistent hunger, flushed and dry skin, weakness, fatigue, and drowsiness indicate impending diabetic coma.

Rationale: Diabetic coma (ketoacidosis) indicates a lack of insulin, which causes inadequate metabolic breakdown of glucose and excess production of acetone bodies and requires immediate treatment.

Fulfilled Needs: Protection from physical harm, increased learning

Describe the manifestations of impending insulin shock Explain that sweating, dizziness, palpitations, pale and moist skin, shallow breathing, trembling, blurred or double vision, hunger, and confusion (if on NPH insulin) indicate impending insulin shock.

Rationale: Excessive insulin in the blood lowers the level of blood sugar to a dangerous degree and requires immediate treatment.

Fulfilled Needs: Protection from physical harm, increased learning

Describe the manifestations of labor onset Explain that the onset of labor is indicated by lightening, in which the infant moves down into the pelvis, thus relieving the pressure against the maternal diaphragm, as well as by a pink vaginal mucous plug discharge, uterine membrane rupture, and labor pains.

Rationale: Awareness of what to expect promotes comfort and safety.

Fulfilled Needs: Protection from psychologic threat, increased learning

Describe the manifestations of pregnancy Explain that the early signs of pregnancy include nausea, vomiting, frequent voiding, breast tenderness, fullness, and increased pigmentation, as well as cessation of menstruation.

Rationale: Awareness of normal physiologic changes promotes comfort.

Fulfilled Needs: Comfort, increased learning

Describe the manifestations of premenstrual tension Explain that certain discomforts are normal a few days before the onset of menstruation: nervousness, irritability, mild depression, dull backache and headache, temporary edema (especially of fingers and ankles), breast tenderness, restlessness, abdominal bloating, urinary frequency, increased thirst and appetite, fatigue, inability to concentrate, and hyperactivity or underactivity. There may be emotional outbursts or weeping without cause.

Rationale: Knowledge of normal physiologic responses promotes safety and comfort.

Fulfilled Needs: Comfort, protection from psychologic threat, increased learning

Describe the normal behavioral pattern common during labor Explain that there is a wide range of normal emotional reactions as labor progresses: happy anticipation, fear, anxiety, frustration, discouragement. and overwhelming delight. Expressive reactions to pain are normal and acceptable and should not cause feelings of shame and guilt.

Rationale: Awareness that the normal emotional outlets are culturally accepted promotes comfort.

Fulfilled Needs: Comfort, protection from psychologic threat, increased learning

Describe the normal behavioral pattern common during male puberty Explain that during male puberty the normal youth becomes increasingly interested in the opposite sex. He develops a consciousness of his own identity, but experiences contradictory desires for independence and for peer group identity. He becomes irritable, has difficulty with emotional adjustments, and expresses inconsistent attitudes.

Rationale: Knowledge of normal behavioral patterns during puberty promotes comfort.

Fulfilled Needs: Comfort, protection from psychologic threat, increased learning

Describe the normal behavioral pattern common during pregnancy Explain that most pregnant women experience joy, but also fear of death, fear of losing the baby, fear of child abnormalities, and superstitious fears. In some instances a mother rejects her child. A woman should know that such emotions are normal and are common to most pregnant women.

Rationale: Awareness that such feelings are culturally accepted promotes comfort and helps reduce the physiologic side effects that result from emotional tension.

Fulfilled Needs: Comfort, protection from physical harm, increased learning

Describe normal changes associated with male climacteric Explain that between the ages of 50 and 60 years men can expect to experience decreased sexual desire, fatigue and muscle weakness, emotional depression or excessive emotional response, hot or cold flushes, rapid heartbeat and palpitations, dizziness, profuse perspiration, numbness and tingling of toes and fingers, nervousness, irritability, shortness of breath, spots before the eyes, tinnitus, flatulence and abdominal distention after meals, inability to sleep well, headaches at the base of the neck and top of the head, decreased physical energy, poor concentration, and feelings of inadequacy.

Rationale: Awareness of normal physiologic processes promotes comfort and safety.

Fulfilled Needs: Comfort, protection from psychologic threat, increased learning

Describe the normal changes associated with male puberty Explain that the developements in male secondary sex characteristics between the ages of 14 and 15 years include appearance of pubic, axillary, and facial hair, onset of rapid growth, ejaculation, accentuation of the Adam's apple, voice huskiness, diminished pulse rate, skin disorders, and increased biologic tensions.

Rationale: Knowledge of normal physiologic processes promotes comfort.

Fulfilled Needs: Comfort, protection from psychologic threat, increased learning

Describe the normal changes associated with menopause Explain that permanent cessation of menstruation usually occurs between the ages of 40 and 50 years. The usual pattern involves scanty periods at first, then occasionally absent periods, and finally cessation of menstruation altogether. As the production of estrogen diminishes, one can expect facial and body flushing, sweating, chills, excitability, irritability, dyspnea, vertigo, headaches, fatigue, depression, urinary frequency, joint pain and stiffness, sparsity of scalp and pubic hair, hair growth on the upper lip and chin, loss of skin elasticity, increased wrinkling, breast sagging, skin dryness, brittle nails, perineal

pruritus, vaginal discharge, painful intercourse as a result of atrophy of genital mucous membranes, palpitations with constrictive chest pressure, cold hands and feet, and numbness and tingling. Sedentary life may lead to excessive weight gain. Complacency often leads to less concern with physical appearance. Many women have feelings of worthlessness or of being unneeded because their children have become independent. Many women fear change-of-life pregnancy, but they also may find sexual activity more pleasurable because of decreased fear of pregnancy.

Rationale: Knowledge of normal physiologic processes promotes comfort.

Fulfilled Needs: Comfort, protection from psychologic threat, increased learning

Describe the normal changes associated with premenopause   Explain that during premenopause certain bodily changes occur, such as weight gain around the hips, abdomen, thighs, waist, and breasts. Normal discomforts include nervousness, weakness, fatigue, depression, insomnia, palpitations, irritability, headache, and numbness and tingling. The person may experience excessive emotional responses and tearfulness as well. Explain that during premenopause many normal variations in the menstrual cycle can occur: the regular menstrual cycle may continue to occur for a time and then suddenly stop, menstruation may stop for 6 or 8 months and then reappear, the cycle may remain regular in regard to date of onset but with gradual decreasing flow, the cycle may remain regular in regard to date of onset but with a decrease in the number of days of flow, menstruation may occur for the same number of days and the same amount of flow but with an increase in the length of time between two onsets, the cycle may be regular but with longer and more profuse flow, cyclic onsets may change to 2–3 weeks apart or 7–8 weeks apart, there may be total irregularity of onset, or the cycle may occur now and then without ovulation.

Rationale: Awareness of normal physiologic responses promotes safety and comfort.

Fulfilled Needs: Comfort, protection from psychologic threat, increased learning

Describe the normal psychic changes common during menopause   Explain that emotional instability, weeping, melancholia, insomnia, worry, fatigue, self-depreciation, and sometimes suicidal thoughts are common during menopause.

Rationale: Awareness of normal behavior reduces psychologic threat and promotes comfort.

Fulfilled Needs: Comfort, protection from psychologic threat, increased learning

Describe the normal stages of grief[279]   Explain that grief is a normal emotional phenomenon and that it follows certain patterns. During the initial stage of grief there exists a state of shock and disbelief. Gradually the person comes to a realization of his loss. During the period called grief work, he focuses on the lost person almost continuously and mentally relives experiences that were shared with the lost person. The period of resolving grief involves a gradual change of focus from the lost person to other interests. During this period the grieving person attempts to reestablish stable life patterns and form new relationships.

Rationale: Knowledge of normal behavioral patterns reduces anxiety and threat, promotes comfort and increased reality perception, and supports mature growth.

Fulfilled Needs: Comfort, protection from psychologic threat, personal growth and maturity, increased learning, increased reality perception and problem-solving ability

Describe the normal stages of tooth development   Explain that teeth appear between the ages of 6 and 9 months. At 12 months there are usually 6 teeth, at 18 months 12 teeth, at 24 months 16 teeth, and at 2½ years 20 teeth. Explain that teeth should come in straight.

Rationale: Knowledge of normal physiologic processes promotes comfort and safety.

Fulfilled Needs: Comfort, protection from physical harm, increased learning

Describe the predisposing factors   Enumerate those risk factors that increase the probability that a problem could occur. Such factors include age, sex, race, lifestyle, and environmental factors.

Rationale: Knowledge of high-risk factors provides the opportunity to alter changeable risk factors and reduces the potential for illness.

Fulfilled Needs: Protection from physical harm, increased learning

Describe the process of labor and delivery   Explain to the pregnant woman the normal course of labor. During the first stage of labor, labor pains gradually increase in intensity. There is a marked increase in show, and cervix dilatation occurs. At this point, bearing down accomplishes nothing and may exhaust the mother. During the second stage of labor, pain is severe and long, occurring every 2–3 minutes. The membranes rupture with a gush of amniotic fluid from the vagina. By bearing down, the mother assists in the child's birth. The infant's head causes pressure against the vagina, finally become visible. The infant then passes through the birth canal and is born. During the third stage of labor, the placenta drops into the lower uterus and, with applied pressure, is expelled from the uterus.

Rationale: Knowledge of what to expect promotes human comfort.

Fulfilled Needs: Comfort, increased learning

Contraindications: Delay if the explanation severly heightens anxiety.

Describe the signs and symptoms that indicate the need for taking the temperature   Explain that when a person has hot dry skin, a flushed face, malaise, a rash, or respiratory distress, his temperature should be taken. Such signs indicate a rise in the body heat level.

Rationale: Knowing when to take a person's temperature reduces the risk of overlooking a high fever and the significant illness it represents.

Fulfilled Needs: Protection from physical harm, increased learning.

Describe the signs of infant readiness to be weaned   Explain that when a child begins to shorten the periods of time that he breast-feeds or bottle-feeds, or when he is restless because of his mother's hold on him, he is demonstrating a desire for independent feeding. At that time a gradual introduction to the cup should be started, with decreased feeding from breast or bottle.

Rationale: The joy of independent feeding replaces the pleasure of breast or bottle feeding when developmental skills allow for independence.

Fulfilled Needs: Comfort, independence, increased learning

Describe the specific dangerous effects of poor health practices   Explain that poor health practices can have potentially dangerous effects on health. For example, excessive consumption of alcohol impairs liver function, insufficient rest inhibits adequate healing, and poor nutrition impairs normal growth.

Rationale: Recognition of the potentially dangerous effects of certain health practices can minimize unhealthy practices and provide motivation toward the practice of better health.

Fulfilled Needs: Protection from physical harm, increased learning, increased reality perception

Describe the symptoms commonly associated with tobacco withdrawal   Explain that the following symptoms frequently occur when one is attempting to stop smoking: For several days a week the person may experience occasional dizziness, headache, irritability, tremor, sweating, constipation or diarrhea, inability to sleep, inability to concentrate, impaired memory, anxiety, restlessness, craving for tobacco, gnawing stomach, and mouth soreness or blisters. At the end of 2 weeks the desire to smoke is greatly relieved, except when seeing others smoking. Gradually, over a 3–6 month period, the craving decreases and subsides.

Rationale: Awareness of the normal symptoms associated with tobacco withdrawal reduces anxiety and supports completion of the withdrawal phase.

Fulfilled Needs: Comfort, protection from psychologic threat, increased learning

Describe the undesirable effects of (name the specific therapy) Describe the side effects of specific therapies that the person can expect to experience: the urine turns orange when on pyridium therapy, the stools become black when taking iron, hair falls out when taking chemotherapy or radiation therapy, diuretics produce urinary frequency, and thyroid drugs increase activity level.

Rationale: Awareness of what to expect reduces needless anxiety and promotes comfort.

Fulfilled Needs: Comfort, protection from psychologic threat, increased learning

Describe those behaviors that usually occur in communication impairment Explain that persons unable to communicate usually display frustration, embarrassment, irritation with the listener, depression, and agitation.

Rationale: Awareness that certain uncharacteristic behavior by a patient is to be expected reduces the sensitivity of his loved ones to behavior that would ordinarily be perceived as threatening.

Fulfilled Needs: Comfort, protection from psychologic threat, increased learning

Describe those factors that intensify fear/helplessness/anxiety/etc. Explain that being alone and being in the dark tend to magnify fear and anxiety. Relatively mild, but deep-rooted, fears and anxieties may grow out of proportion when one encounters situations that require considerable emotional adaptation or change in normal living patterns, such as relocation for a new job or the occurrence of pregnancy.

Rationale: Awareness of the factors that intensify fear and anxiety supports control and prevention of the emotions.

Fulfilled Needs: Comfort, protection from psychologic threat, personal growth and maturity, increased learning, increased reality perception and problem-solving ability

Describe those persons who have a decreased tolerance for stress Persons who have a low tolerance for stress include premature or underweight infants, ill or injured persons, and the aged. The more serious the illness, the less stress can be endured.

Rationale: By recognizing those persons who cannot tolerate stress, one can take measures to reduce their stress to a minimum.

Fulfilled Needs: Comfort, protection from physical harm, protection from psychologic threat, increased learning

Describe those symptoms/problems that should be reported/expected Explain the specific signs and symptoms that may be related to the patient's particular health problem or that are expected to occur. Explain which problems should be reported without delay.

Rationale: Prompt care can minimize the harmful effects of unhealthy conditions.

Fulfilled Needs: Comfort, protection from physical harm, increased learning

Emphasize that children need guidance Emphasize that because the judgment of a child is not developed and he has no experience to fall back on, he requires guidance by those who are more experienced.

Rationale: Guidance from his elders keeps the child safe from physical and psychologic harm.

Fulfilled Needs: Protection from physical harm, protection from psychologic threat, increased learning, increased reality perception and problem-solving ability

Emphasize that contaminated clothing should be changed immediately Emphasize that whenever dust particles, bacteria, vapors, fumes, or other harmful products come in contact with clothing, the clothing should be changed as soon as possible and properly cleaned.

Rationale: Contaminated clothing can cause skin or respiratory disorders.

Fulfilled Needs: Protection from physical harm, increased learning

Emphasize that food in bulging cans and jars with bulging lids should be discarded   Emphasize that when a food can bulges or when a jar has a lid that bulges, the container and contents should be thrown away.

Rationale: A bulging can or jar lid is usually the result of gas formed by the action of pathogenic microorganisms within the container.

Fulfilled Needs: Protection from physical harm, increased learning

Emphasize that food wastes should be burned in animal-inhabited outdoor areas   Emphasize that anyone living or camping in outdoor areas where there are bears or raccoons should burn food wastes.

Rationale: Raccoons and bears can smell buried food and dig it up. They leave what they do not eat to the flies, which in turn transmit disease.

Fulfilled Needs: Protection from physical harm, increased learning

Emphasize that garbage should be covered   Emphasize that garbage should be placed in tightly covered containers, preferably inside sealed bags.

Rationale: Tightly sealed garbage containers prevent flies and rats from transmitting infection.

Fulfilled Needs: Protection from physical harm, increased learning

Emphasize that in outdoor living, human wastes should be buried   Emphasize that when people are living outdoors, human excreta and food wastes should be placed in the ground and covered with dirt.

Rationale: Uncovered human excreta and food wastes attract flies, which in turn transmit disease.

Fulfilled Needs: Protection from physical harm, increased learning

Emphasize that outdated foods/drugs should be discarded   Emphasize that dated foods, which spoil easily, should not be used after the expiration date. Drugs should always be discarded when outdated.

Rationale: Foods and drugs are dated for the purpose of assuring their fitness for consumption. Discarding foods after the expiration date assures safety from food poisoning. Since time, light, and moisture alter the chemical composition of drugs, discarding them after the expiration date prevents drug side effects.

Fulfilled Needs: Protection from physical harm, increased learning

Emphasize that play areas should be fenced   Emphasize that small children should play only in fenced areas.

Rationale: Small children are not sufficiently experienced to recognize many dangers, and their distraction during play further decreases their perception of danger.

Fulfilled Needs: Protection from physical harm, increased learning

Emphasize that potentially unsafe water should be boiled for 10 minutes   Emphasize that outdoor water or water in foreign countries should be boiled for 10 minutes to make it safe for consumption. If it has a flat taste after boiling, vigorously shake it in a container to aerate it. Keep it well covered at all times.

Rationale: Boiling water drives off air and gases and destroys bacteria.

Fulfilled Needs: Protection from physical harm, increased learning

Emphasize that small children should always be attended   Emphasize that small children should never be left alone for extended periods.

Rationale: The perception and judgment of small children are not sufficiently developed for them to recognize potential danger.

Fulfilled Needs: Protection from physical harm, increased learning

Emphasize the danger of breathing cold air   Explain that in very cold weather the mouth should be covered with a scarf, and breathing should be nasal rather than oral in order to prevent injury to respiratory tissue.

Rationale: Breathing cold air through the mouth burns respiratory passages, increases the chance of infection, and stimulates the cough reflex. Nasal breathing is preferable because the nasal mucous membranes warm the air as it passes through.

Fulfilled Needs: Comfort, protection from physical harm, increased learning

Emphasize the danger of cutting calloused skin   Explain that thick, hardened skin should not be cut off with scissors but should be softened with skin lubricants.

Rationale: Cutting calloused skin traumatizes underlying tissue; it can cut into vessels and cause bleeding and can introduce bacteria into the open wound.

Fulfilled Needs: Protection from physical harm, increased learning

Emphasize the danger of diving into shallow water   Explain that the potential for hitting one's head on the bottom of the pool and compressing the cervical vertebrae is great when diving into shallow water. Young children should be warned of the danger when first learning to swim.

Rationale: Cervical trauma can result in paralysis.

Fulfilled Needs: Protection from physical harm, increased learning

Emphasize the danger of excessive body weight   Explain that excessive body weight places stress on all body systems, thereby increasing the potential for a system breakdown.

Rationale: Excessive weight increases the heart's work load and the potential for impaired oxygenation of tissues. Excessive weight imposes strain on spinal disks, increases weight-bearing pressure on bones, and weakens the muscular supportive structures of the body.

Fulfilled Needs: Comfort, protection from physical harm, increased learning

Emphasize the danger of excessive coffee consumption   Explain that drinking five or more cups of coffee a day increases blood pressure, intraocular pressure, and stomach acid. It causes arteriosclerosis and disguises fatigue.

Rationale: The caffeine in coffee has a stimulating effect. Taken in excess, it is detrimental to health.

Fulfilled Needs: Protection from physical harm, increased learning

Emphasize the danger of excessive exposure to noise   Explain that loud, prolonged, and high-frequency noise can cause diminished hearing or deafness and can place stress on the nervous system.

Rationale: Sound waves more intense than 80 decibels cause auditory damage and overstimulate the nervous system.

Fulfilled Needs: Protection from physical harm, increased learning

Emphasize the danger of excessive use of nose drops   Explain that excessive use of nose drops can injure nasal tissue and cause addiction to the chemicals in the drops.

Rationale: Injury to nasal mucous membrane interferes with the olfactory and filtering functions of the membrane.

Fulfilled Needs: Protection from physical harm, increased learning

Emphasize the danger of exposure to x-rays during the first 3 months of pregnancy   Explain that women in the first 3 months of pregnancy should avoid exposure to any type of x-ray therapy.

Rationale: X-ray therapy may cause injury to the fetus or may interfere with fetal development.

Fulfilled Needs: Protection from physical harm, increased learning

Emphasize the danger of fad dieting Explain that attempting to lose a large amount of weight in a short time places severe stress on the body's adaptive mechanisms. Eating a poor nutritional diet decreases the body's nutritional resources.

Rationale: The severe stress placed on the body by crash dieting increases susceptibility to illness.

Fulfilled Needs: Protection from physical harm, increased learning

Emphasize the danger of induced abortion Explain that abortion induced by external means can cause vaginal infection and hemorrhage.

Rationale: Induced abortion that results in vaginal infection and hemorrhage can cause serious and sometimes fatal illness.

Fulfilled Needs: Protection from physical harm, increased learning

Emphasize the danger of massaging a painful calf/frostbitten tissue Explain that rubbing or kneading a painful calf poses the danger of dislodging a thrombus. Massaging frostbitten tissue can damage the tissue.

Rationale: Calf tenderness often results from blood vessel obstruction caused by blood clot formation and localization. Frostbitten tissue should be gradually warmed in water to prevent tissue injury.

Fulfilled Needs: Protection from physical harm, increased learning

Emphasize the danger of mixing drugs and alcohol Explain that simultaneous use of drugs and alcohol can cause dangerous chemical reactions that often result in death.

Rationale: Both drugs and alcohol have sedative effects. When they are mixed, the sedation can be so severe that respiratory depression and death can occur.

Fulfilled Needs: Protection from physical harm, increased learning

Emphasize the danger of self-regulation of intravenous fluids Explain to the person that he must not release the regulating clamp on an intravenous infusion in order to facilitate more rapid flow; doing so could overload the circulatory system with fluid. This problem is sometimes encountered with anxious persons who want to get the intravenous infusion completed and be rid of it.

Rationale: Knowledge that rapid flow of intravenous fluid can overload the heart and cause circulatory failure promotes safety.

Fulfilled Needs: Protection from physical harm, increased learning

Emphasize the danger of sharing drugs between persons Explain that a drug that affects one person in a certain way may affect another person in another way, not in the intended therapeutic manner, but with serious side effects. Therefore drugs should never be shared.

Rationale: Chemical reactions within the body that result from the combination of incompatible elements can produce a poisoning effect.

Fulfilled Needs: Protection from physical harm, increased learning

Emphasize the danger of using excessive hair dye Explain that excessive use of hair dye irritates the scalp and damages the hair follicles, making them coarse and brittle.

Rationale: Many hair dyes contain silver nitrate or aniline dyes, which are chemically irritating to the skin and eyes.

Fulfilled Needs: Protection from physical harm, increased learning

Emphasize the importance of follow-up care Verbally stress the importance of keeping follow-up appointments. Follow-up care should not be considered unnecessary or only an added financial burden. Explain the reasons such care is needed.

Rationale: Follow-up care is essential for evaluation of the progress from illness toward wellness. It also relates concern by the health care provider, providing support for continued compliance to therapy.

Fulfilled Needs: Comfort, protection from physical harm, increased learning

Emphasize the importance of planning and anticipating future activities

Emphasize the importance of planning activities in advance so that some pleasant event or situation can be looked forward to in the near future.

Rationale: Planned use of time encourages a positive attitude. It allows for development of creative talents, skills, and interests and helps maintain social contacts. Looking forward to something offers a psychologic lift for the present and provides a predictable and orderly world.

Fulfilled Needs: Comfort, protection from psychologic threat, predictable and orderly world, personal growth and maturity, increased learning, increased pleasantness

Emphasize the importance of recognizing tension within oneself   Emphasize that reduction of tension can be accomplished only by conscious recognition of tension. Irritability, nervousness, and tight muscles indicate the presence of tension.

Rationale: Recognizing and relieving tension can promote comfort, since there is decreased demand placed on the body to respond to stimuli.

Fulfilled Needs: Protection from physical harm, protection from psychologic threat, personal growth and maturity, increased learning, increased reality perception and problem-solving ability

Emphasize the need to avoid certain drugs and/or chemicals   Explain that certain drugs and chemicals can cause specific diseases or can adversely affect persons with existing diseases. This is especially true of medications that have toxic effects on the liver, kidneys, or heart. Emphasize that persons with ulcers should not take aspirin. In renal disease, nephrotoxic drugs are to be avoided. In thyroid disease, ephedrine is dangerous.

Rationale: Knowledge of drugs and chemicals that are potentially dangerous can prevent injury and complications.

Fulfilled Needs: Protection from physical harm, increased learning

Emphasize the need to develop self-reliance   Explain that each person must learn that he can rely on his internal and external resources when meeting life's challenges.

Rationale: Self-confidence is based on the conviction that one's internal and external resources are adequate for any task.

Fulfilled Needs: Protection from psychologic threat, self-reliance, personal growth and maturity, increased learning, increased reality perception and problem-solving ability

Emphasize the need to fly only in pressurized airplanes   Emphasize that persons in poor health should fly only in airplanes that have controlled barometric pressure. Light private planes should be avoided.

Rationale: The lowered barometric pressure that is encountered at high altitudes decreases the pressure and amount of oxygen going to the lungs, which can cause anoxia, pneumothorax, or cardiac impairment. Unequal internal and external pressures may cause the ear's tympanic membrane to rupture. Unequal abdominal pressures may cause fecal contents to be expelled from a colostomy.

Fulfilled Needs: Protection from physical harm, increased learning

Emphasize the need to use only an approved sewage facility   Emphasize that drainage systems for toilets, sinks, and tubs should be approved and should meet sanitation standards.

Rationale: Safe waste disposal prevents the spread of infection.

Fulfilled Needs: Protection from physical harm, increased learning

Emphasize the need to use only an approved water supply   Emphasize that only water that has been inspected and approved by government agencies should be used for drinking.

Rationale: Water that has not been decontaminated is a potential source of disease.
Fulfilled Needs: Protection from physical harm, increased learning

Emphasize what the person can rather than cannot eat When a person is expected to adhere to a diet, focus on those foods that can be eaten rather than on those that are forbidden.
Rationale: When the positive approach is used in initiating dietary changes, the potential for compliance is increased.
Fulfilled Needs: Comfort, increased learning

Explain about normal sexual tensions[471] Explain that sexual tensions begin in adolescence. The person becomes aware of a stirring within himself and an attraction to the opposite sex. These tensions are easily aroused and although strongest during adolescence and young adulthood, such tensions prevail throughout life. The need for sexual satisfaction is as important as the need for eating and sleeping.
Rationale: Knowledge of normal sexual tensions promotes mature sexuality and reduces the potential for feelings of inadequacy.
Fulfilled Needs: Comfort, sexuality, protection from psychologic threat, increased learning

Explain about the unique personality of each individual/person/child Explain that no two persons have the same qualities or characteristics. Note that we often expect certain behaviors from individuals but that such behaviors are more a reflection of ourselves rather than of them. Encourage others to accept the person for his unique qualities.
Rationale: Recognizing and accepting the uniqueness of another, promotes understanding, and personal growth.
Fulfilled Needs: Personal growth and maturity, increased learning.

Explain and offer hope that the emotional pain will decrease with time Explain that intensely severe emotional pain that may seem unbearable at the moment will gradually decrease in intensity and be more endurable as time goes on and adjustment occurs.
Rationale: An awareness that severe emotional pain will gradually subside in the future promotes comfort and strength as the person realizes it is a temporary stress.
Fulfilled Needs: Comfort, protection from psychologic threat, endurance, increased learning

Explain how and where organ donations are made Explain that organs for transplant come from two major sources: unrelated persons who have recently died and living relatives. Recommend those organizations or physicians whose prime function is to secure such donations.
Rationale: Inquires about organ donation can result in the giving of an organ needed to preserve life or improve body function.
Fulfilled Needs: Increased learning

Explain how emotional responses occur[105] Explain that emotions are the result of a complex process: the perception and evaluation of a situation in terms of its significance to the individual, the experience of an emotional response to the perception, and physiologic changes accompanying the emotional response.
Rationale: Awareness of how emotions occur gives the person insight into his emotional life. This knowledge increases the potential for more appropriate emotional responses and greater emotional control.
Fulfilled Needs: Personal growth and maturity, increased learning

Explain how impending insulin shock can be interrupted Explain that when a person is going into insulin shock, he should be given one of the following: sugar, a piece of candy, a carbonated beverage, or fruit juice with sugar in it. This should be followed by a regular meal or by high-protein food.

Rationale: Excessive insulin in the blood lowers the level of blood sugar. A normal level of blood sugar can be rapidly reestablished by giving foods or fluids containing sugar.

Fulfilled Needs: Protection from physical harm, increased learning

Explain how the equipment works Explain as simply as possible how the specific equipment associated with the patient's care functions. If there are flashing lights, buzzer signals, etc., explain their meanings.

Rationale: Knowledge of the functioning of devices associated with one's care reduces anxiety and promotes comfort.

Fulfilled Needs: Comfort, protection from psychologic threat, increased learning

Explain how the infant grows in utero[527] Explain the sequence of child development in utero. At the end of the *first month*, the embryo head is very prominent, as is the backbone. It is only 1/4 inch long. At the end of the *second month*, the fetus has a human face and arms and legs. It is about 1 inch long and weighs 1/30 ounce. At the end of the *third month*, sex can be distinguished and nails appear, as well as teeth buds. Kidneys develop and secrete small amounts of urine into the bladder. The fetus is 3 inches long and weights 1 ounce. At the end of the *fourth month*, downy hair appears, and faint fetal movements are sometimes felt. The fetus is 6 1/2 inches long and weighs 4 ounces. At the end of the *fifth month*, fetal heart tones can be heard and fetal movements felt. It is 10 inches long and weighs 6 ounces. At the end of the *sixth month*, the fetus begins to resemble an infant. It develops a skin coating called vernix caseosa. It is 12 inches long and weighs 1 1/2 lb. At the end of the *seventh month*, the fetus is 15 inches long and weights 2 1/2 lb. At the end of the *eight month*, the fetus is 16 1/2 inches long and weighs 4 lb. At the end of the *ninth month*, the infant becomes mature; it is 19 inches long and weighs about 6 lb.

Rationale: Knowledge of physiologic processes promotes comfort.

Fulfilled Needs: Comfort, increased learning

Explain how the loss of an organ will affect the living donor's future health Explain that if a living person sacrifices one of duplicate organs within his body, there is always the possibility that the remaining organ could develop impaired function. Explain that in most cases the donor enjoys a lifetime of good health.

Rationale: Knowledge of what to expect reduces anxiety and permits realistic assessment of whether to donate the organ.

Fulfilled Needs: Comfort, protection from psychlogic threat, increased learning, increased reality perception and problem-solving ability

Explain how thinking occurs[34,471] Explain that thinking is a process involving many factors. Incoming information is perceived. This information is interpreted on the basis of a preexisting inner frame of reference that includes language skills (symbols such as words and numbers), sensorimotor development, remembering, reasoning, imagining (mental pictures that stand for events), and evaluation. Thinking is based on an inner tendency to organize and adapt to incoming information. Early thinking is concrete or specific. As thought processes mature, the person learns to think in abstract or general terms. The person's frame of reference may change if new information is perceived as indicating a need for change, or may remain constant if new information is simply added.

Rationale: Knowledge of how thinking occurs increases understanding of thinking deficits.

Fulfilled Needs: Comfort, increased learning, increased problem-solving ability

Explain how to adjust clothing to meet health needs/problem(s) Explain that some clothing is more appropriate in certain health conditions than in others.

High-necked clothing, long sleeves, and scarves can cover wounds and scars. After mastectomy, clothing worn before surgery can be filled in with soft materials, or seams can be adjusted to accommodate the current body shape. Women who breast-feed should wear nursing bras and clothes that open down the front. When one is wearing a brace, culottes, wide pants, shift dresses, and A-line dresses offer freedom of movement; loosely knit underwear should be avoided, and the inside seams of trousers should be finished off so that they are not caught in the brace. Patients with limited range of motion should use clothing one size too large when dressing themselves. Wide sleeves and pants legs should be worn over casts. Oversize clothing is needed for body casts, and clothes that button down the front are needed for body and neck casts. A heavy sock instead of a shoe is necessary on a casted foot.

Rationale: The proper use of clothing for comfort, reduction of fatigue, and safety during movement supports positive health action.

Fulfilled Needs: Comfort, protection from physical harm, independence, increased learning

Explain how to apply elastic stockings or an elastic bandage

Explain that elastic hose and elastic bandages should be applied in the morning before getting out of bed. A wrinkle-free application that provides an evenly distributed and moderate amount of pressure is the goal. To apply an elastic stocking, turn it inside out down to the heel, fit the foot part on snugly, and then gradually work the length of the stocking up onto the leg, making sure no tourniquet effect is created. To apply elastic bandages to the leg, begin wrapping at the foot, enclosing the foot, heel, and ankle with the figure-eight wrap. Continue with a smooth spiral wrap to midthigh, making sure that the second or third bandage is not placed over or too close to the knee joint. To bandage the arm, use the same technique, beginning at the hand.

Rationale: Evenly distributed, moderate external pressure applied to the extremity diverts the venous blood from the smaller veins into the large veins that lie deeper; this increases the flow rate and decreases the chance of thrombosis. The superficial veins must be relatively empty as a result of having been in an elevated position prior to application of pressure; otherwise, blood will be trapped and thrombi will form.

Fulfilled Needs: Tissue oxygenation or perfusion, comfort, protection from physical harm, mastery and competence in skills, increased learning.

Contraindications: Circulatory thrombus or embolus

Explain how to attach the drainage system to the appliance/tube

Demonstrate how the drainage system is attached to an appliance or tube. Be sure sterile technique is used, especially with urinary catheters.

Rationale: Attaching drainage systems to an appliance or tube reduces the discomfort of wetness and ensures a sealed system, preventing bacterial invasion into the body.

Fulfilled Needs: Comfort, protection from physical harm, increased learning

Explain how to budget

Explain how to plan for health needs and how to judge the comparable values of health essentials such as bandages and food. Teach a realistic approach from the standpoint of priorities and the available budget.

Rationale: Budgeting for health essentials supports improved health care.

Fulfilled Needs: Increased learning, increased problem-solving ability

Explain how to calculate the delivery date

Explain that the approximate date of delivery can be determined as follows: count back 3 calendar months from the first day of the last menstrual period; add 7 days; this will give the anticipated date of delivery.

Rationale: Knowledge of the anticipated birth date of a child promotes comfort.

Fulfilled Needs: Comfort, increased learning

Explain how to care for a leg brace   Explain that a leg brace should be stored in an aligned position, that the brace locks and joints should be oiled once a week with one drop of machine oil, that the brace straps should be washed with soap and water and replaced when frayed, that lint should be removed from the locks and joints, and that the brace shoe heels should be kept in good repair to maintain a balanced walking surface.

Rationale: A therapeutic brace kept in good repair effectively supports weakened muscles, joints, and bones and facilitates motion or temporarily reduces motion while healing occurs.

Fulfilled Needs: Protection from physical harm, increased learning

Explain how to channel emotional/sexual energy and obtain release from stress   Explain that emotional tension (involving fear, anxiety, sex drive, etc.) can be channeled into accomplishments. When such energy is diverted toward work, hobbies, sports, travel, or other activities, the emotional tension is weakened.

Rationale: Emotion stimulates energy resources. If the energy is not used, muscular tension increases. Body movements can absorb and decrease tension and at the same time channel the energy into successful endeavors.

Fulfilled Needs: Comfort, protection from psychologic threat, personal growth and maturity, increased learning

Explain how to clean the external part of the indwelling urinary catheter   Explain that the external portion of the urinary catheter should be kept clean with soap and water. Clean especially well where the catheter enters the meatus.

Rationale: Cleanliness minimizes the potential for urinary tract infection.

Fulfilled Needs: Cleanliness, protection from physical harm, increased learning

Explain how to collect a specimen   Explain how to collect the specific specimens that are required for analysis.

Rationale: Employing the correct procedures in collecting and transporting specimens can contribute to the accuracy of the analysis.

Fulfilled Needs: Increased learning

Explain how to control weight gain during pregnancy   Explain that during pregnancy the total weight gain should not exceed 25 lb, although weight gain will depend on the mother's size. Weight gain should be limited to ½ lb/each week from the fourth month through the sixth month and ¾ lb/a week from the seventh month through the ninth month.

Rationale: Excessive weight gain enhances the potential for difficult labor and delivery. Excessive pregnancy weight places unnecessary pressure on the leg and back muscles and may cause backache, leg pain, and fatigue.

Fulfilled Needs: Protection from physical harm, increased learning

Explain how to correctly wash diapers   Explain that mild soap should be used when washing diapers. They should be rinsed thoroughly and, if possible, allowed to dry in the sunshine.

Rationale: Removal of all foreign particles from diapers decreases skin irritation.

Fulfilled Needs: Cleanliness, protection from physical harm, increased learning

Explain how to counteract the theories of drug users   When a drug user justifies his habit by stating that he has the right of free choice, the right to destroy his body, or the right to manipulate reality, be prepared to rebut such statements. Suggest that free choice is based on the intent of man to improve himself. Free choice also implies compromise in consideration of the rights of the majority. If the drug user claims the right to destroy his body because he sees destruction of human life throughout the world, agree that destruction does exist, but emphasize that it is not acceptable behavior. If there are destructive elements significant in the user's own life, perhaps a change can be brought about. When the drug user claims the right to manipulate reality because he sees people manipulating one another for their own gain, agree that manipulation does exist, but emphasize that it diminishes human dignity.

Rationale: Recognition and discussion of social problems promote realistic solutions and release of socially imposed tensions.

Fulfilled Needs: Protection from psychologic threat, increased learning

Explain how to describe pain Explain that there are standard terms used to express the intensity, duration, and quality of pain and that use of these terms clarifies the patient's problem.

Rationale: Comfort and safety can derive from an ability to communicate personal needs.

Fulfilled Needs: Protection from physical harm, protection from psychologic threat, increased learning

Explain how to detect pacemaker failure Explain that the average pacemaker battery has a life of 30–36 months. Signs that a battery is beginning to fail may include chest pain, dizziness, pulse rate increase or decrease, and loss of consciousness.

Rationale: Since pacemakers are usually essential to maintenance of adequate cardiac output, they must be kept in optimum working order.

Fulfilled Needs: Protection from physical harm, increased learning

Explain how to determine proper cane length[108] Explain that a cane is the proper length when the person's arm is at a 30° angle as the cane is held a few inches in front of and to the side of his foot.

Rationale: Proper cane length is essential for safe and comfortable mobility.

Fulfilled Needs: Comfort, protection from physical harm, increased learning

Explain how to determine proper crutch length[108] Explain that the following measurements will determine whether crutch length is correct. For an axillary crutch, have the patient lie in bed or stand; then measure the length from the axilla to a point 6 inches out from the side of the foot. When the person's hand is on the handbar, the elbow should be bent at a 30° angle. When a forearm (Lofstrand) crutch fits properly, the elbows will be bent at a 30° angle and the crutch tips will be 6-8 inches to the side of and in front of the foot. When crutches are too short, the head, shoulders, and body will be bent forward and downward in a stooped-shoulder crutch-walking posture. When crutches are too long, the shoulders will be bent into an arch in a hunched-shoulder crutch-walking posture, and there will be pain in the axilla from crutch pressure.

Rationale: Correct crutch length is essential for adequate body support, mobility, and comfort. Crutches that are too long can cause nerve damage under the axilla.

Fulfilled Needs: Comfort, protection from physical harm, increased learning

Explain how to determine proper walker height[108] Explain that if the walker height is correct, the patient's elbows will be bent at a 30° angle. When the walker is too short, the shoulders will be bent in a slumped position. When the walker is too tall, the shoulders will be bent slightly backward.

Rationale: Correct walker height is essential for adequate body support, mobility, and comfort.

Fulfilled Needs: Comfort, protection from physical harm, increased learning

Explain how to determine the optimum time for conception Explain that the best time to attempt conception is 7–10 days after menstrual bleeding stops.

Rationale: Ovulation usually occurs between the 10th day and the 16th day after menstrual bleeding begins. If pregnancy is to occur, there must be discharge of ovum and male germ cell impregnation.

Fulfilled Needs: Comfort, increased learning

Explain how to dispose of infectious expectoration Explain that infectious expectorated material should be burned or disposed of through the sewer system.

Rationale: Removing infectious microorganisms from locations where they might contact other people reduces the potential for transfer of disease.

Fufilled Needs: Cleanliness, protection from physical harm, increased learning

Explain how to dispose of soiled dressings Explain that soiled dressings should be placed in paper or plastic sacks, tightly sealed, and then burned or placed in the container for city or institution garbage collection.

Rationale: Isolating infectious objects prevents the spread of infection.

Fulfilled Needs: Cleanliness, protection from physical harm, increased learning

Explain how to distinguish crying because of hunger and other causes Explain that babies can cry for many reasons, such as a wet or soiled diaper, discomfort or need for attention. When crying because of hunger, the cry is usually associated with finger or fist sucking.

Rationale: Correct determination of why an infant cries provides rapid and correct need resolution.

Fulfilled Needs: Nutritional balance, comfort, increased learning

Explain how to escape a fire[728,729] Explain that preplanning escape routes and meeting places for family members is very important. If caught in a burning building, recommend the following: Leave the fire scene immediately. Crawl along the floor if the room is smoke filled. If a door feels hot or smoke is seeping under it, do not open it, and use an alternate escape route. Do not use elevators for escape. If unable to escape, close all doors and seal off all cracks with clothing or rags. Signal by hanging a sheet from the window, flashing a flashlight, etc. Do not return to the fire scene once outside the burning building.

Rationale: Knowledge of how to escape a fire can save lives.

Fulfilled Needs: Protection from physical harm, increased learning

Explain how to estimate temperature by touch Explain that when a thermometer is not available, one can estimate fever by touching the skin, especially the forehead and face. Temperature estimation is as follows:

Very hot skin	Dangerous fever
Hot skin	High fever
Very warm skin	Slight fever
Warm skin	Normal
Cool skin	Slightly subnormal temperature
Cold skin	Moderately low temperature
Very cold skin	Dangerously low temperature

Rationale: Abnormal body temperature may indicate excessive heat production or loss or a poor temperature regulating mechanism.

Fulfilled Needs: Protection from physical harm, increased learning

Explain how to evaluate the pulse after exercise[746] Explain that pulse should be counted for 10 minutes and multiplied by 6 immediately upon stopping exercise. If the pulse falls below or within the normal range for the person's age, it is safe to continue the exercise. If it is above the normal age or if the person has chest pain, irregular heartbeats, or shortness of breath, the exercise should be stopped. Less vigorous pursuit of the exercise may maintain the pulse within the normal range.

Age	*Normal Postexercise Pulse Range Not to Be Exceeded*
20	140–170
25	137–165

Age	*Normal Postexercise Pulse Range Not to Be Exceeded*
30	133–160
35	130–157
40	125–153
45	123–150
50	120–145
55	115–140
60	110–136
65	108–130
70	105–128
75	100–125

Rationale: Keeping the pulse within the normal range during exercise prevents the danger of overtaxing the heart with physiologic stress.

Fulfilled Needs: Protection from physical harm, increased learning

Explain how to extinguish fires[728,729] Explain ways to put out a fire. If clothing catches on fire, have the person drop to the floor and roll over until the fire is out. Pan fires should be covered with a lid. Use water to put out paper, cloth, wood or trash fires. Do not use water on flammable liquids or electrical fires. Use dry chemical, carbon dioxide or foam extinguishers on flammable liquid (gasoline, paint, oil) fires. Use carbon dioxide on electrical (motors, wiring) fires. Multipurpose dry chemical fire extinguishers can be used on any fire.

Rationale: A fire which is immediately extinguished will prevent burn injury.

Fulfilled Needs: Protection from physical harm, increased learning

Explain how to file the nails correctly Explain that nails should be shaped by filing only the undesirable areas and by filing in only one direction. A metal file should be used for shaping long, hard nails. The coarse side of an emery board should be used for shaping normal nails, with the fine side being used to finish off the shaping.

Rationale: Proper nail shaping prevents nail splitting and tearing of nails.

Fulfilled Needs: Protection from physical harm. Increased learning

Explain how to give medications to children Explain that although children may be irritable and fussy when ill, medicines can be given successfully. Infants accept medicines well from a plastic dropper. Young children do better if allowed some independence, such as choosing between tablet and liquid, putting the tablet into a gelatin capsule, choosing the flavor of syrup to mix with the medicine, or drinking the medicine from a doll's teacup. Avoid restraining the child unless it is absolutely necessary. Children appreciate explanations of why the medication is necessary.

Rationale: Successful administration of medications to children increases the potential for improved health.

Fulfilled Needs: Comfort, protection from physical harm, increased learning

Explain how to handle contaminated linen Explain that linens contaminated with infectious material should be either boiled or burned.

Rationale: Disinfection or destruction of contaminated articles prevents the spread of infection.

Fulfilled Needs: Cleanliness, protection from physical harm, increased learning

Explain how to illuminate a room correctly Explain that proper lighting involves both immediate illumination of the work area and distant illumination from a second light in the room. Explain that light should come over the left shoulder if the person is right-handed and over the right shoulder if the person is left-handed.

Rationale: Proper room illumination promotes visual acuity.

Fulfilled Needs: Comfort, protection from physical harm, increased learning

Explain how to interpret food/product contents listed on container labels
Explain how the contents of food or other products are listed on their container. Emphasize the need to check for content, amounts of ingredients, and contents listed under unfamiliar names. Relate how the food or product content affects the individual's health problem.

Rationale: Knowledge of food contents is important to health maintenance, especially when a diet low in sodium, sugar, fat, cholesterol, etc., will improve health. Knowledge of chemical contents in commercial products can affect the health of the skin and respiratory systems.

Fulfilled Needs: Protection from physical harm, increased learning

Explain how to keep a positive emotional family relationship[471] Explain that ways of maintaining positive relationships within a family include frequent phone calls, letters and visits, remembrances on special occasions, maintaining emotional control rather than reacting emotionally, avoiding emotional triangles during visits.

Rationale: Positive family relationships promote the personal growth of each family member and are a source of support throughout life.

Fulfilled Needs: Increased learning, personal growth and maturity

Explain how to keep urine within the desired pH range Explain that the normal pH range of urine is acid (average pH 6). When the urine is alkaline with a pH greater than 7, acid–ash fluids and vitamin C can be taken to acidify the urine. This should bring the urine pH to below 7 (5.5–6.5).

Rationale: Acid urine reduces the potential for bacterial infection of the genitourinary tract, since bacteria fail to thrive in an acid environment. Calcium tends to precipitate and form stones in alkaline urine.

Fulfilled Needs: Acid–base balance, protection from physical harm, increased learning

Explain how to maintain a correct sitting position Explain that when one is sitting, the body weight should be equally distributed on the thighs and buttocks. The lower back should rest against the back of the chair, with the feet flat on the floor.

Rationale: Proper body alignment keeps organs in their correct positions and functioning well. It can favor gravity pull or provide support against gravity; it reduces fatigue and maintains skeletal balance, which in turn promotes effective circulation and respiration.

Fulfilled Needs: Comfort, protection from physical harm, increased learning

Explain how to maintain a diabetic diet when away from home Explain that diabetics can eat any time and anywhere without worry. When traveling, they can take along nonperishable foods if meals are delayed or unavailable on trains or airplanes. They should take the following precautions: Eat only clear broths and consomme soups. Eat only unglazed, unbuttered, and uncreamed meat, poultry, fish, and vegetables. Eat leafy salads containing celery, lettuce, tomatoes, cucumbers, or pickles. Eat fresh fruits for dessert. Avoid casseroles, since their contents vary. Use only lemon and vinegar for salad dressings.

Rationale: Knowing how to manage a diabetic diet away from home can support good health and allow the diabetic increased social comfort.

Fulfilled Needs: Comfort, protection from physical harm, increased learning

Explain how to maintain body alignment Explain the various methods used to position and support the extremities and other body parts in a normal line for functioning.

Rationale: Functional body alignment promotes circulation and comfort; it helps prevent joint deformities, painful stretching or shortening of tendons, and further damage to vital tissues by fractured bones.

Fulfilled Needs: Tissue oxygenation or perfusion, comfort, protection from physical harm, increased learning

Explain how to maintain cleanliness of the ostomy appliance Explain that the ostomy bag and tubing should be cleaned daily with soap and water, rinsed in cold water, and dried.

Rationale: A clean ostomy appliance minimizes the potential for infection, promotes comfort, and supports independent self-care.

Fulfilled Needs: Comfort, cleanliness, protection from physical harm, increased learning

Explain how to maintain environmental cleanliness Explain that a clean environment is essential for health. Cleaning should include the following: damp-dusting of furniture, uncarpeted floors, baseboards, pictures, doors, and drapes, washing of floors, baseboards, windows, cabinets, tables, and shelves with antiseptic solutions, daily rug vacuuming and periodic vacuuming of stuffed furniture and drapes.

Rationale: Cleanliness inhibits the growth of harmful microorganisms.

Fulfilled Needs: Cleanliness, protection from physical harm, increased learning

Explain how to maintain ileostomy/colostomy cleanliness Explain that the ileostomy or colostomy stoma and the surrounding skin should be kept clean with mild soap and water.

Rationale: Cleansing of an ostomy stoma prevents skin excoriation, decreases offensive odor, promotes comfort, and supports independent self-care.

Fulfilled Needs: Comfort, cleanliness, protection from physical harm, increased learning

Explain how to maintain maximum nutrients in food Explain that the maximum nutrient value of foods can be retained by employing slow cooking methods rather than rapid boiling, by steaming rather than cooking in water, and by broiling and baking.

Rationale: Conservation of nutrients in food promotes improved nutrition.

Fulfilled Needs: Nutritional balance, protection from physical harm, increased learning

Explain how to manage insulin therapy on sick days[376] When a diabetic is ill with common upper respiratory or gastric disorders, instruct him to use the following procedure: Take the prescribed dose of insulin. Check urine glucose and ketones four times daily. If urine glucose is high, call the doctor for an increased insulin dose. If urine ketones are present, the insulin dose remains the same. Increase fluid intake if there is no nausea or vomiting. Keep an accurate record of the fluid intake, urine glucose and ketones, and insulin dosage.

Rationale: Insulin requirements for management of diabetes varies when illness places additional stress on the body. Early attention to this need can prevent ketoacidosis.

Fulfilled Needs: Protection from physical harm, increased learning

Explain how to manage seizure episodes Explain that when seizures occur, the person's clothing should be loosened. He should not be restrained, nor should there be interference with seizure movements. All surrounding objects that might cause harm to the patient should be removed. If the patient's mouth is open, place something soft between the jaw teeth on one side only. If the teeth are tightly clenched, do not attempt to force anything between them. Allow the person to rest once the seizure is over.

Rationale: Knowledge of the methods for safe handling of persons having seizures promotes comfort and safety.

Fulfilled Needs: Comfort, protection from physical harm, increased learning

Explain how to massage Explain that bony prominences such as the heels, ankles, knees, iliac crest, scapula and clavicle, wrists, and elbows should be frequently massaged with rhythmic, stimulating strokes.

Rationale: Prolonged pressure of bone against skin can result in decreased circulation, with increased potential for irritation and necrosis. Stimulation of the bony prominences prevents tissue damage.

Fulfilled Needs: Protection from physical harm. Increased learning

Explain how to measure the intake and output Explain how to measure and record the volume of fluids taken in and excreted from the body in a 24 hour period.

Rationale: Assistance from the patient and family in measuring intake and output promotes accuracy.

Fulfilled Needs: Protection from physical harm, increased learning

Explain how to observe respirations Explain that respiration count is the number of times a person breathes in 1 minute. Explain the need to watch for deviations from normal respiratory patterns.

Rationale: Normal oxygen and carbon dioxide exchange through respiration is essential to tissue cell life.

Fulfilled Needs: Protection from physical harm, increased learning

Explain how to obtain supplies/drugs or therapeutic supplies/drugs When therapeutic supplies are needed, tell the person where and how to obtain them at minimum cost.

Rationale: Having the appropriate supplies supports continuity of health therapy.

Fulfilled Needs: Comfort, protection from physical harm, increased learning

Explain how to pad bony prominences Explain that all bony prominences should be padded with soft materials whenever they are subject to prolonged pressure. This procedure is essential for persons undergoing prolonged rest, for those with paralyzed limbs, etc.

Rationale: Pressure on bony prominences causes irritation and impaired circulation, which can result in necrosis.

Fulfilled Needs: Comfort, protection from physical harm, increased learning

Explain how to pad rough cast edges Explain that all rough or ragged cast edges should be padded (petaled) so as to minimize pressure against the skin and prevent plaster particles from falling under the cast and causing decubitus ulcer.

Rationale: Small rough particles rubbed into the skin can cause abrasion and infection.

Fulfilled Needs: Comfort, protection from physical harm, increased learning

Explain how to prepare for the procedure/diagnostic study Explain what the person needs to do to prepare himself for a particular study or procedure. This includes such preparations as limiting food and fluids for a specified time, eating special diets, taking special drugs or dyes, taking laxatives and enemas, and collecting specimens. Be sure that the person understands when, how, and why the preparations should be carried out.

Rationale: Adequate preparation for studies facilitates accurate diagnostic findings.

Fulfilled Needs: Comfort, increased learning

Explain how to prepare the breasts during pregnancy for postdelivery breast-feeding Explain that breast care during pregnancy can bring the breast to optimum condition for breast-feeding after delivery. Instruct the woman to massage her breasts once or twice daily, apply lanolin to her breasts, gently pull on the nipples, and rub the nipples with a terrycloth towel.

Rationale: Massaging and rubbing the breasts will toughen the nipples and prevent cracking, bleeding, and pain during breast feeding. Lubricating the breasts makes them more elastic so that they will stretch and the nipple will not split.

Fulfilled Needs: Comfort, cleaniness, protection from physical harm, increased learning

Explain how to prevent coughing   Explain that coughing may be deferred by taking slow, gentle deep breaths when the cough reflex seems imminent.

Rationale: Coughing causes increased intrathoracic, intraocular, intraabdominal, and intracranial pressure. Unproductive coughing wastes energy.

Fulfilled Needs: Protection from physical harm, freedom from pain, increased learning

Explain how to prevent crossinfection   Explain that crossinfection can be reduced by room and article decontamination, limited direct human contact, hand washing, and wearing a gown and mask.

Rationale: Removing infectious microorganisms from surfaces and preventing contact with organisms can decrease the potential for disease transfer from one person to another.

Fulfilled Needs: Protection from physical harm, increased learning

Explain how to prevent sneezing   Explain that sneezing may be prevented by exerting finger pressure above the lip and under the nose or by taking deep breaths through the mouth. The nares should not be squeezed together in an attempt to prevent sneezing.

Rationale: Since sneezing causes increased intranasal pressure and can dislodge blood clots that have sealed off bleeding, sneezing should be avoided when there has been nasal bleeding or trauma.

Fulfilled Needs: Protection from physical harm, increased learning

Explain how to prevent the common cold   Explain that good basic health practices such as adequate rest and balanced nutrition make one less susceptible to colds. In addition, other measures include wearing warm clothing to protect against chill, maintaining good room ventilation, staying away from persons with colds and persons who are sneezing or coughing, wearing a mask when one has a cold and is caring for others, preventing the drying out of respiratory mucous membrane linings, avoiding dieting during the cold season, avoiding breathing cold air, and avoiding sudden temperature changes.

Rationale: Prevention of the common cold preserves health and reduces suffering.

Fulfilled Needs: Comfort, protection from physical harm, increased learning

Explain how to recognize when a brace has been outgrown   Explain that brace joints should coincide with body joints. When it is noticed that brace joints do not coincide with body joints, the patient is outgrowing his brace.

Rationale: A brace that does not fit properly causes pressure on skin areas and does not provide the intended support.

Fulfilled Needs: Protection from physical harm, increased learning

Explain how to reduce muscular tension   Explain that muscular tension can be reduced by stretching the muscles, yawning, and suddenly letting the muscles go limp. It can also be accomplished by assuming a lying or sitting position and allowing all muscles to become limp.

Rationale: Stretching brings the muscles to peak contraction, and this is followed by relaxation. Muscle contraction during illness consumes energy that is vital for healing. Relief of muscular tension promotes comfort.

Fulfilled Needs: Sleep, rest, and relaxation, energy, comfort, protection from physical harm, increased learning

Explain how to remove earwax   Explain that earwax may be softened by placing a few drops of warmed glycerin in the ear; this is followed by gentle removal with a small piece of twisted gauze or tissue gently inserted, not packed, into the canal to absorb the solution.

Rationale: Removal of earwax promotes cleanliness and can improve impaired hearing when impacted cerumen is its cause.

Fulfilled Needs: Comfort, cleanliness, protection from physical harm, increased learning

Contraindications: Ear infection, inflammation, or drainage, ruptured tympanic membrane, presence of a myringotomy tube.

Explain how to remove hair lice   Explain that lice can be removed from the hair and scalp by moistening the hair with hot vinegar and combing the ova out with a fine-tooth comb; there are also prescription shampoos.

Rationale: Head lice cause scalp inflammation, which has the potential for bacterial infection.

Fulfilled Needs: Cleanliness, protection from physical harm, increased learning

Explain how to set behavioral limits   Explain that limits are set on another person's behavior by clearly stating what constitutes acceptable and unacceptable behavior.

Rationale: External control of behavior supports internal control when the latter cannot be maintained. Limitations protect against future shame that can result from uncontrolled behavior.

Fulfilled Needs: Protection from psychologic threat, personal growth and maturity, increased learning, increased reality perception and problem-solving ability.

Explain how to shampoo the hair/scalp   Explain how to shampoo hair so that optimum cleanliness is attained. The technique may include shampooing in bed as well as out of bed.

Rationale: Cleanliness prevents infection and promotes comfort.

Fulfilled Needs: Comfort, cleanliness, protection from physical harm, increased learning

Explain how to splint an incision   Explain that patients who experience discomfort while coughing should splint or support the painful site with a pillow while coughing.

Rationale: Supporting a painful site during coughing decreases tension and stretching of the severed muscles.

Fulfilled Needs: Comfort, protection from physical harm, increased learning

Explain how to sterilize contaminated dishes   Explain that contaminated dishes can be sterilized by submerging them in a large pan of disinfecting solution, by boiling them, or by placing them in a dishwasher that attains the proper temperature.

Rationale: Sterilization destroys all surface microorganisms and helps prevent infection.

Fulfilled Needs: Protection from physical harm, increased learning

Explain how to stimulate an infant to remain awake during feeding   Explain that some infants fall asleep during feeding time. Changing the infant's position or moving his bottle will usually awaken him.

Rationale: Knowledge that infants may go to sleep before receiving adequate nourishment increases the parent's ability to ensure proper nourishment.

Fulfilled Needs: Protection from physical harm, increased learning

Explain how to strain urine   Explain how to filter urine output through a gauze or strainer to catch urinary stones.

Rationale: Catching urinary stones provides evidence that the stones have been passed. Analysis of urinary stones facilitates the prescription of measures to prevent future stone formation.

Fulfilled Needs: Protection from physical harm, increased learning

Explain how to take allergy precautions Suggest that persons with allergies take the following precautions: travel in air-conditioned vehicles, do not bring cut flowers indoors, stay out of smoke-filled rooms, avoid using perfumes and scented cosmetics, do not engage in water sports that necessitate swimming under water, avoid excessive sun, get adequate rest, avoid fog, rain, and road dust as much as possible, have a short-haired dog instead of a long-haired one, do not keep birds in the house, avoid eating fish, nuts, chocolate, oranges, and tomatoes, use hypoallergenic cosmetics, avoid fuzzy blankets and wool clothing, do not use insecticides, do not apply dust-catching oils to the skin, avoid sudden temperature changes, especially becoming overheated.

Rationale: Avoidance of allergic stimuli promotes safety and comfort.

Fulfilled Needs: Comfort, protection from physical harm, increased learning

Explain how to use a bed rope Teach a person to use a rope or a strong piece of sheeting attached to the foot of the bed so that he can pull himself from a lying position to a sitting position.

Rationale: The ability to move about prevents stasis of secretions, stimulates circulation, restores strength, and promotes independence.

Fulfilled Needs: Activity and exercise, comfort, protection from physical harm, independence, increased learning

Explain how to use a paper bag to reduce hyperventilation Teach persons who experience dizziness because of rapid breathing to breathe into a paper bag for about 5 minutes, or until the dizziness and rapid breathing cease.

Rationale: When the patient rebreathes the exhaled carbon dioxide collected in the paper bag, the level of carbon dioxide in his blood is raised to normal, reestablishing respiratory acid–base balance.

Fulfilled Needs: Acid–base balance, protection from physical harm, increased learning

Contraindications: Elevated blood levels of carbon dioxide, emphysema

Explain how to use nondrug methods for pain relief Explain that pain relief methods other than drugs can be used: heat or cold therapy, positioning, tension reduction, therapeutic soaks, elastic bandage support, body alignment, supportive garments. Discuss which of these is applicable to the person's specific situation.

Rationale: Relieving pain without using drugs reduces the potential for drug habituation and drug side effects.

Fulfilled Needs: Comfort, protection from physical harm, freedom from pain, increased learning

Explain how to use the stop-and-think technique Teach the person that when unwanted thoughts occur, he can shout "stop" to himself and then think about something new.

Rationale: By shouting "stop" to himself, the original thought is interrupted. New thoughts are then able to replace the unwanted thoughts. This also gives the person a feeling of control over his thought processes.

Fulfilled Needs: Protection from psychologic threat, increased learning

Explain how to use toilet tissue correctly by cleansing from front to back Explain that when cleansing the perineal area with toilet tissue, wiping should begin at the anterior (front) perineum and continue to the posterior (back) perineum. Never wipe toward the front or wipe twice with the same piece of tissue.

Rationale: Bacteria-containing fecal matter can cause urinary tract infection when spread from the posterior to the anterior perineum.

Fulfilled Needs: Cleanliness, protection from physical harm, increased learning

Explain how venereal disease is transmitted Explain that venereal diseases are transmitted primarily by sexual intercourse and that persons who frequently change sexual partners run a high risk because they do not always know the health status of these partners. Explain that venereal disease can be transmitted to the fetus through the placenta or through contact in an infected birth canal. If there are lip lesions, venereal disease can be contracted by kissing.

Rationale: Prevention of venereal disease preserves health and reduces suffering.

Fulfilled Needs: Protection from physical harm, increased learning

Explain methods for position change when in pain Explain that when the person has an abdominal incision and wants to sit up, he should first raise the bed, turn on his side (lateral position) and slowly push himself up with his arm until he is in a sitting position.

Rationale: When a person has an abdominal incision, raising the bed and turning to the lateral position before sitting up reduces tension on the abdominal musculature and reduces pain.

Fulfilled Needs: Comfort, freedom from pain, increased learning

Explain normal organ (kidney, heart, liver, etc.) function/normal body function Explain in detail how the specific body organ and the body as a whole functions. When appropriate, use organ models, charts and drawings to illustrate function.

Rationale: Knowledge of how an organ or the body functions increases the understanding of the body, which supports improved health practices.

Fulfilled Needs: Increased learning

Explain that a cast should not be painted with nonporous paint Explain that when a cast is painted for decorative reasons, only porous paint should be used. All forms of sealers such as varnish and plastic spray should be avoided.

Rationale: Cast material is porous, allowing air to reach the skin through the minute holes in the plaster. Nonporous paint seals the holes, preventing the skin from "breathing," resulting in skin maceration.

Fulfilled Needs: Protection from physical harm, increased learning

Explain that a child should become accustomed to dry diapers during toilet training Explain that toilet training is facilitated if the child's diaper is changed frequently so that he becomes accustomed to a dry diaper.

Rationale: Children accustomed to dry diapers find wet diapers uncomfortable and are more amenable to toilet training.

Fulfilled Needs: Comfort, increased learning

Explain that care should be taken to prevent scratching of the contact lenses Explain that contact lenses should be handled gently and never placed on a rough surface where scratching can occur.

Rationale: A scratched contact lens impairs vision and causes discomfort.

Fulfilled Needs: Comfort, protection from physical harm, increased learning

Explain that change must come from within the person/family Explain that any change in behavior must come from within the person or group. There must be recognition of a need for change, knowledge of what changes to make, and activity that will actually produce the change. Change does not occur by changing others.

Rationale: An awareness that change must come from within rather than from without supports positive behavioral change.

Fulfilled Needs: Increased learning, increased reality perception and problem solving

Explain that childbirth is a normal process Explain that childbirth is not a disease, but a natural physiologic process, just as are the processes of breathing and digestion.

Rationale: Awareness that physiologic processes are normal promotes comfort.

Fulfilled Needs: Comfort, protection from psychologic threat, increased learning

Explain that clothes should be laid out in the order of dressing for persons with impaired cerebral function/for small children Explain that small children and confused or retarded persons should have their clothes laid out in the proper order of dressing when attempting to dress themselves.

Rationale: Orderliness reduces confusion and supports the development of skill and self-reliance.

Fulfilled Needs: Comfort, self-reliance, mastery and competence in skills, independence, increased learning

Explain that commode sittings should be scheduled during toilet training Explain that during toilet training the child should be placed on the commode every day at the same time.

Rationale: Placing the child on the commode at the same time every day facilities adaptation to routine physiologic functioning.

Fulfilled Needs: Comfort, increased learning

Explain that communication should be encouraged despite impairment Teach the family to assist the patient to communicate in any way possible, whether it be by speech, writing, or symbols, and to select the method that causes the least frustration and self-depreciation.

Rationale: Comfort is promoted by a sense of effective communication with others.

Fulfilled Needs: Comfort, caring and communicating relationships, increased learning

Contraindications: When a person is relearning speech, he should not be encouraged to use short-cut methods to communicate.

Explain that controlled elimination should be praised during toilet training Explain that toilet training is facilitated by words of approval and appreciation when elimination control is successful.

Rationale: Praise gives the child a sense of satisfaction and a desire to master the behavior that precipitates praise.

Fulfilled Needs: Comfort, increased learning

Explain that corrective eye lenses require periodic adjustment Explain that persons wearing glasses or contact lenses should have their eyes checked for visual changes at least every 2 years and should have their glasses or contact lenses adjusted to meet these changes.

Rationale: Periodic readjustment of eye lenses supports improved vision.

Fulfilled Needs: Protection from physical harm, increased learning

Explain that daily bowel elimination is not essential Explain that as long as feces are not hard and dry, daily elimination is not necessary. Elimination is dependent on body routine and food consumption.

Rationale: Awareness that daily bowel elimination is not essential can prevent the use of poor health practices to stimulate elimination.

Fulfilled Needs: Comfort, protection from physical harm, increased learning

Explain that drug or alcohol abuse/dependence is an illness Explain that the excessive use of drugs or alcohol indicates a basic psychologic disorder that must be dealt with in order to overcome the problem. Although addicts may commit criminal acts to obtain drugs, addiction itself is not a crime. Addiction is an illness.

Rationale: Recognizing that drug dependence is an illness supports a realistic approach to solution of the problem.

Fulfilled Needs: Comfort, protection from physical harm, protection from psychologic threat, increased learning, increased reality perception and problem-solving ability

Explain that drug/alcohol use is not socially essential   Explain that one does not have to use drugs or alcohol to be accepted within a peer group. Those who prefer not to use drugs are generally held in equal, if not higher, esteem than those who do.

Rationale: The mistaken notion that one must conform to every peer pressure in order to be accepted frequently overrides intelligent recognition of the inadvisability of an activity.

Fulfilled Needs: Comfort, protection from physical harm, protection from psychologic threat, personal growth and maturity, increased learning, increased reality perception and problem-solving ability

Explain that extreme cold cracks and heat warps contact lenses   Explain that if a contact lens is stored in solution and left in an extremely cold environment, the lens will crack. Explain that a contact lens should never be placed near a stove or heater because it will change shape.

Rationale: Proper care of contact lenses assures their availability as a visual aid.

Fulfilled Needs: Protection from physical harm, increased learning

Explain that fatigue should be recognized as a stress factor   Help families recognize that high percentages of disagreements occur when family members are fatigued. This is especially true in the evening, when the father comes home from a hard day's work, the children are tired from school, and the mother, who has been housekeeping or working at outside employment, has the additional stress of meal preparation.

Rationale: Understanding stress factors promotes preventive behavior and acceptance of the behavior of others.

Fulfilled Needs: Protection from physical harm, protection from psychologic threat, increased learning, increased reality perception and problem-solving ability

Explain that fear/anxiety often disguises itself   Explain that an expressed fear or anxiety is often a substitute for another fear or anxiety that is not socially acceptable. Disguising fear or anxiety can convert the original fear or anxiety into a form that is socially approved.

Rationale: Facing fear or anxiety in its original form reduces the complexity of the fear situation.

Fulfilled Needs: Comfort, protection from psychologic threat, personal growth and maturity, increased learning, increased reality perception and problem-solving ability

Explain that fluids should not be given to persons unable to swallow   Explain that nothing should be given by mouth to persons who are unable to swallow. This includes those who are unconscious or stuporous, those with throat paralysis, and those who cough and spit up when attempting to swallow.

Rationale: Difficulty in swallowing or inability to swallow poses the threat of food or liquid aspiration into the lungs and consequent airway obstruction.

Fulfilled Needs: Protection from physical harm, increased learning

Explain that hair lost during illness usually returns   Explain that hair loss resulting from high fever or drug reactions is temporary and that hair will return when body processes are restored to normal.

Rationale: Awareness that lost hair will return to normal promotes comfort.

Fulfilled Needs: Comfort, increased learning

Explain that ill persons/aged persons/adolescents/pregnant women/ small children are often hypersensitive   Explain that in certain instances, many persons are highly susceptible to emotional upsets inadvertently caused by others. The person becomes keenly aware of others' responses regarding the acceptability of his situation, and he often prefers that his problems not be discussed outside the family. Persons may also be sensitive to environmental confusion and noise.

Rationale: Awareness of the hypersensitivity of persons supports behavior modification on the part of others to meet the needs of the person.

Fulfilled Needs: Comfort, protection from psychologic threat, personal growth and maturity, increased learning, increased reality perception and problem-solving ability

Explain that immobility related to pain causes increased pain Explain that despite the pain involved, noninflamed arthritis and age-stiffened joints should be moved as much as possible; otherwise, greater pain and stiffness will be experienced.

Rationale: Maintenance of joint mobility promotes comfort.

Fulfilled Needs: Comfort, protection from physical harm, freedom from pain, increased learning

Explain that it is acceptable to admit the existence of pain Explain that admitting the existence of pain is culturally acceptable and that when it is reported relief measures can be taken.

Rationale: Psychologic safety requires that the person experience acceptance by others.

Fulfilled Needs: Comfort, protection from psychologic threat, acceptance, increased learning

Explain that it is essential to foster healthy drinking attitudes Explain that it is the family's responsibility to their children to communicate moderate and positive attitudes toward alcohol consumption.

Rationale: Moderate and positive attitudes taught during early childhood support healthy behavior in adult life.

Fulfilled Needs: Protection from physical harm, protection from psychologic threat, personal growth and maturity, increased learning, increased reality perception and problem-solving ability

Explain that long-term drug/alcohol abuse reduces the pleasures derived from drug/alcohol abuse Explain to persons taking drugs or alcohol for their pleasurable effects that the experience becomes less and less pleasurable with time. As drug or alcohol dosage is increased to stimulate ecstasy, the quality of the experience gradually deteriorates.

Rationale: Awareness that drugs and alcohol cannot maintain a heightened pleasurable experience indefinitely supports recognition that abuse for the sake of pleasure is futile.

Fulfilled Needs: Protection from psychologic threat, personal growth and maturity, increased learning, increased reality perception and problem-solving ability

Explain that mothers have a choice of single or double breast-feeding Explain that once lactation is well established, the mother may alternate breasts with each feeding or may use both breasts for each feeding. The decision depends on the milk flow, on infant demand for feeding, and on the mother's comfort.

Rationale: Proper breast-feeding supports maternal and infant health.

Fulfilled Needs: Comfort, protection from physical harm, increased learning

Explain that nails should be soaked before trimming Explain that nails should be soaked in warm soapy water before being cut.

Rationale: Soaking softens the nail, making trimming easier and reducing the potential for nail injury.

Fulfilled Needs: Protection from physical harm, increased learning

Explain that nursing the infant on alternate breasts reduces tenderness

Explain that during the first few days of breast feeding, if the mother experiences breast tenderness or soreness, she may prefer to alternate breasts with each feeding.

Rationale: Alternating breasts with each feeding decreases irritation from infant sucking and promotes comfort.

Fulfilled Needs: Comfort, protection from physical harm, increased learning

Explain that objects should be consistently placed in the same location for the visually impaired Explain that when persons have difficulty in seeing, objects should always be kept in their accustomed places according to individual needs.

Rationale: Consistently keeping objects in their usual places reduces the stress of adapting to an unfamiliar situation; it promotes comfort, meets dependency needs, supports independent mobility, and reduces the potential for injury.

Fulfilled Needs: Comfort, protection from physical harm, dependence, predictable and orderly world, independence, increased learning

Explain that one's face should be kept visible when speaking to a hearing-impaired person Explain that in speaking to a hearing-impaired person, the speaker should directly face the hearing-impaired person and maintain a position such that light falls on the face of the speaker.

Rationale: Hearing-impaired persons depend on facial expressions to clarify messages.

Fulfilled Needs: Comfort, caring and communicating relationships, increased learning

Explain that one's rank and sex among siblings affect how one interrelates Explain that being a male or female and being youngest, oldest, or in the middle has a definite effect on how we interrelate with others. A male who is younger than his three sisters may project his anger for his sisters toward his spouse. A male who is older than his three sisters may feel very responsible for the females in his life.

Rationale: Awareness that rank and sex in a family affect behavior supports insight into and change of behavior.

Fulfilled Needs: Increased learning, increased reality perception and problem-solving ability

Explain that parental attitudes affect child development Explain that the attitudes parents communicate to children, both verbally and nonverbally, affect the child's perception of himself and his world and result in child behavior that reflects that perception.

Rationale: Awareness of the effect that attitudes have on others supports favorable behavior toward others.

Fulfilled Needs: Protection from physical harm, protection from psychologic threat, personal growth and maturity, increased learning, increased reality perception and problem-solving ability

Explain that persons must make adjustments at their own pace Explain that persons who are making emotional adjustments should not be forced into activities and contacts with other people, but should be allowed to participate as they desire.

Rationale: Forcing rapid adaptation and adjustment increases the threat of internal tension, especially when the person feels inadequate to cope with the situation.

Fulfilled Needs: Comfort, protection from psychologic threat, increased learning, increased reality perception and problem-solving ability

Explain that persons wearing leg braces should avoid contact sports Explain that persons wearing braces should not participate in sports that bring them into physical contact with others, such as football, basketball, and soccer. Tennis, volleyball, baseball, and swimming are safer.

Rationale: Severe injury can result from impact with the steel brace frame.

Fulfilled Needs: Protection from physical harm, increased learning

Explain that persons with impaired cerebral function require close observation   Explain that persons whose cerebral functioning is impaired are often not responsible and should not be left alone; they require constant and close supervision.

Rationale: Persons with impaired cerebral function require close supervision because of their increased potential for accidental injury.

Fulfilled Needs: Protection from physical harm, increased learning, increased reality perception and problem-solving ability

Explain that persons with limited attention span require message repetition   Explain that messages should be repeated to a person whose attention span is limited.

Rationale: Repetition enhances communication by reinforcing perception of the intended ideas and thoughts.

Fulfilled Needs: Caring and communicating relationships, increased learning

Explain that pregnancy can result from sexual activity   Explain that sexual intercourse, when occurring at ovulation, may result in pregnancy.

Rationale: Knowledge of physiologic processes promotes comfort.

Fulfilled Needs: Comfort, increased learning

Explain that premature infants require at-home supervision   Explain that premature infants discharged from the hospital cannot be taken to nurseries or left in the care of babysitters. They must be kept at home and supervised by family members specifically instructed in their care.

Rationale: Since the health status of the premature infant is more fragile than that of the full-term baby, early care must be carefully supervised to assure health maintenance.

Fulfilled Needs: Protection from physical harm, increased learning, increased reality perception and problem-solving ability

Explain that premature infants require prescribed foods   Explain that premature infants at home must have specifically prescribed foods for proper growth and development.

Rationale: Since premature infants are not as well developed physiologically as full-term infants, they cannot digest the same foods at the same age.

Fulfilled Needs: Protection from physical harm, increased learning

Explain that proper storage of insulin ensures drug potency[376]   Explain that insulin should preferably be stored in the refrigerator, but can be stored at room temperature. Insulin should never be frozen or left in an environmental temperature over 100° F. Expiration dates should be noted, and bottles discarded on such dates.

Rationale: Insulin remains stable in potency when stored in the refrigerator or at room temperature. Freezing clumps the insulin and heat destroys its potency.

Fulfilled Needs: Increased learning

Explain that questions need to be phrased for yes and no answers when there is impaired speech delivery   Explain that when a person has difficulty in speaking, he is most comfortable when he is able to give a yes or no answer to a question, rather than having to respond in detail to conversation.

Rationale: Simple and direct communication reduces frustration and anxiety and promotes comfort.

Fulfilled Needs: Comfort, protection from psychologic threat, caring and communicating relationships, increased learning

Explain that recreation aids total health, supports personal growth, and is not an escape mechanism   Explain that recreation provides a balance between pleasure and work. Recreation should not be considered an escape, but rather a growth factor that gives personal satisfaction.

Rationale: The movement and motor coordination experienced in recreational activities stimulate physical and mental processes. Growth results from positive attitudes that enrich and develop the personality, often by recreational means.

Fulfilled Needs: Comfort, personal growth and maturity, increased learning, increased reality perception and problem-solving ability, increased pleasantness or pleasure

Explain that relaxation is essential for a successful sexual response   Explain that an important aspect of successful sexual activity involves relaxing and allowing natural responses to occur.

Rationale: The body performs best when relaxed.

Fulfilled Needs: Relaxation, sexuality, increased learning, increased reality perception and problem-solving ability

Explain that rhythmic and repetitive exercises are most effective[746]   Explain that rhythmic, or aerobic, exercise involving continuous movement of the arms and legs is most beneficial. Such exercise must be performed over and over again.

Rationale: Rhythmic, repetitive exercise involves motion and the use of large muscles, resulting in improved circulation and oxygenation of tissues.

Fulfilled Needs: Tissue oxygenation or perfusion, exercise, protection from physical harm, mastery and competence in skills, independence, increased learning

Contraindications: Fever, states of severe energy depletion or increased metabolic rate, and acute illness are conditions under which such exercise should not be performed. Any person who has elevated blood pressure, elevated serum cholesterol or triglyceride levels, elevated uric acid levels, an abnormal electrocardiogram, a known cardiac condition for which he is on cardiac drugs, chest pain, a family history of heart disease, diabetes, asthma or emphysema, any condition such as arthritis or gout in which muscle or joint motion would aggravate the condition, dyspnea or intermittent claudication (leg cramping when walking), or any chronic illness should be seen and evaluated by a physician before starting an exercise program.

Explain that sexual activity is not always an expression of intimacy   Explain that sexual activity can be engaged in for purposes other than the expression of love. It can be the end result of anger, anxiety, or conflict. Ideally, sexual activity results from or promotes deep intimacy between partners.

Rationale: Knowledge of the motivation for sexual activity can help the person evaluate the relationship with a partner.

Fulfilled Needs: Protection from psychologic threat, increased reality perception, increased learning

Explain that sexual activity should be temporarily limited   Explain that when recovering from cardiac disease, the patient should refrain from sexual activity for several months. During pregnancy, sexual activity should be avoided if the membrane has ruptured or if there is vaginal bleeding. Intercourse should be avoided when a vaginal infection exists.

Rationale: Sexual intercourse increases the heart rate, respirations, blood pressure, and cardiac output and can result in cardiac overload. Sexual activity after the membrane has ruptured can cause vaginal infection, placenta previa, or perforation of the placenta. When vaginal infection exists, sexual activity can extend the infection in the female and cause infection of the male's genitourinary tract.

Fulfilled Needs: Protection from physical harm, increased learning

Explain that sexual function may be slow to return   Explain that after surgery, such as a prostatectomy, erection may be difficult for a few weeks. Temporary impotence takes time to resolve itself.

Rationale: Explanations of temporary impotence keeps the person from becoming discouraged and possibly developing a psychogenic impotence. It encourages a return to normal sexual function.

Fulfilled Needs: Sexuality, protection from psychologic threat, increased learning

Explain that sexual response normally varies Explain that the degree of sexual satisfaction varies from day to day and is dependent on fatigue level, mood, current life problems, muscular tension caused by anxiety, and other such factors.

Rationale: Awareness that sexual response varies promotes comfort and reality perception.

Fulfilled Needs: Comfort, sexuality, protection from psychologic threat, increased learning, increased reality perception and problem-solving ability

Explain that sexuality is but one part of human development Explain that there are other significant areas of human development besides sexuality, such as all the developmental tasks throughout life, of which sexuality is but one part. Relate that human achievement includes all areas of life.

Rationale: Knowledge of the broad basis of human development raises the potential for a higher level of personal maturity.

Fulfilled Needs: Increased reality perception, increased learning

Explain that socialization depletes the ill person's energy Explain that socializing with visitors fatigues sick persons and therefore should be limited.

Rationale: Socializing consumes energy that ill persons need for healing and recovery.

Fulfilled Needs: Protection from physical harm, protection from psychologic threat, increased learning

Explain that some tension is normal Explain that one normally experiences a certain amount of tension and should not expect to feel tension free.

Rationale: Normal tension gives pleasure and stimulates activity.

Fulfilled Needs: Comfort, protection from psychologic threat, increased learning, increased reality perception and problem-solving ability

Explain that the behavior of one family member is not a reflection on other family members Explain that the abnormal behavior of a family member does not reflect negatively on other family members. Despite family ties, each person is independently responsible for his behavior.

Rationale: Awareness that each person is solely responsible for his behavior reduces the anxiety commonly experienced when the values and behavior of one family member are in conflict with the basic values of the family.

Fulfilled Needs: Comfort, protection from psychologic threat, increased learning, increased reality perception and problem-solving ability

Explain that the common cold is contagious for 48 hours after symptom onset Explain that the common cold can be given or contracted from others during the first 48 hours after symptoms (heightened sneezing) appear.

Rationale: Reduced contact with those who have colds for the first 48 hours after their symptoms appear can prevent the spread of infection.

Fulfilled Needs: Protection from physical harm, increased learning

Explain that the fluid intake and output should be balanced Explain that maintenance of balance in body fluids requires daily consumption of approximately 2,000 cc (six to eight 240-cc glasses of liquid), with about equal output.

Rationale: Water balance is essential for normal cell function, production of secretions, elimination of urine and feces, maintenance of electrolyte balance, and other important physiologic functions.

Fulfilled Needs: Fluid and electrolyte balance, protection from physical harm, increased learning

Explain that the pacemaker's electrical current is not strong enough to electrocute Explain that the electrical current in a pacemaker is not sufficient to do harm, only to stimulate the heart.

Rationale: Assurance that pacemakers are safe reduces anxiety.

Fulfilled Needs: Comfort, protection from psychologic threat, increased learning

Explain that the person's response/emotional response is appropriate and commonly experienced Explain that the emotion the person is experiencing is considered a normal response in the particular situation and that other persons often experience the same emotion in similar situations.

Rationale: Feelings of adequacy and comfort evolve from an awareness that one's emotions are normal and are similarly experienced by others.

Fulfilled Needs: Comfort, protection from psychologic threat, sense of adequacy, increased learning, increased reality perception and problem-solving ability

Explain that the situation is temporary Explain to the person that the current illness or other life crisis is temporary and will pass in time. Acknowledge that this difficult period will eventually end.

Rationale: The knowledge that a painful situation is temporary provides comfort and the hope of relief.

Fulfilled Needs: Comfort, protection from psychologic threat, endurance, increased learning, increased reality perception

Explain that the teeth should not be brushed with potentially unsafe water Explain that the teeth should not be brushed with contaminated water. Boiled, chlorinated, or carbonated water can be used.

Rationale: Brushing the teeth with contaminated water introduces bacteria into the mouth that can eventually enter the intestinal tract.

Fulfilled Needs: Protection from physical harm, increased learning

Explain that the tracheostomy must be covered in order to speak Teach the person who has had a tracheostomy to cover the tracheostomy opening for a few moments, with sterile mesh, if he wants to speak.

Rationale: The ability to communicate by speech reduces anxiety and promotes comfort.

Fulfilled Needs: Comfort, protection from psychologic threat, increased learning

Contraindications: Severe respiratory distress, after laryngectomy

Explain that the urinary catheter should be taped to the abdomen of males Explain that a male having an indwelling catheter for a prolonged period should tape the end of the catheter to his abdomen.

Rationale: Taping the urinary catheter to the abdomen prevents ulceration at the penile-scrotal junction by keeping pressure off the glans and urethra.

Fulfilled Needs: Protection from physical harm, increased learning

Contraindications: An unhealed abdominal surgical incision

Explain that the use of drugs/alcohol to solve problems is dangerous Explain that drugs and alcohol should not be taken in an effort to resolve problems. Not only does drug use fail to resolve problems, it also creates new ones.

Rationale: Drugs and alcohol have damaging effects on the body. They deaden a person's perception of any solution to the problem that is causing the drug use.

Fulfilled Needs: Protection from physical harm, protection from physiologic threat, increased learning

Explain that there are nondrug methods available for pain relief Explain that pain relief methods other than drugs can be used, such as heat or cold therapy, positioning, tension reduction, therapeutic soaks, elastic bandage support, body alignment, and supportive garments. Discuss which of these is applicable to the person's specific situation.

Rationale: Relieving pain without using drugs reduces the potential for drug habituation and drug side effects.

Fulfilled Needs: Comfort, protection from physical harm, freedom from pain, increased learning

Explain that undesirable thoughts and feelings are normal Explain that every person occasionally has thoughts, feelings, and impulses whose consequences he would consider wrong if he were to act upon them.

Rationale: Awareness that undesirable thoughts and feelings are normal promotes comfort in persons who have difficulty accepting such thoughts and feelings within themselves.

Fulfilled Needs: Comfort, protection from psychologic threat, personal growth and maturity, increased learning, increased reality perception and problem-solving ability

Explain that unpleasant conversation increases stress Explain to visitors that the stress of unpleasant conversation depletes the energy that the patient needs for healing purposes. Therefore conversation should be pleasant.

Rationale: Awareness that unpleasant conversation increases stress encourages behavior that can reduce stress.

Fulfilled Needs: Protection from physical harm, protection from psychologic threat, increased learning

Explain that yawning and swallowing will equalize ear pressure Explain that if pressure, pain, or hearing loss occurs as an airplane descends for a landing, one should yawn or swallow several times. Chewing gum will promote swallowing.

Rationale: As an airplane descends, the air pressure in the passenger's middle ear is less than the increasing atmospheric pressure. Yawning or swallowing opens the eustachian tube and allows the outside air at higher pressure to enter the ear, with resulting equalization of pressure.

Fulfilled Needs: Comfort, protection form physical harm, increased learning

Explain the advantages and disadvantages of breast-feeding Explain that breast-feeding has several advantages. Breast milk contains the best nutritional composition known for infants. It is the correct temperature, it is free from bacteria, and it seldom causes allergic reactions. Breast-feeding reduces formula preparation, and fewer women who breast-feed their infants have breast cancer.

There are also disadvantages to breast-feeding, such as being committed to a rigid home schedule in order to be available for infant feeding and breast discomforts associated with lactation.

Rationale: Awareness of the advantages and disadvantages of breast-feeding assists in making the proper choice of whether to breast-feed.

Fulfilled Needs: Comfort, increased learning, increased reality perception and problem-solving ability

Contraindications: Insufficient lactation, breast infection or irritation

Explain the body alterations associated with the illness/surgical procedure Explain the physiologic and anatomic body changes expected to occur during an illness or surgical procedure. Give sufficient detail so the person understands the changes in body structure and/or function.

Rationale: Knowledge of expected changes in body function or structure reduces the element of surprise, in turn eliminating unnecessary anxiety and increasing the time available for adaptation and the quality of adaptation.

Fulfilled Needs: Comfort, protection from psychologic threat, increased learning

Explain the cause(s) of the problem/the health problem Explain the significant factors that brought about the person's problem.

Rationale: Awareness of the causes of problems reduces fear associated with the unknown. It decreases the potential for recurrence of the problem and helps the person seek correct solutions for the problem.

Fulfilled Needs: Comfort, protection from physical harm, protection from pyschologic threat, increased learning, increasd reality perception and problem-solving ability

Contraindications: Delay explanation if it appears to heighten anxiety.

Explain the contraindications for various family planning methods Explain that some family planning methods are not advised in certain health conditions. Oral contraceptives are not recommended if the woman has or has had cancer of the breast or uterus, is pregnant, has active liver disease, hyperlipidemia, hypertension, diabetes mellitus, or coronary artery disease, or during lactation if she intends to nurse her baby. Intrauterine devices are not to be used during a vaginal infection, etc.

Rationale: Knowledge of when not to practice certain family planning methods reduces the potential for health complications.

Fulfilled Needs: Protection from physical harm, increased learning

Explain the criteria for acceptance of an organ donor Explain that close relatives, especially identical twins, are usually the most compatible kidney donors. The process of determing compatibility is as follows: Blood types are determined; they must be compatible. When the blood types are cross-matched, agglutination (clumping) of the cells must not occur. Tissue typing is performed; if any one of the 11 known antigens is present in the donor but not in the recipient, the tissues are incompatible. If an antigen is present in the recipient but not in the donor, there is only minor incompatibility. It is preferable that the donor be living and well and that he have no history of urinary tract disease. Pyelography, renal function studies, and renal arteriograms are performed. Corneal donations are acceptable as long as the cornea is healthy.

Rationale: Knowledge of what to expect promotes feelings of comfort and safety.

Fulfilled Needs: Comfort, protection from psychologic threat, increased learning

Explain the dangers of incorrect use of equipment/drugs/therapy Explain the possible adverse effects when equipment, drugs, or therapy are not used according to specified instructions. Emphasize that increasing or decreasing equipment pressures, doses of drugs, frequency of therapy, etc., can drastically change the intended results.

Rationale: Knowledge of the end results of tampering with prescribed treatment can prevent injury or complications.

Fulfilled Needs: Protection from physical harm, increased learning

Explain the difference between freedom from fear/anxiety and freedom from problems Explain that when a person is free of fear, there are no feelings of dread or doubt as he attempts to solve a problem; instead, he approaches the problem with positive solutions. As long as we live we will never be free of problems.

Rationale: Some persons perceive fears and problems as being the same, because the challenge of a problem evokes fear in them. Awareness that the two are different and that problems can be solved by a sound, fearless approach supports good mental health.

Fulfilled Needs: Protection from psychologic threat, personal growth and maturity, increased learning, increased reality perception and problem-solving ability.

Explain the difference between salt and sodium diet restriction Explain that since salt consists of 40% sodium and 60% chloride, a dietary restriction of salt limits only the intake of sodium chloride. But sodium is not found only in salt (sodium chloride); it occurs in a variety of chemical compounds: sodium bicarbonate, sodium phosphate, sodium bromide, sodium carbonate, sodium citrate, sodium sulfate. A sodium-restricted diet restricts all these forms of sodium, and it necessitates very careful reading of product labels.

Rationale: In the presence of certain circulatory and renal disorders, excess sodium is not excreted effectively, resulting in edema, excess vascular fluid, and electrolyte imbalance.

Fulfilled Needs: Fluid and electrolyte balance, protection from physical harm, increased learning

Explain the difference between true and false labor pains   Explain that true labor pains occur at regular intervals that gradually become shorter; the pains increase in intensity, they are intensified by walking, they are located mainly in the back, and they are accompanied by bloody show. Explain that false labor pains occur at irregular long intervals, do not increase in intensity, are located mainly in the abdomen, are either relieved or unaffected by walking, and are not accompanied by bloody show.

Rationale: Knowledge that helps differentiate one problem from another promotes comfort.

Fulfilled Needs: Comfort, increased learning

Explain the dysfunctional family system of fixed triangles[471]   Explain that an emotional triangle consists of three people or two people and a group or issue. The person(s) can then focus on the third party or issue in the triangle rather than focus on the tension-producing conflict within themselves. In many dysfunctional families, one person or issue of the triangle is consistently used as a focus (scapegoat) for reducing stress. Parents often put their child in the triangle space that they were in as a child. This prevents them from constructively dealing with their own uncomfortable emotions.

Rationale: When persons want to distance themselves from uncomfortable closeness, they use the triangle method to avoid looking at and discussing emotionally charged subjects. This allows the person to focus on a more comfortable issue. Such behavior is dysfunctional in that it is used to avoid the real issue.

Fulfilled Needs: Increased learning, personal growth and maturity, increased reality perception and problem-solving ability

Explain the effects of the specific type pacemaker   Explain the specific effects of the type of pacemaker being used. An asynchronous pacemaker stimulates the ventricle at a preset rate regardless of the person's activity. A synchronous pacemaker stimulates the ventricle at a specific rate according to the person's activity and is often used by young persons. A demand pacemaker stimulates the ventricle if there is delayed natural stimulation.

Rationale: Awareness of the effects of therapeutic devices supports effective use of the devices.

Fulfilled Needs: Comfort, increased learning

Explain the emotional causes of reduced sexual response   Explain that the emotional causes of reduced sexual response are fear of motherhood, fear of venereal disease, fear of organic damage, fear that passionate appetite will cause self-degradation and loss of love, perception of sex as disgusting, inability to give oneself to another, homosexual tendencies, feeling dominated by a partner, feeling that it is wrong to enjoy sexual activity because of its procreative purpose, feeling inadequate as a person, feeling guilty because of extramarital relations, feeling that the sexual relationship with the husband indicates disloyalty to one's father.

Rationale: Awareness of causes of a situation frequently resolves the problem.

Fulfilled Needs: Comfort, sexuality, protection from psychologic threat, personal growth and maturity, increased learning, increased reality perception and problem-solving ability

Explain the essential factors that affect memory[774]   Explain that certain factors affect the ability to recall information: we must understand what we are trying to remember, we remember only what is important to us, what we learn must be reinforced if it is to be remembered, we remember things best that are outstanding and unique, we must focus on what we want to remember, and we must unclutter and relax our minds and allow time for assimilation of the information.

Rationale: An understanding of the essential factors that affect memory will improve the memory.

Fulfilled Needs: Increased learning, increased reality perception and problem-solving ability

Explain the genetic factors involved in the disease   Explain that certain diseases are passed from parents to children by transmission of genes in chromosomes. Explain to the parents the degree of probability that their child will inherit their disease. Make it clear to the parents that transmission of genes has not yet been brought under scientific control. Keep them informed of any medical breakthrough involving their particular disease.

Rationale: Knowledge of the genetic factors involved in disease transmission promotes understanding and offers some degree of comfort.

Fulfilled Needs: Comfort, protection from psychologic threat, increased learning

Explain the hazards of flat positioning/bottle propping during infant feeding   Explain that during bottle feedings, infants should not be laid flat or have the bottle propped with a pillow, etc. The child should be held in a head-elevated position or be sitting up when sucking a bottle.

Rationale: Propped bottles and flat positioning cause choking, ear infections. Dental caries occur when the infant goes to sleep sucking a bottle.

Fulfilled Needs: Protection from physical harm, increased learning

Explain the high-risk factors and how to reduce them   Provide a list of the factors that increase the risk of a person developing a familial or an environmental disease, or becoming injured. Explain what can be done to reduce those risks. For example, the risks of lung cancer include smoking, pollution. The risks can be reduced by not smoking.

Rationale: Knowledge of high-risk factors and how to prevent them, reduces the potential for disease or injury.

Fulfilled Needs: Protection from physical harm, increased learning

Explain the importance of blood replacement after transfusion   Explain that in order for health facilities to have adequate blood supplies, blood should be replaced by donations of family or friends when a transfusion is administered.

Rationale: Blood is available only through human donations, and a standby supply is essential to community health.

Fulfilled Needs: Protection from physical harm, increased learning

Explain the importance of continuing therapy   Explain that it is important to continue therapy for such reasons as preventing recurrence of signs and symptoms, achieving desired control or eradication of disease, and promoting comfort for the person.

Rationale: Explanations of why therapy should be continued promote understanding and acceptance of the therapy and reinforce compliance to prescribed self-therapy.

Fulfilled Needs: Protection from physical harm, increased learning

Explain the importance of correct message interpretation   Explain that the person communicating a message must be certain that the receiver has interpreted the message correctly. If the interpretation is inconsistent with the message, the misinterpretation must be corrected immediately.

Rationale: Correct message interpretation is essential to human understanding and good interpersonal relationships.

Fulfilled Needs: Protection from psychologic threat, caring and communicating relationships, increased learning

Explain the importance of developing and/or maintaining a positive self-attitude   Explain that each person must have a consistent, positive attitude toward himself. At some time each day, he should briefly reflect on what is good about himself.

Rationale: Positive attitudes toward oneself promote positive behavior.

Fulfilled Needs: Comfort, protection from psychologic threat, high self-evaluation, personal growth and maturity, increased learning

Explain the importance of eating on time   Emphasize that it is essential for the person to eat at the prescribed times. Point out that eating on time should take priority over other important activities.

Rationale: Diabetics must consistently eat at the specified time so as not to disrupt carbohydrate metabolism as it relates to insulin dosage.

Fulfilled Needs: Protection from physical harm, increased learning

Explain the importance of giving insulin on schedule[376]   Explain that insulin should be given before meals so that it will take effect during and after carbohydrate ingestion.

Rationale: When short-acting insulin is given before meals, the onset of insulin action will occur at about the same time as glucose intake. Since intermediate- and long-acting insulin have a delayed onset, they should be given before the intake of glucose in order to be available when the glucose reaches the bloodstream.

Fulfilled Needs: Protection from physical harm, mastery and competence in skills, independence, increased learning

Explain the importance of individual use of a comb and brush   Explain that each person should use only his own comb and brush.

Rationale: Individual use of a comb and brush prevents the transfer of scalp bacteria, parasites, dirt particles, and dandruff to other persons.

Fulfilled Needs: Cleanliness, protection from physical harm, increased learning

Explain the importance of learning and practicing health principles   Explain that by learning and practicing health principles, the potential for good health will be increased.

Rationale: Awareness of the importance of health information supports improved health.

Fulfilled Needs: Protection from physical harm, increased learning, increased reality perception and problem-solving ability

Explain the importance of meeting one's own needs as well as those of a significant other   Explain that when a person is meeting dependent or crisis needs of a significant other, he should determine his own needs at the time and see that they too are fulfilled.

Rationale: When a supportive person or care provider has his own needs meet, he can more adequately meet the needs of another. Disregarding his own needs in favor of another, reduces the competency with which the provider can function.

Fulfilled Needs: Protection from physical harm, protection from psychologic threat, sense of adequacy, increased learning

Explain the importance of periodic breast inspection/examination   Explain that the breasts should be inspected because early detection and treatment of breast abnormalities can save the person's life.

Rationale: Knowledge of the importance of an examination supports good health practice.

Fulfilled Needs: Protection from physical harm, increased learning

Explain the importance of persons offering emotional support to one another Explain that every person needs to feel that family and friends will support him during times of stress or crisis. This support should be freely offered between significant persons.

Rationale: Psychologic comfort and safety are promoted by support from significant persons who help meet physical and psychologic needs in times of stress.

Fulfilled Needs: Protection from psychologic threat, unity with loved ones, caring and communicating relationships, personal growth and maturity, increased learning, increased reality perception

Explain the importance of recognizing tension within oneself Explain that the person needs to be aware of when uncomfortable tension is occurring within him. Irritability, anxiousness, rushing about, clasping hands tightly are some signs of increased body tension.

Rationale: Early awareness of increased body tension provides the opportunity for decreasing the tension before it becomes a significant problem.

Fulfilled Needs: Comfort, protection from psychologic threat, increased learning

Explain the importance of remaining calm Explain that the ability to control emotions in a stressful situation is extremely important both for the person and for others.

Rationale: Calmness reduces internal tension, conserves the energy needed for action, supports realistic problem solving, and sets an example for others less likely to remain calm. If one person seeks self-gratification by attempting to cause another person emotional upset, only to find that the second person remains calm, he receives the communication that his attempt has served no purpose. This usually leads to calm, favorable behavior on the part of the instigator.

Fulfilled Needs: Energy, protection from psychologic threat, personal growth and maturity, increased learning, increased reality perception and problem-solving ability

Explain the importance of staying well informed on drug abuse Advise parents of teenage children to keep up with the latest scientific information on drug abuse.

Rationale: Well-informed parents can give accurate information to their children and make realistic decisions if drug problems arise.

Fulfilled Needs: Comfort, increased learning, increased reality perception and problem-solving ability

Explain the importance of testing cosmetics for skin irritation Explain that before new cosmetics are applied to the face, they should be tested on other skin areas such as the inner arm. If no irritation occurs, then it is probably safe to use them on the face.

Rationale: Early detection of potential skin irritants reduces the possibility of severe skin disorders.

Fulfilled Needs: Protection from physical harm, increased learning

Explain the importance of wearing a Medic Alert tag Explain that persons with chronic illnesses or diseases should wear Medic Alert tags in case they are in accidents or other situations in which they are unable to communicate.

Rationale: A .Medic Alert tag assures the person of prompt and accurate treatment for his chronic illness, and it minimizes the potential for adverse reactions to treatments used for his other injuries.

Fulfilled Needs: Protection from physical harm, increased learning

Explain the long-term effects of suicide on children Explain that when a significant other attempts or commits suicide, it affects the child for a lifetime. Children feel abandoned when left, but when left after a suicide, they feel they have been abandoned because of some wrongdoing that makes them deserving of abandonment, as a punishment. Such feelings often prevail for years or a lifetime.

Rationale: Knowledge of the effects of behavior on others often alters the behavior.

Fulfilled Needs: Protection from psychologic threat, increased learning, increased reality perception

Explain the meaning of premature birth Explain that an infant is considered premature if he weighs less than 5½ lb and is born sooner than 37 weeks after conception.

Rationale: Knowing the factors associated with prematurity clarifies the perception of the special needs of the infant.

Fulfilled Needs: Increased learning, increased reality perception

Explain the meaning of the diagnostic report/test(s) Explain to the person what x-ray reports, laboratory findings, and other studies mean in relationship to his specific problem.

Rationale: An understanding of the health problem promotes comfort, safety, and confidence in handling the problem.

Fulfilled Needs: Comfort, protection from physical harm, caring and communicating relationships, increased learning

Contraindications: Delay the explanation if it appears to heighten anxiety.

Explain the need for family restructuring during developmental stages[471] Explain that during different life phases, the structure of the family is changed to meet the changing needs of its members. When a grown child marries, the parents restructure by adjusting to the separation from the child, by including the child's spouse in the family, and by recognizing a new subsystem in the family. The young couple restructures by adjusting to parenting when their child is born, etc.

Rationale: Knowledge that family restructuring during developmental phases is a normal process and supports positive family changes.

Fulfilled Needs: Increased learning, increased reality perception and problem solving

Explain the need for frequent hair shampooing Explain that the hair should be shampooed once a week.

Rationale: Cleanliness prevents infection of hair and scalp.

Fulfilled Needs: Cleanliness, protection from physical harm, increased learning

Contraindications: Severe head trauma

Explain the need for increased nutrition during specific conditions Explain that during blood loss or anemia there is an increased need for high iron and protein foods, during tissue healing there should be an increased protein intake, during pregnancy a higher protein and calcium intake is desirable, during lactation the need for calories and calcium increases, during high fever an increased metabolic rate is needed, during high energy-consuming activity the body needs increased carbohydrates, during growth periods increased protein intake is necessary, and smokers require an increased intake of vitamins B and C.

Rationale: Knowledge of the need for increased nutritional requirements helps maintain and promote health.

Fulfilled Needs: Nutritional balance, protection from physical harm, increased learning

Explain the need for maintaining a firm surface under the hip of an amputated leg Explain that a firm mattress should be placed under the hips of a patient who has had a leg amputated, to prevent hip sagging.

Rationale: Hip sagging will cause flexion contracture of the amputation stump, which will impair the effective use of a prosthesis.

Fulfilled Needs: Protection from physical harm, increased learning

Explain the need for nail cleanliness Explain that fingernails and toenails should be cleaned daily by brushing or soaking in soap and water.

Rationale: Cleanliness prevents infection in body areas that come in contact with the fingers.

Fulfilled Needs: Cleanliness, protection from physical harm. Increased learning

Explain the need for pleasant mealtimes Explain that mealtime conversation should revolve around pleasant subjects. The atmosphere should be unhurried and relaxed.

Rationale: Unpleasant conversation causes muscular tension, reduces appetite, and impairs digestion.

Fulfilled Needs: Protection from physical harm, increased learning

Explain the need for properly fitting dentures Explain that dentures that do not fit properly should be readjusted.

Rationale: Dentures that do not fit properly irritate the mouth and prevent effective chewing of food.

Fulfilled Needs: Protection from physical harm, increased learning

Explain the need for realistic expectations of others Explain that in many cases in which a person feels he is not being treated with the consideration he deserves, he is expecting more from others than he should realistically expect.

Rationale: Some persons perceive the normal self-concerns of others to be threatening to their own self-concerns. Realizing that most people are normally preoccupied with their own problems supports realistic perception that this normal concern is not an expression of rejection by others.

Fulfilled Needs: Comfort, protection from psychologic threat, personal growth and maturity, increased learning, increased reality perception and problem-solving ability

Explain the need for scheduled bowel eliminations Explain that it is advisable to set a time for daily bowel elimination, preferably at an unhurried hour of the day.

Rationale: Body systems function best when a regular schedule is followed.

Fulfilled Needs: Waste elimination of food residue, comfort, protection from physical harm, increased learning

Explain the need to avoid contaminated soil Explain that soil contaminated with parasites or worms should be kept away from the hands and face.

Rationale: Parasites and worms promote disease.

Fulfilled Needs: Protection from physical harm, increased learning

Explain the need to avoid overexertion Explain that exercising beyond normal limits, exercising strenuously when unaccustomed to doing so, becoming involved in very heavy activity, or overexerting when one is recuperating and feeling reasonably well places stress on the body. If the body cannot accommodate to the stress, one or more systems may fail to function.

Rationale: Strenuous exercise increases tissue requirements for oxygen as well as the rate and amount of blood that must be pumped through the heart to the muscles, causing elevated arterial and venous pressures and possibly inadequate tissue oxygenation. Overexertion taxes the body's energy supply.

Fulfilled Needs: Tissue oxygenation or perfusion, energy, protection from physical harm, increased learning

Explain the need to avoid sudden movements of an extremity having an arteriovenous shunt Explain that an extremity containing an arteriovenous shunt should not be moved suddenly and forcefully, especially not in a twisting motion. It should be moved slowly and smoothly.

Rationale: Sudden extremity movements can pull an arteriovenous shunt joint apart and cause hemorrhage.

Fulfilled Needs: Protection from physical harm, increased learning

Explain the need to avoid trauma/mechanical trauma Explain that body injury of any type should be avoided, including activities that tend to result in trauma, such as skateboard riding and climbing up on high objects. Explain that mechanical trauma in which there is forceful body contact with other objects should be avoided, such as contact sports, dropping heavy objects on oneself, accidentally cutting oneself, and running into doors, chairs, table corners, or other potentially harmful objects.

Rationale: Avoiding trauma prevents bodily injury that could precipitate crisis situations in existing disease states. Avoiding trauma prevents injury.

Fulfilled Needs: Protection from physical harm, increased learning

Explain the need to predict and plan for change Explain that anxiety can be reduced by admitting that certain changes probably will occur and by making definite plans to meet those changes. For instance, we are reasonably sure of growing old and can realistically plan for it.

Rationale: Anxiety results from a sense of helplessness. Helplessness can be overcome through prediction and planning.

Fulfilled Needs: Comfort, protection from psychologic threat, predictable, orderly world, personal growth and maturity, increased learning, increased reality perception and problem-solving ability

Explain the need to recognize highly stressful situations Explain the importance of being aware of situations that place one under intense stress. Each person should learn to recognize which situations cause him stress. Significant others should avoid causing situations that place undue stress on a person.

Rationale: Recognition of highly stressful situations gives the person and his significant others an opportunity to avoid such situations or modify the degree of stress.

Fulfilled Needs: Comfort, protection from physical harm, protection from psychologic stress, increased learning

Explain the options available for family planning Explain that there are options for controlling conception, such as drugs, the rhythm method, intrauterine devices, and condoms. Include a discussion of the person's religious and cultural beliefs and practices regarding family planning.

Rationale: Knowledge of family planning methods provides choices suitable to the person's religious and cultural beliefs.

Fulfilled Needs: Protection from physical harm, increased learning

Explain the physical causes of reduced sexual response Explain that the physical causes of reduced sexual response include pathology of sex organs or nearby organs, external genital lesions, endocrine disorders, drug- or alcohol-induced anesthesia, and fatigue.

Rationale: Awareness of the causes of sexual problems reduces anxiety and supports solution of the problem.

Fulfilled Needs: Comfort, sexuality, protection from psychologic threat, increased learning, increased reality perception and problem-solving ability

Explain the physical/behavioral changes that occur during the developmental phases[105,148,149]
Explain that normal physical changes and functioning abilities or developmental tasks occur as the person moves through different phases of life. Give examples:

Early childhood: Ages 0-6 years   Rapid physical growth, developing motor coordination, acquiring trust in self and others, achieving a self-concept, learning to live in a group, learning personal care, and developing use of language.

Middle childhood: Ages 6-12 years   Learning both physical and intellectual skills, social roles, and sharing responsibility, living in a wider physical and social world, and establishing values.

Adolescence: Ages 12-18 years   Development of secondary sex characteristics, adjusting to body changes, becoming more independent with a clearer sense of identity and self-confidence, and preparing for an occupation, marriage, and family life.

Early adulthood: Ages 18-35 years   Assuming an occupation, marrying, starting a family, and managing a home, and assuming civic responsibilities.

Middle age: Ages 35-60 years   Adjusting to physiologic changes of the menopause and climacteric, helping children to mature and become independent, assuming occupational, civic, and social responsibilities, preparing for later financial security, and adjusting to aging parents.

Old age: Over age 60   Adjusting to physiologic changes of decreased strength, to retirement and reduced income, and to loss of spouse and friends.

Rationale: Knowledge of the expected level of functioning during different life phases helps the person set goals for normal development.

Fulfilled Needs: Personal growth and maturity, increased learning

Explain the psychologic causes of organic pain
Explain that organic pain can result from muscle tension and nerve stimulation caused by stress situations.

Rationale: Awareness that stress can produce organic pain should support attempts at reducing stress situations, with emphasis on relaxation.

Fulfilled Needs: Protection from physical harm, protection from psychologic threat, personal growth and maturity, increased learning, increased reality perception and problem-solving ability

Contraindications: Delay explanation if it appears to heighten anxiety.

Explain the reason for and intended effect of the therapy/study/examination/hygienic care/methods used/agency services/preventive therapy/assistive therapy/wellness behavior
Explain why certain specific treatments, studies, examinations, etc., are recommended or are being incorporated into the patient's plan of care. Let him know what effects they will have on his health condition.

Rationale: Knowledge of why treatments, studies, examinations, etc., are performed and their intended effects reduces anxiety and promotes comfort.

Fulfilled Needs: Comfort, protection from psychologic threat, increased learning

Explain the reason for delaying the prosthesis application
Explain that applying a stump prosthesis is often delayed to allow for deep tissue healing, which takes about 6 weeks. If pressure is applied to the tissue before healing is complete, tissue injury and excessively long inactivity may result.

Rationale: Knowledge of why treatments are delayed reduces anxiety and promotes comfort.

Fulfilled Needs: Comfort, protection from psychologic threat, increased learning

Explain the reason for the delay in giving a pain relief drug
Explain that the administration of pain relief drugs is often delayed because of the possibility of side effects occurring from frequent drug dosage. Be sure that the patient understands that staff apathy is not the reason for the delay.

Rationale: Knowledge of why treatments are delayed reduces anxiety and promotes comfort.

Fulfilled Needs: Comfort, protection from psychologic threat, increased learning.

Explain the relationship between conflict and psychogenic pain
Explain that psychogenic pain is a symbolic means of attempting to solve emotional conflict and that it occurs at the subconscious level.

Rationale: Awareness of behavioral mechanisms supports healthy behavioral responses.

Fulfilled Needs: Protection from psychologic threat, personal growth and maturity, increased learning, increased reality perception and problem-solving ability

Explain the reproductive process[169]
Explain that pregnancy results from union of a female egg with a male spermatozoon. One egg is discharged from the ovary each month; it then works its way into the fallopian tube. If intercourse occurs at the right time, the spermatozoon penetrates the egg in the fallopian tube and fertilization takes place. The fertilized egg then moves itself into the uterus and embeds itself in the uterine lining, where fetal development begins.

Rationale: Knowledge of physiologic processes promotes comfort and safety.

Fulfilled Needs: Comfort, protection from physical harm, increased learning

Explain the side effects of various family planning methods
Explain that methods of contraception have some adverse side effects. Oral contraceptives can cause breast tenderness, bleed-through, amenorrhea after the pill has been stopped, altered thyroid function, fluid retention, hypertension, an elevated glucose level, or mood changes. Intrauterine devices can cause pain, bleeding, vaginal infection, etc.

Rationale: Knowledge of the side effects of various family planning methods gives the person a broader base of knowledge from which to choose.

Fulfilled Needs: Protection from physical harm, increased learning

Explain the significance of premature membrane rupture and that it does not indicate difficult labor
Explain that once the uterine membrane ruptures, labor onset will follow within 24–46 hours. Reassure the patient that early rupture of the membrane does not mean that labor will be difficult. Even though the bulk of amniotic fluid is lost at membrane rupture, the fluid is continuously being produced until delivery occurs. Its lubricating quality facilitates ease of birth.

Rationale: Knowledge of normal physiologic responses promotes comfort.

Fulfilled Needs: Comfort, increased learning

Explain the significance of regressive behavior in illness
Explain that return to an earlier behavioral pattern is the patient's way of coping with the anxiety and insecurity of illness or hospitalization. When a child displays regressive behavior, the parents may need help in accepting his behavior until he is ready to resume behavior appropriate for his developmental stage. Adults often display regressive behavior by desiring more attention and wanting to be waited on.

Rationale: Significant others are often embarrassed by the regressive behavior of a loved one. If such behavior occurs in a child, they may scold or punish the child, increasing his feelings of insecurity and inadequacy. Loving acceptance during the stressful period will help the person adjust more quickly.

Fulfilled Needs: Protection from psychologic threat, dependence, increased learning

Explain the various types of insulin and their effects[376]   Explain that there are three different kinds of insulin. Regular and Semilente (short-acting) are quickly absorbed and last for a short duration. NPH, Globin, and Lente (intermediate-acting) are absorbed with moderate speed and lasts for a moderate duration. PZI and Ultralente (long-acting) are slowly absorbed and have a long duration. Explain that all types of insulin come in three concentrations: 40 units/ml (U40), 80 units/ml (U80), and 100 units/ml (U100).

Rationale: Understanding the various types of insulin and their effects increases the probability of correct insulin dosage.

Fulfilled Needs: Protection from physical harm, mastery and competence in skills, independence, increased learning

Explain those menstrual variations that indicate abnormality   Explain that menstruation is considered abnormal if it occurs more frequently than every 21 days, if it occurs less frequently than every 35 days, if its duration is less than 3 days or more than 7 days, or if more than 12 perineal pads are used within a 24-hour period.

Rationale: Knowledge of normal physiologic processes promotes safety.

Fulfilled Needs: Protection from physical harm, increased learning

Explain to families the importance of role modeling through abstinence from drug use   Explain that if the family does not want its children to use drugs, alcohol, or tobacco, they must set an example by not using them. This also applies to those in the presence of anyone struggling to curtail habituation.

Rationale: Children who grow up in families where drugs, alcohol, and tobacco are not used are less likely to indulge in them. Seeing others use drugs for pain relief can cause an automatic expectation of relief of distress through drugs. Alcoholics frequently resent seeing others drink when they are struggling not to, and this often precipitates a drinking episode.

Fulfilled Needs: Increased learning

Explain what is considered justifiable aggression   Explain that in most cultures aggression is justified when self-defense is necessary.

Rationale: Healthy adjustment maintains a balance between appropriate assertiveness and antisocial aggressive impulses.

Fulfilled Needs: Protection from psychologic threat, personal growth and maturity, increased learning, increased reality perception and problem-solving ability

Explain when to perform the procedure   Give the person information as to the time of day and length of each treatment.

Rationale: Specific information about the time for performing procedures supports compliance and a more accurate therapy.

Fulfilled Needs: Protection from physical harm, increased learning

Explain when showering should be substituted for tub bathing during pregnancy   Explain that pregnant women may bathe in a tub until such time as the membrane ruptures, the mucus plug is passed, or bleeding occurs. Showering is recommended after any one of these occurs.

Rationale: After the membrane ruptures or the mucus plug is passed or bleeding occurs, tub bathing heightens the potential for vaginal infection because of vaginal exposure to unclean water. Showering provides constantly running clean water, which reduces the chance of vaginal infection.

Fulfilled Needs: Comfort, cleanliness, protection from physical harm, increased learning

Explain when the postpartum flow normally resumes Explain that when a mother is not breast feeding her infant, menstruation usually resumes about 8 weeks after delivery. Mothers who are breast feeding usually do not resume menstruation until breast feeding has stopped. However, both menstruation and pregnancy have been known to occur during the period of breast feeding.

Rationale: Knowledge of normal physiologic processes promotes comfort.

Fulfilled Needs: Comfort, increased learning

Explain which drugs and foods have adverse interactions[212,565] Explain specifically which foods and drugs should not be mixed. Included here are some of the more common interactions. For a complete listing, refer to a drug reference book.

Alcohol: Avoid drinking alcohol, which increases the drug effect of all drugs listed except those with other effects noted: antihistamines, antihypertensive drugs, aspirin (causes stomach bleeding), barbiturates, Flagyl (causes nausea, cramps), hypnotics, MAO inhibitors, muscle relaxants, narcotics (codiene, Demerol) sedatives, tranquilizers (Valium).

Antacids: Avoid taking antacids, which decrease drug absorption and the therapeutic effect of all oral drugs listed: antibiotics (tetracycline, oral penicillins), digitalis, Dulcolax, Lomotil, quinidine, time-release capsules.

Antibiotics: Taking antibiotics with the following decreases the antibiotic absorption and therapeutic effect: antacids, cheese (specific to penicillin), citrus juices, high-calcium foods/fluids, iron or zinc compounds, magnesium-containing laxatives. Mixing penicillin and tetracycline decreases the effect of the penicillin. For maximum absorption, antibiotics should be taken 1 hour before or 2 hours after eating

Anticoagulants: To avoid increased bleeding, do not take anticoagulants with aspirin, cimetidine (Tagamet) Orinase or Tolinase, vitamin E. To avoid decreased anticoagulant effectiveness, do not take anticoagulants with estrogen, oral contraceptives. To avoid decreased anticoagulant effectiveness, do not mix with high-fat or high-protein foods or raw vegetables such as cabbage and okra. Do not go on a diet without first discussing it with a physician. To avoid decreased effectiveness of other drugs, do not take anticoagulants with vitamins B_6, C, or K or levodopa.

Antidepressants: To avoid a toxic reaction, do not take antidepressants with any other drug.

Antihypertensive drugs: Avoid taking antihypertensive drugs with the following, which increase the hypotensive effect: alcohol, barbiturates, levodopa, Levoprome, MAO inhibitors (Pargyline), phenothiazines, procainamide (Pronestyl), quinidine, tricyclic antidepressants. Concurrent use of the following could increase the hypertensive state: amphetamines, ephedrine, norepinephrine, phenylephrine (Neo-Synephrine).

Aspirin: Alcohol, anticoagulants, and Indocin, when mixed with aspirin, will increase the potential for bleeding. Oral diabetic drugs (Orinase, Tolinase), when taken with aspirin, result in a·dangerously low blood sugar. The therapeutic effect of Motrin or iron compounds is decreased when combined with aspirin.

Corticosteroids: Cortisone, when taken with the following drugs, decreases drug absorption: calcium, iron, magnesium, vitamin A. Cortisone, when taken with a thiazide diuretic, increases potassium loss.

Digitalis: To avoid a toxic reaction, do not take the following with digitalis: corticosteroids, diuretics without potassium replacement, laxatives, sympathometics (Afrin, Bronkosol, Neo-Synephrine, etc.). To avoid severe bradycardia, do not take digitalis with propranolol.

Diuretics: To avoid a toxic reaction, do not take the following with diuretics: digitalis, dyazide and potassium, lithium. To avoid severe potassium loss, do not combine the following: Thiazides and corticosteroids, thiazides and licorice.

Licorice: To avoid sodium retention and potassium loss, do not ingest licorice with digitalis or diuretics. To avoid a toxic reaction, do not ingest licorice with MAO inhibitors.

Tagamet (cimetidine):   To avoid adverse effects, do not take Tagamet with the following: aminophyllin (causes anxiety or depression), Coumadin (causes stomach bleeding), Inderal (causes severe bradycardia), Valium (causes oversedation).

Monoamine oxidase (MAO) inhibitors: To avoid a toxic reaction, do not take MAO inhibitors with any other drug (while taking the MAO inhibitor and for 3 weeks after the drug is discontinued) or with any foods containing tyramine (cheese, alcohol, yeast, yogurt, caffeine, liver, chicken livers, pickled herring, broad beans, figs, licorice).

Oral hypoglycemic (or antidiabetic) drugs (Orinase, Tolinase):   To avoid an accentuated hypoglycemia, do not take oral hypoglycemic drugs with aspirin, Coumadin, butazolidine, propranolol (Inderal). Concurrent use of oral hypoglycemic drugs and anticoagulants results in an increased or decreased effect of the anticoagulant drug.

Rationale: Knowledge of expected drug and food interactions prevents adverse effects.

Fulfilled Needs: Protection from physical harm, increased learning

Explain which foods are or are not recommended for the diet   Give the person a list of foods that are and are not recommended for his specific diet.

Rationale: Only when the person knows exactly what foods comprise a diet can he successfully carry out a therapeutic plan.

Fulfilled Needs: Nutritional balance, protection from physical harm, increased learning

Explain why persons resort to drug/alcohol abuse   Explain that persons take drugs and alcohol for group acceptance, for excitement, to cope with emotional problems, as a means of rejecting and shaming parents by whom they feel rejected, and as a stimulant to increase efficiency.

Rationale: Knowledge of the causes of drug or alcohol abuse facilitates understanding the problem as an illness.

Fulfilled Needs: Increased learning, increased reality perception and problem-solving ability

Explain why persons should maintain self-control   Explain that self-control is maintained out of respect for other persons and to obtain social approval.

Rationale: Awareness of the reasons for behavior supports healthy behavioral responses.

Fulfilled Needs: Personal growth and maturity, increased learning, increased reality perception and problem-solving ability

Explain why the potential problem could become actual   Give reasons why a nonexisting problem could occur. Be specific in terms of what the actual problem could be.

Rationale: Knowledge of why a problem could occur increases one's understanding of the problem and reasons for preventive measures.

Fulfilled Needs: Protection from physical harm, protection from psychologic threat, increased learning

Familiarize the person with the component parts of the equipment   Show the person all parts of the equipment. Explain how each part functions. Demonstrate how pieces come apart and fit back together. Explain the purpose of and how to use the equipment.

Rationale: Knowledge of how therapeutic equipment functions increases the probability of correct and independent use of that equipment.

Fulfilled Needs: Protection from physical harm, independence, increased learning

Inform about various assistive devices for the wheelchair

Inform the person of special devices that can be used on a wheelchair, such as hand grips on the wheel rims, which make it easier to propel the chair, apparatus for narrowing the chair as it goes through doorways, and motors that move the chair with the touch of a switch.

Rationale: Assistive devices on a wheelchair can increase the person's independent mobility.

Fulfilled Needs: Independence, increased learning

Inform as to the correct terminology used for elimination

Explain that the proper terms to describe defecation are stool, feces, and bowel movement. Explain that the proper terms for passing urine are voiding and urinating.

Rationale: Small children being toilet trained should be taught the proper terminology for elimination.

Fulfilled Needs: Increased learning

Inform family members of the need for both emotional closeness and separateness[471]

Explain that while people need to feel emotionally close to others, they also need a separate identity as an individual person apart from others in the family. Excessive emotional fusion destroys this separateness and interferes with mature personal growth.

Rationale: Knowledge of needs of family members supports the probability that needs will be met.

Fulfilled Needs: Increased learning, personal growth and maturity, increased reality perception and problem-solving ability.

Inform of the American Heart Association's recommended exercise schedule[746]

Explain the American Heart Association's recommended schedule for specific exercises:

Walking, running, and jogging: Recommend the wearing of thick-soled shoes and exercise on grass, dirt road, or running track rather than pavement. For all the following time limits, the person should continue the exercise until pulse reaches the maximum rate for the person's age: walk briskly 1 mile in 30 minutes, then walk 1 mile in 20 minutes, then walk 2 miles in 40 minutes, then walk 3 miles in 60 minutes, then walk 3.5 miles in 1 hour, then jog 4–5 miles in 1 hour, then run 6 miles in 1 hour.

Swimming: Do the breast stroke for 5 minutes for warmup, swim vigorously for 5–20 minutes, stay in the water resting for 5 minutes for cooling period.

Cycling: Cycle slowly on flat land or in low gear for 5 minutes for warmup, cycle rapidly on flat land in high gear or up and down hills in normal gear for 20 minutes, cycle slowly on flat land or in low gear for 5 minutes for cooling period.

Jumping rope: *First week:* Jump in place 100 times for warmup, jump 50 times at a comfortable speed for conditioning period, add 10 skips a day for 4 days so that the person will be jumping 90 times at the end of the 4th day. *Second week:* Hop 50 times for warmup, skip 100 times for conditioning period, add 10 skips a day for 4 days. *Third week:* Hop 50 times for warmup, skip 100 times for conditioning period, rest 15–30 seconds, skip again 100 times. *Fourth week and after:* Same schedule as for third week, only add skips until breathless, or until the person reaches 500 skips per minute.

Rationale: Muscular exertion through exercise enhances free joint movement, strengthens muscle tone, develops coordination, and promotes increased blood circulation, which supports lowered blood pressure and decreased oxygen needs of the cardiopulmonary system. It improves carbohydrate metabolism and reduces the amount of adrenal hormones secreted by the body during emotional stress. It increases the endurance of the body to undergo physical and emotional stress with less fatigue and better performance. Exercise uses up excessive body calories, thereby supporting healthy weight management. Exercise improves pelvic circulation and stretches pelvic ligaments, reducing menstrual pain.

Fulfilled Needs: Tissue oxygenation or perfusion, exercise, protection from physical harm, mastery and competence in skills, independence, increased learning

Contraindications: Fever, states of severe energy depletion or increased metabolic rate, and acute illness. Any person who has an elevated blood pressure, elevated serum cholesterol, triglycerides or uric acid, abnormal electrocardiogram, known cardiac condition, chest pain, is on cardiac drugs, has a family history of heart disease, has diabetes, asthma or emphysema, has any condition such as arthritis or gout in which muscle or joint motion would aggravate the condition, has dyspnea or intermittent claudication (leg cramping when walking), or any chronic illness should be seen and evaluated by a physician before starting an exercise program.

Inform of the contraindications for exercising[746] Explain that there are conditions during which exercise is not recommended: fever, states of severe energy depletion or increased metabolic rate, during acute illness. Any person who has an elevated blood pressure, elevated serum cholesterol, triglycerides or uric acid, abnormal electrocardiogram, known cardiac condition, chest pain, is on cardiac drugs, has a family history of heart disease, has diabetes, asthma or emphysema, has any condition such as arthritis or gout in which muscle or joint motion would aggravate the condition, has dyspnea or intermittent claudication (leg cramping when walking), or any chronic illness should be seen and evaluated by a physician before starting an exercise program.

Rationale: Knowledge of the contraindications for exercising reduces the potential for physical injury.

Fulfilled Needs: Protection from physical harm, independence, increased learning

Inform of the factors that affect growth and development Relate those factors that affect growth and development, such as state of health, nutrition, emotional love and security, education, and exposure to positive reinforcement.

Rationale: Knowledge of growth and development factors supports the use of such factors for positive growth and development.

Fulfilled Needs: Protection from physical harm, protection from psychologic threat, increased learning

Inform of the recommended length of infant nursing periods Explain that the length of infant nursing period varies with each baby and mother. Much depends on the comfort or discomfort the mother experiences. When infants are first fed by the breast, the usual time is from 1 to 10 minutes, with gradual daily increases up to 20 minutes. If the mother's breasts are cracked, nursing should be limited to short periods.

Rationale: Adequate nursing periods are essential for the comfort and safety of the mother and infant.

Fulfilled Needs: Comfort, protection from physical harm, increased learning

Inform of the recommended minimum hours of sleep[371] Explain that it is recommended that average healthy persons obtain these amounts of sleep each day, although sleep requirements are individualized somewhat:

Infants	10–20 hours
Children	10–14 hours
Adults	7– 9 hours
Aging persons	5– 7 hours

Ill persons require more sleep than healthy persons.

Rationale: Adequate daily sleep is essential to the replacement of energy within tissue cells.

Fulfilled Needs: Sleep and rest, energy, protection from physical harm, increased learning

Inform of the resources available for health care Make known to the person the health agencies and institutions that are available to assist in solving his particular health problem, such as rehabilitation and financial resources.

Rationale: Knowledge and use of available health resources promote improved health status and independent self-care.

Fulfilled Needs: Protection from physical harm, independence, increased learning

Inform of the therapies available for the specific condition Provide information on the different therapeutic approaches that can be used to improve the person's specific condition.

Rationale: Awareness of the therapies available for improving health reduces anxiety and provides factual information that can support optimum decision-making.

Fulfilled Needs: Comfort, protection from psychologic threat, increased learning, increased reality perception and problem-solving ability

Inform of the time-zone changes that cause jet lag Explain that jet lag does not occur when flying north or south because the time zones are not changed, that jet lag does occur when flying east or west because of multiple time zones, that time zone changes cause a discrepancy between the actual time of day and the time according to the person's circadian rhythm thus adding hours to or taking from the person's normal cycle, and that adjustment is more difficult on flights away from home than on flights toward home because the person is moving toward an unfamiliar environment, which in itself causes stress.

Rationale: Knowledge of time-zone changes assists the person in adjusting to the environmental changes.

Fulfilled Needs: Comfort, increased learning

Inform of the warning signs to exercise less vigorously[746] Explain that the following physical manifestations indicate that exercise should be pursued less vigorously: an elevated heart rate that persists for 5–10 minutes after stopping the exercise, symptoms of arthritis or gout, nausea or vomiting, severe breathlessness, prolonged fatigue, shin splints (front or side leg pain), acute insomnia, muscle cramps in the calves, stitch (pain) under the ribs.

Rationale: Exercise that causes moderately unfavorable side effects must be decreased in terms of degree of exertion to prevent tissue damage and impaired body function.

Fulfilled Needs: Protection from physical harm, independence, increased learning

Inform of the warning signs to stop exercising[746] Explain that the following physical manifestations indicate that exercise should be stopped immediately: irregular, rapid, or very slow heartbeat, abnormal heart rhythm such as fluttering or palpitations, pain or pressure in the arm, throat, or center of the chest, dizziness, lightheadedness, impaired coordination, confusion, cold sweats, pallor, cyanosis, or fainting.

Rationale: Exercise that causes severe unfavorable side effects must be stopped immediately to prevent tissue damage and impaired body function.

Fulfilled Needs: Protection from physical harm, independence, increased learning

Inform of those conditions that precipitate seizures Explain that certain conditions should be avoided because they tend to stimulate epileptic seizures. They include excessive food or liquid intake, excitement, overexertion, inadequate rest, fever, infection, an irregular daily schedule, and flashing light patterns.

Rationale: Avoiding conditions that precipitate seizures reduces the potential for seizures.

Fulfilled Needs: Protection from physical harm, increased learning

Inform of when to do the breast examination[73] Explain that breast inspection for tumors should be done once a month, 1–2 days after completion of menstruation.

After menopause occurs, the examination should be done once a month, at the same time each month.

Rationale: Early detection of breast abnormalities reduces the potential for severe and advanced breast diseases.

Fulfilled Needs: Protection from physical harm, increased learning

Inform that a brown vaginal discharge often indicates uterine carcinoma

Explain that a foul-smelling, watery, dark brown vaginal discharge is indicative of a cancerous lesion and should be reported immediately.

Rationale: Malignant cells within an organ cause tissue damage.

Fulfilled Needs: Protection from physical harm, increased learning

Inform that a child should be diapered only at night during toilet training

Explain that during toilet training, a child should be diapered only at night and should wear pants during the day.

Rationale: Diapers imply elimination without heed to time or place. Gradually discontinuing the use of diapers supports accommodation to more acceptable patterns of elimination and introduces the child to greater feelings of comfort.

Fulfilled Needs: Comfort, increased learning

Inform that a child should be dressed in easily removable clothes for toileting

Explain that toilet training can be facilitated if the child is dressed in pants that slip down easily, in trousers with a few large buttons, and in easily removed playsuits.

Rationale: Hard-to-remove clothing results in frustration and rebellion, which retard learning.

Fulfilled Needs: Comfort, increased learning

Inform that a child should be fully awakened during nightime toileting

Explain that when a child is taken to the bathroom at night, he should be fully awakened so that he knows that toileting is taking place.

Rationale: To learn conscious sphincter control, full awareness is necessary.

Fulfilled Needs: Comfort, increased learning

Inform that a clear, mucoid vaginal discharge occurs with ovulation

Explain that a clear, stringy vaginal discharge indicates that ovulation is occurring.

Rationale: Knowledge of normal physiologic processes promotes comfort.

Fulfilled Needs: Comfort, increased learning

Inform that a predisposition to the illness exists

Inform the patient that inherited factors passed from parents to children make the children susceptible to certain diseases. Explain that frequent physical examinations should be scheduled as a precautionary measure when a certain disease is prevalent in a family.

Rationale: Recognition of a predisposition to specific diseases should support early detection and treatment of the disease.

Fulfilled Needs: Protection from physical harm. Increased learning.

Inform that a yellow, purulent vaginal discharge indicates inflammation

Explain that a yellow, puslike vaginal discharge is indicative of inflammation and infection in the reproductive system. It should be reported immediately.

Rationale: Infection or inflammation of organs causes tissue damage.

Fulfilled Needs: Protection from physical harm. Increased learning.

Inform that afterbirth pains following delivery are normal

Explain that for 24 to 48 hours after delivery, spasm-type abdominal pains will normally be felt.

Rationale: Awareness that afterbirth pains are normal involuntary uterine contractions produced to expel lochia and return the uterus to normal size promotes comfort.

Fulfilled Needs: Comfort, increased learning

Inform that airway noise indicates obstruction   Explain that snoring or wheezing breath sounds indicate that an obstruction is preventing optimal ventilation of the lungs.

Rationale: A patent airway is essential for respiratory exchange of oxygen and carbon dioxide.

Fulfilled Needs: Protection from physical harm, increased learning

Inform that artificial larynxes are available   Explain to the person who has had a laryngectomy that several kinds of electronic and mechanical larynx devices are available.

Rationale: The use of an artificial larynx device supports verbal communication.

Fulfilled Needs: Comfort, caring and communicating relationships, increased learning.

Inform that bathing is permitted when wearing a pacemaker   Teach the patient wearing a pacemaker that he may bathe so long as he keeps the wires and generator box dry.

Rationale: Knowledge of how to use therapeutic equipment promotes safety.

Fulfilled Needs: Protection from physical harm, increased learning

Inform that battery monitors should be disconnected during tub bathing or showering   Teach the patient who has a battery-operated monitor to disconnect the monitor from the leads when taking a tub bath or shower and reconnect them later. Disconnecting the monitor is not necessary for sponge bathing.

Rationale: If a battery-operated monitor becomes wet, it can damage the monitoring equipment. Knowledge that there is no danger of electrocution from a wet monitor promotes comfort.

Fulfilled Needs: Comfort, increased learning

Inform that bearing down aids the progress of second stage labor   Teach the patient to strain, as if to force a bowel movement, during the second stage of labor.

Rationale: Bearing down assists in pushing the infant through the vaginal canal.

Fulfilled Needs: Protection from physical harm. Increased learning.

Contraindications: First stage of labor

Inform that bribing and threatening are ineffective child discipline methods   Explain that in disciplining children, the use of material rewards and gifts leads the child to believe that favorable behavior earns him a reward, whereas it should be seen as merely a part of social interaction. Expressed intentions to inflict injury do not gain the child's cooperation; they result in hostility. The child begins to perceive the adult–child relationship with resentment, and he comes to feel threatened because his previously secure relationship has been weakened.

Rationale: Effective methods of discipline support child socialization while maintaining a secure child-parent relationship and a sense of adequacy.

Fulfilled Needs: Protection from psychologic threat, sense of adequacy, growth and maturity, increased learning, increased reality perception and problem-solving ability

Inform that carbonated beverages are safe to drink in foreign countries   Explain that it is safe to drink carbonated soft drinks, mineral water, and beer in foreign countries.

Rationale: The carbonation process makes liquids safe from contamination.

Fulfilled Needs: Protection from physical harm, increased learning

Inform that children are receptive to stages of toilet training at different ages   *Bladder control:*   Explain that the infant's bladder has minimal urine retention capacity until the age of *12–18 months*. At *15–16 months* the bladder is sufficiently developed that the child will stay dry for about 2 hours at a time. At *18–24 months* the child is aware of his full bladder. He notifies adults when he is wet, he may want to go to the bathroom frequently because of pride of accomplishment, and he needs assistance with dressing and getting on the seat. He wears training pants. At age *2–2½ years* the child goes alone to the bathroom; he stays dry most of the day, but he still has occasional accidents. At age *3–3½ years* the child usually stays dry at night but has occasional accidents.

Bowel control: Beginning at *7 or 8 months* of age, the child has no voluntary control, but he may have bowel movements at the same time every day. At age *12–18 months* the child is irregular. He can verbally identify the bowel movement, he is proud of his accomplishment, and he may have a movement immediately after getting off the commode. If he fusses about being placed on the commode, this indicates that training should be delayed. At age *18–24 months* the child will notify adults that his diaper is soiled. Dirtiness bothers him, and he may show aversion to the stool. He likes to flush the commode, but he may have the fear that he will be flushed down the commode. He wears training pants. At age *2 years* the child has developed control, with only occasional accidents. At age *2½ years* the child uses the toilet alone.

Rationale: Knowledge of what to expect in the way of normal behavior promotes comfort and realistic expectations.

Fulfilled Needs: Comfort, increased learning

Inform that clean cooking utensils are essential
Explain that cooking utensils must be free of food, dust, or grime before they are used. If necessary, they should be washed before use.

Rationale: Cleanliness inhibits the growth of bacteria and reduces the potential for infection and disease.

Fulfilled Needs: Cleanliness, protection from physical harm, increased learning

Inform that clean linens are essential
Explain that bed linens should be washed at least once a week, and towels and washcloths should be washed several times a week. If possible, a clean towel and washcloth should be used for each bath, especially when bating infants.

Rationale: Cleanliness reduces the potential for infection.

Fulfilled Needs: Cleanliness, protection from physical harm, increased learning

Inform that cleanliness is basic to health/essential to infection prevention
Explain that cleanliness inhibits the growth of bacteria and therefore reduces the potential for disease.

Rationale: Cleanliness prevents infection.

Fulfilled Needs: Cleanliness, protection from physical harm, increased learning

Inform that clothing should be worn between the brace and the skin
Explain that socks or stockings should be worn under a leg brace. A T-shirt should be worn under the body brace. Long lightweight sleeves should be worn under an arm brace.

Rationale: Clothing between a brace and the skin prevents skin irritation by the steel brace frame.

Fulfilled Needs: Comfort, protection from physical harm, increased learning

Inform that coughing should be avoided
Explain that it is important that the patient avoid coughing as much as possible.

Rationale: Coughing should be avoided in situations where increased pressure within the body can lead to tissue damage, bleeding, or pain. This is especially true when intravascular, intraocular, intracranial, intraabdominal, and intrathoracic pressures need to be kept to a minimum.

Fulfilled Needs: Protection from physical harm, freedom from pain, increased learning

Inform that elimination is advisable before abdominal examinations and procedures Explain that physical examinations and procedures are more successful if the patient has a bowel elimination and voids shortly before the procedure.

Rationale: Bowel and bladder elimination before an examination or procedure makes for easier palpation and reduces the potential for organ rupture.

Fulfilled Needs: Protection from physical harm, increased learning

Inform that elimination straining should be avoided Explain that it is important that the patient avoid straining when attempting to eliminate stool.

Rationale: Elimination straining should be avoided, because increased pressure within the body can lead to tissue damage, bleeding, or pain. This is especially true when intravascular, intraocular, intracranial, intraabdominal, and intrathoracic pressures need to be kept to a minimum.

Fulfilled Needs: Protection from physical harm, freedom from pain, increased learning

Inform that esophageal speech therapy is available Explain to the patient who has had a laryngectomy that esophageal speech can be learned. It is basically a method of speaking by regurgitating swallowed air.

Rationale: Knowledge of available methods for improved communications promotes comfort.

Fulfilled Needs: Comfort, caring and communicating relationships, increased learning

Inform that extended breast sucking indicates hunger Explain that when an infant sucks at the breast 30–45 minutes or longer, this may be an indication that he is still hungry.

Rationale: Awareness that the breast milk may not be sufficient to satisfy the infant can facilitate use of a supplementary formula.

Fulfilled Needs: Protection from physical harm, increased learning

Inform that eyeglasses should be kept clean, rested on their rims to prevent lens scratching, and placed in a case when unused Explain that eyeglasses should be kept clean at all times, that they should be set to rest on their rims and not on their lens, and that they should be put in a cushioned case.

Rationale: Eyeglass cleanliness promotes visual acuity, which is essential to safety and comfort. Resting eyeglasses on their rims prevents lens scratching, which can result in distorted vision. Undamaged eyeglasses are essential for optimum vision.

Fulfilled Needs: Comfort, protection from physical harm, increased learning

Inform that foods causing allergies fall into specific categories[12] Explain that foods that cause allergic reactions fall into specific groupings: chicken, turkey, duck, and fowl; chocolate and cola drinks; radishes, cabbage, Brussels sprouts, turnips, cauliflower, broccoli, and lettuce; strawberries and raspberries; peanuts, peas, soybeans, and lima beans; cantaloupe, cucumbers, and watermelons; shrimp and oysters; potatoes and sweet potatoes; ginger and cinnamon; buckwheat and wheat; corn, salad oils, and cottonseed; apricots, peaches, plums, and nectarines. Other foods that cause allergic reactions are milk, eggs, pork, spicy foods, shellfish, and tomatoes.

Rationale: Knowledge of the specific items to avoid when one has an allergic condition promotes comfort and safety.

Fulfilled Needs: Comfort, protection from physical harm, increased learning

Inform that halazone tablets should be added to potentially unsafe water Explain that halazone tablets, which are found in most first-aid kits, may be used to chlorinate potentially contaminated water. Allow the treated water to stand 30 minutes before drinking.

Rationale: Knowledge that chlorination of water destroys bacteria promotes safety.

Fulfilled Needs: Protection from physical harm, increased learning

Inform that handwashing is essential before touching the laryngectomy stoma   Teach the patient who has had a laryngectomy to avoid touching the stoma until he has first washed his hands.

Rationale: Cleanliness prevents infection of the laryngectomy stoma and respiratory tract.

Fulfilled Needs: Cleanliness, protection from physical harm, increased learning

Inform that heavy lifting should be avoided   Explain that one should not lift heavy objects. If objects must be moved, it is preferable to slide them across the floor.

Rationale: Lifting heavy weights strains muscles, increases cardiac load, and uses large quantities of energy reserves. Heavy lifting causes increased intravascular, intraocular, intrathoracic, intracranial, and intraabdominal pressures.

Fulfilled Needs: Energy, comfort, protection from physical harm, increased learning

Inform that immunity does not occur with venereal infection   Explain that having a venereal disease does not confer immunity from future contagion.

Rationale: Persons who believe that having had a disease makes them immune tend to neglect precautions against future contagion.

Fulfilled Needs: Protection from physical harm, increased learning

Inform that isolation, loss of treat, and restitution are effective child discipline methods   Explain that the most effective forms of child discipline include the following: temporary removal of the child from the pleasure of social contacts, so long as the isolation does not include the threat of or the actual loss of parent or parental love; depriving the child of special treats, especially if peers are receiving the treats; requiring that the child make up for his misbehavior. For instance, if he breaks another child's toy, he must give up one of his toys, or he must be required to apologize.

Rationale: Isolation from others forces the child to realize that it is his own fault that he is missing the pleasure of human relationships. Loss of treats forces the child to realize the advantages of being good. When compensating for misbehavior requires more time and effort than behaving, the child realizes that good behavior is easier than bad. Discipline should put emphasis on the misbehavior, not on the child.

Fulfilled Needs: Sense of adequacy, personal growth and maturity, increased learning

Inform that large-print reading material is available   Explain that popular reading material can be obtained in very large print from public libraries.

Rationale: Large-print reading material supports ease of reading for persons with impaired vision.

Fulfilled Needs: Comfort, protection from physical harm, increased learning

Inform that menopause does not interfere with sex life   Explain that sex life is not affected by menopause, since sexual desire and response are of psychologic, emotional, and sensory origin.

Rationale: An awareness that menopause does not interfere with sex life supports comfort.

Fulfilled Needs: Comfort, increased learning

Inform that new foods should be introduced to children at the beginning of the meal   Explain that when new foods are to be introduced to a child, they should be presented at the beginning of the meal.

Rationale: Since the appetite is greatest at the beginning of a meal, the child is more likely to accept the food at that time.

Fulfilled Needs: Nutritional balance, increased learning

Inform that seizures are not contagious Explain that epilepsy is not a contagious disease and that it indicates a neurologic lesion or disorder. Explain that touching the froth on the mouth of seizuring epileptics does not transfer the disease.

Rationale: Awareness that seizures are not contagious can reduce the fear commonly associated with the disorder.

Fulfilled Needs: Comfort, protection from psychologic threat, increased learning

Inform that spinal injury often impairs sexual potency Explain that sexual potency after spinal cord injury depends on the level and the amount of cord injury. Future sexual capacity cannot be predicted early. If the reflex arcs are intact, there will be contraction of the external sphincter when a rectal examination is done. Sensation in the penile skin, scrotal skin, and saddle area is also a favorable sign. Reflex erections are not indicative of sexual potency. If there has been complete transection of the cord, both voluntary and reflex impulses are abolished. When the lumbar and sacral regions are affected, erection is not possible, except occasionally by psychic stimulation. When the upper lumbar region or a region below that is affected, ejection of seminal fluid from the urethra (ejaculation) is rare. When the third or fourth sacral region or a region above that is affected, male discharge of semen (or female orgasm) cannot occur. If there is incomplete transection of the cord, some reflex impulses may be possible. When the lumbar and sacral regions are affected, erection occurs from both organic and psychic stimulation most of the time, but not necessarily with every stimulation. When the upper lumbar region or a region below that is affected, ejection of seminal fluid from the urethra (ejaculation) is possible 30–70% of the time. When the third or fourth sacral region or a region above that is affected, male discharge of semen (or female orgasm) may, but seldom does, occur.

Rationale: Factual information about physical limitations promotes reality perception and supports adaptation to the affected phase of life.

Fulfilled Needs: Sexuality, increased learning, increased reality perception and problem-solving ability

Inform that stooping and lowering the head should be avoided Explain that it is inadvisable to bend forward and downward or to lower the head.

Rationale: Stooping and lowering the head should be avoided when intraocular and intracranial pressures need to be kept to a minimum. This precaution will help to prevent tissue damage, bleeding, and pain.

Fulfilled Needs: Comfort, protection from physical harm, freedom from pain. Increased learning.

Inform that the color and taste of outdoor water do not indicate its safety Explain that although water coming from springs and rivers may be clear and may taste fresh and cool, it may be contaminated.

Rationale: Since people use outdoor water for bathing, wading, dumping wastes, etc., there is always the possibility of contamination.

Fulfilled Needs: Protection from physical harm, increased learning

Inform that the extremities should be kept warm when the circulation is impaired Explain that when there is poor circulation in the extremities, loosely fitting soft wool socks or gloves and lightweight blankets can be used to maintain natural warmth. Heavy blankets should be avoided because their pressure on the extremities may further reduce circulation. Heat applications should also be avoided, since they increase metabolism, which in turn reduces the blood supply to the extremities.

Rationale: Natural body warmth helps maintain circulation in the extremities through vasodilatation.

Fulfilled Needs: Protection from physical harm, increased learning

Inform that the laryngectomy stoma should be protected against sunburning   Teach the patient who has had a laryngectomy to be careful that the stoma does not become sunburned. The area should be covered when exposed to sunlight.

Rationale: If a laryngectomy stoma becomes sunburned, it will swell and decrease the airway size.

Fulfilled Needs: Protection from physical harm, increased learning

Inform that the skin should be protected from windburn   Explain that the skin should be covered with a protective scarf when the wind is either cold or hot and dry.

Rationale: Wind at high velocity and extremes of temperature dries the skin and results in tissue irritation.

Fulfilled Needs: Comfort, protection from physical harm, increased learning

Inform that the use of a lightweight wheelchair is preferable   Explain that it is wise to purchase a lightweight wheelchair.

Rationale: Lightweight wheelchairs are easily handled independently, and they minimize fatigue in patients whose muscle strength is limited.

Fulfilled Needs: Energy, comfort, protection from physical harm, independence, increased learning

Inform that the use of a walker without wheels is preferable   Explain that it is best to use a walker that does not have wheels.

Rationale: Wheels on a walker make it less stable for supporting body weight.

Fulfilled Needs: Protection from physical harm, increased learning

Inform that the use of nonadjustable crutches for heavy persons is preferable   Explain that a person who weighs a great deal should use crutches that are not adjustable and are made of a solid piece of wood.

Rationale: Weight puts stress on the bolts, nuts, and holes in adjustable crutches, whereas a solid piece of wood has greater strength and is therefore safer.

Fulfilled Needs: Protection from physical harm, increased learning

Inform that toilet training should be delayed until the child can sit up   Explain that toilet training should be delayed until a child can sit up comfortably.

Rationale: If sitting is beyond the child's physiologic capability, he will experience anxiety and discomfort when placed in a sitting position.

Fulfilled Needs: Comfort, protection from psychologic threat, increased learning

Inform that toilet training should be limited to short periods daily   Explain that the child should be placed on the commode seat for only a short period each day.

Rationale: If prolonged sitting results in discomfort, the child will develop antagonism toward the training situation.

Fulfilled Needs: Comfort, protection from psychologic threat, increased learning

Inform that toys should be small enough to hold   Teach parents to provide children with toys compatible with the size of the child's hands.

Rationale: Small toys help the child develop fine motor skills.

Fulfilled Needs: Comfort, protection from physical harm, increased learning

Inform that underweight persons require additional sleep   Explain that persons who weigh less than normal usually require more sleep than do those of normal weight. This is especially true of children who are failing to thrive satisfactorily.

Rationale: Underweight persons have less energy reserve than those of normal weight. They require more energy restoration through sleep.

Fulfilled Needs: Sleep and rest, energy, protection from physical harm, increased learning

Inform that vegetables should be fed to children before fruits at the meal
Explain that when feeding a child both fruits and vegetables at the same meal, give the vegetable first. Recommend the selection of nonsweetened baby foods.

Rationale: The natural sweetness of fruits, if eaten before other foods, tends to deaden the appetite for less sweet foods.

Fulfilled Needs: Nutritional balance, increased learning

Inform that water should be kept out of the ears/out of the infected ear
Explain that water must be kept out of the ears when one has a fungus infection or is susceptible to fungal infections or when there has been rupture of the tympanic membrane.

Rationale: Water, when mixed with hard earwax, promotes fungal and bacterial growth. The force of water rushing into the ears may push earwax farther into the ear.

Fulfilled Needs: Protection from physical harm, increased learning

Inform that when there is limited movement, the affected body side should be dressed first
Teach patients with impaired mobility to put the affected limb into an armhole or pant leg first and then to dress the unaffected limb.

Rationale: Since the unaffected limb has the greatest mobility, moving it into the strained positions often associated with the final stages of dressing is easier than moving the affected limb.

Fulfilled Needs: Comfort, mastery and competence in skills, independence, increased learning

Instruct how to keep a daily apnea chart
Teach the parents how to keep a day-by-day record of apnea spells experienced by the infant in the home.

Rationale: The physician uses the home apnea record to determine when it is safe to take the child off the monitor.

Fulfilled Needs: Protection from physical harm, increased learning

Instruct not to blow the nose
Explain that whenever there is nasal bleeding or trauma, nose blowing should be avoided until healing occurs.

Rationale: Nose blowing increases intranasal pressure, traumatizing sensitive tissue and dislodging blood clots.

Fulfilled Needs: Protection from physical harm, increased learning

Instruct not to dangle the legs
Instruct the person not to sit with feet and legs hanging off the side of the bed. Advise that pressure not be placed under the back of the knee.

Rationale: The force of gravity on the dangling leg causes fluid to be pulled into the interstitial tissue spaces, causing edema. It also decreases venous return from the extremities to the heart. Pressure behind the knees impairs arterial and venous circulation.

Fulfilled Needs: Tissue oxygenation or perfusion, protection from physical harm, increased learning

Instruct not to insert foreign objects into body orifices/into the mouth
Explain that objects other than food and fluids should be kept out of the mouth. Beads, pins, and buttons should never be put in the mouth, nose, or ears. Such objects should be kept away from small children.

Rationale: Foreign objects irritate internal mucosa and can cause fatal airway obstruction.

Fulfilled Needs: Protection from physical harm, increased learning

Instruct not to kill animals suspected of being infected
Explain that when an animal has injured a person, the animal should not be destroyed, but should be cap-

tured and held for observation. An exception is that snakes should be killed and brought to medical authorities.

Rationale: A diseased animal that is alive will develop evidence of disease. Such evidence will not be observable if the animal is killed.

Fulfilled Needs: Protection from physical harm, increased learning

Instruct not to massage the breasts or use a breast pump   Explain that when attempting to dry up lactating breasts, the person should avoid rubbing, stroking, kneading, or pumping the breasts.

Rationale: Breast massage stimulates the mammary glands and promotes lactation. If a tumor is present, massaging the breast can spread tumor cells.

Fulfilled Needs: Protection from physical harm, increased learning

Instruct not to pick the nose   Explain that picking the nose should be avoided because it traumatizes nasal tissue and causes bleeding.

Rationale: Injury to nasal mucosa membranes interferes with the olfactory and filtering functions of the membrane.

Fulfilled Needs: Protection from physical harm, increased learning

Instruct not to pull out cast padding   Teach that the padding beneath the cast should not be pulled out or rearranged.

Rationale: Cast padding is designed to protect the skin against irritation from plaster. Removal of padding increases the potential for skin irritation and may cause the cast to fit too loosely.

Fulfilled Needs: Comfort, protection from physical harm, increased learning

Instruct not to swallow blood during epistaxis   Tell the person who has a bleeding nose not to swallow the blood but to lean forward and allow the blood to drain from the nose.

Rationale: Swallowing blood leads to vomiting.

Fulfilled Needs: Comfort, protection from physical harm, increased learning

Instruct not to use a drinking straw   Explain that the patient should not use a drinking straw for transporting liquids to the mouth.

Rationale: Sucking on a straw creates a vacuum within the oral cavity and can cause bleeding by disrupting clots formed around healing tissue. Sucking on a straw increases air swallowing, which can increase the discomfort of flatulence.

Fulfilled Needs: Comfort, protection from physical harm, increased learning

Instruct not to use a scratching device under the cast   Explain that putting such scratching devices as coat hangers and sticks inside a cast should be avoided. Instead, instruct the person to set a hand hair dryer on cool air and to direct the cool air toward the skin under the cast.

Rationale: Scratching devices inside a cast can injure the skin and wad the cast padding. Cool blowing air will relieve itching and remove skin debris under the cast.

Fulfilled Needs: Protection from physical harm, increased learning

Instruct not to use rubber rings and doughnuts   Explain that inflated rubber rings or doughnuts should not be used in the treatment of existing or potential decubitus ulcer.

Rationale: Pressure from rubber rings impairs circulation, increasing the potential for decubitus ulcer.

Fulfilled Needs: Protection from physical harm, increased learning

Instruct not to vigorously rinse the mouth   Instruct the person who has had oral surgery or who has suffered trauma to oral mucous membranes not to rinse out his mouth unless he does so very gently.

Rationale: Pressure applied to the oral mucous membrane when rinsing out the mouth may cause bleeding.

Fulfilled Needs: Protection from physical harm, increased learning

Instruct that contact lenses should not be worn beyond the prescribed time, during an eye disorder, or while sleeping Explain that contact lenses should not be worn any longer than 10–16 hours a day and should not be worn when the eyes are infected or traumatized. Contact lenses should be removed during sleep or naps because of the danger of eye injury.

Rationale: Improper use of contact lenses can cause corneal irritation, laceration, and ulceration.

Fulfilled Needs: Protection from physical harm, increased learning

Instruct that diabetics should not fry foods[376] Teach the diabetic that unless he uses the amount of fat allowed in his diet for cooking instead of eating, he cannot have fried foods. Meats, fish, potatoes, etc., should be baked, boiled, or broiled. It is preferable to use the fat allowance for salad dressings and spreads on bread.

Rationale: The stability of diabetic metabolism is dependent on a limited caloric intake.

Fulfilled Needs: Protection from physical harm, increased learning

Instruct that douching should be avoided Explain that douching should be avoided during pregnancy, before a vaginal examination, during puerperium healing, when abortion is habitual, and during a vaginal infection, unless it is ordered for therapeutic reasons.

Rationale: Vaginal irrigations disrupt the natural vaginal flora and pH, which increases susceptibility to infection in the vagina and can further spread existing infection. The pressure of vaginal irrigations can precipitate abortion. Douching before a vaginal examination may remove bacteria and cells that have diagnostic value.

Fulfilled Needs: Protection from physical harm, increased learning

Instruct that it is essential to carry an arteriovenous shunt clamp Explain that arteriovenous shunt clamps must be carried by the patient at all times in case the shunt comes apart.

Rationale: Hemorrhage from a disconnected arteriovenous shunt can result in death.

Fulfilled Needs: Protection from physical harm, increased learning

Instruct that only water, not milk or juice, be given in the infant's bottle at bedtime Explain that when a child prefers a bottle before going to sleep, the bottle should be filled with nothing but plain water.

Rationale: Carbohydrates that are allowed to remain in the mouth will cause tooth decay. Water, a noncarbohydrate, will not cause tooth decay.

Fulfilled Needs: Protection from physical harm, increased learning

Instruct that pillows, blankets, or trochanter rolls not be placed under the knee Explain that pillows, blankets, and trochanter rolls should not be placed under the knee, especially after a below-knee amputation. If a pillow must be placed under the knee to prevent hemorrhage, it should be removed as soon as possible.

Rationale: The flexion position of an amputation stump causes contractures. Pressure behind the knee (popliteal area) can impair circulation in the lower legs.

Fulfilled Needs: Tissue oxygenation or perfusion, protection from physical harm, increased learning

Instruct that premature infants require a moderate environmental temperature Explain that premature infants at home require a consistently moderate environmental temperature and should not be exposed to extreme heat or cold.

Rationale: Premature infants require a moderate environmental temperature because their poorly developed internal temperature control system cannot protect them from temperature extremes.

Fulfilled Needs: Normal temperature, protection from physical harm, increased learning

Instruct that premature infants require protection against infection Explain that the premature infant at home must be protected from infection by a clean, uncrowded environment. Stress the necessity for handwashing before touching the infant.

Rationale: The premature infant has poor resources for fighting infection. Cleanliness minimizes the potential for infection.

Fulfilled Needs: Cleanliness, protection from physical harm, increased learning

Instruct that several stump socks should not be worn simultaneously Teach amputees that it is unwise to wear several stump socks in order to obtain a snug prosthesis fit. Suggest that the prosthesis be adjusted to fit properly.

Rationale: An improperly fitting prosthesis impairs mobility and irritates the skin.

Fulfilled Needs: Protection from physical harm, increased learning

Instruct that soap should not be used on the laryngectomy stoma Teach the patient who has had a laryngectomy not to use soap for cleaning the stoma.

Rationale: Soap will damage the mucosa and stimulate coughing if it gets into the stoma.

Fulfilled Needs: Protection from physical harm, increased learning

Instruct that the amputation stump should not be rested on the crutch handrail Teach the amputee to avoid resting his amputation stump on the handrail of his crutch.

Rationale: The flexion position of an amputation stump causes contractures, which make the use of a prosthesis impossible. Pressure from resting the stump on the hard handrail will impair circulation to the stump.

Fulfilled Needs: Protection from physical harm, increased learning

Instruct that the drainage container should be kept below the bladder/ kidney/stomach/or chest level Explain that any drainage container should be kept below the level of the insertion site of the tube that is draining.

Rationale: A drainage apparatus kept below the level of its drain tube prevents backflow of the drainage into the tubing insertion site, reducing the potential for infection and promoting better drainage.

Fulfilled Needs: Protection from physical harm, increased learning

Instruct that the flexion stump position be avoided Teach the amputee not to let his amputation stump hang over the edge of a bed, wheelchair, or chair.

Rationale: The flexion position of an amputation stump results in contractures.

Fulfilled Needs: Protection from physical harm, increased learning

Instruct that the nonhemiplegic leg be placed down first when getting out of bed Teach the patient with one-sided paralysis to put his strong foot down first when getting out of bed.

Rationale: The strong side of the body can support body weight, but the affected side cannot.

Fulfilled Needs: Comfort, protection from physical harm, mastery and competence in skills, independence, increased learning

Instruct the person to empty his bladder/bowel before the procedure Explain that physical examinations and procedures are more successful if the patient has a bowel elimination and voids shortly before the procedure.

Rationale: Bowel and bladder elimination before an examination or procedure makes for easier palpation and reduces the potential for organ rupture.

Fulfilled Needs: Protection from physical harm, increased learning

Instruct the person to use his tongue to move food from the buccal pockets When a person has difficulty chewing and controlling food because of unilateral paralysis, explain that the tongue can be used to move food from the paralyzed side to the functioning side of the mouth, where chewing can be performed.

Rationale: Knowing substitute methods for manipulating food when there is unilateral paralysis aids in supporting adequate nutrition and hygiene.

Fulfilled Needs: Nutritional balance, comfort, increased learning

Instruct to align brace joints with body joints when applying a brace Explain that when applying a brace, the joints of the brace should not be allowed to twist. They should be aligned with the body joints.

Rationale: A properly applied therapeutic brace will effectively support weakened muscles, joints, and bones and facilitate motion.

Fulfilled Needs: Protection from physical harm, increased learning

Instruct to allow the cast to dry 2–3 days before approved weight bearing Teach that it takes a full 2–3 days for a cast to dry. Plaster of Paris will set within 5–10 minutes after water is applied and the warm chemical reaction occurs. The complete drying process of the total cast takes several days, however, and the person should not walk on it until drying is complete.

Rationale: Placing weight on an undried cast may crack the cast or distort alignment, causing improper healing.

Fulfilled Needs: Protection from physical harm, increased learning

Instruct to anchor the urinary catheter securely Explain that the urinary catheter should be taped to the inner thigh. The extended tubing should then be pinned to the sheet or mattress.

Rationale: Anchoring the urinary catheter will prevent tension on the catheter and will minimize the potential for pulling it out and causing pain.

Fulfilled Needs: Comfort, protection from physical harm, increased learning

Instruct to apply a warm, moist nonobstructive compress to the laryngectomy stoma for dyspnea If the patient who has had a laryngectomy becomes short of breath, teach him to place a warm moist compress over the stoma and breathe quietly. This will ease those breathing difficulties caused by dried secretions.

Rationale: Warm moist air liquefies secretions and promotes comfortable breathing.

Fulfilled Needs: Waste elimination of bronchopulmonary secretions, comfort, protection from physical harm, increased learning

Instruct to avoid activities that increase intracranial pressure Teach the person to avoid activities that increase pressure in the brain, such as coughing, straining on defecation, bending the head down, and straining to reach for objects.

Rationale: Avoiding activities which increase intracranial pressure keep the intracranial pressure at a minimal level.

Fulfilled Needs: Protection from physical harm, increased learning

Instruct to avoid artificial leg abduction Teach the person wearing a lower limb prosthesis to avoid moving his leg to the side and outward from his body when walking.

Rationale: Poor body alignment impairs body balance and mobility.

Fulfilled Needs: Protection from physical harm, increased learning

Instruct to avoid foods that have strong odors Explain that foods with strong

odors should not be eaten. This includes onions, cauliflower, Brussels sprouts, garlic, strong cheese, sausage, corned beef, and fish.
Rationale: Foods with strong odors tend to increase the odor from a colostomy, ileostomy, ureterostomy, or ureteroileostomy stoma. When intake of such foods is reduced, the odor decreases.
Fulfilled Needs: Comfort, increased learning

Instruct to avoid heat applications Explain that heat should not be applied to body areas when there is paralysis or sensation loss, edema, inadequate peripheral circulation, vasodilatation, or localized allergic reaction, in areas of hemorrhage or trauma, after heart surgery, or to persons with fever. Diabetics, having sensitive skin, need to take special precaution not to use heat applications.
Rationale: Heat applied to body areas during the above-mentioned conditions can cause tissue damage.
Fulfilled Needs: Protection from physical harm, increased learning

Instruct to avoid hiking the shoulder when walking with a leg prosthesis
Teach the patient wearing a lower limb prosthesis to avoid raising one shoulder higher than the other when walking.
Rationale: Poor body alignment impairs body balance and mobility.
Fulfilled Needs: Protection from physical harm, increased learning

Instruct to avoid/limit direct contact with infected persons Teach the person to limit direct physical contact of the infected patient with noninfected persons.
Rationale: Pathogen transfer from person to person is decreased by limiting human contact.
Fulfilled Needs: Cleanliness, protection from physical harm, increased learning

Instruct to avoid pushing and pulling activities Explain that fatigue can be reduced by abstaining from pushing or pulling heavy objects.
Rationale: Fatigue results from energy-depleting activity.
Fulfilled Needs: Energy, comfort, protection from physical harm, increased learning

Instruct to avoid rubbing the eyes Explain that eye rubbing should be avoided because foreign and infectious material can be transferred to the eyes from the fingers and because rubbing causes friction and pressure against the eyelids and eye tissue.
Rationale: Foreign objects in the eyes or pressure on the eyes can cause tissue infection or trauma.
Fulfilled Needs: Comfort, cleanliness, protection from physical harm, increased learning

Instruct to avoid self-defeating thoughts Teach the person to avoid thoughts of self-depreciation, such as belittling himself for nonaccomplishments, failing to forgive himself for being human or for committing human errors, thinking negatively about his self-worth, and thinking of himself as "poor me."
Rationale: Self-defeating thoughts support activity that leads to failure and diminishes the potential for growth toward emotional maturity.
Fulfilled Needs: Protection from psychologic threat, personal growth and maturity, increased learning

Instruct to avoid storing insulin in a syringe[376] Teach the person not to draw up insulin and leave it in the syringe.
Rationale: After a period of time, insulin will cling to glass or plastic syringes, altering the available dose.
Fulfilled Needs: Protection from physical harm, mastery and competence in skills, independence, increased learning

Instruct to avoid taking diet pills Teach that diet pills should not be taken as a means of weight reduction. This is especially true for persons who are ill or on other medication.

Rationale: Amphetamines used to reduce appetite cause poor concentration, nervousness, and difficulty sleeping. Such drugs can have harmful effects on existing physical disorders.

Fulfilled Needs: Protection from physical harm, increased learning

Instruct to avoid the Valsalva maneuver Instruct the person not to take a deep breath, hold the nose and mouth closed, and make a forceful effort to exhale. Also instruct not to hold the breath while straining the abdominal muscles, such as in turning over in bed, sitting up, lifting legs while in bed, and picking up a heavy object from the floor.

Rationale: Performing the Valsalva maneuver puts a strain on the cardiovascular system that should be avoided when there is cardiovascular pathology.

Fulfilled Needs: Protection from physical harm, increased learning

Instruct to bring crutches when the leg cast is removed When the cast is scheduled to be removed, instruct the person to bring his crutches with him.

Rationale: Since the person cannot walk immediately after a cast is removed, crutches are needed to support the body during the transition period.

Fulfilled Needs: Comfort, protection from physical harm, increased learning

Instruct to change position frequently Explain that a person who is bedridden should be moved from one position to another, from side to side, and from back to abdomen at least every 2 hours day and night.

Rationale: Changing body positions prevents congestion of respiratory secretions, facilitates expectoration, promotes circulation, provides comfort by preventing prolonged pressure on body areas, reduces fatigue, and prevents contractures.

Fulfilled Needs: Comfort, protection from physical harm, increased learning

Instruct to change position gradually Explain that when the body position is changed from lying to sitting or from sitting to standing, it should be done slowly. The head should be gradually elevated upward, and there should be a rest period between each position change. This is especially true when there are blood pressure abnormalities, when there is bleeding or when there could be bleeding, when there are injured bones, and when an arteriovenous cannula is in place.

Rationale: Changing position gradually minimizes blood pressure adaptations in arteries and veins, promotes good circulation, and decreases the pressure placed on the body part by another.

Fulfilled Needs: Comfort, protection from physical harm, increased learning

Instruct to change wet diapers immediately Explain that as soon as an infant's diaper is wet, it should be changed and replaced with a dry diaper. Explain that the child should be checked frequently to determine whether the diaper is wet.

Rationale: Acidic urine in contact with the skin causes skin irritation.

Fulfilled Needs: Comfort, cleanliness, protection from physical harm, increased learning

Instruct to check the cane/crutch safety tip regularly for needed replacement Instruct the person to notice if the safety tip at the bottom of the cane or crutch is worn on one side and is securely attached. If worn, it should be replaced.

Rationale: A firm base of support with a cane or crutch is essential for safe ambulation.

Fulfilled Needs: Protection from physical harm, increased learning

Instruct to check the pulse daily when wearing a pacemaker Teach the person who has a pacemaker to check his pulse rate twice a day and to report any increase or decrease of more than five beats/minute.

Rationale: In the person who is wearing a pacemaker, an increase or decrease in pulse rate usually indicates battery failure or a weakening battery.

Fulfilled Needs: Protection from physical harm, increased learning

Instruct to clean the nails with a cotton-tipped stick Explain that a soft cotton-tipped orange stick should be used to clean the nails and that sharp objects should be avoided.

Rationale: Use of sharp objects increases the chance of tissue puncture and resulting infection.

Fulfilled Needs: Comfort, cleanliness, protection from physical harm, increased learning

Instruct to comb the dandruff up from the scalp Explain that dandruff can be removed by gently pressing the comb against the scalp and pushing the dandruff up and away from the hair roots.

Rationale: Dandruff causes hair dullness and itching.

Fulfilled Needs: Comfort, cleanliness, protection from physical harm, increased learning

Instruct to cover the mouth when coughing Explain that the mouth should be covered with a handkerchief, a tissue, or a hand when coughing.

Rationale: Covering the mouth when coughing minimizes the spread of droplets that can carry infection.

Fulfilled Needs: Cleanliness, protection from physical harm, increased learning

Instruct to cover the nose when sneezing Explain that the nose should be covered with a handkerchief or tissue when sneezing.

Rationale: Covering the nose when sneezing minimizes the spread of droplets that can carry infection.

Fulfilled Needs: Cleanliness, protection from physical harm, increased learning

Instruct to cut the toenails straight across Explain that nails should be cut straight across. They should never be cut shorter than the tips of the toes and should be rounded gently with an emery board.

Rationale: Cutting the nails straight across prevents ingrown nails, which can become infected.

Fulfilled Needs: Protection from physical harm, increased learning

Instruct to decrease the frequency of bathing Explain that bathing the entire body daily should be avoided when there is skin irritation or when there are abnormal conditions. Complete bathing several times a week is sufficient.

Rationale: Daily bathing can remove too much of the natural oils from the skin, resulting in skin dryness and irritation.

Fulfilled Needs: Comfort, protection from physical harm

Instruct to do the Valsalva maneuver Instruct the person to take a deep breath, to hold his nose and keep his mouth closed, and to make a forceful effort to exhale.

Rationale: The Valsalva maneuver increases pressure on the tympanic membrane and within the thoracic cavity. It may relieve auditory tube obstruction, certain arrhythmias, and hiccoughs.

Fulfilled Needs: Protection from physical harm, increased learning

Instruct to do wheelchair pushups Teach the person confined to a wheelchair to place the palms of his hands against the chair seat or chair arms and to push himself off the wheelchair cushion every 30 minutes.

Rationale: Wheelchair pushups relieve pressure on areas of diminished circulation and reduce the potential for decubitus ulcers.

Fulfilled Needs: Protection from physical harm, increased learning

Instruct to eat only at mealtime   Teach the person to eat only at mealtime. The person should refrain from snacking between meals and at bedtime.

Rationale: When diabetics eat unprescribed foods between meals, they disrupt carbohydrate metabolism and heighten the potential for diabetic coma. When patients with gastric ulcers eat between meals, they stimulate gastric acidity, increasing the potential for further ulceration and reducing the potential for healing.

Fulfilled Needs: Protection from physical harm, increased learning

Contraindications: If between-meal or bedtime snacks are prescribed, as in diabetic diets

Instruct to eat only prescribed foods and amounts of foods   Explain that it is not advisable to substitute unprescribed foods and amounts of foods in a therapeutic diet.

Rationale: Indiscriminate experimentation with a prescribed therapeutic diet can have adverse effects and can cause recurrence or complication of the nonhealth condition.

Fulfilled Needs: Protection from physical harm, increased learning

Instruct to eat 25% of the daily calories at breakfast, 50% at lunch, and 25% at supper to achieve weight loss[110]   Explain that 25% of daily calorie intake should be eaten at breakfast, 50% at lunch, and 25% at supper. The largest portion of calories should be eaten before 1 o'clock PM.

Rationale: Research has indicated that the proportion in which calories are consumed affects the maintenance of weight loss. It is believed that food consumed early in the day is more readily processed.

Fulfilled Needs: Nutritional balance, increased learning

Instruct to eat yogurt or to drink buttermilk   Recommend that the person drink buttermilk or eat yogurt daily.

Rationale: Buttermilk and yogurt contain lactobacilli that increase the absorption of nutritional substances, such as vitamins. During and after antibiotic therapy or diarrhea, buttermilk or yogurt will restore normal intestinal bacteria, improving digestion and preventing yeast infection. Yogurt is a good source of calcium, riboflavin, and protein.

Fulfilled Needs: Protection from physical harm, increased learning

Instruct to elevate the body part   Explain that an injured, inflamed, or infected body part should be positioned above other adjacent body parts.

Rationale: Elevation of a body part reduces edema and promotes circulation.

Fulfilled Needs: Tissue oxygenation or perfusion, comfort, protection from physical harm, increased learning

Instruct to elevate the head   Explain that the head should be raised higher than the chest level. This is done by raising the head and shoulders on pillows or raising the head of a mechanical bed.

Rationale: Elevation of the head supports the easy intake of food and fluids and reduces cerebral edema and pressure.

Fulfilled Needs: Comfort, protection from physical harm, increased learning

Instruct to exercise at least three times a week on nonconsecutive days[746]

Teach that exercise should be accomplished a minimum of three times each week. If not performed every day, the person should skip 1 or 2 days between sessions, but no more than 1 or 2 days.

Rationale: For the body to maintain healthy function, exercise should be done in a consistent pattern. When periods of more than 2 days elapse before reexercise occurs, unnecessary stress is placed on the body, which has to readjust to the increased activity.

Fulfilled Needs: Tissue oxygenation or perfusion, exercise, protection from physical harm, mastery and competence in skills, independence, increased learning

Contraindications: Fever, states of severe energy depletion, or increased metabolic rate, during acute illness. Any person who has an elevated blood pressure, elevated serum cholesterol, triglycerides or uric acid, abnormal electrocardiogram, known cardiac condition, chest pain, is on cardiac drugs, has a family history of heart disease, has diabetes, asthma or emphysema, has any condition such as arthritis or gout in which muscle or joint motion would aggravate the conditions, has dyspnea or intermittent claudication (leg cramping when walking), or any chronic illness should be seen and evaluated by a physician before starting an exercise program.

Instruct to exercise 20–30 minutes each session[746] Teach that exercise should be performed as follows: There should be a warmup or light exercise period of 3–5 minutes, a conditioning or heavy exercise period of 10–20 minutes, and a cooling or light exercise period of 3–5 minutes.

Rationale: In order to reduce excess stress on the body, light exercise is first attempted. Then strenuous exercise is performed. Before stopping exercise completely, light exercise is employed to facilitate the body's adjustment to reduced activity.

Fulfilled Needs: Tissue oxygenation or perfusion, exercise, protection from physical harm, mastery and competence in skills, independence, increased learning

Contraindications: Fever, states of severe energy depletion, or increased metabolic rate, during acute illness. Any person who has an elevated blood pressure, elevated serum cholesterol, triglycerides or uric acid, abnormal electrocardiogram, known cardiac condition, chest pain, is on cardiac drugs, has a family history of heart disease, has diabetes, asthma or emphysema, has any condition such as arthritis or gout in which muscle or joint motion would aggravate the condition, has dyspnea or intermittent caludication (leg cramping when walking), or any chronic illness should be seen and evaluated by a physician before starting an exercise program.

Instruct to feed unhurriedly Explain that a person needs to be fed slowly. Adequate time should be allowed for chewing, swallowing, and pausing between food bites. With chewing or swallowing problems, there may be a need to feed very slowly.

Rationale: Knowledge of appropriate feeding methods prevents choking and aspiration of food and fluids. Relaxed eating promotes comfort and normal digestive functioning.

Fulfilled Needs: Relaxation, comfort, protection from physical harm, increased learning

Instruct to increase exercise tolerance gradually[746] Explain that exercise should be increased gradually to the desired level of exertion over a period of several months. One should never begin exercising vigorously.

Rationale: In order to reduce excess stress on the body, light exercise is first attempted. As the body adjusts to new levels of activity, the exercise can be increased without tissue damage.

Fulfilled Needs: Protection from physical harm, mastery and competence in skills, independence, increased learning

Instruct to increase/maintain fluid intake Explain that the amount of fluid taken each day should be increased by whatever amount is appropriate to the situation or is maintained at the same level.

Rationale: Increased fluid intake in certain situations ensures adequate hydration of body tissues. During jet travel, increased fluid intake offsets the potential for dehydration caused by atmospheric pressure changes.

Fulfilled Needs: Fluid and electrolyte balance, protection from physical harm, increased learning

Instruct to increase the wearing time of the prosthesis gradually Explain that the length of time the prosthesis is worn should be increased gradually each day.

Rationale: Gradually increasing the prosthesis wearing time allows for slow, comfortable adjustment of the stump to pressure.

Fulfilled Needs: Comfort, protection from physical harm, increased learning

Instruct to inspect the skin/scalp/hair Explain that patients, especially diabetics and patients confined to bed or wheelchair, should inspect the skin for redness, irritation, duskiness, and intactness. The back, buttocks, and soles of the feet can be inspected with a hand mirror. Explain that where there is the possibility of lice, etc., the scalp should be inspected periodically.

Rationale: Skin inspection facilitates early detection and treatment of skin disorders. Infestation can cause scalp inflammation and facilitates bacterial infection.

Fulfilled Needs: Protection from physical harm, increased learning

Instruct to introduce infants to only one new food each week and note allergic responses Explain that when feeding an infant, no more than one new food should be given to the child each week. Note if the infant develops a rash, nasal stuffiness, wheezing, or diarrhea after the new food is introduced.

Rationale: Giving only one new food each week allows time for determining if the infant is allergic to the newly introduced food.

Fulfilled Needs: Protection from physical harm, increased learning

Instruct to keep the cast dry with a plastic wrap when bathing Explain that the cast should be covered with some form of plastic wrap when the person bathes or showers.

Rationale: Wetness weakens the cast, heightening the potential for distorted alignment. The result is improper healing.

Fulfilled Needs: Protection from physical harm, increased learning

Instruct to lean forward or sit up for improved ventilation Teach the orthopneic person to sit up or to lean forward and rest his arms on a table for easier breathing.

Rationale: Good positioning facilitates lung ventilation and improved oxygenation and promotes comfort.

Fulfilled Needs: Tissue oxygenation or perfusion, comfort, increased learning

Instruct to lie in the prone position Teach the person with an amputated lower extremity to lie on his abdomen several times a day and to place the stump in a straightened (extended) position. Teach the mother to sleep and lie on her abdomen after child delivery.

Rationale: Using the prone position to extend the hip after amputation will reduce flexion contractures. Abdominal positioning helps the uterus resume its normal position.

Fulfilled Needs: Comfort, protection from physical harm, increased learning

Contraindications Delay until caesarean section incision is well healed.

Instruct to limit weight loss to 3 lb/week Teach persons attempting to lose weight that weight loss should be limited to 3 lb/week.

Rationale: Rapid weight loss places severe stress on energy reserves and on the function of body systems, increasing the susceptibility to illness.
Fulfilled Needs: Protection from physical harm, increased learning

Instruct to lock the wheelchair before transferring   Explain that the wheelchair brake should be locked before the patient attempts to get in or out of the chair.
Rationale: Locking the wheelchair provides a stable base for weight bearing when getting in and out of the chair and prevents accidental injury.
Fulfilled Needs: Protection from physical harm, increased learning

Instruct to lubricate the skin/scalp/nails   Explain that dry skin should be moistened daily with a soothing, lubricating solution or cream. Recommend oil treatments for a dry, scaling scalp.
Rationale: Lubrication prevents skin and scalp drying.
Fulfilled Needs: Comfort, protection from physical harm, increased learning
Contraindications: Excessively oily skin or hair, acned skin

Instruct to maintain a moist laryngectomy bib   Teach the patient who has had a laryngectomy to keep the bib moist at all times.
Rationale: Maintaining a moist laryngectomy bib prevents crusting around the stoma and promotes comfort.
Fulfilled Needs: Comfort, protection from physical harm, increased learning

Instruct to maintain skin dryness   Explain that as soon as the skin becomes wet from any body discharge, the excretion should be removed with mild soap and water and the skin thoroughly dried. Persons who are incontinent or who experience profuse perspiration or drainage should be checked frequently to determine skin wetness.
Rationale: Prolonged wetness irritates the skin.
Fulfilled Needs: Comfort, protection from physical harm, increased learning

Instruct to maintain skin/scalp cleanliness   Explain that the skin should be thoroughly cleansed periodically with soap and water, and the scalp with shampoo, so that dirt and bacteria are removed.
Rationale: Removal of dirt and bacteria from the skin and scalp promotes comfort and reduces the potential for infection.
Fulfilled Needs: Comfort, cleanliness, protection from physical harm, increased learning

Instruct to measure foods after cooking   Explain that food should be weighed or measured after it has been cooked in order to assure accuracy of allowable amounts.
Rationale: Cooking alters the fluid content and weight of food, precise diet measurements are essential to maintaining many health states, especially stable diabetic metabolism.
Fulfilled Needs: Protection from physical harm, increased learning

Instruct to move the injured body part carefully   Explain that an injured body area, if movable, may be moved slowly and gently with extreme care during mobility or position change.
Rationale: Carefully moving injured body parts can reduce pain and prevent further injury.
Fulfilled Needs: Comfort, protection from physical harm, increased learning

Instruct to place a pillow between the thighs in below-knee amputation
Teach the patient who has had a below-knee amputation to place a pillow between his thighs when lying in bed.

Rationale: Placing a pillow between the thighs promotes extension and alignment of the amputation stump.

Fulfilled Needs: Protection from physical harm, increased learning

Instruct to place food into the unaffected side of the mouth of the hemiplegic When a person has difficulty chewing and controlling food because of unilateral paralysis, explain that he should place the food into the side of the mouth that is not paralyzed.

Rationale: By placing food into the nonparalyzed side of the mouth, food can be properly chewed, supporting nutrition and decreasing the potential for choking.

Fulfilled Needs: Nutritional balance, comfort, increased learning

Instruct to position correctly Teach the correct position for the specific situation. Give clear details so that appropriate positioning is achieved.

Rationale: Correct positioning promotes circulation and respiratory exchange, reduces or eliminates pain, supports secretion drainage, and prevents pressure against skin and organs.

Fulfilled Needs: Comfort, protection from physical harm, increased learning

Instruct to protect the laryngectomy opening/tracheostomy from water Explain that the patient who has had a laryngectomy or tracheostomy should not swim. When he takes a shower, he should shield the opening from the water.

Rationale: The potential for drowning is high if water enters a laryngectomy or tracheostomy stoma.

Fulfilled Needs Protection from physical harm, increased learning

Instruct to remove dentures Explain that dentures should be removed from persons who are unconscious, from those who are having seizures, and from those who have obstructed airways.

Rationale: Removing dentures when a person is unable to control their movement prevents airway obstruction and injury to the oral mucosa.

Fulfilled Needs: Protection from physical harm, increased learning

Instruct to report any/all serious/early signs/symptoms immediately Explain that certain symptoms should be reported as soon as they occur, with no delay.

Rationale: Certain symptoms indicate serious threats to health, and any lapse of time before treatment is begun can greatly affect outcome.

Fulfilled Needs: Protection from physical harm, increased learning

Instruct to respond immediately to the elimination reflex Explain that it is advisable to respond to the bladder and bowel elimination reflexes as soon as they occur.

Rationale: Prolonged retention of feces in the lower colon causes pressure and discomfort. Water continues to be absorbed from the feces, making them harder and more difficult to expel. Prolonged retention of urine in the bladder causes discomfort because of distention and promotes urinary tract infection.

Fulfilled Needs: Waste elimination of food residue and urine, comfort, protection from physical harm, increased learning

Instruct to restrict children to a fenced play area Stress the need to keep small children in a fenced-in area during playtime.

Rationale: Children can wander from a safe area if there is no fence. They are then vulnerable to automobile or other injury.

Fulfilled Needs: Protection from physical harm, increased learning

Instruct to sit down whenever possible Explain that when performing usual daily activities, it is best to sit down whenever possible. The person can talk with others, iron clothes, peel potatoes, etc., just as well sitting down as standing up.

Rationale: The sitting position gives the body a few moments of rest, especially when a person feels weak and has limited energy reserves.

Fulfilled Needs: Comfort, protection from physical harm, increased learning

Instruct to take medications immediately after meals Recommend that medications be taken immediately after the meal is finished.

Rationale: Drugs taken after a meal are less likely to cause gastric irritation because of the fullness of the intestinal tract.

Fulfilled Needs: Comfort, protection from physical harm, increased learning

Contraindications: Drugs such as penicillin G should be taken on an empty stomach because food interferes with their absorption.

Instruct to toilet frequently Recommend that the patient go to the bathroom at frequent intervals. This is especially important for patients who have bladder infections or who are recovering from bladder infections.

Rationale: Frequent toileting reduces the amount of urine that the bladder must handle at one time, minimizes the chance of accidental or uncontrolled voiding, and helps to prevent prolongation or recurrence of infection.

Fulfilled Needs: Comfort, increased learning

Instruct to use a footboard Explain that a board should be placed at the foot of the bed, with the feet positioned against the board at a right angle to the legs with the person in the prone position.

Rationale: Placing the feet against a footboard prevents footdrop and keeps pressure from covers off the feet. It can promote circulation when pressing exercises are performed against the board.

Fulfilled Needs: Protection from physical harm, increased learning

Instruct to use a soft, new toothbrush and to apply only mild toothbrush pressure Explain that a new (not old or bent) soft toothbrush should be used when gums are easily injured, degenerating, or bleeding. The pressure applied should be gentle but firm, never excessive.

Rationale: Bent toothbrush bristles cannot be controlled. They can puncture soft gum tissue. Excessive toothbrush pressure causes gum surface irritation. A new soft toothbrush minimizes trauma to gums and oral mucosa but provides gum stimulation and the comfort of clean teeth.

Fulfilled Needs: Comfort, cleanliness, protection from physical harm, increased learning

Instruct to use a water-base lubricant around the laryngectomy stoma Instruct the person to use a lubricant (K-Y jelly or Lubafax) that has a water base rather than an oil base around the laryngectomy stoma. Instruct the patient to apply small amounts of lubricant twice a day. It should be allowed to soak in for 2 minutes and then removed. Caution against applying lubricant into the stoma.

Rationale: Lubricating a stoma can prevent crusting and promote comfort. A water-base lubricant is preferred, since oil-base lubricants can be inhaled into the lungs and cause pneumonia.

Fulfilled Needs: Comfort, protection from physical harm, increased learning

Instruct to use a wide supportive stance for good body balance Explain that when the body is erect, the feet should be placed at equal distances from the body midline.

Rationale: Equal support on both sides of the body promotes balanced movement.

Fulfilled Needs: Protection from physical harm, increased learning

Instruct to use ice applications to control bleeding Explain that applying ice or an ice bag or pack to a bleeding site will stop bleeding and prevent or minimize the formation of hematomas.

Rationale: Cold applications cause vasoconstriction, which reduces blood supply to the area.

Fulfilled Needs: Protection from physical harm, increased learning

Contraindications: Decubitus ulcers, gangrenous tissue, recent skin graft, varicose veins, areas of paralysis or sensation loss

Instruct to use pressure applications to control bleeding Explain that bleeding can be stopped by applying finger pressure or a tight bandage to the bleeding area.

Rationale: Pressure obstructs blood flow.

Fulfilled Needs: Protection from physical harm, increased learning

Instruct to use simple words when speaking with persons having impaired communication reception Explain that short, simple statements are best for communicating with persons who have impaired communication reception.

Rationale: Short, simple statements are most easily understood and promote effective communication.

Fulfilled Needs: Comfort, caring and communicating relationships, increased learning

Instruct to use vagal stimulation methods to terminate dysrhythmias[327] Explain that the following methods can be used to stimulate the vagus nerve: hold a deep breath for 6–8 seconds after inspiration, bend the body at the waist and hold the chest parallel to the floor for a few seconds, hold the breath after inspiration and press the right or left carotid artery, stimulate the gagging reflex by inserting the finger down the throat, drink ice water.

Rationale: Heart rate is regulated by an inhibiting nervous system and an accelerating nervous system, each working against the other. When the vagus nerve, which is part of the inhibiting nervous system, is stimulated, it slows the heart rate.

Fulfilled Needs: Tissue oxygenation or perfusion, comfort, protection from physical harm, increased learning

Instruct to use wide crutch tips Explain that the tips on crutches should be as wide as is comfortable for the user.

Rationale: A firm, stable base is essential to safe ambulation. The larger the crutch tip, the greater the friction and stability.

Fulfilled Needs: Protection from physical harm, increased learning

Instruct to wash combs and brushes with each shampoo Explain that each time the hair is cleansed by shampooing, the person's comb and brush should be cleaned with soap and water.

Rationale: Cleanliness prevents infection.

Fulfilled Needs: Cleanliness, protection from physical harm, increased learning

Instruct to wash the stump sock frequently Explain that the stump sock should be washed thoroughly with soap and water daily.

Rationale: Unclean perspiration residue on the stump sock causes skin irritation.

Fulfilled Needs: Comfort, cleanliness, protection from physical harm, increased learning

Instruct to wear well-fitting shoes Explain that one should wear shoes that are not tight, do not rub against the skin, give good support, and are comfortable.

Rationale: Friction causes skin pressure and irritation, which can result in tissue injury. A firm supportive base promotes stability of body movement and comfort.

Fulfilled Needs: Comfort, protection from physical harm, increased learning

Instruct to wear white socks Explain that the person should wear white, not colored, socks.
Rationale: Dyes from colored socks irritate the skin and lesions. White socks contain no dye.
Fulfilled Needs: Protection from physical harm

Recommend a daily change of clean clothing Suggest that clean clothing be worn each day.
Rationale: Clean clothing promotes comfort and reduces the potential for infection.
Fulfilled Needs: Comfort, cleanliness, protection from physical harm, increased learning

Recommend a habitual positive mental attitude Suggest that the person avoid dwelling on possible failure and unpleasantness. Suggest that he develop positive approaches to problems, plan for the success he hopes to attain, and have a definite alternative plan in case failure does occur. If negative thinking has been his approach in the past, he will encounter considerable difficulty in developing a positive approach.
Rationale: A positive mental attitude supports self-confidence, which overcomes fear and anxiety and leads to success.
Fulfilled Needs: Comfort, protection from psychologic threat, personal growth and maturity, increased learning, increased reality perception and problem-solving ability

Recommend a preadmission visit to a nursing home/institution/maternity area Recommend that the person visit a nursing home, institution, etc., before being admitted. Allow time for the individual to become familiar with the environment.
Rationale: Preadmission visits to institutions familiarize the person with the unknown environment. It provides information for making choices and gives the person control of the situation.
Fulfilled Needs: Comfort, protection from psychologic threat, control over a situation

Recommend a regular meal/feeding schedule Suggest that meals be served at approximately the same time each day so that a regular eating pattern is established.
Rationale: Body systems adapt more readily to routine functioning than to unrelated phenomena and activity. Scheduled feeding reduces the visceral hunger sensation and promotes comfort.
Fulfilled Needs: Nutritional balance, comfort, protection from physical harm, increased learning

Recommend a regular sleeping schedule Suggest that the patient make it a habit to go to bed at the same time each night.
Rationale: Stable sleep habits promote physical and emotional health.
Fulfilled Needs: Sleep and rest, protection from physical harm, protection from psychologic threat, increased learning

Recommend a trial period before making a final decision Suggest that institutionalization, therapy, etc., be given a trial period before the person decides to accept or reject such.
Rationale: A trial period reduces the threat of adjustment because of the temporary nature of the situation. It gives more realistic data from which to make a decision. Having confronted the anxiety of the situation, decisions are more apt to be sound.
Fulfilled Needs: Comfort, protection from psychologic threat, increased learning, increased reality perception and problem-solving ability

Recommend activities that improve circulation Teach the person to perform exercises, to walk briskly, or to rock in a chair.
Rationale: Activities that alternately cause vasodilatation and vasoconstriction improve circulation.

Fulfilled Needs: Tissue oxygenation or perfusion, activity and exercise, protection from physical harm, increased learning

Recommend adequate food refrigeration Suggest that perishable foods and foods labeled as requiring refrigeration be kept cold in a tightly closed refrigerator.

Rationale: Adequate refrigeration prevents bacterial growth in food.

Fulfilled Needs: Protection from physical harm, increased learning

Recommend adherence to a pace of living with which the person is comfortable Explain that it is essential to control pace of living so that stress is kept to a minimum, but productivity is satisfactory. This can be done by starting the day unhurriedly, by allowing extra time for activities, and by not becoming involved in more activities than one can comfortably perform.

Rationale: Living at a rapid pace consumes the energy vital to healing or depletes limited amounts of energy. Prolonged stress caused by a rapid pace breaks down the health of vital body organs and diminishes the capacity for healthy emotional adaptation.

Fulfilled Needs: Energy, comfort, protection from physical harm, protection from psychologic threat, increased learning

Recommend alternative approaches to sexual activity Make suggestions for other ways that the person can make love. Include precoital activities, different coital positions, assistive devices for the physically impaired, etc.

Rationale: Increased knowledge of how to achieve sexual satisfaction supports a more fulfilling and lasting sexual relationship. It increases self-esteem as the persons grow in in-depth relatedness.

Fulfilled Needs: Comfort, sexuality, love and affection, caring and communicating relationships, high evaluation of self, personal growth and maturity, increased learning, increased pleasure

Recommend an appropriate breast prosthesis Depending on the stage of recovery, give advice regarding a breast prosthesis. Shortly after surgery the person will not be able to tolerate a commercial prosthesis. Suggest that she fill her regular brassiere with cotton or a sanitary pad as a temporary measure. Later recommend a professional prosthesis fitter for a prosthesis filled with air, fluid, or sponge and designed to order.

Rationale: A breast prosthesis provides a feeling of body balance and a symmetric appearance.

Fulfilled Needs: Comfort, increased learning

Recommend behavior modification for changing eating habits[110,471] Suggest methods of behavior modification for eating habits such as the following: avoid eating while performing another activity frequently engaged in, eat only sitting down and at a table that has been set, establish a pattern of eating only at mealtime before attempting to reduce food intake, purchase only foods that must be prepared, store foods in less accessible places, reduce the rate of eating by chewing thoroughly and by putting new food on the fork after swallowing and not while chewing. Recommend that if the person knows he will be in a situation in which high-calorie foods will be served, that he eat low-calorie foods before entering the situation. Suggest substituting a noneating activity for snacking between meals, such as writing a letter instead of chewing on a candy bar.

Rationale: If a person eats whenever engaging in a frequent activity, then the frequency of eating will clearly be increased. By being specific about the setting in which we eat, we reduce the environmental stimuli for eating. Well-established eating patterns reduce the potential for snacking. Having food out of sight, and having to cook it, decreases the frequency of consumption. By reducing the rate of eating, the person exerts control over the amount eaten and satisfaction in eating. Eating low-calorie foods before entering a situation in which high-calorie foods will be served increases the feeling of fullness and reduces the desire to eat.

Fulfilled Needs: Protection from physical harm, increased learning

Recommend closed shoes for foot protection   Suggest that shoes closed at the toes and heels be worn to protect against foot injury.

Rationale: A protective shoe can prevent trauma to an injured foot or to the stump of an amputated toe.

Fulfilled Needs: Comfort, protection from physical harm, increased learning

Recommend communication by gesture   Teach the person who is unable to communicate by speech to convey messages by using hand movements, such as pointing, making signs, and drawing in the air.

Rationale: Effective communication promotes comfort.

Fulfilled Needs: Comfort, caring and communicating relationships, increased learning

Recommend eating and drinking in moderation   Suggest that the patient eat and drink moderately and not indulge in excessive food or drink.

Rationale: Overconsumption distends the stomach wall and causes pain and discomfort. It accelerates the digestive process, which increases heart rate and makes sleeping difficult. Excessive intake of food (calories) causes obesity.

Fulfilled Needs: Comfort, protection from physical harm, increased learning

Recommend eating methods suggested for the visually impaired   Explain that by gently touching food, the blind person can learn to distinguish food differences. The liquid level in a glass can be found by bending the forefinger into the glass and determining the distance between the liquid and the top of the glass. A piece of bread can be used to scoop food onto an eating utensil. Food for the blind person can be placed on the plate according to a system similar to the hours on a clock face. For example, the meat can be at 5 o'clock, the salad at 9 o'clock, the potatoes at 1 o'clock.

Rationale: Special techniques for eating support independence for the blind person.

Fulfilled Needs: Sense of adequacy, independence, mastery and competence in skills, increased learning

Recommend eating only well-cooked meat and vegetables in foreign countries   Explain that meat should be ordered well done, not rare, when one is visiting a foreign country. Vegetables should also be well cooked.

Rationale: Thorough cooking decreases the potential for infection from bacteria or infestation (blood flukes, trichina).

Fulfilled Needs: Protection from physical harm, increased learning

Recommend energy-conserving methods for lifting and moving objects   Explain that the entire body weight should be employed in pushing or pulling, rather than just the arms or legs. Objects should be lifted with the arms close to the body, rather than extended outward from the body, and the weight of an object should be borne equally by both arms.

Rationale: Fatigue results from energy-consuming activity. The use of efficient methods conserves strength, promotes comfort, and supports independent activity.

Fulfilled Needs: Energy, comfort, protection from physical harm, independence, increased learning

Recommend fluid restriction   Suggest that no fluids or limited fluids be taken as appropriate to the person's health needs or situations.

Rationale: Limiting fluid intake after the evening meal reduces the amount of urine produced by the kidneys after the bladder is emptied at bedtime. This practice decreases the reflex stimulation to void during the night.

Fulfilled Needs: Comfort, increased learning

Recommend home adaptations appropriate to the health problem   Offer

ideas as to how home adjustments may be made to fit the health problem. Suggest
methods that support independence of the ill person and reduce stress on those caring
for him. Suggest methods such as attaching hand rails in bathrooms and putting a chair
lift on a stairway.

Rationale: Home adaptations can assist the person to achieve greater independence.

Fulfilled Needs: Comfort, sense of adequacy, independence, increased learning, increased problem-solving ability.

Recommend home adaptations appropriate for persons in a wheelchair[108]   Recommend adaptations such as living in a single-level, ground-floor dwell-

ing, using outdoor carpeting instead of deep carpeting or tile floor coverings, removing
unnecessary doors when possible, having hallways at least 48 inches wide, using a narrow wheelchair, having windowsills, doorknobs, and light switches no higher than 36
inches from the floor, placing electrical outlets 18 inches above the floor, using polyethylene instead of wood or metal doorsills, using front-loading washers and dryers, and
front stove controls, having low storage cabinets and revolving cabinet shelves, and installing low clothing racks.

Rationale: Proper adaptation of the home environment promotes safe and easier use
of a wheelchair for mobility.

Fulfilled Needs: Protection from physical harm, increased learning

Recommend home adaptations appropriate for persons unable to stoop[108]

Recommend adaptations such as high electrical outlets, top-loading washers and dryers,
top stove controls, and high storage cabinets.

Rationale: Proper adaptation of the home environment promotes safety and efficiency for persons who are unable to stoop.

Fulfilled Needs: Protection from physical harm, increased learning

Recommend limiting jet flying time to five consecutive hours when possible   Suggest that a person engaging in jet travel plan stopovers after 4 or 5 hours of

flight whenever possible.

Rationale: Interrupting lengthy jet flights can reduce fatigue and the stress imposed
by time-zone changes.

Fulfilled Needs: Energy, protection from physical harm, increased learning

Recommend methods for achieving total relaxation   Suggest that total re-

laxation can be accomplished by setting aside some time each day when one is totally
free from all mental and physical activity. Explain that the person should not feel that
doing nothing is a waste of time, since relaxation is essential to health. Controlled
breathing, involving a conscious and gradual decrease in respirations below 10 times a
minute, promotes relaxation. Quietly listening to soft music is also recommended.
These methods should be practiced daily.

Rationale: Sitting and relaxing can reduce the muscular contraction and tension associated with activity. Soothing music aids relaxation because of its calming effect on the
nervous system and because it distracts the mind from other mental activity. Slow,
rhythmic breathing lowers oxygen intake, which slows the nervous system and general
body function, quiets the emotions, and reduces muscular contraction.

Fulfilled Needs: Relaxation, energy, comfort, protection from physical harm, protection from psychologic threat, increased learning

Contraindications: Respiratory distress

Recommend methods for distraction from pain   Relate the methods that can

be used to distract attention from pain, such as watching television, listening to music,
counting, praying, and imagining pleasant scenes.

Rationale: Distraction from pain temporarily reduces the perception of pain severity.

Fulfilled Needs: Comfort, protection from psychologic threat

Recommend methods for increasing sensory stimulation
Suggest that there are many ways in which sensory stimulation can be increased: avoid monotonous tasks; increase room lighting; use bright room colors; add background sound by turning on a radio, television, or tape recorder; open windows to admit street noises; use unfamiliar routes to and from places; find employment in a large organization; mingle with crowds; attend exciting entertainment such as disaster movies, horse races, and competitive sports; use many nonpermanent articles; travel; seek out a variety of friends; live in a big city.

Rationale: Adequate sensory stimulation is essential for sound physical and mental health. Sensory stimulation increases motivation and encourages creativity.

Fulfilled Needs: Comfort, stimulation, protection from physical harm, protection from psychologic threat, increased learning, increased creativity

Recommend methods for noise reduction
Suggest that noise can be reduced by closing doors and windows, using heavy drapes, turning radios, recorders, or televisions off or to low volume, wearing earplugs or mufflers, and carpeting areas where noisy equipment is used.

Rationale: Sound waves at intensities above 80 decibels irritate the human ear. The noise level inside the home should be limited to 35 or 40 decibels. Excessive environmental stimuli increase stress.

Fulfilled Needs: Comfort, protection from physical harm, protection from psychologic threat, increased learning

Recommend methods for preparing a sick room at home
Suggest ways in which the sick room can be prepared or improved: room location, equipment needed, furniture placement, and the like.

Rationale: A properly located and equipped sick room meets the patient's needs and facilitates ease in caring for the patient.

Fulfilled Needs: Comfort, protection from physical harm, increased learning

Recommend methods for reducing sensory stimulation
Suggest ways in which sensory stimulation can be limited: use subdued room light; decrease the noise level by turning off radios and televisions; close windows to reduce street noises; avoid offensive environmental odors; use familiar routes to and from places; find employment in a small, quiet office; remain away from crowds; attend light entertainment that does not involve tension and excitement; participate in noncompetitive games; dismiss unimportant matters so that the mind is not overstressed; delegate decision-making to other capable persons; reduce change by using permanent articles instead of throwaway articles; minimize travel or limit travel to only familiar places; keep the same job, the same car, and several very close friends; limit change to one change at a time whenever possible; live in a small or moderate-size community; become involved only up to a comfortable level, not to a higher level that might please others.

Rationale: Reduction of sensory stimulation decreases the amount of physical and psychologic adaptation to be made in order to deal with stress, which in turn supports good health.

Fulfilled Needs: Comfort, protection from physical harm, protection from psychologic threat, increased learning, increased pleasantness

Recommend methods used to stop smoking
Explain that there are many different methods used to stop smoking: withdrawing gradually by cutting one's smoking in half each day; stopping suddenly; keeping cigarettes in a pocket or purse so that they are available if one feels desperate; delaying each smoke by an hour; quitting while on vacation, when normal pressures are decreased; promising to stop smoking, but keeping it private so as to reduce the social pressures; puffing on an empty cigarette holder; chewing on a pipe; chewing on root ginger, which will cause a bad taste if one resumes smoking; letting a cigarette burn unsmoked; smoking only part of a cigarette; smoking bad-tasting cigarettes; chewing gum or eating candy; treating oneself each time one

avoids smoking; changing the habits of living associated with smoking, such as going for a walk after meals instead of having a cigarette.

Rationale: Smoking increases the carbon monoxide content in hemoglobin and reduces its capacity to carry oxygen; it contracts airway muscles thus narrowing respiratory passages and reducing air flow; it constricts and thickens blood vessels, which decreases circulation, especially to the extremities; it increases the catecholamine level, which increases the heart's need for oxygen; it irritates the intestines, causing ulceration; it retards healing of peptic ulcers because of vasoconstriction; it causes paralysis of respiratory cilia, which prevents the cilia from expelling foreign particles from the respiratory system; it thickens the respiratory mucous membranes and obstructs them with secretions; it causes growth of abnormal lung cells and produces tissue inflammation.

Fulfilled Needs: Protection from physical harm, increased learning

Recommend new options for effective methods of coping   If the person is not coping in the most effective manner, suggest coping mechanisms that will lead to greater success in the struggle. For instance, if a person is angrily venting frustration on loved ones, suggest that these frustrations can better be vented on the tennis court.

Rationale: Effective coping methods are essential to good mental health and happiness.

Fulfilled Needs: Comfort, protection from psychologic threat, psychologic stability, increased learning

Recommend putting one or two drops of oil of wintergreen in the vacuum cleaner bag   Suggest that the person place one or two drops of oil of Wintergreen in the vacuum cleaner bag before using the vacuum cleaner.

Rationale: Oil of wintergreen in the vacuum cleaner bag will freshen the air when the carpet is being cleaned.

Fulfilled Needs: Comfort, increased learning

Recommend rough-textured food to stimulate swallowing   Suggest that the person select foods that have a rough texture, such as toast instead of soft bread, baked instead of mashed potatoes, and apple slices instead of applesauce.

Rationale: Rough-textured food tends to stimulate swallowing in persons with hemiplegia, whereas soft foods have little stimulating quality.

Fulfilled Needs: Comfort, increased learning

Recommend safety measures to prevent a burn injury   Recommend measures such as keeping fireplaces and open heaters screened, storing matches in a metal container, keeping stoves free of grease, not wearing long sleeves or plastic aprons around open flames, using well-padded pot holders, turning pot handles toward the back of the stove, not smoking around oxygen or in bed, and avoiding the danger of fireworks and chemicals.

Rationale: Knowledge of how to reduce the potential for burn injury prevents human suffering.

Fulfilled Needs: Protection from physical harm, increased learning

Recommend safety measures to prevent electrical injury   Recommend measures such as disconnecting unused electrical equipment, immediately repairing worn electrical cords and hot equipment switches or plugs, placing safety guards over electrical outlets, standing on dry surfaces and wearing insulated rubber gloves and rubber-soled shoes when working with electricity, never using electrical appliances near or in water, using only grounded electrical equipment and appliances, never plugging a two-prong adaptor into a three prong plug, not overloading extension cords or wall outlets, and never standing in an open field during an electrical storm.

Rationale: Knowledge of preventive measures reduces the danger of electrical injury.

Fulfilled Needs: Protection from physical harm, increased learning

Recommend safety measures to prevent eye injury   Recommend measures

such as wearing safety goggles, avoiding sungazing even when wearing sunglasses, never wiping the eyes with soiled towels or hands, properly focusing the television picture, viewing the television from the front and not side angles, putting a light on in the room while viewing television, viewing television from a moderate distance, and preventing children from playing with toys that could injure the eye.

Rationale: Knowledge of preventive measures reduces the potential for eye injury, impaired vision, or blindness.

Fulfilled Needs: Protection from physical harm, increased learning

Recommend safety measures to prevent falling Recommend measures such as using suction mats in tubs, securing extension cords in place, keeping the floors and stairways litterfree and wax free, removing snow and ice from stairways, maintaining sturdy stair rails, using only sturdy ladders, using stairgates to prevent tumbles down stairs, and using safety straps for poorly coordinated persons and in hazardous occupations.

Rationale: Knowledge of preventive measures diminishes the potential for injury from falling.

Fulfilled Needs: Protection from physical harm, increased learning

Recommend safety measures to prevent motor vehicle injury Recommend measures such as always fastening seat belts, placing small children in safety seats, keeping the vehicle in good repair, driving no faster than the speed limit, respecting stop and yield signs, and driving defensively.

Rationale: Knowledge of preventive measures reduces the potential for injury from motor vehicles.

Fulfilled Needs: Protection from physical harm, increased learning

Recommend safety measures to prevent poisoning Recommend measures such as storing dangerous products out of reach, locking medicine cabinets, clearly and correctly labeling all containers, and using safety caps on drugs and chemicals.

Rationale: Knowledge of safety measures assists the person to practice preventive health.

Fulfilled Needs: Protection from physical harm, increased learning

Recommend safety measures to prevent suffocation Recommend measures such as never starting a car in a closed garage, using fume-producing substances only in open air, venting heaters to the outside, shredding or discarding plastic bags, locking unused refrigerators or removing the doors, placing infants in a pillow-free crib, never sleeping in the same bed with an infant, never smoking in bed, not hanging a pacifier around an infant's neck, keeping clotheslines high enough to prevent strangulation, and using protective measures against unattended entry into pools.

Rationale: Knowledge of preventive measures reduces the potential for suffocation.

Fulfilled Needs: Protection from physical harm, increased learning

Recommend safety measures to prevent wound injuries Recommend measures such as discarding cracked or broken dishware, using only covered knife racks, storing unloaded guns and ammunition in a locked cabinet or drawer, removing large icicles before they melt and fall, wearing a hard hat for head protection, and discarding or not giving children any toys with sharp edges or that are sharp when broken.

Rationale: Knowledge and practice of preventive measures diminishes the potential for wound injury.

Fulfilled Needs: Protection from physical harm, increased learning

Recommend strict adherence to safety rules Explain that safety rules should be followed without exception.

Rationale: Safety rules are devised to protect against accidental injury or disease.

Fulfilled Needs: Protection from physical harm, increased learning

Recommend that a high glucose source be carried at all times Teach the person who is likely to develop low blood sugar to carry a ready source of glucose, such as sugar packets or candy.

Rationale: Ingestion of glucose will raise a low blood sugar level to normal and maintain body cell activity and energy production. Prolonged and severe low blood sugar levels can result in brain damage.

Fulfilled Needs: Protection from physical harm, increased learning

Recommend that alkalis be used conservatively Explain that when alkalis are taken in large doses, they disturb acid–base balance. Foods such as milk, cream, and buttermilk and antacid and alkali medications should be taken in moderation.

Rationale: Normal body function is dependent on acid–base balance.

Fulfilled Needs: Acid–base balance, protection from physical harm, increased learning

Contraindications: When large doses of alkali are prescribed as an ulcer regimen.

Recommend that behavioral limits be set Suggest that there are times to set limits on how far to go to meet the demands of another person. It should be made clear that excessive demands cannot be met, and an explanation or a reason should be given.

Rationale: Setting limits gives the demanding person a guideline by which to control behavior. Giving a reason for not meeting a person's demand reduces the possibility that the refusal will be perceived as rejection.

Fulfilled Needs: Protection from psychologic threat, personal growth and maturity, increased learning, increased reality perception and problem-solving ability

Recommend that bones be removed from food before eating Explain that bones should be removed before food is placed in the mouth, not after.

Rationale: Once bones are in the mouth, they can easily be aspirated, which can cause lung or tracheal injury.

Fulfilled Needs: Protection from physical harm, increased learning

Recommend that children be introduced to a wide variety of food Suggest that a child taste as many different foods as possible at the earliest appropriate time.

Rationale: Exposing children to a wide variety of food supports taste development and good nutrition.

Fulfilled Needs: Nutritional balance, comfort, protection from physical harm, increased learning

Recommend that extra therapeutic supplies/drugs be carried Suggest that the person carry an additional supply of whatever he might need to carry out self-care or prescribed treatment, such as an extra ostomy appliance, absorbent dressings, or medications.

Rationale: Extra supplies provide the comfort of being ready for accidents or delays in returning home.

Fulfilled Needs: Comfort, increased learning

Recommend that families not financially support the drug user's habit Explain that money should not be given to drug users to buy drugs. But it should be made known that love and emotional support are always available to the drug user.

Rationale: Financial support of a drug habit perpetuates drug use. Giving love and emotional support makes the person feel significant and may help overcome the drug abuse.

Fulfilled Needs: Comfort, protection from psychologic threat, increased learning

Recommend that food be cut in small bite-size pieces Suggest that food be cut into small bite-size portions rather than into large chunks.

Rationale: If small bites of food are aspirated, they are less likely to cause fatal airway obstruction than large bites.

Fulfilled Needs: Protection from physical harm, increased learning

Recommend that food servings be in proportion to the appetite   Suggest that the size of the food serving be appropriate to the person's appetite. Never serve more food than a person wants and can eat.

Rationale: Serving large portions of food to the person with a poor appetite has a discouraging effect and further diminishes his desire to eat.

Fulfilled Needs: Comfort, increased learning

Recommend that high altitudes be avoided   Explain that persons with heart disease, sickle cell anemia, or hemoglobin below 10 g avoid traveling to areas high above sea level, especially areas higher than 6,000 feet.

Rationale: The partial pressure of oxygen in the blood is decreased at high altitudes, placing extra stress on the heart. Altitudes above 6,000 feet cause hypoxia. In sickle cell anemia, such altitudes sometimes result in increased sickling of erythrocytes, causing splenic infarction.

Fulfilled Needs: Tissue oxygenation or perfusion, protection from physical harm, increased learning

Recommend that independence be encouraged   Explain that every person needs freedom from control by others and should have the opportunity to try new things.

Rationale: Balancing dependence and independence needs is essential to growth, maturity, adequacy, and self-reliance. Independence supports the development of a person's potential.

Fulfilled Needs: Protection from psychologic threat, sense of adequacy, self-reliance, independence, personal growth and maturity, awareness of potential, increased learning, full development of potential, increased reality perception and problem-solving ability

Recommend that infants be fed on a self-demand schedule   Suggest that infants be fed when they indicate hunger through crying. Most babies will put themselves on a regular schedule.

Rationale: An infant fed on a self-demand schedule is most likely to obtain adequate nutrition, since his food demand is based on physiologic needs.

Fulfilled Needs: Nutritional balance, comfort, protection from physical harm, increased learning

Recommend that jet travelers reduce stress by arriving 24 hours before scheduled activity[564,657]   Suggest that the person engaged in extensive jet travel arrive at his destination 24 hours before planned meetings or sightseeing activities.

Rationale: Arriving 24 hours before scheduled activity allows time for rest and adjustment to time-zone changes. This is particularly important for a job in which major decisions have to be made.

Fulfilled Needs: Energy, protection from physical harm, protection from psychologic threat, increased learning

Recommend that passive activities be avoided   Explain that passive activities such as sleeping, reading, watching television, and listening to radio should be avoided as much as possible by healthy persons. Explain that active activities are preferable.

Rationale: Passive activities lead to boredom and frustration and reduce involvement in healthy activity and exercise.

Fulfilled Needs: Protection from physical harm, protection from psychologic threat, increased learning

Recommend that perfumed vaginal products be avoided   Suggest that perfumed products for vaginal hygiene not be used. Such products include feminine hygiene sprays, prepackaged douches, deodorants, powders of any kind, and perfumed tampons or sanitary pads.

Rationale: Products containing perfume can cause skin and mucosal irritation. They also disguise odors that may be signs of disease.

Fulfilled Needs: Protection from physical harm, increased learning

Recommend that self-medication be avoided

Explain that prescribing drugs for oneself or one's children can result in serious side effects, because faulty determination of the cause of the problem will result in taking the wrong drug.

Rationale: Chemical reactions within the body resulting from combination of incompatible elements can produce poisoning effects. Drugs taken during pregnancy can cause birth defects or impair fetal development.

Fulfilled Needs: Protection from physical harm, increased learning

Recommend that the approximate eating schedule be maintained despite long jet trips[564,657]

Suggest that the person engaged in extensive jet travel eat three times a day at 5–6-hour intervals, or as near to his normal schedule as possible.

Rationale: Adequate nutrition reduces the fatigue associated with travel.

Fulfilled Needs: Nutritional balance, protection from physical harm, increased learning

Recommend that the tongue be brushed

Suggest using a toothbrush to brush the tongue gently.

Rationale: Brushing the tongue cleans its surface and removes food particles from cracks in the tongue.

Fulfilled Needs: Comfort, cleanliness, protection from physical harm, increased learning

Contraindications: Tongue inflammation or pain.

Recommend that toys be washable

Suggest that parents provide children with toys that can be washed or cleaned. Plush unwashable toys can be cleaned by sprinkling them with corn meal, letting them stand awhile, and then brushing out the corn meal.

Rationale: Unclean toys can carry bacteria and lead to infection.

Fulfilled Needs: Cleanliness, protection from physical harm, increased learning

Recommend that two ostomy appliances be used alternately

Suggest that the person have two ostomy appliances so that one can be used while the other is being prepared for use.

Rationale: Having two ostomy appliances allows for one appliance to be thoroughly cleaned and dried while the other is in use.

Fulfilled Needs: Comfort, cleanliness, increased learning

Recommend that windows be screened

Suggest that screens be put on windows to keep insects out.

Rationale: Insects carry microorganisms from one person to another and transmit disease.

Fulfilled Needs: Energy, comfort, protection from physical harm, independence, increased learning

Recommend the carrying of extra undergarments when away from home

When a person has a colostomy, incontinence, or heavy menstrual flow, suggest that he carry extra undergarments when at work, shopping, etc. Underpants can be tucked into the purse or briefcase without notice by others.

Rationale: Having a change of undergarments promotes comfort when unsuspected accidents occur.

Fulfilled Needs: Comfort, increased learning

Recommend the continued practice of wellness behavior Recommend that even though the person has achieved wellness, he should continue those practices that lead to even higher levels of health.

Rationale: Wellness is not a consistent state unless the person practices wellness behavior from day to day and from year to year.

Fulfilled Needs: Protection from physical harm, increased learning

Recommend the installation of a smoke alarm Suggest the installation of an alarm that signals when a fire is still in the smoldering stage.

Rationale: If a person is unable to detect odors easily, a smoke alarm can warn that a fire is in its early stages. Smoke alarms will wake a sleeping person in time to escape a fire.

Fulfilled Needs: Protection from physical harm, increased learning

Recommend the person have a pet Suggest that the person obtain a pet of his choice to live with him. Dogs and cats are preferred in-house pets.

Rationale: Pets give the person a feeling of responsibility for a significant other, promoting a feeling of self-worth. Pets can be talked to and seem to listen with full attention, providing unqualified acceptance of the person's comments. They provide company for persons who are alone. The warmth and affection with which pets respond meet the needs of persons seeking comfort in relatedness.

Fulfilled Needs: Comfort, caring and communicating relationships, love and affection, acceptance, increased learning

Recommend the preferable age for introducing specific foods to children[460] Explain that certain solid foods should be introduced to young children at certain ages. At *age 1–4 months* the child should begin to eat cereals, at *age 2–4 months* stewed or strained fruits and very ripe bananas, *age 3–5 months* strained vegetables, *age 2–6 months* pureed egg yolk, *age 6 months and older* puddings, potatoes, and finger foods such as toast and zwieback, *age 7–12 months* lumpy foods, *age 9 months* soft-boiled eggs or scrambled whole eggs and mashed foods, *age 10–12 months*, boiled or broiled fish that has been boned.

Rationale: Sound nutrition is essential to healthy growth and development.

Fulfilled Needs: Comfort, nutritional balance, protection from physical harm, increased learning

Recommend the pursuit of only one activity at a time Explain that muscular tension can be reduced by engaging in only one activity at a time. When that activity is completed, then one can move on to the next task.

Rationale: Performing only one activity at a time reduces the number of stimuli to which the body must respond, promoting relaxation and decreasing energy consumption.

Fulfilled Needs: Relaxation, energy, comfort, protection from physical harm, protection from psychologic threat, increased learning

Recommend the use of a back-support garment Suggest that snugly fitting garments be worn to give back support.

Rationale: Back-support garments reduce muscle strain and promote body alignment and comfort.

Fulfilled Needs: Comfort, freedom from pain, increased learning

Recommend the use of a brassiere for breast support Suggest that during pregnancy and lactation, or after a mastectomy, a comfortable supportive brassiere be worn. The brassiere should have a sufficiently large cup; it should cover all breast tissue in the underarm area and should have wide supportive straps.

Rationale: Use of a supportive brassiere during pregnancy, lactation, or breast engorgement can relieve discomfort from breast weight, shield the breast for cleanliness, and minimize fluid congestion. Breast support prevents overstretching and tearing of muscle fibers, thus forestalling premature breast sagging. Since the absence of one breast tends to pull the body to one side, breast support after mastectomy brings the body into normal alignment.

Fulfilled Needs: Comfort, cleanliness, protection from physical harm, increased learning

Recommend the use of a car backrest
Suggest that the person with back problems use a backrest, especially designed for automobiles, when driving.

Rationale: A car backrest offers firm support, which promotes comfort.

Fulfilled Needs: Comfort, freedom from pain, increased learning

Recommended the use of a face mask
Suggest that whenever dust, bacteria, vapor, or fumes come in contact with the face, a mask should be worn.

Rationale: A face mask protects the skin and respiratory system against injurious foreign objects.

Fulfilled Needs: Protection from physical harm, increased learning

Recommend the use of a fluoride toothpaste
Suggest that a toothpaste containing fluoride be used every day.

Rationale: Trace amounts of the element fluorine in water or toothpaste help prevent tooth decay.

Fulfilled Needs: Protection from physical harm, increased learning

Recommend the use of a laryngectomy bib
Suggest that the patient who has had a laryngectomy wear a cotton or crocheted bib to keep clothing clean.

Rationale: Expulsion of mucus from the laryngectomy stoma will stain clothing. A bib helps maintain cleanliness and offers protection from irritants.

Fulfilled Needs: Comfort, cleanliness, increased learning

Recommend the use of a mouthwash
Suggest the use of salt solution or commercial mouthwash to rinse the mouth. When oral bleeding occurs, mouthwash should be used gently, or a padded tongue blade may be soaked in mouthwash and swabbed around the mouth.

Rationale: Use of a mouthwash removes food particles from the teeth, refreshes the breath, and provides a pleasant taste.

Fulfilled Needs: Comfort, cleanliness, protection from physical harm, increased learning

Contraindications: Avoid using mouthwash when there are blood clots in the mouth or when oral mucosa is inflamed or irritated.

Recommend the use of a night light
Suggest that a night light be kept on when a person has visual or mobility impairment.

Rationale: Use of a night light prevents accidents. It keeps sleep disturbance to a minimum when the person must get up during the night, and it prevents distorted perception.

Fulfilled Needs: Protection from physical harm, increased learning

Recommend the use of a nipple shield or nipple padding
Suggest that when a breast is cracked or irritated, a soft protective shield be placed over the nipple, especially while the infant is nursing. Suggest that pads be placed over the breast nipple or inserted into the brassiere when lactation secretion threatens to soil clothes.

Rationale: A nipple shield prevents irritation of breast nipple tissue, facilitates healing, promotes cleanliness, and permits continued breast-feeding. Nipple padding promotes comfort and cleanliness by preventing seepage of breast secretions onto clothes.

Fulfilled Needs: Comfort, cleanliness, protection from physical harm, increased learning

Recommend the use of a pacemaker shirt Suggest that an undershirt with a pocket large enough to hold a pacemaker be worn.

Rationale: An undershirt can hold a pacemaker in place and prevent skin irritation from the pacemaker.

Fulfilled Needs: Comfort, protection from physical harm, increased learning

Recommend the use of a sheepskin Suggest that sheep's wool be placed under a person who must lie or sit for prolonged periods.

Rationale: The air spaces in a sheepskin help keep the person's skin dry. Its softness eases pressure on the skin and helps prevent decubitus ulcer.

Fulfilled Needs: Comfort, protection from physical harm, increased learning

Recommend the use of a shower chair Suggest that the weak patient sit on a waterproof chair or stool in the shower.

Rationale: Using a chair or stool in the shower can reduce the potential for falling and can conserve energy.

Fulfilled Needs: Energy, comfort, protection from physical harm, increased learning

Recommend the use of a typewriter when unable to write Suggest that the person who is unable to write but who still has coarse finger movements use a typewriter.

Rationale: Use of a typewriter can facilitate communication with others.

Fulfilled Needs: Caring and communicating relationships, increased learning

Recommend the use of a water-soluble lubricant Suggest that, before sexual intercourse, the woman lubricate the vaginal orifice with a water-soluble jelly (K-Y jelly).

Rationale: When there is vaginal dryness, the lubrication of the vaginal orifice allows for easier and less painful penile penetration during sexual intercourse.

Fulfilled Needs: Comfort, protection from physical harm, increased learning

Recommend the use of absorbent padding Suggest that padding made of a material that will soak up liquid excretions and drainage be placed under the patient and around draining wounds.

Rationale: Many materials can absorb wetness that would otherwise remain in contact with the skin and cause skin irritation.

Fulfilled Needs: Comfort, cleanliness, protection from physical harm

Recommend the use of an abdominal-support garment Suggest that a girdle or binder be worn when the patient is out of bed.

Rationale: Supportive garments prevent muscle sagging.

Fulfilled Needs: Comfort, protection from physical harm, increased learning

Contraindications: Impaired circulation

Recommend the use of an antiperspirant Suggest the use of commercial antiperspirants on the axilla after bathing for control of sweating and skin odor.

Rationale: Body odor may be controlled by oxidizing odoriferous material or by inhibiting bacterial growth.

Fulfilled Needs: Comfort, cleanliness, increased learning

Contraindications: Axillary skin irritation or inflammation, allergy

Recommend the use of an antiperspirant foot powder Explain that foot odor can be controlled by a thin application of a commercial foot powder that prevents sweat secretion.

Rationale: Inhibiting sweat secretion reduces skin odor and promotes cleanliness and comfort.

Fulfilled Needs: Comfort, cleanliness, increased learning

Contraindications: Skin irritation or inflammation, allergy

Recommend the use of bed rails Suggest that young children, old persons and irresponsible persons be protected with side rails on their beds.

Rationale: Side rails minimize the potential for falling.

Fulfilled Needs: Protection from physical harm, increased learning

Recommend the use of dental floss Suggest that dental floss be used to clean between the teeth at least once a day.

Rationale: Dental floss removes food particles and plaque from between the teeth and reduces the potential for decay.

Fulfilled Needs: Protection from physical harm, increased learning

Recommend the use of denture adherent Suggest that an adherent be used to assure snug-fitting dentures.

Rationale: Properly fitting dentures are necessary for comfort, for normal chewing, and for prevention of oral mucosa injury.

Fulfilled Needs: Comfort, protection from physical harm, increased learning

Contraindications: Oral mucosal infection, inflammation, or irritation, or allergy

Recommend the use of disposable dishes for contagious diseases Suggest that paper or plastic disposable dishes and utensils be used when caring for the person with a communicable disease.

Rationale: Disposable dishes minimize the possibility of transmitting infection.

Fulfilled Needs: Cleanliness, protection from physical harm, increased learning

Recommend the use of double-thickness tissue for infectious sputum Suggest that when infectious sputum is expectorated, double-thickness tissue should be used.

Rationale: It is difficult for microorganisms to penetrate double-thickness tissue. This reduces the potential for transmitting infection.

Fulfilled Needs: Protection from physical harm, increased learning

Recommend the use of dry shampoo Suggest that dry shampoo may be used to clean and freshen the hair when it cannot be washed.

Rationale: Dry shampoo cleans superficial dirt and oil from the hair by absorbing greasy materials that hold dirt.

Fulfilled Needs: Comfort, cleanliness, protection from physical harm, increased learning

Contraindications: Scalp infection, abrasions, or bleeding

Recommend the use of eye shields for sleeping Suggest that persons traveling by airplane use eye shields for sleeping especially when flying all night and into the dawn.

Rationale: Eye shields provide darkness, which is conducive to sleep.

Fulfilled Needs: Sleep and rest, protection from physical harm, increased learning

Recommend the use of individual dishes, utensils, and drinking glasses Suggest that each person have his own dishes, utensils, and glasses and that dishes not be shared between persons.

Rationale: Use of separate dishes minimizes the potential for transfer of infectious microorganisms.

Fulfilled Needs: Cleanliness, protection from physical harm, increased learning

Recommend the use of individual towels and washcloths   Suggest that each person have his own towel and washcloth and not use linens used by others.

Rationale: Using individual towels and washcloths promotes cleanliness and minimizes the spread of disease.

Fulfilled Needs: Cleanliness, protection from physical harm, increased learning

Recommend the use of iodized salt   Suggest that salt containing sodium iodide or potassium iodide be used to season food.

Rationale: Use of iodized salt will prevent iodine deficiency, and its use during early iodine deficiency will usually correct the problem. Iodine is essential to the production of thyroxine, which is necessary for normal metabolism.

Fulfilled Needs: Protection from physical harm, increased learning

Recommend the use of knots to distinguish clothing color for the visually impaired   Suggest that different numbers of embroidery knots placed inside of clothing can designate the color. For example, two knots might indicate brown, three knots green, and so on.

Rationale: Coding clothes by knots enables persons with impaired vision to know the colors of their clothing and to dress independently.

Fulfilled Needs: Comfort, mastery and competence in skills, independence, increased learning

Recommend the use of lightweight clothing   Suggest that the person wear clothing made of cool material, such as cottons instead of polyesters. Also, recommend clothing that weighs as little as possible.

Rationale: Lightweight clothing can help maintain a cool body temperature, decrease pressure on irritating lesions, and reduce the weight a weakened body must carry.

Fulfilled Needs: Normal body temperature, energy, comfort, protection from physical harm, increased learning

Recommend the use of low-heeled shoes   Suggest that shoes having no heels or slight heels be worn in preference to high-heeled shoes.

Rationale: Low-heeled shoes maintain correct body alignment. High-heeled shoes throw the skeleton and abdominal organs forward and increase the potential for falling.

Fulfilled Needs: Protection from physical harm, increased learning

Recommend the use of rubber gloves   Suggest that rubber gloves be worn whenever the hands are placed in harsh detergents.

Rationale: Harsh detergents irritate the skin and cause chapping, cracking, and allergic responses.

Fulfilled Needs: Comfort, cleanliness, protection from physical harm, increased learning

Recommend the use of safety lens in eyeglasses   Suggest that eyeglasses with shatterproof lenses be purchased.

Rationale: Shatterproof eyeglasses reduce the potential for eye injury.

Fulfilled Needs: Protection from physical harm, increased learning

Recommend the use of slow, distinct speech with persons having impaired communication reception   Suggest that slow, clear speech be used when talking to persons who have difficulty receiving messages.

Rationale: Slow, distinct speech enhances communication perception.

Fulfilled Needs: Comfort, protection from psychologic threat, caring and communicating relationships, increased learning

Recommend the use of sun-screening lotion   Suggest that when out in the sun for long periods, the person use a lotion that protects the skin. The lotion should contain padimate O and PABA. Lotions containing padimate A should not be used because it causes severe burns.

Rationale: Sunscreening lotion prevents ultraviolet sunrays from reaching and burning the skin.

Fulfilled Needs: Protection from physical harm, increased learning

Recommend the use of warm clothing   Suggest that adequately warm clothing be worn in cold weather, including hat and gloves.

Rationale: Warm clothing protects the body from the harmful effects of cold weather. Warm clothing in bed prevents chilling, which stimulates bed-wetting.

Fulfilled Needs: Comfort, protection from physical harm, increased learning

Recommend the wearing of cotton underpants   Suggest that underpants be worn that are made of cotton instead of synthetic fibers.

Rationale: Cotton, being more absorbent than synthetics, will confine odors and drainage. Synthetics, being less absorbent, permit distribution of drainage and odor over a larger area.

Fulfilled Needs: Comfort, increased learning

Recommend things to do when the person begins to feel out of control

Sit down with the person and make a list of things he can do when he feels he is beginning to lose emotional control. Such activities include washing the hands and face in cold water, taking slow, deep breaths to promote relaxation, temporarily withdrawing from the situation, counting to 500 while considering the outcome of loss of control, beating a pillow, and taking a walk. Individualize the list for the person.

Rationale: When experiencing an emotion, having something to do defuses the emotion and gives the person something to do besides feel. By maintaining self-control, the person has increased control of the situation. Self-control prevents future feelings of guilt, low self-esteem, etc.

Fulfilled Needs: Protection from psychologic threat, psychologic stability, personal growth and maturity, increased learning

Recommend thorough food chewing   Suggest that food be chewed slowly and thoroughly before swallowing.

Rationale: The first step toward adequate digestion is chewing food into small particles. Thorough chewing helps offset deficient digestive secretion if saliva production is diminished, and it enhances digestive enzyme activity when food reaches the stomach and intestines.

Fulfilled Needs: Comfort, protection from physical harm, increased learning

Recommend throat gargling   Suggest the use of a salt gargle or medicated gargle whenever the throat feels scratchy or painful.

Rationale: Warm isotonic saline gargles are cleansing and soothing. Antiseptic gargles are astringent and cleansing. Anesthetic gargles have analgesic effects.

Fulfilled Needs: Comfort, cleanliness, protection from physical harm, increased learning

Contraindications: Impaired swallowing

Recommend voiding after sexual intercourse   Suggest that a woman void after having sexual intercourse.

Rationale: Voiding after sexual intercourse flushes bacteria from the external urinary meatus that could be transferred into the urethra and upward.

Fulfilled Needs: Protection from physical harm

Recommend work methods for decreasing human energy consumption

Recommend methods such as eliminating unnecessary work, combining work activities, dividing time between high-energy and low-energy consuming activities, distributing heavy tasks throughout the week, duplicating equipment in work areas, using a cannister or self-propelled vacuum, using rolling tables, using lightweight household items, installing push-bar windows and electric garage doors, and living in a single-level ground-floor home.

Rationale: Knowledge of how to conserve human energy improves the performance efficiency of daily tasks.

Fulfilled Needs: Sense of usefulness, increased learning

Relate specific methods for improving communications with speech-impaired persons   Explain that the person with impaired communication ability must be allowed time for thought comprehension, that misinterpreted messages should be corrected immediately, that nonverbal communications should be limited to only one person at a time, that discussions should be short, that assistive devices such as alphabet letters, words, and phrases cards, and writing pad and pencil are helpful, that the person should not be asked to repeat the message too often, that shouting at the person should be avoided, that messages may have to be repeated frequently, that the person should wait for a response to one message before delivering another.

Rationale: Communication abilities are essential to meeting basic human needs.

Fulfilled Needs: Comfort, caring and communicating relationships, protection from physical harm, increased learning

Relate the accepted criteria for commitment of drug or alcohol abusers or the mentally ill   Explain that confinement is considered when a person is unable to function normally, breaks with reality, or is in danger of harming himself or others.

Rationale: Legal action for confinement taken by one person against another should be instigated for the well-being of the sick person and should be based on sound reasoning so as to reduce the potential for guilt.

Fulfilled Needs: Protection from psychologic threat, increased learning

Relate the accepted criteria for notifying authorities of drug abuse   Explain that notifying legal authorities of drug abuse is basically a matter of conscience. It is generally accepted that if a person is a minor or is a drug pusher, he should be reported to the authorities.

Rationale: Law-enforcement action taken by one person against another should be for the well-being of the sick person and should be based on sound reasoning so as to reduce the potential for guilt.

Fulfilled Needs: Protection from psychologic threat, increased learning

Relate the criteria for a successful sexual response   Explain that the experience of satisfaction, completeness, euphoria, or contentment indicates that the sexual relationship is successful.

Rationale: Awareness of enjoying successful sexual relationships supports comfort and feelings of adequacy.

Fulfilled Needs: Comfort, sexuality, protection from psychologic threat, sense of adequacy, increased learning

Relate the criteria for determining mental illness   Explain that some of the signs indicating mental illness are severe behavioral changes, periodic confusion or memory loss, feelings of persecution or grandiose feelings, talking to oneself, hearing voices, seeing visions, complaints of strange odors or tastes, bodily complaints that are physically not possible, severe depression, and physical abuse of others.

Rationale: Awareness of the manifestations of mental illness can support early and effective treatment.

Fulfilled Needs: Protection from physical harm, protection from psychologic threat, increased learning, increased reality perception and problem-solving ability

Relate the criteria for successful child-rearing[94] Explain that certain factors are necessary for successful child-rearing. They include frequent physical contact with the child, constant exposure of the child to emotional support in the form of positive reinforcement, and discipline based on informing the child of what is and is not acceptable and pleasing. Correction should be in the form of suggesting alternative activities or approaches, of providing good examples, and of insisting on an absolute minimum of "do nots." Punishment should be dealt at the time of the unacceptable behavior, should be appropriate to the child's age, should not inflict physical harm, and should be consistent. There should be a gradual lessening of adult restraint with a greater assumption of behavior control and responsibility by the child.

Rationale: Knowledge of successful child-rearing practices serves as a guide for positive parenting.

Fulfilled Needs: Personal growth and maturity, increased learning

Relate ways in which the person can enhance his self-image Enumerate ways that the person can feel good about his inner picture of himself. They include making his own decisions, assuming responsibility for his actions, being independent and not relying on others, being an individual and not copying others, accepting all of his limitations, feelings, senses, appetites, and physiologic changes as part of the self, and maintaining control of feelings, which heightens the ego.

Rationale: As self-image improves, the person becomes more confident and self-assured, more consistently productive, and less disturbed by negative comments from others.

Fulfilled Needs: High evaluation of self, self-reliance, personal growth and maturity

Suggest participation in group plans for weight reduction Suggest that the person who wishes to lose weight join an organized group of persons who are doing the same.

Rationale: Most groups working toward weight reduction support good nutrition. They emphasize gradual but steady weight loss and avoid harmful methods such as diet pills, one-food diets, etc. Groups also offer emotional support among persons working toward the same goal.

Fulfilled Needs: Comfort, group companionship, goal achievement, endurance, increased learning

Teach correct weight bearing on the crutch handbar Teach the person to bear weight on the crutch handbar. He should not lean on the crutches or suspend his weight from the point where his axillae meet the tops of the crutches.

Rationale: The pressure of the person's weight against the crutches at the axillae can cause nerve damage, with resulting paralysis of the hand or arm.

Fulfilled Needs: Protection from physical harm, increased learning

Teach decubitus ulcer care Explain how to take care of a decubitus ulcer. Include skin cleansing, use of toughening and healing agents, frequent turning, and use of sheepskin.

Rationale: Decubitus ulcer care promotes healing of pressure-damaged tissue.

Fulfilled Needs: Protection from physical harm, mastery and competence in skills, increased learning

Teach diabetic foot care[376,510] Teach the diabetic that foot care is essential. Explain that care of the foot requires the following steps: Washing the feet gently in warm, not hot, water, patting the skin dry between the toes, applying a light coating of lanolin to the feet immediately after drying, lightly applying mild foot powder between the toes and to the socks and shoes if the feet are sweaty, lightly rubbing the feet with alcohol instead of lanolin if there is extreme foot perspiration, lightly rubbing callouses and corns with a towel after bathing and avoiding trimming callouses and corns or applying corn removal pads, alternating socks and shoes daily and allowing them to dry thoroughly, and not walking barefooted.

Rationale: Diabetics are susceptible to hardening and narrowing of the arteries, which causes poor circulation in the skin. Washing the feet gently and using a soft towel on the feet reduces friction and decreases the potential for irritation of easily traumatized tissue. Keeping the skin dry between the toes minimizes the chance of fungal infection. The use of alcohol on the skin has a drying effect and prevents the irritation of perspiration wetness. Good foot care helps maintain intact, healthy feet and promotes healing when injury and lesions exist.

Fulfilled Needs: Comfort, protection from physical harm, increased learning

Teach diabetic nail care[376,510] Teach the diabetic that nail care is essential. Explain that care of the nails requires the following steps: washing the nails thoroughly in warm, soapy water, cleaning them with softened orange sticks, filing the nails frequently to keep them smooth and short, filing the toenails straight across and keeping the length even with the end of the toe, applying lanolin to brittle nails, and drying cuticles immediately after soaking them in warm water and patting them dry.

Rationale: The nails of the diabetic are susceptible to injury and infection. Lanolin softens the nails and surrounding tissue. It decreases skin cracking and facilitates healing. Soaking softens the nails for easier trimming. A cotton-tipped orange stick is used for cleaning instead of a sharp instrument to prevent injury to sensitive diabetic skin. By cutting the nails straight across, ingrown nails and infection are prevented. Filing the nails in one direction prevents splitting and tearing of nails.

Fulfilled Needs: Comfort, protection from physical harm, increased learning

Teach good body mechanics Explain that lifting an object from the ground should be accomplished with both the back muscles and leg muscles. In carrying a heavy object, the muscles of the shoulders, back, legs, and arms should be used. Stooping should be avoided. The person should squat by bending the knees and keeping the back straight.

Rationale: Good body mechanics can prevent injury to the skeletal system.

Fulfilled Needs: Comfort, protection from physical harm, increased learning

Teach good crutch-walking posture Teach the person walking with crutches to stand with his chest high, to extend fully (straighten) his hips and knees, and to look forward rather than down at his feet.

Rationale: Comfort, protection from physical harm, mastery and competence in skills, increased learning.

Fulfilled Needs: Comfort, protection from physical harm, mastery and competence in skills, increased learning

Teach good posture when walking with a leg prosthesis Teach the person wearing a lower-extremity prosthesis to avoid taking longer steps with the prosthesis foot than with the natural foot, to avoid walking with his feet far apart, and to avoid hip and shoulder hiking with each prosthetic step. The body should be held in good alignment.

Rationale:. Proper use of a prosthesis is essential for maximum weight-bearing and mobility.

Fulfilled Needs: Comfort, protection from physical harm, mastery and competence in skills, increased learning

Teach how and when to administer medications Explain the proper dosage and method for administering prescribed drugs. Include information about the purpose of the drug and the potential for side effects.

Rationale: Knowledge of correct drug administration increases the potential for effectiveness of therapy, reduces the potential for drug side effects, and supports independence.

Fulfilled Needs: Protection from physical harm, independence, increased learning

Teach how and when to irrigate a colostomy Teach the person who has had a colostomy to irrigate the stoma while sitting up in bed or on a commode. Explain that a 50–1,500-cc solution of soap, plain water, or saline at about 105° F is used. A catheter is inserted 2–3 inches into the colostomy stoma, and the irrigating can is placed about 2 feet above the colostomy opening to allow for solution flow. Explain that colostomy irrigations should be done daily or on alternate days.

Rationale: Colostomy irrigations empty the colon of fecal material and gases and provide the comfort of cleanliness.

Fulfilled Needs: Waste elimination of food residue, cleanliness, mastery and competence in skills, increased learning

Contraindications: Delay if the patient is not psychologically ready.

Teach how to adjust the diet Help the person adjust his diet to his particular lifestyle and food preferences. Make it as easy as possible for the person to follow the diet.

Rationale: When a diet is adjusted to a person's lifestyle, there is a greater chance for compliance.

Fulfilled Needs: Comfort, nutritional balance, increased learning

Teach how to adjust the hearing aid for optimum sensory intake Explain how the hearing aid is adjusted for sound reception according to the instructions of the specific type of hearing aid. Adjustments are usually made by simply turning a knob.

Rationale: A properly functioning hearing aid is essential for optimum hearing.

Fufilled Needs: Comfort, protection from physical harm, increased learning

Teach how to administer tube feeding Explain how to determine whether the tube is correctly placed in the stomach. Have the person check for residual food in the stomach before each feeding by aspirating the contents of the stomach into a syringe, measuring the residual and returning it to the stomach. The feeding and fluid intake should be adjusted according to the residual. When the residual is 150 ml, subtract that amount from the total to be given; when the residual approaches the same amount as the feeding, omit that feeding. Administer the tube feeding according to the basic need of 35 ml/kg of body weight with a minimum of 7 cc of water per 1 g of protein in the formula. During fever states, increase the water by 10–15% per 1° C of fever. If receiving 150 g protein or more per day, observe for hypertonic dehydration. Explain that the prescribed tube feeding formula should be of a moderate temperature and should be given by slow drip followed by a small amount of water. Explain the proper attachment and adjustment of the tube feeding set. Teach how to provide afterfeeding tube care. For a retention tube, either clamp or leave it open as needed for decompression. Use gentle traction on the balloon type tube. For an intermittent tube, clamp and remove the tube, and apply a sterile dressing to the gastrostomy site. Demonstrate how to clean the tube feeding set.

Rationale: Adequate nutritional intake is essential to cellular activity and energy production for food.

Fulfilled Needs: Nutritional intake, protection from physical harm, mastery and competence in skills, independence, increased learning

Teach how to apply a bandage Teach the basic methods of bandaging: circular method, spiral, spiral reverse, figure-eight, and recurrent method. Teach which methods are most appropriate to different parts of the body and different injuries.

Rationale: Correct performance of health procedures increases the potential for effectiveness of the procedure.

Fulfilled Needs: Protection from physical harm, mastery and competence in skills, increased learning

Teach how to apply a breast binder Explain how a wide binder (8-inch Ace bandage or muslin binder) is encircled around the breasts. The breasts should be held in normal position while the binder is being applied snugly, but not too tightly. It is best to pin the binder from the bottom up.

Rationale: The application of a breast binder to an engorged or lactating breast aids in preventing fluid congestion. It shields the breast for cleanliness, relieves discomfort from breast weight by offering support, and prevents backache by enhancing good posture.

Fulfilled Needs: Comfort, protection from physical harm, mastery and competence in skills, increased learning

Teach how to apply a stump sock Explain that a clean stump sock should be applied smoothly over the stump without any wrinkles.

Rationale: Wrinkles or creases in a stump sock can cause skin irritation, with resulting decubitus ulcers.

Fulfilled Needs: Protection from physical harm, mastery and competence in skills, increased learning

Teach how to apply a urinary collection container Explain how to connect a plastic or waterproof bag and tubing to the urinary drainage tubing for collecting urinary output.

Rationale: A collection apparatus for urine assures accurate output measurement, maintains dryness and thus prevents skin irritation, and provides the comfort of cleanliness.

Fulfilled Needs: Comfort, cleanliness, protection from physical harm, mastery and competence in skills, increased learning

Teach how to apply an arm sling Explain how a triangular bandage is laid flat across the chest with one tail over the shoulder opposite the injury and the pointed end across the elbow of the injured arm. Position the forearm a little higher than at a right angle. Lift the hanging tail up under the arm and around the neck. Tie the two tails behind the unaffected shoulder. Support the hand and wrist in the sling. Fold the point of the sling smoothly around the elbow and pin it in the front.

Rationale: Support of a traumatized body part prevents further injury and promotes comfort.

Fulfilled Needs: Comfort, protection from physical harm, mastery and competence in skills, increased learning

Teach how to apply an external urinary catheter Explain how to apply a balloon-type catheter to the external male genitalia. Caution against anchoring the catheter too tightly, and explain how to attach it to a drainage container.

Rationale: An external urinary catheter assures accurate output measurement, maintains dryness and thus prevents skin irritation, and provides the comfort of cleanliness.

Fulfilled Needs: Comfort, cleanliness, protection from physical harm, mastery and competence in skills, increased learning

Teach how to apply and remove a leg brace Explain the procedure for putting on a leg brace: Sit in a chair and place the unaffected leg midline in front of the body. Cross the affected leg over the unaffected leg. Pull up the tongue of the shoe. Hold the brace at the top, swinging the shoe far enough forward so the toes can be inserted into the shoe. Turn the shoe slightly inward so that the toes can be inserted at a slight angle. Pull the brace up as far as possible onto the leg. If a shoehorn is needed, hold the brace between the two legs. Move the shoehorn back and forth until the foot fits into the shoe. Fasten the laces and straps. Also explain the procedure for removing a leg brace: Cross the affected leg over the unaffected leg. Unfasten the laces and straps on the brace. Push downward until the shoe is off the foot.

Rationale Proper application and removal of a leg brace assure correct use of the device.

Fulfilled Needs: Protection from physical harm, mastery and competence in skills, increased learning

Contraindications: Delay brace application if severe skin irritation exists.

Teach how to apply and remove the hearing aid Explain how the ear piece, cord, and transmitter are placed in or about the ear, depending on the type hearing aid used. Explain the printed directions accompanying the aid.

Rationale: Correctly applying a hearing aid supports maximum utilization of the aid for improved hearing and reduces the potential for ear injury.

Fulfilled Needs: Comfort, protection from physical harm, increased learning

Teach how to apply and remove the ostomy appliance Explain the methods for applying an ostomy collection apparatus. This applies to the appliances used following colostomy, ileostomy, and ureteroileostomy. Emphasize skin care and cleanliness of the immediate and surrounding areas. Acquaint the patient with the disposable bags, which are not reused, and the reusable permanent bags, which require daily soap and water cleaning and exposure to fresh air.

Rationale: Proper application of a collection apparatus assures accurate output measurement, maintains dryness and thus prevents skin irritation, and provides the comfort of cleanliness.

Fulfilled Needs: Comfort, cleanliness, protection from physical harm, mastery and competence in skills, increased learning

Teach how to apply cold therapy Explain how and when to administer cold applications to body areas. This includes ice collars, cold packs, ice bags, and soaks in cold water. Explain that extremities should not be immersed in ice water or kept in ice packs for long periods because of the danger of frostbite.

Rationale: Cold applications decrease circulation by means of mild vasoconstriction; they relieve pain and congestion and reduce pus formation, swelling, and bleeding. Correct application of therapeutic measures assures their effectiveness and promotes safety.

Fulfilled Needs: Protection from physical harm, increased learning

Contraindications: Do not apply cold applications to decubitus ulcers, gangrenous tissue, skin graft areas, varicose veins, areas of paralysis or sensation loss, or aged or debilitated skin.

Teach how to apply disinfecting solutions Explain how to use cleansing products to disinfect household surfaces.

Rationale: Cleanliness inhibits bacterial and viral growth and minimizes infection.

Fulfilled Needs: Cleanliness, protection from physical harm, increased learning

Teach how to apply heat therapy Explain how and when to apply heating pads, hot-water bottles, and warm, moist compresses. Explain that whenever heat, wet or dry, is applied to the body surface, it should first be tested against the inner wrist to determine if the degree of heat is comfortable to the skin. If not, the application should be allowed to cool.

Rationale: Heat applications cause mild vasodilatation, which increases skin circulation; they relieve pain and congestion, promote muscle relaxation, and bring the pus of an abscess to the skin surface. Correct application of therapeutic measures assures their effectiveness and promotes safety.

Fulfilled Needs: Comfort, protection from physical harm, increased learning

Contraindications: Do not apply heat to areas of paralysis, sensation loss, edema, vasodilatation, or allergic response. Do not apply heat to any body part after heart surgery or to areas of hemorrhage or trauma. Do not apply heat after a head injury.

Teach how to apply preventive splints   Explain that preventive splints should be put on with the body part in the functional position and should fit securely.

Rationale: Proper use of preventive splints will hold affected body parts in functional positions so that muscles can be used after healing. Their use can also prevent contractures.

Fulfilled Needs: Protection from physical harm, mastery and competence in skills, increased learning

Teach how to apply sanitary pads   Explain the method for applying sanitary pads. Explain that most sanitary pads have adhesive strips down the center. The pad is pressed against a panty undergarment that is then pulled up so that the pad fits snugly against the perineum. Sanitary pads may also be held in place with a belt appliance. During heavy flow, two sanitary pads may be used together, or a sanitary pad and a tampon may be used simultaneously. Sanitary pads should be changed at least every 4 hours, and more often if heavily saturated.

Rationale: Sanitary pads absorb menstrual flow so as to prevent soiled clothing. Frequent changing of pads reduces odor and prevents bacterial growth that could cause infection.

Fulfilled Needs: Comfort, protection from physical harm, mastery and competence in skills, increased learning

Teach how to apply the prescribed topical agent   Explain how to apply the prescribed drug, usually in cream or ointment form.

Rationale: Correct application of topical agents to the skin reduces pain and infection, promotes comfort, and supports healing.

Fulfilled Needs: Comfort, protection from physical harm, mastery and competence in skills, independence, increased learning

Teach how to bathe an infant   Explain that infants should be bathed at the same time each day. Clean bathing equipment and clean hands are essential. The infant should never be left alone during a bath. Sponge baths are usually given before the umbilical cord is shed. Bath water should be checked for moderate temperature. One should avoid splashing water because it tends to startle the infant. Once undressed, the infant should be kept warm with a towel. It is easier to hold and bathe a baby if one wears clean white cotton gloves. This prevents the baby from slipping out of one's grasp, and one glove can serve as a washcloth. Cleansing proceeds as follows: The nose, outer ear, and face are washed with plain water. Hair and scalp are washed with soap and water, followed by body and limbs, uncovering only one area at a time and giving special attention to creases and areas between toes and fingers. The genital area is washed last. The infant is wrapped in an absorbent towel and thoroughly dried. Since the towel will become wet, the child should be placed in a cotton receiving blanket until dressed. Lotion can be applied around fingernails, toenails, and genitals. Powder should be used sparingly, if at all.

Rationale: Bathing cleans the skin, promotes comfort, and stimulates circulation.

Fulfilled Needs: Comfort, cleanliness, protection from physical harm, mastery and competence in skills, increased learning

Teach how to blow the nose correctly   Explain that one side of the nose should be blown at a time and that the mouth should be kept open while blowing.

Rationale: Proper nose blowing prevents excessive pressure in the middle ear and facilitates removal of secretions.

Fulfilled Needs: Comfort, cleanliness, protection from physical harm, increased learning

Teach how to bottle-feed an infant   Explain that infants should be fed at reasonable intervals and that the amount of feeding depends on the child's needs during different growth stages. Bottle feedings should be at room temperature or warm—never cold. The infant should be held with his head supported and turned slightly to one side. The neck of the bottle should be full at all times.

Rationale: Proper bottle feeding increases comfort, provides adequate nutrition, and reduces the potential for aspiration.

Fulfilled Needs: Nutritional balance, comfort, protection from physical harm, mastery and competence in skills, increased learning

Contraindications: Vomiting, high fever, diarrhea

Teach how to breast-feed an infant Explain how to feed an infant with milk from the mother's breast. After the mother has rested from the delivery, the infant is usually breast fed. If the mother prefers to lie down, she should lie on her side with the arm on that side raised and a pillow under her head. The baby should be placed on his side, either flat or supported with pillows. If the mother prefers to sit up, she should sit in a comfortable chair and support the infant with her arm or a pillow. The infant should be fed at a moderate pace and should be bubbled every 5 minutes. The breasts should be washed with warm water before feeding.

Rationale: Proper breast-feeding supports maternal and infant comfort and provides adequate infant nutrition.

Fulfilled Needs: Nutritional balance, comfort, protection from physical harm, mastery and competence in skills, increased learning

Contraindications: Breast infection or inflammation

Teach how to brush and floss the teeth correctly Explain that the toothbrush bristles should be pointed toward the roots of the teeth. The brush should be rotated so that the bristles sweep over the gums and teeth in the direction of the biting surface. The teeth should be brushed in the following sequence: the chewing surfaces of the upper and lower teeth, the outside surfaces of the upper and lower back teeth, and inside surfaces of the upper and lower back teeth, the front teeth, the outer surfaces of the upper and lower front teeth. The teeth should be brushed after every meal.

Rationale: Brushing the teeth properly reduces bacterial action and decay through cleansing and provides the comfort of a clean mouth.

Fulfilled Needs: Comfort, cleanliness, protection from physical harm, mastery and competence in skills, increased learning

Teach how to calculate a diet Explain that special diets are based on daily need for the four basic food groups. Help the person or family to select foods from the exchange lists and to interchange them in quantities specified so that the special diet needs are met along with the essential food requirements.

Rationale: Proper calculation of a therapeutic diet is essential if the diet is to be effective for improved health.

Fulfilled Needs: Protection from physical harm, mastery and competence in skills, increased learning

Teach how to care for a hearing aid Explain that when a hearing aid is not in use, it should be placed where it will not be damaged, and the batteries should be removed. The hearing aid should be checked for efficiency at least every 2 years.

Rationale: A properly functioning hearing aid is essential for optimum hearing.

Fulfilled Needs: Comfort, protection from physical harm, increased learning

Teach how to care for an arteriovenous shunt Teach the person to clean the shunt connection sites and the skin of the entire extremity, to change the dressing daily, and to observe for kinks in the joint and slipping of the rings that hold the joint together.

Rationale: Cleaning an arteriovenous shunt prevents infection. Proper care of the shunt assures its availability for hemodialysis.

Fulfilled Needs: Cleanliness, protection from physical harm, mastery and competence in skills, increased learning

Teach how to care for an artificial eye Explain that normal saline solution or tap water may be used to soak and clean an artificial eye.

Rationale: A clean artificial eye minimizes the potential for eye socket infection and promotes comfort.

Fulfilled Needs: Comfort, cleanliness, protection from physical harm, increased learning

Teach how to clean a nondisposable thermometer Explain that soap, cool water, and friction are used to clean a thermometer. The soap and water should be brought from the top of the thermometer down to the bulb with rotating friction on the glass. Caution against cleaning with boiling water.

Rationale: Thermometer cleanliness helps prevent the spread of infection to others and reduces the potential for reinfection of the patient.

Fulfilled Needs: Cleanliness, protection from physical harm, increased learning

Teach how to clean a soiled cast with a moist cloth and Bon Ami cleanser Explain that a cast can be cleaned with a small amount of Bon Ami cleanser on a slightly damp rag. Do not use other brands of cleansers for this purpose.

Rationale: Bon Ami's gentle abrasion cleans, but does not damage the cast. A clean cast promotes comfort.

Fulfilled Needs: Comfort, increased learning

Teach how to clean a tracheostomy/laryngectomy tube Explain that the tracheostomy or laryngectomy tube outer cannula is cleaned by suctioning. The inner cannula is soaked in hydrogen peroxide. Pipe cleaners or sterile gauze may be inserted in the center hole of the inner cannula for further cleaning and to assure patency. After the cannula is clean, it should be soaked for a few minutes in sterile water to remove any cleansing agent that might irritate tracheal tissue. The skin around the tracheostomy or laryngectomy stoma should be cleaned with hydrogen peroxide or saline, and the dressing should be changed frequently.

Rationale: A clean tracheostomy or laryngectomy tube is essential to provide adequate respiratory gas exchange and to prevent infection.

Fulfilled Needs: Tissue oxygenation or perfusion, comfort, cleanliness, protection from physical harm, increased learning

Teach how to clean an elastic bandage or stockings Explain that elastic bandages and stockings should be washed daily with mild soap and warm (not hot) water, laid flat for drying, and rolled loosely when dry.

Rationale: Cleaning removes perspiration residue on stockings and bandages that might irritate the skin. Hanging elastic bandages and stockings when they are wet or rolling them tightly after they dry decreases their elasticity.

Fulfilled Needs: Comfort, cleanliness, protection from physical harm, increased learning

Teach how to clean an infant's ears Explain that extreme care must be exercised when cleaning an infant's ear. The head must be held still. The creases of the auricle should be cleaned with a washcloth, and a few drops of mineral oil may be put into the ear before cleaning in order to soften earwax.

Rationale: Cleaning the ear promotes comfort and minimizes the potential for infection and impaired hearing from wax accumulation.

Fulfilled Needs: Comfort, cleanliness, protection from physical harm, increased learning

Teach how to clean an infant's nose   Explain that an infant's nose should be cleaned gently with a washcloth, with flexible cotton-tipped sticks moistened with warm water, or by suctioning with a bulb syringe.

Rationale: Cleanliness of the nares assures a patent airway.

Fulfilled Needs: Comfort, cleanliness, protection from physical harm, increased learning

Teach how to clean and dress a/the wound/surgical site   Teach the patient how to clean a wound and how to use sterile technique when doing so. The specific method of cleaning and bandaging will depend on the particular condition.

Rationale: Cleaning and covering a wound with a sterile dressing help to minimize infection, prevent trauma, restrict motion, and absorb secretions.

Fulfilled Needs: Comfort, protection from physical harm, mastery and competence in skills, increased learning

Teach how to clean contact lenses   Explain that contact lens should be cleaned frequently with a noncaustic, sterile solution.

Rationale: Keeping contact lenses clean promotes visual acuity and minimizes the potential for eye infection. A caustic, nonsterile solution on a contact lens could cause ulceration or abrasion of the cornea.

Fulfilled Needs: Comfort, cleanliness, protection from physical harm, increased learning

Teach how to clean dental braces   Explain that when people have braces on their teeth, they should use a soft toothbrush and a water jet to clean between the braces.

Rationale: A soft toothbrush prevents gum damage. The pulsation of a water jet removes food particles which adhere to the teeth and braces.

Fulfilled Needs: Cleanliness, protection from physical harm, increased learning

Teach how to clean dentures: Explain that dentures should be cleaned with denture powder or solution at least twice a day.

Rationale: Denture cleaning provides a clean breath and refreshing mouth and prevents gum tissue injury from hardened food particles on dentures.

Fulfilled Needs: Comfort, cleanliness, protection from physical harm, increased learning.

Teach how to control breathing to aid the labor process[405]   Explain that breathing during uterine contractions should consist of slow, deep breathing at the beginning of the contraction, shallow breathing during the peak of the contraction, and renewed slow, deep breathing as the contraction subsides. Be certain that the person does not hyperventilate.

Rationale: By tensing abdominal muscles and relaxing the perineum, controlled breathing helps the progress of labor.

Fulfilled Needs: Relaxation, comfort, increased learning

Teach how to control ileostomy–colostomy odor by deodorization   Disagreeable odors from an ileostomy or colostomy can be controlled by keeping the person, his clothes, and the appliance clean, by inserting deodorant tablets such as charcoal, chlorophyll, and aspirin into the bag after each emptying, by placing an alcohol-saturated cloth or tissue in the bag, by using spray deodorant, or by applying an extra plastic covering such as kitchen wrap over the bag.

Rationale: Freedom from body odor promotes comfort.

Fulfilled Needs: Comfort

Teach how to detriangle dysfunctional fixed triangles[471]   In order to break up the fixed triangle system, at least one person in the triangle must identify the behavior or verbalizations of other person(s) that are causing him to react in a particular way. He must then change his responses to that behavior.

Rationale: When the person recognizes his own responses to the behavior of others, and changes those responses, he gains control of the situation. This process changes the triangle system.

Fulfilled Needs: Increased learning, personal growth and maturity, increased reality perception and problem-solving ability

Teach how to dilate the stoma with a sterile catheter   In the patient who has an ileal conduit, it is possible for the orifice to become obstructed; teach the patient how to insert a sterile catheter gently into the orifice.

Rationale: The ileal conduit orifice can become plugged with mucus produced by mucosa of the ileum. Insertion of a sterile catheter into the orifice removes the mucus and allows for adequate urine drainage.

Fulfilled Needs: Waste elimination of urine, increased learning

Teach how to do a catheterization   Explain how to insert an indwelling catheter. Explain correct positioning, how to maintain sterile technique, cleaning of the genitalia, catheter insertion into the meatus, and how to attach the catheter to a drainage system.

Rationale: Self-catheterization facilitates urine flow, ensures accurate output measurement, maintains dryness and thus prevents skin irritation, and provides the comfort of cleanliness.

Fulfilled Needs: Comfort, cleanliness, waste elimination of urine, protection from physical harm, mastery and competence in skills, increased learning

Teach how to do abdominal breathing   Instruct the person to place one hand on his abdomen and the other on his chest. As he takes a deep breath, have him watch his abdomen rise. As he exhales, have him contract the abdominal muscles. During abdominal breathing, the chest will remain still.

Rationale: When lung elasticity is lost or lung alveoli become distended (as in emphysema), breathing places stress on the thoracic muscles. Abdominal breathing can reduce the stress placed on the thorax.

Fulfilled Needs: Tissue oxygenation or perfusion, protection from physical harm, increased learning

Teach how to do above-knee stump exercises   Instruct the person who has had an above-knee amputation to move the stump inward (adduction) toward the body centerline and then outward (abduction) or away from the body and to straighten the stump (extension) in alignment with the hip.

Rationale: Stump exercises prepare the stump for a prosthesis and for future mobility.

Fulfilled Needs: Activity and exercise, protection from physical harm, mastery and competence in skills, increased learning

Teach how to do back exercises[721]   Explain that there are several exercises the person can do to relieve back discomfort:

Knee-to-chest exercise: In the supine position with knees flexed, raise the right knee to the chest, then the left knee, then both knees. Hold the position while counting to five and repeat each movement five times.

Pelvic-tilt exercise: In the supine position with knees flexed, firmly tighten the buttock muscles. Hold the position while counting to five and repeat five times.

Single-leg-raise exercise: In the supine position, slowly raise the right leg straight up. Hold the position while counting to five. Repeat five times. Do the same with the left leg.

Half-situp exercise: In the supine position, with the knees flexed, slowly raise the head and neck to the top of the chest. Place both hands on the knees and count to five. Repeat five times.

Nose-to-knee touch exercise: In the supine position, with the knees flexed, raise the left knee to the chest, pulling with both hands. Raise the head, and touch the nose to the knee. Hold the position while counting to five, and repeat five times. Do the same with the right leg.

Hamstring stretch exercise: In the sitting position, tuck the right leg back and reach to touch the left toe with one's hands. Repeat five times. Do the same with the right side.

Rationale: The *knee-to-chest exercise* decreases stiffness in the back. The *pelvic-tilt exercise* strengthens the front and back muscles. The *single-leg-raise exercise* decreases stiffness and stretches the hamstring muscle. The *half-situp exercise* strengthens the back and abdominal muscles. The *nose-to-knee touch exercise* stretches the hip muscles and strengthens the abdominal muscles. The *hamstring stretch exercise* decreases tightness in the hamstring muscles.

Fulfilled Needs: Protection from physical harm, freedom from pain, increased learning

Contraindications: Do not do back exercises only on occasion. They must be done every day to prevent injury. Do not exercise if the person is having pain or is recovering from a back problem and the doctor has not ordered therapeutic exercises yet.

Teach how to do below-knee stump exercises Instruct the person who has had a below-knee amputation to move the straightened leg upward as much as possible and then return the leg to the neutral position (hip extension). Have him move the stump outward (abduction) or away from the body by contracting the large muscles on the anterior thigh (quadriceps sitting).

Rationale: Stump exercises prepare the stump for a prosthesis and for future mobility.

Fulfilled Needs: Activity and exercise, protection from physical harm, mastery and competence in skills, increased learning

Teach how to do blood sampling Teach the person how to do studies on blood at home. Such studies are especially needed during home dialysis, when the person needs to determine the microhematocrit. Include instructions on how to use the centrifuge and how to store blood plasma in the freezer.

Rationale: Knowledge of how to do blood sampling promotes independent self-therapy and supports self-protection against unfavorable blood levels.

Fulfilled Needs: Protection from physical harm, independence, increased learning

Teach how to do breath-holding Teach the person who is hyperventilating or experiencing atrial tachycardia to take a deep breath and hold it for a few seconds.

Rationale: Holding the breath prevents carbon dioxide exhalation and increases the level of carbon dioxide in the blood to normal. Holding the breath causes vagal stimulation, which reduces cardiac rate and interrupts tachycardia.

Fulfilled Needs: Comfort, protection from physical harm, increased learning

Contraindications: Elevated blood level of carbon dioxide, emphysema

Teach how to do bronchopulmonary hygiene measures Explain how to perform measures such as coughing, positioning for pulmonary drainage, thoracic percussion, airway suctioning, nebulization methods, and maintaining fluid intake.

Rationale: Bronchopulmonary hygiene maintains a clear airway by removing thick secretions. It increases ventilation and prevents pulmonary infection.

Fulfilled Needs: Tissue oxygenation or perfusion, waste elimination of bronchopulmonary secretions, protection from physical harm, increased learning

Teach how to do home dialysis[71,84]   Explain how to assemble an artificial kidney, how to mix hemodialysis fluid, and how to run and clean the machine. Explain that the following procedure is carried out in preparing the hemodialysis machine. Coils are sterilized if they are not presterilized. Check for membrane tears or leaks by introducing air pressure into the blood compartment. If the pressure does not decrease, there are no leaks. Prepare the dialysate solution in a batch. Set gauges and monitors, and check them. Begin anticoagulation therapy. Attach the patient's access tube to the blood lines. Regulate the machine during the procedure. Disconnect the blood lines at completion of the procedure. Include how to clean the machine and what to do in case of power failure.

Rationale: Competence in hemodialysis therapy is essential to maintaining life in a patient experiencing renal failure.

Fulfilled Needs: Fluid and electrolyte balance, waste elimination of nitrogenous and other toxic substances, comfort, protection from physical harm, mastery and competence in skills, increased learning

Teach how to do isometric exercises   Teach the person how to exercise his muscles without moving the injured body part. If his leg is in a cast, the nurse's hand may be placed under his knee while he pushes downward. If his arm is in a cast, he may open and close his hand for several minutes each hour. He also may be taught to move his fingers and toes for several minutes every half-hour. Teach the cardiac patient to perform mild leg exercises while in bed by bending his foot up (dorsiflexion) and down (extension) 10 times each hour.

Rationale: Exercises stimulate circulation and prevent muscle atrophy.

Fulfilled Needs: Tissue oxygenation or perfusion, activity and exercise, protection from physical harm, increased learning

Contraindications: Circulatory thrombus

Teach how to do perineal care   Teach the person with perineal stitches that after voiding she should pour a moderate amount of warm water over the sutured area and gently pat the area dry.

Rationale: Perineal care cleans the area of urine and reduces the potential for infection. Warm water provides comfort to the healing area.

Fulfilled Needs: Comfort, cleanliness, protection from physical harm, increased learning

Teach how to do postmastectomy exercises[722]   Explain that after removal of a breast, the affected arm must be exercised:

Hair-brushing exercise: Involves brushing the hair with the affected arm while keeping the head erect. The person should start brushing at one side of the head and slowly work around to the other side.

Jump rope exercise: A rope ½ yard long is attached to a doorknob or dresser knob. The person stands with her affected side toward the rope, keeping her feet apart, and places her unaffected hand on her hip. She then swings the rope from the affected shoulder as one would swing a jump rope, alternating directions, without bending her waist or arm.

Rod rope exercise: A rope 5 feet long is tossed over a shower rod. A knot is tied at each end of the rope. Sitting in a chair under the rod, with a knot held between the second and third fingers of each hand, the person pulls down on the rope, alternating the unaffected and affected sides. Pulling down on the rope with the unaffected arm pulls the affected arm up. This should be done five times in the morning and evening, with gradual increases to 25 times.

Rubber ball exercise: A rubber ball with a string is needed. The ball is held in the hand of the affected arm. The hand is alternately squeezed and relaxed. The ball can also be thrown against a wall with the affected arm from gradually increasing distances.

Shoulder rotating exercise: The person bends her elbows to shoulder level and then rolls her shoulders as far back and around as possible. The rotation should occur in both directions, five times on each side. Then, with elbows bent, she rolls both arms back and around until the shoulder blades almost meet.

Wall-climbing exercise: The person faces a wall with the palms and forearms resting against the wall. Slowly the fingers of the affected arm climb the wall, reaching higher and higher each time. This exercise should be done several times a day, keeping the climbing arm as close to the head as possible.

Window shade exercise: The person raises or lowers window shades or blinds many times each day, reaching the top and bottom of the window.

Rationale: Postmastectomy exercises prevent muscle shortening, preserve muscle tone, extend the range of motion, and promote lymphatic drainage from the arm.

Fulfilled Needs: Activity and exercise, protection from physical harm, increased learning

Contraindications: Incisional bleeding or infection

Teach how to do postpartum exercises[527] Explain how to do the various postpartum exercises:

Back and pelvis strengthening exercise: The person lies on her back, places her feet slightly apart, and draws her knees up until her legs almost form a right angle. Then she raises her buttocks so that her body rests only on the soles of her feet and on her shoulders. Next she presses her knees together, contracting the gluteal muscles, and then relaxes.

Gluteal and pelvic strengthening exercise: The person lies on her back, bends one knee sharply toward her abdomen, brings her head down toward her buttocks, then straightens her leg and lies flat. She then alternates legs.

Knee–chest postpartum exercise: The person takes a kneeling position with knees widely separated and head turned to one side. She bends her body forward until her shoulders and chest touch a bed or the floor as close to her knees as possible, all the while keeping her back straight.

Monkey-trot postpartum exercise: The person walks along on her feet and hands simultaneously.

Rationale: Postpartum exercises strengthen the lower back muscles and the gluteal and pelvic muscles and assist the uterus to resume the prepregnant pelvic position.

Fulfilled Needs: Exercise, protection from physical harm, mastery and competence in skills, increased learning

Contraindications: Delay until caesarean section incision is well healed.

Teach how to do pre-crutch-walking exercises In anticipation of using crutches, teach the person to do pushups while lying on his abdomen, to do pushups on the palms of his hands while in a sitting position, to lift weights or sandbags while lying on his back, and to do straight elbow pushups in bed with crutches sawed off just below the handbars.

Rationale: Pre-crutch-walking exercises strengthen the arm and shoulder muscles for crutch walking.

Fulfilled Needs: Activity and exercise, protection from physical harm, increased learning

Teach how to do range-of-motion exercises Teach the patient exercises that move the joints through the functional range so that function will not be low. Cover active assistance, active, passive, and resistive range of motion.

Rationale: Range-of-motion exercises promote joint mobility, strengthen muscle tone, develop coordination, prevent nonfunctional contractures, and increase blood circulation.

Fulfilled Needs: Tissue oxygenation or perfusion, activity and exercise, comfort, protection from physical harm, mastery and competence in skills, increased learning

Teach how to do resistive breathing exercises[205] Instruct the person to lie on his back without a pillow and with his legs elevated. Then have him place a book or some other object weighing about 1 lb on his abdomen. Have him breathe and try to push with his abdomen against the weight. This should be done five to 10 times twice a day. Every third day, ½ lb of weight should be added until the weight reaches 5 lbs and the patient can comfortably do the exercise for 30 minutes. Another resistive exercise involves having the patient blow out a candle at gradually increasing distances or blow a pencil or pen to various spots on the top of a table.

Rationale: The person who has emphysema has a tendency to let the chest muscles do most of the breathing work, with the diaphragm doing less and less. Resistive breathing exercises help restore the normal breathing function of the diaphragmatic and abdominal muscles.

Fulfilled Needs: Tissue oxygenation or perfusion, waste elimination of carbon dioxide, protection from physical harm, increased learning

Teach how to do therapeutic soaks   Explain how to apply a warm, moist compress or immerse a particular body part in warm water.

Rationale: Moist heat applications cleanse, relieve the edema and pain of inflammation, and remove necrotic tissue.

Fulfilled Needs: Comfort, cleanliness, protection from physical harm, mastery and competence in skills, increased learning

Teach how to do umbilical care   Explain how to clean the newborn's umbilical area by wiping it gently with alcohol.

Rationale: Proper umbilical care promotes comfort and reduces the potential for infection. Alcohol dries the cord.

Fulfilled Needs: Comfort, cleanliness, protection from physical harm, increased learning

Teach how to dress an infant   Explain that when dressing an infant, the garment should be gathered from the bottom to the neck so that the infant's head can be slipped easily into the opening before his arms are dressed. Explain that clothing on infants should not be restrictive.

Rationale: Proper infant dressing promotes comfort and safety.

Fulfilled Needs: Comfort, protection from physical harm, mastery and competence in skills, increased learning

Teach how to elevate from a sitting to a standing position with crutches[108]   Teach the person who must use crutches to rise. He should back his chair against a stable surface, then move his body to the chair's edge and place his unaffected leg against the chair's edge. Then he should hold both crutches together at the handpiece with one hand and place the other hand on the chair armrest. Pushing upward with both hands, he should straighten his strong leg and stand up. Balancing on the crutches and his strong leg, he should then transfer one crutch at a time to the underarm position.

Rationale: Safe mobility is essential to carrying out daily activities and maintaining independence.

Fulfilled Needs: Activity and exercise, comfort, protection from physical harm, mastery and competence in skills, independence, increased learning

Teach how to elevate from a sitting to a standing position with leg braces[108]   Teach the person with a brace to rise. He should back his chair against a stable surface, move his body to the chair's edge, and lock one brace at the knee. Then he should cross the locked and braced leg over the foot of the other leg and turn his body at the waist toward the unlocked and braced leg until his head and shoulders face the back of the chair. Then he should grasp the chair armrests with both hands and push the body upward until the leg with the locked brace is supporting the body. After locking the brace of the other leg at the knee, he should place the crutches, one at a

time, under his arms, bearing weight on the crutches while coming to a standing position. He should back a few steps away from the chair before turning to move forward.

Rationale: Safe mobility is essential to carrying out daily activities and maintaining independence.

Fulfilled Needs: Activity and exercise, comfort, protection from physical harm, mastery and competence in skills, independence, increased learning

Teach how to get into a bathtub when hemiplegic[108]
Teach the person with one-sided paralysis to get into the bathtub so that his weak side is next to the wall. This will allow him to emerge from the tub putting his strong leg out first.

Rationale: Safe mobility is essential to carrying out daily activities and maintaining independence.

Fulfilled Needs: Activity and exercise, comfort, protection from physical harm, mastery and competence in skills, independence, increased learning

Teach how to give a bed bath
Explain how to bathe the person confined to bed. Include draping the person, washing with soap and water, drying, and maintaining a warm environment during the bath.

Rationale: A bed bath cleans the skin, promotes comfort, stimulates circulation, and reduces energy consumption.

Fulfilled Needs: Circulation, energy, comfort, cleanliness, protection from physical harm, increased learning

Teach how to give a douche
Explain that a douche is given in the reclining position with the knees flexed and thighs separated. The external genitalia are cleaned with soap and water. The irrigating nozzle is gently inserted into the vagina. An irrigating solution at approximately 105° F is allowed to flow slowly in and out of the vagina by careful nozzle rotation. The perineum is then wiped dry.

Rationale: Vaginal irrigations discourage bacterial growth, remove foul and irritating discharges, and provide heat therapy.

Fulfilled Needs: Comfort, cleanliness, protection from physical harm, mastery and competence in skills, increased learning

Contraindications: Vaginal bleeding

Teach how to give an enema
Explain that before giving an enema, the bladder should be emptied. The person should lie on his left side with his right leg flexed. He should be properly draped and have adequate privacy. After preparation of the appropriate solution at 105° F, the enema tubing should be lubricated and inserted 2–3 inches into the rectum. The enema container should be held no more than 2 feet above the person, and the person should take several deep breaths while the fluid flows into his colon. If the person complains of abdominal cramping, the tubing should be clamped for a few minutes and then unclamped until all the solution is given. The tube should be removed slowly. The person should retain the solution as long as possible. Then he should be placed on a bedpan or commode. The results of the enema should be checked, and it should be determined that the person is dry.

Rationale: Proper administration of an enema promotes elimination of food residue and gases from the intestinal tract.

Fulfilled Needs: Waste elimination of food residue, comfort, stimulation, cleanliness, protection from physical harm, increased learning

Teach how to give oxygen therapy
Teach the person who has been prescribed oxygen therapy how and when to use the equipment and how to make regulatory adjustments specific to his problem.

Rationale: Oxygen therapy provides a higher intake of oxygen than normal, which can ease difficult breathing. Oxygen toxicity is less likely to occur if the patient knows the correct use of oxygen equipment.

Fulfilled Needs: Tissue oxygenation or perfusion, comfort, protection from physical harm, mastery and competence in skills, independence, increased learning

Contraindications: Oxygen toxicity

Teach how to give/take positive-pressure breathing   Teach the person who has been prescribed positive-pressure breathing how and when to use the equipment and how to make regulatory adjustments specific to his problem.

Rationale: Intermittent positive-pressure breathing inflates the lungs, pushes pressurized air past mucus secretions, and stimulates coughing for secretion elimination.

Fulfilled Needs: Waste elimination of bronchopulmonary secretions, protection from physical harm, mastery and competence in skills, independence, increased learning

Contraindications: Cardiac insufficiency, pulmonary hemorrhage

Teach how to give vaporized-solution inhalation   Explain how to use a vaporizing apparatus for breathing moistened air. Explain that many household objects can be used for inhalation of humidified air, such as an electric percolator, a teakettle, or a funnel made from a newspaper or a paper bag and attached to a kettle.

Rationale: Inhalation of heated humidified air decreases respiratory tissue dryness, prevents tissue friction during respirations, and loosens and thins mucus secretions.

Fulfilled Needs: Comfort, protection from physical harm, increased learning

Teach how to handle an infant   Explain that infants should be handled in a gentle but firm manner. They require good body support, especially of the head and neck, and they should be made to feel safe at all times.

Rationale: Proper infant handling is essential to infant safety, comfort, and security.

Fulfilled Needs: Comfort, protection from physical harm, mastery and competence in skills, increased learning

Teach how to inflate and deflate an airway cuff   Explain how to insert air into and remove air from an airway cuff. Emphasize the importance of suctioning the trachea during cuff deflation to remove secretions. Explain that the cuff should be inflated while the person is eating or taking inhalation therapy and should then be deflated.

Rationale: Deflating an airway cuff relieves pressure from the tracheal and laryngeal mucosa, which decreases the potential for tissue necrosis. Inflation of an airway cuff provides a tight seal between the tube and the trachea. It prevents air leakage during ventilation procedures and food aspiration during meals.

Fulfilled Needs: Comfort, protection from physical harm, increased learning

Teach how to insert a vaginal suppository   Explain that insertion of a vaginal suppository involves the following steps: handwashing before insertion, douching when ordered before insertion, positioning herself lying down with the hips elevated on a pillow, use of the longest finger to insert the suppository gently upward and back or use of a suppository applicator, and remaining in the same position for 10–15 minutes after insertion. The same procedure is used for vaginal cream applications.

Rationale: Vaginal suppositories and creams reduce vaginal irritation, inflammation, and infection.

Fulfilled Needs: Comfort, protection from physical harm, mastery and competence in skills, increased learning

Contraindications: Abnormal vaginal bleeding

Teach how to insert and remove an artificial eye   For insertion of an artificial eye, have the person pull down on his lower eyelid and gently slip the eye into position. For removal, have him place gentle pressure below the eye with the index finger until the prosthesis slips out of the socket. A suction cup may be used instead of the fingers to hold the artificial eye for insertion and removal.

Rationale: Artificial eye replacement promotes comfort and prevents eye socket shrinkage. Removal of the artificial eye permits prosthesis cleansing, prevents orbit irritation, and promotes comfort.

Fulfilled Needs: Comfort, cleanliness, protection from physical harm, mastery and competence in skills, increased learning

Contraindications: Eye socket irritation, inflammation, or infection

Teach how to insert and remove contact lenses Explain that the proper way to insert a contact lens is as follows: Pull the upper lid up and the lower lid down with the index finger and thumb of one hand. Place wetting solution on the inner side of the lens. With the index finger of one hand, gently place the lens over the cornea of the opposite eye. Be careful to place the left lens on the left cornea and the right lens on the right cornea. The right contact lens is identified by a black dot. Explain that the proper way to remove a contact lens is as follows: Pull the side of the eye (near the ear) outward with one hand. With the other hand, gently pull the lids together; the lens should then pop out. Place the lens, with fluid, safely in its container. Be sure to place the right lens in its receptacle and vice versa.

Rationale: Proper contact lens insertion promotes visual acuity; proper contact lens removal prevents corneal injury.

Fulfilled Needs: Comfort, protection from physical harm, mastery and competence in skills, increased learning

Contraindications: During eye irritation, inflammation, or infection

Teach how to insert tampons Explain that the insertion of a tampon should be done according to the directions on the package. This includes handwashing before the procedure and positioning on a commode or bed with the legs separated. The labia are then separated by the fingers and the tampon is inserted by using the cardboard or plastic applicator as a guide. After insertion, the applicator is removed, while the absorbent cotton remains in the vagina. The attached cord remains outside the vagina and is used to later remove the tampon. Instruct young girls to use water-soluble lubricating jelly on the tampon tip so it will slide in easily. Explain that when there is difficulty removing a tampon, it is easy to remove when one is in the bathtub and the tampon is wet. Warn that if tampons increase menstrual cramps, sanitary pads should be substituted. During heavy flow, a tampon and a sanitary pad may be used simultaneously. The tampon should be changed at least every four hours and more often if heavily saturated.

Rationale: Tampons absorb menstrual flow so as to prevent soiled clothing. Frequent changing of tampons reduces odor and prevents bacterial growth which could cause infection. Correct use of tampons reduces the potential for injury or irritation of the vaginal muscles.

Fulfilled Needs: Comfort, protection from physical harm, mastery and competence in skills, increased learning

Contraindications: Abnormal vaginal bleeding or discharge, symptoms of toxic shock (fever, vaginal odor, discharge)

Teach how to instill eardrops Explain that when eardrops are to be instilled, the person should lie so that the ear to be medicated is facing upward. The person instilling the drops should straighten the adult auditory canal by gently pulling the ear auricle (lobe) upward, backward, and outward. The ears of children should be gently pulled down and back. When drainage is present, it should be wiped clean. Warm drops should then be placed into the ear. The person should remain on his side for approximately 5 minutes. Cotton may be gently inserted into the ear if desired.

Rationale: Correct instillation of eardrops support effective drug therapy.

Fulfilled Needs: Comfort, protection from physical harm, mastery and competence in skills, increased learning

Teach how to instill eyedrops Explain that when instilling eyedrops, the person should tilt his head back, look up, gently pull down his lower eyelid, place the drops just inside his lower lid, and close his eyes. Explain that the eyedropper should never come in contact with eye tissue.

Rationale: Correct instillation of eyedrops supports effective drug therapy.

Fulfilled Needs: Comfort, protection from physical harm, mastery and competence in skills, increased learning

Teach how to irrigate a urinary catheter Explain how to introduce sterile normal saline, 0.25% acetic acid, or another prescribed solution into the urinary catheter at periodic intervals. Explain how to use sterile technique and how to use gravity flow for return of the solution.

Rationale: A patent catheter facilitates urine output. Irrigation with an acetic acid solution destroys microorganisms and dissolves calcium precipitates.

Fulfilled Needs: Protection from physical harm, mastery and competence in skills, increased learning

Teach how to irrigate a wound Explain how to flush a wound with sterile solution until the injured tissue appears clean and free of debris.

Rationale: Flushing a wound with a sterile solution promotes comfort and healing by cleaning the tissue and removing foreign particles.

Fulfilled Needs: Comfort, cleanliness, protection from physical harm, mastery and competence in skills, increased learning

Teach how to locate and count a pulse Explain that when taking a pulse, the person should be sitting or lying down. Forefingers should be placed on the thumb side of the person's wrist, and the pulse beats should be counted for 1 minute using a watch with a second hand. The thumb should not be used to count the person's pulse, because it is possible to feel one's own pulse in the thumb.

Rationale: Pulse abnormalities may indicate cardiac or circulatory pathology.

Fulfilled Needs: Protection from physical harm, mastery and competence in skills, increased learning

Teach how to make an occupied bed Explain that changing the bed linen of a person confined to bed involved the following steps: loosening all linen tucked under the mattress, rolling the person to one side of the bed, rolling the soiled linen up to the person's back, placing the fresh sheet folded in half lengthwise on the mattress at the person's back, tucking in half the sheet and rolling the other half up to the person's back, turning the person onto the clean sheet, going to the other side of the bed and pulling off the soiled sheets, pulling the clean sheets over the mattress and tucking them in, turning the person on his back.

Rationale: Changing the bed linen of the person who cannot get out of bed promotes cleanliness and comfort.

Fulfilled Needs: Comfort, cleanliness, increased learning

Teach how to manually express breast milk Explain that when breast milk is expressed by hand, the breast should be gently massaged for a few moments. One hand is placed on top of the other above the breast. The hands are then brought down over the breast and the fingers turned downward as the hands are drawn apart to encircle the breast. Three fingers should cup and support under the breast as well as bring the breast forward and upward. The forefinger is then placed below the alveoli and the thumb above the alveoli with gentle pressure until the milk flows in a stream. The fingers should be gently rotated around the alveoli until all milk is expressed. The opposite hand is used for holding a sterile collecting container. Handwashing is essential before breast milk expression.

Rationale: When breast-feeding is temporarily curtailed, breast milk must be re-moved manually so that lactation will not cease.

Fulfilled Needs: Comfort, protection from physical harm, mastery and competence in skills, increased learning

Contraindications: Intentional suppression of lactation

Teach how to massage the gums   Explain that gums can be stimulated by eating fibrous foods or by using a water jet.

Rationale: Gum stimulation strengthens the gum tissue so that it can hold the teeth firmly in the mouth.

Fulfilled Needs: Protection from physical harm, increased learning

Teach how to massage the uterine fundus   Teach the person to place her hand on her abdomen, grasp the body of the uterus, and externally massage by applying moderate pressure.

Rationale: Uterine fundus massage reduces hemorrhage.

Fulfilled Needs: Protection from physical harm, mastery and competence in skills, in-creased learning

Teach how to mechanically express breast milk   Explain that breast milk may be expressed by use of a hand pump or an electric pump. When using a hand pump, the suction cup is applied to the nipple, and the suction bulb is alternately squeezed and released. When using an electric pump, the suction cup is applied to the nipple, and a low degree of vacuum is applied. Breast suctioning should be gradual and inter-mittent. It should be continued for no more than 15 minutes and should be stopped earlier if the breast is empty. The milk should be measured and saved in a sterile con-tainer for later infant feeding. Handwashing is essential before milk expression.

Rationale: When breast-feeding is temporarily curtailed, breast milk must be re-moved manually so that lactation will not cease.

Fulfilled Needs: Comfort, protection from physical harm, mastery and competence in skills, increased learning

Contraindications: Intentional suppression of lactation

Teach how to move from a bed to a chair when hemiplegic[108]   Teach the person with one-sided paralysis to place a chair on the same side of the bed as his unaf-fected (strong) side. He should move into a dangling position and place his strong hand on the far armrest of the chair. Then, bearing most of his weight on the strong hand and leg, he can pivot and lift his body into the chair.

Rationale: Safe mobility is essential for carrying out daily activities and maintaining independence.

Fulfilled Needs: Activity and exercise, comfort, protection from physical harm, mas-tery and competence in skills, independence, increased learning

Teach how to move from a chair to a bed when hemiplegic[108]   Teach the person with one-sided paralysis to place his chair so that his unaffected (strong) body side is nearest the bed. He then moves to the edge of the chair and places his strong hand on the bed. Then, bearing most of his weight on his strong hand and leg, he can pivot and lift his body onto the bed.

Rationale: Safe mobility is essential for carrying out daily activities and maintaining independence.

Fulfilled Needs: Activity and exercise, comfort, protection from physical harm, mas-tery and competence in skills, independence, increased learning

Teach how to move from a sitting to a standing position when hemiple-gic[108]   Teach the person with one-sided paralysis to sit on a bed or chair edge with his feet flat on the floor. The person assisting him should face the hemiplegic and grasp him under the arms. The patient leans forward and supports his affected (weak) leg by bracing his foot and knee against the foot and knee of the assisting person. When the assisting person pulls the patient to a standing position, the patient should bear most of his weight on the unaffected (strong) leg and as much weight as possible on the affected (weak) leg.

Rationale: Safe mobility is essential for carrying out daily activities and maintaining independence.

Fulfilled Needs: Activity and exercise, comfort, protection from physical harm, mastery and competence in skills, independence, increased learning

Teach how to percuss the amputation stump   Teach the amputee to gently tap his stump against a soft pillow or his hand. He should gradually increase the pressure by tapping on firmer surfaces until a hard surface can be used. Percussion must be done in proportion to the gradual decrease in stump pain.

Rationale: Stump percussion toughens the skin, gradually decreases nerve sensitivity, and prepares the stump for the pressure of a prosthesis.

Fulfilled Needs: Comfort, protection from physical harm, increased learning

Contraindications: Nonhealing of the stump wound, stump hemorrhage

Teach how to prepare a formula   Explain the several methods for preparing a formula. For the presterilized method, clean and sterilize the bottles, nipples, and formula equipment. Add formula to the bottles and store them in a refrigerator. For the thermal heat method, clean the bottles, nipples, and formula equipment, then pour the formula into the bottles, sterilize them, cool them, and store them in the refrigerator. Explain what is available in the prepackaged formulas. Explain how to prepare various tube feeding formulas.

Rationale: Correctly prepared and stored formulas are less likely to cause problems of digestion, absorption, or infection and are more likely to provide the essentials for food and fluid balance.

Fulfilled Needs: Fluid and electrolyte balance, nutritional balance, comfort, protection from physical harm, mastery and competence in skills, increased learning

Teach how to prepare balanced meals   Assist the person in planning a series of meals, each of which provides good nutrition. Plan a variety of foods, even where there are dietary limitations.

Rationale: Well-balanced meals contribute to better health and good nutritional habits and increase appetite.

Fulfilled Needs: Nutritional balance, protection from physical harm, increased learning

Teach how to propel the wheelchair   Suggest that the best method of propelling a wheelchair is to push both wheels forward simultaneously, using long, even, intermittent strokes.

Rationale: Use of efficient means to propel a wheelchair reduces energy consumption, minimizing fatigue.

Fulfilled Needs: Energy, comfort, protection from physical harm, increased learning

Teach how to remember to take medications   Explain that there are specific ways to remember to take medications. They include the following steps: planning to take the medications at the same time the person plans to perform other routine activities such as getting out of bed, meals, taking a coffee break, or before going to bed; placing a written reminder on the mirror, the refrigerator, the desk, or the calendar; making a check-off chart; setting an alarm on a clock or wristwatch; and taking the medications along instead of leaving them at home. If there are multiple drugs to be taken each day, it is a good idea to place each day's supply, for a week, in small, separate plastic bags, and the night before, the person should place the next day's supply in a purse, wallet, pillbox, etc.

Rationale: Unless a person remembers to take his medication, the drug cannot have a therapeutic effect. Taking medications should fit into the daily routine and should not cause a disruption of routine.

Fulfilled Needs: Protection from physical harm, increased learning

Teach how to suction an airway Explain the proper method for suctioning the nose, mouth, tracheostomy stoma, endotracheal tube, etc. Explain how to insert catheters and prevent tissue trauma, as well as appropriate suctioning techniques.

Rationale: Removal of secretions maintains a patent airway.

Fulfilled Needs: Tissue oxygenation or perfusion, protection from physical harm, mastery and competence in skills, increased learning

Teach how to take a blood pressure Explain the method for reading blood pressure. Include proper cuff application, differentiation of systolic and diastolic blood pressures, undelayed cuff release, and accepted norms.

Rationale: Knowledge of blood pressure status is necessary for persons with hypertension and for those who are receiving home hemodialysis therapy.

Fulfilled Needs: Protection from physical harm, mastery and competence in skills, increased learning

Teach how to take a sitz bath Teach the person to sit in a tub of hot water (96–106° F) with the tub filled so that the water comes up to the umbilicus. Caution the person to rise slowly when getting out of a hot sitz bath because of the potential for hypotension.

Rationale: Moist heat promotes relaxation and healing by cleansing and increases circulation to the pelvic area through vasodilatation.

Fulfilled Needs: Tissue oxygenation or perfusion, relaxation, comfort, cleanliness, protection from physical harm, increased learning

Contraindications: New abdominal surgical incision, menstruation.

Teach how to take a temperature and accurately read a thermometer Explain that before taking a temperature, the thermometer should read 95° F or below. For oral temperature, the thermometer bulb should be placed well under the tongue with the lips kept closed for at least 3 minutes. For rectal temperature, the thermometer bulb should be inserted about 1½ inches into the rectum for 3–5 minutes. For axillary temperature, the thermometer bulb should be placed in the axilla, with the arm pressed against the body for 5 minutes. When the thermometer is removed, the temperature should be read and recorded and the thermometer wiped clean.

Rationale: Knowledge of temperature status is necessary to determine excessive body heat production or loss or poor temperature control.

Fulfilled Needs: Protection from physical harm, mastery and competence in skills, increased learning

Teach how to test the blood for glucose using the finger-stick method Explain how to use Dextrostix to determine the glucose level in blood.

Rationale: Knowledge of the glucose level in blood promotes safety for diabetics and for persons with hypoglycemia.

Fulfilled Needs: Protection from physical harm, mastery and competence in skills, increased learning

Teach how to test the urine by dipstick (Multistix) Explain how the urine can be tested for urobilinogen, blood, nitrate, sugar acetone, protein, and pH levels by placing a dipstick into a urine specimen and reading the results. Have the person make a return demonstration.

Rationale: Knowledge of how to treat urine can make the person aware of significant clinical findings that can be reported to health personnel.

Fulfilled Needs: Protection from physical harm, increased learning

Teach how to test the urine for pH Explain how to check the urine acid level with litmus or Nitrazine paper or other appropriate chemical agents.

Rationale: Urinary pH (acidity or alkalinity) affects urinary stone formation.

Fulfilled Needs: Protection from physical harm, mastery and competence in skills, increased learning

Teach how to test the urine for protein Explain how to use Combistix or Urostix to determine the protein level in urine.

Rationale: Protein in the urine indicates impaired renal function, prostatitis, epididymitis, or impending pregnancy toxemia, or kidney transplant rejection.

Fulfilled Needs: Protection from physical harm, mastery and competence in skills, increased learning

Teach how to test the urine for sugar acetone/glucosuria Explain how to use Clinitest, Diastix, or Tes-Tape to determine the level of urine sugar (glucose) and how to use Acetest or Ketostix to determine the level of acetone (ketone bodies) in the urine. Explain the specific directions for each test and how to match the results of the test with the color chart provided and to record results.

Rationale: Testing the urine for sugar acetone provides information as to the current degree of control of carbohydrate–fat metabolism in the diabetic. Sugar in the before-meal urine of a diabetic indicates inadequate insulin or excess carbohydrate intake. Acetone in the urine indicates abnormal metabolism of fat.

Fulfilled Needs: Protection from physical harm, mastery and competence in skills, independence, increased learning

Teach how to transfer from a bathtub to a wheelchair[108] When a person who is in a bathtub wants to get into a wheelchair, he should place the front of the wheelchair toward the side of the bathtub as close to the bathtub as possible and lock the wheelchair. Making sure that his hands are dry, he places one hand on each side of the tub and carefully raises his body to sit on the edge of the tub. Then he moves his body backward into the wheelchair.

Rationale: Safe mobility is essential for carrying out daily activities and maintaining independence.

Fulfilled Needs: Activity and exercise, comfort, protection from physical harm, mastery and competence in skills, independence, increased learning

Teach how to transfer from a bed to a wheelchair[108] When a person who is in bed wants to get into a wheelchair, he should place the front of the wheelchair toward the side of the bed as close to the bed as possible and lock the brakes. In a sitting position, with his back facing the chair, he should move his body to the edge of the bed. He should place his hands on the arms of the chair and slide his body backward off the bed into the wheelchair. Then he should lift his legs off the bed into the chair.

Rationale: Safe mobility is essential for carrying out daily activities and maintaining independence.

Fulfilled Needs: Activity and exercise, comfort, protection from physical harm, mastery and competence in skills, independence, increased learning

Teach how to transfer from a chair to a wheelchair[108] When a person who is in a regular chair wants to move into a wheelchair, he should place the regular chair and the wheelchair so that they face each other as close together as possible. Then he should lock the wheelchair brakes. He should move his body to the edge of the chair, place one hand on the chair seat and the other on the wheelchair arm, and pivot his body into the wheelchair.

Rationale: Safe mobility is essential for carrying out daily activities and maintaining independence.

Fulfilled Needs: Activity and exercise, comfort, protection from physical harm, mastery and competence in skills, independence, increased learning

Teach how to transfer from a wheelchair to a bathtub[108]   When a person who is in a wheelchair wants to get into a bathtub, he should place the front of the wheelchair toward the side of the bathtub as close to the bathtub as possible and lock the wheelchair. He should lift his feet and legs into the tub, place each hand on an arm of the wheelchair, and move his body forward off the wheelchair to a sitting position on the edge of the tub. Then he should place one hand on the near side of the tub and the other hand on the far side and carefully lower his body into the water.

Rationale: Safe mobility is essential for carrying out daily activities and maintaining independence.

Fulfilled Needs: Activity and exercise, comfort, protection from physical harm, mastery and competence in skills, independence, increased learning

Teach how to transfer from a wheelchair to a bed[108]   When a person who is in a wheelchair wants to get into bed, he should place the front of the wheelchair toward the bed as close to the bed as possible and lock the wheelchair brakes. He should put his feet on the floor, place one hand firmly on the mattress and the other on the nearest wheelchair arm, and then pivot his body onto the bed.

Rationale: Safe mobility is essential for carrying out daily activities and maintaining independence.

Fulfilled Needs: Activity and exercise, comfort, protection from physical harm, mastery and competence in skills, independence, increased learning

Teach how to transfer from a wheelchair to a chair[108]   When a person who is in a wheelchair wants to get into a regular chair, he should place the wheelchair and the regular chair so that they face each other as close together as possible and lock the wheelchair brakes. He should move his body to the edge of the wheelchair, place one hand on the wheelchair arm and the other on the seat of the regular chair, and pivot his body onto the chair.

Rationale: Safe mobility is essential for carrying out daily activities and maintaining independence.

Fulfilled Needs: Activity and exercise, comfort, protection from physical harm, mastery and competence in skills, independence, increased learning

Teach how to transfer from a wheelchair to an automobile[108]   When a person who is in a wheelchair wants to move into a car, he should open the car door as far as possible and move the wheelchair close to the side of the car facing the car. Then he should lock the wheelchair brakes. He should move his body to the edge of the wheelchair, turning it in the direction of the front of the car, and place one hand on the window ledge of the car door and the other on the wheelchair arm. Then he should lift his body onto the car seat and lift his legs and feet into the car.

Rationale: Safe mobility is essential for carrying out daily activities and maintaining independence.

Fulfilled Needs: Activity and exercise, comfort, protection from physical harm, mastery and competence in skills, independence, increased learning

Teach how to transfer from an automobile to a wheelchair[108]   When a person who is in a car wants to get into a wheelchair, he should open the car door as far as possible and place the wheelchair close to the car facing the side of the car. He should lock the wheelchair brakes and then move to the edge of the car seat. Then he can swing his legs out of the car, place one hand on the car window ledge and the other on the farthest wheelchair arm, and lift his body into the wheelchair.

Rationale: Safe mobility is essential for carrying out daily activities and maintaining independence.

Fulfilled Needs: Activity and exercise, comfort, protection from physical harm, mastery and competence in skills, independence, increased learning

Teach how to turn over when hemiplegic[108] When a person with one-sided paralysis wants to turn on his affected (weak) side, he should bend the unaffected (strong) leg and pull on the bedrail with his strong arm. This will turn his body onto the affected side. If he wants to turn on his unaffected (strong) side, he should grasp the pajama leg of the affected (weak) side and pull the paralyzed leg across the strong leg. Then, placing his paralyzed arm on his chest, he can grasp the bedrail and pull his body onto his strong side.

Rationale: Frequent turning prevents fluid congestion in the lungs, stimulates circulation, and promotes comfort. Safe mobility encourages independence.

Fulfilled Needs: Activity and exercise, comfort, protection from physical harm, mastery and competence in skills, independence, increased learning

Teach how to use a cane/walker for balancing and weight bearing Explain that body balance can be maintained by holding a cane in the hand opposite the weak leg and moving the cane forward at the same time the weak leg moves forward. A walker can be used by holding it with two hands and slowly moving it ahead of oneself. Explain that weight bearing can be accomplished by holding a cane in the hand of the side of the weak leg as one bears weight on that leg and steps forward with the good leg. A walker can also be used for weight bearing as one moves along.

Rationale: Knowledge of how to use a cane or walker can provide the body support and stability necessary for active locomotion.

Fulfilled Needs: Activity, comfort, protection from physical harm, mastery and competence in skills, increased learning

Teach how to use a hand nebulizer Explain how to use a hand nebulizer: Keep the mouth open and simultaneously breathe in and squeeze the nebulizer so that the medication is inhaled.

Rationale: Medication by hand nebulizer can reduce respiratory spasm or loosen secretions.

Fulfilled Needs: Protection from physical harm, increased learning

Teach how to use a hydraulic hoist Explain the use of a hoist to make lifting the body easier.

Rationale: Use of a hydraulic hoist can provide even weight distribution and limit skin pressure when the body is moved, and it supports independent activity.

Fulfilled Needs: Protection from physical harm, mastery and competence in skills, independence, increased learning

Teach how to use a systematic desensitization technique[471] Teach the person the muscle-relaxing and anxiety-reducing technique of deep breathing and exhaling. When the person feels no anxiety, talk about the anxiety-provoking situation in his life. Do this until the person is able to talk about the subject without feeling anxious. Continue to introduce the anxiety-provoking situation gradually by engaging in sessions of imagining it occurring, confronting it at a distance, moving in closer, and finally confronting it outright. Stay at the current level of desensitization until the person can meet the situation without anxiety. Have him return to the relaxation technique if fear recurs. For example, if a person fears dogs, teach the relaxation technique. Then have the person talk about dogs until he can do this without experiencing fear. Then have him look at pictures of dogs. Next have him look at a dog from inside the house. Then have him sit on the porch with the dog in the yard. Gradually, have him approach and finally pet the dog.

Rationale: Since tension causes anxiety, a relaxed confrontation with a situation will reduce the anxiety response. Systematic desensitization assists the person to change his response to a threatening stimulus.

Fulfilled Needs: Comfort, protection from psychologic threat, personal growth and maturity, increased learning

Teach how to use a temporary prosthesis   Explain that when a temporary prosthesis is used shortly after amputation surgery, only 10% of the body weight should be borne on the prosthesis. A stump wrap should be applied at night to prevent swelling.

Rationale: Use of a temporary prosthesis supports early ambulation.

Fulfilled Needs: Activity, comfort, protection from physical harm, mastery and competence in skills, increased learning

Teach how to use assistive dressing devices   Explain how to use self-help devices for dressing, such as buttonhooks, Velcro clothing closures, and long-handled shoehorns.

Rationale: Use of assistive dressing devices promotes independence.

Fulfilled Needs: Comfort, mastery and competence in skills, independence, increased learning

Teach how to use assistive eating/drinking devices   Explain how to use self-help devices for eating, such as a feeder cuff for spoon and fork, long straws, removable handles to make a cup from a glass, one-handed rocking knives for easy cutting, plate guards, extension forks, swivel spoons, and suction plates.

Rationale: Use of assistive eating devices promotes independence.

Fulfilled Needs: Comfort, mastery and competence in skills, independence, increased learning

Teach how to use assistive grooming devices   Explain how to use self-help devices for grooming, such as a suction nailbrush, a suction brush for cleaning dentures, a long-handled bath brush, soap mits, a feeder cuff to hold the toothbrush, and a long-handled hairbrush.

Rationale: Use of assistive grooming devices promotes the comfort of being refreshed and having a pleasant appearance and encourages independence.

Fulfilled Needs: Comfort, cleanliness, protection from physical harm, independence, increased learning

Teach how to use assistive toileting devices   Teach the patient how to use such devices as the bedpan, urinal, bedside commode, and heightened commode seat. Explain how they are most comfortably used and how to clean them.

Rationale: The use of assistive toileting devices supports hygiene elimination when a person is unable to use standard toilet facilities.

Fulfilled Needs: Comfort, cleanliness, independence, increased learning

Teach how to use the forearm to push up from a lying position when hemiplegic[108]   Teach the person with one-sided paralysis to use his unaffected (strong) arm to lift his body from the bed and then push up with his forearm and hand to move his body to a sitting position.

Rationale: Safe mobility is essential for carrying out daily activities and maintaining independence.

Fulfilled Needs: Activity and exercise, comfort, protection from physical harm, mastery and competence in skills, independence, increased learning

Teach how to use the problem-solving method   Explain that a systematic method for solving problems should include defining the problem, gathering and analyzing data related to the problem, examining the possible solutions, and evaluating the effectiveness of the chosen solution.

Rationale: Successful problem solving is essential to mental health.

Fulfilled Needs: Comfort, protection from psychologic threat, mastery and competence in skills, personal growth and maturity, increased learning, increased reality perception and problem-solving ability

Teach how to use the unaffected leg to move the hemiplegic leg[108]
Teach the person with one-sided paralysis to place his unaffected (strong) leg under his affected (weak) leg and lift his affected (weak) leg to the edge of the bed and over the side.
Rationale: Safe mobility is essential for carrying out daily activities and maintaining independence.
Fulfilled Needs: Activity and exercise, comfort, protection from physical harm, mastery and competence in skills, independence, increased learning

Teach how to weigh   Explain how to measure and record body weight.
Rationale: Changes in body weight may indicate loss or retention of fluid, changes in appetite, abnormalities of food absorption or metabolism, or poor nutrition.
Fulfilled Needs: Protection from physical harm, increased learning

Teach how to wrap an amputation stump   Teach the amputee that a stump wrapping is applied by beginning at the mid-anterior thigh and bringing one length of bandage down to the stump end, under the stump, and over the anterior stump and thigh. A crisscross or figure-eight pattern is used, never a circular pattern. The bandage must be applied with even pressure, and it should be changed in the morning, in the afternoon, and before bedtime.
Rationale: Wrapping shrinks and shapes the stump in preparation for the prosthesis, supports soft tissue, and decreases edema.
Fulfilled Needs: Comfort, protection from physical harm, mastery and competence in skills, increased learning

Teach hygiene methods   Explain and demonstrate the specific hygiene methods appropriate to the situation.
Rationale: Hygiene promotes the comfort of cleanliness and protection from infection and disease.
Fulfilled Needs: Comfort, cleanliness, protection from physical harm

Teach measures to prevent apnea   Suggest ways to prevent the infant from having absent respirations, such as making sure that the infant does not become too hot or too cold and not overfeeding the infant, which causes stomach distention and puts pressure on the diaphragm. Burping the infant adequately will avoid distention. Dehydration can be prevented by giving adequate fluids especially during fever, high activity levels, and environmental heat. The child should be positioned to keep his airway clear.
Rationale: The use of preventive measures reduces the potential for the actual occurrence of apnea.
Fulfilled Needs: Protection from physical harm, increased learning

Teach menstrual cycle physiology   Explain that menstruation is the monthly discharge of uterine blood, mucus, and epithelial cells. It occurs at intervals of approximately 28 days between the ages of 12 and 45 years. The menstrual cycle begins on the 1st day of menstruation, when the discharge of blood, mucus, and epithelial cells occurs. At the end of this period, or approximately 5 days later, the uterine membrane becomes very thin. From the fifth day to about the 10th or 12th day, estrogen secretion causes the uterus lining to become thick and cushiony. Around the 12th or 14th day ovulation occurs, during which a small body in the ovaries (the graafian follicle) ruptures, releasing an egg and then forming the corpus luteum, which secretes progesterone. The egg moves into the fallopian tube and down into the uterus. The progesterone stimulates increased blood supply to the uterine lining, making it even thicker in preparation for a fertilized egg. If fertilization does not occur by about the 25th day, the corpus luteum stops its activity and the uterine lining degenerates and is shed. Bleeding occurs because of the rupture of the small blood vessels in the uterine lining.
Rationale: Knowledge of physiologic body processes promotes comfort and safety.
Fulfilled Needs: Comfort, protection from physical harm, increased learning

Teach menstrual hygiene   Explain that during menstrual flow, bathing, shampooing, exercise, and other normal activities are important to good health. Answer questions specific to the person's needs.

Rationale: Good menstrual hygiene promotes comfort and health.

Fulfilled Needs: Comfort, cleanliness, increased learning

Teach methods for improving the memory[774]   Teach the specific methods that improve memory, such as linking and connecting ideas together, paying strict attention to the information being received, and not dividing attention between several subjects at the same time. Teach the person how to reinforce the memory by using the five senses to increase imagery. For example, to remember the name of a particular flower, it helps to touch, smell, and visualize the flower. Recommend that the person review the information he wants to recall within 10 minutes, and then again within 24 hours, to review the information when going to sleep, and to make lists of what should be remembered. He should avoid disorganized thinking and should organize information well. Exercise can improve cerebral circulation, which improves memory. Recommend the use of memory games to have fun remembering and that he improve the memory by rereading, retelling, rehearing, reviewing, and reinforcing the information. Finally, teach the person to think positively that he will remember and to ignore the times he forgets.

Rationale: An improved memory maintains self-esteem and independent functioning.

Fulfilled Needs: Comfort, protection from psychologic threat, increased learning, increased reality perception and problem-solving ability.

Teach mobility down a curb with crutches[108]   Teach the person to approach the curb, stand still, move his crutches down off the curb, and then move his affected (weak) leg down, followed by his unaffected (strong) leg.

Rationale: Safe mobility is essential for carrying out daily activities and maintaining independence.

Fulfilled Needs: Activity and exercise, comfort, protection from physical harm, mastery and competence in skills, independence, increased learning

Teach mobility down stairs and curbs with leg braces[108]   Teach the person to place one hand on the stair rail and both crutches under his opposite arm. He should move the crutches down to the next step, place as much weight as possible on his hands, and swing both braced legs down to that step. He should repeat the procedure for each step.

Rationale: Safe mobility is essential for carrying out daily activities and maintaining independence.

Fulfilled Needs: Activity and exercise, comfort, protection from physical harm, mastery and competence in skills, independence, increased learning

Teach mobility down stairs with crutches[108]   Teach the person to place one hand on the stair rail and both crutches under his opposite arm. He should place as much weight as possible on his hands and arms, move the crutches to the step below, and then move his affected (weak) leg down, followed by his unaffected (strong) leg. He should repeat the procedure at each step.

Rationale: Safe mobility is essential for carrying out daily activities and maintaining independence.

Fulfilled Needs: Activity and exercise, comfort, protection from physical harm, mastery and competence in skills, independence, increased learning

Teach mobility from a standing to a sitting position with crutches[108]   Teach the person to back a chair against a stable surface. He should move as close to the chair as possible, hold both crutches together at the handpiece with one hand, and place his other hand on the chair arm. Then he can slide into the chair.

Rationale: Safe mobility is essential for carrying out daily activities and maintaining independence.

Fulfilled Needs: Activity and exercise, comfort, protection from physical harm, mastery and competence in skills, independence, increased learning

Teach mobility from a standing to a sitting position with leg braces[108]
Teach the person to back a chair against a stable surface. He should move as close to the chair as possible, unlock one brace at the knee, grasp the chair arms with both hands, and slide into the chair. He should then unlock the other leg brace.

Rationale: Safe mobility is essential for carrying out daily activities and maintaining independence.

Fulfilled Needs: Activity and exercise, comfort, protection from physical harm, mastery and competence in skills, independence, increased learning

Teach mobility up a curb with crutches[108]
Teach the person to use his crutches to maintain balance as he approaches a curb. Then he should step up on the curb with his strong leg, straighten that leg, and lift his weak leg and his crutches onto the curb.

Rationale: Safe mobility is essential for carrying out daily activities and maintaining independence.

Fulfilled Needs: Activity and exercise, comfort, protection from physical harm, mastery and competence in skills, independence, increased learning

Teach mobility up a curb with leg braces[108]
Teach the person to use his crutches to maintain balance as he backs up to the curb. He should swing one leg back and up onto the curb while leaning on both crutches. Then he should shift his weight to the leg on the curb and swing the other leg back and up onto the curb. He should balance his body on one crutch and both legs and bring first one crutch and then the other up onto the curb.

Rationale: Safe mobility is essential for carrying out daily activities and maintaining independence.

Fulfilled Needs: Activity and exercise, comfort, protection from physical harm, mastery and competence in skills, independence, increased learning

Teach mobility up stairs with crutches[108]
Teach the person to place one hand on the stair rail and both crutches under his opposite arm. He should place as much weight as possible on his hands and arms and then step up with his strong leg, straighten that leg, and lift his weak leg and crutches. He should repeat the procedure at each step.

Rationale: Safe mobility is essential for carrying out daily activities and maintaining independence.

Fulfilled Needs: Activity and exercise, comfort, protection from physical harm, mastery and competence in skills, independence, increased learning

Teach mobility up stairs with leg braces[108]
Teach the person to place one hand on the stair rail and both crutches under his opposite arm. He should place as much weight as possible on his hands and arms and step up by lifting his legs and then bringing the crutches up to that step. He should repeat the procedure at each step.

Rationale: Safe mobility is essential for carrying out daily activities and maintaining independence.

Fulfilled Needs: Activity and exercise, comfort, protection from physical harm, mastery and competence in skills, independence, increased learning

Teach muscle-strengthening exercises
Teach the person how to do exercises that strengthen muscles. Recommend doing pushups off a chair or firm surface to strengthen triceps and lifting the body weight with a trapeze bar to strengthen biceps and shoulder muscles, in preparation for crutch-walking or moving from bed to wheelchair.

Rationale: Exercise strengthens weak muscles, improving the capacity to function.

Fulfilled Needs: Activity and exercise, increased learning

Contraindications: Severe cardiac or respiratory disorders, wounds or incisions that have not completely healed

Teach positive parenting behavior[47,259] Teach methods for rearing children in a positive, supportive way. Instruct in methods of constructive discipline and loving care. Teach that permissiveness is necessary for the child to develop his full potential and to become eventually independent, but it must be balanced with reasonable and consistent discipline (limit setting). Loving acceptance and approval contribute to the development of a positive self-concept and effective interpersonal relationships.

Rationale: Positive parenting behavior results in physical and mental child health. It provides rewarding parenting for adults.

Fulfilled Needs: Comfort, protection from physical harm, personal growth and maturity, increased learning

Teach postural drainage After determining which lobe of the lung needs draining, teach the patient proper positioning for drainage.

Rationale: Postural drainage removes secretions from the lung by using the force of gravity.

Fulfilled Needs: Protection from physical harm, increased learning

Contraindications: Do not place the patient in the head-down position if he has increased intracranial or intraocular pressure or hypertension.

Teach precautions after back injury[721] Explain that there are certain measures for preventing injury to back muscles, which include avoiding certain activities: lifting heavy objects above the shoulder, reaching far distances to retrieve objects, pulling heavy objects, maintaining one position for a prolonged period, assuming a stooped position, lifting objects weighing more than 20 lb, bending over at the waist with the knees straight to lift something off the ground, being overweight, and pushing tight windows open. Recommend that the person use a firm mattress, adjust the car seat so it is close to the steering wheel with the person's hips flexed at approximately a 90° angle, move to the front of the chair before getting up, use long-handled equipment to prevent stooping, and that he do appropriate exercises to strengthen back muscles.

Rationale: Use of preventive measures reduces the potential for reinjury.

Fulfilled Needs: Protection from physical harm

Teach prenursing nipple hygiene Explain that immediately before breast-feeding, the nipples should be washed with warm water.

Rationale: Cleanliness helps prevent infection and promotes comfort.

Fulfilled Needs: Comfort, cleanliness, protection from physical harm, increased learning

Teach proper care of equipment Teach the person how to clean and maintain the functioning of equipment. Explain the simplest and safest ways to care for equipment.

Rationale: Clean and well-functioning equipment more effectively provides its intended effect. It also prevents physical injury such as infection.

Fulfilled Needs: Comfort, protection from physical harm, increased learning

Teach reverse isolation Explain that persons who are highly susceptible to infection can be protected somewhat if those with whom they come in contact wash their hands and wear gowns and masks.

Rationale: Wearing gowns and masks and washing the hands help protect the susceptible person from infectious organisms carried by others.

Fulfilled Needs: Protection from physical harm, increased learning

Teach safety measures to be practiced when wearing a pacemaker Teach the person wearing a pacemaker to avoid high-frequency signals (microwaves), to use battery-operated appliances, etc., instead of electrical. The person should not use ungrounded electrical equipment when wearing a pacemaker and should avoid using worn electrical cords, plugs, or outlets.

Rationale: Since the pacemaker is designed to maintain cardiac function, safety measures are needed to protect against dysfunction of the pacemaker.

Fulfilled Needs: Protection from physical harm, increased learning

Teach skin care after cast removal   After the cast has been removed, explain that the underlying skin should be treated. Instruct the person to apply vegetable or mineral oil generously to the area and to leave the oil on for several hours and then wash gently with mild soap and water.

Rationale: Skin that has been casted and without air exposure for some time becomes dry and flaky. Oil applications help restore skin integrity.

Fulfilled Needs: Comfort, protection from physical harm, increased learning

Teach sterile technique   Teach methods for maintaining sterility of equipment, dressings, etc. Include methods of opening sterile packages, handling sterile equipment, and maintaining sterility while performing procedures.

Rationale: The use of sterile technique minimizes the entrance of microorganisms into catheters, wounds, etc.

Fulfilled Needs: Cleanliness, protection from physical harm, mastery and competence in skills, independence, increased learning

Teach that weight bearing should be done on the unaffected side   Explain that in almost any injury, weight should be borne by the unaffected side of the body.

Rationale: Use of the body's strongest side helps prevent further injury to the weak side. It promotes healing and provides support for the total body.

Fulfilled Needs: Protection from physical harm, increased learning

Teach the common factors that will cause a false positive or inaccurate glucose reading   Explain that certain factors can cause the urine glucose test to register a false reading. Such factors include excess salicylate ingestion, a large intake of vitamin C, shaking the solution during processing, and certain antibiotics such as cephalosporins.

Rationale: Correct readings of urine glucose levels are essential to determining a correct insulin dosage.

Fulfilled Needs: Protection from physical harm, increased learning

Teach the precautions to be taken in bandaging   Teach that bandages should be applied evenly and snugly but not too tightly, that bony prominences should be padded when applying a bandage, and that the body part should be in correct alignment when bandaging. Explain the need to watch for danger signs of swelling, skin pallor, redness, or blueness, pain, tingling sensation, numbness, or coldness.

Rationale: Precautions taken in bandaging promote good circulation, protect against skin, joint, and muscle injury, and support correct body alignment.

Fulfilled Needs: Protection from physical harm, increased learning

Teach the principles of good nutrition   Explain the daily need for the basic foods in every diet: one or more servings of leafy green or yellow vegetables, one or more servings of cirtus fruit, tomatoes, or raw cabbage, two or more servings of potatoes and other vegetables and.fruits, 2–4 cups of milk or the equivalent in cheese or ice cream, one or more servings of meat, poultry, fish, eggs, or dried peas or beans, one or more servings of bread, flour, or cereals; and some butter or margarine.

Rationale: A balanced nutritional intake is essential to cellular activity and energy production from food.

Fulfilled Needs: Nutritional balance, energy, protection from physical harm, increased learning

Teach the proper gait to use with a walker[108] Explain that the standard gait pattern used with a walker involves moving the walker forward first, followed by the right foot and then the left foot.

Rationale: Proper use of a walker promotes safe mobility.

Fulfilled Needs: Protection from physical harm, increased learning

Teach the proper gait to use with crutches[108] Teach the person the crutch-walking gait appropriate for his condition. For *two-point crutch-walking*, the person should move forward by advancing the right crutch and the left foot together and the left crutch and right foot together at a reasonable pace. In *three-point crutch walking*, the person should stand on his good leg and place both crutches the same distances ahead of him. He should swing himself forward ahead of the crutches, then place his body weight on his good leg, and regain his balance before advancing the crutches again. For *four-point crutch-walking*, the person should employ the pattern of right crutch, left foot, left crutch, right foot. In *swing-through crutch-walking*, the person should place the crutches ahead of him and then raise his entire body off the floor and up to and through the crutches. For *tripod crutch-walking*, the person should place the crutches slightly ahead of him and drag his body up to the crutches, then repeat the process.

Rationale: The ability to move about is essential to daily living activities. Three-point crutch-walking facilitates walking after an amputation or a fractured hip. Four-point crutch-walking is best for patients who can manipulate both lower extremities. Swing-through crutch-walking facilitates movement where there is severe lower-extremity involvement, such as in paraplegia. Tripod crutch-walking facilitates movement for the person who cannot lift his body off the floor.

Fulfilled Needs: Protection from physical harm, mastery and competence in new skills, increased learning

Teach the specific procedure/method When a person needs to perform a certain health procedure, teach him which supplies he will need and how to perform the procedure. After the explanation, have him give a return demonstration.

Rationale: Correct performance of health procedures increases the potential for effectiveness of the procedure.

Fulfilled Needs: Protection from physical harm, mastery and competence in skills, increased learning

Teach the types of bandages to be used Teach that several types of bandages are used: *stretch gauze* (Kling or Kerlex) molds to the body, *flannel* is a soft bandage that helps retain the body's warmth, *crinoline* is a coarse gauze used in applying casts, *muslin* is a heavy cotton used for support as in splints, *elasticized bandages* (Ace bandages) are used to apply pressure and support, *elastic adhesive* (Elastoplast or Coban) is a combined elastic and adhesive bandage used to give support and *plastic adhesive* is a combined waterproof and adhesive bandage designed to provide support and maintain dryness.

Rationale: Knowledge of the types of bandages and their usefulness increases the potential for effectiveness of the bandaging procedure.

Fulfilled Needs: Protection from physical harm, mastery and compentence in skills, increased learning

Teach which drugs and chemicals have the potential for habituation Explain that the following drugs can lead to drug habituation: sleeping pills and barbiturates (Amytal, Nembutal, phenobarbital), amphetamine pep pills and diet pills (Benzedrine, Dexedrine, Methedrine), opiates and narcotics (morphine, heroin, codeine, paregoric), tranquilizers (Valium, Meprobamate, Librium), marijuana, and deliriants such as airplane glue, gasoline, lighter fluid, paint thinner, varnish, shellac, and Freon.

Rationale: Accurate knowledge about drugs that can lead to habituation can result in abstinence or cautious use of such drugs.

Fulfilled Needs: Protection from physical harm, increased learning

Teach which drugs and foods have potential adverse interactions[212,299,565]

Explain that certain drugs need to be taken with or without certain foods to minimize undesirable interactions. Drugs such as Furadantin, Macrodantin, Fulvicin, Grifulvin, Tagamet, Morax, and Tedral should be taken with or immediately after meals. Antibiotics should be taken 1 hour before or 2–3 hours after meals. Certain drugs, such as tetracycline, Vibramycin, Minomycin, Dulcolax, Declomycin, Achromycin, and Ecotrin, should not be taken with milk or dairy products. Sulfonamide antibiotics and drugs such as Benemid, which potentiates the excretion of uric acid in the urine, are taken with a full glass of water. Anticholinergic drugs should be taken 30–45 minutes before meals. When taking monoamine oxidase (MAO) inhibitors such as Marplan, Nardil, and Parnate, foods high in tyramine (aged cheese, chicken livers, beer, bananas, dried fish, fermented sausage, red wines, and sherry) should be avoided. When taking anticoagulants, leafy green vegetables such as spinach, Brussels sprouts, and turnip greens should be avoided.

Rationale: Taking drugs with or immediately after meals reduces the possibility of gastric irritation. When antibiotics are taken with food, the amount of drug absorption is decreased. Maximum absorption is more likely when the drug is taken on an empty stomach. The calcium in dairy products can cause fecal excretion of a drug, or it can raise the pH level of the stomach to a degree that enteric coatings are dissolved while the drug is still in the stomach, causing gastric irritation or ulceration. Large amounts of water taken with drugs prevents precipitation of the drug in the renal tubules. Anticholinergic drugs are taken before meals so that their antacid effect is activated at about the same time food stimulation of gastric secretions begins. Tyramine increases the secretion of norepinephrine, the metabolism of which is inhibited by MAO drugs. Leafy green vegetables contain high levels of vitamin K, which counteracts the effect of anticoagulants.

Fulfilled Needs: Protection from physical harm, increased learning

MEDICAL TREATMENTS PERFORMED BY NURSES

Administer a blood transfusion   Infuse typed and crossmatched blood into the vein.

Rationale: A blood infusion increases circulating blood volume, red cell volume, and hemoglobin content, and these facilitate oxygen transport to cells. It provides protein and essential nutrient elements. Freshly drawn blood also restores platlets and white blood cells.

Fulfilled Needs: Tissue oxygenation or perfusion, fluid and electrolyte balance, protection from physical harm

Contraindications: Known allergies, polycythemia vera, circulatory overload

Administer a medicated enema   Dispense a medicated solution into the colon. Encourage the person to retain the solution for 30 minutes to 1 hour.

Rationale: In the presence of liver damage, the intestinal flora increase ammonia production. Cleaning the bowel with neomycin or lactulose decreases intestinal bacteria and reduces the ammonia level.

Fulfilled Needs: Protection from physical harm

Administer aerosol mist by nebulizer   Dispense a fine mist of liquid particles suspended in air by running oxygen or compressed air through a nebulizer to produce a spray.

Rationale: Aerosol mist can liquefy mucus secretions and promote their elimination from the respiratory tract.

Fulfilled Needs: Waste elimination of bronchopulmonary secretions, comfort, protection from physical harm

Administer controlled positive-pressure breathing   Dispense intermittent positive-pressure breathing, which completely controls the breathing pattern.

Rationale: When normal respirations cannot be maintained, controlled positive-pressure breathing supports respirations at normal rate, depth, and rhythm; it prevents respiratory failure, promotes carbon dioxide elimination, and supports acid–base balance.

Fulfilled Needs: Tissue oxygenation or perfusion, acid–base balance, waste elimination of carbon dioxide, protection from physical harm

Contraindications: Pulmonary hemorrhage

Administer heated humidified oxygen (ET)   (listed under Nursing Treatments)

Administer humidified oxygen (ET)   (listed under Nursing Treatments)

Administer intermittent positive-pressure breathing (ET)   (listed under Nursing Treatments)

Administer intermittent positive-pressure by expiratory positive-pressure mask   When giving IPPB for pulmonary edema, use an expiratory positive-pressure mask that has a multihole valve with disks of varying diameters.

Rationale: The expiratory positive-pressure mask maintains positive pressure in the alveoli and airway. The smaller the disk hole, the greater the positive pressure. It re-

1783

tards blood flow back to the heart during exhalation, which decreases blood flow to the lungs.

Fulfilled Needs: Tissue oxygenation or perfusion, protection from physical harm

Contraindications: Pulmonary embolus, pulmonary hemorrhage

Administer intravenous fluids (ET)   (listed under Nursing Treatments)

Administer manual or mechanical ventilation   Give the person manual ventilation with a bag-valve-mask apparatus or mechanical ventilation with positive end-expiratory pressure (PEEP).

Rationale: Assistive ventilation is essential to life during severe respiratory distress and supports improved gas exchange.

Fulfilled Needs: Tissue oxygenation or perfusion, acid–base balance, waste elimination of carbon dioxide, comfort

Administer oxygen by nasal cannula/nasal catheter/facial mask/tent/croupette/incubator   Give oxygen with a double-prong nasal cannula, or with a small plastic tube inserted through the nose to the oropharynx at a flow rate of 2–4 liters/minute, or with a nonrebreathing mask having a safety inlet valve between the mask and oxygen-reservoir bag, or with a partial rebreathing mask having no valve between the mask and oxygen-reservoir bag. When giving oxygen to a person who requires environmental control, use an oxygen tent, croupette, or incubator in which oxygen and humidified air are circulated.

Rationale: The nasal cannula provides high-oxygen concentrations and the comfort of freedom of movement. A nasal catheter provides highly concentrated oxygen. A nonrebreathing mask prevents rebreathing of the same air, thus providing fresh oxygen concentration. A partial rebreathing mask allows for one-third of the exhaled air to be rebreathed. In severe oxygen deficiency, a very high therapeutic oxygen concentration elevates the body's oxygen level to normal.

An oxygen tent, a croupette, or an incubator provides high-oxygen concentrations and controls environmental humidity and temperature. Humidified air prevents tissue friction during respirations, loosens secretions, and promotes comfort.

Fulfilled Needs: Tissue oxygenation or perfusion, comfort, protection from physical harm

Administer oxygen by venturi mask   Give oxygen with a mask that delivers precise oxygen concentrations.

Rationale: When respirations have been depressed by oxygen excess or carbon dioxide retention, it is essential that precise amounts of oxygen be given for maintenance of normal blood levels and prevention of further respiratory depression.

Fulfilled Needs: Tissue oxygenation or perfusion, waste elimination of carbon dioxide, protection from physical harm

Administer phototherapy treatment   Expose jaundiced skin to ultraviolet rays (bili light) and protect the person's eyes with bandages during exposure to the light.

Rationale: Exposure of jaundiced skin to ultraviolet rays reduces the yellow skin color.

Fulfilled Needs: Comfort, protection from physical harm

Contraindications: Sensitivity of skin or eyes to light

Administer the hemodialysis treatment   Give the hemodialysis treatment according to the physician's prescribed order.

Rationale: Hemodialysis removes those body wastes that are not being removed because of renal failure. Hemodialysis is essential to maintenance of life when renal failure occurs.

Fulfilled Needs: Waste elimination of nitrogenous and toxic substances, protection from physical harm

Advance the intestinal tube as ordered Gently push the intestinal tube farther into the intestinal tract. Insert as frequently as ordered and the number of inches ordered for each insertion.

Rationale: Slow advancement of an intestinal tube opens blocked areas of the intestinal tract.

Fulfilled Needs: Protection from physical harm

Apply a biologic dressing[49] Apply skin from another human (homograft) or pig skin (heterograft) to the burned area. This skin is available from skin banks.

Rationale: Biologic dressings are applied to burned skin because they provide a barrier to reduce water vaporization, decrease protein and exudate loss, protect against infection, relieve pain, support joint movement, help in debridement, and support the growth of epithelium and granulation tissue.

Fulfilled Needs: Activity, comfort, protection from physical harm

Apply a medicated dressing Apply a sterile dressing dampened with medicinal solution. Most medication solutions are not heated because heat destroys the active properties of most drugs.

Rationale: A wet medicated wound dressing soothes and cools by moisture evaporation from the dressing; it allows for slow medication penetration into the wound; it softens wound discharges, promotes drainage, localizes the area of infection, and has a bacteriostatic–bactericidal effect.

Fulfilled Needs: Comfort, cleanliness, protection from physical harm

Contraindications: Known medication allergy

Apply the prescribed preventive splint Apply to the limb a prescribed supportive splint. Such splints are applied primarily at night, but occasionally during the day.

Rationale: Preventive splints hold limbs in functional positions, thus preventing contractures and supporting future muscle use after healing.

Fulfilled Needs: Protection from physical harm

Apply the prescribed prosthesis Put the artificial body part that the physician has prescribed on the person.

Rationale: A prescribed prosthesis provides the person with a means of functioning and substitutes for the loss of a body part that has impaired normal function.

Fulfilled Needs: Activity, independence

Apply the prescribed topical agent[49] Apply to the skin the prescribed drug usually in salve or ointment form. In burn therapy, topical agents include Sulfadiazine, silver nitrate, Sulfamylon cream, Betadine, Cerium Nitrate.

Rationale: Topical agents applied to the skin reduce pain, infection, promote comfort, and support healing.

Fulfilled Needs: Comfort, protection from physical harm

Apply the prescribed traction Exert weighted pulling pressure against designated bones and establish their alignment, as prescribed by the physician.

Rationale: Skeletal traction helps to disengage bone fragments, position and immobilize bones for healing, decrease muscle spasms, prevent deformities, and increase future mobility of currently injured and immobile bones.

Fulfilled Needs: Protection from physical harm

Attach the gastric tube to suction Remove gastric contents from the stomach or duodenum by attaching the gastric tube to a suction device.

Rationale: Removal of gastric fluids and gas decreases gastric activity and pressure and promotes healing and comfort.

Fulfilled Needs: Waste elimination of food residue, comfort, protection from physical harm

Bivalve and spread the cast to relieve pressure (ET) (listed under Nursing Treatments)

Defibrillate the heart muscle (ET) (listed under Nursing Treatments)

Encourage the prescribed exercise(s) Exercise the person as prescribed by the physician. Prescribed exercises include those specific to cardiac conditions and Buerger–Allen exercises. The Buerger–Allen exercise involves placing the person in the flat position and elevating the legs above the heart level for 2 minutes. Then have the person dangle his legs, exercise his feet for 3 minutes, and lie flat for 5 minutes.

Rationale: Prescribed exercises improve arterial blood flow, which supports better circulation.

Fulfilled Needs: Tissue oxygenation or perfusion, exercise, stimulation, protection from physical harm

Give/apply the prescribed drugs Give medicinal substances that require a physician's prescription in specified doses at specified times.

Rationale: Drugs consist of chemicals that combine with body processes to alter or improve body function, promote comfort, or balance body fluid, salts, and acid–base levels. They promote elimination, stimulate body functions, regulate body temperature, and protect from inflammatory or infectious conditions.

Fulfilled Needs: Fluid and electrolyte balance, acid–base balance, waste elimination, normal temperature, sleep, rest, relaxation, comfort, stimulation, protection from physical harm, freedom from pain

Contraindications: Drug intolerance, drug allergy

Give the prescribed diet Give diets explicitly calculated for a specific disease.

Rationale: Certain nutritional elements, when given in proper amounts, can correct certain diseases and imbalances.

Fulfilled Needs: Nutritional balance, fluid and electrolyte balance, acid–base balance, protection from physical harm

Give the prescribed fluids Give the specific amounts and kinds of fluids prescribed by the physician.

Rationale: Prescribed fluids assist in the maintenance of fluid and electrolyte balance, especially in such conditions as edema, ascites, renal insufficiency, and congestive heart failure.

Fulfilled Needs: Fluid and electrolyte balance, comfort, protection from physical harm

Give the prescribed hyperalimentation feeding Administer the hyperalimentation feedings as prescribed by the physician.

Rationale: Hyperalimentation feedings provide additional nutrients essential to health and healing that cannot be ingested or absorbed.

Fulfilled Needs: Fluid and electrolyte balance, nutritional balance, energy, protection from physical harm

Give the prescribed number of peritoneal dialysis exchanges Give the number of dialysis treatments the physician has ordered. This includes instillation, leaving the fluid in the abdomen, and drainage. Most treatments are given every hour for 24–36 hours.

Rationale: The numbers of peritoneal dialysis exchanges are ordered according to blood levels of electrolytes and urea.

Fulfilled Needs: Waste elimination of nitrogenous and toxic substances, protection from physical harm

Give the prescribed tube-feeding   Administer food and fluids through a gastric, gastrostomy, or jejunostomy (enterostomy) tube.

Rationale: Balanced nutritional intake is essential to cellular activity and energy production from food products. Relief of the visceral hunger sensation promotes comfort.

Fulfilled Needs: Fluid and electrolyte balance, nutritional balance, comfort, protection from physical harm

Immunize against infectious disease   Inject immunizing drugs into the body to bring about resistance to disease.

Rationale: Resistance against disease prevents needless suffering and maintains a healthier society.

Fulfilled Needs: Protection from physical harm

Contraindications: Viral infections, pregnancy, special situations as stated in the drug brochures

Instill dialysate into the peritoneum, allow it to remain in the abdomen, then drain the dialysate   Instill the dialysate fluid, leave it in the peritoneal cavity, and drain according to the physician's prescription for amount and length of each stage of treatment.

Rationale: The effectiveness of removal of waste material by the dialysate fluid depends on the amount of fluid and the length of time it is left in the peritoneum.

Fulfilled Needs: Waste elimination of nitrogenous and toxic substances, protection from physical harm

Irrigate the bladder by tidal drainage   Gradually fill the bladder with irrigating solution and periodically empty the solution from the bladder.

Rationale: Gradual bladder distention increases muscle tone. Periodic bladder filling stimulates bladder emptying and conditions the bladder for activity not controlled by the central nervous system. The flow of irrigating fluid into the catheter prevents obstruction by clots, facilitates the application of warmth to the mucous lining, and allows for medication instillations.

Fulfilled Needs: Waste elimination of urine, protection from physical harm

Irrigate the ostomy   Dispense a water solution into the colon through an artificial anus or stoma surgically placed in the anterior abdominal wall and stimulate the defecation reflex.

Rationale: Distention and irritation of the colon stimulate fecal elimination. Colostomy irrigation maintains cleanliness by preventing defecation at socially inappropriate times.

Fulfilled Needs: Waste elimination of food residue, comfort, cleanliness

Lavage the stomach (ET)   (listed under Nursing Treatments)

Mobilize with the prescribed brace   Apply to the limb the prescribed supportive brace.

Rationale: A therapeutic brace supports weakened muscles, joints, and bones; it facilitates motion or temporarily reduces motion during healing.

Fulfilled Needs: Activity and exercise, protection from physical harm

Contraindications: Delay if severe skin irritation exists

Mobilize with the prescribed crutches   Help the person move about with crutches specifically ordered and fitted to him.

Rationale: Crutches facilitate good body balance and independent mobility

Fulfilled Needs: Activity and exercise, comfort, protection from physical harm, independence

Contraindications: Severe energy depletion

Place on a hypothermia/hyperthermia blanket   Maintain a low, normal, or elevated body temperature by placing the person on a temperature-regulating blanket.

Rationale: Lowering the body temperature decreases metabolic demand for oxygen, reduces blood pressure, and decreases fever. Raising the body temperature can gradually bring the level to normal following exposure to severe cold.

Fulfilled Needs: Normal temperature, comfort, protection from physical harm

Place on the prescribed bed rest   Encourage the person to adhere to the amount of bed rest the physician has prescribed. The amount of rest needed each day will be determined by the nature of the disease or injury being treated.

Rationale: Rest is essential to maintenance of body function; it replenishes the cell energy that the body uses for maintenance of life and activity and promotes healing and comfort.

Fulfilled Needs: Sleep and rest, energy, comfort, protection from physical harm

Resuscitate breathing (ET)   (listed under Nursing Treatments)

Resuscitate mouth-to-neck when the patient has a laryngectomy (ET) (listed under Nursing Treatments)

Soak in a medicated bath   Apply medication to the skin by placing the medication in a tub of water and soaking the person's body in it.

Rationale: Use of a tub provides for overall and equal body coverage of medications.

Fulfilled Needs: Comfort, cleanliness, protection from physical harm

Contraindications: Known allergy to the medication

Soak in a medicated solution   Immerse the arm, hand, fingers, leg, foot, or toes in a warm medicated solution for approximately 20–30 minutes three to four times a day.

Rationale: Local application of a warm medicated solution promotes comfort by relieving inflammation; it removes necrotic tissue and has cleansing or bacteriostatic-bactericidal effects.

Fulfilled Needs: Comfort, cleanliness, protection from physical harm

Contraindications: Known allergy to the medication

Appendix 1:
COMMON ETIOLOGY AND STRESSORS

The following is a list of causes or stress factors identified as applicable to the nursing diagnoses in this study. It is not a classification of etiology.

BIRTH DEFECTS

Birth defects are physical or mental abnormalities evident at birth or during early childhood.

Conditions of Birth Defects

Acrocephaly
Adrenal hyperplasia
Albinism
Anencephaly
Aortic insufficiency, congenital
Aortic stenosis
Apert's syndrome
Atopy
Atrial septal defect
Blindness
Cerebral palsy
Chylothorax
Cleft lip
Cleft palate
Clubfoot
Clubhand
Coarctation of the aorta
Congenital heart disease (cardiac anomalies)
Congenital hip dislocation
Congenital kidney disease
Congenital rubella
Craniostenosis
Cretinism
Crouzon's syndrome
Cystic fibrosis
Cystinuria
Deafness
Developmental deficit (mental retardation)
Down's syndrome
Duchenne's muscular dystrophy
Dwarfism
Dyslexia
Erythroblastosis fetalis
Esophageal atresia
Familial amyloidosis
Galactosemia
Gastrointestinal tract atresia
Giantism

Hemophilia
Hyaline membrane disease
Hydatidiform mole
Hydrocephalus
Kyphosis
Lordosis
Meningomyelocele (myelomeningocele)
Microcephaly
Microtia (ear deformity)
Omphalocele
Orbital hypertelorism
Osteogenesis imperfecta
Patent ductus arteriosus
Pectus carcinatum (pigeon chest)
Pectus excavatum (funnel chest)
Phenylketonuria
Polycystic kidney disease
Pyloric stenosis
Red-green color blindness
Schizophrenia
Sickle cell anemia
Sickle cell trait
Scoliosis
Spina bifida
Subaortic stenosis
Tay-Sachs disease
Tetralogy of Fallot
Thalassemia
Tracheoesophageal fistula
Treacher-Collins syndrome (face deformity)
Tricuspid atresia
Truncus arteriosus
Turner's syndrome
Ventricular septal defect
XYZ syndrome

Infants, Children, and Adults

Being a person with a birth defect
Birth of an imperfect child
Giving birth to an imperfect infant
Imperfect infant, child, or adult
Maternal drug addiction effects on a child
Previously having given birth to an imperfect child

BIRTH STATUS

Birth status is an infant's condition at birth.

Low-birth-weight infants
Multiple births or multiple gestation infants
Premature infant
   Potential premature infant
Sick newborn

INHERITED FACTORS

Inherited factors are not acquired but are received from one's ancestors.

Genetic Abnormalities

Known genetic or chromosomal abnormality in the person or spouse
Maternal genetic Rh-negative factor
Transmission of genetic abnormalities from self to child

Familial Tendency

Familial history of birth defects
Familial tendency for the disease
Familial tendency for the disorder
Infant of a diabetic mother

Stature

Short stature
Tall stature

Sex

Female
Male

Blood Type

Type A

Race and Ethnic Background

Black (Negro)
Oriental
Puerto Rican
Spanish
White (Caucasian)

DISEASES

A disease is a pathologic condition of the body identified by a specific group of signs and symptoms.

Diseases, Nonspecific

Any disease
Any prolonged disease
Any severe disease
Central nervous system infection or disorder
Cerebral lesions or disease

Communicable disease
Emotional disorders
Epidemic of disease
Having transmitted disease to others
Infectious disease
   Bacterial infection
   Infection of any kind
   Viral infection
Possibly transmitting disease

Diseases, Specific

Abortion, natural (miscarriage, spontaneous abortion)
Abruptio placentae
Abscess
Acidosis
   Diabetic acidosis
   Metabolic acidosis
   Renal tubular acidosis
   Respiratory acidosis
Acne vulgaris
Acoustic nerve tumor
Acquired immune deficiency syndrome (AIDS)
Acromegaly
Actinomycosis
Addison's disease (addisonian crisis)
Adenitis
Adenoiditis
Adrenal insufficiency
Adrenal tumor
Adult respiratory distress syndrome (ARDS)
Agnosia
Agraphia
Air sickness
Alcoholism
Aldosteronism
   Hyperaldosteronism
   Hypoaldosteronism
   Primary
Alkalosis
Allergic disorder
Allergic rhinitis
Alopecia
Alzheimer's dementia
Amblyopia
Amenorrhea
Amyloidosis
Amyotrophic (lateral) sclerosis
Anaphylactic shock
Anemia
   Aplastic anemia
   Hemolytic anemia
   Iron deficiency anemia
   Pernicious anemia
Aneurysm
   Abdominal aneurysm
   Aortic aneurysm
   Cerebral aneurysm, leaking or ruptured
   Dissecting aneurysm
   Thoracic aneurysm
Angina pectoris
Angioneurotic edema

Anthrax
Ankylosing spondylitis
Anxiety reaction
Aortic coarctation
Aortic insufficiency
Aortic regurgitation
Aortic stenosis
Aphasia
Appendicitis
Apraxia
Arrhythmias
Arteriosclerosis
Arteriosclerosis obliterans
Arteriosclerotic heart disease
Arteriovenous fistula
Arteritis
Arthralgia
Asbestosis
Asthma
Astigmatism
Atelectasis from airway obstruction
Atherosclerosis
Atrial fibrillation or flutter
Autism
Bacteremia
   Gram-negative bacteremia
Bacteremic shock
Bacterial endocarditis
Bartter's syndrome
Bell's palsy
Benign prostatic hypertrophy
Beriberi
Biliary cirrhosis
Bladder calculi
Bladder prolapse
Blindness
Boil
Bottle-mouth syndrome (in toddlers)
Botulism
Brain abscess
Brain tumor
Bronchiectasis
Bronchitis
Bronchopneumonia
Brucellosis
Bubonic plague
Budd-Chiari syndrome
Buerger's disease
Bulbar palsy
Bundle branch block
Bursitis
Cachexia
Car sickness
Carbuncle
Carcinoma (cancer)
  Adenocarcinoma
  Bronchogenic carcinoma
  Gastrointestinal carcinoma
  Hepatic, or liver, carcinoma
  Metastatic carcinoma
  Pancreatic carcinoma
  Prostatic carcinoma

Cardiac arrest
Cardiac insufficiency or failure
Cardiac tamponade
Cardiovalvular disease
Cardiovascular disease
Carditis
Carpal tunnel syndrome
Cataracts
Celiac disease (Sprue)
Cellulitis
Cerebral ischemia
Cerebrovascular accident
Cervicitis
Chicken pox
Chiggers
Chilblain
Cholangitis
Cholecystitis
Choledocholithiasis
Cholelithiasis
Cholera
Cholesterolesis
Chronic obstructive pulmonary disease (COPD)
Coccidioidomycosis
Colitis
  Spastic colitis
  Ulcerative colitis
Colorado tick fever
Congestive heart failure (CHF)
Conjunctivitis
Contact dermatitis
Conversion hysteria
Corneal ulcer
Coronary occlusion
Crohn's disease
Croup
Cushing's syndrome
Cyst
Cystitis
Cytomegalovirus infection
Deafness
Decalcification of bone
Decompression sickness
Degenerative disc disease
Degenerative joint disease of the spine
Dengue fever
Dental caries
Depression, major or depressive reaction
Dermatitis
Diabetes insipidus
Diabetes mellitus
Diabetic ketoacidosis
Diphtheria
Diplopia
Discoid lupus erythematosus
Diverticulitis
Diverticulosis
Drug addiction
Duodenal ulcer
Dysarthria
Dysentery
  Amebic dysentery

Bacillary dysentery
Dyshidrosis
Dysmenorrhea
Eclampsia (toxemia of pregnancy)
Ectopic pregnancy
Eczema
Elephantiasis
Emotional crisis
Emphysema
Empyema
Encephalitis
Endocarditis
Endometriosis
Endometritis
Enteritis
Epidemic louse-born typhus
Epidemic neuromyasthenia
Epididymitis
Epilepsy
Epistaxis (nosebleed)
Erythema multiforme
Esophageal abscess
   Ruptured esophageal abscess
Esophageal hernia (hiatal hernia)
Esophageal stricture
Esophageal varices
   Ruptured esophageal varices
Farsightedness
Fasciolopsiasis
Fecal impaction
Femoral hernia
Fibroid tumor
Fibromyositis
Fibrosarcoma
Filariasis
Fissure
   Anal fissure
Fistula
   Anal fistula
   Colon fistula
   Draining fistula
   Rectal fistula
   Small bowel fistula
   Vaginal fistula
Folic acid deficiency
Folliculitis
Friedreich's ataxia
Furuncle
Gallstone ileus
Ganglion
Gangrene
Gas gangrene
Gastric ulcer
Gastritis
Gastroenteritis
Giardiasis
Gingivitis
Glaucoma
   Acute or chronic closed-angle glaucoma
   Chronic open-angle glaucoma
Glomerulonephritis
Gonococcal pharyngitis

Gonorrhea
Gout
Guillain-Barré syndrome
Hand-Schüller-Christian disease
Hansen's disease
Hemangiosarcoma
Hemolytic jaundice or disease
Hemophilia
Hemorrhage
   Intracranial hemorrhage
   Subcapsular hemorrhage
Hemorrhoids
Hepatic failure or insufficiency
Hepatic granulomata
Hepatitis
Hernia
   Inguinal hernia
   Strangulated hernia
   Umbilical hernia
Herpes genitalia
Herpes simplex
Herpes zoster
Hirsutism
Histoplasmosis
Hodgkin's disease
Hookworm disease
Hordeolum
Horner's syndrome
Huntington's chorea
Hydronephrosis
Hyperadrenalism
Hyperbilirubinemia
Hypercalcemia
Hypercapnia
Hyperemesis
   Hyperemesis gravidarum
Hyperemia
Hyperglycemia
Hypernephroma
Hyperparathyroidism
Hypertension
   Essential hypertension
   Malignant hypertension
   Portal hypertension
Hypertrophic adenoids
Hyperventilation
Hypervitaminosis
Hypocalcemia
Hypochondriasis
Hypoglycemia
   Ketotic hypoglycemia (age 18 months through 5 years)
Hypogonadism
Hypoparathyroidism
Hypopituitarism
Hypotension
Hypothroidism (myxedema)
Hypovolemic shock
Ileitis
Impacted cerumen
Impetigo
Impotence

Indigestion (dyspepsia)
Infection
  Acute infection
  Chronic infection
  Fecal infection
  Puerperal infection
  Viral infection
  Wound infection
Infectious mononucleosis
Infestation, parasitic
Influenza
Intermittent claudication
Intestinal obstruction
Intussusception
Iritis
Kala-azar
Keratitis
Kernicterus
Korsakoff's syndrome
Kwashiorkor
Kyphoscoliosis
Labyrinthitis
Laennec's cirrhosis
Laryngitis
Laryngotracheitis
Laryngotracheobronchitis
Legg-Calvé-Perthes disease
Legionnaire's disease
Leukemia
Leukorrhea
Liver abscess
Lupus erythematosis
Lymphadenitis
Lymphoblastoma
Lymphosarcoma
Malabsorption syndrome (dumping syndrome)
Malaria
Malnutrition
Malocclusion
  Jaw malocclusion
  Teeth malocclusion
Mammary abscess
Manic–depressive psychosis
Mastitis
Mastoiditis
Measles
Meatal stenosis
Mediastinitis
Meniere's disease
Meningioma
Meningitis
Mental illness
Mesenteric vascular occlusion
Migraine headache
Miliaria
Milk-alkali syndrome
Milroy's disease
Mitral insufficiency
Mitral regurgitation
Mitral stenosis
Mitral valve prolapse (Barlow's disease)
Monilia infection

Moniliasis
Multiple myeloma
Multiple sclerosis
Mumps
Myasthenia gravis
Mycosis fungoides
Myocardial infarction
Myocarditis
Myopia
Myositis
Nasopharyngitis
Necrosis, tubular
Nephritis
  Interstitial nephritis
Nephroblastoma
Nephrolithiasis
Nephrosclerosis
Nephrosis
Nephrotic syndrome
Nerve root irritation or inflammation
Neuralgia
Neurasthenia
Neuritis
  Peripheral neuritis
Neurologic deficit
Neuropathy
  Peripheral neuropathy
Neurosis
Neurosyphilis
Nystagmus
Obesity
Obsessive–compulsive neurosis
Optic atrophy
Organic brain syndrome
Osteoarthritis
Osteoma
Osteomalacia
Osteomyelitis
Osteoporosis
Otitis externa
Otitis media
Otosclerosis
Ovarian cyst (cystic ovary)
Paget's disease
Pancreatitis
Paralytic ileus (ileus)
Paranoid state
Paratyphoid fever
Parkinson's disease
Parotitis
Pediculosis
Pellagra
Pemphigus
Peptic ulcer
Perforated appendix
Perforated intestines
Perforated ulcer
Pericarditis
Peridontal disease
Peripheral vascular disease
Peritonitis
Personality disorder

Pertussis
Pharyngitis
Pheochromocytoma
Phlebitis
Phlebothrombosis
Photodermatitis
Pickwickian syndrome
Pilonidal cyst
Pinworm
Pityriasis rosea
Placenta previa
Placental insufficiency
Pleural effusion
Pleurisy
Pneumoconiosis
Pneumonia
  Pneumococcal pneumonia
Pneumonitis
Pneumothorax
Poison ivy
Poison oak
Poliomyelitis
Polyarteritis nodosa
Polycythemia vera
Polymyocitis
Polyp
  Anal polyp
  Rectal polyps
Posterolateral sclerosis
Postural hypotension
Preeclampsia
Presbyopia
Proctitis
  Ulcerative proctitis
Prostatic hypertrophy
Prostatitis
Psoriasis
Psychoneurosis
Psychosexual disorder
Psychosis
Pulmonary edema
Pulmonary embolus
Pulmonary stenosis
Purpura
Pyelonephritis
Pyorrhea
Rabies
Rat-bite fever
Raynaud's disease
Rectocaval ureter
Rectocele
Renal calculi
Renal failure
Renal glucosuria
Renal insufficiency
Rendu-Osler-Weber disease
Respiratory distress syndrome
Respiratory insufficiency
Restless leg syndrome
Retinal detachment
Retinitis
Retroperitoneal fibrosis

Reye's syndrome
Rheumatic fever
Rheumatic heart disease
Rheumatoid arthritis
Rhinitis
  Allergic rhinitis (hay fever)
  Chronic rhinitis
  Vasomotor rhinitis
Rickets
Rickettsialpox
Ringworm
Rocky Mountain spotted fever
Roseola infantum
Rubella
Rubeola
Salmonella gastroenteritis
Salpingitis
Sarcoidosis
Scabies
Scarlet fever
Schizophrenia
Scleroderma
Scurvy
Seborrhea dermatitis
Senility
Septicemia
Serous otitis media
Shigellosis
Sickle cell anemia
Sickle cell trait
Simmonds' disease
Sinusitis
Spinal shock
Splenic infarction
Spondylitis
Staphylococcus infection
Sterility
Stillbirth
Stokes-Adams syndrome
Stomatitis
Strabismus
Streptococcal pharyngitis
Streptococcus infection
Stress reaction
Stricture
  Anal stricture
  Rectal stricture
  Ureter stricture
  Urethral stricture
Strongyloidiasis
Subarachnoid hemorrhage
Subdural hematoma
Sudden infant death
Sydenham's chorea
Syphilis
  Central nervous system syphilis
Tabes dorsalis
Tachycardia
  Paroxysmal atrial tachycardia (PAT)
Tapeworm
Telangiectasia, hemorrhagic
Tendinitis

Tension headache
Tentorial herniation
Tetanus
Thrombocytopenia
Thrombophlebitis
Thrush
Thyroiditis
Thyrotoxicosis (Graves' disease, hyperthyroidism, thyroid storm)
Tic doulourex
Tinea
Tonsilitis
Toxoplasmosis
Tracheitis
Tracheobronchitis
Tracheoesophageal fistula
Trench mouth
Trichinosis
Trichomoniasis
Trichuriasis
Tricuspid insufficiency
Tricuspid regurgitation
Tricuspid stenosis
Trigeminal neuritis
Tuberculosis
    Meningitis tuberculosis
    Osteotuberculosis
    Pericarditis tuberculosis
    Pulmonary tuberculosis
    Pyelonephritis tuberculosis
    Spinal tuberculosis
Tularemia
Tumor
    Abdominal tumor
    Extrapancreatic tumor
    Pancreatic tumor
    Spinal cord tumor
    Thoracic tumor
Typhoid
Typhus fever
Ulcer
    Anal ulcer
    Rectal ulcer
Undulent fever
Urethral calculi
Urethritis
Urinary tract infection
Urinary tract obstruction
Urticaria
Uterine retroversion
Uterus prolapse
Vaginitis
Varicose veins
Ventricular failure, left or right
Ventricular fibrillation
Vesicoureteral reflux
Vincent's angina
Viral pharyngitis
Vitamin A deficiency
Vitiligo
Volvulus
Von Gierke's disease

Von Willebrand's disease
Vulvitis
Wegener's granulomatosis
Weil's disease
Whipple's disease
Wilms' tumor
Wilson's disease
Winter pruritis
Yellow fever
Zollinger-Ellison syndrome

Disease Effects

Disfigurement from disease
Disfiguring disease

INJURIES

An injury consists of trauma or damage to the human body.

Injuries, Nonspecific

Any injury that has broken the skin
Any self-inflicted trauma
Any trauma inflicted on others
Any trauma occurring to others
Birth injuries
Blunt and penetrating wounds to the chest
Injuries to the central nervous system
Joint injury
Multiperson trauma
Severe trauma of any kind
Trauma of any kind
    Abdominal trauma
    Cranial trauma
    Spinal trauma
    Peripheral nerve trauma

Injuries, Specific

Abortion
    Self-induced abortion
Aorta, ruptured
Bites
    Animal bite
    Human bite
    Insect bite or sting
    Tick bite
Bruising or hematoma
Burn wound scars
Cerebral (brain) injury
    To the medulla
    To the hypothalamus
Child, parent, or spouse abuse or neglect
Concussion
    Cerebral concussion
Contusion
    Cerebral contusion
    Cerebral hematoma
    Lung contusion
    Myocardial contusion

Corneal abrasion
Crushing injury
Dislocation
Drowning (near drowning)
Electric shock
Flail chest
Foreign body
  Foreign body in the ear
  Foreign body in the eye
  Foreign body in the larynx
  Foreign body in the nose
  Foreign body in the pharynx
  Foreign body in the rectum
  Foreign body in the skin
  Foreign body in the upper airway
  Swallowed foreign body
Fracture, bone
  Basal skull fracture
  Fracture and compression of the spinal cord
  Fracture of the rib and sternum
  Fractured neck
  Nasal fracture
  Skull or cranial fracture
Fracture or tear of the liver and spleen
Frostbite
Heat exhaustion
Heat stroke
Herniated intervertebral disc
Perinatal trauma
Poisoning
  Carbon monoxide poisoning
  Drug overdose
Rape-trauma syndrome
Rupture of the tympanic membrane
Severed tendon or nerve
Snakebite
  Nonvenemous snakebite
  Venomous snakebite
Sprains
  Joint lumbosacral sprain
Starvation
Strains
  Lumbosacral strain
Subungual hemorrhage
Sunburn
Tendon or ligament damage
Traumatic amputation
Traumatic disfigurement
Vascular injury, or damage
Venomous marine-life sting
Wounds
  Abrasion wound
  Avulsion or tear wound
  Burn wound
    Chemical burn wound
    Electrical burn wound
    Thermal burn wound
  Gunshot wound
  Incision wound
  Laceration wound
  Penetrating wound
  Puncture wound
  Sucking chest wound

SIGNS AND SYMPTOMS

Signs and symptoms include objective evidence of illness and the person's perception of illness.

Signs and Symptoms, Nonspecific

The absence of signs and symptoms

Signs and Symptoms, Specific

Aching
Air swallowing
Alkaline urine (pH above 6.5)
Amnesia (fugue state)
Anesthesia sensation
Anorexia
Anosmia (lack of sense of smell)
Anoxia
Anuria
Anxiety
Ascites
Ataxia
Backache
Belching (eructation)
Bladder spasms
Bleeding
Blurred vision
Bradypnea
Breathing difficulty
Breathing, mouth
Bruising
Chest tightness
Choking
Coma
  Diabetic coma
  Eclamptic coma
  Epileptic coma
  Hepatic coma
  Open eyes when in a coma
  Uremic coma
Concentrating, difficulty
Confusion
Constipation
Convulsions
Coordination, poor
Coughing
  Forceful paroxysms of coughing
Dehydration
Delirium
Delusions
  Response to delusions
Depression
  Depressed mood
Diarrhea
Difficulty swallowing
Diplopia
Distention
  Abdominal distention
  Gastric dilatation
Dizziness
Drooling
Dysphagia
Dyspnea

Dysuria
Earache
Edema (swelling)
   Eye edema
   Joint edema
   Laryngeal edema
   Tonsillar edema
Electrolyte imbalance
Enuresis
Excess cerumen
Exophthalmia
Fatigue
Fetal movements
Fever
Flatulence
Flushing
Frequency
Fullness sensation
Gait, unsteady
Gnawing sensation
Hair loss
Hallucinations
   Responses to hallucinations
Headache
Hearing loss
Heartburn
Heat sensitivity
Hematuria
Hemiplegia
Hemoptysis
Hiccough
Hoarseness
Hot flashes
Hunger
Hyperactivity
Hyperhidrosis
Hyperkalemia
Hypernatremia
Hypokalemia
Hyponatremia
Hypothermia
Hypoventilation (hypercapnia)
Hypoxia
Immobility
   Prolonged immobility
Inappropriate affect
Incontinence
Increased intracranial pressure
Inflammation
Irritability
Ischemia
Itching sensation
Jaundice
   Obstructive jaundice
Laryngeal spasm
Lassitude
Lid lag
Limping
Lump in the throat
Malaise
Memory loss
Muscle spasm (tetany)
Myalgia

Nasal congestion
Nausea
Nervousness
Night sweats
Nightmares
Numbness
Oliguria
Orthopnea
Pain
   Chronic pain
   False labor pain
   Ovulation pain
   Phantom pain
   The threat of a hurting sensation
Palpitations
Paralysis
Paresthesia (numbness, tingling)
Photophobia
Plaque accumulation
Polyuria
Priapism
Prickling sensation
Quadriplegia
Rash
Regurgitation
Residual urine (urine retention)
Restlessness
Seizures
Semiconsciousness
Shock
Sinus congestion
Sleeplessness
Smell loss
Sneezing
Somnolence
Sore throat
Soreness
Sputum
Steatorrhea
Stiffness
Stridor
Sucking difficulty
Swallowing difficulty
Sweating (diaphoresis)
Syncope
Taste loss
Taste, unusual
Tinnitus
Tongue soreness
Toothache
Touch-sensation loss
Tremor
Tunnel vision
Unconsciousness
Uremia
Vertigo
Vision loss
Voice loss
Vomiting
Weakness
Weight, body
Weight loss or gain
Wheezing

PSYCHOSOCIAL FACTORS

Psychosocial factors are related to both the psychologic (mental and emotional) and the social (interaction of persons) elements in a person's life.

Activity

An attempt to redirect feelings into activity

Adaptive Reserves

Exhaustion of adaptive reserves

Affection (Love)

Lack of affection
The substitution of food for the absence of love

Attachment

An attempt to lessen one's attachment to another
Impending loss of a normal attachment
Loss of a normal attachment

Attention

An attempt to gain attention

Attitudes

Lack of self-reinforcement of positive self-attitudes

Autonomy

Lack of achievement of developmental autonomy (age 2–4)
Lack of autonomy or freedom in self-direction
Lack of skill in self-direction
Loss of autonomy or freedom in self-direction

Behavior

The use of passive–aggressive behavior
Unlearned alternative behavior

Behavior of a Significant Other

Changes in the behavior of a significant other

Burdens

The threat of burdens placed on one person by another

Change

An attempt to adjust to change
An attempt to change the direction of one's life
An attempt to maintain the present status, to avoid moving forward
The threat of change
The threat of forced adaptation to change from a dependent to an independent role
The threat of forced adaptation to change from being socially undesirable to desirable

Closeness

The threat of physical closeness

Communication with Others

Lack of communication with others

Conscience

An excessively rigid conscience
Failure to follow one's conscience by not doing what should be done
Lack of achievement of developmental conscience (age 4–5)
The threat of violating one's conscience by doing wrong

Control

An attempt to prove that one can regain control of one's self-destructive habits
Lack of emotional control
Lack of external limits or control
The threat of being overly controlled (restricted or dominated)

Control by Others

An attempt to resist control by others

Control of a Life Situation

An attempt to control a life situation
Lack of control of a life situation
Loss of control of a life situation
The threat of lack of control of a life situation
The threat of loss of control of a life situation

Control of Others

An attempt to control others or another
Lack of control of others
Loss of control of others
The threat of loss of control of others

Coping

Lack of competence in coping with everyday problems
Lack of competence in using effective coping mechanisms

Danger (Threat)

A possible threat of real or imagined danger
Lack of the perception of danger or threat
The threat and arousal of two or more incompatible choices requiring a decision
The threat of abandonment
The threat of danger not clearly identified or perceived
The threat of danger not clearly identified or perceived that is redirected into an object outside oneself
The threat of dependency
The threat of failure to make the right choices

The threat of real or imagined danger

The threat of a specific, clearly identified danger

Deception

The threat of deception by a significant other or health care provider

Defense Mechanisms

The use of exaggerated defense mechanisms

The use of ineffective defense mechanisms

Developmental Phase or Stage

The threat of change in a developmental phase

Disapproval

The threat of disapproval from others

Discipline (Limit Setting)

Excessive discipline

Lack of consistent discipline

The threat of discipline

Ego

The threat of the ego being overtaken by the id

Emotional Support (Positive Reinforcement)

Lack of emotional support from others

Loss of emotional support from others

Emotions

A direct or indirect expression of conflict

An attempt to control (painful) emotions

An attempt to express an emotion indirectly (anger, anxiety, guilt, dependency, fear, hate, hopelessness, rejection, ambivalence)

Lack of emotional expression

Lack of emotional stimuli from others

The indirect expression of guilt feelings

The threat of having to deal with strong emotions

The threat of powerful, opposing simultaneous emotions

Unresolved emotions (feelings) about a situation

Equilibrium

The person attempting to maintain his own equilibrium is unable to give love or to guide others

Excitement

Excessive emotional excitement

Expectations

An attempt to achieve unrealistic expectations of self (parents or a significant other)

Failure to achieve unrealistic expectations of self (parents or a significant other)

Failure of one person to meet the expectations of another

Lack of the expected, positive infant response to mothering

Loss of the expected, normal child

Experiences

An attempt to recreate a pleasurable experience

Failure to Achieve

The threat of failure to achieve

The threat of repeated failure to achieve

Goal Achievement

The threat of delayed goal achievement

The threat of frustration

The threat of frustration regardless of the course chosen

Goals

An attempt to achieve one's own goals by using others

Lack of a definite goal

Lack of achievement of unrealistic or unattainable goals

Lack of resources to achieve a goal

Harm

The threat of anticipation of harm

The threat of possibly harming another

History

A history of aggression

Hope

Lack of hope for the present or future

Hostility

The threat of hostility from another

Identity

Lack of achievement of developmental identity (age 12–18)

The threat of loss of identity

Impulses

An attempt to conceal unacceptable impulses

Lack of impulse control

Inadequacy

The threat of inadequacy

The threat of inadequacy as a mother

Independence

Lack of encouragement and motivation toward independence

Loss of independence

Loss of independence in old age

Loss of physiologic independence
The threat of being unable to manage independently

Industry

Lack of achievement of developmental industry (age 6–11)

Integrity (Completeness and Unity of the Self)

Lack of achievement of developmental integrity (old age)

Interests

Lack of mutual interests

Intimacy

An attempt to avoid intimacy
Lack of achievement of developmental intimacy (young adulthood)
Lack of intimacy
The threat of intimacy

Learning

Incorrect learning that aggression is a normal response to threat
Lack of early learning of effective coping mechanisms

Loss

Any loss

Meaning and Purpose

Lack of meaning and purpose in one's life

Motivation

Lack of motivation toward standards of high performance

Needs

Changes in one's needs
Differences between the essential needs of the persons involved
Lack of need gratification from a role
Loss of any kind that deprives one of need gratification
The threat of being unable to meet one's own needs
The threat of having needs unfulfilled through constructive behavior, which results in negative or destructive behavior
The threat of, or deprivation of, essential needs

Omnipotence

An attempt to test one's own omnipotence

Options

The threat of multiple options available

Peer Pressure

The threat of peer pressure

Personality

A highly dependent personality
Type A personality

Play

Lack of opportunity for play

Pleasure

An attempt to obtain pleasure
The pleasure of the sedative, relaxing effect, and satisfaction gained from food

Pregnancy

The threat of pregnancy

Problem Solving

The threat of ineffective problem-solving efforts
Lack of problem-solving skills

Punishment

Lack of fear of punishment
The threat of punishment

Reality

Differences between maternal prebirth fantasies and postbirth realities about the infant
Lack of a realistic perception
Lack of reinforcement of reality by the masking of facts
The threat of unpleasant reality

Reinforcement

The presence of reinforcing stimuli that maintain maladaptive behavior

Rejection

The threat of previous rejection
The threat of rejection

Relationships

Lack of an affectionate, rewarding relationship with the parent of the same sex
Lack of unity in a relationship
Loss of a relationship
The threat of a deteriorating relationship
The threat of loss of an ideal or imagined relationship
The threat of termination of a relationship by another

Responsibility

An attempt to reduce present life responsibilities and assume a less demanding personal status

Excessive responsibility
Lack of achievement of developmental power and responsibility (middle years)
Lack of responsibility
The threat of responsibility beyond or incompatible with one's developmental phase

Ridicule

The threat of ridicule

Role Behavior

Differences in expected role behavior between two or more people

Role Demands

Lack of opportunity for normal dependency
The threat of incompatible role demands

Role Expectations

Differences in personal and social or cultural role expectations
Lack of knowledge about role expectations

Role Models

Exposure to a role model who practiced poor coping skills
Exposure to a substance-abuser role model
Exposure to an abusive or violent suspicious role model.
Exposure to an impulse-directed role model.
Exposure to parental aggression
Lack of a consistent role model
Lack of a role model

Role Performance

Lack of resources for role performance
The threat of inadequacy in role performance

Roles

Change of a vital life role
Lack of enjoyment of a particular role with another person
Lack of flexibility of other family members to change roles
Lack of personality qualities suitable to the role
Lack of resources for role performance
Loss of a role
Loss of the child role in adolescence
Loss of the parent role in middle age
Role changes with a significant other

Security

The threat of loss of security

Self (Being or Existence)

The threat of not being able to preserve oneself

Self-Concept

An attempt to maintain a favorable self-concept
Failure to act in accordance with one's self-concept
The threat to the person's self-concept

Self-Confidence

Lack of confidence in the body's ability to sustain itself
Lack of self-confidence

Self-Discipline

Lack of training in self-discipline

Self-Esteem (Self-Value)

An attempt to enhance one's own self-esteem
Lack of self-esteem
Loss of self-esteem
The threat of loss of self-esteem

Sensory Deprivation

Decreased sensory input
The threat of acute sensory deprivation

Sensory Overload

The threat of sensory overload

Significant Other

An attempt by one person to reinforce the illness role of another
An attempt to punish a significant other
An attempt to test the love of a significant other
Exposure to an alcoholic, dependent significant other
Exposure to an antisocial significant other
Exposure to the negative attitudes of a significant other
Gain of a significant other
Impending loss of a significant other
Impending separation from a significant other
Lack of a care-providing significant other
Lack of affection from significant others
Lack of appreciation from a significant other
Lack of attention from a significant other
Lack of guidance from and control by a significant other (parents)
Lack of interest shown by a significant other
Lack of respect from a significant other
Lack of unity with a significant other
Loss of a significant other
Separation from a significant other
The absence of a significant other
The threat of abuse from a significant other
The threat of an unusually successful significant other (parent or sibling)
The threat of being expected to care for a significant other
The threat of chronic family discord

The threat of desertion by a significant other
The threat of social pressure from a significant other or peers
The threat of upsetting a significant other

Situation

Loss of a significant or valued situation

Social Skills

Lack of training in social skills

Socialization

Lack of early training in socialization

Stress

An attempt to relieve stress through eating
The threat of chronic stress
The threat of overwhelming stress
The threat of severe stress

Therapeutic Relationship

Lack of an adequate therapeutic relationship

Thoughts

The threat of compelling thoughts
The threat of painful, unconscious thoughts emerging into consciousness

Threat

See *Danger*

Touch

Lack of touch contact with others

Trust

Lack of achievement of developmental trust (birth to 1 year)

Valued Concept

Loss of a valued concept
Loss or gain of a valued concept of self
The valued concept of self-control

Valued or Significant Objects

Loss of a valued or significant objects
Separation from a significant or valued object

Values

Changes in cultural practices and values
Differences in parental and childrens' values
Differences in parental and community values
Differences in personal, peer, and community values
Failure to live up to one's ethical and moral values
Lack of clearly defined values

HUMAN BODY

The body is the physical aspect of a human being.

Anatomic Abnormalities

Abnormal formation of the mouth or teeth
Deformed body part
Incompetent cervix
Small pelvis

Body Adjustment

Adjustment of the infant to a sleep cycle
As the body strives toward wellness, it reaches a plateau, and from that point, progress toward greater health is very slow

Body Appearance

Appearance changes occurring during puberty
Body changes that seem different from changes in the bodies of peers
Body distortion during pregnancy
Changes in body appearance
A deformed body part
A disfigured body

Body Energy

The use of body energy for healing

Body Function

Changes in body function
Improved body function
Loss of body function
Loss of control of body function

Body Function, Natural

Birth
    The transition to extrauterine life
Breast-feeding
    Breast-feeding after childbirth
    Breast-feeding an infant
    Prolonged breast-feeding of an infant
Childbirth
    Impending childbirth
    Loss of the fetus from the maternal body at childbirth
    Maternal energy depletion after childbirth
    Membrane rupture before or during childbirth
    Natural childbirth
    The labor of childbirth
    The pain of childbirth
Conception of a child
    Attempts at conception of a child
Defecation
Growth
    Normal body growth
Sexual activity

Body Part and Body Structure

Changes in body structure
Loss of a body part

Body Size

Changes in body size during growth
Delayed body growth

Body States

Climacteric, male
  Onset of the male climacteric
Developing body
Lactation
  Excessive lactation
  Lactation after childbirth
Menopause
  The onset of menopause
Menstrual cycle
Menstruation or menses
  The onset of menstruation
Pregnancy
  Loss of the prepregnancy body
Teething

HEALTH CARE FACTORS

Health care, or iatrogenic, factors are stressors within or concerned with the health care system.

Health Care Consent Forms

Signing a health care consent form

Health Care Costs

High health care costs

Health Care Decisions for Self

Decision about the choice of (high-risk) treatment options
Decision made independently of a significant other
Decision to continue or discontinue health therapy
Decision to die naturally
Decision to donate a body organ
Decision to donate blood
Decision to donate one's body to science
Decision to seek diagnosis and treatment

Health Care Decisions for a Significant Other

Decision to donate a significant other's body organ
Decision to institutionalize a significant other
Decision to prolong life mechanically
Decision to seek diagnosis and treatment for a significant other
Decision to withdraw life-support systems

Health Care Delivery

Low-quality health care delivery

Health Care Environment

Contact with sick or very sick persons in the health care environment
Coronary care unit
  Admittance to a coronary care unit
Crisis-oriented health care environment
Crowding in the health care environment
Emergency room
Excessive stimuli in the health care environment
Exposure to intense human suffering of persons in the health care environment
Holding room for surgery
Hospital bed
Hospital or clinic gown
Insufficient stimuli in the health care environment
Intensive care unit
  Admittance to an intensive care unit
Isolation unit
Lack of food or kitchen privileges
Lack of or limited phone privileges
Lack of privacy
Locked psychiatric unit
Noise in the health care environment
Radiology unit or department
Stretcher
Surgical suite
The absence of natural light and dark in the health care environment
Uncleanliness of the health care environment
Unfamiliar health care environment
Unsuitable health care facilities

Health Care Procedures for a Significant Other

Having to perform health care procedures for a significant other
The threat of incorrectly performing a health care procedure for a significant other

Health Care Providers

Health care provider misplacing the patient's personal property
Lack of a health care provider
Lack of recognition or attention from a health care provider
Misinterpretation of a nurse's or physician's comments
Nonprivate health care discussions by a health care provider
Suggestion by a health care provider that symptoms are not real
Suggestion by a health care provider that the condition is the result of the person's inadequacy
The absence of a health care provider
The focus of the health care provider on equipment, routine, treatment, and pathology
The security of having a dependable health care provider
Unfavored by a health care provider

Health Care Surveillance

Decreased health care surveillance
Intensive health care surveillance

Health Care System

Delayed entry into the health care system
Entry into the health care system
Inefficient health care system
Rigid health care system

Health Instruction and Information

Incorrect health instruction
Lack of correct information
Lack of health instruction

Health-Skill Experience

Lack of health-skill experience

Health Therapy for Self or a Significant Other

Body exposure for therapy
Controlling but not curative effects of medical, drug, or surgical therapy
Controlling effects of medical, drug, or surgical therapy
Curative effects of medical, drug, or surgical therapy
Delayed therapy
Experimental therapy
Frequent medical, drug, or surgical therapy
Frequent, painful medical, drug, or surgical therapy
Group therapy
Impending medical, drug, or surgical therapy
Irreversible medical, drug, or surgical therapy
Lack of follow-through with prescribed therapy
Long-term therapy
Loss of body heat during therapy
Loss of on-the-job time because of therapy
Loss of physiologic independence during medical, drug, or surgical therapy
Painful medical, drug, or surgical therapy
Physical contact during therapy
Recommended medical, drug, or surgical therapy
Sleep interruption for therapy
Successful therapy
Termination of therapy
The threat of unwanted therapy
The uncertain outcome of therapy
Time-consuming therapy
Transporting a significant other to therapy
Undignified positioning for therapy
Unfamiliar therapy
Unsuccessful or ineffective medical, drug, or surgical therapy
Urgency of the therapy

Hospitalization of Self

Admittance procedure for hospitalization

Arrangements for family care during hospitalization
Prolonged hospitalization
Recommendation for hospitalization
Separation from significant other during hospitalization
The threat of hospitalization
The welfare of the family during hospitalization

Hospitalization of a Significant Other

Prolonged hospitalization of a significant other
Separation during hospitalization of a significant other

Identification Band

Delayed attachment of the identification band
Incorrectly labeled identification band

Institutional Policies

Enforced exclusion from the care of a significant other
Restrictive institutional policies

Institutional Routine

Inflexible institutional routine

Institutionalization

Institutionalization by a significant other
Institutionalization of a significant other
Institutionalization of self

Patient Overload

Patient overload limiting the health care provider's availability

Patients

Disruptive patients
Sexually familiar or provocative patients

Physicians and Physicians' Visits

Frequent physician visits
Infrequent physician visits
Multiple consultant physicians
The absence of physician contact immediately before surgery or during delivery
The absence of the physician

Visiting Hours

Limited and restrictive visiting hours

Visitors

Disturbing visitors
Restriction of visitors
The absence of visitors

Welfare and Human Resource Services

Dehumanizing welfare services
Inadequate welfare services

Well Persons
Wellness of others or significant others

History of . . .

Name specifics of the history

Diagnostic Equipment
Audiometer booth
CAT scanner
Otoscope and ophthalmoscope
Sphygmomometer
Stethoscope
Tilt table or somersault chair in x-ray
X-ray machine

Diagnostic Procedures and Studies
Any diagnostic procedure
Body exposure for a diagnostic procedure
Dyes used in diagnostic studies (radiographic contrast media)
Extensive diagnostic procedures
Frequent diagnostic procedures
Fequent, painful diagnostic procedures
High-risk diagnostic procedures
Impending diagnostic procedures
Invasive diagnostic procedures
Nasal intubation for a diagnostic procedure
Painful diagnostic procedure
Physical contact during a diagnostic procedure
Prediagnostic-study preparation
    Bowel preparation
    Skin preparation
Removal of a prosthesis for a diagnostic procedure
Specimen collection for diagnostic studies
Uncertain outcome of a diagnostic procedure
Undignified positioning for a diagnostic procedure
Unfamiliar diagnostic procedure

Diagnostic Procedures, Specific
Amniocentesis
Angiography
Anoscopy
Arterial blood gases
Barium enema
Biopsy of the kidney, liver, lung, muscle, or skin
Blood analysis sampling by venipuncture
Bone marrow
Breast examination
Bronchoscopy
Cardiac catheterization
Chest x-ray
Cholangiogram, oral
Cholangiography, transhepatic or T-tube
Cholecystography, oral or IV

Cisternal puncture
Colonoscopy
Corneal staining
Culdoscopy
Cystometry
Cystoscopy
Cystourethrography, voiding
Dilation and curettage (D and C)
Electrocardiogram
Electroencephalogram
Electromyelogram
Electronic evaluation of urinary flow rate
Gastric analysis
Gastroscopy
Gonioscopy
Hysterosalpingography
Laryngoscopy
Lumbar puncture
Lymphangiography
Mammography
Myelography
Pancreatocholangiography, endoscopic
Papanicolaou smear
Pelvic examination
Perimetry
Physical examination
Pneumoencephalogram
Proctoscopy
Proctosigmoidoscopy
Radioisotope scanning
Rectal examination
Residual capacity pulmonary function test by mask or nose clip
Retrograde pyelogram
Slit lamp examination with pupil dilatation
Tomography
Tonometry
Upper GI series
Urethrography, retrograde
Urinary catheterization
Urography, excretory (IVP)
Ventriculogram
Vital capacity pulmonary function test by mask or nose clip
X-ray
    Exposure to x-ray procedures
    X-ray during the first trimester of pregnancy
    X-ray of any kind

Medical Diagnosis for Self or a Significant Other
Differing opinions as to the medical diagnosis
Disclosure of the medical diagnosis
Impending medical diagnosis
Inconclusive medical diagnosis
Unfavorable medical diagnosis

Medical and Nursing Nonsurgical Therapy, Nonspecific
Any medical therapy

Impending therapy
Invasive medical therapy

Medical and Nursing Nonsurgical Therapy and Procedures, Specific

Acupuncture
Ambulation
  Therapeutic ambulation
Apheresis, therapeutic
Back rub
Bed bath
Bed rest
  Prolonged bed rest
  Therapeutic bed rest
Biofeedback
Breast pump therapy
Carbonic anhydrase inhibitor therapy
Cardioversion (defibrillation)
Casting or cast
  Bivalve of a cast
  Body casting
  Removal of a cast
Compressed air
  Unhumidified compressed air
Continuous or intermittent positive-pressure breathing (mechanical ventilation)
  Mask application during intermittent positive-pressure breathing
  Prolonged continuous or intermittent positive-pressure breathing
  Use of the same intermittent positive-pressure breathing machine by more than one person
Coughing and deep breathing
Delivery procedure
Diathermy
Diet
  Limitations visible when eating outside the home
  Prolonged absence of food intake
  Significant others' therapeutic diet
  Therapeutic diet
Drainage
  Chest-tube drainage
  Drainage by tube
  Gastrointestinal drainage
  Genitourinary drainage/suction
  Interrupted closed-chest drainage
  Odor from drainage
  T-tube drainage
  Urinary catheter drainage
  Wound drainage
Dressing change
  Therapeutic dressing change
Dressings
  Draining wound dressings
  Removal of dressings
  Therapeutic dressings
  Tight dressings
Douche
Elastic bandages or stockings
  Application of elastic bandage or stockings

Electroconvulsive therapy
  Recovery from electroconvulsive therapy
Enema
Exercise
  Postmastectomy exercise
  Therapeutic exercise
Feeding
  Gastrostomy feeding
  Jejunostomy feeding
  Nasogastric feeding
Fluid intake
  Limited or restricted fluid intake NPO
Gastric lavage (gavage feedings)
Heat
  Application of heat (hot packs, heating pad, etc.)
Hemodialysis
  Bovine shunt for hemodialysis
  AV cannula for hemodialysis
  Change from institutional to home hemodialysis
  Venipuncture for hemodialysis
Hygiene
  Body exposure for hygiene
Infusion
  Dextrose infusion without potassium
  Hyperalimentation infusion
  Intravenous infusion
    Intravenous infusion with large doses of bicarbonate and potassium (K)
    Intravenous infusion with large doses of potassium penicillin G
    Intravenous infusion with potassium
    Intravenous infusions containing drugs
    Lactated infusion
    Lactated Ringer's infusion
    Overload of intravenous infusion
    Prolonged normal saline or dextrose infusion
    10% dextrose infusion
    Withdrawal of the intravenous infusion needle
Inhalation
  Heated mist inhalation therapy
  Mask application during inhalation therapy
Injection
  Needle injection
  Nerve block injection
Irrigation
  Bladder irrigation
  Colonic irrigation
  Ear irrigation
  Eye irrigation
  Mouth irrigation
Isolation
  Placement in therapeutic isolation
  Preventive isolation (prevents others from getting the disease)
  Protective isolation (protects the person from getting diseases from others)
  Psychiatric isolation
Mechanical ventilation
  Hyperventilation from mechanical ventilation

Monitoring
    Frequent monitoring of vital signs
Nasal packing
Oxygen/oxygen therapy
    The administration of high concentrations of oxygen
    Unhumidified oxygen
Paracentesis
Patching the eye
Perineal care
Peritoneal dialysis
    Abdominal catheter for peritoneal dialysis
    Continuous ambulatory peritoneal dialysis
Phlebotomy
Phototherapy
Physical therapy
    Tilt table for physical therapy
Plasmaphoresis
Positioning
    Painful positioning
Psychotherapy
Radiation therapy
    Hair loss from radiation therapy
    Loss of hair growth from radiation therapy
Radioactive iodine therapy
Radioisotope therapy
Rehabilitation therapy
    Painful or long-term rehabilitation therapy
Speech therapy
Splintering
    Corrective splinting
Suction
    Airway suction
    Disrupted wound suction
    Nasogastric suction
Thoracentesis
Traction
    Disrupted spinal or cervical traction
    Disrupted traction
    Nonaligned traction
Transfusion
    Blood exchange on newborn
    Blood transfusion
    Large volume of blood
    Rapid or excessive blood transfusion
    Withdrawal of the blood transfusion needle
Tubes (intubation)
    Endotracheal intubation
    Nasogastric tube
Turning
    Therapeutic turning
Urinary catheterization
Withdrawal
    Alcohol withdrawal
    Drug withdrawal
    Narcotic withdrawal
    Tobacco withdrawal

Drug Therapy, Nonspecific

Adverse effects of drugs
Adverse interactions of drugs
Any drug therapy

Cold or headache compounds
Distasteful drugs
Drug interactions
Exposure to toxic drugs
Impending drug therapy
Incorrectly administering drugs
Infiltration of drugs into tissue
Injections in the buttocks
Intake of foods that alter the chemical components of the drug
Intake of multiple drugs
Known sensitivity to or intolerance for a drug
Large supplies of drugs available
Need to use life-maintenance drugs
Neuromuscular blocking drugs
Prescribed or over-the-counter drugs
Prolonged drug therapy
Use of life maintenance drugs
Use of pain medication

Drug Therapy, Specific

Amphetamines
Antacids
    Antacids containing magnesium
Antibiotics
Anticholinergics
Anticoagulant therapy
Anticonvulsants
Antidepressants
    Tricyclic antidepressants
Antihistamines
Antihypertensive drugs
Antineoplastics
Aspirin
    Large doses of aspirin or drugs containing aspirin
Atropinelike drugs
Barbiturates
Belladonna or atropine optic solution
Bromides
Bronchodilators
Caffeine
Calcium
Carbenicillin
Carbonic anhydrase inhibitors
Cardiac drugs
Cathartics
Chemotherapy
Chloramphenicol
Cocaine
Codeine (opium)
Contraceptive drugs
Corticosteroids
    Withdrawal of corticosteroids
Demerol
Digitalis
Diuretic(s)
    Potassium-sparing diuretics
Epinephrine
Gentamicin
Glucagon
Hallucinogenic drugs
Hormone drugs

Hydantoin therapy
  Dilantin
Hypnotics
Immunosuppressive therapy
Immunization therapy and vaccines
Immunization therapy
  Bone marrow suppressing drugs
Insulin
Iodides
Iron compounds
Ketamine (as an anesthetic)
Laxatives
L-dopa
Mephenytoin
Mithramycin
Morphine (opium)
Narcotics
Nephrotoxic drugs
Neuroleptic drugs
Phenylbutazone
Placebos, use of
Potassium chloride salt tablets
Pro-Banthine
Procainamide
Purgatives
Quinidine
Rectal instillations
Scopolamine
Sedatives
Sodium bicarbonate
Streptomycin
Sulfonamides
Suppositories
Tagamet
Testosterone
Thiouracil
Thyroid preparations
Tranquilizers
  Phenothiazine
Vaginal inserts or suppositories

Surgical Therapy

Any surgical therapy

Presurgical Prepararation

Abdominal preparation
Bowel preparation
Cranial preparation
Genitalia preparation
Ingrowing hair after presurgical preparation

Surgical Anesthesia

Daytime anesthesia followed by a wakeful night
General anesthesia
Impending anesthesia
Induction of anesthesia
Local anesthesia
Recovery from anesthesia
Spinal anesthesia
Unconsciousness from anesthesia

Surgery, Nonspecific

Abdominal surgery
Any surgery
Body exposure during surgery
Brain surgery
Emergency surgery
Lying on a hard table during surgery
Major surgery of any kind
Multiple surgeries
Positioning during surgery
Removal of prosthesis before surgery (dentures,
  breast or limb prosthesis, hearing aid, eye-
  glasses)
Surgery of any kind
Surgery requiring an incision
Unscheduled organ transplant

Surgical Procedures

Abortion, therapeutic
Adrenalectomy
Amputation
  Surgical amputation
Angioplasty
Appendectomy
Arterial bypass surgery
Arterioplasty
Arthroplast
  Hip arthroplasty
  Knee arthroplasty
Bunionectomy
Burr holes
Bursectomy
Cataract extraction
Cauterization by electrocautery
Cesarean section
Cholecystectomy
Circumcision
Colectomy
Colostomy
Cosmetic operation
Craniofacial surgery
Cranioplasty
Craniotomy
Cryosurgery
Cystectomy
Cystostomy
Debridement
Decompression of the spinal cord
Decortication
Dermoplasty
Dilation and curettage (D and C)
Diverticulectomy
Duraplasty
Embolectomy
Enucleation of the eyeball
Episiotomy
Esophagectomy
Esophagogastrectomy
Evisceration of the eyeball
Excision of lymphatics
Face lifting
Fallopian tube ligation

Fasciotomy
Fissurectomy
Fistulectomy
Fixation of bone
Forceps delivery
Fusion of bone
Fusion of joint
Ganglionectomy
Gastrectomy
Gastrostomy
Gingivectomy
Gingivoplasty
Glossectomy (tongue excision)
Graft of artery
Graft of bone
Graft of skin
Hemipelvectomy
Hemorrhoidectomy
Hernioplasty
Hysterectomy
Ileectomy
Ileocolostomy
Ileostomy
Implant of artery
Implant of breast (silicone)
Implant of cornea
Incision and drainage (I and D)
Iridectomy (cataract extraction)
Jejunostomy
Jejunotomy
Keratoplasty
Laminectomy
Laparotomy
Laryngectomy
Laryngotomy
Ligation of vein
Lobectomy of brain
Lobectomy of liver
Lobectomy of lung
Lobotomy
    Prefrontal lobotomy
Mammoplasty
Mastectomy
Mastoidectomy
Myringotomy (ear)
Nephrectomy
Nephrostomy (drainage tube)
Nephrotomy
Oophorectomy (ovaries)
Orchidectomy (testes)
Paracentesis
Parotidectomy
Pharyngotomy
Phlebotomy
Photocoagulation (for retina reattachment)
Pneumonectomy
Proctectomy
Proctotomy
Prostatectomy, suprapubic
Reconstruction procedure for cleft lips or palate
    Harelip reconstruction
    Mouth reconstruction

Reduction of dislocation
Reduction of fracture
Reimplantation of ureters
Replantation of digits
Replantation of extremity
Resection
    Neck resection
    Skin tumor resection
    Small bowel resection
Rhinoplasty
Salpingectomy
Scleral buckling
Sclerotomy
Sigmoidostomy
Splenectomy
Stabilization of joint
Surgical incision
    Painful surgical incision
    Fragile surgical incision
Sutures
    Removal of sutures
Sympathectomy, lumbar
Tamponade
Tenoplasty (hand)
Thoracentesis
Thoracotomy
Thrombectomy
Thyroidectomy
Tonsillectomy
Tooth extraction
Tracheostomy
Transplantation of bone
Transplantation of cornea
Transplantation of hair
Transplantation of heart
Transplantation of kidney
Transplantation of liver
Transplantation of muscle
Transplantation of skin
Tympanoplasty
Ureterocolostomy
Ureteroileostomy (ileal conduit)
Ureterosigmoidostomy
Ureterostomy
Ureterotomy
Valvotomy
Valvuloplasty
Vasectomy
Vocal cordectomy
Wiring of a mandible fracture

Surgical Incision

Disfiguring surgical incision
Facial surgical incision
Painful surgical incision
Visualization of the surgical incision

Surgical Postoperative Period

Postoperative inactivity
    First 24–48 hours after major surgery

Adverse Effects of Medical Therapy

Blood transfusion

Blood transfusion reaction

Use of citrated blood for transfusion that binds the calcium and reduces the blood calcium level

Cast

    Circulatory constriction from a cast

    Knee flexion after prolonged use of a cast

    Nonaligned healing of a bone when a cast is indented or incorrectly applied

Dressing

    Circulatory constriction from a dressing

Elastic bandages or stockings

    Circulatory constriction from an elastic bandage or stockings

Endotracheal intubation

    Loss of speech from endotracheal intubation

Hemodialysis

    Loss of libido (decreased sexual arousal) from hemodialysis

    Hypocalcemia due to hemodialysis

Radiation therapy

    Loss of hair from radiation therapy

Traction

    Immobility from traction

    Loss of mobility from traction

Adverse Effects of Drug Therapy

Anticholenergic drugs

    Hesitancy of urination from anticholinergic drugs

Antihypertensive drugs

    Loss of libido (decreased sexual arousal) from antihypertensive drugs

Bicarbonates

    Excessive use of bicarbonates to correct acidosis, resulting in alkalosis

Chemotherapy

    Hair loss from chemotherapy

    Immunosuppressive effects of chemotherapy

Contraceptives

    Thrombus formation from estrogen contraceptives

Corticosteroids

    Edema from corticosteroids

    Decreased sexual arousal of a significant other

Epinephrine

    Irritability from epinephrine

Hallucinogenic drugs

    Images perceived after drug ingestion

Hormones

    Moodiness and weeping from hormones

Levadopa and antipsychiatric drugs

    Jerking, involuntary movements from drugs

Persons receiving drugs such as curare, Syncurine, Pavulon,

    Anectine may have exacerbation of paralysis if certain antibiotics are given too soon, such as kanamycin, neomycin, tetracycline, lincomycin, streptomycin, colistin

Sedatives

    Total fetal central nervous system depression from maternal sedation

    Heavy drug sedation from sedatives

Tagamet

    Loss of libido from Tagamet

Thyroid preparations

    Irritability from thyroid preparations

Adverse Effects of Surgical Therapy

Abortion, therapeutic

    Loss of the fetus from therapeutic abortion

Amputation

    Hip flexion after amputation

    Loss of body part from amputation

Cholecystectomy

    Loss of body part from cholecystectomy

Colostomy

    Loss of elimination control from colostomy

    Loss of natural elimination from colostomy

Enucleation of eyeball

    Loss of vision from enucleation of eyeball

    Loss of body part from enucleation of eyeball

Esophagectomy

    Loss of normal food intake from esophagectomy

Evisceration of eyeball

    Loss of body part from evisceration of eyeball

    Loss of vision from evisceration of eyeball

Fallopian tube ligation

    Loss of reproductive ability from fallopian tube ligation

Gastrectomy

    Loss of body part from gastrectomy

Glossectomy

    Loss of speech from glossectomy

Hemipelvectomy

    Loss of body part from hemipelvectomy

Hysterectomy

    Loss of body part from hysterectomy

    Loss of reproductive ability from hysterectomy

Ilectomy

    Loss of body part from ilectomy

Ileocolostomy

    Loss of elimination control from ileocolostomy

    Loss of natural elimination from ileocolostomy

Ileostomy

    Loss of elimination control from ileostomy

    Loss of natural elimination from ileostomy

Laryngectomy

    Loss of speech from laryngectomy

Lobectomy of brain, liver, lung

    Loss of body part from lobectomy

Mastectomy

    Loss of body part from mastectomy

Nephrectomy

    Loss of body part from nephrectomy

Oophorectomy
  Loss of reproductive ability from oophorectomy
Orchidectomy
  Loss of reproductive ability from orchidectomy
Prostatectomy
  Loss of reproductive ability from prostatectomy
Salpingectomy
  Loss of reproductive ability from salpingectomy
Splenectomy
  Loss of body part from splenectomy
Thyroidectomy
  Loss of body part from thyroidectomy
Tongue excision
  Loss of body part from tongue excision
  Loss of speech from tongue excision
Tonsillectomy
  Loss of body part from tonsillectomy
Tracheostomy
  Loss of speech from tracheostomy
Ureterocolostomy
  Loss of elimination control from ureterocolostomy
  Loss of natural elimination from ureterocolostomy
Ureteroileostomy
  Loss of elimination control from ureteroileostomy
  Loss of natural elimination from ureteroileostomy
Ureterosigmoidostomy
  Loss of elimination control from ureterosigmoidostomy
  Loss of natural elimination from ureterosigmoidostomy
Ureterostomy
  Loss of elimination control from ureterostomy
  Loss of natural elimination from ureterostomy
Ureterotomy
  Loss of elimination control from ureterotomy
  Loss of natural elimination from ureterotomy
Vasectomy
  Loss of reproductive ability from vasectomy
Vocal cordectomy
  Loss of speech from vocal cordectomy

Therapeutic Equipment, Devices, and Products

Apheresis equipment
Artificial eye
Artificial limb (leg or foot or hand or arm prosthesis)
  Use of an artificial limb
Bandage (dressing)
Bedpan
Bedside commode

Bed covers
  Tight bed covers
Bypass machine
  Extracorporeal circulation by bypass machine
  Failure of the bypass machine
  Placement on a bypass machine
Brace
  Use of a brace
Breast prosthesis
Cane
  Use of a cane
Cannula for hemodialysis
  Previous or potential loss of the cannula site
  Cannula clotting
Cardiac pacemaker
  Failure of the cardiac pacemaker
  Malfunctioning cardiac pacemaker
  Use of a cardiac pacemaker
Cast
  Body cast
  Hip-spica cast
  Soiled cast
  Wet cast
Catheter
  Intravenous catheter
  Obstructed urinary catheter
  Urinary catheter
Cervical collar
CircOlectric bed
  Placement on a CircOlectric bed
  Prone positioning on a CircOlectric bed
Contact lenses
  Use of contact lenses
Crutches
  Use of crutches
Defibrillation
Defibrillator
Dental bridge
Dentures
  Plastic dentures
  Poor-fitting dentures
Electrocautery
Electroconvulsive shock equipment
Eyeglasses
  Use of eyeglasses
Hearing aid
Hemodialyzer
  Use of the hemodialyzer
  Use of the same hemodialyzer by more than one person
Hyperalimentation setup
Internal prosthesis
  Arterial prosthesis
  Hip prosthesis
  Knee prosthesis
Intermittent positive-pressure breathing machine
  Use of an intermittent positive-pressure breathing machine
Isolette
Monitor readouts
  Incorrect person or family interpretation of monitor readouts

Monitoring equipment
Nursing bottle
  Nursing bottle with a hard nipple
Oxygen
  Use of an oxygen cannula, mask, or tent
Penile prosthesis
Respirator
  Failure of the respirator
  Use of a respirator
Rotating tourniquets
Safety restraints
  Enforced confinement with safety restraints
Side rails
Stryker frame
  Placement on a Stryker frame
  Prone positioning on a Stryker frame
Suction apparatus
  Malfunctioning nasogastric suctioning
Tubes
  Laryngectomy tube
  Therapeutic tubes
  Tracheostomy tube
Tubes and drainage apparatus
  Chest tube and drainage apparatus
  Genitourinary tube drainage apparatus
  Nasogastric tube
  T-tube
Unconventional toileting receptacles
  Use of a bedpan
  Use of a bedside commode
  Use of a urinal
Unfamiliar therapeutic equipment, devices, and
  products
Urinal
Vaginal tampons
  Use of vaginal tampons
Walker
  Use of a walker
Wheelchair
  Prolonged sitting in a wheelchair
  Use of a wheelchair

Complications

Complicated pregnancy or delivery, previous or
  current
Unforseen health complications

Prognosis

Inconclusive prognosis
Unfavorable prognosis
Unknown prognosis

Hospital Leave

Trial hospital leave

Hospital or Medical Discharge

Delayed hospital discharge
Hospital discharge without the expected infant
Impending hospital discharge

Convalescence

Arrangements for family care during convales-
  cence
Reduced human contact during convalescence
Resumption of physical activity during conva-
  lescence
Slow recovery during convalescence
Unknown length of convalescence

Recovery from Illness

Delayed recovery from illness
Renewed physical activity after recovery
Renewed sexual activity after recovery

Follow-up Evaluation or Care

Delayed follow-up care
Impending follow-up care and evaluation
Infrequent follow-up care
Ongoing follow-up care and evaluation

DEVELOPMENTAL PHASES

Developmental phases are the stages of life
from conception to old age.

Developmental Phases, Nonspecific

Age
Increases with age
Nonoccurrence of or complications of develop-
  mental stages or changes
Persons being in different developmental
  phases

Developmental Phases, Sequence of

Prenatal (conception to birth)
Infancy (newborn, birth to the end of the sec-
  ond week)
Toddler or babyhood (end of the second week
  to the end of the second year)
Childhood
  Preschooler (early childhood, age 3–6)
  School age (late childhood, age 6–10)
Puberty or preadolescence (age 10 or 12–age
  13 or 14)
Adolescence (age 13 or 14–18)
Early adulthood (age 18–40)
Middle age (age 40–60)
Old age or senescence
  Early old age (age 60–70)
  Advanced old age (age 70 and above)

LIFESTYLE

Lifestyle consists of a person's habits of daily
living.

Activity Level

Decreased activity level

Involvement in too many activities above the person's comfort level

Alcohol Intake

Alcohol abuse
Alcohol dependence
High alcohol intake

Clothing

Unclean clothing
Wearing constrictive clothing

Communal Living

Participation in communal living

Culture

Cultural and family habits of overeating
Cultural changes, unacceptable
Cultural expectations, norms, and mores
Cultural inhibitors and prohibitions
Cultural superstitions
Cultural traditions
Lack of conformity to cultural mores
Varied cultural backgrounds

Diet

Fad diet and fad dieting
High caffeine intake
High calcium intake
High calorie intake and diet
High carbohydrate intake and diet
High cholesterol intake and diet
High fat intake and diet (saturated)
High gas-forming food intake
High meat intake
High milk intake
High salt or sodium intake diet
High sugar intake
High triglyceride diet
Insufficient iodine intake
Low acid/ash food intake
Low bulk/fiber intake
Low calcium intake
Low carbohydrate intake
Low protein intake
Low sodium intake
Low vitamin D intake
Prolonged bottle-feeding of an infant with homogenized milk instead of milk and food
Spicy food intake

Drug Dependence and Abuse

Drug dependence
 Amphetamines or sympathomimetics
 Barbiturates
 Cannabis (marijuana)
 Cocaine
 Opioids
 Sedatives or hypnotics
Lysergic acid diethylamide (LSD) drug abuse

Marijuana drug abuse
Phencyclidine (PCP) drug abuse
Arylcyclohexylamine drug abuse
Cocaine drug abuse
Hallucinogen drug abuse

Education

Disrupted education
Lack of education

Employment

Change of employment
Employment requiring heavy lifting
Excess time and effort at employment
Mother becomes employed

Exercise

Increased exercise
Lack of exercise
Marked decrease in exercise or activity
Overvigorous exercise
Sporadic exercise

Gambling

Excessive gambling

Hygiene

Lack of dental hygiene
Lack of hygiene

Language

Foreign language

Leisure Time

Abundance of leisure time
Misuse of leisure time
Nonallocation of leisure time

Lifestyle

Loss of preillness lifestyle
Loss of preretirement lifestyle
Loss of the quality of lifestyle

Occupation

Hazards

Peers

Peer expectations

Relaxation

Insufficient relaxation

Religious and Spiritual Beliefs

Any religious and spiritual beliefs

Rest and Sleep

Insufficient rest and sleep
Prolonged lack of sleep

Sexual Activity, Performance, and Response

Changes in sexual activity/performance or response
Normal sexual activity
Promiscuous sexual activity
Resumed sexual activity
Sexual intercourse
Variant sexual preferences

Smoking

Cigarette or tobacco smoking or chewing
High nicotine intake
Marijuana smoking
Snuff dipping

Social Status

Change of social status

Socialization

Excessive socialization
Little socialization
No socialization

Sports

Participation in contact sports

Standing or Sitting

Prolonged standing or sitting (at work, etc.)

Transportation

Lack of transportation

Work

Heavy exertion
Overwork

SITUATIONAL FACTORS

Situational factors include life events and experiences.

Abuse

Having been abused as a child
Physical abuse by a significant other

Accident

Being a survivor of an accident

Adolescent

Runaway adolescent

Adoption

Adoption of a child
Being adopted or available for adoption
Child being put up for adoption
Placing a child up for adoption
Unable to adopt a child

Arson

Loss of property by arson

Care Provider

Death of the care provider
Employment of the care provider
Hospitalization of the care provider
Old age of the care provider
Prolonged illness or injury of the care provider
Youth of the care provider

Child

Being a foster child
Being a stepchild
Child–parent difficulties
Child–peer difficulties
Giving up a foster child
Having had a previous imperfect child

Childbirth

Impending childbirth
Multiple births
Separation from a significant other during childbirth
The birth of the first child

Childlessness

The situation of being childless

Child Rearing

First experience with child rearing
The curtailment of a parent's activities and freedom during the child-rearing years

Children

Launching grown children

Confinement

Confinement in prison

Death of or Dying Significant Other

Death of a spouse
Death of one parent
Disclosure of the death of a significant other
Forced discussion of the death of a significant other
Impending death of oneself or of a significant other
Recent death of a significant other
Significant other dying alone
Unexpected death of a significant other

Death of Self, Dying Self

Impending death
Impending death of oneself
The experience of dying

Disaster

Loss of property by disaster

Natural or human-caused disaster
Surviving a disaster

Divorce

Divorce and its effect on children
Divorce from a spouse
Divorce of parents
Impending divorce

Economic Factors

Unfavorable economic factors

Employment

A new job
Financial needs requiring maternal employment
Job demotion
Job promotion
Loss of employment
The threat of loss of employment
Uncertain employment
Working night shifts

Family

Geographically distant family
Large family

Finances

Lack of finances
Lack of finances to replace material possessions

Grandparenthood

The situation of being a grandparent

Holidays

Holidays without a significant other
Pharmacy closure on holidays
The stress of holidays

Home

Establishing a home
Lack of privacy in the home
Loss of a home
Relocation of a home
Selling a home

Illness or Injury of a Significant Other

Acute illness of a significant other
Chronic illness of a significant other
Critical illness of a significant other
Disabling illness of a significant other
Maternal or newborn illness
Mental illness of a significant other
Stress of the illness of a significant other

Illness or Injury to Self

Acute illness
Chronic illness
Controlled but incurable illness
Critical illness (life-threatening illness)
Disabling illness

Disclosure of an illness
Energy depletion after illness or injury
Fantasized illness
Loss of property through illness
Mental illness
Poor personal grooming due to illness or injury
Reduced human contact during illness
Socially unacceptable illness
Terminal illness

Illness to Wellness

Change from a state of illness to wellness

Infant

A new baby
Newborn infant
Unborn infant
Unregulated sleep schedule of the infant

Insurance Coverage

Insufficient insurance coverage
Lack of insurance coverage
Restrictions and limitations on insurance coverage

Legal Restrictions

Legal termination of parental rights
Limited visiting rights of a child or parent
One-parent custody of a child

Living Alone

The situation of living alone

Marriage

Forced marriage
Impending marriage
Marriage of a significant other
Never married
Reconciliation of a marriage
Remarriage of a parent
Unmarried

Military Service

The situation of being in military service

Neglect

Child neglect
Elderly parent neglect

Outstanding Achievement

Outstanding achievement by oneself
Outstanding achievement by a significant other

Parenting (Child Rearing)

Fatherhood
Foster parenting (parenthood)
Motherhood
Single parenting
Stepparenting

Parents

Frequent change of foster parents
Frequent change of parents
Runaway parent(s)
Unwed parents

Poverty

The situation of being poor

Pregnancy, as an Event

Beyond-term pregnancy status
Multiple pregnancy of twins, triplets, etc.
Planned pregnancy
Termination of pregnancy
Unplanned pregnancy
Unwanted pregnancy

Relative

Aged relative in the home

Relocation

Being relocated in a distant city

Retirement

Impending retirement
Retirement of a family member

School

Change of school
Dropping out of school
End of school
Entry into school
Failure in school

Separation (Marital Separation)

Impending marital separation
Separation from spouse
Separation of parents

Situations

Intolerable situations
Maturational crisis or stress situations
Multiple crisis situations
Situational crisis or stress

Suicide

Attempted suicide
History of attempted suicide

Theft

Loss of property by theft

Time

Lack of time

Travel

Air travel

Extensive travel by a significant other
Foreign travel
Travel to a time-zone change

Victim

Victimized by combative assault
Victimized by previous sexual assault
Victimized by sexual assault

Violence

Use of violence
Victimized by violence
Violence on television

War

Exposure to war

Widowhood

The situation of being a widow

Wellness to Illness

Change from a state of wellness to illness

ENVIRONMENTAL FACTORS

Environmental factors include all external forces.

Altitude

Altitude changes in an aircraft
High altitude

Biologic Agents

Animals such as cats, dogs, rabbits, rats, horses, cows
  Bites of animals
  Dander from animals
  Exposure to animals
  Exposure to infected animals
Infectious agents such as viruses, bacteria, fungi, protozoa, moles, yeast, *Clostridium tetani*
  Exposure to infectious agents
Insects such as spiders, mosquitos, ants, chiggers, ticks, lice, mites
  Bites of insects
  Exposure to infected insects
  Exposure to insects
Microspores
  Grass
  Pollen
  Ragweed
  Tree
Snakes
  Bites of snakes
  Exposure to snakes
  Nonpoisonous snakes
  Poisonous snakes

Blast or Explosion
Exposure to a blast or explosion

Cataclysm
Exposure to a cataclysm such as avalanche, cyclone, dust storm, earthquake, flood, hailstorm, hurricane, tidal wave, tornado, torrential rain, or volcanic eruption

Chemical Substances
Nonspecific chemical agents
  Allergenic chemicals and substances in disposable diapers
  Corrosive acids
  Corrosive alkalis
  Disinfectants
  Drugs
  Fertilizers
  Food additives
  Harsh detergents
  Household cleaning and polishing agents
  Household gas
  Industrial chemicals and solvents
  Insulation
  Paints and varnishes
  Pesticides
  Petroleum products
  Plastic bags
  Poison
  Pollution
Specific chemical agents
  Ammonia
  Arsenic
  Asbestos
  Chromate nickel
  Mine dust
  Uranium
Miscellaneous
  Absorption of chemical substances
  Availability of chemical substances
  Contact with chemical substances
  Excessive powdering of the skin
  Exposure to toxic gases or vapors
  Exposure to urban air pollution
  Ingestion of chemical substances
  Inhalation of chemical substances
  Injection of chemical substances
  Lack of prevention against the ingestion of chemical substances
  Sensitivity to mouthwashes or toothpaste
  Splashing chemical agents
  The use of new cosmetics
  Unknown chemical agents

Color
Dull environmental color

Crushing
By building collapse
By cave-in

By a falling object
Exposure to crushing

Darkness
Exposure to darkness

Electricity
Exposure to ungrounded electrical currents

Environmental Cold
Freezing external temperature
Low external temperature
Prolonged exposure to environmental cold

Environmental Disorder
Clutter, noise, moving persons

Environmental Heat
Burning building or home
Fire and flames
High external temperature
Indoor heating
Prolonged exposure to environmental heat
Sitting in a hot bath

Environmental Percipitation
Rain
Snow

Food Substances
Adverse effect of poorly tolerated formula
Availability or abundance of food
Food contaminated by bacteria or toxic agents
Inadequate food storage or refrigeration
Insufficient amounts of food available
Plain poorly seasoned food

Foreign Bodies
Any foreign body

Drink
Food
Propelled foreign bodies

Friction or Rubbing
Exposure to friction

Geographic Location
Name specific location

Housing
Overcrowded housing
Peeling paint on housing

Humans, Persons
Bite of a human
Exposure to a sexually aroused person
Exposure to an agitated person
Exposure to an infected person

Humidity

Dry climate
High environmental humidity
Low environmental humidity
Prolonged exposure to environmental humidity

Light

Bright light
Inadequate environmental light
Prolonged exposure to light

Lightning

Exposure to lightning

Machinery or Equipment

Injury from machinery or equipment
Mechanical breakdown of machinery or equipment

Moving Vehicles

Impact and collision of moving vehicles
Involvement in a moving vehicle accident
Propulsion of the body into the air upon the collision of moving vehicles
Riding in a moving vehicle
Whiplash neck movements during the collision of moving vehicles

Noise

Loud noise
Prolonged exposure to noise
The absence of noise

Objects

Blunt objects
Extension cords
Falling objects
　Rocks
　Stones
　Timber
Heavy objects
Hot objects
　Heaters
　Hot liquids
　Steam
　Stoves
　Torches
Particles
　Dander from animals
　Dirt or dust particles
　Glass particles
　Metal particles
　Oil particles
　Wood particles
Plastic bags
Pointed objects
Ropes
Round objects
Rusty, wound-causing objects
Sharp objects
　Availability of sharp objects

Contact with sharp objects
　Exposure to sharp objects
Sheets

Odors

Obnoxious odors
The absence of a variety of odors

Plants

Adverse effect of plants
Poison ivy, poison oak, poison sumac

Pollen

Dust
Grass
Ragweed

Pressure

Air pressure
Changes in atmospheric pressure
Underwater pressure

Quiet

Excessive quiet

Sanitation

Substandard sanitation

Sights

Obnoxious sights

Stimulation

Lack of maternal stimulation
Lack of sensory stimulation

Radiation, Environmental

Exposure to radiation
Infrared rays
Microwaves, exposure to damaging
Ultraviolet light from the sun
X-rays

Soil

Contaminated soil

Television

Scary or violent movies on television

Tools

Powered and nonpowered tools

Waste Disposal

Substandard waste disposal

Water

Deprivation of water
Exposure to contaminated water
Inaccessibility of water

Prolonged exposure to water
Submersion and drowning in water

Weapons

BB guns
Clubs
Guns
Knives
Nuclear weapons

Wind

High wind
Prolonged exposure to high wind

Windows

High unscreened windows
The absence of windows

HUMAN ERROR

Human error includes mistakes made in human practices or decisions.

Air

Swallowing large amounts of air

Alcohol

Excessive alcohol intake

Batteries

Improperly maintaining pacemaker battery replacements

Beds and Cribs

Infant is placed in bed with an adult
Pillows are placed in an infant's crib

Chemicals

Person experiments with chemicals or gasoline
Takes little or no precaution when near or using acids or alkalis

Childbirth

Miscalculation of the stages of childbirth

Circulation

Prolonged impairment of venous flow by garters, girdles, elastic-topped stockings or from sitting with legs crossed or with pressure on the backs of knees or thighs

Clotheslines

Clotheslines are placed at a low level

Clothing

Overdressing an infant in excessively warm clothing

Cold

Excessive cooling of an infant by baths or from exposure
Exposure of a premature infant to the cold
Person fails to wear gloves when handling ice
Large icicles are left hanging from the roof

Contact Lens

Wearing contact lens while sleeping, during eye infections or disorders, or for prolonged periods

Cooking

Allowing frying pans to catch fire from cooking fat
Allowing grease to collect on stoves
Facing pot handles toward the front of the stove
Knives are placed uncovered in drawers
Tripping and falling while carrying hot liquids
Using thin, worn pot holders or mits
Wearing plastic aprons or long sleeves around an open flame

Dangerous Substances

Sniffing dangerous substances such as glue, benzene, or gasoline

Diet

Bottle-feeding an infant with milk before the infant's bedtime
Insisting that a child always eat everything on his plate
The introduction of protein (eggs, meat) in a baby's diet before the age of 6–8 months

Dishware

Cracked dishware or glasses are used

Doors

Catching a finger in a door or tight place

Douches

Chronic and excessive use of douches

Dressings

Airtight dressing
Infrequent dressing changes
Unclean dressings
Wet, unsterile dressing

Drugs and Medications

Accidental or intentional drug ingestion or overdose
Containers are poorly labeled
Dangerous products have been placed within the reach of children or confused persons
Drug ingestion during the first trimester in pregnancy

Duplication of drugs

Excessive intake of salicylic acid, bicarbonates, antacids, laxatives, licorice, or vitamins

Excessive insulin dosages

Improper dosage of insulin

Ingestion of duplicate drugs

Incorrect use of diuretics

Incorrect use of eye medications

Medicinal products or drugs prescribed for another person are being used for self-medication

Medicines stored in unlocked cabinets are accessible to children and confused persons

Not taking maintenance dosages of corticosteroids

Outdated drugs are used

Overdose of respiratory depressants

Products have been placed in containers that are marked and intended for other products

Self-treatment with over-the-counter drugs

Taking incorrect doses of insulin or drugs

Taking incorrect drug dosages

Using contaminated needles to inject drugs

Electricity

Allows electrical equipment to become wet or places wet objects on such equipment

Disregards warm or hot equipment switches or switch plates

Does not avoid arcing machinery on power lines

Does not use safety guards on electrical outlets to protect small children

Leaves extension cords unanchored and loose

Leaves hot, sparking, or smoking electrical equipment plugged in

Leaves unused electrical equipment plugged in

Overloads extension cords or outlets

Touches faucets or metal pipes while simultaneously touching an electrical appliance

Uses cut, frayed or exposed electrical cord or wiring

Uses electrical appliances when showering or when otherwise wet

Uses faulty plugs

Uses loose or broken wall outlets

Uses two-prong adaptors to plug in three-prong plugs

Elimination

Excessive straining at stool

Inattention to the defecation reflex

Incomplete cleansing after elimination

Enemas

Chronic use of enemas

Chronic use of tap-water enemas

Multiple tap-water enemas

Exercise

Inadequate exercise (stretching)

Increased exercise without insulin or diet adjustment (diabetics)

Eyeglasses

Nonuse of safety eyeglasses

Eyes

Engaged in prolonged, close eye work

Person does not have regular eye examinations or seek treatment for eye disorders

Falling

Accidental falling

Fireworks

Plays with fireworks or gunpowder

Floors

Polishes floors with slippery wax

Fluids

Excessive water intake

Fluid intake of less than 1,200–1,500 cc daily

Insufficient fluid intake

Prolonged, vigorous activity causing heavy perspiration without fluid or sodium replacement

Rapid ingestion of liquids

Refusal to drink fluids

Food and Feeding

Diabetic eating high-carbohydrate meals or snacks

Eating incompatible food combinations

Excess intake of vegetables containing carotene

Feeding an infant in the flat position

Laughing or talking while eating or drinking

Overeating

Overfeeding an infant

Rapid eating or drinking

Swallowing food whole

Fractures

Failure to have bone fractures treated

Fumes

Paint or lacquer are used in closed areas

Heaters

Fails to screen fireplace and heaters that can ignite clothing

Heaters have not been vented to the outside

Hygiene

Inadequate or incorrect hygiene methods of toileting

Incorrect trimming of nails

Infrequent changing of soiled diapers or sheets

Infrequent or inadequate oral hygiene

Use of bubble bath and fragrances in bath water

Withholding hygiene in order to avoid injuring the infant's fontanelle (soft spot)

Immunizations

No initial tetanus immunizations or no tetanus booster within the past 5 year

Ladders

Uses unsteady ladders

Licorice

Excessive ingestion of licorice

Lifting

Heavy lifting

Using incorrect lifting methods

Lighting

Walks into an unlighted room

Machinery

Takes little or no precaution when near rapidly moving machinery, industrial pulleys, or machine belts

Massaging

Massaging a hot, tender, reddened calf area

Matches

Holds matches near gas leaks

Plays with matches

Stores matches in paper or wood containers

Metal

Allows oneself to be splattered by hot metal being poured

Milk

High intake of milk

Moving Vehicles

Driving a car more than 8 years old

Driving a mechanically unsafe vehicle

Driving at a speed greater than 55 miles per hour

Falls or slides on concrete or other hard surfaces when riding a bicycle or motorcycle

Warms an automobile in a closed garage

Pacifier

Hangs a pacifier around an infant's neck

Plastic Bags

Placing plastic bags over the face

Small children are allowed to play with plastic bags

Play Area

Children are allowed to play in unfenced play areas

Poisons

Accidental or intentional overdose or ingestion of chemical substances

Accidental or intentional poisoning

Ingestion of acids

Ingestion of poisonous substances

Pools

Children are left unattended in pools or bathtubs

Positioning

Nonaligned positioning

Pressure

Infrequent relief of pressure on skin surfaces

Refrigerators

Children are allowed to play near discarded refrigerators or freezers

Crawling into and closing abandoned refrigerators

Rugs

Uses slippery throw rugs or tub mats

Safety Helmets

Nonuse of safety helmets or hard hats

Seatbelts

Failure to use seatbelts or child restraints

Shoes

Wearing improperly fitting shoes

Smoking

Smoking in bed or around oxygen

Solutes

Excessive ingestion of solutes such as nasogastric feedings, of milk and cream for peptic ulcers, or of a very-high-carbohydrate diet

Speech

Excessive use of the voice as in giving speeches or teaching

Prolonged shouting and cheering

Stairs

Allowing children to play at the top of the stairs without a stair gate

Allowing snow to collect on stairs and walkways

Does not clean up litter or liquid spills on floors and stairways

Does not repair nonsturdy stair rails

Sun

Looking directly at the sun or sun eclipse

Overexposes self to sun, heat or ultraviolet lamps

Suntanning

Prolonged sunbathing or suntanning

Swimming

Swimming and diving while having an ear infection

Teeth

Applies excess friction or heavy abrasives when brushing the teeth

Disregards dental prophylaxis

Toys

Children are allowed to play with sharp-edged toys

Gives children toys made from flammable materials

Ventilation

Improperly ventilating gas or wood stoves or furnaces

Uncontrolled use of gases in industry

Ventilator

Improper settings on a mechanical ventilator

Walking

Walking barefooted

Walking on a thrombosed leg

Water

Bathes in very hot water

Water Safety

Disregards water safety methods

Weapons

Guns and ammunition are within easy reach

Wound

Inadequate cleaning of a wound or skin surface

Placing tension on a wound

ETIOLOGY OF WELLNESS

Etiology of wellness includes the causes of attaining a high level of health.

Defense Mechanisms

The use of previously successful defense mechanisms

Developmental Factors

The achievement of one's developmental tasks

Health Care Factors

Correct and sufficient health information or instruction

High-quality health care delivery

Human Body

A physiologic and psychosocial state of maximum function

A state of physiologic and psychosocial homeostasis

Inherited Factors

The inheritance of normal genes and chromosomes

Lifestyle

The consistent practice of sound health principles

Psychosocial Factors

Exposure to a role model who demonstrates competence

Exposure to a role model who practices or practiced wellness behavior

Positive health attitudes

Positive self-attitudes

Situational Factors

Experience in handling the situation or problem

The presence of adequate resources for the gratification of basic physiologic and psychologic needs

The presence of adequate resources to achieve a task

Therapy

Adherence to prescribed health therapy

Appendix 2:
CODING DIAGNOSES
AND INTERVENTIONS
FOR DATA PROCESSING

The nursing diagnoses in this text have been coded for use in computerized processing systems. First, a basic code number was assigned to each nursing diagnosis pattern. All the nursing diagnoses that fell within each pattern were alphabetized and coded accordingly. Then, they were listed under the specific categories that appear in Parts Two and Three. This may give the impression that the coded numbers are not in order, but the entries are in order alphabetically. The letter *N* was placed before each code number to signify the profession of nursing. Dual diagnoses that are currently coded in the *International Classification of Diseases (ICD-9)* and the *Diagnostic and Statistical Manual of Mental Disorders*, 3rd edition, *(DSM-3)* were given the same code numbers here for the purpose of consistency. Dual diagnoses not listed in those taxonomies were assigned code numbers identified by *A* (additions). In the following lists, basic codes for the diagnosis patterns are divided into two categories: general and psychological. Codes for specific diagnoses are listed under the categories used in this text.

Categories of nursing interventions have also been coded for use in data processing systems.[73,86,313,362,451,471,486,779] The coding of categories of interventions expands the options for their use. It provides a means of specifically identifying nursing services rendered when nurses are being paid on a fee-for-service rather than salaried basis. The coding of nursing intervention categories is also applicable to the federal government cost-containment program for Diagnostic Related Groups (DRGs), in which nurses perform interventions in conjunction with medical diagnoses. The input of these nursing interventions into a computerized retrieval system will facilitate documentation of nursing care. As with the diagnoses, a code number was assigned to each category of nursing intervention. Again, the letter *N* was placed before each code number to signify the profession of nursing. Codes for specific intervention categories are listed under four main headings: "General Nursing Interventions," "Psychological Interventions," "Nursing Observation Interventions," and "Health Teaching Interventions."

GENERAL NURSING DIAGNOSIS PATTERNS

N1.000	Discomfort of . . .
N2.000	Difficulty . . .
N3.000	Inability to . . .
N4.000	Incapacity to . . .
N5.000	Partial incapacity to . . .
N6.000	Instability of . . .
N7.000	Potential for . . .
N8.000	Positive screening cues for . . .
N9.000	Spiritual awareness . . .
N10.000	Spiritual distress . . .
N11.000	Unknowledgeable about . . .
N12.000	Unskilled at . . .
N13.000	Competence in . . .
N14.000–N30.000	Reserved for additional general patterns

PSYCHOLOGICAL NURSING DIAGNOSIS PATTERNS

N31.000	Abandoned feeling . . .
N32.000	Loneliness/isolated feeling . . .
N33.000	Ambivalence . . .
N34.000	Anger . . .
N35.000	Anxiety . . .
N36.000	Conflict . . .
N37.000	Depression . . .
N38.000	Dependency feelings . . .
N39.000	Embarrassment . . .
N40.000	Fear of . . .
N41.000	Frustration . . .
N42.000	Grief reaction . . .
N43.000	Guilt . . .
N44.000	Helplessness/powerlessness . . .
N45.000	Hopelessness . . .

N46.000	Feeling rejected . . .
N47.000	Rejection of . . .
N48.000	Denial of . . .
N49.000	Regression . . .
N50.000	Withdrawal from . . .
N51.000	Bonding interruption . . .
N52.000	Disengagement/detachment . . .
N53.000	Role conflict . . .
N54.000	Role modification . . .
N55.000	Low self-esteem . . .
N56.000	Threatened body image . . .
N57.000	Body-image modification . . .
N58.000	Self-identity modification . . .
N59.000– N100.000	Reserved for additional psychological patterns

COMFORT DEFICITS

Discomforts Associated with Hearing Sensation

N1.100	Discomfort of noise

Discomforts Associated with the Olfactory Sensation

N1.010	Discomfort of body odor

Discomforts Associated with Tactile Sensation

N1.040	Discomfort of dry mouth/lips/nares
N1.050	Discomfort of dry skin
N1.130	Discomfort of thirst
N1.170	Discomfort of wetness

Discomforts Associated with Pressure Sensation

N1.060	Discomfort of intra-abdominal pressure
N1.070	Discomfort of intranasal pressure
N1.080	Discomfort of intrapulmonary pressure
N1.120	Discomfort of skin pressure

Discomforts Associated with Taste Sensation

N1.030	Discomfort of diminished taste
N1.140	Discomfort of unpleasant taste

Discomforts Associated with Thermal Sensation

N1.020	Discomfort of cold body sensation
N1.150	Discomfort of warm body sensation

Discomforts Associated with Visual Sensation

N1.090	Discomfort of light sensitivity
N1.110	Discomfort of restricted vision

Discomforts Associated with Energy Sensations

N1.160	Discomfort of weakness

Self-Care Deficit in Managing Comfort

N4.060	Incapacity to manage pain
N5.080	Partial incapacity to manage pain

COMMUNICATION DEFICITS

Self-Care Deficits in Managing Communications

N4.010	Incapacity to communicate needs
N5.030	Partial incapacity to communicate needs

HYGIENE DEFICITS

Self-Care Deficits in General Hygiene

N4.100	Incapacity to perform personal hygiene
N5.130	Partial incapacity to perform personal hygiene
N12.430	Unskilled at personal hygiene
N12.270	Unskilled at hygiene methods for a dependent person

Self-Care Deficits in Hygiene for Specific Body Parts

N4.080	Incapacity to perform hair care
N5.100	Partial incapacity to perform hair care
N12.250	Unskilled at hair care
N4.090	Incapacity to perform nail care
N5.110	Partial incapacity to perform nail care
N12.390	Unskilled at nail care
N4.100	Incapacity to perform oral hygiene
N5.120	Partial incapacity to perform oral hygiene
N12.410	Unskilled at oral hygiene
N4.120	Incapacity to perform skin care
N5.140	Partial incapacity to perform skin care
N12.510	Unskilled at skin care

N4.070	Incapacity to perform feminine hygiene
N5.090	Partial incapacity to perform feminine hygiene
N12.230	Unskilled at feminine hygiene

Self-Care Deficits in Urinary/Bowel Elimination Hygiene

| N4.130 | Incapacity to perform toileting |
| N5.150 | Partial incapacity to perform toileting |

Self-Care Deficits in Environmental Hygiene

| N12.170 | Unskilled at environmental cleanliness |

Self-Care Deficits in Clothing the Body

N4.020	Incapacity to dress self
N5.040	Partial incapacity to dress self
N12.160	Unskilled at dressing self

Self-Care Deficits in Hygiene Specific to Child Care

N12.050	Unskilled at bathing/dressing infant
N12.530	Unskilled at toilet training a child
N12.550	Unskilled at umbilical cord care

Family Self-Care Deficits in Providing Physical Care

| N3.020 | Family inability to provide physical care |
| N2.020 | Family difficulty providing physical care |

MOBILITY DEFICITS

Self-Care Deficits in Mobility

N5.010	Partial incapacity to ambulate
N4.150	Incapacity to sit up
N5.170	Partial incapacity to sit up
N5.180	Partial incapacity to stand up
N5.200	Partial incapacity to transfer body

Self-Care Deficits in Exercise

| N4.030 | Incapacity to exercise |
| N5.050 | Partial incapacity to exercise |

SELF-NUTRITION DEFICITS

Self-Care Deficits in Food/Fluid Intake

N4.040	Incapacity to feed/hydrate self
N5.060	Partial incapacity to feed/hydrate self
N12.210	Unskilled at feeding/hydrating self
N12.200	Unskilled at feeding/hydrating a dependent person
N5.020	Partial incapacity to chew/swallow food and fluids
N5.190	Partial incapacity to suck fluids

Self-Care Deficits in Nutrition Specific to Child Care

N12.060	Unskilled at bottle-feeding infant
N12.070	Unskilled at breast-feeding infant
N12.220	Unskilled at feeding infant solid food
N12.460	Unskilled at preparing infant formula

SELF-PROTECTION DEFICITS

Actual threats of Acid–Base Nonhomeostasis

| N6.010 | Instability of acid-base status (acid–base instability) |

Actual Threats of Body-Temperature Nonhomeostasis

| N6.110 | Instability of thermoregulation (thermoregulation instability) |

Actual Threats of Cardiovascular Nonhomeostasis

N6.020	Instability of arterial pressure (arterial pressure instability)
N6.030	Instability of cardiac rate/rhythm (cardiac rate/rhythm instability)
N6.120	Instability of tissue perfusion (tissue perfusion instability)

Actual Threats of Fluid and Electrolyte Nonhomeostasis

| N6.050 | Instability of fluid and electrolyte status (fluid and electrolyte instability) |

Actual Threats of Neurologic Nonhomeostasis

N6.060	Instability of intracranial pressure (intracranial pressure instability)
N6.070	Instability of neuromuscular function (neuromuscular instability)

Actual Threats of Pulmonary Nonhomeostasis

N6.080	Instability of pulmonary function (pulmonary function instability)

Actual Threats of Renal Nonhomeostasis

N6.100	Instability of renal clearance (renal clearance instability)

Actual Threats of Reproductive Nonhomeostasis

N6.040	Instability of fetus status (fetus instability)

Actual Threats of Psychosocial Behavior Nonhomeostasis

N6.090	Instability of psychosocial behavior (psychosocial instability)

Potential Threats to Acid–Base Homeostasis

N7.608	Potential for metabolic acidosis
N7.616	Potential for metabolic alkalosis
N7.752	Potential for respiratory acidosis
N7.760	Potential for respiratory alkalosis

Potential Threats to Body Temperature Homeostasis

N7.496	Potential for hypothermia (potential for subnormal temperature)
N7.336	Potential for fever (potential for pyrexia) (potential for elevated body temperature)

Potential Threats to Cardiovascular Homeostasis

N7.088	Potential for bleeding/hemorrhage
N7.096	Potential for blood transfusion reaction

N7.288	Potential for dysrhythmia
N7.312	Potential for epistaxis
N7.328	Potential for fat embolus
N7.512	Potential for impaired peripheral circulation (potential for venous stasis, potential for blood pooling)
N7.728	Potential for rectal bleeding
N7.808	Potential for shock
N7.888	Potential for thrombus displacement
N7.896	Potential for thrombus formation

Potential Threats to Cognitive Homeostasis

N7.208	Potential for confusion
N7.272	Potential for disorientation

Potential Threats to Electrolyte Homeostasis

N7.400	Potential for hypercalcemia
N7.456	Potential for hypocalcemia
N7.416	Potential for hyperkalemia
N7.472	Potential for hypokalemia
N7.424	Potential for hypermagnesemia
N7.480	Potential for hypomagnesemia
N7.432	Potential for hypernatremia
N7.488	Potential for hyponatremia

Potential Threats to Endocrine Homeostasis

N7.408	Potential for hyperglycemia
N7.464	Potential for hypoglycemia
N7.016	Potential for adrenal crisis
N7.904	Potential for thyroid crisis

Potential Threats to Fluid Homeostasis

N7.344	Potential for fluid depletion
N7.352	Potential for fluid overload
N7.584	Potential for localized edema

Potential Threats to Gastrointestinal Homeostasis

N7.008	Potential for abdominal distention
N7.216	Potential for constipation/fecal impaction
N7.264	Potential for diarrhea
N7.368	Potential for gastroenteritis
N7.832	Potential for stomatitis
N7.840	Potential for stress ulcer
N7.944	Potential for vomiting

Potential Threats to Genitourinary Homeostasis

N7.920	Potential for urinary tract infection
N7.936	Potential for voiding difficulty

Potential Threats to Hemopoietic Homeostasis

N7.824	Potential for spleen rupture

Potential Threats to Immunologic Homeostasis

N7.560	Potential for infection
N7.912	Potential for transmitting infection
N7.736	Potential for rejection of transplanted organ

Potential Threats to Integument Homeostasis

N7.232	Potential for delayed wound healing
N7.816	Potential for skin breakdown
N7.952	Potential for wound dehiscence
N7.960	Potential for wound infection

Potential Threats to Musculoskeletal Homeostasis

N7.104	Potential for bone deformity
N7.112	Potential for bone demineralization
N7.576	Potential for joint contracture
N7.632	Potential for muscle spasm
N7.640	Potential for muscle weakness

Potential Threats to Neurologic Homeostasis

N7.144	Potential for central nervous system depression
N7.384	Potential for headache
N7.536	Potential for increased intracranial pressure
N7.648	Potential for nerve injury
N7.784	Potential for seizures

Potential Threats to Reproductive Homeostasis

N7.192	Potential for complicated pregnancy
N7.184	Potential for complicated labor and delivery
N7.200	Potential for complicated puerperium

Potential Threats to Respiratory Homeostasis

N7.040	Potential for airway obstruction
N7.064	Potential for aspiration
N7.080	Potential for atelectasis
N7.440	Potential for hyperoxia
N7.504	Potential for hypoxia
N7.552	Potential for infant apnea
N7.680	Potential for pneumothorax
N7.704	Potential for pulmonary congestion
N7.712	Potential for pulmonary edema
N7.768	Potential for respiratory depression/arrest
N7.776	Potential for respiratory infection

Potential Threats to Sensory Homeostasis

N7.544	Potential for increased intraocular pressure
N7.792	Potential for sensory deprivation
N7.800	Potential for sensory overload

Potential Threats of Pain During Illness

N7.672	Potential for pain

Potential Threats to Physical Strength and Strength Restoration

N7.376	Potential for generalized weakness
N7.528	Potential for inadequate sleep/rest

Potential Threats to Communications During Illness

N7.520	Potential for impaired verbal communications

Potential Threats from Drug Therapy

N7.024	Potential for adverse response related to drug intake
N7.032	Potential for adverse response related to drug interactions

Potential Threats to Psychologic Homeostasis

N7.056	Potential for anxiety/fear
N7.072	Potential for assaultive/violent behavior
N7.280	Potential for distrust
N7.304	Potential for emotional deprivation
N7.224	Potential for delayed maternal/infant bonding
N7.696	Potential for psychologic decompensation

SELF-RESTORATIVE DEFICITS

Self-Care Deficits in Sleep/Rest

N4.140	Incapacity to promote sleep readiness

N5.160   Partial incapacity to promote sleep readiness

Self-Care Deficits in Energy Needs

N12.120   Unskilled at conserving physical energy

SELF-THERAPY DEFICITS

Self-Care Deficits in Managing/Performing Health Therapy

N4.050	Incapacity to manage health therapy
N5.070	Partial incapacity to manage health therapy
N12.010	Unskilled at amputation stump care
N12.020	Unskilled at arteriovenous shunt care
N12.040	Unskilled at bandaging
N12.080	Unskilled at burn wound care
N12.090	Unskilled at cast care
N12.100	Unskilled at circumcision care
N12.110	Unskilled at colostomy/ileostomy care
N12.130	Unskilled at continuous ambulatory peritoneal dialysis
N12.140	Unskilled at diabetic insulin therapy
N12.150	Unskilled at diabetic skin/foot/nail care
N12.190	Unskilled at esophagostomy feeding
N12.240	Unskilled at gastrostomy feeding
N12.260	Unskilled at hemodialysis
N12.280	Unskilled at hyperalimentation infusion
N12.290	Unskilled at intravenous infusion
N12.300	Unskilled at jejunostomy feeding
N12.310	Unskilled at laryngectomy care
N12.340	Unskilled at managing drugs
N12.350	Unskilled at monitoring blood pressure
N12.360	Unskilled at monitoring blood/urine glucose
N12.370	Unskilled at monitoring pulse
N12.380	Unskilled at monitoring temperature
N12.400	Unskilled at nasogastric feeding
N12.420	Unskilled at peritoneal dialysis
N12.440	Unskilled at postmastectomy care
N12.450	Unskilled at postpartum perineal care

N12.480	Unskilled at retraining in elimination control
N12.520	Unskilled at therapeutic traction
N12.540	Unskilled at tracheostomy care
N12.560	Unskilled at ureteroileostomy care
N12.570	Unskilled at ureterosigmoidostomy care
N12.580	Unskilled at ureterostomy care
N12.590	Unskilled at urinary catheter care
N12.700	Unskilled at wound care

Family Self-Care Deficits in Providing Therapeutic Care

N3.030	Family inability to provide therapeutic care
N2.030	Family difficulty providing therapeutic care

PSYCHOSOCIAL ADAPTATION

Adaptive Responses of Emotion (Affect): Aloneness

N31.010	Abandoned feeling related to absent health care provider
N31.020	Abandoned feeling related to absent significant other
N32.010	Loneliness/isolated feeling related to loss of a significant other
N32.020	Loneliness/isolated feeling related to physical loss
N32.030	Loneliness/isolated feeling related to separation from significant other

Adaptive Responses of Emotion (Affect): Ambivalence

N33.010	Ambivalence related to health care termination
N33.020	Ambivalence related to recovery from illness
N33.030	Ambivalence related to removal of life-support systems
N33.040	Ambivalence related to significant other

Adaptive Responses of Emotion (Affect): Anger

N34.010	Anger related to approaching death
N34.020	Anger related to family burdens

N34.030	Anger related to health care delivery
N34.040	Anger related to inflicted physical pain
N34.050	Anger related to loss of a significant other
N34.060	Anger related to loss of personal freedom
N34.070	Anger related to material loss
N34.080	Anger related to physical loss
N34.090	Anger related to role loss
N34.100	Anger related to separation from a significant other

Adaptive Responses of Emotion (Affect): Anxiety

N35.010	Anxiety related to undefined threat
N35.020	Anxiety related to physiologic imbalance

Adaptive Responses of Emotion (Affect): Conflict

N36.010	Conflict related to differences between significant others
N36.020	Conflict related to health decisions for a significant other
N36.030	Conflict related to health decisions for self

Adaptive Responses of Emotion (Affect): Dependency Feelings

N37.010	Dependency feelings related to life-support systems
N37.020	Dependency feelings related to natural body changes
N37.030	Dependency feelings related to physical loss

Adaptive Responses of Emotion (Affect): Depression

N38.010	Depression related to approaching death
N38.020	Depression related to loss of a significant other
N38.030	Depression related to material loss
N38.040	Depression related to physical loss
N38.050	Depression related to role loss
N38.060	Depression related to separation from a significant other
N38.070	Depression related to physiologic imbalance

Adaptive Responses of Emotion (Affect): Embarrassment

N39.010	Embarrassment related to body exposure
N39.020	Embarrassment related to health devices
N39.030	Embarrassment related to natural body function

Adaptive Responses of Emotion (Affect): Fear

N40.010	Fear of abandonment
N40.020	Fear of abnormal child development
N40.030	Fear of adverse drug effects
N40.040	Fear of aloneness/isolation
N40.050	Fear of bearing a child with a birth defect
N40.060	Fear of becoming ill
N40.070	Fear of becoming infected
N40.080	Fear of brain damage
N40.090	Fear of burdening others
N40.100	Fear of burn injury
N40.110	Fear of castration
N40.120	Fear of confinement
N40.130	Fear of confiscation of personal belongings
N40.140	Fear of death
N40.141	Fear of death of a significant other
N40.150	Fear of dependency
N40.160	Fear of disfigurement
N40.170	Fear of disruption of personal/family/life plans
N40.180	Fear of disturbing ideation
N40.190	Fear of drug dependency
N40.200	Fear of dysfunction of an internal prosthesis
N40.210	Fear of dysfunction of a life-support system
N40.220	Fear of electrocution
N40.230	Fear of emotional pain
N40.240	Fear of exsanguination
N40.250	Fear of failure
N40.260	Fear of falling
N40.270	Fear of fetal injury
N40.280	Fear of financial loss
N40.290	Fear of harming another
N40.300	Fear of hearing loss
N40.310	Fear of impotence
N40.320	Fear of incision rupture
N40.330	Fear of internal organ injury
N40.340	Fear of involuntary institutionalization
N40.350	Fear of loss of a body part
N40.360	Fear of loss of body function
N40.370	Fear of loss of consciousness
N40.380	Fear of loss of control of body function
N40.390	Fear of loss of decisional control

N40.400	Fear of loss of emotional control
N40.410	Fear of loss of employment
N40.420	Fear of loss of lifestyle
N40.430	Fear of loss of marital integrity with spouse
N40.440	Fear of loss of parental control of children
N40.450	Fear of loss of parental integrity with children
N40.460	Fear of loss of personal identity
N40.470	Fear of loss of sexuality
N40.480	Fear of loss of social integrity with friends
N40.490	Fear of loss of the ability to communicate
N40.500	Fear of mutilation
N40.510	Fear of pain
N40.520	Fear of paralysis
N40.530	Fear of physical injury
N40.540	Fear of pregnancy
N40.550	Fear of recurrence of an illness
N40.560	Fear of rejection
N40.570	Fear of retaliation
N40.580	Fear of role loss
N40.590	Fear of separation from a significant other
N40.600	Fear of sexual assault
N40.610	Fear of social stigma
N40.620	Fear of a strange environment
N40.630	Fear of strange equipment
N40.640	Fear of strangers
N40.650	Fear of suffocation
N40.660	Fear of termination of life-support systems
N40.670	Fear of the unavailability of prescribed drugs
N40.680	Fear of the uncertain diagnosis
N40.690	Fear of the uncertain outcome of a procedure/therapy
N40.700	Fear of the unknown health care routine
N40.710	Fear of the unknown health procedure/therapy
N40.720	Fear of transmitting disease by contact
N40.730	Fear of transmitting familial disease
N40.740	Fear of unfamiliar developmental changes
N40.750	Fear of unfamiliar/unexpected body sensations
N40.760	Fear of unreal images/voices
N40.770	Fear of vision loss

Adaptive Responses of Emotion (Affect): Frustration

N41.010	Frustration related to a dependent significant other
N41.020	Frustration related to physical limitations

Adaptive Responses of Emotion (Affect): Grief (Mourning)

N42.010	Grief reaction related to anticipatory loss
N42.020	Grief reaction related to approaching death
N42.030	Grief reaction related to loss of a significant other
N42.040	Grief reaction related to material loss
N42.050	Grief reaction related to physical loss
N42.060	Grief reaction related to role loss

Adaptive Responses of Emotion (Affect): Guilt

N43.010	Guilt related to being a survivor
N43.020	Guilt related to harm inflicted on self/others
N43.030	Guilt related to the birth of an imperfect child
N43.040	Guilt related to the burden placed on others
N43.050	Guilt related to unacceptable thoughts/emotions/behavior
N43.060	Guilt related to unintentional neglect of others
N43.070	Guilt related to unsanctioned health therapy

Adaptive Responses of Emotion (Affect): Helplessness

N44.010	Helplessness related to a life situation
N44.020	Helplessness related to health care/health therapy
N44.030	Helplessness related to natural body function
N44.040	Helplessness related to physical loss

Adaptive Responses of Emotion (Affect): Hopelessness

N45.010	Hopelessness related to a life situation
N45.020	Hopelessness related to approaching death
N45.030	Hopelessness related to physical loss

Adaptive Responses of Emotion (Affect): Rejection Feelings

N46.010	Feeling rejected related to a life situation

| N46.020 | Feeling rejected related to physical loss |
| N47.010 | Rejection of a significant other related to physical loss |

Adaptive Ego Defense Responses

N48.010	Denial of a life situation
N48.020	Denial of approaching death
N48.030	Denial of emotions
N48.040	Denial of habituation
N48.050	Denial of loss of a significant other
N48.060	Denial of pain
N48.070	Denial of physical loss
N48.080	Denial of role loss
N49.010	Regression related to physical loss
N50.010	Withdrawal from a life situation
N50.020	Withdrawal from a signifiant other
N50.030	Withdrawal from socialization

Adaptive Responses of Closeness in Interpersonal Interrelatedness

N51.010	Bonding interruption related to a life situation
N51.020	Bonding interruption related to health care/health therapy
N52.010	Disengagement/detachment related to approaching death
N52.020	Disengagement/detachment related to physical loss

Adaptive Responses to Role Relationships

N53.010	Role conflict related to a developmental phase
N53.020	Role conflict related to loss/gain of a significant other
N53.030	Role conflict related to physical loss/gain
N54.010	Role modification related to a developmental phase
N54.020	Role modification related to loss/gain of a significant other
N54.030	Role modification related to physical loss/gain
N54.040	Family role modification related to a disrupted lifestyle

Adaptive Responses in Self-Esteem (Self-Evaluation, Self-Ideal)

N55.010	Low self-esteem related to adaptive behavior change
N55.020	Low self-esteem related to health care/therapy/devices
N55.030	Low self-esteem related to loss of emotional control
N55.040	Low self-esteem related to natural body changes
N55.050	Low self-esteem related to physical loss
N55.060	Low self-esteem related to unattained goals

Adaptive Responses in Self-Identity (Self-Image)

N56.010	Threatened body image related to natural body changes
N56.020	Threatened body image related to physical loss
N57.010	Body-image modification related to improved health status
N57.020	Body-image modification related to natural body changes
N57.030	Body-image modification related to physical loss
N58.010	Self-identity modification related to a developmental phase
N58.020	Self-identity modification related to loss/gain of a significant other
N58.030	Self-identity modification related to physical loss

EMERGENCY CONDITIONS

Emergency Conditions of Acid-Base Balance

276.2	(ICD-9)	Metabolic acidosis
276.3	(ICD-9)	Metabolic alkalosis
276.2	(ICD-9)	Ketoacidosis
276.2	(ICD-9)	Respiratory acidosis
276.3	(ICD-9)	Respiratory alkalosis

Emergency Conditions of the Cardiovascular System

411	(ICD-9)	Acute cardiac ischemia
999.8	(ICD-9)	Blood transfusion reaction
427.5	(ICD-9)	Cardiac arrest
276.6	(ICD-9)	Circulatory overload (fluid overload)
992.5	(ICD-9)	Heat exhaustion
992.0	(ICD-9)	Heat stroke
459.0	(ICD-9)	Hemorrhage (nontraumatic)
998.1	(ICD-9)	Hemorrhage (postoperative)
904.9	(ICD-9)	Hemorrhage (injury–trauma)

995.0	(ICD-9)	Anaphylactic shock (allergic shock)
785.59	(ICD-9)	Bacteremic shock (septic shock, endotoxic shock, exotoxic shock)
785.51	(ICD-9)	Cardiogenic shock
994.8	(ICD-9)	Electrical shock
785.59	(ICD-9)	Hypovolemic shock (hemorrhagic shock, hematogenic shock, surgical shock, traumatic shock, oligemic shock)

Emergency Conditions of the Endocrine System

255.4	(ICD-9)	Adrenal shock (adrenal crisis, Addisonian crisis)
251.0	(ICD-9)	Insulin shock (hypoglycemic shock)
242.9	(ICD-9)	Thyrotoxic shock (thyrotoxic storm)

Emergency Conditions of the Gastrointestinal System

998.3	(ICD-9)	Abdominal evisceration (dehiscence)
789.0	(ICD-9)	Acute abdominal pain (acute abdomen)
536.1	(ICD-9)	Acute gastric dilatation
005.9	(ICD-9)	Food poisoning
977.9	(ICD-9)	Ingestion poisoning
868.00	(ICD-9)	Nonpenetrating abdominal injury
868.10	(ICD-9)	Penetrating abdominal injury (internal abdominal injury)

Emergency Conditions of the Integument

E906.3	(ICD-9)	Animal bite
949.0	(ICD-9)	Burn injury
991.3	(ICD-9)	Frostbite
E968.9	(ICD-9)	Human bite
879.8	(ICD-9)	Laceration
989.5	(ICD-9)	Venomous snakebite (poisonous snakebite)
989.5	(ICD-9)	Venomous spider bite (poisonous spider bite)

Emergency Conditions of the Musculoskeletal and Neurologic Systems

829.0	(ICD-9)	(Closed) Bone fracture
829.1	(ICD-9)	(Open) Bone fracture
952.00	(ICD-9)	Cervical injury (spinal cord injury)
839.8	(ICD-9)	Dislocation
854.0	(ICD-9)	Intracranial injury (brain tissue injury)
959.0	(ICD-9)	Scalp injury

Emergency Conditions of a Psychiatric Nature

309.29	(ICD-9)	Emotional crisis

Emergency Conditions of the Reproductive System

623.8	(ICD-9)	Abnormal vaginal bleeding (hemorrhage)
73.59	(ICD-9)	Emergency childbirth
959.9	(ICD-9)	Rape-trauma syndrome

Emergency Conditions of the Respiratory System

518.4	(ICD-9)	Acute pulmonary edema
519.8	(ICD-9)	Airway obstruction
807.4	(ICD-9)	Flail chest
799.0	(ICD-9)	Hypoxia (oxygen insufficiency)
987.9	(ICD-9)	Inhalation poisoning
994.1	(ICD-9)	Near drowning (drowning)
875	(ICD-9)	Open chest wound (sucking chest wound)
799.1	(ICD-9)	Respiratory arrest (failure of respiration)

Emergency Conditions of the Sensory Systems

931	(ICD-9)	Foreign body in the ear
930.9	(ICD-9)	Foreign body in the eye
932	(ICD-9)	Foreign body in the nose
940.9	(ICD-9)	Chemical eye burn
940.9	(ICD-9)	Heat eye burn

MINOR HEALTH PROBLEMS

Minor Health Problems Associated with Body Temperature Regulation

780.9	(ICD-9)	Chills
780.6	(ICD-9)	Fever (pyrexia, elevated body temperature)
991.6	(ICD-9)	Hypothermia (subnormal temperature)

Knowledge Deficits Associated with Body Temperature Regulation

N11.140	Unknowledgeable about coping with environmental cold
N11.150	Unknowledgeable about coping with environmental heat
N11.260	Unknowledgeable about fever

Minor Health Problems Associated with the Cardiovascular System

443.9	(ICD-9)	Arterial peripheral insufficiency

459.0	(ICD-9)	Bleeding
784.7	(ICD-9)	Epistaxis
523.8	(ICD-9)	Gum bleeding
924.9	(ICD-9)	Hematoma (bruising)
401.9	(ICD-9)	Hypertension (high blood pressure, not to be confused with hypertensive disease)
458.9	(ICD-9)	Hypotension (low blood pressure)
457.1	(ICD-9)	Lymphatic edema (lymphadema)
528.9	(ICD-9)	Oral mucosa bleeding (mouth bleeding)
A11.00		Pacemaker failure
458.0	(ICD-9)	Postural hypotension
569.3	(ICD-9)	Rectal bleeding
427.81	(ICD-9)	Sinus tachycardia
459.81	(ICD-9)	Venous peripheral insufficiency

Knowledge Deficits Associated with the Cardiovascular System

N11.040	Unknowledgeable about bleeding and hemorrhage
N11.230	Unknowledgeable about dysrhythmias
N11.300	Unknowledgeable about health restrictions on air travel
N11.310	Unknowledgeable about hypertension
N11.570	Unknowledgeable about sickle cell anemia
N11.700	Unknowledgeable about vein varicosities
N12.320	Unskilled at managing a pacemaker

Minor Health Problems Associated with the Ears, Nose, and Throat

380.4	(ICD-9)	Impacted cerumen
478.1	(ICD-9)	Nasal congestion
462	(ICD-9)	Pharyngitis
472.0	(ICD-9)	Rhinitis
381.4	(ICD-9)	Serous otitis (eustachian tube obstruction)
784.9	(ICD-9)	Sneezing
462	(ICD-9)	Sore throat
388.30	(ICD-9)	Tinnitus

Knowledge Deficits Associated with the Ears, Nose, and Throat

N11.440	Unknowledgeable about otitis externa

Minor Health Problems Associated with the Endocrine System

240.0	(ICD-9)	Simple goiter

Knowledge Deficits Associated with the Endocrine System

N11.190	Unknowledgeable about diabetes mellitus

Minor Health Problems Associated with Fluid Balance

276.5	(ICD-9)	Fluid volume depletion (fluid loss)
782.3	(ICD-9)	Localized edema

Knowledge Deficits Associated with Fluid and Electrolyte Balance

N11.270	Unknowledgeable about fluid balance
N11.240	Unknowledgeable about electrolyte balance

Minor Health Problems Associated with the Gastrointestinal System

783.0	(ICD-9)	Anorexia
564.0	(ICD-9)	Constipation
558.9	(ICD-9)	Diarrhea
787.3	(ICD-9)	Eructation (belching)
560.39	(ICD-9)	Fecal impaction
787.3	(ICD-9)	Flatulence
536.9	(ICD-9)	Gastrointestinal irritation
536.8	(ICD-9)	Gastrointestinal spasms
787.1	(ICD-9)	Heartburn (pyrosis)
787.9	(ICD-9)	Hemorrhoid pain
786.8	(ICD-9)	Hiccough
536.8	(ICD-9)	Indigestion (dyspepsia)
787.0	(ICD-9)	Morning sickness
787.0	(ICD-9)	Nausea
787.9	(ICD-9)	Painful defecation
527.2	(ICD-9)	Parotitis
564.2	(ICD-9)	Postmeal diarrhea (dumping syndrome)
787.0	(ICD-9)	Regurgitation, chronic
787.0	(ICD-9)	Rumination, chronic
521.8	(ICD-9)	Sensitive dentin (sensitive teeth)
535.5	(ICD-9)	Simple gastritis
520.7	(ICD-9)	Teething syndrome
112.0	(ICD-9)	Thrush
525.9	(ICD-9)	Toothache
787.0	(ICD-9)	Vomiting

Knowledge Deficits Associated with the Gastrointestinal System

N11.050	Unknowledgeable about bowel elimination

Minor Health Problems Associated with the Genitourinary System

596.8	(ICD-9)	Bladder spasms

788.1	(ICD-9)	Dysuria (painful urination)
788.2	(ICD-9)	Retention of urine

Knowledge Deficits Associated with the Genitourinary System

N11.340	Unknowledgeable about juvenile enuresis
N11.430	Unknowledgeable about organ donation
N11.090	Unknowledgeable about chronic renal disease
N11.510	Unknowledgeable about renal calculi
N11.680	Unknowledgeable about urinary tract infection

Minor Health Problems Associated with the Immunologic System

682.9	(ICD-9)	External abscess
682.9	(ICD-9)	Limited cellulitis

Knowledge Deficits Associated with the Immunologic System

N11.320	Unknowledgeable about infection prevention
N11.220	Unknowledgeable about drug allergy
N11.280	Unknowledgeable about food allergy
N11.520	Unknowledgeable about respiratory allergy
N11.580	Unknowledgeable about skin allergy
N11.560	Unknowledgeable about sexually transmitted diseases

Minor Health Problems Associated with the Integument

924.9	(ICD-9)	Contusion
707.0	(ICD-9)	Decubitus ulcer (skin breakdown, bedsore)
691.0	(ICD-9)	Diaper dermatitis
278.3	(ICD-9)	Dietary carotenemia
709.4	(ICD-9)	Foreign body in the skin
054.9	(ICD-9)	Herpes simplex
053.9	(ICD-9)	Herpes zoster (shingles)
684	(ICD-9)	Impetigo
782.9	(ICD-9)	Incisional pain
691.8	(ICD-9)	Infantile seborrhea dermatitis (cradle cap)
703.0	(ICD-9)	Ingrowing nail
919.4	(ICD-9)	Insect bite
782.4	(ICD-9)	Jaundice
705.1	(ICD-9)	Militaria (prickly heat)
E906.2	(ICD-9)	Nonvenomous snakebite
E906.2	(ICD-9)	Nonvenomous spider bite
132.9	(ICD-9)	Pediculosis

692.6	(ICD-9)	Poison ivy/poison oak dermatitis
698.9	(ICD-9)	Pruritus
133.0	(ICD-9)	Scabies
690	(ICD-9)	Seborrheic dermatitis (dandruff)
686.9	(ICD-9)	Skin sloughing
707.9	(ICD-9)	Skin ulcer
454.0	(ICD-9)	Stasis ulcer
703.8	(ICD-9)	Subungual hemorrhage
989.5	(ICD-9)	Tick bite
110.9	(ICD-9)	Tinea (ringworm)
782.9	(ICD-9)	Uremic frost
708.9	(ICD-9)	Urticaria (hives)

Knowledge Deficits Associated with the Integument

N11.590	Unknowledgeable about skin cancer
N11.600	Unknowledgeable about skin protection

Minor Health Problems Associated with the Musculoskeletal/Neurologic Systems

733.90	(ICD-9)	Bone pain
780.4	(ICD-9)	Dizziness
736.79	(ICD-9)	Footdrop
784.0	(ICD-9)	Headache
346.2	(ICD-9)	Cluster headache
784.0	(ICD-9)	Hypertensive headache
784.0	(ICD-9)	Meningeal headache
346.9	(ICD-9)	Menstrual migraine headache
346.9	(ICD-9)	Migraine headache
349.0	(ICD-9)	Postspinal headache
307.81	(ICD-9)	Tension headache
781.0	(ICD-9)	Involuntary muscle twitching
799.2	(ICD-9)	Irritability
718.40	(ICD-9)	Joint contracture
719.40	(ICD-9)	Joint pain (arthralgia)
846.0	(ICD-9)	Lumbosacral strain
994.6	(ICD-9)	Motion sickness
728.85	(ICD-9)	Muscle spasm
848.9	(ICD-9)	Muscle strain
729.2	(ICD-9)	Neuralgia
353.6	(ICD-9)	Phantom limb
353.8	(ICD-9)	Phantom pain
333.99	(ICD-9)	Restless leg syndrome
848.9	(ICD-9)	Sprain
780.2	(ICD-9)	Syncope
780.4	(ICD-9)	Vertigo
736.05	(ICD-9)	Wristdrop

Knowledge Deficits Associated with the Musculoskeletal/Neurologic Systems

N11.460	Unknowledgeable about physical growth and development

N11.540		Unknowledgeable about seizures

Minor Health Problems Associated with the Reproductive System and Reproduction

625.8	(ICD-9)	Afterbirth pain
676.2	(ICD-9)	Breast engorgement
611.71	(ICD-9)	Breast tenderness (breast pain)
676.1	(ICD-9)	Cracked nipple
625.3	(ICD-9)	Dysmenorrhea
676.4	(ICD-9)	Failure of lactation (agalactia)
644	(ICD-9)	False labor
644.1	(ICD-9)	Labor pain
625.2	(ICD-9)	Ovulation pain (mittelschmerz)
625.5	(ICD-9)	Pelvic congestion
625.9	(ICD-9)	Postpartal perineum pain

Knowledge Deficits Associated with the Reproductive System and Reproduction

N11.010	Unknowledgeable about abnormal vaginal bleeding
N11.470	Unknowledgeable about postsurgical vaginal bleeding
N11.070	Unknowledgeable about childbirth
N11.350	Unknowledgeable about lactation suppression
N11.360	Unknowledgeable about male climacteric
N11.370	Unknowledgeable about male puberty
N11.380	Unknowledgeable about managing a normal pregnancy
N11.390	Unknowledgeable about managing a normal puerperium
N11.400	Unknowledgeable about menopause
N11.410	Unknowledgeable about menstruation
N11.480	Unknowledgeable about premenopause
N11.250	Unknowledgeable about family planning
N11.670	Unknowledgeable about the reproductive process
N11.060	Unknowledgeable about breast cancer
N11.490	Unknowledgeable about prostate cancer
N11.690	Unknowledgeable about uterine cancer
N11.730	Unknowledgeable about yeast infections

N11.500		Unskilled at self-breast examination

Minor Health Problems Associated with the Respiratory System

987.8	(ICD-9)	Carbon dioxide retention
786.2	(ICD-9)	Cough
784.49	(ICD-9)	Hoarseness
786.09	(ICD-9)	Hypoventilation
464.0	(ICD-9)	Laryngitis
786.52	(ICD-9)	Painful respiration (ponopnea)
786.09	(ICD-9)	Respiratory distress
514	(ICD-9)	Pulmonary congestion
A13.00		Sinus congestion

Knowledge Deficits Associated with the Respiratory System

N11.500	Unknowledgeable about pulmonary disease
N12.640	Unskilled at using a respiratory device

Minor Health Problems Associated with the Sensory System

368.13	(ICD-9)	Eyestrain
782.0	(ICD-9)	Sensory deprivation
782.0	(ICD-9)	Sensory overload

Knowledge Deficits Associated with Sensory Responses

N12.030	Unskilled at artificial eye care
N12.670	Unskilled at using contact lenses
N12.690	Unskilled at using eyeglasses
N12.620	Unskilled at using a hearing aid

Minor Health Problems Associated with Sleep

780.52	(ICD-9)	Insomnia
307.47	(ICD-9)	Nightmares
780.55	(ICD-9)	Sleep rhythm inversion
307.46	(ICD-9)	Sleep terror disorder (night terrors)
307.46	(ICD-9)	Sleepwalking

Knowledge Deficits Associated with Sleep

N11.330	Unknowledgeable about jet lag
N11.610	Unknowledgeable about sleep/rest
N12.470	Unskilled at relaxation methods

Knowledge Deficits Associated with Procedures for Diagnosing and Treating Health Problems

N11.630	Unknowledgeable about the diagnostic study
N11.650	Unknowledgeable about the medical/surgical procedure
N11.660	Unknowledgeable about the physical examination

Knowledge Deficits Associated with Diseases or Conditions

N11.640	Unknowledgeable about the disease/condition

PAIN PROBLEMS

Types of Pain

A12.01		Aching pain
782.0	(ICD-9)	Burning pain
A12.02		Constrictive pain
729.82	(ICD-9)	Cramping pain
A12.03		Gnawing pain
A12.04		Stabbing pain
A12.05		Throbbing pain

Knowledge Deficits Associated with Pain

N11.450	Unknowledgeable about pain relief methods

HEALTH MAINTENANCE AND PREVENTIVE HEALTH PROBLEMS

At-Risk Factors for Accidental Injury

N7.128	Potential for burn injury
N7.296	Potential for electrical injury
N7.320	Potential for fall injury
N7.624	Potential for motor vehicle injury
N7.688	Potential for poisoning
N7.720	Potential for radiation injury
N7.864	Potential for suffocation
N7.960	Potential for wound injury
N11.710	Unknowledgeable about waste sanitation
N11.720	Unknowledgeable about water sanitation

At-Risk Factors for Cardiovascular Disease

N7.136	Potential for cardiovascular disease
N7.152	Potential for cerebrovascular disease
N7.448	Potential for hypertensive disease

At-Risk Factors for Dental Disease

N7.240	Potential for dental disease

At-Risk Factors for Endocrine Disease

N7.256	Potential for diabetes mellitus
N7.656	Potential for nontoxic goiter (potential for simple goiter)

At-Risk Factors for Gastrointestinal Disease

N7.176	Potential for colorectal cancer
N7.360	Potential for gastric or duodenal ulcer

At-Risk Factors for Genitourinary Disease

N7.744	Potential for renal calculi

At-Risk Factors for Hematologic Disease

N7.568	Potential for iron deficiency anemia

At-Risk Factors for Immunologic Disease

N7.048	Potential for allergic reaction

At-Risk Factors for Neurologic Disease

N7.880	Potential for tetanus

At-Risk Factors for Nutritional Disease

N7.600	Potential for malnutrition
N7.664	Potential for obesity

At-Risk Factors for Psychosocial Disorders

N7.168	Potential for child abuse
N7.248	Potential for depression
N7.848	Potential for substance (alcohol or drug) abuse
N7.856	Potential for substance (alcohol or drug) dependence
N7.876	Potential for suicide

At-Risk Factors for Reproductive Disease

N7.120	Potential for breast cancer
N7.160	Potential for cervical cancer

At-Risk Factors for Respiratory Disease

N7.592	Potential for lung cancer

At-Risk Factors for Sensory Disorders

N7.392	Potential for hearing loss
N7.928	Potential for vision loss

SUSPECTED DISEASE PROBLEMS

Screening for Cardiovascular Disorders

N8.060   Positive screening cues for abnormal newborn apgar

N8.090   Positive screening cues for cardiovascular disease

N8.140   Positive screening cues for congenital heart disease

N8.280   Positive screening cues for hypertensive disease

N8.380   Positive screening cues for peripheral vascular disease

Screening for Dental Disorders

N8.160   Positive screening cues for dental disease

Screening for Gallbladder or Hepatic Disorders

N8.190   Positive screening cues for gallbladder disease

N8.250   Positive screening cues for hepatic disease

N8.270   Positive screening cues for hyperbilirubinemia

Screening for Gastrointestinal Disorders

N8.200   Positive screening cues for gastrointestinal disease

N8.360   Positive screening cues for oral cancer

N8.400   Positive screening cues for pinworm disease

Screening for Genitourinary Disorders

N8.420   Positive screening cues for renal disease

N8.530   Positive screening cues for urinary tract infection

Screening for Hematologic Disorders

N8.070   Positive screening cues for anemia

N8.460   Positive screening cues for sickle cell disease

Screening for Infectious Disorders

N8.220   Positive screening cues for gonorrhea

N8.260   Positive screening cues for herpes genitalia

N8.290   Positive screening cues for infectious mononucleosis

N8.370   Positive screening cues for otitis media

N8.470   Positive screening cues for streptococcal infection

N8.500   Positive screening cues for syphilis

N8.520   Positive screening cues for tuberculosis

Screening for Integument Disorders

N8.460   Positive screening cues for skin cancer

Screening for Metabolic Disease

N8.150   Positive screening cues for cystic fibrosis

N8.180   Positive screening cues for diabetes mellitus

N8.510   Positive screening cues for thyroid disease

Screening for Musculoskeletal Disorders for Thyroid Disease

N8.080   Positive screening cues for arthritic disease

N8.230   Positive screening cues for growth disturbance

N8.300   Positive screening cues for lumbar disc disorder

N8.320   Positive screening cues for musculoskeletal disorder

N8.440   Positive screening cues for scoliosis

Screening for Neurologic Disorders

N8.170   Positive screening cues for developmental delay

N8.330   Positive screening cues for neurologic disorder

N8.340   Positive screening cues for newborn neuromuscular deficit

N8.350   Positive screening cues for newborn neuromuscular overstimulation

N8.390   Positive screening cues for phenylketonuria

Screening for Pregnancy and Pregnancy Disorders

N8.410   Positive screening cues for pregnancy

N8.030   Positive screening cues for a complicated pregnancy

N8.020   Positive screening cues for a complicated labor and delivery

N8.040   Positive screening cues for a complicated puerperium

Screening for Psychosocial Disorders

N8.120   Positive screening cues for child abuse

N8.130   Positive screening cues for child abuser

N8.310   Positive screening cues for maladaptive behavior

N8.480   Positive screening cues for substance (alcohol or drug) abuse

N8.490   Positive screening cues for substance (alcohol or drug) dependence

Screening for Reproductive System Disorders

N8.010   Positive screening cues for a breast mass

N8.110   Positive screening cues for cervical cancer

N8.050   Positive screening cues for a vaginal infection

Screening for Respiratory Disorders

N8.430   Positive screening cues for respiratory disorder

Screening for Sensory Disorders

N8.100   Positive screening cues for cataracts

N8.210   Positive screening cues for glaucoma

N8.240   Positive screening cues for hearing loss

N8.540   Positive screening cues for vision loss

DRUG PROBLEMS

Untoward Reactions to Drugs

995.2   (ICD-9)   Adverse drug effect

Knowledge Deficits About Drugs

N11.020   Unknowledgeable about alcohol abuse

N11.160   Unknowledgeable about coping with the alcohol abuser

N11.210   Unknowledgeable about drug abuse

N11.170   Unknowledgeable about coping with the drug abuser

NUTRITION AND FOOD PROBLEMS

Nutrition-Related Disorders/Problems

269.9   (ICD-9)   Malnutrition (deficient nutrition)

278.0   (ICD-9)   Obesity

Knowledge Deficits About Nutrition

N11.030   Unknowledgeable about balanced nutrition

N11.200   Unknowledgeable about dieting

N12.330   Unskilled at managing a prescribed diet

Knowledge Deficits About Food

N12.490   Unskilled at safe food handling

N11.290   Unknowledgeable about foreign food hazards

PSYCHOSOCIAL NONADAPTATION

Nonadaptive Responses of Emotion (Affect): Anger

312.0   (ICD-9)   Acting-out behavior

312.23   (ICD-9)   Aggressive behavior
       (DSM-3)   (aggressive disorder)

312.34   (DSM-3)   Explosive behavior (explosive disorder)

301.84   (ICD-9)   Passive–aggressive behavior
       (DSM-3)   (passive–aggressive disorder)

Nonadaptive Responses of Emotion (Affect): Anxiety

301.40   (ICD-9)   Compulsive behavior
       (DSM-3)   (compulsive disorder)

306.90   (ICD-9)   Obsessive thoughts
       (DSM-3)   (obsessive disorder, rumination)

300.30   (ICD-9)   Obsessive–compulsive
       (DSM-3)   behavior (obsessive-compulsive disorder)

313.00   (ICD-9)   Overanxious behavior
       (DSM-3)   (overanxious disorder)

300.01   (ICD-9)   Panic disorder (anxiety
       (DSM-3)   attack)

309.21   (ICD-9)   Separation anxiety
       (DSM-3)

Nonadaptive Responses of Emotion (Affect): Attachment

A8.00   Maternal–child nonbonding

A8.01   Significant-other nonbonding

Nonadaptive Responses of Emotion (Affect): Depression

309.0	(ICD-9)	Depression reaction (acute, situational)
309.1	(DSM-3)	Depressive reaction (prolonged)

Nonadaptive Responses of Emotion (Affect): Fear

300.29	(ICD-9) (DSM-3)	Simple phobia

Nonadaptive Responses of Emotion (Affect): Grief

A1.00		Delayed grief reaction
309.1	(ICD-9) (DSM-3)	Prolonged grief reaction

Nonadaptive Responses of Emotion (Affect): Guilt

A10.00		Nonadaptive guilt

Nonadaptive Responses of Emotional (Affect): Fluctuation

312.30	(ICD-9) (DSM-3)	Impulse-control disorder
301.59	(ICD-9) (DSM-3)	Labile affect (labile personality)
296.0	(DSM-3)	Manic behavior (manic reaction)

Nonadaptive Responses Associated with Self-Esteem/Self-Evaluation

300.9	(ICD-9)	Self-destructive behavior
300.9	(ICD-9)	Suicidal threats
300.9	(ICD-9)	Suicidal attempt/gesture

Nonadaptive Responses Associated with Self-Identity

A3.00		Disturbed body image
302.60	(ICD-9)	Gender identity disorder
313.82	(ICD-9) (DSM-3)	Identity disorder

Nonadaptive Responses of Psychosexual Function

302.76	(ICD-9) (DSM-3)	Functional Dyspareunia
306.51	(DSM-3)	Functional vaginismus
302.71	(ICD-9) (DSM-3)	Inhibited sexual desire
302.72	(ICD-9) (DSM-3)	Inhibited sexual excitement (frigidity, impotence)

312.0	(ICD-9)	Sexual acting out (excessive libido)

Nonadaptive Responses Associated with Stress

309	(ICD-9)	Adjustment reaction

Knowledge Deficits Associated with Psychosocial Problems

N11.180	Unknowledgeable about coping with the mentally ill
N11.080	Unknowledgeable about child socialization/discipline
N11.420	Unknowledgeable about mental health principles
N11.550	Unknowledgeable about sexuality
N11.620	Unknowledgeable about stress management

Nonadaptive Ego Defense Responses

301.60	(ICD-9) (DSM-3)	Dependency reaction (dependent personality disorder)
300.7	(ICD-9) (DSM-3)	Hypochondriasis
300.10	(ICD-9) (DSM-3)	Hysteria (conversion disorder)
A7.00		Manipulative behavior (manipulation)
A9.00		Nonadaptive denial
297.1	(ICD-9) (DSM-3)	Paranoia (paranoid (disorder)
307.80	(ICD-9) (DSM-3)	Psychogenic pain disorder
306.9	(ICD-9)	Somatic reaction (somatization reaction, psychosomatic pain)
A14.00		Suspiciousness

Nonadaptive Responses of Families

A4.00	Faltering family
A4.01	Troubled, dominated family
A4.02	Troubled, conflicted family
A4.03	Troubled, chaotic family

Altered Responses in Thought Process

314.00	(ICD-9) (DSM-3)	Attention deficit disorder
298.9	(ICD-9)	Confusion
A2.00		Disorientation
A5.00		Illogical thought process
312.9	(ICD-9)	Impulsiveness

Altered Responses in Thought Content

297.9	(ICD-9)	Delusional thinking (delusions)
780.9	(ICD-9)	Memory loss

Altered Responses in Perception

780.1	(ICD-9)	Hallucinations
A6.00		Illusional thinking

Knowledge Deficits Associated with Cognitive Functioning

N11.481	Unknowledgeable about problem-solving methods

PHYSICAL AND SPEECH REHABILITATION

Knowledge Deficits Associated with Physical Rehabilitation

N11.130	Unknowledgeable about coping with architectural barriers
N12.600	Unskilled at using a brace
N12.610	Unskilled at using a cane
N12.680	Unskilled at using crutches
N12.630	Unskilled at using a limb prosthesis
N12.650	Unskilled at using a walker
N12.660	Unskilled at using a wheelchair
N12.191	Unskilled at exercise methods

Knowledge Deficits Associated with Speech Impairment

N12.180	Unskilled at esophageal speech
N11.110	Unknowledgeable about coping with a speech-impaired person

SPIRITUAL CARE

Spiritual Problems Associated with Illness and Suffering

N9.010	Spiritual awareness related to a life situation
N10.010	Spiritual distress related to disrupted spiritual practices
N10.020	Spiritual distress related to a life situation

WELLNESS

Wellness Responses of Children

A15.01	Well baby/infant

A15.02	Well toddler
A15.03	Well preschool child
A15.04	Well school-age child
A15.05	Well adolescent

Wellness Responses of Young Adults

A15.06	High-level well, young adult
A15.07	Moderate-level well, young adult
A15.08	Low-level well, young adult

Wellness Responses of Middle-Aged Adults

A15.09	High-level well, middle-aged adult
A15.10	Moderate-level well, middle-aged adult
A15.11	Low-level well, middle-aged adult

Wellness Responses of Aged Adults

A15.12	High-level well, aged adult
A15.13	Moderate-level well, aged adult
A15.14	Low-level well, aged adult

Wellness Responses of Women in Pregnancy

650	(ICD-9)	Normal pregnancy
V22	(ICD-9)	Normal labor and delivery
A15.15		Normal puerperium

Wellness Responses of the Family

A15.16	Well family

Wellness Responses of Competencies

N13.010	Competence in health knowledge/skills
N13.020	Competence in managing health therapy
N13.030	Competence in managing psychologic adaptation
N13.040	Competence in parenting
N13.050	Competence in self-care
N13.060	Competence in utilizing community resources

Knowledge Deficits Associated with Well Persons

N11.120	Unknowledgeable about coping with aged persons

HEALTH RESOURCE PROBLEMS

Deficits in Utilizing Health Care Resources

N2.010	Difficulty utilizing community resources

N3.010   Inability to utilize community resources

Knowledge Deficits in Utilizing Health Care Resources

N11.100   Unknowledgeable about community resources

GENERAL NURSING INTERVENTIONS

N120.000   Admission of patient
N130.000   Airway patency maintenance
 N130.005   Esophageal
 N130.010   Nasal
 N130.015   Nasopharyngeal
 N130.020   Oral
 N130.025   Tracheostomy
N140.000   Alignment, body
N150.000   Ambulation of client
N160.000   Ambulation of client with mechanical aids
 N160.005   Brace
 N160.010   Cane
 N160.015   Crutches
 N160.020   Walker
 N160.025   Wheelchair
N170.000   Amputation stump care
N180.000   Arm sling, application of an
N190.000   Artificial eye care
N200.000   Assessment
 N200.005   Of client problem
 N200.010   Of client status (level of progress toward health)
N210.000   Bath, administration of a
 N210.005   Cleansing bath
 N210.010   Medicated bath
 N210.015   Sitz bath
 N210.020   Sponge bath for fever
 N210.025   Towel bath
 N210.030   Whirlpool bath
N220.000   Bed, making a
 N220.005   Occupied bed
 N220.010   Postoperative bed
 N220.015   Unoccupied bed
N230.000   Binder, application of a
 N230.005   Abdominal binder
 N230.010   Breast binder
 N230.015   Chest binder
 N230.020   Scultetus binder
 N230.025   T binder
N240.000   Bladder training
N250.000   Blood transfusion, administration of a
N260.000   Bowel training
N270.000   Breast care

N280.000   Case finding
 N280.005   Behavioral (emotional) disorder
 N280.010   Cardiovascular disorder
 N280.015   Cognitive function disorder
 N280.020   Communicable disease
 N280.025   Ear, nose, and throat disorder
 N280.030   Endocrine disorder
 N280.035   Eye disorder
 N280.040   Gastrointestinal disorder
 N280.045   Gynecologic disorder
 N280.050   Hematologic disorder
 N280.055   Hepatobiliary disorder
 N280.060   Immune disorder
 N280.065   Infection disorder
 N280.070   Integument disorder
 N280.075   Musculoskeletal disorder
 N280.080   Neurologic disorder
 N280.085   Nutritional disorder
 N280.090   Obstetric disorder
 N280.095   Renal disorder
 N280.100   Respiratory disorder
 N280.105   Sexual disorder
 N280.110   Trauma
 N280.115   Urologic disorder
N290.000   Cast care
N300.000   Catheter care, urinary
N310.000   Catheter clamping
N320.000   Catheterization
 N320.005   External catheter application
 N320.010   Indwelling (retention) catheter
 N320.015   Nonretention (intermittent) catheterization
 N320.020   Removal of retention catheter
N330.000   Cecostomy care
N340.000   Charting/record keeping
N350.000   Chest drainage system, management of
N360.000   CircOlectric frame, management of client on
N370.000   Circumcision care

N380.000 Cold application(s)
    N380.005   Cold/cool moist compress
    N380.010   Cold/ice pack
    N380.015   Cool, damp cloth to face
    N380.020   Ice bag
    N380.025   Ice collar
N390.000 Colostomy care
N400.000 Communications, facilitating client
N410.000 Consultation on client's behalf
    N410.005   With chaplain
    N410.010   With dietition
    N410.015   With nurse/nurse specialist
    N410.020   With occupational therapist
    N410.025   With pharmacist
    N410.030   With physical therapist
    N410.035   With physician
    N410.040   With radiology personnel
    N410.045   With social worker
    N410.050   With others
N420.000 Contact lens care
N430.000 Coughing and deep breathing exercises
N440.000 Crutch walking, preparation for
N450.000 Debridement compress, application of
N460.000 Decubitus-ulcer care
    N460.005   Decubitus ulcer prevention
N470.000 Deep breathing exercises
N480.000 Denture care
N490.000 Dialysis management
    N490.005   Continuous ambulatory peritoneal dialysis
    N490.010   Hemodialysis
    N490.015   Peritoneal dialysis
N500.000 Diet, assistance with
    N500.005   Assistance with food preferences
    N500.010   Diet calculation
    N500.015   Nonprescription nutritional supplements
    N500.020   Providing a balanced diet
N510.000 Discharge of patient
N520.000 Dressing (bandage) application
    N520.005   Elastic bandage application
    N520.010   Subclavian catheter/CVP linedressing change

N530.000 Dressing and undressing the client
N540.000 Ear hygiene
N550.000 Elastic stockings, application of
N560.000 Electrolyte balance, maintenance of
    N560.005   By fluid supplements
    N560.010   By food supplements
    N560.015   By food and fluid supplements
N570.000 Elimination, assistance with
N580.000 Enema, administration of an
N590.000 Environmental control
    N590.005   Environmental barriers, minimizing
    N590.010   Environmental cleanliness, maintaining
    N590.015   Environmental humidity, regulating
    N590.020   Environmental safety, maintaining
    N590.025   Environmental temperature, regulating
    N590.030   Environmental ventilation, regulating
N600.000 Exercise, therapeutic
    N600.005   Isometric exercise
    N600.010   Moderate physical exercise
    N600.015   Range-of-motion exercise
N610.000 Feeding of client
    N610.005   Bottle feeding
    N610.010   Spoon feeding
    N610.015   Syringe feeding
    N610.020   Tube feeding
N620.000 Fluid balance, maintenance of
    N620.005   Assistance with fluid intake
    N620.010   Calculation of fluid replacement
    N620.015   Regulation of fluid intake/fluid volume
    N620.020   Restriction of fluid intake
N630.000 Gastric drainage system, management of
N640.000 Growth chart percentile, calculation of
N650.000 Hair care
N660.000 Heat application(s)
    N660.005   Heat cradle

	N660.010	Heat lamp		N810.005	Controlled positive-pressure breathing
	N660.015	Heating pad			
	N660.020	Hot food bath			
	N660.025	Hot pack			
	N660.030	Hot water bottle		N810.010	Intermittent positive-pressure breathing
	N660.035	Warm, moist compress			
	N660.040	Whirlpool bath			
N670.000	Heel protectors, application of		N820.000	Medication, administration of	
N680.000	Home visit		N820.005	Inhalation	
N690.000	Hyperalimentation, management of		N820.010	Intamuscular	
N700.000	Hypodermaclysis, management of		N820.015	Intravenous	
	N700.005	Hypodermaclysis, administration of		N820.151	Continuous infusion pump system
N710.000	Ileostomy care			N820.152	Heparin lock
N720.000	Incubator, management of infant in an			N820.153	Intravenous, piggyback
N730.000	Intravenous infusion, management of			N820.154	Intravenous push
	N730.005	Intravenous infusion, administration of		N820.155	Volume infusion system
N740.000	Irrigation(s)		N820.020	Oral	
	N740.005	Bladder		N820.025	Rectal
	N740.010	Ear		N820.030	Subcutaneous
	N740.015	Eye		N820.035	Topical (nasal, ophthalmic, otic)
	N740.020	Gastric lavage			
	N740.025	Nasogastric tube			
	N740.030	Nose			
	N740.035	Urinary catheter		N820.040	Transdermal
	N740.040	Wound		N820.045	Vaginal
N750.000	Isolation, management of therapeutic		N830.000	Mobility, management of client	
	N750.005	Communicable disease precautions		N830.005	Mobility, assisting client with
			N840.000	Nail care	
				N840.005	Diabetic nail care
	N750.010	Radiation precautions	N850.000	Oral hygiene	
			N860.000	Oxygen therapy, management of	
	N750.015	Reverse (protective) isolation		N860.005	Heated humidified oxygen
	N750.020	Strict isolation		N860.010	Humidified oxygen
N760.000	Jejunostomy care				
N770.000	Labor and delivery, management of	N870.000	Pacemaker, management of a	
			N880.000	Pack, removal of a	
N780.000	Laryngectomy care		N880.005	Nasal pack	
N790.000	Linen, changing		N880.010	Oral pack	
	N790.005	Clean gown		N880.015	Rectal pack
	N790.010	Clean pillow case		N880.020	Vaginal pack
	N790.015	Protective pads		N880.025	Wound pack
N800.000	Massage		N890.000	Perineal care	
	N800.005	Back massage	N900.000	Pheresis therapy, management of	
	N800.010	Bony prominence massage	N910.000	Physical examination	
			N920.000	Positioning of the body	
	N800.015	Full body massage		N920.005	Extremity elevation
	N800.020	Gum massage		N920.010	For comfort
	N800.025	Uterine massage		N920.015	Frequent position change (turning)
N810.000	Mechanical ventilation, management of				

N920.020	Functional position
N920.025	Head elevation
N920.030	Knee–chest position
N920.035	Lithotomy position
N920.040	Prone position
N920.045	Semi-Fowler's position
N920.050	Semi-Trendelenburg position
N920.055	Side-lying position
N920.060	Sitting position
N920.065	Supine position
N920.070	Trendelenburg position

N930.000	Postmortem care
N940.000	Postpartum care
N950.000	Postural drainage
N960.000	Predeath care
N970.000	Predischarge planning conference
N980.000	Prenatal care
N990.000	Procedures and/or examinations
	N990.005	Nonsurgical procedure, providing assistance with
	N990.010	Obtaining client/family permission for procedures
	N990.015	Radiology procedure, preparing client for
	N990.020	Surgical procedure, preparing client for
	N990.025	Surgical procedure, providing assistance with
N1000.000	Referral
	N1000.005	To community agency
	N1000.010	To dietician
	N1000.015	To nurse specialist
	N1000.020	To physician
	N1000.025	To social worker
	N1000.030	To other
N1010.000	Rest and sleep, promotion of
N1020.000	Resuscitation, management of
	N1020.005	Cardiopulmonary resuscitation
	N1020.010	Defibrillation (cardioversion)

	N1020.015	Heimlich maneuver
N1030.000	Rotating tourniquets, management of
N1040.000	Safety measures, promotion of
	N1040.005	Bed netting
	N1040.010	Chest restraint
	N1040.015	Crib dome
	N1040.020	Limb restraint
	N1040.025	Safety helmet to head
	N1040.030	Safety strap to waist
	N1040.035	Side rails
	N1040.040	Side rail padding
	N1040.045	Other
N1050.000	Skin care
	N1050.005	Diabetic foot care
	N1050.010	Skin cleansing
	N1050.015	Skin lubrication
N1060.000	Sleep, preparation for bedtime/nightime (H S care)
N1070.000	Soaks, administration of
	N1070.005	Foot soaks
	N1070.010	Hand soaks
N1080.000	Specimen(s), collection of
	N1080.005	Blood
	N1080.010	Drainage
	N1080.015	Sputum
	N1080.020	Stool
	N1080.025	Urine
N1090.000	Spiritual care, provision of
	N1090.005	Assistance with spiritual rituals
	N1090.010	Providing spiritual articles
	N1090.015	Providing spiritual dietary needs
N1100.000	Splint, application of a
N1110.000	Stryker frame, management of client on
N1120.000	Sutures, removal of
N1130.000	T-tube care
N1140.000	Tracheostomy care
N1150.000	Traction, management of therapeutic
N1160.000	Transcription of physician's orders
N1170.000	Transfer/transport of client
	N1170.005	To community agency
	N1170.010	To extended-care facility
	N1170.015	To in-house department
	N1170.020	To hospital from home, work, or accident site
	N1170.025	To home from hospital or institution
	N1170.030	To nursing home

	N1170.035	To rehabilitation facility	N1430.000		Reinforcement (provocative) therapy, negative
N1180.000	Tube insertion		N1440.000		Reinforcement therapy, positive
	N1180.005	Colon tube	N1450.000		Relaxation therapy
	N1180.010	Endotracheal tube	N1460.000		Role modeling
	N1180.015	Nasogastric tube	N1470.000		Self-exploration therapy
N1190.000	Tube removal		N1480.000		Self-responsibility therapy (nondirective psychotherapy)
	N1190.005	Colon tube	N1490.000		Sensitivity training
	N1190.010	Endotracheal tube	N1500.000		Sexual counseling
	N1190.015	Nasogastric tube	N1510.000		Silence therapy
N1200.000	Umbilical cord care		N1520.000		Social isolation
N1210.000	Urine, racking (six-bottle regime)		N1530.000		Stress management therapy
			N1540.000		Suicide prevention therapy
N1220.000	Urine, straining		N1550.000		Support, psychologic
N1230.000	Vaginal douche, administration of a			N1550.005	To client
				N1550.010	To family
N1240.000	Vaporized air, administration of (nebulization)			N1550.015	To significant others
N1250.000	Weighing the client				
N1260.000	Wound care		N1560.000		Therapeutic touch
N1270.000	Wound closure		N1570.000		Therapeutic weaning
	N1270.005	Butterfly closure		N1570.005	From life-saving devices
	N1270.010	Wound closure strips		N1570.010	From long-term therapy
	N1270.015	Wound suturing		N1570.015	From therapeutic relationship

PSYCHOLOGICAL INTERVENTIONS

N1280.000	Activities therapy	
	N1280.005	Art
	N1280.010	Dance
	N1280.015	Music
	N1280.020	Play
	N1280.025	Recreational
	N1280.030	Other
N1290.000	Attending therapy	
	N1290.005	Constant attendance
	N1290.010	Intermittent attendance
N1300.000	Bonding therapy	
	N1300.005	Client and family
	N1300.010	Client and visitors (nonfamily)
	N1300.015	Infant and parents
N1310.000	Confrontation therapy ·	
N1320.000	Crisis therapy	
N1330.000	Family therapy	
N1340.000	Group therapy	
N1350.000	Limit setting	
N1360.000	Listening therapy	
N1370.000	Milieu therapy	
N1380.000	Orientation therapy	
	N1380.005	To events
	N1380.010	To persons
	N1380.015	To places
	N1380.020	To time
N1390.000	Problem-solving therapy	
N1400.000	Rape counseling	
N1410.000	Reality therapy/orientation	
N1420.000	Reflecting (feedback) therapy	

NURSING OBSERVATION INTERVENTIONS

N1580.000	Observing for significant signs	
	N1580.005	Airway, nonpatent
	N1580.010	Apgar, abnormal infant
	N1580.015	Apnea
	N1580.020	Arrhythmias
	N1580.025	Ascites
	N1580.030	Attention deficit
	N1580.035	Babinski sign, positive
	N1580.040	Battle's sign
	N1580.045	Bleeding/ hemorrhage
	N1580.050	Blood pressure, abnormal
	N1580.055	Body temperature, abnormal
	N1580.060	Cardiac output, abnormal
	N1580.065	Central venous pressure, abnormal
	N1580.070	Cerebral perfusion pressure, abnormal
	N1580.075	Cerebrospinal fluid leakage
	N1580.080	Chvostek's sign

N1580.085	Circulation, impaired		N1580.300	Odor, abnormal body
N1580.090	Confusion		N1580.305	Organ enlargement
N1580.095	Consciousness, impaired level of		N1580.310	Pallor
			N1580.315	Papilledema
N1580.100	Coughing		N1580.320	Placenta, abnormal
N1580.105	Cyanosis			
N1580.110	Dehiscence		N1580.325	Pulmonary artery pressure, abnormal
N1580.115	Dehydration			
N1580.120	Delirium		N1580.330	Pulmonary capillary wedge pressure, abnormal
N1580.125	Depression			
N1580.130	Disorientation			
N1580.135	Distention, abdominal			
			N1580.335	Pulmonary edema
N1580.140	Distention, bladder		N1580.340	Pulse pressure
			N1580.345	Pulses, abnormal or absent
N1580.145	Edema			
N1580.150	Epistaxis		N1580.350	Pulsus paradoxicus
N1580.155	Fetal heart sounds, abnormal			
			N1580.355	Pupils, abnormal
			N1580.360	Reflex responses, abnormal deep
N1580.160	Gait, abnormal			
N1580.165	Halo sign		N1580.365	Restlessness
N1580.170	Healing, delayed		N1580.370	Seizures
N1580.175	Hemoptysis		N1580.375	Shock
N1580.180	Hiccoughs		N1580.380	Skin breakdown
N1580.185	Homan's sign, positive		N1580.385	Skin lesions
			N1580.390	Sleep patterns, abnormal
N1580.190	Hyperactivity			
N1580.195	Hypersensitivity response		N1580.395	Speech loss
			N1580.400	Suicidal threats
N1580.200	Incontinence		N1580.405	Tetany
N1580.205	Infant head rolling		N1580.410	Tracheal deviation
N1580.210	Inflammation		N1580.415	Tremors
N1580.215	Intake, excessive		N1580.420	Trousseau's sign
N1580.220	Intake, inadequate		N1580.425	Venous distention
			N1580.430	Umbilical cord, abnormal
N1580.225	Output, excessive			
N1580.230	Output, inadequate		N1580.435	Voiding, abnormal
N1580.235	Irritability			
N1580.240	Jaundice		N1580.440	Vomiting
N1580.245	Laryngeal edema		N1580.445	Water intoxication
N1580.250	Lethargy			
N1580.255	Mean arterial pressure, abnormal		N1580.450	Weight changes, body
		N1590.000	Observing for significant symptoms	
N1580.260	Mobility, impaired		N1590.005	Anorexia
N1580.265	Motor function, impaired		N1590.010	Anxiety
			N1590.015	Chills
			N1590.020	Constipation
N1580.270	Mouth breathing		N1590.025	Diarrhea
N1580.275	Muscle or motor strength, impaired		N1590.030	Dizziness
			N1590.035	Dyspnea
			N1590.040	Dysuria
N1580.280	Muscle twitching/jerking		N1590.045	Euphoria
			N1590.050	Flatulence
N1580.285	Nasal flare		N1590.055	Fatigue
N1580.290	Necrosis		N1590.060	Headache
N1580.295	Neurologic signs			

N1590.065	Hearing, diminished		N1660.005	Braces
N1590.070	Itching		N1660.010	Cane
N1590.075	Lightheadedness		N1660.015	Crutches
N1590.080	Malaise		N1660.020	Prosthesis
N1590.085	Menstrual cycle abnormalities		N1660.025	Walker
			N1660.030	Wheelchair
		N1670.000	Evaluating environmental safety	
N1590.090	Nasal congestion		N1670.005	Housing safety
N1590.095	Nausea		N1670.010	Institutional safety
N1590.100	Nervousness			
N1590.105	Nocturia		N1670.015	Occupational safety
N1590.110	Noise sensitivity			
N1590.115	Numbness and tingling	N1680.000	Checking the mechanical or correct functioning of equipment or devices	
N1590.120	Orthopnea			
N1590.125	Pain		N1680.005	Airfloat system, Lapidus
N1590.130	Pain, the sudden absence of			
			N1680.010	Blood transfusion setup
N1590.135	Thirst		N1680.015	CircOlectric frame
N1590.140	Tinnitus			
N1590.145	Urinary frequency		N1680.020	Drainage systems (urinary, water-seal, etc.)
N1590.150	Visual disturbance			
N1590.155	Warmth, excessive		N1680.025	Ear oximeter or transcutaneous monitor
N1590.160	Weakness			
N1600.000	Evaluating cognitive functioning			
N1600.005	Attention span		N1680.030	External counterpulsation pressure suit apparatus
N1600.010	Judgment			
N1600.015	Learning ability			
N1600.020	Memory			
N1600.025	Orientation to time, place, persons, and events		N1680.035	Fetal/maternal ultrasound monitor
			N1680.040	Hemodialyzer
N1600.030	Thinking processes		N1680.045	Hemodynamic monitoring system/telemetry
N1610.000	Evaluating behavioral/emotional responses			
N1610.005	Adaptive		N1680.050	Hyperalimentation setup
N1610.010	Nonadaptive			
N1620.000	Determining adherence to recommended therapy		N1680.055	Hypodermaclysis setup
N1630.000	Observing for adverse effects of therapy		N1680.060	Hypothermia/hyperthermia blanket
N1640.000	Monitoring and interpreting lab results		N1680.065	Incubator
N1640.005	Blood		N1680.070	Intermittent positive-pressure breathing machine
N1640.0051	Dextrose Stix test			
N1640.010	Gastric analysis			
N1640.015	Papanicolaou smear		N1680.075	Internal counterpulsation intra-aortic balloon apparatus
N1640.020	Sputum			
N1640.025	Stool			
N1640.030	Urine			
N1640.0301	Clinitest and Acetest test		N1680.080	Intracranial pressure monitor
N1650.000	Monitoring patient recovery from anesthesia			
N1660.000	Checking for correct utilization of devices		N1680.085	Intravenous infusion setup

N1680.090	Irrigating equipment		N1690.175	Catheter care, urinary
N1680.095	Mechanical ventilators		N1690.182	Catheterization
			N1690.189	Child socialization
N1680.100	Oxygen equipment		N1690.196	Circumcision care
			N1690.203	Climacteric, male
N1680.105	Pacemaker		N1690.210	Clothing adjustments for health needs
N1680.110	Peritoneal dialysis setup			
N1680.115	Pheresis equipment		N1690.217	Cold applications
			N1690.224	Colostomy care
N1680.120	Stryker frame		N1690.231	Communication methods
N1680.125	Suction equipment			
			N1690.238	Contact lenses, use and care of
N1680.130	Swan-Ganz catheter		N1690.245	Continuous ambulatory peritoneal dialysis
N1680.135	Tube feeding setup			
N1680.140	Traction apparatus		N1690.252	Coping methods for adaptation, effective

HEALTH TEACHING INTERVENTIONS

			N1690.259	Coughing and deep breathing
N1690.000	Health teaching, specific to		N1690.266	Crutch walking
N1690.007	Activity level, appropriate		N1690.273	Dangers of poor health practices
N1690.014	Airway patency management		N1690.280	Decubitus ulcer care
N1690.021	Alcohol abuse		N1690.287	Dependent person, care of a
N1690.028	Alcohol abuser, coping with the			
N1690.035	Allergic responses		N1690.294	Diabetic foot and nail care
N1690.042	Amputation stump care		N1690.301	Diabetic skin care
N1690.049	Apnea monitoring		N1690.308	Diet instructions, specific
N1690.056	Artificial eye care			
N1690.063	Assistive devices, utilization of		N1690.315	Disease, information about any
N1690.070	Bandaging			
N1690.077	Bedmaking, occupied		N1690.322	Drug abuse
			N1690.329	Drug abuser, coping with the
N1690.084	Behavior modification techniques		N1690.336	Ear hygiene
			N1690.343	Elimination hygiene
N1690.091	Behavioral limits			
N1690.098	Binder applications		N1690.350	Elimination practices, healthy
N1690.105	Bladder training			
N1690.112	Blood pressure, measuring		N1690.357	Enema administration
N1690.119	Bowel training		N1690.364	Environmental cold, coping with
N1690.126	Brace, use of a			
N1690.133	Breast care			
N1690.140	Breast examination, self		N1690.371	Environmental heat, coping with
N1690.147	Breast–feeding		N1690.378	Equipment, how to use and maintain health- or illness-related
N1690.154	Breathing exercises, deep			
N1690.161	Cane, use of a			
N1690.168	Cast care			

N1690.385	Exercise, therapeutic	N1690.623	Menopause
N1690.392	Eye care	N1690.630	Memory improvement
N1690.399	Eyeglasses, care and use of	N1690.637	Mental health principles
N1690.406	Family planning	N1690.644	Mentally ill, coping with the
N1690.413	Feminine hygiene		
N1690.420	Fluid balance	N1690.651	Menstruation
N1690.427	Fluid restriction	N1690.658	Mobility methods
N1690.434	Food preparation and storage, safe	N1690.665	Nail care
		N1690.672	Normal organ function
N1690.441	Genetic factors/influences	N1690.679	Nutrition, balanced
N1690.448	Growth and development, normal	N1690.686	Odor control
		N1690.693	Oral hygiene
		N1690.700	Organ donation
N1690.455	Hair care	N1690.707	Oxygen therapy
N1690.462	Hearing aid use and maintenance	N1690.714	Pacemaker management
		N1690.721	Pain management
N1690.469	Heat applications	N1690.728	Parenting, positive
N1690.476	Hemodialysis		
N1690.483	Home adaptations, methods for	N1690.735	Peritoneal dialysis
		N1690.742	Postural drainage
		N1690.749	Premenopause
N1690.490	Hygiene, personal	N1690.756	Prenatal care
N1690.497	Hyperalimenta-tion therapy	N1690.763	Preventive measures for health maintenance
N1690.504	Ileostomy care		
N1690.511	Illness, information about any	N1690.770	Problem-solving methods
N1690.518	Immunizations	N1690.777	Procedures, diagnostic or therapeutic
N1690.525	Infant care, premature		
N1690.532	Infant or child care	N1690.784	Prosthesis, management of a
N1690.539	Infant or child feeding	N1690.791	Puberty
N1690.546	Intermittent positive-pressure breathing	N1690.798	Pulse, counting a
		N1690.805	Reproductive process, the
		N1690.812	Respirations, counting
N1690.553	Irrigations		
N1690.560	Isolation technique	N1690.819	Rest and sleep
		N1690.826	Resuscitation
N1690.567	Jejunostomy care	N1690.833	Safety measures to prevent accident or injury
N1690.574	Jet lag		
N1690.581	Labor and delivery		
N1690.588	Laryngectomy care	N1690.840	Self-care in health promotion
N1690.595	Massage, body	N1690.847	Sexuality
N1690.602	Mechanics, body	N1690.854	Signs and symptoms to be reported
N1690.609	Medications, administration of		
		N1690.861	Sitz bath
N1690.616	Medications, general information about	N1690.868	Skin care
		N1690.875	Smoking
		N1690.882	Specimen collecting

N1690.889	Stocking applications, elastic	N1690.931	Transferring, body
N1690.896	Stress management	N1690.938	Trauma, information about any
N1690.903	Temperature, measuring body	N1690.945	Umbilical cord care
N1690.910	Testing techniques for monitoring one's health	N1690.952	Walker, use of a
		N1690.959	Weight control
		N1690.966	Wheelchair, use of a
N1690.917	Toilet training	N1690.973	Wound care
N1690.924	Tracheostomy care	N1690.980	Wound care, burn
		N1690.987	Other

GLOSSARY

The following is a list of terms and definitions as used in this text.

ABANDONED FEELING. . . : a feeling of having been deserted by another person, whether the desertion is real or imagined.

ACCEPTANCE: a need to feel that one is worthy of love in the eyes of others.

ACID–BASE BALANCE: a need for a constant hydrogen ion level which is neither acid or alkali.

ACTIVITIES OF DAILY LIVING (ADL): self-maintenance activities pursued as a daily routine, such as bathing, toileting, oral hygiene, dressing, hair care, self-feeding and hydration.

ACTIVITY: a need for bodily action or movement.

AMBIVALENCE. . . : the existence of two or more opposing emotions directed at an object.

ANGER. . . : a feeling of resentment or hostility.

ANXIETY. . . : a vague, ill-defined feeling of apprehension and uneasiness.

APPROVAL FROM OTHERS: a need for the expression of positive attitudes and support from others.

ASSESSMENT: "a systematic method of data collection, which consists of the appraisal of the individual, the family, or the community for the purpose of identifying potential and actual health needs."[89:43]

ASSISTIVE NURSING INTERVENTION: a nursing measure that provides help or aid in the carrying out of normal daily activities that cannot be carried out by the individual due to illness, injury, or disease.

ATTENTION: a need for the concentration and focusing of one person onto another.

AWARENESS OF POTENTIAL: the need to be conscious of the capabilities one can achieve.

BODY-IMAGE MODIFICATION. . . : adjusting one's concept of the body as a result of body changes.

BONDING INTERRUPTION. . . : feeling cut off, from relating to a significant other, expressions of emotional closeness and caring.

CARING AND COMMUNICATING RELATIONSHIPS: a need for the expression of concern and warmth, which results in positive feelings between persons.

CLEANLINESS: a need for freedom from body dirt or soil as is necessary for the maintenance of health.

COMFORT: a need for a state of physical or psychologic contentment.

COMPETENCE IN. . . : adequate ability, knowledge, or proficiency in handling a problem or task.

COMPLAINT PROBLEM: the problem the person presents to the professional.[125:16–17]

CONFLICT. . . : a conscious or unconscious struggle between opposing choices or persons.

CONTINUED COMPETENCE IN SKILLS: a need to maintain, over a period of time, proficiency in the performance of a particular skill.

CONTROL OVER OTHERS, SELF, OR SITUATION: a need to have power or mastery over oneself, others or a situation.

DATA ANALYSIS: putting collected data in order, selecting essential information, discarding nonessential data, and interpreting the meaning of the data.

DATA COLLECTION: the gathering of relevant information.

DENIAL OF. . . : being unable to admit the existence of facts.

DEPENDENCE: a need to rely on others to meet one's needs.

DEPENDENCY FEELINGS. . . : feeling the need to rely on others for support.

DEPRESSION. . . : a mental state of gloom and sadness.

DIAGNOSTIC LABEL: the title of the nursing diagnostic pattern or full nursing diagnosis statement.

DIFFICULTY. . . : the person or family is only partially effective in achieving whatever the person wishes to achieve.

DIGNITY: a need for respect from others regarding one's intrinsic worth.

DIRECT AND COMMUNICATING RELATIONSHIPS: a need to express feelings, ideas, or information in a straightforward manner so that the communication is clearly understood.

1851

DISCOMFORT OF. . . : experiencing as distressful the physical sensation of cold, heat, dryness, wetness, pressure, loudness, etc.

DISENGAGEMENT/DETACHMENT. . . : an attempt to release oneself or others from personal attachments or responsibilities.

DUAL DIAGNOSIS: patient problems commonly solved or treated by more than one health discipline.

EDUCATIVE NURSING INTERVENTION: a nursing measure in which the nurse provides satisfactory and accurate health information and explanations of treatment.

EMBARRASSMENT. . . : a state of self-conscious uneasiness or noncomposure.

ENDURANCE: a need for the capacity to tolerate suffering, pain, or misfortune and to continue on despite such situations.

ENERGY: a need for physical strength.

ESSENTIAL CRITERIA: the subjective and objective data that distinguish one diagnostic pattern from another and that are required to be present for the diagnosis of that pattern.

ET: emergency treatment.

ETIOLOGY: all the factors that bring about a result, effect, or response[524:124]: the causes of a problem; stressors.

EVALUATION: an appraisal of the effectiveness of nursing interventions.

EXERCISE: a need for vigorous or energetic body exertion for the purpose of improving or strengthening health.

FEAR OF. . . : a feeling of alarm and fright directed at a specific object.

FEELING REJECTED. . . : feeling that one is not acceptable to another or others.

FOOD BALANCE: nutritional balance; a need for the ingestion and utilization of nutritional products appropriate for human consumption in adequate amounts of protein, carbohydrates, fat, vitamins, and minerals.

FREEDOM FROM PAIN: a need to be without any distressful hurting sensation.

FRUSTRATION. . . : feelings of irritation and tension when a desired goal is blocked.

FULL OR CONTINUED DEVELOPMENT OF POTENTIAL: a need to develop existing or latent capabilities to their maximum level; a need to consistently develop one's capabilities.

GOAL ACHIEVEMENT: the need to achieve a desired end.

GREATER SATISFACTION IN BEAUTY: the need to increase one's contentment through exposure to that which is beautiful and which inspires pleasure to the senses, mind, and soul.

GRIEF REACTION. . . : feelings of deep sorrow and distress.

GROUP UNITY AND COMPANIONSHIP: the need for association, identification, and togetherness with a number of persons who are joined for a mutual purpose.

GUILT. . . : blaming oneself for a particular action or omission.

HEALTH TEACHING: a nursing measure that provides health information and explanations.

HELPLESSNESS/POWERLESSNESS. . . : feeling that one has no power or resources to control a situation and is unable to manage alone.

HOMEOSTASIS: the normal integration of all body systems resulting in harmony of the whole being.[328]

HOPELESSNESS. . . : the feeling that efforts are useless and ineffective.

HUMAN NEED: an essential component of the human system that must be gratified if there is to be a healthy existence.[328] "A requirement within a person that creates tension which, in turn, creates energy that is transformed into some form of behavior." [410:53]

HUMAN RESPONSE: a person's reaction or behavior aroused by a stimulus.

HUMAN STRENGTHS: qualities, resources, and conditions that favor the ability of a person to cope with problems.

HYGIENCE NURSING INTERVENTION: a nursing measure designed to maintain cleanliness as thoroughly and completely as required for health.

IDENTIFICATION OF PRIORITIES: a need to rank persons, situations, or tasks according to their significance in one's life or goal achievement.

IDENTIFICATION OF VALUES: a need to select modes of behavior that one sees as desirable and that serve as a guide for actions.

ILLNESS: the interaction of disease as it affects a person, his surroundings, life patterns, human relationships, attitudes, and capabilities.

IMPORTANCE-INFLUENCE: the need to be significant to or have an effect on other persons or situations.

INABILITY TO. . . : being ineffective in achieving whatever the person wishes to achieve.

INCAPACITY TO. . . : being incapable of performing activities of daily living and requiring total assistance with such activities.

INCREASED OR CONTINUED LEARNING: the need for a higher level of knowledge and skill or the need for consistent learning.

INCREASED CREATIVITY: the need for a higher level of productivity in which a person develops new ideas or objects.

INCREASED PLEASANTNESS OR PLEASURE: the need for a higher level of delight and enjoyment.

INCREASED REALITY PERCEPTION AND/ OR PROBLEM-SOLVING ABILITIES: the need for a higher level of awareness of what is true or actually exists and the capacity to find and act upon solutions to problems.

INDEPENDENCE: the need for freedom from the control of others.

INDEPENDENT NURSING INTERVENTION: a single-action nursing treatment that is ordered by a professional nurse and carried out by a professional nurse or by a nursing assistant under professional nursing supervision, without physician direction.

INSTABILITY OF. . . : unstable physiologic signs indicating a physiologic imbalance that threatens the integrity of the specific body system.

LESS OF THE FAMILIAR, MORE OF THE NOVEL: the need for reduced exposure to that which one is accustomed to and increased exposure to that which is different.

LESS OF THE SIMPLE, MORE OF THE COMPLEX: the need for reduced exposure to that which is uncomplicated and increased exposure to that which is challenging.

LESS RIGID CONVENTIALITY: the need for reduced adherence to strict conformity.

LIFE-SUPPORT SYSTEM: any assistive method that maintains life and without which life would cease or be seriously threatened.

LONELINESS/ISOLATED FEELING. . . : feeling separate and remote from others.

LOSS OF A SIGNIFICANT OTHER: being permanently parted from a person important to oneself.

LOVE AND AFFECTION: the need to give and receive strong emotional attachment (love), or moderate emotional warmth (affection).

LOW SELF-ESTEEM. . . : having feelings of negative self-worth.

MASTERY AND COMPETENCE IN SKILLS: the need to be capable of proficiently performing a particular skill.

MATERIAL LOSS: loss of tangible, valued objects.

MEDICAL DIAGNOSIS: "the determination of what kinds of a disease a patient is suffering from, especially the art of distinguishing between several possibilities."437:27

MEDICAL INTERVENTION: a treatment that is ordered by a physician and carried out by

the physician or by someone under the supervision of the physician.

MEDICAL TREATMENTS PERFORMED BY NURSES: medical treatments that have been delegated by the physician to the nurse.

NORMAL TEMPERATURE: the need to maintain a normal level of internal and external warmth and coolness.

NURSING DIAGNOSIS: a clinical diagnosis made by a professional nurse to "describe actual or potential health problems which nurses, by virtue of their education and experience, are capable of and licensed to treat."196:2

NURSING DIAGNOSIS PATTERN: a set of essential criteria, a definition of the response, and a diagnostic label that, together, describe the characteristics of the human response.

NURSING GOAL: a statement of the expected and desired change in a person's response or behavior.

NURSING INTERVENTION: a single-action nursing measure designed to fulfill the unmet needs that are inferred from the person's problem.

NURSING OBSERVATIONS: single-action nursing measures of examining, checking, inspecting, monitoring, and testing.

NURSING PLAN: determining the course of action to be used by the nurse to assist in solving the person's problem.

NURSING PROBLEM: any difficulty the nurse has in solving the defined patient problems.

NURSING PROCESS: a step-by-step system of thought used to identify and solve problems that nurses treat.

NURSING TREATMENT: a single-action nursing measure that provides assistance, regulates the internal or external environment, supports functioning, comforts, facilitates hygiene, provides improved or independent activity, and prevents illness or injury through protective and precautionary measures.

OBJECTIVE DATA: signs; overt manifestations that can be observed or discovered through examination or testing in which the examiner uses the senses of seeing, hearing, feeling, smelling or touching. 125

OBSERVATIONAL NURSING INTERVENTION: a nursing measure in which the nurse examines, inspects, monitors, and tests behavioral and physical responses to illness, injury, and disease and their associated therapies.

OPTIMUM FUNCTION: the need for the highest possible level of self- direction and activiy.

OXYGEN, CIRCULATION: tissue oxygenation or perfusion; the need for the presence of a colorless, odorless, tasteless gas in the blood that moves through the blood vessels and into body tissue and organs in sufficient quantity to maintain human life and support human activity.

PARTIAL INCAPACITY. . . : being capable of but needing assistance with the performance of activities of daily living.

PATIENT PROBLEM: that which the professional nurse determines to be the person's difficulty, synonymous with the nursing diagnosis statement.[333:7]

PERSONAL GROWTH AND MATURITY: the need for progressive development of the person leading to qualities of maturity such as self- direction, competence, confronting reality, acquiring knowledge, and becoming moral and other-centered.

PHYSICAL LIMITATIONS: bodily characteristics that impose activity restrictions on the person.

PHYSICAL LOSS: being without a positive, balanced state of health, including loss of a body part or body function.

PHYSIOLOGIC STABILITY: the need for a state of homeostasis of all body systems.

POSITIVE SCREENING CUES FOR. . . : a human response in which the person exhibits significant, abnormal clinical findings during brief testing.

POTENTIAL FOR. . . : the presence of stressors that increase the possibility of the occurrence of a problem.

PREDICTABLE AND ORDERLY WORLD: the need for a life situation in which one can anticipate what will happen next and in which one's world is well ordered.

PREDOMINANT NURSING DIAGNOSIS: patient problems more often solved or treated by professional nurses than by any other professionals.

PRESCRIBED MEDICATION: any drug that can only be legally obtained through the written prescription of a licensed physician.

PREVENTIVE NURSING INTERVENTION: protective and precautionary nursing measures designed to avert physical or behavioral illness, injury, disease, or threat and to prevent complications or recurrences of physical or behavioral disorders, malfunctioning of therapeutic devices, or adverse effects of treatments.

PROBLEM LIST: a composite of identified nursing and medical problems listed on the health care record.[507]

PROBLEM-ORIENTED CHARTING: a systematic method of organizing health care records devised by Weed.[507]

PROFESSIONAL PERSON: a person employed in an intellectual occupation based on long-term, formal training in a systematic, theoretical body of knowledge upon which professional activity is based; the person has intellectual expertise unknown to the general public, has autonomy, uses theoretical judgment, has professional commitment, and assumes full responsibility for the welfare of the client.[373]

PROTECTION FROM PHYSICAL HARM: the need to be safeguarded against disease, injury, spread of infection, or hypersensitivity responses.

PROTECTION FROM PSYCHOLOGIC THREAT: the need to be safeguarded against feelings that threaten internal emotional harmony or significant relationships.

PSYCHOLOGIC STABILITY: the need for a state of emotional homeostasis.

RECOGNITION/APPRECIATION FROM OTHERS: the need to be acknowledged as an individual or to receive expressions of gratitude from others.

REGRESSION. . . : an attempt to protect oneself by using coping behavior appropriate at an earlier developmental level.

REHABILITATIVE NURSING INTERVENTION: a nursing measure that supports improved or independent activity and function in mobility, management of specific devices, supplies, and body alterations, retraining for bowel and bladder function, measures to ease work and conserve physical energy, clothing adjustments specific to health problems, budgeting, planning with the family and agencies, referral to resource persons, and involvement of the person in community and social affairs.

REJECTION OF. . . : feeling that a significant other or situation is not acceptable to oneself.

RELATED DATA: data that include such information as age, race, geographic location, occupation, nationality, environmental influences, or specifics to a particular group.

RELAXATION: the need for a decreased stress level achieved by relieving the normal tension of structured living through pleasurable activity.

REPUTATION OF GOOD CHARACTER: the need to be known for having favorable personal traits.

REST: the need for freedom from physical or psychologic disturbance with a resulting feeling of refreshment after the period of rest.

ROLE BEHAVIORS: that which the person actually does in response to role expectations;

the actual actions of the person in a particular role.[414]

ROLE EXPECTATIONS: that which is expected in a certain role by oneself or others.[414]

ROLE LOSS: being without a previously held position or responsibility.

SELF-IDENTITY MODIFICATION. . . : adjusting the beliefs, attitudes, ideas, and feelings one has about oneself.

SELF-RELIANCE: the need to depend on oneself rather than on others.

SENSE OF ADEQUACY: the need to feel capable of and confident in meeting demands or responsibilities.

SENSE OF USEFULNESS: the need to feel that one is serving some meaningful purpose.

SEPARATION FROM A SIGNIFICANT OTHER: being temporarily apart from a person important to oneself.

SEX: the need to perform sexual activity with distinctive functions of the male and female in reproduction.

SEXUALITY: the need to possess those characteristics that make up the personality structure of being a whole man or woman.

SLEEP: the need for a temporary loss of perception of conscious life from which one can be easily aroused.

SOCIAL PROBLEMS: those difficulties that arise in regard to interaction between persons and groups of persons in relationship to cultural expectations.

SPIRITUAL: that which includes a relationship with a Supreme Being, a life philosophy, or a system of faith.

SPIRITUAL AWARENESS. . . : an ongoing consciousness of a need for a more positive, spiritual force in one's life.

SPIRITUAL DISTRESS. . . : troubled concern about threats to one's belief system.

SPIRITUAL, RELIGIOUS, OR PHILOSOPHIC SATISFACTION: the need for the internal integration of principles of spirituality, religion, and philosophy that bring contentment to the inner self.

STANDARDS OF NURSING PRACTICE: criteria set by the American Nurses' Association for the expected level of achievement of nursing practice, as a means of guaranteeing the quality of nursing service.[754]

STATUS: the need for position in society.

STIMULATION: the need to be aroused to response.

SUBJECTIVE DATA: those symptoms perceived and reported by the person that indicate present abnormal sensations or conditions not observable to the examiner and information regarding past events, abnormalities, and treatments that is not available except through patient or family confirmation.

SUPPORTIVE NURSING INTERVENTION: a nursing measure in which the nurse provides needed objects (oxygen, nutrition, fluids), facilitates processes or activities (elimination, body alignment exercise, rest, sleep, entertainment), provides physical or psychologic comfort or healing measures, or maintains a healthy environment.

TECHNICAL SKILL: a step-by-step measure involving the use of manual treatment, machinery, or tools, based on knowledge of "methods" of performance and for which the technician assumes responsibility for correctness of performance but is reliant on professional judgment regarding responsibility for appropriateness and therapeutic effect.[373]

THERAPEUTIC ENVIRONMENT: those conditions or surroundings that promote healing and/or the maintenance, maximum function or improvement of physical or behavioral function.

THREATENED BODY IMAGE. . . : feeling endangered by changes in one's body that alter one's concept of the body.

UNITY WITH LOVED ONES: the need for identification with specific significant persons who one loves and is loved by.

UNKNOWLEDGEABLE ABOUT. . . : lacking sufficient information.

UNMET NEEDS: the absence of essential components that are vital to an integrated or homeostatic body system.[328:35-38]

UNSKILLED AT. . . : being nonproficient, with or without knowledge, in performing a specific task.

WATER–SALT BALANCE: fluid and/or electrolyte balance; the need to maintain a constant state of equilibrium between the amount of liquid and the level of sodium, potassium, chloride, calcium, and magnesium within body tissues and cells.

WITHDRAWAL FROM. . . : moving away from interactions with persons or situations.

BIBLIOGRAPHY

BOOKS

1. AACN Manual. *Methods in Critical Care.* Philadelphia: W.B. Saunders Co., 1980.

2. Abbott Laboratories. *Fluid and Electrolytes.* Chicago: Abbott Laboratories, 1969.

3. Abdellah, Faye, and Eugene Levine. *Better Patient Care Through Nursing Research.* London: Macmillan & Co., 1965.

4. Abdellah, Faye, Irene Beland, Almeda Martin, and Ruth Matheney. *New Directions in Patient-Centered Nursing: Guidelines for Systems of Service, Education and Research.* New York: Macmillan Publishing Co., 1973.

5. Abdellah, Faye, Irene Beland, Almeda Martin, and Ruth Matheney. *Patient-Centered Approaches to Nursing.* New York: Macmillan Publising Co., 1964.

6. Abels, Linda Feiwell. *Mosby's Manual of Critical Care: 1979.* St. Louis: C.V. Mosby Co., 1979.

7. Abrahamsen, David. *The Road to Emotional Maturity.* Englewood Cliffs, N.J.: Prentice-Hall, Inc., 1966.

8. Abrahamson, E.M., and A.W. Pezet. *Body, Mind and Sugar.* New York: Holt, Rinehart and Winston, 1972.

9. Adams, John. *Viruses and Colds.* New York: American Elsevier Publishing Co., 1967.

10. Aldrich, C. Knight. *An Introduction to Dynamic Psychiatry.* New York: McGraw-Hill Book Co., 1966.

11. Allen, James H. *May's Diseases of the Eye.* Baltimore: Williams & Wilkins Co., 1963.

12. Allergy Foundation of America. *Allergy: Its Mysterious Causes and Modern Treatment.* New York: Grossett & Dunlap, 1967.

13. Allport, Gordon W. *Pattern and Growth in Personality.* New York: Henry Holt & Co., 1937.

14. Allport, Gordon W. *Personality: A Psychological Interpretation.* New York: Henry Holt & Co., 1937.

15. Alvarez, Walter. *Live at Peace with Your Nerves.* Englewood Cliffs, N.J.: Prentice-Hall, Inc., 1961.

16. American Medical Association. *Current Medical Terminology.* Chicago: American Medical Association, 1966.

17. American Medical Association. *Drug Dependence: A Guide for Physicians.* Chicago: American Medical Association, 1961.

18. American Pharmaceutical Association. *Handbook of Nonprescription Drugs.* Washington, D.C.: American Pharmaceutical Association, 1979.

19. American Psychiatric Association. *Diagnostic and Statistical Manual of Mental Disorders,* 3rd edition *(DSM-3)*Washington, D.C.: American Psychiatric Association, 1980.

20. American Red Cross. *Advanced First Aid and Emergency Care.* Garden City, N.Y.: Doubleday & Co., Inc., 1979.

21. American Red Cross. *Family Health and Home Nursing.* Garden City, N.Y.: Doubleday & Co., Inc., 1979.

22. American Red Cross. *Standard First Aid and Personal Safety.* Garden City, N.Y.: Doubleday & Co., Inc., 1973.

23. Anthony, Elwyn James, and Theresa Benedek. *Parenthood: Its Psychology and Psychopathology.* Boston: Little, Brown & Co., 1970.

24. Ardell, Donald B. *High-Level Wellness: An Alternative to Doctors, Drugs and Diseases.* Pa: Rodale Press, 1977.

25. Armed Forces Information Service, Department of Defense. *Drug Abuse: Game Without Winners.* Washington, D.C.: U.S. Government Printing Office, 1969.

26. Armstrong, Margaret, Elizabeth Dickason, and Jeanne Howe. *McGraw-Hill Handbook of Clinical Nursing.* New York: McGraw-Hill Book Co., 1979.

27. Arnold, Magda. *Feelings and Emotions.* New York: Academic Press, 1960.

28. Artz, Curtis, and John Moncrief. *The Treatment of Burns.* Philadelphia: W.B. Saunders Co., 1969.

29. Bailey, June, and Karen Claus. *Decision Making in Nursing.* St. Louis: C.V. Mosby Co., 1975.

30. Baker, Charles. *Physician's Desk Reference,* 37th edition. Oradell, N.J.: Medical Economics, Inc., 1983.

31. Barbata, Jean, Deborah Jensen, and William Patterson. *A Textbook of Medical-Surgical Nursing.* New York: G.P. Putnam's Sons, 1964.

32. Barber, Janet, Lillian Stokes, Diane Billings. *Adult and Child Care: A Client Ap-*

proach to Nursing. St. Louis: C.V. Mosby Co., 1977.

33. Bates, Barbara. *A Guide to Physical Examination.* Philadelphia: J.B. Lippincott Co., 1979.

34. Beardsley, Monroe C. *Thinking Straight.* Englewood Cliffs, N.J.: Prentice-Hall, Inc., 1975.

35. Beland, Irene. *Clinical Nursing: Pathophysiological and Psychosocial Approaches.* New York: Macmillan Publishing Co., 1981.

36. Belgum, David. *Guilt: Where Religion and Psychology Meet.* Englewood Cliffs, N.J.: Prentice-Hall, Inc., 1963.

37. Bellet, Samuel. *Clinical Disorders of the Heart Beat.* Philadelphia: Lea & Febiger Co., 1971.

38. Berger, Milton H. *Working with People Called Patients.* New York: Brunner/Mazel Publishers, 1977.

39. Bergman, B. Abraham, J. Bruce Beckwith, and C. George Ray. *Sudden Infant Death Syndrome.* Seattle: University of Washington Press, 1970.

40. Bergmann, Klaus. *The Aged: Their Understanding and Care.* London: Wolfe Publishing Limited, 1972.

41. Bergstrom, Doris. *Care of Patients with Bowel and Bladder Problems: A Nursing Guide.* Minneapolis: American Rehabilitation Foundation, 1968.

42. Berkow, Robert. *The Merck Manual of Diagnosis and Therapy.* Rahway, N.J.: Merck Sharp & Dohme Research Laboratories, 1977.

43. Berland, Theodore, and Alfred Seyler. *Your Children's Teeth.* New York: Meredith Press, 1968.

44. Bernard, Jessie, and Deborah Jensen. *Sociology.* St. Louis: C.V. Mosby Co., 1962.

45. Bernard, Jessie, and Lida Thompson. *Sociology: Nurses and Their Patients in a Modern Society.* St. Louis: C.V. Mosby Co., 1970.

46. Berne, Eric. *A Layman's Guide to Psychiatry and Psychoanalysis.* New York: Simon and Schuster, 1968.

47. Berry, Mildred Freburg. *Language Disorders of Children: The Basis and Diagnosis.* New York: Appleton-Century-Crofts, 1969.

48. Beutner, Karl, and Nathan Hale. *Emotional Illness: How Families Can Help.* New York: G.P. Putnam's Sons, 1957.

49. Beyers, Marjorie, and Susan Dudas. *Medical Surgical Nursing,* Chapter 15: "Nursing Care Delivery for the Thermally Injured Patient." Boston: Little, Brown & Co., 1977.

50. Bleier, Inge J. *Bedside Maternity Nursing.* Philadelphia: W.B. Saunders Co., 1979.

51. Block, Marvin. *Alcohol and Alcoholism.* Belmont, Calif.: Wadsworth Publishing Co., 1970.

52. Bogert, L. Jean, George Briggs, and Doris Callaway. *Nutrition and Physical Fitness.* Philadelphia: W.B. Saunders Co., 1966.

53. Bollinger, Rick L., Patricia F. Waugh, and Anita F. Zatz. *Communication Management of the Geriatric Patient.* Danville, Ill.: Interstate Printers & Publishers, Inc., 1977.

54. Bonney, Merl. *Mental Health in Education.* Rockleigh, N.J.: Allyn and Bacon, Inc., 1960.

55. Bookmiller, Mae, George Bowen, and Dolores Carpenter. *Textbook of Obstetrics and Obstetric Nursing.* Philadelphia: W.B. Saunders Co., 1967.

56. Bordicks, Katherine. *Patterns of Shock.* New York: Macmillan Publishing Co., 1965.

57. Botwinick, Bob. *Aging and Behavior: A Comprehensive Integration of Research Findings.* New York: Springer Publishing Co., 1978.

58. Bower, Fay L., and Marie Scott Brown. *Health Maintenance.* New York: John Wiley & Sons, Inc., 1980.

59. Brain, Lord, and John N. Walton. *Brain Diseases of the Nervous System.* New York: Oxford University Press, 1969.

60. Brainard, John B. *Control of Migraine.* New York: W.W. Norton and Co., Inc., 1979.

61. Brams, William. *Managing Your Coronary.* Philadelphia: J.B. Lippincott Co., 1966.

62. Brauer, Earle. *Your Skin and Hair.* London: Macmillan Publishing Co., 1969.

63. Braun, Carl, and Gerald Diettert. *Coronary Care Unit Nursing, Part I.* Missoula, Mont.: Montana Clinic Foundation, 1968.

64. Braverman, Irvin. *Skin Signs of Systemic Disease.* Philadelphia: W.B. Saunders Co., 1970.

65. Bray, Patrick. *Neurology in Pediatrics.* Chicago: Year Book Medical Publishers, Inc., 1969.

66. Breckenridge, Marina E., and Margaret N. Murphy. *Growth and Development of the Young Child.* Philadelphia: W.B. Saunders Co., 1969.

67. Brichall, Ellen, and Noll Gerson. *Sex and the Adult Woman.* New York: Gilbert Press, 1965.

68. Brighthill, Charles. *Man and Leisure.* Englewood Cliffs, N.J.: Prentice-Hall, Inc., 1961.

69. Brown, Jason W. *Aphasia, Apraxia and Agnosia.* Springfield, Ill.: Charles C. Thomas Publisher, 1972.

70. Brughera-Jones, Antonella. *Manual of Laboratory Medicine.* New York: Harper & Row, Publishers, Inc., 1970.

71. Brundage, Dorothy. *Nursing Management of Renal Problems.* St. Louis: C.V. Mosby Co., 1976.

72. Brunner, Lillian, Charles Emerson, L. Kraeer Ferguson, and Doris Suddarth. *Textbook of Medical-Surgical Nursing.* Philadelphia: J.B. Lippincott Co., 1980.

73. Brunner, Lillian, and Doris Suddarth. *The Lippincott Manual of Nursing Practice.* Philadelphia: J.B. Lippincott Co., 1982.

74. Bryant, Richard, and Anna Overland. *Obstetric Management and Nursing.* Philadelphia: F.A. Davis Co., 1964.

75. Buckley, Joseph. *The Retirement Handbook.* New York: Harper & Row, Publishers, Inc., 1967.

76. Burd, Shirley, and Margaret Marshall. *Some Clinical Approaches to Psychiatric Nursing.* New York: Macmillan Publishing Co., 1963.

77. Burgess, Ann, and Aaron Lazare. *Psychiatric Nursing in the Hospital and the Community.* Englewood Cliffs, N.J.: Prentice-Hall, Inc., 1973.

78. Burrell, Lenette Owens, and Zeb L. Burrell, Jr. *Critical Care.* St. Louis: C.V. Mosby Co., 1982.

79. Buscaglia, Leo F. *Personhood: The Art of Being Fully Human.* New York: Fawcett Columbine, 1978.

80. Byers, Virginia. *Nursing Observation.* Dubuque, Iowa: William C. Brown Co., 1971.

81. Byrd, Oliver. *Health.* Philadelphia: W.B. Saunders Co., 1971.

82. Byrne, Marjorie, and Lydia Thompson. *Key Concepts for the Study and Practice of Nursing.* St. Louis: C.V. Mosby Co., 1978.

83. Callahan, Sidney Cornelia. *Parenting, Principles and Politics of Parenthood.* Baltimore: Penguin Books, Inc., 1974.

84. Cameron, Stewart, Allison Russell, and Diana Sale. *Nephrology for Nurses.* New York: Medical Examination Publishing Co., Inc., 1976.

85. Cammer, Leonard. *Up from Depression.* New York: Simon and Schuster, 1971.

86. Campbell, Claire. *Nursing Diagnosis and Intervention in Nursing Practice.* New York: John Wiley & Sons, Inc., 1978.

87. Cannon, Walter. *The Wisdom of the Body.* New York: W.W. Norton & Co., Inc., 1939.

88. Capell, Peter T., and David B. Case. *Ambulatory Care Manual for Nurse Practitioners.* New York: J.B. Lippincott Co., 1976.

89. Carlson, Judith H., Carol A. Craft, and Anne D. McGuire. *Nursing Diagnosis.* Philadelphia: W.B. Saunders Co., 1982.

90. Castles, Mary Reardon, and Ruth Beckmann Murray. *Dying In An Institution: Nurse/Patient Perspectives.* New York: Appleton-Century-Crofts, 1979.

91. Chapman, Frederick. *Recreation Activities for the Handicapped.* New York: Ronald Press, 1960.

92. Chess, Stella, Alexander Thomas, and Herbert Berch. *Your Child Is a Person.* New York: Viking Press, 1965.

93. Child Study Association of America, Inc. *You, Your Child and Drugs.* New York: Child Study Press, 1971.

94. Chinn, Peggy L. *Child Health Maintenance: Concepts in Family-Centered Care.* St. Louis: C.V. Mosby Co., 1974.

95. Chinn, Peggy L. *Child Health Maintenance: A Guide to Clinical Assessment.* St. Louis: C.V. Mosby Co., 1979.

96. Chinn, Peggy. *Advances in Nursing Theory Development.* Rockville, Md.: Aspen Systems Corp., 1983.

97. Chyatte, Samuel. *On Borrowed Time: Living With Hemodialysis.* Oradell, N.J.: Medical Economics Co., 1979.

98. Clark, Ann L. *Culture, Child rearing, Health Professionals.* Philadelphia: F.A. Davis Co., 1978.

99. Clark, Marguerita. *Why So Tired? The Ways of Fatigue and the Ways of Energy.* New York: Duell, Sloan and Pearce, 1962.

100. Clements, H. *What to Do about a Bad Back and Disc Trouble.* New York: Drake Publishers, 1972.

101. Coffin, Margaret. *Nursing Observations of the Young Patient.* Dubuque, Iowa: William C. Brown Co., 1970.

102. Cohen, Sidney. *The Drug Dilemma.* New York: McGraw-Hill Book Co., 1969.

103. Cohen, Yehudi. *Social Structure and Personality.* New York: Holt, Rinehart and Winston, 1961.

104. Cole, Warren H., and Charles B. Puestow. *Emergency Care: Surgical and Medical.* New York: Appleton-Century-Crofts, 1972.

105. Coleman, James. *Psychology and Effective Behavior.* Glenview, Ill.: Scott, Foresman & Co., 1969.

106. Collins, Daniel. *Your Teeth*. Garden City, N.Y.: Doubleday & Co., Inc., 1967.

107. Colman, Arthur, and Libby Coleman. *Pregnancy: The Psychological Experience*. New York: Herder and Herder, 1971.

108. Colorado State Department of Public Health. *Elementary Rehabilitation Nursing Care*. Washington, D.C.: U.S. Department of Health, Education and Welfare, 1967.

109. Conway, Barbara Lang. *Carini and Owen's Neurological and Neurosurgical Nursing*. St. Louis: C.V. Mosby Co., 1978.

110. Cooper, Kenneth H. *The Aerobics Program for Total Well-Being*. New York: M. Evans and Co., Inc., 1982.

111. Cooper, Kenneth H. *The Aerobics Way*. New York: M. Evans and Co., Inc., 1978.

112. Cooper, Signe Skott. *Contemporary Nursing Practice*. New York: McGraw-Hill Book Co., 1970.

113. Cope, Sir Zackery. *The Early Diagnosis of the Acute Abdomen*. London: Oxford University Press, 1972.

114. Craig, William Stuart. *Care of the Newly Born Infant*. Baltimore: Williams & Wilkins Co., 1969.

115. Creighton, Helen. *Law Every Nurse Should Know*. Philadelphia: W.B. Saunders Co., 1981.

116. Crenshaw, Andrew Hoyt. *Campbell's Operative Orthopedics*, Vol. 1. St. Louis: C.V. Mosby Co., 1971.

117. Crews, Eli Rush. *A Practical Manual for the Treatment of Burns*. Springfield, Ill.: Charles C. Thomas Publisher, 1967.

118. Crohn, Burrell. *Understand Your Ulcer*. New York: Sheridan House Publishers, 1969.

119. Culver, Vivian. *Modern Bedside Nursing*. Philadelphia: W.B. Saunders Co., 1969.

120. Danforth, David. *Textbook of Obstetrics and Gynecology*. New York: Harper & Row Publishers, Inc., 1966.

121. Dangott, Lillian R., and Richard A. Kalish. *A Time to Enjoy the Pleasures of Aging*. Englewood Cliffs, N.J.: Prentice-Hall, Inc., 1979.

122. Davis, Maxine. *Every Woman's Book of Health*. New York: McGraw-Hill Book Co., 1969.

123. Davis, M. Edward, and Reva Rubin. *Obstetrics for Nurses*. Philadelphia: W.B. Saunders Co., 1966.

124. DeBeauvoir, Simone. *The Coming of Age*. New York: G.P. Putnam's Sons, 1972.

125. DeGowin, Elmer, and Richard DeGowin. *Bedside Diagnostic Examination*. New York: Macmillan Publishing Co., 1981.

126. Delacato, Carl H. *The Diagnosis and Treatment of Speech and Reading Problems*. Springfield, Ill.: Charles C. Thomas Publisher, 1965.

127. De Levita, David. *The Concept of Identity*. Paris: Mouton and Co., 1965.

128. Delp, Mahlon, and Robert Manning. *Major's Physical Diagnosis*. Philadelphia: W.B. Saunders Co., 1968.

129. DeMyer, William. *Technique of the Neurological Examination*. New York: McGraw-Hill Book Co., 1969.

130. Dennis, Lorraine. *Psychology of Human Behavior for Nurses*. Philadelphia: W.B. Saunders Co., 1967.

131. De Ropp, Robert. *Drugs and the Mind*. New York: Grove Press, Inc., 1961.

132. Dewey, John. *How We Think*. Boston: D.C. Heath & Co., 1933.

133. Dickason, Elizabeth J., and Martha Olsen Schult. *Maternal and Infant Care*. New York: McGraw-Hill Book Co., 1975.

134. Diehl, Harold S., and Stewart Thompson. *Textbook of Healthful Living*. New York: McGraw-Hill Book Co., 1960.

135. Diehl, Harold S., and Willard Dalrymple. *Healthful Living*. New York: McGraw-Hill Book Co., 1968.

136. Diekelmann, Nancy. *Primary Health Care of the Well Adult*. New York: McGraw-Hill Book Co., 1977.

137. Dolger, Henry, and Bernard Seeman. *How to Live with Diabetes*. New York: Pyramid Publications, Inc., 1970.

138. DuGas, Beverly Witter. *Introduction to Patient Care: A Comprehensive Approach to Nursing*. Philadelphia: W.B. Saunders Co., 1977.

139. Duke-Elder, Sir Stewart. *Parson's Diseases of the Eye*. London: J.&A. Churchill Co., 1970.

140. Dunn, Halbert. *High-Level Wellness*. Arlington, Va.: R.W. Beatty Co., 1961.

141. Dushkin, David. *Psychology Today: An Introduction*. Del Mar, Calif.: CRM Books, 1970.

142. Duvall, Evelyn Millis. *Parent and Teenager, Living and Loving*. Nashville, Tenn.: Broadman Press, 1976.

143. Eckelberry, Grace. *Administration of Comprehensive Nursing*. New York: Appleton-Century-Crofts, 1971.

144. Elhart, Dorothy. *Scientific Principles in Nursing*. St. Louis: C.V. Mosby Co., 1978.

145. Elliott, Frank. *Clinical Neurology*. Philadelphia: W.B. Saunders Co., 1964.

146. Engeelberg, Hyman, and Henry F. Greenberg. *The Doctor's Modern Heart At-*

tack Prevention Program. New York: Funk & Wagnalls, 1974.

147. Epp, Theodore. *Why Do Christians Suffer?* Lincoln, Neb.: Good News Broadcasting Association, Inc., 1970.

148. Erikson, Erik. *Childhood and Society.* New York: W.W. Norton & Co., Inc., 1963.

149. Erikson, Erik. *Adulthood.* New York: W.W. Norton & Co., Inc., 1976.

150. Erven, Lawrence W. *First Aid and Emergency Rescue.* Beverly Hills, Calif.: Glencoe Press, 1970.

151. Fabricant, Noah D. and Groff Conklin. *The Dangerous Cold.* New York: Macmillan Publishing Co., 1965.

152. Falk, Abraham. *Diagnostic Standards and Classification of Tuberculosis.* New York: National Tuberculosis and Respiratory Disease Association, 1969.

153. Farley, John, and Howard Mold. *The Teaching Role.* St. Paul, Minn.: College of St. Thomas, 1968.

154. Feifel, Herman, *The Meaning of Death.* New York: McGrawHill Book Co., 1965.

155. Finnerty, Frank, Jr., and Shirley Motter Linde. *High Blood Pressure.* New York: David McKay Co., Inc., and Pavilion Publishing Co., Inc., 1975.

156. Fischer, Valentia, and Arlene Connolly. *Promotion of Physical Comfort and Safety.* Dubuque, Iowa: W.C. Brown Publishers, 1970.

157. Fish, Sharon, and Judith Shelly. *Spiritual Care: The Nurse's Role.* Downer's Grove, Ill.: Varsity Press, 1979.

158. Fishbein, Anna Mantel, *Modern Woman's Medical Encyclopedia.* Garden City, N.Y.: Doubleday & Co., Inc. 1966.

159. Fishbein, Morris, and Justin Fishbein. *Fishbein's Illustrated Medical and Health Encyclopeida: Family Health Guide Edition.* New York: H.S. Stuttman, 1978.

160. Fitzpatrick, Elise, Sharon Reeder, and Luigi Mastroianni. *Maternity Nursing.* Philadelphia: J.B. Lippincott Co., 1980.

161. Fleming, Mary, and Marion Benson. *Home Nursing Handbook.* Boston: D.C. Heath and Co., 1961.

162. Flynn, Patricia Anne Randolph. *Holistic Health: The Art and Science of Care.* Bowie, Md.: Prentice-Hall Publishing and Communications Co., 1980.

163. Foa, Edna B. *Handbook of Behavioral Interventions: A Clinical Guide.* New York: John Wiley & Sons, Inc., 1980.

164. Fordtran, John S., and Marvin H. Sleisenger. *Gastrointestinal Disease.* Philadelphia: W.B. Saunders Co., 1978.

165. Foreyt, John Paul. *Behavioral Treatments of Obesity.* New York: Pergamon Press, 1977.

166. Foster, Daniel W. *A Layman's Guide to Modern Medicine.* New York: Simon and Schuster, 1980.

167. Fowler, Noble O. *Cardiac Diagnosis and Treatment.* Hagerstown, Md.: Harper & Row Publishers, Inc., 1976.

168. Francis, Gloria, and Barbara Munjas. *Promoting Psychological Comfort.* Dubuque, Iowa: William C. Brown Co., 1968.

169. Francone, Clarice, and Stanley Jacob. *Laboratory Manual of Structure and Function in Man.* Philadelphia: W.B. Saunders Co., 1970.

170. Freedman, Alfred, and Harold Kaplan. *Comprehensive Textbook of Psychiatry.* Baltimore: Williams & Wilkins Co., 1974.

171. Freeman, Ruth, and Janet Heinrich. *Community Health Nursing Practice.* Philadelphia: W.B. Saunders Co., 1981.

172. Freeman, Ruth. *Public Health Nursing Practice.* Philadelphia: W.B. Saunders Co., 1957.

173. French, Ruth. *Guide to Diagnostic Procedures.* New York: McGraw-Hill Book Co., 1980.

174. Fried, Barbara. *The Middle-Age Crisis.* New York: Harper & Row, Publishers, Inc., 1967.

175. Friel, John P., editor. *Dorland Illustrated Medical Dictionary,* 26th edition. Philadelphia: W.B. Saunders Co., 1981.

176. Frohlich, Edward. *Pathophysiology: Altered Regulatory Mechanism in Disease.* Philadelphia: J.B. Lippincott Co., 1972.

177. Fromm, Erich. *The Art of Loving.* New York: Bantam Books, Inc., 1963.

178. Fromme, Allan. *The Ability to Love.* New York: Farrar, Straus and Giroux, 1963.

179. Fuerst, Elinor, LuVerne Wolff, and Marlene H. Weitzel. *Fundamentals of Nursing.* Philadelphia: J.B. Lippincott Co., 1974.

180. Galton, Lawrence. *Don't Give Up on an Aging Parent.* New York: Crown Publishers, Inc., 1975.

181. Galton, Lawrence. *The Silent Disease: Hypertension.* New York: Crown Publishers, Inc., 1973.

182. Ganong, William. *Review of Medical Physiology.* Los Altos, Calif.: Lange Medical Publishers, 1969.

183. Garb, Solomon. *Laboratory Tests in Common Use.* New York: Springer Publishing Co., Inc., 1976.

184. Gardner, A. Ward, and Peter Roylance. *New Essential First Aid.* Boston: Little, Brown & Co., 1971.

185. Gebbie, Kristine, and Mary Ann Lavin. *Classification of Nursing Diagnosis: Proceedings of the First National Conference.* St. Louis: C.V. Mosby Co., 1975.

186. Gebbie, Kristine M. *Summary of the Second National Conference: Classification of Nursing Diagnosis.* St. Louis: Clearinghouse, National Group for Classification of Nursing Diagnoses, 1976.

187. George, Julia B., and Nursing Theories Conference Group. *Nursing Theories: The Base for Professional Nursing Practice.* Englewood Cliffs, N.J.: Prentice-Hall, Inc., 1980.

188. Gesell, Arnold Lucius. *Gesell and Amatruda's Developmental Diagnosis: The Evaluation and Management of Normal and Abnormal Neuropsychologic Development in Infancy and Early Childhood.* Hagerstown, Md.: Harper & Row, Publishers, Inc., 1975.

189. Gifford-Jones. *Hysterectomy.* Toronto: University of Toronto Press, 1961.

190. Gilbert, Arlene. *You Can Do It from a Wheelchair.* New York: Arlington House Publishers, 1973.

191. Gilmer, B. von Haller. *Applied Psychology: Problems in Living and Work.* New York: McGraw-Hill Book Co., 1967.

192. Given, Barbara, and Sandra Simmons. *Nursing Care of the Patient with Gastrointestinal Disorders.* St. Louis: C.V. Mosby Co., 1971.

193. Goode, William. *The Dynamics of Modern Society.* New York: Atherton Press, 1968.

194. Goodrich, Frederick. *Infant Care.* Englewood Cliffs, N.J.: Prentice-Hall, Inc., 1968.

195. Gordon, David. *Overcoming the Fear of Death.* New York: Macmillan Publishing Co., 1970.

196. Gordon, Marjorie. *Nursing Diagnosis: Process and Application.* New York: McGraw-Hill Book Co., 1982.

197. Gray, Madeline. *The Normal Woman.* New York: Charles Scribner's Sons, 1967.

198. Greenhill, Jacob Pearl, and Emanuel Friedman. *Biological Principles and Modern Practice of Obstetrics.* Philadelphia: W.B. Saunders Co., 1974.

199. Grenard, Steve, Gustav Beck, and George Rich. *Introduction to Respiratory Therapy: Workbook Study Guide.* New York: Glenn Educational Medical Services, Inc., 1971.

200. Guitar, Mary Anne. *The Young Marriage.* New York: Doubleday & Co., 1968.

201. Gutch, C.F., and Martha H. Stoner. *Review of Hemodialysis for Nurses and Dialysis Personnel.* St. Louis: C.V. Mosby Co., 1975.

202. Guthrie, Diana W., and Richard A. Guthrie. *Nursing Management of Diabetes Mellitus.* St. Louis: C.V. Mosby Co., 1977.

203. Guyton, Arthur. *Textbook of Medical Physiology.* Philadelphia: W.B. Saunders Co., 1976.

204. Gyetvan, Mary, and Barbara McVan. *Documenting Patient Care Responsibility: Nursing Skillbook.* Horsham, Pa: Intermed Communications, Inc., 1978.

205. Haas, Albert. *Essentials of Living with pulmonary Emphysema.* New York: Institute of Physical Medicine and Rehabilitation, 1963.

206. Hall, Joanne E., and Barbara R. Weaver. *Distributive Nursing Practice: A Systems Approach to Community Health.* Philadelphia: J.B. Lippincott Co., 1977.

207. Hall, Joanne E., and Barbara R. Weaver. *Nursing of Families in Crisis.* Philadelphia: J.B. Lippincott Co., 1974.

208. Hall, Robert. *Nine Months' Reading: A Medical Guide for Pregnant Women.* Garden City, N.Y.: Doubleday & Co., Inc., 1982.

209. Halpern, Susan, Dorothy Hicks, and Theresa Crenshaw. *Rape: Helping the Victim.* Oradell, N. J.: Medical Economics Co., 1978.

210. Hamilton, James Alexander. *Post-Partum Psychiatric Problems.* St. Louis: C.V. Mosby Co., 1962.

211. Hampers, Constantine L., and Eugene Schupak. *Long-Term Hemodialysis.* New York: Grune & Stratton, 1967.

212. Hansten, Philip D. *Drug Interactions.* Philadelphia: Lea & Febiger Co., 1979.

213. Harris, Ann C., and Kathleen McCarthy. *Mental Health Practice for Community Nurses.* New York: Springer Publishing Co., 1981.

214. Hawkins, Joellen Watson, and Loretta Pierfedeici Higgins. *Maternity and Gynecological Nursing: Women's Health Care.* Philadelphia: J.B. Lippincott Co., 1981.

215. Hays, Samhammer Joyce, and Kenneth Larson. *Interacting with Patients.* New York: Macmillan Publishing Co., 1965.

216. Head, Henry. *Aphasia and Kindred Disorders of Speech.* London: Hafner Publishing Co., 1963.

217. Heather, Arthur. *Manual of Care for the Disabled Patient.* New York: Macmillan Publishing Co., 1960.

218. Heidgerken, Loretta. *Teaching and Learning in Schools of Nursing.* Philadelphia: J.B. Lippincott Co., 1965.

219. Henderson, John. *Emergency Medical Guide*. St. Louis: McGraw-Hill Book Co., 1973.

220. Henderson, Virginia. *Basic Principles of Nursing Care*. New York: S. Karger Basil, 1970.

221. Henderson, Virginia. *The Nature of Nursing*. London: Macmillan & Co., 1970.

222. Hess, Patricia A., and Candra Day. *Understanding the Aging Patient*. Bowie, Md.: Robert J. Brady Co., 1977.

223. Hoff, Ebbie Curtis. *Alcoholism: The Hidden Addiction*. New York: Seabury Press, 1974.

224. Hoff, Lee Ann. *People in Crisis: Understanding and Helping*. Menlo Park, Calif.: Addison-Wesley Publishing Co., Inc., 1978.

225. Hofling, Charles, and Joan J. Kyes. *Basic Psychiatric Concepts in Nursing*. Philadelphia: J.B. Lippincott Co., 1980.

226. Hogeman, Karen, and Warp Eha. *Adaptations and Techniques for the Disabled Homemaker*. Minneapolis, Minn.: Sister Kenny Institute, 1976.

227. Holtgrew, Marian. *A Guide for Public Health Nurses Working with Mentally Retarded Children*. Washington, D.C.: U.S. Government Printing Office, 1964.

228. Holvey, David. *The Merck Manual*. Rahway, N.J.: Merck Sharp & Dohme Research Laboratories, 1972.

229. Horracks, John. *The Psychology of Adolescence*. Boston: Houghton Mifflin Co., 1962.

230. Hudak, Carolyn M., Editor. *Critical Care Nursing*. Philadelphia: J.B. Lippincott Co., 1977.

231. Hull, Edgar, and Cecilia Perrodin. *Medical Nursing*. Philadelphia: F.A. Davis Co., 1960.

232. Hunt, Robert. *Personalities and Culture*. New York: Natural History Press, 1967.

233. Hurlock, Elizabeth. *Adolescent Development*. New York: McGraw-Hill Book Co., 1973.

234. Hurlock, Elizabeth. *Child Growth and Development*. New York: McGraw-Hill Book Co., 1970.

235. Hurst, J. Willis, and R. Bruce Logue. *The Heart*. New York: McGraw-Hill Book Co., 1974.

236. Hurst, J. Willis, and Robert Schlant. *Examination of the Heart: Inspection and Palpitation of the Anterior Chest*. New York: American Heart Association, 1967.

237. Illingworth, Ronald. *Common Symptoms of Disease in Children*. Philadelphia: F.A. Davis Co., 1969.

238. Illingworth, Ronald, and Cynthia Illingworth. *Babies and Young Children*. London: Churchill Livingston, Inc., 1972.

239. Ingalls, A. Jay, and M. Constance Salerno. *Maternal and Child Health Nursing*. St. Louis: C.V. Mosby Co., 1979.

240. Ingram, Madeline. *Principles and Techniques of Psychiatric Nursing*. Philadelphia: W.B. Saunders Co., 1960.

241. Iorio, Josephine. *Childbirth: Family-Centered Nursing*. St. Louis: C.V. Mosby Co., 1975.

242. Irving, Susan. *Basic Psychiatric Nursing*. Philadelphia: W.B. Saunders Co., 1978.

243. Israel, S. Leon. *Menstrual Disorders and Sterility*. New York: Harper & Row Publishers, Inc., 1967.

244. Jackson, Eugene. *Nursing Skillbook: Assessing Vital Functions Accurately*. Horsham, Pa.: Intermed Communications, Inc., 1978.

245. Jackson, Eugene. *Nursing Skillbook: Giving Cardiovascular Drugs Safely*. Horsham, Pa.: Intermed Communications, Inc., 1978.

246. Jackson, Eugene. *Nursing Skillbook: Giving Emergency Care Competently*. Horsham, Pa.: Intermed Communications, Inc., 1978.

247. Jackson, Eugene. *Nursing Skillbook: Monitoring Fluid and Electrolytes Precisely*. Horsham, Pa.: Intermed Communications, Inc., 1978.

248. Jackson, Eugene. *Using Crisis Intervention Wisely*. Horsham, Pa.: Nursing 81 Books, Intermed Communications, Inc., 1980.

249. Johanson, Brenda Crispell, Consuelo Urtula Dungca, Denise Hoffmeister, and Sara Jeanne Wells. *Standards for Critical Care*. St. Louis: C.V. Mosby Co., 1981.

250. Johnson, Mae, Mary David, and Mary Bilitch. *Problem Solving in Nursing Practice*. Dubuque, Iowa: William C. Brown Co., 1970.

251. Johnson, Suzanne Hall. *High-Risk Parenting: Nursing Assessment and Strategies for the Family At-Risk*. Philadelphia: J.B. Lippincott Co., 1979.

252. Jones, W. Gifford. *On Being a Woman: The Modern Woman's Guide to Gynecology*. New York: Macmillan Publishing Co., 1969.

253. Judge, Richard D., and George D. Zuidema. *Physical Diagnosis: A Physiologic Approach to the Clinical Examination*. Boston: Little, Brown & Co., 1974.

254. Kalmer, John. *Clinical Diagnosis by Laboratory Examination*. New York: Appleton-Century-Crofts, 1961.

255. Kaplan, Norman, and Ellin Lieberman. *Clinical Hypertension*. Baltimore: Williams & Wilkins Co., 1982.

256. Kark, Robert, and James Lawrence. *A Primer of Urinalysis*. New York: Harper & Row, Publishers, Inc., 1964.

257. Kelly, Lucie Young. *Dimensions of Professional Nursing.* New York: Macmillan Publishing Co., 1975.

258. Kempe, C. Henry, Henry K. Silver, and Donough O'Brien. *Current Pediatric Diagnosis and Treatment,* 2nd edition. Los Altos, Calif.: Lange Medical Publications, 1972.

259. Kempe, Ruth S., and C. Henry Kempe. *Child Abuse.* Cambridge, Mass.: Harvard University Press, 1978.

260. Kendig, Edwin. *Disorders of the Respiratory Tract in Children.* Philadelphia: W.B. Saunders Co., 1967.

261. Kendler, Howard. *Basic Psychology.* New York: Appleton-Century-Crofts, 1968.

262. Kennedy, Eugene. *Sexual Counseling.* New York: The Seabury Press, 1977.

263. Kennedy, Joseph. *Relax and Live.* Englewood Cliffs, N.J.: Prentice-Hall, Inc., 1961.

264. Kenyon, Herbert. *The Prostate Gland.* New York: Random House, 1970.

265. Keuhnelian, John, and Virginia Sanders. *Urologic Nursing.* New York: Macmillan Publishing Co., 1970.

266. Kim, MiJa, and Derry Ann Mortiz. *Classification of Nursing Diagnosis: Proceedings of the Third and Fourth National Conferences.* New York: McGraw-Hill Book Co., 1982.

267. King, Imogene. *Toward a Theory of Nursing: General Concepts of Human Behavior.* New York: John Wiley & Sons, Inc., 1971.

268. Kirk, Samuel, Merle Karnes, and Winifred Kirk. *You and Your Retarded Child.* Palo Alto, Calif.: Pacific Books Publishers, 1968.

269. Knight, James. *Conscience and Guilt.* New York: Appleton-Century-Crofts, 1969.

270. Knopf, Olga. *Successful Aging: The Facts and Fallacies of Growing Old.* New York: Viking Press, 1975.

271. Kordels, Lelord. *Natural Folk Remedies.* New York: G.P. Putnam's Sons, 1974.

272. Kozier, Barbara, and Glenora Lee Erb. *Fundamentals of Nursing Concepts and Procedures.* Reading, Mass.: Addison Wesley Publishing Co., 1979.

273. Krantzler, Mel. *Creative Divorce.* New York: M. Evans and Co., Inc., 1974.

271. Kraus, Hans. *Backache: Stress and Tension.* New York: Simon and Schuster, 1965.

275. Krause, Marie. *Food, Nutrition and Diet Therapy.* Philadelphia: W.B. Saunders Co., 1979.

276. Kroger, William. *Psychosomatic Obstetrics, Gynecology and Endocrinology.* Springfield, Ill.: Charles C. Thomas Publisher, 1962.

277. Krueger, Judith Amerkan, and Janis Compton Ray. *Endocrine Problems in Nursing.* St. Louis: C.V. Mosby Co., 1976.

278. Krupp, Marcus, and Milton Chatton. *Current Medical Diagnosis and Treatment.* Los Altos, Calif.: Lange Medical Publications, 1982.

279. Kubler-Ross, Elizabeth. *Living with Death and Dying.* New York: Macmillan Publishing Co., 1981.

280. Laing, J. Ellsworth, and Joyce Harvey. *The Management and Nursing of Burns.* London: English Universities Press, 1967.

281. Lally, James. *The Over 50 Health Manual.* Englewood Cliffs, N.J.: Prentice-Hall, Inc., 1961.

282. Lamb, Carolyn editor. *Patient Care Flow Chart Manual.* Conn.: Patient Care Publications, Inc., 1980.

283. Lamb, Lawrence. *Your Heart and How to Live with It.* New York: Viking Press, 1969.

284. Lamb, Tony, and Dave Duffy. *The Retirement Threat.* Los Angeles: J.P. Tarcher, Inc., 1977.

285. Landis, Judson, and Mary Landis. *Personal Adjustment, Marriage, and Family Living.* Englewood Cliffs, N.J.: Prentice-Hall, Inc., 1972.

286. Larson, Carroll, and Marjorie Gould. *Orthopedic Nursing.* St. Louis: C.V. Mosby Co., 1978.

287. Lascelles, P.T., and D. Donaldson. *Diagnostic Tests.* New York: G.P. Putnam's Sons, 1971.

288. Latham, Helen C. *Pediatric Nursing.* St. Louis: C.V. Mosby Co., 1977.

289. Lekoff, William, Bernard Segal, and Lawrence Galton. *Your Heart.* Philadelphia: J.B. Lippincott Co., 1972.

290. Lennard, Henry, Leon Epstein, Arnold Bernstein, and Donald Ransom. *Mystification and Drug Abuse.* San Francisco: Jossey-Bass, Inc., 1971.

291. Lerch, Constance. *Maternity Nursing.* St. Louis: C.V. Mosby Co., 1978.

292. Lesnik, Milton, and Bernice Anderson. *Nursing Practice and The Law.* Philadelphia: J.B. Lippincott Co., 1969.

293. Lewis, Jerry. *How's Your Family: A Guide to Identifying Your Family's Strengths and Weaknesses.* New York: Brunner/Mazel, Inc., 1979.

294. Lewis, Lucile. *Planning Patient Care.* Dubuque, Iowa: William C. Brown Co., 1970.

295. Lewy, Robert. *Preventive Primary Medicine.* Boston: Little, Brown & Co., 1980.

296. Lidz, Theodore. *The Person: His Development Throughout the Life Cycle.* New York: Basic Books, 1968.

297. Lipkin, Gladys, and Robert Cohen. *Effective Approaches to Patient's Behavior.* New York: Springer Publishing Co., Inc., 1973.

298. Little, Dolores, and Doris Carnevali. *Nursing Care Planning.* Philadelphia: J.B. Lippincott Co., 1976.

299. Loebl, Suzanne, George Spratto, and Estelle Heckheime. *The Nurses' Drug Handbook,* 3rd edition. New York: John Wiley & Sons, Inc., 1983.

300. Louria, Donald. *Overcoming Drugs.* New York: McGraw-Hill Book Co., 1971.

301. Lowsley, Oswald, and Thomas Kirwin. *Clinical Urology,* vol. 2. Baltimore: Williams & Wilkins Co., 1956.

302. Luce, Gay Gaer, and Julius Segal. *Sleep.* New York: Coward-McCann, Inc., 1966.

303. Luce, Gay Gaer, and Julius Segal. *Insomnia: The Guide for Troubled Sleepers.* Garden City, N.Y.: Doubleday & Co., Inc., 1969.

304. Luce, Henry. *The World's Great Religions.* New York: Golden Press, 1965.

305. Luckmann, Joan, and Karen Creason Sorensen. *Medical-Surgical Nursing: A Psychophysiologic Approach.* Philadelphia: W.B. Saunders Co., 1974.

306. Lyght, Charles. *The Merck Manual of Diagnosis and Therapy.* Rahway, N.J. Merck Sharp & Dohme Research Laboratories, 1956.

307. Lynn, David B. *The Father: His Role in Child Development* Monterey, Calif.: Brooks/Cole Publishing Co., 1974.

308. Lysaught, Jerome P. *An Abstract for Action.* St. Louis: McGraw-Hill Book Co., 1970.

309. MacBryde, Cyril M. *Signs and Symptoms: Applied Pathologic Physiology and Clinical Interpretation.* Philadelphia: J.B. Lippincott Co., 1964.

310. McCaffery, Margo. *Nursing Management of the Patient with Pain.* Philadelphia: J.B. Lippincott Co., 1972.

311. McDonald, Linda. *Contact Lenses: How to Wear Them Successfully.* Garden City, N.Y.: Doubleday & Co., Inc., 1972.

312. McDougall, Deborah, and Marjorie Cantor. *Achieving Nursing Care Standards: Internal and External.* Wakefield, Mass.: Nursing Resources, 1978.

313. McFarlane, Judith M., Betty Jo Whitson, and Lucy M. Hartley. *Contemporary Pediatric Nursing: A Conceptual Approach.* New York: John Wiley & Sons, Inc., 1980.

314. McVan, Barbara. *Nursing Skillbook: Helping Cancer Patients Effectively.* Horsham, Pa.: Intermed Communications, Inc., 1977.

315. Magda, Arnold. *Emotion and Personality,* vol. 1. New York: Columbia University Press, 1960.

316. Mager, Robert F. *Preparing Instructional Objectives.* Palo Alto, Calif.: Fearon Publishers, 1962.

317. Maier, Norman. *Frustration: The Study of Behavior Without a Goal.* New York: McGraw-Hill Book Co., 1949.

318. Maloney, Elizabeth. *Interpersonal Relations.* Dubuque, Iowa: William C. Brown Co., 1966.

319. Maltz, Maxwell. *Creative Living for Today.* New York: Pocket Books, 1970.

320. Maltz, Maxwell. *Psycho-Cybernetics.* Englewood Cliffs, N.J.: Prentice-Hall, Inc., 1960.

321. Manfreda, Marguerita, and Sydney D. Krampetz. *Psychiatric Nursing.* Philadelphia: F.A. Davis Co., 1977.

322. Marlow, Dorothy. *Textbook of Pediatric Nursing.* Philadelphia: W.B. Saunders Co., 1973.

323. Marlow, Dorothy, and Gladys Sellew. *Textbook of Pediatric Nursing.* Philadelphia: W.B. Saunders Co., 1977.

324. Maroon, Joseph. *What You Can Do About Cancer.* Garden City, N.Y.: Doubleday & Co., Inc., 1969.

325. Marriner, Ann. *Guide to Nursing Management.* St. Louis: C.V. Mosby Co., 1980.

326. Marriner, Ann. *The Nursing Process.* St. Louis: C.V. Mosby Co., 1979.

327. Marvin, H.M. *Your Heart.* Garden City, N.Y.: Doubleday & Co., Inc., 1960.

328. Maslow, Abraham. *Motivation and Personality.* New York: Harper & Brothers, 1970.

329. Matheney, Ruth, Breda Nolan, Alice Hogan, and Gerald Griffin. *Fundamentals of Patient-Centered Nursing.* St. Louis: C.V. Mosby Co., 1972.

330. May, Elizabeth Eckhardt, Neva R. Waggoner, and Eleanor Boethke. *Homemaking for the Handicapped.* New York: Dodd, Mead and Company, 1966.

331. May, Rollo. *Psychology and the Human Dilemma.* Princeton, N.J.: D. Van Nostrand Co., Inc., 1966.

332. May, Rollo. *The Meaning of Anxiety.* New York: W.W. Norton and Co., Inc., 1977.

333. Mayers, Marlene Glover. *A Systematic Approach to the Nursing Care Plan.* New York: Appleton-Century-Crofts, 1978.

334. Mayers, Marlene G., Ronald B. Norby, and Anita B. Watson. *Quality Assurance for Patient Care: Nursing Perspectives.* New York: Appleton-Century-Crofts, 1977.

335. Mayers, Marlene, and El Camino Hospital Nursing Staff. *Standard Nursing Care Plans*, vol 1. San Jose, Calif.: K/P Company Medical Systems, 1974.

336. Mayers, Marlene, and El Camino Hospital Nursing Staff. *Standard Nursing Care Plans*, vol 2. San Jose, Calif.: K/P Company Medical Systems, 1975.

337. Meares, Ainslie. *Relief Without Drugs*. Garden City, N.Y.: Doubleday & Co., Inc., 1967.

338. Megargie, Edwin, and Jack Hokanson. *The Dynamics of Aggression*. New York: Harper & Row, Publishers, Inc., 1970.

339. Meltzer, Lawrence, Faye Abdellah, and Roderick Kitchell. *Concepts and Practices of Intensive Care for Nurse Specialists*. Philadelphia: Charles Press, 1970.

340. Meltzer, Lawrence, Rose Pinneo, and Roderick Kitchell. *Intensive Coronary Care: A Manual for Nurses*. Philadelphia: Charles Press, 1968.

341. Menard, Richard. *Introduction to Arrhythmia Recognition*. San Francisco: California Heart Association, 1968.

342. Mendelson, Jack H., and Nancy K. Mello. *The Diagnosis and Treatment of Alcoholism*. New York: McGraw-Hill Book Co., 1979.

343. Meng, H.C., and David Law. *Parenteral Nutrition*. Springfield Ill.: Charles C. Thomas, Publisher, 1970.

344. Merton, Robert King. *Social Theory and Social Structure*. New York: The Free Press, 1968.

345. Miller, Ashton, W. Slade, and H.M. Leather. *A Synopsis of Renal Diseases and Urology*. London: John Wright and Sons, 1966.

346. Miller, Benjamin, Lawrence Galton, and Daniel Brunner. *Freedom from Heart Attacks*. New York: Simon and Schuster, 1972.

347. Miller, Robert. *How to Live with a Heart Attack*. Radnor, Pa.: Chilton Book Co., 1971.

348. Mims, Fern H., and Melinda Swenson. *Sexuality: A Nursing Perspective*. New York: McGraw-Hill Book Com., 1980.

349. Mitchell, Helen, Henderika Rynbergen, Linnea Anderson, and Marjorie Dibble. *Nutrition in Health and Disease*. Philadelphia: J.B. Lippincott Co., 1976.

350. Mitchell, J.B. *Urology for Nurses*. John Wright and Sons, 1976.

351. Mitford, Jessica. *The American Way of Death*. New York: Simon and Schuster, 1963.

352. Moidel, Harriet, Gladys Sorensen, Elizabeth Giblin, and Margaret Kaufmann. *Nursing Care of the Patient with Medical-Surgical Disorders*. New York: McGraw-Hill Book Co., 1976.

353. Molloy, Julia. *Teaching the Retarded Child to Talk*. New York: John Day Co., 1961.

354. Montag, Mildred, and Ruth Swenson. *Fundamentals in Nursing Care*. Philadelphia: W.B. Saunders Co., 1959.

355. Morgan, William, and George Engel. *The Clinical Approach to the Patient*. Philadelphia: W.B. Saunders Co., 1969.

356. Morressey, Alice. *Rehabilitation Nursing*. New York: G.P. Putnam's Sons, 1951.

357. Mowbray, A.Q. *The Transplant*. New York: David McKay Co., Inc., 1974.

358. Muir, Bernice L. *Pathophysiology: An Introduction to the Mechanisms of Disease*. New York: John Wiley & Sons, Inc., 1980.

359. Mullen, Robert. *The Latter-Day Saints: The Mormons Yesterday and Today*. Garden City, N.Y.: Doubleday & Co., Inc., 1966.

360. Murchison, Irene, Thomas S. Nichols, and Rachel Hanson. *Legal Accountability in the Nursing Process*. St. Louis: C.V. Mosby Co., 1978.

361. Murray, Ruth, and Judith Zenter. *Nursing Concepts for Health Promotion*. Englewood Cliffs, N.J.: Prentice-Hall, Inc., 1979.

362. Narrow, Barbara W., and Kay B. Buschle. *Fundamentals of Nursing Practice*. New York: John Wiley & Sons, Inc., 1982.

363. Naish, John Mitchell, and Alan E. Read. *Basic Gastroenterology Including Diseases of the Liver*. Chicago: A. John Wright and Sons, Ltd., Publication, 1974.

364. National League for Nursing Council of Associate Degree Programs. *Associate Degree of Education for Nursing 1982–1983*. New York: National League for Nursing, 1982.

365. National League for Nursing Council of Baccalaureate and Higher Degree Programs. *Baccalaureate Education in Nursing: Key to a Professional Career in Nursing 1982–1983*. New York: National League for Nursing, 1982.

366. National League for Nursing Council of Diploma Program. *Education for Nursing: The Diploma Way 1982–1983*. New York: National League for Nursing, 1982.

367. Neisser, Edith G. *Primer For Parents of Preschoolers*. New York: Parents' Magazine Press, 1972.

368. Nelson, Waldo, Victor Vaughn, and R. James McKay. *Nelson Textbook of Pediatrics*. Philadelphia: W.B. Saunders Co., 1979.

369. Newman, Margaret. *Theory Development in Nursing*. Philadelphia: F.A. Davis Co., 1979.

370. Nightingale, Florence. *Notes on Nursing: What It Is and What It Is Not.* Philadelphia: J.B. Lippincott Co., 1966 reprint of 1860 edition.

371. Nordmark, Madelyn, and Anne Rohweder. *Scientific Foundations of Nursing.* Philadelphia: J.B. Lippincott Co., 1975.

372. Nose, Yukihiko. *The Artificial Kidney,* vol. 1. St. Louis: C.V. Mosby Co., 1969.

373. Nosow, Sigmund, and William Form. *Man, Work, and Society.* New York: Basic Books, 1962.

374. Novak, Edmund, and J. Donald Woodruff. *Gynecologic and Obstetric Pathology.* Philadelphia: W.B. Saunders Co., 1962.

375. Nurenberg, Gerard, and Henry Calero. *How to Read a Person Like a Book.* New York: Hawthorn Books, Inc., 1971.

376. Nursing 80. *Managing Diabetes Properly: Nursing Skillbook.* Horsham, Pa.: Intemed Communications, Inc., 1977.

377. Ochsner, Alton. *Smoking: Your Choice Between Life and Death.* New York: Simon and Schuster, 1970.

378. Olsen, Paul, James L. Fosshage, and Kenneth A. Frank. *Healing: Implications for Psychotherapy.* New York: Human Sciences Press, 1978.

379. Orem, Dorothea, and the Nursing Development Conference Group. *Concept Formalization in Nursing: Process and Product.* Boston: Little, Brown & Co., 1979.

380. Orem, Dorothea. *Nursing Concepts of Practice.* New York: McGraw-Hill Book Co., 1971 and 1980 editions.

381. Orton, Samuel Torrey. *Reading, Writing, and Speech Problems in Children.* New York: W.W. Norton & Co., Inc., 1964.

382. Page, Irvine H. *Strokes.* New York: E.P. Dutton & Co., Inc., 1961.

383. Papper, Solomon. *Clinical Nephrology.* Boston: Little, Brown & Co., 1978.

384. Parcel, Guy S. *First Aid in Emergency Care.* St. Louis: C.V. Mosby Co., 1977.

385. Parker, Elizabeth. *The Seven Ages of Woman.* Baltimore: Johns Hopkins University Press, 1967.

386. Patterson, Roy. *Allergic Diseases Diagnosis and Management.* Philadelphia: J.B. Lippincott Co., 1972.

387. Peplau, Hildegard. *Aspects of Psychiatric Nursing: Therapeutic Concepts.* New York: National League for Nursing, 1957.

388. Perez, Rosanne Harrigan. *Protocols for Perinatal Nursing Practice.* St. Louis: C.V. Mosby Co., 1981.

389. Phaneuf, Maria C. *The Nursing Audit: Self-Regulation in Nursing Practice.* New York: Appleton-Century-Crofts, 1976.

390. Phillips, Raymond, and Mary Feeney. *The Cardiac Rhythms.* Philadelphia: W.B. Saunders Co., 1973.

391. Phipps, Wilma J., Barbara C. Long, and Nancy Fugate Woods. *Medical-Surgical Nursing Concepts and Clinical Practice.* St. Louis: C.V. Mosby Co., 1979.

392. Pirenne, M.H. *Vision and the Eye.* London: Chapman and Hall, Ltd., 1967.

393. Pitorak, Elizabeth, Carolyn Hudak, Joan O'Gureck, and Patricia Hanusz. *Nurses Guide to Cardiac Surgery and Nursing Care.* New York: McGraw-Hill Book Co., 1971.

394. Pohl, Margaret L. *The Teaching Function of the Nursing Practitioner.* Dubuque, Iowa: William C. Brown Co., 1973.

395. Porter, Joseph. *Stamford Curriculum Guide for Drug Abuse Education.* Chicago: J.G. Ferguson Publishing Co., 1971.

396. Price, Alice. *The Art, Science and Spirit of Nursing.* Philadelphia: W.B. Saunders Co., 1965.

397. Pritchard, Jack A., and Paul C. MacDonald. *Williams Obstetrics.* New York: Appleton-Century-Crofts, 1976.

398. Quigley, Edward, editor. *Diagnostics.* Springhouse, Pa.: Nursing 81, Intermed Communications, Inc., 1981.

399. Quigley, Edward, editor. *Diseases.* Horsham, Pa.: Nursing 81, Intermed Communications, Inc., 1981.

400. Race, George. *Laboratory Medicine,* vol. 1. New York: Harper & Row, Publishers, Inc., 1973.

401. Rapaport, Howard G., and Shirley Motter Linde. *The Complete Allergy Guide.* New York: Simon and Schuster, 1970.

402. Ratner, Herbert. *The Womanly Art of Breastfeeding.* Franklin Park, Ill.: La Leche League International, 1969.

403. Ravin, Abe. *Cardiac Auscultation: An Audio Presentation.* Philadelphia: Merck, Sharp, & Dohme Research Laboratories, 1969.

404. Redman, Barbara Klug. *The Process of Patient Teaching in Nursing.* St. Louis: C.V. Mosby Co., 1968.

405. Reeder, Sharon, Luis Mastroianni, Jr., Leonide L. Martin, and Elsie Fitzpatrick. *Maternity Nursing.* Philadelphia: J.B. Lippincott Co., 1976.

406. Regnier, Edme. *There Is a Cure for the Common Cold.* New York: Parker Publishing Co., Inc., 1971.

407. Reich, Nathaniel, and Rudolph Fremont. *Chest Pain: Systematic Differentiation and Treatment.* New York: Macmillan Publishing Co., 1961.

408. Reinhardt, Adina M., and Mildred Quinn. *Current Practice in Family-Centered Community Nursing.* St. Louis: C.V. Mosby Co., 1977.

409. Richardson, Frank Howard. *Grandparents and Their Families.* New York: David McKay Company, Inc., 1964.

410. Riehl, Joan P., and Sister Callista Roy. *Conceptual Models for Nursing Practice.* New York: Appleton-Century-Crofts, 1980.

411. Rines, Alice, and Mildred Montag. *Nursing Concepts and Nursing Care.* New York: John Wiley & Sons, Inc., 1976.

412. Robinson, Corinne. *Proudfit-Robinson's Normal and Therapeutic Nutrition.* New York: Macmillan Publishing Co., 1967.

413. Robinson, John, and Phillip Shaver. *Measures of Social Psychological Attitudes.* Ann Arbor, Mich.: Survey Research Center, Institute for Social Research, 1969.

414. Rodgers, Roy H. *Family Interaction and Transaction: The Developmental Approach.* Englewood Cliffs, N.J.: Prentice-Hall, Inc., 1973.

415. Rodman, Morton J., and Dorothy Smith. *Pharmacology and Drug Therapy in Nursing.* Philadelphia: J.B. Lippincott Co., 1968.

416. Roeske, Nancy, Clare Assue, Richard French, and Toner Overley. *Examination of the Personality.* Philadelphia: Lea & Febiger Co., 1972.

417. Rogers, Carl. *Client-Centered Therapy.* Boston: Houghton Mifflin Co., 1951.

418. Rogers, Carl, and Barry Stevens. *Person to Person: The Problem of Being Human.* Calif.: Real People Press, 1967.

419. Rogers, Martha. *An Introduction to the Theoretical Basis of Nursing.* Philadelphia: F.A. Davis Co., 1970.

420. Rogers, Martha. *Educational Revolution in Nursing.* New York: Macmillan Publishing Co., 1967.

421. Roscoe, John T. *Fundamental Research for the Behavioral Sciences.* New York: Holt, Rinehart, and Winston, 1969.

422. Rossman, Isadore. *Clinical Geriatrics.* Philadelphia: J.B. Lippincott Co., 1979.

423. Rothweiler, Ella, Jean White, and Doris Geitgey. *The Art and Science of Nursing.* Philadelphia: F.A. Davis Co., 1959.

424. Roy, Sister Callista. *Introduction to Nursing: An Adaptation Model.* Englewood Cliffs, N.J.: Prentice-Hall, Inc., 1976.

425. Roy, Sister Callista. *Theory Construction in Nursing: An Adaptation Model.* Englewood Cliffs, N.J.: Prentice-Hall, Inc., 1981.

426. Rubinstein, Max. *You and Your Hormones.* New York: Twayne Publishers, 1960.

427. Runyan, John W., Jr. *Primary Care Guide.* New York: Harper & Row Publishers, 1975.

428. Ruslink, Doris. *Family Health and Home Nursing.* New York: Macmillan Publishing Co., 1963.

429. Saba, Virginia K. *A Classification Scheme for Client Problems in Community Health Nursing.* Hyattsville, Md.: U.S. Department of Health and Human Services, 1980.

430. Sanford, Nevitt. *Self and Society.* New York: Atherton Press, 1966.

431. Sarason, Irwin. *Personality: An Objective Approach.* New York: John Wiley & Sons, Inc., 1967.

432. Sartain, A.O., A.J. North, J.R. Strange, and H.M. Chapman. *Understanding Human Behavior.* Dallas: Southern Methodist University Press, 1955.

433. Sauer, Gordon C. *Manual of Skin Diseases.* Philadelphia: J.B. Lippincott Co., 1980.

434. Sawyer, Janet. *Nursing Care of Patients with Urologic Diseases.* St. Louis: C.V. Mosby Co., 1963.

435. Saxton, Dolores F., and Phyllis W. Haring. *Care of Patients with Emotional Problems.* St. Louis: C.V. Mosby Co., 1971.

436. Scheie, Harold, and Daniel Albert. *Textbook of Ophthalmology.* Philadelphia: W.B. Saunders Co., 1977.

437. Schmidt, Jacob. *Attorneys' Dictionary of Medicine and Word Finder.* New York: Matthew Bender & Co., Inc., 1962. Cumulative supplement and revision, May 1975.

438. Schmitt, Barton. *The Child Protection Team Handbook: A Multidisciplinary Approach to Managing Child Abuse and Neglect.* New York: Garland STMP, 1977.

439. Schneider, F. Richard. *Cast Care.* Daly City, Ca.: Physician's Art Service, Inc., 1976.

440. Schultz, Duane. *Sensory Restriction.* New York: Academic Press, 1965.

441. Seyle, Hans. *The Stress of Life.* New York: McGraw-Hill Book Co., 1956.

442. Shaffer, Martin. *Life After Stress.* New York: Plenum Press, 1982.

443. Sharp, LaVaughn, and Beatrice Rabin. *Nursing in the Coronary Care Unit.* Philadelphia: J.B. Lippincott Co., 1970.

444. Sheehy, Gail. *Passages.* New York: E.P. Dutton & Co., Inc., 1976.

445. Shipp, Thomas. *Helping the Alcoholic and His Family.* Englewood Cliffs, N.J.: Prentice-Hall, Inc., 1963.

446. Shires, George Thomas. *Care of the Trauma Patient.* New York: McGraw-Hill Book Co., 1979.

447. Silverman, Harold M., and Gilbert I. Simon. *The Pill Book.* New York: Bantam Books, 1979.

448. Simonson, Josephine. *According to the Aphasic Adult.* Dallas: University of Texas Medical School, 1971.

449. Skydell, Barbara, and Anne Crowder. *Diagnostic Procedures.* Boston: Little, Brown & Co., 1975.

450. Smith, Christine. *Maternal-Child Nursing.* Philadelphia: W.B. Saunders Co., 1963.

451. Smith, Dorothy, Carol Germain, and Claudia Gips. *Care of the Adult Patient: Medical-Surgical Nursing.* Philadelphia: J.B. Lippincott Co., 1971.

452. Smith, Henry Clay. *Sensitivity to People.* New York: McGraw-Hill Book Co., 1966.

453. Smith, Henry Clay. *Personality Development.* New York: McGraw-Hill Book Co., 1968.

454. Smithers, R. Brinkley. *Biochemical and Nutritional Aspects of Alcoholism.* New York: Clayton Foundation Biochemical Institute, 1964.

455. Soreff, Stephen M. *Management of the Psychiatric Emergency.* New York: John Wiley & Sons, Inc., 1981.

456. Southard, Samuel. *Religion and Nursing.* Nashville, Tenn.: Broadman Press, 1959.

457. Spencer, Marietta. *Blind Children: In Family and Community.* Minneapolis: University of Minnesota Press, 1960.

458. Spencer, Roberta T. *Patient Care in Endocrine Problems.* Philadelphia: W.B. Saunders Co., 1973.

459. Spielberger, Charles. *Anxiety and Behavior.* New York: Academic Press, 1966.

460. Spock, Benjamin. *Baby and Child Care.* New York: Pocket Books, 1981.

461. Spotnitz, Hyman, and Lucy Freeman. *How to Be Happy Though Pregnant.* New York: Coward-McCann, Inc., 1969.

462. Stangler, Sharon R., Cathee J. Huber, and Donald K. Routh. *Screening Growth and Development of Preschool Children.* New York: McGraw-Hill Book Co., 1980.

463. Steele, Harold, and Charles Crow. *High Blood Pressure: Cholesterol and You.* Huntsville, Ala.: Strode Publishers, 1969.

464. Stein, Edward. *Guilt: Theory and Therapy.* Philadelphia: Westminister Press, 1969.

465. Steincrohn, Peter. *How to Get a Good Night's Sleep.* Chicago: Henry Regnery Company, 1968.

466. Stern, Edith, and Mabel Ross. *You and Your Aging Parents.* New York: Harper & Row Publishers, Inc., 1965.

467. Stevens, Barbara. *Nursing Theory: Analysis, Application, Evaluation.* Boston: Little, Brown & Co., 1979.

468. Stewart, Gary K., and Robert A. Hatcher. *Contraceptive Technology 1976–1977.* New York: Irvington Publishers, Inc., 1976.

469. Storlie, Francis. *Principles of Intensive Nursing Care.* New York: Appleton-Century-Crofts, 1969.

470. Strang, Ruth. *Helping Your Child Develop His Potentialities.* New York: E.P. Dutton & Co., Inc., 1965.

471. Stuart, Gail, and Sandra Sundeen. *Principles and Practice of Psychiatric Nursing.* St. Louis: C.V. Mosby Co., 1979.

472. Sutton, Audrey. *Bedside Nursing Technique.* Philadelphia: W.B. Saunders Co., 1969.

473. Sutton, Audrey. *Bedside Nursing Techniques in Medicine and Surgery.* Philadelphia: W.B. Saunders Co., 1964.

474. Sutton, Maurice. *Cancer Explained.* New York: Hart Publishing Co., Inc., 1966.

475. Swatz, Harry. *The Allergy Guide Book.* New York: Frederick Unger Publishing Co., 1961.

476. Taber, Clarence. *Taber's Cyclopedic Medical Dictionary.* Worcester, Mass.: F.A. Davis Co., 1978.

477. Terry, Florence, Gladys Benz, Dorothy Mereness, and Frank Kleffner. *Principles and Techniques of Rehabilitation Nursing.* St. Louis: C.V. Mosby Co., 1961.

478. Thompson, Edward, and Adaline Hayden. *Standard Nomenclature of Diseases and Operations.* New York: McGraw-Hill Book Co., 1967.

479. Thompson, Lloyd. *Reading Disability: Developmental Dyslexia.* Springfield, Ill.: Charles C. Thomas, Publisher, 1966.

480. Tinkham, Catherine W., and Eleanor F. Voorhies. *Community Health Nursing: Evolution and Process.* New York: Appleton-Century-Crofts, 1977.

481. Toch, Hans. *Violent Men: An Inquiry into the Psychology of Violence.* Chicago: Aldine Publishing Co., 1969.

482. Toole, James. *Diagnosis and Management of Stroke.* New York: American Heart Association, 1968.

483. Townsend, Carolynn. *Nutrition and Diet Modification for the Nurse.* New York: Delmar Publishers, Inc., 1966.

484. Travelbee, Joyce. *Interpersonal Aspects of Nursing.* Philadelphia: F.A. Davis Co., 1966.

485. Travis, John. *Wellness Workbook.* Mill Valley, Ca.: Wellness Resource Center, 1981.

486. Tucker, Susan, Mary Ann Breeding, Mary Canobbio, Eleanor Paquette, Marjorie

Wells, and Mary Willmann. *Patient Care Standards.* St. Louis: C.V. Mosby Co., 1980.

487. Tuft, Louis. *Allergy Management in Clinical Practice.* St. Louis: C.V. Mosby Co., 1973.

488. Tyler, Edward T. *Birth Control: A Continuing Controversy.* Springfield, Ill.: Charles C. Thomas Publisher, 1967.

489. United States Department of Health, Education and Welfare. *International Classification of Diseases,* 8th revision (ICD-9), vol. 1. Washington, D.C.: National Center for Health Statistics.

490. United States Department of Health, Education and Welfare. *Nursing Problem Classification for Children and Youth.* Rockville, Md.: U.S. Government Printing Office, 1976.

491. United States Department of Health, Education and Welfare. *Detection, Evaluation, and Treatment of High Blood Pressure.* Rockville, Md.: U.S. Department of Health, Education and Welfare, 1977.

492. United States Department of Health and Human Services. *A Classification Scheme for Client Problems in Community Health Nursing.,* Rockville, Md.: U.S. Department of Health and Human Services, 1980.

493. United States Department of Labor. *Job Descriptions and Organizational Analysis for Hospitals and Related Health Services.* Washington, D.C.: U.S. Government Printing Office, 1970.

494. Van Riper, Charles. *Your Child's Speech Problems.* New York: Harper & Row, Publishers, Inc., 1961.

495. Vaughn, Daniel, Robert Cook, and Asbury Taylor. *General Ophthalmology.* Los Altos, Calif.: Lange Medical Publications, 1965.

496. Victor, Diana. *Care of the Maternity Patient.* New York: McGraw-Hill Book Co., 1971.

497. Villaverde, Manuel M., and C. Wright MacMillan. *Ailments of Aging: From Symptom to Treatment.* New York: Van Nostrand Reinhold Co., 1980.

498. Waechter, Eugenia, and Florence G. Blake. *Nursing Care of Children.* Philadelphia: J.B. Lippincott Co., 1976.

499. Wagman, Richard, and J.G. Ferguson. *The New Concise Family Health and Medical Guide.* Chicago: J.G. Ferguson Publishing Co., 1972.

500. Wallach, Jacques. *Interpretation of Diagnostic Tests.* Boston: Little, Brown & Co., 1978.

501. Walraven, Gail. *Basic Arrhythmias.* Bowie, Md.: Robert J. Brady Co., 1980.

502. Walter, Judith Bloom, Geraldine P. Pardee, and Doris M. Morbo. *Dynamics of Problem-Oriented Approaches: Patient Care and Documentation.* New York: J.B. Lippincott Co., 1978.

503. Watson, Jeannette. *Medical-Surgical Nursing and Related Physiology.* Philadelphia: W.B. Saunders Co., 1972.

504. Watson, Robert. *Psychology of the Child.* New York: John Wiley & Sons, Inc., 1965.

505. Wattenberg, William. *The Adolescent Years.* New York: Harcourt Brace Jovanovich, Inc., 1973.

506. Wayler, Thelma, and Rose Klein. *Applied Nutrition.* New York: Macmillan Publishing Co., 1965.

507. Weed, Lawrence. *Medical Records, Medical Education, and Patient Care.* Chicago: Case Western Reserve University Press, 1971.

508. Weinberg, George. *The Action Approach.* New York: World Publishing Co., 1969.

509. Weller, Charles, and Brian Boylan. *How to Live with Hypoglycemia.* Garden City, N.Y.: Doubleday & Co., Inc., 1968.

510. Weller, Charles, and Brian Boylan. *The New Way to Live with Diabetes.* Garden City, N.Y.: Doubleday and Co., Inc., 1966.

511. Wenar, Charles. *Personality Development.* Boston: Houghton Mifflin Co., 1971.

512. Wepman, Joseph M. *Asphasia and the Family.* New York: American Heart Association, 1969.

513. White, Dorothy, Edith Rubino, and Philip DeLorey. *Fundamentals: The Foundation of Nursing.* Englewood Cliffs, N.J.: Prentice-Hall, Inc., 1972

514. Whitehead, Sylvia. *Nursing Care of the Adult Urology Patient.* New York: Appleton-Century-Crofts, 1970.

515. Wiebe, Anne. *Orthopedics in Nursing.* Philadelphia: W.B. Saunders Co., 1961.

516. Wiedenbach, Ernestine, and Caroline Falls. *Communication: Key to Effective Nursing.* New York: Tiresias Press, 1978.

517. Wiggins, Jerry, Edward Renner, Gerald Clare, and Richard Rose. *The Psychology of Personality.* Reading, Mass.: Addison-Wesley Publishing Co., 1971.

518. Wilson, Eva, Katherine Fisher, and Mary Fuqua. *Principles of Nutrition.* New York: John Wiley & Sons, Inc., 1966.

519. Wilson, J. Robert, Clayton Beechan, and Elsie Reid Carrington. *Obstetrics and Gynecology.* St. Louis: C.V. Mosby Co., 1971.

520. Winter, Chester, and Marilyn Roehm. *Nursing Care of Patients with Urologic Diseases.* St. Louis: C.V. Mosby Co., 1977.

521. Winter, Ruth. *Do You Have Sinus Trouble* New York: Grosset & Dunlap, 1973.

522. Wintrobe, Maxwell Mayer, George Thorn, Raymond Adams, Ivan Bennett, Eugene Braunwald, Kurt Isselbacher, and Robert Petersdorf *Harrison's Principles of Internal Medicine.* New York: McGraw-Hill Book Co., 1971.

523. Wood, Lucile A. *Nursing Skills for Allied Health Services,* vol. 1–3. Philadelphia: W.B. Saunders Co., 1975.

524. Woolf, Henry B., editor. *Webster's New Collegiate Dictionary.* Springfield, Mass.: G & C Merriam Co., 1979.

525. Wu, Ruth. *Behavior and Illness.* Englewood Cliffs, N.J.: Prentice-Hall, Inc., 1973.

526. Yura, Helen, and Mary Walsh. *The Nursing Process: Assessing, Planning, Implementing, Evaluating.* New York: Appleton-Century-Crofts, 1978.

527. Ziegel, Erna, and Mecca S. Cranley. *Obstetric Nursing.* New York: Macmillan Publishing Co., 1978.

528. Zschoche, Donna A. *Mosby's Comprehensive Review of Critical Care.* St. Louis: C.V. Mosby Co., 1981.

529. Zubek, John P. *Sensory Deprivation: Fifteen Years of Research.* New York: Appleton-Century-Crofts, 1969.

ARTICLES

530. Alexander, Leo. "Differential Diagnosis Between Psychogenic and Physical Pain." *Journal of American Medical Association* (September 8, 1962), 149–155.

531. Alford, Dolores M. "Tips for Teaching Older Adults." *Nursing Life,* vol. 2, no. 5 (September–October 1982), 60–63.

532. American Heart Association, Committee on Cardiopulmonary Resuscitation and Emergency Cardiac Care. "Standards for Cardiopulmonary Resuscitation and Emergency Cardiac Care." *Journal of American Medical Association,* vol. 227, no. 7 (February 1974), 837–868.

533. Baer, Eva, Lois Jean Davitz, and Renee Lieb. "Inferences of Physical Pain." *Nursing Research,* vol. 19, no. 5 (September–October 1970), 388–401.

534. Baker, J.B., and H. Merskey. "Pain in General Practice." *Journal of Psychosomatic Residence,* vol. 10 (1967), 383–387.

535. Barnard, Jan. "Understanding and Treating the Patient in Pain." *R.N. Magazine* (May 1967), 73–75.

536. Baxter, Charles, R.P. William Curreri, and Janet A. Marvin. "The Control of Burn Wound Sepsis by the Use of Quantitative Bacteriologic Studies and Sebeschar Clysis With Antibiotics." *Surgical Clinics of North America,* vol. 53 (December 1973), 1,509–1,517.

537. Bayless, Colin E., et al. "The Pacemaker—Twiddler's Syndrome: A New Complication of Implantable Transvenous Pacemakers." *Canadian Medical Association Journal* (August 24, 1968), 371–373.

538. Beecher, Henry. "The Powerful Placebo." *Journal of American Medical Association* (December 24, 1955), 1,602–1,606.

539. Bell, Janice. "Stressful Life Events and Coping Methods in Mental Illness and Wellness Behavior." *Nursing Research,* vol. 26, no. 2 (March–April 1977), 136–410.

540. Benjamin, Harry, and Charles Ihlenfeld. "Transsexualism." *American Journal of Nursing* (March 1973), 457–461.

541. Berry, Margaret, and Colette Kerlin. "The Drops of Life: Fluids and Electrolytes." *R.N. Magazine,* vol. 33, no. 9 (September 1970), 35–67.

542. Betson, Carol. "Blood Gases." *American Journal of Nursing* (May 1968), 1,010–1,012.

543. Billars, Karen. "You Have Pain? I Think This Will Help." *American Journal of Nursing,* vol. 70, no. 10 (October 1970), 2,113–2,145.

544. Billing, Dorothy. "Nursing Care of Patients with Mechanical Cardiac Pacemakers." *Nursing Clinics of North America,* vol. 7, no. 3 (September 1972), 509–515.

545. Blaylock, Jerry. "Nursing Functions and the Tradition of Nursing." *The Bulletin: Texas Nurses Association (October 1970),* 8–11.

546. Blaylock, Jerry. "The Psychological and Cultural Influences on the Reaction to Pain." *Nursing Forum,* vol. 7, no. 3 (1968), 263–274.

547. Bloom, Judith. "Problem-Oriented Charting." *American Journal of Nursing,* vol. 19 (November 1971), 2,144–2,148.

548. Bloom, Stephen G. "Debunking the Ulcer Myths." *The Dallas Morning News* (August 24, 1982), Section C, 1C and 3C.

549. Bonkowsky, Marilyn. "Adapting the POMR to Community Child Health Care." *Nursing Outlook* (August 1972), 515–518.

550. Boylan, Ann, and Bernard Marback. "Dehydration: Subtle, Sinister, Preventable." *R.N. Magazine,* vol. 42, no. 8 (August 1979), 37–41.

551. Brabenstetter, Joan. "Synthetic Fat Helps Prevent Pressure Sores." *American Journal of Nursing* (July 1968), 1,521.

552. Bruegel, Mary Ann. "Relationship of Preoperative Anxiety to Perception of Postoperative Pain." *Nursing Research*, vol. 20, no. 1 (January–February 1971), 26–31.

553. Bullough, Bonnie. "Discovery of the First Signs and Symptoms of Breast Cancer." *Nurse Practitioner.* vol. 5, no. 6 (November–December 1980), 31–47.

554. Bush, Helen. "Models for Nursing." *Advances in Nursing Science*, vol. 1, no. 2 (January 1979), 13–21.

555. Bush, James. "Cervical Esophagostomy to Provide Nutrition." *American Journal of Nursing*, vol. 79, no. 1 (January 1979), 107–109.

556. Busse, Ewald. "How to Handle Problems of Aging." *Today's Health* (July 1969), 29–31, 58.

557. Campbell, Margaret. "Identifying Nursing Problems." *Canadian Nurse* (February 1965), 96–99.

558. Carbeil, Madeline. "Nursing Process for a Patient with a Body-Image Disturbance." *Nursing Clinics of North America*, vol. 6, no. 1 (March 1971), 155–163.

559. Castleberry, Vivian. "A Journey Through Cancer." *Dallas Times Herald* (October 22, 1978), Section H, 1 and 5; (October 23, 1978), Section B, 1 and 8; (October 24, 1978), Section B, 1 and 3.

560. Chambers, Wilda. "Nursing Diagnosis." *American Journal of Nursing* (November 1962), 102–104.

561. Chernov, Merrill, Harry Hale, and MacDonald Wood. "Prevention of Stress Ulcers." *The American Journal of Surgery*, vol. 122 (November 1971), 674–677.

562. Clark, Nancy Fairchild. "Pump Failure." *Nursing Clinics of North America*, vol. 7, no. 3 (September 1972), 529–539.

563. Clearinghouse, National Group for Classification of Nursing Diagnosis. "Nursing Diagnosis Resources." *Advances in Nursing Science*, vol. 2, no. 1 (October 1979), 99–100.

564. Dallas Times Herald. "Doctor Offers These Tips on Conquering Jet Lag." *Dallas Times Herald*, August, 22, 1976), Section J7, 1

565. Davidson, Bill. "Drugs That Don't Mix." *Family Circle Magazine* (April 6, 1982).

566. Davis, Anne. "The Skills of Communication." *American Journal of Nursing* (January 1963), 66–70.

567. Davis, Barbara. "Until Death Ensues." *Nursing Clinics of North America*, vol. 7, no. 2 (June 1972), 303–309.

568. Decker, Deborah. "Grief: In the Valley of the Shadow." *American Journal of Nursing* (March 1978), 416–418.

569. Denniston, Donna J., and Kathryn T. Burns. "Home Peritoneal Dialysis." *American Journal of Nursing*, vol. 80, no. 11 (November 1980), 2,022–2,026.

570. Donald, Paul J. "Guide to the Diagnosis and Management of Eustachian Otitis." *Hospital Medicine* (March 1976), 44–46.

571. Drake, Virginia Koch. "Battered Women: A Health Care Problem in Disguise." *Images*, vol. 14, no. 2 (June 1982), 40–47.

572. Draye, Mary, and Betty Pesznecker. "Diagnostic Scope and Certainty: An Analysis of FNP Practice." *Nurse Practitioner*, vol. 4, no. 1 (January–February 1979), 15–51.

573. Dunn, Halbert. "High-Level Wellness for Man and Society." *American Journal of Public Health*, vol. 49, no. 6 (June 1959), 786–792.

574. Durand, Mary, and Rosemary Prince. "Nursing Diagnosis: Process and Decision." *Nursing Forum*, vol. 5, no. 4 (1966), 50–64.

575. Engel, George. "Grief and Grieving." *American Journal of Nursing* (September 1964), 93–98.

576. Farabee, Ray. "What Nurses Need to Know About the Texas Natural Death Act." *Texas Nursing*, vol. 51, no. 10 (November–December 1977), 10–11.

577. Favorito, John, Joan Orchardo Pernice, and Patricia Ruggiero. "Apnea Monitoring to Prevent SIDS." *American Journal of Nursing*, vol. 79, no. 1 (January 1979), 101–104.

578. Fellows, Barbara. "Hemodialysis at Home." *American Journal of Nursing*, vol. 66 (August 1966), 1,775–1,778.

579. Flaskerud, Jacquelyn, and Edward J. Halloran. "Areas of Agreement in Nursing Theory Development." *Advances in Nursing Science*, vol. 3, no. 1 (October 1980), 1–7.

580. Foley, Mary F. "Air Travel for Patients." *American Journal of Nursing* (June 1973), 1,020–1,023.

581. Gadboys, H.L., et al. "Long-Term Follow-up of Patients with Cardiac Pacemakers." *American Journal of Cardiology* (January 1968), 55–59.

582. Garofano, Catherine D. "Helping Diabet-

ics Live with Their Neuropathies." *Nursing 80*, vol. 10, no. 6 (June 1980), 42–44.

583. Garrison, Webb. "Pain: Your Body's Early Warning System." *Today's Health* (October 1969), 29–66.

584. Gebbie, Kristine, and Mary Ann Lavin. "Classifying Nursing Diagnosis." *American Journal of Nursing*, vol. 74 (February 1974), 250–253.

585. Geiderman, Joel M., and Larry J. Baraff. "Infectious Disease Emergencies." *Topics in Emergency Medicine* (April 1982), 72–77.

586. Giovannitti, Christine, and Terry Schwinghammer. "Food and Drugs: Managing the Right Mix for Your Patient." *Nursing 81*, vol. 11, no. 7 (July 1981), 26–31.

587. Golub, Sharon. "Recognizing the Drug Abuser." *R.N. Magazine* (July 1969), 44–45.

588. Goosen, Geraldine M., and Helen A. Bush. "Adaptation: A Feedback Process." *Advances in Nursing Science*, vol. 1, no. 4 (July 1979), 51–64.

589. Gordon, Marjorie. "Classification of Nursing Diagnoses." *Journal New York State Nurses' Association* (March 1978), 5–9.

590. Gordon, Marjorie. "Nursing Diagnosis and the Diagnostic Process." *American Journal of Nursing*, vol. 76 (August 1976), 1,298–1,300.

591. Graffam, Shirley R. "Nurse Response to the Patient in Distress: Development of an Instrument." *Nursing Research*, vol. 19, no. 4 (July–August 1970), 331–336.

592. Graham, Jory. "Doctor's Can't Predict." *Dallas Times Herald* (April 23, 1978), D-3.

593. Grant, Jo Ann Nallinger. "Patient Care in Parenteral Hyperalimentation." *Nursing Clinics of North America*, vol. 8, no. 1 (March 1973), 165–181.

594. Haferkorn, Virginia. "Assessing Individual Learning Needs as a Basis for Patient Teaching." *Nursing Clinics of North America*, vol. 6, no. 1 (March 1971), 199–209.

595. Hamdi, Mary, and Carol Hutelmyer. "A Study of the Effectiveness of an Assessment Tool in the Identification of Nursing-Care Problems." *Nursing Research*, vol. 19 (July–August 1970), 354–358.

596. Harris, Elizabeth. "The Dexamethasone Suppression Test." *American Journal of Nursing*, vol. 82, no. 5 (May 1982), 784–785.

597. Hoffman, M., S. Donckers, and M. Hauser. "The Effect of Nursing Intervention on Stress Factors Perceived by Patients in a Coronary Care Unit." *Heart Lung*, vol. 7, no. 5 (September–October 1978), 804.

598. Hoppe, Mary. "The New Tube-Feeding Sets." *Nursing 80*, vol. 10, no. 3 (March 1980), 79–85.

599. Hubert, Sister Mary. "Spiritual Care for Every Patient." *The Journal of Nursing Education*, vol. 2, no. 2 (May–June 1963), 9–11.

600. Hunter, John. "The Mark of Pain." *American Journal of Nursing*, vol. 61, no. 10 (October 1961), 96–99.

601. Hutchinson, Rosemary. "The Common Cold Primer." *Nursing 79*, vol. 9, no. 3 (March 1979), 57–62.

602. Jense, Hellene N., and Gene Tillotson. "Dependency in Nurse–Patient Relationships." *American Journal of Nursing* (February 1961), 81–84.

603. Johnson, JoAnn Rao. "Discharge Planning." *Texas Nursing* (November 1976), 9–10.

604. Jones, Phyllis E. "A Terminology for Nursing Diagnosis." *Advances in Nursing Science*, vol. 2, no. 1 (October 1979), 65–71.

605. Jones, Phyllis E., and Dorothea Fox Jacob. "An Investigation of the Definition of Nursing Diagnosis: Report of Phase One." University of Toronto Faculty of Nursing (1977).

606. Kanner, Leo. "Judging Emotions from Facial Expressions." *Psychological Review*, vol. 61, no. 3 (1931), 16–20.

607. Karlsberg, Florence. "The Prevention of Malignant Melanoma." National Cancer Institute Fact Sheet (March 1981).

608. Kaufmann, Margaret, and Dorothy Brown. "Pain Wears Many Faces." *American Journal of Nursing*, vol. 61, no. 1 (January 1961), 48–51.

609. Kelly, Katherine. "Clinical Inference in Nursing." *Nursing Research* (Winter 1966), 23–26.

610. Komarita, Nori. "Nursing Diagnosis." *American Journal of Nursing* (December 1963), 83–86.

611. Kotsubo, Carol Zinger. "Helping Families Survive S.I.D.S." *Nursing 83*, vol. 13, no. 5 (May 1983), 94–96.

612. Kryschyshen, Patt L., and David A. Fischer. "External Fixation for Complicated Fractures." *American Journal of Nursing*, vol. 80, no. 2 (February 1980), 256–259.

613. Langford, Teddy. "The Evaluation of Nursing: Necessary and Possible." *Supervisor Nurse* (November 1971), 65–75.

614. Larson, Duane, and Rita Gaston. "Current Trends in the Care of Burned Patients." *American Journal of Nursing*, vol. 67, no. 2 (February 1967), 319–327.

615. Lasagna, Louis, Fredrick Mosteller, John M. Von Felsinger, and Henry Beecher. "A Study of Placebo Response." *American Journal of Medicine* (June 1954), 770–779.

616. Law, Jane. "The Fat Embolism Syndrome." *The Journal of Bone and Joint Surgery*, vol. 13 (March 1971), 58.

617. Lawson, Betty. "Clinical Assessment of Cardiac Patients in Acute Care Facilities." *Nursing Clinics of North America*, vol. 7, no. 3 (September 1972), 431–444.

618. Lehmann, Sister Janet. "Auscultation of Heart Sounds." *American Journal of Nursing* (July 1972), 1,242–1,246.

619. Leslie, Flora M. "Nursing Diagnosis: Use in Long-Term Care." *American Journal of Nursing*, vol. 81, no. 5 (May 1981), 1,012–1,014.

620. Levin, Nathaniel, John E. McClear, Vitus F. Pekarek, and James Shanks. "Rehabilitation: Sound the Way for Laryngectomees." *Patient Care* (August 15, 1972), 58.

621. Levine, Rhoda. "Disengagement in the Elderly: Its Causes and Effects." *Nursing Outlook* (October 1969), 28–30.

622. Littmann, David. "Stethoscopes and Auscultation." *American Journal of Nursing* (July 1972), 1,239–1,241.

623. Lundin, Dorothy V. "Reporting Urine Test Results: Switch from Plus to Percent." *American Journal of Nursing*, vol. 78, no. 5 (May 1978), 878–879.

624. McBride, Mary. "Additive to the Analgesic." *American Journal of Nursing* (May 1969), 974–976.

625. McBride, Mary Angela. "Nursing Approach, Pain and Relief: An Exploratory Experiment." *Nursing Research*, vol. 16, no. 4 (Fall 1967), 337–340.

626. McCaffery, Margo. "Understanding Your Patient's Pain." *Nursing 80*, vol. 10, no. 9 (September 1980), 26–31.

627. McCaffery, Margo. "Patients Shouldn't Have to Suffer: How to Relieve Pain with Injectable Narcotics." *Nursing 80*, vol. 10, no. 10 (October 1980), 34–39.

628. McCaffery, Margo. "How to Relieve Your Patient's Pain Fast and Effectively with Oral Analgesics." *Nursing 80*, vol. 10, no. 11 (November 1980), 58–63.

629. McFarland, Mary Brambilla. "Fat Embolism Syndrome." *American Journal of Nursing*, vol. 76, no. 12 (December 1976), 1,942–1,944.

630. McKay, Rose P. "What is the Relationship Between the Development and Utilization of a Taxonomy and Nursing Theory?" *Nursing Research*, vol. 26 (May–June 1979), 222–224.

631. McQuade, Anne, and Alvin I. Goldfarb. "Coping with Feelings of Helplessness." *American Journal of Nursing* (May 1963), 77–79.

632. Martin, Harry W., and Arthur J. Prange. "The Stages of Illness: Psychosocial Approach." *Nursing Outlook* (March 1962), 169–170.

633. Maslow, Abraham. "Deficiency Motivation and Growth Motivation." *Personality Dynamics and Effective Behavior*. Edited by James Coleman. Glenview, Ill.: Scott, Foresman & Co., 1960, 475–485.

634. Mastal, Margaret Fisk, and Helen Hammond. "Analysis and Expansion of the Roy Adaptation Model: A Contribution to Holistic Nursing." *Advances in Nursing Science*, vol. 2 no. 4 (July 1980), 71–81.

635. Matthews, Carol Ann, and Alice LeVeille Goul. "Nursing Diagnosis from the Perspective of Concept Attainment and Critical Thinking." *Advances in Nursing Science*, vol. 2, no. 1 (October 1979), 17–25.

636. Mazzara, James, and Stephen Ayres. "Fluid, Electrolytes, and Acid–Base Disturbances in the Coronary Care Unit." *Nursing Clinics of North America*, vol. 7, no. 3 (September 1972), 549–562.

637. Metheny, Norma. "Renal Stones and Urinary pH." *American Journal of Nursing*, vol. 82, no. 95 (September 1982), 1,372–1,375.

638. Metheny, Norma A., and William Snively. "Perioperative Fluids and Electrolytes." *American Journal of Nursing*, vol. 78, no. 5 (May 1978), 840–845.

639. Miller, D.L., and G.A. Friday. "Allergic Diseases of the Nose and Middle Ear in Children." *Pediatric Annals*, vol. 5, no. 5 (May 8, 1976), 23–49.

640. Moncrief, Jack. "Continuous Ambulatory Peritoneal Dialysis." *Dialysis and Transplantation*, vol. 7, no. 8 (August 1978), 809–810.

641. Moncrief, Jack, Mullins-Blackson, Carol, and Nursing Staff at ACORN Research Lab. "Exchange Instructions." The Austin Diagnostic Clinic and Association, (1981).

642. Moss, Faye, and Burton Meyer. "The Effects of Nursing Interaction upon Pain

Relief in Patients." *Nursing Research*, vol. 15, no. 4 (Fall 1966), 303–306.

643. Mundinger, Mary O'Neil, and Grace Dotterer Jauron. "Developing a Nursing Diagnosis." *Nursing Outlook* (February 1975), 94–98.

644. Nalls, Sandra. "Developing a Therapeutic Relationship." *American Journal of Nursing* (December 1965), 114–118.

645. Nehren, Jeanette, and Naomi Gilliam. "Separation Anxiety." *American Journal of Nursing* (January 1965), 109–112.

646. Neylan, Margaret. "The Nurse in a Healing Milieu." *American Journal of Nursing* (April 1964), 72–74.

647. Norris, Catherine. "The Professional Nurse and Body Image." *Behavioral Concepts and Nursing Intervention.* Philadelphia: J.B. Lippincott Co., 1970, 39–60.

648. Norris, Catherine. "Toward a Science of Nursing." *Nursing Forum*, vol. 3, no. 3 (1964), 10–45.

649. O'Donnell, D.R. "The Internal Clock of the International Jet Traveler." *The Medical Journal of Australia* (June 5, 1971), 1,227–1,230.

650. Okoniewski, Gail A. "Sexual Activity Following Myocardial Infarction." *Cardiovascular Nursing*, vol. 15, no. 1 (January–February 1979), 1–4.

651. Osoba, Kathy. "Hospital Visitors May Create Anxiety in Patients, Say Medical Researchers." *Dallas Times Herald* (July 13, 1979), Section E, E-3.

652. Paris, Paul M. "Urinary Tract Infection." *Topics in Emergency Medicine*, vol. 4, no. 1 (April 1982), 26–33.

653. Patterson, Edith, and Frances Stence. "Thinking Together to Solve Care Problems." *American Journal of Nursing* (August 1970), 1,703–1,706.

654. Payne, D. "Effectiveness of Milk Products in Dietary Management of Lactose Malabsorption." *American Journal of Clinical Nutrition*, vol. 34 (December 1981), 2,711–2,715.

655. Peplau, Hildegard E. "Talking with Patients." *American Journal of Nursing* (July 1960), 964–966.

656. Pisarcik, Gail. "Pacing the Violent Patient." *Nursing 81* (September 1981), 62–65.

657. Plorde, James J. "Advice to Foreign Travelers." *Postgraduate Medicine* vol. 51 (January 1972), 179–183.

658. Pohl, Margaret. "Teaching Activities of the Nurse Practitioner." *Nursing Research*, vol. 14 (1965), 4–11.

659. Popovich, Robert, Jack Moncrief, Karl Nolph, Ahad Ghods, Zbylut Twardowski, and W.K. Pyle. "Continuous Ambulatory Peritoneal Dialysis." *Annals of Internal Medicine*, vol. 88, no. 4 (April 1978), 449–456.

660. Puder, Barbara. "What You Should Know About Nursing Diagnosis." *Medical Records News* (August 1975), 87–90.

661. Richardson, Jamie I. "The Manipulative Patient Spells Trouble." *Nursing 81*, vol. 11, no. 1 (January 1981), 48–53.

662. Rinear, Charles, and Eileen Rinear. "Emergency Bandaging." *Nursing 75*, vol. 5, no. 1 (January 1975), 29–35.

663. Ripley, Herbert. "Psychological Factors in Pain." *Nebraska State Medical Journal*, vol. 9, no. 4 (April 1964), 166–169.

664. Rogers, Martha. "Nursing: To Be or Not to Be." *Nursing Outlook*, vol. 20 (January 1972), 42–46.

665. Rossi, Laura P., and Virginia M. Haines. "Nursing Diagnoses Related to Acute Myocardial Infarction." *Cardiovascular Nursing*, vol. 15, no. 3 (May–June 1979), 11–15.

666. Rothberg, June. "Why Nursing Diagnosis?" *American Journal of Nursing* (May 1967), 1,040–1,042.

667. Rowan, Noel M. "New Systems for Supporting the Patient in the Management of Decubitus Ulcer: Preliminary Report." *Journal of the American Geriatrics Society* (May 1970), 422–424.

668. Roy, Sister Callista. "Adaptation: A Conceptual Framework of Nursing." *Nursing Outlook*, vol. 18, no. 3 (March 1970), 42–43.

669. Roy, Sister Callista. "Adaptation: A Basis for Nursing Practice." *Nursing Outlook*, vol. 19, no. 4 (April 1971), 254–256.

670. Roy, Sister Callista. "Adaptation: Implications for Curriculum Change." *Nursing Outlook*, vol. 21, no. 3 (March 1973), 163–168.

671. Roy, Sister Callista. "A Diagnostic Classification System for Nursing." *Nursing Outlook*, vol. 23, no. 2 (February 1975), 90–92.

672. Rubin, Reva. "Body Image and Self-Esteem." *Nursing Outlook* (June 1968), 20–23.

673. Scalzi, C.C. "Nursing Management of Behavioral Responses Following An Acute Myocardial Infarction." *Heart Lung*, vol. 2, no. 1 (January–February 1973), 62.

674. Schell, Pamela L., and Alla T. Campbell. "POMR: Not Just Another Way to

Chart." *Nursing Outlook*, vol. 20 (August 1972), 510–511.

675. Schulmeister, Lisa. "Screening for Skin Cancer." *Nursing 81*, vol. 2, no. 10 (October 1981), 42–45.

676. Schumann, Delores. "How to Help Wound Healing in Your Abdominal Surgery Patient." *Nursing 80*, vol. 10, no. 4 (April 1980), 34–10.

677. Searcy, Laurel. "Nursing Care of the Laryngectomy Patient." *R.N. Magazine* (October 1972), 35–41.

678. Skalka, Patricia. "Solving the Mystery of the Decaying Teeth." *Today's Health* (January 1974), 27–28, 70.

679. Skipper, James, Daisy Tagliacazzo, and Hans Mauksch. "What Communication Means to Patients." *American Journal of Nursing* (April 1964), 101–103.

680. Smitherman, Colleen. "Dealing With the Patient's Denial: What Should You Do?" *Nursing 81*, vol. 2, no. 12 (December 1981), 70–71.

681. Solak, Sandra. "Assessment of Psychogenic Stresses in the Coronary Patient." *Cardiovascular Nursing*, vol. 15, no. 4 (July–August 1979), 16–20.

682. Tapia, Jayne Anitila. "The Nursing Process in Family Health." *Nursing Outlook*, vol. 20 no. 4 (April 1972), 267–270.

683. Traver, Gayle. "Assessment of Thorax and Lungs." *American Journal of Nursing* (March 1973), 466–471.

684. Ullman, Montague. "Disorders of Body Image After Stroke." *American Journal of Nursing* (October 1964), 89–91.

685. University of Texas at Arlington. "Community Health Nursing Family Coping Index." University of Texas, (1978).

686. VanMeter, Margaret, and Romaine Hart. "Chest Tubes: Basic Techniques for Better Care." *Nursing 74* (December 1974), 48–55.

687. Varma, Surendra. "Sick Day Management." *American Diabetes Association Newsletter*, vol. 1, no. 1 (1981), 1.

688. Varvaro, Filomena Fanelli. "Teaching the Patient About Open Heart Surgery." *American Journal of Nursing* (October 1965), 111–115.

689. Verwoerdt, Ardian. "Communications with the Fatally Ill." *A Cancer Journal for Clinicians*, vol. 15 (1965), 105–111.

690. Volicer, Beverly J., and Mary W. Burns. "Preexisting Correlates of Hospital Stress." *Nursing Research*, vol. 26, no. 6 (November–December 1977), 408.

691. Walleck, Constance Anne. "A Neurologic Assessment Procedure That Won't Make You Nervous." *Nursing 82*, vol. 12, no. 12 (December 1982), 50–57.

692. Washington State Board of Nursing. "Statement on Advanced Registered Nurse/Specialized Registered Nurse Rules and Regulations." *Washington State Journal of Nursing* (Winter 1975), 15–16.

693. Weaver, Barbara, and Elsie Williams. "Teaching the Tuberculosis Patient." *American Journal of Nursing*, vol. 63 (December 1963), 80–82.

694. Weed, Lawrence L. "Medical Records That Guide and Teach." Part 1. *New England Journal of Medicine* vol. 278, no. 11 (March 14, 1968), 593–600.

695. Weed, Lawrence L. "Medical Records That Guide and Teach." Part 2. *New England Journal of Medicine* vol. 278, no. 12 (March 21, 1968), 652–657.

696. Wenkler, Gerald, and Robert Young. "Efficacy of Chronic Propranolol Therapy in Action Tremors of the Familial, Senile, or Essential Varieties." *The New England Journal of Medicine*, vol. 290 (May 2, 1974), 984–988.

697. Western Pennsylvania Regional Medical Program. "The Nursing Process." University of Pittsburgh School of Nursing, 1973.

698. William, Mary. "The Patient Profile." *Nursing Research*, vol. 9, no. 3 (Summer 1960), 122–124.

699. Wilson, W.P. and B.S. Nashold. "Pain and Emotion." *Postgraduate Medicine* (May 1970), 182–187.

700. Winstead-Fry, Patricia. "The Scientific Method and Its Impact on Holistic Health." *Advances in Nursing Science*, vol. 2 no. 4 (July 1980), 1–7.

701. Woods, Susan L. "Monitoring Pulmonary Artery Pressure." *American Journal of Nursing*, vol. 76, no. 11 (November 1976), 1,765–1,771.

702. Wu, Ruth. "Explaining Treatments to Young Children." *American Journal of Nursing*, vol. 65 (July 1965), 71–73.

703. Zimmerman, Dorothy, and Carol Gohrke. "The Goal-Directed Nursing Approach: It Does Work." *American Journal of Nursing* (February 1970), 306–310.

PAMPHLETS, BOOKLETS, AND MANUALS

704. Abata, Russell M. "How to Develop a Better Self-Image." Liquori, Mo.: Liquori Publications, 1980.

705. American Cancer Society. "First Aid for Laryngectomees." New York: American Cancer Society, 1973.

706. American Cancer Society. "Helping Words for the Laryngectomee." New York: American Cancer Society, 1972.

707. American Cancer Society. "Rehabilitating Laryngectomees." New York: American Cancer Society, 1971.

708. American Diabetes Association. "Calorie Control for You." New York: The Upjohn Company, 1966.

709. American Diabetes Association. "Facts About Diabetes." New York: American Diabetes Association, 1966.

710. American Heart Association. "Advanced Cardiac Life-Support Manual." Dallas, Texas: American Heart Association, 1975.

711. American Heart Association. "An Active Partnership for the Health of Your Heart." Dallas, Texas: American Heart Association, Communications Division, 1978.

712. American Heart Association. "Heart Facts." Dallas, Texas: American Heart Association, Communications Division, 1981.

713. American Heart Association. "Standards for Emergency Cardiac Care in Advanced Life-Support Units." Dallas, Texas: American Heart Association, Committee on Emergency Cardiac Care, 1976.

714. DeJong, Russell, A.L. Sahs, C.K. Aldrich, and John Milligan. "Essentials of the Neurological Examination." Philadelphia: Smith, Kline and French Laboratories, 1962.

715. Department of Health, Education and Welfare. "Patient Classification For Long-Term Care: User's Manual." Publication No. HRA-74-3107. Washington, D.C.: Department of HEW, Health Resources Administration, Bureau of Health Services Research and Evaluation, December 1973.

716. Eli Lilly and Company. "A Guide for the Diabetic." Indianapolis: Eli Lilly and Company, 1971.

717. Epilepsy Foundation of America. "Epilepsy." Washington, D.C.: Epilepsy Foundation of America, 1972.

718. Epilepsy Foundation of America. "Teacher Tips." Washington, D.C.: Epilepsy Foundation of America, 1972.

719. Hurst, J. Willis, Robert Schlant, W. Dallas Hall, and H. Kenneth Walker. "The Problem-Oriented Medical System." Atlanta: Emory University School of Medicine, 1972.

720. Johnson and Johnson. "Narcotic Addiction in the Newborn." New York: Medical Programs Incorporated, 1972.

721. Krames, Lawrence A., Richard F. Schneider, and Leland H. Johnson. "Back Owner's Manual." Daly City, Calif.: PAS Publishing Co., 1977.

722. Lasser, Terese. "Reach to Recovery." American Cancer Society, 1953.

723. Leonard, James, and Frank Kroetz. "Examination of the Heart: Auscultation." New York: American Heart Association, 1967.

724. Mental Health Association. "Eighteen Ways to Deal with Stress. Mental Health Association Pamphlet, undated.

725. Moncrief, Jack. "Continuous Ambulatory Peritoneal Dialysis Procedure." Austin, Texas, 1980.

726. National Association for Mental Health. "How to Deal with Mental Problems. New York: National Association for Mental Health, undated.

727. National Association for Mental Health. "Mental Health is 1, 2, 3." Arlington, Va.: National Association for Mental Health, 1976.

728. National Fire Protection Association. "Fire Escape Where You Work." Boston: National Fire Protection Association, 1977.

729. National Fire Protection Association. "Fire Safety for You. Quincy, Mass.: National Pire Protection Association, 1977.

730. National Fire Protection Association. "Know Your ABCDs of Portable Fire Extinguishers." Boston: National Fire Protection Association, 1970.

731. National Society for the Prevention of Blindness, Inc. "Cataract: Fact and Fancy." New York: National Society for the Prevention of Blindness, Inc., 1971.

732. National Society for the Prevention of Blindness, Inc. "Television and Your Eyes." New York: National Society for the Prevention of Blindness, Inc., 1968.

733. National Society for the Prevention of Blindness, Inc. "Your Eyes for a Lifetime of Sight." New York: National Society for the Prevention of Blindness, Inc., 1968, 1971.

734. National Tuberculosis Association. "Homemaking Hints." New York: National Tuberculosis Association, 1954.

735. Normand, Hal. "A Procedure Manual for the Voluntary or Involuntary Commitment of the Mentally Ill." Dallas: Beddoe Printing Co., undated.

736. Reynolds, William. "Home Care Programs in Arthritis." New York: The Arthritis Foundation, 1969.

737. Roche Laboratories. "Facts at Your Fingertips." Nutley, N.J.: Roche Laboratories, udated.

738. Rosenthal, Helen, and Joseph Rosenthal. "Diabetic Care in in Pictures." Philadelphia: J.B. Lippincott Co., 1960.

739. Ross Laboratories. "Clinical Education Aid No. 7: Congenital Heart Abnormalities." Columbus, Ohio: Ross Laboratories, November 1975.

740. Ross Laboratories. "Your Child Goes to the Hospital." Columbus, Ohio: Ross Laboratories, 1971.

741. Snyder, Michael T. "Drug Interactions." Presented to American Association of Occupational Health Nurses, April 12, 1978.

742. Sprague, Howard. "Examination of the Heart: History Taking." New York: American Heart Association, 1967.

743. Unnamed author. "What Everyone Should Know About Stress." Channing L. Bette Co., Inc., 1982.

744. Van Allen, M.W. "Pictorial Manual of Neurologic Tests." Chicago: Year Book Medical Publications, Inc., 1969.

745. Vazuka, Francis. "Essentials of the Neurological Examination." Philadelphia: Smith, Kline and French Laboratories, 1962.

746. Zohman, Lenore R. "Exercise Your Way to Fitness and Heart Health." New York: American Heart Association in cooperation with Best Foods, 1974.

PAPERS

747. American Druggist Association. "Counterdoses for the Home." 1965.

748. American Heart Association "High Blood Pressure Screening Clinic Instructions." Dallas County Chapter, 1976.

749. American Heart Association and National Academy of Sciences, National Research Council. "Standards for Cardiopulmonary Resuscitation (CPR) and Emergency Cardiac Care (ECC)." Washington, D C., 1973.

750. American Medical Association Committee on Nursing. "Medicine and Nursing in the 1970s: A Position Statement." Chicago: American Medical Association, June 1970, 2.

751. American Nurses Association. "A Position Paper." New York: American Nurses Association, 1965.

752. American Nurses Association. "H.E.W. report on Licensure and Related Health Personnel Credentialing." New York: American Nurses Association, 1972.

753. American Nurses Association. Task Force for Review and Revision of ANA's Model Practice Act of the ANA Congress for Nursing Practice. "Legal Barriers to Expanded Nursing Role Responsibilities." New York: American Nurses Association, 1973.

754. American Nurses Association. "Standards of Nursing Practice." Kansas City, Mo.: American Nurses Association, 1973.

755. American Nurses Association. "Practice of Nursing Defined in State Nursing Practice Acts." New York: American Nurses Association, 1973.

756. American Nurses Association. "The American Nurse," vol. 8, no. 11. Kansas City, Mo.: American Nurses Association, September 1, 1976, 9.

757. Barnett, E. Kathryn. "The Development of a Theoretical Construct of the Concepts of Touch as They Relate to Nursing." Ph.D. dissertation, North Texas State University, Denton, Texas, 1970.

758. Cardiac Alert. Exercise and the Heart," vol. 3, no. 12. Bethesda, Md.: Phillips Publishers, Inc., December 1981,

759. Christian Fellowship, Nurses. "The Nurse's Role in Spiritual Care." Workshop, Baylor University Medical Center, Dallas, Texas, March 1980.

760. Cross, Harold. "Teaching Methods and Patient Care with Emphasis on the Weed Method." Paper presented at the University of Medicine Symposium at Emory University, Atlanta, Ga., September 10–11, 1971.

761. Fish, Sharon, Judy Van Heukelem, Judy Hoff, and Mary Berg. "Nursing Diagnosis: Lassen Pines Conference." Nurses Christian Fellowship, Madison, Wis., June 1977.

762. Gottleib, Laurie. "Categories for Health-Related Concerns/ Problems." Demonstration grant from the Research Directorate of Health and Welfare, Canada, McGill University School of Nursing, Canada, July 1977.

763. Health, Education and Welfare. "Extending the Scope of Nursing Practice." Washington, D.C.: November 1971, 12.

764. Health, Education and Welfare. "Guidelines for the Utilization of Nurse Practitioners." Public Law 91–63.

765. Health, Education and Welfare. "Report on Licensure and Related Health Personnel Credentialing." Presented at the Educational Conference Council of

State Boards of Nursing, Detroit, Mich., 1972, 2–3.

766. Henderson, Betty. "Physical Assessment of the Respiratory System." Texas Woman's University, Denton, Texas, 1973.

767. Jones, Phyllis, and Dorothea Jakob. "An Investigation of the definition of *Nursing Diagnoses.*" University of Toronto, Toronto, Ontario, March 1977.

768. Kenner, Cornelia. "Assessment of the Thermally Injured." Texas Woman's University, Denton, Texas, 1973.

769. Kuempel, Anne. "Individual Reaction to Pain." Unpublished paper, Texas Woman's University, Denton, Texas, April 1971.

770. Kuempel, Anne. "Categories of Nursing Care Needs of Patients." Unpublished paper, St. David's Hospital, Austin, Texas, 1982.

771. Neal, Kathleen Brown. "Spiritual Values of Nurses and Identifying a Patient's Spiritual Need." Master's thesis, Texas Woman's University, Denton, Texas, August 1979.

772. Olson, Mary. "Postoperative Patients Evaluate Preoperative? Teaching." Master's thesis, Texas Woman's University, Denton, Texas, December 1971.

773. Pinterich, Shirley, "Deliberate Nursing Care for the Quiet Patient." Unpub-lished paper, Texas Woman's University, Denton, Texas, December 1970.

774. Robinson, Ann D. "Teaching Your Geriatric Client How to Improve His/Her Memory." Workshop for Advanced Nurse Practitioners, Texas Nurses' Association, Austin, Texas, March 18, 1983.

775. University of Texas at Arlington School of Nursing. "Community Health Nursing Family Coping Index." Arlington, Texas, 1979.

776. Vance, Maxine L. "Nursing Observations of Maternal Attachment in Relation to Postpartum Separation." Masters thesis, Texas Woman's University, Denton, Texas, 1978.

777. Watt, Nancy B. "Management Reporting System: Patient Classification System." Irving Community Hospital, Irving, Texas, 1981.

778. Western Pennsylvania Regional Medical Program. "The Nursing Process." University of Pittsburgh School of Nursing, Pittsburgh, 2.

779. "Huguley Hospital Policy and Procedure Manual." Huguley Hospital. Fort Worth, Texas, 1983.

780. Book: Neilson, Terry E. Tippett, and Donna M. Behler. *Pediatric Nurse Practitioner Certification Review.* New York: John Wiley & Sons, 1983.

Index

Index entries are classified according to the following abbreviations: *NDx* = nursing diagnoses; *NT* = nursing treatments; *NO* = nursing observations; *HT* = health teaching; *MDRx* = medical treatments performed by nurses.

ABANDONED FEELING . . . (NDx pattern)

NDx
Abandoned feeling related to an absent health care provider, 404
Abandoned feeling related to an absent significant other, 405

ABANDONMENT

NDx
Fear of abandonment, 474

ABDOMEN

NDx
Abdominal evisceration (dehiscence), 743
Acute abdominal pain (acute abdomen), 744
Discomfort of intraabdominal pressure, 85
Nonpenetrating abdominal injury, 750
Penetrating abdominal injury (internal abdominal injury), 752
Potential for abdominal distention, 254
NO
Inspect the abdomen for ascites, 1587
Inspect the abdomen for distention, 1587
Inspect the abdomen for vein engorgement, 1587
Inspect the abdomen for visible peristalsis, 1588
Palpate the abdomen for tenderness, rigidity, and masses, 1632
Palpate the abdominal aorta for increased pulsation, 1633
Percuss the abdomen for abnormal resonance, 1636

ABORTION

HT
Emphasize the danger of induced abortion, 1670

ABSCESS

NDx
External abscess, 892

ACCEPTANCE

NT
Accept and attempt to relieve unexplainable body complaints, 1417
Provide an atmosphere of acceptance, 1528
HT
Advise acceptance of the drug user's return home, 1645
Advise that significant persons express acceptance of one another, 1657

ACETONE

NO
Test the urine for sugar and/or acetone/ketones, 1643

ACHIEVEMENT

NT
Encourage the desire for satisfactory achievement, 1473
Explore with the person previous achievements of success, 1479

ACHING

NDx
Aching pain, 1050
Neuralgia, 960

ACID–ASH

NT
Encourage decreased acid–ash food intake, 1459
Encourage increased acid–ash food intake, 1464

ACID–BASE

NDx
Instability of acid–base status (acid–base instability), 180
NT
Encourage increased acid–ash food intake, 1464
NO
Monitor blood studies for abnormal acid–base, 1597

ACIDOSIS

NDx
Ketoacidosis, 713
Metabolic acidosis, 710
Potential for metabolic acidosis, 210
Potential for respiratory acidosis, 213
Respiratory acidosis, 715

ACTING OUT

NDx
Acting-out behavior, 1214
Sexual acting out (excessive libido), 1267

ACTIVITY/ACTIVITIES

NT
Avoid placing the person on enforced inactivity, 1435

INDEX

INSTABILITY OF . . . (NDx Pattern)

NDx

INSTITUTIONALIZATION

NDx

INSULIN

NDx

KNEE(S)

NT
Place a knee rest under the knees, 1514
Place a pillow between the knees, 1514
Refrain from placing a pillow under the knee, 1543

LABILE

NDx
Labile affect (labile personality), 1248

LABOR AND DELIVERY

NDx
False labor, 980
Labor pain, 981
Normal labor and delivery, 1390
Positive screening cues for a complicated labor and delivery, 1166
Potential for complicated labor and delivery, 292

NT
Facilitate the delivery by gently guiding the infant through the vulva, 1481

HT
Describe the manifestations of labor onset, 1663
Describe the normal behavior pattern common during labor, 1664
Describe the process of labor and delivery, 1666
Explain that childbirth is a normal process, 1685
Explain the difference between true and false labor pains, 1696
Explain the significance of premature membrane rupture and that it does not indicate difficult labor, 1704
Inform that bearing down aids the progress of second stage labor, 1712
Teach how to control breathing to aid the labor process, 1758

LABORATORY RESULTS

NO
Interpret laboratory results and notify the physician of abnormalties, 1595
Obtain standard laboratory studies and evaluate for normal levels, 1632

HT
Explain how to calculate the delivery date, 1674

LABORATORY STUDIES
See Studies, Blood, Gastric, Sputum, Urine etc.

LACERATION

NDx
Laceration, 760

LACTATION

NDx
Failure of lactation (agalactia), 979
Unknowledgeable about lactation suppression, 990

LANOLIN

NT
Clean with castile or lanolin soap, 1443

HT
Advise that lanolin be applied to brittle nails, 1656

LARYNGEAL EDEMA

NO
Observe for laryngeal edema, 1624

LARYNGECTOMY

NDx
Unskilled at laryngectomy care, 369

NT
Clean the tracheostomy (or laryngectomy) tube inner cannula, 1442
Defer speech communications for 72 hours after a partial laryngectomy, 1448
Shield the tracheostomy (or laryngectomy stoma) from water, 1554
Ventilate the person mouth-to-stoma or bag-to-stoma when the person has a laryngectomy/tracheostomy (ET), 1565

HT
Inform that artificial larynxes are available, 1712
Inform that handwashing is essential before touching the laryngectomy stoma, 1715
Inform that the laryngectomy stoma should be protected against sunburning, 1717
Instruct that soap should not be used on the laryngectomy stoma, 1721
Instruct to apply a warm, moist, nonobstructive compress to the laryngectomy stoma for dyspnea, 1722
Instruct to maintain a moist laryngectomy bib, 1729
Instruct to protect the laryngectomy opening/tracheostomy from water, 1730
Instruct to use a water-base lubricant around the laryngectomy stoma, 1731
Recommend the use of a laryngectomy bib, 1744
Teach how to clean a tracheostomy/laryngectomy tube, 1757

MDRx
Resuscitate mouth-to-neck when the patient has a laryngectomy (ET), 1788

LARYNX

NDx
Laryngitis, 1014

LAUGHTER

NT
Encourage laughter, 1468

LAVAGE

NT
Refrain from administering gastric lavage, 1537

MDRx
Lavage the stomach (ET), 1787

Potential for malnutrition, 1097

MANIC

NDx
Manic behavior (manic reaction), 1249

MANIPULATION

NDx
Manipulative behavior (manipulation), 1275

NT
Avoid assuming that all behavior is manipulative, 1434

MASK

NT
Refrain from strapping the ventilator mask in place, 1544
Wear a clean gown and mask, 1566
Wear a mask when suctioning, 1566

HT
Recommend the use of a face mask, 1744

MASSAGE

NT
Do not massage, 1454
Massage bony prominences, 1509
Massage gently, 1509
Massage the gums, 1509
Massage the uterine fundus, 1509
Massage vigorously, 1509

HT
Emphasize the danger of massaging a painful calf/frostbitten tissue, 1670
Explain how to massage, 1680
Instruct not to massage the breasts or use a breast pump, 1719
Teach how to massage the gums, 1768
Teach how to massage the uterine fundus, 1768

MASTECTOMY

NDx
Unskilled at postmastectomy care, 382

HT
Teach how to do postmastectomy exercises, 1761

MATTRESS

NT
Place on a flotation mattress, 1519
Place on a polyurethane foam pad, 1519
Place on a silicone pad, 1520
Place on a split-foam mattress, 1520
Place on an alternating pressure mattress, 1520
Provide a firm mattress, 1526
Turn the mattress frequently, 1563

MEALS/MEALTIME

HT
Advise handwashing before meals/before meal preparation, 1652
Explain the need for pleasant mealtimes, 1701

Recommend a regular meal/feeding schedule, 1733
Teach how to prepare balanced meals, 1769

MEAN ARTERIAL PRESSURE

NO
Monitor the mean arterial pressure, 1608

MEANINGFULNESS

NT
Assist the person to set standards of a meaningful existence, 1433
Encourage meaningful activity, 1468

MEASURING

NO
Measure the body weight, 1595
Measure the chest drainage after clamping the chest tube, and attaching a new drainage system, 1595
Measure the girth/circumference of the (specific body part), 1596
Measure the height, 1596
Measure the intake, 1596
Measure the output, 1596
Measure the pelvic size, 1596
Measure the residual urine, 1596
Measure the urine output hourly, 1597

MECHANICAL VENTILATION

MDRx
Administer mechanical ventilation (ET), 1420
Administer manual or mechanical ventilation (ET), 1784

MECONIUM

NO
Inspect the amniotic fluid for meconium, 1588
Observe the time of the first meconium stool, 1631

MEDIC ALERT TAG

HT
Explain the importance of wearing a Medic Alert tag, 1699

MEMORY

NDx
Memory loss, 1317

NT
Encourage the person to write down what he wants to remember, 1475
Stimulate the memory by repeating the person's last expressed thought, 1557

NO
Observe for memory impairment, 1624

HT
Explain the essential factors that affect memory, 1697
Teach methods for improving the memory, 1776

OBSESSION

ODOR

OIL

OINTMENT

Withhold the oxygen therapy, 1567

NO

Check the oxygen flow rate, 1575

HT

Teach how to give oxygen therapy, 1764

MDRx

Administer heated humidified oxygen (ET), 1783

Administer humidified oxygen (ET), 1783

Administer oxygen by nasal cannula/nasal catheter/facial mask/tent/croupette/incubator, 1784

Administer oxygen by venturi mask, 1784

PACE OF LIVING

HT

Recommend adherence to a pace of living with which the person is comfortable, 1734

PACEMAKER, CARDIAC

NDx

Pacemaker failure, 817

Unskilled at managing a pacemaker, 831

NT

Position the pacemaker generator box comfortably, 1523

Protect the person wearing a pacemaker by practicing safety measures, 1524

Record the battery-change date on the pacemaker generator box, 1536

Replace the pacemaker batteries, 1549

Tape the pacemaker wire to the person, 1562

NO

Check the pacemaker for pacing rate, 1575

HT

Explain how to detect pacemaker failure, 1676

Explain that the pacemaker electrical current is not strong enough to electrocute, 1693

Explain the effects of the specific type pacemaker, 1696

Inform that bathing is permitted when wearing a pacemaker, 1712

Instruct to check the pulse daily when wearing a pacemaker, 1725

Recommend the use of a pacemaker shirt, 1745

Teach safety measures to be practiced when wearing a pacemaker, 1778

PACIFIER

NT

Give a pacificer to the infant, 1483

PACKING

NT

Pack the draining wound with fine-mesh gauze, 1512

Pack sterile cotton between the ingrown nail and the skin, 1512

PADS AND PADDING

NT

Apply a heating pad, 1422

Place absorbent pad(s) under the person, 1515

Place on a polyurethane foam pad, 1519

Place on a silicone pad, 1520

Place the infant on an apnea pad, 1522

Protect with absorbent padding, 1524

HT

Explain how to pad bony prominences, 1681

Explain how to pad rough cast edges, 1681

Recommend the use of absorbent padding, 1745

PAIN/PAIN MANAGEMENT

NDx

Aching pain, 1050

Acute abdominal pain (acute abdomen), 744

Afterbirth pain, 972

Anger related to physical pain, 423

Bone pain, 936

Breast tenderness/breast pain, 975

Burning pain, 1052

Constrictive pain, 1055

Cramping pain, 1057

Denial of pain, 652

Dysmenorrhea, 978

Dysuria (painful urination), 884

Fear of pain, 558

Gnawing pain, 1059

Headache, 940

Hemorrhoid pain, 863

Incapacity to manage pain, 97

Incisional pain, 911

Joint pain (arthralgia), 954

Labor pain, 981

Ovulation pain (mittelschmerz), 983

Painful defecation, 869

Painful respiration (ponopnea), 1015

Partial incapacity to manage pain, 99

Phantom pain, 963

Postpartal perineum pain, 985

Potential for pain, 314

Stabbing pain, 1061

Throbbing pain, 1063

Toothache, 879

Unknowledgeable about pain-relief methods, 1066

NT

Ask the person to relate the onset of returning pain, before the pain becomes severe, 1431

Communicate nurse sensitivity to the person's pain/problem, 1444

Discuss possible pain-reducing measures, 1451

Offer assurance of other measures if the pain-relief method fails, 1511

Prepare the person for a/the painful experience, 1523

Provide a pain-relief measure of the person's choice, 1527

Reassure that the pain will subside or be relieved, 1536

Refrain from equating sleep with the absence of pain, 1538

NO

Determine the influence of culture on the pain reaction, 1578

Provide a paper bag for tissue disposal, 1527

HT

Explain how to use a paper bag to reduce hyperventilation, 1684

PAP SMEAR

NT

Do a Papanicolaou (Pap) test, 1452

NO

Monitor the Papanicolaou smear results for positive findings, 1608

PAPILLEDEMA

NO

Inspect the eyes for papilledema, 1589

PARALYSIS

NDx

Fear of paralysis, 560

PARANOIA

NDx

Paranoia (paranoid disorder), 1278

PARASITICIDE

NT

Wash the brush and comb with a parasiticide, 1566

PARENTING

NDx

Competence in parenting, 1399

HT

Teach positive parenting behavior, 1778

PAROTID GLAND

NDx

Parotitis, 870

NO

Palpate the parotid gland for swelling, 1635

PARTIAL INCAPACITY . . . (NDx Pattern)

NDx

Partial incapacity to ambulate, 152

Partial incapacity to chew/swallow food and fluids, 169

Partial incapacity to communicate needs, 105

Partial incapacity to dress self, 140

Partial incapacity to exercise, 160

Partial incapacity to feed/hydrate self, 165

Partial incapacity to manage health therapy, 339

Partial incapacity to manage pain, 99

Partial incapacity to perform feminine hygiene, 132

Partial incapacity to perform hair care, 116

Partial incapacity to perform nail care, 120

Partial incapacity to perform oral hygiene, 124

Partial incapacity to perform personal hygiene, 111

Partial incapacity to perform skin care, 128

Partial incapacity to perform toileting, 136

Partial incapacity to promote sleep readiness, 333

Partial incapacity to sit up, 154

Partial incapacity to stand up, 156

Partial incapacity to suck fluids, 171

Partial incapacity to transfer body, 157

PELVIC SIZE

NO

Measure the pelvic size, 1596

PELVIS

NDx

Pelvic congestion, 984

PERCEPTIONS

NO

Identify abnormal perceptions, 1582

Test for heat and cold perception, 1638

Test for impaired smell perception, 1639

Test for impaired taste perception, 1639

Test the skin for impaired feeling perception, 1642

HT

Advise against denouncing erroneous perceptions, 1646

PERCUSSION

NO

Percuss the abdomen for abnormal resonance, 1636

Percuss the chest for abnormal resonance, 1636

Percuss the posterior chest for decreased diaphragmatic descent, 1637

PERFORMANCE

NT

Encourage self-performance, 1471

NO

Observe performance level and problems involved in completing the task/activities of daily living, 1628

PERINEAL CARE

NDx

Unskilled at postpartum perineal care, 384

NT

Give perineal care, 1491

HT

Teach how to do perineal care, 1761

PERINEUM

NDx

Postpartal perineum pain, 985

PERISTALSIS

NO

Inspect the abdomen for visible peristalsis, 1588

PERITONEAL DIALYSIS

NDx

Unskilled at continuous ambulatory peritoneal dialysis, 352

POSITIVE-PRESSURE BREATHING

NT

HT

MDRx

POSITIVE SCREENING CUES FOR . . .
(NDx Pattern)

NDx

POSTPARTUM PERIOD

NDx

Recommend the use of iodized salt, 1747

SALT SOLUTION

NT

Give a salt solution orally, 1484

SALT-SODA SOLUTION

NT

Give a salt-soda solution orally, 1483

SANDBAGS

NT

Position with sandbags, 1523

Restrict head movements with a cervical collar, pillows, or sandbags, 1550

SANITARY PADS

NT

Change the sanitary pads/tampons frequently, 1440

NO

Count the number of sanitary pads used, 1577

HT

Advise frequent sanitary pad/tampon change, 1652

Teach how to apply sanitary pads, 1755

SCABIES

NDx

Scabies, 924

SCALP (Also see HAIR)

NDx

Infantile seborrhea dermatitis (cradle cap), 912

Scalp injury, 771

NT

Comb the dandruff up from the scalp, 1444

Shampoo the hair/scalp, 1554

HT

Advise against prolonged skin/scalp exposure to the sun and/or the water, 1649

Instruct to comb the dandruff up from the scalp, 1725

Instruct to inspect the skin/scalp/hair, 1728

Instruct to lubricate the skin/scalp/nails, 1729

Instruct to maintain skin/scalp cleanliness, 1729

SCOLIOSIS

NDx

Positive screening cues for scoliosis, 1156

SCRATCHING/SCRATCHING DEVICES

HT

Advise against scratching, 1650

Instruct not to use a scratching device under the cast, 1719

SECLUSION

NT

Provide seclusion, 1534

SECRETIONS, RESPIRATORY

HT

Advise against drawing secretions to the back of the throat, 1646

SEDATION

NO

Observe for oversedation, 1625

SEIZURES

NDx

Unknowledgeable about seizures, 971

Potential for seizures, 289

NO

Observe for convulsions/seizures, 1619

Observe for seizure characteristics, 1631

HT

Describe the manifestations of an impending seizure, 1663

Explain how to manage seizure episodes, 1680

Inform of those conditions that precipitate seizures, 1710

Inform that seizures are not contagious, 1716

SELF-ATTITUDES

NT

Observe for impaired self-attitudes, 1623

HT

Explain the importance of developing and/or maintaining a positive self-attitude, 1698

SELF-CARE

NDx

Competence in self-care, 1396

NT

Provide assistance until the person is fully able to assume self-care, 1529

NO

Observe for readiness to assume self-care/infant care, 1626

SELF-CONTROL

HT

Explain why persons should maintain self-control, 1707

SELF-IDEAL

NT

Encourage the differentiation between self-ideal and actual self, 1473

SELF-IDENTITY MODIFICATION . . . (NDx Pattern)

NDx

Self-identity modification related to a developmental phase, 701

Self-identity modification related to loss/gain o a significant other, 702

Self-identity modification related to physical lo 704

UNKNOWN, THE

NDx

UNSKILLED AT . . . (NDx Pattern)

NDx

UREMIA

URETEROILEOSTOMY

URETEROSTOMY

URETEROSIGMOIDOSTOMY

URINAL

URINARY CATHETER

URINARY DRAINAGE/CONTAINER/ SYSTEM

URINARY FREQUENCY